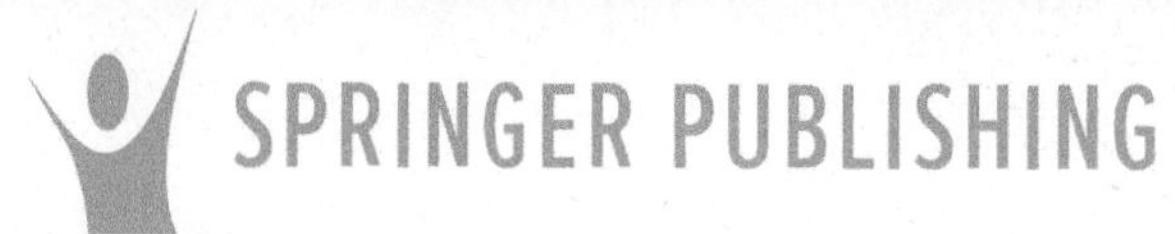

MW00852403

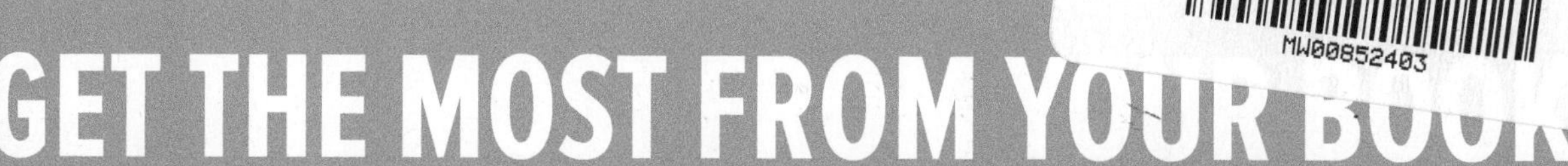

Access your included eBook and educator resources today!

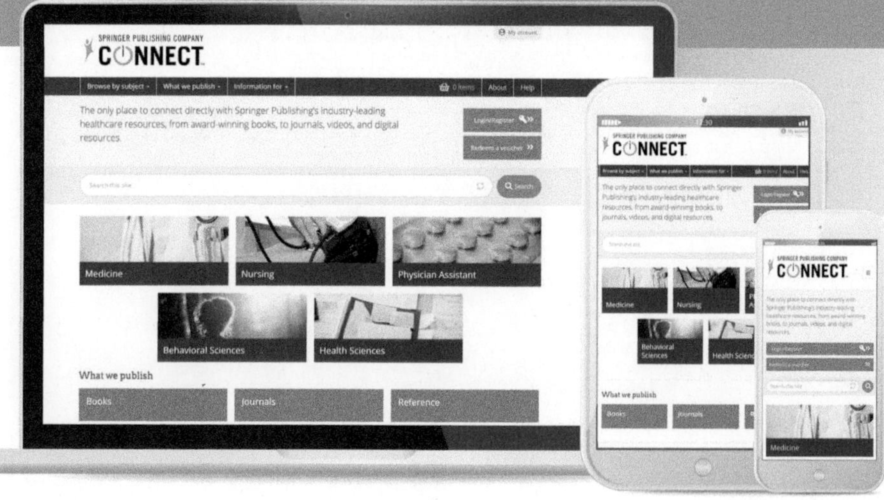

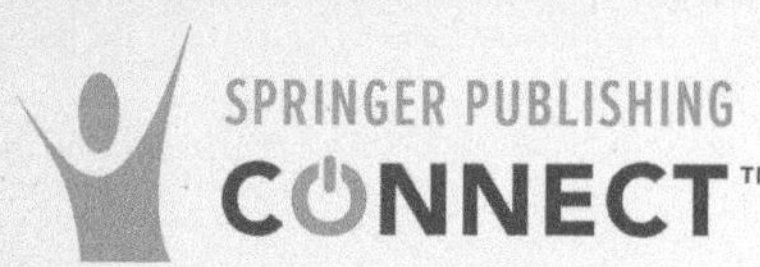

GHBTFM7S

eBook Access

Your print purchase of *Clinical Medicine for Physician Assistants* includes **online access via Springer Publishing Connect**™ to increase accessibility, portability, and searchability.

Insert the code at http://connect.springerpub.com/content/book/978-0-8261-8243-2 today!

Educator Resource Access

Let us do some of the heavy lifting to create an engaging classroom experience with a variety of educator resources included in your textbooks SUCH AS:

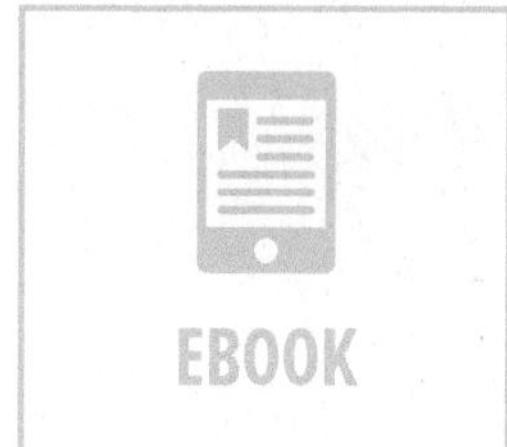

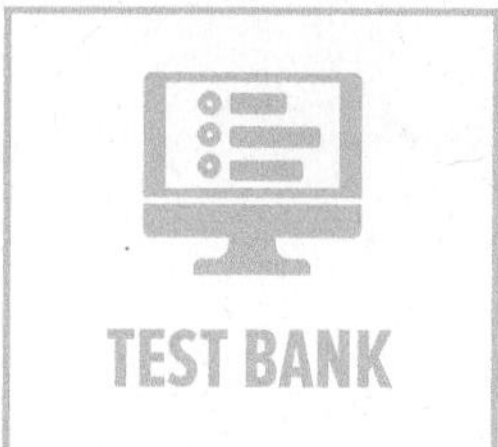

Visit **https://connect.springerpub.com/** and look for the **"Show Supplementary"** button on your **book homepage** to see what is available to you! First time using Springer Publishing Connect?

Email **textbook@springerpub.com** to create an account and start unlocking valuable resources.

CLINICAL MEDICINE *for* PHYSICIAN ASSISTANTS

James Van Rhee, MS, PA-C, DFAAPA

James A. Van Rhee, PA-C, MS, the Program Director for the Yale University School of Medicine Physician Assistant Online Program, is a graduate of Grand Valley State University, 1982, with a BS in Medical Technology and a BS in Medicine, 1989, from the University of Iowa, where he completed his training as a physician assistant. In 1997, he received a MS in Physician Assistant Studies from Rosalind Franklin University.

Van Rhee has been involved in physician assistant education for over 20 years. He was the academic coordinator at the physician assistant program at Grand Valley State University. Then he spent nine years as Department Chair and Program Director of the Department of Physician Assistant Studies at Western Michigan University, in Kalamazoo. He then was a tenured associate professor and Department Chair and Program Director of the Department of Physician Assistant Studies at Wake Forest University School of Medicine. He then was appointed by Northwestern University Feinberg School of Medicine to start a new physician assistant program and served as program director and associate professor. In 2013, joined Yale School of Medicine and became the program director for the Yale School of Medicine Physician Associate program and in 2016 became the founding program director for the Yale School of Medicine Physician Assistant Online Program.

Van Rhee has also spent 10 years as the project director and as an item-writer for the Physician Assistant Education Association's (PAEA) Physician Assistant Clinical Knowledge Rating Assessment Tool (PACKRAT). He also spent nine years on the Accreditation Review Commission for Physician Assistant Education (ARC-PA) as a commissioner, having served as chair for two years. For 17 years, Mr. Van Rhee has been the course director for an on-line Kaplan Medical PANCE/PANRE board review course. He is author of the Physician Assistant Certification and Recertification Board Review, and consulting editor for Physician Assistant Clinics. He has authored several articles and been a presenter at the local, state, and national levels on various clinical medicine and education topics.

Christine Bruce, DMSc, MHSA, PA-C, DFAAPA

Christine Bruce, DMSc, MHSA, PA-C, DFAAPA, is a clinically active physician assistant for the St. Luke's University Health Network and an Associate Professor and founding Program Director of the Penn State University Physician Assistant Program. Prior to her appointment at Penn State, Bruce was the founding Program Director and Full Professor at DeSales University's PA Program. She served as visiting scholar and faculty member for the Harvard Macy Health Education Professors Program. She has practiced for 38 years in hospitalist medicine, cardiology, and general internal medicine. She graduated from the St. Francis University PA Program in 1983, completed her Master of Health Services Administration from St. Joseph's University, and a Doctor of Medical Science from Lynchburg University. In 2017, Bruce was honored by the NCCPA as one of 50 PAs who has made a significant contribution to the profession. Dr. Bruce's PA graduates have had 100% first-time PANCE pass rates for over 20 consecutive years while having less than 1% attrition and 100% employment within 4 months of graduation. She has served as a clinical preceptor for PA students during her 38 years of clinical practice. She is the senior editor for the *Kaplan PA Review* and has served on multiple PAEA committees and the ARC-PA as a site visitor. She also served on the PACKRAT test writing committee for a decade.

Stephanie Neary, MPA, MMS, PA-C

Stephanie Neary, MPA, MMSc, PA-C, joined the Yale School of Medicine PA Online Program 2017. She is an assistant professor adjunct, the director of didactic education for the program, and course director for Behavioral and Preventive Medicine I, II, and III while also serving on the admissions committee. Stephanie is an academic advisor for incoming and current students. Neary is a physician assistant who graduated with an MMS from Midwestern University-Glendale in 2015. She began practicing clinically in refugee and urban underserved family medicine clinics in Phoenix, Arizona, and now works in inpatient endocrinology on the Diabetes Management Service at the Medical University of South Carolina (MUSC). In 2012, she became adjunct faculty at Grand Canyon University in the College of Science, Engineering and Technology and the College of Nursing and Health Care Professions. She has been a member of the Physician Assistant Education Association's (PAEA) Future Educator Development Steering Committee and has presented multiple times at the American Academy of PAs (AAPA) national conferences, the PAEA Forums, and the IAMSE Annual Meeting. Neary also earned Master of Public Administration in Health Care Management from Grand Canyon University in 2013 and a Bachelor of Science in Exercise Science from the George Washington University in 2010. She was a 2020 PAEA Research Fellow and currently pursuing a PhD in Nursing Science at MUSC.

CLINICAL MEDICINE *for* PHYSICIAN ASSISTANTS

James Van Rhee, MS, PA-C, DFAAPA

Christine Bruce, DMSc, MHSA, PA-C, DFAAPA

Stephanie Neary, MPA, MMS, PA-C

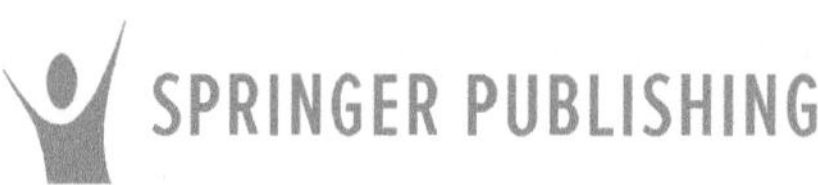

Springer Publishing Company, LLC
11 West 42nd Street, New York, NY 10036
www.springerpub.com
connect.springerpub.com/

Acquisitions Editor: Suzanne Toppy
Director, Content Development: Taylor Ball
Production Manager: Kris Parrish
Compositor: Amnet Systems

ISBN: 978-0-8261-8242-5
ebook ISBN: 978-0-8261-8243-2
DOI: 10.1891/9780826182432

SUPPLEMENTS:
Instructor Materials:

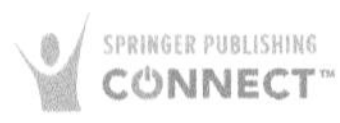

A robust set of instructor resources designed to supplement this text is located at **http://connect.springerpub.com/content/book/978-0-8261-8243-2.** Qualifying instructors may request access by emailing **textbook@springerpub.com.**

Instructor's Manual ISBN: 978-0-8261-8297-5
Instructor's Test Bank ISBN: 978-0-8261-8298-2 (Also available on Respondus®.)
Instructor's PowerPoints ISBN: 978-0-8261-8299-9

22 23 24 25 / 5 4 3 2 1

Medicine is an ever-changing science. Research and clinical experience are continually expanding our knowledge, in particular our understanding of proper treatment and drug therapy. The authors, editors, and publisher have made every effort to ensure that all information in this book is in accordance with the state of knowledge at the time of production of the book. Nevertheless, the authors, editors, and publisher are not responsible for any errors or omissions or for any consequence from application of the information in this book and make no warranty, expressed or implied, with respect to the content of this publication. Every reader should examine carefully the package inserts accompanying each drug and should carefully check whether the dosage schedules therein or the contraindications stated by the manufacturer differ from the statements made in this book. Such examination is particularly important with drugs that are either rarely used or have been newly released on the market.

Library of Congress Cataloging-in-Publication Data

Names: Van Rhee, James, editor. | Bruce, Christine (Christine H.), editor. | Neary, Stephanie, editor.
Title: Clinical medicine for physician assistants / [edited by] James Van Rhee, Christine Bruce, Stephanie Neary.
Description: First Springer Publishing edition. | New York, NY : Springer Publishing Company, 2022. | Includes bibliographical references and index.
Identifiers: LCCN 2021033011 | ISBN 9780826182425 (paperback) | ISBN 9780826182432 (ebook)
Subjects: MESH: Clinical Medicine | Physician Assistants
Classification: LCC R697.P45 | NLM WB 102 | DDC 610.73/72069--dc23
LC record available at https://lccn.loc.gov/2021033011

Publisher's Note: **New and used products purchased from third-party sellers are not guaranteed for quality, authenticity, or access to any included digital components.**

Printed in the United States of America.

This book is dedicated to my family, who had to put up with me during all the hours spent writing and reviewing this manuscript. Thanks to all the physician assistant students I have had contact with over the years—without all of you this book would not have been possible.

—James Van Rhee

To all the PA students I have had the privilege working with over the past 38 years, who have taught me as much as I have taught them! Also, to my nephew Doug, who was taken from this earth much too early—your life mattered and my memories of you will continue as long as I live.

—Christine Bruce

To my daughters, Emily, Caroline, and Nora, and to my husband, who continuously supports my ideas and efforts… like writing a textbook while we raise toddlers. To all parents who are trying to balance having a family with pursuing your passions.

—Stephanie Neary

Contents

Contributors

Mark Aksamit, MPAS, PA-C, CAQ-Psych
Assistant Professor
Division of Physician Assistant Education
College of Allied Health Professions
Physician Assistant
Department of Psychiatry
University of Nebraska Medical Center
Omaha, Nebraska
Chapter 9: Nutrition

Analisa Ambrosi, PA-C
Physician Assistant–Hospital Medicine
Main Line Health
Bryn Mawr Hospital
Bryn Mawr, Pennsylvania
Chapter 4: Pulmonary System

Jonathan Baker, MPAS, PA-C
Laser Surgery Care
New York, New York
Chapter 19: Care of the Sexual and Gender Minority Patient

Thomas Balga, PA
Lecturer in Emergency Medicine
Lead Physician Assistant–SRC Campus
Yale School of Medicine
New Haven, Connecticut
Chapter 21: Abuse and Violence Identification

John Bastin, DMSc, PA-C, EM-CAQ
Assistant Professor, PA Principal Faculty
School of Physician Assistant Practice
Florida State University College of Medicine
Tallahassee, Florida
Chapter 20: Preventive Medicine

Carrie Beebout, PsyD, MPAS, PA-C
Chair, Department of Physician Assistant Science
Associate Professor
St. Francis University
Loretto, Pennsylvania
Chapter 14: Rheumatology

Laura E. Beerman, RD, CNSC
Intestinal Rehabilitation and Transplant Dietitian
Department of Pharmaceutical and Nutrition Care
Intestinal Rehabilitation Program
Small Bowel and Liver Transplant
Courtesy Faculty College of Allied Health Professions
Nebraska Medicine/University of Nebraska Medical Center
Omaha, Nebraska
Chapter 9: Nutrition

Ashley Bell, DMSc, PA-C, CHSE
Arcadia University Hybrid PA Program
Glenside, Pennsylvania
Chapter 15: Neurologic System

Richard D. Bennett, PhD, MMSc, PA-C
Associate Professor
Physician Assistant Studies Program
University of Utah Department of Family & Preventive Medicine
St. George, Utah
Chapter 9: Nutrition

Nana Bernasko, CRNP, DNP, WHNP-BC
Assistant Professor of Medicine
Penn State Health
Division of Gastroenterology and Hepatology
Hershey, Pennsylvania
Chapter 8: Gastrointestinal System

Richard Bottner, DHA, PA-C
Assistant Professor
Department of Internal Medicine
Dell Medical School
University of Texas at Austin
Austin, Texas
Chapter 18: Psychiatry

David Brissette, MMSc, PA-C
Yale Physician Associate Program
Department of Internal Medicine
Yale University School of Medicine
New Haven, Connecticut
Chapter 3: Ears, Nose, and Throat Disorders

Christine Bruce, DMSc, MHSA, PA-C, DFAAPA
Program Director, Physician Assistant Program
St. Luke's University Health Network
Associate Professor
Division of General Internal Medicine
Department of Medicine
College of Medicine
Penn State University
Hershey, Pennsylvania
Chapter 5: Cardiovascular System
Chapter 13: Muscoloskeletal System
Chapter 14: Rheumatology
Chapter 22: Surgery

Diane Bruessow, MPAS, PA-C, DFAAPA
Instructor, PA Online Program
Department of General Internal Medicine
Yale School of Medicine
New Haven, Connecticut
Healthy Transitions
Montclair, New Jersey
Chapter 19: Care of the Sexual and Gender Minority Patient

Laura D. Buch, MSPAS, PA-C
Certified Physician Assistant
General and Biochemical Genetics
Greenwood Genetic Center
Greenville, South Carolina
Chapter 23: Genetic Disorders

Rachel Byrne, MA, PA-C, Psych CAQ
Faculty Instructor University of Colorado Physician Assistant Program
Aurora, Colorado
Chapter 18: Psychiatry

Rebecca Orsulak Calabrese, MHS, PA-C, CPAAPA
Surgical PA
APP Clinical Manager
Department of Surgery
Yale New Haven Hospital
New Haven, Connecticut
Chapter 3: Ears, Nose, and Throat Disorders

Jill Cavalet, DHSc, PA-C
Clinical Professor
Department of Physician Assistant Science
Saint Francis University
Loretto, Pennsylvania
Chapter 18: Psychiatry

Ryan C. Chaney, MMS, PA-C
FastMed Urgent Care
Candler, North Carolina
Chapter 2: Ocular System

Brigitta Cintron, DMSc, CTTS, PA-C
Assistant Professor
School of Physician Assistant Practice
College of Medicine
Florida State University
Tallahassee, Florida
Chapter 20: Preventive Medicine

Jesse A. Coale, DMin, PA-C, DFAAPA
Associate Professor
Program Director, Physician Assistant Studies
Thomas Jefferson University
Philadelphia, Pennsylvania
Chapter 4: Pulmonary System

Marci Contreras, MPAS, PA-C
Franklin Pierce University
Physician Assistant Studies
Goodyear, Arizona
Chapter 18: Psychiatry

Christa Cooper, PA-C, MMS, MPH
Rush University Medical Center
Chicago, Illinois
Chapter 15: Neurologic System

Jill Cowen, MSPAS, PA-C
Penn State Health Children's Hospital
Pediatric Cardiology
The Milton S. Hershey Medical Center
The Pennsylvania State University
Hershey, Pennsylvania
Chapter 5: Cardiovascular System

Jacqueline Cristini, PA-C, MMSc
Director, Deep Brain Stimulation Program
Barnabas Health Medical Group
Department of Neurology, Movement Disorders
Livingston, New Jersey
Chapter 15: Neurologic System

Jessica Dahmus, MD
Penn State Health
Division of Gastroenterology and Hepatology
Hershey, Pennsylvania
Chapter 8: Gastrointestinal System

Deanna L. Denault, PhD, MA, MEd
Professor of Practice
Physician Assistant Program
Assumption University
Worcester, Massachusetts
Chapter 4: Pulmonary System

Julie DesMarteau, MPAS, PA-C
Clinical Instructor
Department of Neurology
Medical University of South Carolina
Charleston, South Carolina
Chapter 15: Neurologic System

Shannon N. Diallo, MMS, PA-C, CAQ-HM
Program Director–Physician Assistant Program
Delaware Valley University
Doylestown, PA
Physician Assistant–Hospital Medicine
Lehigh Valley Health Network
Allentown, Pennsylvania
Chapter 4: Pulmonary System

Lauren Eisenbeis, PA
Johns Hopkins Center for Transgender Health
Baltimore, Maryland
Chapter 19: Care of the Sexual and Gender Minority Patient

Stephanie Elko, PA
The Emily Program
St. Paul, Minnesota
Chapter 12: Reproductive System

Sylvie M. Fadrhonc, PA-C
Physician Assistant
Division of Pediatric Rheumatology
Department of Pediatrics
University of Utah School of Medicine
Salt Lake City, Utah
Chapter 14: Rheumatology

Lori Fauquher, MS, PA-C
Assistant Professor
Department of Physician Assistant Studies
College of Pharmacy and Health Sciences
Butler University
Indianapolis, Indiana
Chapter 15: Neurologic System

Taylor L. Fischer, MMS, PA-C
Associate Professor
Department of Physician Assistant Studies
Wingate University
Clinical Provider Mission Health/HCA NC Division
Wingate University Hendersonville Health Sciences Center
Hendersonville, North Carolina
Chapter 2: Ocular System

Blakely A. Garrity, MMS, PA-C
The Vancouver Clinic
Vancouver, Washington
Chapter 2: Ocular System

Brooke Jackson Gerlach, MS, PA-C, RD
Department of Neurology
College of Health Professions
Medical University of South Carolina
Charleston, South Carolina
Chapter 15: Neurologic System

Rena Godfrey, PA-C
Physician Assistant
Undiagnosed Diseases Program
National Human Genome Research Institute
National Institutes of Health
Bethesda, Maryland
Chapter 23: Genetic Disorders

Daniel Goldstein, MPAS, PA-C
Bethesda, Maryland
Chapter 23: Genetic Disorders

Melinda Moore Gottschalk, DMSc, PA-C, DFAAPA
Adjunct Faculty-Master of Physician Assistant Studies
Mayborn College of Health Science
University of Mary Hardin-Baylor
Belton, Texas
Chapter 15: Neurologic System

Shaun Grammer, DMSc, PA-C
Chair, Department of Medical Sciences
Associate Professor and Program Director
Physician Assistant Education
College of Alied Health Professions
University of Nebraska Medical Center
Omaha, Nebraska
Chapter 9: Nutrition

Samuel L. Gurevitz, PharmD
Associate Professor
Butler University College of Pharmacy and Health Sciences
Indianapolis, Indiana
Chapter 18: Psychiatry

Gretchen L. Hackett, DO, MS
Penn State Health Children's Hospital
Pediatric Cardiology
The Milton S. Hershey Medical Center
The Pennsylvania State University
Hershey, Pennsylvania
Chapter 5: Cardiovascular System

Brandon Headlee, MS, PA-C
Penn State Health
Division of Gastroenterology and Hepatology
Hershey, Pennsylvania
Chapter 8: Gastrointestinal System

Michael Higbee, PA-C
Scottsdale Mental Health and Wellness Institute
Connections Arizona Urgent Psychiatric Center
Phoenix, Arizona
Chapter 18: Psychiatry

Gina Hogg, MSPAS, PA-C
Geriatrics Physician Assistant
Medical University of South Carolina
Charleston, South Carolina
Chapter 16: Endocrine System

Traci Hornbeck, MS, PA-C
Department of Neurosurgery
Stanford University
Stanford, California
Chapter 15: Neurologic System

Mia J. Hyde, MPAS, PA-C
Assistant Professor
Director of Clinical Development
Physician Assistant Education
College of Allied Health Professions
University of Nebraska Medical Center
Kearney, Nebraska
Chapter 9: Nutrition

Mariah K. Jackson, MMN, RDN, LMNT
Instructor
Medical Nutrition
College of Allied Health Professions
University of Nebraska Medical Center
Omaha, Nebraska
Chapter 9: Nutrition

Julie Jones, MSPAS, PA-C
Penn State Hershey Medical Center
Harrisburg, Pennsylvania
Chapter 5: Cardiovascular System

Julia Karnoski, PA-C
Orange, California
Chapter 15: Neurologic System

JONATHAN KILSTROM, MPAS, PA-C, NRP
Instructor, Physician Assistant Online Program
Yale School of Medicine
Yale University
New Haven, Connecticut
Chapter 9: Nutrition
Chapter 15: Neurologic System

PAUL KUHLMAN, PA-C
Fort Collins, Colorado
Chapter 13: Musculoskeletal System

LINDA LANG, RN, MPAS, PA-C, DFAAPA
Instructor
Physician Assistant Online Program
Yale School of Medicine
New Haven, CT
Chapter 11: Genitourinary System

RAYNE LODER, MHS, PA-C
Assistant Professor of Public Health and Community Medicine
Physician Assistant Program
Tufts University School of Medicine
Boston, Massachusetts
Chapter 15: Neurologic System

BRITTANY R. LUEKING, MPAS, PA-C
Physician Assistant
Department of Neurology
Medical University of South Carolina
Charleston, South Carolina
Chapter 15: Neurologic System

LINDSAY LYON, MPA, PA-C
Assistant Professor
Department of Physician Assistant Studies
Wingate University Hendersonville Health Sciences Center
Hendersonville, North Carolina
Chapter 2: Ocular System

AMY MAURER, MS, MMS, PA-C
Assistant Professor
Department of PA Medicine
North Greenville University
Greer, South Carolina
Chapter 23: Genetic Disorders

ANNE M. MCRAE, MMS, CGC, PA-C
Ann & Robert H. Lurie Children's Hospital of Chicago
Chicago, Illinois
Chapter 23: Genetic Disorders

RYAN MULLANE, DO
Assistant Professor, Internal Medicine
Division of Nephrology
College of Medicine
University of Nebraska Medical Center
Omaha, Nebraska
Chapter 9: Nutrition

MELISSA MURFIN, PHARMD, BCACP, PA-C
Department of Physician Assistant Studies
Elon University
Elon, North Carolina
Chapter 23: Genetic Disorders

STEPHANIE NEARY, MPA, MMS, PA-C
Assistant Professor Adjunct and Director of Didactic Education
Physician Assistant Online Program
Yale School of Medicine
New Haven, Connecticut
Chapter 12: Reproductive System
Chapter 15: Neurologic System
Chapter 16: Endocrine System
Chapter 18: Psychiatry

MARNIE I. O'DONNELL, MS, PA-C
Penn State Health Children's Hospital
Pediatric Cardiology Electrophysiology Division
The Milton S. Hershey Medical Center
The Pennsylvania State University
Hershey, Pennsylvania
Chapter 5: Cardiovascular System

NGUYEN H. PARK, MS, PA-C, DFAAPA
President and Founder
Society of Physician Assistants in Genetics/Genomics
Great Falls, Virginia
Chapter 23: Genetic Disorders

WESLEY PATTERSON, PHD(C), MS, PA-C
Genetics Physician Assistant
Greenwood Genetic Center
Greenwood, South Carolina
Chapter 23: Genetic Disorders

NATHAN PAYNE, MPAS, PA-C
Clinical Director
ADHD Clinic of Arizona
Phoenix, Arizona
Chapter 18: Psychiatry

KATHY PEDERSEN, PA-C, MPAS
Associate Professor, Emeritus
Division of Physician Assistant Studies
Department of Family and Preventive Medicine
School of Medicine
University of Utah
Salt Lake City, Utah
Chapter 15: Neurologic System

SARAH PRYOR, MMS, PA-C
Clinical Assistant Professor
Sacred Heart University
Physician Assistant Studies
Fairfield, Connecticut
Chapter 18: Psychiatry

JOHN RAMOS, MMS, PA-C, EM-CAQ
Raleigh, North Carolina
Chapter 15: Neurologic System

Jannelle Reynolds, MPAS, PA-C
Assistant Professor
Academic Director, Physician Assistant Education
College of Allied Health Professions
University of Nebraska
Kearney, Nebraska
Chapter 9: Nutrition

Catherine Roden, MHS, PA-C
Penn State Health Children's Hospital
Hershey, Pennyslvania
Chapter 5: Cardiovascular System

Chris Roman, MA, MMS, PA-C
Associate Professor
Physician Assistant Studies Program
Butler University
Indianapolis, Indiana
Chapter 11: Genitourinary System

Mary Ruggeri, MMSc, PA-C
Clinical Coordinator
Physician Assistant Online Program
Yale School of Medicine
New Haven, Connecticut
Chapter 11: Genitourinary System
Chapter 12: Reproductive System

Erin Salcido, MPAS, PA-C
Associate Professor
Director of Didactic Education
Marshall B. Ketchum University
Fullerton, California
Chapter 15: Neurologic System

Elizabeth Schmidt, MS, PA-C
Assistant Professor, Assistant Program Director
Department of Physician Assistant Studies
Butler University
Indianapolis, Indiana
Chapter 11: Genitourinary System

Tad Schrader, PA-C, MSPAS
Physician Assistant
Berthoud, Colorado
Chapter 13: Musculoskeletal System

Aniqa Shahrier, MD
Penn State Health Children's Hospital
Pediatric Cardiology
The Milton S. Hershey Medical Center
The Pennsylvania State University
Hershey, Pennsylvania
Chapter 5: Cardiovascular System

Marie Shaner, PA-C, MMS
Penn State Health Children's Hospital
Pediatric Cardiology
The Milton S. Hershey Medical Center
The Pennsylvania State University
Hershey, Pennsylvania
Chapter 5: Cardiovascular System

Kenneth D. Sherry, PA-C, CPAAPA
Surgical Advanced Practice Services
St. Luke's University Health Network
Bethlehem, Pennsylvania
Chapter 22: Surgery

Benjamin J. Smith, DMSc, PA-C, DFAAPA
Director of Didactic Education
Assistant Professor
School of Physician Assistant Practice
Florida State University College of Medicine
Tallahassee, Florida
Chapter 14: Rheumatology

Jina Stephen, PA-C, MBA
GI Medical Oncology Physician Assistant
MD Anderson Cancer Center
Houston, Texas
Chapter 23: Genetic Disorders

Daniel Sturm, MMS, PA-C
Associate Professor
Physician Assistant Studies
College of Pharmacy and Health Sciences
Butler University
Indianapolis, Indiana
Chapter 15: Neurologic System
Chapter 18: Psychiatry

Diana M. Sukup, MMS, PA-C
Pardee Hospital, UNC Health Care
Southeastern Sports Medicine & Orthopedics
Hendersonville, North Carolina
Chapter 2: Ocular System

Anna Swanson, MPAS, PA-C
Dementia Care Coordinator
Department of Neurology
Medical University of South Carolina
Charleston, South Carolina
Chapter 15: Neurologic System

Ashley Taylor, MHS, PA-C
University of Oklahoma Health Science Center
Oklahoma City, Oklahoma
Chapter 23: Genetic Disorders

Elizabeth Thompson, MS, RD, PA-C
Penn State Health
Division of Gastroenterology and Hepatology
Hershey, Pennsylvania
Chapter 8: Gastrointestinal System

Megan Timmerman, MPA, RD, LMNT
Assistant Professor and Clinical Education Coordinator
Medical Nutrition Education Division
College of Allied Health Professions
University of Nebraska Medical Center
Omaha, Nebraska
Chapter 9: Nutrition

James Van Rhee, MS, PA-C, DFAAPA
Program Director
Physician Assistant Online Program
Yale School of Medicine
New Haven, Connecticut
Chapter 1: Dermatologic System
Chapter 6: Hematologic System
Chapter 7: Oncology
Chapter 10: Renal System
Chapter 11: Genitourinary System
Chapter 13: Msucoloskeletal System
Chapter 17: Infectious Diseases

Elesea Villegas, MPAS, PA-C
Assistant Professor
Texas Tech University Health Sciences Center
Midland, Texas
Chapter 18: Psychiatry

Joshua Wageman, PA-C, DPT, CSCS
Treasure Valley Metabolic Medicine
Eagle, Idaho
Chapter 12: Reproductive System
Chapter 15: Neurologic System

Elyse J. Watkins, DHSc, PA-C, DFAAPA
University of Lynchburg School of PA Medicine
Lynchburg, Virginia
Florida State University School of PA Practice
Tallahassee, Florida
Chapter 12: Reproductive System

Heidi Webb, MMS, PA-C
Physician Assistant
Bahl and Bahl Medical Associates
Pittsburgh, Pennsylvania
Chapter 9: Nutrition

Jeniece Wert, PA-C, MEd
McAllen, Texas
Chapter 12: Reproductive System
Chapter 18: Psychiatry

Carey A. Wheelhouse, MSPAS, PA-C
Assistant Professor
Director of Clinical Assessment
Physician Assistant Education
College of Allied Health Professions
University of Nebraska Medical Center
Omaha, Nebraska
Chapter 9: Nutrition
Chapter 13: Musculoskeletal System

Sampath Wijesinghe, DHSc, PA-C, AAHIVS
Principal Faculty, MSPA Program
Stanford School of Medicine
Stanford University
Stanford, California
Chapter 17: Infectious Diseases

Anne Wildermuth, MMS, PA-C, EM-CAQ, RD
Associate Program Director & Assistant Professor
Division of PA Education
University of Nebraska Medical Center
Omaha, Nebraska
Chapter 9: Nutrition

Courtney Wilke, MPAS, PA-C
Assistant Professor
School of Physician Assistant Practice
College of Medicine
Florida State University
Tallahassee, Florida
Chapter 20: Preventive Medicine

Morgan Wilson, MSPAS, PA-C, ATC
Loveland, Colorado
Chapter 13: Musculoskeletal System

Jennifer Simms Zorn, DMS, PA-C
Doctor of Medical Science Program Director
Butler University
College of Pharmacy and Health Sciences
Department of Physician Assistant Studies
Indianapolis, Indiana
Chapter 18: Psychiatry

Reviewers

Heather P. Adams, MPAS, PA-C
Associate Professor
Gannon University
Erie, Pennsylvania

Kathleen M. Barta, MPAS, PA-C
Senior Physician Assistant
Infectious Disease Specialists of Southeastern Wisconsin
Brookfield, Wisconsin

Megan Fitzgerald, PA-C
Physician Assistant
Sacramento, California

Kristi E. Gruber, MEd, PA-C
Physician Assistant, Orthopaedic Trauma Surgery
Instructor, Department Orthopaedic Surgery
Penn State Health
Hershey, Pennsylvania

Kristine A. Himmerick, PhD, PA-C, DFAAPA
Director of Assessment and Accreditation
University of the Pacific, School of Health Sciences
Sacramento, California

Gerald Kayingo, PhD, PA-C
Associate Clinical Professor
Physician Assistant Studies
Betty Irene Moore School of Nursing
University of California–Davis
Davis, California

Jonathan Kilstrom, MPAS, PA-C, NRP
Instructor, Physician Assistant Online Program
Yale School of Medicine
Yale University
New Haven, Connecticut

David Knechtel, MPAS, PA-C
Assistant Professor and Clinical Coordinator
Physician Assistant Program
Milligan University
Elizabethton, Tennessee
Pulmonology PA
Pulmonary Associates of East Tennessee
Johnson City, Tennessee

Joshua Leslie, PA-C
Physician Assistant
President, Ascend Telemedicine
Chandler, Arizona

Kevin Michael O'Hara, MMSc, MS, PA-C
Memorial Sloan Kettering Cancer Center
Adjunct Faculty
Department of PA Studies
Pace University
New York, New York

Alicia Ottman, MMS, PA-C
Director of Advanced Practice, Neighborhood Outreach
Access to Health
Phoenix, Arizona

Dipu Patel, MPAS, PA-C
Director of Clinical Pathways
DayToDay Health
Bengaluru, India

Kylie Pont, PA-C
Abdominal Transplant Organ Advanced Practitioner
Team Lead
Mayo Clinic Arizona
Phoenix, Arizona

Cody Randel, PA-C
Physician Assistant
Vice President, Ascend Telemedicine
Chandler, Arizona

Joanne Rolls, MPAS, MEHP, PA-C
Associate Professor, Clinical
University of Utah School of Medicine
Salt Lake City, Utah

Ashley Ryan, MS, CGC
Clinical Research Coordinator/Genetic Counselor
Translational Genomics Research Institute (TGen)
Phoenix, Arizona

Benjamin J. Smith, DMSc, PA-C, DFAAPA
Director of Didactic Education,
Assistant Professor
Florida State University College of Medicine School
of Physician Assistant Practice
Tallahassee, Florida

Shelby Springer, PA-C
Physician Assistant
Ascend Telemedicine
Chandler, Arizona

Eric Vangsnes, PhD, PA-C
Professor Emeritus
Western Michigan University
Department of Physician Assistant
Kalamazoo, Michigan

Deborah Vaughan, MMSc., PA-C
Physician Assistant
Connecticut Ear Nose and Throat Associates
Hartford, Connecticut

Foreword

Over 50 years have passed since the first Physician Assistant (PA) program—at Duke University—graduated its first cohort of students in 1967. Since that time, the number of programs across the country has increased tremendously to meet the rapidly growing demand for primary care clinicians. As a result, PAs have established themselves not only as expert clinicians, but as educators and mentors responsible for directing the education and training of future clinicians according to standards and competencies unique to the PA profession. Comprehensive clinical medicine textbooks covering all organ systems across the life span and providing guidance on patient evaluation, diagnosis, management, and patient counseling and education are critically important to the successful clinical training of PA students. However, until *Clinical Medicine for Physician Assistants*, no such textbook has been written *by* PAs *for* PAs. This innovative textbook provides a much-needed comprehensive approach to the clinical education of PA students specifically designed according to PA standards and competencies. Providing PA students with a single, go-to clinical medicine resource in *Clinical Medicine for Physician Assistants* will benefit the PA profession by supporting clinical education and practice alike.

Editors James Van Rhee, Christine Bruce, and Stephanie Neary—themselves accomplished PA educators—and the nearly 100 contributing authors they have assembled have carefully crafted 23 chapters into this comprehensive clinical textbook. Each chapter is written in clear and concise language, includes summary tables and figures that are easily understood, and photos and diagrams that enhance understanding of the topics. This work will surely become a standard future addition to PA curricula in the United States and around the world. Each chapter is well-referenced, and the chapters collectively follow a standardized format for ease of use in obtaining needed information by students and practicing clinicians alike.

To date, we have not encountered such a robust and thorough systems-based clinical education product that goes beyond the textbook alone. We commend the editors for their creative approach to supporting both the teaching and learning process throughout the textbook and in accompanying supplements. The textbook includes clear learning objectives for each chapter and innovative "knowledge checks" to prompt student reflection and discussion. The inclusion of an instructor manual featuring case studies, a robust test bank, and lecture PowerPoints will meaningfully support busy educators throughout their courses. By following a systems-based approach, using the NCCPA blueprint as a guide, and addressing the relevant ARC-PA standards, the content in *Clinical Medicine for Physician Assistants* ensures that all clinical medicine topics PAs need to master are covered in accessible detail relevant to clinical practice.

In light of the COVID-19 pandemic's recent major upheaval to the global health care delivery system, it is critical to ensure that all clinicians—students and educators both—have access to state-of-the-art clinical information within their course curriculum. *Clinical Medicine for Physician Assistants* provides that content and is a most welcome addition to the PA educator's toolbox.

P. Eugene Jones, PhD, PA-C Emeritus
Professor Emeritus
Department of Physician Assistant Studies
UT Southwestern Medical Center
Dallas, Texas

Donald M. Pedersen, PhD, PA
Professor Emeritus
Utah Physician Assistant Program
University of Utah School of Medicine
Salt Lake City, Utah

PREFACE

Clinical medicine, internal medicine, primary care. These are all course titles used by Physician Assistant (PA) programs throughout the United States to describe didactic or clinical year courses covering the essentials of evaluation, diagnosis, and management of clinical problems across clinical settings.

Our overall goal with *Clinical Medicine for Physician Assistants* is to provide—in a single, comprehensive resource—the information and strategies required by students and clinicians alike to successfully learn and practice medicine. Organized and designed to support the clinical year courses, *Clinical Medicine for Physician Assistants* provides the foundation for evaluating a patient—including the assessment of pertinent history and physical examination findings—building a differential diagnosis, ordering and performing diagnostic studies, and treating and managing patients with a wide variety of clinical presentations and diagnoses, covering all of the clinical topics on the current NCCPA PANCE blueprint and more.

Covering in detail the current ARC-PA standards and competencies for clinical medicine courses, *Clinical Medicine for Physician Assistants* further aims to support the major themes that are core to our approach as clinical educators. The information in this textbook has been carefully written and edited to promote evidence-based practice in patient evaluation and patient management to ensure that clinicians base decisions on valid and reliable information. Furthermore, we emphasize an approach to patient care that encompasses cultural competency, social determinants of health, and a wellness perspective. Finally, we support the readers' understanding and development of cost-effective approaches to patient care. As we complete development of this first edition, the American Academy of Physician Assistants House of Delegates has recently voted to approve a professional title change from Physician Assistant to Physician Associate. While implementation of this change is expected to be a multi-year process, we acknowledge that this change is forthcoming, and the content covered and materials presented here are designed to be valuable for the PA regardless of title.

Clinical Medicine for Physician Assistants is organized by body system and provides the in-depth, head-to-toe foundation a PA student needs as they move through the didactic and clinical years of education. Covering hundreds of clinical conditions, each chapter follows a digestible and methodical review of conditions, in which discussions are preceded by overviews that cover epidemiology and pathophysiology, introducing specific clinical disorders through their clinical presentation, reviewing physical examination steps and associated findings, and diagnosis details—differentials and tests—for each condition. Also included are treatment options along with important patient education information. Common chief complaints are located at the end of each chapter with useful algorithms to guide you through a patient visit. Key points and special considerations for specific patient populations are highlighted throughout the text, and knowledge checks appear at the end of each chapter helping students synthesize and apply what they have learned.

In addition, this textbook offers chapters dedicated to specific populations or topics that are often overlooked in medical texts. Entire chapters are dedicated to the following topics:

- Chapter 19: Care of the Sexual and Gender Minority Patient
- Chapter 20: Preventive Medicine
- Chapter 21: Abuse and Violence Identification
- Chapter 22: Surgery
- Chapter 23: Genetic Disorders

Clinical Medicine for Physician Assistants is accompanied by an Instructor's Manual and comprehensive instructor resources, which include learning objectives, case studies, assessment questions—including multiple-choice questions with rationales—and PowerPoint slides.

We are grateful to the many colleagues who have joined us in this project as contributing writers. We are particularly proud of the result and hope you enjoy using *Clinical Medicine for Physician Assistants* as much as we enjoyed creating it.

James Van Rhee
Christine Bruce
Stephanie Neary

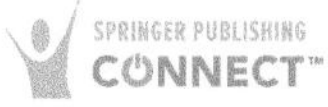

A robust set of instructor resources designed to supplement this text is located at **http://connect.springerpub.com/content/book/978-0-8261-8243-2**. Qualifying instructors may request access by emailing **textbook@springerpub.com**.

Instructor Resources

A robust set of resources designed to supplement this text is located at http://connect.springerpub.com. Qualifying instructors may request access by emailing textbook@springerpub.com.

Available resources include:

- **Instructor's Manual:**
  - Case Studies
  - Knowledge Check Discussion Questions and Answers/Rationales
- **Test Bank:**
  - Multiple-Choice Questions with Answers/Rationales
- **Chapter-Based PowerPoint Presentations**

CHAPTER 1

DERMATOLOGIC SYSTEM

JAMES VAN RHEE

LEARNING OBJECTIVES

- Define the following key terms: macule, papule, patch, plaque, wheal, pustule, vesicle, bulla, cyst, nodule, purpura, petechiae, and ulcer.
- Review the pathophysiology, clinical presentation, diagnosis, and management of drug reactions and anaphylaxis.
- Discuss the pathophysiology, clinical presentation, diagnosis, management, and prognosis of contact dermatitis, atopic dermatitis (AD), seborrhea (seborrheic dermatitis), irritant dermatitis, pityriasis rosea, and psoriasis.
- Discuss the epidemiology, pathophysiology, clinical presentation, diagnosis, management, and prognosis of common bacterial, viral, parasitic, and fungal infections of the skin.
- Describe the clinical presentation, diagnosis, and management of the various forms of alopecia.
- Describe the epidemiology, clinical presentation, diagnosis, management, and prognosis of acne vulgaris, rosacea, and hidradenitis suppurativa.
- Compare and contrast the epidemiology, clinical presentation, diagnosis, management, and prognosis of actinic keratosis (AK), basal cell carcinoma (BCC), squamous cell carcinoma (SCC), and malignant melanoma.

INTRODUCTION

The skin consists of distinct layers. The most superficial layer is the epidermis. Below the epidermis is the dermis. The epidermis consists of stratified squamous epithelium and keratinocytes. Among the keratinocytes there are melanocytes and Merkel cells. The keratinocytes provide the structure and maintain the barrier function of the skin. Melanocytes make protective pigment. Merkel cells function as mechanoreceptors. The dermis layer contains subcutaneous fat, pilosebaceous unit, apocrine and eccrine glands, and structural proteins.

The primary functions of skin include protection, sensory function, thermoregulation, and vitamin D synthesis.

The secondary functions of skin include immune functions, such as dryness, desquamation, and normal flora, and antigen presenting cells such as Langerhans cells and keratinocytes; solar and heat interaction including UV radiation protection with melanin, thermoregulation, and vitamin D metabolism.

Several terms are used to describe the morphology of skin lesions. See Table 1.1 for the description of the various terms.

1.1 ACNE DISORDERS

OVERVIEW

Acne is a common disorder in adolescents and adult acne is more prevalent than previously thought. The hallmark of acne vulgaris is the presence of inflammatory papules and pustules along with comedones involving the face, chest, shoulders, and back. Nodules and cystic lesions are noted in more severe disease. Secondary changes such as scarring and postinflammatory hyperpigmentation or erythema are common and may impact both management and disease outcomes.

EPIDEMIOLOGY

Acne affects up to 85% of 12- to 24-year-olds. The prevalence in women age 30 to 39 years is 35%.[1] Adolescent acne appears slightly more often in males, while post-adolescent acne mostly affects women. Genetic influences may impact risk. Several hormonal abnormalities, such as polycystic ovary syndrome (PCOS), hyperandrogenism, hypercortisolism, and precocious puberty, increase risk for development of acne.

PATHOPHYSIOLOGY

Four primary factors are involved in the pathophysiology of acne vulgaris.

- **Increased sebum production:** At puberty, increased sebum production occurs in conjunction with enlarging sebaceous glands. This provides an environment for *Propionobacterium acnes* (*P. acnes*) to grow.
- **Follicular hyperkeratinization:** Hyperkeratinization of the follicle leads to the development of a hyperkeratotic plug, which can cause impaired sebum excretion and the induction of local inflammatory mediators.

TABLE 1.1 Definitions of Dermatology Terms

Term	Definition	Example
Macule	Circumscribed, flat lesion without elevation or depression, <1.0 cm in diameter	Petechiae
Patch	Circumscribed, flat lesion without elevation or depression, >1.0 cm in diameter	Vitiligo
Papule	Elevated solid lesion, <1.0 cm in diameter, may become confluent and form a plaque	Angioma
Plaque	Circumscribed, flat elevated lesion, >1.0 cm in diameter	Psoriasis
Nodule	Circumscribed, elevated firm lesion, >1.0 cm in diameter; resides in dermal layer	Lipoma
Vesicle	Circumscribed, elevated lesion, filled with fluid or semi solid material, usually <1.0 cm	Herpes
Bulla	Elevated, fluid-filled lesion, usually >1.0 cm	Bullous pemphigoid
Pustule	Circumscribed, elevated, pus-filled lesion, usually <1.0 cm	Acne
Wheal	Firm, elevated, pink to red swelling, size and shape vary, itchy, duration <24 hours	Urticaria

- **Increased colonization of *P. acnes*:** *P. acnes* gram-negative bacilli are normal flora of the skin. The organism is proinflammatory.
- **Inflammation:** This is caused by a variety of factors, including the proliferation of *P. acnes*, the proinflammatory cascade, and hyperkeratinization.

1.1A ACNE VULGARIS

Acne is common, especially in adolescents and young adults. Approximately 50 million people in the United States have acne vulgaris.[2] Acne affects approximately 85% of teenagers but can occur in any age group and can persist into adulthood.[1] While there is no mortality associated with acne, there is often significant physical and psychological morbidity, such as permanent scarring, poor self-image, depression, and anxiety.

Acne fulminans is a severe, eruptive form of acne that primarily occurs in teenage males. It appears abruptly on the face and upper body with papules and nodules that can coalesce, suppurate, and bleed. It may also be accompanied by fever, joint pain, and malaise. Scarring is often severe and is inevitable. Acne conglobata is a form of severe, nodulocystic acne. The nodules coalesce into suppurative plaques. Neonatal acne, occurring from birth to 3 months of age, affects about 20% of healthy newborns and presents as small inflamed papules and pustules on the cheeks and nasal bridge.[3] Comedones are not present and neonatal acne resolves spontaneously. Infantile acne occurs between 3 and 6 months of age, lasting through the first and second year of life. Comedones are present, along with variable inflammatory lesions.

MEDICAL HISTORY AND CLINICAL PRESENTATION

A complete medication history should be obtained, including any prescription and over-the-counter medications used for acne. Several medications can cause acne or acneiform eruptions, including corticosteroids, anabolic steroids, phenytoin, lithium, and isoniazid. Menstrual and oral contraceptive history should be obtained to determine any hormonal influences related to the acne. There are reports of acne flares related to certain foods (e.g., high fat foods and chocolate) and diets high in dairy products. High glycemic foods have been shown to exacerbate acne flares.

Negative psychological findings, anxiety, depression, and social withdrawal are common among patients with acne and acne scars. If noted, the patient should be referred to a psychologist or psychiatrist.

SIGNS AND SYMPTOMS

There are numerous grading systems for acne. One example is noted in Table 1.2. Moderate to severe acne is depicted in Figure 1.1.

TABLE 1.2 Acne Grading System

Grade	Severity	Description
I	Mild	Open and closed comedones with few inflammatory papules and pustules. Also considered mild if only a few or small pimples.
II	Moderate	Inflammatory lesions present as a small papule or pustule with erythema, mainly on face.
III	Moderately severe	Numerous papules and pustules with occasional inflamed nodules, also noted on chest and back.
IV	Severe	Many papules, pustules, and nodules. Nodules are often reddish and painful. May lead to scarring.

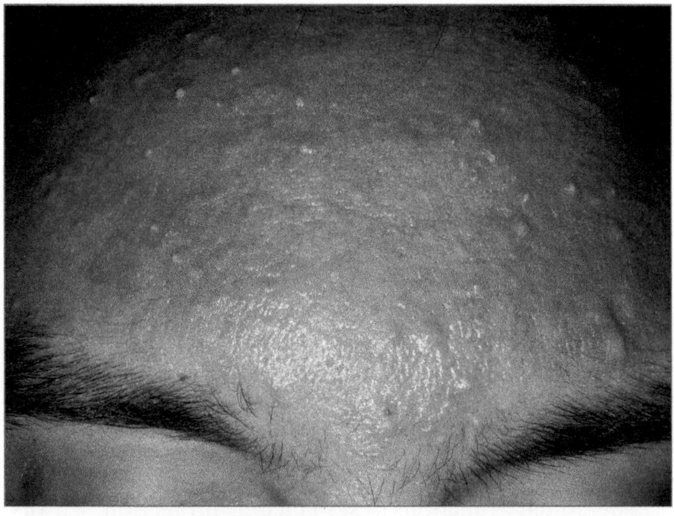

Figure 1.1 Moderate to severe acne in an adolescent male.
(Source: Image courtesy of Roshu Bangal.)

PHYSICAL EXAMINATION

On physical examination, lesion morphology, presence of comedones, inflammatory lesions, and nodules should be noted.

Lesions of acne include open and closed comedones. Open comedones are small, 1 mm papules with a dilated follicular outlet that is black. Closed comedones are 1 mm papules without an apparent follicular opening. Both lack any associated erythema.

The clinically inflammatory lesions seen in acne vary from papules and pustules (filled with thick purulent fluid) to more severe nodules and nodulocystic lesions. Nodules can combine to form large plaques that can result in scarred sinus tracts.

DIFFERENTIAL DIAGNOSIS

The differential diagnosis for acne is noted in Box 1.1.

DIAGNOSTIC STUDIES

The diagnosis of acne is based on clinical findings, and laboratory studies are typically not needed.

EVALUATION

Acne or acneiform eruptions may be the common presenting feature in several syndromes.

- PCOS is the most common syndrome associated with acne, and is characterized by polycystic ovaries, oligo- and/or anovulation, and biochemical and/or clinical signs of hyperandrogenism. PCOS presents with acne, central obesity, hirsutism, alopecia, and infertility.
- Seborrhea and acne with hirsutism and/or androgenic alopecia (SAHA syndrome) is a result of either elevated androgen levels or increased sensitivity of the pilosebaceous unit to androgens.

TREATMENT

Treatment for acne is based on the severity of disease. See Table 1.3.

Retinoids (tretinoin, adapalene, and tazarotene) are anti-comedogenic, are comedolytic, have significant direct and indirect anti-inflammatory effects, and prevent the formation of new microcomedos. Enhanced efficacy is noted when retinoids are used in combination with benzoyl peroxide (BP) or other topical antibiotics. Side effects include local erythema, dryness, and itching within the first weeks of usage but decrease with continued, more regular use. Sunscreen use is indicated because of increased susceptibility to sunburn due to thinning of the skin. Retinoids are known teratogens, so use during pregnancy is strongly discouraged.

BP is a bactericidal agent that works by reducing *P. acnes* within the follicle. It is effective when used alone or when combined with topical retinoids. Side effects include bleaching of clothing, towels, and bedding.

Topical dapsone has anti-inflammatory properties and is more effective in treating inflammatory acne lesions than comedones. When used with BP, topical dapsone can cause a yellow-orange staining of skin and hair. Topical use is safe in those with sulfa allergies.

Salicylic acid is a comedolytic and mild anti-inflammatory agent. Side effects are mild and include erythema and scaling.

Several antibiotics are used in the treatment of acne. Tetracyclines are the centerpiece of antibiotic treatment. All tetracyclines can cause photosensitivity and teeth staining and should be avoided in pregnancy because of a negative effect on bone and cartilage growth in the fetus. Minocycline is

BOX 1.1 Differential Diagnosis for Acne

Keratosis pilaris	Drug-induced acne	Sebaceous hyperplasia
Perioral dermatitis	Tropical acne	Milia
Folliculitis	Radiation acne	Milaria rubra
Sebaceous hyperplasia	Acne cosmetica	
Papulopustular rosacea	Acne mechanica	
Pseudofolliculitis barbae	Occupational acne	

TABLE 1.3 Treatment Options for Acne

	Mild	Moderate	Severe
First-line treatment	Benzoyl peroxide (BP) *or* Topical retinoid *or* Topical combination therapy of BP + antibiotic *or* BP + retinoid *or* BP + retinoid + antibiotic	Topical combination therapy BP + antibiotic *or* Retinoid + BP *or* BP + retinoid plus antibiotic *or* Oral antibiotic + topical retinoid + BP *or* Oral antibiotic + topical retinoid + BP *or* Oral antibiotic + topical retinoid + BP + topical antibiotic	Oral antibiotic + topical combination therapy BP + antibiotic or retinoid + BP *or* Retinoid + BP + antibiotic *or* Oral isotretinoin
Alternative treatment	Add topical retinoid *or* BP (if not already used) *or* Consider alternative retinoid *or* Consider topical dapsone	Consider alternative combination therapy *or* Consider change in oral antibiotic *or* Add combined oral contraceptive or oral spironolactone (females) *or* Consider oral isotretinoin	Consider change in oral antibiotic *or* Add combined oral contraceptive *or* Oral spironolactone (females) *or* Consider oral isotretinoin

associated with blue pigmentation of the skin or gums, lupus-like reaction, and autoimmune hepatitis.

Tetracycline absorption is affected by substances containing calcium, aluminum, iron, and zinc and should not be taken with dairy products or antacids.

Several other oral antibiotics have been used for the treatment of acne. They include trimethoprim-sulfamethoxazole, amoxicillin and other penicillins, cephalosporins, and azithromycin. Data on their efficacy and safety are not well established and their use in the treatment of acne is generally discouraged.

Isotretinoin works by normalizing epidermal differentiation, markedly decreasing sebum production, reducing the presence of *P. acnes,* and exerting anti-inflammatory effects. It is approved for severe, nodulocystic acne and recalcitrant acne. Mild side effects are often noted and include chelitis, xerosis, and dryness of the oral and nasal mucosa. Isotretinoin is a potent teratogen. Two negative pregnancy test results are required before therapy can begin. Contraception counseling should also be discussed, and two effective forms of birth control should be used in women who are sexually active.

Baseline laboratory testing before isotretinoin therapy is also recommended and generally includes cholesterol and triglyceride assessment and hepatic transaminase levels. These values should be rechecked once the patient is at a steady dosing.

PATIENT EDUCATION

- Follow-up will depend on acne severity. Mild to moderate disease should be followed up at 3- to 4-month intervals once treatment is initiated. Severe cases should be followed up at 2- to 3-month intervals.
- Use of cosmetics can be very beneficial in covering up active acne and improving patient quality of life. Water-based, non comedogenic formulations should be used.
- Sunscreen is indicated in patients on medications that can cause photosensitivity, such as retinoids or doxycycline.
- In most patients with acne, specific changes to diet are not recommended.

1.1B ROSACEA

Rosacea is a common disorder that affects over 45 million people worldwide.[4] There is equal prevalence in both males and females. Age of onset is typically between 30 and 50 years of age and occurs more commonly in patients with fair skin and chronic solar damage.

Etiology is multifactorial. Some patients with rosacea have an increased number of *Demodex* mites (*Demodex folliculorum*), mainly in those patients with steroid-induced rosacea. Genetics may also pay a role. Alcohol has been linked to flushing of the skin and is a trigger for rosacea.[5]

There are four identified rosacea subtypes and patients may have more than one subtype present.

1. **Erythematotelangiectatic rosacea:** Presents with permanent redness and a tendency to flush or blush easily. Telangiectasias are visible near the surface of the skin and burning or itching sensations are noted.
2. **Papulopustular rosacea:** Some permanent redness with red papules and some pus-filled pustules.
3. **Phymatous rosacea:** Most commonly associated with rhinophyma. Symptoms include thickening skin, irregular surface nodularities, and enlargement. Telangiectasias may be visible near the surface of the skin.
4. **Ocular rosacea:** Presents with red, dry, and irritated eyes and eyelids. Other symptoms include foreign body sensations, itching and burning.

MEDICAL HISTORY AND CLINICAL PRESENTATION

Rosacea starts as erythema on the central face and across the cheeks, nose, or forehead, but can also affect the neck and chest. As the disease progresses there may be other symptoms such as semi permanent erythema, telangiectasia, red domed papules and pustules, red eyes, burning and stinging sensations, and rhinophyma. The presence of rash on the scalp or ears suggests a different or coexisting diagnosis, as rosacea is primarily a facial presentation.

PHYSICAL EXAMINATION

Primary clinical features include flushing, non transient erythema, papules, pustules, and telangiectasias usually in a central facial distribution (Figure 1.2). There is a tendency for the periocular skin to be spared.

DIFFERENTIAL DIAGNOSIS

Differential diagnosis includes polycythemia vera, connective tissue disease, mastocytosis, photosensitivity, periorificial dermatitis, and chronic steroid application.

DIAGNOSTIC STUDIES

Biopsy is typically not necessary in patients responsive to treatment. Histopathology shows vascular dilation of the upper and mid-dermal vessels with perivascular and perifollicular lymphocytic inflammation. There are no typical laboratory findings.

TREATMENT

General treatment includes mild cleansers and moisturizers as well as sunscreens. The various subtypes of disease have more specific treatments. See Table 1.4 for treatment.

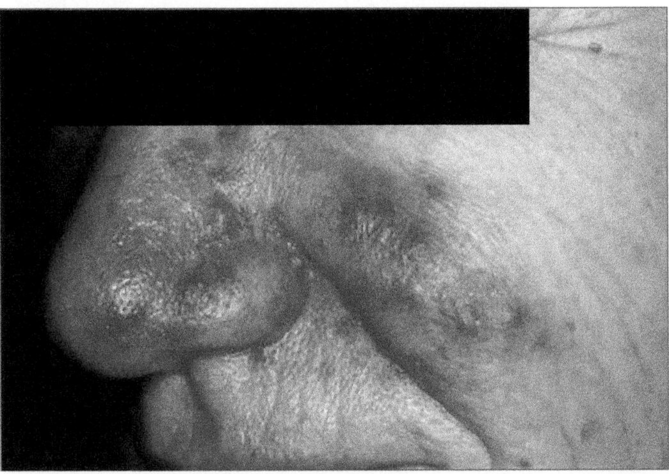

Figure 1.2 Rosacea.
(Source: Image courtesy of Michael Sand, Daniel Sand, Christina Thrandorf, Volker Paech, Peter Altmeyer, and Falk G. Bechara.)

TABLE 1.4 Treatment of Rosacea

Subtype	Treatment
Erythematotelangiectatic rosacea	Topical azelaic acid or sodium sulfacetamide-sulfur or mild to high-potency steroid ointment Low-dose carvedilol for refractory flushing and persistent erythema
Papulopustular rosacea	Topical metronidazole, sodium sulfacetamide-sulfur, azelaic acid, tretinoin or ivermectin cream daily Systemic tetracycline, macrolides, or isotretinoin
Phymatous rosacea	Topical benzoyl peroxide, benzoyl peroxide plus antibiotics (clindamycin or erythromycin), tretinoin, sodium sulfacetamide-sulfur, or tretinoin Systemic tetracycline or macrolides, spironolactone, or oral contraceptives for women Patients with phymatous changes can be treated with isotretinoin or surgical options (laser ablation, dermabrasion, cryosurgery)
Ocular rosacea	Topical warm compresses, baby shampoo scrubs Systemic tetracyclines or macrolides, omega-3 fatty acid supplements

PATIENT EDUCATION

- Rosacea is a chronic inflammatory disease and may be associated with other inflammatory conditions such as atherosclerosis, gastroesophageal reflux disease, diabetes mellitus type 1, celiac disease, multiple sclerosis, and rheumatoid arthritis.
- Cutaneous complications include phymatous skin changes, skin fibrosis, and a purplish red color spread to the central facial skin.
- Reassessment should occur every 2 to 3 months to evaluate therapy. More aggressive reassessment is needed with the use of isotretinoin.

SPECIAL CONSIDERATIONS

- Because of teratogenicity, patients on isotretinoin should be provided with pregnancy-prevention measures and monitoring guidelines.

KEY POINTS

- The negative psychological effect of acne vulgaris can be profound and long-lasting.
- Combination therapy with a retinoid and a BP–containing antimicrobial agent is used to control mild-to-severe inflammatory acne.
- For moderate-to-severe cases, an oral antibiotic agent is also recommended.
- Combined oral contraceptive therapy and spironolactone are effective hormonal therapies for inflammatory acne in female patients.

1.2 DESQUAMATION DISORDERS

OVERVIEW

While there are several desquamation disorders, this section will focus on three major disorders: erythema multiforme (EM), Stevens-Johnson syndrome (SJS), and toxic epidermal necrolysis (TEN). These three disorders were thought to be on a continuum, but now it is felt that EM is different from the other two disorders. All are characterized by confluent epidermal necrosis with minimal associated inflammation.

EPIDEMIOLOGY

The annual incidence of EM is about 1% and EM occurs most frequently in young adults.[6] Incidence of SJS is 5.3 cases per 1 million person-years and for TEN is 0.4 case per 1 million person-years.[7]

PATHOPHYSIOLOGY

EM is a skin condition of unknown etiology but may be mediated by deposition of immune complex in the superficial microvasculature of the skin and oral mucous membranes. The exact pathophysiology of SJS/TEN is not completely understood but it is believed it may be immune mediated because of a major histocompatibility complex (MHC) class I restricted T-cell mediated cytotoxic reaction to drug antigens leading to cell death.

1.2A ERYTHEMA MULTIFORME

EM is an acute, self-limiting disorder due to a hypersensitivity reaction. The hallmark finding is targetoid lesions of the skin with or without bullae or erosions. EM can be grouped into two categories based on severity. EM minor is noted in patients with little to no mucosal involvement while EM major is noted in patients with mucosal involvement of the oral, genital, or ocular mucosa.

MEDICAL HISTORY AND CLINICAL PRESENTATION

With EM there is acute development over days of erythematous papules on the skin, extremities, and oral/genital or ocular mucosa. The lesions are often painful and pruritic. They may become bullous and erode. Associated symptoms might include fever, malaise, or myalgias with pulmonary symptoms (e.g., cough, shortness of breath, sputum production) noted in patients with underlying *Mycoplasma pneumoniae* infection.

The majority of cases of EM are induced by acute or chronic infections with acute herpes simplex virus (HSV) infections being the most common. Several common medications (e.g., antibiotics, antiepileptics, sulfonamides, and nonsteroidal anti-inflammatory drugs [NSAIDs]) are linked to the development of EM.

PHYSICAL EXAMINATION

The most common physical findings in EM include:

- Targetoid lesions with associated concentric color zones, bullae, and/or necrosis symmetrically on the skin (trunk, back, extremities or face), palms, and/or soles with or without oral, genital, and ocular mucosa involvement
- Associated conjunctivitis and/or ciliary flush

TABLE 1.5 Differential Diagnosis for Erythema Multiforme

Differential Diagnosis	Description
Stevens-Johnson syndrome	Mucosal involvement and macular lesions on the skin, with the most common cause being drugs
Bullous pemphigus	Blistering disorder involving the skin and can involve the mucous membranes, differentiated by presence of autoimmune antibodies and/or skin biopsy
Paraneoplastic pemphigus	Blistering disorder associated with lymphoma, leukemia; differentiated by the presence of autoimmune antibodies to plakin proteins and skin biopsy
Urticaria	Acute erythematous pruritic plaques that last up to 24 hours with new lesions appearing continuously over the outbreak period
Fixed drug eruption	Single or multiple erythematous plaques with or without necrosis or bullae in association with drug therapy
Systemic lupus erythematosus	Lesions in patient with cutaneous lupus; differentiated by clinical picture and presence of antinuclear antibodies

DIFFERENTIAL DIAGNOSIS

Conditions that might mimic EM are noted in Table 1.5.

DIAGNOSTIC STUDIES

The diagnosis of EM is clinical, and biopsy can be used to exclude other possible diagnoses.

TREATMENT

The management of EM consists of the following: determine the severity of the disease, evaluate for possible causes and treat any that may be life-threatening, discontinue any possible etiologic medication, and treat any secondary skin infections.

1.2B STEVENS-JOHNSON SYNDROME

SJS is a severe reactive blistering disease. The condition is rare in the general population with increased incidence in the HIV-positive population. Though SJS is most commonly associated with exposure to medications, it is also associated with herpesvirus or *Mycoplasma*. The onset of the disease ranges from 1 to 3 weeks after exposure to the medication.

MEDICAL HISTORY AND CLINICAL PRESENTATION

Most of cases of SJS are caused by exposure to a medication. See Box 1.2 for a list of common medications linked to SJS. Fewer than half of cases of SJS are caused by infections, with herpes or *Mycoplasma* being the most common.

SIGNS AND SYMPTOMS

SJS starts with a prodrome of fever, sore throat, malaise, and influenza-like symptoms. The prodrome starts 2 to 3 days before skin manifestations. Skin manifestations include pain, blisters, and rash involving the two or more mucous membranes. Arthralgias may also be noted.

BOX 1.2 Drugs Implicated in Stevens-Johnson Syndrome and Toxic Epidermal Necrolysis

- Sulfonamides
- Nevirapine
- Anticonvulsants (e.g., lamotrigine, carbamazepine, phenytoin, barbiturates)
- Allopurinol
- Aminopenicillins
- Nonsteroidal anti-inflammatory drugs (e.g., ibuprofen, naproxen)

PHYSICAL EXAMINATION

Skin findings include erythematous, dusky, or purpuric macules that progress to atypical targetoid lesions with purpuric centers followed by desquamation. These purpuric atypical targets develop into bullae followed by desquamation. The face and trunk are often the initial sites of involvement along with palms and soles. SJS covers <10% of the patient's body surface area (BSA); the maximum BSA is reached within 4 days. Slight rubbing of intact skin results in exfoliation; this is called a positive Nikolsky sign.

Other findings include shock due to hypovolemia, toxic appearance, lymphadenopathy, hepatosplenomegaly, and swollen, tender joints.

DIFFERENTIAL DIAGNOSIS

Differential diagnosis includes:

- **Staphylococcal scalded skin syndrome:** Commonly noted in newborns and young children, spares the mucous membranes and palms and soles
- **Acute graft-versus-host disease (GVHD):** Noted most commonly in allogeneic stem cell transplantation recipients
- **Paraneoplastic pemphigus:** Noted in patients with non-Hodgkin lymphoma, chronic lymphocytic leukemia, sarcoma, or thymoma; severe oropharyngeal erosions/ulcerations
- **Erythema multiforme:** Target lesions that may be pruritic or burning, involving palms and soles

DIAGNOSTIC STUDIES

Routine laboratory studies are not needed. White blood cell count can vary, with about a fifth of patients having eosinophilia. Elevated aspartate aminotransferase and/or alanine transaminase, glucose, and creatinine may be noted. Sedimentation rate is elevated. The diagnosis of SJS is most commonly made clinically. When the diagnosis is unclear a skin biopsy may be helpful.

TREATMENT

Treatment consists of discontinuing the offending agent as soon as possible. Care in a burn unit may be needed if

>15% of BSA is involved. Drug treatment is controversial. Cyclosporine has been shown to decrease disease duration. Systemic corticosteroids may increase risk of mortality and, if used, should be used early. Other treatment options include plasma exchange or intravenous (IV) immune globulin (IVIG). Systemic antibiotics are reserved for documented infections.

PATIENT EDUCATION

- The most common cause of death in patients with SJS/TEN is infection.

1.2C TOXIC EPIDERMAL NECROLYSIS

TEN is a severe reactive blistering disease. It is an uncommon to rare condition in the general population with increased incidence in the HIV-positive population. TEN is most commonly associated with exposure to medications and typically develops 1 to 3 weeks after starting the medication.

MEDICAL HISTORY AND CLINICAL PRESENTATION

Nearly all cases of TEN are caused by exposure to a medication, prescribed or over-the-counter. See Box 1.2 for a list of common medications.

SIGNS AND SYMPTOMS

Within 1 to 3 weeks of starting the offending drug, the patient develops a prodrome of malaise, fever, headache, cough, and keratoconjunctivitis. Macules, often targetoid, appear suddenly on the face, neck, and upper trunk. These macules appear elsewhere on the body, coalesce into large bullae, and slough over a period of 1 to 3 days. Nails and eyebrows may also be lost. The palms and soles may be involved. In severe cases, large sheets of epithelium slide off the entire body at pressure points—a positive Nikolsky sign—exposing weepy, painful, and erythematous skin.

PHYSICAL EXAMINATION

Skin findings include erythematous, dusky, or purpuric macules that progress to atypical targetoid lesions with purpuric centers followed by desquamation. These purpuric atypical targets develop into bullae followed by desquamation. The face and trunk are often the initial sites of involvement along with palms and soles. TEN covers more than 30% of the patient's BSA. Other findings include shock due to hypovolemia, toxic appearance, lymphadenopathy, hepatosplenomegaly, and swollen, tender joints.

DIFFERENTIAL DIAGNOSIS

The differential diagnosis is the same as for SJS as noted above.

DIAGNOSTIC STUDIES

The diagnosis of TEN is most commonly made clinically. When the diagnosis is unclear a skin biopsy may be helpful. Biopsy will reveal scattered necrotic keratinocytes to full-thickness epidermal necrosis with a lymphocytic inflammatory infiltrate.

TREATMENT

Treatment is most successful when started early. Stop the offending agent. Supportive care is essential and treatment in a burn unit or ICU may be needed. Drug treatment is controversial. Cyclosporine has been shown to decrease disease duration. Systemic corticosteroids may increase mortality risk and, if used, should be used early. Other treatment options include plasma exchange or IVIG.

Prognosis of TEN can be determined by the SCORTEN (Score of Toxic Epidermal Necrosis) scale.[8] This score is based on several factors including BSA involved, comorbidities, age, and signs of systemic disease at the time of admission.

PATIENT EDUCATION

- Overall mortality rate is approximately 10% in SJS and more than 30% in TEN.[9]
- Respiratory tract involvement is a poor prognostic indicator.
- The most common cause of death in patients with SJS/TEN is infection.

SPECIAL CONSIDERATIONS

- Ophthalmology consult is indicated with eye involvement.

KEY POINTS

- EM is usually caused by HSV but can be caused by medications.
- Target lesions and lesions on the palms and soles are noted in EM.
- Drugs are the cause of most cases of SJS and TEN.

1.3 HAIR AND NAIL DISORDERS

OVERVIEW

Nail and hair disorders are diseases distinct from other diseases of the skin. Many changes to the hair and nails may be related to other medical conditions. See Table 1.6 for nail changes related to systemic disease.

1.3A HAIR LOSS

There are two major types of alopecia to be discussed here: androgenetic alopecia and alopecia areata. Androgenetic alopecia is caused by genetic follicular sensitivity to androgens, particularly dihydrotestosterone (DHT), in select regions of the scalp. The intracellular enzyme 5α-reductase converts circulating testosterone to DHT, which then acts on specific intracellular receptors within the follicle and shortens the anagen phase, resulting in follicular atrophy. The role of androgens in the pathogenesis of female pattern hair loss is unknown.

Alopecia areata is thought to be caused by an autoimmune attack at the base of the hair follicle that spares the stem cell compartment of the follicle, so regrowth of hair remains possible.

TABLE 1.6 Nail Changes Noted With Systemic Diseases

Nail Finding	Definition	Systemic Disease
Beau lines	Horizontal lines on nail plate due to interrupted nail bed mitosis	Pemphigus Chemotherapy Raynaud disease
Pitting	Pinpoint depressions in the nails	Psoriasis Lichen planus Alopecia areata
Clubbing	Thickening of nail bed soft tissue with angle between nail plate and soft tissue >180 degrees, due to altered vasculature	Cystic fibrosis Pulmonary fibrosis Celiac sprue Bronchiectasis COPD
Koilonychia	Spoon nails with concavity of the nail	Iron deficiency Hemochromatosis Hypothyroidism SLE
Mees lines	White bands traversing the nail bed, running parallel to the lunula across the entire nail bed	Arsenic poisoning Heavy metal poisoning
Muehrcke lines	Transverse white lines within the nail bed	Hypoalbuminemia Nephrotic syndrome Malnutrition
Pincer line	Transverse line over the curvature of the nail plate	SLE Psoriasis Onychomycosis Kawasaki disease
Splinter hemorrhage	Red-brown longitudinal lines due to leaking capillaries in the nail bed	Endocarditis Psoriasis

COPD, chronic obstructive pulmonary disease; SLE, systemic lupus erythematosus.

MEDICAL HISTORY AND CLINICAL PRESENTATION

Both males and females of all races are equally affected, and it is estimated that 50% of males and females have some degree of pattern hair loss by age 50.[10] Male and female pattern hair loss can express itself any time after puberty, most often between 20 and 30 years of age, and again during or after the fifth decade in both genders. Male and female pattern hair loss is considered an autosomal dominant disease with variable penetrance.

Ninety-five percent of cases of alopecia areata involve the scalp, but any hair-bearing area can be affected. All races and males and females are affected equally. Alopecia totalis is defined as a loss of 100% of scalp hair and alopecia universalis is loss of 100% of body hair.

SIGNS AND SYMPTOMS

Androgenetic alopecia presents with gradual hair loss over time.

Alopecia areata presents with a sudden onset of asymptomatic patchy, nonscarring hair loss. Recurrence is common. A prodrome consisting of mild paresthesia, pruritus, tenderness, or a burning sensation may precede hair loss.

PHYSICAL EXAMINATION

In androgenetic alopecia with the male pattern hair loss the frontal hairline will take on a classic "M" shape or have thinning of the vertex, crown, and frontal scalp. The peripheral scalp is often unaffected. Female pattern hair loss characteristically spares the anterior hairline and patients typically first notice an increase in the width of their part over the crown. Few females have diffuse thinning of the entire scalp.

Alopecia areata presents with 1- to 4-cm well-demarcated round to oval patches of hair loss with exclamation point hairs at the periphery. A hair pull test is positive, with greater than five hairs shed with pulling small tufts of hair near the area of alopecia. Nail changes are found in up to two-thirds of cases, including linear pitting.

DIFFERENTIAL DIAGNOSIS

The diagnosis of androgenetic alopecia is straightforward, so developing a differential diagnosis is not needed. Trichotillomania can present in a pattern like female pattern hair loss and present with broken hairs and hairs of variable length.

The differential diagnosis for alopecia areata includes trichotillomania, tinea capitis, secondary syphilis, and telogen effluvium. Trichotillomania presents with irregularly shaped areas of alopecia, with broken hairs and a negative hair pull test. Tinea capitis presents with inflamed, scaling patches of alopecia with characteristic black dot hairs. Secondary syphilis presents with a moth-eaten pattern of irregular, diffuse patches of alopecia. Telogen effluvium is a form of temporary hair loss that usually happens after stress, a shock, or a traumatic event. It usually occurs on the top of the scalp.

DIAGNOSTIC STUDIES

Androgenetic alopecia in females with signs of excess androgens should be worked up with serum-free and total testosterone, serum dehydroepiandrosterone sulfate (DHEAS), serum prolactin, and thyroid-stimulating hormone.

TREATMENT

Androgenetic alopecia treatment in men consists of topical minoxidil and oral finasteride. It may take 6 to 12 months before results are noted. The most common side effect is scalp irritation, which generally improves with repeated applications. Oral finasteride may need to be used for 6 months before change is noted. Males over the age of 40 years need a baseline prostate-specific antigen (PSA) level as finasteride will decrease the PSA level by half. Sexual side effects such as impotence are rare and often recede with treatment continuation.

Androgenetic alopecia treatment in women is treated with minoxidil. Side effects include symmetric facial hypertrichosis that reverses once the medication is stopped. Scalp irritation can develop but lessens with continued treatment.

Antiandrogen therapy, with spironolactone, is used when systemic androgen excess is associated with female pattern hair loss but may be used in conjunction with topical minoxidil in resistant cases. Side effects include breast tenderness and menstrual irregularity. Use of an oral contraceptive can limit these side effects.

Nonpharmacologic treatments include follicular unit hair transplant and hair pieces.

Treatment of alopecia areata consists of observation, since regrowth can occur in 1 to 3 months, or intralesional triamcinolone acetonide injections. Triamcinolone acetonide is the therapy of choice and if no response is seen within 6 months, consider alternative treatment.

PATIENT EDUCATION

- The course of alopecia areata is unpredictable. Most patients will experience regrowth of hair in 1 to 3 months with or without therapy, but relapse is common.
- Patients should be counseled that hair washing and styling will not expedite loss.

1.3B ONYCHOMYCOSIS

Onychomycosis is a fungal infection of the nail. It is common and makes up over half of all nail abnormalities. Toenails are affected ten times more frequently than fingernails, and onychomycosis presents in males three times more frequently than females. Predisposing factors include diabetes mellitus, peripheral vascular disease, immunosuppression, genetic predisposition, occlusive footwear, repeated nail microtrauma, use of communal showers, and older age.

Dermatophytes are the most common cause of onychomycosis, followed by yeasts. Dermatophytes include *Trichophyton* and *Epidermophyton*. The most common yeast etiology is *Candida albicans*.

MEDICAL HISTORY AND CLINICAL PRESENTATION

Onychomycosis presents with nail discoloration, brittleness, or thickening. Disfigured nails can cause local pain. Predisposing factors include diabetes mellitus, older age, peripheral vascular disease, and immunosuppression.

PHYSICAL EXAMINATION

On physical examination white/yellow or orange/brown longitudinal streaks in the nail plate are noted. Nonspecific clinical findings include onycholysis, subungual hyperkeratosis, and nail thickening

DIFFERENTIAL DIAGNOSIS

The differential diagnosis includes dermatologic disorders such as psoriasis and lichen planus (LP), genetic disorders such as pachyonychia congenita, nail unit neoplasms, repeated trauma, drugs, bacterial infections, and systemic diseases.

DIAGNOSTIC STUDIES

The most common diagnostic studies are potassium hydroxide (KOH) smear, fungal culture, and histopathologic examination. KOH smear may reveal septate hyphae and/or arthroconidia and fungal culture may be positive for dermatophytes or *Candida* organisms. *Candida albicans* may be a contaminant and clinical correlation is critical.

TREATMENT

There are several topical and systemic antifungal medications used in the treatment of onychomycosis.

Terbinafine is an allylamine oral antifungal used in the treatment of dermatophyte onychomycosis. Side effects are mild and transient, and include gastrointestinal disturbances, liver function abnormalities, and dermatologic effects. Hepatotoxicity, exacerbation of systemic lupus erythematosus, and SJS have been reported.

Itraconazole is a triazole antifungal used in the treatment of dermatophyte onychomycosis. Itraconazole is fungistatic. Itraconazole is contraindicated in patients with heart failure. Hepatic injury has been reported during and after treatment completion. Liver function tests should be monitored monthly.

Griseofulvin is fungistatic against dermatophytes, but ineffective against molds and *Candida* species. It has a low affinity for keratin and requires long-term therapy. Griseofulvin should be avoided in pregnancy, systemic lupus erythematosus, hepatocellular failure, and porphyria.

Fluconazole, a triazole, is fungistatic against dermatophytes, *Candida*, and some nondermatophytes. Fluconazole is well tolerated.

PATIENT EDUCATION

- The infected nail plate will continue to grow out after the completion of oral therapy.
- May take 6 to 9 months for fingernails and 12 to 18 months for toenails to completely grow out.
- Nails may not appear normal even after the eradication of fungi.
- Recurrence is common.

1.3C PARONYCHIA

Paronychia is an infection of the nail bed. Acute and chronic paronychia are best separated by a detailed history. Acute paronychia is most commonly due to *Staphylococcus aureus*, followed by *Streptococcus*, *Pseudomonas,* or *Proteus* species. Chronic paronychia is most commonly due to habitual hand washing, extensive manicure with cuticle destruction, and infection with *Candida* species or molds.

Acute paronychia is an acute dermatitis due to bacteria just beneath the proximal and/or lateral nail folds, leading to inflammation. Pus formation can develop.

Chronic paronychia is due to repeated inflammatory processes due to different detergents causing chronic dermatitis. Pus formation is uncommon.

MEDICAL HISTORY AND CLINICAL PRESENTATION

History may include excessive hand washing with water and soaps, detergents, and other chemicals; recurrent manicure or pedicure that injures the nail folds; allergic contact dermatitis; or irritation due to certain nail polish or latex. Pain, swelling, and increased warmth may be noted.

PHYSICAL EXAMINATION

Acute infection presents with redness, with or without pus, and swelling around the lateral or proximal nail plates. Acute paronychia causes warmth and variable pain along the nail margin; mild pressure on the nail folds may provoke severe pain.

Chronic infection presents with findings consistent with acute paronychia, but no pus accumulation. In the chronic phase, nail changes such as thick, rough ridges or other nail deformations may be noted.

DIAGNOSTIC STUDIES

Diagnosis is based on the clinical appearance and the clinical history of the paronychia. Ultrasound examination and culture from purulent material will help determine if and what systemic antibiotic should be given.

TREATMENT

Prevention is key with chronic paronychia. Prevention includes avoiding excessive hand and/or foot washing, proper nail care including cutting of the nails, avoidance of nail biting or picking, and avoidance of nail irritants.

Medical treatment is based in severity and cause of the infection. If pus is present it should be drained. If a systemic antibiotic is indicated, treatment options include dicloxacillin or clindamycin. If methicillin-resistant *S. aureus* (MRSA) is a concern, doxycycline or trimethoprim/sulfamethoxazole should be used. If *Pseudomonas* infection is a concern, ofloxacin should be given.

Surgical treatment may be recommended as monotherapy in mild cases. In severe cases surgical treatment is recommended with an antibiotic.

SPECIAL CONSIDERATIONS

- Spironolactone and finasteride use in alopecia is contraindicated in pregnancy.

KEY POINTS

- Onychomycosis treatment is warranted if severe; first-line therapy is terbinafine.
- Paronychia presents with severe redness, pain, and warmth along the nail margin.
- Androgenetic alopecia is the most common type of hair loss.

1.4 INSECT BITES

OVERVIEW

Stinging insects are members of the order Hymenoptera. Hymenoptera venoms cause local reactions in all people and allergic reactions in those previously sensitized. Severity depends on the dose of venom and degree of previous sensitization. The average unsensitized person can safely tolerate 22 stings/kg body weight.

The major Hymenoptera subgroups are as follows:

- Apids (e.g., honeybees, bumblebees)
- Vespids (e.g., wasps, yellow jackets, hornets)
- Formicids (e.g., nonwinged fire ants)

Other insect bites to consider are black widow and brown recluse spider bites.

EPIDEMIOLOGY

Honeybees are the most common insect sting and can lead to severe allergic reactions. According to the American Association of Poison Control Centers, there were 7,140 single exposures to insects (ants, bees, wasps, hornets, mosquitos, and other) with 435 moderate reactions, 14 serious reactions, and 3 deaths in 2018.[11]

Black widow spiders (*Latrodectus mactans*) are most commonly found from southern New England to the southern United States. The spider is 3 to 4 cm in length and has a red hourglass-shaped marking on the ventral surface of the abdomen. Only the female spider is capable of envenomation.

Brown recluse spiders (*Loxosceles rectusa*) are typically noted in south central United States. The spider is yellow, tan, or brown with a 10 to 15 mm body length and has a dark brown, violin-shaped marking on its back.

PATHOPHYSIOLOGY

The most common response is a local allergic reaction to proteins in insect saliva, as noted with mosquito bites. The more severe anaphylactic reaction is a IgE-mediated systemic allergic reaction and occurs with insects from the order Hymenoptera.

Black widow venom is a neurotoxin that causes acetylcholine depletion at the motor nerve ending and catecholamine release from adrenergic nerve endings. With a brown recluse spider bite, there is release of sphingomyelinase D, which is cytotoxic and is responsible for the necrosis.

SIGNS AND SYMPTOMS

Local apid and vespid reactions present as immediate burning, transient pain, and itching, with erythema, swelling, and induration up to a few centimeters across. Swelling and erythema peak at 48 hours but can persist for weeks. Allergic reactions manifest with urticaria, angioedema, bronchospasm, refractory hypotension, or a combination of these symptoms.

Symptoms and signs of a formicid bite are immediate pain followed by a wheal and flare lesion. This typically resolves in 45 minutes and may give rise to a sterile pustule. The lesions can become infected.

Black widow spider bites present with a mildly painful target-lesion bite reaction along with crampy abdominal pain, hypertension, muscle complaints, and irritability or agitation. The abdominal pain may mimic an acute surgical abdomen.

Brown recluse spider bites may go unnoticed or present with a localized hive-like reaction with minimal redness and swelling. A localized pain, burning, and stinging occur at the bite site 6 to 8 hours after the bite. Systemic symptoms may occur including fever, chills, nausea and vomiting, weakness, and muscle pain within 12 to 24 hours.

PHYSICAL EXAMINATION

A pink hive or raised wheal with a central pinpoint opening appears about 20 minutes after the bite or sting. Angioedema develops, with a localized reaction that appears thick, hard, and edematous over an area 10 to 50 cm.

The physical examination findings in black widow bites are variable and include a mild erythema or swelling at the bite sites. Red-brown fang marks may be noted.

Brown recluse spider bites present with a localized hive-like reaction with minimal redness and swelling. This is followed by a cyanotic color and expanding necrosis. A small percentage go on to develop significant necrosis. Most severe reactions occur in tissue with high fat content, such as the thighs, abdomen, and buttocks.

DIFFERENTIAL DIAGNOSIS

The differential diagnosis for insect bites includes hives, angioedema, and bites from other insects. The differential diagnosis for spider bites includes the acute abdomen, black widow spider bite, brown recluse spider bite, necrotizing fasciitis, and pyoderma gangrenosum.

DIAGNOSTIC STUDIES

Diagnosis is clinical. Apid stings are checked for the stinger. Upper and lower airways are assessed for signs of allergic reaction. Secondary bacterial cellulitis is rare but is considered when erythema and swelling begin a day or two after the sting (rather than immediately), there are systemic signs of infection (e.g., fever, chills), and pain is significant.

TREATMENT

Localized care includes removal of any stinger. The pain, burning, and itching can be reduced with ice packs or cold compress over the sting and with oral H_1 blockers and/or NSAIDs. For allergic reactions IV antihistamines can be used and for severe anaphylaxis parenteral epinephrine is given. Alert bracelets should be provided to all patients with a history of anaphylaxis or a known allergy to insect bites.

Treatment of black widow spider bites consists of ice to limit spread of the venom and intramuscular (IM) or IV antivenom for severe envenomation with pain poorly controlled with opioid analgesics. Muscle relaxants may be needed.

Most brown recluse spider bites heal with supportive care only. Treatment, if needed, of brown recluse spider bites consists of localized ice, cold compresses, elevation, and pain medications. Necrotic tissue may need local wound care or surgical debridement. Antibiotics and tetanus toxoid may be indicated. Dapsone can be used to prevent severe necrosis.

PATIENT EDUCATION

- People who have had anaphylaxis are at risk from subsequent stings.
- Desensitization immunotherapy can be considered as venom immunotherapy is highly effective.
- A high degree of suspicion is needed to make the diagnosis of spider bites.

SPECIAL CONSIDERATIONS

- Venom immunotherapy seems to be safe for use during pregnancy.

KEY POINTS

- Apid and vespid stings cause immediate pain, burning, itching, erythema, and swelling.
- Allergic reaction symptoms include urticaria, angioedema, bronchospasm, and possibly hypotension.
- Local treatment consists of ice, oral H_1 blockers, and/or NSAIDs.

1.5 EXANTHEMS

OVERVIEW

An exanthem is any eruptive skin rash that can be associated with systemic symptoms, such as fever. Etiologies include infectious pathogens, medication reactions, or a combination of both.

Viral exanthems are common in childhood. Diagnosing a exanthem is based on the characteristic morphology, distribution and time course of the eruption, as well as an assessment of infectious contacts, immunization status, and physical examination. See Table 1.7 for a summary of the viral exanthems.

TABLE 1.7 Summary Review of the Viral Exanthems

Syndrome	Agent	Description	Epidemiology
Roseola	Human herpesvirus-6	Erythematous macules and papules surrounded by white halos	Infant-preschool
Erythema infectiosum (fifth disease)	Parvovirus B19	Erythematous cheeks (slapped cheek) followed by reticular red rash on the body	School age
Hand-foot-and-mouth disease	Coxsackie virus A16 Enterovirus 71	Vesicles on palms, soles, and buttocks; oral erosions	Infant-preschool
Measles	Measles	Erythematous macules and papules with white lesions on the buccal mucosa	Most cases in the United States are imported or lack of vaccination
Rubella	Rubella	Pruritic pink macules and papules with petechial lesions on the soft palate	Lack of vaccination

1.5A ERYTHEMA INFECTIOSUM

Erythema infectiosum (EI) is due to infection with parvovirus B19.

Most infections occur in children between the ages of 4 and 10 years and occur most commonly in late winter and spring. Transmission is most common via the respiratory route with an incubation period of 4 to 15 days. Although most individuals become infected, most persons with infection are asymptomatic.

MEDICAL HISTORY AND CLINICAL PRESENTATION

The diagnosis of EI is a clinical diagnosis, made after a careful history and physical examination. Classically there are three stages of the disease:

1. Mild prodromal illness characterized by low-grade fever, headache, malaise, myalgia, and gastrointestinal complaints
2. Erythematous exanthem on the face that involves the malar eminences and spares the nasal bridge and perioral area, giving the characteristic "slapped cheek" appearance
3. Lacy, erythematous, maculopapular exanthem on the trunk and extremities

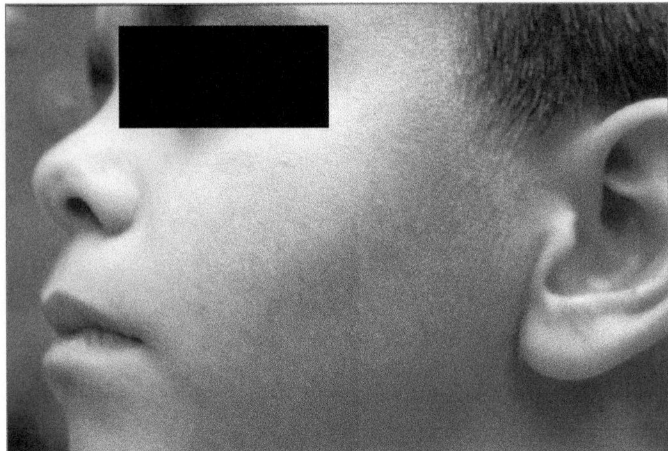

Figure 1.3 Erythema infectiosum, facial erythema ("slapped cheek"). *(Source: Centers for Disease Control and Prevention/Dr. Philip S. Brachman.)*

PHYSICAL EXAMINATION

The facial exanthem occurs 3 to 7 days after the prodrome, while the lacy, reticular exanthem develops 1 to 4 days after the appearance of the facial rash (Figure 1.3). The facial rash may be become more pronounced with exposure to sunlight, while the lacy reticular rash on the trunk and extremities may be pruritic.

Patients typically appear well, and do not appear toxic. A low-grade fever may be present in the prodromal stage but is not present during the exanthematous stages.

A symmetric polyarthropathy of the knees and fingers is common in adults and an asymmetric involvement of the knees is most common in children.

DIFFERENTIAL DIAGNOSIS

The differential diagnosis of EI includes measles, rubella, roseola, streptococcal scarlet fever, drug reactions, and vasculitis.

DIAGNOSTIC STUDIES

Diagnostic studies for EI are not needed.

TREATMENT

In healthy patients the infection is self-limited, and no specific therapy is warranted.

PATIENT EDUCATION

- Children with EI are not contagious. The period of contagion is 1 to 2 weeks before the appearance of the exanthem. Children with EI can attend school or child care, because they are no longer contagious at the time that the rash appears.

1.5B HAND-FOOT-AND-MOUTH DISEASE

Hand-foot-and-mouth disease is caused by group A coxsackievirus, particularly serotypes A16, A5, and A10. Enterovirus 71 can cause a similar illness with more neurologic symptoms. Infants and young children have the highest rate of infection, although all age groups can be affected. The disease peaks in the summer and fall.

Transmission is by fecal-oral route primarily, so persons involved in diaper changing and young children with poor toilet hygiene are at risk The virus sheds from the upper respiratory tract for 1 to 3 weeks and from the feces for 3 to 8 weeks. Patients are most contagious in the first 1 to 2 weeks of illness, when the rash is present.

MEDICAL HISTORY AND CLINICAL PRESENTATION

Three to 6 days after infection, symptoms develop. The exanthem is typically accompanied by fever, which may precede the rash. Other symptoms include cough, sore throat, myalgias, malaise, mild abdominal pain, nausea, vomiting, and diarrhea. Oral lesions can be painful and may cause diminished appetite or refusal to eat or drink.

PHYSICAL EXAMINATION

Hand-foot-and-mouth disease presents with small, tender, gray-white, ovoid papules, papulovesicles, and vesicles on the palms of the hands and soles of the feet. Dorsal and lateral surfaces of the hands, feet, and digits may also be involved. The vesicles are surrounded by an erythematous border. Painful macular or vesicular lesions develop in the mouth several days after onset of fever (Figure 1.4).

Eruption of erythematous macules, papules, and vesicles may be observed on the buttocks, thighs, and genitalia.

DIFFERENTIAL DIAGNOSIS

The differential diagnosis includes infections with adenovirus, Epstein-Barr virus, group A streptococcus, HSV, human herpesvirus 6, measles, EI, and rubella.

DIAGNOSTIC STUDIES

Diagnostic studies are rarely needed in outpatient practice.

TREATMENT

Most patients require supportive care only. Adequate fluid intake should be assured, topical analgesia can provide temporary relief of pain, and fever can be controlled with oral ibuprofen and/or acetaminophen. The rash is self-resolving over a period of days and requires no specific therapy.

PATIENT EDUCATION

- Good hand hygiene should be practiced in order to avoid disease spread. Alcohol-based hand sanitizers may provide better antiviral activity than standard soap and water.
- Hospitalized patients should be placed under contact precautions.

1.5C MEASLES

Measles is caused by the measles virus. This virus is transmitted person to person via droplets to the respiratory tract and is highly contagious. Patients with measles are infectious 3 to 5 days before the onset of rash to about 4 days after the onset of rash. The incubation period for measles is about 10 days to onset of symptoms. Measles transmission peaks in late winter and early spring.

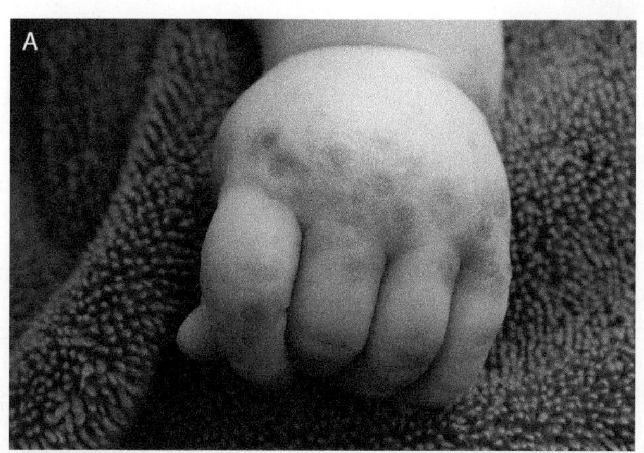

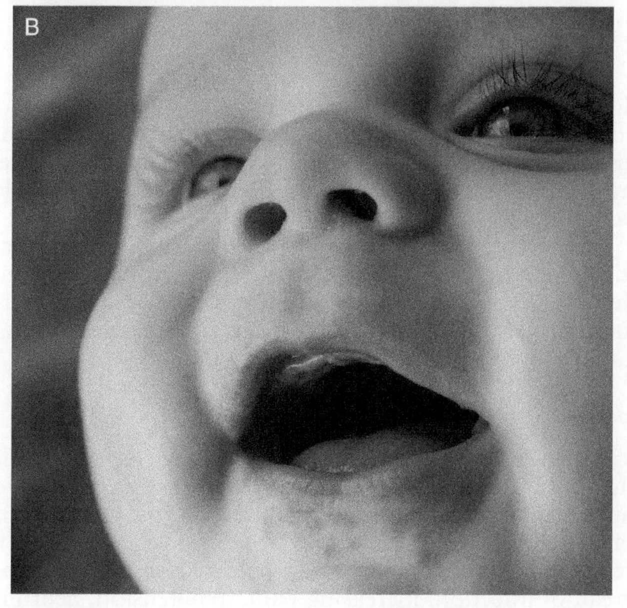

Figure 1.4 **Hand-foot-and-mouth disease. Top photo shows vesicles on the hand and bottom photo shows oral vesicles.**

(Source: Ousley LE, Gentry RD. Evidence-based assessment of skin, hair and nails. In: Gawlik KS, Melnyk BM, Teall AM, eds. Evidence-Based Physical Examination. *Springer Publishing Company; 2021:242.)*

Infants become susceptible to measles infection when passively acquired maternal antibody is lost. During the incubation period, measles virus replicates and spreads within the infected host. Replication occurs first in the upper respiratory tract and spreads to the lymphatic tissue. Viremia then develops and the virus spreads to the rest of the body.

MEDICAL HISTORY AND CLINICAL PRESENTATION

Measles symptoms begin 7 to 14 days after a person has been infected. Clinical presentation includes fever of at least 3 days and least one of the following: cough, coryza, and conjunctivitis. The fever may reach up to 104 °F. The erythematous maculopapular rash begins on the head and spreads to the trunk and extremities

The respiratory tract is a frequent site of complication, with pneumonia accounting for most measles-related deaths. Pneumonia is caused by secondary viral or bacterial infections or the measles virus in immunocompromised persons.

Serious complications can develop that involve the central nervous system. They include encephalomyelitis, measles inclusion body encephalitis, and subacute sclerosing panencephalitis.

PHYSICAL EXAMINATION

Three to 5 days after the start of symptoms, a red, pruritic, blanching, maculopapular erythematous rash appears. The rash first appears on the face, at the hairline, and spreads downward to the neck, trunk, and extremities. It disappears in the same fashion in 5 to 7 days. The rash may coalesce, becoming plaques and patches. The patient's fever may spike at the appearance of the rash. Koplik spots (small white papules) are seen on the buccal mucosa before the onset of rash.

DIFFERENTIAL DIAGNOSIS

The differential diagnosis includes rubella, enterovirus infection, roseola, scarlet fever, and dengue fever.

DIAGNOSTIC STUDIES

Diagnosis is typically made by history and physical examination. Serologic test for measles IgM antibodies can be used to confirm the diagnosis. A positive test indicates acute measles virus infection.

False negative test results may be noted if testing is done within 72 hours of rash onset. In this case if measles is suspected, the test should be repeated.

TREATMENT

Treatment of uncomplicated measles is symptomatic and includes bed rest, hydration, and antipyretic agents.

The World Health Organization recommends administration of two daily doses of 200,000 IU of vitamin A to children with measles who are 12 months of age or older, 100,000 IU is recommended for children 6 to 12 months of age, and 50,000 IU for children younger than 6 months of age.[12]

PATIENT EDUCATION

- The Centers for Disease Control and Prevention (CDC) recommends children receive the measles, mumps, and rubella (MMR) vaccine at age 12 to 15 months, and again at 4 to 6 years.

1.5D ROSEOLA

Roseola disease is caused by human herpesvirus 6 (HHV6). It is acquired via respiratory droplets. It is a disease of infants and characterized by an abrupt rise in body temperature to as high as 40 °C (104 °F) followed by a rapid drop to normal within the next 2 to 4 days with the appearance of an erythematous maculopapular rash that lasts for 1 to 3 days. It is a benign disease that resolves without complications.

MEDICAL HISTORY AND CLINICAL PRESENTATION

The infection is most common in infants and toddlers between 6 months and 3 years of age and is more common in the spring. Roseola presents with a nonpruritic maculopapular rash preceded for 3 to 5 days by high fever (40–40.5 °C) in an otherwise healthy appearing infant.

PHYSICAL EXAMINATION

The rash is a blanching, nonpruritic maculopapular rash starting on the trunk, neck, and spreading to the extremities. The rash can be vesicular and last from a few hours to 3 days.

Other findings include upper respiratory injection of the tympanic membranes and cervical or occipital lymphadenopathy. Red papules on the soft palate may be seen, called Nagayama spots.

DIFFERENTIAL DIAGNOSIS

Differential diagnosis includes other viral exanthems such as adenovirus, enterovirus, parvovirus B19, rubella, and parainfluenza.

DIAGNOSTIC STUDIES

Diagnostic studies are rarely needed to make the diagnosis.

TREATMENT

The disease is typically mild and self-limiting, and treatment is supportive using antipyretics, such as acetaminophen, during the febrile stage. In more severe cases, ganciclovir or foscarnet have activity against HHV-6.

1.6 BACTERIAL INFECTIONS

OVERVIEW

Bacterial skin infections are grouped as skin and soft tissue infections and as acute bacterial infections and skin structure infections. Skin and soft tissue infections include carbuncles, ecthyma, folliculitis, furuncles, impetigo, and lymphadenitis. Acute bacterial infections and skin structure infections include cellulitis, erysipelas, lymphangitis, and necrotizing soft tissue infection.

EPIDEMIOLOGY

Skin and soft tissue infections are one of the most common infections seen in all healthcare settings. From 2005 to 2009 the incidence of skin and soft tissue infections was between 45.5 and 50.0 episodes per 1,000 person-years.[13] This is much higher than urinary tract infections (17.3–20 episodes/1,000 person-years) and pneumonia (4.5–5.1 episodes/1,000 person-years).[13]

PATHOPHYSIOLOGY

Skin infections may be either primary or secondary. Primary infections are initiated by single organisms and usually occur in normal skin. They are most frequently caused by *Staphylococcus aureus*, *Streptococcus pyogenes*, and coryneform bacteria. Impetigo, folliculitis, boils, and erythrasma are examples. Systemic infections may also have skin manifestations. Secondary infections originate in diseased skin as a superimposed condition. Intertrigo and toe web infections are examples of secondary infections

1.6A CELLULITIS

Cellulitis is a diffuse acute inflammatory infectious process that involves the dermal and subcutaneous layers of the skin. Cellulitis develops when infectious organisms gain access and spread through the dermal and subcutaneous tissue layers, causing tissue damage and initiating an inflammatory response.

Streptococcal infections generally present as diffuse tissue infections without discrete abscess formation, while staphylococcal infections often start in the hair follicles, causing a neutrophilic response that results in a small abscess. Cellulitis can also develop from the contiguous infection spread from deeper focal processes such as osteomyelitis, septic arthritis, dental abscesses or enteric abscesses and fistulas.

MEDICAL HISTORY AND CLINICAL PRESENTATION

Medical history should focus on possible exposures or preceding events. Preceding events may include recent trauma, surgery, animal bites or scratches, environmental exposures, and contact with patients with streptococcal or staphylococcal infections.

The host's predisposition to infection should be evaluated. Review the history for chronic skin disorders, chronic edema or lymphedema, chronic open wounds, peripheral vascular disease, or systemic diseases that increase the risk of more severe infection.

SIGNS AND SYMPTOMS

Skin infections are most common in the lower extremities and usually unilateral. Signs and symptoms include fever, chills, tachycardia, headache, hypotension, and delirium and may precede cutaneous findings by several hours. A possible life-threatening infection should be considered when rapid spread of infection, increasing pain, hypotension, delirium, or skin sloughing is noted.

PHYSICAL EXAMINATION

Physical examination findings include induration and swelling, erythema, warmth, and tenderness that may be accompanied by fever and varying degrees of systemic toxicity. The skin is hot, red, and edematous. The infection borders are usually indistinct. Petechiae are common; large areas of ecchymosis are rare. Vesicles and bullae may develop and rupture. Tender regional lymph nodes and lymphangitic streaking may be noted.

DIFFERENTIAL DIAGNOSIS

The differential diagnosis includes superficial and deep venous thromboses, dermatologic conditions (such as contact dermatitis, eczema, urticaria, and angioedema), insect bites/stings, foreign body reactions, cutaneous drug reactions, rheumatologic inflammatory processes such as gout and lupus, and a variety of panniculitis syndromes.

DIAGNOSTIC STUDIES

Diagnosis is typically made based on history and physical examination. Laboratory findings in uncomplicated cellulitis include leukocytosis and elevated C-reactive protein (CRP).

Cultures can identify responsible pathogens but may also recover surface-colonizing organisms, making culture interpretation difficult. Blood cultures may be useful, but yield is typically low. Imaging results in cellulitis are nonspecific but may be helpful in diagnosing deeper, necrotizing soft tissue infections or underlying osteomyelitis.

TREATMENT

Patients with uncomplicated cellulitis can be safely managed with oral antimicrobial therapy. Oral antibiotics are targeted at beta-hemolytic streptococci and/or *S. aureus* including MRSA depending on clinical features.

Inpatient parenteral antimicrobial therapy is indicated in severely ill patients with more systemic toxicity, underlying immune compromise or multiple comorbidities. Approximately one-fifth of patients will require hospitalization and parenteral antibiotic therapy. Initial antibiotic regimens in these patients are often broader in spectrum than those used in less severely ill or immunocompromised patients and usually include streptococcal and staphylococcal activity. Typical total durations of antimicrobial therapy are 7 to 14 days, but durations are often determined by clinical response.

Local care such as limb elevation or compressive stockings can decrease edema and swelling. Surgical treatment, including abscess drainage or surgical debridement, may be indicated in severe infections.

Fasciotomy may be necessary with cellulitis and marked tissue edema that results in compartment syndrome.

Nonpurulent cellulitis treatment should cover both group A streptococci and *S. aureus*. Oral therapy is adequate for mild infections, typically with dicloxacillin or cephalexin. Levofloxacin or moxifloxacin can also be used if a single daily dose is needed. Bacteria resistant to the fluoroquinolones are becoming more prevalent. In patients allergic to penicillin, clindamycin or a newer macrolide are alternatives.

If the mild cellulitis is caused by mammalian bites, outpatient treatment with amoxicillin-clavulanate is indicated. If penicillin allergic, clindamycin plus either an oral fluoroquinolone or trimethoprim-sulfamethoxazole is indicated.

For suspect MRSA without high-risk symptoms, empiric outpatient treatment with trimethoprim-sulfamethoxazole, clindamycin, or doxycycline can be used. Patients with more serious infections, or if oral therapy has failed, or patients who are hospitalized can be treated with oxacillin or nafcillin or a cephalosporin, such as cefazolin. For penicillin-allergic patients or those with suspected or confirmed MRSA infection, drug options include vancomycin, linezolid, or daptomycin.

Cellulitis in a patient with neutropenia requires empiric antipseudomonal antibiotics, such as tobramycin, until blood culture results are available.

1.6B IMPETIGO

Impetigo is a superficial skin infection that may follow any type of break in the skin. Risk factors include a moist environment, poor hygiene, or chronic nasopharyngeal carriage of staphylococci or streptococci. Impetigo may be bullous or nonbullous. *Staphylococcus aureus* is the predominant cause of nonbullous impetigo and the cause of all bullous impetigo. Up to 70% of impetigo cases are nonbullous.[14]

MEDICAL HISTORY AND CLINICAL PRESENTATION

Nonbullous impetigo presents with honey-colored or light brown crusts around the mouth, nose, chin, and face. The infection can spread to other parts of the body through autoinoculation. The infection begins with an erythematous macule or papule that becomes a vesicle or pustule that ruptures leaving behind a honey-colored crust. Bullous impetigo begins as a vesicle that enlarges into a flaccid bulla filled with fluid. The bullae then rupture and leave behind fluid that also crusts over and develops an orange-brown color.

PHYSICAL EXAMINATION

Honey-colored crusts around the mouth, nose, chin, and other parts of the face are noted in nonbullous impetigo. (Figure 1.5) Underneath the dried liquid debris or crusts is a superficial, shining base. In bullous impetigo there are flaccid bullae with well-defined margins; they may be intact or may have ruptured leaving honey-colored crusts. Regional lymphadenopathy may occur but is not common.

DIFFERENTIAL DIAGNOSIS

The differential diagnosis for nonbullous disease includes ecthyma, superficial fungal infections, candidiasis, AD, contact dermatitis, and insect bites. The differential diagnosis for bullous disease includes bullous pemphigoid, pemphigus vulgaris, and staphylococcal scaled skin syndrome.

DIAGNOSTIC STUDIES

Diagnosis of impetigo is by characteristic appearance and laboratory studies are not required. The following laboratory findings may be noted:

- Complete blood count (CBC) shows mild leukocytosis.
- Erythrocyte sedimentation rate (ESR) and antistreptolysin O (ASO) titers are elevated.
- Anti-DNAse B and direct and indirect immunofluorescence of the skin are positive for infection.

Cultures are indicated only if the patient does not respond to empiric therapy. Patients with recurrent impetigo should have a nasal culture obtained to determine carrier status.

TREATMENT

Local care involves gentle washing of the area with soap and water several times a day to remove any crusts.

Treatment for localized impetigo is topical mupirocin ointment. Oral antibiotics, dicloxacillin or cephalexin, may be needed in immunocompromised patients, or those with extensive or resistant impetigo lesions. In penicillin-allergic patients clindamycin or erythromycin can be used, but resistance to both drugs is increasing.

Treatment of MRSA should be directed by culture and sensitivity test results, but typically clindamycin, trimethoprim/sulfamethoxazole, or doxycycline can be used.

Prompt recovery usually follows timely treatment.

PATIENT EDUCATION

- Prognosis is usually good, with complete resolution of the symptoms.
- Patients may have postinflammatory hyper- or hypopigmentation of the affected skin, but this should fade with time.

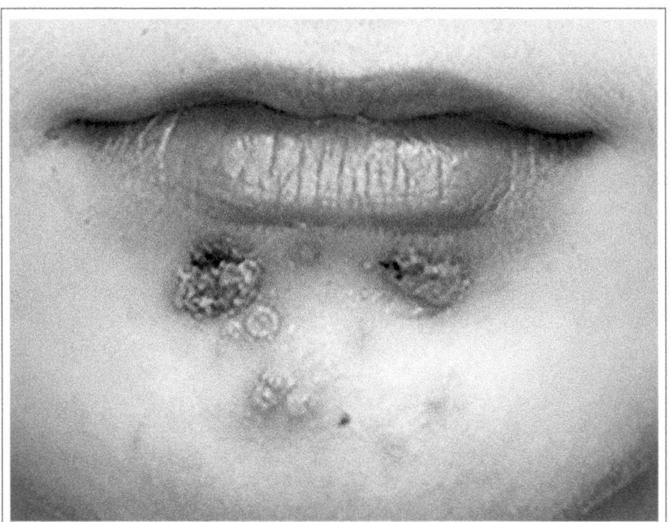

Figure 1.5 Impetigo. Note honey-crusted lesions around the mouth.
(Source: Ousley LE, Gentry RD. Evidence-based assessment of skin, hair and nails. In: Gawlik KS, Melnyk BM, Teall AM, eds. Evidence-Based Physical Examination. *Springer Publishing Company; 2021:242.)*

1.6C ERYSIPELAS

Erysipelas is an acute inflammatory epidermal infection. It is most often caused by group A (rarely group C or G) beta-hemolytic streptococci and occurs most frequently on the legs and face. Other etiologic organisms include *Staphylococcus aureus* (including MRSA), *Klebsiella pneumoniae, Haemophilus influenzae*, *Escherichia coli*, *Streptococcus pneumoniae*, *S. pyogenes*, and *Moraxella*. MRSA is more common in facial erysipelas than lower-extremity erysipelas.

Erysipelas may be recurrent and may result in chronic lymphedema. Erysipelas should not be confused with erysipeloid, a skin infection caused by *Erysipelothrix*. Erysipeloid is acquired by direct contact with infected animals.

MEDICAL HISTORY AND CLINICAL PRESENTATION

Erysipelas patients may present with blisters, fever, fatigue, vomiting, and pain and swelling of the infected area. Medical history should be reviewed to identify risk factors such as obesity, venous insufficiency, lymphedema, chronic skin ulcers, occupational or recreational exposures via mild trauma, and breast cancer.

PHYSICAL EXAMINATION

Erysipelas manifests with a characteristic rash involving the epidermis, typically on the face, torso, hands, and feet. Findings include erythema, edema, bullae, or vesicles. The patient may also be ill-appearing with systemic findings of fever and chills.

Erysipelas has a characteristic rash. The area is red and swollen, with a sharp, demarcated border between inflamed and normal tissue (Figure 1.6).

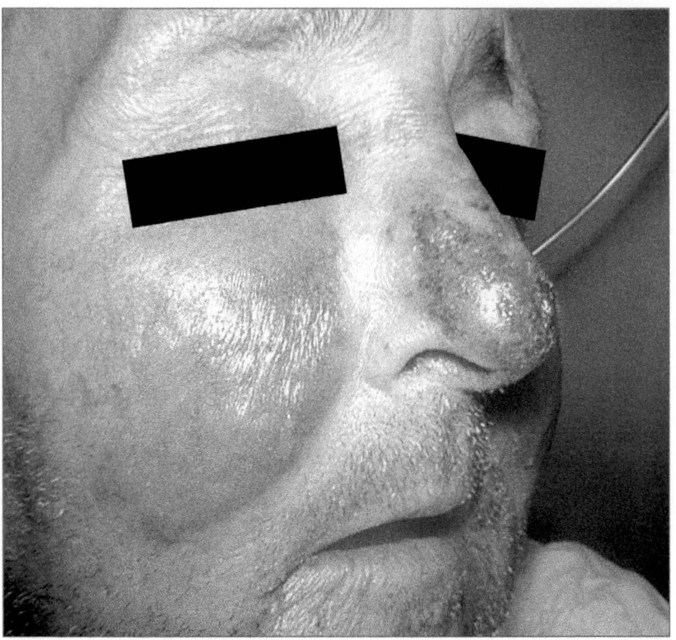

Figure 1.6 Erysipelas.
(Source: Centers for Disease Control and Prevention/Dr. Thomas F. Sellers, Emory University.)

DIFFERENTIAL DIAGNOSIS

The differential diagnosis of erysipelas includes chronic venous insufficiency, acute deep venous thrombosis, filariasis, and causes of generalized edema.

DIAGNOSTIC STUDIES

Diagnosis of erysipelas is by characteristic appearance and laboratory studies are not required.

TREATMENT

The treatment of choice is penicillin V for lower-extremity erysipelas and vancomycin or dicloxacillin for facial erysipelas or if MRSA is suspected. In the penicillin-allergic patient erythromycin, ceftriaxone, or cefazolin is given. Duration of treatment is based mainly on clinical response rather than a fixed interval.

PATIENT EDUCATION

- With treatment the prognosis is excellent.
- Complications of untreated erysipelas include sepsis, gangrene, glomerulonephritis, lymphedema, and streptococcal toxic shock syndrome.

KEY POINTS

- The most common pathogens for cellulitis are *S. pyogenes* and *S. aureus*.
- Do not culture skin or wounds.
- *S. aureus* causes most cases of impetigo and presents with honey-crusted lesions.
- Erysipelas presents with shiny, raised, indurated, and tender plaques with distinct margins. Systemic symptoms are common.

1.7 FUNGAL INFECTIONS

OVERVIEW

Fungi are typically noted in moist areas of the body where skin surfaces meet, such as between the toes, genital area, and under the breasts. Common fungal skin infections are caused by yeasts, including *Candida* or *Malassezia*; or dermatophytes, including *Epidermophyton*, *Microsporum*, and *Trichophyton*. Many fungi live in the topmost layer of the epidermis and do not penetrate deeper. Increased risk of infection is noted in obesity because of excessive skin folds and broken-down areas of skin and diabetes due to increased susceptibility.

EPIDEMIOLOGY

A study from South Korea looking at mycoses infection from 2009–2013 showed the annual prevalence of all-type mycoses is approximately 7.0%.[15] Dermatophyte infection was 5.2% annually, opportunistic mycoses 1.7%, and superficial mycoses 0.2%.[15] The prevalence of subcutaneous mycoses and generalized mycoses is very low.

PATHOPHYSIOLOGY

Mycoses are classified according to the tissue level they colonize. Superficial infections are limited to the outermost layers of the skin and hair. Cutaneous infections extend deeper into the epidermis and invade the hair and nails but are restricted to the keratin layers. Subcutaneous infections involve the dermis, subcutaneous tissues, muscle, and fascia. These infections are chronic and can be initiated by piercing trauma to the skin, which allows the fungi to enter.

1.7A CANDIDIASIS

Candida intertrigo is a superficial infection of the skin with *Candida* species. *Candida albicans* is the most commonly encountered pathogenic species but infections with other species can occur including *C. galbrata, C. tropicalis, C. parapsilosis,* and *C. krusei.*

Infections typically arise in areas with persistent moisture. This includes skin folds of the breasts, pannus, axilla, groin, perineum, and genitals. Infections of the hands and nails can be noted in patients whose hands are in frequent contact with water or wear occlusive gloves.

MEDICAL HISTORY AND CLINICAL PRESENTATION

Candida is not considered normal flora of the skin. Predisposing factors include loss of local tissue integrity, alterations in normal flora of the skin, and impaired immune response to infection. Risk factors include obesity, use of occlusive dressings, diaper use, inadequate self-care, and poor nutritional status. Antibiotic use can alter the normal flora of the skin and allow for the growth of *Candida*. Several immunocompromised states can predispose to *Candida* skin infection including diabetes, malignancy, chemotherapy, steroids, immune modulating medications, radiation treatments, HIV/AIDS, and autoimmune disease.

SIGNS AND SYMPTOMS

Patients present with redness, itching, burning, and discomfort at the site of infection.

PHYSICAL EXAMINATION

Physical examination reveals areas of erythematous, macerated skin along skin folds. Whitish or gray areas may be seen on the inflamed skin. Infected skin may be demarcated by a scaly border along the edge of infection. Satellite pustules separate from the primary lesion can occur. *Candida* balanitis presents with persistent scaly patches and ulceration of the glans penis.

DIFFERENTIAL DIAGNOSIS

Differential diagnosis includes tinea infections, bacterial cellulitis, scabies, AD, contact dermatitis, psoriasis, herpes, seborrheic dermatitis, viral exanthema, and drug reactions.

DIAGNOSTIC STUDIES

Diagnostic testing includes KOH preparations and culture of skin scrapings and swabs. KOH is positive with appearance of the fungal elements of *Candida* including budding yeast and pseudohyphae. Culture of skin swabs from the affected area may allow for identification of specific *Candida* species.

TREATMENT

Initial management of *Candida* skin infections includes topical antifungals and local care to reduce moisture and skin contact. Topical antifungals include imidazoles, terbinafine, and ciclopirox. They should be applied twice daily for 2 to 4 weeks.

Systemic antifungals, fluconazole and itraconazole, are effective treatments for *Candida* skin infections.

Limiting use of occlusive dressings, regular bathing, changing soiled diapers, and frequent repositioning may help to resolve the infection.

PATIENT EDUCATION

- Preventive measures should be taken to reduce moisture and friction including keeping areas clean and dry and wearing absorbent, nonocclusive clothing.

1.7B TINEA INFECTIONS

Tinea infections are skin infections of the stratum corneum of the epidermis or to the hair and nails. The most common types of superficial mycoses are dermatophytosis.

Dermatophyte infections are caused by three fungi, *Microsporum*, *Trichophyton,* and *Epidermophyton*. Infections caused by these organisms are referred to as tinea infections. Tinea versicolor is due to the yeast *Malassezia furfur*.

MEDICAL HISTORY AND CLINICAL PRESENTATION

Dermatophytes grow best in warm and humid environments and are more common in tropical and subtropical regions.

Infections are most common in young adults, except for tinea capitis, which is more common in children, with an incubation period of typically 1 to 3 weeks. Predisposing factors include household exposure to an infected family member, immunosuppression, diabetes mellitus, and atopy.

Infection occurs by direct contact with spores on infected hosts or from indirect contact with conidia found in the environment or on fomites. Infective elements can remain viable in the environment for months to years depending on the species.

Tinea versicolor is common in warm and humid environments.

SIGNS AND SYMPTOMS

Symptoms vary depending on the location of the infection. In most cases there is little or no inflammation and the infected areas are mildly itchy with a scaling, slightly raised border. The patches can come and go intermittently.

PHYSICAL EXAMINATION

The clinical presentation is variable depending upon several factors, including the site of infection, the species of the fungus, the host's response, and the immunologic status of the patient.

Tinea capitis (scalp) is most common in children after the first year of life but can be seen in adults. Clinically it presents as dry scaly patches of alopecia with broken hairs. Since hairs break off close to the scalp this is referred to as "black dot" tinea capitis. Tinea capitis is often associated with posterior cervical and auricular lymphadenopathy.

Tinea faciei (face) is a regional form of tinea corporis that involves the face, but not the beard area. The primary lesions resemble those on the body and present as plaques that have an annular configuration with scale or pustules at the border.

Tinea barbae (beard) involves the beard region of the face and neck and is seen in postpubertal males. It is acquired through contact with infected animals and can be spread through use of contaminated razors. It presents with erythematous plaques studded with pustules pierced by terminal hairs. Abscesses, sinus tracks and bacterial superinfection are common, and the patient may have malaise, fever, and lymphadenopathy.

Tinea corporis (body) occurs on the exposed hairless skin of the trunk and extremities. It is most frequently noted in those who have close contact with other people, such as in military housing, contact sports, locker rooms, and in those who are immunosuppressed. Domestic animals are a source of transmission. Lesions appear as erythematous, annular to serpiginous growing plaques that have a peripheral scale and central clearing (Figure 1.7).

Tinea cruris (groin) infection involves the inguinal region and may spread to buttocks, waist, and thighs, but spares the scrotum. It is most frequently seen in men since the scrotum encourages a moist, warm environment, which allows for fungal growth. Lesions can be unilateral or bilateral and have sharply demarcated erythematous plaques with a scaling advancing border. At times the area can contain pustules. Cutaneous candidiasis should be considered if the scrotum is involved or if there are satellite lesions.

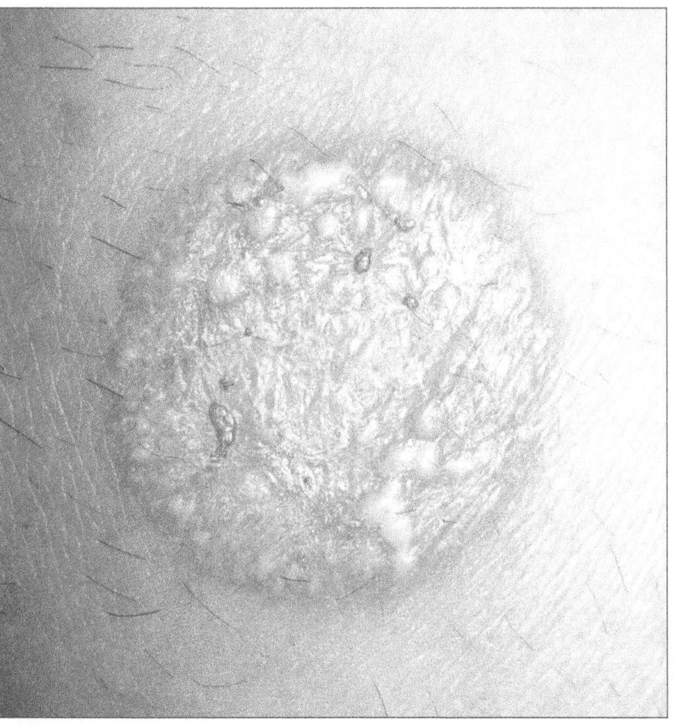

Figure 1.7 Tinea corporis infections (ringworm).
(Source: Ousley LE, Gentry RD. Evidence-based assessment of skin, hair and nails. In: Gawlik KS, Melnyk BM, Teall AM, eds. Evidence-Based Physical Examination. *Springer Publishing Company; 2021:258, Fig. 9.31.)*

Tinea versicolor presents with hypo- and hyperpigmentation of oval spots that may merge into larger patches. The most commonly involved areas are the back, underarm, upper arm, and chest.

DIFFERENTIAL DIAGNOSIS

The differential diagnosis of tinea infections includes contact dermatitis, nummular eczema, urticaria, pityriasis rosea, erythema chronicum migrans, EM, and subacute cutaneous lupus erythematosus.

DIAGNOSTIC STUDIES

KOH prep will show hyphae interspersed among the epithelial cells, or within or on the hair shaft. In patients with tinea versicolor the wet prep will reveal yeast with a "spaghetti and meatball appearance."

Fungal culture is used for positive identification of the species. Usually fungal growth is noted in 5 to 14 days.

TREATMENT

Tinea may be treated topically or orally.

Tinea pedis can be treated with prescription or over-the-counter medications. Medications include butenafine (Lotrimin), terbinafine (Lamisil), econazole (Ecoza), and sertaconazole (Ertaczo). Aluminum acetate (Domeboro, Burow's solution) can also be used as a drying agent for bullous tinea pedis. Keeping feet dry, wearing breathable shoes, and using moisture-wicking socks should be part of a treatment plan.

Tinea cruris is treated topically since it is a localized infection. Over-the-counter products are available and are effective. Butenafine and the imidazole class of medications including clotrimazole (Desenex), ketoconazole (Nizoral), and econazole can also be used. Terbinafine topically can also be used one to two times a day in those over 12 years of age for 1 to 2 weeks. It is uncommon to require oral antifungal medications.

Tinea corporis is treated with topical therapy since it is a localized infection. Common medications include clotrimazole, miconazole (Cruex), econazole, butenafine, and terbinafine.

Systemic therapy may be necessary for disseminated disease or in immunocompromised individuals. Griseofulvin (Grifulvin V) or systemic azoles, like fluconazole (Diflucan), can be used.

Tinea faciei can usually be treated with topical antifungal therapy such as the azoles or terbinafine.

Tinea versicolor is treated with antifungal agents such as selenium sulfide or ketoconazole.

PATIENT EDUCATION

- Prevention is key and involves keeping the area dry, avoiding touching the infected area, and not sharing towels or socks.

SPECIAL CONSIDERATIONS

- In children and adults (including pregnant women) with tinea infection that is not extensive, topical treatment with terbinafine or miconazole should be used.
- Griseofulvin should be avoided in pregnancy as it may be teratogenic.

KEY POINTS

- Mucocutaneous candidiasis is best treated with the azoles such as clotrimazole, miconazole, or nystatin.
- Topical agents are not able to penetrate the hair shaft, so systemic therapy with agents like griseofulvin or terbinafine is needed for tinea capitis.
- Dermatophyte infections present with pruritus, scaling, and erythema; they are best diagnosed with a KOH prep.

1.8 VIRAL INFECTIONS

OVERVIEW

Viral skin infections can produce localized or disseminated disease. The diagnosis is based on pattern of presentation and occasionally laboratory testing is required.

Patients can present with localized complaints or systemic symptoms (e.g., malaise, fever), followed by a maculopapular or vesicular rash. Vesicular rashes contain replicating viral organisms and are infectious.

EPIDEMIOLOGY

The prevalence of the various viral skin infections varies around the world. In the United States the prevalence of HSV type 1 (HSV-1) was 47.8% in 2015 to 2016 in adults age 14 to 49.[16] The prevalence of condyloma acuminatum is 10% to 20% in the United States.[17] The prevalence of molluscum contagiosum is estimated to be <5% of children in the United States.[18]

1.8A HERPES SIMPLEX INFECTIONS

Herpes simplex infections are caused by HSV-1, which is commonly associated with oral herpes and is primarily spread by contact with infected saliva or other secretions; and HSV type 2 (HSV-2), which is more commonly associated with genital herpes and is primarily spread by sexual contact.

The virus replicates at the site of infection, travels retrogradely to the dorsal root ganglion, and establishes latent infection. Recurrent lesions occur with reactivation of latent disease. Triggers for reactivation include stress, fever, immunocompromised state, damage to local tissue, and UV light. This section will focus on HSV-1 infections.

MEDICAL HISTORY AND CLINICAL PRESENTATION

HSV can be spread by infected individuals who are asymptomatic or symptomatic during times of viral shedding. HSV-1 is more commonly associated with oral herpes and is primarily spread by contact with infected saliva or other secretions. The disease is commonly acquired in childhood and most young adults are HSV-1 antibody positive.

HSV infection may be asymptomatic. For primary infections, symptoms occur approximately 3 to 7 days after exposure to infection. In primary infection the patient may present with prodromal symptoms, which include fever, malaise, loss of appetite, and localized pain and/or burning at the site of the lesions. The prodrome may occur in patients with recurrent lesions, but the symptoms are often decreased in severity and duration. Orolabial herpes can cause edema and pain that may lead to dysphagia.

PHYSICAL EXAMINATION

For orolabial herpes the mouth (buccal and gingival mucosa) and lips are the most common site of infection. Recurrent lesions are commonly found on the vermilion border. Other sites may include perioral skin, nasal mucosa, and hard palate.

The skin lesions typically start as painful clustered vesicles on an erythematous base; they may progress to pustules and ulcerate. These ulcerations may cluster to form one large ulcer with a scalloped border.

Lymphadenopathy may be noted before and during the outbreak.

Resolution of the ulceration typically occurs in 1 to 2 weeks in immunocompetent patients but may take longer in immunocompromised patients.

DIFFERENTIAL DIAGNOSIS

The differential diagnosis includes:

- **Varicella zoster virus infection:** The appearance is very similar, but varicella tends to be in a dermatomal pattern.
- **Stevens–Johnson syndrome (SJS)/toxic epidermal necrolysis (TEN):** SJS/TEN may present with oral ulcerations but differ in that they also present with ocular involvement, subepidermal blisters, epidermal sloughing, and involvement of the palms and soles.

- **Aphthous ulcers:** Occurring in the mouth on the mucosal inner lips, tongue, floor of the mouth, and inner cheeks, they present as small round ulcers with a yellow or gray ulcer floor.

DIAGNOSTIC STUDIES

Diagnosis is typically made based on history and physical examination findings. If the diagnosis needs to be confirmed, a Tzanck smear would reveal multinucleated epithelial giant cells; other tests are tissue culture, HSV deoxyribonucleic acid detection by polymerase chain reaction (PCR), and direct fluorescent antibody.

Serologic testing can show primary seroconversion for HSV-1 infection but does not definitively diagnose active disease.

TREATMENT

Treatment is typically not needed in most patients. Antiviral medications, such as acyclovir, famciclovir, and valacyclovir, are the effective medications in the treatment of HSV; however, they reduce the severity and frequency of symptoms but cannot cure the infection.

Prevention of outbreaks is best accomplished by avoiding contact with infected patients. This includes avoidance of oral contact with others and sharing objects that have contact with saliva and abstaining from oral sex to avoid transmitting herpes to the genitals of a sexual partner.

PATIENT EDUCATION

- People with a history of HSV-1 infection can have recurrence of flares.
- Complications of severe oral herpes include dysphagia, severe pain, and inability to take oral medications.

1.8B CONDYLOMA ACUMINATUM

Condyloma acuminatum, genital warts, is most commonly caused by human papillomavirus (HPV) types 6 and 11. HPVs are small, nonenveloped, and double-stranded DNA viruses.

Infection begins with inoculation of virus into the epithelium through microabrasions. HPV infects basal keratinocytes and then replicates and integrates into the host DNA. Assembly of the virus particles occurs in the upper layer of the epithelium and then the virus is released to infect other tissue. The exophytic appearance of condyloma acuminatum is a result of those viral effects on the epithelium.

MEDICAL HISTORY AND CLINICAL PRESENTATION

A complete sexual history from the patient should include history of sexually transmitted diseases (STDs), gender of sex partners, and anatomic areas that have been exposed during sexual contact. A general medical history should assess whether immunosuppression might be present and should include a social history.

PHYSICAL EXAMINATION

Condyloma acuminatum is usually diagnosed clinically via visual examination. Lesions are papules, 2 mm to 5 mm in diameter, although size can vary. Lesions can be either papilliform or sessile.

The surface of the lesions can be verrucous or flat, with flat lesions more common for mucosal lesions. The color of lesions can vary from flesh-colored to darker or lighter. More than one lesion may be present and can be grouped in the anogenital area.

Lesions in men occur on and around the penis or anus. Intraurethral lesions can occur; the patient may present with hematuria, altered urinary stream, or frank bleeding. Lesions in women occur on the vulva, cervix, perineum, or anus. Condyloma acuminatum can also appear in the oral or nasopharyngeal cavity.

DIFFERENTIAL DIAGNOSIS

The differential diagnosis includes molluscum contagiosum, which presents with smooth, dome-shaped lesions with a central umbilication. Condyloma latum, seen in secondary syphilis, presents as plaques in the anogenital area that have a moist, sometimes weepy surface. Vulvar papillomatosis, which can be a normal variant in women, is characterized by smooth papillary projections, each arising from an individual base, proximal to the vaginal introitus. Pearly penile papules are monomorphic papules noted along the penile corona or coronal sulcus in uncircumcised men; skin tags are smooth and pedunculated; and SCC presents with ulcerating lesions.

DIAGNOSTIC STUDIES

Diagnosis is typically made by visual examination. If confirmation is needed, then histopathologic examination of biopsied tissue can be used. Biopsy may be needed in the following:

- Uncertain diagnosis
- Failure to respond or worsening during therapy
- Atypical lesions, including pigmentation, induration, bleeding, or ulceration
- Immunocompromised patient

TREATMENT

The goal of treatment is removal of the wart. If left untreated, anogenital warts can resolve spontaneously within a year, remain unchanged, or increase in size or number. Because warts might spontaneously resolve an accepted plan is to have patients forgo treatment and wait for spontaneous resolution.

Treatment of should be guided by size, number, and anatomic site of the lesions; patient preference; convenience; and adverse effects. No one treatment is better than another and no single treatment is ideal for all patients.

Recommended, patient-applied, treatments for external anogenital warts include imiquimod, podofilox, or sinecatechins. Clinician-applied treatments include cryotherapy with liquid nitrogen or cryoprobe and surgical removal by tangential scissor excision, tangential shave excision, curettage, laser, electrosurgery, trichloroacetic acid, or bichloracetic acid.

PATIENT EDUCATION

- Women with genital warts do not need Pap tests more often than other women.
- Genital warts may cause considerable psychosocial impact after receiving this diagnosis.
- Although genital warts can be treated, such treatment does not cure the virus.

- Because genital warts can be sexually transmitted, patients with genital warts benefit from testing for other STDs.
- The Gardasil vaccine is available for males and females to prevent genital warts, but it will not treat existing HPV infection or genital warts.

1.8C MOLLUSCUM CONTAGIOSUM

Molluscum contagiosum is the most common poxvirus infection in humans. It is acquired from skin-to-skin spread, including sexual transmission, casual contact, autoinoculation, and less commonly, fomites. The virus contacts skin and infects epidermal keratinocytes.

MEDICAL HISTORY AND CLINICAL PRESENTATION

Molluscum contagiosum most commonly affects sexually active adults, patients with impaired cellular immunity, and children. It is most commonly noted in patients between 15 and 29 years of age. It is important to ask about contact with people with similar lesions and sexual history. Patients may note pruritus.

PHYSICAL EXAMINATION

The lesions are dome-shaped, smooth, and often shiny. Lesions often have a central umbilication, but it is not always clinically obvious. (Figure 1.8)

The papules are often grouped together and range in size from 1 mm to 1 cm in diameter. Individual lesions may have surrounding erythema and there may be associated itching of the lesions. Lesions in adults are most often sexually transmitted and are located on the genitals, suprapubic area, and/or inner thighs. Widespread lesions may occur in immunocompromised patients.

DIFFERENTIAL DIAGNOSIS

The differential diagnosis includes verruca, benign adnexal tumors, pyoderma, and condyloma acuminatum. In the immunocompromised hosts, molluscum may mimic disseminated deep fungal infections.

DIAGNOSTIC STUDIES

Laboratory studies are not typically needed to make the diagnosis. If the diagnosis needs to be confirmed a skin biopsy may be helpful.

TREATMENT

Molluscum contagiosum may resolve spontaneously and treatment may not be required. In patients with extensive disease, or in immunocompromised patients who may be at risk for extensive or persistent disease, there are several treatment options. These options include topical therapies, such as topical acids, podophyllotoxin, cantharidin, imiquimod, tretinoin, adapalene, and topical cidofovir. Destructive methods such as curettage, pulsed laser, cryotherapy, and photodynamic therapy can be used.

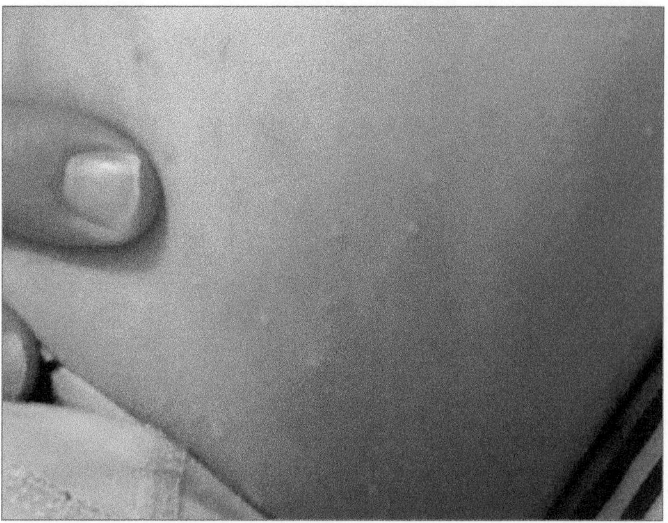

Figure 1.8 **Molluscum contagiosum. Note numerous white, pink, or flesh-colored umbilicated lesions.**
(Source: Ousley LE, Gentry RD. Evidence-based assessment of skin, hair and nails. In: Gawlik KS, Melnyk BM, Teall AM, eds. Evidence-Based Physical Examination. *Springer Publishing Company; 2021:243.)*

Molluscum contagiosum can be prevented by avoiding skin-to-skin contact with infected individuals.

PATIENT EDUCATION

The prognosis for molluscum infection is good, since it is an infection that only involves the skin.

SPECIAL CONSIDERATIONS

- In the treatment of condyloma acuminatum in pregnant women, imiquimod, sinecatechins, podophyllin, and podofilox should not be used during pregnancy.
- Although removal of warts during pregnancy can be considered, resolution might be incomplete or poor until pregnancy is complete.
- Cesarean delivery is indicated for women with anogenital warts if the pelvic outlet is obstructed or if vaginal delivery would result in excessive bleeding.

KEY POINTS

- Molluscum contagiosum spreads via direct contact, such as sexual contact and wrestling.
- Genital warts are caused by human papillomavirus.
- Herpes simplex remains dormant in the dorsal root ganglia.

1.9 PARASITIC INFECTIONS

OVERVIEW

Epidermal parasitic skin diseases are a group of infectious diseases in which parasite–host interactions are confined to the upper layer of the skin. The six major epidermal parasitic skin diseases are scabies, pediculosis capitis (head lice), pediculosis corporis (body lice), pediculosis pubis (pubic lice), sand flea, and hookworm-related cutaneous larva migrans.

EPIDEMIOLOGY

Scabies, pediculosis capitis, and pediculosis pubis occur worldwide but pediculosis corporis is restricted to cold-climate countries and is absent in the tropics

PATHOPHYSIOLOGY

Scabies goes through four stages in its life cycle: egg, larva, nymph, and adult. The female deposits eggs under the skin. The eggs hatch and the larvae migrate to the skin surface and burrow into the intact stratum corneum. The larvae molt resulting in nymphs. The nymph molts into an adult.

Pediculosis has three stages: egg, nymph, and adult. The adult lays eggs (nits) and eggs hatch to release nymphs. The nymph matures and molts into the adult form.

1.9A SCABIES

Scabies is caused by the human mite, *Sarcoptes scabiei* var. hominis. Transmission is most often through direct skin-to-skin contact.The mite may be viable for 2 or 3 days away from its host.

MEDICAL HISTORY AND CLINICAL PRESENTATION

The major symptom of scabies is pruritus. The combination of severe pruritus, often worse at night, and rash present in other members of the household is strong evidence for scabies infestation.

PHYSICAL EXAMINATION

Characteristic findings of scabies on physical examination include nonspecific erythematous papules, excoriations, and burrows. Burrows, tunnels in the epidermis, are pathognomonic for scabies.

The lesions are commonly noted in the interdigital webs, periumbilical and periareolar areas, anterior and posterior axillary fold areas, wrists, elbows, intergluteal areas, genitalia, and buttocks. Excoriation in these areas is common. The scalp is rarely involved, but intense itching associated with extensive scaling may be a clue to the diagnosis.

DIFFERENTIAL DIAGNOSIS

The differential diagnosis of scabies includes AD, atypical folliculitis or impetigo, arthropod bites, and dermatitis herpetiformis.

DIAGNOSTIC STUDIES

Diagnosis is made by microscopic examination of scrapings of skin with direct visualization of the mite. The scraping may not reveal the mite, but discovery of ova or even fecal particles also confirms the diagnosis.

TREATMENT

Scabicides are used to kill scabies mites. No nonprescription products have been tested and approved to treat human scabies.

The following medications are used in the treatment of scabies. Permethrin cream (Elimite) is the drug of choice used to treat scabies in patients over the age of 2 months. It kills both mites and eggs. Crotamitin cream or lotion (Eurax) is used only in adults. Sulfur ointment is safe for use in children, including under 2 months of age. Lindane lotion, while approved for use in the treatment of scabies, is not first-line therapy. Its use is limited to those who have failed treatment because of the neurologic toxicity.

PATIENT EDUCATION

- Itching may continue after treatment because of the patient having a hypersensitivity reaction to the mites and their feces.

1.9B LICE

Lice are parasitic insects that can be found on a patient's head, body, and pubic area. Human lice survive by feeding on human blood. Lice found on each area of the body are different organisms. The three types of lice live on humans:

- ***Pediculus humanus capitis* (head louse):** These lice are 2.1 mm to 3.3 mm in length, infest the head and neck, and attach their eggs to the base of the hair shaft. They move by crawling.
- ***Pediculus humanus corporis* (body louse, clothes louse):** These lice are 2.3 mm to 3.6 mm in length, live and lay eggs on clothing, and only move to the skin to feed. Only the body louse is known to spread disease.
- ***Pthirus pubis* ("crab" louse, pubic louse):** These lice are 1.1 mm to 1.8 mm in length, are found attached to hair in the pubic area but at times can be found on coarse hair of the eyebrows, eyelashes, beard, mustache, chest, and armpits.

Lice infestations are spread most commonly by close person-to-person contact.

MEDICAL HISTORY AND CLINICAL PRESENTATION

Head lice are not known to transmit any disease and are not considered a health hazard.

Head lice infestations can be asymptomatic. Itching is the most common symptom of head lice infestation and is caused by an allergic reaction to louse bites. It may take 4 to 6 weeks for itching to appear the first time a person has head lice. Other symptoms may include a sensation of something moving in the hair, irritability and sleeplessness, and sores on the head caused by scratching.

Body lice presents with intense itching pruritus) and rash caused by an allergic reaction to louse bites. As with other lice infestations, intense itching leads to scratching, which can cause sores and secondary bacterial infection of the skin. Body lice are known to transmit disease, such as epidemic typhus and epidemic relapsing fever.

Pubic lice present with itching in the pubic and groin area. Itching can lead to scratching, which can cause sores and secondary bacterial infection of the skin. Visible lice eggs or lice crawling or attached to pubic hair are other signs of pubic lice infestation. Pubic lice on the head of a child may be an indication of sexual exposure or abuse.

Persons infested with pubic lice should be evaluated for other sexually transmitted infections.

PHYSICAL EXAMINATION

On physical examination nits may be noted cemented to the hair shaft. Nits are fluorescent, so a Wood's light can be used to screen children.

DIFFERENTIAL DIAGNOSIS

The differential diagnosis includes seborrheic dermatitis, impetigo, and insect bites.

DIAGNOSTIC STUDIES

Combing using the conditioner and nit comb technique is the gold standard for diagnosis.

TREATMENT

Many head lice medications are available without a prescription. Treatment options include:

- **Permethrin lotion (Nix):** This is the drug of first choice. It is safe and effective when used as directed. Permethrin kills live lice but not unhatched eggs but may continue to kill newly hatched lice for several days after treatment. A second treatment often is necessary on day 9 to kill any newly hatched lice before they can produce new eggs. Permethrin is approved for use on children 2 months of age and older.
- **Lindane:** This prescription medication can kill lice and lice eggs. Lindane is not recommended as a first-line therapy because of neurologic toxicity and is restricted to patients who have failed treatment or cannot tolerate other medications. Lindane should not be used to treat premature infants, persons with a seizure disorder, women who are pregnant or breastfeeding, infants, children, the elderly, and persons who weigh less than 110 pounds.
- **Malathion lotion (Ovide):** This prescription medication can kill lice and some lice eggs; malathion lotion currently is approved by the U.S. Food and Drug Administration (FDA) for treatment of pubic lice.

A body lice infestation is treated by improving the personal hygiene of the infested person, including assuring a regular change of clean clothes. Clothing, bedding, and towels used by the infested person should be laundered using hot water and machine dried using the hot cycle.

PATIENT EDUCATION

- Management of head lice can be complicated. The patient should follow treatment instructions carefully.
- Recurrent infections may occur due to incorrect treatment, resistance, failure to kill the nymphs emerging from eggs, and reinfection.

SPECIAL CONSIDERATIONS

- Lindane is contraindicated in pregnancy.

KEY POINTS

- Risk factors for scabies includes crowded living conditions and immunosuppression.
- The key symptom with scabies is intense itching.
- Head and pubic lice live on people; body lice live in garments.

1.10 KERATOTIC DISORDERS

1.10A ACTINIC KERATOSIS

AK, or solar keratosis, is the most common precancerous lesion on the skin and due to chronic exposure to UV rays from the sun and/or indoor tanning. AK can develop into SCC.

Fair-skinned individuals are six times more likely to develop AKs than dark-skinned individuals.[19] AKs are most prevalent in countries close to the equator, and less prevalent in countries in the Northern Hemisphere. The prevalence of AKs increases with advancing age; AKs are more common in men than women.

Chronic exposure to UV rays (particularly UVB in the spectrum of 290–320 nm) has been implicated in keratinocyte DNA damage, leading to skin carcinogenesis.

MEDICAL HISTORY AND CLINICAL PRESENTATION

Risk factors for AK include Fitzpatrick skin types I to III, past sun exposure, advancing age, geographic location, history of immunosuppression, and history of certain genetic disorders, such as xeroderma pigmentosum and albinism.

Most patients are asymptomatic or may note a scaly lesion on the sun-exposed areas of the skin.

PHYSICAL EXAMINATION

The AK lesion typically appears as circumscribed, rough, scaly patches on sun-exposed skin, ranging from flesh-colored to reddish brown. Most are asymptomatic, but some may show signs and symptoms such as thickening, burning, tenderness, or itching (Figure 1.9).

Other clinical presentations include hyperkeratotic AKs, scaly lesions with a hyperkeratotic surface; pigmented AKs, well-defined scaly brown lesions resembling solar lentigo; spreading pigmented AKs, lesions resembling seborrheic keratosis (SK), melanocytic nevus, and early malignant melanoma; and lichenoid AKs, violaceous well-defined papules with fine white lines on the surface.

DIFFERENTIAL DIAGNOSIS

The differential diagnosis includes several different skin disorders. See Table 1.8 for a list of the differential diagnosis of AKs.

DIAGNOSTIC STUDIES

Diagnosis is usually made based on clinical appearance. A biopsy may be needed to rule out a SCC or other advanced lesions. Dermoscopy may reveal a "strawberry" pattern with an erythematous background, a pink-red network of vessels surrounding hair follicles, white-yellow scale, and a surrounding white halo.

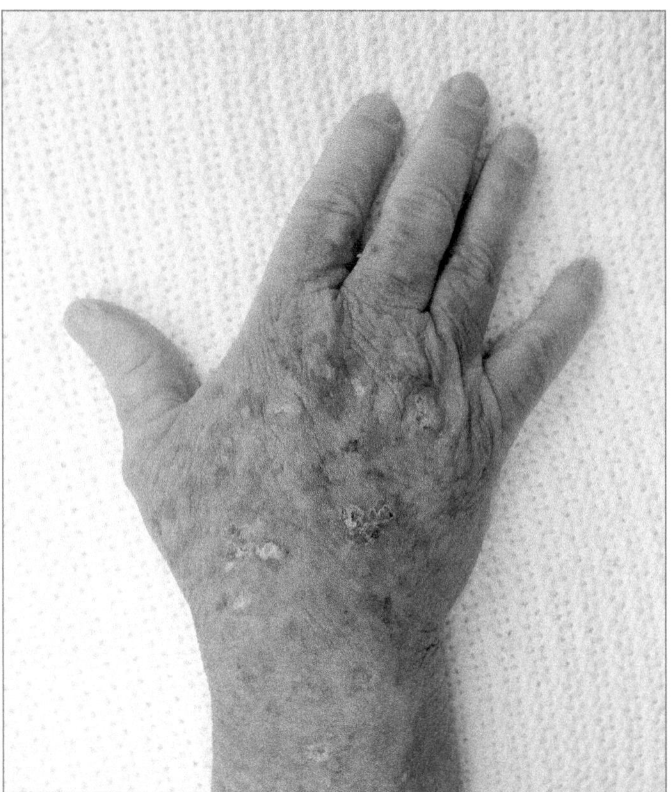

Figure 1.9 **Actinic keratosis. Note rough, scaly lesions on the back of the hand.**
(Source: Image courtesy of James Heilman, MD.)

TABLE 1.8 Differential Diagnosis of Actinic Keratosis

Disorder	Description
Squamous cell carcinoma	Larger red ulcer with a granular base and thick border
Squamous cell carcinoma in situ (Bowen disease)	Larger, solitary lesion in the same distribution as actinic keratoses; can ulcerate and bleed
Basal cell carcinoma	Smooth, pearly papule with telangiectasias mostly on the face
Keratoacanthoma	Rapidly growing, flesh-colored dome-shaped lesions with central keratinous crater
Warts	Benign proliferations of skin and mucosa caused by the human papillomavirus
Seborrheic keratosis	Greasy yellowish plaques with a nonerythematous base that occur on the face
Cutaneous horn	Accumulation of compacted keratin in a projection above the skin surface
Lichen planus	Pruritic, violaceous, polygonal lesions with scaling
Psoriasis	Salmon-pink plaques; often with distinct nail changes

TREATMENT

Several medical options are available for the treatment of AKs.

Imiquimod cream is an immune response modifier used to treat clinically typical, nonhyperkeratotic, nonhypertrophic AKs on the face or scalp in immunocompetent adults. Imiquimod induces immune memory, minimizing the recurrences of AKs. Adverse events are localized and include erythema, scabbing or crusting, flaking, erosion, and edema. Use in patients with autoimmune disease, while not absolutely contraindicated, should be avoided or applied with caution.

5-Fluorouracil (5-FU), a chemotherapeutic agent, is commonly used for patients with multiple lesions. 5-FU inhibits thymidylate synthetase and causes cell death in actively proliferating cells. 5-FU selectively targets the damaged skin, causing an inflammatory response with erythema, necrosis, and erosion. Side effects include pain, irritation, tenderness, burning, ulceration, and inflammation. Pulse therapy can be used in patients who have difficulty tolerating treatment.

Diclofenac in hyaluronan gel is an NSAID that is less effective than other treatment but is also associated with the fewest and most tolerable side effects, due to its anti-inflammatory properties. Diclofenac has a higher affinity for COX-2, which is overexpressed in AKs. Hyaluronic acid in the topical diclofenac gel formulation aids in decreasing the diffusion time through the skin, allowing a greater exposure of the epidermis to the medication.

Medium-depth chemical peel with 30% to 50% trichloroacetic acid has been shown to be as effective as topical 5-FU, but it is better tolerated and preferred by patients.

Ingenol mebutate (Picato) is an extract from sap of the milkweed plant and is an inducer of cell death. It is used topically, and adverse effects include local skin irritation, periorbital edema, pigment change at site of application, and allergic reaction.

Surgical options include cryosurgery with liquid nitrogen, which is the most common treatment for AKs and is most appropriate when discrete AKs are present. The liquid nitrogen is applied directly to AK lesions as a method of destruction; both atypical and typical keratinocytes are destroyed. The procedure involves only mild pain and minor side effects, such as temporary postprocedure erythema.

Other surgical options include curettage with or without electrosurgery, dermabrasion, chemical peels, laser resurfacing by carbon dioxide laser, and full-thickness elliptical excision for AKs.

PATIENT EDUCATION

- All AKs on the lip, ear, or eyelid and those in immunocompromised patients should be removed.
- While progression to SCC is rare, it is advocated that AKs be treated early before invasive or metastatic disease can become a concern.
- Patients should be educated on avoidance of sun exposure and the use of protective clothing and sunblock.

- Patients in high-risk groups should perform self-examinations to detect changes in addition to having regular dermatologic examinations.

1.10B SEBORRHEIC KERATOSIS

SK is a benign epithelial skin tumor. The incidence of SK rises with age and they typically appear after the age of 50. SK is found at sun-exposed body sites, suggesting that UV light and additional risk factors such as genetics may play a role in the development of SK.

MEDICAL HISTORY AND CLINICAL PRESENTATION

SK is usually asymptomatic, but occasionally itching, bleeding, pain, redness, and crusting is observed after trauma or irritation.

SK can be found anywhere on the body except for palms, soles, and mucous membranes. The back, chest, head, and neck are the most commonly affected areas.

PHYSICAL EXAMINATION

SKs are sharply demarcated, round or oval tumors. They range in size from a few millimeters to several centimeters, with average size of 0.5 to 1 cm. The color of the lesions varies from yellow and brown to black. SKs are typically elevated on the skin surface and have a "stuck on" appearance. Their surface can be smooth, uneven, dull, punched-out, or verrucous (Figure 1.10).

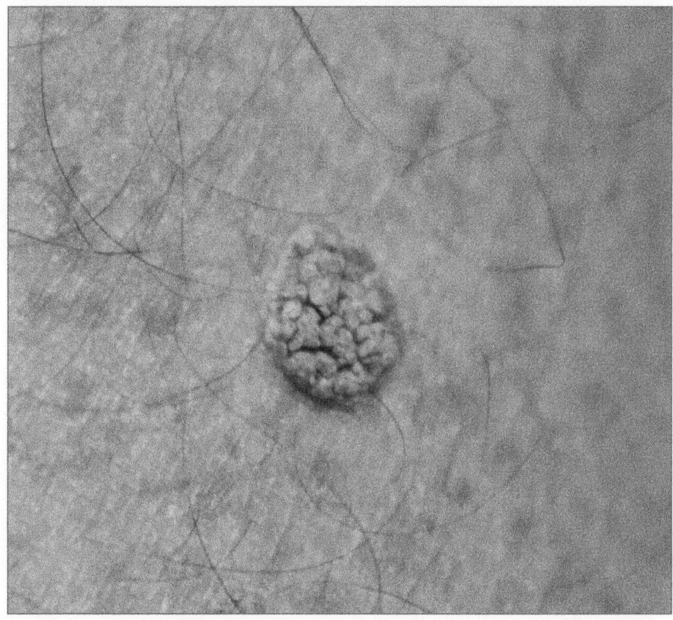

Figure 1.10 Seborrheic keratosis. Note the stuck-on appearance. *(Source: Ousley LE, Gentry RD. Evidence-based assessment of skin, hair and nails. In: Gawlik KS, Melnyk BM, Teall AM, eds.* Evidence-Based Physical Examination. *Springer Publishing Company; 2021:246, Fig. 9.10.)*

DIFFERENTIAL DIAGNOSIS

The differential diagnosis includes BCC, Bowen disease, AK, viral wart, condyloma acuminatum, and adnexal tumors. Pigmented SKs can be mistaken for melanoma or pigmented BCC.

DIAGNOSTIC STUDIES

The diagnosis of SK is easily made by their typical clinical appearance. Dermatoscopy may be needed to exclude malignant tumors. A biopsy or complete removal of a clinically suspicious lesion with histologic evaluation is strongly recommended to rule out possible malignancy.

TREATMENT

Since SKs are benign tumors, no treatment is usually necessary. Removal of an SK lesion may be indicated if mechanical irritation of the lesions causes itching, bleeding, and inflammation; to exclude malignancy; or for cosmetic reasons. Surgical treatment represents the standard therapy.

PATIENT EDUCATION

- Since SKs have no malignant potential, there is no need for long-term monitoring.

SPECIAL CONSIDERATIONS

- 5-FU can cause fetal harm, so its use is contraindicated in pregnant and nursing mothers.

KEY POINTS

- AK can be a precursor to the development of SCC.
- SK is a benign lesion, with no risk of malignancy.

1.11 MALIGNANCIES

OVERVIEW

Skin cancer is the most common type of cancer and develops in sun-exposed areas of skin. It is most common among outdoor workers, farmers, outdoorsmen, and sunbathers. The risk of skin cancer is inversely related to the amount of melanin skin pigmentation; a fair-skinned person is more susceptible than a dark-skinned person.

At presentation there is often an irregular red or pigmented lesion that does not go away; the lesion may bleed, be painful, and pruritic. Any lesion that appears to be enlarging should be biopsied.

EPIDEMIOLOGY

Over 5.4 million new cases of skin cancer are diagnosed in over 3.3 million people in the United States yearly.[20] The most common skin cancers are BCC (80%), SCC (16%), and melanoma (4%).[21] Rare forms of skin cancer include Paget disease of the nipple, Kaposi sarcoma, Merkel cell carcinoma, and cutaneous T-cell lymphoma (CTCL).

PATHOPHYSIOLOGY

The pathophysiology of BCC is not completely understood. BCC may arise from stem cells in the hair follicle bulge or interfollicular epidermis rather than basal keratinocytes. The most common causative factor of BCC is UV radiation.

1.11A BASAL CELL CARCINOMA

BCC is the most common cancer in humans, with over 4 million new cases a year in the United States.[21] It is more common in fair-skinned people with a history of sun exposure. The incidence of BCC is increasing. BCC is most common among elderly men and the incidence is increasing among young women, due to lifestyle factors leading to increased sun exposure.

MEDICAL HISTORY AND CLINICAL PRESENTATION

Patients often present with a history of a slow-growing or persistent sore that will not heal. They may also note frequent bleeding with minor trauma such as picking, shaving, washing, or drying with a towel. Most patients report a significant history of recreational or occupational sun exposure.

BCCs occur most commonly on the head and neck; but 20% of BCCs occur at non-sun-exposed sites.

The primary risk factors for BCC are fair skin, extensive intermittent or cumulative lifetime UV exposure, and history of prior non-melanoma skin cancer. Other risk factors include red or blond hair, light eye color, and sensitivity to UV radiation.

BCCs rarely metastasize; rates of metastases are <0.1%.[22] Metastases most commonly occur with large, ulcerated, or neglected tumors. The prognosis is poor, with a median survival of only 8 months.

PHYSICAL EXAMINATION

The classic finding in BCC is an erythematous, pearly, telangiectatic papule or plaque, often with a central erosion or ulcer (Figure 1.11).

The clinical manifestations of BCCs vary with type.[23]

- **Nodular (79%):** Small, shiny, firm, translucent to pink nodules with telangiectases, usually on the face. Ulceration and crusting are common.
- **Superficial (15%):** Red or pink, thin papules or plaques, commonly on the trunk.
- **Morpheaform (6%):** Flat, scar-like, indurated plaques that can be flesh-colored or light red and have vague borders.

DIFFERENTIAL DIAGNOSIS

The differential diagnosis includes dermal nevi, sebaceous hyperplasia, lichenoid keratoses, actinic keratoses, SCCs, fibrous papules, and amelanotic melanomas.

DIAGNOSTIC STUDIES

In most cases, no other diagnostic studies are needed. CT or MRI may be indicated if there is suspicion of metastatic disease.

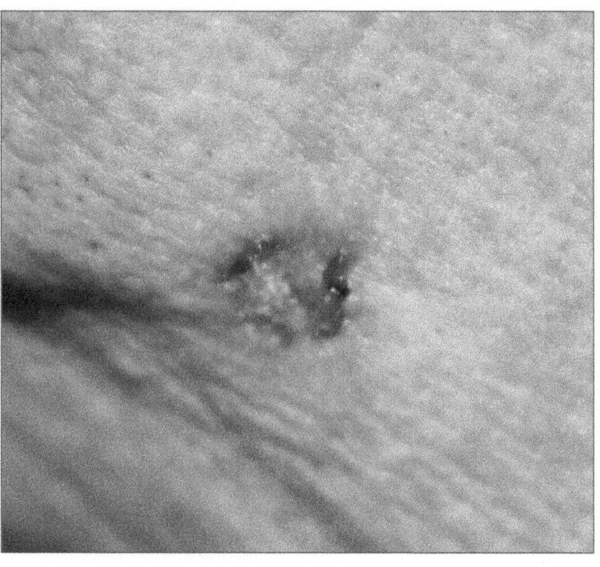

Figure 1.11 Basal cell carcinoma.
(Source: Ousley LE, Gentry RD. Evidence-based assessment of skin, hair and nails. In: Gawlik KS, Melnyk BM, Teall AM, eds. Evidence-Based Physical Examination. *Springer Publishing Company; 2021:256, Fig. 9.24.)*

TREATMENT

Several treatments are available for BCC. Surgical options, which are first-line and definitive therapy, include electrodesiccation and curettage, excision, and Mohs micrographic surgery. Medical treatments, such as imiquimod and fluorouracil, and physical modalities, including cryosurgery, photodynamic therapy, and radiation may be used in certain settings. Vismodegib, a systemic therapy, is available for metastatic and inoperable BCCs.

Surgical treatments generally have higher cure rates than medical therapies. Mohs surgery offers the highest long-term cure rate of any treatment modality; primary nodular BCCs under 2 cm in diameter on the trunk and extremities are most commonly treated by electrodesiccation and curettage or excision.

Topical medical treatments include topical chemotherapy agents and immune-modulating agents. These treatments are best reserved for small, superficial BCCs on the trunk and extremities. Both topical imiquimod and topical fluorouracil are FDA approved for treatment of superficial BCCs <2 cm in diameter.

Physical modalities including photodynamic therapy, cryosurgery, and radiation therapy may be effective for treating BCC in certain settings. These treatment options are less invasive than surgery but offer no pathologic evaluation to confirm clear margins.

PATIENT EDUCATION

- The recommended follow-up for patients with skin cancer is a complete skin examination every 6 to 12 months.
- Patients with a prior history of BCC have a greater risk of developing another BCC.
- All patients should be counseled regarding UV avoidance and protection. Broad-spectrum sunscreens with sun protection factor of 30 or higher with reapplication every 2 hours, wearing a broad-brimmed hat during outdoor activities, and engaging in outdoor activities before 10 am and after 4 pm should be encouraged.

1.11B SQUAMOUS CELL CARCINOMA

SCC, the second most common type of skin cancer, has been reported on all parts of the body and in all races. The highest incidence is noted in patients with fair skin, increased cumulative UV exposure, and immunosuppression.

Tanning booth usage correlates with a higher incidence of SCC. Using a tanning device increases the risk of SCC by 67%.[24]

Other risk factors include immunosuppression, older age, certain chemical exposures, ionizing radiation, viral infection (HPV), chronic scarring or inflammation, and genetic disorders.

MEDICAL HISTORY AND CLINICAL PRESENTATION

Patients may present with a tender or scaly growth, often on sun-exposed surfaces such as the face or hand. They may describe the lesions as being present "for years" or rapidly increased in size over 2 to 3 weeks. The lesions may bleed following minimal trauma and do not seem to ever completely heal.

PHYSICAL EXAMINATION

SCCs can develop anywhere on the skin and mucosal surfaces, but are most often found on the head, neck, and sun-exposed surfaces of the arms, hands, and legs. Lesions are pink to red, hyperkeratotic, and tender. They range in size from a few millimeters to several centimeters (Figure 1.12).

DIFFERENTIAL DIAGNOSIS

The differential diagnosis varies based on the lesion's appearance. With the presentation of nonhealing ulcers, the differential diagnosis includes pyoderma gangrenosum and venous stasis ulcers. With nodular and hyperkeratotic lesions, the differential diagnosis includes verruca vulgaris. With scaling plaques, the differential diagnosis includes BCC, AK, SK, psoriasis, and nummular eczema.

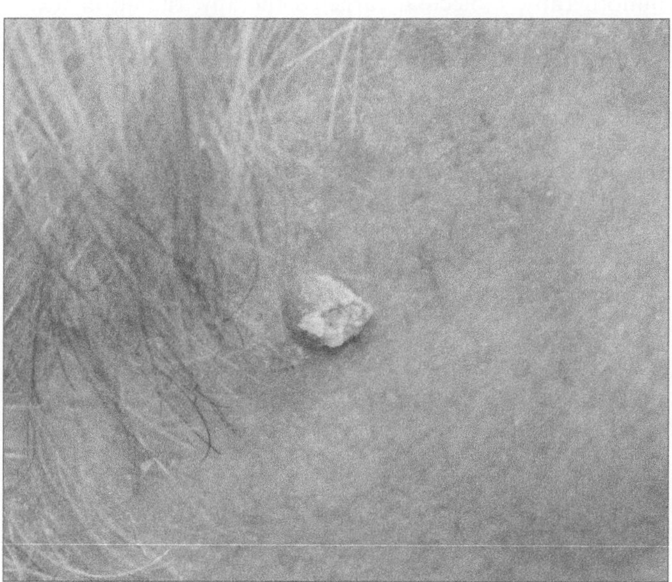

Figure 1.12 Squamous cell carcinoma.
(Source: Ousley LE, Gentry RD. Evidence-based assessment of skin, hair and nails. In: Gawlik KS, Melnyk BM, Teall AM, eds. Evidence-Based Physical Examination. *Springer Publishing Company; 2021: 256, Fig. 9.25)*

DIAGNOSTIC STUDIES

Dermoscopic examination reveals surface scale, blood spots, white structureless zones, and coiled vessels.

The gold standard for diagnosing SCC is a skin biopsy for histopathologic examination. Punch biopsy, shave biopsy, or excisional biopsy are appropriate techniques.

TREATMENT

Treatment of SCC is the same as for BCC and includes curettage and electrodesiccation, surgical excision, cryosurgery, topical chemotherapy, or radiation therapy. Treatment and follow-up must be monitored closely because of the greater risk of metastasis compared with BCC. For most SCCs, a surgical modality is the treatment of choice.

The prognosis for small lesions removed early and adequately is excellent. Regional and distant metastases of SCCs on sun-exposed skin are uncommon but do occur. The characteristics of aggressive tumors include poorly differentiated, size >2 cm in diameter, invasion depth >2 mm, perineural invasion, and location near the anogenital region, ear, or vermilion border.

PATIENT EDUCATION

- SCC is an extremely common type of cancer and, when caught early and treated effectively, has a limited chance of metastasis and significant morbidity.
- Once diagnosed with a primary SCC of the skin, there is a 30% chance that a second primary SCC of the skin will develop within 5 years.[25]
- Ninety percent of recurrences and metastases will develop in the first 5 years following treatment.[26]

1.11C MELANOMA

Melanomas occur mainly on the skin but also on the mucosa of the oral, genital, and rectal regions, conjunctivae, and nail beds. Melanomas vary in size, shape, and color and in their likelihood to invade and metastasize. Metastasis occurs via lymphatics and blood vessels.

Melanoma has the fastest growing incidence of any cancer in the United States. It is the fifth most common cancer in men and sixth most common cancer in women. In 2021, just over 100,000 new cases of melanoma will be diagnosed in the United States, causing about 7,100 deaths.[20] Melanoma accounts for <5% of total skin cancers diagnosed in the United States but causes most skin cancer deaths.[20]

Melanocytes, located in the basal layer of the epidermis, produce melanin to absorb UV radiation and prevent further DNA damage through absorption of UV rays. UV-induced DNA damage is repaired by DNA repair mechanisms. Any errors within DNA repair mechanisms may lead to the formation of an invasive melanoma.

MEDICAL HISTORY AND CLINICAL PRESENTATION

Evaluation of the patient with melanoma centers on the ABCDE (asymmetry, border irregularity, color variation, diameter

>6 mm, and evolution of the lesion) system for describing and evaluating suspicious skin lesions. Patient history should focus on these features of the lesion and how they have changed over time.

The presence of inflammation can be determined by features such as itching, crusting, or bleeding. Most melanomas are asymptomatic. The most common symptom is itching.

The patient should also be evaluated for possible metastatic disease by obtaining a complete review of systems related to sites of potential metastasis.

Risk factors for melanoma include genetic and environmental causes or a combination of the two. Genetic traits include fair skin, light hair, and light eye color.

UV sun exposure is the most important and most potentially modifiable risk factor. A history of intermittent, intense exposure to the sun is a greater risk than that for those with chronic, continuous exposure. A history of sunburns, specifically blistering sunburns, should also be obtained, as risk may be doubled with these factors. Artificial UV exposure in tanning salons exposes people to a higher dose of UVA over a shorter period compared to sun exposure. The risk of melanoma increases with age, especially in men. A positive family history is a strong risk factor for the development of melanoma.

PHYSICAL EXAMINATION

A complete skin exam should be completed to evaluate for other suspicious lesions, including scalp, subungual regions, genitals, and perineum. All lymph node basins should be palpated for lymphadenopathy and the abdomen assessed for hepatosplenomegaly.

The ABCDE characteristics should be utilized when evaluating lesions on physical examination. The characteristics that suggest malignancy on dermoscopy include the presence of pigmented networks, globules, dots, blue-gray veil, or streaks (Figure 1.13).

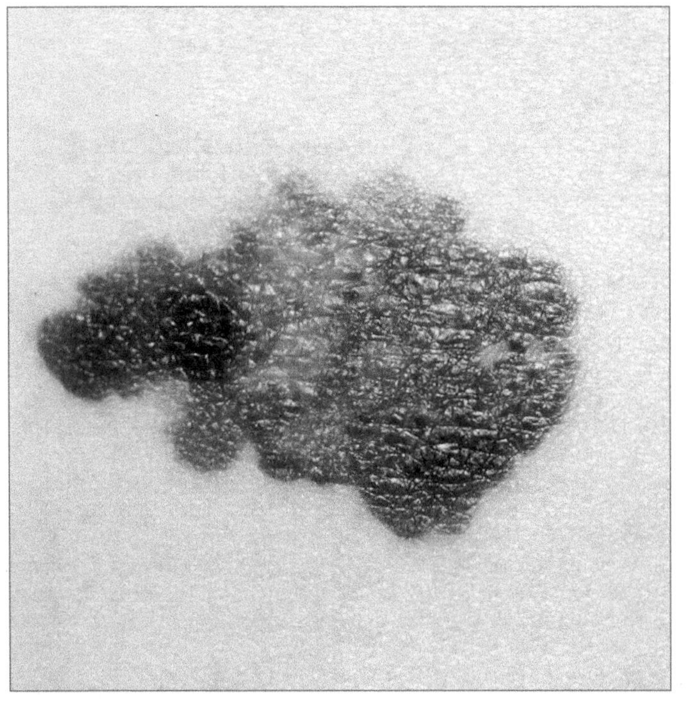

Figure 1.13 Melanoma.
(Source: National Cancer Institute. Visuals online. 1985. https://visualsonline.cancer.gov)

DIFFERENTIAL DIAGNOSIS

The differential diagnosis includes BCC, SCC, SK, atypical moles, moles, venous lakes, and hematomas of the hands and feet.

DIAGNOSTIC STUDIES

The staging of melanoma is based on clinical and pathologic criteria. The staging system classifies melanomas based on local, regional, or distant disease:

- **Stages I and II:** Localized primary melanoma
- **Stage III:** Metastasis to regional lymph nodes
- **Stage IV:** Distant metastatic disease

Stage strongly correlates with survival. Recommended staging studies depend on the Breslow depth and histologic characteristics of the melanoma. Staging studies may include sentinel lymph node biopsy, laboratory tests, chest x-ray, CT, and PET scan.

TREATMENT

Treatment of melanoma is primarily by wide local surgical excision. In tumors <0.8 mm thick but with ulceration, sentinel lymph node biopsy should be considered. Thicker lesions may deserve larger margins, more radical surgery, and sentinel lymph node biopsy.

Topical therapies for melanoma include imiquinod, local ablation therapy, and intralesional injection with bacillus Calmette-Guerin (BCG) or interferon. These treatment options are not first-line options but may be considered in patients with positive margins after surgical resection and patients with in-transit metastasis.

External beam radiation can be used in the treatment of melanoma. Adjuvant radiation treatment to the primary excision site should be considered if surgical margins are not adequate due to the location of the lesion. Definitive radiation treatment may be considered if surgical treatment is not possible.

Treatment of metastatic melanoma typically includes immunotherapy, molecular targeted therapy, radiation therapy, and occasionally surgical resection.

Metastatic disease is generally inoperable, but in certain cases, localized and regional metastases can be excised to help eliminate residual disease. For metastatic or unresectable melanoma, immunotherapy with pembrolizumab, nivolumab, or ipilimumab; targeted therapy with vemurafenib, dabrafenib, or encorafenib; and radiation therapy should be considered.

Chemotherapeutic options for patients with metastatic melanoma include dacarbazine and temezolamide. Interferon alpha 2b is an FDA-approved adjuvant treatment regimen for patients with stage IIb or stage III melanoma.

Median survival for metastatic melanoma is 11 to 12 months, and no systemic treatment options currently offer a significant survival advantage.

All patients diagnosed with melanoma should have annual skin examination and surveillance for life.

PATIENT EDUCATION

- Prevention is obtained by reducing exposure to both natural and artificial UV radiation. Patients should be advised to avoid sun exposure during the mid-day hours, use clothing protection such as hats with broad brims, and use sunscreen.

SPECIAL CONSIDERATIONS

- In pregnant women the clinical course, prognosis, and overall survival is like that for nonpregnant women.
- Thicker lesions are associated with pregnancy, likely due to delay in diagnosis and possibly response of the melanoma to systemic hormones.
- Prompt biopsy of suspicious lesions and wide local excision of confirmed melanoma is safe in pregnant patients. Biopsy and wide local excision should not be delayed until after delivery.

KEY POINTS

- Because many skin cancers seem to be related to UV exposure, exposure should be limited.
- SCC should be considered in any nonhealing lesion in a sun-exposed area.
- Melanoma accounts for <5% of all skin cancers but causes most skin cancer deaths.[20]

1.12 PAPULOSQUAMOUS DISORDERS

OVERVIEW

Papulosquamous diseases are characterized by well-demarcated areas of papules and scale on an erythematous background.

1.12A CONTACT DERMATITIS

Contact dermatitis is an eczematous skin dermatitis characterized by inflammation. Patients develop erythematous and pruritic skin lesions after contact with a foreign substance. Contact dermatitis is divided into two groups: irritant and allergic. Irritant contact dermatitis is due to exposure to a foreign substance that causes a nonimmunologic reaction in the skin, while allergic contact dermatitis is caused by a hypersensitivity reaction.

Only the superficial regions of the skin are affected in contact dermatitis, including epidermis and outer dermis.

MEDICAL HISTORY AND CLINICAL PRESENTATION

A detailed exposure history should be obtained. This includes the patient's occupation, hobbies, household duties, vacations, clothing, topical drug use, cosmetics and skin care products, and spouse's activities.

Irritant contact dermatitis is more painful than pruritic. Signs range from mild erythema to hemorrhage, crusting, erosion, pustules, bullae, and edema. The pain is typically described as burning.

In allergic contact dermatitis intense pruritus is more common than pain. Pain is the result of excoriation or infection. Skin changes range from transient erythema through vesiculation to severe swelling with bullae, ulceration, or both. Changes often occur in a pattern, distribution, or combination that is suggestive of a specific exposure, such as linear streaking on an arm or leg due to brushing against poison ivy or circumferential erythema due to nickel exposure under a wristwatch or waistband.

Any surface may be involved, but hands are the most common surface due to handling and touching potential allergens.

PHYSICAL EXAMINATION

In allergic contact dermatitis the findings depend on the degree of sensitivity and amount of exposure. Typical skin findings include vesicles, edema, erythema, and intense pruritus. The pattern of the rash can indicate the allergen.

Irritant contact dermatitis presents with erythema, dryness, painful cracking, and scaling. Acute irritant contact dermatitis may show papules or vesicles on an erythematous base with weeping and edema. Chronic disease presents with lichenification, patches of erythema, fissures, excoriations, and scaling.

DIFFERENTIAL DIAGNOSIS

The differential diagnosis of contact dermatitis includes AD, dyshidrotic eczema, palmoplantar psoriasis, scabies, and tinea pedis or manus.

DIAGNOSTIC STUDIES

The diagnosis of contact dermatitis is made based on skin changes and exposure history. The suspected agent can be tested by applying the possible agent far from the original area of dermatitis and evaluating for a reaction. This may be helpful when perfumes, shampoos, or other home agents are suspected.

Patch testing for possible allergens is indicated when allergic contact dermatitis is suspected and does not respond to treatment. Definitive diagnosis requires a positive test result and a history of dermatitis in the area where the tested agent contacted the skin.

TREATMENT

Treatment focuses on three areas: avoidance of offending agents, supportive care such as cool compresses and antihistamines, and topical corticosteroids.

Topical treatment includes cool compresses (saline solution) and corticosteroids. Patients with mild to moderate allergic contact dermatitis may need mid- to high-potency topical corticosteroids, such as triamcinolone 0.1% ointment or betamethasone valerate cream 0.1%. Oral corticosteroids, such as prednisone, can be used for severe blistering or extensive disease. Systemic antihistamines, hydroxyzine or diphenhydramine, help relieve pruritus; low-sedating H_1 blocker antihistamines with low anticholinergic potency are not as effective.

PATIENT EDUCATION

- Resolution may take up to 3 weeks and reactivity is usually lifelong.

1.12B ATOPIC DERMATITIS (ECZEMA)

AD or eczema is a chronic, relapsing, pruritic dermatitis that presents in early infancy or childhood. Diagnosis depends on a careful history and physical examination.

In the United States, 15% of children and 7% of adults are thought to be affected by AD.[27]

Disease onset occurs by 1 year of age in about 60% of affected infants and by age 5 years of age in about 85% of affected children.[28]

AD develops because of a complex interplay of genetic, immune, metabolic, infectious, neuroendocrine, and environmental factors. The two main causes of AD are defects in the epidermal barrier function and cutaneous inflammation.

MEDICAL HISTORY AND CLINICAL PRESENTATION

Onset occurs in the first year of life in 60% of patients, with most developing signs and symptoms between the third and sixth months of age.[29] About 85% of patients develop the disease before 5 years of age.[29] Patients may have another atopic disorder such as asthma or allergic rhinitis.

Most patients have a family history of atopy. Parents should be questioned regarding any family history of asthma, allergic rhinitis (hay fever), or AD, as the absence of an atopic family history makes the diagnosis of AD less likely.

There are three different clinical phases of AD: infantile, childhood, and adulthood. Each phase has a typical distribution pattern and lesion morphology, although there may be some overlap of phases. The infantile phase occurs from infancy up to 2 to 3 years of age, childhood phase from approximately 2 years of age to puberty, and the adult phase from puberty onward.

PHYSICAL EXAMINATION

Infantile AD is commonly found on the cheeks and scalp; other areas that can be involved include the trunk, wrists, extensor surfaces of the legs, neck, and periauricular areas. The diaper area is usually spared. The lesions are symmetric, scaly, erythematous patches, with weeping and crusting prominent in severe cases. Lichenification is not a prominent feature in this phase.

Pruritus is common. Infants may rub themselves against objects and the pruritus often leads to sleep disturbance and/or secondary infection (Figure 1.14).

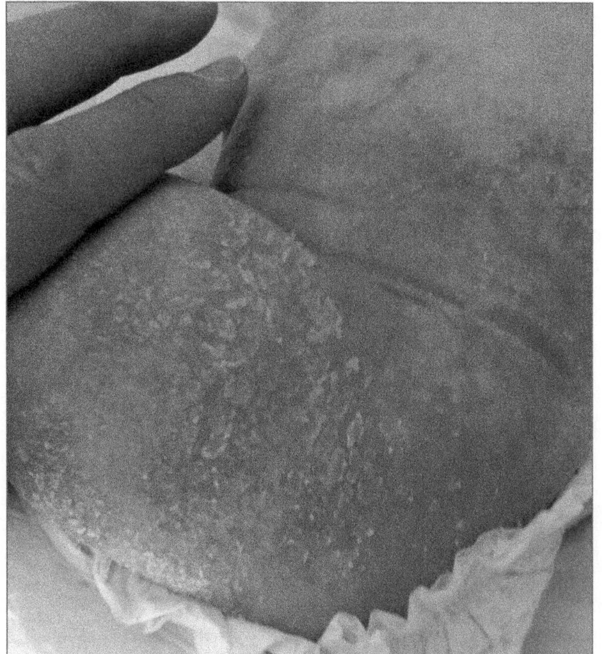

Figure 1.14 Atopic dermatitis (eczema) on the thigh of an infant. *(Source: Image courtesy of GZ.)*

Childhood AD is commonly noted on the flexural surfaces of the extremities and the antecubital and popliteal fossae. Other sites include the neck, flexures of the wrist and ankle, and the creases between the thighs and buttocks. The lesions tend to be ill-defined, scaly, erythematous patches with or without crusting and excoriation. Lichenification becomes prominent.

Adult AD also involves the flexural areas of the extremities and can be focal or diffuse. Chronic hand and foot dermatitis become prominent and may be the only manifestation of AD for some patients. Neck and facial involvement also tends to be more prominent, with severe periocular disease noted. Adults have more scaling and less crusting than infants and children.

DIFFERENTIAL DIAGNOSIS

The differential diagnosis includes:

- **Seborrheic dermatitis:** Greasy scale, involvement of the diaper area, and less pruritus
- **Scabies:** Papules, nodules, pustules, or urticarial lesions in addition to eczematous lesions
- **Allergic/irritant contact dermatitis:** Rash suggesting an external source or history of a common inciting agent
- **Psoriasis:** Red, sharply demarcated papules and plaques often located on the scalp, lower back, and extremities
- **Tinea corporis**

DIAGNOSTIC STUDIES

Laboratory studies are not typically needed to make the diagnosis. Patients with AD may have elevated serum immunoglobulin E (IgE) levels, but a normal serum IgE level is possible.

TREATMENT

Treatment plans vary depending on the patient's age, the extent and localization of AD, overall disease course, previous response to treatment, disease persistence, frequency of flares, and susceptibility to and past history of infection. Long-term therapy should include patient/family education, trigger avoidance, excellent skin care, and medical and physical treatment.

Education regarding the care of dry skin is the cornerstone of management. Use of an emollient/moisturizer without topical sensitizers, such as fragrance, neomycin, or benzocaine, should be encouraged.

Topical corticosteroids remain first-line therapy for inflammation and pruritus. Treatment depends on the location and severity of the AD.

Wet wraps, commonly utilizing corticosteroids applied to wet skin and covered with wet gauze or clothing, are a useful tool to intensify treatment of severe AD and/or disease that is refractory to standard topical therapies.

Topical calcineurin inhibitors, such as tacrolimus and pimecrolimus, are second-line therapy. Topical calcineurin inhibitors may benefit those with disease persistence and/or frequent flares. They are also indicated in sensitive or thin skin areas, such as around the eye, face, neck, and genital area. These medications have minimal side effects with no significant evidence of systemic immunosuppression or increase for skin cancer.

Sedating systemic antihistamines, such as diphenhydramine or hydroxyzine, do not appear to have direct effects on pruritus, but may be useful in improving sleep. Topical antihistamines are not recommended because of potential cutaneous sensitization.

Phototherapy is thought to suppress proinflammatory cytokines found in AD and induce T-cell apoptosis. Phototherapy may be useful for widespread or recalcitrant disease.

Systemic therapy should be considered in patients with severe AD that does not respond to topical treatments.

Dupilumab, a monoclonal antibody, is used to treat AD. Side effects include allergic reactions, conjunctivitis, and keratitis.

Azathioprine can be effective monotherapy for severe AD. Marrow suppression and liver toxicity are major concerns.

Cyclosporine may be used as a short-term treatment or as a bridge between other steroid-sparing alternatives. Flares can occur after discontinuation of therapy, so gradual tapering is recommended. Hypertension, renal toxicity, and the risk of malignancy are limitations to long-term therapy.

Methotrexate, at low doses, is used to treat AD, and is less immunosuppressive than other systemic therapies. Hepatotoxicity and pulmonary toxicity are noted side effects.

PATIENT EDUCATION

- Common complications of AD include superinfection with *S. aureus*, HSV, and molluscum contagiosum.
- Majority of the infants and children with AD usually grow out of the disease during childhood.
- AD is a lifelong disease with periods of waxing and waning skin lesions.

1.12C LICHEN PLANUS

LP is a papulosquamous disorder of the skin, mucous membranes, hair, and nails. There are multiple subtypes and depending on subtype and area of involvement, lesions may range from asymptomatic to pruritic and erosive. The prevalence of LP is estimated to be approximately 1%.[30] Females and males are equally affected.

LP is thought to be due to a T-cell–mediated autoimmune reaction against epithelial keratinocytes. Drugs, especially beta blockers, NSAIDs, ACE inhibitors, sulfonylureas, gold, antimalarial drugs, and thiazides, can cause LP. Drug-induced LP may be indistinguishable from nondrug-induced LP.

Associations with hepatitis, particularly hepatitis C and primary biliary cirrhosis, have been reported.

MEDICAL HISTORY AND CLINICAL PRESENTATION

Symptoms are limited in most patients. Oral lesions may be asymptomatic but other patients may complain of pain, difficulty eating, odynophagia, or bleeding gums. If the hair is involved the symptoms can range from a scarring alopecia of the scalp to nonscarring alopecia of the axilla and pubic hair.

PHYSICAL EXAMINATION

In LP the lesions are pruritic, violaceous, polygonal, flat-topped papules and plaques. Lesions initially are 2 to 4 mm in diameter, with angular borders and a distinct sheen in cross-lighting. They are usually symmetrically distributed, most common on the flexor surfaces of the wrists, legs, trunk, glans penis, and oral and vaginal mucosa. The face is rarely involved. Onset may be abrupt or gradual.

During the acute phase, new papules may appear at sites of minor skin injury (Koebner phenomenon), such as a superficial scratch.

The oral mucosa is involved in about half of cases; oral lesions may occur without cutaneous lesions. Reticulated, lacy, bluish white, linear lesions (Wickham striae) are a hallmark of oral LP, especially on the buccal mucosae.

DIFFERENTIAL DIAGNOSIS

The differential diagnosis of LP includes:

- **Lichenoid drug eruptions:** Presents with eosinophilia, noted on photo-exposed areas, history of exposure to ACE inhibitors, antimalarials, betablockers, methyldopa, NSAIDs, or penicillamine
- **Lupus erythematosus:** Will note a positive antinuclear antibody (ANA) text
- **Lichen nitidus:** Presents with pinpoint-sized, flesh-colored, nonpruritic papules
- **Guttate psoriasis:** Prominent extensor surface involvement, no oral lesions, white silvery scale

DIAGNOSTIC STUDIES

Laboratory studies are typically not necessary. Eosinophilia may be present in drug-induced LP. An ANA test may be needed to separate LP from systemic lupus erythematosus.

Because of the association between hepatitis C and LP, hepatitis C testing may be indicated.

TREATMENT

Asymptomatic LP does not require treatment. Drugs suspected of causing LP should be stopped; it may take weeks to months after the offending drug has been stopped for the lesions to resolve.

Most LP on the trunk or extremities can be treated topically. Topical corticosteroids are first-line treatment for most cases of localized disease. High-potency ointments or creams may be used on the thicker lesions on the extremities; lower-potency drugs may be used on the face, groin, and axillae.

Local therapy is not feasible for generalized LP so oral drugs or phototherapy is indicated. Oral corticosteroids may be used for severe cases. The disease may rebound when therapy ends.

Oral retinoids are indicated for otherwise recalcitrant cases. Cyclosporine can be used when corticosteroids or retinoids fail. Light therapy using psoralen plus UVA (PUVA) or narrowband UVB (NBUVB) is an alternative to oral therapies.

Treatment of oral LP consists of viscous lidocaine, which may relieve symptoms of erosive ulcers.

PATIENT EDUCATION

- Isolated cutaneous LP is a self-limited disease that may resolve spontaneously between 1 month and 7 years, with a mean duration of 5 years.
- Mucosal LP is a chronic disease that rarely resolves spontaneously.
- Treatment can result in substantial improvement, but recurrence is common when discontinued.

1.12D PITYRIASIS ROSEA

Pityriasis rosea presents with a pink, oval rash. The exact cause is unknown. Pityriasis rosea can affect members of either sex of any age, but it is most common in females between the ages of 8 and 35. It tends to be seen more frequently in the spring and fall.

Pityriasis rosea-like eruptions have been reported with several gastric and bronchogenic neoplasms, T-cell lymphomas, Hodgkin disease, and bone marrow transplantation.

MEDICAL HISTORY AND CLINICAL PRESENTATION

Although classically asymptomatic, there may be differing degrees of pruritus as well as a prodrome of constitutional symptoms including malaise, nausea, gastrointestinal and respiratory symptoms, headache, irritability, difficulty in concentration, loss of appetite, joint pain, sore throat, and mild fever. Relapse is uncommon but may occur.

PHYSICAL EXAMINATION

Pityriasis rosea begins with a single, primary, 2 cm to 10 cm herald patch that appears on the trunk or proximal limbs. This is followed in 7 to 14 days by a general centripetal eruption of 0.5- to 2-cm rose-colored oval papules and plaques. The lesions orient along skin lines giving the rash a Christmas tree–like distribution. The lesions have a scaly, slightly raised border. Most patients itch, occasionally severely. Children commonly have inverse pityriasis rosea with lesions in the axillae or groin that spread centrifugally.

DIFFERENTIAL DIAGNOSIS

The differential diagnosis of pityriasis rosea includes tinea corporis, tinea versicolor, guttate psoriasis, syphilis, nummular eczema, subacute cutaneous lupus erythematosis (SCLE), benign pigmented purpura, AD, digitate dermatoses, CTCL, and pityriasis lichenoides.

DIAGNOSTIC STUDIES

Diagnosis is based primarily on history and physical examination alone. A skin biopsy may be necessary to confirm the diagnosis as it can mimic many other conditions.

Syphilis testing is indicated when the palms or soles are affected, when a herald patch is not seen, or when lesions occur in an unusual sequence or distribution.

TREATMENT

No specific treatment is necessary because the eruption typically resolve within 5 weeks and recurrence is rare. Artificial or natural sunlight may hasten resolution.

PATIENT EDUCATION

- Patients should be advised to return if the rash does not disappear in 3 months or if there are severe constitutional symptoms.
- Harsh soaps should be discontinued, and bathing should be minimal with just water or bath oils.

1.12E PSORIASIS

Psoriasis is a hyperproliferative disorder of the epidermal keratinocytes combined with inflammation of the epidermis and dermis. It affects about 0.5% to 11% of the population worldwide; light-skinned people are at higher risk.[31] Peak onset is at ages 16 to 22 and ages 57 to 60. There is equal sex distribution, but early onset is more often seen in girls. Psoriasis can also affect the joints and contribute to cardiovascular disease.

Psoriasis is a T-cell mediated autoimmune condition. Infectious diseases, upper respiratory tract infections, and streptococcal infections that can attract T-cells to the skin are found to be triggering factors.

MEDICAL HISTORY AND CLINICAL PRESENTATION

Lesions are either asymptomatic or pruritic and often localized to the scalp, extensor surfaces of the elbows and knees, sacrum, buttocks, and genitals. The nails, eyebrows, axillae, umbilicus, and perianal region may also be affected. The disease can be widespread, involving confluent areas of skin extending between these regions.

PHYSICAL EXAMINATION

The rash is raised, erythematous plaques >10 mm in diameter covered with thick, silvery, shiny scales. The plaques are located over the extensor surfaces of large joints, face, scalp, buttocks, and umbilical area. Pinpoint bleeding (Auspitz sign) may be noted at the base of a removed scale (Figure 1.15).

DIFFERENTIAL DIAGNOSIS

Differential diagnosis of psoriasis includes atopic/nummular dermatitis, tinea, pityriasis rubra pilaris, pityriasis rosea, and CTCL/mycosis fungoides.

DIAGNOSTIC STUDIES

Diagnosis is made based on clinical presentation. Skin biopsy can be used to confirm the diagnosis.

TREATMENT

Treatment options include topical treatments to UV light therapy to systemic treatments.

Topical treatment includes corticosteroids, vitamin D3 analogs, calcineurin inhibitors, emollients salicylic acid, coal tar, and anthralin.

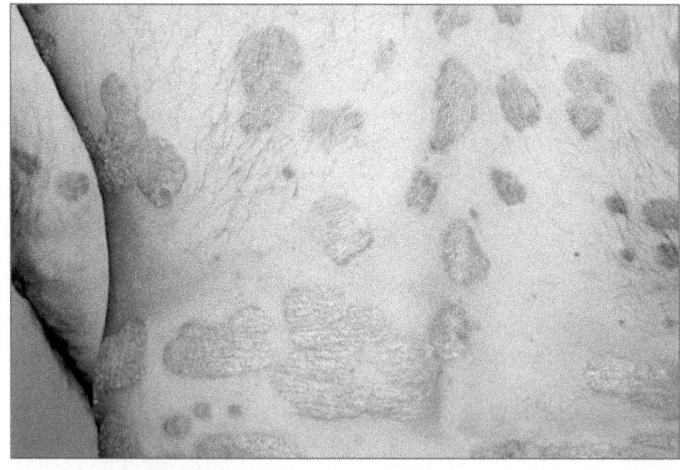

Figure 1.15 Psoriasis.

(Source: Ousley LE, Gentry RD. Evidence-based assessment of skin, hair and nails. In: Gawlik KS, Melnyk BM, Teall AM, eds. Evidence-Based Physical Examination. *Springer Publishing Company; 2021:257, Fig. 9.28.)*

Systemic corticosteroids may precipitate exacerbations or development of pustular psoriasis and should not be used to treat psoriasis. Corticosteroids are most effective when used overnight under occlusive coverings and without occlusion during the day.

Topical vitamin D3 analogs, such as calcipotriol and calcitriol, induce normal keratinocyte proliferation and differentiation. They can be used alone or in combination with topical corticosteroids.

Calcineurin inhibitors, tacrolimus and pimecrolimus, are available in topical form and are well tolerated. They are not as effective as corticosteroids but may avoid the complications of corticosteroids when treating facial and intertriginous psoriasis.

Emollients include creams, ointments, petrolatum, and paraffin. Emollients reduce scaling. Lesions may appear redder as scaling decreases or becomes more transparent. Emollients are safe and should probably always be used for mild to moderate plaque psoriasis.

Salicylic acid is a keratolytic that softens scales, facilitates their removal, and increases absorption of other topical agents. It is especially useful as a component of scalp treatments.

Coal tar preparations are anti-inflammatory and decrease keratinocyte hyperproliferation via an unknown mechanism. Coal tar products can be used in combination with topical corticosteroids or with natural or artificial broadband UVB light.

Anthralin is a topical antiproliferative, anti-inflammatory agent. Its mechanism of action is unknown. It may be irritating and should be used with caution in intertriginous areas; it also stains.

Phototherapy typically consists of UV light therapy. It is used in patients with extensive psoriasis. The mechanism of action is unknown, although UVB light reduces DNA synthesis and can induce mild systemic immunosuppression.

Immunosuppressants such as methotrexate, cyclosporine, and mycophenolate are also used. Methotrexate is used for severe disabling psoriasis.

Cyclosporine is used for severe psoriasis. Its use should be limited and alternated with other therapies. Side effects include renal dysfunction and long-term effects on the immune system. Mycophenolate is an alternative option when another option fails.

Immunomodulatory agents include the tumor necrosis factor (TNF) inhibitors etanercept, adalimumab, and infliximab. TNF inhibitors lead to clearing of psoriasis.

PATIENT EDUCATION

- Psoriasis is usually a chronic or chronic-relapsing disease. In children there is a high rate of spontaneous improvement to even clearing.

1.12F STASIS DERMATITIS

Stasis dermatitis occurs in patients with chronic venous insufficiency. Pooled venous blood in the legs causes a decrease in endothelial integrity in the microvasculature, which results in fibrin leakage, local inflammation, and local cell necrosis.

MEDICAL HISTORY AND CLINICAL PRESENTATION

Early in the disease there are eczematous changes. Hyperpigmentation and red-brown discoloration occur secondary to venous stasis and may be present before or after stasis dermatitis develops. If not inadequately treated, stasis dermatitis progresses to ulceration, chronic edema, and thickened fibrotic skin.

PHYSICAL EXAMINATION

Chronic stasis dermatitis appears as fibrotic skin thickening and hyperpigmentation. Central weeping ulcerations surrounded by chronic changes may develop. If not adequately treated venous stasis ulcers and secondary infections can develop.

DIFFERENTIAL DIAGNOSIS

The differential diagnosis of stasis dermatitis includes AD, irritant and allergic contact dermatitis, lichen simplex chronicus, hypertrophic LP, eczema, psoriasis, and tinea corporis.

DIAGNOSTIC STUDIES

Diagnosis of stasis dermatitis is based on clinical appearance of the skin lesions and signs of chronic venous insufficiency.

TREATMENT

In stasis dermatitis the key to treatment is the treatment of the chronic venous insufficiency with leg elevation and compression stockings.

For acute stasis dermatitis tap water compresses should be applied. For less acute dermatitis, a corticosteroid cream or ointment should be applied or incorporated into zinc oxide paste.

Ulcers are best treated with compresses and bland dressings. Regardless of the dressing used, reduction of edema, usually with compression, is paramount for healing.

Oral antibiotics, cephalosporins or dicloxacillin, are used to treat superimposed infection. Topical antibiotics, mupirocin, or silver sulfadiazine are useful for treating erosions and ulcers.

Complex or multiple topical drugs or over-the-counter remedies should not be used.

PATIENT EDUCATION

- In stasis dermatitis the skin is vulnerable to direct irritants and to potentially sensitizing topical agents.

SPECIAL CONSIDERATIONS

- Pityriasis rosea in the first 15 weeks of pregnancy is associated with premature birth and fetal death. Pregnant women should be offered antiviral therapy, even though this is not proved to reduce obstetric complications.

KEY POINTS

- Contact dermatitis can be caused by irritants or allergens. Symptoms are pain or pruritus.
- LP is an autoimmune disorder or may be caused by drugs. It presents with pruritic, polygonal, purple papules and may be associated with hepatitis C.
- Psoriasis has several disease triggers and presents with well-circumscribed, red plaques covered with silvery scales.

- Pityriasis rosea presents with a herald patch followed by centripetal eruption of oval papules and plaques along skin lines.
- Stasis dermatitis is due to chronic venous insufficiency and presents with erythema, scaling, and weeping lesions.

1.13 PIGMENT DISORDERS

OVERVIEW

Pigmentation disorders involve hypopigmentation, depigmentation, or hyperpigmentation. Areas involved may be focal or diffuse. In hypopigmentation, pigment is decreased, whereas in depigmentation, pigment is completely lost, leaving white skin.

Focal disease is typically due to injury, inflammatory dermatoses, burns, or chemical exposure.

Focal hypopigmentation or depigmentation is a feature of vitiligo, leprosy, nutritional deficiencies, genetic disorders, tinea versicolor, lichen sclerosis, and pityriasis alba. Diffuse hypopigmentation is noted in albinism and vitiligo. Hyperpigmentation may also be caused by a systemic disorder, drug, or cancer; distribution is usually more diffuse.

PATHOPHYSIOLOGY

Melanin, produced by melanocytes, is the brownish pigment responsible for the color of skin, hair, and the iris. Color shades of human skin is due to the amount of melanin produced and not the number of melanocytes. UV radiation, as in sunlight, stimulates melanin production, as do several pathologic processes.

1.13A VITILIGO

Vitiligo is an acquired autoimmune disorder in which melanocytes are destroyed causing depigmented areas on the skin. Vitiligo is most commonly noted in fair-skinned persons on the face, hands, arms, or other exposed skin. Patients with dark skin will note that skin is turning light or white.

The prevalence of vitiligo is up to 1% in the United States.[32]

The cause of vitiligo is unknown but three factors are involved: melanocyte susceptibility to destruction, hyperactive immune system, and environmental factors.

MEDICAL HISTORY AND CLINICAL PRESENTATION

Vitiligo affects males and females equally and often begins early in life before the age of 10 years. Between 70% and 80% of adult patients develop vitiligo by age 30.[32] This disorder primarily affects young people, although it can begin much later in life.

Patients with vitiligo vulgaris or bilateral or generalized vitiligo early in the disease will have depigmentation of the fingertips, knuckles, ventral side of the wrist, axillae, toes, ankles, around the eyes and mouth, and along the hair line. It can be incited by trauma.

PHYSICAL EXAMINATION

Vitiligo is characterized by hypopigmented or depigmented areas, sharply demarcated and symmetric. Depigmentation may be localized or cover entire body segments. Vitiligo commonly involves the face, digits, dorsal hands, flexor wrists, elbows, knees, shins, dorsal ankles, armpits, inguinal area, anogenital area, umbilicus, and nipples. Cosmetic disfigurement can be especially severe and emotionally devastating in dark-skinned patients.

DIFFERENTIAL DIAGNOSIS

The differential diagnosis includes pityriasis alba, tinea versicolor, halo nevus, tuberous sclerosis, and albinism.

DIAGNOSTIC STUDIES

The diagnosis is made on clinical findings. The pattern of depigmentation noted above is usually characteristic. Laboratory testing may be indicated to rule out associated conditions such as pernicious anemia, Addison's disease, and thyroid disease.

TREATMENT

Treatment of vitiligo should be supportive and cosmetic; it can be treated medically or occasionally surgically. Topical medication options include topical steroids, calcipotriene, or calcineurin inhibitors such as tacrolimus. All these uses are off label and not approved by the FDA for vitiligo but have been used for many years. Treatment should be given for at least 3 to 4 months.

Oral and topical psoralen PUVA therapies are often successful, but over a hundred treatment sessions may be necessary, which can increase risk of skin cancer. NBUVB is as effective as topical PUVA and has few adverse effects, making NBUVB preferable to PUVA.

Surgery, micrografting and tattooing, is reasonable only for patients with stable, limited disease when medical therapy has failed.

1.13B MELASMA

Melasma, also known as the mask of pregnancy, is a dark facial discoloration. It is common in women, especially pregnant women and those taking oral contraceptives or hormone replacement therapy medications.

The pathophysiologic mechanism is still largely debated. It is thought that UV B irradiation causes an increase alpha-melanocyte-stimulating hormone (alpha-MSH) and adrenocorticotropic hormone (ACTH). These hormones lead to proliferation of melanocytes and an increase in melanin synthesis in the affected skin.

MEDICAL HISTORY AND CLINICAL PRESENTATION

Melasma is more common in young to middle-aged females, especially those of Asian, Hispanic, African American, and Middle Eastern ancestry. It is also associated with an increased estrogen state. Pregnancy, use of oral contraceptives, or hormone replacement therapies are well-known risk factors.

Hyperpigmentation may resolve spontaneously in the postnatal period. Thyroid disease has also been shown to be a risk factor for the development of melasma.

Medication history should be obtained. Phenytoin has been implicated in the development of melasma, as has recent exposure to heavy metals such as mercury.

PHYSICAL EXAMINATION

On physical examination, melasma presents as well-demarcated light to dark brown hyperpigmented and often symmetrically distributed macules or patches with a predilection for the face.

DIFFERENTIAL DIAGNOSIS

The differential diagnosis of melasma includes drug induced hyperpigmentation, actinic LP, solar lentigines, heavy metal deposition, and phytophotodermatitis.

DIAGNOSTIC STUDIES

Diagnosis is made based on history and physical examination findings.

TREATMENT

Monotherapy with hydroquinone remains the gold standard of treatment. It works by decreasing the formation of melanin. It is safe with side effects including allergic or irritant contact dermatitis and postinflammatory hyperpigmentation.

To optimize any treatment, sun avoidance and protection strategies must be initiated, including the use of broad-spectrum sunscreen with an SPF of at least 30, wide brimmed hats, and protective clothing.

1.13C ACANTHOSIS NIGRICANS

Acanthosis nigricans (AN) is a brown to black, poorly defined, velvety hyperpigmentation of the skin, typically present in the posterior and lateral folds of the neck, axilla, groin, and umbilicus. It generally is due to insulin resistance resulting in abnormal skin growth. The most common cause of AN is insulin resistance from diabetes mellitus type 2.

Obese patients with associated insulin resistance are the most likely population to develop AN and it may be a sign of developing metabolic syndrome.

MEDICAL HISTORY AND CLINICAL PRESENTATION

AN is a skin disease that may occur in any location of the body. Because of the association between AN and various systemic abnormalities, a complete review of medical history should be obtained. A history of insulin resistance, obesity, hyperandrogenism, and malignancy should be obtained.

Symptoms of cutaneous virilism due to hyperandrogenism include hirsutism, acne vulgaris, hidradenitis suppurativa, and androgenic alopecia. Because several medications are linked to AN a complete drug history is important. Likely medications include nicotinic acid, oral contraceptives, heroin, corticosteroids, diethylstilbestrol, methyltestosterone, and fusidic acid. A history of unintentional weight loss, fevers, night sweats, or a constellation of other nonspecific symptoms should alert a malignancy workup.

PHYSICAL EXAMINATION

AN is a skin disease characterized by symmetric, velvety, hyperpigmented plaques that may occur in any location of the body. Lesions are most commonly found on the lateral and posterior neck, axilla, groin, elbows, knuckles, and face. AN may be benign or malignant. The benign types include idiopathic or benign, obesity-related, syndromic, unilateral/nevoid, acral, drug-induced, and mixed.

DIAGNOSTIC STUDIES

Diagnosis is typically made by physical examination. A skin biopsy may be needed in unusual cases.

TREATMENT

Treatment varies depending on the underlying etiology. For obesity-related disease, metformin is utilized. Topical treatment options include retinoic acid, calcipotriol, or tretinoin cream with ammonium lactate cream. If due to malignancy, the approach is to treat the malignancy.

PATIENT EDUCATION

- The importance of diet and exercise should also be stressed to patients.
- People with AN should be screened for diabetes and cancer.

SPECIAL CONSIDERATIONS

- Melasma fades slowly and incompletely after childbirth or cessation of hormone use.

KEY POINTS

- Vitiligo is due to loss of skin melanocytes, can be focal or segmental, and is diagnosed by skin examination.
- Melasma is linked to pregnancy, oral contraceptives, and hormone replacement therapy.
- AN is linked to obesity, diabetes, and certain malignancies.

1.14 VASCULAR ABNORMALITIES

OVERVIEW

Vascular malformations are due to abnormal development of blood and lymphatic vessels. Table 1.9 summarizes various vascular malformation.

TABLE 1.9 Vascular Malformations

Type of Vessel	Description
Capillary	Macular staining; occur on eyelids (angel kiss), forehead, and nuchal area (stork bite); often resolve in early childhood
Venous	Appear blue and spongy, enlarge with Valsalva maneuver
Lymphatic	Composed of microcystic and macrocystic channels
Arterial	Minimal skin findings but can cause swelling, ulceration, and necrosis; most common in head and neck region

1.14A ANGIOMAS

Cherry angiomas are benign vascular neoplasms found most commonly in people over the age of 50. They occur equally in both sexes and all ethnicities but are more common in Caucasians. Most Caucasians obtain a few cherry angiomas by their 30s to 40s, and the number of lesions increase over time. The etiology of these lesions is unknown.

MEDICAL HISTORY AND CLINICAL PRESENTATION

Lesions appear gradually in adulthood and are asymptomatic.

PHYSICAL EXAMINATION

Cherry angiomas are round to oval, dome-shaped papules ranging in size from pinpoint to several millimeters. They are found mainly on the trunk and proximal extremities but can be found anywhere on the body. They are usually bright cherry red in color but can become thrombosed and become black.

DIFFERENTIAL DIAGNOSIS

The differential diagnosis of cherry angiomas includes melanoma, bacillary angiomatosis, and petechiae.

DIAGNOSTIC STUDIES

Diagnosis is made by physical examination. No laboratory testing is needed.

TREATMENT

Treatment is seldom needed unless they become irritated; patients may request cosmetic removal.

PATIENT EDUCATION

- Presence of numerous cherry angiomas should lead to the investigation of possible malignancies.

1.14B TELANGIECTASIAS

Telangiectasias are asymptomatic, dilatations of capillaries, venules, and arterioles. They occur in a variety of settings with little variation in appearance. It is important to separate those that are from a primary disorder from those that arise secondarily.

MEDICAL HISTORY AND CLINICAL PRESENTATION

Certain aspects of the patient's history will aid in identifying the various etiologies. Primary etiologies include rosacea, Osler-Rendu-Weber syndrome, hereditary benign telangiectasia, ataxia telangiectasia, generalized essential telangiectasia, and unilateral nevoid telangiectasia. Secondary causes include BCC, rosacea, collagen vascular disease, corticosteroid atrophy, scleroderma, and CREST (calcinosis, Raynaud phenomenon, esophageal dysmotility, sclerodactyly, and telangiectasia) syndrome.

PHYSICAL EXAMINATION

The lesion appears as a dilated dermal vessel with a diameter of 1 mm or less. They are not palpable and easily blanch. Distribution varies with underlying condition.

DIFFERENTIAL DIAGNOSIS

The differential diagnosis includes petechiae.

DIAGNOSTIC STUDIES

Diagnosis is based on physical examination findings and history.

TREATMENT

Treatment typically is not indicated but these lesions can be removed with laser surgery for cosmetic reasons.

1.15 VESICULOBULLOUS DISORDERS

OVERVIEW

Vesiculobullous disease is a mucocutaneous disease characterized by vesicles and bullae. Both are fluid-filled lesions and are distinguished by size. Vesicles are <5 mm to 10 mm, and bullae are >5 mm to 10 mm. Examples of vesiculobullous disease include infectious etiologies such as herpes simplex, varicella-zoster, and hand-foot-and-mouth disease. Immune disorders include pemphigoid and pemphigus vulgaris.

1.15A PEMPHIGOID

Bullous pemphigoid is more common than pemphigus. It is a rare autoimmune condition that occurs more commonly with increasing age, with a median age of 80. The incidence of occurrence in women and men is approximately the same. The risk of death is significantly less than that of pemphigus.

The bullae in pemphigoid are generated when IgG autoantibodies attack bullous pemphigoid antigen 2, which is a component of hemidesmosomes.

MEDICAL HISTORY AND CLINICAL PRESENTATION

Bullous pemphigoid usually involves pruritic bullae and/or urticarial plaques that occur most commonly in the groin, axillae, and flexural areas. Involvement of the oropharyngeal mucosa occurs in only one-third of cases. It is important to rule out a drug-induced etiology, so that the drug can be removed.

PHYSICAL EXAMINATION

Bullous pemphigoid lesions are large, tense fluid-filled blisters, which can rupture and form erosions. The lesions can be localized to one area or widespread on trunk and proximal limbs. Pruritic lesions can be found in flexural areas such as the groin and axilla.

DIFFERENTIAL DIAGNOSIS

The differential diagnosis includes pemphigus vulgaris. If ulcers of the oropharyngeal mucosa are most common the differential diagnosis includes HSV, aphthous ulcers, LP, and EM.

DIAGNOSTIC STUDIES

When typical bullae are present the diagnosis of bullous pemphigoid is based on clinical findings. The diagnosis can be confirmed by skin biopsy.

TREATMENT

The mainstay of treatment is topical or oral glucocorticoid therapy, which works by reducing autoantibody production. Oral glucocorticoids are reserved for patients with disease extending to the mucous membranes that has not responded to topical therapy. Azathioprine has also been used as monotherapy in patients with mild to moderate disease who are unable to tolerate steroid therapy. Other treatments include oral doxycycline and niacinamide supplementation.

PATIENT EDUCATION

- Bullous pemphigoid can take 1 to 2 years to resolve.

1.15B PEMPHIGUS

Pemphigus vulgaris is an autoimmune disorder in which blistering of the skin is the primary symptom. Autoantibodies against desmoglein cause the intraepidermal blistering seen in pemphigus.

Pemphigus vulgaris is a rare condition that occurs more commonly with increasing age, with a median age of 71. It occurs in women nearly twice as much as in men and has a high risk of death.

Three major types of pemphigus have been defined, of which pemphigus vulgaris is the most common. Pemphigus is unique from pemphigoid in that the blistering can involve the mucous membranes as well as skin.

MEDICAL HISTORY AND CLINICAL PRESENTATION

The primary lesions of pemphigus vulgaris are flaccid bullae that cause widespread and painful skin, oral, and other mucosal erosions. About half of patients have only oral erosions, which rupture and remain as chronic, painful lesions. Dysphagia and poor oral intake are common because lesions also may occur in the upper esophagus. Cutaneous bullae typically arise in normal-appearing skin, rupture, and leave a raw area with crusting. Itching is usually absent. Erosions often become infected. If large portions of the body are affected, fluid and electrolyte loss may become an issue.

PHYSICAL EXAMINATION

Pemphigus has flaccid, thin-walled bullae that generally originate on the oropharyngeal mucosa. Then the bullae can spread to involve other parts of the skin, including the face, scalp, chest, axilla, and groin. The bullae rupture easily, and patients develop open erosions that can become infected. The superficial layer of skin in affected individuals can be separated from the deeper layers by mechanical pressure; this is called Nikolsky sign.

DIFFERENTIAL DIAGNOSIS

The differential diagnosis includes bullous pemphigoid. If ulcers of the oropharyngeal mucosa are most common the differential includes HSV, aphthous ulcers, LP, or EM.

DIAGNOSTIC STUDIES

The gold standard for diagnosis of pemphigus vulgaris is skin lesion biopsy. A deep-shave or punch biopsy from the edge of a newly formed erosion will show histologic evidence of loss of intercellular connections between keratinocytes.

TREATMENT

The mainstay of treatment is oral glucocorticoid therapy, which works by reducing autoantibody production. Immunosuppressants, such as rituximab, can reduce the need for corticosteroids and reduce the side effects of long-term corticosteroid use.

Treatment of open lesions consists of cleaning and dressing, similar to the treatment of partial-thickness burns, with reverse isolation and silver sulfadiazine dressings.

PATIENT EDUCATION

- Pemphigus is a chronic and potentially fatal disease and patients may require hospitalization and treatment in a burn unit.

KEY POINTS

- Bullous pemphigoid is noted in patients over the age of 60 and is autoimmune and idiopathic. Pruritus is the initial symptom.
- Pemphigus vulgaris predominately presents with oral lesions. Nikolsky sign aids in differentiating it from other bullous disorders.

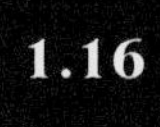

1.16 DRUG/PHOTOSENSITIVITY REACTIONS

OVERVIEW

Drugs can cause multiple skin eruptions and reactions. The most serious include SJS and TEN. For more information see desquamation disorders in this chapter. Other reactions include hypersensitivity syndrome, serum sickness, exfoliative dermatitis, angioedema, anaphylaxis, and drug-induced vasculitis. Drugs are also linked to hair loss, LP, erythema nodosum, skin pigment change, systemic lupus erythematosus, photosensitivity reactions, pemphigus, and pemphigoid.

Many drugs have been implicated in causing skin reactions. The most common include the antibiotics, anticonvulsants, NSAIDs, and allopurinol. See Table 1.10 for a summary of the common drug reactions.

EPIDEMIOLOGY

Adverse skin reactions to drugs are frequent, affecting 2% to 3% of all hospitalized patients.[33] Only about 2% of adverse skin reactions are severe and very few are fatal.[33]

PATHOPHYSIOLOGY

Morbilliform drug reactions are a T-cell mediated eruption of the delayed hypersensitivity (type IV) type. Morbilliform reactions has been classified both as type IVb (eosinophils) and type IVc (T-cell mediated apoptosis).

TABLE 1.10 Types of Common Drug Reactions

Type of Reaction	Description	Typical Agents
Acneiform eruptions	Looks like acne but lacks comedones, sudden onset	Corticosteroids, iodines, hydantoins, lithium, isoniazid, phenytoin, phenobarbital
Blistering eruptions	Widespread vesicles and bullae	Penicillamine, thiol-containing medications
Cutaneous necrosis	Demarcated, painful red lesions that progress to necrosis	Warfarin, heparin, epinephrine, vasopressin
Drug-induced lupus	Appears as a lupus-like syndrome, often without rash	Hydralazine, procainamide, hydrochlorothiazide
Erythema nodosum	Tender, red nodules, mainly pretibial region	Sulfonamides, oral contraceptives
Exfoliative dermatitis	Red, scaly lesions	Penicillin, sulfonamides
Morbilliform	Most common; pruritic, morbilliform disease	Almost any drug
Mucocutaneous eruptions	Small oral lesions or painful oral ulcers	Penicillin, barbiturates, sulfonamides
Photosensitivity eruptions	Dermatitis or gray-blue hyperpigmentation on sun-exposed skin	Phenothiazines, tetracyclines, sulfonamides, chlorothiazide
Serum sickness	Type III immune complex reaction; urticaria and angioedema	Penicillin, insulin, foreign proteins
Urticaria	Common, IgE mediated; well-defined edematous wheals	Penicillin, aspirin, sulfonamides, ACE inhibitors

ACE, angiotensin-converting enzyme; IgE, immunoglobulin E.

MEDICAL HISTORY AND CLINICAL PRESENTATION

The onset of a morbilliform eruption typically occurs within 7 to 10 days after the initiation of the culprit drug. When challenged with a drug that the patient has been sensitized to in the past, the eruption may occur within 24 hours.

PHYSICAL EXAMINATION

Initially, there are erythematous blanching macules and papules, which may coalesce to form larger macules and plaques. Pruritus is common. The rash begins on the trunk and upper extremities and progresses caudally. Mucous membranes are typically spared.

DIFFERENTIAL DIAGNOSIS

The differential diagnosis includes viral exanthems, toxin-mediated erythemas, graft-versus-host disease, and SJS/TEN.

DIAGNOSTIC STUDIES

The diagnosis is made based on the typical clinical appearance in concert with drug history and the absence of systemic involvement.

TREATMENT

The offending medication should be discontinued if possible. If this is not possible to do, symptomatic and supportive treatment while continuing the drug therapy is a feasible option.

Mid- or high-potency topical steroid or antihistamines may help to relieve pruritus.

KEY POINTS

- Because drugs can cause a variety of reactions, drugs should be considered as causes of almost any unexplained skin reaction.

1.17 URTICARIA

OVERVIEW

Urticaria is a vascular reaction of the skin with the transient appearance of smooth, slightly elevated pale or erythematous patches, often attended by severe pruritus or itching. The wheals vary in size and are raised above the surface of the surrounding skin.

There are three types of urticaria: acute urticaria (onset <6 weeks), chronic urticaria (lasting >6 weeks from onset), and physical urticaria.

EPIDEMIOLOGY

Up to 20% of the population will experience urticaria at some point in their life.[34] The incidence varies with age, with most cases noted in preschool and school-age children.

PATHOPHYSIOLOGY

Urticaria results from the release of vasoactive substances, such as histamine, from mast cells and basophils in the superficial dermis. This results in edema caused by vasodilation and leukocyte infiltration. This process is immune mediated or nonimmune mediated.

Immune-mediated reactions include type I hypersensitivity reactions and autoimmune disorders. Nonimmune-mediated reactions include direct nonallergic activation of mast cells by certain drugs, drug-induced cyclooxygenase inhibition, or activation by physical or emotional stimuli.

MEDICAL HISTORY AND CLINICAL PRESENTATION

The first step is a detailed history to review any potential exposure that may have caused allergic urticaria within 48 hours prior to the onset of the urticaria. The list of items of possible allergic exposure should include foods (e.g., dairy, nuts, fish, shellfish), drugs (e.g., antibiotics, NSAIDs), insect sting or bite, and latex.

Chronic urticaria is less likely to have an identifiable cause. With physical urticaria the history provides clues to the cause of the skin rash.

PHYSICAL EXAMINATION

There are two classic findings: itching and wheal formation. Patients with urticaria will complain of severe itching from the onset. It may start with the first appearance of skin lesions and may spread. Scratching exacerbates spread of the rash.

The onset of skin lesions, welt, or wheal is sudden. The lesions are pruritic and characterized by a pale, slightly red color. The size of the lesions ranges from 2 mm to 15 mm, and their appearance is that of flat-topped wheals scattered over the body.

DIFFERENTIAL DIAGNOSIS

The differential diagnosis includes angioedema, mastocytosis, urticaria pigmentosa, AD (eczema), contact dermatitis, juvenile idiopathic arthritis, pityriasis rosea, serum sickness, and urticarial vasculitis.

DIAGNOSTIC STUDIES

Laboratory testing may be useful in patients with allergenic urticaria. IgE allergic antibody tests (RAST [radioallergosorbent test] or skin test for IgE) for specific foods may be useful.

Laboratory evaluation for chronic urticaria includes selective testing to evaluate possible underlying conditions. No laboratory testing is indicated with physical urticaria.

EVALUATION

The first step in the evaluation is to differentiate between acute urticaria, duration <6 weeks; chronic urticaria, duration >6 weeks; and physical urticaria. This is followed by a detailed history to identify possible offending agents. Suspected offending agents should be removed immediately. The next step is to rule out food allergy, drug sensitivity, insect sting allergy, latex allergy, or contact allergy by requesting appropriate testing like RAST or the skin test for IgE antibody.

TREATMENT

Any identified offending agent should be stopped. Nonspecific symptomatic treatment, such as cool baths, avoiding scratching, and wearing loose clothing may be helpful.

Antihistamines remain the mainstay of treatment. They must be taken on a regular basis at higher than normal doses. Newer oral antihistamines (cetirizine, desloratadine, fexofenadine) are preferred because of daily dosing and they are less sedating.

Systemic corticosteroids (prednisone) are used for severe symptoms, but long-term treatment should be avoided due to side effects. Topical corticosteroids or topical antihistamines are not beneficial.

Patients who have angioedema involving the oropharynx or any involvement of the airway should receive epinephrine subcutaneously and be admitted to the hospital. Patients should be supplied with an autoinjectable epinephrine pen once discharged from the hospital.

If concerned about the development of anaphylaxis, epinephrine should be given immediately, followed by corticosteroid treatment and a short-acting antihistamine.

PATIENT EDUCATION

- The patient and family should be instructed about emergency symptoms to be aware of including angioedema of the face, tongue, and lips; stridor, wheezing, or respiratory distress; or urticaria that lasts more than 48 hours.

SPECIAL CONSIDERATIONS

- The older oral antihistamines are sedating and can cause confusion, urinary retention, and delirium. They should be used with caution in elderly patients.

KEY POINTS

- Acute urticaria is caused by allergic reaction while chronic urticaria is idiopathic or autoimmune disease.

1.18 BURNS

OVERVIEW

Burns are the fourth most common cause of injury worldwide. The first 48 hours after a thermal burn offers the greatest opportunity to impact survival.

EPIDEMIOLOGY

According to the CDC, each year there are about 1.1 million burn injuries that require medical attention; of these, 50,000 require hospitalization and up to 10,000 people in the United States die every year of burn-related infections.[35] Approximately 86% of burns are thermal, 4% electrical, and 3% chemical.[35]

PATHOPHYSIOLOGY

Burns of the skin involve two main layers: the outer epidermis and the thicker, deeper dermis. There are various types of burns. Chemical burns are either acid or alkali burns. Alkali burns are more severe with deeper penetration into the skin by liquefying the skin. Acid burns have less penetration due to coagulation injury. Electrical burns may have small entry and exit wounds, but there may be extensive internal organ injury and associated traumatic injuries. Thermal burns are the most common type of burn.

Burn depth is classified into three types based on how deep into the epidermis or dermis the injury extends.

- Superficial burns (previously called first degree) involve only the epidermis and are warm, painful, red, soft, and blanch when touched. Usually, there is no blistering. An example is a sunburn.
- Partial thickness burns (previously called second degree) extend through the epidermis and into the dermis. The depth into the dermis can vary, being superficial or deep dermis. They are usually very painful, red, blistered, moist, and blanch when touched. Examples include burns from hot surfaces, hot liquids, or flame.
- Full-thickness burns (previously called third degree) extend through the epidermis and dermis into the subcutaneous fat or deeper. There is little or no pain, they can be white, brown, or charred and feel firm and leathery with no blanching. These occur from a flame or hot liquids.

When calculating the extent of burn, only partial thickness and full thickness burns are considered, and superficial burns are excluded.

MEDICAL HISTORY AND CLINICAL PRESENTATION

If the patient has burns classified as severe, the approach to the patient should be like that of a major trauma patient. Key information to obtain include the type of burn, possible inhalation injury, and associated injuries. If there was prolonged smoke exposure consider carbon monoxide poisoning, cyanide poisoning, or lung injury. Examination of the burn can be done in the patient's secondary survey.

PHYSICAL EXAMINATION

Along with determining the depth of the burn and identifying any secondary trauma, the extent of the burns should be determined. There are several methods to determine the extent of the burn.

Rule of nines: The head represents 9%, each arm is 9%, the anterior chest and abdomen are 18%, the posterior chest and back are 18%, each leg is 18%, and the perineum is 1%. For children, the head is 18%, and the legs are 13.5% each (see Figure 1.16).

Palmar surface: For small burns, the hand surface (including the palm and fingers) represents about 1% of their BSA.

DIAGNOSTIC STUDIES

The diagnosis is made based on physical assessment. Laboratory assessment is needed for the care of the burn patient. CBC is needed to evaluate for occult blood loss and determining oxygen-carrying capacity.

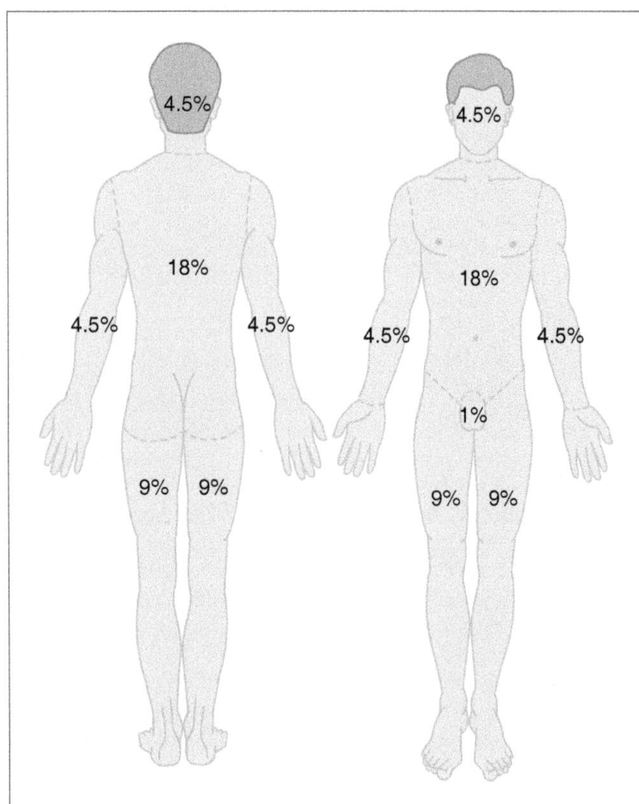

Figure 1.16 **Rule of nines.**

Basic metabolic panel including electrolytes and renal function is helpful because of the fluid shifts and metabolic changes that occur. Carbon monoxide level should be obtained if the patient was in a fire.

TREATMENT

Minor burns can be approached using the following four Cs of burn care:

- **Cooling:** Cool small areas of burn with tap water or saline solution to prevent progression of burning and to reduce pain.
- **Cleaning:** Clean the burn with mild soap and water or mild antibacterial wash. Large blisters should be debrided and small blisters and blisters involving the palms or soles are left intact.
- **Covering:** Cover with topical antibiotic ointments or cream with absorbent dressing or specialized burn dressing materials.
- **Comfort:** Give over-the-counter pain medications or prescription pain medications when needed.

For burns classified as severe (>20% TBSA), fluid resuscitation should be initiated to maintain urine output >0.5 mL/kg/hour. One fluid resuscitation formula is the Parkland formula. The total amount of lactated Ringer's fluid to be given during the initial 24 hours = 4 mL × patient's weight (kg) × % TBSA. Half of the calculated amount is administered during the first 8 hours. This is only an estimate and more or less fluid may be needed based on vital signs, urine output, other injuries, or other medical conditions.

In patients with moderate to severe flame burns and with suspicion for inhalation injury, carboxyhemoglobin levels should be checked, and patients should be placed on high-flow oxygen until carbon monoxide poisoning is ruled out. If carbon monoxide poisoning is confirmed, continue treatment with high-flow oxygen and consider hyperbaric oxygen in select cases. Cyanide poisoning can occur from smoke inhalation and can be treated with hydroxocobalamin or nitrites plus thiosulfate.

PATIENT EDUCATION

- Prognosis is determined on the extent and location of the burn tissue damage, associated injuries, comorbidities, and complications.

KEY POINTS

- Estimates of the burn location, size, and depth determine treatment plan.
- The first 48 hours after a thermal burn offers the greatest opportunity to impact survival.

1.19 HIDRADENITIS SUPPURATIVA

OVERVIEW

Hidradenitis suppurativa is a chronic inflammatory condition of the hair follicle and associated structures. Follicular inflammation and occlusion cause rupture of the follicle and development of abscesses, sinus tracts, and scarring.

Hidradenitis suppurative is often mistaken for boils, delaying diagnosis and leading to progression of a chronic, disabling scarring condition that negatively impacts quality of life.

EPIDEMIOLOGY

Prevalence has been estimated at 0.1%.[36] It is more common in women in their early 20s. It rarely occurs prior to puberty and is unusual following menopause.

PATHOPHYSIOLOGY

The development is linked to genetic factors with many patients reporting a positive family history.

Hormonal factors (the androgens) obesity, and nicotine are linked to the development of hidradenitis suppurativa.

SIGNS AND SYMPTOMS

The onset of disease is insidious. Early in disease there is development of random small, red indurated papules, pustules, or nodules that may resolve, persist, or drain. Early symptoms consist of mild pruritus and burning, although lesions may be deep seated and very painful. Lesions are generally found in intertriginous areas, axilla, groin, and under the breast.

PHYSICAL EXAMINATION

Physical examination findings include swollen, tender masses resembling cutaneous abscesses. These lesions are sterile. In chronic disease pain, fluctuance, discharge, and sinus tract formation are common. If bacterial infection develops there may be development of deep abscesses and sinus tracts. Drainage from these lesions may be serous, purulent, and/or bloody, and an odor may be present. Sinus tracts can be single or multiple and will range from being barely visible to swollen, painful and inflamed with multiple areas of drainage. With healing, hypertrophic scars develop and fibrotic bands can be seen crisscrossing the areas of involvement and can lead to skin contractures.

DIFFERENTIAL DIAGNOSIS

Differential diagnosis includes infections such as carbuncles, furuncles, abscesses, ischiorectal/perirectal abscess, Bartholin duct abscess, erysipelas, granuloma inguinale, and lymphogranuloma venereum. Other possibilities include epidermoid, Bartholin, and pilonidal cysts; Crohn disease; and anal or vulvovaginal fistula.

DIAGNOSTIC STUDIES

The diagnosis is made clinically. Laboratory testing is not helpful.

EVALUATION

The severity of hidradenitis suppurativa can be classified using Hurley clinical staging. Staging is also used to direct management. The stages are:

- **Stage I:** Abscess formation, single or multiple without sinus tracts and scarring
- **Stage II:** Recurrent abscesses with tract formation and scarring, single or multiple separated lesions
- **Stage III:** Diffuse or near-diffuse involvement, or multiple interconnecting tracts and abscesses across entire area

TREATMENT

Hidradenitis suppurativa treatment goals are to prevent new lesions, reduce inflammation, and remove sinus tracts and is based on Hurley staging.

For stage I disease, typical treatment includes topical clindamycin, topical resorcinol, or oral zinc gluconate, intralesional corticosteroids, and a short course of oral antibiotics. Tetracycline, doxycycline, minocycline, or erythromycin can be used.

Stage II disease is treated with a longer course of the same oral antibiotics used to treat stage I disease. Adding antiandrogen therapy, with oral estrogen or combination oral contraceptives, spironolactone, or finasteride may be useful in some cases. Incision and drainage may reduce the pain of an abscess but are insufficient for disease control. Sinus tracts should be unroofed and debrided.

Stage III disease is treated with aggressive medical and surgical therapy. Options include infliximab, adalimumab, or oral retinoids. Wide surgical excision and repair or grafting of the affected areas is often necessary if the disease persists.

Recommended adjunctive measures for all patients include maintaining good skin hygiene, minimizing trauma, and providing psychological support.

PATIENT EDUCATION

- The prognosis strongly depends on the stage of hidradenitis suppurativa at the time of presentation and the patient's response to therapy/therapies used.
- Mild disease which can be adequately controlled with antiandrogen and anti-inflammatory medication.
- The severe and chronic disease may have an impact on mental health. Long-standing untreated hidradenitis suppurativa can result in depression, withdrawal, and isolation.

SPECIAL CONSIDERATIONS

- Complications may include chronic pain and discomfort, restricted mobility, fistula formation, odor, significant lymphedema, and concomitant decreased quality of life.

KEY POINTS

- Lesions are usually sterile except for deep abscesses.
- Treatment is based on the Hurley staging system.

1.20 PILONIDAL DISEASE

OVERVIEW

Pilonidal disease is an acute abscess or chronic draining sinus in the sacrococcygeal area.

EPIDEMIOLOGY

Pilonidal disease usually occurs in young, hairy, males but can also occur in women.

PATHOPHYSIOLOGY

It is usually considered to be an acquired condition but may be congenital. A traumatic event is not a cause of a pilonidal cyst but may inflame an existing cyst.

MEDICAL HISTORY AND CLINICAL PRESENTATION

Some people with a pilonidal cyst will be asymptomatic. Pilonidal cysts are often very painful, and typically occur between the ages of 15 and 35. Although usually found near the coccyx, other areas that can be affected include the navel, armpit, or genital region.

PHYSICAL EXAMINATION

On physical examination a sinus tract may originate from the source of infection and open to the skin surface. Material from the cyst may drain through the pilonidal sinus. One or more midline or adjacent sinuses occur in the skin of the sacral region and may form a cavity, often containing hair.

DIFFERENTIAL DIAGNOSIS

The differential diagnosis includes hidradenitis suppurativa, dermoid cyst, germ cell tumor, and granulomatous diseases related to syphilis and tuberculosis.

DIAGNOSTIC STUDIES

Biopsy may be needed to rule out malignancy.

TREATMENT

Pilonidal disease is treated with both operative and nonoperative techniques. The method of intervention is determined by the extent of the disease and history of previous intervention. Recurrent disease after surgical intervention requires a more invasive approach with wide excision and flap closure. Asymptomatic pits do not require surgical intervention. Surgical techniques include pit excision, incision, or excision with or without marsupialization, and wide excision with rotational flap closure.

PATIENT EDUCATION

- The key to preventing recurrence is ensuring that hair remains out of, and away from, the healing wound, with weekly clipping or shavings.

KEY POINTS

- Pilonidal disease is a common condition that is acquired.
- Initial management of infection is to drain any abscess off the midline and allow the infection to resolve before commencing definitive therapy for the pilonidal pits.
- Asymptomatic pilonidal pits do not require therapy, but symptomatic disease should be surgically managed.

COMMON CHIEF COMPLAINTS

APPROACH TO RASH AND FEVER IN CHILDREN

Children frequently present with a fever and rash. While the differential diagnosis is broad, adequate history and physical examination can help narrow down a list of etiologies. See Figure 1.17 for the evaluation algorithm for fever and rash.

While there is a strong link between the presentation of fever and rash and infectious disease, it is important to keep in mind that other noninfectious diseases can also have similar presentations, such as drug reactions, lupus erythematosus, and inflammatory bowel disease. See Table 1.11 for characteristics of the common childhood rashes.

A complete history should include onset of symptoms, duration, and evolution of the rash and fever. History related to the rash includes distribution sequence of the rash, blanching or nonblanching, associated symptoms, recent medications, or exposure to allergens. Recent travel or close contact with others who are ill should be noted. The age of the patient can provide an idea of possible etiologies.

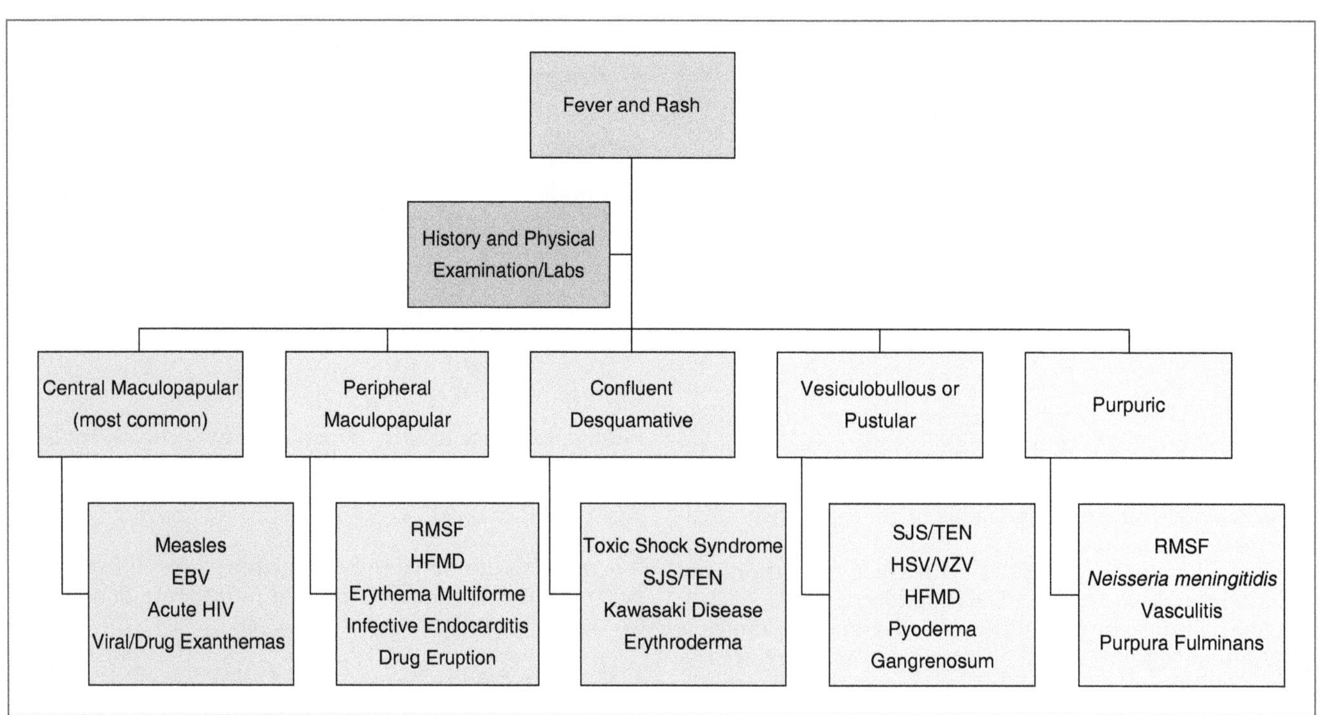

Figure 1.17 Evaluation algorithm for fever and rash. EBV, Epstein-Barr virus; HFMD, hand-foot-and-mouth disease; HSV, herpes simplex virus; RMSF, Rocky Mountain spotted fever; SJS, Steven-Johnson syndrome; TEN, toxic epidermal necrolysis; VZV, Varicella-zoster virus.

TABLE 1.11 Characteristics of Common Childhood Rashes

Disease	Location	Description
Atopic dermatitis	Young children: extensor surface, chest, scalp Older children: flexor surfaces	Erythematous plaques, itching, scaling, dry skin
Erythema infectiosum	Face and thighs	Red "slapped cheek" then pink papules and macules in lacy pattern
Impetigo	Face and extremities	Vesicles or pustules with thick, yellow crust
Molluscum contagiosum	Anywhere, oral mucosa rare	Flesh-colored, small papules with central umbilication
Pityriasis rosea	Trunk, bilateral and symmetric	Herald patch, followed by rose-colored patches with scale in Christmas tree pattern
Roseola	Trunk, peripheral spread	Macular to maculopapular
Scarlet fever	Upper trunk, spares palms and soles	Red, blanching, macules, sandpaper-like
Tinea infection	Anywhere	Red annular patch or plaque with raised border and central clearing

Physical examination is key to the evaluation of the rash. It is important to note the morphology of the rash, if the rash is petechial or palpable purpura; associated clinical features; relationship of the rash with onset of the fever; and presence of prodrome respiratory symptoms.

KNOWLEDGE CHECKS

1. Skin infections due to bacteria, viruses, and fungi are common. Compare and contrast the various causes of skin infections, grouped according to whether they are bacterial, viral, or fungal.
2. The viral exanthems are common in children and may present with similar rashes. Develop a focused approach based on an understanding of the etiologies, pathophysiology, and presentation of the various exanthems.
3. Acne is common disorder in the adolescent patient. Describe the various presentations of acne including treatment options.
4. Compare and contrast the different types of skin cancer.
5. There are three major desquamation disorders. Create a table outlining the presentation, etiologies, and treatment.
6. Dermatitis is very common in primary care. Create a table outlining the various types of dermatitis including presentation and treatment.

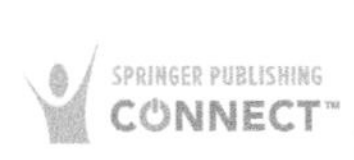

A robust set of instructor resources designed to supplement this text is located at **http://connect.springerpub.com/content/book/978-0-8261-8243-2.** Qualifying instructors may request access by emailing **textbook@springerpub.com.**

REFERENCES

The complete reference list for this chapter appears in the digital version of the chapter, accessible at https://connect.springerpub.com/content/book/978-0-8261-8243-2/chapter/ch01.

CHAPTER 2

OCULAR SYSTEM

TAYLOR L. FISCHER, RYAN C. CHANEY, BLAKELY A. GARRITY, LINDSAY LYON, AND DIANA M. SUKUP

LEARNING OBJECTIVES

- Recognize ocular emergencies and urgencies. Integrate clinical findings to appropriately determine initial management and when to refer to a higher medical specialty.
- Establish a plan for the evaluation and differential diagnosis of the "red eye."
- Identify infectious conditions involving the lid, lacrimal apparatus, conjunctiva, and cornea. Establish a plan to diagnose and treat each of these conditions.
- Identify the ocular signs and symptoms of various systemic diseases.
- Describe the physical findings of diabetic retinopathy and hypertensive retinopathy.
- Establish a plan for the diagnosis and initial management of vascular injuries to the eye: central and branch retinal artery occlusions and retinal vein occlusions.
- Differentiate the presentation and management of orbital cellulitis and preseptal cellulitis.
- Compare and contrast cataracts, macular degeneration, and glaucoma with regard to epidemiology, pathophysiology, presentation, and management.

INTRODUCTION

Disorders of the eye are a common occurrence across the spectrum of care settings. They can range from benign conditions like conjunctivitis to vision threating conditions like angle closure glaucoma. Onset of eye disease can also occur across the life span, from pediatrics to geriatrics. The ability to take in and process visual stimuli is critical to daily life. As such, knowledge of the normal ocular system and the ability to appropriately evaluate patients with eye complaints is essential.

This chapter presents the common eye disorders. Their pathologies, clinical presentations, diagnoses, and management strategies will be addressed.

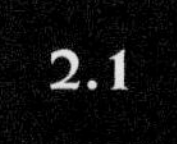

2.1 DISORDERS OF THE LIDS/ LACRIMAL APPARATUS

OVERVIEW

Disorders of the lid and lacrimal apparatus represent a heterogeneous set of disorders that affect the supporting structures of the eye and eye surface. Generally, complaints are benign but can represent significant irritation to the patient, prompting presentation to the medical clinic. Clinicians must understand the dynamics of lid and lacrimal anatomy and function to properly manage and reassure patients.

EPIDEMIOLOGY

Disorders of the lid and lashes occur across the spectrum of ages and may or may not be related to other underlying disorders, such as eczema or infection. Some diagnoses are specific to certain populations. For example, issues arising from the lacrimal gland such as dacrocystitis are more common in infants. Congenital dysfunction of the nasolacrimal duct may be seen in approximately 20% of newborns, resolving spontaneously by age 6 months.[1] Others are not age specific, as blepharitis and hordeola, for example, are seen across age groups.

PATHOPHYSIOLOGY

The purpose of the lacrimal apparatus is to produce tears for lubrication of the eye and debris removal. Tears are produced in the lacrimal gland located above and lateral to the globe (Figure 2.1). They flow down and medial across the eye into the puncta where they then move through the lacrimal canals into the lacrimal sac, ultimately being deposited into the nose by way of the nasolacrimal duct.

The lids and eyelashes play similar roles in relation to protection of the eye and surface lubrication. A detailed diagram of lid anatomy can be seen in Figure 2.2. Note the meibomian glands, which secrete oil that mixes with tears to increase moisture spread across the eye surface.

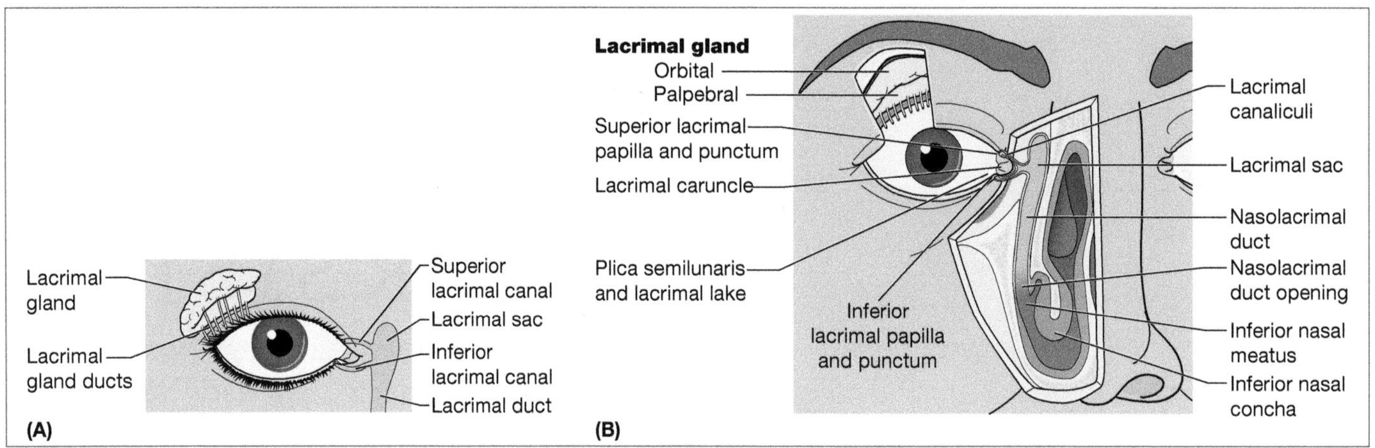

Figure 2.1 The lacrimal apparatus of the eye. (A) External anatomy and anterior view of the lacrimal apparatus of the eye. (B) External anatomy and dissection of the lacrimal apparatus of the eye.

(Source: Guida KM. Advanced health assessment of the eyes and ears. In: Myrick KM, Karosas LM, eds. Advanced Health Assessment and Differential Diagnosis. *Springer Publishing Company; 2021:58, Fig. 4.2.)*

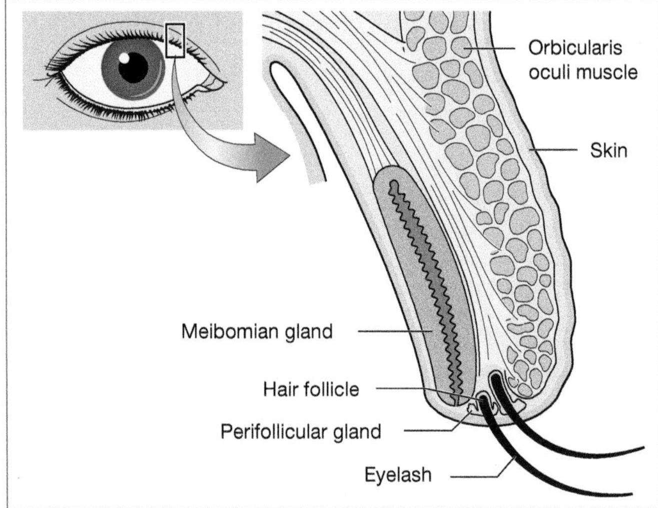

Figure 2.2 Glands associated with the palpebrae.

(Source: Guida KM. Advanced health assessment of the eyes and ears. In: Myrick KM, Karosas LM, eds. Advanced Health Assessment and Differential Diagnosis. *Springer Publishing Company; 2021:58, Fig. 4.3.)*

2.1A BLEPHARITIS

Blepharitis is characterized by inflammation of the eyelid margins. There are two subtypes based on anatomic location, anterior and posterior, or by duration of symptoms, acute or chronic. Blepharitis can be caused by bacteria, *Staphylococcus* species, or by dysfunction of the meibomian gland.

MEDICAL HISTORY AND CLINICAL PRESENTATION

Blepharitis involves inflammation of the lid margin. This may be the result of irritation from environmental factors such as cigarette smoke or associated skin conditions, for example, rosacea or psoriasis. Posterior blepharitis leads to disruption of the normal function of the meibomian glands. Anterior blepharitis often results from bacterial overgrowth and chronic infection. There is some evidence that infestation with the parasite *Demodex folliculorum* plays a role.[2]

SIGNS AND SYMPTOMS

The resultant symptom profile is very similar between anterior and posterior blepharitis, making the exact diagnosis irrelevant to the initial treating clinician.

Patients generally present with ongoing eye irritation, lid scaling, dry eyes, and itching. Symptoms and signs are usually bilateral in nature.

PHYSICAL EXAMINATION

Lid scaling and erythema should be present on examination. There may also be evidence of excoriation due to itching.

DIFFERENTIAL DIAGNOSIS

The diagnosis is made clinically by identification of classic history and the appearance of erythematous lids with an apparent crust visible on inspection. The differential diagnosis includes conjunctivitis, hordeolum, and chalazion.

DIAGNOSTIC STUDIES

There are no laboratory findings. Diagnosis is made based on clinical features.

EVALUATION

The different types of blepharitis and symptoms vary as noted below:

- Staphylococcal blepharitis presents with mildly sticking eyelids, thickened lid margins, and missing and misdirected eyelashes.
- Seborrheic blepharitis presents with greasy flakes or scales around the base of eyelashes and a mild redness of the eyelids.
- Ulcerative blepharitis presents with matted, hard crusts around the eyelashes, eyelash loss, and chronic tearing. Removal the crusts leaves sores that ooze and bleed.
- Meibomian blepharitis presents with blockage of the oil glands in the eyelids, poor quality of tears, and redness of the lining of the eyelids.

TREATMENT

- Management involves education on lid hygiene to include washing the lids with warm water and a mild, nonstinging shampoo.

- Application of warm compresses and lid massage can prevent backup of meibomian gland secretions.
- Artificial tears can help reduce the sensation of dryness.
- In refractory cases, topical antibiotics such as erythromycin ointment may help lubricate the eyelid and resolve concurrent bacterial infection.
- Patients should be referred when symptoms fail to respond to topical antibiotics or if symptoms suggest an alternative problem, such as vision loss, photosensitivity, or pain with eye movement.
- Treat underlying conditions and manage modifiable risk factors.

PATIENT EDUCATION

- Patients should be assured of the benign but frustrating nature of blepharitis along with the importance of adhering to hygiene advice.
- Preventive strategies include lid hygiene and antidandruff shampoo.

2.1B HORDEOLUM

A hordeolum, or sty, is a painful infection of the sebaceous gland at the base of the eyelid, or inside under the eyelid. The usual cause is *Staphylococcus aureus* and it can be triggered by stress, poor nutrition, or lack of sleep. It may also develop secondary to blepharitis.

MEDICAL HISTORY AND CLINICAL PRESENTATION

Hordeolum is a benign lesion of the eyelid, an abscess on either the upper or lower lid. Clinically, it may be confused with a chalazion, which is a lid nodule that is more chronic in its nature yet appears similar to hordeolum. Hordeola are described as either external, on the lid margin, or internal, just below the lid margin based on the involvement with either the meibomian glands (internal) or hair follicles (external). Clinical delineation is not necessary. Patients suffering from other dermatologic conditions such as rosacea or blepharitis may be more prone to development of hordeola.[3]

SIGNS AND SYMPTOMS

Patients will usually present with a painful, tender, erythematous bump on the lid that has arisen and progressively worsened over a few days (Figure 2.3). They may complain of pain with blinking, watering of eye, and light sensitivity.

PHYSICAL EXAMINATION

The physical examination will reveal a localized, tender area with a pointing eruption in the affected area. The lesion may appear yellow.

DIFFERENTIAL DIAGNOSIS

The differential diagnosis includes chalazion, xanthelasma, papilloma, and cyst.

DIAGNOSTIC STUDIES

Although cultures are not routinely indicated or performed, *Staphylococcus aureus* is the most likely causative pathogen and may be cultured.

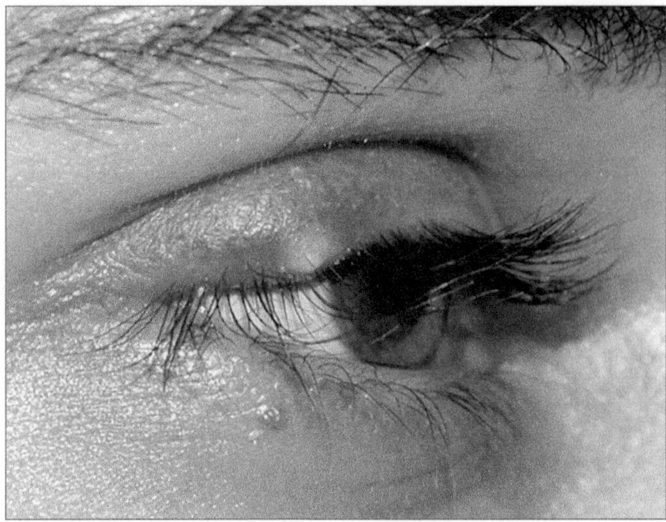

Figure 2.3 **Hordeolum.**
(Source: Guida KM. Advanced health assessment of the eyes and ears. In: Myrick KM, Karosas LM, eds. Advanced Health Assessment and Differential Diagnosis. *Springer Publishing Company; 2021:79, Fig. 4.30.)*

EVALUATION

Evaluation is based on clinical findings.

TREATMENT

- Hordeola are generally self-resolving and patients should be instructed to apply a warm compress multiple times per day to facilitate draining and pain relief.
  Draining of a hordeolum can be done if it is superficial or presents with an obvious "head."
  - This can be accomplished by simple eversion of the lid followed by pressure applied to the base by a sterile, cotton-tipped applicator.
  - If unsuccessful, needle drainage with an 18G needle may also be accomplished.
- Incision and drainage is not recommended and should be performed by an opthalmologist. Lesions that are large or fail to resolve in 1–2 weeks should be referred accordingly.

PATIENT EDUCATION

- Patients should be advised against attempting to "lance" lesions themselves given the proximity to the eye.
- If there is no improvement, patients should return in 2 weeks to facilitate a specialist referral.

2.1C CHALAZION

Chalazion is a cyst in the eyelid caused by inflammation of a blocked meibomian gland, typically on the upper eyelid. The lesions are typically painless and will disappear on their own in a few months.

MEDICAL HISTORY AND CLINICAL PRESENTATION

Chalazion is very similar in size, shape, and appearance to hordeolum. Chalazia, however, are noninflammatory, and therefore lack inflammatory signs and symptoms such as erythema, pain, and tenderness. In some cases, they may result from the resolution of acute hordeola or they may present independently by obstruction of the meibomian or Zeis glands.

SIGNS AND SYMPTOMS

Signs and symptoms include eyelid swelling and tenderness, light sensitivity, and excessive tearing. A large chalazion may present with astigmatism due to pressure on the cornea.

PHYSICAL EXAMINATION

The physical examination reveals a nonerythematous, nontender nodule without any purulence.

DIFFERENTIAL DIAGNOSIS

The differential diagnosis includes hordeolum and cysts.

DIAGNOSTIC STUDIES

Diagnosis is made based on history and physical examination. No diagnostic studies are needed.

TREATMENT

- Chalazia may be self-resolving; warm compresses may soften the hardened oils and promote drainage and healing.
- In cases of large or cosmetically displeasing lesions, referral to an ophthalmologist is appropriate for discussion of incision and drainage or glucocorticoid injection.

PATIENT EDUCATION

- As with hordeola, patients should be cautioned against lancing lesions themselves given the proximity to the eye.

2.1D DACRYOCYSTITIS

Dacryocystitis is the inflammation of the lacrimal sac. It is commonly due to a bacterial infection that leads to obstruction of the nasolacrimal duct and sac and is common in neonates and females over the age of 40. It is classified as acute, subacute, or chronic. Congenital obstruction occurs most often in term infants and is due to blockage by epithelial debris or incomplete canalization. Acquired obstruction is primary with idiopathic inflammatory stenosis or secondary due to trauma, infection, inflammation, tumor, or mechanical obstruction.

MEDICAL HISTORY AND CLINICAL PRESENTATION

Refer to the Overview (Section 2.1) for information on the anatomy and function of the lacrimal apparatus. When the nasolacrimal duct is obstructed, which can happen congenitally, tears are prevented from draining into the nose, thus causing stagnation in the lacrimal sac and nasolacrimal duct. Complications include the development of a cystic mass in the nasolacrimal duct (dacrocystocele) and infection (acute dacrocystitis). The most common pathogens responsible for dacrocystitis are alpha-hemolytic streptococci, *Staphylococcus epidermidis,* and *Staphylococcus aureus.*[4] Dacrocystocele appears as a blue-tinted swelling adjacent to the bridge of the nose.

SIGNS AND SYMPTOMS

More often seen in infants and toddlers, signs of acute dacrocystitis include erythema, swelling, and tenderness over the nasolacrimal duct. This may be accompanied by purulent drainage from the medial canthus of the eye, fever, and other signs of infection, such as increased agitation, fussiness, and poor feeding. Traumatic disruption of the nasolacrimal apparatus may be a cause for presentation in older populations including adolescents and adults. In adults there may be pain, erythema, swelling, and excessive watering of the eye.

PHYSICAL EXAMINATION

The physical examination reveals signs of infection in the eye and around the nose where the nasolacrimal apparatus is located. Excessive tearing and swelling may be noted. Signs of systemic infection like fever and altered mental status should concern clinicians for sepsis, orbital cellulitis, or meningitis. If the infection spreads posteriorly to the orbital septum orbital cellulitis may develop.

DIFFERENTIAL DIAGNOSIS

The initial diagnosis should be made based on the history and physical examination noted above. The differential diagnosis includes dacrocystocele, erysipelas, and periorbital cellulitis.

DIAGNOSTIC STUDIES

The diagnosis of dacryocystitis is clinical; laboratory studies are not needed. Orbital CT scan may be needed to rule out orbital cellulitis. Blood cultures and cultures of nasolacrimal drainage should be obtained to guide definitive management.

TREATMENT

- Medical treatment consists of warm compresses and pain medication. Empiric antibiotics such as ampicillin-sulbactam or cephalosporins may be needed.
- Suspicion of dacrocystitis should prompt referral to an ophthalmologist and possible hospital admission if signs and symptoms of systemic infection are present.
- Accompanying orbital cellulitis or meningitis must be ruled out.
- Surgical probing of the nasolacrimal duct is first-line therapy and is accompanied by empiric antibiotic therapy either in the hospital or on an outpatient basis.
  - Antibiotics of choice include clindamycin and vancomycin.

PATIENT EDUCATION

- Patients should be instructed on the need for prompt referral and management by a specialist for disorders of the eye lid and lacrimal system. It is reasonable to inform parents that treatment will involve antibiotics and a procedure to open the tear duct.

KEY POINTS

- Common symptoms of blepharitis include itching and burning of the eyelid margins and conjunctival irritation with lacrimation, photosensitivity, and foreign body sensation.
- Supportive treatments for blepharitis include warm compresses and eyelid cleansing as needed.

- Hordeola cause redness and edema of the eyelid, swelling, and pain.
- Treatment of a hordeolum consists of hot compresses and possibly incision and drainage.
- Chalazion causes eyelid hyperemia and swelling.
- Treatment of a chalazion consists of hot compresses and possibly intralesional corticosteroids.

2.2 CONJUNCTIVITIS

OVERVIEW

Conjunctivitis, or inflammation of the conjunctiva, is one of the most common acute complaints seen in primary care. It also represents one of the major causes of "red eye," as will be discussed at the end of this chapter. Conjunctivitis is almost always benign and either self-resolving or easily treatable on an outpatient basis.

EPIDEMIOLOGY

Conjunctivitis is seen across the life span. Infective conjunctivitis is easily spread by direct contact with eye secretions and contact with contaminated surfaces. As such, the diagnosis is commonly made in children and can present public health concerns in the school or daycare environment.

PATHOPHYSIOLOGY

The anatomic structure of the conjunctiva is broken into two thin layers: an epithelial layer and a substantia propria, which contains vasculature. The conjunctiva covers the inside of both lids and the anterior aspect of the globe up to the limbus. These are known as the palpebral and bulbar conjunctivae, respectively. The conjunctiva acts to protect and lubricate the eye and inner surfaces of the lid. Compromise of this structure either by trauma or infection can cause significant discomfort, leading patients to seek care.

Conjunctivitis is divided into four categories based on origin: bacterial infection, viral infection, noninfectious allergic, and nonallergic/chemical. Infection, either bacterial or viral, makes up the vast majority of cases.[5] The common finding of "pink eye," or engorgement of the vessels in the substantia propria, can make the diagnosis and treatment confusing to both the clinician and the patient.

See Table 2.1 for the features that differentiate the several types of acute conjunctivitis.

TABLE 2.1 Differentiating Signs and Symptoms of Acute Conjunctivitis

Type	Discharge	Eyelid Edema	Lymph Node Involvement	Itching
Bacterial	Purulent	Moderate	Typically none	None
Viral	Clear, watery	Minimal	Typically present	None
Allergic	Clear, mucoid	Severe to moderate	None	Moderate to severe

2.2A VIRAL CONJUNCTIVITIS

MEDICAL HISTORY AND CLINICAL PRESENTATION

Viral conjunctivitis is more common than bacterial.[5] Adenovirus is responsible for the majority of viral conjunctivitis cases.[6] Point of care testing for adenovirus is commercially available but is unnecessary in patients with a classic history and physical examination.

SIGNS AND SYMPTOMS

In addition to conjunctival injection, patients may have other signs and symptoms of adenovirus infection such as rhinorrhea, sore throat, and low-grade fever. Redness may be in one or both eyes, especially after the first 24 hours. Patients also note the presence of lid crusting in the morning and a thin, mucoid or watery discharge. Blinking may cause a stinging or gritty sensation.

PHYSICAL EXAMINATION

Physical examination reveals conjunctival hyperemia, watery discharge, and ocular irritation. Preauricular lymphadenopathy may be present. Photophobia may also be present.

DIFFERENTIAL DIAGNOSIS

The differential diagnosis includes other forms of conjunctivitis (e.g., bacterial and allergic). As noted above, the diagnosis is clinical and confirmed by the absence of red flags (see Box 2.1) that may be indicative of more serious pathology causing the red eye.

DIAGNOSTIC STUDIES

Diagnostic studies are not required to make the diagnosis of viral conjunctivitis. Cultures may be needed to identify bacterial etiologies, such as chlamydia or gonococci, as they are part of the differential diagnosis and can lead to complications.

A rapid antigen test is available for the diagnosis of viral conjunctivitis, but typically it is not needed as the condition is self-limiting.

EVALUATION

Evaluation should focus on the various causes of conjunctivitis. The type of eye discharge is the first step. A purulent

BOX 2.1 Red Flag Signs and Symptoms

- Pain with or limitation of extraocular movements
- Foreign body sensation
- History of ocular injury
- Change in vision
- Photophobia
- Severe headache or neurologic deficits
- Alteration in pupillary response to light

discharge suggests a bacterial infection. A watery discharge suggests viral or allergic conjunctivitis. The next step is to determine if itching is present. The presence of itching of the eye suggests allergic conjunctivitis. The lack of itching suggests dry eye disease or viral conjunctivitis.

TREATMENT

- Treatment is supportive.
- Warm compresses can provide soothing pain relief.
- Topical antihistamines may be used to reduce redness and irritation.
- Patients should be instructed to maintain good hygiene practices including frequent hand washing and avoidance of sharing towels, bedding, cups, and eating utensils.

PATIENT EDUCATION

- Patients remain contagious for approximately 1 week, and symptoms may persist for 2 to 3 weeks.
- Patient education on the etiology and expected course is critical, as is accurate characterization of discharge as mucus rather than "pus."

2.2B BACTERIAL CONJUNCTIVITIS

MEDICAL HISTORY AND CLINICAL PRESENTATION

The presentation of bacterial conjunctivitis parallels viral conjunctivitis in many respects. The usual upper respiratory pathogens are responsible for most cases: *Staphylococcus aureus, Streptococcus pneumoniae, Haemophilus influenzae,* and *Moraxella catarrhalis.*[7]

SIGNS AND SYMPTOMS

Patients will complain of the presence of pink eye or eyes (Figure 2.4). Symptoms typically are unilateral but spread to the other eye in a few days.

PHYSICAL EXAMINATION

Discharge is purulent. The conjunctiva is hyperemic and edematous. Lid crusting and pain with blinking are also common in bacterial infections. There is no preauricular lymphadenopathy.

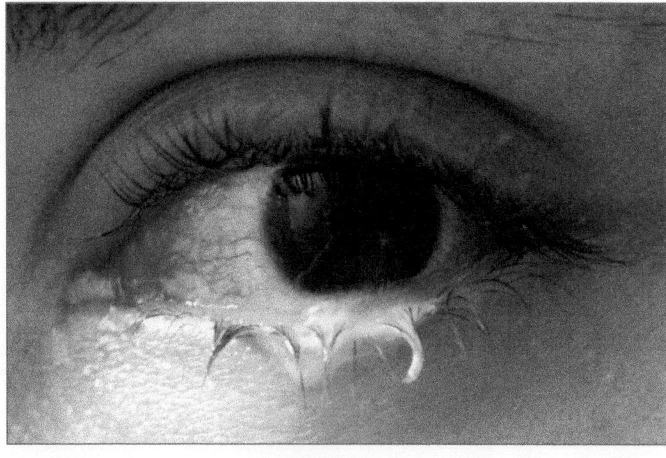

Figure 2.4 Bacterial conjunctivitis.
(Source: Image courtesy of Tanalai.)

DIFFERENTIAL DIAGNOSIS

The differential diagnosis includes other forms of conjunctivitis (e.g., bacterial and allergic). The absence of red flags (Box 2.1) must be assured; otherwise the diagnosis is clinical. Cultures are unnecessary.

DIAGNOSTIC STUDIES

Diagnostic studies are typically not required to make the diagnosis of bacterial conjunctivitis. Cultures can be used to identify bacterial agents.

EVALUATION

Evaluation should focus on the various causes of conjunctivitis. The type of eye discharge is the first step. A purulent discharge suggests a bacterial infection. A watery discharge suggests viral or allergic conjunctivitis. The next step is to determine if itching is present. The presence of itching of the eye suggests allergic conjunctivitis. The lack of itching suggests dry eye disease or viral conjunctivitis.

TREATMENT

- Empiric treatment involves topical antibiotic preparations such as erythromycin and tobramycin. Ointment is preferred in pediatric populations while drops are sufficient for older children, adolescents, and adults.

PATIENT EDUCATION

- Patients should be instructed on the importance of completing the full antibiotic regimen and of not sharing drops within the household because containers may become vectors for the spread of infection.
- To avoid transmission patients should wash hands frequently or use hand sanitizer, avoid touching the infected eye, and avoid sharing towels or pillows.
- Improvement should be noticed in a few days. Any worsening, including increased pain, photophobia, or pain with eye movement, should cause prompt follow-up.

2.2C ALLERGIC CONJUNCTIVITIS

MEDICAL HISTORY AND CLINICAL PRESENTATION

Allergic conjunctivitis results from a type I hypersensitivity reaction to common allergens such as dust mites or cat dander. Contact between the conjunctiva and these substances leads to the release of histamine, eosinophils, and other immune mediators. There are three types of allergic conjunctivitis:

- **Seasonal:** Also called hay fever conjunctivitis, this type is caused by airborne spores or pollen. It peaks in spring and late summer and disappears during the winter months.
- **Perennial:** Also called atopic conjunctivitis, this is caused by dust mites and animal dander. Symptoms tend to occur year-round.
- **Vernal keratoconjunctivitis:** This severe disease is most common in young males with a history of eczema, asthma, or seasonal allergies. It typically appears every spring and subsides in the fall. Children outgrow the condition in early adulthood.

SIGNS AND SYMPTOMS

Patients typically present with bilateral eye redness, watery discharge, and marked itching. Patients may also have a history of seasonal allergies or known environmental allergy. Itching is the primary differentiator from viral conjunctivitis as the two problems are otherwise very similar. Patients may have other symptoms of allergies including rhinorrhea and sneezing.

PHYSICAL EXAMINATION

The physical examination is consistent with the history, with injection and scant, mucoid discharge.

DIFFERENTIAL DIAGNOSIS

The differential diagnosis includes other forms of conjunctivitis (e.g., bacterial and viral). The diagnosis is clinical, and clinicians should document the absence of red flags (Box 2.1) and purulent discharge.

TREATMENT

- Although the process is self-limited, symptomatic therapy with antihistamine or mast cell stabilizing eye drops can provide relief.

PATIENT EDUCATION

- Patients should be instructed on the likely etiology.
- Patients suffering from concomitant allergic rhinitis must be made aware that oral antihistamines will not be as effective for symptoms as topical agents.

2.2D CHEMICAL CONJUNCTIVITIS

MEDICAL HISTORY AND CLINICAL PRESENTATION

Chemical conjunctivitis, also known as toxic conjunctivitis or toxic keratoconjunctivitis, is a less commonly seen form of conjunctivitis that results from exposure to topical ocular medications, particularly those that contain preservatives. Topical antibiotic preparations, glaucoma medications, and contact lens solutions have all been implicated.

SIGNS AND SYMPTOMS

Patients will present with eye redness, discharge, burning, and/or itching.

PHYSICAL EXAMINATION

The eyes will appear as described above, with chemosis and lid swelling. These findings may be accompanied by punctate epithelial defects or large corneal ulcers seen with fluorescein staining.

DIFFERENTIAL DIAGNOSIS

The differential diagnosis includes other forms of conjunctivitis (e.g., infectious and allergic). The diagnosis is clinical and made evident by a history of exposure to a likely causative agent.

DIAGNOSTIC STUDIES

The diagnosis is made by history and physical examination findings. No laboratory testing is needed.

TREATMENT

- Treatment involves removal of the offending agent, which makes identification of prior eye medications an imperative part of the patient history.
- Cool compresses, preservative-free rewetting drops, and topical steroids are all helpful in management.
- Suspicion of chemical keratoconjunctivitis should prompt referral to ophthalmology.

PATIENT EDUCATION

- Referral for keratoconjunctivitis should be made as soon as possible, and patients should be advised not to delay treatment or attempt management at home with over-the-counter topical agents prior to discussion with a specialist.

SPECIAL CONSIDERATIONS

- Commonly, schools and daycare centers treat all conjunctivitis cases as bacterial, requiring 24 hours of topical antibiotic treatment before returning to school or work. The decision to treat should only be made after thorough patient education. Inexpensive preparations, such as erythromycin or tobramycin ointment, with low penetration and acidity are well suited for treatment.
- Gonococcal conjunctivitis must be identified as a sight-threatening process. Most instances present with significant redness, chemosis, lid swelling, and eye tenderness. The volume of purulent discharge is significant and often patients will have concurrent urethritis or vaginitis. Suspicion of infection with *Neisseria gonorrhoeae* should prompt immediate referral to an ophthalmologist for inpatient intravenous (IV; ceftriaxone) and oral antibiotics (azithromycin). Topical antibiotics, bacitracin or gentamicin ointments, can be used in addition to systemic treatment.
- Contact lens wearers should be treated with topical fluoroquinolones to cover for infections with *Pseudomonas aeruginosa.* Clinicians should maintain a high degree of suspicion for keratitis and a threshold for performing a fluorescein stain. Ulcerations or corneal infiltrates should prompt referral to an ophthalmologist. Contact lenses should be left out of the eyes until symptoms resolve, and disposable lenses should be discarded in favor of a fresh pair.
- Neonatal conjunctivitis is due to maternal gonococcal or chlamydial infection. Infected is spread via the birth canal. Prevention is by treatment with silver nitrate eye drops or erythromycin ointment at birth.

KEY POINTS

- Conjunctivitis typically results from infection, allergy, or irritation.
- Infectious conjunctivitis is usually highly contagious.
- Typical findings are redness and various types of discharge, without pain or vision loss.
- Treatment includes measures to prevent spread and treatment of the cause, including antibiotics for bacterial infections.

2.3 CORNEAL DISORDERS

OVERVIEW

Unlike conjunctival diseases, disorders of the cornea are often vision-threatening and a cause for many referrals to an

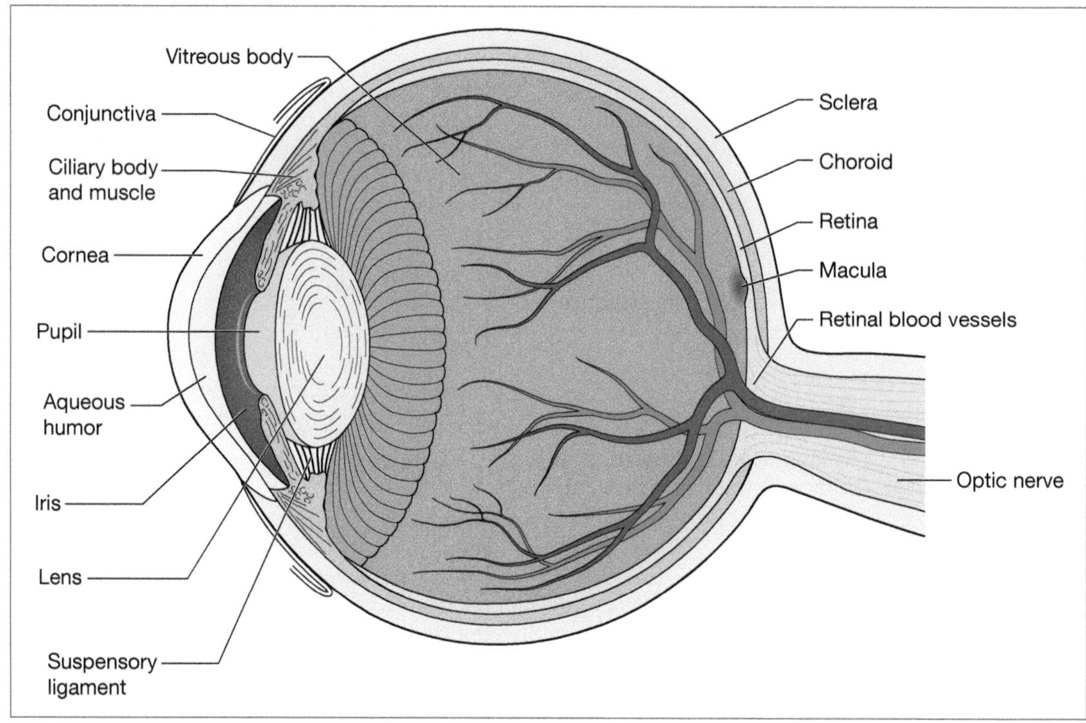

Figure 2.5 Internal eye structures.
(Source: Guida KM. Advanced health assessment of the eyes and ears. In: Myrick KM, Karosas LM, eds. Advanced Health Assessment and Differential Diagnosis. *Springer Publishing Company; 2021:60, Fig. 4.5.)*

ophthalmologist. The primary role of the PA in corneal disease is proper identification followed by coordination with eye specialists to prevent further destruction and scarring of the cornea. Corneal involvement is suggested by unilateral involvement, foreign body sensation, pain, photophobia, and decreased visual acuity.

EPIDEMIOLOGY

Epidemiologic data regarding corneal disorders is lacking. Contact lens wearing is more common in adults; this suggests that corneal disorders such as ulceration and keratitis are more common in adults. Mild traumatic abrasions are seen in the clinic across the patient life span.

PATHOPHYSIOLOGY

The cornea is a translucent, collagen fiber matrix that sits on the anterior surface of the eye flush with the sclera (Figure 2.5). It allows light into the pupil, focusing it onto the lens. There are five layers of corneal tissue, the outermost of which is the epithelium. This is followed by Bowman's layer, the stroma, Descemet's membrane, and the endothelium. The epithelium obtains nutrients and oxygen from tears as the cornea is avascular. The cornea is also heavily innervated, making pain a primary characteristic to many corneal processes.

2.3A CORNEAL ABRASION

MEDICAL HISTORY AND CLINICAL PRESENTATION

Corneal abrasions are common self-limited, superficial epithelial defects that are noted across the patient life span. Infants can cause abrasions by scratching their own eyes. Adults may develop abrasions spontaneously from improper contact lens wear or traumatically from work-related injuries.

SIGNS AND SYMPTOMS

Disruption of the corneal epithelium can be very painful, and patients will often be reluctant to open the affected eye. They may have a significantly more irritated eye following repeated rubbing, washing, or attempts to remove a suspected foreign body.

Clinicians should confirm specific trauma, if possible, to identify the risk of penetrating injury. The shape of the globe, reactivity of the pupil, and absence of other red flag signs and symptoms (Box 2.1) should be documented.

PHYSICAL EXAMINATION

The physical examination should include eversion of the lids to look for retained foreign bodies, especially if this is suggested by the history. Fluorescein staining should also be performed to evaluate the size, shape, and location of the abrasion. Seidel's sign, the appearance of aqueous humor "waterfalling" from a corneal puncture, should be noted and is an indication of penetrating eye trauma.

Of note, topical anesthetic agents may be used to assist with discomfort from the physical examination (Exhibit 2.1). Preparations including proparacaine and tetracaine are readily available and rapidly improve pain prior to eye manipulation.

DIFFERENTIAL DIAGNOSIS

The differential diagnosis includes penetrating injury, corneal ulcer, infection, and retained foreign body. Foreign body sensation and injury history should be expected, but otherwise red flags (Box 2.1) should be ruled out.

EXHIBIT 2.1 Topical Anesthetic Animal Study

An animal study completed in 1994 comparing the use of topical proparacaine, topical saline, and topical morphine sulfate showed that repeated use of topical anesthetics delayed wound healing and increased likelihood of scarring. Some clinicians are reluctant to use these agents as a result, but the data from this study were limited: four of six rabbits showed incomplete corneal healing after 8 days.[6] Furthermore, no human studies have been performed to back up the results. Conservative use of anesthetic drops in clinic to facilitate proper evaluation is unlikely to cause harm.

DIAGNOSTIC STUDIES

A slit-lamp examination should be done to evaluate for abrasions and detection of Seidel's sign. The patient with intraocular injury or globe rupture should have a CT scan done to evaluate for intraocular foreign body. An MRI should not be obtained if a metallic foreign body is suspected due the metal moving and causing more damage.

EVALUATION

After an anesthetic is instilled, each lid should be everted, and the entire conjunctiva and cornea are inspected with a binocular lens or a slit lamp. Fluorescein staining should be done to identify any corneal abrasions. Patients with multiple vertical linear abrasions should have their eyelids everted to search for a foreign body under the upper lid. Patients with possible intraocular injury or globe perforation should undergo CT to rule out intraocular foreign body.

TREATMENT

- Most abrasions are healed within 24 hours due to the rapid growth rate of corneal epithelium and patients can be treated expectantly with warm compresses and over-the-counter analgesics.
- An antibiotic ointment (bacitracin/polymyxin B or ciprofloxacin) should be given for 3–5 days while the abrasion heals. Contact lens wearers require treatment with ciprofloxacin to prevent infection with *Pseudomonas*. Patching the eye is not indicated and unhelpful in most cases.
- The presence of corneal infiltrates, purulent eye drainage, or lack of healing after 72 hours should prompt referral to an ophthalmologist.
- Large, central abrasions may be referred as well to evaluate for risk of scarring.

PATIENT EDUCATION

- Patients should be advised not to utilize over-the-counter patches and that repeated flushing at home may exacerbate symptoms.

2.3B CORNEAL ULCER

A corneal ulcer is a corneal epithelial defect with underlying inflammation usually due to invasion by bacteria, fungi, viruses, or *Acanthamoeba*. Corneal ulcer may be due to mechanical trauma or nutritional deficiencies. Symptoms include conjunctival redness, foreign body sensation, photophobia, and lacrimation. Diagnosis is by slit-lamp examination, fluorescein staining, and culture. Treatment consists of topical antimicrobials and referral to an ophthalmologist.

MEDICAL HISTORY AND CLINICAL PRESENTATION

A corneal ulcer starts as an epithelial defect. Severe ulcers may spread the width of the cornea and penetrate deeply. A layer of white blood cells, a hypopyon, may be noted in the anterior chamber. There are four major etiological categories for corneal ulcers: nontraumatic corneal abnormalities such as with viral keratitis and primary dry eyes; corneal injury secondary to foreign body or contact lenses; eyelid abnormalities secondary to chronic blepharitis and entropion; and nutritional deficiencies secondary to vitamin A deficiency.

SIGNS AND SYMPTOMS

Signs and symptoms include conjunctival redness, eye pain, foreign body sensation, photophobia, and watery eyes. Ulcers due to *Acanthamoeba* are very painful and may show a ring-shaped infiltrate.

PHYSICAL EXAMINATION

Physical examination will reveal conjunctival redness and excessive lacrimation. Fluorescein staining and slit-lamp examination are required to make the diagnosis. A corneal infiltrate with epithelial defect that stains with fluorescein is diagnostic.

DIFFERENTIAL DIAGNOSIS

The differential diagnosis includes penetrating injury, corneal abrasion, infectious keratitis, and retained foreign body.

DIAGNOSTIC STUDIES

All but the small ulcers should be cultured. Microscopic examination of corneal scrapings can identify *Acanthamoeba*.

EVALUATION

After an anesthetic is instilled, the eye should be evaluated for a foreign body. Fluorescein staining should be done to identify any corneal ulcers or evaluate for possible keratitis.

TREATMENT

- For ulcers treatment may include a cycloplegic to decrease the pain of a corneal ulcer and to reduce the formation of posterior synechiae. In severe cases, debridement of the infected epithelium may be required.
- Treatment for corneal ulcers, regardless of cause, begins with moxifloxacin or gatifloxacin for small ulcers and tobramycin and cefazolin for more significant ulcers, particularly those near the center of the cornea. Patching is contraindicated because it creates a stagnant, warm environment that favors bacterial growth and prevents the administration of topical drugs.
- Herpes simplex is treated with trifluridine, ganciclovir, valacyclovir, or acyclovir for about 14 days.
- Fungal infections are treated with topical antifungal drops, such as natamycin, amphotericin B, or voriconazole. Deep infections may require addition of oral voriconazole, ketoconazole, fluconazole, or itraconazole.

- If *Acanthamoeba* is identified, therapy includes topical propamidine, neomycin, and polyhexamethylene biguanide or chlorhexidine supplemented with miconazole, clotrimazole, or oral ketaconazole or itraconazole.

PATIENT EDUCATION

- Contact lens wearers should play close attention to hand washing and maintaining cleanliness of the lens.
- Eye infections should be treated early to prevent the development of ulcers.

2.3C BACTERIAL KERATITIS

Keratitis is a condition in which the cornea is inflamed. There are two types of keratitis. Superficial disease involves the superficial layers of the cornea and after healing this form does not leave a scar. Deep disease involves the deeper layers of the cornea and typically leaves a scar after healing. This scar may impair vision if on or near the visual axis.

MEDICAL HISTORY AND CLINICAL PRESENTATION

Bacterial keratitis is most commonly caused by gram-negative bacteria, notably *Pseudomonas aeruginosa*.[8] Bacterial invasion of the cornea results from a breakdown in the patient's normal immune barrier. Contact lens wearing is the most significant risk for bacterial keratitis (Exhibit 2.2).[9] Poor contact lens hygiene can act as a bacterial vector, and prolonged wear can deprive the corneal surface of oxygen.

SIGNS AND SYMPTOMS

Patients generally present with rapid onset of eye redness, photophobia, and foreign body sensation. Symptoms and signs may extend beyond the corneal surface and include purulent drainage, lid edema and redness, and hypopyon.

PHYSICAL EXAMINATION

Physical examination with fluorescein staining may reveal an infiltrate or opacified area of stain uptake. This is a response from the immune system involving the collection of white blood cells. Infiltrates may be isolated or multiple depending on the variety of keratitis, with larger infiltrates (>1 mm) more common from bacterial causes. *Pseudomonas* infections often involve large, central infiltrates.[8]

EXHIBIT 2.2 Keratitis Versus Corneal Ulcer

Keratitis is a broad term used to describe inflammation of the cornea from various sources, often infectious. Once this process involves a loss of corneal tissue, the more appropriate term is corneal ulcer. This can create some confusion in the literature of two diagnoses that essentially fall along a single pathway, have similar presentations, and involve identical management options for the treating PA.

DIFFERENTIAL DIAGNOSIS

Definitive diagnosis should be made by an eye specialist with the ability to thoroughly evaluate the cornea. Corneal scraping and culture are not always done prior to initial treatment, but this decision should be left to the ophthalmologist. Keratitis can be confused with allergic conjunctivitis.

DIAGNOSTIC STUDIES

Corneal scraping and culture may be needed to make the diagnosis.

TREATMENT

- Keratitis requires urgent management and prompt referrals to an ophthalmologist.
- Treatment involves same-day referral to an ophthalmologist for slit-lamp examination and proper measurement of infiltrate size.
- Topical antibiotics, most commonly fluoroquinolones, are used with or without steroids.
- Left untreated, corneal ulcers may penetrate the anterior chamber or cause significant corneal scarring and vision loss.
- Corneal transplant is an option in extreme cases.

PATIENT EDUCATION

- Patients should not delay evaluation by an eye specialist. They should be counseled on the potential complications of untreated keratitis, including permanent vision loss.

2.3D VIRAL KERATITIS

MEDICAL HISTORY AND CLINICAL PRESENTATION

Viral keratitis most often refers to corneal inflammation due to either herpes simplex virus (HSV) or varicella-zoster virus (VSV). Other viral pathogens, such as adenovirus and measles, may also infect the cornea, but they are less common and typically self-limited.

SIGNS AND SYMPTOMS

HSV infection of the cornea presents similarly to bacterial keratitis with eye redness, photophobia, and foreign body sensation. Bilateral keratitis may present in an immunocompromised patient, but the majority of cases are unilateral. Ophthalmic involvement of HSV infection is rare, with most cases involving a recurrent outbreak from a previous exposure, rather than representing primary infection. The disease may manifest as blepharitis or conjunctivitis.

Varicella-zoster ophthalmicus is a reactivation of the chickenpox virus that attacks the ophthalmic division of the fifth cranial nerve. Signs and symptoms may not directly involve the eye initially. Patients may experience headache, burning pain, or hyperesthesia along the path of the ophthalmic division prior to the development of a rash or any ocular symptoms.

PHYSICAL EXAMINATION

The hallmark of HSV corneal involvement is a lacey, dendritic lesion seen on fluorescein stain (Figure 2.6).

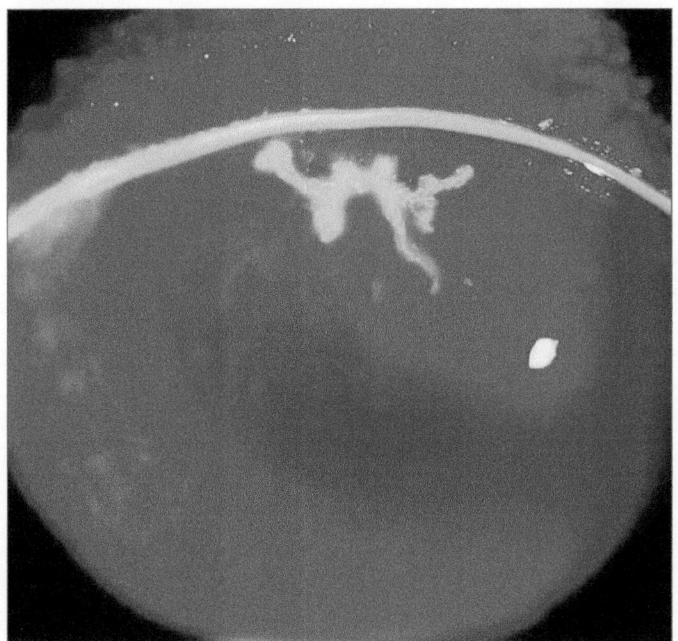

Figure 2.6 **The hallmark of herpes simplex virus corneal involvement is a lacey, dendritic lesion seen on fluorescein stain.**
(Source: Courtesy of Imrankabirhossain)

VSV will typically reveal a vesicular rash unilaterally along the forehead and possibly involve the eyelid. Lesions on the tip of the nose, known as Hutchinson's sign, are predictive of ocular involvement.[10]

DIFFERENTIAL DIAGNOSIS

The differential diagnosis includes other causes of keratitis including bacteria and parasites.

DIAGNOSTIC STUDIES

Fluorescein staining may reveal punctate corneal opacities or even dendrites, which may confuse the diagnosis with HSV infection.

TREATMENT

- This is a vision-threatening condition that requires urgent referral to an ophthalmologist.
- Patients with suspected HSV infection of the eye require ophthalmologic investigation. Treatment involves topical antiviral agents, such as ganciclovir or trifluridine, combined with topical steroids.
- Suppressive therapy may be necessary to reduce the likelihood of corneal scarring and vision loss.
- Patients with VZV ophthalmicus should be treated with oral antivirals, such as acyclovir or valacyclovir, within 72 hours of rash eruption as with other VZV infections.
- Topical steroids can be used adjunctively to reduce corneal inflammation. As such, patients are best treated by an ophthalmologist.

PATIENT EDUCATION

- Patients should be counseled on the need for prompt evaluation by an eye specialist. It may be pertinent to discuss suppressive therapy in patients with HSV keratitis.

SPECIAL CONSIDERATIONS

- Topical corticosteroids are contraindicated in epithelial keratitis but may be effective with an antiviral for stromal keratitis or uveitis.
- All cases of keratitis should be referred to an ophthalmologist.

KEY POINTS

- Symptoms of corneal abrasion or foreign body include foreign body sensation, tearing, and redness; visual acuity is typically unchanged. Diagnosis is usually by slit-lamp examination with fluorescein staining.
- Suspect an intraocular foreign body if fluorescein streams away from a corneal defect, if the pupil is teardrop shaped, or if the mechanism of injury involves a high-speed machine, hammering, or explosion.
- Causes of corneal ulcers include infection of the cornea, overwearing of contact lenses, eye trauma, abnormalities of the eyelid, and nutritional deficiencies.
- Herpes simplex keratitis is due to a recurrence of primary herpes simplex eye infection.
- Characteristic findings of herpes keratitis include a branching dendritic or serpentine corneal lesion, disc-shaped, localized corneal edema and haze plus anterior uveitis, or stromal scarring.
- Treatment of herpes keratitis requires antivirals, usually topical ganciclovir or trifluridine or oral acyclovir or valacyclovir.

2.4 GLAUCOMA

OVERVIEW

Glaucoma is considered a progressive optic neuropathy leading to visual field defects and blindness. Inability to appropriately manage the outflow of aqueous humor from the front of the eye puts pressure on the posterior structures, including the retina. As the pressure tries to escape, it does so at the weakest point, the optic disc, thus damaging the optic nerve leading to blindness.

EPIDEMIOLOGY

Glaucoma is the second leading cause of blindness in the world. The risk of glaucoma increases with age and cases under the age of 55 are exceedingly rare.[11] Glaucoma has also long been associated with systemic diseases like hypertension and diabetes.

PATHOPHYSIOLOGY

Understanding the anatomy of the anterior eye and the normal flow of aqueous humor is paramount to understanding the pathophysiology of glaucoma. Figure 2.7 shows aqueous humor being produced within the ciliary body and secreted into the posterior chamber. Aqueous humor helps maintain normal eye pressure and provides nutrients to the lens and cornea. It travels from the posterior chamber to the anterior chamber by way of the pupil. From there it moves through the trabecular meshwork and Schlemm's canals into the venous drainage of the sclera. Normal intraocular pressure (IOP) is from 8 to 21 mm Hg. As aqueous humor is constantly produced, if production and drainage are not properly balanced, problems ensue.

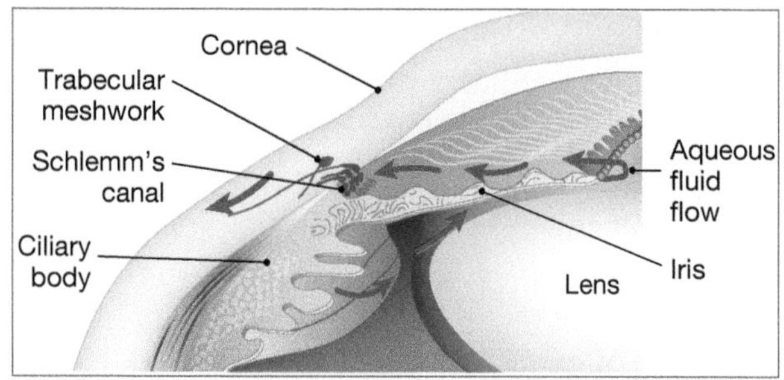

Figure 2.7 **Flow of aqueous humor.**
(Source: Melnyk J, Zeno R, Teall AM. Evidence-based assessment of the eye. In: Gawlik KS, Melnyk BM, Teall AM, eds. Evidence-Based Physical Examination. *Springer Publishing Company; 2021:311, Fig. 12.9.)*

Glaucoma results from improper drainage of humor and can be divided into two categories based on the cause of the blockage and the resultant clinical presentation: angle closure glaucoma and open angle glaucoma.

2.4A ANGLE CLOSURE GLAUCOMA

MEDICAL HISTORY AND CLINICAL PRESENTATION

Angle closure glaucoma occurs when there is contact between the lens and iris, disrupting the normal flow of aqueous humor into the anterior chamber. Primary angle closure glaucoma is the result of an anatomic defect whereby the lens rests too closely to the iris. Over time, this changes the angle at which the iris sits, making the patient susceptible to pupillary blockage. Patients may present with repeated episodes of angle closure, subsequent resolution, and spontaneous resolution of symptoms. Secondary angle closure glaucoma results when the iris is deformed, compressing the angle and trabecular meshwork. This may result from medical conditions such as iritis or a tumor in the posterior eye. It may result from medications, notably topiramate, which cause iritis. Disruption of the lens via surgery or ocular trauma also plays a role.

SIGNS AND SYMPTOMS

Complete disruption of flow causes rapid onset of extreme eye pain and blurry vision. Pain may be so severe that the patient has associated headache, nausea, and vomiting. IOP may be 30 mm Hg or higher. The blurry vision may be accompanied by halos around lights.

PHYSICAL EXAMINATION

Initial physical examination should reveal a red eye with a cloudy cornea with a mid-dilated pupil.

DIFFERENTIAL DIAGNOSIS

The differential diagnosis includes iritis, traumatic hyphema, conjunctivitis, episcleritis, corneal abrasion, and infectious keratitis.

DIAGNOSTIC STUDIES

Tonometry can be performed to measure IOP >18 mm Hg and can be conducted in the clinic using a tanopen. The presentation is striking and although other causes of red eye need to be considered, patients with sudden, excruciating eye pain need immediate referral to the ED.

EVALUATION

Acute closure glaucoma can be distinguished from other disorders by the presence of severe eye pain, headache, nausea and vomiting, dilated pupil, and decreased vision. Secondary angle closure glaucoma should be evaluated by an ophthalmologist.

TREATMENT

- Treatment involves rapid lowering of IOP with IV acetazolamide and topical preparations such as pilocarpine or timolol.
- Ultimately, peripheral iridotomy in both the symptomatic and asymptomatic eyes is performed once IOP is successfully reduced.

PATIENT EDUCATION

Patients with glaucoma should be warned about medications that are contraindicated in patients with glaucoma. These medications include glucocorticoids, systemic sympathomimetics, and systemic anticholinergics.

2.4B OPEN ANGLE GLAUCOMA

MEDICAL HISTORY AND CLINICAL PRESENTATION

Unlike angle closure glaucoma, open angle glaucoma generally presents as a slowly progressive peripheral vision loss. The pathophysiology of open angle glaucoma is not well understood, and as such, the diagnosis is less straightforward than angle closure glaucoma (Figure 2.8). Risk factors include race, as glaucoma is much more common in African

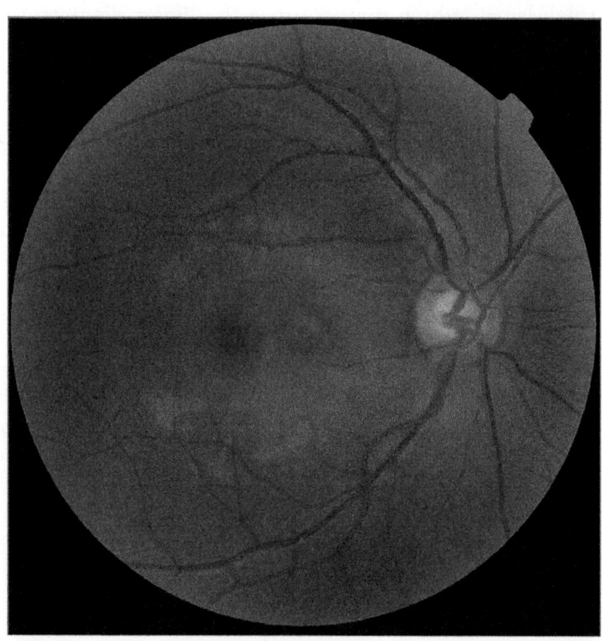

Figure 2.8 **Open angle glaucoma.**
(Source: Ske)

Americans. Family history of glaucoma, hypertension, diabetes, and advancing age are also significant risk factors.

SIGNS AND SYMPTOMS

Early glaucoma is asymptomatic. Vision loss does not always correlate to severity of IOP elevation, nor is asymptomatic IOP a direct predictor of glaucoma development.

PHYSICAL EXAMINATION

Patients rarely present due to symptoms, but clinicians may identify physical exam findings consistent with glaucoma that warrant documentation and referral. Optic disc cupping, or indentation of the optic disc is particularly indicative of glaucoma. A disc-to-cup ratio >50% should alert the clinician of possible glaucoma and the need for subsequent referral.

DIFFERENTIAL DIAGNOSIS

The differential diagnosis includes other forms of glaucoma, myopia, and ocular hypertension.

DIAGNOSTIC STUDIES

Given the potentially devastating effects of untreated glaucoma as well as the known associated risk factors, screening for disease has been investigated. However, there is no gold standard for screening, and the U.S. Preventive Services Task Force does not recommend screening for the general population. The American Academy of Ophthalmology (AAO) recommends a baseline comprehensive eye examination for all individuals at age 40, and resultant examination needs are based on risk factors.[12] Diabetic patients are recommended to have yearly eye exams following diagnosis.

The definitive diagnosis should be reserved for an ophthalmologist, but the diagnostic criteria suggested by the AAO are illustrated in Box 2.2.

TREATMENT

- The goal of glaucoma treatment is vision preservation and may involve pharmacologic agents or procedures that alter the trabecular meshwork.
- Topical prostaglandins are the preferred therapy. Other options include beta blockers, alpha-adrenergic agonists, and topical carbonic anhydrase inhibitors.

BOX 2.2 Open Angle Glaucoma Diagnostic Criteria

Absence of known (e.g., secondary) causes of open angle glaucoma.
Evidence of optic nerve damage from either or both of the following: • Optic disc or retinal nerve fiber layer structural abnormalities (e.g., thinning, cupping, or notching of the disc rim, progressive change, nerve fiber layer defects) • Reliable and reproducible visual field abnormalities (e.g., arcuate defect, nasal step paracentral scotoma, generalized depression) in the absence of other causes or explanations for a field defect
Open, normal appearing anterior chamber angles
Adult onset

- Another treatment option is laser therapy or trabeculoplasty, which increases aqueous outflow by improving drainage of aqueous humor through the trabecular meshwork.

PATIENT EDUCATION

- The primary care PA should educate at-risk patients on the importance of eye examinations and perform and document thorough funduscopic exams on appropriate patients.
- Patients with glaucoma should be warned about medications that are contraindicated in patients with glaucoma. These medications include glucocorticoids, systemic sympathomimetics, and systemic anticholinergics.

KEY POINTS

- Glaucoma is common, often asymptomatic, and contributes to blindness worldwide.
- Suspect glaucoma if patients have elevated IOP, optic nerve abnormalities on ophthalmoscopy, or a family history of glaucoma.
- Screen patients >40 years old and patients with risk factors every 1 to 2 years.
- Treatment consists of pharmacologic or surgical options.

2.5 CATARACTS

OVERVIEW

Cataracts are a leading cause of blindness worldwide, affecting 20 million individuals in 2010.[13] Surgical management has been performed for centuries. Twentieth century advancements in surgical technique have made cataracts a readily treatable condition.[14]

EPIDEMIOLOGY

Cataracts are an important cause of blindness. Worldwide, cases of blindness secondary to cataracts have increased from 12.3 million in 1990 to 20 million in 2010. The proportion of blindness due to cataract ranges from 12.7% in North America to 42% in Southeast Asia.[15]

Risk factors for cataract development include advancing age, smoking, alcohol intake, sunlight exposure, malnutrition, diabetes mellitus, HIV/AIDS, and systemic corticosteroids.

PATHOPHYSIOLOGY

The lens is a highly organized, transparent structure that pushes dead cells toward its center rather than shedding them as with other body tissues. As these nonviable cells accumulate, they lose their transparency causing the lens to become cloudy (Figure 2.9). This process becomes more prominent as individuals age. It can also be accelerated by trauma to the eye, inflammatory diseases of the eye such as uveitis, and certain medications like systemic or topical corticosteroids.

MEDICAL HISTORY AND CLINICAL PRESENTATION

Cataracts generally present as slowly progressive, bilateral decrease in vision. Night vision may diminish first and may be accompanied by increased glare from lights. Patients over the age of 60 are at higher risk of cataract development,

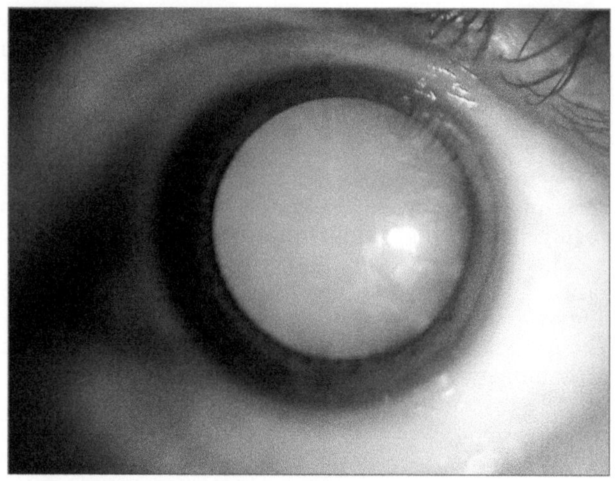

Figure 2.9 Pearly gray appearance of a cataract.
(Source: Courtesy of Imrankabirhossain)

as are patients with a history of smoking, diabetic patients, and patients with a history of topical and oral steroid use.

There may be an increase in nearsightedness before the lens opacity affects the vision.

PHYSICAL EXAMINATION

PAs should note patients with cloudy appearing lens, decreased red reflex, or obscured funduscopic examination.

DIFFERENTIAL DIAGNOSIS

The differential diagnosis includes glaucoma, refractive errors, macular degeneration, diabetic retinopathy, and retinitis pigmentosa.

DIAGNOSIS

The diagnosis of cataract is based on the findings of opacity on ophthalmic examination. A diagnosis of visually significant cataract is made if no other pathology is detected and the degree of lens opacity correlates with the patient's complaints and best-corrected visual acuity. Patients with noted abnormalities should be referred to an ophthalmologist for further evaluation. The diagnosis, however, is often made incidentally during routine eye examinations.

TREATMENT

- The treatment of cataracts involves surgical removal of the opacified lens and replacement with an artificial lens.
- The process is remarkably straightforward and generally performed in an outpatient setting with only topical anesthetics. Complications of surgery include retinal detachment and endophthalmitis.
- Candidates for surgery are identified based on the impact of vision loss on daily activities.
- Visual acuity does not play a role in the determination, and no standardized criteria currently exist.

PATIENT EDUCATION

- Patients should be counseled on the need to discuss changes in vision at routine visits, particularly when those changes affect daily activities like driving or reading.
- Surgical management of cataracts, as noted, is a very common procedure that can drastically improve quality of life.

KEY POINTS

- Modifiable risk factors for cataract include exposure to UV light; use of alcohol, tobacco, and systemic corticosteroids; and poor diabetes management.
- Symptoms include loss of contrast, glare or halos around lights, and visual blurring.
- Surgical removal and placement of an intraocular lens are usually indicated if the cataract contributes to visual loss that interferes with activities of daily living, causes bothersome glare, or reaches certain degrees of severity.

2.6 UVEITIS

OVERVIEW

Uveitis refers to inflammation of the middle portion of the eye, the uveal tract. The anterior segment of the uveal tract includes the iris and ciliary body. The posterior segment is known as the choroid (see Figure 2.5). Uveitis can be classified based on the involvement of a particular segment, the chronicity, the underlying cause, and the presence or absence of granulomas.

EPIDEMIOLOGY

Uveitis is associated with a wide variety of both infectious and autoimmune inflammatory conditions. As many as half of cases are due to an underlying disease. For example, uveitis is a potential consequence of multiple sclerosis (MS), psoriatic arthritis, sarcoidosis, and infections such as tuberculosis, syphilis, and toxoplasmosis. Certain medications, notably bisphosphonates and fluoroquinolones, can also cause uveitis. Advancing age and smoking are also risks for development of uveitis.[14] The prevalence of uveitis ranges from 69 to 204 per 100,000 persons.[16]

PATHOPHYSIOLOGY

The exact pathophysiology of uveal inflammation is defined by the underlying cause rather than by a singular process across the spectrum of disease.

Uveitis is classified anatomically as

- **Anterior uveitis:** Localized primarily to the anterior segment of the eye, includes iritis and iridocyclitis
- **Intermediate uveitis:** Localized to the vitreous cavity
- **Posterior uveitis:** Any form of retinitis, choroiditis, or inflammation of the optic disc
- **Panuveitis:** Inflammation involving anterior, intermediate, and posterior structures

MEDICAL HISTORY AND CLINICAL PRESENTATION

A thorough history of any patient complaining of red eye should include past medical history and current medications, which may reveal history of underlying infection or inflammatory disorder.

SIGNS AND SYMPTOMS

Signs and symptoms will be discussed in terms of anterior and posterior uveitis. Anterior uveitis, also called iritis, is more common than posterior uveitis. Patients may present with pain, redness, photophobia, and vision loss (Figure 2.10).

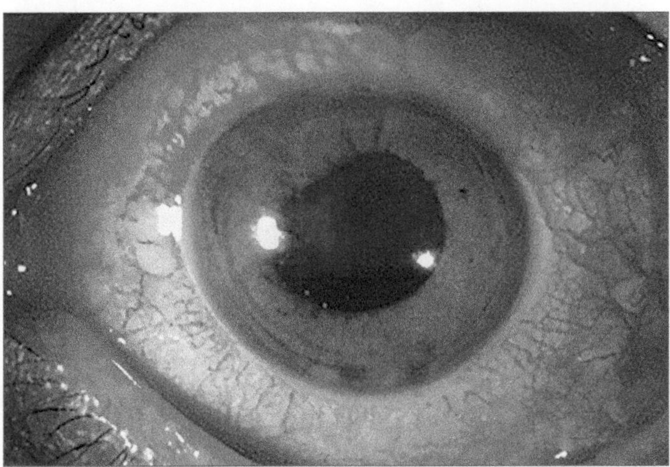

Figure 2.10 **Iritis.**
(Source: Courtesy of Jonathan Trobe.)

Symptoms are most often unilateral. The presentation of posterior uveitis is less readily apparent to the clinician and includes vision loss and complaints of floaters in the visual fields. Redness may not be present.

Although the presentation is typically acute, it may be indolent and difficult to detect depending on the underlying cause. Slit-lamp examination reveals leukocytes in the anterior chamber. Hypopyon may also be present. Posterior uveitis is typically bilateral. Funduscopic exam reveals leukocytes in the vitreous humor.

PHYSICAL EXAMINATION

The classic picture of anterior uveitis involves a red eye and a fixed, constricted pupil. The redness may be concentrated around the limbus, a limbic flush. The pupil may be irregularly shaped because of adhesions between the iris and lens.

DIFFERENTIAL DIAGNOSIS

Uveitis must be differentiated from other diseases that cause conjunctival injection, eye pain, photophobia, or visual changes. This list includes corneal ulcer or abrasion, conjunctivitis, closed angle glaucoma, keratitis, scleritis, and endophthalmitis.

DIAGNOSTIC STUDIES

There are no diagnostic lab findings noted with uveitis. Laboratory studies may be needed to identify the underlying condition.

EVALUATION

In both anterior and posterior uveitis, the presence of red flag signs and symptoms, specifically pain and vision loss, should prompt referral to an ophthalmologist. Complications of uveitis include cataracts, glaucoma, retinal edema, and bend keratopathy, which involves calcium deposition in the corneal epithelium.

TREATMENT

- Initial treatment of anterior uveitis involves topical glucocorticoids. Panuveitis and posterior uveitis do not respond to topical steroids. Topical cycloplegics may be needed.
- Ophthalmologists may choose to use periocular steroid injections.
- Resistant cases can be treated with immunosuppressive therapy and systemic steroids. Infectious causes should be treated with the appropriate antimicrobial agents.
- Referral to ophthalmology is indicated.

PATIENT EDUCATION

- Patients with autoimmune disorders in which uveitis is a potential complication should be counseled on the basic signs and symptoms of disease along with advice to seek evaluation if they occur.
- Patients should also be kept informed on any screening recommendations that accompany specific diseases.

KEY POINTS

- Inflammation of the uveal tract can affect the anterior segment, intermediate uveal tract, or posterior uvea.
- Most cases are idiopathic, but known causes include infections, trauma, and autoimmune disorders.
- Findings in acute anterior uveitis include aching eye pain, photophobia, redness closely surrounding the cornea (ciliary flush), and, on slit-lamp examination, cells and flare.
- Diagnosis is confirmed by slit-lamp examination and ophthalmoscopic examination.
- Treatment should be managed by an ophthalmologist and includes corticosteroids and a cycloplegic-mydriatic drug.

2.7 ORBITAL CELLULITIS

OVERVIEW

Orbital cellulitis describes an infection within the orbit of the eye, involving the periorbital musculature and fat. Clinically, this can be difficult to differentiate from other infections near the eye, specifically periorbital cellulitis.

EPIDEMIOLOGY

Children are affected by orbital cellulitis more than adults.[17] Incidence is higher in the winter months. Bacterial rhinosinusitis is the most common cause of orbital cellulitis.

PATHOPHYSIOLOGY

The orbit is bound by aspects of seven different bones and their periosteum. It is surrounded by the frontal, maxillary, paranasal, and ethmoid sinuses. The ethmoid sinus is separated from the orbit by a thin membrane through which many nerves and blood vessels travel. The orbit is protected anteriorly by the orbital septum, a membrane that projects forward from the periosteum to the tarsal plate. This can be seen in Figure 2.11.

The orbital septum is a critical divider. Orbital cellulitis—infection behind the septum—generally results from bacterial spread through the ethmoid sinus into the orbit. Preseptal cellulitis—infection anterior to the septum—is often the result of superficial bacterial inoculation, perhaps through a scratch or insect bite. Orbital cellulitis most often occurs in

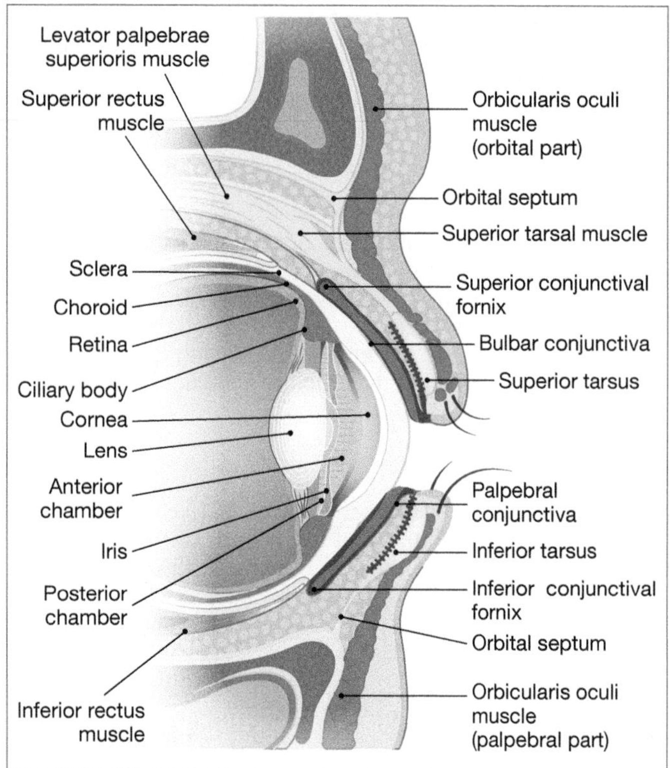

Figure 2.11 **Anatomy of the eyelid.**
(Source: Melnyk J, Zeno R, Teall AM. Evidence-based assessment of the eye. In: Gawlik KS, Melnyk BM, Teall AM, eds. Evidence-Based Physical Examination. *Springer Publishing Company; 2021:308, Fig. 12.3.)*

younger patients, and although it is a rare complication of rhinosinusitis, studies show a high rate of co-occurrence, up to 91%.[18] Other potential causes include orbital trauma, dental infections, and infections following eye surgery. The most common pathogens identified are *Staphylococcus aureus,* and streptococci species, including *S. pneumoniae, S. anginosus,* and *S. pyogenes.*[19,20] Culture is often difficult to obtain and antibiotic coverage should be directed at the most likely causative agents.

MEDICAL HISTORY AND CLINICAL PRESENTATION

The clinical presentations of both preseptal and orbital cellulitis include eye pain and lid swelling. Historical clues can help differentiate the two. As noted above, a history of external trauma, insect bite, or even poison ivy should lead the clinician away from orbital cellulitis. Associated upper respiratory symptoms favor this diagnosis.

SIGNS AND SYMPTOMS

Symptoms and signs of preseptal cellulitis include tenderness, swelling, warmth, redness of the eyelid, and fever. Patients may be unable to open their eyes because of eyelid swelling. Visual acuity is not affected, ocular movement is intact, and there is no proptosis.

Symptoms and signs of orbital cellulitis include swelling and redness of the eyelid and surrounding soft tissues, conjunctival hyperemia and chemosis, decreased ocular motility, pain with eye movements, decreased visual acuity, and proptosis due by orbital swelling.

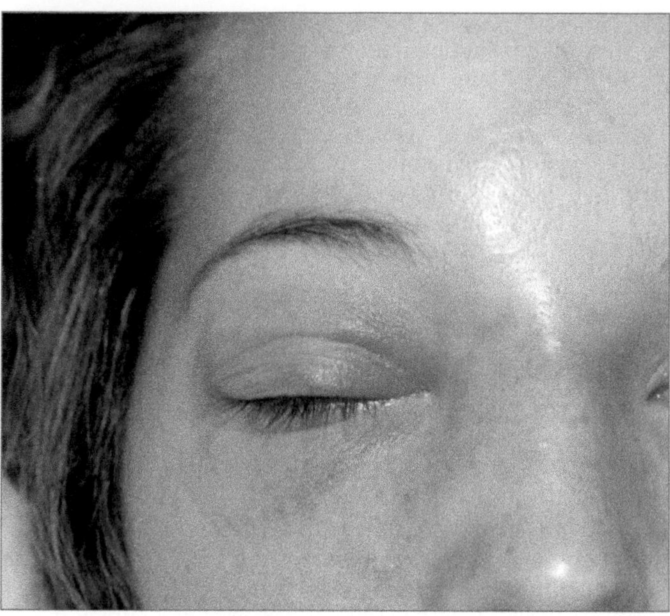

Figure 2.12 **Orbital cellulitis.**
(Source: Centers for Disease Control and Prevention/Dr. Thomas F. Sellers, Emory University.)

PHYSICAL EXAMINATION

Physical examination findings for orbital cellulitis include proptosis and pain with extraocular movements. See Box 2.1 for red flags of the eye examination.

Preseptal cellulitis presents with tenderness, swelling, and erythema. Visual acuity is normal, there is no proptosis, and ocular movements are intact (Figure 2.12).

DIFFERENTIAL DIAGNOSIS

The differential diagnosis includes cavernous sinus thrombosis, neoplasms, use of bisphosphonates, mucocele, dermoid cyst, exophthalmos, sarcoidosis, and numerous infectious etiologies.

DIAGNOSTIC STUDIES

CT scan of the head is used to separate preseptal cellulitis from orbital cellulitis. In orbital cellulitis there are hyperdensities with low-density periorbital fat and elevation of the periorbital region. Blood cultures are needed in patients with orbital cellulitis.

EVALUATION

The diagnosis is made clinically based on history and physical examination. If left untreated, infection can damage the optic nerve and spread to the surrounding bony structure and brain making recognition and referral of the utmost importance.

TREATMENT

- Clinicians should consult an ophthalmologist for any individual presenting with eye pain and lid swelling with painful eye movement, decreased visual acuity, ophthalmoplegia, proptosis, or fever.
- With orbital cellulitis patients should be hospitalized and started on second- or third-generation cephalosporin, such as cefotaxime or ceftriaxone. Other options

include imipenem or piperacillin/tazobactam. Vancomycin should be added if related to trauma or foreign body. Surgical drainage may be necessary if an orbital abscess is identified.

- If these signs and symptoms are absent, a trial of oral antibiotics for preseptal cellulitis may be considered, with follow-up in 24–48 hours.
- Preseptal cellulitis generally improves rapidly with appropriate antibiotics (amoxicillin/clavulanate) and failure to improve at follow-up should prompt referral as above.

PATIENT EDUCATION

- Patients treated presumptively for preseptal cellulitis should be given strict precautions for returning to the clinic for evaluation. These include painful eye movement, decreased visual acuity, ophthalmoplegia, proptosis, or fever.
- If there is any concern regarding the patient's ability to follow treatment directions, a same-day referral to an ophthalmologist is reasonable.

KEY POINTS

- Preseptal and orbital cellulitis are differentiated by whether infection is anterior or posterior to the orbital septum.
- Orbital cellulitis is usually caused by contiguous spread of ethmoid or frontal sinusitis, while preseptal cellulitis is caused by contiguous spread from local facial or eyelid injuries, conjunctivitis, and chalazion.
- Orbital cellulitis is likely if there is decreased ocular motility, pain with eye movements, proptosis, or decreased visual acuity.
- Antibiotic therapy is indicated, with surgery reserved for complicated orbital cellulitis.

2.8 MUSCLE PALSIES

OVERVIEW

Eye function is controlled by four cranial nerves. Damage to any of these can result in significant impairment and may indicate serious disease processes ranging from orbital cellulitis to occipital stroke. The following section will address palsies of cranial nerves III (oculomotor), IV (trochlear), and VI (abducens).

2.8A CRANIAL NERVE III PALSY

EPIDEMIOLOGY

Oculomotor palsies are more frequent in individuals over 60 years old and are less common in children and young adults.[21]

PATHOPHYSIOLOGY

Cranial nerve III, the oculomotor nerve, supplies motor innervation to the pupil and lens, the upper eyelid, and seven eye muscles that allow for visual tracking and gaze fixation. It has somatic and autonomic nerve fibers bundled deep inside that allow for voluntary and involuntary movement. The oculomotor nerve originates in the midbrain and must pass by multiple sinuses and arteries before reaching the orbit and the multiple muscles surrounding the eye.

The somatic fibers within the nerve innervate five muscles: levator palpebrae superioris muscle (elevates the upper eyelid), superior rectus muscle (elevates the eye to primary position/looking straight ahead), medial rectus muscle (adducts the eye from primary position), inferior rectus muscle (moves the eye down from primary position), and inferior oblique muscle (elevates the eye when the eye is adducted). Parasympathetic fibers innervate the sphincter pupillae (allowing constriction of the pupil) and the ciliary muscles (altering the curvature of the lens for focus on near objects).

Cranial nerve III palsies result from lesions disrupting the nerve pathway, causing a disconnect from the oculomotor nucleus in the midbrain to the extraocular muscles in the orbit. Lesions may be the result of vascular ischemia, trauma, intracranial neoplasm, hemorrhage, congenital defect, or a medical cause like diabetes mellitus or hypertension.

MEDICAL HISTORY AND CLINICAL PRESENTATION

The signs and symptoms a patient will present with depend on the etiology, the location of the lesion in the brain, and the fibers that are affected. Compression from a tumor, an aneurysm of the posterior communicating artery, or supratentorial brain herniation affect the nerve blood supply as well as resultant superficial pupillomotor fibers. This leads to extraocular motor disfunction and pupillary dysfunction. If the endoneurial sheath is damaged, an aberrant regeneration phenomenon may develop leading to lid and pupillary dyskinesis. Vascular lesions caused by diabetes mellitus, hypertension, giant cell arthritis, or herpes zoster often spare the pupil because of their effects on the microvasculature.

PHYSICAL EXAMINATION

Patients generally present with ptosis, restricted extraocular movements, diplopia, and a divergent, slightly depressed gaze ("down and out").

The pupil may or may not be affected. If the pupil is affected, such as with compressive lesions, the eye is generally painful, and the pupil will not constrict to light or accommodation.

DIFFERENTIAL DIAGNOSIS

When evaluating a patient with this presentation, the following diagnoses should also be considered: ophthalmoplegic migraine, ptosis in adults, anisocoria, myasthenia gravis, and thyroid ophthalmopathy.

Giant cell arteritis (GCA) can be considered as well, particularly in the geriatric population. Clinical evidence of a third nerve palsy warrants urgent consult with both an ophthalmologist and neurologist.

DIAGNOSTIC STUDIES

CT angiography and MRI may be useful when there is high suspicion of an aneurysm. Complete blood count (CBC), serum glucose, hemoglobin A1c, and erythrocyte sedimentation rate (ESR) may be helpful if an ischemic cause is suspected based on lack of pupillary dysfunction.

TREATMENT

- Conservative management for cranial nerve III palsies is appropriate for patients over 50 years old and with a history of diabetes or hypertension.
- Patients should be followed closely for signs of improvement. In patients with diplopia, an eye patch may help with disconjugate gaze.
- Surgical treatment is recommended in patients with pupil-sparing palsy lasting longer than 6 months.

PATIENT EDUCATION

- Some patients may see improvements within the first month, but it may take up to 3 months or longer to fully recover.

2.8B CRANIAL NERVE IV PALSY

EPIDEMIOLOGY

Fourth nerve palsies most commonly occur from congenital developmental anomalies of the nerve, superior oblique muscle, or surrounding tendons. There is no dominance of age or gender.[22] Because of the extensive intracranial length of the fourth cranial nerve compared to the other nerves that control eye movement, it is more likely to be injured from blunt head trauma (even mild blows to the head), microvascular disease, brain tumor, increased intracranial pressure, or any type of swelling.[23]

PATHOPHYSIOLOGY

The fourth cranial nerve, also called the trochlear nerve, is a pure motor nerve that originates as fascicles in the fourth nerve nucleus of the midbrain. The trochlear nerve exits the anterior medulla dorsally, and then crosses with its contralateral partner before passing between the superior and posterior cerebellar arteries into the subarachnoid space and then into the cavernous sinus. It then enters the superior orbital fissure, where it innervates the superior oblique muscle. A lesion can occur anywhere along that pathway, causing paralytic strabismus, loss of abduction, and intorsion of the eye.

MEDICAL HISTORY AND CLINICAL PRESENTATION

Patients with mild fourth cranial nerve palsy will usually complain of sudden onset of pain or pupillary involvement with difficulty focusing, blurred vision, dizziness, or neurologic abnormalities. These symptoms can be unilateral or bilateral. More severe cases of cranial nerve IV palsy will involve binocular vertical diplopia and/or torsional diplopia (subjective tilting of objects) bilaterally.

PHYSICAL EXAMINATION

On physical examination, there may be ipsilateral hypertropia (upward deviation of the eye) with failure of depression on adduction, and a loss of inward rotation, forcing outward rotation (excyclotorsion) of the affected eye. Patients may develop a conscious or unconscious head tilt to the opposite side of the paralyzed muscle as a response to the torsional and vertical diplopia.

The Parks-Bielschowsky three-step test is used to confirm the diagnosis of isolated unilateral fourth nerve palsy.

- First, determine which is the hypertrophic (higher) eye so as to narrow down which group of four muscles are paralyzed: two depressors from one eye and two elevators of the other eye (ipsilateral superior oblique or inferior rectus on one side, and the contralateral inferior oblique or superior rectus).
- Then, decide if the hypertropia is worse in right or left gaze to narrow which two of the four muscles are involved. For example, worsening hypertropia with right gaze in a patient with left hypertropia suggests the left superior oblique or the right superior rectus.
- Lastly, resolve if the hypertropia is worse in right or left head tilt. The direction of the head tilt that worsens the hypertropia highlights the involved muscle. Therefore, right hypertropia that worsens with left gaze and a right head tilt is from a right superior oblique palsy.

Bilateral fourth nerve palsy is suspected in a physical exam with alternating hypertropia on head tilt or horizontal gaze, positive head tilt to both sides, >10 degrees of excyclotorsion, a decreased abduction of superior obliques in depression and overaction of inferior obliques, or a slight hypertropia of both eyes in primary position.

DIFFERENTIAL DIAGNOSIS

Restrictive vertical strabismus, other paretic vertical strabismus, myasthenia gravis, ocular tilt reaction with skew deviation, and thyroid ophthalmopathy are part of the differential diagnosis.

DIAGNOSTIC STUDIES

Neuroimaging is only necessary for patients with nonisolated fourth nerve palsies with neurologic signs or symptoms. MRI is the gold standard for evaluation, due to its sensitivity of detecting intracranial lesions. A CT scan may be used in patients who cannot undergo an MRI or with suspicion of acute bleeding.

TREATMENT

- In symptomatic patients with isolated palsies, the focus of treatment is on the underlying cause, to maximize visual function and ocular alignment.
- Patients with microvascular lesions are likely to see improvement of symptoms in a few weeks to months.
- Patching one eye by an ophthalmologist is often used to treat binocular diplopia.
- Those with an asymptomatic palsy are observed over several months before considering treatment.
- If there is no improvement, then prism therapy is considered. If the patient fails prism therapy, they may find success with strabismus surgery.

2.8C CRANIAL NERVE VI PALSY

EPIDEMIOLOGY

A recent study found the overall incidence of sixth nerve palsy among the general Korean population to be 4.66 per 100,000 with a slight prevalence for males, and greater prevalence for older individuals, particularly those over 60.[24]

PATHOPHYSIOLOGY

The sixth cranial nerve, also called the abducens nerve, is the most common ocular cranial nerve to be involved in an isolated palsy. Each sixth cranial nerve nucleus begins in the dorsal pons, where the nerve fascicles leave to travel within the pontine tegmentum, eventually leaving the brainstem at the pontomedullary junction, and entering the subarachnoid space. Cranial nerve VI has the longest course within the subarachnoid space before entering the cavernous sinus and into the orbital fissure to innervate the ipsilateral lateral rectus, allowing for eye abduction/horizontal gaze. Additionally, the sixth nerve contains all the interneurons to the contralateral third nerve medial rectus muscle subnucleus.

Sixth nerve palsy is often labeled as an isolated event. The location of the lesion on the nerve pathway dictates the dysfunction that will incur. There are multiple possible etiologies for sixth nerve palsy, but the most common are neoplasia, tumors, vascular disease, inflammatory and infectious disorders (e.g., meningitis), and trauma.[25]

MEDICAL HISTORY AND CLINICAL PRESENTATION

The most typical symptom of sixth nerve palsy is binocular horizontal diplopia, which worsens when both eyes are open, looking into the distance, or with horizontal gaze toward the weak lateral rectus muscle. Other common symptoms include nonpainful, blurred vision, unable to abduct affected eye, facial weakness, droopy eyelid, difficulty focusing, and dizziness.

PHYSICAL EXAMINATION

Strabismus may be present early on when staring straight ahead or gazing toward the paretic side. In nonisolated palsies, accompanying clinical manifestations may be present and are specific to the location of the lesion on the nerve. These include ipsilateral horizontal gaze palsy, ipsilateral facial nerve palsy, hemiparesis, central Horner syndrome, proptosis, facial pain, and involvement of fifth, seventh, and eighth cranial nerves.

DIFFERENTIAL DIAGNOSIS

Other conditions should be considered with isolated abduction deficits, including restrictive orbitopathy, orbital myositis, myasthenia gravis, childhood esotropia, convergence spasm, and sagging eye syndrome.

DIAGNOSTIC STUDIES

Neuroimaging is necessary for most children and adults with isolated nerve palsy and always indicated if other neurologic findings are present. Older patients with vascular issues may wait up to 3 months before having imaging completed since their palsy may improve after a couple of weeks or months. MRI is the gold standard for imaging due to its superior capability to illustrate the posterior fossa. A CT scan is a secondary option if the MRI cannot be used for some reason.

TREATMENT

- Whether it is infectious, inflammatory, or neoplastic, the underlying cause of sixth nerve palsy should be treated with appropriate therapy.
- Patients with isolated, unilateral, or nontraumatic palsy will likely recover spontaneously on their own.
- Symptomatic isolated congenital or acquired palsies may be treated with patching, prism therapy, strabismus therapy, and botulinum toxin injections to maximize visual function and alignment.

KEY POINTS

- Symptoms of cranial nerve III palsy include diplopia, ptosis, and impaired adduction and upward gaze. If the pupil is affected, consider aneurysms and transtentorial herniation; if the pupil is spared, consider ischemia of the nerve.
- Cranial nerve IV palsy is often idiopathic; it may affect one or both eyes. Symptoms include double vision, worse when going down the stairs.
- Cranial nerve VI palsy typically results from small-vessel disease, particularly in diabetics. Symptoms include impaired abduction and horizontal diplopia. Sixth cranial nerve palsy usually resolves whether a cause is identified or not.
- Treat the disorder causing the cranial nerve palsy.

2.9 VASCULAR DISEASES

OVERVIEW

The retinal vasculature is delicate and highly susceptible to insult. Several systemic and ocular disorders involve changes to the retinal blood supply. This topic will primarily focus on the acute forms of occlusive retinal artery and vein disease.

EPIDEMIOLOGY

Vision loss related to retinal artery occlusion, both central and branch, is rare, with an annual prevalence of <0.001%.[26] Patients are typically older with risk factors for atherosclerosis such as hypertension, diabetes, and a history of smoking. Similarly, retinal venous disease is rare, with patients having the same risk factors as with arterial disease.

PATHOPHYSIOLOGY

The internal carotid artery branches to the ophthalmic artery, which supplies the central retinal artery. The central retinal artery then branches into smaller arteries that spread out across the retina. The central retinal artery directly feeds the central portion of the retina and the optic nerve. Occlusion of the retinal arteries may result from emboli that develop locally because of microvascular disease or from distant emboli originating in the internal carotid or heart. Cardiac origin of embolus should be suspected if there is a history of underlying valve disease or atrial fibrillation. Hypercoagulable patients are also at risk of retinal vessel occlusion.

The branch retinal veins drain from the capillary beds into the central retinal artery. The central retinal artery drains into the superior ophthalmic artery. The pathophysiology of retinal vein occlusion involves one of two mechanisms: embolus as with retinal artery occlusion, or compression by a crossing retinal artery. Vision loss develops in a less straightforward manner than with arterial occlusion. Venous blood backs up into the vein causing increased ocular pressure and hemorrhaging into the vitreous. Furthermore, as blood continues to backflow, it limits arterial flow into the capillary beds leading to ischemia.

2.9A RETINAL ARTERY OCCLUSION

MEDICAL HISTORY AND CLINICAL PRESENTATION

Patients with central retinal artery occlusion present with sudden, severe monocular vision loss. Pain is absent. Branch retinal artery occlusions have a similar presentation with less severe vision loss, typically restricted to a particular aspect of the visual field.

SIGNS AND SYMPTOMS

A hallmark sign of retinal artery occlusion is painless vision loss. Visual acuity will be diminished in central retinal artery occlusion, but not necessarily with branch artery occlusions. Visual field testing is typically abnormal.

PHYSICAL EXAMINATION

Central occlusions will be accompanied by an afferent pupillary defect. The funduscopic exam may reveal the site of the embolus. With central artery occlusions, the retina will appear pale with a "cherry red" macula. The retina is thinner over the macula, allowing the underlying choroidal blood supply to be visualized. Loss of color in the retina will be more segmental in a branch retinal vein occlusion.

DIFFERENTIAL DIAGNOSIS

The differential diagnosis includes all causes of painless monocular vision loss. The differential diagnosis includes exposure to intense light (welder's flash), ischemic optic neuropathy (ION), occipital lobe costovertebral angle (CVA), optic neuritis, hyphema, and retinal detachment.

DIAGNOSTIC TESTING

Carotid ultrasonography, echocardiography, temporal artery biopsy, and lab tests to evaluate for hypercoagulable states may all be indicated depending on the associated symptoms and presenting history. Fluorescein angiography is often done and shows absence of perfusion in the affected artery.

EVALUATION

Diagnostic workup to investigate the cause of the embolus is indicated. This should be driven by the history, but involves carotid artery ultrasound which, if negative, prompts the need for an echocardiogram to investigate for valvular defects or vegetation.

TREATMENT

- Thrombolytic agents may be considered within the first 24 hours after onset. Other treatment mechanisms involve anterior chamber paracentesis to reduce ocular pressure and possibly push the embolus downstream, ocular massage, and IV acetazolamide, both of which are also directed at altering ocular pressure.

PATIENT EDUCATION

- Patients should be encouraged to control modifiable risk factors. This include smoking cessation, decreasing blood pressure, and managing lipids and blood sugar.

2.9B RETINAL VEIN OCCLUSION

MEDICAL HISTORY AND CLINICAL PRESENTATION

Patients with a central retinal vein occlusion typically present with sudden, monocular blurry vision. Branch retinal vein occlusions may be asymptomatic, discovered on routine examination. Eye pain is not common and should cause the clinician to suspect an alternative diagnosis.

SIGNS AND SYMPTOMS

As noted, painless vision blurring in one eye is the typical presentation of central retinal vein occlusion. Visual field testing may be abnormal. If the macula is involved, the blurriness will be centrally located.

PHYSICAL EXAMINATION

The physical examination may be unremarkable aside from diminished acuity or abnormal visual field testing. Funduscopic examination should reveal retinal edema, retinal hemorrhages, dilated retinal veins, and optic disc swelling.

DIFFERENTIAL DIAGNOSIS

The differential diagnosis includes other causes of monocular vision loss. The differential diagnosis includes exposure to intense light (welder's flash), ION, occipital lobe CVA, optic neuritis, hyphema, and retinal detachment.

EVALUATION

The evaluation of monocular vision loss begins with the key indicators including the absence of pain and blurry vision rather than complete vision loss. The consulting eye specialist may perform fluorescein angiography to quantify the amount of retinal ischemia.

TREATMENT

- Treatment by an opthalmologist is dependent upon three factors: involvement of the macula, the presence of neovascularization, and the location of the occlusion (i.e., either a branch retinal vein or the central vein).
- Branch retinal vein occlusions and central retinal vein occlusions that do not involve the macula are usually monitored with routine eye exams at varying intervals depending on the amount of vision loss.
- Macular edema is treated with intravitreal anti-vascular endothelial growth factor (VEGF). Neovascularization is treated with photocoagulation.

PATIENT EDUCATION

- Patients should be encouraged to manage modifiable risk factors to decrease the likelihood of ocular complications like vision loss.
- Patients with hypertension and diabetes should be advised to maintain healthy numbers, follow up routinely with primary care, and improve unhealthy lifestyles.

KEY POINTS

- Central or branch retinal artery occlusion can be caused by an embolus, thrombosis, or GCA. Painless, severe loss of vision affects part or all the visual field.

- Central or branch retinal artery occlusion is diagnosed by funduscopic examination, revealing a pale, opaque fundus with a red fovea and arterial attenuation).
- Central or branch retinal artery occlusion workup includes color fundus photography and fluorescein angiography and search for an embolic source by Doppler ultrasonography and echocardiography.
- Retinal vein occlusion involves blockage by a thrombus and presents with painless loss of vision that is typically sudden and may have risk factors.
- Retinal vein occlusion funduscopic examination demonstrates macular edema with dilated veins and hemorrhages; additional tests include color fundus photography, fluorescein angiography, and optical coherence tomography.

2.10 PINGUECULA/PTERYGIUM

OVERVIEW

Pinguecula and pterygium are both benign, superficial, fleshy masses that evolve over time. While the pathophysiology is very similar between the two, there are some slight differences in clinical presentation and prognosis.

EPIDEMIOLOGY

The epidemiologic data on both pingueculas and pterygiums are limited. Studies indicate wide variation among population groups. The prevalence of pinguecula is around 48% and the prevalence of pterygium is around 6%. Pingueculas are more common in males over the age of 50 who have had long-term exposure to UV radiation or irritants like dust. Contact lens wearers have a higher incidence of pinguecula as well.[27]

Pterygiums are also common in older males with outdoor jobs. They are more common in areas of the world with higher UV exposure, such as countries closer to the equator.

PATHOPHYSIOLOGY

Pingueculas are a type of corneal degenerative disorder of the collagen fibers within the conjunctival stroma. Granular deposits lead to hyalinization (deterioration of normal tissue) with periodic calcifications causing a thinning of the overlying epithelium.[27]

Like pingueculas, pterygiums are a corneal degenerative disorder, but the pathology is more directly related to UV damage. Prolonged exposure of UV radiation causes cellular damage to DNA, RNA, and extracellular matrix composition.

2.10A PINGUECULA

MEDICAL HISTORY AND CLINICAL PRESENTATION

Often patients will be older males with an occupation in outdoor landscaping or construction, possibly welding. Patients are usually asymptomatic but may present with inflammation or a foreign body sensation.

PHYSICAL EXAMINATION

It is common for the lesions to appear white to yellowish with an elevated flat texture (Figure 2.13). The lesions are typically bilateral, presenting medially in the 3 or 9 o'clock positions without crossing the limbus or involving the cornea.

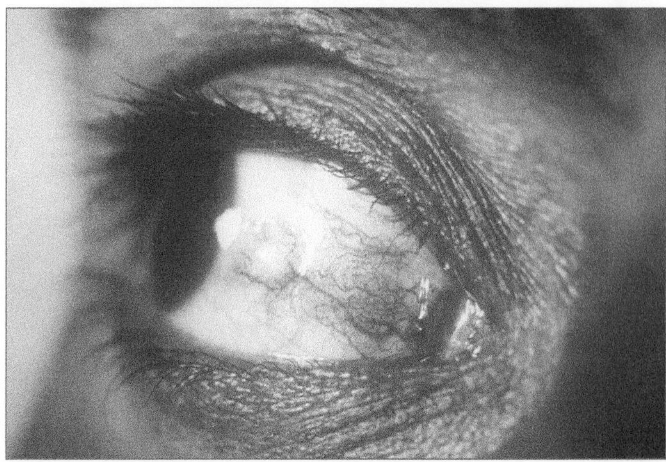

Figure 2.13 Pinguecula.
(Source: Centers for Disease Control and Prevention.)

If there is inflammation, sometimes described as "pingueculitis," there will be erythema and swelling of the conjunctiva. The patient will also complain of dry, itchy, burning eyes with blurry vision and foreign body sensation.

DIFFERENTIAL DIAGNOSIS

Pingueculas are clinically diagnosed, but other disorders should be ruled out, such as pterygium, conjunctival intraepithelial neoplasia, episcleritis, or conjunctivitis.

DIAGNOSTIC STUDIES

No diagnostic studies are needed. The diagnosis is made clinically.

TREATMENT

Reassurance that lesions are benign is important. If symptoms exist, a cold compress and lubricant eye drops are used as a first line to relieve irritation. In the unlikely instance that this is not adequate, referral to an ophthalmologist may be indicated, and a corticosteroid eye drop may be added to the regiment to decrease redness and swelling.

PATIENT EDUCATION

- Patient education is imperative to prevent self-inflicted irritation and inflammation.
- Patients should also be encouraged to wear sunglasses when outside, avoid dust and debris with proper eye protection, and apply artificial tear eye drops to keep eyes from drying.

2.10B PTERYGIUM

MEDICAL HISTORY AND CLINICAL PRESENTATION

Pterygiums have an insidious onset from months to years and are typically seen in older males with outdoor jobs. Their presentation is typically bilateral. They can become

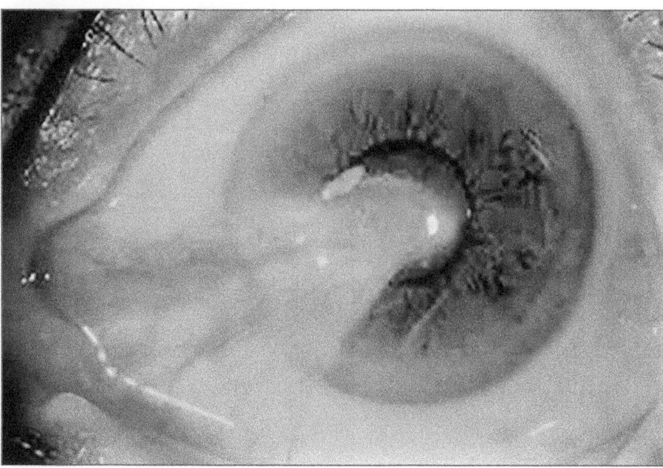

Figure 2.14 Pterygium.
(Source: Image courtesy of Jmvaras)

inflamed from prolonged UV damage and will continue to grow and thicken over time. When inflamed, the most common symptoms are redness and irritation.

PHYSICAL EXAMINATION

A pterygium will appear as a white, triangular, wing-shaped wedge of fleshy fibrovascular tissue that is soft and nearly flat (Figure 2.14). It begins on the nasal side of the cornea and extends laterally. There is no limit to the size to which it can progress, sometimes growing over the cornea and leading to vision problems including blurriness, impairment, severe ocular irritation, and astigmatism.

DIFFERENTIAL DIAGNOSIS

Similar to pinguecula, pterygiums are diagnosed clinically based on their classic shape and location on the eye. On examination other similar conditions should be considered including pinguecula, neoplastic lesion, pseudo-pterygium, episcleritis, conjunctivitis, and blepharitis.

DIAGNOSTIC STUDIES

No diagnostic studies are needed. The diagnosis is made clinically.

TREATMENT

- Treatment involves lubricant drops or artificial tears to relieve irritation and keep the eye moist. When the lesion is inflamed and swollen, topical decongestants, topical NSAIDs, or topical glucocorticoids may be used for a limited amount of time. These should be prescribed by an ophthalmologist.
- Surgery to remove pterygiums is reserved for complications such as the development of astigmatism, intractable irritation, visual impairment, opacity in the visual axis, restriction of eye movement, or a significant cosmetic impact.

PATIENT EDUCATION

- It is important to counsel the patient that pterygium surgery has a 30–80% recurrence of lesion regrowth, often with increased size and symptoms.[28]
- Patients should be counseled on proper eye protection to decrease the amount of UV exposure. Counsel all patients with outdoor jobs or high UV exposure.

KEY POINTS

- Pinguecula is a raised yellowish white mass within the bulbar conjunctiva, adjacent to the cornea. It does not tend to grow onto the cornea.
- Pterygium is a fleshy triangular growth of bulbar conjunctiva that may spread across and distort the cornea.

2.11 RETINAL DISORDERS

OVERVIEW

Disorders of the retina are some of the most challenging to recognize and treat. As the retina is positioned at the back of the eye, which is a closed, pressured structure, adequate assessment is difficult. The retina must be visualized through the pupil at the front of the eye. The volume of sensitive neurologic tissues that make up the retina leave this structure susceptible to insult and catastrophic vision loss for the patient.

EPIDEMIOLOGY

With the exception of retinoblastoma, most retinal diseases are seen in adults, particularly older adults. Retinal detachment, for example, involves liquefaction of the vitreous humor, which is a product of age. Macular degeneration also has a clear predilection for older adults.

PATHOPHYSIOLOGY

As light enters the eye, it is refracted first by the cornea, followed by the aqueous humor, and then the lens, all components of the anterior chamber. The amount of light entering the eye is controlled by the iris, which constricts and dilates. Of the anterior structures, the lens is the primary mode of light refraction, and is controlled by the ciliary muscles, changing shape to alter refraction. Light then enters the posterior chamber where it passes through vitreous humor before reaching the retina. The retina is the light sensitive portion of the eye, containing a layer of photoreceptors that convert light into nerve impulses. Photoreceptors can be divided into two types: rods and cones, which function more in dim light and bright light, respectively. There are significantly more rods than cones, over 100 million as compared to 6 million.[29] Cones are further subdivided by color and the sequencing of cone stimulation determines color vision. Signals are transmitted from the retina to the brain via the optic nerve. The two optic nerves cross over the optic chiasm, with medial fibers traveling to the contralateral side of the brain and lateral fibers proceeding to the ipsilateral side. The retina is a multilayered structure, with the various layers having different blood supply. The internal layers obtain blood supply from the central retinal artery and the outermost layers are adherent to the choroid and receive blood supply from diffusion across the choroid blood vessels.

2.11A RETINAL DETACHMENT

MEDICAL HISTORY AND CLINICAL PRESENTATION

Retinal detachment is the process where by the neural retina separates from the underlying retinal pigment epithelium and choroid, leading to ischemia and rapid photoreceptor degeneration. Detachment often involves injury to the eye, or increased traction of collagenous fibrils within the vitreous humor leading to fluid or blood collecting between the retina and the pigment epithelium.

Retinal detachments can be broken down by severity and type. A full-thickness break (hole or tear) in the retina, causing the retina to detach from the underlying retinal pigment and choroid, is referred to as a rhegmatogenous retinal detachment. Rhegmatogenous retinal detachments are caused by posterior vitreous detachment or a traumatic event that increases pressure where the retina meets the choroid. A nonrhegmatogenous retinal detachment is caused by an accumulation of fluid between the retina and underlying retinal pigment and choroid, due to exudative fluid or vitreous traction. Risk factors include myopia, age over 50, ocular trauma, ocular inflammation, or systemic inflammatory disorders.

SIGNS AND SYMPTOMS

Holes or tears in the retina may be symptomatic or asymptomatic. Symptoms of a rhegmatogenous retinal detachment caused by spontaneous posterior vitreous detachment include sudden onset of floaters, photopsias, and acutely progressive peripheral visual field loss in the affected eye. Vitreous hemorrhaging may cause a "shower of black spots." Progression of the retinal detachment that impedes on the macula results in enlarged visual field defects. Eventually, reading is compromised as the central retina is affected.

PHYSICAL EXAMINATION

All patients presenting with eye complaints should have visual acuity evaluated. A decrease in visual acuity may be appreciated but is not specific to retinal detachment. Visual fields should also be checked. It is reasonable for the initial treating clinician to perform a funduscopic exam looking for gross abnormalities in the retina or vitreous, but the lack of findings should not delay referral to ophthalmology (Figure 2.15).

DIFFERENTIAL DIAGNOSIS

The differential diagnosis should include vitreous hemorrhage, vitreous inflammation, intraocular foreign body, and ocular lymphoma. If the patient is found to have a monocular decreased visual field on exam, urgent referral to an ophthalmologist or retinal surgeon to undergo a more extensive ophthalmic examination to view the retina is warranted.

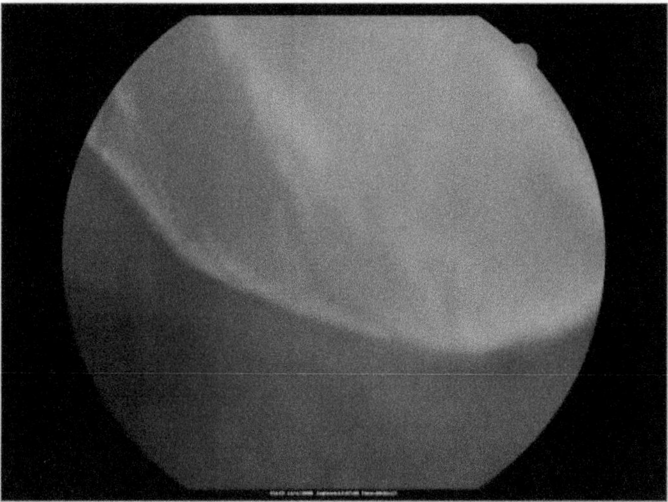

Figure 2.15 Funduscopic examination of retinal detachment.

DIAGNOSTIC STUDIES

No diagnostic studies are needed. The diagnosis is made clinically.

TREATMENT

- Treatment may include retinopexy, cryoretinopexy, scleral buckle, or vitrectomy.
- Traction retinal detachments related to diabetic retinopathy, ocular trauma, or vitreomacular syndrome are treated with surgical vitrectomy.
- Smaller and more peripheral retinal detachments may be treated with cryoretinopexy or photocoagulation. These methods involve surgically replacing the retina to its normal location against the choroid.
- If treatment is not initiated in a timely fashion, the ischemic retina will be unable to function despite surgical intervention.
- Surgical treatment is not recommended for exudative retinal detachment; instead, the cause should be identified and treated.

PATIENT EDUCATION

- Patients may present complaining of new-onset floaters, concerned for the diagnosis of retinal detachment. Although referral to and evaluation by a specialist is the standard of care, patients can be reasonably reassured that not all floaters are signs of active retinal detachment.
- In the absence of all other signs and symptoms, floaters may indicate changes to the vitreous structure known as lattice degeneration, a breakdown in the collagenous structure of the vitreous humor that pulls traction on the retina.

2.11B MACULAR DEGENERATION

MEDICAL HISTORY AND CLINICAL PRESENTATION

Age-related macular degeneration (AMD) is an age-related degenerative disease of the macula, the central portion of the retina, that leads to central vision loss. It is classified into two categories: atrophic, also referred to as dry, and neovascular, referred to as wet or exudative. It is the leading cause of adult blindness in industrialized countries and the risk increases substantially with age.[12] Other aspects of a patient's medical history that may pose a risk for macular degeneration include a history of smoking and the presence of complement factor H genetic polymorphism.[30]

The pathophysiology of dry AMD is not clear. Lipid deposits known as drusen and retinal atrophy lead to progressive vision loss. Dry AMD may progress to wet AMD, which involves the formulation of new blood vessels beneath the retina, pulling it away from the choroid. These vessels are fragile and leaky, giving this form of AMD its characteristic name "wet." The vision loss associated with wet AMD may be substantially more acute in onset and profound.

SIGNS AND SYMPTOMS

In the primary care setting, a detailed history including when vision loss began and which eyes are involved, should be documented. Patients presenting with dry macular degeneration may report gradual vision loss in one or both eyes. Patients may also note scotomas; difficulty reading, driving, or watching television; needing brighter lights to do normal activities; worsening night vision; or needing magnification to read.

The earliest visual change with wet macular degeneration is distortion of straight lines. Wet macular degeneration may also present as acute central vision loss, typically in one eye, though disease is usually present in both eyes. Progression of macular degeneration results in significant vision loss, but does not typically result in total blindness. These findings are summarized in Table 2.2.

PHYSICAL EXAMINATION

The initial physical examination may reveal drusen, appearing as small, yellow plaques on the retinal surface, but given the limitations of funduscopy in the primary care setting, the absence of abnormalities should not delay referral. If an Amsler grid is available, patients may note line distortion (Figure 2.16).

Ophthalmologic evaluation should include a dilated, slit-lamp eye examination. Dry macular degeneration will reveal drusen. Wet macular degeneration will appear as subretinal fluid or hemorrhage with neovascularization appearing as grayish green discoloration of the macula.

DIFFERENTIAL DIAGNOSIS

Macular degeneration is a clinical diagnosis based on ophthalmologic evaluation. Patients presenting with acute vision loss in the primary care setting should have an urgent referral to an ophthalmologist. Differential diagnosis includes presbyopia, cataracts, glaucoma, and retinopathy as they are other common causes of visual impairment in older adults.

DIAGNOSTIC STUDIES

No diagnostic studies are needed. The diagnosis is made clinically.

EVALUATION

Both types of age-related macular degeneration are diagnosed by funduscopic examination. Visual changes can often be detected with an Amsler grid. Color photography and fluorescein angiography are needed if wet AMD is considered.

TABLE 2.2 Characteristics of Dry and Wet AMD

Dry AMD	Wet AMD
Slowly progressive vision loss	Acute central vision loss
Symptoms in both eyes	Symptoms in one eye
Difficulty reading, driving, watching television	Distortion of straight lines
Need for more light and magnification	
Worsening night vision	

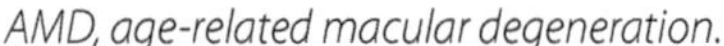

AMD, age-related macular degeneration.

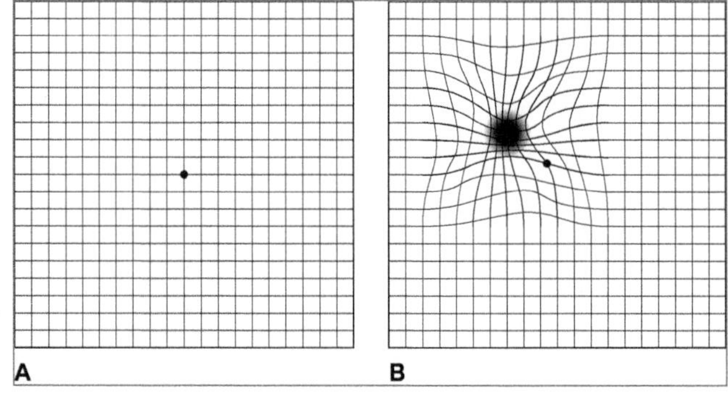

Figure 2.16 **Loss of central vision with macular degeneration. (A) Amsler grid. (B) Amsler grid as seen by a patient with macular degeneration.**

(Source: Guida KM. Advanced health assessment of the eyes and ears. In: Myrick KM, Karosas LM, eds. Advanced Health Assessment and Differential Diagnosis. *Springer Publishing Company; 2021:81, Fig. 4.34.)*

TREATMENT

- Treatment of dry macular degeneration includes a daily oral vitamin supplement that contains vitamin C, vitamin E, lutein, zeaxanthin, zinc, and copper.
- If the patient does not smoke and has never smoked, they can substitute a vitamin supplement containing beta-carotene rather than lutein or zeaxanthin.
- Wet macular degeneration is treated with intravitreal VEGF inhibitors, photodynamic therapy, and antioxidant vitamin and zinc supplementation.

PATIENT EDUCATION

- Patients diagnosed with AMD should be educated on the use of Amsler grids, testing each eye daily and reporting any line distortions or changes from previous tests.
- All patients who smoke should be counseled on the risk of AMD and advised to quit. Patients previously diagnosed with AMD who smoke should be counseled in smoking cessation to help prevent progression.

2.11C DIABETIC RETINOPATHY

OVERVIEW

Retinopathy is a broad term that encompasses diseases that directly affect vision through damage of the retina. Development and progression of diabetic retinopathy are caused by chronic hyperglycemia. Chronically elevated blood sugar causes bodily end-organ damage through many complex mechanisms, particularly by damaging blood vessels. These effects occur no less on the eyes, where findings primarily consist of abnormal permeability in the retinal vessels as well as retinal ischemia and neovascularization.

EPIDEMIOLOGY

Diabetic retinopathy is a leading cause of new-onset blindness, and evidence of retinopathy is found in as many as one third of diabetic patients over the age of 40.[31] The risk of diabetic retinopathy increases progressively with duration of underlying disease. This single fact makes screening eye examinations in patients with diabetes imperative.

MEDICAL HISTORY AND CLINICAL PRESENTATION

Diabetic retinopathy is divided into two categories based on examination findings: proliferative and nonproliferative. Proliferative retinopathy is so named for the involvement of neovascularization. Vision loss related to proliferative retinopathy may be sudden and severe depending on the exact mechanism. New blood vessels may involve the optic disc. Vitreous hemorrhaging may cause blindness itself or lead to fibrosis, vitreous traction, and retinal detachment. Nonproliferative retinopathy involves blindness through the more typical mechanisms, such as vascular ischemia, increased permeability and bleeding, retinal thickening, and macular edema.

SIGNS AND SYMPTOMS

PAs should ensure all diabetic patients are routinely following up with an ophthalmologist for dilated eye examinations. Although findings like cotton wool spots, representing intraretinal infarcts, as well as neovascularization may be seen, the primary care examination is not sensitive enough to make decisions on management. The ophthalmologic examination may include dilated funduscopy or fluorescein angiography, revealing small, flame-shaped and blot hemorrhages, or cotton wool spots surrounding a retinal occlusion. Tortuous loops and increased retinal veins may be present. Vasoproliferation and neovascularization are obviously associated with proliferative retinopathy. If macular edema is present, it will appear as yellow exudates due to diffuse capillary leakage.

DIFFERENTIAL DIAGNOSIS

Diagnosis of diabetic retinopathy is clinical and based on the presence of the above signs. The AAO recommends patients with type 1 diabetes be screened starting 3 to 5 years after diagnosis.[32] Patients with type 2 diabetes should be screened with dilated funduscopy starting near the time of diagnosis due to the possibility of chronic, undiagnosed hyperglycemia.[32]

DIAGNOSTIC STUDIES

No diagnostic studies are needed. The diagnosis is made clinically via ophthalmoscopy on a dilated fundus.

TREATMENT

- From a primary care perspective, treatment revolves around improving hemoglobin A1c and controlling blood pressure.
- The American Diabetes Association recommends treating patients to a systolic blood pressure of <140 mm Hg and diastolic blood pressure of <90 mm Hg.[33]
- If macular edema with impaired visual acuity is present, intravitreal injections of anti-VEGF are recommended.
- Treatment of macular edema without visual impairment is determined on a case-by-case basis to observe or implement therapy of intravitreal injections or laser photocoagulation.

PATIENT EDUCATION

- Patients need to understand the importance of good glycemic control in the prevention of retinopathy. For patients with established retinal disease, glycemic control should be highlighted as a means of slowing progression. Patients should also be advised on the need for good blood pressure control.

2.11D HYPERTENSIVE RETINOPATHY

OVERVIEW

Hypertension has widespread consequences on most organ systems including the eyes. Retinal microvascular changes due to hypertension are referred to collectively as hypertensive retinopathy. Although high blood pressure has direct effects on the retina, hypertension's effects on vision are primarily through coexisting diagnoses like diabetes.

MEDICAL HISTORY AND CLINICAL PRESENTATION

Patients with evidence of retinopathy typically have a long-standing history of uncontrolled hypertension, and the ability to directly observe the retinal vessels serves as an indicator for blood pressure management. Funduscopy should be part of the routine examination of patients with hypertension who are otherwise unlikely to have symptoms related to disease. Patients who have evidence of retinopathy in the absence of demonstrated hypertension have been shown to be at risk of developing elevated blood pressure in the future.[34]

SIGNS AND SYMPTOMS

The effects of hypertension on vision are primarily through other diseases as noted above. Hypertensive retinopathy, in and of itself, rarely causes vision loss. When vision loss does occur, retinopathy is typically severe and accompanied by more pressing symptoms to include chest pain, shortness of breath, headache, or altered level of consciousness. These represent increased intracranial pressure or hypertensive crisis.

PHYSICAL EXAMINATION

A funduscopic examination revealing microvascular changes is diagnostic and allows the retinopathy to be classified as mild, moderate, or severe. Patients with mild to moderate retinopathy typically do not have visual symptoms. Findings of mild hypertensive retinopathy include retinal arteriolar narrowing, arteriolar wall thickening, and arteriovenous nicking (AV nicking). AV nicking occurs when a dilated arteriole crosses over a vein, compressing it and leading to appreciable engorgement on either side of the compression. Moderate disease includes flame hemorrhages, cotton wool spots, and microaneurysms. Optic disc edema separates moderate from severe retinopathy. Severely hypertensive patients will have signs and symptoms of end-organ damage elsewhere as noted above.

DIFFERENTIAL DIAGNOSIS

The diagnosis is clinical based on the presence of absence of the signs discussed above. It is then classified as mild, moderate, or severe. Although there is some overlap with diabetic retinopathy, a thorough history should make the likely culprit more readily apparent.

DIAGNOSTIC STUDIES

No diagnostic studies are needed. The diagnosis is made clinically. Laboratory testing may be needed to identify secondary causes of hypertension.

TREATMENT

- Adequate control of hypertension may allow for regression of retinopathy, which should be used by the treating PA as a tool for encouragement and reassurance to hypertensive patients.
- Treatment of severe disease is emergent and involves rapidly lowering the patient's mean arterial pressure by 10% to 15% in the first hour via a parenteral antihypertensive agent, with the stipulation that blood pressure should not be lowered by more than 25% of baseline at 24 hours.[35]
- Once blood pressure is controlled using an IV hypertensive agent, the patient can be switched to oral therapy with the aim to reduce systolic blood pressure to <130 mm Hg and diastolic blood pressure to <80 mm Hg over 2 to 3 months.

PATIENT EDUCATION

- Hypertensive patients should be educated on lifestyle changes that can improve high blood pressure and the consequences of uncontrolled hypertension. Lifestyle modifications include dietary changes such as reduced sodium intake, reduced alcohol consumption, and following the DASH eating plan. Patients should be counseled on the benefits of exercise, weight loss, and smoking cessation.
- Routine follow-up of hypertension and medication compliance should also be stressed.

SPECIAL CONSIDERATIONS

- Women who develop gestational diabetes are not at increased risk for diabetic retinopathy and do not need screening. Pregnant females with preexisting retinopathy should have a retinal screening in the first trimester and possibly throughout pregnancy up until 1 year post partum.
- Hypertension increases the risk of other ocular diseases, including diabetic retinopathy, retinal vein and retinal artery occlusion, retinal occlusion, and anterior ION; hence controlling hypertension is vital to reduce end-organ damage and cardiovascular events.

KEY POINTS

- Risk factors for retinal detachments include myopia, previous cataract surgery, ocular trauma, and lattice retinal degeneration and presents with blurry vision and a curtain or veil across the visual field.
- Macular degeneration, dry (nonexudative) or wet (exudative), is the leading cause of permanent vision loss in older adults.
- Funduscopic changes in dry macular degeneration include drusen, areas of chorioretinal atrophy, and changes to the retinal pigment epithelium.
- Features of diabetic retinopathy include microaneurysms, intraretinal hemorrhage, exudates, cotton wool spots, macular edema, macular ischemia, neovascularization, vitreous hemorrhage, and traction retinal detachment.
- Screen all diabetic patients with an annual dilated ophthalmologic examination.

2.12 OPTIC DISC DISORDERS

OVERVIEW

The optic nerve carries visual information received from the retina to the occipital lobe of the brain (Figure 2.17). Damage to this nerve related to disease is broadly categorized as optic neuropathy. In most cases, optic neuropathy involves monocular vision loss and optic nerve swelling seen on funduscopic examination. Multiple systemic diseases affect the optic nerve to include systemic lupus erythematosus (SLE), sarcoidosis, and MS. A list of systemic conditions and medications that have ocular manifestations such as optic neuropathy may be found in Section 2.15 Ocular Disorders and Systemic Disease, and Table 2.3.

EPIDEMIOLOGY

Optic neuritis is the most common form of optic neuropathy, particularly in younger adults.[33] This is due to its close association with MS, which usually presents in the third or fourth decade of life. ION, on the other hand, is seen more frequently in older individuals.

PATHOPHYSIOLOGY

The optic nerve is divided into four segments based on location. Moving in the direction from the globe to the brain, the intraocular region contains the optic disc, defined by unmyelinated retinal ganglion cell axons. This is the aspect seen on funduscopy. The intraocular section is followed by the intraorbital section as the nerve exits the globe. It becomes myelinated and surrounded by the meningeal layers, which are contiguous from the sclera to the brain. Entering the optic foramen, the intracanalicular segment passes through the optic canal at the back of the orbit into the cranial vault. The intracranial section crosses

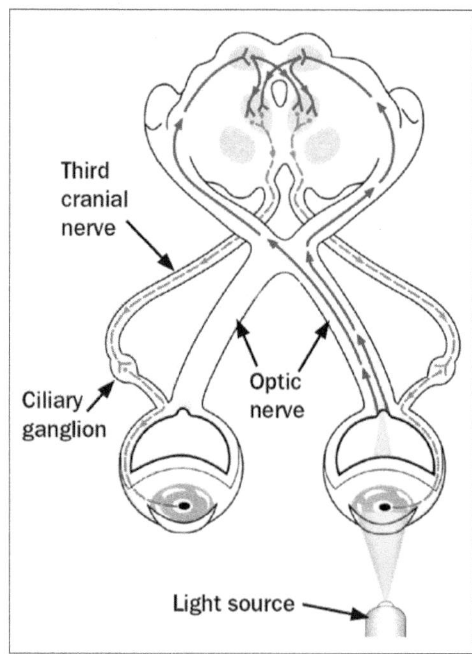

Figure 2.17 Pupil reflex pathway.

(Source: Reproduced with permission from the American Academy of Ophthalmology)

TABLE 2.3 Systemic Diseases and Their Ocular Manifestations

Systemic Disease	Ocular Manifestation
Toxoplasmosis	Posterior uveitis, vitreal leukocytosis
Migraine	Scintillating scotomas, visual field defects, homonymous hemianopia
Polycythemia vera	Retinal vein dilation, retinal hemorrhages, conjunctival injection
Metastatic carcinoma	Vision loss from tumor growth
Sjögren syndrome	Dry eyes, corneal ulcerations
Rheumatoid arthritis	Dry eyes, scleritis, uveitis
Juvenile rheumatoid arthritis	Anterior uveitis, cataract formation
Polyarteritis or periarteritis nodosa	Dry eyes, corneal ulcers, scleritis
Systemic lupus erythematosus	Dry eyes, anterior uveitis, retinal vasculitis, vision loss related to optic neuritis
Sarcoidosis	Anterior uveitis, posterior uveitis, dry eyes, eyelid granulomas, optic neuropathy
Giant cell (temporal) arteritis	Acute vision loss
Leukemia	Edema of optic disc, retinal hemorrhages
Sickle cell anemia	Retinal arterial occlusions, retinal ischemia, retinal neovascularization
Ankylosing spondylitis	Anterior uveitis, vision loss
Thyroid disorders	Exophthalmos/proptosis
Myasthenia gravis	Diplopia, ptosis
Intracranial hypertension	Papilledema, vision loss
Multiple sclerosis	Optic neuritis
AIDS	Cytomegalovirus retinitis
Stroke, basilar artery	Horizontal gaze palsy, horizontal conjugate gaze palsy, ophthalmoplegia
Stroke, posterior vertebral artery	Hemianopia
Syphilis	Uveitis, posterior and panuveitis
Medications	
Thioridazine	Retinitis pigmentosa, corneal infiltrates
Chloroquine	Amblyopia, loss of accommodation, decreased vision, retinopathy, visual field defects, corneal opacity, macular degeneration (may be irreversible)
Hydroxychloroquine	Retinopathy
Tamoxifen	Cataract formation
Ethambutol	Optic neuropathy, specifically red-green color blindness
Isoniazid	Optic neuritis, atrophy
Fluoroquinolones	Retinal detachment (direct relationship not established)
Infliximab	Optic neuropathy

the optic chiasm with fibers from the medial aspect of the nerve crossing over to the contralateral side of the brain. Insult to any aspect of the optic nerve can lead to symptomatic vision loss and ocular nerve palsy.

2.12A OPTIC NEURITIS

MEDICAL HISTORY AND CLINICAL PRESENTATION

Optic neuritis is a demyelinating condition highly associated with MS. More than half of all patients with MS will have an episode of optic neuritis during their lifetime. Neuritis is often the first presenting sign of MS and thus warrants a thorough investigation for this disease once it is identified. Patients are generally younger at presentation and female.

SIGNS AND SYMPTOMS

The classic presentation involves monocular vision loss that worsens over days to weeks. Vision loss is rarely complete, but rather a noticeable decrease in acuity. Patients may also complain of visual scotomas. Bilateral neuritis is possible but not common. Mild pain may be noted, which is often worse with eye movement.

PHYSICAL EXAMINATION

The hallmark physical examination finding is the Marcus Gunn pupil. This is an afferent pupillary defect identified when a light is sequentially shined in both eyes and a sluggish response to direct light and alternative brisk response to consensual light is noted in the affected eye. This is accompanied by diminished visual acuity. Visual field defects may also be appreciated. Disturbed color vision may also be noted.

DIFFERENTIAL DIAGNOSIS

The differential diagnosis includes other causes of monocular vision loss such as retinal vein occlusion, retinal artery occlusion, angle closure glaucoma, tumor, and stroke. As with many of the conditions noted throughout this chapter, suspicion of optic neuritis should prompt a same-day referral to an ophthalmologist for detailed eye examination.

DIAGNOSTIC STUDIES

Optic neuritis is a clinical diagnosis made by a thorough history and physical examination. Contrast-enhanced MRI of the orbits and brain should still be a standard part of the workup. Imaging may reveal optic nerve inflammation and cerebral white matter lesions. Lumbar puncture (LP) may also be indicated if the diagnosis of MS is in doubt or if the MRI is normal. CSF analysis revealing oligoclonal IgG bands is highly indicative of MS.

TREATMENT

- IV corticosteroids are the mainstay of therapy for acute optic neuritis, lasting up to 2 weeks.
- Further management of MS with immune modulating agents should be considered by neurology.

PATIENT EDUCATION

- Patients can be reassured that recovery of vision is common, even in the absence of treatment.

2.12B ISCHEMIC OPTIC NEUROPATHY

MEDICAL HISTORY AND CLINICAL PRESENTATION

The best example of ION is GCA. ION may be idiopathic with no appreciable underlying cause despite optic disc edema and evidence of ischemia on exam. GCA is a vasculitis primarily affecting the large and medium sized arteries of the body. It primarily affects elderly patients and is exceedingly rare in patients under the age of 50.

SIGNS AND SYMPTOMS

Patients with GCA will complain of headache, scalp tenderness, and vision loss. They may also have polyarthritis and jaw stiffness. GCA is associated with polymyalgia rheumatica.

PHYSICAL EXAMINATION

On physical examination, the scalp should be tender on the same side as the affected eye. A funduscopic examination should be completed and may reveal a pale, swollen optic disc. Absence of these findings by the primary care PA should not delay management if suspicion is high. Prompt treatment is critical to maintenance of vision.

DIFFERENTIAL DIAGNOSIS

The differential diagnosis includes all other causes of acute, monocular vision loss as noted under Section 2.12A Optic Neuritis, subsection Differential Diagnosis.

DIAGNOSTIC STUDIES

Biopsy of the temporal artery is the mainstay of definitive diagnosis, but elevation of ESR or C-reactive protein (CRP) is suggestive of disease. Given the risk of permanent vision loss, delaying treatment for a biopsy is not recommended.

TREATMENT

- Treatment involves high-dose corticosteroids tapered over 6 to 12 months.
- Low-dose aspirin may prevent ischemic events and should be used unless contraindicated.
- Tocilizumab, an interleukin 6 receptor antagonist, can be used alone or in combination with corticosteroids.
- Prognosis is based on the amount of vision loss determined on presentation prior to initiation of steroids.
- Patients with normal vision at initial evaluation usually do not suffer any permanent vision abnormalities.

SPECIAL CONSIDERATIONS

- Bilateral GCA is rare at presentation but GCA may evolve to include both eyes. Conversely, bilateral symptoms should not preclude the diagnosis.

KEY POINTS

- Optic neuritis is most common among adults 20 to 40 years of age; the most common causes are demyelinating diseases, such as MS.
- Findings in optic neuritis include mild pain with eye movement, visual disturbances, and afferent pupillary defect.
- Treatment of optic neuritis includes corticosteroids.

- GCA is a common large artery vasculitis and manifestations include headache, jaw claudication, temporal artery tenderness, and constitutional symptoms.
- In GCA an elevated ESR is noted, and diagnosis is made by temporal artery biopsy.
- Treatment of GCA consists of immediately starting corticosteroids, low-dose aspirin, and tocilizumab.

2.13 TRAUMA

OVERVIEW

Ocular trauma is a common chief complaint in urgent and emergency care settings. Furthermore, ocular trauma is often overlooked as a cause of vision loss due to delay in treatment, misdiagnosis, or lack of follow-up, particularly if other injuries are present concomitantly. When assessing a patient for ocular trauma, it is important to understand the basic anatomic structures of the eye as well as how to tell if they are damaged (Figure 2.18). Identification of emergent diagnoses requiring early ophthalmology involvement is critical to the prevention of long-term disability.

EPIDEMIOLOGY

In the United States, ocular trauma is far more prevalent in men with a male-to-female ratio of 4.6:1, reaching 7.4:1 in the fourth decade of life. Ocular trauma is seen throughout all ages, with a prevalence in young adult and adolescent males.[36] Common mechanisms include direct impact from baseballs, softballs, and even bats.

PATHOPHYSIOLOGY

Traumatic ocular injuries result from blunt or penetrating trauma impacting the globe, orbit, or supporting structures of the eye. For a detailed discussion on the internal structures of the eye, see Section 2.11 Retinal Disorders, subsection Pathophysiology. The lid and lacrimal apparatus, which may also be injured by trauma, are discussed in Section 2.1 Disorders of the Lids/Lacrimal Apparatus. The orbit is composed of the frontal, zygomatic, maxillary, sphenoid, ethmoid, palatine, and lacrimal bones. The weakest of these structures is the orbital floor, made up of the maxillary and zygomatic bones. Although fractures can occur anywhere along the orbit, the relative thinness of the maxillary bone causes this to be a common site of disruption during trauma. The orbit is protected anteriorly by the orbital septum, a membrane that projects forward from the periosteum to the tarsal plate. The space between the globe and the bony structure is occupied by fat, the seven extraocular muscles, and the ocular nerve exiting the back of the orbit.

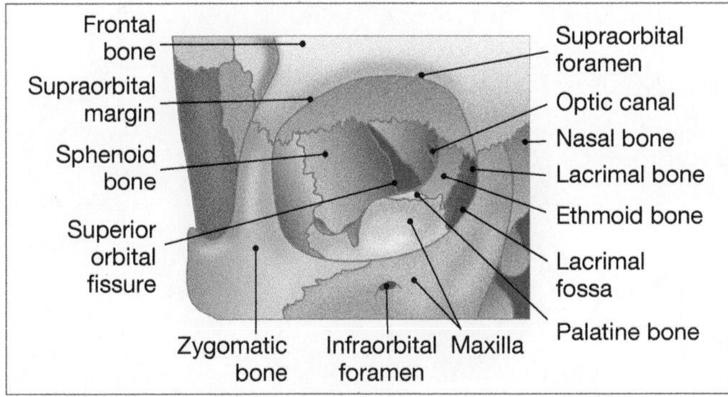

Figure 2.18 Bones of the orbit.

(Source: Melnyk J, Zeno R, Teall AM. Evidence-based assessment of the eye. In: Gawlik KS, Melnyk BM, Teall AM, eds. Evidence-Based Physical Examination. *Springer Publishing Company; 2021:308, Fig. 12.2.)*

2.13A BLOWOUT FRACTURES

MEDICAL HISTORY AND CLINICAL PRESENTATION

A blowout fracture refers specifically to an orbital fracture involving the orbital floor. As noted above, the orbital floor comprises the zygoma and maxillary bones, and is relatively weak when compared to the other aspects of the orbit. As such, anterior force from an object is directed inferiorly leading to a "blowout" of the orbital floor. The inferior rectus muscle runs across the orbital floor. It is important to recognize this injury early, as a delay in diagnosis can lead to permanent damage secondary to the entrapped inferior rectus muscle and increased edema and hemorrhage resulting in loss of muscle function.[37]

Patients will often present to the ED immediately for evaluation of this injury, complaining of pain, swelling, possible change in vision, and difficulty with extraocular movements. As in any other patient assessment, obtaining a detailed history of present illness will help aid in identifying a blowout fracture. Depending on the patient's clinical condition, the history may be obtained from the patient, a witness to the incident, or the emergency medical team that transported the patient.

For patients able to participate in the examination, specific questions may help reveal the extent of injury. Asking where the pain is located may help identify an orbital hematoma, which will cause pain globally across the eye and orbit, as opposed to localized pain in a region of the orbit, which may accompany a corresponding orbital rim fracture. Numbness, tingling, or vision loss are clues to nerve damage. Vision loss obviously implies insult to the ocular nerve, but numbness to the superior or inferior regions of the orbit should raise concern respectively for a supra- or infraorbital nerve injury. Double vision, particularly when associated with movement, is indicative of an extraocular muscle injury.

SIGNS AND SYMPTOMS

The list of signs and symptoms present depend on the severity of the injury and the presence or absence of other ocular trauma. Orbital pain with and without palpation, swelling, and periorbital ecchymosis may be present even with relatively minor injuries. Crepitus could indicate fracture or orbital emphysema due to significant injury and sinus involvement. Decreased sensation, inability to look up with affected eye, and diplopia are markers of neuromuscular damage. The patient may also have a hyphema, discussed further below. Enophthalmos is the term for posterior displacement of the eye. The patient may complain of nausea and vomiting. This is due to the oculovagal reflex (oculocardiac reflex) which can induce nausea, vomiting, hypotension, and bradycardia as secondary to ocular muscle swelling or tight entrapment putting pressure on the globe.[38]

PHYSICAL EXAMINATION

The initial step of this physical examination should be assessment of visual acuity. With time and increased swelling, the patient may be unable to open their eye to adequately test vision. The clinician should assess for swelling, periocular ecchymosis, obvious deformity, and enophthalmos. Hypotropia may also be evident. This is an inferior positioning of the affected eye, a sunken appearance from the globe falling into the inferior orbital floor defect.

Assessing pupillary reactivity, size, and shape should be assessed and documented. Attention should then turn to evaluation of extraocular movements, specifically looking for muscle entrapment. The inferior rectus muscle can be presumed entrapped when the affected eye has a limited upgaze. If there is evidence of muscle entrapment, this makes the diagnosis more urgent, whereas a blowout fracture without muscle entrapment often results in nonoperative or delayed surgical management.[39]

DIFFERENTIAL DIAGNOSIS

The differential diagnosis should include alternative or additional orbital fractures and disruptions of the globe such as hyphema.

DIAGNOSTIC STUDIES

A CT scan of the orbits is necessary to confirm the presence of a fracture (Figure 2.19).

TREATMENT

- The role of the clinician is to identify potential vision-threatening trauma and to consult an eye specialist accordingly.
- While many blowout fractures are treated nonoperatively, this decision is ultimately made by the ophthalmologist and/or maxillofacial surgeon.
- The presence of muscle entrapment, enophthalmos, or an oculovagal reflex means the need for urgent surgical fixation is more likely. In most cases, however, surgical fixation is delayed 7–10 days.
- Patients should be instructed to avoid nose blowing, straining, or any other maneuvers that increase pressure in the face and orbit.
- Medication for pain control and antiemetics should be distributed if necessary.
- Tetanus prophylaxis should be provided in the ED.[40]

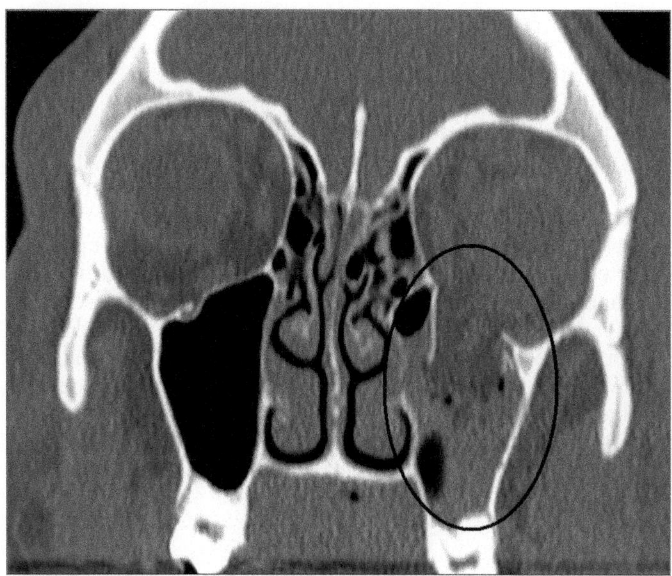

Figure 2.19 CT scan of the orbits revealing orbital fracture. *(Source: James Heilman, MD.)*

PATIENT EDUCATION

- It is important for patients to maintain close follow-up with the ophthalmologist and/or maxillofacial surgeon for ongoing management and monitoring.
- The patient must also understand the importance of updating their ophthalmologist with any changes in symptoms, especially new vision changes, pain with eye movement, or loss of eye movement, as these things suggest acute worsening.

2.13B GLOBE RUPTURE

MEDICAL HISTORY AND CLINICAL PRESENTATION

Globe rupture is defined as a splitting or tearing of the cornea and/or sclera due to blunt eye trauma. Ruptures involve rapid change in intraocular pressure. Like blowout fractures above, pressure escapes at areas of weakness. These include the limbus, insertion of the optic nerve, and locations of previous eye surgery.[41] Although rupture can occur anywhere along the eye, these are the more common sites. Penetrating injuries are generally discussed alongside globe ruptures. Penetrating injuries, as the name suggest, result from a sharp object or projectile piercing the surface of the eye.

Patients with open globe injuries will typically present with a history of blunt trauma or a penetrating injury. Common mechanisms include shrapnel or pellet fragments from a shotgun, worksite accidents, and blunt force from a ball. Patients may be unable to provide the detailed information due to the traumatic nature of the injury; thus, the clinician should obtain information from family members or bystanders when possible.

SIGNS AND SYMPTOMS

The presentation of a globe injury may be rather striking. Pupillary distortion, a "teardrop pupil," may be seen and typically points toward the wound. Intraocular contents may also be visible (Figure 2.20). Patients will likely complain of pain and vision alteration.

The pupils should be closely evaluated for their size, shape, and symmetry as well as their response to direct and consensual light. The patient may require conscious sedation for evaluation of the eye injury, specifically in the pediatric population. It is important to be aware during the physical

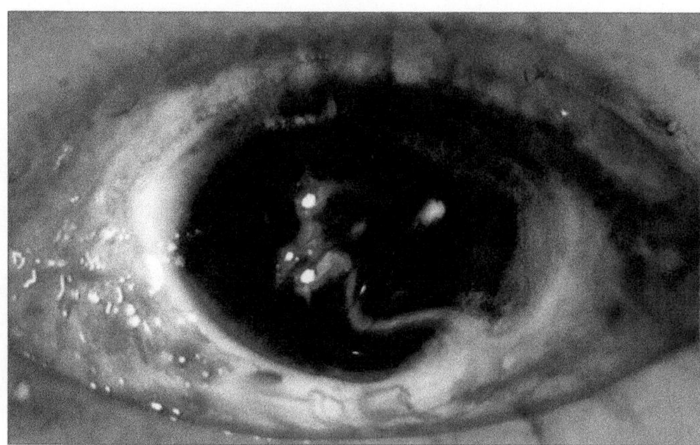

Figure 2.20 Pupillary distortion following orbital globe injury. *(Source: S. Bhimji, MD.)*

examination to exclude anything that would increase IOP such as attempting to obtain ocular pressure with tonometry or performing lid retraction. The clinician should avoid using any eye drops or stains as well as applying any direct pressure to the eye if a globe rupture is suspected.

PHYSICAL EXAMINATION

As with any trauma, the assessment of the patient should always start with identifying and treating any life-threatening injuries. Once this has been completed, the clinician can then focus attention on the specific eye trauma. If the patient's clinical status allows, visual acuity should be obtained from each eye using the Snellen acuity chart. If a Snellen chart is not available, the clinician may ask the patient to identify a number of fingers or motion of fingers.

Obvious signs of an open globe include a flat anterior chamber, extraocular protrusion of uveal tissue, a profoundly soft eye, extrusion of vitreous humor, retained foreign body, ecchymosis, proptosis, or visible lacerations.[41] Other signs include hemorrhagic chemosis, intraocular blood (hyphema or vitreous hemorrhage), and low IOP. Extreme caution should be taken to avoid further damage to the eye or loss of intraocular volume. Certain aspects of the exam, including palpation and manipulation of the lids, should be delayed for suspected globe injury. Instillation of anesthetic agents or fluorescein stain should be likewise avoided.

DIFFERENTIAL DIAGNOSIS

The differential diagnosis includes subconjunctival hemorrhage, nontraumatic bloody chemosis, and corneal-scleral laceration.[42] Emergent consultation with an ophthalmologist for patients with globe injury, both blunt and penetrating, is very important.

DIAGNOSTIC STUDIES

A non-contrast CT of the head should be obtained if assessing for intraorbital foreign body. Such a decision can be guided by the history of injury.

TREATMENT

- Globe rupture requires emergent consultation with an ophthalmologist for evaluation and surgical repair.
- In the emergency setting, the clinician should place a protective eye shield over the eye.
- IV antibiotics are administered, including vancomycin plus ceftazidime or vancomycin plus a fluoroquinolone.[41]
- Tetanus vaccine should be administered.
- Antiemetic and analgesic medications should be administered to prevent vomiting and control pain.
- The patient should then be placed on strict bed rest with head of bed elevated 30 degrees if not contraindicated from any other traumatic injuries.
- In the operating room, depolarizing agents (e.g., succinylcholine) should be avoided as they can lead to increased IOP and extrusion of intraocular contents.[1]
- Once general anesthesia has been induced the ophthalmologist will then closely inspect the injury to obtain a better understanding of the extent of the injury and to make the appropriate surgical decisions.
- Any tissues outside the wound may be replaced inside the eye if there is no evidence of necrosis or gross contamination.
- Corneal ruptures are then closed, and antibiotics and corticosteroids are often injected subconjunctivally.
- Eye drops are typically prescribed postoperatively.[43]

PATIENT EDUCATION

- Patients need to be informed of the signs and symptoms of potential postoperative complications, which include, but are not limited to, infection, recurrent bleeding, and leaking from the wounds.
- It is important to remind the patient and those involved in patient care to avoid any increase in IOP, especially from direct external pressure of the eye, as this can increase the risk of further extrusion of ocular contents.

2.13C HYPHEMA

MEDICAL HISTORY AND CLINICAL PRESENTATION

A hyphema describes an accumulation of blood in the anterior chamber of the eye due to injury of the blood vessels supplying the iris or ciliary body (Figure 2.21). This injury is often the result of blunt trauma to the eye but can also be atraumatic (spontaneous) in nature due to sickle cell disease, ocular tumors, blood thinning medications, and other bleeding diathesis. In young children, the mechanism is often from contact by a blunt object such as a baseball or soccer ball to the eye. In teenagers and adults, a traumatic hyphema more often occurs from a direct blow to the eye from an assault. They can also occur from other mechanisms like paintballs (in the absence of eye protection), airbag deployment, projectiles resulting in penetrating trauma, and bungee cords.[44]

Patients will present with pain, vision changes (often blurred vision), and light sensitivity.[37] In most cases, there is obvious accumulation of blood in the anterior chamber of the eye. However, a microhyphema may be present, with blood being visible only on slit-lamp examination. Inquiring about a personal or family history of sickle cell disease, use of anticoagulants, or any personal or family history of bleeding disorders is imperative even in the setting of known trauma. The clinician should ask about previous episodes and, if so, how recent. Traumatic hyphemas are at risk for rebleeding, with the greatest risk occurring 3–5 days after initial injury.

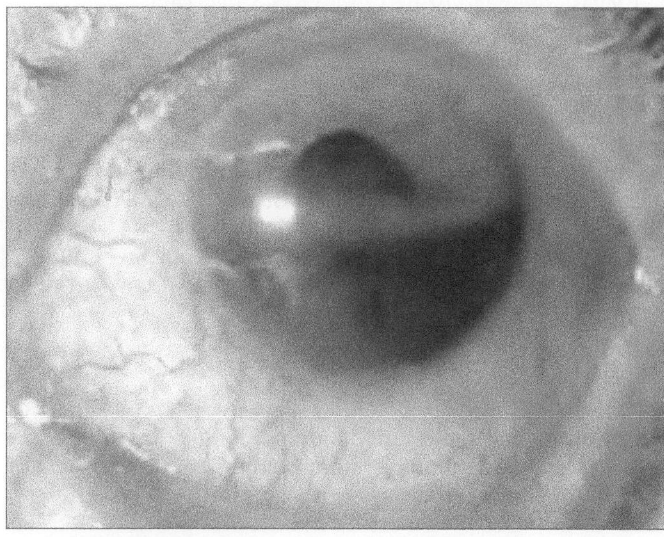

Figure 2.21 Hyphema.
(Source: Courtesy of Rakesh Ahuja.)

SIGNS AND SYMPTOMS

As noted previously, eye pain (especially with pupillary constriction), vision changes (depending on height of hyphema), and light sensitivity are the three primary symptoms. A visible accumulation of blood in the anterior chamber may be accompanied by abnormal IOP.

PHYSICAL EXAMINATION

Assuming a hyphema is readily identified by inspection, it can be graded I–IV (IV being the most severe) based on the percentage of anterior chamber filling.[44] If possible, the patient should be evaluated in an upright position when assessing for a hyphema, as they tend to level out when supine, making the diagnosis more challenging. If a hyphema is suspected but difficult to visualize on clinical exam, it is possible the patient has a microhyphema, which can be visualized on slit-lamp examination. The slit-lamp examination also allows for exact measurement of the height of the hyphema in millimeters. The height of the hyphema will determine the severity of injury. Hyphemas may be evidence of an open globe injury and examination, particularly any palpation, should be done with caution.

DIFFERENTIAL DIAGNOSIS

The differential diagnosis includes traumatic iritis, open globe injury, vitreous hemorrhage, iridodialysis, scleral rupture, and corneal abrasion.

DIAGNOSTIC STUDIES

The diagnosis is clinical based on the mechanism of injury and physical examination findings. However, additional head, ocular, or facial injuries may require further evaluation to include a CT of the head or ultrasound of the eye. For spontaneous hyphemas, laboratory studies should be obtained to include CBC, prothrombin time (PT), activated partial thromboplastin time (aPTT), and international normalized ratio (INR).

TREATMENT

- The goal of treatment is to prevent increased IOP and rebleeding. This includes placement of an eye shield over the affected eye.
- Identification of hyphema should prompt a consultation with an ophthalmologist.
- Elevate the head of bed to 30 to 45 degrees.
- Achieve pain control with topical analgesics such as tetracaine or proparacaine, for short term use only.
- Avoid oral analgesia with antiplatelet properties such as NSAIDs.
- The ophthalmologist may recommend treatment with topical corticosteroids, cycloplegic agents (dilating eye agents) such as cyclopentate 1% or scopolamine 0.25%, antifibrinolytics, and surgery.[42,44]
- The patient may require admission to the hospital for close observation or daily follow-up in the outpatient setting to monitor for any rebleeding.

PATIENT EDUCATION

- Patients must understand the risks as well as the signs and symptoms of rebleeding and maintain close follow-up with the ophthalmologist as rebleeding can often be worse than the initial bleed.
- Any activities that increase eye straining such as screen time and reading should be avoided.

SPECIAL CONSIDERATIONS

- Antibiotic prophylaxis may be indicated for blowout fractures if the fracture involves a sinus. All blowout fractures with a normal initial eye examination in the ED warrant close follow-up with an ophthalmologist to ensure there is no evidence of a retinal tear or detachment.[37]
- If a hyphema is suspected but difficult to see on supine examination, sit the patient in an upright position and you will see filling of the anterior chamber if a hyphema is present. If the trauma patient is unable to sit upright, then evaluate for any slight differences in iris color as this can be indicative of a hyphema.

KEY POINTS

- Globe trauma may cause globe laceration, lens dislocation, glaucoma, vitreous hemorrhage, or retinal damage.
- Globe rupture should be suspected if trauma results in a visible corneal or scleral laceration, leaking aqueous humor, an unusually shallow or deep anterior chamber, or an irregular pupil.
- Hyphema is diagnosed by slit-lamp examination, requires bed rest with head elevation at 30 to 45 degrees, and monitoring of IOP.
- Refer patients for surgical repair of blowout fractures that cause diplopia or unacceptable enophthalmos.

2.14 VISION ABNORMALITIES

OVERVIEW

Vision is one of the five senses, and alterations or decreases in the ability to see will have dramatic effects on daily living and interpersonal interactions. As an example, decrease in night vision from cataracts (see Section 2.5 Cataracts) may lead to hesitancy around driving at night, which in turn may make an individual with cataracts reluctant to plan activities at or near the end of the day. While most of this chapter focuses on acquired forms of vision loss in adults, this topic will focus on vision loss related to developmental abnormalities and amblyopia.

EPIDEMIOLOGY

The majority of vision loss occurs in the later stages of life as acquired disease. Both cataracts and macular degeneration—two of the leading causes of blindness—have predilections for older patients. Problems like strabismus or even retinoblastoma may, on the other hand, lead to diminished visual acuity at younger ages. Below is a description of just some of the causes of abnormal vision along with their associated examination findings and treatment recommendations. Discussion of vision changes or loss of vision should be a component of every eye examination.

PATHOPHYSIOLOGY

For a detailed discussion on the physiology of vision, see Section 2.11 Retinal Disorders. Any disruption along the visual pathway can alter vision, either acutely or chronically, temporarily or permanently.

2.14A AMAUROSIS FUGAX

MEDICAL HISTORY AND CLINICAL PRESENTATION

The term amaurosis fugax (AF) refers to transient vision loss. AF can affect one or both eyes and can result from a variety of conditions. AF is not a diagnosis, but rather a symptom. Clues to the underlying cause may be identified in the history: monocular versus binocular vision loss, duration of vision loss, complete loss versus visual field defects.

Many clinicians discuss AF exclusively as an aspect of cerebral ischemia, specifically transient ischemic attacks (TIAs). Patients with underlying vascular risks including diabetes, hypertension, and previous TIA are believed to be at risk of developing AF. Conversely, diagnosis of AF is a risk factor for cerebrovascular disease. As many as 18% of patients with AF have concomitant carotid artery stenosis.[45] Nevertheless, the investigation of AF should include nonvascular causes of vision loss.

SIGNS AND SYMPTOMS

Transient vision loss is usually monocular, but this needs to be established by visual acuity and visual field testing. Homonymous hemianopia involves a binocular visual field defect on the medial side of one eye and the temporal side of the other eye. Bipolar hemianopia involves binocular visual field defects along the temporal regions of both eyes. Binocular vision loss suggests origin of disease behind the optic chiasm. The duration of vision loss is also important. Fleeting vision loss may be evidence of intracranial hypertension and optic disc swelling. Longer durations of vision loss may be due to TIA. Localized symptoms such as eye pain indicate a source within the globe, whereas systemic signs and symptoms like fever or altered mental status may be more indicative of an intracranial process.

PHYSICAL EXAMINATION

The physical examination should be directed by the history, but at a minimum it should involve pupillary response to light and accommodation, extraocular muscle function, and funduscopic evaluation to detect optic disc swelling (papilledema), retinal ischemia, or vitreous hemorrhage.

DIFFERENTIAL DIAGNOSIS

The differential diagnosis includes such problems as GCA, angle closure glaucoma, retinal artery occlusion, retinal vein occlusion, optic neuritis, TIA, carotid artery disease, intercranial tumor, orbital abscess or tumor, migraine, and retinal detachment. A detailed history and physical examination may help narrow the list and provide for a sound referral when consulting an ophthalmologist. All patients with transient vision loss should have an evaluation by an ophthalmologist. Consultations should also involve a neurologist and cardiologist if evidence points toward an ischemic disorder.

DIAGNOSTIC STUDIES

The workup should include an evaluation of possible vascular causes. ESR and platelet count are used to evaluate for possible GCA. Ultrasound is used to evaluate blood flow in the carotids and retina blood flow. MRI is needed to evaluate neurologic etiologies, such as MS.

TREATMENT

- Treatments are guided by underlying disorder.

PATIENT EDUCATION

- Patients with transient vision loss should be encouraged to follow all instructions regarding follow-up and referrals.
- Despite being transient, AF may be a predictor of future events and should not be ignored.

2.14B STRABISMUS

MEDICAL HISTORY AND CLINICAL PRESENTATION

Strabismus refers quite simply to misalignment of the eyes. It can be intermittent or constant, acquired or congenital, and affects roughly 2% of the pediatric population. For the vast majority of clinicians practicing outside ophthalmology, the primary goal is to recognize such a misalignment, and to make a referral to an ophthalmologist when appropriate.[46]

The specific causes of strabismus are myriad and depend on the direction of strabismus. Duane syndrome, for instance, is a congenital problem that results from abnormal development of the sixth cranial nerve. Type I causes an esotropic deviation, while type II causes an exotropic deviation. The vast majority of cases of strabismus are horizontal.[46] Vertical strabismus (hyper- and hypotropic) may be attributed to muscle palsies, acute fracture of the bony orbit, and even Graves disease in adults.

Risk factors include family history of strabismus, low birth weight, associated vision disorders, cerebral palsy, and muscular dystrophy.

SIGNS AND SYMPTOMS

Parents may note the appearance of "crossed eyes" at the routine wellness exams of preverbal children (Figure 2.22). This must be distinguished from pseudostrabismus, the illusion of eye misalignment caused by a wide nasal bridge or overlapping epicanthal folds. Vision abnormalities may be noted on older children during Snellen eye test.

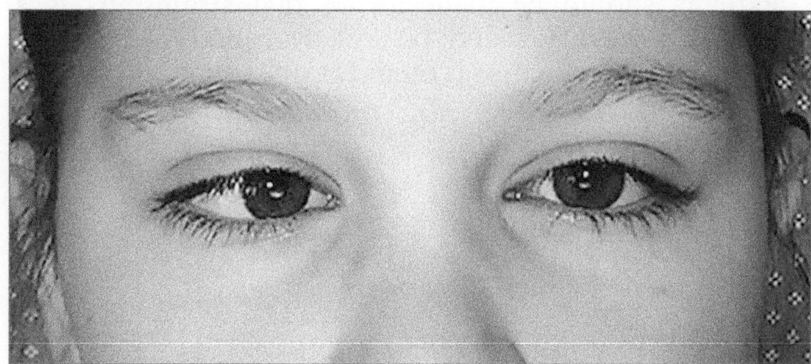

Figure 2.22 Strabismus.
(Source: Guida KM. Advanced health assessment of the eyes and ears. In: Myrick KM, Karosas LM, eds. Advanced Health Assessment and Differential Diagnosis. *Springer Publishing Company; 2021:82, Fig. 4.37.)*

PHYSICAL EXAMINATION

The normal pediatric wellness examination should include the corneal light reflex, or Hirschberg test. In this test, a light is held centrally a few feet from the patient's eyes. Light reflecting off the corneas should do so at approximately the same locations if both eyes are aligned properly. If light reflects closer to the medial aspect of the cornea, this indicates a lateral deviation of the eye and vice versa.

Additional to the corneal light reflex, the cover test may be performed. Here, the patient fixates on a target (a toy) held directly ahead. One eye is covered for 1–2 seconds while the uncovered eye is observed for movement. Movement indicates refocusing and the presence of a tropia. If the covered eye refocuses once the cover is removed, this is more indicative of a phoria. This second aspect is also known as the cover/uncover test.

DIFFERENTIAL DIAGNOSIS

The differential diagnosis includes pseudostrabismus. This is a false appearance of strabismus typically noted in infants with a bridge of the nose that wide and flat causing the appearance of strabismus.

DIAGNOSTIC STUDIES

This is a clinical diagnosis. No laboratory testing is required.

EVALUATION

Any abnormality of either the cover, cover/uncover, or corneal light reflex test should prompt referral to a pediatric eye specialist in a patient over the age of 6 months. Infants from newborn to 6 months may have intermittent deviation known as ocular instability of infancy and need continued monitoring rather than immediate referral. The ophthalmologist examination should be comprehensive and include more detailed testing of refraction and the need for correction

TREATMENT

- Treatment of strabismus varies based on the exact cause and amount of deviation present.
- Current strategies include regular follow-up and monitoring if both depth perception and binocular vision are intact, occlusion of the unaffected eye, correction of refractive errors with glasses, and surgery to alter extraocular muscles.

PATIENT EDUCATION

- Patients should be made aware that strabismus is a treatable condition and very likely will resolve. If left untreated, the major complication of strabismus is amblyopia.

2.14C AMBLYOPIA

MEDICAL HISTORY AND CLINICAL PRESENTATION

Amblyopia refers to a reduction in visual acuity that results from developmental abnormalities. If both eyes are presented with different pictures that cannot be aligned, the brain in turn "shuts off" signals from the weaker, nonaligned eye. The term amblyopia is often confused with strabismus. Furthermore, some references note that amblyopia causes strabismus, a factual error that highlights the need for proper understanding of medical terminology as it relates to the eyes. In fact, amblyopia can result from several problems that are divided into three categories: refractive amblyopia, strabismic amblyopia, and deprivational amblyopia.

SIGNS AND SYMPTOMS

For a detailed discussion of the signs, symptoms, and clinical presentation of strabismus, see the preceding Section 2.14A Strabismus. Refractive amblyopia occurs in the setting of asymmetric refractive error, leading to image discrepancy between eyes. Patients often have no symptoms so long as the other eye is compensating. Deprivational amblyopia is the result of vision loss related to pathology along the visual axis. In other words, a retinoblastoma or congenital cataract may cause a deprivational amblyopia. Patients presenting with this form of vision loss will have signs and symptoms related to the underlying disease (see Section 2.12 Optic Neuropathy).

PHYSICAL EXAMINATION

The physical findings associated with amblyopia vary by age and the patient's ability to communicate verbally. Patients over the age of 3 will be able to adequately perform visual acuity testing with an eye chart either with letters, numbers, or recognizable shapes. Clinicians should suspect amblyopia if either eye is 20/40 in a child between the ages of 3 and 5, or 20/30 in a child age 6 or older.[47] Additionally, a difference in acuity of greater than two lines between eyes is suggestive of amblyopia.

Visual acuity in children under 3 is tested by visual fixation. Similar to the test for strabismus, an object is held in front of the patient and moved slowly while the clinician monitors for visual fixation. The ability to maintain a fixed gaze suggests adequate acuity. Alternatively, monitoring a child's response to covering each of the child's eyes can help identify an amblyopic eye. Patients may become agitated or upset when the functioning eye is covered leaving only the weaker eye for vision.

DIFFERENTIAL DIAGNOSIS

The differential diagnosis includes acquired or congenital exotropia, acquired or accommodative esotropia, or congenital ptosis.

DIAGNOSTIC STUDIES

No laboratory studies are indicated; the diagnosis is based on clinical findings.

EVALUATION

Screening for amblyopia is recommended in all children before starting school, typically before age 3.

Photoscreening can be used in young children and those unable to undergo subjective testing because of learning or developmental disorders. In older children screening consists of acuity testing with figures, which do not require knowing the alphabet, or Snellen eye charts.

TREATMENT

- Treatment depends on the underlying cause of the amblyopia but includes correction in any deprivational issues, such as cataracts or tumors, for example.

- This is followed by correction of any refraction error with prescription lenses and a detailed patching routine that encourages use of the amblyopic eye by removing visual input from the stronger eye.

PATIENT EDUCATION

- Astute clinicians should discuss examination techniques as they are being performed so parents better understand the results. For example, explaining the purpose of the fixation test and what is being evaluated will facilitate a more productive conversation when lack of fixation in an eye is identified, and a referral must be made.
- The potential consequences of withholding or delaying treatment when problems are identified is also critical. When parents are involved in the treatment plan, they are more likely to comply with modalities like intermittent patching throughout the day or glasses wearing.

2.14D SCLERITIS

MEDICAL HISTORY AND CLINICAL PRESENTATION

Scleritis is an aptly named condition that involves inflammation of the sclera. Patients with scleritis complain of intense, deep-seated eye pain that is worse with movement and worse at night. Like uveitis (Section 2.6), scleritis has a strong association with underlying inflammatory disease, such as rheumatoid arthritis, systemic lupus erythematous, or polyarthritis nodosa.[48] Scleritis can be broken down into four subcategories: necrotizing anterior scleritis, nodular anterior scleritis, diffuse anterior scleritis, and posterior scleritis. The diagnosis of posterior scleritis is often more difficult due to location. Diffuse and nodular anterior scleritis are the most common varieties with diffuse being the least severe. Necrotizing is the most severe.

SIGNS AND SYMPTOMS

Patients with diffuse or nodular anterior scleritis generally present as described above with intense eye pain and redness. Necrotizing anterior scleritis pain is often accompanied by globe tenderness. The pain may also be worse in the morning. Posterior scleritis involves intense eye pain like the other forms but lacks eye redness. Patients may also complain of vision loss.

PHYSICAL EXAMINATION

Diffuse anterior scleritis involves scleral erythema and painful extraocular movements, whereas nodular anterior scleritis is identified by localized, erythematous nodules and notable dilation of the scleral blood vessels (Figure 2.23). Necrotizing scleritis is best seen by an ophthalmologist who, using a slit lamp, may identify scleral thinning. Clinicians may appreciate corneal involvement in the form of ulcerations as well. Inspection for posterior scleritis will be unremarkable, but patients will have painful eye movements as with other forms. Vision loss may also be apparent.

DIFFERENTIAL DIAGNOSIS

The differential diagnosis of scleritis involves all other causes of red eye, including conjunctivitis, uveitis, and angle closure glaucoma. Patients presenting with intense eye pain, tenderness, and pain with movement need immediate consultation with an ophthalmologist and should be referred accordingly.

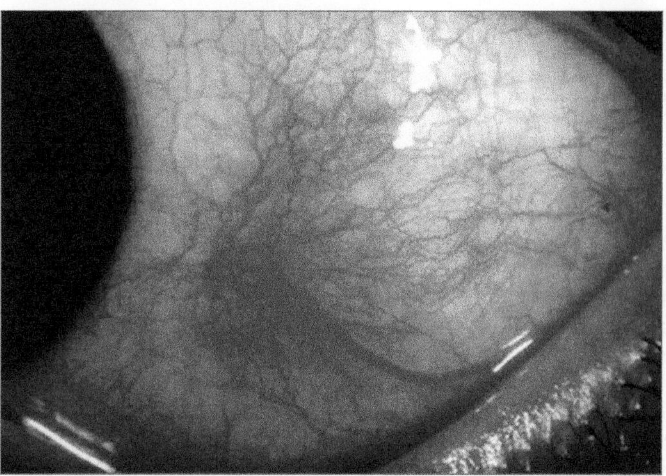

Figure 2.23 Scleritis.
(Source: Image courtesy of Kribz)

DIAGNOSTIC STUDIES

Diagnosis of scleritis is made clinically and with slit-lamp examination. Smears or biopsies may be needed to diagnosis infectious scleritis. CT or ultrasonography may be needed for posterior scleritis.

TREATMENT

- Control of inflammation is paramount to management and generally involves NSAIDs.
- Glucocorticoids may be utilized in more severe cases or when NSAIDs are proving ineffective.
- Immunosuppressive agents, such as cyclophosphamide, methotrexate, or rituximan, are also utilized for severe or unrelenting cases or when systemic symptoms are present.

PATIENT EDUCATION

- Patients diagnosed with scleritis must understand the close association with underlying rheumatologic disease and the need for extensive investigation of such disease even when no prior symptoms or diagnosis were present. This typically involves consultation or follow-up with a rheumatologist.

KEY POINTS

- Strabismus is misalignment of the eyes and causes some vision loss (amblyopia).
- Most cases of strabismus are caused by refractive error or muscle weakness but sometimes due to retinoblastoma or cranial nerve palsy.
- Amblyopia is visual loss in an eye caused by lack of clearly focused, properly aligned input to the visual cortex from each eye during early childhood prior to maturation of the visual pathways. It is diagnosed by screening tests, including photoscreening.
- Scleritis is a severe, vision-threatening inflammation. Treatment is systemic corticosteroids.

2.15 OCULAR DISORDERS AND SYSTEMIC DISEASE

OVERVIEW

The eye structure is an intersection among multiple anatomic systems, ranging from nervous to integumentary, to musculoskeletal, to cardiovascular. A variety of tissue types and smaller, delicate structures must work together to provide vision. As such, the eye is sensitive to insult, and systemic conditions often involve ocular disease manifestations. In some cases, the source of eye symptoms is readily apparent. For example, optic neuritis is strongly associated with MS. In other instances, the list of associated systemic diseases is broad (see Section 2.6 Uveitis). Furthermore, many commonly employed medications cause significant eye side effects.

EPIDEMIOLOGY

There is no unified epidemiologic data representing the entirety of systemic disease and its relationship to the eye. Throughout this chapter, statistical relationships between diseases and eye manifestations are discussed.

PATHOPHYSIOLOGY

The pathophysiology of ocular manifestations is disease specific. For a detailed description of vision, see Section 2.11 Retinal Disorders, subsection Pathophysiology.

MEDICAL HISTORY AND CLINICAL PRESENTATION

Table 2.3 summarizes a brief list of systemic diseases and their ocular manifestations. This list does not include diagnoses discussed elsewhere in this chapter such as diabetic retinopathy or hypertensive retinopathy.

COMMON CHIEF COMPLAINTS

APPROACH TO THE RED EYE

Ocular complaints, such as a "red eye," are common in the primary care setting. Most red eye complaints are benign and can be managed in the clinic. Eye redness can represent serious and sight threatening conditions that require urgent or even emergent referrals to ophthalmology. The best approach to a red eye uses a focused history and physical examination to reveal or rule out alarm symptoms, to assess the acuity of the illness, and to make appropriate management decisions.

The initial history should include the basic facts of the present illness. This includes questions about duration, severity, relieving and aggravating factors, and associated symptoms. Involvement of one or both eyes is also important to document. A review of the red flag signs and symptoms is appropriate (see Box 2.1). Some of these items can be addressed in the history.

Ask the patient or the mother about the following items:

- Was there trauma involved?
  - A positive response should prompt further questions regarding the mechanism and other bodily injuries.
- Is the eye pain severe?
  - The answer to this question should be contextualized to the patient's age. Furthermore, observation for signs of discomfort can provide support for reported pain level. Patients in extreme pain may be tachycardic, diaphoretic, or unable to find a comfortable position. A distressed patient may be holding their eye, may be reluctant to open it, or may even be vomiting.
- Is there any decrease in vision?
  - A careful approach to this question is important. Vision loss should be thoroughly differentiated from blurry vision associated with drainage.
- Is there a foreign body sensation?
  - Patients may detail having tried to flush dirt or sand from the eye.
- Is there any photophobia?
  - This may be evident if the patient is reluctant to open the eye or is wearing dark glasses.

Positive red flags in the history help narrow the differential diagnosis and better guide the physical examination.

- If the patient experiences a foreign body sensation without other alarm symptoms, a noncentral corneal abrasion or ulcer should be suspected. Visual acuity is usually not affected. The patient may be only slightly sensitive to light. Penlight exam may reveal a pinpoint pupil that is reactive to light and accommodation. Fluorescein staining will reveal the size and location of the lesion.
- A foreign body sensation accompanied by decreased vision indicates a more severe corneal process such as a central corneal abrasion or ulcer, uveitis, or keratitis. Visual acuity is usually decreased with keratitis but often normal with a corneal abrasion unless the lesion is central or has an associated iritis. Keratitis or a corneal ulcer will generally be associated with moderate to severe pain. Photophobia is more common in keratitis compared to a corneal abrasion.
  - A foreign body sensation should prompt the clinician to perform a fluorescein exam. Corneal defects are easier to visualize as the fluorescein pools in areas of tissue loss. Lesion characteristics may give further clues to diagnosis. Viral keratitis may involve branching lesions (e.g., herpes simplex) or punctate lesions (e.g., adenovirus). Bacterial keratitis is associated with spherical white opacities on the cornea, and hypopyon, purulent material in the anterior chamber, in severe cases.
- Photophobia is indicative of a corneal or uveal process. In the absence of foreign body sensation, iritis should be higher on the differential diagnosis. The clinician should identify the pattern of redness, pupil shape, and pupil size. Limbic flush is the hallmark sign of iritis (anterior uveitis). Uveal inflammation may alter the shape of the iris, deforming the round shape of the pupil.
- Severe deep, boring pain is suspicious for scleritis. Patients will have constant, severe, boring pain worse at night and early morning. An intensely injected sclera is commonly seen in scleritis.
- Severe eye pain, with associated nausea, vomiting, abdominal pain, and/or visual halos are all alarming findings of angle closure glaucoma. A fixed mid-dilated pupil may be present. Although severe eye pain is more commonly associated with acute angle closure glaucoma, a patient may present with a severe headache instead.

In the absence of red flag items requiring emergent management and referral, the history and physical examination should focus on detailing associated ocular signs and symptoms.

- Is there discharge from the eye? Is it purulent or watery?
  - Self-limiting conditions such as viral and allergic conjunctivitis are associated with a morning crusting followed by watery discharge throughout the day. The discharge may be reported as white, yellow, or purulent that changes to watery discharge as the day progresses. Viral conjunctivitis may present alone or with a prodrome of signs and symptoms to include pharyngitis, runny nose, and sinus congestion. Preauricular lymphadenopathy may be found on physical exam. Bacterial conjunctivitis is associated with white, green, or yellow discharge that is thick and rapidly reappears after wiping. Profuse purulent discharge should prompt the clinician to obtain a sexual history and look for associated signs of sexually transmitted illness. Infections with *N. gonorrhoeae* lead to a hyperacute form of bacterial conjunctivitis that is an ophthalmic emergency.
- Is there any itching?
  - Allergic conjunctivitis is usually associated with itching while viral and bacterial conjunctivitis are not.
- Is there swelling of the eyelid?
  - Focal eyelid swelling that is painful and erythematous should point the clinician toward a hordeolum as the likely diagnosis. In contrast, focal eyelid swelling that is painless and lacks erythema should point the clinician toward a chalazion as the likely diagnosis. Both hordeolum and chalazion can be treated without referral to ophthalmology.
  - Generalized lid swelling and erythema are suspicious for preseptal (periorbital) cellulitis or orbital cellulitis. Pain with eye movement, proptosis, ophthalmoplegia, and diplopia suggest involvement of the orbital structures, particularly orbital abscess or cellulitis.
  - Recurrent subconjunctival hemorrhages should make a clinician suspicious for a bleeding disorder.
- Is the redness generalized or focal?
  - A clinician should be concerned for a scleral process if the redness is focal. Both episcleritis and scleritis are associated with systemic and rheumatologic diseases. An ophthalmology referral may be warranted during a first suspected episode of episcleritis to help differentiate it from the sight-threatening condition scleritis.
- Did an episode of coughing or straining precede the redness?
  - Subconjunctival hemorrhage occurs with trauma to the eye, sneezing, coughing, vomiting, straining, and less commonly, bleeding disorders. It is a painless collection of blood between the sclera and the conjunctiva that results from disruption of the conjunctival blood vessels. The clinician should rule out child abuse in children <12 months old without an identifiable cause.

TABLE 2.4 Differential Diagnosis of a Red Eye

Corneal abrasion	Episcleritis
Corneal ulcer	Orbital cellulitis
Keratitis (bacterial, viral, or fungal)	Preseptal cellulitis
Conjunctivitis (bacterial, viral, or allergic)	Iritis (anterior uveitis)
Endophthalmitis	Hordeolum
Acute angle closure glaucoma	Chalazion
Scleritis	Subconjunctival hemorrhage

DIFFERENTIAL DIAGNOSIS

The presence of any red flag signs or symptoms should prompt consultation with ophthalmology (Table 2.4). In their absence, the diagnosis is guided by a detailed history and physical examination. All patients presenting with eye complaints should have vision assessed prior to examination. Appropriate treatment for each diagnosis can be found by reviewing the specific chapter topics.

See Table 2.5 for a comparison of the common etiologies of the red eye.

TABLE 2.5 Comparison of Common Etiologies of the Red Eye

Disorder	Pupil	Conjunctiva	Pain	Discharge	Cornea	Vision
Allergic conjunctivitis	Normal	Diffuse vessel dilation	Itching	Watery	Normal	Normal
Infectious conjunctivitis	Normal	Diffuse vessel dilation	Mild	Bacterial-purulent	Normal	Normal
Uveitis	Small	Vessel dilation around cornea	Marked photophobia	None	Cloudy anterior chamber	Decreased
Angle closure glaucoma	Mid-dilated	Vessel dilation around cornea	Marked	None	Steamy, shallow angle	Decreased with halos
Subconjunctival hemorrhage	Normal	Hemorrhage	Painless	None	Normal	Normal
Episcleritis	Normal	Dilated vessels	Moderate	None	Normal	Normal
Acute iritis	Sluggish, irregular	Normal	Photophobia	Watery	Variable	Impaired
Corneal abrasion	Normal	Normal	Severe	Watery	Irregular light reflex	Varies

KNOWLEDGE CHECKS

1. Lid disorders are common. Compare and contrast the various disorders related to the eyelid and lacrimal region.
2. Conjunctivitis has a variety of causes. Compare the signs and symptoms, physical examination, and treatment of bacterial, viral, and allergic conjunctivitis.
3. Loss of vision has a wide variety of etiologies and may be due to disorders of a variety of eye structures. Describe the various causes of vision loss, along with signs and symptoms and physical examination findings.
4. Describe the approach to the patient with the red eye, differentiating between vision-threatening and benign conditions.

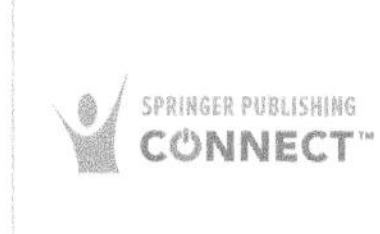

A robust set of instructor resources designed to supplement this text is located at **http://connect.springerpub.com/content/book/978-0-8261-8243-2.** Qualifying instructors may request access by emailing **textbook@springerpub.com.**

REFERENCES

The complete reference list for this chapter appears in the digital version of the chapter, accessible at https://connect.springerpub.com/content/book/978-0-8261-8243-2/chapter/ch02.

CHAPTER 3

EARS, NOSE, AND THROAT DISORDERS

DAVID BRISSETTE AND REBECCA ORSULAK CALABRESE

LEARNING OBJECTIVES

- Compare and contrast the common causes of the red eye with regard to epidemiology, pathophysiology, clinical presentation, diagnosis, and management.
- Discuss the clinical presentation, physical exam findings, diagnosis, and management of maxillofacial trauma.
- Compare and contrast sensorineural and conductive hearing loss with regard to epidemiology, pathophysiology, clinical presentation, diagnosis, and management.
- Compare and contrast acute otitis media (AOM), chronic otitis media, and otitis externa with regard to epidemiology, pathophysiology, clinical presentation, diagnosis, management, and complications.
- Discuss the clinical presentation and management of foreign body of the nose, eye, and ear.
- Discuss the clinical presentation, differential diagnosis, diagnostic workup, and management plan for a patient presenting with vertigo.
- Compare and contrast acute and chronic sinusitis with regard to risk factors, epidemiology, pathophysiology, clinical presentation, diagnosis, and management.
- Compare and contrast rhinitis and rhinosinusitis with regard to epidemiology, pathophysiology, clinical presentation, diagnosis, and management.
- Discuss the pathophysiology, clinical presentation, diagnosis, and management of epistaxis.
- Compare and contrast the various causes of pharyngitis with regard to epidemiology, pathophysiology, clinical presentation, diagnosis, and management.
- Compare and contrast croup and epiglottitis with regard to epidemiology, pathophysiology, clinical presentation, diagnosis, and management.
- Describe the symptoms and manifestations of various oral cavity disorders.

INTRODUCTION

Otolaryngology disorders are very common in primary care, accounting for 20% to 50% of presenting complaints to a primary care clinician. Management of common conditions of the ear, nose, and throat, such as sinusitis, otitis media, and acute neck lesions, may require referral to an otolaryngologist for expert medical and, when necessary, surgical interventions.

Conditions that affect the ears, nose, and throat are among the most common causes for patients to seek primary care.

3.1 DISEASES OF THE EAR

OVERVIEW

The ear is made up of three main parts: outer, middle, and inner ear.

The ear canal functions mainly to facilitate the process of transmission of sound for hearing while also providing various protections to the middle and inner ear from the external environment. As the first line of defense, the ear canal is susceptible to disorders that can cause pain, pruritus, swelling, and difficulty hearing. These disorders may be related to infection, exposure, masses/tumors, or trauma, or even may be self-induced.

The middle ear is made up of the tympanic membrane (TM) as well as an air-filled chamber containing a chain of three bones (ossicles) that connect the eardrum to the inner ear. The main function of the middle ear is to amplify sound. The inner ear converts mechanical sound waves into electrical signals that are sent to the brain via the acoustic nerve. Middle and inner ear disorders can cause similar symptoms, and because of their proximity to each other, a disorder in one may lead to a disorder in the other. Middle ear disorders include infections, dysfunction of the eustachian tube, and trauma.

The inner ear is composed of three main parts: cochlea, semicircular canals, and the vestibule. The cochlea is the auditory area that changes nerve sound waves into nerve signals. The semicircular canals sense head position and posture to assist in balance and equilibrium. The vestibule lies between the cochlea and the semicircular canals, also assisting in balance and equilibrium. Many conditions affect the inner ear such as vertigo, vestibular neuritis, labyrinthitis, eustachian tube dysfunction (ETD), vestibular schwannoma, and tinnitus.

EPIDEMIOLOGY

Hearing Loss

Approximately 30 million people in the United States are affected by hearing loss in some form. Hearing loss can affect patients at any age; however, it is most prevalent in older individuals. Approximately 50% of people in their 70s experience some hearing loss; the proportion increases to 80% by the age of 85 or older.[1]

Ear Canal Disorders

Patients of all ages are subject to disorders of the ear canal. Accumulation of cerumen resulting in narrowing or blockage of the ear canal occurs in all age groups affecting 10% of children, 5% of adults, and 33% of the elderly as well as those who have delayed development. Approximately 12 million patients per year seek medical care for problems related to cerumen impaction.[2] Foreign bodies in the external auditory canal are more common in young children due to the number of small objects that can be placed in the canal. Adults may present with foreign bodies in the ear canal; however, these are more commonly insects.[3] Otitis externa is a common infection usually seen in younger adults but can affect older adults as well. Most often it occurs in warmer months in colder climates but could be year-round in warmer climates. Pruritus of the ear can affect patients of all ages and is very common due to its association with many conditions related to otolaryngologic processes as well as other systemic diseases.[4]

Eustachian Tube Dysfunction

ETD is estimated to be fairly common in the U.S. population with a prevalence of 4.6% among adults[5] and 6.1% among children 12 to 19 years old.[6] In U.S. adults, ETD is more common in males than females.[7]

Middle Ear Disorders

Middle ear disorders affect patients of all ages. The majority of cases of AOM occur in children age 6 to 24 months in whom the peak is 9 to 15 months, and overall incidence decreases significantly after the age of 5. AOM occurs in adolescence and adulthood but it is less common for those age groups.[8] While chronic suppurative otitis media (CSOM) is more common in children than adults, the World Health Organization (WHO) estimates that about 65 to 330 million people are affected by CSOM. The true cholesteatoma incidence is not known; however, retrospective studies have estimated that it is about 9.2 cases per 100,000 persons of all ages.[9] The true incidence of TM perforations is not known because the vast majority heal on their own.

Inner Ear Disorders

Vestibular schwannoma is an inner ear disorder with an incidence of 1 per 100,000 person-years in the United States and all sexes are affected equally.[10] The median age at diagnosis is about 50 years.[11] Tinnitus is an inner ear disorder that can be associated with many disease processes that involve the ear and others that are nonotologic. It affects about 15% of the general population and prevalence is about 20% in older individuals.[12]

Vertigo

Dizziness—including vertigo and nonvestibular dizziness—accounts for one of the most common presenting complaints in medicine, affecting about 20% to 30% of the general population. The lifetime prevalence of vertigo in adults ages 18 to 79 is 7.4%. It is more common in females than males and it is about three times more prevalent in elderly populations as compared to younger individuals.[13]

PATHOPHYSIOLOGY

Hearing Loss

Hearing loss results from a conductive problem, a sensorineural problem, or a combination of both (mixed hearing loss). Conductive hearing loss is due to dysfunction of the external or middle ear where the movement of sound vibration to the inner ear is impaired. Causes include impaction of cerumen, infections of the ear (otitis externa and otitis media), and otosclerosis (fixation of the bones of the middle ear, most commonly the stapes). Sensorineural hearing loss can be divided into sensory and neural causes. Sensory hearing loss occurs when there is damage to the organ of Corti or the stria vascularis, which supports function of the organ of Corti and transduction of sound by hair cells. The most common form is high-frequency hearing loss (presbycusis) as an individual ages. Other causes include acute exposure to loud noise (e.g., explosions), chronic exposure to loud noise (e.g., concerts), trauma to the head, exposure to pharmaceutical agents with ototoxic side effects, genetic mutations, and systemic diseases. Neural hearing loss is a result of damage to the auditory nerve (e.g., tumors such as meningioma or acoustic neuroma), impaired message signaling along ascending tracts (e.g., auditory neuropathy), or lesions in the auditory cortex of the temporal lobe (e.g., infections, hemorrhage, tumors, or trauma).[1]

Ear Canal Disorders

Cerumen production is a normal physiologic process of the outer two-thirds of the ear where it is usually expelled as a self-cleaning process. The canal can become either partially or completely obstructed owing to failure of the self-cleaning process or ineffective attempts to clean the ear manually. Obstruction can lead to the development of pressure, fullness, or hearing loss.

Otitis externa is an infection of the external ear canal that is usually caused by gram-negative rods (e.g., *Pseudomonas*) or gram-positive cocci (e.g., *Staphylococcus*) and may be related to recent water exposure or manual trauma from scratching or cleaning the ear.

Foreign bodies in the ear canal occur more commonly in children. Common findings are beads, cotton or tissues, and hearing aid parts.

Pruritus is a common dermatologic issue that can affect the ear. Conditions that may result in pruritus include otitis externa, allergic contact dermatitis, seborrheic dermatitis, psoriasis, and eczema.

Tumors of the ear canal may be isolated to the canal but may also spread to adjacent structures such as the temporal bone, parotid gland, dura, and brain. Squamous cell carcinoma (SCC) is the most common type.[14] Adenomatous tumors can originate from cerumen glands of the external canal but tend to follow a more indolent course.

Eustachian Tube Dysfunction

There are three functions of the eustachian tube: pressure regulation through ventilation, which allows for normal function of the TM; protection of the middle ear from pathogens; and drainage of the middle ear cleft. When this tube fails or functions

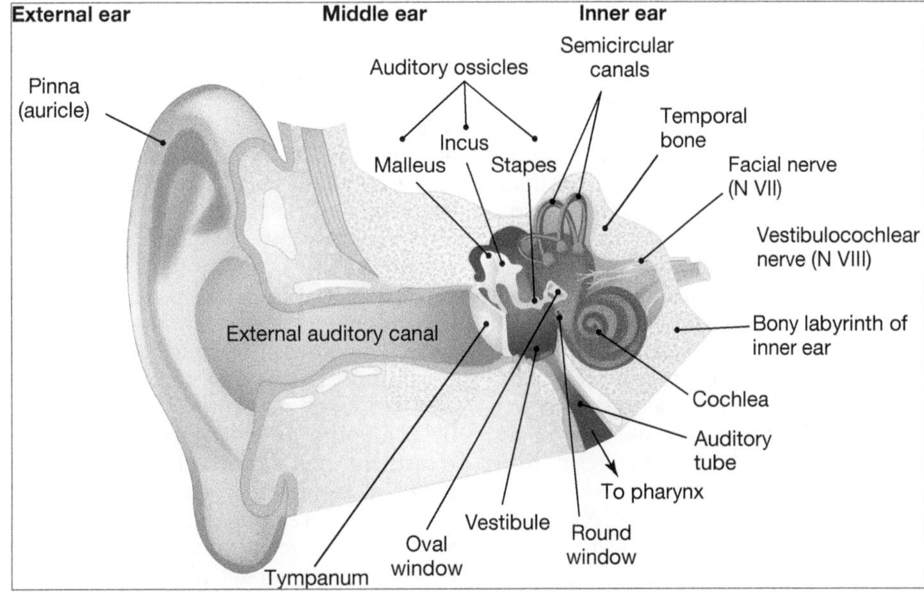

Figure 3.1 **Anatomy of the ear.**

(Source: With permission from Colandrea M, Raynpor EM. Evidence-based assessment of the ears, nose, and throat. In: Gawlik KS, Melnyk BM, Teall AM, eds. Evidence-Based Physical Examination. *Springer Publishing Company; 2021:337, Fig. 13.2.)*

improperly, the dysfunction can cause disease in the middle ear such as otitis media with effusion (OME), chronic otitis media, and retraction of the eardrum. Those with poor eustachian tube function can develop pain in the ear due to the stress of barotrauma, or negative pressure in the middle ear caused by rapid change in altitude during air travel or underwater diving.

Middle Ear Disorders

Otitis media is inflammation of the middle ear and can be acute or chronic. AOM is usually caused by bacteria resulting in fluid buildup behind the TM. More common in children, it often begins after an upper respiratory infection (URI). If the URI is bacterial, these bacteria can spread to the middle ear; if the URI is caused by a virus, bacteria may be drawn to the microbe-friendly environment and move into the middle ear as a secondary infection. As a result, fluid accumulates behind the TM (Figure 3.1). In children, the most common bacterial causes are *Streptococcus pneumoniae*, *Haemophilus influenzae*, and *Moraxella catarrhalis*. These organisms can also cause AOM in adults.[15] Group A streptococcus (GAS) and *Staphylococcus aureus* are less common causes of AOM in children and are more likely to affect adults. Fluid can accumulate behind the TM without infection and is known as OME or serous otitis media (Figure 3.2). This condition may occur after an episode of AOM or may result from ETD. Some patients may develop a chronic middle ear infection called CSOM, which involves otorrhea through a perforation of the TM persisting for at least 6 weeks. This usually results from an initial episode of AOM that is not diagnosed promptly or treated adequately. Pathogens associated with CSOM include aerobes, anaerobes, and fungi. *Pseudomonas aeruginosa* and *Staphylococcus aureus* are the common aerobes, with *Klebsiella, Escherichia coli*, and *Proteus* occurring less often. *Candida* and *Aspergillus* species have been reported as fungal causes but are rare. A complication of otitis media is mastoiditis that occurs after several weeks of inadequately treated AOM resulting in pain and erythema over the mastoid bone and spiking fever. The mastoid may also be involved in patients with CSOM. Inadequately treated or untreated mastoiditis can lead to deafness, sepsis, brain abscess, meningitis, or even death. Other complications of acute or chronic otitis media include facial palsy and central nervous system (CNS) infections from hematogenous spread of bacteria (*S. pneumoniae* or *H. influenzae)* causing epidural abscess, brain abscess, meningitis, or death.[16]

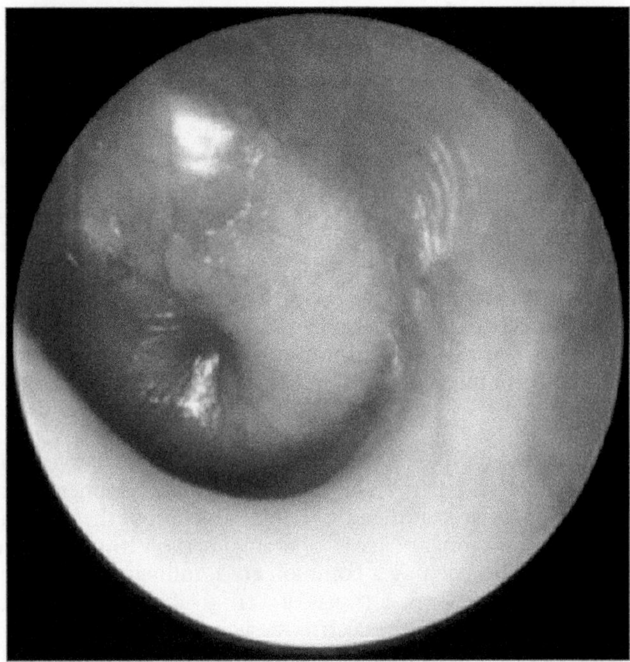

Figure 3.2 **Serous otitis media.**

(Source: With permission from Guida KM. Advanced health assessment of the eyes and ears. In Myrick KM, Karosas LM, eds. Advanced Health Assessment and Differential Diagnosis. *Springer Publishing Company; 2021:102, Fig. 4.48.)*

Cholesteatoma is a benign collection of keratinized epithelium within the middle ear and can be either congenital or acquired. Congenital cholesteatomas are derived from the remnants of epithelium that become trapped behind the TM during development. They usually present as a white mass behind the TM in a patient with no previous history of otitis media.[17] The acquired form results from pathologic changes causing uncontrolled growth of squamous epithelium in the middle ear. The most common cause is prolonged ETD that results in inward migration of the upper flaccid portion of the TM. The pathogenesis is not fully understood. Once present, they can continue to grow and damage surrounding structures in the middle ear such as the mastoid and ossicular chain and can also erode into the inner ear.

TM perforation typically results from infection in the middle ear or trauma. Infection causes inflammation and fluid accumulation with pressure on the membrane in the setting of AOM or CSOM. Perforations may also be due to trauma. A foreign body (FB) placed into the ear can directly rupture the membrane; a direct blow to the head can result in fracture of the temporal bone and dislocation and fracture of the ossicular chain. Membrane rupture from explosions or barotrauma result from the increase in ambient pressure external to the body—either atmospheric or hydrostatic pressure—causing negative pressure that is exerted on the membrane. Rupture of the TM results in conductive hearing loss, which may be temporary.

Inner Ear Disorders

Vestibular schwannoma is a benign, usually slow–growing tumor that develops from the balance and hearing nerves that supply the inner ear. The tumor results from overproduction of Schwann cells. As the tumor grows, it can result in unilateral hearing loss, tinnitus, and loss of balance or dizziness. The trigeminal nerve may also be affected with facial weakness or palsy. If it enlarges enough to press against structures in the brain, it may become life-threatening.

Tinnitus is defined as the perception of sound in the absence of external sound input. Most patients describe a ringing sensation in the ear, which can be unilateral or bilateral. The cause of tinnitus is often multifactorial, but in many cases, it is a response by the CNS to insufficient or abnormal input from the ear. It is often associated with sensorineural hearing loss caused by noise exposure or presbycusis. Other causes include conductive hearing loss, effusions of the middle ear, otosclerosis, and certain medications that can also cause hearing loss.[18]

Vertigo

Vertigo is a symptom experienced as illusions of movement and can relate to a peripheral or central cause. Peripherally, it is a result of a disruption in the normal function of the vestibular system, semicircular canals, or cranial nerve VIII. Any cause of inflammation such as a common cold, influenza, or bacterial infections may cause transient vertigo if the inner ear is involved. Chemical insults such as medications (e.g., aminoglycosides) or physical trauma (e.g., skull fractures) can also result in vertigo. Centrally, vertigo occurs when there is dysfunction or a lesion of vestibular structures of the CNS. Central causes of vertigo most commonly result from ischemic or hemorrhagic insult to the vestibular structures of the brainstem. Other central causes include CNS tumors, infection, or trauma.[19]

3.1A HEARING LOSS

MEDICAL HISTORY AND CLINICAL PRESENTATION

Hearing loss is defined as the partial or complete inability to hear sound. It occurs across the lifespan; however, the prevalence increases with age. Hearing loss is a result of dysfunction of the outer ear, middle ear, inner ear, acoustic nerve, or the auditory system from a variety of conditions, which can be temporary or permanent. According to the WHO, hearing loss is classified as mild, moderate, severe, or profound (see Table 3.1). Any degree of hearing loss can have a significant impact on the ability to communicate and can adversely affect the quality of life of the affected individual. As a result, it is a common reason for patients to seek medical care. It is important to be able to recognize the many conditions that are treatable by the primary care clinician and those that may require further evaluation by an otolaryngologist.

Episodes of hearing loss can be short-lived and resolve on their own without intervention; however, some episodes can have a significant impact on the patient's ability to hear or communicate and may require evaluation.

Obtaining important characteristics at presentation can help identify potential causes and guide evaluation and treatment. It is important to ask the patient to describe what is meant by hearing loss, when it was first noticed, how it progressed over time, and whether one or both ears are affected. The severity of the hearing loss can be elucidated by exploring the impact it has on the patient's ability to hear usual sounds and how they are able to communicate with others. Eliciting the presence or absence of associated symptoms can be helpful as well to include a sensation of ear fullness, drainage from the ear, pain, or ringing. A review of any over-the-counter or prescription medications taken in relation to the onset of symptoms should be obtained as some can have ototoxic side effects (see Box 3.1).[20] A review of the patient's overall health is essential to identify a related cause such as recent infections, chronic medical conditions, recent barotrauma, or physical trauma to the head.

TABLE 3.1 WHO Classification of Hearing Loss

Classification	Sound Equivalent	Decibel (dB) Range
Normal	Whisper	0–25 dB
Slight/mild	Soft voice	26–40 dB
Moderate	Normal voice	41–60 dB
Severe	Loud voice	61–80 dB
Profound	Shout	>81 dB

WHO, World Health Organization.
Source: Modified from the WHO Grades of Hearing Impairment. https://www.who.int/pbd/deafness/hearing_impairment_grades/en

BOX 3.1 Medications With Ototoxic Side Effects

- Aminoglycoside antibiotics
- Loop diuretics
- NSAIDs
- Platinum-based chemotherapeutic agents
- Salicylates
- Quinine-based medications

NSAIDs, nonsteroidal anti-inflammatory drugs.
Source: Data from Michels TC, Duffy MT, Rogers DJ. Hearing loss in adults: differential diagnosis and treatment. Am Fam Physician. *2019;100(2):98–108. https://www.aafp.org/afp/2019/0715/p98.html*

SIGNS AND SYMPTOMS

Patients with hearing loss may describe sound as muffled, or express difficulty in understanding some consonants or voices when in a crowd. Affected individuals may find themselves asking others to speak slower, talk louder, or repeat themselves. Patients may note a need to listen to audio or TV at higher volumes. Some may withdraw from conversations and even avoid some social settings because of difficulty hearing.

PHYSICAL EXAMINATION

Examination begins with inspection of the external ears for any signs of trauma or drainage. Gross hearing ability is assessed by asking the patient to repeat words that are whispered, spoken in normal voice, or shouted into both ears. A 512-Hz tuning fork can help in differentiating between conductive and sensorineural hearing loss. In performing the Weber test, the tuning fork is vibrated and placed on the patient's forehead. When conductive hearing loss is present, the sound transmitted by the vibration is louder in the affected ear. In sensorineural hearing loss the sound is louder in the unaffected ear. The Rinne test is used primarily in the evaluation of hearing loss in one ear by comparing the perception of sounds transmitted through bone conduction at the mastoid and comparing that to sound transmitted by air. A vibrating tuning fork is placed on the mastoid bone and then repeated in front of the external auditory canal. When conductive hearing loss >25 dB is present, bone conduction exceeds air conduction. In sensorineural hearing loss, air conduction exceeds bone conduction. In the normal ear, air conduction should exceed bone conduction. Palpate the external ear to check for pain or tenderness. Assess the external auditory canal and TM via otoscope to evaluate for cerumen impaction, otitis externa, or otitis media.

DIFFERENTIAL DIAGNOSIS

Table 3.2 summarizes the differential diagnosis for hearing loss.[20]

TABLE 3.2 Differential Diagnosis for Hearing Loss

Type of Hearing Loss	Differential Diagnosis
Conductive hearing loss (external ear)	Cerumen impaction
	Otitis externa
	Foreign body Mass
Conductive hearing loss (middle ear)	Cholesteatoma: growth behind TM
	Otitis media with effusion
	Otosclerosis: abnormal remodeling of bones of the inner ear
	Perforated TM: infections, barotrauma, loud noises, foreign body, head trauma
Sensorineural hearing loss	Medications with ototoxic side effects
	Idiopathic
	Infections: bacterial/viral
	Ménière disease
	Noise exposure
	Presbycusis
	Trauma
	Tumor

TM, tympanic membrane.

Source: Data from Michels TC, Duffy MT, Rogers DJ. Hearing loss in adults: differential diagnosis and treatment. Am Fam Physician. *2019;100(2):98–108. https://www.aafp.org/afp/2019/0715/p98.html*

DIAGNOSTIC STUDIES

Not all causes of hearing loss will require further diagnostic testing. Pneumoscopy—insufflation of air into the external auditory canal during otoscopic evaluation—can assess if the TM moves normally or if it is immobile because of fluid or a mass. Audiometric evaluation in a soundproof room can be performed to determine the severity and frequency of hearing loss. Based on the possible causes of the hearing loss, laboratory workup with complete blood count (CBC), serum glucose, thyroid function tests, serologic test for syphilis, or autoimmune markers may be necessary. Neuroimaging with CT or MRI may be warranted based on the history if a mass or central cause is suspected.

Auditory brainstem response (ABR) testing, also known as the auditory evoked potential (AEP), can be used to evaluate infants or adults who cannot cooperate with traditional testing to assess the function of the cochlea and brain pathways for hearing.

EVALUATION

Evaluation should include a detailed history and physical examination to include assessment of gross hearing and performance of Weber and Rinne tests. If conductive hearing loss is identified, the auricle and the external auditory canal should be evaluated by otoscopy for obstruction or mass. The TM should also be examined for abnormalities such as fluid or perforation. Pneumoscopy can be used to evaluate for mobility of the TM. Patients with sensorineural hearing loss or hearing loss without an identifiable cause should be referred for formal audiologic evaluation as well as evaluation by an otolaryngologist.

TREATMENT

- Conductive hearing loss affecting the external ear
  - **Cerumen impaction:** Instill detergent ear drops with carbamide peroxide into the ear canal at home or extract cerumen with irrigation or mechanical removal by a clinician.
  - **Otitis externa:** Patients should be advised to avoid moisture in the ear or physical trauma by touching or scratching; instill topical antibiotics (e.g., fluoroquinolones or aminoglycosides) with or without topical glucocorticoids, which may help with decreasing swelling; and take anti-inflammatory medications for pain. In cases of severe otitis externa, when swelling of the external canal prevents the instillation of antibiotic drops, a wick may need to be inserted to facilitate treatment. Cases that do not resolve with treatments above may require the addition of oral antibiotics. Patients with impaired immunity who are not improving with standard treatments above may require referral for further evaluation, especially if there is concern

for malignant otitis externa, which may require a prolonged course of systemic antibiotics and possibly surgical intervention.
  - **Foreign body:** Requires removal. Based on the shape and type of FB, equipment may include various types of curettes or forceps. Catheters may be used for irrigation or suction. Irrigation with water should be avoided when there is an organic object in the canal to avoid swelling. Insects may be paralyzed before removing by instilling mineral oil or lidocaine into the ear canal. If an attempt is unsuccessful, a specialist referral may be necessary.
- Conductive hearing loss affecting the middle ear
  - **Cholesteatoma:** May require surgical intervention
  - **ETD:** Treat any underlying causes of dysfunction such as sinusitis, allergic rhinitis (AR), laryngopharyngeal reflux, adenoid hypertrophy, or tumors.
  - **OME:** Antibiotics, surgical intervention with myringotomy if persistent effusion
  - **Otosclerosis:** May benefit from a hearing aid, surgical intervention
  - **Perforated TM:** Treat with antibiotics if infection present, surgical repair if healing does not occur
- Sensorineural hearing loss
  - **Medications:** Discontinue/avoid offending agent, audiology referral for hearing test, consideration for hearing aids if indicated
  - **Idiopathic:** Trial of glucocorticoids; sudden sensorineural hearing loss should be referred immediately to an audiologist and otolaryngologist.
  - **Infections:** Appropriate infectious workup, antibiotics for bacterial causes; vestibular labyrinthitis may need vestibular rehabilitation.
  - **Ménière disease:** Thiazide diuretics, antihistamines, vestibular rehabilitation; may require surgical intervention
  - **Noise exposure:** Noise prevention, audiology referral, otolaryngology referral; consider hearing aids, cochlear implant if profound hearing loss
  - **Presbycusis:** Referral to audiologist, otolaryngologist; consider hearing aids, cochlear implant if profound hearing loss
  - **Trauma:** Manage trauma
  - **Tumor:** Appropriate oncologic or surgical referral

PATIENT EDUCATION

- Patients should be informed about causes of hearing loss and various treatment options.
- For those chronically exposed to noise or who experience noise-related hearing loss, education should include hearing protection and strategies to reduce exposure (safe sound levels with headphones, earbuds or use of hearing protection devices).

3.1B EAR CANAL DISORDERS

MEDICAL HISTORY AND CLINICAL PRESENTATION

Patients with cerumen impaction may complain of hearing loss, a sensation of fullness in the ear, pruritus, ear pain, discharge, or tinnitus. Older patients may have a previous history of impaction.

A FB in the ear canal can lead to clinical manifestations such as pain, decreased hearing, itching, or drainage from the ear. A parent or caregiver may state that they saw a child place an object in the ear. Patients with an insect in the ear may hear or feel the insect moving inside the ear.

Pruritus of the external auditory canal may be secondary to a history of excessive cleaning of the ear or dermatologic conditions such as psoriasis or seborrheic dermatitis.

Those with otitis externa may give a history of swimming recently or trauma due to aggressive cleaning with cotton swabs or other objects that may result in trauma to the external canal. They may complain that there is a fullness, swelling, drainage, or decreased hearing in the affected ear.

Masses from bony overgrowth or tumors in the ear may be an incidental finding; however, they can result in drainage, a sensation of fullness or decreased hearing in the affected ear.

SIGNS AND SYMPTOMS

Disease processes of the external ear include discomfort with movement of the jaw, bloody discharge, mucopurulent drainage that may or may not be foul smelling, edema, erythema, fever, pain, pruritus, possible conductive hearing loss, edema, or erythema.

PHYSICAL EXAMINATION

Physical examination begins with inspection of the external ear and the external meatus for masses, lesions, erythema, or drainage. This is followed by palpation of the external ear for any areas of tenderness. Active movement and palpation of the jaw should be assessed if there is a complaint of ear pain. Assessment of gross hearing and Weber and Rinne tests should be performed if there is a history of hearing loss. This is followed by otoscopic evaluation of the ear canal as well as the TM.

Cerumen impaction may be visible in the external canal and appears as a yellowish, brown, or dark waxy material that partially or completely obstructs the canal (Figure 3.3). FBs can be visible in the canal and may include food, insects,

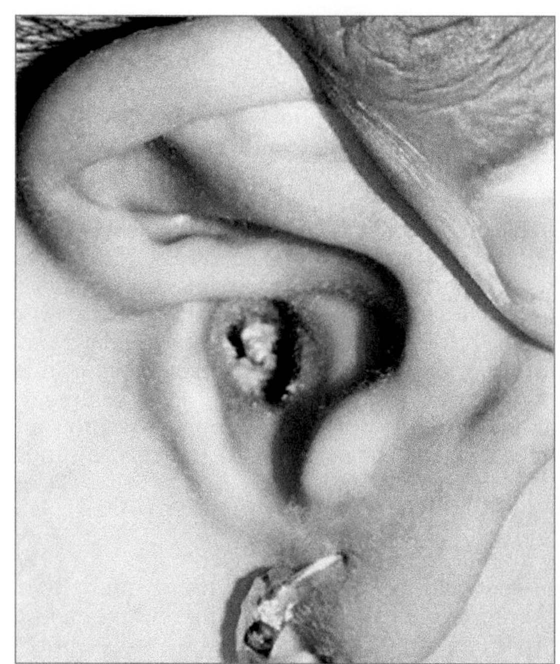

Figure 3.3 Excessive cerumen.
(Source: Courtesy of Annand2022)

toys, crayons, batteries, or buttons. Pruritus cannot be observed but skin conditions such as psoriasis and seborrheic dermatitis may be seen. Bony overgrowths or tumors can be seen from direct visualization with otoscopy (Figure 3.4).

DIFFERENTIAL DIAGNOSIS

Table 3.3 summarizes the differential diagnosis of ear canal disorders.

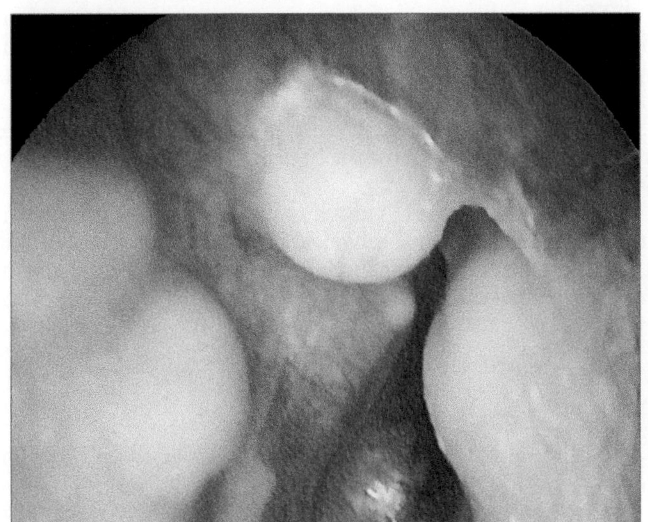

Figure 3.4 Osteoma.
(Source: Courtesy of Didier Descouens.)

TABLE 3.3 Differential Diagnosis of Ear Canal Disorders

Condition	Description
Cerumen impaction	Waxy discharge from the ear, pruritus, conductive hearing loss.
Exostoses	Bony skin-covered mounds that project into the ear canal and are usually bilateral. There is may be a history of chronic exposure to cold water (e.g., "surfer's ear").
Foreign body	Painless conductive hearing loss, most likely unilateral; patient is likely a young child.
Neoplasia	Mass in the ear canal. May cause otalgia, hearing loss, drainage from the ear. Occurrence is rare but most common type is squamous cell.
Osteomas	Bony skin-covered neoplasm, usually unilateral.
Otitis externa	May be painful or painless conductive hearing loss with swelling of the external canal. May have purulent drainage, history of water exposure/swimming or pruritus. Usually a result of infection with fungi (*Aspergillus*) or bacteria *Proteus* or *Pseudomonas*. Persistent external otitis may result in malignant external otitis in diabetic or immunocompromised patient when the infection (usually *Pseudomonas*) invades the surrounding bone causing osteomyelitis.
Pruritus	Commonly occurs at the meatus, may be associated with skin disorders such as psoriasis, eczema, or seborrheic dermatitis.

Source: Data from Roland PS, Marple BF. Disorders of the external auditory canal. J Am Acad Audiol. *1997;8:367–378.*

DIAGNOSTIC STUDIES

Audiology should be performed in the case of hearing loss that does not resolve with intervention such as cerumen impaction removal or treatment of otitis externa with topical or systemic antibiotics. CT scan is indicated for the evaluation of suspected malignant otitis externa.

EVALUATION

If conductive hearing loss is identified, the auricle and the external auditory canal should be evaluated for obstruction or mass. The TM should also be examined for abnormalities such as fluid or perforation. Pneumoscopy can be used to evaluate for mobility of the TM. Patients with sensorineural hearing loss or hearing loss without an identifiable cause should be referred for formal audiologic evaluation as well as evaluation by an otolaryngologist.

TREATMENT

- **Cerumen impaction:** See treatment for hearing loss.
- **Exostoses:** May require surgical removal if they result in infection or obstruction of the ear canal.
- **Foreign body:** See treatment for hearing loss.
- **Neoplasia:** Requires referral to an otolaryngologist for further evaluation and treatment, which may include biopsy or surgical removal.
- **Osteomas:** May require surgical removal if they result in infection or obstruction of the ear canal.
- **Otitis externa:** See treatment for hearing loss.
- **Pruritus:** Advise avoidance of excessive cleaning if that is the cause. Application of mineral oil may help if the patient has naturally dry skin within the ear canal. Treatment of inflammatory dermatologic conditions may be required.

PATIENT EDUCATION

- Patients should be instructed to avoid excessive cleansing of the ear canal.

3.1C EUSTACHIAN TUBE DISORDERS

MEDICAL HISTORY AND CLINICAL PRESENTATION

Dysfunction of the eustachian tube related to obstruction from inflammation or edema of the tubal lining usually occurs in the setting of AR, a recent URI, or previous history of otitis media. Patients may have a sensation of pressure in the ear, tinnitus, or an alteration in their ability to hear. Patients may state that they have tried a few maneuvers such as opening and closing the jaw or blowing air out of the nose with the nose blocked and mouth closed (Valsalva maneuver).

When dysfunction is due to an overly patent eustachian tube, patients may experience ear fullness with the ability to hear one's own breathing or voice loudly. Symptoms may improve when the patient is in the supine position or if a URI is present. Some patients may develop these symptoms if there is a history of rapid weight loss, or they may be idiopathic.

Some patients develop ETD from changes in barometric pressure that result in fullness, pain, or a popping sensation in the ears. There may be a history of swimming or diving underwater or symptom development while descending from an elevated altitude during air travel.

SIGNS AND SYMPTOMS

Eustachian tube disorders that accompany obstructive dysfunction result in fullness or "plugged" feeling in the ear, muffled sounds, mild to moderate hearing loss, tinnitus, otalgia, hearing one's own voice loudly, and problems with balance.

ETD from patulous etiology may result in autophony, ear blockage, or fullness in the ear that may be relieved when in the supine position, or hyperacusis. Swallowing, chewing, and yawning are not effective in relieving symptoms.

Patients with poor eustachian tube function under barometric stress from air travel with rapid change in altitude or underwater diving may have ear pain due to negative pressure in the middle ear.

PHYSICAL EXAMINATION

Physical examination should include examination of the ear with assessment of gross hearing and otoscopic evaluation of the ear to evaluate the TM for effusion or signs of infection. If hearing loss is evident, Weber and Rinne tests should be performed to evaluate for conductive or sensorineural hearing loss. Conductive hearing loss may occur with obstructive ETD but not with patulous ETD.

Examination of the head and neck is usually normal; however, some pertinent findings may include a retracted or hypomobile TM, especially in the pars flaccida area, or a serous otitis media. When the patient breathes vigorously there may be respiratory excursions of the TM. Findings in the nose may be inflammation, allergic changes, bleeding, polyps, or masses. In the setting of nasopharyngeal neoplasm, lymphadenopathy may be present.

DIFFERENTIAL DIAGNOSIS

Table 3.4 summarizes the differential diagnosis of ETD.

DIAGNOSTIC STUDIES

Audiometric evaluation can be used to assess pressure in the middle ear and for loss of hearing with a tympanogram and pure tone audiometry. CT or MRI studies with the use of contrast can be helpful to rule out a neoplasm as the cause of ETD. Nasal endoscopy by an otolaryngologist can assist with a complete nasopharyngeal examination.

TABLE 3.4 Differential Diagnosis for Eustachian Tube Dysfunction

Condition	Description
Acute otitis media	Aural fullness with fever, otalgia, hearing loss, pressure in the ear
Chronic suppurative otitis media	Aural fullness with otorrhea and hearing loss
Cerumen impaction	Can result in a sense of aural fullness and hearing loss that usually improve promptly upon removal of cerumen
Ménière disease	Aural fullness associated with vertigo, hearing loss, and tinnitus
Otitis externa	Aural fullness with pain on palpation of the pinna, external ear pruritus, conductive hearing loss
Otitis media with effusion	Aural fullness with reduced hearing, may have sensation of imbalance

Source: Data from Shan A, Ward BK, Goman AM, et al. Prevalence of eustachian tube dysfunction in adults in the United States. JAMA Otolaryngol Head Neck Surg. *2019;145(10):974–975. doi:10.1001/jamaoto.2019.1917*

EVALUATION

If otoscopic evaluation shows TM retraction and/or tympanogram shows that there is negative pressure in the middle ear, the patient has an obstructive cause.

ETD due to barometric change mostly relies on the patient history as physical examination is usually normal. Otoscopy and tympanometry may be normal; however, some cases may have evidence of middle ear effusion or TM rupture.

ETD due to patulous dysfunction will show that there is movement of the TM with breathing during otoscopy or tympanometry.

The diagnosis of ETD is made clinically through a comprehensive history and physical examination. Audiologic studies, nasal endoscopy, or CT or MRI may be helpful in the diagnostic process.

TREATMENT

Obstructive ETD:

- **AR:** Treatment begins with avoidance of the offending agent if possible. Pharmacologic treatments include a combination of antihistamines, intranasal steroid sprays, and leukotriene inhibitors.
- **Laryngopharyngeal reflux:** Avoidance of offending agents that may trigger symptoms such as alcohol, caffeine, mints, spicy foods, carbonated beverage, and nicotine. Eating smaller meals may be helpful.
- **Mass lesions:** Treatment varies depending on the type of mass causing the obstruction. In the case of hypertrophy of the adenoids, surgical resection is indicated. If the mass is due to nasopharyngeal carcinoma, radiation is the usual treatment.
- **Rhinosinusitis:** For moderate to severe acute cases of rhinosinusitis, narrow-spectrum antibiotics are used. In the case of chronic rhinosinusitis, antibiotics may be used along with intranasal saline, intranasal and systemic steroids, leukotriene inhibitors, and antifungals.
- When medical management is not effective, surgical management may be indicated with tympanostomy tube placement to correct negative pressure in the middle ear, tuboplasty to reduce the thickness of the mucosal lining of the eustachian tube, or balloon dilation of the eustachian tube.

Patulous ETD:

- In cases of mild symptoms, reassurance should be the mainstay of treatment.
- For more severe cases lasting more than 6 weeks it is important to ensure proper hydration. Nasal saline drops placed may also be helpful.
- If the above is not effective, thickening of the mucus with 8 to 10 drops of potassium iodide in juice three times a day may be helpful. Recommend weight gain if the patient is underweight.
- Surgical management may be necessary in severe cases that are not responsive to the above treatments.

Barotrauma:

- Prevention of barotrauma
  - Avoid precipitants if possible.
  - Oral decongestants, antihistamines, and nasal decongestants may help with pressure equalization.

  - Swallowing, opening/closing the mouth, or performing a Valsalva maneuver (blowing air out the nose against a closed nasal airway) may also help equalize pressure.
- Most injuries heal with time and require no intervention.
- Surgical repair may be required for severe cases resulting in ossicular disruption and perilymphatic fistula.

PATIENT EDUCATION

- It is important to manage underlying causes of ETD such as allergies or a cold as this can help to keep the eustachian tubes clear and prevent infection from developing.
- Smoking and exposure to second-hand smoke should be avoided.
- Prevention of blockage of the eustachian tube can be done during takeoff and landing when in an airplane by chewing gum, yawning, drinking liquids, or gently blowing with the mouth closed and the nose blocked.

3.1D MIDDLE EAR DISORDERS

MEDICAL HISTORY AND CLINICAL PRESENTATION

AOM is a bacterial infection of the middle ear behind the TM that can affect patients of any age. It is usually the result of a URI caused by a virus that causes inflammation and obstruction of the eustachian tube. In young children or those who cannot communicate, ear pain may manifest as pulling or rubbing of the ear. Parents may say their child has been febrile, is irritable, and has difficulty sleeping. Children with OME can be asymptomatic. Others will present with hearing loss or developmental delays. In adults, AOM is characterized by acute onset of ear pain that may follow a recent URI as well. Otalgia is usually continuous and worsens over time. In some cases, the infection will cause the TM to rupture, which will relieve the pain but will result in purulent otorrhea. Some patients may experience transient conductive hearing loss. Unusual symptoms such as persistent high fever, confusion, severe pain behind the ear, neck pain, neck stiffness, or facial paralysis may signal complications of otitis media and warrant urgent attention.

Cholesteatoma is a benign cystic lesion arising from abnormal growth of epithelial tissue in the middle ear which. If left untreated, it can progressively expand and destroy surrounding structures through necrosis and cause secondary infections. Those at risk for the development of cholesteatoma have ETD, history of acute or chronic ear infections, cleft palates, craniofacial anomalies, Turner syndrome, Down syndrome, or a positive family history of cholesteatoma.[17] Some patients are asymptomatic while others will present with a history of drainage from the ear. They may also experience a sense of fullness within the ear and possibly decreased hearing in the affected ear (conductive hearing loss if ossicular erosion has occurred). Pain may develop as well as dizziness in some cases.

Patients with TM perforation can have a history of having placed something in the ear for cleaning, trauma such as a fall or blow to the head, episodic ear infections, or loud noise exposure such as an explosion. Once the rupture has occurred patients will complain of hearing loss in the affected ear. If there is fluid accumulation behind the membrane, there may be clear, bloody, or purulent drainage from the ear.

SIGNS AND SYMPTOMS

Patients with AOM typically have fever and otalgia. Children may not be able to convey what they are experiencing but may be noted to be irritable, tug on the ear, or have a fever. Adults with AOM may have varying degrees of otalgia ranging from mild to severe. In some cases when the TM ruptures there may be relief from the otalgia, but they will experience purulent drainage from the affected ear. Some patients may experience impaired or loss of hearing. Chronic otitis media symptoms include otorrhea, aural fullness, otalgia, hearing loss, and sometimes vertigo.

Cholesteatomas can cause no symptoms, although some may have otorrhea, conductive hearing loss, or dizziness.

Symptoms of TM perforation may include ear pain that subsides suddenly and may be followed by bleeding or purulent drainage from the affected ear. There may also be tinnitus or hearing loss.

PHYSICAL EXAMINATION

The examination for otitis media should include assessment for fever, inspection of the auricle and preauricular region, and otoscopic evaluation. The TM suggestive of AOM may appear retracted or bulging (Figure 3.5). There may be fluid behind the ear with air bubbles suggestive of purulent otitis media (Figure 3.6). Small vesicles on the TM can be seen in bullous myringitis as a result of *Mycoplasma* or a viral infection. Rupture of bullous myringitis may result in serous or serosanguineous otorrhea. There may also be erythema, yellowish/clear fluid behind the membrane, impaired mobility of the TM on pneumatic otoscopy, and in rare cases perforation of the TM with purulent drainage (Figure 3.7). Chronic otitis media may cause partial or complete TM perforation, purulent drainage, and evidence of mucosal inflammation.

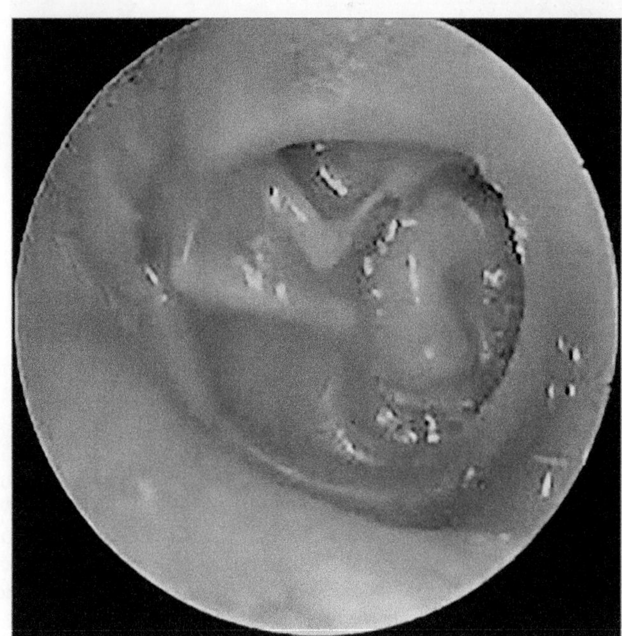

Figure 3.5 Retracted tympanic membrane.
(Source: With permission from Guida KM. Advanced health assessment of the eyes and ears. In: Myrick KM, Karosas LM, eds. Advanced Health Assessment and Differential Diagnosis. *Springer Publishing Company; 2021:101, Fig. 4.47.)*

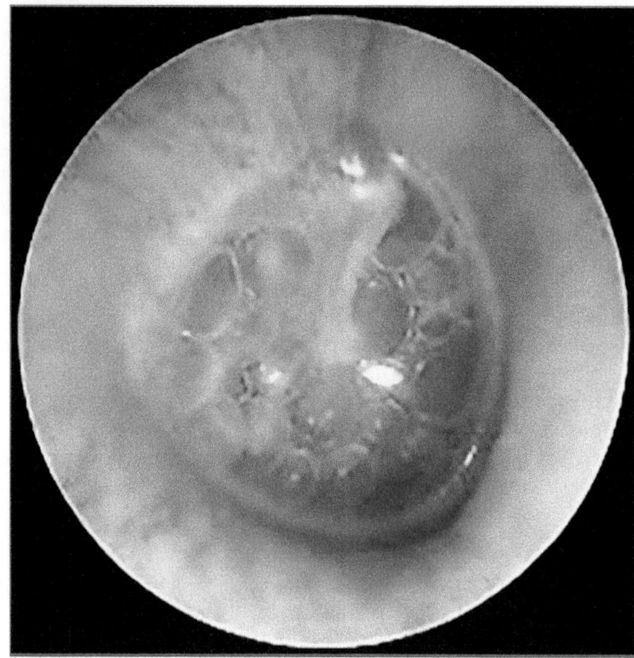

Figure 3.6 Acute purulent otitis media. Note distinctive air bubbles.
(Source: With permission from Guida KM. Advanced health assessment of the eyes and ears. In: Myrick KM, Karosas LM, eds. Advanced Health Assessment and Differential Diagnosis. *Springer Publishing Company; 2021:103, Fig. 4.49.)*

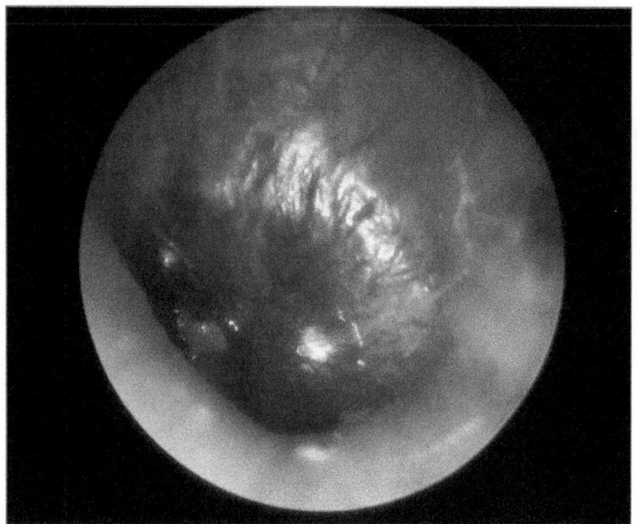

Figure 3.7 Bullous myringitis.
(Source: Courtesy of B. Wellescik.)

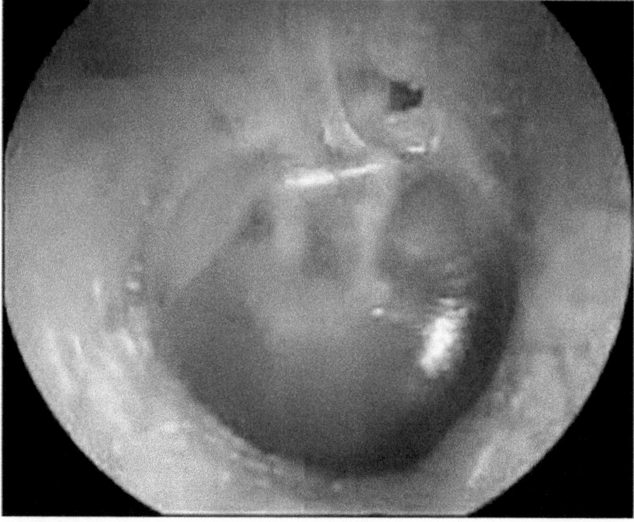

Figure 3.8 Cholesteatoma.
(Source: With permission from Guida KM. Advanced health assessment of the eyes and ears. In: Myrick KM, Karosas LM, eds. Advanced Health Assessment and Differential Diagnosis. *Springer Publishing Company; 2021:104, Fig. 4.51.)*

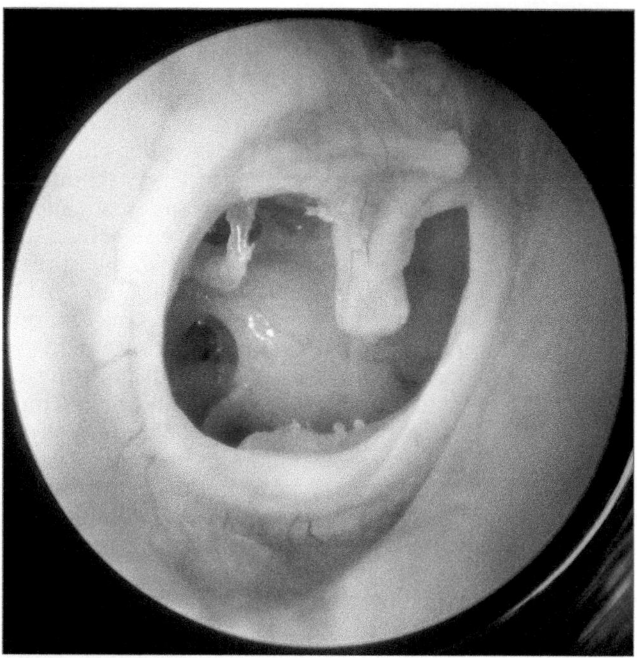

Figure 3.9 Perforated tympanic membrane.
(Source: Courtesy of Michael Hawke.)

Examination for cholesteatoma should include careful otoscopic evaluation. Primary cholesteatoma may show TM retraction (pars flaccida or pars tensa) and the presence of debris or tissue that appears inflamed (Figure 3.8). In secondary cholesteatoma, there will be evidence of a healed TM with visible whitish material behind the membrane.

TM perforations are diagnosed by routine otoscopic evaluation of the ear. Occasionally cerumen or drainage may occlude the ear canal so the eardrum cannot be completely visualized. Attempts to clear the ear canal can be attempted. When a TM perforation is found, it is important to note how much of the TM is involved (Figure 3.9).

DIFFERENTIAL DIAGNOSIS

Table 3.5 summarizes the differential diagnosis for otitis media. Table 3.6 summarizes the differential diagnosis for cholesteatoma.

DIAGNOSTIC STUDIES

AOM can be evaluated with pneumatic otoscopy and tympanometry.

Chronic otitis media can be evaluated with Gram stain and culture to help guide treatment if initial topical therapy fails. If there is hearing loss, audiometry is indicated. CT imaging should be obtained if there is a concern for

TABLE 3.5 Differential Diagnosis for Otitis Media

Condition	Description
Acute Otitis Media	
Barotrauma	Severe otalgia with history of air travel, scuba diving, or other trauma to ear.
Bullous myringitis	Can be associated with viral, *Mycoplasma*, or usual AOM pathogens. There is usually severe otalgia, component of sensorineural hearing loss.
Cholesteatoma	May be asymptomatic in early disease but some will develop otorrhea and hearing loss. Visible white keratinous debris or mass in the middle ear cavity.
Exacerbation of chronic OM	History of chronic ear infections, perforation of the TM, purulent drainage. Hearing loss may be present.
Otitis externa	Ear canal is usually edematous and erythematous resulting in decreased ability to see the TM. There is usually tenderness to palpation of the tragus.
Mastoiditis	Symptoms of AOM but pain and tenderness on palpation of the mastoid bone.
Serous/mucous tympanic effusion	No pain, erythema, or purulent drainage.
Chronic Otitis Media	
Otitis externa	Ear canal is usually edematous and erythematous resulting in decreased ability to see the TM. There is usually tenderness to palpation of the tragus.
Foreign body	May cause otorrhea and conductive hearing loss but will lack other classic signs of OM. Visible FB should be seen on physical examination.
Nasopharyngeal carcinoma	Common complaints include headache, diplopia, and facial numbness. Patients with nasopharyngeal carcinoma can also have OM.

AOM, acute otitis media; FB, foreign body; OM, otitis media; TM, tympanic membrane.
Source: Data from Harmes KM, Blackwood RA, Burrows HL, Cooke JM, Harrison RV, Passamani PP. Otitis media: diagnosis and treatment. Am Fam Physician. *2013;88(7):435–440. https://www.aafp.org/afp/2013/1001/p435.html Erratum in:* Am Fam Physician. *2014;89(5):318. Dosage error in article text. https://www.aafp.org/afp/2014/0301/p318*

TABLE 3.6 Differential Diagnosis for Cholesteatoma

Condition	Description
Bulging otitis media	May mimic cholesteatoma in appearance but in the setting of symptoms of OM it may resolve with treatment of OM.
Exostoses	Bony outgrowth into the external ear canal.
Inclusion cyst	Involves the TM but moves with the TM on pneumatic endoscopy; cholesteatomas are not mobile.
White foreign body	There may be a history of placing objects in the ear. Visible in front of the TM and is removable, whereas cholesteatoma requires surgical removal.

OM, otitis media; TM, tympanic membrane.
Source: Data from Isaacson G. Diagnosis of pediatric cholesteatoma. Pediatrics. *2007;120(3):603. doi:10.1542/peds.2007-0120*

extracranial complications. MRI is better for evaluation of suspected intracranial complications.

Cholesteatomas can be evaluated with CT or MRI.

Perforations of the TM may result in drainage from the ear that, if thought to be bacterial, may be sent for culture. Tympanometry can be used to assess for perforation in the case of inability to visualize the membrane. Audiogram can be used to assess the degree of hearing loss.

EVALUATION

The diagnosis of AOM requires acute onset of signs and symptoms as described above, physical examination finding of a middle ear effusion that may include erythema of the TM, bulging of the TM, decreased or no mobility of the TM, air-fluid level behind the TM, or drainage from the ear. Focal neurologic signs or facial paralysis may require an otolaryngology or neurosurgical referral and CT or MRI evaluation.

The evaluation of cholesteatoma should include a careful examination of the head and neck with focus on the ear. Patients with suspected cholesteatoma or findings suggestive of cholesteatoma should be referred to an otolaryngologist.

TM perforation is diagnosed by otoscopic evaluation. Audiometry is recommended to assess the degree of hearing loss.

TREATMENT

AOM

- In the pediatric population, a conservative approach with watchful waiting is common for those with symptoms that are not severe. This requires shared decision-making with the parents, analgesics, close follow-up, and plans for starting antibiotics in 48 to 72 hours if symptoms do not improve. Children over age 2 years with mild to moderate symptoms may be treated with amoxicillin for 5 to 7 days with 10 days of treatment for those under age 2 years with severe symptoms. Patients with mild penicillin

delayed hypersensitivity may be treated with cephalosporins. Those with a severe allergy to penicillin can be treated with macrolides or clindamycin.
- In adults, the standard of care treatment is oral antibiotics with amoxicillin, cephalosporins, or quinolones.

Chronic otitis media

- Medical treatment with topical antibiotics (quinolones) is the first-line therapy for uncomplicated otorrhea. Systemic antibiotics based on culture results are indicated for those who fail topical antibiotics or have resistant organisms.
- Surgical treatment with reconstruction of the TM may be indicated.

Complications of otitis media

- **Mastoiditis:** This requires intravenous (IV) antibiotics and myringotomy. Mastoidectomy may be indicated for treatment failure.
- **Facial palsy:** In the setting of AOM treatment requires urgent myringotomy with or without tube insertion, culture of fluid, and IV antibiotics. IV corticosteroids, although controversial, are routinely used. In the setting of chronic otitis media, treatment is IV antibiotics and mastoidectomy.

Cholesteatoma

- Surgical resection is typically performed with tympanoplasty. A mastoidectomy may be indicated if the lesion extends beyond the middle ear space.

TM perforation

- Most cases of perforations will usually heal spontaneously in a few weeks.
- In the case of perforation due to AOM, topical otic antibiotics are indicated for 10 to 14 days with specialist follow-up to evaluate healing and an assessment of hearing.
- In the case of perforation due to barotrauma, noise trauma, or blunt trauma, patients should see an otolaryngologist as soon as possible after the trauma. In the case of penetrating trauma, it is suggested that the patient should see an otolaryngologist urgently (within 24 hours).
- If the TM fails to heal, surgical repair may be required. A referral to a specialist is necessary for consideration of tympanoplasty. This procedure is reserved for those 7 years of age or older to allow for proper positioning of the eustachian tube.

PATIENT EDUCATION

- Patients with TM perforation should be instructed to avoid getting water in the ears and to use earplugs when swimming or bathing.

3.1E INNER EAR DISORDERS

MEDICAL HISTORY AND CLINICAL PRESENTATION

Disorders that affect the inner ear include vestibular schwannoma (acoustic neuroma), barotrauma, ETD, labyrinthitis, tinnitus, and vertigo. This section will focus on vestibular schwannoma and tinnitus as ETD is covered in Section 3.1C; labyrinthitis and vertigo are covered in Section 3.1F.

Vestibular schwannoma presents classically with progressive, unilateral hearing loss. Tinnitus is another common presenting symptom, and some may experience ataxia and vertigo as well. Atypical presenting symptoms may include headache, otalgia, facial pain, and alteration in facial sensation.

Risk factors for the development of tinnitus include exposure to loud noise, barotrauma, head trauma, history of ear infections or use of medications associated with the development of tinnitus. Patients will often describe a perceived quiet background noise to a noise that is audible over louder external sounds. Tinnitus can be divided into objective and subjective categories. Objective is audible to another person and subjective is audible only to the patient. Most patients describe tinnitus as a hissing, buzzing, or ringing sound although in some cases patients may hear musical sound or voices. Some may have an intermittent or continuous sensation of tinnitus that varies in intensity and it may be unilateral or bilateral. The main risk factor for developing tinnitus is hearing loss; however, some patients with hearing loss do not experience it. Those who have had occupational or recreational noise exposure are more likely to have tinnitus. Several diseases of the ear including otosclerosis, Ménière disease, and acoustic neuroma can be associated with tinnitus. Additionally, various drugs such as salicylates, aminoglycoside antibiotics, and some antineoplastic agents have been associated with tinnitus.

SIGNS AND SYMPTOMS

Common signs and symptoms of acoustic neuroma include gradual or sometimes sudden unilateral hearing loss, tinnitus, loss of balance, vertigo, and facial numbness or weakness.

Tinnitus may be experienced as an intermittent or constant ringing, buzzing, roaring, hissing, clicking, or humming sound. It may vary in pitch from a low roar to a high squeal and it may be present in one or both ears. Some patients may experience tinnitus so loud that it impedes ability to concentrate.

PHYSICAL EXAMINATION

Physical examination in the workup of acoustic neuroma should include evaluation of cranial nerve VIII with assessment of gross hearing as well as Weber and Rinne tests, which may show unilateral sensorineural hearing loss. Additional cranial nerve testing may reveal decreased or absent ipsilateral corneal reflex, facial weakness, or facial numbness.

The physical examination for tinnitus should focus on the ear and the nervous system. The ear canal may show cerumen impaction, drainage, or presence of a FB. The TM may show signs of acute infection, chronic infection, TM perforation or tumor. If there is a central nervous cause, cranial nerves relating to vestibular function may be abnormal along with strength, sensation, or reflexes. Auscultation over the carotid arteries or jugular veins may reveal a bruit or venous hum, which is an objective finding that may explain the sensation of tinnitus.

DIFFERENTIAL DIAGNOSIS

Table 3.7 summarizes the differential diagnosis for acoustic neuroma (vestibular schwannoma). Table 3.8 summarizes the differential diagnosis for tinnitus.

DIAGNOSTIC STUDIES

Audiometry and MRI are used in the evaluation of acoustic neuroma. High-resolution CT scanning can be used for those who cannot tolerate MRI.

TABLE 3.7 Differential Diagnosis for Acoustic Neuroma (Vestibular Schwannoma)

Condition	Description
Benign paroxysmal positional vertigo (BPPV)	Vertigo may occur in different positions but there is no hearing loss
Ménière disease	Episodic vertigo, sensorineural hearing loss, and tinnitus
Meningioma	Intracranial tumor that can cause double vision, headaches, hearing loss, tinnitus, memory loss, seizure, weakness in arms or legs, or language difficulty
Multiple sclerosis	Plaques seen on MRI
Ototoxic medications	Aminoglycosides, salicylates, diuretics
Vertebrobasilar insufficiency	Risk factors for vascular disease; vertigo, dizziness, double vision, paresthesia, change in mental status, headache ataxia, motor weakness

Source: Data from McDonald R. Acoustic neuroma: what the evidence says about evaluation and treatment. J Fam Pract. *2011;60(6):E1–E4.*

TABLE 3.8 Differential Diagnosis for Tinnitus

Condition	Description
Acoustic neuroma (schwannoma)	Benign tumor of the vestibular nerve causing unilateral hearing loss, tinnitus, dizziness, and facial numbness or weakness
Acoustic trauma	Known noise trauma resulting in ringing sensation in the ear, may be unilateral but more likely bilateral
Acute otitis media	Aural fullness with fever, otalgia, hearing loss, pressure in the ear
Cerumen impaction	Can result in a sense of aura fullness and hearing loss, which usually resolve promptly upon removal
Chronic suppurative otitis media	Aural fullness with otorrhea and hearing loss
Foreign body	May cause otorrhea and conductive hearing loss. Visible FB should be seen on physical examination.
Ménière disease	Episodic vertigo, sensorineural hearing loss, and tinnitus
Ototoxic medications	Aminoglycosides, salicylates, diuretics causing hearing loss and tinnitus

FB, foreign body.
Source: Data from Yew KS. Diagnostic approach to patients with tinnitus. Am Fam Physician. *2014;89(2):106–113. https://www.aafp.org/afp/2014/0115/p106.html*

For the diagnostic evaluation of tinnitus, audiometry can be used to assess for associated hearing loss. MRI or CT can be used to evaluate the anatomy and pathologic process.

EVALUATION

Acoustic neuroma in early stages may be difficult to detect due to subtle symptoms or the similarity of symptoms with other disease processes. If suspected, a thorough examination of the ear should be performed along with audiometry. If there is asymmetric hearing loss, MRI or high-resolution CT can be used to evaluate the size and location of the tumor for monitoring or surgical planning.

All patients with tinnitus should undergo audiometry. Additional investigation can be guided by the history, physical examination, and audiometry results. Patients with unilateral or pulsatile tinnitus may require specialist referral for evaluation of a serious underlying process. If imaging is indicated, MRI or CT of the brain should be obtained.

TREATMENT

Acoustic Neuroma

- Observation with periodic MRI studies, radiation, or surgical excision are the three mainstays of treatment.
- Gamma knife may have a role in reducing the size or limiting the growth of the tumor as an alternative to invasive surgical techniques.

Tinnitus

- Identifiable causes (e.g., Ménière disease) should be treated. For patients with hearing loss and tinnitus, hearing aids or cochlear implants may be beneficial. Offending drugs that are associated with tinnitus should be discontinued. In the absence of a treatable underlying condition, the goal of treatment is to lessen the impact on the patient with cognitive behavioral therapy, acoustic therapy, biofeedback, and stress reduction.

PATIENT EDUCATION

- Patients with acoustic neuroma should be advised to monitor their symptoms and report any change to their clinician. They should understand that periodic follow-up will be required to monitor the size of the tumor.
- Patients with tinnitus should be encouraged to avoid exposure to loud noises and sounds as well as stimulants such as coffee, tea, soda, and tobacco. Exercise, adequate rest, and stress reduction should be encouraged.

3.1F VERTIGO

MEDICAL HISTORY AND CLINICAL PRESENTATION

A detailed history with a clear description of the symptoms can help the clinician determine if the origin of the vertiginous symptoms is central (cerebellar or brainstem), peripheral (inner ear or the vestibular nerve), or located on the left or the right side. A description of the onset, duration, severity, and aggravating and alleviating factors as well as any other symptoms that may occur along with the sensation of vertigo should be evaluated. Sensation of spinning that occurs when the head has moved to a new position or the sensation of self-motion when not moving may suggest vertigo.

Peripheral defects are often associated with nausea, vomiting, hearing loss, recent or current URI, or trauma. A change in the position of the head can trigger symptoms of room spinning. Hyperventilation in the setting of stress, anxiety, or a panic attack may cause one to experience vertigo. Medications that affect the vestibular system such as

TABLE 3.9 Differential Diagnosis of Vertigo

Condition	Description
Peripheral Causes	
Benign paroxysmal positional vertigo (BPPV)	The onset and duration are seconds to minutes, usually brought on by movement or change in position of the head. Some patients may have associated nausea, but vomiting is rare. Nystagmus is peripheral. Dix-Hallpike maneuver is positive.
Labyrinthitis	Onset of vertigo is seconds to minutes that is severe and can last many days with associated nausea, vomiting, and gait instability. There may be a history of current or recent URI symptoms. Hearing loss is present.
Ménière disease	Onset of vertigo is spontaneous. Duration is minutes to several hours with associated unilateral sensorineural hearing loss and tinnitus. Symptoms result from pressure in the inner ear from an excess of endolymphatic fluid.
Vestibular neuritis	Onset of vertigo is seconds to minutes that is severe and can last many days with associated nausea, vomiting, and gait instability. There may be a history of current or recent URI symptoms. There is no associated hearing loss.
Otosclerosis	Onset of vertigo is spontaneous with associated conductive hearing loss. Symptoms result from excess bone growth in the middle ear.
Central Causes	
Cerebrovascular disease	Onset of vertigo is spontaneous. Duration is variable. Impairment or occlusion of blood flow to the vertebrobasilar system results in symptoms.
Vestibular migraine	Onset of vertigo is spontaneous in the setting of classic migraine headache symptoms. Duration is variable.

URI, upper respiratory infection.

Source: Data from Post RE, Dickerson LM. Dizziness: a diagnostic approach. Am Fam Physician. *2010;82(4):361–369. https://www.aafp.org/afp/2010/0815/p361.html*

furosemide, salicylates, and some antihypertensive agents may also trigger vertigo.

Certain symptoms that occur together such as otalgia, ear drainage, and hearing loss can also indicate that the problem originates in the ear and which ear is affected. A fast heart rate, irregular heart rate, or loss of consciousness may imply that the symptoms are cardiac in origin. Vision loss, slurred speech, extremity weakness, or loss of consciousness could indicate that the cause is neurologic. Past medical history as well as a previous history of ear infections or head trauma should be obtained. History of prescribed and over-the-counter medications as well as illicit substance use should be obtained.

SIGNS AND SYMPTOMS

Vertigo is most commonly described by patients as a sensation of "spinning"; however, some may describe a sensation of falling backward or forwards or listing to one side. It is important to differentiate vertigo from lightheadedness or loss of consciousness.

Vertigo that is peripheral in origin usually has a sudden onset when patients sometimes have significant difficulty walking or even standing. Some patients may complain that they run into walls or doorways when walking. They may have associated nausea, vomiting, hearing loss, or tinnitus. In contrast, vertigo that arises from a central cause develops gradually, then becomes progressively more severe over time and can become debilitating.

PHYSICAL EXAMINATION

Examination of a patient with vertigo should include vital signs with assessment of orthostatic blood pressure and pulse in the supine and standing positions. Examination of the ear should include assessment of gross hearing and otoscopic evaluation. The eye should be examined for nystagmus and papilledema. Cardiac examination should include evaluation of the blood pressure, heart rate and rhythm. The carotid arteries should be examined to evaluate for bruits. Neurologic examination should include gait, balance, and coordination.

DIFFERENTIAL DIAGNOSIS

Table 3.9 summarizes the differential diagnosis for vertigo.

DIAGNOSTIC STUDIES

Laboratory analysis is usually not performed in the evaluation of vertigo; however, checking serum electrolytes and glucose in patients with hypertension or diabetes who present with dizziness may be considered. Symptoms suggestive of a cardiac etiology should have an EKG performed. If the patient's history or physical examination point toward an acoustic neuroma or central cause, imaging with CT, MRI, or magnetic resonance angiography of the brain is indicated. Neuroimaging should be pursued if the vertigo is accompanied by a headache. If hearing loss is present, audiometry should be performed to quantify the hearing loss. Specialists may use electronystagmography and video nystagmography (VNG) to help distinguish between central and peripheral causes of vertigo.

EVALUATION

It is important to elicit a history that confirms that the symptoms are related to vertigo as opposed to another type of dizziness. Next it is helpful to differentiate the cause of vertigo based on history and physical exam that can help to localize the pathology as peripheral or central.

Peripheral causes are generally considered to be benign; however, central causes may require urgent evaluation and treatment. If vertigo is the only symptom it may be challenging to differentiate. Peripheral defects are often associated with nausea, vomiting, hearing loss, recent or current URI, or trauma. A change in the position of the head can trigger a sensation of room spinning. Hyperventilation related to stress, anxiety, or a panic attack may cause a patient to experience vertigo. Medications that affect the vestibular system such as furosemide, salicylates, and some antihypertensive agents may also trigger vertigo.

Evaluation of the head-impulse, nystagmus, and test of skew (HINTS) can also assist in differentiating a peripheral from central etiology. HINTS testing is as follows:

- Head-Impulse. With the patient in the sitting position and their eyes fixed on the clinician's nose at all times during the test, the clinician who is holding the patient's head at the ears, thrusts the patient's head 10 degrees to the left and then to the right. If the clinician observes rapid movement of both eyes the ideology is likely peripheral. If there is no eye movement it strongly suggests a central cause.[21]
- Nystagmus. The clinician moves a finger slowly in front of the patient's eyes left to right while the patient follows the movement of the finger. Spontaneous unidirectional horizontal nystagmus that worsens with gaze in the direction of the nystagmus is suggestive of a peripheral cause. Spontaneous nystagmus that is vertical or torsional or that changes direction with the gaze suggests a central cause.[21]
- Test of Skew. With the patient looking straight ahead, the clinician covers and then uncovers each eye. Vertical deviation of the covered eye upon uncovering is considered an abnormal result. Although less sensitive for central pathology, it is fairly specific for brainstem involvement.[21]

Evaluation for benign paroxysmal positional vertigo (BPPV) can be evaluated using the Dix-Hallpike maneuver. Patient faces forward with the head turned to the right at 45 degrees and the eyes open. While the patient's head is supported, the patient is placed in the supine position, allowing the head to hang 20 degrees over the edge of the examination table. The patient remains here for 30 seconds then is returned to the upright position and observed for another 30 seconds. The test is repeated on the left. If the maneuver to the right or the left causes vertigo with nystagmus that has an initial latency before onset, is rotational, and fatigues after 30 to 40 seconds or with repeat testing, it is considered a positive test for BPPV. Patients who develop vertigo symptoms with Dix-Hallpike testing but do not have nystagmus do not have BPPV, and patients with vertigo due to a central cause can develop nystagmus with Dix-Hallpike testing but there is no latency or fatiguability and it is rarely accompanied by nausea.[22]

TREATMENT

Vertigo from peripheral lesions:

- BPPV is best treated with the Epley maneuver rather than with medications that can cause sedation and increase risk of falls.
  - Epley maneuver begins with the patient sitting on the edge of the examination table, facing forward with the head turned to the right at 45 degrees and the eyes open. The clinician then supports the patient's head and lies the patient back in the supine position, allowing the head to hang 20 degrees over the edge of the examination table. The patient's head is then turned 90 degrees to the left where it remains for 30 seconds. The clinician then rotates the patient's head to the left another 90 degrees while the patient's body turns 90 degrees in the same direction and remains there for 30 seconds. Then the patient sits up on the left side of the table. The procedure may be repeated on each side until relief of symptoms is achieved.
- Labyrinthitis is treated with meclizine or diazepam for control of vertiginous symptoms. Antibiotics may be prescribed in the setting of fever or suspected bacterial infection.
- Ménière disease (endolymphatic hydrops) is treated with lifestyle changes such as sodium restriction to 2 g/day, reduction of caffeine intake, and limiting alcohol intake to 1 drink per day or none at all. When lifestyle changes are not effective, the addition of a diuretic (acetazolamide) may be helpful. For vertiginous symptom control, oral meclizine or diazepam (Valium) can be used. Refractory cases may benefit from intratympanic injections of steroids or gentamicin. As gentamicin can cause hearing loss, this should be avoided in those patients who have preserved hearing.
- Vestibular neuritis is treated with meclizine or Valium. If there is associated nausea, an antiemetic may be helpful. In addition to pharmacologic treatments, vestibular rehabilitation is helpful

Vertigo from central lesions:

- Vestibular migraine is treated with avoidance of triggers of migraine symptoms, stress relief, exercise, sleep hygiene, and antimigraine medications.
- Vertebrobasilar ischemia is treated with risk factor reduction, antiplatelet therapy. Oral anticoagulation may be used in the case of severe vertebral or basilar artery stenosis.

PATIENT EDUCATION

It is important for patients to know that vertigo is a type of dizziness that results in the sensation of spinning, swaying, or tilting when staying still. It can result from medications, trauma, infection, or diseases that affect the inner ear. Patients should be advised to see a clinician if they have fever, severe headache, difficulty hearing, persistent vomiting, inability to walk, symptoms of stroke, or a history of stroke in the past.

SPECIAL CONSIDERATIONS

- Patients with hearing loss that is not readily identifiable or treatable should be offered a referral for audiometric evaluation by an audiologist and formal evaluation by an otolaryngologist.
- Sudden idiopathic hearing loss should be assessed with history and physical examination to determine if it is conductive or sensorineural in origin. Sudden hearing loss that affects one or both ears that is sensorineural in origin occurring within a 72-hour period of at least 30 dB that involves three consecutive frequencies without identifiable cause or is related to trauma is considered an emergency. A referral to an otolaryngologist should be obtained in this case for formal audiometric studies and for consideration of a trial of oral glucocorticoids.[1]
- Geriatric patients with dementia or depression may not report concerns about hearing. These patients should be screened for hearing loss and evaluated if it is evident.
- Recurrent episodes of BPPV may warrant MRI of the brain as BPPV can mimic symptoms of CNS events such as vertebrobasilar insufficiency.

3.2 DISEASES OF THE NOSE AND SINUSES

OVERVIEW

Disorders of the nose and sinuses are common among the general population and result in infections, pain, headache, bleeding, breathing difficulties, and loss of the sense of smell. Acute and chronic rhinosinusitis, AR, nosebleeds, airway obstruction, and tumors will be discussed in this section.

EPIDEMIOLOGY

Sinusitis can affect about 1 in every 8 adults in the United States, which translates to over 30 million diagnoses per year. Sinusitis is the fifth most common diagnosis that results in the prescribing of antibiotic therapy.[23]

AR is the most prevalent chronic noncommunicable disorder affecting 10% to 20% of the entire population.[24] In the United States, the prevalence of AR is about 15% on review of actual documented diagnoses but can be as high as 30% based on patient self-reported nasal symptoms. AR has significant impact on those who are affected to include missed or less productive time at work or school, interrupted sleep, and decreased involvement in outdoor activities. Sensitization to inhaled allergens is known to begin during the first year of life but due to viral respiratory infections having similar symptoms as AR that occur frequently in young children in the first few years of life, it can be challenging to diagnose AR in young patients. The prevalence of AR peaks in the second to fourth decades of life and diminishes from there.[25]

Epistaxis is a common occurrence in the general population. Everyone will have experienced at least one nosebleed in their lifetime; however, nosebleeds are most common in children under 10 years of age and in those 70 years and older. Patients taking blood thinners and antiplatelet therapies also have increased incidence of nosebleed.[26]

Nasal foreign bodies account for approximately 40,000 ED visits annually. The majority of patients are younger than 5 years old with females having more visits than males. Foreign bodies recovered include jewelry (beads accounted for almost 50% of cases) but also food, toys, coins, buttons, crayons, pens/pencils, and button batteries.[27]

Benign tumors of the nasal cavity include nasal polyps, which affect up to 4% of the population and present in adulthood. Incidence of inverted papillomas (IPs) is 0.2 to 0.6 people per 100,000 per year. IP is more common in the fifth and sixth decades of life and males are affected more than females at a ratio of 3:1.[28]

According to the American Cancer Society, tumors of the nasal cavity and paranasal sinuses are rare, affecting about 2,000 people in the United States annually. The incidence becomes more common with age and about 80% occur in patients who are 55 years or older. Men are more likely to be diagnosed with this type of cancer than women. The majority occur in the nasal cavity or the maxillary sinuses; tumors occur less often in the ethmoid sinuses and rarely in frontal and sphenoid sinuses.

PATHOPHYSIOLOGY

Acute rhinosinusitis is the most common infection in the maxillary sinus, the largest of the sinuses with only one single drainage pathway that can be easily obstructed. Viruses cause most sinus infections, and acute rhinosinusitis usually begins as a viral respiratory infection. Chronic rhinosinusitis is more often caused by inflammation and blockage due to allergies or a physical obstruction including deviated septum, nasal polyps, bone or cartilage abnormalities, tumors, or foreign objects.[29] Sinus infections occur when fluid builds up in the sinuses, allowing growth of viruses or bacteria. In cases of bacterial sinusitis in adults the common pathogens are *S. pneumoniae, H influenzae, M catarrhalis*, and *S. aureus*.[30]

The process of AR involves an early and late phase response resulting from exposure to allergens such as pollen or animal dander that are recognized by the antigen-specific immunoglobulin E (IgE) receptors that are located on mast cells and basophils. The early phase is characterized by mast cell degranulation, which over a period of minutes causes acute nasal symptoms (sneezing or rhinorrhea) or ocular symptoms (itchy, watery eyes and redness). The late phase develops over a period of hours after the patient has had an allergen exposure. This is characterized by recruitment of basophils, neutrophils, T-lymphocytes, monocytes, and eosinophils as well as by the release of cytokines, prostaglandins, and leukotrienes, which exacerbate the inflammatory response.[31]

The blood supply and vasculature of the nose is complex; epistaxis can be classified as anterior or posterior based on location of the bleeding vessel. Ninety percent of all cases of epistaxis arise in the anterior portion of the nose, with the most common site being anteroinferior or the Kiesselbach plexus. Anterior bleeds can be self-limiting but can also allow for visualization of the source for proper treatment. Posterior bleeds account for about 10% of cases of epistaxis and arise from the sphenopalatine arteries. Posterior bleeding may be severe enough to cause hypotension, nausea, hematemesis, hemoptysis, or anemia.[26]

Most foreign bodies of the nasal cavity occur in young children or those with intellectual disability and are found along the nasal floor below the first turbinate or anterior to the middle turbinate. Nasal foreign bodies should be removed promptly to avoid the risk of aspiration. Button batteries can be harmful as they can result in chemical burns if they leak, causing significant damage to the mucosa, necrosis, and septal perforation.[32] Magnets can also lead to tissue necrosis and should be removed promptly.

Nasal cavity tumors can be benign, as in the case of nasal polyps. Their etiology is unclear, but they are associated with conditions that cause chronic inflammation such as allergies, asthma, infection, cystic fibrosis, and aspirin sensitivity. SCC is the most common type of nasal cavity tumor. Nonsquamous types can be present including adenocarcinoma and melanoma.[33]

3.2A INFECTIOUS DISORDERS

MEDICAL HISTORY AND CLINICAL PRESENTATION

Rhinosinusitis involves not only the sinuses but also the nasal passages. Of the different types of rhinosinusitis acute viral rhinosinusitis (AVRS) is the most common and usually improves or resolves in 7 to 10 days; acute bacterial rhinosinusitis (ABRS) can persist beyond 10 days and up to 4 weeks. When symptoms last beyond 12 weeks, it is considered chronic rhinosinusitis. Purulent drainage or facial pain do not distinguish bacterial from viral as they can be present in both.[23]

Patients who are at risk for sinus infections include those who have had a recent cold, experience seasonal allergies, smoke or have exposure to second-hand smoke, or have structural problems (e.g., nasal polyps) or weakened immune systems.

SIGNS AND SYMPTOMS

Major symptoms of sinusitis include fever, runny nose with drainage, nasal congestion, alteration in smell, facial pain, facial pressure, and cough. Minor symptoms include fatigue, headache, otalgia, and maxillary tooth pain.

PHYSICAL EXAMINATION

The physical examination includes evaluation for swollen turbinates, purulent drainage, nasal polyps, and local sinus pain when the patient bends over. Pain induced by percussion of the sinus is less reliable than focal pain experienced in the bent-over position. Examination of the patient with sinusitis may reveal fever, inflamed mucosa of the nasal passages, purulent drainage from the nose, tenderness to palpation over the sinuses, and possible lymphadenopathy.

DIFFERENTIAL DIAGNOSIS

Table 3.10 summarizes the differential diagnosis for sinusitis.

DIAGNOSTIC STUDIES

Uncomplicated sinusitis may be diagnosed by history and physical examination alone and in these cases no diagnostic studies are necessary. In patients who experience sinusitis that persists despite treatment with antibiotics or recurrent episodes of sinusitis, x-ray or CT scan of the sinuses may be helpful. A CBC may correlate with a bacterial cause. Culture of nasal discharge may identify responsible organisms in cases of chronic infections or complications.

TABLE 3.10 Differential Diagnosis for Sinusitis

Condition	Description
Acute invasive fungal sinusitis	More common in profoundly immunocompromised patients. Symptoms include fever, nasal congestion and facial pain but also changes in vision and mentation.
Common cold	May have some symptoms in common but usually lack facial pain. Patients often have cough, sore throat, sneezing, or rhinorrhea.
Headache	Cluster, migraine, and tension headaches can cause pain in the frontal sinuses, but these patients will lack most of the other typical symptoms.
Rhinitis (noninfectious)	May have some symptoms in common but usually lack facial pain and purulent drainage. Predominant symptoms include nasal congestion, sneezing, nasal itching, and rhinorrhea.
Temporomandibular joint disorder	Facial pain that usually is exacerbated by movement or with palpation of the TMJ.

TMJ, temporomandibular joint.
Source: Data from Bernstein JA, Fox RW, Martin VT, Lockey RF. Headache and facial pain: differential diagnosis and treatment. J Allergy Clin Immunol Pract. *2013;1:242–251. doi:10.1016/j.jaip.2013.03.014*

EVALUATION

The first step in the evaluation is to distinguish acute rhinosinusitis from a viral infection. If there is nasal obstruction and/or facial pain/pressure, a sinus infection is more likely to be present. If symptoms improve in 7 days after diagnosis, AVRS is likely. If the illness is worsening, bacterial rhinosinusitis should be considered. Acute rhinosinusitis unresponsive to therapy or chronic sinusitis requires further investigation with otolaryngology referral and imaging.

Patients with suspected fungal rhinosinusitis should have early nasal endoscopy with biopsy to identify the organism, which is required to make the diagnosis and guide treatment. CT and MRI findings may suggest disease but are not used for confirmation of the diagnosis.

TREATMENT

- **AVRS:** Treatment is mostly observational with symptomatic therapies to include saline irrigation, intranasal steroids, analgesics, and antipyretics. Oral decongestants may be helpful if related to ETD; however, caution should be used in those patients with cardiac disease, glaucoma, and urinary retention. Antihistamines may be helpful for symptom relief by drying the nasal passages, but they may cause drowsiness.
- **ABRS:** Treatment options can be observational or antibiotics in addition to symptomatic therapies noted above. For 7 days observation plus symptomatic treatment are recommended for those patients who can return in 7 days for a follow-up evaluation. If there is improvement in 7 days after the diagnosis, no further treatment is needed. For those who may not be able to return in 7 days for follow-up evaluation, they can be started on oral antibiotics along with symptomatic therapies.
  - Antibiotic options include amoxicillin or amoxicillin-clavulanate with high-dose amoxicillin-clavulanate if the patient is at risk for pneumococcal resistance.
  - For penicillin-allergic patients who can tolerate cephalosporins, third-generation options include cefuroxime, cefixime, or cefpodoxime.
  - Fluoroquinolones levofloxacin or moxifloxacin can also be effective options in penicillin-allergic patients.
  - Owing to high resistance rates for *S. pneumoniae*, macrolides and trimethoprim-sulfamethoxazole are not indicated for treatment.
  - Duration of therapy is usually 5 to 7 days.
  - For initial treatment failures in the setting of uncomplicated ABRS, a broader spectrum antibiotic or an alternative class can be tried for 7 to 10 days.
  - Glucocorticoids are not recommended.
  - Treatment failures after a second course of antibiotics should be imaged with CT and referred to a specialist.
- **Invasive fungal sinusitis:** Treatment can be challenging due to the profound degree of immunosuppression and is considered a medical and surgical emergency. Options for antifungal treatment include amphotericin B, voriconazole, or isavuconazole. Echinocandins (caspofungin or micafungin) may be added to the above for treatment of *Aspergillus* species.
  - Duration of therapy ranges from weeks to 3 months based on the clinical course. Treatment begins with IV formulations but can be transitioned to oral once improvement is achieved.
  - Those with persistent immunosuppression may require lifelong suppressive therapy.

- Sinus surgery should be considered as part of the treatment in order to remove necrotic tissue and decrease the overall fungal burden; however, some patients may not be surgical candidates due to extent of their underlying immunosuppressive disease (e.g., malignancy or AIDS).

PATIENT EDUCATION

- Patients should be educated about proper hand hygiene to prevent self-inoculation with viruses or bacteria. They should also be encouraged to avoid contact with people who have colds or URIs and avoid smoking or smoke exposure.
- Sinusitis can progress into more serious illness so patients should be made aware of when to contact a medical professional such as fever >102 °F (38.9 °C), severe facial or head pain, visual changes, confusion, swelling or redness around one or both eyes, or neck stiffness.

3.2B ALLERGIC RHINITIS

MEDICAL HISTORY AND CLINICAL PRESENTATION

AR symptoms can be like those of viral rhinitis; however, they are usually persistent or may show activation in certain seasons (seasonal AR). Nasal symptoms of congestion, clear rhinorrhea, and frequent sneezing are frequently accompanied by irritation of the eyes, pruritus, conjunctival erythema, and excessive tearing. Often there is a positive family history of allergies or atopy. Those with persistent AR may be affected by dust mites or cockroaches, although it may not be apparent in the history.

SIGNS AND SYMPTOMS

Common complaints of AR include runny nose that is clear, nasal congestion, sneezing, sinus pressure, eye itching, ear irritation, hives, cough, or an itchy throat. Fever is not associated with AR.

PHYSICAL EXAMINATION

Physical examination findings may include scleral injection, watery drainage, infraorbital swelling with darkening or swelling of the conjunctivae of the eyes; bluish/pale swelling of the nasal mucosa with clear drainage; hyperplastic lymphoid tissue lining the posterior pharynx (cobblestoning); and in patients with ETD there may be retraction of the TM with or without fluid accumulation behind the membrane. In children, "allergic facies" may be seen, which is open mouth with a recessed lower jaw and a highly arched palate.

DIFFERENTIAL DIAGNOSIS

Table 3.11 summarizes the differential diagnosis for AR.

DIAGNOSTIC STUDIES

Routine laboratory studies are typically normal. Imaging is usually not indicated unless there is an associated condition that requires investigation such as obstruction or chronic rhinosinusitis.

TABLE 3.11 Differential Diagnosis for Allergic Rhinitis

Condition	Description
Acute infectious rhinitis	May be similar to allergic symptoms but usually isolated or sporadic occurrence associated with an infectious source, most likely viral.
Chronic nonallergic rhinitis	Symptoms are perennial and exacerbated by odors, alcohol, or changes in temperature or humidity. Headaches, sinus congestion, and anosmia are common but sneezing and nasal itching are uncommon.
Drug-induced rhinitis	Medications such as ACE inhibitors, beta blockers, aspirin, and NSAIDs causing rhinitis symptoms.
Hormonal induced rhinitis	Pregnancy, oral contraceptive use, and hypothyroidism may cause rhinitis symptoms.
Nonallergic rhinitis with eosinophilia syndrome	Allergic rhinitis symptoms with nasal eosinophilia but no source of the allergic source on skin testing.
Rhinitis medicamentosa	Rhinitis is induced by the overuse of over-the-counter nasal decongestant sprays.

ACE, angiotensin-converting enzyme; NSAIDs, nonsteroidal anti-inflammatory drugs.
Source: Data from Quillen DM, Feller DB. Diagnosing rhinitis: allergic vs. nonallergic. Am Fam Physician. *2006;73(9):1583–1590. https://www.aafp.org/afp/2006/0501/p1583.html*

EVALUATION

The diagnosis of AR is a clinical diagnosis when the typical symptoms, clinical history, and physical examination findings are present. Some patients may require allergy testing to confirm the allergic trigger, but this is not required to make the diagnosis of AR.

TREATMENT

- The goal of treatment is to decrease or eliminate symptoms for improved quality of life.
- Over-the-counter medications to decrease the incidence of sneezing, rhinorrhea, and nasal itching include cetirizine, loratadine, fexofenadine, and diphenhydramine. Also available are intranasal corticosteroids such as fluticasone or mometasone, which can decrease nasal inflammation and congestion.
- For patients who cannot tolerate intranasal corticosteroids or for those with asthma and AR, leukotriene receptor agonists may be helpful.
- Nonpharmacologic treatment with neti pots or nasal saline rinses using sterile or distilled water may be helpful prior to administration of intranasal corticosteroids. These devices require regular cleaning to avoid contamination risk.
- Referral to an allergist should be considered when above therapies are unsuccessful, overall symptoms are severe, or the patient has severe asthma or recurrent sinusitis.

PATIENT EDUCATION

- Patients with AR should be educated on how to avoid exposure to allergens. They should understand indoor allergens (mold, pet dander, and dust mites) and outdoor allergens (various tree and grass pollens) that can trigger symptoms and ways to control them.

- Patients may also require counseling on which medications would be most beneficial based on their symptoms and those that may be combined safely for improved management.

3.2C EPISTAXIS/FOREIGN BODIES

MEDICAL HISTORY AND CLINICAL PRESENTATION

Approximately 40% of cases of epistaxis are idiopathic while others result from nasal mucosa dryness, trauma (picking), nasal polyps, infections, neoplasms, environmental irritants, cocaine use, and other medical conditions.[26] These other conditions include those that require anticoagulants such as warfarin or direct oral anticoagulants (DOACs) to prevent or treat thrombosis; bleeding disorders such as hereditary hemorrhagic telangiectasia (Osler-Weber-Rendu disease); hereditary blood dyscrasias such as von Willebrand disease and hemophilia; vitamin deficiencies (A, C, D, E, and K); aneurysm of the carotid artery; and nasal neoplasms.

Patients may present with a history of a witnessed insertion of a FB, but others will not have a clear history. Children may present with foul unilateral nasal discharge. Rarely, patients may complain of pain, headaches, intermittent nosebleeds, or sneezing.[34]

SIGNS AND SYMPTOMS

Patients with epistaxis usually experience spontaneous, unilateral or bilateral bleeding from the nares that may be mild, moderate, or severe. In severe cases it may result in dizziness, lightheadedness, nausea, and vomiting.

Patients with a nasal FB may not have any symptoms but were observed to have inserted an object into the nose. Some may have nasal obstruction with resultant mouth breathing, unilateral nasal drainage, foul odor, or epistaxis from subsequent trauma.

PHYSICAL EXAMINATION

Epistaxis requires initial assessment of vital signs, patency of the airway, and mental status. The nose should be examined to identify the source of bleeding if possible. Suction may be helpful to clear blood or clots that may impede ability to identify a source. Topical mucosal vasoconstriction may also assist in achieving some control of bleeding to improve visualization. Anesthesia using cotton swabs soaked with an anesthetic and a vasoconstrictor (lidocaine and epinephrine) may ease any discomfort and facilitate the examination. Inspection should focus on Kiesselbach's plexus first for bleeding, ulceration, or erosion because most bleeds begin there. The nasal vestibule, septum, and turbinates should also be examined for bleeding sources. If the source cannot be found, the cause may be a posterior bleed, mass, or trauma.

Examination of the patient with a nasal FB should include evaluation of the ear and nose with an otoscope as patients with a nasal FB may also have a FB in the ear canal as well. Patients usually have unilateral nasal obstruction (bilateral obstruction is possible), purulent and foul-smelling drainage from the nose, sneezing, epistaxis, or facial pain. FB button batteries in the nose may result in epistaxis and purulent nasal discharge that can be black if there is associated tissue necrosis.

DIFFERENTIAL DIAGNOSIS

Table 3.12 summarizes the differential diagnosis for epistaxis.

Unilateral nasal discharge can result from sinusitis, but this is a diagnosis of exclusion and a FB must be ruled out. The differential diagnosis for bilateral nasal FB can look similar to that for a URI, AR, and sinusitis; however, unilateral nasal symptoms is classic for FB.

DIAGNOSTIC STUDIES

Because the majority of foreign bodies are not radiolucent, plain films are not indicated. When known or suspected foreign bodies are difficult to visualize or there is concern

TABLE 3.12 Differential Diagnosis for Epistaxis

Condition	Description
Nonsystemic Causes	
Chronic sinusitis	Inflammation leading to bleeding
Foreign bodies	Nasal obstruction results with drying effect leading to mucosal disruption or direct trauma
Medications	Intranasal steroids, antihistamines with drying effect
Nasal cavity neoplasm	Bleeding related to malignancy
Nasal cavity polyp	Inflammation and drying effect leading to bleeding
Rhinitis	Inflammation leading to bleeding
Septal perforation	Anatomic deformity causing turbulence and drying effect, predisposing to bleeding
Trauma, nose picking	Most common cause of epistaxis
Trauma, other	Cocaine-induced erosions, nasogastric tube placement, facial trauma
Systemic Causes	
Hemophilia	Hemophilia A (deficiency in factor VIII) and hemophilia B (deficiency in factor IX)
Leukemia	Hematologic malignancy predisposing affected patients to mucosal bleeding including epistaxis
Liver disease	Thrombocytopenia and vitamin K deficiency predispose to bleeding
Renal disease	Uremia can result in platelet dysfunction
Medications	Aspirin, clopidogrel, warfarin
Platelet dysfunction	Poorly functioning platelets
Thrombocytopenia	Low platelets
von Willebrand disease	Genetic bleeding disorder, lack of von Willebrand factor to help blood form clots

Source: Data from Kucik CJ, Clenney T. Management of epistaxis. Am Fam Physician. *2005;71(2):305–311. https://www.aafp.org/afp/2005/0115/p305.html*

for metal FB placement, x-rays may be helpful, especially if there is pain, facial swelling, or epistaxis.

EVALUATION

Initial evaluation of the patient with epistaxis should focus on assessment of hemodynamic stability and the status of the airway given that cases of severe bleeding can cause hypotension and compromise the airway, especially posterior nosebleeds. In the case of hemodynamic instability with hypotension, normal saline boluses should be administered while obtaining a CBC, type and crossmatch, and preparing for blood transfusion if clinically indicated. Symptoms of hematemesis or hemoptysis may indicate a posterior bleed, which tends to be more voluminous than anterior bleeds, although some anterior bleeds can be quite significant. Comprehensive history should focus on conditions that could contribute to nosebleeds or make them worse. A physical examination of the nose can help to identify the source of bleeding.

Most foreign bodies in the nose are diagnosed by direct visualization with a light source or otoscopic evaluation. In the setting of purulent drainage, suctioning may be required to assist in direct visualization of the object. When objects are too high up in the nasal vault to be seen, fiberoptic endoscopy may be required for diagnosis.

TREATMENT

- Treatment of epistaxis:
  - Begin with the patient sitting up and leaning forward. Instruct the patient to blow their nose to remove clots and blood. Instillation of oxymetazoline into the side that is bleeding may help to constrict the blood vessels to achieve hemostasis. The patient should apply firm pressure to the nares for 10 to 15 minutes. This alone can control a majority of cases. If no recurrent bleeding after 30 minutes, the patient can be discharged with an antibiotic ointment to be placed with a cotton swab three times a day for 3 days
  - If a visible bleeding vessel is identified, chemical or electric cautery may be used to achieve hemostasis. If cautery is not successful, nasal packing with antibiotic-coated tampon is indicated. Nasal balloon packing can also be effective. Antibiotics should be prescribed for the duration of nasal packing using amoxicillin-clavulanate or a first-generation cephalosporin. Follow up in 24 to 48 hours with a specialist.
  - If bleeding persists after nasal packing, the contralateral nares may need packing as well. For bleeding that persists with both nares packed, the likelihood of a posterior bleed is almost certain and otolaryngology referral and hospitalization are indicated.
- Treatment of a nasal FB:
  - Removal of the object can be done in the office or emergency setting. Batteries or magnets require urgent removal.
  - Referral to an otolaryngologist for removal of a FB may be required for impacted, posterior, penetrating foreign bodies or difficult removals.

PATIENT EDUCATION

- Patients should be educated on risk factors for the development of nosebleeds to include avoidance of trauma to the nasal mucosa (e.g., nose picking) and maintenance of hydration of the nasal mucosa with the use of humidifiers or saline nasal spray.
- Patients should also understand ways to control nosebleeds that can be performed at home and when they should seek medical attention (bleeding unresponsive to manual compression of the nose for 15 to 20 minutes or profuse bleeding resulting in dizziness, lightheadedness, or shortness of breath).

3.2D TUMORS

MEDICAL HISTORY AND CLINICAL PRESENTATION

Benign tumors such as nasal polyps are sometimes seen in patients with AR, chronic rhinosinusitis, asthma, cystic fibrosis, and aspirin-exacerbated respiratory disease. They typically cause nasal obstruction and decreased sense of smell. IPs resulting from infection with human papillomavirus (HPV) cause nasal obstruction and sometimes hemorrhage. Although benign, IP can be associated with SCC in about 10% of cases.[32]

Patients with malignant nasal or sinus tumors typically present with signs and symptoms that can be nonspecific but mimic rhinosinusitis. They describe persistent unilateral nasal, sinus, or ear congestion with or without pain that have failed to improve with either symptomatic or antibiotic treatments. Vascular tumors may present with obstructive symptoms of the nose and epistaxis. Advanced lesions can result in anosmia, diplopia, visual disturbance, facial swelling, or facial pain.

SIGNS AND SYMPTOMS

There may be no signs or symptoms in early stages of nasal cavity tumors as they may appear only as the tumor grows. Patients may have nasal obstruction, sinus pressure, headaches, runny nose, nosebleeds, facial pain, facial swelling, double vision, or protrusion of the eye.

PHYSICAL EXAMINATION

Patients with nasal cavity tumors should have a complete physical examination of the head and neck including anterior rhinoscopy. Nasal endoscopy may be indicated in the examination. Examination may also include assessment of cranial nerves, ophthalmologic examination, and assessment of hearing with audiometry.

Benign polyps appear as pale, edematous, watery appearing, mucosa-covered masses. IPs are cauliflower-like masses on the lateral nasal wall or pale polypoid lesions. Malignant tumors may result in findings of unilateral nasal obstruction, otitis media, and discharge along with evidence of hemorrhage. Some cases of advanced disease can reveal proptosis or facial swelling.

DIFFERENTIAL DIAGNOSIS

Table 3.13 summarizes the differential diagnosis for nasal tumors.

DIAGNOSTIC STUDIES

Nasal polyps or IPs can be seen on anterior rhinoscopy; however, endoscopy may be required to make the diagnosis.

CT scan or MRI is indicated to define the location and extent of malignant tumors. Tissue biopsy is required to confirm the diagnosis and the type of neoplasm. PET

TABLE 3.13 Differential Diagnosis for Nasal Tumors

Condition	Description
Inverting papilloma	Typically presents in males, arises in lateral aspect of nasal cavity close to middle turbinate. Benign but can become malignant in about 10% of cases.
Nasal polyp	Benign, usually presents in adulthood with nasal obstruction, rhinorrhea, and facial pain. Appears as pale, edematous watery-appearing mucosa-covered mass.
Squamous cell carcinoma	Most common, accounts for about 60% of cases. Presents as nasal mass, obstruction, or epistaxis. Maxillary sinus and nasal cavity are common location of the tumor.
Melanoma	Typically occurs in males in fifth to seventh decades. Occurs in the nasal septum and turbinates.
Lymphoma	Can occur in the nasal cavity or paranasal sinuses.

Source: Data from Lathi A, Syed MM, Kalakoti P, Qutub D, Kishve SP. Clinicopathological profile of sinonasal masses: a study from a tertiary care hospital of India. Acta Otorhinolaryngol Ital. *2011;31(6):372–377. https://www.ncbi.nlm.nih.gov/pmc/articles/PMC3272868*

scan along with CT can assist in the detection of nodal and metastatic disease.

EVALUATION

Benign tumors of the nasal cavity can usually be easily seen with anterior rhinoscopy. If rhinoscopy is unrevealing, nasal endoscopy is indicated.

If a nasal cavity malignancy is found, evaluation should proceed with a biopsy for histopathology to accurately diagnose and classify the nasal cavity tumor. Biopsies are obtained endoscopically, or a fine-needle aspirate biopsy may be required. Imaging studies should include CT and MRI to evaluate for the extent of disease.

TREATMENT

- Benign nasal tumors:
  - The first line of treatment for nasal polyps is intranasal corticosteroid therapy (fluticasone, budesonide, or mometasone) for 1 to 3 months. For larger polyps or those refractory to intranasal corticosteroids oral prednisone may be helpful. Surgery is for those cases that are refractory to medical treatment, although relief may only be temporary as recurrence is possible.
  - IPs require surgical excision.
- Malignant nasopharyngeal and paranasal sinus tumors:
  - Treatment depends on the type of tumor and the extent of the disease. Early stage disease can be treated with radiation therapy (RT) alone.
  - Advanced disease is generally treated with RT and chemotherapy.
  - Some SCC s may be treated with RT and surgery if they are amenable to resection.

PATIENT EDUCATION

- Patients with nasal polyps should continue intranasal steroids even if they have had surgical resection to prevent recurrence. Those with nasal papillomas should be informed that there is a 20% recurrence rate after resection, and they will require periodic follow-up.
- Patients with malignant nasopharyngeal or paranasal sinus tumors should be informed that the treatment options and chance of recovery vary based on tumor location, type, size, and whether it has spread. After treatment, it is important to have close follow-up to monitor for recurrence.

SPECIAL CONSIDERATIONS

- Hospitalized patients are at risk for the development of sinusitis, especially patients who have had head injuries or who require prolonged nasogastric tube placement, antibiotics, or steroids. The risk for development of maxillary sinusitis is increased in patients who are on mechanical ventilators.[29]
- Pregnant women with ABRS may be treated with amoxicillin or amoxicillin-clavulanate. Those who are allergic to penicillin may be treated with clindamycin plus cefixime or cefpodoxime.[23]
- Immunocompromised patients with ABRS are more likely to have resistant bacteria and should receive amoxicillin-clavulanate as first-line therapy.[23]

3.3 DISEASES OF THE ORAL CAVITY AND PHARYNX

OVERVIEW

The oral cavity can be a window into the general health of an individual. Many disease processes can manifest in the oral cavity and pharynx and adversely affect quality of life of some patients. Examination of the oral cavity and pharynx may reveal signs and symptoms of nutritional deficiencies, hematologic disorders, immunologic diseases, oncologic diseases, and systemic infections. Being able to identify the various conditions that affect the oral cavity and pharynx can allow for disease prevention or early diagnosis and treatment.

EPIDEMIOLOGY

Candida is a fungus that is present in the normal microflora of the oral cavity and oropharynx of approximately 30% to 50% of the general population and this rate increases as patients age. In those over the age of 60, the species *Candida albicans* has been recovered from the oral cavity in approximately 60% of patients.[35]

Acute pharyngitis accounts for approximately 15 million visits per year to pediatricians and primary care clinicians in the United States.[36] It is prevalent in the late winter through early spring. Incidence of acute pharyngitis peaks in childhood and adolescence when about 50% of all cases occur before the age of 18. In adults, most cases occur before the age of 40, with declining incidence thereafter.[37]

Overall, 30 cases of peritonsillar abscess are identified per every 100,000 people annually in the United States.[38] It is the most common deep head and neck infection. While it can occur in all age groups, the highest incidence is in those age 20 to 40 years old.[38] Teenagers, young adults, smokers, and patients with recurrent tonsillitis are all at increased risk for developing peritonsillar abscesses.[39]

Epiglottitis was initially seen more commonly in adults. In the 1960s, predominance shifted to children, particularly those between 3 and 5 years old.[40] With the development of the *Haemophilus influenzae* type b vaccine in 1985, cases of acute epiglottitis in children have decreased in developed countries where the vaccine is routinely available.[40,41] Although there has been a sharp decline in epiglottitis cases since the development of the vaccine, it still does occur in both pediatric and adult populations; infection in adults is once again on the rise. This is due in part to varying vaccination rates and the efficacy of the vaccine (and possible diminished efficacy over time). Additionally, while group A ß-hemolytic *Streptococcus* is now the most common cause of epiglottitis, other respiratory pathogens not covered by the current vaccine have been implicated in its development.[41]

The prevalence of oral leukoplakia is estimated to range from 1.49% to 4.11% worldwide.[6,7] Predisposing factors include trauma, mechanical irritation, dentures, and exposure to various forms of tobacco use.

The prevalence of ulcerative disorders varies by the type of ulceration. Necrotizing ulcerative gingivitis (NUG) incidence is low in developed countries. If NUG is present, it is usually found in adults age 18 to 30.[42] Aphthous ulcers are quite common and affect about 25% of the general population and are more common among females.[43] According to the CDC, the herpes simplex virus (HSV-1) that can result in painful oral blisters has a prevalence in the United States of 47.8% and is more common in females than males.

The National Cancer Institute reports that there are approximately 11.1 new cases of oral cavity and pharyngeal cancer per 100,000 men and women per year. In 2017, there were an estimated 396,900 people living with cancer of the oral cavity and pharynx in the United States (https://seer.cancer.gov/statfacts/html/oralcav.html).

Deep neck infections are most common in patients who smoke or chew tobacco, use IV drugs, have poor oral health, lack proper nutrition, and are of low socioeconomic status. They tend to occur between the second and fourth decades of life, but elderly patients are also highly susceptible. Patients with underlying systemic diseases such as diabetes, HIV, and hypertension are at increased risk.

PATHOPHYSIOLOGY

Candida is normally found in the mouth, throat, and digestive tract; however, in healthy individuals it does not create symptoms. When conditions are favorable, *Candida* can multiply and cause infection in the oral cavity, oropharynx, or the esophagus.

Pharyngitis, or tonsillitis, is any inflammation of the pharyngeal or tonsillar tissue. Most episodes of acute pharyngitis are caused by viruses and affect all age groups. Various bacterial infections can also result in acute pharyngitis. The most common bacterial source of acute pharyngitis is GAS.[36] GAS pharyngitis has a predominance in children between 5 and 15 years of age and accounts for 15% to 30% of pediatric cases.[45] GAS pharyngitis is very contagious and is transmitted through close person-to-person contact via respiratory or salivary droplets. Infections are increased in crowded areas, within schools and families. Patients often present with a sore throat, headache, and fever after a 2- to 5-day incubation period.[45]

Peritonsillar abscess, or quinsy, is an acute infection caused by a collection of pus in the space between the tonsillar capsule and the superior pharyngeal constrictor muscle.[39] The majority of peritonsillar abscesses form posterior to the upper tonsillar pole, in the supratonsillar space. There are two pathophysiologic thoughts regarding peritonsillar abscesses: They develop as a complication of acute tonsillitis or in association with minor salivary glands superior to the tonsil, referred to as Weber glands.[39] Bacteria identified in peritonsillar abscesses are most frequently *Fusobacterium necrophorum* and GAS, both of which have been identified in acute tonsillitis.[39] Patients with recurrent tonsillitis are four times more likely to develop recurrent peritonsillar abscesses. Some theories suggest that tonsillar infections spread retrogradely through Weber glands salivary ducts and into the peritonsillar space.[38,39] High levels of amylase, a main component in saliva, have been identified in drainage from peritonsillar abscesses.[39]

Epiglottitis is an acute, rapidly progressing infection of the epiglottis and surrounding tissue. When severe, edema narrows the airway, compresses the vocal cords, and can result in sudden airway compromise and death. *H. influenzae* type b and group A ß-hemolytic *Streptococcus* are the most common pathogens causing epiglottitis. *S. pneumoniae, S. aureus,* and *Klebsiella pneumoniae* are other bacterial causes that should be kept in mind when choosing an antibiotic.[41]

Leukoplakia is a condition in which thick, white patches or plaques form on the oral mucosa that can be found on the tongue, oral mucosa, or the floor of the mouth. These lesions can be benign but have the potential for malignant transformation making it an oral potentially malignant disorder (OPMD). Leukoplakia can be classified into two different types: homogeneous and nonhomogeneous. The homogeneous type is thin and uniformly white with well-defined borders, whereas the nonhomogeneous type may be white with speckles of red (erythroleukoplakia) or white with a granular, nodular, or verrucous texture. Malignant transformation to SCC is more common in the nonhomogeneous type than in the homogeneous type but does occur with both.[46] The annual malignant transformation rate of leukoplakia is 2% to 3%.[47]

Ulcerative disorders of the oral cavity result from defects in the epithelium, underlying connective tissue, or both. These lesions may be solitary or multiple. The cause of these can be attributed to malnutrition, poor dentition, viruses (herpes virus), trauma, and tobacco use.

The most common oral cancer is SCC (90%), which arises from the epithelial lining of the oral cavity. The diagnosis of carcinoma requires evidence of invasion of epithelial cells through the basement membrane into the superficial connective tissues. Invasion results from breaches by a few cells or small epithelial islands and progresses to gross infiltration of the underlying submucosa or bone by malignant cells. This process of invasion gives rise to classic clinical signs of cancer: The lesion becomes hard (induration) and is fixed to the underlying tissues (fixation). As lesions enlarge, they may outgrow their blood supply, or become traumatized, giving rise to a third important clinical sign—ulceration of the tumor surface.[48]

A deep neck infection is defined as an infection in the potential spaces and actual facial planes of the neck. When an infection overtakes the natural resistance of the facial planes, infection can spread along communicating boundaries. Infection may manifest as cellulitis, abscess formation, or necrotizing fasciitis.[49]

3.3A INFECTIOUS DISORDERS: CANDIDIASIS

MEDICAL HISTORY AND CLINICAL PRESENTATION

Oral candidiasis, also known as thrush, is a very common fungal infection (the causative agent is *Candida albicans* but can also be *C. glabrata*, *C. krusei*, or *C. tropicalis*) of the oral cavity resulting in white patches on the oral mucosa, tongue, or throat. These patches can be easily removed with gauze. Those at risk for candidiasis include patients with compromised immune systems, diabetes, or HIV infection; those who use or oral or inhaled steroids; or those who wear dentures.

SIGNS AND SYMPTOMS

Some patients may be asymptomatic while others may feel as though they have a burning sensation, or a feeling of cotton in their mouth, or loss of their sense of taste. Pain with eating or swallowing can also occur.

PHYSICAL EXAMINATION

Examination of the oral cavity usually shows thick white plaques of *Candida* on the mucosa. These lesions can be easily removed with gauze. Some patients can develop erythematous or ulcerative lesions on the oral mucosa. Denture wearers may have a stomatitis around the tissue in contact with the dentures. The clinician may also see *Candida*-induced fissuring at the corners of the mouth referred to as angular cheilitis (Figure 3.10).

DIFFERENTIAL DIAGNOSIS

Table 3.14 summarizes the differential diagnosis for candidiasis.

DIAGNOSTIC STUDIES

A potassium hydroxide (KOH) prep can be used to evaluate for budding yeast with or without pseudohyphae.

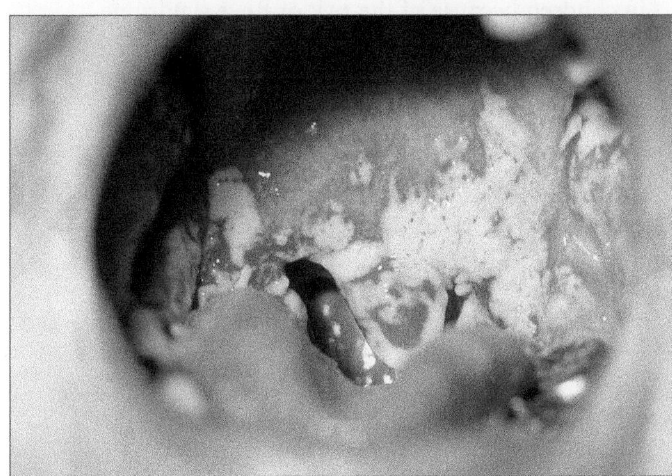

Figure 3.10 This condition is known as oral thrush, which manifested as a result of a *Candida albicans* infection. Note the yellowish beige oral ulcers known as aphthae.

(Source: Courtesy of the Centers for Disease Control and Prevention. https://phil.cdc.gov/details.aspx?pid=1217)

TABLE 3.14 Differential Diagnosis for Candidiasis

Condition	Description
Leukoplakia	White patches or plaques on the oral mucosa that cannot be removed with gauze.
Oral lichen planus	Inflammatory autoimmune-mediated disease resulting in white papules, plaques—typically bilateral or multifocal and lacy in appearance—or patches that can be found on the gingiva, buccal mucosa, or tongue. More common after age 40 and more common in females than males. May be painful or symptomatic discomfort may occur with certain foods. Can look similar to candidiasis, hyperkeratosis, or squamous cell cancer.
Squamous cell carcinoma	White lesions within the oral cavity that are ulcerated, raised, firm, patches and usually tender to palpation. Associated with human papillomavirus (HPV) (most commonly type 16) infection as well as tobacco and alcohol use.

Source: Data from Singh A, Verma R, Murari A, Agrawal A. Oral candidiasis: an overview. J Oral Maxillofac Pathol. *2014;18(suppl 1):S81–S85. doi:10.4103/0973-029X.141325*

Fungal culture may be obtained if looking to identify the organism but generally it is not indicated.

EVALUATION

Diagnosis is made clinically. Oral candidiasis may be the first manifestation of HIV infection. Patients with HIV and oral candidiasis should also be evaluated for possible concomitant *Candida* esophagitis.

TREATMENT

- Nystatin oral rinse and swallow three times per day for 7 to 10 days, Fluconazole orally daily for 7 days or ketoconazole daily for 7 to 14 days.
- Patients with HIV infection may require longer courses of treatment with fluconazole.
- Itraconazole therapy may be required in cases of fluconazole resistance.

PATIENT EDUCATION

- Patients who use steroid inhalers should be encouraged to rinse their mouths or brush their teeth after each use.
- Diabetics should be educated about maintaining good blood glucose control.

3.3B INFECTIOUS DISORDERS: PHARYNGITIS/TONSILLITIS

MEDICAL HISTORY AND CLINICAL PRESENTATION

The medical history should focus on differentiating viral etiologies from bacterial (GAS) to guide the need for GAS testing. Fever, sore throat, and tonsillar exudate are nonspecific findings. Associated cough, rhinorrhea, hoarseness, diarrhea, or the presence of oropharyngeal vesicles can be suggestive of a viral etiology. The presence of a scarlatiniform rash, petechiae of the palate, tonsillar exudate, vomiting, and tender cervical lymph nodes can, in combination, increase the likelihood of the presence of GAS to more than 50%.[50]

SIGNS AND SYMPTOMS

Bacterial and viral pharyngitis may have overlapping signs and symptoms of sore throat, pain with swallowing, and general malaise. Other associated signs and symptoms may aid in distinguishing between the two causes. Patients with viral pharyngitis are often afebrile and have associated conjunctivitis, nasal congestion, rhinorrhea, oral ulcers, hoarseness, cough, or diarrhea.[36] Those with bacterial pharyngitis, in particular GAS pharyngitis, have sudden onset of high fever (above 101.3 °F or 38.5 °C), sore throat, headache, nausea, vomiting and abdominal pain.[36,45]

PHYSICAL EXAMINATION

Direct visualization of the oropharynx often reveals diffuse tonsillopharyngeal erythema and inflammation. Tonsillar exudates, a swollen, erythematous uvula, and petechiae on the hard and soft palate may also be present. Examination of the anterior neck may reveal tender cervical lymphadenopathy. In cases of viral pharyngitis, oral ulcers might be found on examination of the oral cavity. In some cases, a diffuse scarlatiniform rash is present.

DIFFERENTIAL DIAGNOSIS

Viral and bacterial etiologies should be considered in the differential diagnosis of acute pharyngitis or tonsillitis. Table 3.15 lists common and uncommon viral and bacterial causes.[36,45] *Neisseria gonorrhoeae* is seen in sexually active patients or children subjected to sexual abuse. Group C *Streptococcus* is commonly seen in college-aged young adults. Any potential causes of sore throat or tonsillar hypertrophy should also be considered, such as trauma, ingestion or inhalation of caustic agents, recent surgery or intubation, thyroiditis, laryngeal reflux, lymphoma, and tonsillar malignancy.[36,45]

DIAGNOSTIC STUDIES

Diagnosis of acute pharyngitis is clinical; however, certain testing can help guide treatment. A rapid antigen detection test for GAS pharyngitis infection is highly specific and can provide results within 5 to 20 minutes.[45] Rapid antigen detection testing for GAS infection should not be performed if there is high suspicion for viral etiology, in children younger than 3 years old (unless they have had sick contacts), after completion of treatment, or in asymptomatic household contacts.[36] While rapid antigen detection testing is highly specific, it is only moderately sensitive and false negative results do occur.[36]

Obtaining a throat culture is the gold standard. Throat cultures are highly sensitive; however, they require between 24 and 48 hours to produce a result. Throat cultures should be performed if rapid antigen detection testing is negative for GAS, yet clinical suspicion is high.[36]

Measurements of antistreptococcal antibody titers are useful in managing rheumatic fever or glomerulonephritis associated with GAS infections. Because antibody levels do not reach their maximum until 3 to 8 weeks after GAS infection, they are not useful for the diagnosis of acute pharyngitis.[36]

Other diagnostics, such as heterophile antibody test (monospot) to diagnose infectious mononucleosis, and throat cultures to rule out gonorrhea or *Chlamydia* infection should be performed if clinical suspicion is high.[36]

EVALUATION

A diagnosis of acute pharyngitis can often be made through history and physical examination alone. All patients should be evaluated for exposure to close sick contacts and any predisposing factors. Rapid antigen detection testing provides quick information that can guide treatment to mitigate the risk of complications.

TREATMENT

- Supportive therapy should be provided to all patients. Saltwater gargles, adequate hydration, and humidification can provide symptomatic relief. Nonsteroidal anti-inflammatory agents or acetaminophen can be used as antipyretics or pain relievers. Aspirin should be avoided in children because of the risk of Reye syndrome.

TABLE 3.15 Common and Uncommon Viral and Bacterial Causes of Acute Pharyngitis or Tonsillitis

Viral		Bacterial	
Common	**Less Common**	**Common**	**Less Common**
Adenovirus	Coxsackievirus	Group A *Streptococcus*	*Corynebacterium diphtheriae*
Influenza A or B	Echoviruses	Group C *Streptococcus*	*Neisseria gonorrhoeae*
Parainfluenza	Herpes simplex virus 1 and 2		*Arcanobacterium haemolyticum*
Rhinovirus	Cytomegalovirus		*Francisella tularensis*
Respiratory syncytial virus	Rubella		*Yersinia enterocolitica*
Epstein-Barr virus (mononucleosis)	Measles		*Mycoplasma pneumoniae*
			Chlamydia pneumoniae
			Fusobacterium necrophorum

Source: Data from Shulman ST, Bisno AL, Clegg HW, et al. Clinical practice guideline for the diagnosis and management of group A streptococcal pharyngitis: 2012 update by the Infectious Diseases Society of America. Clin Infect Dis. *2012;55(10):e86–e102. doi:10.1093/cid/cis629; Shulman ST. Acute streptococcal pharyngitis in pediatric medicine: current issues in diagnosis and management.* Pediatr Drugs. *2003;5(suppl 1):13–23*

- Most cases of acute pharyngitis, including GAS cases, are self-limited, resolving within a few days.
- Antibiotic therapy is used for GAS pharyngitis in order to prevent transmission to close contacts and complications such as rheumatic fever.[45] A 10-day course of oral penicillin V is first-line antibiotic treatment for GAS pharyngitis.[36] A single intramuscular injection of benthazine penicillin G can be used as an alternative.[36] Patients allergic to penicillins may be treated with a 10-day course of first- or second-generation cephalosporins such as cephalexin, cefadroxil, or cefprozil. If noncompliance with a 10-day regimen is of concern, a third-generation cephalosporin, such as cefdinir, cefixime, or cefpodoxime proxetil can be prescribed for 5 days.[45] Azithromycin can also be prescribed for a 5-day course. Other macrolides, such as clarithromycin, should be prescribed for 10 days. A 10-day course of clindamycin is also effective against GAS pharyngitis.
- Patients typically see clinical improvement of their symptoms within 24 to 48 hours after initiation of antibiotic therapy.[36]

PATIENT EDUCATION

- It is important for patients to be aware that not all episodes of acute pharyngitis require antibiotic therapy.
- If antibiotics are prescribed, common side effects include diarrhea, gastrointestinal upset, rash, and allergy. Patients and clinicians should monitor for complications of GAS or non-GAS acute pharyngitis, such as acute rheumatic fever, poststreptococcal glomerulonephritis, peritonsillar abscess, cervical lymphadenitis, mastoiditis, and other systemic infections.

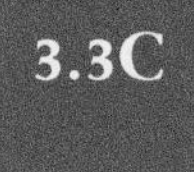

3.3C INFECTIOUS DISORDERS: PERITONSILLAR ABSCESS

MEDICAL HISTORY AND CLINICAL PRESENTATION

Peritonsillar abscess most commonly occurs after an episode of acute tonsillitis but may develop after infectious mononucleosis or spontaneously without a previous history of a sore throat. Patients with peritonsillar abscess generally complain of progressively increasing unilateral throat pain. Some may also experience a referred earache on the same side as the throat pain. The pain can be severe enough to result in the inability to swallow one's own saliva. Some may develop severe halitosis. As the abscess increases in size, it may cause muffled speech or a "hot potato" voice. Neck pain can result from enlarged cervical lymph nodes. Varying degree of trismus is present in almost all cases of peritonsillar abscess. Some may experience respiratory distress as the enlarging abscess obstructs the airway. Other accompanying features include fever, shaking chills, malaise, body aches, headache, and nausea.

SIGNS AND SYMPTOMS

Patients generally present with overall malaise, fatigue, and fever. The chief complaint is often throat pain that is profoundly worse on one side. Dysphagia, drooling, and odynophagia have also been reported. The throat pain or pain with swallowing is often referred to the ipsilateral ear.

PHYSICAL EXAMINATION

On physical examination, patients are often ill-appearing and febrile. Prominent unilateral swelling and erythema of the tonsil, surrounding soft palate, and oropharynx will be present. The uvula may be deviated to the unaffected side. In severe cases resulting in airway obstruction, patients can have stridor. Palpate the neck to assess for induration, warmth, or associated tender cervical lymphadenopathy.

DIFFERENTIAL DIAGNOSIS

The differential diagnosis should include infections or conditions of the adjacent anatomic structures. These include tonsillitis, peritonsillar cellulitis, retropharyngeal abscess, retromolar abscess, periodontal infection, infectious mononucleosis, epiglottitis, lymphoma, tonsillar cancer, or other head and neck neoplasms.

DIAGNOSTIC STUDIES

A rapid throat antigen detection test should be obtained to evaluate if the peritonsillar abscess is associated with tonsillitis. Intraoral ultrasound or CT scan of head and neck with IV contrast can be considered to identify and determine the extent of the abscess and its relationship to surrounding structures. Imaging should be performed if the swelling or signs of infection on physical examination extend inferior to the angle of the mandible.[38]

Aspiration and culture of the abscess should be performed to guide antibiotic treatment.

EVALUATION

A diagnosis of peritonsillar abscess can often be achieved through physical exam alone. Obtaining a culture from the abscess will guide antibiotic treatment. Mononucleosis has been diagnosed in 1.5% to 6% of cases of peritonsillar abscesses.[38]

TREATMENT

- All patients should receive supportive therapy with hydration, pain control, and antipyretics.
- Broad-spectrum antibiotics are first-line therapy due to the polymicrobial nature of peritonsillar abscesses. All antibiotic courses should be continued for 10 to 14 days. Oral therapy options include[38]:
  - Penicillin VK and metronidazole
  - Augmentin
  - Third-generation cephalosporin and metronidazole
  - Clindamycin
  - Linezolid and metronidazole—if methicillin-resistant *Staphylococcus aureus* is suspected
- The use of macrolides is not recommended because of *Fusobacterium* resistance.[38]
- Smaller abscesses in patients with mild symptoms may not require drainage. Drainage can be achieved through needle aspiration or by incision and drainage. Aspiration should continue until dry. The pus is then sent for culture and sensitivity.
  - If needle aspiration is difficult or unsuccessful, otolaryngology should be consulted. Otolaryngologists can reattempt needle aspiration, perform incision and drainage, or surgically remove the tonsil.
- Most patients with peritonsillar abscess can be treated in the ambulatory setting. Red flags that favor inpatient hospitalization for monitoring are intolerance of oral intake,

dehydration, concern for compromised airway, stridor, failure of prior treatment, or signs of sepsis. Diabetic and immunosuppressed patients should also be closely monitored and considered for inpatient management.
- Corticosteroids remain controversial in the treatment of peritonsillar abscess. Steroids may be used to decrease edema, inflammation, and associated pain, but there is not enough evidence in the literature to support their routine use.[38]

PATIENT EDUCATION

- Patients should be counseled on the importance of fully completing prescribed antibiotics. Proper treatment of acute GAS tonsillitis can reduce the incidence of peritonsillar abscess.
- Patients with peritonsillar abscess are at high risk for recurrence. Peritonsillar abscess can be associated with life-threatening complications that patients should be aware of and monitored for. These include:
  - Airway compromise
  - Extension of infection into the deep neck spaces or mediastinum
  - Carotid blowout secondary to necrosis of abscess into the carotid sheath
  - Pneumonia, lung abscess secondary to aspiration of peritonsillar abscess pus
  - Poststreptococcal glomerulonephritis
  - Rheumatic fever

3.3D EPIGLOTTITIS

MEDICAL HISTORY AND CLINICAL PRESENTATION

The presentation varies significantly between pediatric and adult patients. Children have acute onset of symptoms, and otherwise appear well until sudden manifestation. Epiglottitis in adults is most common between the ages of 42 and 48 years.[41] Adults typically present with a sore throat or trouble swallowing and often do not show initial signs of airway obstruction.[41] Adults with diabetes mellitus or other immunocompromised states are at increased risk for epiglottitis and associated complications.

SIGNS AND SYMPTOMS

Patients of all ages present with generalized malaise, odynophagia, dysphagia, and fevers. Children often have difficulty breathing, a cough, and limited oral intake. Adults will predominately present with sore throat and hoarseness in their voice. Rarely do adults have difficulty breathing.[41]

PHYSICAL EXAMINATION

Pediatric patients are toxic appearing, irritable, febrile, tachycardic, and tachypneic. They are frequently sitting up, leaning forward in a tripod position to assist with their swallowing and breathing. On examination of the oral cavity, the child's mouth is usually open and their tongue protruding to facilitate open mouth breathing. Drooling or pooling of saliva is due to dysphagia and odynophagia. Audible stridor and respiratory distress should raise concern for airway compromise.

Adult patients also appear toxic and are febrile. Drooling, tripoding, dyspnea, and stridor are rarely seen in adults. Infection may spread to the neck, and tender cervical lymphadenopathy may be present. Erythema and warmth over the anterior neck and chest can signify associated cellulitis.

When visualized, the epiglottis is "cherry red."[41] Swelling can range from mild to severe and may extend to tissues beyond the epiglottis, resulting in airway obstruction.

DIFFERENTIAL DIAGNOSIS

Several other URIs, including croup, laryngitis, and peritonsillar abscess can present similarly to epiglottitis. Like epiglottitis, croup causes fever, shortness of breath, and stridor in children. The classic "barking" cough of croup is absent in epiglottitis.

Swelling of the epiglottis can also be caused by airway trauma through inhalation of caustic agents or aspiration of foreign bodies. Allergic reactions resulting in angioedema may present with similar airway compromise.

DIAGNOSTIC STUDIES

Initial laboratory studies should include a CBC and C-reactive protein (CRP). Leukocytosis and elevated CRP are often present and indicate infection. Respiratory and blood cultures should be obtained to properly guide antibiotic treatment. Lateral neck radiographs may reveal an enlarged epiglottis with surrounding edema, frequently referred to as the "thumb-print sign" given its shape.[41] Anesthesiology and otolaryngology should both be consulted early if airway instability is of concern. Visualization of the airway through indirect, direct, or flexible laryngoscopy for diagnostic purposes is not recommended as it may disrupt an already unstable airway. If performed, inflammation and erythema of the epiglottis and aryepiglottic folds are seen in children. In adults, edema and erythema extend to surrounding structures including the uvula, pharynx, base of tongue, and false vocal cords.[41]

EVALUATION

The diagnosis of epiglottitis requires a high degree of clinical suspicion. Patients with tenuous airways need prompt intervention. Early recognition, diagnosis, and management can be lifesaving. Lateral neck radiographs are only moderately sensitive and specific, and the false negative rate is approximately 12%.[41]

TREATMENT

- Ensuring a secured airway is the most critical aspect of treatment. All patients should be admitted for close observation and placed on continuous pulse oximetry monitoring. Any patient with shortness of breath, stridor, respiratory distress, tachycardia, or tachypnea should be considered for airway protection and intervention. Airway assessment is performed in a controlled setting, such as an operating room, with fiberoptic laryngoscopy, videolaryngoscopy, difficult airway cart, and surgical airway kit available. Children should be kept upright as lying them down may result in airway obstruction.
- Treating the underlying bacterial infection is paramount. IV third-generation cephalosporins, such as ceftriaxone, is first-line therapy. Unasyn (ampicillin/sulbactam) is also effective. Levofloxacin or moxifloxacin can be utilized in patients allergic to penicillins.[41]
- Inhaled or IV steroid use is controversial. Most studies have shown they provide no proven benefit.[40]

PATIENT EDUCATION

- Patients and parents should be informed of the importance of vaccination against *H. influenzae* type b. Education about complications of epiglottitis, including epiglottic abscess, necrotizing mediastinitis, airway loss, and death, can illustrate the severe consequences of not vaccinating.

3.3E LEUKOPLAKIA

MEDICAL HISTORY AND CLINICAL PRESENTATION

Oral leukoplakia is usually an asymptomatic condition that presents as white patches on the oral mucosa that cannot be removed with gauze. Although it can be a benign condition, the underlying mechanisms are not well understood and there is a risk of dysplasia to malignant transformation. Risk factors for malignant transformation are similar to those for SCC and include tobacco use in any form and alcohol use. HPV infection can also be associated with this condition.

SIGNS AND SYMPTOMS

Patients may notice a lesion of leukoplakia if it is located in a highly visible area of the mouth; however, these lesions are found during routine examination of the mouth. Most lesions of leukoplakia are asymptomatic; some patients may be able to feel the presence of a raised lesion within the mouth.

PHYSICAL EXAMINATION

Physical examination includes direct visualization of the oral cavity to evaluate the oral mucosa of the mouth and the tongue. Particular attention should focus on the buccal mucosa, gingiva, soft and hard palates, tonsillar fossae, lateral tongue, and the floor of the mouth. Assessment for lymphadenopathy of the neck should also be performed.

Examination may reveal discrete, white plaques, white plaques with red speckles (erythroleukoplakia), or white plaques that are granular, nodular, or verrucous appearing on the mucosa of the oral cavity or tongue and cannot be removed with gauze or gentle scraping.

DIFFERENTIAL DIAGNOSIS

Table 3.16 summarizes the differential diagnosis for leukoplakia.

TABLE 3.16 Differential Diagnosis of Leukoplakia

Condition	Description
Candidiasis	Fungal infection (*Candida*) of the oral cavity resulting in white patches on the oral mucosa, tongue, or throat. These can be easily removed with gauze.
Frictional keratosis	A white keratotic thickening of the buccal mucosa that results from chronic friction (sharp teeth/dentures) or mechanical trauma such as cheek biting. Lesions usually resolve with removal of the friction or cessation of the trauma.
Graft-vs-host disease	Lacy white lines found along the inner cheek or tongue (sides or top) in patients who have had allogenic hematopoietic stem cell transplantation (HSCT). Usually develops 6–24 months after the transplant.
Oral lichen planus	Inflammatory autoimmune-mediated disease resulting in white papules, plaques, or patches that can be found on the gingiva, buccal mucosa, or tongue. More common after age 40 and more common in females than males. May be painful or symptomatic discomfort with certain foods.
Squamous cell carcinoma	White lesions within the oral cavity that are ulcerated, raised, firm, and usually tender to palpation. Associated with human papillomavirus (most commonly type 16) infection as well as tobacco and alcohol use.

Source: Data from van der Waal I. Oral leukoplakia, the ongoing discussion on definition and terminology. Med Oral Patol Oral Cir Bucal. *2015; 20(6):e685–e692. doi:10.4317/medoral.21007*

DIAGNOSTIC STUDIES

The diagnosis is made with history and physical examination; however, the gold standard for diagnosis is biopsy for histopathologic evaluation of the lesion.

EVALUATION

Leukoplakia is a diagnosis that is made clinically by visualization of white plaques, white plaques with speckles of red (erythroleukoplakia), or white plaques with granular, nodular, or verrucous texture that adhere to the oral mucosa.

Multiple biopsy samples are indicated if there is an increase in the size of leukoplakia, the lesion is nonhomogeneous, or the lesion is felt to extend beyond the submucosa on palpation.

TREATMENT

- Frequent monitoring is the mainstay of treatment when patients do not want to proceed with lesion removal or when the lesion is too large. Patients should be encouraged to discontinue habits that may increase the risk of malignant transformation such as the use of alcohol and tobacco products.
    - At follow-up visits, a biopsy is indicated if there is a change in the size or shape of the lesion that is concerning for malignant transformation.
- **Medical therapy:** There are no approved medical regimens; however, retinoids, cyclooxygenase-2 inhibitors (COX-2), beta carotene, and green tea extracts have been tested.
- Resection with a scalpel or CO_2 laser are the most common forms of surgical treatment in cases of smaller nonhomogeneous lesions or those showing epithelial dysplasia. Quarterly follow-up for 1 year then annually after surgery is necessary as recurrence is common and the risk of malignant transformation is not eliminated with surgical resection.

PATIENT EDUCATION

Patients should be educated on the correlation between smoking, alcohol use, the presence of leukoplakia, and the risk of oral cancer. Modifiable risks such as cessation of alcohol and tobacco use should be discussed. Because of the possibility of the development of oral cancer, patients should be informed about the importance of frequent office visits, which may include serial biopsies and excisions.

3.3F ULCERATIVE DISORDERS

MEDICAL HISTORY AND CLINICAL PRESENTATION

Oral ulcerative disorders include NUG (trench mouth or Vincent angina), aphthous ulcer (canker sore or ulcerative stomatitis), and herpes stomatitis.

NUG is a periodontal disease that is felt to result from poor oral hygiene, psychological stress, and malnutrition.[51] It is characterized by pain, interdental necrosis, and bleeding of the gingiva.[42]

Aphthous ulcers are the most common form of lesion in the oral cavity. The cause is uncertain, but it has been suggested that human herpesvirus 6 is associated with these ulcers. Suggested etiologies include changes in hormones, medications, foods that result in hypersensitivity, nutritional deficiency, trauma, stress, and tobacco use.[43]

Herpes stomatitis is an infection of the oral mucosa or lips caused by the HSV-1. Herpetic gingivostomatitis is the most common cause of gingivostomatitis in children before the age of 5 but can also occur in adults where it will often present as severe pharyngitis. Presentation may include fever that is followed by a painful eruption of ulcerative lesions of the gingiva and mucosa. The HSV-1 can spread through direct contact or from droplets from oral secretions or lesions from symptomatic or asymptomatic individuals. After primary infection, virus that is dormant in the trigeminal ganglion can reemerge as herpes labialis. These cold sores can be triggered by stress, fatigue, trauma, or UV light. HSV-1 infection affects about 15% to 45% of the U.S. population.[52]

SIGNS AND SYMPTOMS

Patients with NUG may have fever, malaise, painful and swollen gums that bleed spontaneously or from brushing, purulent drainage from the gums, severe halitosis, or lymphadenopathy.

Patients with aphthous ulcers may experience mild to severe painful ulceration(s) on the nonkeratinized mucosa of the mouth (labial and buccal mucosa or tongue) without systemic symptoms.

Patients with herpes stomatitis will develop a burning sensation then an eruption of painful lesions on the lip or within the mouth. There may be associated fever, chills, anorexia, irritability, and cervical lymphadenopathy.

PHYSICAL EXAMINATION

NUG will appear as ulcerated, swollen, or receding gums that can be painful, bleed easily, or have purulent drainage. There is usually associated severe halitosis. Some patients may also have tooth loss.

Aphthous ulcers are usually found on the nonkeratinized areas of the mouth and will be nonindurated, yellow-white sores with a sloughing base and a surrounding inflammatory erythematous halo. Minor ulcers are <1 cm in diameter. Major ulcers are >1 cm in diameter.

Herpes stomatitis usually involves the gingiva but other oral sites and the skin around the mouth may be involved also. There may be associated lymphadenopathy with initial infection. Examination of the perioral and oral mucosa may show vesicles on the lip border, lip, and adjacent mucosa in the mouth. Outbreaks may also appear on the tongue, buccal mucosa, or soft palate. Lesions will begin as vesicles that will usually rupture, ulcerate, and scab over within 1 to 2 days.

DIFFERENTIAL DIAGNOSIS

Tables 3.17, 3.18, and 3.19 summarize the differential diagnoses for NUG, aphthous ulcer, and herpes stomatitis, respectively.

DIAGNOSTIC STUDIES

No diagnostic studies are indicated for NUG or aphthous ulcers; however, a culture may be obtained for a definitive diagnosis of herpes simplex. Alternatively, a Tzanck smear can be performed in the office for a rapid diagnosis of herpes simplex.

TABLE 3.17 Differential Diagnosis for Necrotizing Ulcerative Gingivitis

Condition	Description
Herpes gingivostomatitis	Edematous gingivae that bleed easily with associated small vesicles. May also have fever, malaise, anorexia, irritability.
Leukemia	May cause bleeding gingiva (particularly acute myelomonocytic leukemia), gingival ulcerations, and gingival enlargement.
Vitamin C deficiency	May cause dental caries as well as bleeding and receding gingiva.

Source: Data from Todescan S, Atout RN. Managing patients with necrotizing ulcerative gingivitis. J Can Dent Assoc. *2013;79:d46.*

TABLE 3.18 Differential Diagnosis for Aphthous Ulcer

Condition	Description
Behçet disease	Rare disease of recurrent oral aphthous ulcers along with systemic manifestations.
Bullous lichen planus	May appear as papular, atrophic, or erosive lesions on the buccal mucosa. Can occur with cutaneous disease or independently.
HIV infection	Recurrent aphthous ulcerations may be associated with HIV infection.
Herpes simplex	May present with extensive oral ulcerations.
Pemphigus	Flaccid bullae of the oral mucosa spreading to the skin (scalp, face, axilla, chest, and groin).
Pemphigoid	Intact bullae or erosions of the oral mucosa and bullous lesions of the skin.
Inflammatory bowel disease (IBD)	Association between oral ulcerations and IBD. Those associated with Crohn disease may have a linear appearance.
Systemic lupus erythematosus (SLE)	Oral ulcers can be associated with lupus in addition to other systemic manifestations (malar rash, photosensitivity, arthritis).
Squamous cell carcinoma (SCC)	White lesions within the oral cavity that are ulcerated, raised, firm, and usually tender to palpation. Associated with human papillomavirus (most commonly type 16) infection as well as tobacco and alcohol use.

Source: Data from Tarakji B, Gazal G, Al-Maweri SA, Azzeghaiby SN, Alaizari N. Guideline for the diagnosis and treatment of recurrent aphthous stomatitis for dental practitioners. J Int Oral Health. *2015;7(5):74–80.*

TABLE 3.19 Differential Diagnosis for Herpes Stomatitis

Condition	Description
Aphthous ulcer	Nonvesicular, round yellow-grayish ulcerations with surrounding halo.
Erythema multiforme	Bullous erosions that may have a target appearance on the oral mucosa. May also involve the skin, genital, and/or ocular mucosae.
Syphilitic chancre	Painless, indurated ulcerative lesion on the oral mucosa or lip. May have associated fever, malaise, skin rashes, pharyngitis, or lymphadenopathy.
Squamous cell carcinoma (SCC)	White lesions within the oral cavity that are ulcerated, raised, firm, and usually tender to palpation. Associated with human papillomavirus (most commonly type 16) infection, tobacco, and alcohol use.

Source: Data from Wiler JL. Diagnosis: recurrent herpes gingivostomatitis. Emerg Med News. *2006;28(9):34. doi:10.1097/01.EEM.0000316937.37487.b3*

EVALUATION

In the evaluation of NUG, a thorough medical history should be obtained to include general health, nutritional habits, tobacco use, and dental history. Primary care clinicians should perform an oral examination for clinical features of NUG that include gingival swelling, gingival bleeding, necrosis or ulceration of the gingiva, and severe halitosis. As NUG can present in patients who are HIV positive, evaluation of the head and neck for lymphadenopathy should also be included.

Aphthous ulcers are usually benign and self-limited and heal within 2 weeks, but those that persist longer than 6 weeks should be evaluated for malignancy.

Herpes stomatitis outbreaks are usually self-limited and heal over the course of 7 to 10 days. In the case of patients who are immunocompromised, outbreaks can be very painful and antiviral therapy should be considered.

TREATMENT

- NUG:
  - Pain control with ibuprofen or acetaminophen
  - Chlorhexidine 0.12% rinses twice a day for 2 weeks
  - Oral antibiotics with metronidazole or penicillin for 7 to 10 days
  - Referral for debridement by a dental professional
- Aphthous ulcers:
  - Some patients with mild ulceration will require no treatment as these lesions will resolve on their own.
  - More severe ulcerations may improve with chlorhexidine gluconate (Peridex) rinses or topical corticosteroids.
- Herpes stomatitis:
  - Some outbreaks will resolve without any intervention. In patients with recurrent outbreaks or who are immunocompromised, antiviral therapy can help to shorten the duration of illness. Antivirals are most effective if started within 1 to 2 days of onset of symptoms. Acyclovir five times per day for 7 to 10 days or valacyclovir twice per day orally for 7 to 10 days may be used.

PATIENT EDUCATION

- Patients with NUG should be educated about good oral hygiene that includes brushing teeth at least two times a day, flossing daily, maintaining a healthy diet, and avoidance of smoking.
- Patients with herpes stomatitis should be educated about the risk of transmission with active cold sores and ways to decrease spreading to others such as avoiding kissing, sharing personal items (e.g., utensils, water bottles, and lip balm), or performing oral sex.
  - They should also be aware that the virus can be transmitted even without active cold sores but that it is more likely to spread with active cold sores.

3.3G ORAL CANCER

MEDICAL HISTORY AND CLINICAL PRESENTATION

Development of oral cancer can affect the lip, oral cavity, and pharynx (nasopharynx, oropharynx, and laryngopharynx). When oral or pharyngeal cancer does occur, 90% of the cases are classified as SCC. Tobacco use in all forms is the greatest risk factor for development of oral cancer. Alcohol use combined with tobacco use is known to increase the risk.[53] According to the CDC, about 70% of cancers of the oropharynx, which includes the tonsils, soft palate, and the base of the tongue, are linked to the HPV, a common sexually transmitted virus. UV light exposure such as exposure to sun or artificial UV rays from tanning beds is a major cause of cancer of the lips. Chewing the areca nut, also called the betel nut, has been linked to the development of SCC of the mouth and esophagus.[54]

Patients should be asked about their current health and previous health conditions as well as risk factors such as health habits and behaviors (tobacco use, alcohol consumption, and sexual practices that may involve oral-genital contact).

SIGNS AND SYMPTOMS

Presenting symptoms of oral cavity tumors are numerous, including mouth pain, nonhealing ulcers, loose teeth, poorly fitting dentures, weight loss, dysphagia, odynophagia, and bleeding. Those who have oropharyngeal tumors may complain of dysphagia, odynophagia, obstructive sleep apnea, bleeding, or a mass in the neck. Hypopharyngeal tumors may be asymptomatic for a longer period of time and may present in later stages with complaints including weight loss, dysphagia, odynophagia, hemoptysis, or a neck mass. Patients with laryngeal cancer may present initially with hoarseness and later with dysphagia, stridor, hemoptysis, cough, and possibly referred otalgia.

PHYSICAL EXAMINATION

Common findings of oral and oropharyngeal cancer can show a wide range of clinical abnormalities that range from a subtle change in surface texture, color, or elasticity to an obvious lesion, ulceration, or mass. Skin or mucosal surface changes may have white, red, or mixed white and red features (e.g., leukoplakia or erythroplakia). Change in mucosal texture may include firmness or induration with palpation. Advanced disease may include lesions that are fixed to surrounding and deeper tissues with or without pain.

TABLE 3.20 Differential Diagnosis for Oral Cancer

Condition	Description
Aphthous ulcer	Nonvesicular, round, yellow-grayish ulcerations with surrounding halo.
Behçet disease	Rare disease of recurrent oral aphthous ulcers along with systemic manifestations.
Candidiasis	Fungal infection (*Candida*) of the oral cavity resulting in white patches on the oral mucosa, tongue, or throat. These can be easily removed with gauze. Patients may be asymptomatic, and some may have associated soreness or difficulty swallowing. Common in patients who are immunosuppressed, are diabetic, and use or oral or inhaled steroids.
Erythroplakia	Red or white-red patches or plaques on the oral mucosa that cannot be removed with gauze.
Frictional keratosis	A white keratotic thickening of the buccal mucosa that results from chronic friction (sharp teeth/dentures) or mechanical trauma such as cheek biting. These lesions usually resolve with removal of the friction or cessation of the trauma.
Leukoplakia	White patches or plaques on the oral mucosa that cannot be removed with gauze.
Oral lichen planus	Inflammatory autoimmune-mediated disease resulting in white papules, plaques, or patches that can be found on the gingiva, buccal mucosa, or tongue. More common after age 40 and more common in females than males. May be painful or symptomatic discomfort may occur with certain foods. Can look similar to candidiasis, hyperkeratosis, or squamous cell cancer.
Leukoplakia	White patches or plaques on the oral mucosa that cannot be removed with gauze.
Syphilitic chancre	Painless, indurated ulcerative lesion on the oral mucosa or lip. May have associated fever, malaise, skin rashes, pharyngitis, or lymphadenopathy.

Source: Data from Gonsalves WC, Chi AC, Neville BW. Common oral lesions: part I. Superficial mucosal lesions. Am Fam Physician. *2007;75(4):501–507. https://www.aafp.org/afp/2007/0215/p501.html*

DIFFERENTIAL DIAGNOSIS

Table 3.20 summarizes the differential diagnosis for oral cancer.

DIAGNOSTIC STUDIES

Biopsy with histopathologic evaluation is indicated for visible lesions suspicious for malignancy. Fine needle aspiration can be used for tissue diagnosis of neck mass or cervical lymphadenopathy.

CT, MRI, and PET scanning are used in the evaluation of oral and oropharyngeal cancers. CT and MRI can be used to stage lymphadenopathy. MRI can better evaluate more superficial tumors or better define tumors of the tongue. CT can evaluate for bone invasion. PET is superior to CT and MRI in detecting metastases or second primary tumors.

EVALUATION

Direct inspection and palpation of the oral cavity is the recommended method for evaluation of oral cancer. Patients who are high risk for the development of oral cancer such as those who use tobacco or alcohol should be screened and suspicious lesions should be referred to an oral surgeon for biopsy. Additional modes of evaluation of lesions outside the mouth may include indirect mirror examination or direct flexible laryngoscopy.

When evaluating for laryngeal and hypopharyngeal malignancies, examination under anesthesia may be required to delineate the extent of tumor and to allow for tissue diagnosis with fine needle aspiration biopsy.

Imaging studies such as CT, MRI, and PET scans can be used to evaluate for local infiltration, regional lymph node involvement, or the presence of distance metastases.

TREATMENT

- **Oral cavity carcinoma:** Tumors detected before they reach 2 cm in diameter are usually treated with local resection. Radiation is prescribed to patients with positive margins or metastatic disease. Larger tumors are treated with resection, dissection of the neck, and RT.
- **Oropharyngeal carcinoma:** For patients who have disease that is resectable, but they prefer organ preservation, chemotherapy and RT are used. Some regimens may include chemotherapy, RT, and surgical resection.

PATIENT EDUCATION

- Patients should be educated about the link between tobacco and alcohol use and the development of oral cancer. They should be encouraged not to use tobacco products in any form and to limit alcohol use so as to decrease the risk of the development of oral cancer as well as other diseases linked to the use of these substances.

3.3H DEEP NECK INFECTIONS

MEDICAL HISTORY AND CLINICAL PRESENTATION

Infections that form in the spaces between fascial planes and structures of the neck range in severity from mild to life-threatening. Deep neck infections can be divided into different categories depending on what space or structures they involve.[44]

Submandibular is the most commonly involved space followed by the peritonsillar space.[44]

The majority of these infections are extensions of dental or tonsillar infections.[44] Other origins include foreign bodies, the salivary glands, malignancy, and trauma to the head or neck. Some infections of the neck, particularly those associated with tonsillitis, pharyngitis, otitis media, or dental caries, have the potential to lead to more life-threatening infections such as Lemierre syndrome and Ludwig angina.[55] Lemierre syndrome is an anaerobic infection leading to septic thrombophlebitis of the internal jugular vein with subsequent sepsis and septic emboli seeding in distant locations.[55] Ludwig angina is a rapidly progressing infection of the bilateral sublingual and submandibular spaces resulting in edema of the floor of mouth with extension into the mediastinum.[44]

SIGNS AND SYMPTOMS

Signs and symptoms associated with deep neck infections depend on the location and involved spaces. Fever, general malaise, and fatigue are commonly present. Varying degrees of dental pain, neck pain, odynophagia, dysphagia, dysphonia, trismus, and otalgia are often seen on initial presentation. If severe, patients may complain of shortness of breath.

PHYSICAL EXAMINATION

Physical examination findings vary from mild to severe and vary according to the structures of the neck that are involved and extent of infection. Patients may be febrile or toxic appearing. Generalized facial and neck edema may be present as well as warmth and erythema over the affected area. Malodorous breath and poor dentition suggest odontogenic source. Drooling and pooling of secretions and trismus may indicate underlying tonsillopharyngeal infection. Likewise, patients with retropharyngeal abscesses often have torticollis, neck stiffness, and oropharyngeal bulging.[55]

Severe, life-threatening deep neck infections are important to recognize early. Patients with Ludwig angina are often tachycardic and tachypneic with visible work of breathing and stridor.[55] The floor of mouth is bulging and edematous. On palpation the patient's neck is swollen, tender, and indurated. Patients with Lemierre syndrome may have fever, neck swelling, difficulty breathing, low oxygen saturations, arthralgias and abdominal pain which are associated with abscesses, or effusions that develop throughout the body due to septic emboli.[55]

DIFFERENTIAL DIAGNOSIS

The differential diagnosis for deep neck space infections should include all head and neck infections. Table 3.21 summarizes the infections that should be considered.

Other disorders that may present similarly to deep neck space infections are angioedema, globus sensation, trauma to the head or neck, and some esophageal conditions.

DIAGNOSTIC STUDIES

Given that deep neck infections are usually polymicrobial, cultures should be obtained from the presumed primary source when possible. *Streptococcus*, *Peptostreptococcus* species, *Staphylococcus aureus*, methicillin-resistant *Staphylococcus aureus*, and anaerobes such as *Fusobacterium* are all common organisms found to cause deep neck infections.[44] Blood cultures should also be obtained if sepsis is of concern.

Neck ultrasound is a readily available, low-cost method for detecting abscesses in the neck spaces. CT scan of the head and neck with IV contrast agent may be preferred if infection is extensive to evaluate for involvement of surrounding structures.

If Lemierre syndrome is suspected, further studies may be warranted depending on the patient's symptoms. Chest radiographs or CT may reveal bilateral necrotic infiltrates, pleural effusions, empyema, and pulmonary abscesses. An echocardiogram can show endocarditis. Abdominal imaging can identify intra-abdominal abscesses and hepatic abscesses. Joint radiographs or cultures may yield septic arthritis or sterile effusions.[55]

EVALUATION

Any infection of anatomic structures of the head and neck can ultimately develop into a deep neck space infection. Many head and neck infections also present with similar signs and symptoms to deep neck infections, but it is important to realize when the infection has progressed and extended into the deep neck spaces.

TREATMENT

- Treatment is centralized on antibiotic therapy, airway management, and surgical intervention. Patients generally require admission to the hospital for monitoring and should initially be started on broad-spectrum IV antibiotics until the results of cultures have been received.

TABLE 3.21 Differential Diagnosis of Deep Neck Space Infections

Differential Diagnosis	Description
Pharyngitis/tonsillitis	Abrupt onset, fatigue, fever, and sore throat.
Peritonsillar abscess	May present with fever, dysphagia, sore throat, trismus, and a "hot potato" voice.
Parapharyngeal abscess	May present with fever, limited neck movement, and neck pain.
Retropharyngeal abscess	Commonly causes fever, sore throat, dysphagia, odynophagia, neck pain, and dyspnea. There is usually a history of trauma (endoscopy, intubation, foreign body).
Salivary gland infections	May include sialadenitis, parotitis, or parotid abscess.
Submandibular space infections (Ludwig angina)	Bilateral infection of the submandibular space (sublingual and submaxillary spaces). Presents as a cellulitis and may obstruct airway.
Submental space infection or abscess	Chin may be erythematous, firm, and swollen.
Dental infection	Infection originating from the teeth or supporting structures causing pain and swelling.
Masticator abscess	Buccal pain swelling and trismus are common symptoms.
Lemierre syndrome	Ill-appearing patient with history of severe pharyngitis, neck pain, and respiratory distress.

Source: Data from Data from Priyamvada S, Motwani G. A study on deep neck space infections. Indian J Otolaryngol Head Neck Surg. *2019;71(suppl 1): 912–917. doi:10.1007/s12070-019-01583-4*

- Patients should be admitted to the ICU if signs of airway compromise, such as trismus, stridor, or upper airway obstruction, are present. Some patients may require temporary tracheostomy. Endotracheal intubations may be difficult, and attempts have the potential to further aggravate a compromised airway.[44]
- Needle aspiration should be performed and sent for culture and sensitivity. Surgical drainage or debridement of necrotic tissue may be required in severe cases.

PATIENT EDUCATION

- Patients should be aware that early diagnosis and intervention are important and can be lifesaving. The neck is a confined space with vital structures. Infection can result in compression, necrosis, and erosion of these structures and lead to profound bleeding, respiratory distress, and rapid demise.

3.4 DISEASES OF THE SALIVARY GLANDS

OVERVIEW

The head and neck contain major and minor salivary glands. The major salivary glands are the bilateral parotid glands, submandibular glands, and sublingual glands while the minor salivary glands exist on the lips, tongue, oral cavity, and pharynx. The purpose of salivary glands is to produce saliva, which is composed of mostly water, but also includes important enzymes, electrolytes and proteins that help to provide lubrication, aid in digestion, alter taste, and protect the oral cavity.[56] Disorders of the salivary glands primarily involve the parotid, submandibular, and sublingual glands and can be categorized as inflammatory, infectious, or neoplastic.

EPIDEMIOLOGY

Inflammatory and infectious disorders of the salivary gland involve all age groups but are most common in children and in elderly, hospitalized patients. Mumps, a highly contagious viral etiology of acute sialadenitis, predominately affects children. Approximately 85% of mumps cases involve pediatric patients under the age of 15.[56]

Salivary gland tumors are relatively rare, accounting for 6% of all head and neck neoplasms.[56] The majority (80%) of salivary gland neoplasms are benign tumors of the parotid gland.[57] Most often, these masses are identified as pleomorphic adenomas.[56] While uncommon, tumors originating from the submandibular, sublingual, and minor salivary glands are usually malignant.[56] Approximately 16% of all salivary masses are malignant in adults.[56] The likelihood of malignancy increases greatly to over 50% for salivary masses found in the pediatric population.[56] Mucoepidermoid carcinoma and adenoid cystic carcinoma are the most commonly identified type on tissue diagnosis.[56]

PATHOPHYSIOLOGY

Most inflammatory or infectious salivary gland disorders are thought to be due to retrograde salivary flow and salivary flow stasis. Retrograde salivary flow introduces pathogens from the oral cavity to the salivary glands, resulting in infection of the gland. Slowed salivary flow can be due to low salivary volume or altered ductal anatomy. Decreased salivary production secondary to dehydration decreased oral intake, malnutrition, and certain medications leads to overall slower flow of saliva through salivary gland ducts. This can easily lead to infection. As a result, infections of the salivary glands frequently occur in conjunction with dental infections.

Salivary stasis also increases the potential for stone, sialolith, formation. Sialoliths, which primarily affect the submandibular gland (80–90%), are made up of salts and proteins. Sialoliths can further impede salivary flow through glandular ducts and result in subsequent infection, fibrosis, and stenosis. Repeated infections or stones can eventually lead to fibrosis and narrowing of the salivary duct, further worsening salivary stasis.[56]

Neoplastic conditions of the salivary glands can be benign or malignant. Over time, some benign masses, including pleomorphic adenomas, may transform into malignant variations.

MEDICAL HISTORY AND CLINICAL PRESENTATION

Patient history and presentation vary widely depending on the type of salivary disorder. Salivary conditions can be acute or chronic. Patients with inflammatory and infectious salivary disorders often have conditions that impair salivary flow including diabetes, hypothyroidism, renal failure, Sjögren syndrome, or dehydration or dysphagia impairing oral intake. Dehydration is a common side effect of antihistamines, anticholinergics, and diuretics. Anatomic variations predisposing patients to sialadenitis involve sialoliths, salivary duct strictures, and recent surgery or dental procedure.[57] Patients with mumps usually have a recent history of close contact with an infected person.

Sialadenitis, infectious or inflammatory, can present gradually or rapidly. It most often affects the parotid gland, causing parotitis.[56] Sialadenitis can also be chronic due to repeated infections. Children and elderly patients are most at risk.[55]

Salivary neoplasms are also seen in all age groups. Benign masses are often slow growing while malignant masses tend to have more rapid growth.[57]

SIGNS AND SYMPTOMS

Inflammatory and infectious salivary conditions such as sialadenitis and parotitis are often associated with unilateral swelling and pain of the cheek. Pain is typically reported at the location of the affected gland and may be exacerbated with eating. Constitutional symptoms may or may not be present; additionally, some patients may report a fever.

Mumps initially presents with unilateral swelling that progresses to bilateral involvement of the salivary glands.[56] Patient with mumps may also complain of referred pain in their ears and trismus. HIV infection may also cause bilateral gland enlargement.

Patients with autoimmune conditions such as Sjögren syndrome often have xerostomia and xeropthalmia.

Sialolithiasis, similar to sialadenitis, is associated with postprandial cheek pain. Patients with sialolithiasis often do not have fever or other signs of infection.

Salivary tumors, whether benign or malignant, are often asymptomatic. Patients may notice swelling or evidence of involvement of surrounding structures such as facial weakness or drooping. While most are painless, some involved or advanced masses may cause discomfort. Patients with metastatic disease may have weight loss, night sweats, fevers, or chills.

TABLE 3.22 Differential Diagnosis of Salivary Gland Disorders

Differential Diagnosis	Description
Infectious/Inflammatory	
Sialolithiasis	Salivary gland stones that can lead to acute sialadenitis but more commonly results in chronic sialadenitis. Submandibular gland affected most commonly.
Salivary stasis	Poor salivary flow in the setting of dehydration or decreased oral intake that leads to acute or chronic sialadenitis.
Sialadenitis, acute	Bacterial infection of the salivary gland causing sudden pain and swelling, most commonly affecting the parotid gland.
Sialadenitis, chronic	Obstructive infection from a stricture or stone resulting in recurrent pain or swelling of the parotid gland.
Mumps	Usually bilateral parotid swelling but can begin unilaterally, can be tender. Most commonly affects children. Otalgia and trismus may also be present.
HIV infection	Usually bilateral parotid swelling but can affect more than one gland, can be tender.
Neoplastic Benign	
Pleomorphic adenoma	Usually present as painless, slow-growing masses of the neck or parotid gland. Can affect both children and adults, may become malignant.
Hemangioma	Usually present as painless, slow-growing masses of the neck or parotid gland. Most common in children.
Lymphatic malformation	Usually present as painless, slow-growing masses of the neck or parotid gland. Most common in children.
Malignant	
Mucoepidermoid carcinoma	Usually present as painless, slow-growing masses of the neck or parotid gland.
Adenoid cystic carcinoma	Usually present as painless, slow-growing masses of the neck or parotid gland. Advanced tumors can be painful or result in nerve paralysis.
Squamous cell carcinoma	Usually results from metastasis to the parotid gland.
Basal cell carcinoma	Usually results from metastasis to the parotid gland.
Melanoma	Usually results from metastasis to the parotid gland.
Other	
Sjögren syndrome	Chronic inflammatory disorder resulting in dry eyes and dry mouth in which autoantibodies affect lacrimal and salivary glands.

Source: Data from Wilson KF, Meier JD, Ward PD. Salivary gland disorders. Am Fam Physician. *2014;89(11):882–888. https://www.aafp.org/afp/2014/0601/p882.html*

PHYSICAL EXAMINATION

In patients with infectious and inflammatory conditions such as sialadenitis or parotitis, visible unilateral swelling and erythema may be present over the affected gland and surrounding area. Localized tenderness, warmth, and edema are commonly felt on palpation of the neck. Induration or fluctuance may also be present if extensive infection or an abscess has formed. Bimanual palpation of Stensen's duct may produce pus in the setting of parotitis. The ductal opening in the oral cavity may be erythematous.

Salivary stones can frequently be identified on physical exam. Palpation of Wharton's ducts in the floor of mouth may yield a small hard mass. If infected, pus may also be expressed on palpation.

On physical examination, benign masses are often freely mobile and painless. Malignant tumors are fixed to the overlying skin and may be tender with palpation. In advanced stages of malignancy, enlarged cervical lymphadenopathy may be noted. The facial nerve courses through the parotid gland and therefore any pathology involving the parotid gland can compress the facial nerve, resulting in facial paresis.

DIFFERENTIAL DIAGNOSIS

Table 3.22 summarizes the differential diagnosis of salivary gland disorders.

DIAGNOSTIC STUDIES

Cultures should be obtained if an infectious etiology is suspected or if pus is expressed from the salivary ducts. *Staphylococcus aureus* is most common bacterial pathogen but *Streptococcus, Haemophilus influenzae,* and other gram-negative rods such as *Escherichia coli* may be found as well. Viral serologic testing for mumps and HIV ought to be done if suspicion is high.[56]

Imaging can be useful in narrowing the differential diagnosis. Ultrasound and contrast-enhanced CT are useful for identifying sialoliths and distinguishing between abscess and mass. Masses should be aspirated or biopsied to obtain a tissue diagnosis.

EVALUATION

In addition to a thorough history and physical exam, it is important to perform a thorough medication reconciliation. Many medications cause dehydration and decreased salivary flow.

TREATMENT

- Acute infections of the salivary glands should be treated with culture-guided antibiotic therapy—often augmentin, cefuroxime, or clindamycin. Warm compresses should be applied to the affected area and adequate hydration should be maintained.
  - Lemon wedges and citrus lozenges are sialagogues and increase the production of saliva, which can aid in treatment. It is imperative to ensure proper oral hygiene to prevent recurrence or worsening of the infection. Parotitis and acute sialadenitis can both be complicated by abscess formation requiring surgical drainage.[56]
- Viral salivary gland infections are treated with supportive measures. Close contacts should be limited for patients diagnosed with mumps.
- Patients with sialoliths can also be treated with sialagogues and hydration.[56] Any associated infection should be managed with antibiotics. Stones that are large, obstructive, or recurrent may require surgical removal. Large stones in difficult to access locations may require surgical excision of the gland.[56]
- Any salivary gland tumor should be surgically resected because of the potential for benign tumors to transform into malignant ones.[56] Complete excision also provides a definitive diagnosis. Patients with malignant tumors should be referred to oncology.

PATIENT EDUCATION

- Patients should be informed that with the introduction of the mumps vaccine in the United States in 1967, cases of mumps have declined by 99%. The vaccine has an 88% efficacy rate after administration of two doses.[58]

3.5 DISEASES OF THE LARYNX

OVERVIEW

Disorders of the larynx are commonly seen by primary care clinicians. Most disorders of the larynx are associated with changes in speaking, breathing, or swallowing due to alterations in the muscle or cartilage of the airway and their overlying mucosa. The larynx protects the airway, produces sound through vocal cord vibration, and facilitates breathing through allowing air passage in and out of the lungs.

EPIDEMIOLOGY

Laryngeal conditions are relatively common. Voice disorders have a yearly prevalence in the United States between 6% and 8% while the lifetime prevalence is 30%.[59] Alterations in voice can have a substantial effect on an individual's quality of life, particularly if they are in an occupation that relies on their voice such as singing, acting, or teaching.

PATHOPHYSIOLOGY

Irritation, infection, inflammation, tumors, neurovascular damage, neuromuscular disorders, and inhalation of pollutants can all cause alteration of the larynx and surrounding structures that result in impairment of the vocal cords. The vocal cords open and close each time a breath is taken to allow for air to enter the lungs. During speech, the vocal cords vibrate as air passes outward to produce sound. Any abnormality of one or both vocal cords can lead to dysphagia, dysphonia, and dyspnea.

3.5A LARYNGITIS

MEDICAL HISTORY AND CLINICAL PRESENTATION

Acute or chronic laryngitis can be due to allergies, bacteria, viruses, or structural causes. Patients who use their voice frequently in their professional occupations, such as teachers, singers, and actors, are at increased risk for laryngitis.[60] Smoking, certain dietary choices, inhalers, medications, and dehydration can also cause laryngeal irritation.[60] It is important to have a high index of suspicion early for patients who present with laryngitis but may have underlying laryngeal cancer. These patients often have a history of weight loss, smoking, and alcohol use.

SIGNS AND SYMPTOMS

Patients often present with changes in their voice including hoarseness, breathiness, difficulty projecting their voice to its normal capacity, and pain or discomfort when speaking. Associated symptoms include postnasal drip, cough, sore throat, difficulty swallowing, and mucus in the throat requiring frequent throat clearing. Fever and myalgias may also be present. Symptoms last <2 weeks in acute laryngitis, whereas cases with symptoms lasting >3 weeks are classified as chronic laryngitis.[60]

PHYSICAL EXAMINATION

Physical examination for laryngitis should start while the clinician is obtaining a patient's history. During this time, attention should be paid to the quality, amplitude, and characteristic of the patient's voice in conversation as well as the amount of effort required for them to speak. Subjective grading systems exist and can be used for evaluating a patient's voice.[60] Some patients may intermittently lose their ability to phonate due to laryngeal swelling. The oral cavity and oropharynx may reveal nonspecific mucosal erythema and edema. Fungal sources of laryngitis may cause small white lesions to develop in the oropharynx.[60] On palpation of the neck, tender cervical lymphadenopathy can be related to acute infection. Any abnormal neck mass is concerning for cancer until proved otherwise. Respiratory effort should be assessed and include the evaluation of accessory muscles use and presence of audible stridor. These findings are concerning and require rapid intervention.

DIFFERENTIAL DIAGNOSIS

Infectious, inflammatory, structural, and neoplastic causes of laryngitis should all be taken into account when evaluating a patient. Viruses are the most common cause of acute laryngitis.[60] Chronic laryngitis is caused by neoplastic, inflammatory, structural, or autoimmune disorders.

DIAGNOSTIC STUDIES

Initially, laryngitis is a clinical diagnosis. If symptoms are persistent beyond treatment or recurrent, further studies are warranted. Flexible laryngoscopy can be performed in the office to directly assess laryngeal tissue. Culture can be obtained if there is concern for bacterial infection and biopsies can be performed if malignancy is suspected. Manometry or 24-hour pH monitoring can help in diagnosing laryngopharyngeal reflux.[59]

EVALUATION

It is difficult to differentiate between bacterial, viral, and allergic laryngitis. Obtaining a thorough history and physical examination is paramount. Most patients with laryngitis have mild symptoms and can be treated in an ambulatory setting. Severe cases of laryngitis may be associated with airway compromise. Anesthesia and otolaryngology should be consulted early for these patients. If dysphagia is present, a speech and language therapy evaluation can be obtained to assess for aspiration risk.

Patients with chronic laryngitis, particularly those with history of significant alcohol or tobacco use, should be referred to an otolaryngologist for further outpatient workup. It is important these patients are evaluated to rule out and treat underlying causes of their laryngeal symptoms. Patients with laryngeal cancer are often initially misdiagnosed with acute laryngitis. Delayed diagnosis increases the morbidity and mortality risks of laryngeal cancer patients.[60]

TREATMENT

- Acute laryngitis is usually self-limiting. Most patients have improvement within 2 weeks.[60] Supportive treatment is focused around voice rest, hydration, humidification, and diet modification. Patients should practice voice rest until they are comfortable humming, usually anywhere from 2 to 7 days.[60] Limiting spicy or acidic foods can improve any reflux-associated symptoms. If laryngopharyngeal reflux is suggested, H2 blocker antagonists or proton pump inhibitors may provide some relief. Mucolytics may assist in thinning and mobilizing mucus. Patients with concern for persistent bacterial infection should be considered for antibiotic treatment.
- It is important to consider the impact that acute or chronic laryngitis can have on a patient's quality of life, particularly if their occupation requires high voice use. Counseling should be offered if these patients are having difficulty coping.

PATIENT EDUCATION

It is important to educate patients that most cases of laryngitis resolve spontaneously and do not require antibiotics. Antibiotic use for laryngitis should be reserved for patients who have been febrile for more than 2 days, have purulent mucus, have signs of distant disease, or have comorbid conditions that put them at higher risk for developing a worsening infection. Patients should be counseled that they should follow up for nonresolving symptoms as this may indicate a more concerning underlying disease.

3.6 FOREIGN BODIES

MEDICAL HISTORY AND CLINICAL PRESENTATION

While more common in the pediatric population, FB aspiration can occur at any age. Children often present with acute, severe, life-threatening symptoms of airway compromise. Because of their smaller airway, any aspirated FB often lodges in the proximal tracheobronchial tree and therefore results in more rapid airway demise.[61] The aspiration of FBs is one of the most common pediatric emergencies and is associated with significant rates of morbidity and mortality.[62]

FB aspiration in adults occurs most frequently in the elderly population or in patients with dysphagia. Adults often present later after aspiration has occurred because of their milder symptoms.[61] FBs become wedged further down the airway in adult patients, in the distal tracheobronchial tree.[61] Therefore, they do not usually have severe difficulty breathing.

Most FBs are food items such as nuts, peas, seeds, and rice. Other frequently aspirated materials include teeth, fish bones, medications, plastic buttons, pen caps, cotton swabs, and metallic objects such as pins, whistles, screws, springs, and nails.[61,62] FBs that are circular or cylindrical in shape have higher risk of airway occlusion.[62] Neuromuscular disease, head injury, intoxication, and altered mental status are risk factors for FB aspiration.[61]

SIGNS AND SYMPTOMS

Pediatric and adult patients with severe airway obstruction have acute onset shortness of breath and difficulty breathing. They may feel as if they are choking. Coughing is common. Throat or chest pain may be present, especially if the aspirated object has sharp or penetrating edges, like push pins or fish bones. Some adults may not recall aspirating the FB.

PHYSICAL EXAMINATION

The examination of a patient with FB aspiration can vary depending on the level and degree of airway obstruction. Patients with acute severe airway obstruction are tachycardic and tachypneic with increased work of breathing and increased oral secretions. They may be sitting up, leaning forward in a tripod position to assist with breathing. Perioral cyanosis and audible stridor are signs of severe airway obstruction requiring immediate intervention. Some patients may have altered mental status or loss of consciousness due to hypoxia.

DIFFERENTIAL DIAGNOSIS

Any cause of airway obstruction can be included in the differential diagnosis for FB aspiration. Comorbid conditions should be considered when treating underlying causes related to FB aspiration. They may include neuromuscular disease, head injury, intoxication, and altered mental status.[61]

DIAGNOSTIC STUDIES

The diagnosis of FB aspiration is often clinical. Radiographs can be obtained but are often initially normal unless the FB is radiopaque.[62] Consolidation, atelectasis, unilateral lung hyperinflation, bronchiectasis, or mediastinal shift may be visible on chest radiographs, but these findings take time to develop.[61]

Bronchoscopy is both diagnostic and therapeutic. It provides direct visualization of foreign bodies and the damage or irritation caused to the surrounding airway structures and tissues. Bronchoscopy may reveal endobronchial stenosis, edema, and formation of granulation tissue.[61]

EVALUATION

A high index of suspicion is crucial in episodes of acute airway obstruction. Patients with unwitnessed FB ingestion and aspiration are at higher risk for complications and poorer outcomes.[62]

TREATMENT

- Many FB aspiration cases can be treated as outpatients once the FB is retrieved or expelled. If the FB is lodged in the upper airway, the Heimlich maneuver can be performed in attempts to dislodge the object. A combination of chest thrusts and back blows should be used for infants.
- Bronchoscopy can be used to remove FBs in the lower airway; they are most frequently found in the right mainstem bronchus.[62] The airway of pediatric patients should be secured prior to performing bronchoscopy. Rigid bronchoscopy is preferred for pediatric patients, whereas flexible bronchoscopy is the first approach used for adults, who tend to have more stable airways.[61] If flexible bronchoscopy is unsuccessful, rigid thoracoscopy should be attempted. Some objects, such as those that are larger, have smooth surfaces, are sharp, or are penetrating the airway, may be difficult to remove.[61] If flexible and rigid bronchoscopy approaches are unsuccessful, surgical thoracotomy may be required.[61]

PATIENT EDUCATION

- Patients should be educated on the severity of FB inhalation or ingestion. Parents should be counseled on how to childproof their homes and how to recognize signs of respiratory distress. It is important to educate parents and all capable patients on how to perform Heimlich and other lifesaving procedures in the event of acute airway obstruction.

3.7 NECK MASSES

OVERVIEW

Neck masses are commonly seen in primary care settings and can be associated with a wide range of benign or malignant conditions. Neck masses can be acute, subacute, or chronic and can be further subdivided based on their anatomic location within the neck.

EPIDEMIOLOGY

Given that neck masses arise from a variety of etiologies it is difficult to track their prevalence. Neck masses in adults are much more frequently associated with malignancy while neck masses in children are often due to infectious or inflammatory causes.[57]

PATHOPHYSIOLOGY

The neck contains a vast network of lymphatic drainage, which predisposes it to infections and metastatic disease. Infections originating in the proximal aerodigestive tract (the oral cavity, dentition, salivary glands, tonsils, pharynx, epiglottis, and larynx) can drain into the lymphatics of the neck and result in neck masses. Cervical lymphadenopathy can be present for 3 to 6 weeks beyond resolution of primary infectious symptoms.[57] Any persistent neck mass in an adult patient should be considered to be malignant until proved otherwise.[57]

MEDICAL HISTORY AND CLINICAL PRESENTATION

History and presentation vary according to the etiology of the neck mass. Patients with infections may have a known exposure. It is important to inquire about recent travel history, sick contacts, recent surgical procedures involving the head or neck, family history, and comorbid conditions. A social history with attention to extracurricular hobbies and substance use is important. Patients who play a musical wind instrument that requires forceful blowing of air and those who blow glass to create artwork are at increased risk for the development of laryngoceles. Laryngoceles are often also found in patients with chronic coughs. Individuals with significant alcohol or tobacco history are more likely to have head and neck cancers. Adults with multiple sexual partners have a higher risk of contracting the HPV, which is also associated with several head and neck malignancies.

SIGNS AND SYMPTOMS

Many neck masses are often asymptomatic. Signs and symptoms vary widely depending on the nature of the neck mass. There may be pain, swelling, dysphagia, or globus sensation. Symptoms of hyperthyroidism or hypothyroidism may also be present if Graves disease or Hashimoto disease is the underlying cause. If the mass is involving the recurrent laryngeal nerve, the patient may have dysarthria. Odynophagia, hoarseness, hemoptysis, night sweats, and weight loss are frequently seen in patients with head and neck cancer. Carotid body tumors may cause generalized flushing, palpitations, and hypertension if functional.[57]

PHYSICAL EXAMINATION

Upon inspection of the neck, the involved area may be prominent or swollen. Overlying erythema and warmth can be present if the mass is infected. Clinicians should have patients swallow and observe and palpate for movement with deglutition, which may identify a thyroglossal duct cyst or thyroid mass. On palpation, diffuse swelling or a defined mass may be palpable. The mass may be mobile or fixed, soft or firm, smooth or irregular, defined or matted. Patients may have localized or generalized tenderness on palpation. Neck masses associated with tuberculosis or certain malignancies such as lymphoma might be nontender.[57] Pulsations can be appreciated in cases of pseudoaneurysm or arteriovenous fistula.[57]

Care should be taken to examine the oral cavity and oropharynx as both infection and malignancy that originate in these areas can initially present as a mass in the neck. Patients may present with a nonhealing oral ulcer suggestive of oral cancer, loose or misaligned teeth, hoarseness, halitosis, or unilateral tonsillar enlargement suggestive of tonsillar infection or malignancy.

DIFFERENTIAL DIAGNOSIS

A common pneumonic to organize the differential diagnosis for neck masses is "kittens" (Figure 3.11).

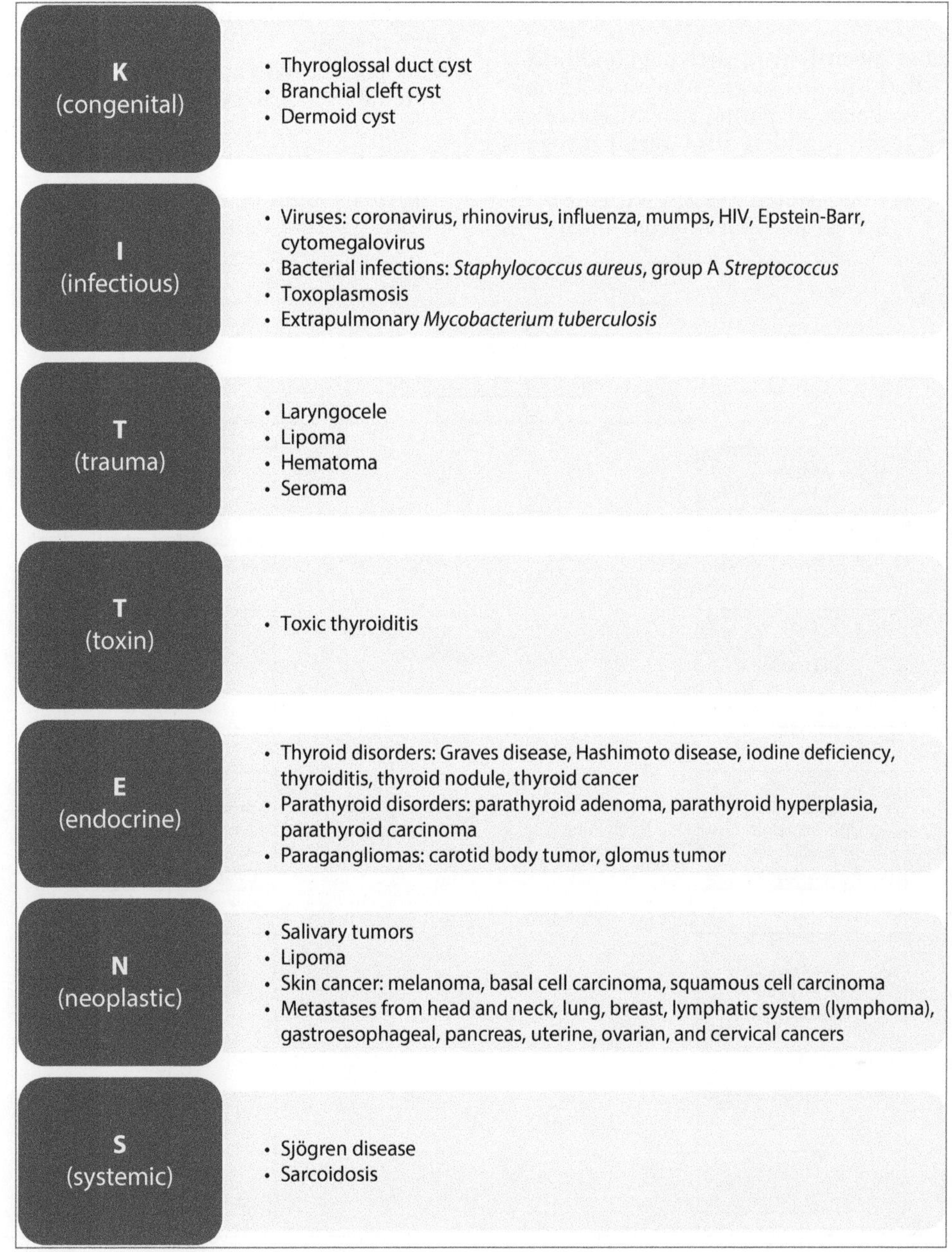

Figure 3.11 The KITTENS pneumonic can be used to organize differential diagnoses for neck masses.

DIAGNOSTIC STUDIES

Diagnostic studies should be obtained based on clinical suspicion. Laboratory studies including CBC, erythrocyte sedimentation rate (ESR), and thyroid function tests are good initial tests. Antibody titers or a tuberculin skin test can be performed if certain viruses or tuberculosis is likely. A 24-hour urine collection and plasma catecholamines may help in diagnosing a paraganglioma.[57]

Ultrasound is the most common imaging study performed to evaluate neck masses. It is low cost and does not require sedation nor does it expose the patient to radiation. Consistency, size, and vascularity of the mass can be distinguished with ultrasound.[57] Suspicious masses are often biopsied through fine needle aspiration biopsy with or without ultrasound guidance. The aspirate is sent for Gram stain, cultures, and cytology. Aspiration should not be performed on vascular lesions.[57]

CT of the neck can further characterize lesions. Contrast agent should be used if malignancy is of concern but should be avoided in those with thyroid disorders. CT angiography should be obtained for pulsatile masses or if vascular injury is suspected.[57]

PET scans may be necessary if malignancy is suspected. This study should be ordered only after consultation with otolaryngologists or oncologists due to its high cost. Laryngoscopy, bronchoscopy, and esophagoscopy can provide direct visualization of the upper aerodigestive tract to assess for abnormalities. Biopsies can be performed during these procedures if suspicious lesions are found.[57]

EVALUATION

A patient's age, history, and the location of their neck mass can help to significantly narrow a differential diagnosis. Most pediatric neck masses are congenital, inflammatory, or infectious. Any neck mass in an adult patient should be considered cancer until proved otherwise. Most often, chronic neck masses are either congenital or due to thyroid disorders.

TREATMENT

- Treatment is targeted toward the underlying condition.
- First-generation cephalosporins, augmentin, or clindamycin often cover most bacterial pathogens.[57] Referral to infectious disease can be considered for rare pathogens or repeated infections.
- Endocrinology should be consulted to assist with the medical management of thyroid and parathyroid disorders. Surgery or otolaryngology should be involved if medical therapy fails.
- Any patient with concern for malignancy should be evaluated by an otolaryngologist, surgeon, or oncologist.

PATIENT EDUCATION

- Patients should be educated on the wide range of disease processes that can cause neck masses. They should be

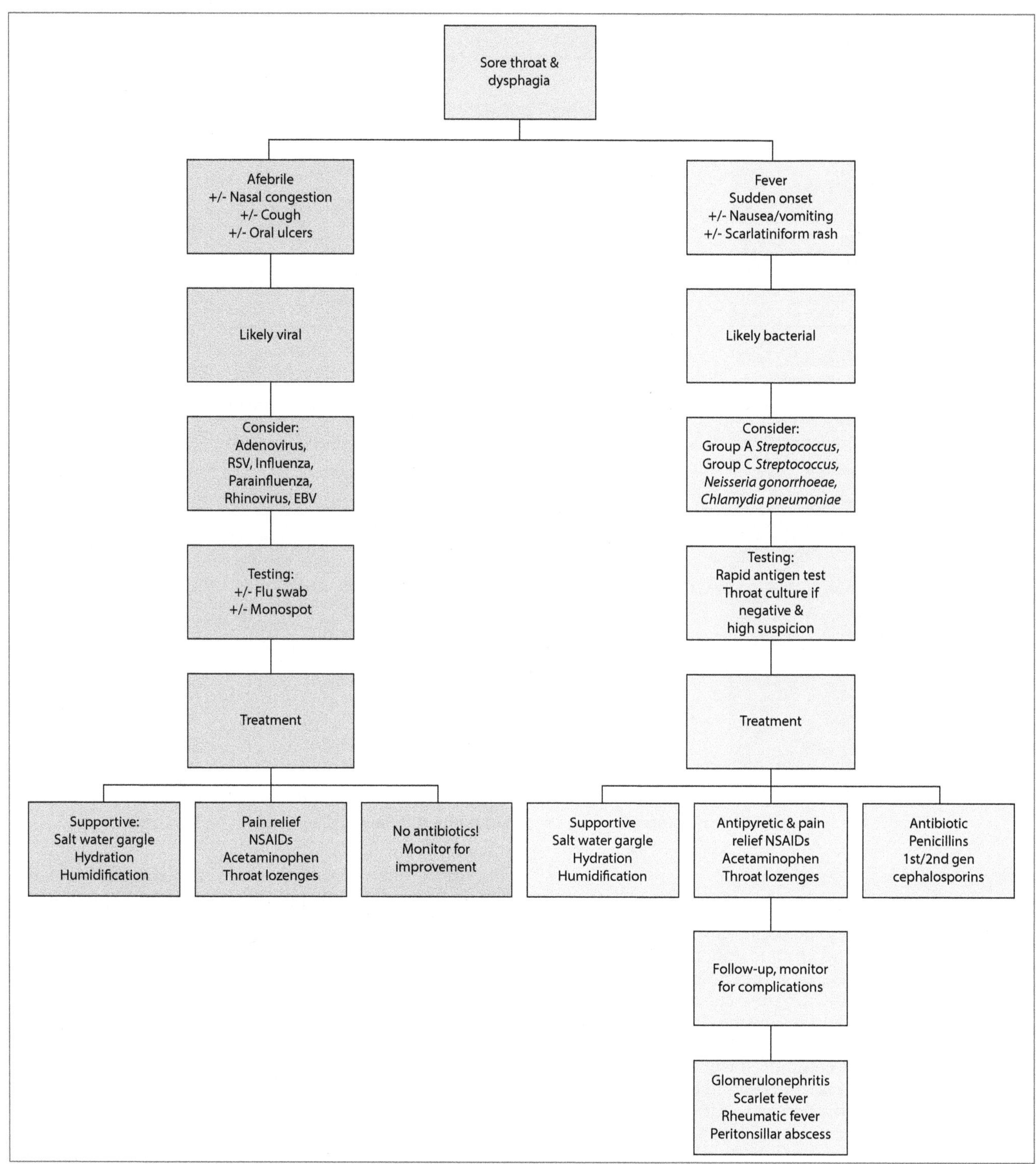

Figure 3.12 **Algorithm for the approach to pharyngitis.** EBV, Epstein-Barr virus; NSAIDs, nonsteroidal anti-inflammatory drugs; RSV, respiratory syncytial virus.

counseled that obtaining a definitive diagnosis is important although it may take time. Clinicians need to inform patients not to ignore any new neck mass, especially in adult patients in whom the most likely cause is cancer.

COMMON CHIEF COMPLAINTS

APPROACH TO PHARYNGITIS

Pharyngitis is one of the most common conditions encountered in clinical practice. The approach for differentiating among various causes of pharyngitis requires a problem-focused history, a physical examination, and appropriate laboratory testing. Identifying the cause of pharyngitis, especially group A beta-hemolytic streptococcus (GABHS), is important to prevent potential life-threatening complications (Figure 3.12).

Red flags for pharyngitis include a hot potato voice, drooling, stridor, and inability to swallow. Airway obstruction or severe unilateral pain several days into the illness suggests epiglottitis, peritonsillar abscess, or retropharyngeal abscess.

Most pharyngitis is viral and therefore antibiotics are not indicated. The primary goal of identifying and treating GAS is the prevention of rheumatic fever. GAS is universally susceptible to penicillin. Patient education and symptomatic treatment are essential in both viral and bacterial pharyngitis.

KNOWLEDGE CHECKS

1. Pharyngitis is a very common complaint. There is much overlap in presentation of the various etiologies. Compare and contrast the various viral, bacterial, and physical etiologies of pharyngitis.
2. The differential diagnosis for vertigo is varied and complex. Develop a focused approach based on an understanding of the pathophysiology of the various etiologies of vertigo.
3. Hearing loss may be central or peripheral. Create a table outlining the various etiologies of hearing loss grouped by central or peripheral types.
4. Ear disorders can be divided by location into those of the external, middle, and inner ear. Compare and contrast the presentation, laboratory findings, and treatment of the various **disorders** of the ear based on location.

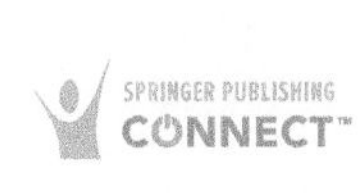

A robust set of instructor resources designed to supplement this text is located at **http://connect.springerpub.com/content/book/978-0-8261-8243-2**. Qualifying instructors may request access by emailing **textbook@springerpub.com.**

REFERENCES

The complete reference list for this chapter appears in the digital version of the chapter, accessible at https://connect.springerpub.com/content/book/978-0-8261-8243-2/chapter/ch03.

CHAPTER 4

PULMONARY SYSTEM

JESSE A. COALE, ANALISA AMBROSI, DEANNA L. DENAULT, AND SHANNON N. DIALLO

LEARNING OBJECTIVES

- Apply epidemiologic information, signs and symptoms, physical examination, and diagnostic studies to diagnose common respiratory diseases.
- Select and interpret the most appropriate diagnostic and/or imaging studies needed to confirm or rule out specific respiratory diseases.
- Develop treatment plans for specific respiratory diseases including pharmacologic and non-pharmacologic interventions.
- Develop appropriate patient education for common respiratory diseases.
- Develop a systematic approach for common respiratory symptoms.

INTRODUCTION

Diseases of the respiratory system are very common in clinical medicine. While the etiology, types of disorders, or vasculature changes may vary, the presenting symptoms of cough and shortness of breath are held in common.

4.1 ASTHMA

OVERVIEW

Asthma is a heterogeneous disease that is characterized by chronic airway inflammation. It is usually defined by a history of respiratory symptoms that include wheezing, shortness of breath, chest tightness, and cough. These symptoms vary in intensity and over time.[1]

EPIDEMIOLOGY

The prevalence of asthma has increased markedly over the past 30 years. Data from the Centers for Disease Control and Prevention (CDC) reveal that asthma affects over 25 million people, including 6 million who are under the age of 18.[2] This makes it a significant health burden to patients, their families, and society. In 2016 almost 1.8 million people visited an ED for asthma-related care and 189,000 people were hospitalized because of asthma.[2] The annual death rate from asthma declined over the period 2001 to 2008 with 15 deaths per 1 million people in 2001 and 11.2 deaths per 1 million people in 2008.[2] The death rate has remained unchanged through 2017.[2]

Some people are more likely to have asthma than others. In 2017, asthma occurred equally among adults and children.[2] Females were noted to have asthma more frequently than males.[2] Asthma prevalence differs across different races and ethnicities. Asthma prevalence was higher among Black persons (10.8%) compared to White persons (8.1%).[2] According to CDC data collected in 2017, asthma prevalence is increased with decreasing annual household income.[2]

PATHOPHYSIOLOGY

Airflow limitation that occurs in asthma is recurrent and caused by a variety of changes in the airway including bronchoconstriction, airway edema, airway hyperresponsiveness, and airway remodeling. The primary physiologic event leading to symptoms in asthma is airway narrowing and subsequent interruption in airflow.[2] During acute asthma exacerbations bronchial smooth muscle contraction occurs in response to exposure to allergens or irritants.[2] This bronchoconstriction occurs quickly and causes acute airflow obstruction. Allergen-induced bronchoconstriction results from an Ig E-dependent release of mediators from mast cells that include histamine, tryptase, leukotrienes, and prostaglandins.[2] These mediators directly contract airway smooth muscle. Additionally, other exposure to other stimuli such as cold air, exercise, and stress may result in acute bronchoconstriction. As asthma becomes more persistent and inflammation progresses, edema, inflammation, and mucus hypersecretion limit airflow. Additionally, structural changes including hypertrophy and hyperplasia of the smooth muscle of the airway play a role. The hypertrophy and hyperplasia of the smooth muscle may not be responsive to the usual treatment.[2]

Airway hyperresponsiveness is defined as an exaggerated bronchoconstrictor response to a wide variety of stimuli and is a major factor contributing to asthma.[2] The mechanisms that influence airway hyperresponsiveness are countless but can be grouped under inflammation, dysfunctional neuro regulation, and structural changes.[2] Treatment of asthma is directed at reducing inflammation and airway hyperresponsiveness to improve asthma control.[2] Additionally, in some patients who have asthma airflow limitation may be only partially reversible.[2] Permanent structural changes can occur in the airway and cannot be prevented or reversed with current therapy.[2] Airway remodeling involves structural changes including thickening of the sub-basement membrane, subepithelial fibrosis, airway smooth muscle hypertrophy and hyperplasia, blood vessel proliferation and dilatation, and mucus gland hypersecretion and hypertrophy.[2] Regulation of this process is not well established but explains the persistent nature of the disease and limitations in treatment response.[2]

MEDICAL HISTORY AND CLINICAL PRESENTATION

Given the mostly nonspecific symptoms of asthma, thorough history taking is essential when patients present with symptoms concerning for asthma. Family history should be obtained including history of asthma, allergies, rhinitis, and eczema. This may indicate a genetic predisposition to atopy and likely an atopic component of the asthma diagnosis.[3] Social history is also important to help determine a patient's particular triggers including potential occupational exposures, environmental exposures, and exposure to tobacco.[3]

Clinical presentation of asthma can vary widely, especially during acute exacerbations. Patients experiencing mild asthma exacerbations may present with end-expiratory wheezing. They will be able to speak in full sentences and lie flat without becoming dyspneic. They may have tachypnea but use of accessory muscles is absent. During moderately severe exacerbations, respiratory distress is present. Patients often have a hard time speaking in full sentences and become breathless when talking. Tachypnea and accessory muscle use are present. It is not uncommon for pulse oximetry to drop into the low 90s on room air at this stage. During severe exacerbations, dyspnea at rest is present. Patients are unable to speak in full sentences and loud inspiratory and expiratory wheezing is present. Patients often assume the tripod position: hunched over with their hands supporting their torso.[3] Imminent respiratory arrest is the most concerning presentation of asthma exacerbation. These patients often have altered mental status. On physical examination wheezing or breath sounds may be absent. Intubation should not be delayed in these patients.

SIGNS AND SYMPTOMS

The four most common presenting symptoms are cough, wheezing, shortness of breath, and a subjective sensation of chest tightness.[3] Wheezing is defined as a high-pitched whistling sound produced by airflow turbulence and is due to air passing through narrowed bronchioles.[3] Patients with asthma often describe their cough as nonproductive and present during nighttime and early morning hours.[3] A subjective sensation of chest tightness may also be present. It is important to thoroughly work up and rule out other potentially serious causes of chest tightness prior to arriving at the diagnosis of asthma.[3] The frequency of asthma symptoms is highly variable between patients. Some patients may experience infrequent symptoms while others may have nearly continuous symptoms. Symptoms may occur after exposure to known triggers, respiratory infections, stress, or weather changes or may occur spontaneously.

PHYSICAL EXAMINATION

Physical examination in people with asthma is often normal, especially when asthma is adequately controlled.[2] The upper respiratory tract, skin, and chest are the focus of the physical examination.[4] The most common physical exam finding is wheezing during auscultation. This is prominent in the expiratory phase of respiration rather than during inspiration and is usually diffuse. A prolonged phase of forced expiration is typical of airway obstruction.[4] However, wheezing during forced expiration is not indicative of airway obstruction. It is important to note that wheezing may be absent in severe asthma exacerbations due to airway obstruction. Other signs of respiratory distress usually present in severe asthma exacerbations include cyanosis, tachypnea, and use of accessory muscles. Wheezing may also be heard with laryngeal obstruction, chronic obstructive pulmonary disease (COPD), respiratory tract infections, or inhaled foreign body.[1] Crackles and inspiratory wheezing are not indicative of asthma.[1] Examination of the nasal mucosa may reveal nasal polyps or signs of allergic rhinitis. Examination of the skin may reveal evidence of atopic dermatitis.

DIFFERENTIAL DIAGNOSIS

The differential diagnosis for asthma is summarized in Table 4.1.

DIAGNOSTIC STUDIES

Diagnostic studies are important in confirming an asthma diagnosis. Asthma is characterized by variable expiratory airflow limitation and lung function testing (spirometry) is used to document this variability. Spirometry should be carried out by well-trained operators using well-maintained and well-calibrated equipment.[1] Forced expiratory volume in 1 second (FEV_1) is more reliable than peak expiratory flow (PEF) when diagnosing asthma. PEF is beneficial as a personal

TABLE 4.1 Differential Diagnostic Possibilities for Asthma

Diagnosis	Description
Foreign body in trachea or bronchus	Cough, dyspnea Inspiratory wheezing (stridor) Confirmation of presence of foreign body via radiography or bronchoscopy Resolution of symptoms with removal of foreign body
Vocal cord dysfunction	Episodic dyspnea and wheezing Diagnosed via direct/indirect visualization of the vocal cord Resolves once the trachea is intubated
Cystic fibrosis	Persistent cough and wheezing present in childhood Confirmation with genetic testing Poor weight gain despite adequate appetite
Pneumonia	Nonproductive or productive cough Fever, tachypnea Wheezing/rhonchi may be present Infiltrate on chest x-ray
Allergic rhinitis	Sneezing, itching/watery eyes Coughing, postnasal drip Symptoms begin after allergen exposure Confirmed with allergy testing

monitoring tool. It may be used to assess response to treatment, to evaluate triggers, or for worsening of symptoms.[1] Generally, in adults with respiratory symptoms typical of asthma, an increase or decrease in FEV_1 of >12% and >200 mL from baseline is accepted as being consistent with asthma.[1] Airflow obstruction is also indicated by a reduced FEV_1/FVC (forced vital capacity) ratio. According to population studies, the normal FEV_1/FVC ratio is usually >0.75 to 0.80 in adults and usually >0.90 in children.[1] Any values less than these benchmarks reflect airflow limitation.[1] Bronchial provocation tests may also be used to document variable airflow limitation. Challenge agents can include inhaled methacholine or histamine.[1] Bronchial provocation tests have a moderate sensitivity for diagnosing asthma, but a limited sensitivity.[1] Therefore, a negative test can help to exclude a diagnosis of asthma, but a positive test does not always confirm a diagnosis of asthma.[1] The pattern of symptoms and other clinical features must be taken into account.[1]

EVALUATION

The National Heart, Lung, and Blood Institute has devised a system for classifying asthma into four categories: mild intermittent, mild persistent, moderate persistent, and severe persistent (Figure 4.1). The classification system takes into account both daytime and nighttime symptoms, frequency of symptoms, and objective data including FEV_1/FVC ratio.

TREATMENT

- Medications for treatment of asthma are classified into two groups: long-term control medications used to achieve and maintain control of persistent asthma and quick relief medications used to treat exacerbations and acute symptoms.[1]
- Long-term control medications
  - **Corticosteroids:** These drugs stop late phase reaction to allergens, reduce airway responsiveness, and inhibit inflammatory cell activation. They are available in both oral and inhaled formulations. Inhaled corticosteroids (ICS) are used in both short- and long-term control of asthma. Short courses of oral systemic steroids are often used during acute exacerbation.[1]
  - **Cromolyn sodium and nedocromil:** These stabilize mast cells and are used as an alternative, but not preferred, medication for the treatment of mild persistent asthma.[1]
  - **Immunomodulators:** These drugs prevent binding of IgE to high-affinity receptors on mast cells and basophils.[1] They are used as an adjunctive therapy in patients ≥12 years of age who have allergies and severe persistent asthma.[1] Omalizumab is an example.
  - **Leukotriene modifiers:** Leukotrienes are potent biochemical mediators that contribute to airway obstruction. Montelukast is available for patients >1 year of age and is used as an alternative, but not preferred therapy, for the treatment of mild persistent asthma.[1]
  - **Long-acting beta$_2$-agonists (LABAs):** LABAs provide 12 hours of bronchodilation after a single dose. They are not to be used as monotherapy for long-term control of asthma.[1] LABAs are used in combination with ICS for long-term control of moderate to severe persistent asthma.[1] The use of LABA for the treatment of acute symptoms or exacerbations is not recommended.[1]
  - **Methylxanthines:** Theophylline is a mild to moderate bronchodilator and may have mild anti-inflammatory effects. This may be used as an alternative, not preferred, adjunctive treatment with ICS.[1] Monitoring of serum concentration of theophylline is essential as there is a narrow toxic-therapeutic window.[1]
- Quick-relief medications
  - **Anticholinergics:** Anticholinergics inhibit muscarinic cholinergic receptors and reduce vagal tone of the airway.[1] They may be used in combination with SABAs (see next) in moderate to severe asthma exacerbations.[1]

Components of Severity		Classification of Asthma Severity (Youths ≥12 years of age and adults)			
			Persistent		
		Intermittent	Mild	Moderate	Severe
Impairment Normal FEV_1/FVC: 8–19 yr 85% 20–39 yr 80% 40–59 yr 75% 60–80 yr 70%	Symptoms	≤2 days/week	>2 days/week but not daily	Daily	Throughout the day
	Nighttime awakenings	≤2x/month	3–4x/month	>1x/week but not nightly	Often 7x/week
	Short-acting beta$_2$-agonist use for symptom control (not prevention of EIB)	≤2 days/week	>2 days/week but not >1x/day	Daily	Several times per day
	Interference with normal activity	None	Minor limitation	Some limitation	Extremely limited
	Lung function	• Normal FEV_1 between exacerbations • FEV_1 >80% predicted • FEV_1/FVC normal	• FEV_1 ≥80% predicted • FEV_1/FVC normal	• FEV_1 >60% but <80% predicted • FEV_1/FVC reduced 5%	• FEV_1 <60% predicted • FEV_1/FVC reduced >5%
Risk	Exacerbations requiring oral systemic corticosteroids	0–1/year (see note)	≥2/year (see note) →		
		← Consider severity and interval since last exacerbation. Frequency and severity may fluctuate over time for patients in any severity category. →			
		Relative annual risk of exacerbations may be related to FEV_1			

Figure 4.1 **Classifying asthma severity and initiating treatment in youths ≥12 years of age and adults who are not currently taking long-term control medications.** EIB, exercise-induced bronchoconstriction; FEV1, forced expiratory volume in 1 second; FVC, forced vital capacity.
(Source: National Heart, Lung, and Blood Institute; National Institutes of Health; U.S. Department of Health and Human Services. Figure 4.2.)

- **Short-acting beta agonists (SABAs):** SABAs are the therapeutic agents of choice for relief of acute symptoms and prevention of exercise-induced bronchospasm.[1]
- **Systemic corticosteroids:** These are used for moderate and severe exacerbations of asthma in conjunction with SABA to speed recovery and prevent recurrence of exacerbation.[1]

- The expert panel recommends a step-wise approach to therapy, in which the dose and number of medications and frequency of administration are increased as necessary and decreased when possible to achieve and maintain adequate control (Figure 4.2).[1] Specific therapy should be tailored to the needs and circumstances of individual patients.[2] Pharmacologic therapy is accompanied at every step by patient education and measures to control comorbid conditions and environmental factors that may make asthma worse.[2]
- The expert panel recommends that initial treatment for asthma exacerbation includes supplemental oxygen, SABA for all patients, multiple doses of ipratropium bromide in the ED for patients with severe exacerbations, and systemic corticosteroids for most patients.[2] For severe refractory exacerbations unresponsive to initial treatments, consideration should be given to adjunct therapies such as magnesium sulfate.[2]
- Intubation is required for those patients with impending respiratory failure.

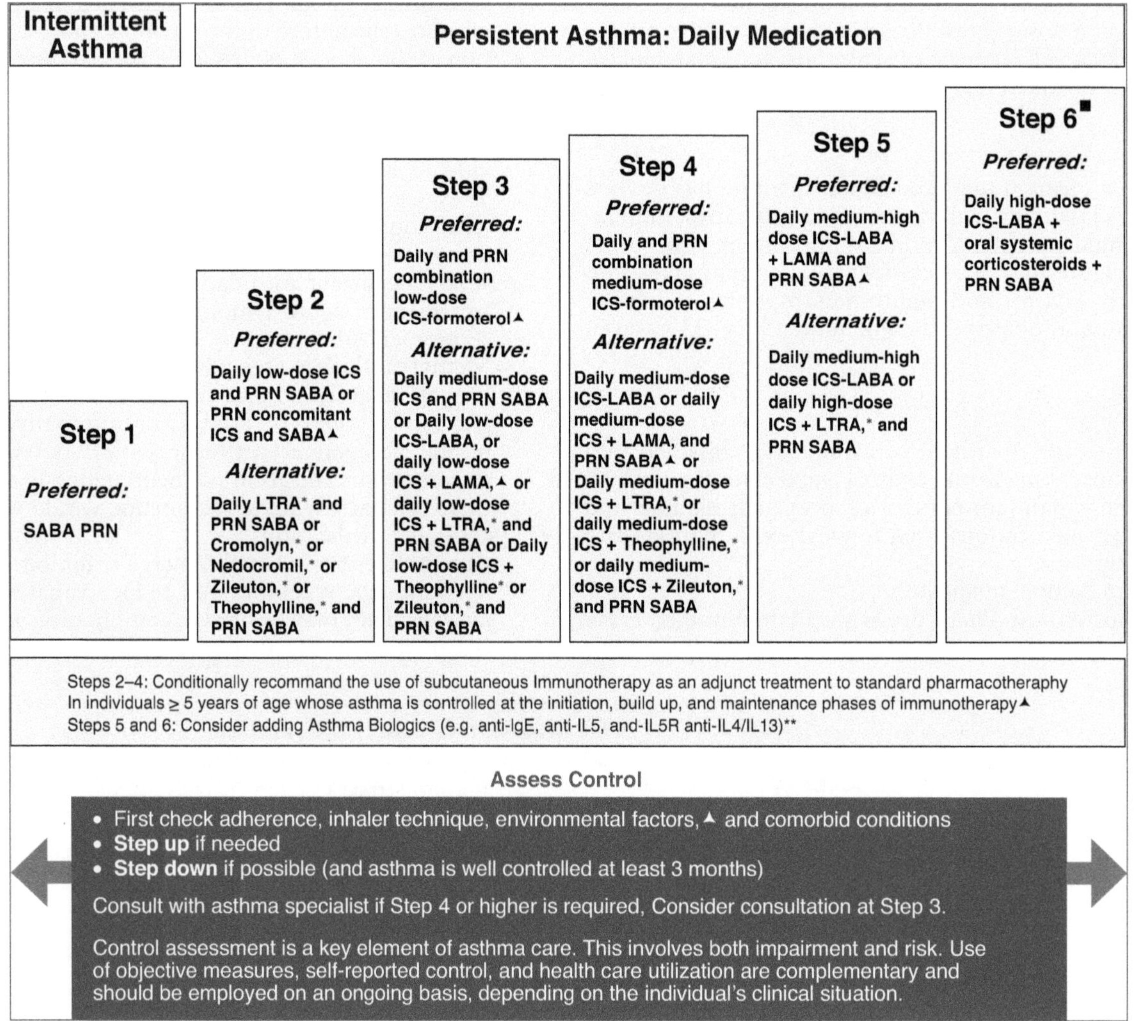

Figure 4.2 **Stepwise approach for management of asthma, ages 12+ years.**

ICS, inhaled corticosteroid; LABA, long-acting beta$_2$-agonist; LAMA, long-acting muscarinic antagonist; LTRA, leukotriene receptor antagonist; SABA, inhaled short-acting beta$_2$-agonist

▲ Updated bsed on the 2020 guidelines.

* Cromolyn, Nedocromil, LTRAs including Zileuton and montelukast, and Theophylline were not considered for this update, and/or have limited availability for use in the United States, and/or have an increased risk of adverse consequences and need for monitoring that make their use less desirable. The FDA issued a Boxed Warning for montelukast in March 2020.

** The AHRQ systematic reviews that informed this report did not include studies that examined the role of asthma biologics (e.g. anti-IgE, anti-IL5, anti-IL5R, anti-IL4/IL13). Thus, this report does not contain specific recommendations for the use of biologics in asthma in Steps 5 and 6.

■ Data on the use of LAMA therapy in individuals with severe persistent asthma (Step 6) were not included in the AHRQ systematic review and thus no recommendation is made.

(Source: National Heart, Lung, and Blood Institute. (2020). 2020 focused updates to the asthma management guidelines: At-a-glance guide. https://www.nhlbi.nih.gov/health-topics/all-publications-and-resources/at-glance-2020-focused-updates-asthma-management-guidelines)

PATIENT EDUCATION

- Clinicians should stress the importance of medication compliance.
- Patients should avoid known triggers.
- Patients should be educated on proper inhaler technique.

4.2 CHRONIC OBSTRUCTIVE PULMONARY DISEASE

OVERVIEW

The Global Initiative for Chronic Obstructive Lung Disease (GOLD) defines chronic obstructive pulmonary disease (COPD) as "a common, preventable and treatable disease that is characterized by persistent respiratory symptoms and airflow limitation due to airway and alveolar abnormalities caused by exposure to noxious particles or gases."[1] Most patients with COPD have features of both emphysema and chronic bronchitis. The natural course of COPD may be peppered by periods of acute worsening of symptoms, referred to as exacerbations.[5]

EPIDEMIOLOGY

COPD is a common and often underdiagnosed problem. The World Health Organization (WHO) estimates that 210 million people suffer from COPD worldwide and that in 2005 it led to 3 million deaths (5% of all deaths). It is known that 90% of COPD-related deaths occur in low- and middle-income countries.[6] Historically, COPD is more common in men. However, as a result of increased tobacco use among women and the higher risk of exposure to indoor air pollution (e.g., biomass fuel used for cooking and heating) in low-income countries, the disease now affects men and women almost equally.[7] A hereditary deficiency of α-1 antitrypsin accounts for approximately 1% of all cases of COPD and is more common in young persons diagnosed with COPD who do not have a history of tobacco use.[6] Those with α-1 antitrypsin are diagnosed with COPD roughly 20 years earlier than those who smoke.[6] By WHO estimates, in 2030 it is predicted that COPD will become the third leading cause of death worldwide.[7]

PATHOPHYSIOLOGY

The term COPD refers to two types of obstructive airway diseases: emphysema and chronic obstructive bronchitis. Emphysema is characterized by enlargement of airspaces and destruction of lung tissue, whereas chronic bronchitis leads to obstruction of small airways. Often, those diagnosed with COPD have overlapping features of both disorders. The mechanisms involved in the pathogenesis of COPD include inflammation of the bronchial wall, hypersecretion of mucus, and loss of alveolar tissue and elastic lung fibers. Inflammation of the bronchial wall along with excess mucus production cause obstruction of airflow, leading to a ventilation/perfusion mismatch. Destruction of alveolar tissue decreases the surface area for gas exchange and leads to airway collapse and air trapping.[6]

There is compelling evidence of an imbalance of proteases and antiproteases in the lungs of those with COPD. Proteases break down connective tissue components and antiproteases work to counteract this action.[5] Proteases, in particular elastase, are released from inflammatory cells such as macrophages, leukocytes and neutrophils. Tobacco smoke and other irritants stimulate the movement of inflammatory cells into the lungs, thus stimulating the release of elastase and other proteases.[5] Increased levels of proteases have been observed in those with COPD.[5] Protease-mediated destruction of elastin, a major connective tissue component of the lung tissue, is an important feature of emphysema.[5]

The best-known genetic association with emphysema, discovered by Carl-Bertil Laurell in 1963, is α-1 antitrypsin deficiency.[6] The α-1 antitrypsin gene is found on chromosome 14; α-1 antitrypsin is a wide-ranging antiprotease that is produced in the liver. Specifically, in the lungs, it acts against neutrophil elastase, which is released from neutrophils at sites of inflammation and in response to tobacco smoke. Mutations of this gene lead to abnormal protein folding with subsequent low circulating blood levels of α-1 antitrypsin due to impaired secretion.[6] A lack of α-1 antitrypsin allows unrestricted elastase activity and subsequent destruction of lung tissue.[6]

There are three recognized subtypes of different pathologic patterns of emphysema: centrilobar, panacinar, and paraseptal.[6] These were first discovered by Gough and colleagues in the 1950s.[6] Centrilobar emphysema is most commonly seen in smokers. It is characterized by the loss of respiratory bronchioles in the central lung and initially spares the distal alveoli. It predominantly affects the upper portions of the lungs.[6] In panacinar emphysema, the distal alveoli are affected as well. Panacinar emphysema affects the entire lung uniformly and is most associated with α-1 antitrypsin deficiency.[6] The third type, paraseptal emphysema (also referred to as distal acinar), is localized around the septae and pleurae.[6] It affects the distal acinar structures and often coexists with centrilobar emphysema in smokers.[6] It can also be an incidental finding in young patients and may lead to spontaneous pneumothorax, particularly if located in the apices.[6]

Chronic bronchitis represents airway obstruction of the large and small airways. Mucus hypersecretion, resulting in chronic cough and subsequent airflow limitation, is an important feature of chronic bronchitis.[5] This is due to an increased number of goblet cells and enlarged submucosal glands.[5] Both enlargement of submucosal glands and the increased number of goblet cells are due to chronic airway irritation secondary to cigarette smoke and other noxious irritants and is thought to be a protective metaplastic reaction.[5]

4.2A CHRONIC BRONCHITIS

MEDICAL HISTORY AND CLINICAL PRESENTATION

A detailed medical history of a patient who is suspected to have COPD is invaluable. Patients with a diagnosis of chronic bronchitis by definition have cough or sputum production present for at least 3 months in each of 2 consecutive years.[5] History taking should include asking a person about exposure to risk factors such as personal history of smoking, exposure to secondhand smoke, family history of COPD or other chronic respiratory diseases, and any environmental or occupational exposures.[5]

As COPD progresses, two symptom patterns tend to emerge. The terms "blue bloater" and "pink puffer" have been used to describe those with chronic bronchitis and emphysema, respectively. For those with chronic bronchitis predominant symptoms, the major presenting complaint is usually chronic cough and shortness of breath with a progressive decline in exercise tolerance. The cough is usually productive of purulent sputum and has been present for more than 3 consecutive months in the last 2 years. In those with chronic bronchitis, the excessive mucus secretion and airway obstruction cause a mismatch of ventilation and perfusion. Therefore, these persons are unable to compensate by increasing their ventilation and hypoxemia and cyanosis occur. Later in the disease course, pulmonary hypertension develops, resulting in right-sided heart failure (cor pulmonale) with peripheral edema. The term "blue bloater" has been historically used to describe these patients who develop cyanosis and edema.

SIGNS AND SYMPTOMS

Chronic bronchitis is characterized by shortness of breath with progressive decrease in exercise tolerance. These patients characteristically present in the fifth or sixth decade of life. Dyspnea is initially noted on exertion, but as disease progresses it is present at rest. COPD patients typically describe their dyspnea as an increased effort to breath, chest heaviness, air hunger, or gasping.[5] Symptoms can vary in intensity from day to day. This can include an increase in sputum production, increased dyspnea, or a change in sputum character. These exacerbations are often precipitated by environmental factors or infection (viral or bacterial). Exacerbations may be severe and require hospitalization for management.

PHYSICAL EXAMINATION

Physical examination is rarely diagnostic in patients with COPD.[5] Physical signs of airflow limitations are not usually present until late in the disease after significant impairment of lung function has occurred.[5] Patients with chronic bronchitis may have a prolonged expiratory phase of respiration. Wheezing or crackles may be present upon auscultation.

4.2B EMPHYSEMA

MEDICAL HISTORY AND CLINICAL PRESENTATION

A detailed medical history of a patient who is suspected to have COPD is invaluable. History taking should include asking a person about exposure to risk factors such as personal history of smoking, exposure to second-hand smoke, family history of COPD or other chronic respiratory diseases, and any environmental or occupational exposures.[5]

Those COPD patients with symptoms that are emphysema predominant have historically been referred to as "pink puffers." In emphysema, there is destruction of lung tissue and thus a proportionate loss of ventilation and perfusion area. Patients with emphysema may present with marked dyspnea. Because of airflow obstruction and prolonged expiratory time, the urge to inspire happens before completion of full expiration.[6] This leads to "stacking" of breaths and hyperinflation of the lung.[6] Air becomes trapped in the lungs causing an increase in the anteroposterior dimension of the chest, resulting in the characteristic barrel chest, typical of those with emphysematous disease.

SIGNS AND SYMPTOMS

Chronic and progressive dyspnea is a cardinal symptom of patients with COPD.[5] Additionally, productive cough is present in up to 30% of patients.[5] Wheezing and chest tightness are common symptoms. They may vary over the course of days or over the course of a single day.[5] Chest tightness often follows physical exertion and is usually muscular in character and poorly localized.[5] An absence of wheezing or chest tightness does not exclude a diagnosis of COPD.

PHYSICAL EXAMINATION

Physical examination is rarely diagnostic in patients with COPD.[5] Physical signs of airflow limitations are not usually present until late in the disease after significant impairment of lung function has occurred.[5] Fatigue, weight loss, and anorexia are common in patients with emphysema. They may appear uncomfortable with pursed lip breathing and accessory muscle use. There is rarely peripheral edema and wheezing may or may not be present during examination.

DIFFERENTIAL DIAGNOSIS

Detailed history taking, imaging, and laboratory findings should help to distinguish COPD from other obstructive airway disorders (Table 4.2). A chest x-ray is not useful in diagnosing COPD but may be helpful in distinguishing alternative diagnoses.[5]

DIAGNOSTIC STUDIES

Spirometry is the most useful and objective measurement for airflow limitation in those in whom a COPD diagnosis is suspected and also those with previously diagnosed COPD.[5] It is a noninvasive and readily available test in most healthcare

TABLE 4.2 Differential Diagnosis for Chronic Obstructive Pulmonary Disease

Diagnosis	Description
Asthma	Early onset (often childhood) Symptoms worse at night and in the morning Family history of asthma Allergy, eczema, atopy also present
Congestive heart failure	Chest radiography revealing pulmonary edema, enlarged heart Peripheral edema Spirometry indicating volume restriction not airflow limitation[5]
Tuberculosis	Infiltrate on chest radiography Confirmation with microbiology testing[5]
Bronchiectasis	Copious purulent sputum Chest radiography/CT revealing bronchial wall thickening and bronchial dilatation[5]
Chronic cough	Presence of postnasal drip, asthma, GERD Due to medication (ACE inhibitors)

ACE, angiotensin-converting enzyme; GERD, gastroesophageal reflux disease.

settings. Spirometry should measure the volume of air expelled forcibly from the point of maximal inspiration (FVC) and the volume of air exhaled during the first second of this maneuver (FEV_1).[5] The ratio of these two measurements (FEV_1/FVC) is then calculated.[5] The spirometric criteria for airflow limitation is a post-bronchodilator fixed ratio of FEV_1/FVC <0.70. This reference has been used in numerous clinical trials that form the evidence from which treatment recommendations have been drawn.[5]

Chest radiography is not useful when establishing a diagnosis of COPD, but it can help to exclude alternative diagnoses. Radiologic changes associated with COPD include lung hyperinflation, hyperlucency of the lungs, and rapid tapering of vascular markings.[5] CT of the chest is not routinely recommended, except for those patients who meet the criteria for lung cancer risk assessment.[5] CT imaging may also be beneficial if surgical intervention is warranted. Additionally, pulse oximetry can be used to evaluate arterial oxygenation and the need for supplemental oxygenation.[5] Arterial blood gases are not routinely checked unless arterial pulse oximetry is <92%.[5]

EVALUATION

GOLD has further classified airflow limitation severity.[5] Those with GOLD stage I disease usually have no signs or symptoms[6] and have mild airflow limitation with $FEV_1 \geq$ 80% of predicted. GOLD stage II represents moderate airflow limitation with 50% $\leq FEV_1$ <80% predicted.[5] These patients have no abnormal signs and often have little or no breathlessness.[6] Symptoms for those in GOLD stage II are often limited to "smoker's cough."[6] Those with GOLD stage III disease have onset of breathlessness without wheezing upon moderate exertion and a productive cough.[6] Abnormal signs in this stage include reduced breath sounds and the presence of wheezing.[6] Airflow limitation in stage III is classified as severe with 30% $\leq FEV_1$ <50% predicted.[5] Very severe airflow limitation is present in GOLD stage IV and is classified as FEV_1 <30% of predicted.[5] Patients with severe airflow limitation characteristically have severe dyspnea at rest and on exertion with prominent wheezing and coughing.[5] Cyanosis and peripheral edema are usually present and worsen during acute exacerbation.[6] Treatment of COPD depends largely on the stage of the disease and requires an interdisciplinary approach.

TREATMENT

- Smoking cessation has the greatest capacity to influence the natural history of COPD. Long-term quit success rates of up to 25% can be achieved with effective resources and time dedicated to smoking cessation.[5] Pharmacologic therapy including nicotine replacement (gum, lozenges, intranasal spray, transdermal patch) has been shown to increase long-term smoking abstinence rates and be significantly more effective than placebo.[5] Varenicline, nortriptyline, and bupropion should never be used alone but rather as a component of a supportive program.[5] Additional content related to tobacco cessation can be found in Chapter 20, on preventive medicine.
- Initial medical treatment of COPD is guided by severity of obstruction, symptom burden, and exacerbation risk with escalation in therapy targeted to control persistent symptoms or further exacerbations.[8]
- Bronchodilators are the mainstay of COPD treatment. They are separated into two major classes based on mechanism of action. Short-acting bronchodilators include short-acting beta agonists (SABAs) and short-acting muscarinic antagonists (SAMAs).[8] Long-acting bronchodilator therapy includes both long-acting $beta_2$-agonists (LABAs) and long-acting muscarinic antagonists (LAMAs) such as tiotropium. SABAs and SAMAs may be used alone or in combination for patients with minimal symptoms or activity-specific symptoms.[8] Long-acting maintenance bronchodilator therapy is recommended for patients using SABAs more than two to three times per week.[8] Combination dual long-acting bronchodilator therapy including both LABA and LAMA provide greater improvement in lung function, symptom scores, and lower exacerbation risk as compared with the individual components.[8]
- Inhaled corticosteroids reduce airway inflammation. In COPD, modest improvements in lung function and significant decreases in exacerbations are seen when corticosteroids are added to combined LABAs or LAMAs therapy.[8]
- There has been a significant increase in the number of pharmacologic compounds and delivery mediums over the past two decades. There have been studies demonstrating differences in FEV_1 among different LAMAs, LABAs, and corticosteroids.[8] However, longer head-to-head studies establishing superiority of individual drugs are not yet available.[8]
- Long-term oxygen therapy improves survival in patients with advanced lung disease who have hypoxemia at rest and is generally indicated for patients whose oxygen drops below 89%.[6]

PATIENT EDUCATION

- Patients should be counseled on smoking cessation.
- Clinicians should stress the importance of medication compliance.

4.3 BRONCHIECTASIS

OVERVIEW

Bronchiectasis is characterized by irreversible dilation and destruction of bronchial walls, resulting in retention of purulent secretions. Patients characteristically present with dyspnea and a chronic cough productive of copious amounts of sputum. While bronchiectasis may be idiopathic, known risk factors include cystic fibrosis, chronic respiratory infections (including pertussis, tuberculosis, and nontuberculosis mycobacteria infection), allergic bronchopulmonary aspergillosis (ABPA), asthma, and impaired humoral defense mechanisms.

EPIDEMIOLOGY

The prevalence of bronchiectasis is estimated at 52/100,000 adults in the United States.[9] An estimated 350,000 to 500,000 U.S. adults are affected by bronchiectasis with an increased prevalence after the age of 60 and women being affected more commonly than men.[10] The overall incidence of bronchiectasis has decreased with better diagnosis and treatment of respiratory infections, though genetic disorders such as cystic fibrosis remain an important cause of bronchiectasis.

PATHOPHYSIOLOGY

A pattern of recurrent airway infection and inflammation in the presence of impaired ciliary clearance or structural abnormalities, leading to dilation and destruction of bronchial walls, is characteristic of bronchiectasis.

Tuberculosis, pertussis, and lung abscesses are common infectious risk factors, while cystic fibrosis and α-1-antitrypsin deficiency represent genetic mechanisms of impaired ciliary clearance predisposing to bronchiectasis. Inherited or acquired immunodeficiencies are additional risk factors that must be considered, along with mechanical airway obstruction, as might be seen with a tumor or foreign body.

The recurrent infectious and inflammatory response results in neutrophils, lymphocytes, and macrophages being released within the bronchial lumen, triggering further release of proinflammatory cytokines that lead to airway destruction and impaired cilia function.[11] This cycle continues until pathologic changes within the bronchi, including transmural inflammation, mucosal edema, cratering, ulceration, and neovascularization, are seen.[9] This ongoing cycle of infection, inflammation, and bronchial destruction results in irreversible thickening and dilation of bronchial walls with retention of secretions and, ultimately, colonization of the bronchial tree by organisms such as *Haemophilus influenzae, Staphylococcus aureus, Streptococcus pneumoniae,* or *Pseudomonas aeruginosa* (Figure 4.3).

MEDICAL HISTORY AND CLINICAL PRESENTATION

Bronchiectasis results from chronic or recurrent lower respiratory infections in the setting of immunodeficiency, anatomic abnormalities, mechanical obstruction, or impaired ciliary clearance. The ongoing infectious and/or inflammatory insult leads to dilation of the bronchi with retention of purulent secretions. The typical clinical presentation is dyspnea and a chronic cough productive of copious amounts of sputum.

In patients for whom bronchiectasis is on the differential diagnosis, medical history should pay particular attention to a history of lung infections. Bacterial pneumonias, tuberculosis, and pertussis are among the respiratory infections that may predispose to bronchiectasis. Any history of immunodeficiency should also be elicited from the patient, as this contributes to the inflammatory response and bronchial remodeling seen with bronchiectasis. Genetic disorders, in particular cystic fibrosis, also represent an important risk factor that should be considered in a patient's history. Finally, causes of impaired ciliary function or mechanical obstruction should be considered. Table 4.3 reviews risk factors for bronchiectasis that should be considered when taking a patient history.

Bronchiectasis is a chronic condition with irreversible lung damage. Over the course of the disease, patients may present with acute exacerbations alternating with periods of relatively good control.

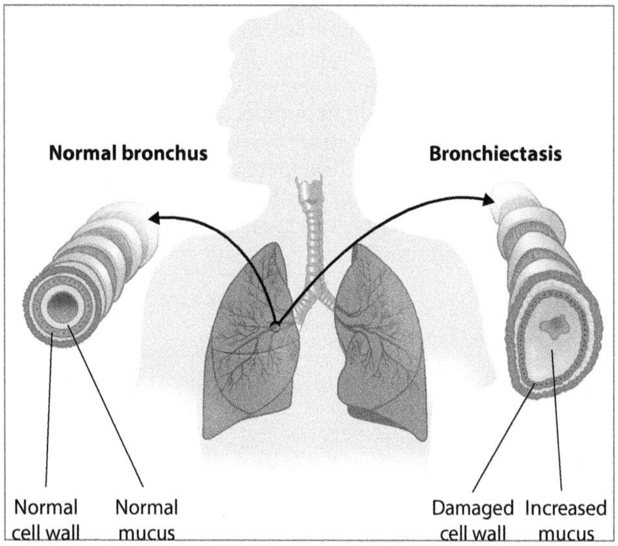

FIGURE 4.3 **Appearance of bronchial tree in patients with bronchiectasis.**

SIGNS AND SYMPTOMS

The classic presenting signs and symptoms of bronchiectasis are a chronic cough with copious amounts of purulent sputum production and dyspnea. Other symptoms patients may present with include hemoptysis, chest pain (often described as pleuritic), and systemic findings such as fever and fatigue. During an acute exacerbation, patients may note fever, increased frequency of cough and increased volume of sputum production, and worsening dyspnea.

PHYSICAL EXAMINATION

Adventitious lung sounds, including wheezing and crackles at the lung bases, may be identified on physical examination. Pulse oximetry should be done to assess for hypoxia. In patients with long-standing, severe disease and chronic hypoxia, digital clubbing may be noted. Fever should raise suspicion for acute infection or exacerbation of bronchiectasis.

DIFFERENTIAL DIAGNOSIS

The differential diagnosis for bronchiectasis includes COPD, specifically the chronic bronchitis subtype, asthma, pneumonia, interstitial lung disease, and pulmonary hypertension (Table 4.4).

DIAGNOSTIC STUDIES

High-resolution chest CT is the imaging modality of choice for confirming a diagnosis of bronchiectasis. The typical finding is airway damage evidenced by dilated and thickened

TABLE 4.3 Risk Factors for Bronchiectasis

Infectious or Inflammatory Insult	Physiologic Abnormality
Bacterial pneumonia Viral pneumonia Pertussis Tuberculosis Lung abscess Cystic fibrosis Aspiration pneumonia or pneumonitis	Ciliary dysfunction • Smoking • Primary ciliary dyskinesia • Cystic fibrosis Obstructing tumor Immunodeficiency Altered mucus production • Cystic fibrosis Anatomic abnormality Alpha-1 antitrypsin deficiency

TABLE 4.4 Differential Diagnosis for Bronchiectasis

Diagnosis	Description
Chronic obstructive pulmonary disease (COPD)	Chronic bronchitis presents with cough and increased sputum production. A history of smoking is common in COPD. Patients with bronchiectasis have increased volume of sputum production compared to patients with COPD.
Asthma	Spirometry will reveal reversible airway obstruction in asthma and patients often have significant improvement with bronchodilators.
Bacterial or viral pneumonia	Patients present with fever and cough. Onset of symptoms is typically more acute.

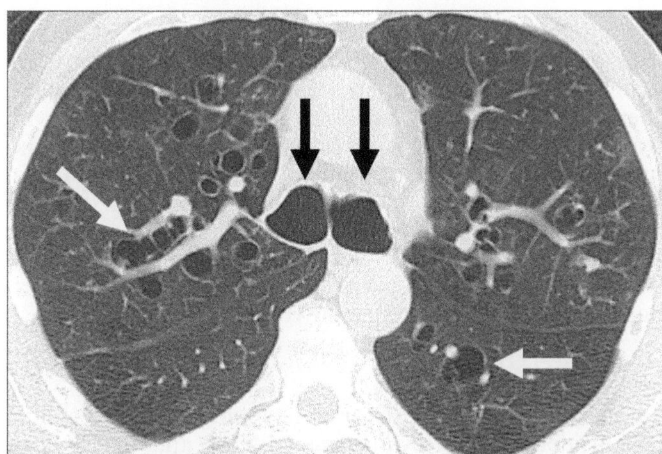

Figure 4.4 **CT imaging of a patient with bronchiectasis. Black arrows point to thickened, dilated bronchi with "tram-track" appearance of the bronchial tree indicated by the white arrows.** *(Source: Mcgfowler)*

bronchi, often described as having a "tram track" appearance (Figure 4.4).

Additional diagnostic studies are focused primarily on identification of the underlying cause and can include serum immunoglobulin levels and HIV serology for identification of immunodeficiencies, sweat chloride and/or genetic testing for cystic fibrosis, or bronchoscopy for anatomic evaluation. Sputum cultures should also be obtained and are useful in guiding treatment.

Spirometry is non specific and may show obstructive or restrictive patterns of lung disease. However, spirometry is useful in monitoring severity and progression of disease, with an FEV_1 60% to 80% of predicted being consistent with mild disease, FEV_1 40% to 59% of predicted indicative of moderate disease, and FEV_1 <40% of predicted indicating severe disease with a poor prognosis.[12] Additionally, an acute decrease in FEV_1% should raise concern for an acute exacerbation of bronchiectasis.[12]

EVALUATION

A wide range of patient presentations is encountered with bronchiectasis. Owing to the variety of initial presentations, severity of disease, and the fact that many cases of bronchiectasis are idiopathic, there is often a delay in diagnosing bronchiectasis, though delayed diagnosis is associated with more rapid disease progression.[12] Thus, clinicians must maintain a high index of suspicion. Generally, any patient with a known predisposing condition, such as cystic fibrosis, immunodeficiency, or chronic lung infections and chronic respiratory symptoms should be evaluated for bronchiectasis. The diagnosis is confirmed radiographically.

TREATMENT

- Acute exacerbations should be treated with antimicrobial therapy targeted to sputum culture results. Long-term prophylactic antibiotics have shown to be effective in cystic fibrosis–associated bronchiectasis. Data are less clear on the role of prophylactic antibiotics in non-cystic fibrosis–related bronchiectasis, though they may decrease frequency of acute exacerbations.
- Supportive therapy with pulmonary hygiene and physiotherapy includes chest percussion (flutter valve devices or high-frequency chest wall oscillation), mucolytic drugs, humidifiers, and supplemental oxygen as needed.
- Smoking cessation
- Appropriate vaccinations

PATIENT EDUCATION

- Bronchiectasis is a chronic, permanent disease state and treatment will be lifelong.
- The goal of chest physiotherapy is to enhance airway clearance and reduce incidence of pneumonia or acute exacerbations; it plays an important role in disease management despite chronic sputum production.
- If symptoms worsen, including increased severity of dyspnea, fever, increased sputum volume, or acute decline in FEV_1, patient should seek medical attention.
- Smoking cessation and preventive care, including typical vaccinations (e.g., influenza and pneumococcal vaccinations) should be encouraged for all patients.

4.4 BRONCHIOLITIS

OVERVIEW

Bronchiolitis is primarily a disorder of infancy and early childhood, with cases most commonly occurring before 2 years of age. While several respiratory viruses have been described in association with bronchiolitis, respiratory syncytial virus (RSV) remains the most important cause, contributing to nearly 70% of cases of bronchiolitis.[13] Infants and young children characteristically present with several days of upper respiratory symptoms followed by lower respiratory manifestations.

EPIDEMIOLOGY

Incidence of bronchiolitis has a seasonal variation, with cases increasing between October and April in the Northern Hemisphere, with a peak incidence from December to March.[14,15] Bronchiolitis is the most common cause of hospital admission in infants <1 year of age in the United States, accounting for 57,500 hospitalizations yearly and 2.1 million outpatient visits.[14,15]

PATHOPHYSIOLOGY

The etiology of bronchiolitis is viral infection, with RSV being the most commonly implicated virus. Direct viral cytotoxic injury is suspected, with resulting necrosis of small airway epithelial cells and ciliary destruction.[14,15] The necrosis and cell destruction trigger an immune and inflammatory response, with neutrophil and lymphocyte infiltration contributing to airway edema and increased mucus secretion.[14] At the same time, the sloughed, necrotic cells plug the bronchioles, leading to obstruction and air trapping, ultimately resulting in airway hyperinflation and atelectasis, as shown in Figure 4.5.[14,15]

MEDICAL HISTORY AND CLINICAL PRESENTATION

While all infants and young children are susceptible to RSV infection and bronchiolitis, infants at particularly high risk for bronchiolitis include those born at <29 weeks' gestation, those with congenital heart disease, and infants with chronic lung disease. Second-hand tobacco exposure also increases the risk for severe bronchiolitis and hospital admission; thus, environmental exposures should be elicited during the medical history.

Several days of upper respiratory symptoms, followed by progression to lower respiratory disease including cough, dyspnea, and increased work of breathing, is the typical presentation. Clinical findings may vary significantly with cough, changes in patient positioning, sleep/wake status, or agitation, with such "minute-to-minute variation" being a hallmark finding of bronchiolitis.[14]

SIGNS AND SYMPTOMS

Patients often have several days of upper respiratory symptoms such as rhinorrhea or nasal congestion followed by progression to lower respiratory symptoms, including cough, dyspnea, and increased respiratory effort. Signs of increased work of breathing may include grunting, retractions, or accessory muscle use. Tachypnea is an important sign that may serve as a predictor of the risk of progression to severe disease.[15]

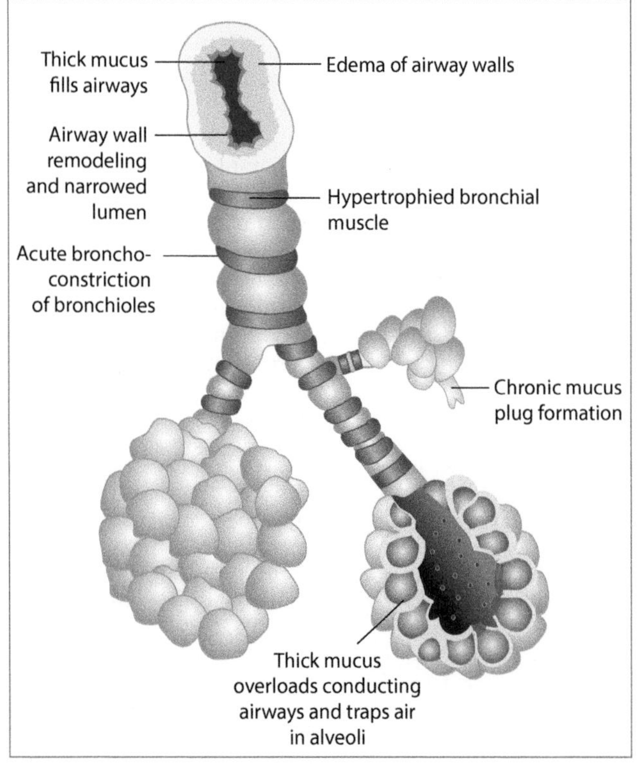

Figure 4.5 **Appearance of bronchioles in patients with bronchiolitis.**

PHYSICAL EXAMINATION

Clinicians should pay particular attention to patients' respiratory effort, noting increased work of breathing if present. Vital signs should be taken to assess for tachypnea, tachycardia, or fever. Tachypnea and tachycardia are associated with more severe presentations.[15] Fever is present in only approximately 30% of patients and, if present in a young infant, should prompt a sepsis workup.[13,14] Adventitious lung sounds, specifically wheezing and crackles, may be identified on physical exam.

DIFFERENTIAL DIAGNOSIS

The differential diagnosis for bronchiolitis is summarized in Table 4.5.

DIAGNOSTIC STUDIES

Bronchiolitis is a clinical diagnosis. No routine laboratory or diagnostic tests, including RSV testing or chest x-ray, are recommended. Pulse oximetry should be used with caution. There is evidence otherwise stable infants and children with bronchiolitis may experience transient hypoxia. If pulse oximetry is used as part of clinical decision-making, a goal oxygen saturation of >90% has been shown to decrease hospitalization and associated complications and morbidity without increasing poor outcomes.[13–15] Viral testing can be considered for admitted patients for the purposes of cohorting patients to reduce secondary transmission.[13]

EVALUATION

Age is the strongest predictor of hospitalization and should be considered when evaluating patients and determining disposition. Patients older than 2 months of age, with no history of intubation, normal respiratory rate, adequate PO intake, and oxygen saturation >90%–94% can be safely discharged with outpatient follow-up, while younger patients who are tachypneic, tachycardic, dehydrated, or showing evidence of respiratory distress should be considered for hospitalization.[15] Patients presenting with a fever, especially in early infancy, should have a sepsis workup.[13]

TREATMENT

- Treatment is supportive in nature.
- No specific therapies have proven benefit. In particular, bronchodilators, steroids, antibiotics, nebulized epinephrine, and nebulized hypertonic saline have not been found to improve outcomes and the risks outweigh the benefits.
- Supplemental oxygen should be used for patients who are persistently hypoxic <90%.

TABLE 4.5 Differential Diagnosis for Bronchiolitis

Diagnosis	Description
Congenital heart or lung disease	Respiratory distress in infants in the absence of upper respiratory symptoms
Foreign body aspiration	Choking, coughing, and wheezing, no upper respiratory symptoms
Pertussis	Paroxysmal cough; known exposure
Pneumonia	Fever and lower respiratory symptoms

PATIENT EDUCATION

- Parents should be educated on strict hand hygiene and avoidance of sick contacts.
- High-risk patients (including premature infants and congenital heart disease patients) may receive prophylactic palivizumab.
- Maintenance of adequate hydration and nutrition should be encouraged.
- Symptoms generally last for approximately 2 weeks.

4.5 INFECTIONS

OVERVIEW

There are numerous respiratory tract infections. Broadly, respiratory infections can be classified as upper or lower respiratory infections and can be caused by various pathogens. Influenza, pneumonia, rhinovirus infection, tuberculosis, RSV infection, and parainfluenza virus infection are just a few of the many common respiratory infections. Collectively, respiratory infections impose a considerable burden to the healthcare system worldwide and are a significant cause of morbidity and death. The severity of respiratory infections varies; while many are asymptomatic, subclinical, or otherwise mild, severe disease can also be seen, with genetic factors, age, smoking, and environmental exposures being some risk factors for severe presentation of respiratory infection.[16] Respiratory infections can be acquired via community spread, exposure in the healthcare system (nosocomial), reactivation of prior infection, or environmental exposures to particular pathogens. This chapter will focus on pneumonias, tuberculosis, and croup.

EPIDEMIOLOGY

The collective incidence of respiratory infection is difficult to classify given the presence of asymptomatic or mild cases that may not present for medical care as well as the number of cases diagnosed clinically without formal laboratory testing.[17] It is generally recognized that pulmonary infections are common worldwide. Pulmonary infections are of particular concern in immunocompromised patients, with opportunistic and atypical organisms presenting in this group. Epidemiologic data for the conditions covered in this chapter are presented in Table 4.6.

PATHOPHYSIOLOGY

The specific mechanism of disease and infection varies based on the causative pathogen. The pathophysiologic mechanisms unique to the infections discussed in this chapter are reviewed in the appropriate sections. In general, microbes can be inhaled via aerosolized spread or respiratory droplets or aspirated from colonized organisms in the oropharyngeal tract. The lungs have an extensive innate immunity system, beginning with physical defenses such as coughing and sneezing. Within the respiratory tract, cilia work to clear infectious particles, mucus contains antimicrobial enzymes, and the alveolar macrophages phagocytose pathogens and release further antimicrobial substances.[18] The innate immune system within the lungs also works to trigger the adaptive immune response. When these defenses are overwhelmed, pulmonary infection occurs.

TABLE 4.6 Incidence and/or Prevalence of Selected Pulmonary Infections

Condition	Incidence/Prevalence
Pneumonia	
Community-acquired	1.7 million ED visits annually with 55,000 deaths in the United States[19]
Nosocomial	
Ventilator-associated	1–2.5 cases/1,000 days of mechanical ventilation[24]
Hospital-acquired	5–20 cases/1,000 admissions[24]
Tuberculosis	Approximately 10 million new cases yearly (133 cases/100,000 population) with approximately 1.5 million deaths[34] South East Asia and Africa account for 70% of worldwide cases[34]
Croup	Affects 3% of children aged 6 months–3 years, accounting for 7% of hospitalizations for respiratory disease/febrile illness in this age range[32]

Source: Data from Kleppin S. Community-acquired pneumonia: treatment options for adults. J Infus Nurs. *2020;43(4):187–190. doi:10.1097/NAN.0000000000000378; Zaragoza R, Vidal-Cortes P, Aguilar G, et al. Update of the treatment of nosocomial pneumonia in the ICU.* Crit Care. *2020;24(383):1–13. doi:10.1186/s13054-020-03091-2; Smith DK, McDermott AJ, Sullivan JF. Croup: diagnosis and management.* Am Fam Physician. *2018;97(9):575–580. https://www.aafp.org/afp/2018/0501/p575.html; MacNeil A, Glaziou P, Sismanidis C, Maloney S, Floyd K. Global epidemiology of tuberculosis and progress toward achieving global targets—2017.* MMWR Morb Mortal Wkly Rep. *2019;68:263–266. doi:10.15585/mmwr.mm6811a3*

4.5A PNEUMONIA

MEDICAL HISTORY AND CLINICAL PRESENTATION

The lungs are a sterile environment with innate immune defenses discussed above. When these mechanisms are overcome by a microbe, pulmonary infection occurs, of which pneumonia is a classic presentation. Pneumonia can be caused by viruses, bacteria, fungi, or yeasts, with viral and bacterial co-infection being a common presentation.[19] Community-acquired pneumonia is the leading cause of death from infectious disease in the United States and primarily affects young children, older adults, and those with underlying comorbidities including chronic heart, lung, liver, or kidney disease; cancer; diabetes mellitus; alcoholism; asplenia; or immunodeficiencies.[20]

Community-Acquired Pneumonia

Community-acquired pneumonia (CAP) is defined as pneumonia occurring in patients who have not been hospitalized or in a long-term care facility for at least 14 days prior to symptom onset. Pathogens can be transmitted via respiratory droplets from person to person or through autoinoculation in patients with naso- or oropharyngeal colonization.[19] Infection leads to inflammation and buildup of purulent secretions within the alveoli.[19] The most common pathogen is *Streptococcus pneumoniae*. Alternate bacterial pathogens causing CAP include *Haemophilus influenzae, Mycoplasma pneumoniae, Staphylococcus aureus, Legionella, Chlamydia pneumoniae, Moraxella catarrhalis,* and *Klebsiella pneumoniae*. Viral pathogens also commonly cause CAP. However, the specific organism is identified in <50% of cases.[20]

Nosocomial Pneumonia

In patients who have been hospitalized or in a long-term care facility within 14 days of symptom onset, or patients in whom pneumonia develops within 48 hours of hospital admission, nosocomial pneumonia is diagnosed. Historically, the term healthcare-associated pneumonia (HCAP) was used. However, the HCAP designation was removed in 2016 as it was found to be poorly evidence-based and neither adequately identified patients at risk of infection with multidrug-resistant organisms nor was it associated with mortality.[21,22] Currently, two distinct entities comprise nosocomial pneumonia: hospital-acquired pneumonia (HAP) and ventilator-associated pneumonia (VAP). Pneumonia in hospitalized patients who are not intubated or mechanically ventilated receives the HAP designation, while pneumonia developing in mechanically ventilated patients is designated VAP. Collectively, HAP and VAP are among the most common hospital-acquired infections.[23]

Risk factors for nosocomial pneumonia are patient-related, infection prevention–related, or procedure-related. Patient-related factors include severe acute or chronic disease, malnutrition, and smoking; infection prevention–related factors include clinician hand hygiene and cleaning/sterilizing of respiratory equipment; and procedural factors include the use of sedative medications, steroids or other immunosuppressants, and prolonged or inappropriate antibiotic usage.[24]

Lung Abscess

Lung abscess is a common complication of pneumonia, though it is most commonly caused by aspiration.[25] Lung abscess is defined as a circumscribed area of pus or necrotic debris in the lung parenchyma.[26] Lung abscesses are further classified as primary (bronchogenic), resulting directly from lung infection or aspiration, or secondary, resulting from hematologic spread from underlying disease states such as endocarditis or postobstructive infection, such as in the case of obstructing lung tumors.[25,26] Patients most at risk are those at increased risk of aspiration, including patients with neuromuscular disease, those with alcoholism, comatose or ventilated patients, and patients with seizure disorders. Immunocompromised patients are also at increased risk of lung abscess formation.

SIGNS AND SYMPTOMS

All causes of pneumonia present with similar signs and symptoms. Fever, chills, productive cough, dyspnea, pleuritic chest pain, generalized weakness, and malaise are common. Though these signs and symptoms may be present in nosocomial pneumonia as well, an increased index of suspicion is necessary in cases of sedated or ventilated patients, or those with altered mental status. Lung abscess initially presents with identical symptoms as well. In later stages, sputum may become particularly foul-smelling and putrid.[25] Hemoptysis may be present in more severe cases of lung abscess.

Atypical CAP, such as that caused by *M. pneumoniae*, may present slightly differently, with nonspecific signs of systemic illness, such as headache, fatigue, and weakness predominating. Sore throat may be present. While cough is typical, respiratory symptoms tend to be less pronounced in cases of atypical pneumonia, leading to the common terminology "walking pneumonia" to describe these cases. However, differentiating infectious organism based on signs and symptoms alone is unreliable.[19]

PHYSICAL EXAMINATION

Physical examination findings in patients with pneumonia are those indicative of consolidation on the lung examination. This includes the presence of crackles, rhonchi, wheezes, increased tactile fremitus, bronchophony, and egophony localized to the affected area. Vital sign abnormalities may include fever, tachycardia, tachypnea, and hypoxia. The most predictive findings are fever and egophony.[27] The presence of pneumonia becomes increasingly unlikely with a normal physical examination.

DIFFERENTIAL DIAGNOSIS

The differential diagnosis for pneumonia is summarized in Table 4.7.

DIAGNOSTIC STUDIES

Radiographic diagnosis is necessary for all causes of pneumonia and recommended prior to initiating antibiotic treatment.[19] Plain-film chest x-ray (CXR) with posteroanterior and lateral views is currently the standard of care. CXR will show an acute infiltrate in cases of CAP and nosocomial pneumonia (Figure 4.6).

Lung ultrasound is an increasingly popular alternative to CXR, with high sensitivity and specificity and the ability to rule out alternate diagnoses such as pleural effusion or pneumothorax.[27] However, lung ultrasound is highly dependent on operator skill.[19] CT is the most sensitive and specific imaging modality but comes with increased cost and radiation exposure that may be unnecessary given the availability of alternate diagnostic radiologic methods.[19] Lung abscess also requires radiographic imaging; CXR will show a cavitating lesion with presence of an air-fluid level indicated communication and drainage with the bronchial tree (Figure 4.7).[25]

CT best defines the anatomic location of the abscess and can rule out alternate diagnoses such as bronchiectasis or infected bullae.[25]

Microbiology testing is not routinely recommended for cases of CAP in the outpatient setting, as it is low yield and difficult to obtain an adequate, noncontaminated sample. Sputum culture remains the gold standard for identifying the causative organism in cases of nosocomial pneumonia.[23] Noninvasive methods of sputum sampling, such as forced expectoration for patients with suspected HAP or endotracheal aspiration in patients with VAP, are preferred to invasive sampling, such as bronchoscopy.[22] Sputum culture is also necessary to guide antimicrobial therapy in cases of lung abscess. Bronchoscopy with bronchoalveolar lavage or ultrasound- or CT-guided fine needle aspiration are preferred methods of obtaining a culture in patients with lung abscess.[25]

Additional laboratory tests that may be indicated in all patients with pneumonia include complete blood count (CBC) assessing presence and degree of leukocytosis, influenza testing, and HIV testing. In hospitalized patients and those with nosocomial pneumonia or lung abscess, blood cultures should be done to assess for bacteremia, though these are not indicated in the outpatient setting. Procalcitonin levels are increasingly being used to assist in differentiating bacterial from viral infections and may be able to guide clinical decision-making related to antibiotic therapy. However, in outpatient cases of radiologically confirmed pneumonia, there is insufficient evidence warranting routine use of procalcitonin.[19] Procalcitonin, along with C-reactive protein, may be elevated in cases of nosocomial pneumonia and lung abscess, though neither

TABLE 4.7 Differential Diagnosis for Pneumonia

Diagnosis	Description
Community-Acquired Pneumonia	
Viral respiratory infection	Common viral symptoms include sore throat, runny nose or nasal congestion, ear discomfort. Low-grade fever may be present. Signs of localized infiltration on physical exam are absent; CXR, if ordered, would be unremarkable.
Acute bronchitis	Inflammation of the bronchi, typically caused by viral infection, causing cough, wheezing, and mild dyspnea and/or pleuritic pain. Fever may be present but is typically low-grade. Wheeze is the typical physical exam finding and may clear with cough.
Influenza	In addition to respiratory signs and symptoms, systemic symptoms including weakness, fatigue, malaise, and headache are often present. Rapid flu testing or PCR test will be positive. Postinfluenza pneumonia is also common with *S. aureus*, and particularly MRSA, representing important pathogens in this subset of patients.
Nosocomial Pneumonia: conditions above, plus:	
Atelectasis	Complete or partial collapse of alveoli common in hospitalized and postoperative patients due to lack of intermittent deep breathing, weakened cough, etc. Often asymptomatic, though dyspnea and hypoxia may be present. CXR reveals loss of lung volume.
Pleural effusion	Excess fluid buildup between pleurae, may cause cough, dyspnea, orthopnea, or chest pain. Characterized as transudative or exudative based on protein in fluid; causes of transudates include heart failure and cirrhosis, while pneumonia or malignancy may cause exudates. Diagnosed with CXR, CT scan, or lung ultrasound.
Pulmonary edema	Excess fluid in lungs commonly caused by heart failure and related conditions presenting with dyspnea, orthopnea, and cough productive of frothy sputum. May also be caused by high altitude. Diagnosis confirmed with CXR.
Lung Abscess	
Cavitary lung cancer	Cavitation can be detected in up to 22% of lung cancers by CT imaging; squamous cell cancers are most likely to cavitate.[35] Smoking is a significant risk factor and other signs and symptoms of malignancy (e.g., weight loss) may be present.
Tuberculosis	Patients often present with fevers, night sweats, weight loss, productive cough, and hemoptysis. Emigration from an endemic region, immunocompromised states, and residents or employees of institutional settings are at highest risk. Acid-fast bacilli and culture will identify presence of *Mycobacterium tuberculosis*.
Emphysematous bullae	Smoking history is the most significant risk factor for development of emphysematous chronic obstructive pulmonary disease. Bullae are air-filled spaces, which may be numerous and adjacent in the case of bullous emphysema. Dyspnea and tachypnea are common, as is a cachectic and barrel-chested appearance.

CXR, chest x-ray; MRSA, methicillin-resistant Staphylococcus aureus; PCR, polymerase chain reaction.
Source: Data from Rendon P, Pizanis C, Montanaro M, Kraai E. What is the best approach to a cavitary lung lesion? Hospitalist. *2015(3). https://www.the-hospitalist.org/hospitalist/article/122550/what-best-approach-cavitary-lung-lesion*

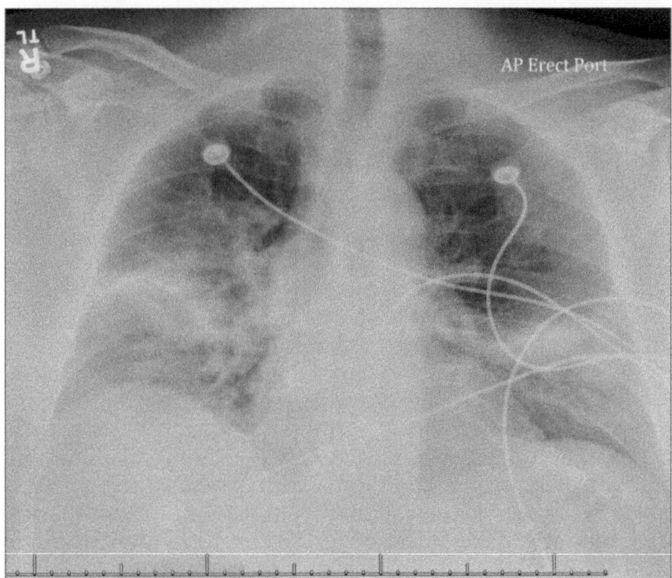

Figure 4.6 **Frontal chest radiograph in a patient with pneumonia. A large right middle lobe infiltrate and smaller left lingular infiltrate are seen with bilateral pneumonia.**

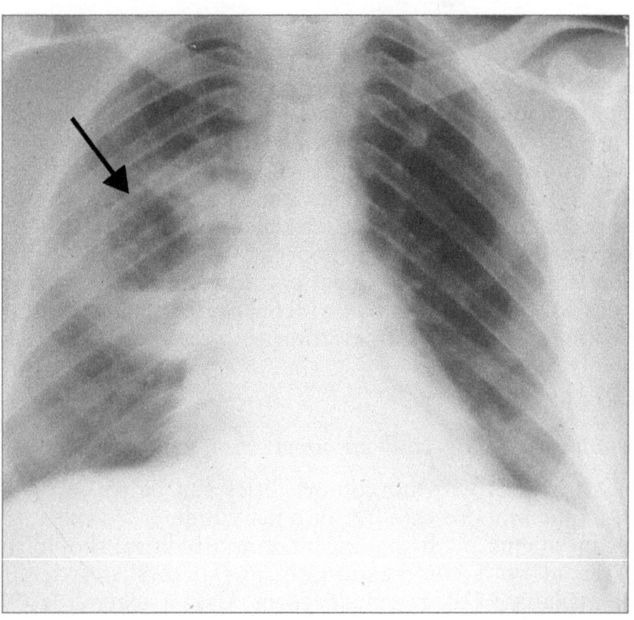

Figure 4.7 **Chest radiograph in a patient with lung abscess. A cavitating lesion, identified by the black arrow, is consistent with lung abscess.**
(Source: Yale Rosen)

are specific and should not be relied upon to make or confirm a diagnosis of HAP or VAP.[23]

EVALUATION

Patients with characteristic signs and symptoms of pneumonia along with abnormal physical examination findings should have further workup with radiographic imaging and laboratory testing to evaluate the possibility of pneumonia. If CXR is unremarkable but the clinician's suspicion remains high, repeat imaging can be obtained in 24 hours.[19]

Community-Acquired Pneumonia

While *S. pneumoniae* is the most common pathogen causing CAP, patients with certain risk factors should be evaluated for alternate pathogens. Patients with alcoholism, history of aspiration, or other risk factors for aspiration may be infected with anaerobic oral flora. *Klebsiella* is also more prevalent among patients with alcoholism. *Legionella* should be considered in patients with recent travel/hotel stays. Patients with recent influenza infection may be at increased risk for methicillin-resistant *Staphylococcus aureus* (MRSA) pneumonia. Finally, those with late-stage HIV disease or who are otherwise immunocompromised should be evaluated for opportunistic pathogens such as *Pneumocystis jirovecii, Aspergillus*, or *Cryptococcus*.

Severity of CAP can be assessed with the pneumonia severity index (PSI) or CURB-65 tool. These scores can further help with clinical decision-making related to patient disposition or need for inpatient treatment. Both tools account for age, comorbidities, and physical exam or diagnostic study findings to assess severity and potential mortality risk associated with CAP.

Nosocomial Pneumonia

Hospitalized patients with new and unexplained fever, leukocytosis, or leukopenia in addition to cough with purulent sputum production, dyspnea, and/or hypoxia should be evaluated for HAP (or VAP, if mechanically ventilated). Chest x-ray should be obtained in those cases to evaluate for new or worsening lung infiltrates.

Lung Abscess

Lung abscess should be considered in patients with a history of pneumonia or aspiration with persistent or progressive symptoms and is of particular concern in immunocompromised individuals. While early signs and symptoms do not differentiate lung abscess from pneumonia, later and more severe findings, including increasing amounts of particularly foul-smelling sputum or hemoptysis, should prompt evaluation with CXR or lung CT. A cavitating lesion, most commonly solitary, is distinctive with the presence of an air-fluid level indicative of communication with the bronchial tree.

TREATMENT

Community-Acquired Pneumonia

- Outpatients with no comorbidities can be treated with amoxicillin, doxycycline, or a macrolide.
- Outpatients with significant comorbidities should be treated with combination therapy: either amoxicillin/clavulanate OR a cephalosporin AND a macrolide OR doxycycline.
- Monotherapy with a respiratory fluoroquinolone may be used for outpatients with significant comorbidities, though black-box warnings must be considered.
- Inpatients should be treated with combination therapy. If MRSA is confirmed or suspected, vancomycin or linezolid should be added. If *Pseudomonas* is confirmed or suspected, piperacillin-tazobactam, cefepime, or another appropriate antipseudomonal agent should be added.

Nosocomial Pneumonia

- Whenever possible, treatment should be guided by local antibiograms.
- Empiric treatment for HAP should be directed at *S. aureus* and most commonly includes a third-generation cephalosporin; MRSA coverage should be added when >20% of *Staphylococcus* isolates locally are MRSA.
- Empiric treatment for VAP should be directed at *S. aureus, Pseudomonas,* and other gram-negative bacilli, and most commonly includes piperacillin/tazobactam or cefepime; MRSA coverage (vancomycin or linezolid) should be added when >10% to 20% of *Staphylococcus* isolates locally are MRSA.

Lung Abscess

- From 85% to 90% of cases will respond to systemic antibiotic therapy, with symptoms improving within 2 to 4 weeks.[25]
- Antibiotic regimen should have substantial anaerobic coverage and may include clindamycin, amoxicillin/clavulanate, ampicillin/sulbactam, or similar regimen.
- Invasive treatment is indicated for patients who failed antibiotic treatment, those with prolonged severe sepsis, and those with empyema. Invasive treatment options include chest tube with drainage, percutaneous drain, endoscopic or bronchoscopic intervention, or surgical resection (VATS or lobectomy).

PATIENT EDUCATION

- Smoking cessation is of utmost importance in preventing and reducing severity of pneumonia.
- Pneumococcal vaccination is indicated for all adults 65 and older and those with diabetes mellitus, chronic heart or lung disease, tobacco or alcohol use, or liver disease.

4.5B TUBERCULOSIS

MEDICAL HISTORY AND CLINICAL PRESENTATION

Tuberculosis is the result of *Mycobacterium tuberculosis* infection. *M. tuberculosis* is spread in an airborne manner, with transmission occurring when aerosolized pathogen, spread by patients with active pulmonary tuberculosis infection, is inhaled. After inhalation, the pathogen moves to the lungs where it encounters alveolar macrophages, which in many cases exert sufficient microbicidal activity to contain the pathogen. If the pathogen survives the alveolar macrophages, most patients will mount an immune response leading to granuloma formation. In those cases, *M. tuberculosis* may remain dormant within a granuloma (latent tuberculosis infection, LTBI) until the patient experiences immune compromise due to age, illness, or other environmental factors leading to disintegration of the granuloma and reactivation of the tuberculosis.[28] The bacilli may disseminate to other organ systems as well, causing extrapulmonary disease. In a minority of cases, the initial immune response is inadequate and progressive primary tuberculosis

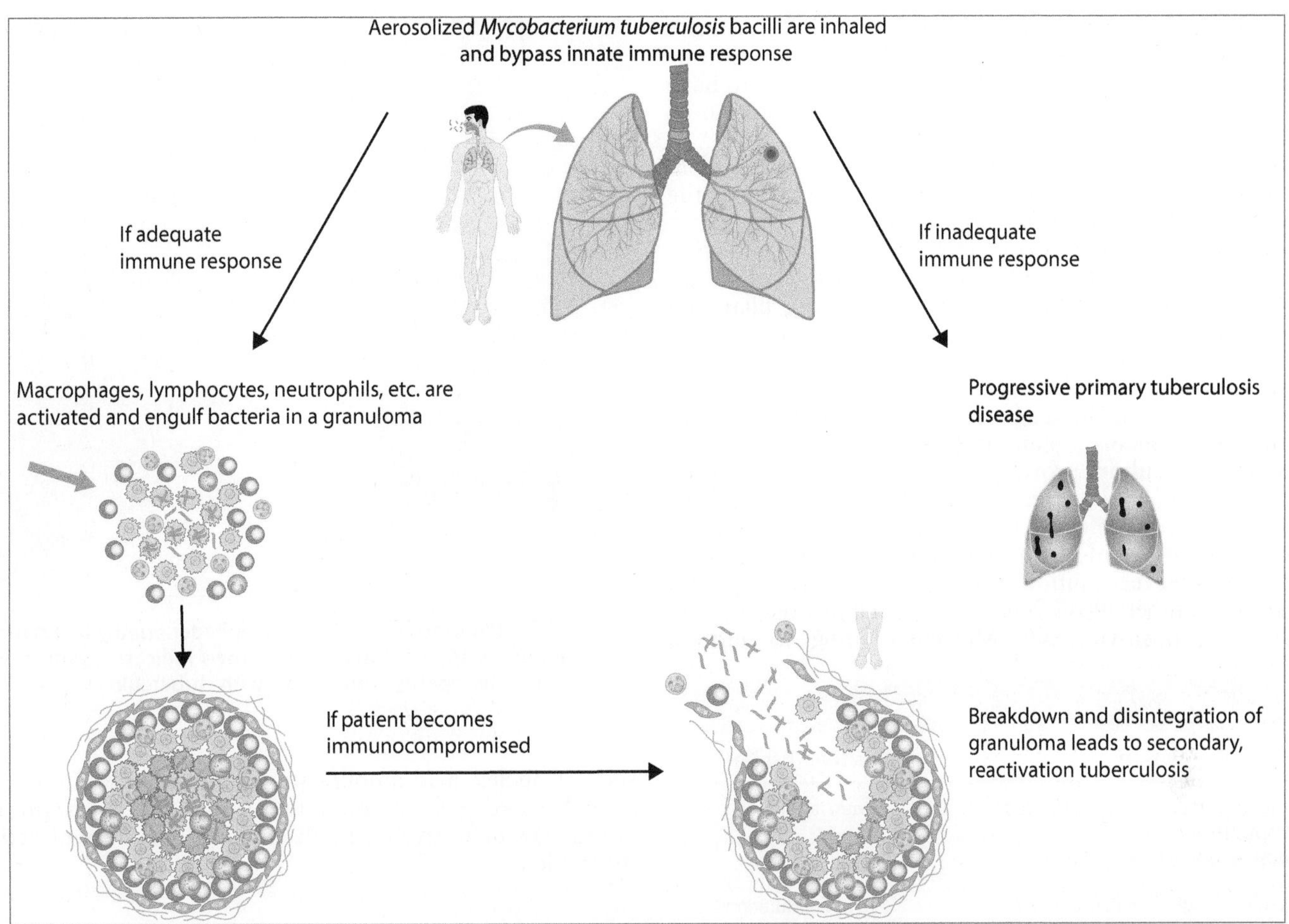

Figure 4.8 **Pathophysiology of pulmonary tuberculosis.**

results after initial infection. Figure 4.8 demonstrates the pathophysiology of pulmonary tuberculosis.

Patients with LTBI are asymptomatic, noninfectious, and typically identified only with screening tests. Patients with active tuberculosis, either primary or reactivation, are symptomatic and infectious.

SIGNS AND SYMPTOMS

Latent tuberculosis is an asymptomatic infection. Classic signs and symptoms of active tuberculosis include persistent cough, which becomes progressively productive of purulent sputum over time, fever, night sweats, and weight loss. Blood-streaked sputum may also be present.

PHYSICAL EXAMINATION

Patients will likely appear chronically ill and frail on general inspection. There are no specific physical exam findings associated with tuberculosis. The lung examination may be unremarkable or findings may be nonspecific such as coarse breath sounds and rales. If pleural effusion is present, associated findings include dullness to percussion and decreased tactile fremitus. In cases of disseminated or extrapulmonary tuberculosis, abnormal physical exam findings may be present and are dependent upon the affected organ systems.

DIFFERENTIAL DIAGNOSIS

The differential diagnosis for tuberculosis is summarized in Table 4.8.

TABLE 4.8 Differential Diagnosis for Tuberculosis

Diagnosis	Description
Nontuberculosis mycobacterial infection	Infection with organisms such as *M. avium, M. abscessus,* etc. often is due to environmental exposures rather than person-person transmission. Patients with chronic lung disease are most at risk. Bronchiectasis and lung nodules are common radiographic findings. Culture or NAAT differentiates from *M. tuberculosis.*
Sarcoidosis	Characterized by noncaseating granulomas (vs. caseating granulomas found in tuberculosis infection) and bilateral hilar lymphadenopathy. Symptoms include dyspnea, fatigue and malaise, joint pain, and skin rash. AFB stain and culture will be negative.
Hodgkin lymphoma	Painless lymphadenopathy is the most common symptom. Systemic symptoms, including fever, night sweats, weight loss may also be present. Biopsy of affected lymph node is diagnostic.

AFB, acid-fast bacilli; NAAT, nucleic-acid amplification test.

DIAGNOSTIC STUDIES

Latent tuberculosis infection is identified through screening tests. The two commonly available options for LTBI screening include the tuberculin skin test with purified protein derivative (PPD) and the interferon-gamma release assay (IGRA). PPD testing is preferred in children younger than 5 years of age. IGRA is recommended for patients who have received the BCG (bacille Calmette-Guérin) vaccination or patients who are unlikely to return for a second visit to have PPD results read. Table 4.9 outlines the interpretation of PPD results based on patient risk.

PPD and IGRA testing do not differentiate latent from active tuberculosis infections; that distinction is made on the basis of symptoms and radiographic findings.

Radiographic evidence of active tuberculosis infection is present on plain film chest x-ray. Findings include alveolar infiltration, cavitary lesions (Figure 4.9), hilar and paratracheal lymphadenopathy (Figure 4.10), and pleural effusions.[29]

Microbiology or molecular biology testing should be performed to confirm the diagnosis. The gold-standard diagnostic study remains a sputum, bronchial aspirate, or tracheal aspirate culture growing *M. tuberculosis*.[29] However, isolating *M. tuberculosis* in culture is a slow process, taking several weeks. Therefore, a need for more rapid methods of detection exists. Acid-fast bacilli (AFB) staining is one such method. However, caution is needed in interpreting AFB stains as nontuberculosis *Mycobacterium* infections may result in a false positive result.[29] Molecular biology techniques, such as nucleic acid amplification testing (NAAT) are also available and yield a result more quickly than a culture but cannot definitively rule in or out a diagnosis of active tuberculosis.

TABLE 4.9 Tuberculin Skin Test Interpretation

Patient Population	Positive Test Result
Immunocompromised (e.g., HIV, organ transplant) Exposure to active tuberculosis	>5 mm induration
Resident of high-prevalence region Intravenous drug users Resident or employee of institutional or other high-risk setting Patients with high-risk medical conditions (DM, CKD, malignancy) Children and infants	>10 mm induration
No known risk factors	>15 mm induration

CKD, chronic kidney disease; DM, diabetes mellitus.

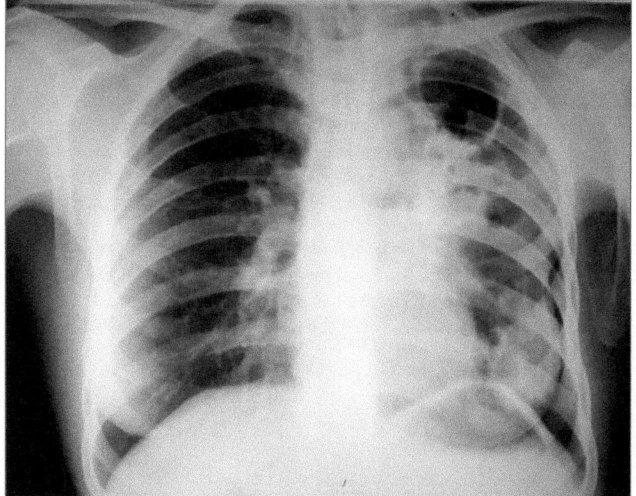

Figure 4.9 **Cavitary lesion on chest radiograph in a patient with pulmonary tuberculosis. A cavitary lesion is seen in the left upper lobe, consistent with pulmonary tuberculosis infection.**
(Source: Giller Borris)

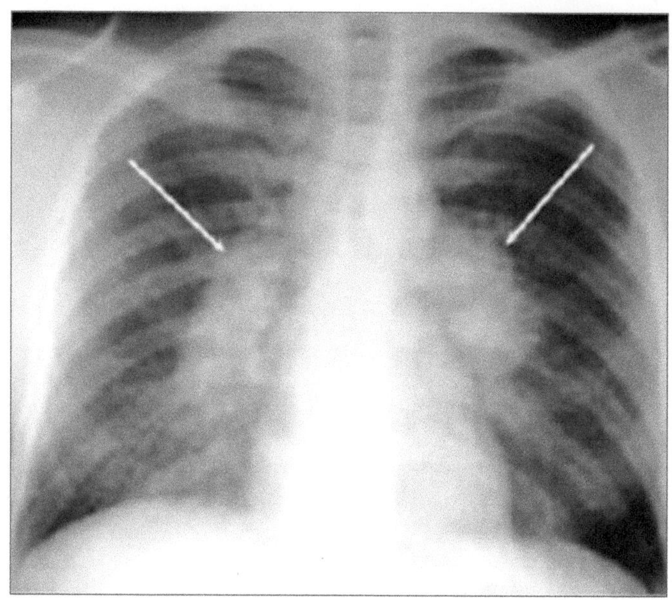

Figure 4.10 **Paratracheal and hilar lymphadenopathy in a patient with pulmonary tuberculosis. White arrows indicate paratracheal, hilar lymphadenopathy consistent with tuberculosis infection.**
(Source: Basem Abbas Al Ubaidi.)

EVALUATION

Screening for LTBI is recommended only for patients with certain risk factors. These patients at increased risk include those who have recently emigrated from a high-incidence area (South East Asia, Africa, etc.), certain healthcare professionals, those living or working in institutional settings, and homeless patients.[30] While all healthcare workers were previously considered high risk for contracting tuberculosis, recent evidence suggests the risk for the majority of healthcare workers is the same as that in the general population, and routine screening for all healthcare workers is no longer recommended.[31]

Multidrug-resistant tuberculosis (MDR-TB) is increasingly becoming a public health concern. Persons with a previous history of tuberculosis, ineffective treatment or treatment non-compliance, those born in or living in countries with high prevalence of MDR-TB, patients who have been exposed to known MDR-TB, and HIV-positive patients are at higher risk for MDR-TB infection. Drug susceptibility testing should be performed in such patients to rule out MDR-TB.[29]

All patients with positive tuberculosis screening tests should be evaluated for active disease and treated as appropriate. Patients presenting with the classic symptoms of tuberculosis (persistent cough, fevers, weight loss, night sweats) and known risk factors should be evaluated for active TB.

TREATMENT

- All patients with LTBI or active tuberculosis should be treated.
- Several antimicrobial regimens are available for the treatment of both latent and active tuberculosis.
- The typical regimen for LTBI is 9 months of isoniazid (INH), though compliance is a concern.

- The classic regimen for active tuberculosis is 2 months of INH, rifampin (RIF), pyrazinamide, and ethambutol, followed by 4 months of INH and RIF.
- Second- and third-line agents, along with novel treatments, are available for MDR-TB.
- Compliance is critical and directly observed therapy may be necessary.

PATIENT EDUCATION

- Tuberculosis is highly infectious and strict isolation is necessary for patients with active disease.
- Compliance with treatment is necessary for cure, prevention of disease transmission, and prevention of MDR-TB strains.
- Side effects and adverse reactions to antitubercular medications should be discussed. In particular, the potential for rifampin to discolor body fluids (sweat, saliva, sputum, and urine), leading to a red-orange tint, may be concerning to patients and should be reviewed.

4.5C CROUP

MEDICAL HISTORY AND CLINICAL PRESENTATION

Croup is most commonly the result of a viral infection, typically with parainfluenza virus, leading to a spectrum of disease states including laryngotracheitis, laryngotracheobronchitis, and laryngotracheobronchopneumonitis.[32] The subglottic region and laryngeal mucosa become inflamed and edematous, resulting in decreased air movement.[32] Figure 4.11 demonstrates the pathophysiology of croup.

Croup is typically a disease of childhood and is a relatively common cause of pediatric ED visits and hospitalizations, particularly in the fall and winter months. While the vast majority of cases are mild and self-limiting, severe disease can occur and is distinguished by hypoxia and associated findings, such as respiratory distress or cyanosis.

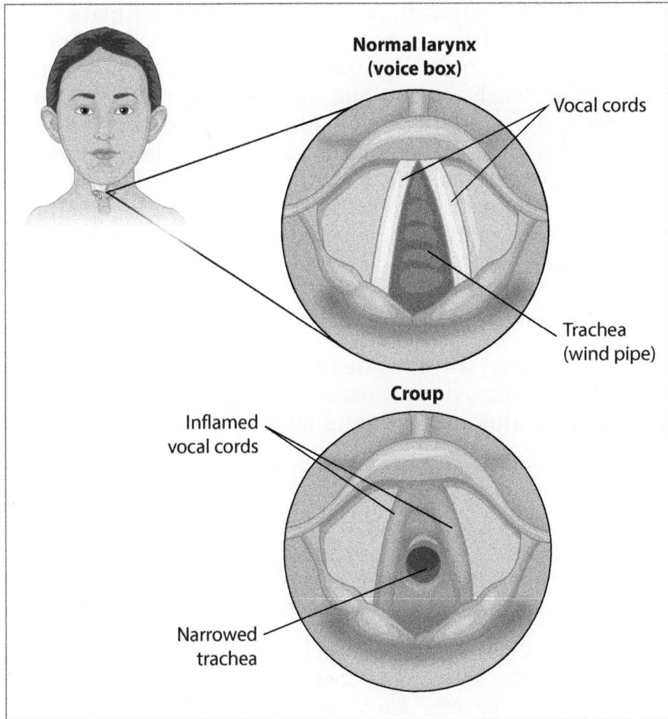

Figure 4.11 **Pathophysiology of croup.**

SIGNS AND SYMPTOMS

Croup typically begins with a low-grade fever and nonspecific viral symptoms such as nasal congestion or rhinorrhea. Those symptoms are followed with an abrupt onset of a harsh cough, often described as having a "bark-like" quality. The cough is typically worse at night. Tachypnea, tachycardia, hypoxia, accessory muscle use and retractions, and cyanosis, if present, indicate more severe disease. Inspiratory stridor is present. While croup is the most common cause of acute stridor in children, stridor is not specific to croup.[33]

PHYSICAL EXAMINATION

The most common physical exam finding is overt inspiratory stridor. Clinicians should note airflow on lung auscultation, as significantly diminished air movement is associated with more severe disease. Vital signs may or may not be abnormal. Fever is common, but the absence of fever does not rule out croup. Tachypnea, tachycardia, and hypoxia indicate more severe disease. Drooling is uncommon in croup. If drooling is noted on general assessment/inspection of the patient, an alternate diagnosis such as epiglottitis or foreign body aspiration should be considered.[32]

DIFFERENTIAL DIAGNOSIS

The differential diagnosis for croup is summarized in Table 4.10.

DIAGNOSTIC STUDIES

Croup is often a clinical diagnosis made on the basis of the typical presentation of a child with stridor and the characteristic bark-like cough. If patients are not improving as expected, or atypical findings are noted on physical examination

TABLE 4.10 Differential Diagnosis of Croup

Diagnosis	Description
Bacterial tracheitis	Most commonly caused by *Staphylococcus* or *Streptococcus* bacteria. Common in children and characterized by sudden onset of high fever, stridor, and copious purulent secretions. Diagnosed with neck x-ray showing tracheal narrowing and irregularities of tracheal wall, differentiating from croup. Laryngoscopy is "gold standard" but not necessary with high index of suspicion.
Epiglottitis	Inflammation of epiglottis classically caused by *Haemophilus influenzae,* though incidence has decreased and alternate organisms now predominate due to vaccination. Signs and symptoms include fever, sore throat, drooling, difficulty swallowing, hoarseness, and stridor. "Thumbprint sign" is characteristic finding on lateral neck x-ray.
Foreign body aspiration	Airway obstruction caused by foreign bodies such as food, toys, or coins, with young children particularly at risk. In symptomatic cases, abrupt onset of choking, dyspnea, coughing, and stridor are present. Localized wheeze on physical exam is typical. Bronchoscopy is indicated for definitive diagnosis and removal of foreign body.

(e.g., wheeze, rales, rhonchi, drooling), diagnostic testing should be considered to rule out alternate causes for the patient's symptoms. CBC may help differentiate croup from bacterial infection, with the CBC being normal or showing lymphocytosis in patients with croup. Respiratory viral testing via PCR may identify parainfluenza virus (typical of croup), or another virus, such as influenza A or B, that may have specific treatment options available.

Radiographic imaging is not routinely indicated. However, if performed, the "steeple sign" on a frontal neck or chest x-ray is often considered the classic finding, though it should be noted this finding is neither sensitive nor specific to croup (Figure 4.12).[32]

EVALUATION

All patients suspected of having croup, even if symptoms are mild and likely to be self-limited, should be evaluated. Corticosteroid treatment is indicated for all patients regardless of severity and decreases duration of symptoms as well as need for subsequent medical care.[32]

The Westley Croup Score can be used to classify the severity of illness in patients with croup. The presence or absence of altered consciousness, cyanosis, stridor, decreased air entry, and retractions are used to characterize illness severity as mild, moderate, severe, or impending respiratory failure. While not a necessary component of patient evaluation, this can be used to assist clinicians' clinical decision-making and disposition determination for patients.

TREATMENT

- Corticosteroids, preferably dexamethasone, are recommended for all patients and have been shown to decrease symptom duration.
- Supplemental oxygen should be reserved for patients with hypoxia.
- Nebulized epinephrine should be given in combination with corticosteroids for patients with moderate-severe disease.
- Humidified air and/or heliox (helium and oxygen) are sometimes used though data on their effectiveness is limited.[32]

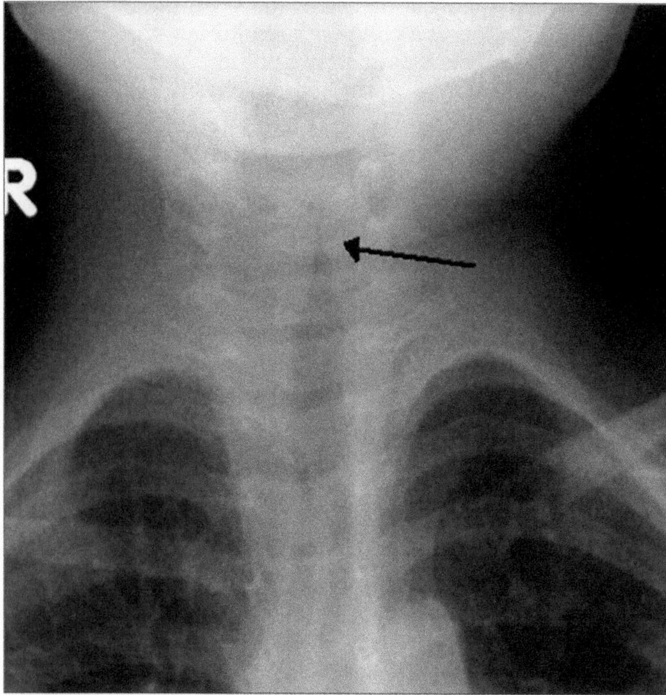

Figure 4.12 **Steeple sign on chest radiograph, classically associated with croup. The black arrow points to the narrowed airway, commonly referred to as the "steeple sign." While neither sensitive nor specific, when present, this finding indicates glottic and subglottic narrowing.** *(Source: Frank Gaillard.)*

PATIENT EDUCATION

- Parents should be reassured that the disease is typically self-limiting and prognosis is favorable even in severe cases.
- Minimizing agitation improves patient symptoms.
- Urgent medical care is required for patients with decreased level of consciousness or signs of respiratory distress.

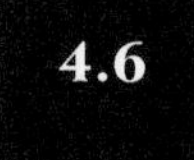

4.6 SOLITARY PULMONARY NODULE

OVERVIEW

A solitary pulmonary nodule (SPN) is defined as a round, well-demarcated lesion ≤3 cm in diameter, surrounded by normal lung tissue. SPNs are frequently found incidentally on routine pulmonary imaging. It is important to recognize and efficiently evaluate the SPN for malignancy because it represents a possibly curable lung cancer.

EPIDEMIOLOGY

The SPN is a very common finding on pulmonary imaging. The incidence of SPNs found on chest radiographs ordered for nonpulmonary indications is 0.09% to 0.2%.[36] Because of its sensitivity, SPNs are seen more commonly on chest CT. The incidence of SPNs on screening chest CTs for high-risk patients enrolled in lung cancer screening ranges from 8% to 51%.[37,38] Overall, in total, it has been estimated that over 1 million SPNs are found on radiographic imaging.[39]

The incidence of malignancy increases with concomitant risk factors, such as smoking and occupational exposure, increasing age, and increasing size of the nodule. The most frequent lung cancer presenting as an SPN is adenocarcinoma. According to Gould et al., 50% of malignant nodules were adenocarcinoma, 20% to 25% were squamous cell carcinoma, and 10% accounted for other etiologies of carcinoma.[40]

PATHOPHYSIOLOGY

An SPN can arise from various etiologies, including neoplastic, inflammatory, infectious, congenital, and other causes. The various etiologies are summarized in Table 4.11.

MEDICAL HISTORY AND CLINICAL PRESENTATION

The medical history may suggest an underlying etiology. Therefore, medical history should include questions that address potential diagnoses. These include:

- Constitutional symptoms including fever, chills, sweats, night sweats, and weight loss
- History of cigarette smoking
- Occupational exposure to carcinogens

- Personal or family history of cancer
- Travel history
- Personal or family history of an underlying autoimmune disorder

SIGNS AND SYMPTOMS

SPN is generally an incidental finding and patients are typically asymptomatic. However, patients can have symptoms of underlying disease that led to the imaging and the incidental finding. For example, a patient could have presented with a cough and as part of the evaluation a chest x-ray was ordered and an SPN was noted.

PHYSICAL EXAMINATION

Typically, the physical examination is unrevealing. Physical examination may suggest underlying causes including infection, malignancy, and autoimmune diseases.

DIFFERENTIAL DIAGNOSIS

The differential diagnosis of solitary pulmonary nodule is summarized in Table 4.12.

DIAGNOSTIC STUDIES

The primary focus of evaluation of the SPN is to assess the characteristics of the nodule and the potential for recognizing a malignant process early. Quite often, a SPN is found on a plain x-ray as an incidental finding. Further evaluation should include comparison of any previous x-rays and evaluating the rate of growth over time and a CT scan of the chest, which can better characterize the nodule.

Several radiographic characteristics would suggest a benign etiology including smooth margins, the presence of calcification, small size (<1 cm), increased nodule density, a pleural location, and a slow rate of growth over time.

Using some of these characteristics, the American College of Radiology has developed a model, the Lung-RADS system, to rate lesions and suggest management recommendations:

- **Categories 1 and 2 (benign):** Annual low-dose CT scan
- **Category 3 (probably benign):** Follow-up low-dose CT scan in 6 months
- **Category 4A (suspicious):** Follow-up low-dose CT in 3 months or PET/CT
- **Category 4B (very suspicious):** Biopsy or PET/CT

Depending upon the etiology, other diagnostic tests could be considered. They include:

- PET scan to evaluate the metabolic activity of the nodule can be helpful in distinguishing neoplastic from benign lesions. The predictability of PET scanning is increased with a higher probability of a neoplastic lesion. False negative results are more likely in smaller lesions (<8 mm) and false-positive results are more likely with infectious and inflammatory etiologies. Also, tumors with slow metabolic rates may be difficult to evaluate by PET scanning.
- Biopsy of the lesion including a radiographic guided needle aspiration, bronchoscopy, or incisional biopsy, depending on the location and size of the nodule, can definitively determine malignancy. The approach is determined by tumor size and location. These are invasive tests, so the malignancy probability and risks/benefits need to be carefully evaluated.
- Laboratory studies are typically not helpful in the evaluation of an SPN. CBC, sputum cultures, PPD, and autoimmune studies may be helpful if the nodule is thought to have an infectious or autoimmune cause.

EVALUATION

The initial evaluation of an SPN begins with an appropriate history and physical examination, which include an assessment of risk factors for malignancy. These factors include advanced age, history of smoking, family history, female sex, occupational exposure to asbestos, personal history of malignancy, and underlying COPD.

Imaging is also important in the evaluation of SPN. It is important to obtain any previous chest imaging for review and comparison. A low-dose CT scan of the chest is the best test initially to evaluate an SPN. It offers valuable information that can categorize the lesion and guide further evaluation as mentioned above.

Several predictive models have been developed that can complement clinical judgment. They include the Brock Model and the Veterans Administrative Cooperative

TABLE 4.11 Etiologies of Solitary Pulmonary Nodule

Neoplastic	Inflammatory	Infectious
Bronchogenic carcinoma Adenocarcinoma Squamous cell carcinoma Large cell lung carcinoma Small cell lung carcinoma Metastatic lung carcinoma Lymphoma Carcinoid tumor Hamartoma Fibromas Neurofibroma Sarcoma	Rheumatoid arthritis Wegener granulomatosis Sarcoidosis Lipoid pneumonia	Granulomas Lung abscess Hydatid cyst Pneumonia

TABLE 4.12 Differential Diagnosis for Solitary Pulmonary Nodule

Diagnosis	Description
Primary lung cancer	This would include squamous cell carcinoma, large cell lung cancer, and small cell carcinoma.
Metastatic cancer	Common primary cancer sites include breast, colon, head and neck, carcinoid tumors, testicular, sarcoma, and renal cancers.
Benign tumors	Includes fibromas and neurofibromas.
Lymphoma	
Autoimmune	Includes rheumatoid nodules, Wegner granulomatosis, and sarcoidosis.
Granulomatous disease	Includes tuberculosis, aspergillosis, blastomycosis, coccidioidomycosis, histoplasmosis, and cryptococcosis.

Model. These predictive models not only take into account radiographic characteristics, but also include historical data such as age, smoking, family history, gender, and past medical history. These predictive models can help to guide further evaluation.

TREATMENT

Treatment is guided by the overall risk of malignancy using clinical judgment and the predicative models mentioned above. The American College of Chest Physicians have given the following recommendations:

- No treatment is needed for lesions that have been stable for 2 years or have benign radiographic characteristics without risk factors.
- Periodic low-dose CT scans are indicated for patients with a very low probability of lung cancer at an interval of 3 to 6 months, 9 to 12 months, and then at 18 to 24 months.
- PET scan for low to moderate probability of lung cancer. If uptake is low, the patient should undergo periodic CT scans, but if uptake is moderate or high, biopsy or section is indicated.
- Surgical resection is indicated for patients with a high probability of lung cancer.

PATIENT EDUCATION

- Patients should be counseled to stop smoking.
- Annual low-dose CT scan for adults 55 to 80 years old with a 30-year pack history and who currently smoke or have quit in the last 15 years.

KEY POINTS

- The SPN is defined as a round, well-demarcated lesion ≤3 cm in diameter, surrounded by normal lung tissue.
- It is commonly an incidental finding.
- Low-dose CT scan is the imaging modality of choice to initially evaluate an SPN.
- The probability of malignancy is determined by risk factors and radiologic characteristics.

4.7 INTERSTITIAL LUNG DISEASE

OVERVIEW

Interstitial lung disease (ILD) or diffuse parenchymal lung disease encompasses a heterogeneous group of disorders that are classified together. They cause inflammation of the alveolar walls and interstitium (collagen and elastic connective tissues) that ultimately leads to fibrosis of the lungs. Though the etiology may be different, as a group they share a common presentation, physical exam, and radiologic findings including dyspnea, inspiratory crackles, and reticulonodular changes ("ground-glass" appearance) on chest radiograph.

The diagnosis of ILD can be difficult due to the overlap of presentation with other collagen vascular diseases and requires the integration of clinical evaluation, laboratory studies, radiographic imaging, pulmonary studies, and at times histopathologyic examination to make the proper diagnosis. Determining the cause is important because treatments vary based upon the etiology. Some forms of ILD are related to exposure to certain drugs. Among the causes are idiopathic pulmonary fibrosis, hypersensitivity pneumonitis, sarcoidosis, eosinophilic pulmonary disease, and occupational lung disease. Patients with idiopathic pulmonary fibrosis have a higher incidence of lung cancer. ILD can also be associated with rheumatologic autoimmune diseases such as rheumatoid arthritis, Sjögren syndrome, systemic lupus erythematosus, and mixed connective tissue disease.

EPIDEMIOLOGY

ILD is primarily a disease of adults. The overall incidence of ILD has been difficult to determine. The most significant registry study was done in Bernalillo County, New Mexico using data from a dedicated ILD registry and chart review, estimating an incidence of 30 per 100,000 per year with approximately one-third in the idiopathic pulmonary fibrosis category.[41] Idiopathic pulmonary fibrosis increases with age with most patients ≥65 years of age, with an estimated 25 per 100,000 per year in 2000.[41] With a tighter classification system, epidemiology studies suggest that ILD is more prevalent than previously thought.[42] The prevalence of ILD was 80.9 per 100,000 in males and 26.1 per 100,000 in females with the most common diagnosis being pulmonary fibrosis and idiopathic pulmonary fibrosis, together accounting for 46.2% of all ILD diagnoses.[43] The mortality rates for patients diagnosed with idiopathic pulmonary fibrosis are increasing in the United States. A mortality study examining death rates from 1992 to 2003 revealed that there was an overall increase of death of 28.4% in men and 41.3% in women.[44] ILD usually affects people 55 to 60 years of age. Approximately, 15% of patients with ILD will have an underlying connective tissue disease.[45]

PATHOPHYSIOLOGY

The exact pathophysiology of ILD is not well understood. It is believed that intestinal lung disease begins with injury to the alveolar epithelium and the interstitium (collagen and elastic connective tissue) from an inciting endogenous or environmental stimulus. The acute injury to the pulmonary parenchyma and the accumulation of immune cells eventually leads to a chronic interstitial inflammation and alveolar thickening and ongoing damage, fibroblast activation, and proliferation leading to fibrosis. Normal functioning tissue is replaced with a fibrotic nonfunctional scar with a marked loss of lung compliance. ILD does not affect the airways directly. It affects the interstitial space including the alveolar walls.

MEDICAL HISTORY AND CLINICAL PRESENTATION

ILD includes a variety of progressive inflammatory diseases that causes irreversible fibrosis of the lungs. ILD can be classified as idiopathic and ILD with an underlying cause, such as an occupational exposure or connective tissue diseases. Obtaining a careful and detailed history can identify potential contributory factors that if addressed can impact the progression of the disease. Careful attention to the patient's past medical history (connective tissue disease, inflammatory bowel disease or malignancy, allergic rhinitis, and asthma), family history (idiopathic interstitial lung disease), social history (smoking, occupational exposure), and associated symptoms can help to determine an underlying etiology.

The age of presentation and gender can be helpful. For those who have sarcoidosis or a connective tissue disorder, the age of onset is between 20 and 40 and patients are typically female. Sarcoidosis is more common in African Americans. Idiopathic causes usually present between the ages of 50 and 65 and is more common in males.

Historically, the progression of the symptoms over time can also shed light into the underlying etiology. Acute eosinophilic ILD and connective tissue lung disease have an accelerated course with a rapid onset and progression of symptoms and radiographic findings. In contrast, idiopathic ILD and sarcoidosis have an insidious onset and progress slowly.

Smoking can be a contributing factor to pulmonary fibrosis. While smoking is strongly associated with COPD, it has been found that a smoking history is common in many patients with ILD. Present smokers and previous smokers are more likely to develop idiopathic pulmonary fibrosis.

Environmental and occupational exposure to possible offending agents should be explored. A detailed occupational history including exposure to dust and chemicals, length of exposure, and use of protective equipment should be noted. Passive exposure should also be considered as well as exposure from hobbies and other family members.

SIGNS AND SYMPTOMS

The primary signs and symptoms of all ILDs are shortness of breath, which can occur either at rest or associated with exertion and cough. Typically, progression is insidious and by the time the patient presents with symptoms, there is significant, irreversible damage to the lung parenchyma. The cough is typically dry. It is usual to have mucus production with ILD. Hemoptysis, chest pain, and wheezing are uncommon.

Patients with underlying connective tissue disease will complain of extrapulmonary symptoms, including constitutional symptoms such as fever, weakness, fatigue, and rheumatologic symptoms involving joint pain, swelling, and stiffness. Although most often, the connective tissue complaints will precede the pulmonary symptoms, it is possible to develop the pulmonary symptoms prior to the frank onset of the rheumatologic symptoms.

PHYSICAL EXAMINATION

The pulmonary examination is usually non specific in patients with ILD. Crackles are common except with granulomatous disease, such as sarcoidosis. The crackles are fine and late inspiratory and found in the basilar area. Early in the course of the disease, the crackles are heard at the base at the posterior axillary line.

The cardiac examination is usually normal except late in the progression of the disease when patients will develop cor pulmonale. Because of rising right ventricular pressures, patients will develop a left parasternal systolic lift, an attenuated pulmonary heart sound (P2), splitting of S2 during inspiration at the apex, a right-sided S3 or S4, and a pansystolic murmur heard best at the right midsternal border with attenuation with inspiration due to tricuspid regurgitation. Other signs of cor pulmonale include hepatomegaly, hepatojugular reflux, and edema.

Clubbing of the digits is common in idiopathic pulmonary fibrosis. It is uncommon in sarcoidosis. It is a late finding that usually indicates advanced disease.

For patients with underlying connective tissue disease associated with ILD, patients will have musculoskeletal changes consistent with that particular disease, which could include stiffness, tenderness, motion pain, swelling, deformity, limited range of motion of the joints, nodules, dry eyes, and xerostomia.

DIFFERENTIAL DIAGNOSIS

The differential diagnosis of ILD is summarized in Table is 4.13.

DIAGNOSTIC STUDIES

Laboratory studies have limited utility in diagnosing ILD. A CBC can assess the patient for a symptomatic anemia, leukocytosis for possible inflammation or infection, and eosinophilia. Serum chemistries evaluate hepatic and renal function, especially for extrapulmonary involvement of sarcoidosis. Rheumatologic studies including a rheumatoid factor (RF), antinuclear antibody (ANA), erythrocyte sedimentation rate (ESR), C-reactive protein (CRP) would be helpful in screening for an underlying connective tissue cause. More specific rheumatologic tests could be ordered for a strong suspicion of an underlying connective tissue cause as guided by the history and physical examination. Angiotensin-converting enzyme (ACE) levels are not specific but may suggest sarcoidosis. It has utility in following the disease course and effectiveness of treatment.

Chest imaging is the mainstay for the initial assessment of ILD. While the chest radiograph is abnormal, in most patients with ILD, its utility is limited due to its lack of specificity. The chest radiograph of idiopathic pulmonary fibrosis will typically reveal a peripheral reticular pattern and reduced lung volumes. As the disease progresses, a course reticular pattern and honeycombed cysts will

TABLE 4.13 Differential Diagnosis for Interstitial Lung Disease

Diagnosis	Description
Chronic obstructive pulmonary disease (COPD)	A group of chronic inflammatory lung diseases that cause an obstructive respiratory pattern on pulmonary function tests, which include chronic bronchitis and emphysema. The major cause of COPD is smoking.
Congestive heart failure (CHF)	A cardiovascular disorder that is caused by weakness or stiffness of the ventricular walls, leading to inefficiency of ventricular stroke volume and a backup of fluid into the lungs and periphery. Major causes of CHF include long-standing hypertension and coronary artery disease.
Coal worker's pneumoconiosis	A pulmonary condition caused by the inhalation of coal dust, which causes the deposition of coal macules leading to focal obstruction changes within the bronchioles.
Hypersensitivity pneumonitis	A rare condition of diffuse inflammation of the lung parenchyma caused by an allergic reaction to inhaled allergens, including microorganisms and plant and animal proteins. Common occupations include farming, bird and animal handlers, lumber milling, and plastic manufacturing.

appear in later stages, which has a poor prognosis. Pleural abnormalities are uncommon and would suggest pleural disease such as mesothelioma. It should be noted that in a small number of patients, symptomatic patients may have a normal chest radiograph. Also, the chest radiograph is limited in its ability to stage the disease. The chest radiograph of chronic eosinophilic lung disease reveals bilateral peripheral or pleural-based opacities in the middle and upper lungs. The chest radiograph of sarcoidosis reveals bilateral hilar lymphadenopathy (classic finding) and parenchymal changes that can include diffuse reticular or ground-glass opacities.

High-resolution CT of the chest will help to suggest particular diseases based upon specific characteristics and distribution in the lung regions:

- **Connective-tissue related ILD reticular pattern** may be seen in the peripheral lung zone.
- **Idiopathic pulmonary fibrosis:** Patchy reticular pattern and honeycombing in the basal and peripheral lung zones. Less commonly, ground-glass opacities are found.
- **Eosinophilic interstitial lung disease:** Ground-glass opacities in the peripheral upper and middle lung zones may be associated with loss of airspace and bronchiectasis.
- **Sarcoidosis** would have a nodular pattern in the central lung zones and granulomatous changes in the upper lung zones with associated hilar adenopathy. The radiographic changes have been staged:
  - **Stage 0:** Normal
  - **Stage 1:** Bilateral hilar adenopathy alone
  - **Stage 2:** Bilateral hilar adenopathy + parenchymal infiltrates
  - **Stage 3:** Parenchymal infiltrates alone
  - **Stage 4:** Pulmonary fibrosis

Pulmonary function tests (PFTs) can be used to differentiate ILD from COPD. COPD would show an obstructive pattern while ILD would have a restrictive pattern. Also, in ILD there would be a decrease in lung volumes and the lung diffusing capacity (DLCO). PFTs can be used to assess the functional severity of disease and monitor the course of the disease. Functionality can also be assessed with a 6-minute walk test, which will also be reduced.

Confirmation of a diagnosis can be made with histopathology, if necessary, with idiopathic pulmonary fibrosis and sarcoidosis. The presence of eosinophils on bronchoalveolar lavage is helpful with the confirmation and to follow the course of the disease.

EVALUATION

The evaluation of a patient presenting with shortness of breath begins with a careful and detailed history and physical examination to assess for COPD, occupational lung disease, and an underlying connective tissue disease. Pulmonary imaging is very important. While a chest radiograph will most likely reveal abnormalities, a high sensitivity CT scan of the chest is more sensitive and based upon the findings can point toward an underlying etiology. Diagnosis can be confirmed by histopathologic findings or, with eosinophilic lung disease, the presence of eosinophils on bronchial lavage. After a diagnosis is made, functional status can be assessed by pulmonary function testing and a 6-minute walk test, which can further guide treatment.

The diagnosis of idiopathic pulmonary fibrosis is a diagnosis of exclusion of other causes of ILD. It is a progressively debilitating disease that is fatal without spontaneous remission. A definitive test does not exist for this disease. The diagnosis is made with radiographic findings that are consistent with pulmonary fibrosis and histopathologic confirmation if necessary.

Sarcoidosis is also a diagnosis of exclusion since a definitive test does not exist. Bronchoscopy with EBUS (endobronchial ultrasound) is typically used to biopsy the mediastinal lymph nodes. The diagnosis is made with the exclusion of other diseases that may present similarly, radiographic findings consistent with sarcoidosis, histopathologic confirmation of noncaseating granulomas and extrapulmonary involvement.

The diagnosis of eosinophilic lung disease is made with the presence of eosinophilia once radiographic findings suggestive of eosinophilic disease is made.

TREATMENT

The treatment of inflammatory lung diseases depends on the underlying etiology. Since they share a similar underlying pathophysiology of progressive destruction of the pulmonary parenchyma, any agents that would exacerbate inflammation, like smoking, should be eliminated. Also, all patients should receive annual influenza vaccine and pneumococcal vaccinations.

- Idiopathic pulmonary fibrosis
  - Pulmonary rehabilitation
  - Supplemental oxygen with a goal of oxygen saturation of >90%
  - Referral to a transplant center
  - First-line medications:
    - Nintedanib
    - Pirfenidone
- Eosinophilic lung disease
  - Systemic corticosteroids for acute symptoms
  - Inhaled or oral corticosteroids for maintenance therapy
  - Treatment is guided by symptoms, eosinophil levels and serial chest x-rays
- Sarcoidosis
  - No treatment is necessary in asymptomatic patients, but treatment may be needed for extrapulmonary manifestations.
  - No treatment may be necessary for symptomatic patients with stage I-III radiographic changes with normal or mildly abnormal PFTs, though patients should have close follow-up. There are no FDA-approved treatments for sarcoidosis.
    - Systemic corticosteroids are first-line medications
    - Second-line medications include:
      - Immunosuppressants (e.g., methotrexate, azathioprine)
      - Antimalarial agents (e.g., chloroquine or hydrochloroquine)
      - Tumor necrosis factor antagonists (e.g., infliximab)

PATIENT EDUCATION

- ILD is a progressive disease that can worsen over time, so regular follow-up is recommended.
- Patients should seek medical attention if they develop shortness of breath, cough, or fever early.

- Patients who smoke should be counseled to quit.
- Patients should be encouraged to get flu and pneumonia vaccines.

KEY POINTS

- ILD is a group of disorders that are classified together due to similar pathology, presentation, and radiographic findings.
- ILD is an insidious and progressing disease that causes dyspnea and a persistent dry cough.
- The diagnosis of a particular inflammatory lung disease is suggested by characteristic changes on high-sensitivity CT scan of the chest and can be confirmed by histopathology.

4.8 VASCULAR DISORDERS

4.8A PULMONARY VENOUS THROMBOEMBOLISM

OVERVIEW

Thrombi can form in any part of the venous system and venous thromboembolism (VTE) is a complex multifactorial disease. Pulmonary embolism (PE), a subset of VTE, is a deadly manifestation associated with substantial risk of morbidity and mortality, often requiring hospitalization. A leading cause of preventable death of hospitalized patients, the presentation of PE is challenging and widely variable, ranging from asymptomatic, incidental discovery to massive, acute presentation leading to sudden death. Although the occurrence may be acute, unpredictable, and underdiagnosed, the fatality rate can be effectively reduced with proper risk stratification, prophylaxis treatment, early diagnosis, and prompt intervention.

EPIDEMIOLOGY

VTE represents a major global health problem that causes significant morbidity and mortality. In the United States, estimates suggest there are over 350,000 annual cases and 100,000 annual deaths related to VTE with an incidence rate of 104 to 183 per 100,000.[46,47] Approximately two-thirds of VTE manifest as a deep vein thrombosis (DVT) and one-third as the more dangerous manifestation, a PE. PE is the third most common cause of cardiovascular death behind myocardial infarction and stroke[48] affecting more than 300,000 people each year in the United States, with reported incidence rates of over 29 to 78 cases per 100,000 people.[47,49] The incidence numbers and hospitalization rates have increased over time in large part because of improved detection and diagnosis.[50,51] The incidence rate rises with age and males have an overall higher incidence compared to females.[52] Some studies revealed that Black patients had ~15% higher incidence rate of hospitalization and higher age-adjusted mortality rate compared to White patients; however, the reason for these disparities is unclear.[53] The increased incidence in the elderly population is likely due to the acquisition of risk factors such as malignancy, heart failure, peripheral vascular disease, surgery and hospitalization, and prolonged bed rest.[54] Pregnancy and use of oral contraceptives are additional factors that increase the risk of developing blood clots.[55,56] Those with previously diagnosed DVT or PE are at increased risk for a second event. Approximately 30% of those with a history of a DVT will have a recurrent event within 10 years, with the greatest risk in the first 2 years.[57]

While the incidence and hospitalizations have increased, until recently, PE-related mortality rates and the age-adjusted death rate for PE in the United States have steadily declined an average of 4.4% per year.[58–60] These decreases are most likely due to early detection and improved thrombolytic therapies.[53,61] Despite advancements in prevention, detection and treatment, PE remains a significant burden for older, sicker adults and pregnant patients.

PATHOPHYSIOLOGY

Thrombi can form in both arteries and veins; however, each have different pathophysiology, outcomes, and treatments. PEs are almost always embolic in origin, most commonly originating from thrombi in the deep veins of the leg. A venous thrombus consists of two components: an inner platelet-rich region and a dense outer fibrin clot. Formation of a venous thrombus typically stems from a combination of three factors from Virchow's triad: venous stasis, endothelial injury, and increased blood coagulation. The clinical conditions closely linked to these factors are prolonged immobility or bed rest, smoking malignancy, congestive heart failure, surgery or trauma, pregnancy, and obesity.

The physiologic effects of a PE depend largely on the size and extent of the obstruction and coexistence of cardiopulmonary disease. Large emboli obstruct the main pulmonary artery and those straddling the bifurcation of the main pulmonary truck are called saddle emboli and have deleterious hemodynamic effects. The clinical consequences involve both the cardiovascular and respiratory systems.

Right ventricular (RV) failure due to an acute increase in pulmonary pressure is largely considered the pathogenic reason for death in severe PE. Hemodynamically, mechanical obstruction of >30% to 50% of the vascular bed flow will lead to increases in pulmonary vascular pressure and right ventricular afterload.[62] In the absence of cardiac disease, compensatory changes in contractility and contraction time will increase in RV workload to maintain cardiac output. The degree of compensation is limited. In the presence of underlying cardiac disease, or with larger obstructions and abrupt increases in pulmonary artery pressures, acute right ventricular dilatation and failure will result. Along with RV failure, there will be a decline in left ventricular (LV) preload, stroke volume, and cardiac output; systemic hypotension; decrease in coronary perfusion; and hemodynamic instability. Large emboli affecting a greater portion of the pulmonary vasculature or small emboli in patients with cardiac disease will cause more severe and acute hemodynamic changes and instability.

Respiratory consequences of PEs are largely due to hemodynamic disturbances, intrapulmonary shunting, and ventilation/perfusion (V/Q) mismatches. Sudden obstruction to vascular blood flow will lead to increased alveolar dead space, hypoxia, and a disruption in pulmonary capillary gas exchange. Additionally, the release of local vasoconstrictive and bronchoconstriction agents including serotonin and thromboxane A2 will further lead to detrimental ventilation-perfusion mismatches and hypoxemia. Collectively, these respiratory and cardiovascular changes result in increased respiratory drive, hypocapnia, hypoxia, and respiratory alkalosis.

MEDICAL HISTORY AND CLINICAL PRESENTATION

PE has a wide variety of nonspecific signs and symptoms that may have a rapid onset or develop over days and week. A thorough history and physical examination should be performed to diagnose or exclude life-threatening causes.

The clinical signs of acute RV failure, including elevated jugular venous pressure, are critical determinants of the severity of disease and the outcomes. PE is suspected in patients with the classic triad of abrupt onset of pleuritic chest pain, dyspnea, and tachycardia; however, all three are rarely seen together and dyspnea is the most common finding. While rare, hypotension, syncope, and hemodynamic instability are the findings of extensive PE due to low cardiac output. Unexplained tachycardia, tachypnea, hypocapnia, or hypoxia may suggest a PE. Chest x-ray is frequently abnormal and EKG may show sinus tachycardia, signs of RV strain, or nonspecific ST-T wave changes. Occasionally, PE is asymptomatic and discovered incidentally.

In addition to the clinical signs and symptoms for PE, identification of predisposing factors for VTE is important in determining clinical probability of the disease. Past medical history should include questions about conditions that increase the risk of thromboembolism including a history of VTE, recent surgery, trauma, cancer, pregnancy, myeloproliferative disorders, and congestive heart failure. Medications associated with thrombi should be noted, especially hormonal contraception, antipsychotic therapy, and fibrates. Smoking and prolonged rest or hospitalization should be included in the social history. Finally, a family history of familial thrombophilia should be documented.

SIGNS AND SYMPTOMS

The most frequent symptom in patients with a PE is the abrupt onset of dyspnea, tachypnea, and pleuritic chest pain. The chest pain is not localized and may be present in any area of the chest but typically is felt as sharp, stabbing, or burning pain that worsens with inspiration.

Symptoms of a pulmonary embolism include:

- Pain in any area of the chest, front or back, upper or lower, typically worse on inspiration
- Sudden shortness of breath
- Unexplained back or shoulder pain
- Cough, sometimes with hemoptysis
- Sinus tachycardia with palpitations
- Anxiety
- Sense of foreboding

Signs of a pulmonary embolism include:

- Rapid respiratory rate
- Shallow breathing and signs of respiratory distress
- Rapid pulse or heart rate
- Low oxygen saturation (normal is 97%–100%)
- Low PaO_2
- Hypocapnia

In patients with massive PE persistent bradycardia, sustained hypotension, syncope, elevated neck veins, a loud P2, right-sided gallop, and right ventricular lift may be present. The patient may be in a shock-like state, cold and diaphoretic.

PHYSICAL EXAMINATION

The physical examination is variable depending on the severity and cardiorespiratory compromise. Vital signs will reveal elevated heart rate, hypotension, and tachypnea. Fever may also be present. In patients in shock, the extremities may be cold and diaphoretic. Lung sounds may be abnormal with rales (crackles) and decreased breath sounds. Accentuated pulmonary component of the second heart sound, elevated jugular venous distention, and right ventricular lift may be seen in patients with pulmonary hypertension and right ventricular involvement. Signs of DVT including unilateral pitting edema, erythema, pain upon deep venous palpation, and prominent superficial veins may be noted on exam.[63]

DIFFERENTIAL DIAGNOSIS

PE should be differentiated from other diseases presenting with similar, nonspecific symptoms of chest pain, dyspnea, tachycardia, and tachypnea (Table 4.14).

DIAGNOSTIC STUDIES

The signs and symptoms of PE, including dyspnea, tachypnea, tachycardia, pleuritic chest pain, and cough, are suggestive but none are sensitive or specific. Therefore, if PE is suspected further testing must be done to confirm or rule out the diagnosis (Table 4.15).

EVALUATION

Careful clinical history, assessment of risk factors, and physical exam are essential in guiding the appropriate diagnostic evaluations. The primary goal of the diagnostic evaluation is to confirm or exclude the diagnosis and identify patients who should be treated with anticoagulant therapy. The evaluation begins with clinical judgment. Clinical judgment is a valuable part of the evaluation process and includes the combination of symptoms, clinical findings from physical exam, and routine tests including CXR, EKG, CBC, coagulation studies and arterial blood gases, and review of predisposing factors. These tests are not specific for making the diagnosis of PE but are helpful in determining the severity of the condition and differential diagnosis.

Despite the value of the clinical judgment, there is a lack of standardization and overtesting for PE and overuse of advanced imaging modalities has long been recognized as a significant and costly problem in the process of ruling out a PE.[64] To avoid the overuse of diagnostic tests, risk stratification using standardized validated prediction rules has been developed. This approach integrates baseline clinical parameters and the patient's history that help guide the diagnostic process and triaging of patients with suspected PE. The practice of determining pretest clinical probability in hemodynamically stable patients is essential since the posttest probability of PE depends not only on the type of diagnostic test but also on the pretest probability.

TABLE 4.14 Differential Diagnosis for Pulmonary Embolus

Diagnosis	Description
Acute coronary syndrome	Spectrum of catastrophic clinical presentations resulting from the rupture of an atherosclerotic plaque within the coronary artery leading to partial or complete obstruction of blood flow to the myocardium
Aortic dissection	The catastrophic separation of laminal planes of the aortic wall
Pericarditis	Inflammation of the pericardium
Acute respiratory distress syndrome	A clinical syndrome caused by diffuse alveolar capillary and epithelial damage resulting in the acute onset of severe respiratory insufficiency, cyanosis, and distress
Aortic stenosis	Structural abnormalities in the aortic valve leading to obstruction to blood flow from the left ventricle to the aorta during ventricular systole
Atrial fibrillation	An arrhythmia characterized by a disorganized irregular and often rapid atrial activation resulting in asynchronous contraction of the myocardium.
Cardiogenic shock	Physiologic state characterized by a decrease cardiac output and tissue hypoxia in the presence of a euvolemic state.
Septic shock	A compromised hemodynamic state characterized by persistent hypotension caused by an abnormal response to infection
Cor pulmonale	An abnormal structure and function of the right ventricle secondarily caused by a primary disorder associated with the respiratory system
Acute congestive heart failure	Sudden dysfunction of the myocardium that reduces the ability of the heart to pump enough blood to the body
Emphysema	Long-term progressive and irreversible airflow obstruction pathologically defined by airspace enlargement distal to the terminal bronchioles accompanied by destruction of their walls in the absence of fibrosis
Fat embolism	Fat globules circulating in the systemic vasculature
Hypersensitivity pneumonitis	Immunologically mediated inflammatory disease of the lungs primarily affecting the alveoli
Mitral stenosis	Structural abnormality of the mitral valve apparatus leading to obstruction to blood flow from the left atrium to the left ventricle during ventricular diastole
Musculoskeletal, chest wall injury and rib fracture	Bruised, cracked, or broken bones of the thorax including the sternum and ribs and associated musculature
Myocardial infarction or ischemia	Imbalance between the coronary blood supply and myocardial oxygen demand leading to reversible tissue injury (ischemia) or irreversible necrosis (infarction)
Pericarditis and cardiac tamponade	Inflammation of the pericardium and subsequent accumulation of fluid in the pericardial cavity resulting in diastolic dysfunction, reduced ventricular filling, and possible hemodynamic instability
Pleuritis and pleural effusion	Inflammation of the pleura and subsequent accumulation of fluid in the pleural cavity
Pneumonia	Broadly defined infection of the lungs
Pneumothorax	The presence of air or gas in the pleural cavity
Pulmonary arterial hypertension	Elevated pulmonary arterial pressure due to sustained increase in pulmonary vascular resistance
Emphysema	Long-term progressive and irreversible airflow obstruction pathologically defined by airspace enlargement distal to the terminal bronchioles accompanied by destruction of their walls in the absence of fibrosis
Pulmonary arteriovenous fistula	Malformation consisting of an abnormal communication between the pulmonary arteries and pulmonary veins
Pulmonary vasculitis	The inflammation and destruction of the pulmonary vasculature and accompanying necrosis
Restrictive cardiomyopathy	Diastolic cardiac dysfunction characterized by impaired diastolic ventricular filling and normal systolic function
Superior vena cava syndrome	A collection of symptoms associated with the obstruction of the blood flow through the superior vena cava

TABLE 4.15 Diagnostic Tests of Pulmonary Emboli

Diagnostic Test	Description
Electrocardiogram (EKG)	Rarely, an EKG will show abnormalities associated with pulmonary embolus (PE), especially if there is right ventricular strain or dysfunction, although these are nonspecific and insensitive in the absence of clinical suspicion. The most common findings are tachycardia and nonspecific ST-T wave changes.
D-dimer	The most frequently used screening test for excluding PE. D-dimer does not detect blood clots but is useful in excluding them in emergency situations. D-dimer can be elevated for many reasons other than blood clots.
Routine chest x-ray	Chest radiographs are abnormal in most PE cases, but the findings are nonspecific. Helpful in diagnosing other conditions including pneumonia, pleural effusions, pneumothorax, or cardiogenic or noncardiogenic pulmonary edema.
Computed tomography pulmonary angiography (CTPA)	CTPA is the initial imaging of choice for stable patients with suspected PE. Direct, noninvasive imaging of the embolus is possible using this technique
Ventilation-perfusion ($\dot{V}/\dot{Q}$) scan	$\dot{V}/\dot{Q}$ scans are useful in confirming the PE diagnosis and will show lung perfusion defect. High probability and low probability criteria are established and used to make the diagnosis.
Echocardiography	Transesophageal echocardiography will identify a central and peripheral PE and also assess right ventricular involvement, strain, and dysfunction. The sensitivity is less than other imaging modalities and is helpful to allow the diagnosis of other conditions including myocardial ischemia, valvular disease, pericardial effusion, and tamponade.
Pulmonary angiogram	Historically, pulmonary angiography was the gold standard for PE diagnosis. Contrast agent is injected through a catheter into the pulmonary artery and identification of a filling defect confirms the presence of a clot. This technique has been largely replaced by CTPA. Catheter-based pulmonary angiography is still performed in patients who require therapeutic interventions and fibrinolysis.

If the clinical suspicion of PE is low, the Pulmonary Embolism Rule-Out Criteria (PERC) was developed to identify avoid further testing for PE in low-risk patients. This "rule-out" tool is based on eight clinical variables. A PERC evaluation is considered positive if any one of the eight criteria are met.[65]

In patients with high clinical probability, hemodynamic stability should be evaluated. Hemodynamically unstable patients and those at high risk for PE should undergo immediate advanced imaging, preferably computed tomography pulmonary angiography (CTPA), to confirm the diagnosis. If CTPA is not immediately available or the patient is too unstable, transthoracic echocardiography is a bedside alternative to evaluate the degree of RV involvement to confirm the diagnosis.[66] High clinical probability patients who are hemodynamically stable with persistent hypotension are also at high risk for PE and should undergo emergent advanced imaging including CTPA or $\dot{V}/\dot{Q}$ scan. In high-risk normotensive PE patients require further (advanced) risk stratification and evaluation of clinical, imaging, and laboratory indicators of PE.

In intermediate or low clinical probability, normotensive patients, a D-dimer test is often used. The D-dimer test is most valuable when used in conjunction with clinical probability and validated clinical decision criteria, such as the Geneva or Wells rule. The scores obtained from these rules may be used to further guide the management and utilization of more extensive diagnostic tests and imaging.

D-dimer measures the plasma levels of a specific derivative of cross-linked fibrin which are elevated in PE but also in patients with cancer, trauma, pregnancy, and inflammatory states. Accordingly, the negative predictive value D-dimer test is high and normal levels safely exclude PE without further testing in most patients. On the other hand, since D-dimer is elevated in a number of conditions, a positive D-dimer test is a nonspecific test and, on its own, is insufficient to confirm a PE diagnosis and further diagnostic imaging is necessary.

TREATMENT

Risk stratification of patients with PE is critical in determining appropriate therapy. The initial treatment should begin with oxygenation and hemodynamic stabilization. Anticoagulation therapy is the mainstay for PE and should be administered immediately in patients with diagnosed PE or in unconfirmed highrisk or intermediate probability patients while awaiting the results of diagnostic tests. Thrombolytic therapy is reserved for patients with high-risk probability and patients who are hemodynamically unstable. Bleeding risk should be considered in patients treated with this type of therapy. Catheter-assisted embolectomy is recommended when there is a contraindication to or failed thrombolysis. Complications of vena cava filters are common and accordingly, their routine use is not recommended. There is, however, a limited use of filters in patients with absolute contraindications to anticoagulant therapy or in cases of recurrence despite therapeutic anticoagulation.

- Hemodynamic and respiratory support
  - Volume
  - Vasopressors
  - Venoarterial extracorporeal membrane oxygenation (ECMO)
- Medical therapies
  - Anticoagulation
  - Thrombolytic
- Surgical therapies
  - Pulmonary embolectomy

PATIENT EDUCATION

- PE is a blood clot in the lungs. The clot blocks flow of blood to the lungs and can interfere with the oxygenation of the blood.
- The signs and symptoms of PE are a sudden shortness of breath, a sharp chest pain that worsens when taking a breath, rapid heartbeat or palpitations, and a cough that may include a small amount of blood. More general symptoms include anxiousness, sweating, and lightheadedness.
- The clots usually are formed in the the lower legs and travel through the bloodstream to the lungs.

- Things that increase the risk of developing these blood clots include smoking, immobility, cancer, surgery, pregnancy, and taking birth control pills.
- Clots can be life threatening and severe. The severity depends on the size of the clot and amount of blockage.
- PE may be diagnosed by a thorough clinical examination, imaging, and blood tests.
- Treatment usually involves medications that prevent clot formation called anticoagulants or medications that dissolve the clot, called thrombolytics. Occasionally, large clots need to be removed by a minimally invasive procedure called an embolectomy.
- Some people with recurrent clots may need a filter placed in a large vein that prevents clots from reaching the lungs.
- Patients who have had a clot form previously are at risk for developing another.

4.8B PULMONARY HYPERTENSION

OVERVIEW

Pulmonary hypertension (PH) is defined by a resting mean pulmonary artery pressure of 25 mm Hg or greater. This abnormal hemodynamic state can impair gas exchange and progressively lead to pathologic tissue remodeling, right-sided heart failure, and death. There are many types of PH that differ widely with respect to etiology, epidemiology, and treatment. Therefore, early identification and precise classification are essential to the selection of appropriate management and improved outcomes.

EPIDEMIOLOGY

The epidemiology of PH is difficult to assess because the definitive diagnosis is based on the gold standard, invasive right heart catherization. Despite this limitation, PH is thought to be a global, heterogeneous disease affecting approximately 1% of the population. While the disease affects all ages, races, and genders the prevalence of PH is highest in those over age 65 years.[67] Death rates for PH as any contributing cause of death have been increasing over time, 5.5 per 100,000 in 2001 and 6.5 per 100,000 in 2010.[68] A PH classification scheme has been recently updated by the 6th World Symposium on Pulmonary Hypertension (WSPS) Task Force. Each group differs considerably in etiology, pathobiology, incidence, and prevalence. The classification is important to help guide a clinician's differential diagnosis, approach, and selection of group-specific therapies. While the classification scheme is helpful, the broad classifications and multiple etiologies limit the ability to obtain accurate estimates on the global prevalence of PH. The most recent, and more accurate epidemiologic studies are based on regional registry data which primarily focused on Group 1, pulmonary arterial hypertension (PAH) due to distinct underlying disorders of the pulmonary vessels, and Group 4, PH due to thromboembolic obstructions.

Group 1, PAH, is a rare, severe disease. The incidence of PAH ranges from 0.9 to 7.6 cases per million adults per year, and the prevalence varies from 5 to 52 cases per 1 million.[69] PAH affects all races including African American, Latinx, and Asian populations.[70] Women are more likely to have PAH, with a female-male ratio of ~3:1, but surprisingly, the severity and mortality rate are greater in men.[71] While thought to be a disease of younger individuals, the age of patients diagnosed with idiopathic or heritable PAH is increasing with a recent study reporting a mean age of 52 compared to 36 years in the 1980s.[72] Infection is also a common global cause and specifically, schistosomiasis-associated PH is the leading type of PH in countries where schistosomiasis is endemic.[73] It is, however, different in regions without endemic schistosomiasis. In the United States, for example, the most common type of PH is idiopathic followed by PH associated with connective tissue disease.[72] PH survival rates have significantly improved with a median survival rate of 6 years compared with 2.8 years in the 1980s.[74–76]

Group 2 is PH due to left-sided heart disease. Owing to the high prevalence of ischemic and structural heart disease, PH due to left-sided heart disease is a frequent cause of PH affecting at least 50% of heart failure patients.[77] These studies also reported a doubling of the mortality rate in these patients.[67]

Group 3 is PH due to lung disease or hypoxia. Hypoxic lung disease, especially COPD and diffuse parenchymal lung diseases (DPLD) including idiopathic and connective tissue disorders, are associated with a high incidence of PH. The prevalence of PH due to hypoxic lung diseases varies with the severity of the disease. For example, the prevalence in patients with COPD and mild PH is 18–50% while the prevalence of severe PH and COPD is 2% to 14%.[78] In all cases, the presence of PH is associated with increased symptoms, exercise limitations, and poorer prognosis.

Group 4, chronic thromboembolic pulmonary hypertension (CTPH), is considered a rare complication; the true incidence and prevalence of this group remain unclear and debated, and thromboembolism is emerging as an important cause of PH due to the considerable mortality and morbidity rates.

Reports have shown that 1.0% to 8.8% of patients with a PE will develop PH.[79] In another study, the cumulative incidence of symptomatic CTPH was 1.0% at 6 months and 3.8% at 2 years.[80]

Group 5, pulmonary hypertension with unclear multifactorial mechanisms, is an important heterogeneous group of PH with multifactorial causes. For many of the diseases and therefore the group, the true incidence, etiology, and treatment remain uncertain. Most studies are small but suggest that PH is common in these cases and its presence is often associated with increased risks of morbidity and mortality.[81]

Despite limited epidemiologic data, heterogeneity of the etiology and pathobiology, a consistent finding for all groups is that PH, independent of the underlying cause, is a concerning complication associated with increased morbidity and mortality rates.

PATHOPHYSIOLOGY

The normal pulmonary vasculature bed is uniquely characterized as a high-flow, low-resistance, and low-pressure system providing an ideal pathway to deliver deoxygenated blood to the pulmonary microcirculation for gas exchange. The extensive capillary network is able to accommodate increases in blood flow with minimal elevation in arterial pressure and has a tremendous capacity to expand and recruit underperfused vessels. Combined, these features play an essential role in the ability of the lungs to respond to exertional stress and increased oxygen demand and optimize gas exchange. Increased pulmonary vascular resistance (PVR) limits the ability of the heart and lungs to respond to stress and remains the common underlying pathogenesis of all types of PH. The increase in afterload is particularly problematic to the heart and right-sided heart failure is a significant unifying consequence of PH. While most cases of PH are due to primary disorders of other systems, Group 1 is unique in that it is a disease of the small pulmonary arteries themselves.

PH is a proliferative vasculopathy characterized by vascular narrowing and increase in pulmonary vascular resistance. The pathophysiologic hallmarks of PH leading to a sustained increase in resistance include endothelial cell dysfunction, endothelial and pulmonary artery smooth muscle cell proliferation, pulmonary vasoconstriction, microthrombosis, and inflammation. These processes, initiated by pulmonary endothelial injury and/or vascular smooth muscle dysfunction, result in long-term cellular changes and vessel remodeling. Pulmonary vascular remodeling is a complex process of hypertrophy and hyperplasia involving all three layers: intima, media, and adventitia. Cellular changes associated with PH include distal extension of smooth muscle into small peripheral, normally nonmuscular pulmonary arteries, formation of a neointima, adventitial neovascularization, endothelial disorganization and proliferation. Structural changes have been noted including perivascular inflammation and inflammatory cell infiltration, although the exact role in the development of PH is unclear.[82] Finally, thrombotic lesions and platelet dysfunction appear to play an important role in the pathogenesis. Intravascular coagulation is upregulated in PH including elevated plasma levels of von Willebrand factor and plasminogen activator inhibitor type 1. Together, along with the increased sheer stress, they generate a procoagulant, thrombogenic state.[83] There is limited evidence of the reversibility of these lesions and the reversibility process remains unclear. Clinically, it is important to note that while significant structural remodeling is a common process in all forms of PH, no single histologic feature leads to a definitive diagnosis of PH. Due in part to the limited understanding of the disease, the pathology and pathobiology describing the extent and type of a pulmonary vascular remodeling have a limited role in establishing a cause and effect, and therefore, adds little prognostic value to the natural history of the disease. There is hope that further pathogenetic insights and understanding of the disease process will not only improve the diagnostic and prognostic power, but also facilitate the development of effective targeted therapies that will reverse the progression.

The pathologic triad of vasoconstriction, cellular proliferation, and thrombosis are thought to be activated early in the disease process through the action of mediators such as thromboxane A2, endothelin-1, and serotonin. Normally, the effects of these vasoconstrictive mediators are counterbalanced by vasodilating agents including prostacyclin, vasoactive intestinal peptide, and nitric oxide. PH is a persistent imbalance of the vasodilators/vasoconstrictors and therapeutic strategies have been directed at correcting this imbalance. While many of these abnormalities are likely secondary, they remain nonetheless interesting and potential therapeutic targets.

In addition to specific mediators, several molecular pathways that contribute to the imbalance of vascular vasoconstriction, vasodilatation and vascular remodeling have been identified as important components (Box 4.1). Transforming growth factor-beta (TGF-β) super family (TGF-β subgroup, bone morphogenic proteins, activins) have emerged as a key mediator of endothelial and smooth muscle dysfunction and proliferation; however, therapeutics targeted at this pathway have yet to be developed. Serotonergic mechanism as well as channelopathies (potassium and calcium) have also been implicated in the development of the disease although the exact mechanisms are unclear.[84]

Clearly, not one factor but rather the converging of many factors and a multifactorial process that will explain the progression of this disease. The progression in the understanding of the entities and interplay has been impressive with results in the development of PH-specific targets. Future work will improve our understanding and perhaps lead to new diagnostic biomarkers for early detection and novel therapeutics aimed at reversing this progressive process.

MEDICAL HISTORY AND CLINICAL PRESENTATION

The primary symptom of every form of PH is dyspnea on exertion. Dyspnea is a nonspecific symptom, the primary manifestation of several diseases including lung disease (asthma, COPD, PE, pneumonia, pneumothorax, aspirations, or

BOX 4.1 Cellular and Molecular Pathobiology: Mediators of Pulmonary Arterial Hypertension

Cellular Processes

- Proliferation
- Migration
- Angiogenesis and neovascularization
- Apoptosis
- Proteolysis
- Inflammation
- Thrombosis

Cellular Determinants

- Smooth muscle cells
- Fibroblasts
- Endothelial cells
- Immune/inflammatory cells
- Thrombocytes

Molecular Determinants

- Nitric oxide (NO)
- Prostacyclin (prostaglandin I2)
- Endothelin (ET-1)
- Vasoactive intestinal peptide (VIP)
- Potassium channels (Kv1.5)
- Serotonin
- TGF-β superfamily
- Growth factors
  - PDGF
  - FGF
  - VEGF
  - EGF
- Proinflammatory cytokines
  - IL-1
  - IL-6
  - RANTES
  - Fractalikine

EGF, epidermal growth factor; FGF, fibroblast growth factor; IL, interleukin; PDGF, platelet-derived growth factor; RANTES, Regulated on Activation, Normal T-cell Expressed and Secreted; TGF-β, transforming growth factor beta; VEGF, vascular endothelial growth factor.

malignancy), heart disease (myocardial ischemia, congestive heart failure, tamponade, arrhythmia, valvular disease, intracardiac shunting), anemia, obesity, deconditioning or other systemic illnesses including metabolic acidosis, shock, cirrhosis and ascites, and thyrotoxicosis. A thorough history qualitatively and quantitatively characterizing the dyspnea is helpful in narrowing the broad etiology. With the progressive nature of the disease the symptoms will become worse over time and may include bendopnea or orthopnea. Syncopal or near syncopal episodes suggest disease progression and are associated with a poorer prognosis. Patients with secondary causes of PH may present with associated signs and symptoms of the causative disorder that provide clues to the primary disorder (e.g., angina, valvular disease, COPD, connective tissue disease). PH should be considered in patients with chronic illnesses, especially cardiac and pulmonary disease, with symptoms disproportionate to the underlying disease or are poorly responsive to therapy. Since PH has a genetic component, a thorough family history of PH is important to rule out familial etiology. All medications should be reviewed with the patient especially the use of prescription amphetamines or diet pills, illicit drugs such as cocaine and methamphetamines, which all have been known to cause PH.

SIGNS AND SYMPTOMS

The diagnosis of PH requires a clinical suspicion based on signs and symptoms, the physical examination, and review of hemodynamic criteria to describe the etiology and severity (Box 4.2). At some time in the progression of the disease, all forms of PH produce symptomatic sequelae. The common symptoms include progressive dyspnea on exertion combined with fatigue, lethargy exertional angina, syncope, and weight gain (from edema). Uncommon symptoms are cough, hemoptysis, and hoarseness, which are due to mechanical complications in the thorax and disruption of the normal distribution of blood. The following signs and symptoms of PH are associated as high risk (>10% 1-year mortality rate).[77]

- Clinical signs of right-sided heart failure
- Rapid progression of symptoms
  - Repeated episodes of syncope, even with little or regular activity
- World Health Organization functional class (WHO FC) IV
- 6-minute walking distance (6MWD) <165 m
- BNP and NT-proBNP plasma levels
  - B-type natriuretic peptide (BNP) level >300 ng/L
  - N-terminal fragment of BNP (NT-proBNP) level >1,400 ng/L
- Abnormal imaging findings (echocardiography, cardiac magnetic resonance)
  - Pericardial effusion
  - Right atrial area >26 cm^2
- Right atrial pressure >14 mm Hg
- Cardiac index of <2 L/m in/m^2
- Mixed venous oxygen saturation of <60%

More specific signs and symptoms will reflect the underlying cause and degree of right ventricular failure.

Signs of PH on physical examination include accentuated and splitting of the pulmonic component of the second heart sound augmented with respiration, systolic ejection murmur on the left parasternal border, third heart sound on the right side, pansystolic murmur of tricuspid regurgitation, a diastolic murmur of pulmonic regurgitation, left parasternal lift and the triad of overt right ventricular decompensation including cervical venous distention, ascites or hepatomegaly and peripheral edema. Signs of right ventricular decompression are associated with late or advanced PH. Splenomegaly is a common finding in infectious PH including schistosomiasis-associated PH.

BOX 4.2 Signs and Symptoms of Pulmonary Hypertension

Symptoms

- Dyspnea on exertion
- Lethargy and fatigue
- Exertional chest pain
- Anorexia
- Cough
- Hemoptysis
- Hoarseness

Signs

Abnormal heart sounds augmented with inspiration

- Enhanced and/or wide-splitting of P2 of the second heart sound
- Systolic ejection murmur on upper left sternal border
- Right-sided third or fourth heart sound
- Holosystolic murmur over the tricuspid valve area
- Diastolic murmur over the upper left sternal border

Right ventricular failure

- Prominent "a" wave in the jugular venous pulse
- Right ventricular heave
- Hepatomegaly
- Pulsatile or tender liver
- Peripheral edema and/or ascites

PHYSICAL EXAMINATION

PH is difficult to diagnose and often unrecognizable. The physical exam of patients with compensated PH may be normal. As the disease progresses, nonspecific physical exam findings usually reflect the degree of right-sided heart failure. Initially, there may be an increased intensity and splitting of the pulmonic component of the second heart sound (P2) at the pulmonic region (second intercostal space, left parasternal border) accompanied by a systolic ejection murmur also heard over the left sternal border. As right ventricular involvement progresses, in the neck, the jugular vein may reveal a prominent or elevated "a" wave signifying resistance to atrial emptying and elevated right ventricular pressure.

DIFFERENTIAL DIAGNOSIS

Since the most common cardinal symptom of PH is dyspnea, the differential diagnosis is broad (Table 4.16). A thorough clinical history of the nature of the dyspnea will guide the initial assessment and the differential narrows considerably in patients with physical examination signs and symptoms of overt right ventricular failure. Additional clinical findings may suggest an underlying cause of dyspnea. Orthopnea may suggest congestive heart failure. Inspiratory crackles points toward interstitial disease. Telangiectasis, digital ulceration,

TABLE 4.16 Differential Diagnosis for Pulmonary Hypertension

Diagnosis	Description
Asthma	Chronic disease characterized by variable airflow obstruction which is usually reversible and caused by inflammation and bronchial hyperresponsiveness that is usually reversible
Congestive heart failure	Dysfunction of the myocardium that reduces the ability of the heart to pump enough blood to the body
Chronic obstructive pulmonary disease (COPD)	A long-term, progressive and irreversible resistance to airflow characterized by persistent respiratory symptoms and airflow limitation
Interstitial lung disease	A large group of diseases leading to the thickening of the pulmonary parenchyma that interferes with lung function
Restrictive lung disease	A disease characterized by the reduced expansion of the lung parenchyma accompanied by a reduction of total lung volume and capacity
Pulmonary emboli	A blood clot in the pulmonary vasculature occludes the pulmonary arteries and obstructs blood flow to the lungs
Congenital heart defects	Structural heart defects that can affect the normal blood flow through the heart and result in abnormal cardiac function and blood flow to the body
Atrial myxoma	Sporadic, primary cardiac tumor of primitive mesenchymal cells in subendocardial tissue of the left atrial septum and can lead to mechanical interference of cardiac blood flow and function
Hypertrophic cardiomyopathy	Increase in the thickness of the left ventricular myocardium in the absence of elevated afterload or systemic vascular resistance
Dilated cardiomyopathy	Disease of the myocardium characterized by ventricular dilation and systolic dysfunction
Restrictive cardiomyopathy	Diastolic cardiac dysfunction characterized by impaired diastolic ventricular filling and normal systolic function
Emphysema	Long-term progressive and irreversible airflow obstruction pathologically defined by airspace enlargement distal to the terminal bronchioles accompanied by destruction of their walls in the absence of fibrosis
Mitral regurgitation	Incompetent mitral valve resulting in abnormal, backward blood flow from the left ventricle to the left atrium during ventricular systole
Mitral stenosis	Structural abnormality of the mitral valve apparatus leading to obstruction to blood flow from the left atrium to the left ventricle during ventricular diastole
Aortic stenosis	Structural abnormality of the aortic valve leading to obstruction to blood flow from the left ventricle to the aorta during ventricular systole
Obstructive sleep apnea	A sleep disorder characterized by recurrent arousals and sleep fragmentation due to the complete or partial obstruction of airflow in the upper airway
Obesity-hypoventilation syndrome	Spectrum of conditions characterized by abnormal breathing patterns characterized by daytime and night-time hypoventilation associated with obesity and increased upper airway resistance or obstruction
Hepatopulmonary syndrome	A lung vascular complication of liver disease characterized by severe dilation of the pulmonary arteries with an accompanied reduction in oxygenation

and sclerodactyly suggest scleroderma. Distal bilateral clubbing is associated with interstitial fibrosis, congestive heart failure, and cyanotic congenital heart disease.

DIAGNOSTIC STUDIES

For all PH groups, diagnostic studies are necessary for three purposes: (1) to confirm the presence of elevated pulmonary artery pressures, (2) to evaluate the severity, and (3) to identify the etiology if possible (Table 4.17). While chest radiograph and EKG should be initially performed for evidence of right ventricular hypertrophy or right ventricular strain, echocardiography is the critical, noninvasive screening diagnostic test to directly evaluate the right ventricular size, function, and strain. Doppler studies will also provide an estimate on pulmonary artery pressure. Right heart catherization (RHC) is the gold standard in the diagnosis of PH since it is the only technique that directly and accurately determines pulmonary artery pressure. RHC will also assess the severity of PH and provide hemodynamic evidence of left-sided heart disease. Electrocardiographic findings will also show evidence of right ventricular strain and hypertrophy including right axis deviation, R to S ratio >1 in V1, increased P-wave amplitude, and conduction abnormalities including complete or incomplete right bundle branch block pattern. Initial laboratory tests include a CBC (for hemoglobin and hematocrit) and BNP or NT-proBNP evidence of ventricular strain. Features on radiograph include right atrial dilatation, prominent pulmonary outflow tract, and enlarged pulmonary arteries. For those with secondary PH, evidence of underlying chronic lung disease or heart failure may be present as well. Chest CT and MRI have a limited role in PH evaluation. CT and MRI show signs of PH but are usually performed when there is a high level of suspicion

TABLE 4.17 Diagnostic Studies for Pulmonary Hypertension

Diagnostic Studies and Rationale	Diagnostic Test and Parameters
Lab studies to assess hypoxemia and underlying causes	Complete blood count (CBC) Chem-7 Coagulation studies PT and aPTT Arterial blood gas (ABG) Antinuclear antibody (ANA) Rheumatoid factor (RF) Anti-Scl-70 Antineutrophil cytoplasmic antibody (ANCA) Liver function Brain natriuretic peptide (BNP or NT-proBNP) HIV Hepatitis serology Urine toxicology
Chest imaging to evaluate radiographic features associated with right-sided or left-sided heart failure and right ventricular enlargement and/or strain	Plain chest x-ray CT MRI
Cardiac studies to evaluate right-sided or left-sided heart failure and right ventricular enlargement and/or strain and evaluate pulmonary pressures	EKG Transthoracic echocardiography Right heart catheterization Cardiac MRI
Pulmonary studies to rule out chronic thromboembolic pulmonary hypertension (CTEPH) and underlying COPD	Ventilation/perfusion scan Pulmonary function tests Pulmonary angiography

aPTT, activated partial thromboplastin time; COPD, chronic obstructive pulmonary disease; NT-proBNP, N-terminal pro-brain natriuretic peptide; PT, prothrombin time.

of a specific etiology that requires increased resolution and detail. V̇/Q̇ scan and/or CT angiogram are useful for evaluating thromboembolic pulmonary hypertension (CTEPH, Group 4). Cardiac MRI is the gold standard for the quantification of RV volumes and function, which may be useful for evaluating response to therapy.[85]

EVALUATION

The clinical course of PH is divided into three phases: asymptomatic compensated, symptomatic decompensating, and advanced decompensated. Early detection and a stepwise approach of PH facilitates earlier treatment, delayed progression, and improved outcomes. Clinicians must hold a good working knowledge of the classification scheme that will guide the stepwise evaluation. Initially, PH should be suspected in all patients who present with dyspnea and a detailed history characterizing the dyspnea. If PH is suspected, a comprehensive evaluation and assessment are required since no single variable provides sufficient diagnostic and prognostic information. Patients presenting with signs and symptoms suggestive of PH should undergo targeted noninvasive tests and an assessment of functional capacity (FC) and exercise capacity. Although associated with variable interobserver reliability, the World Health Organization functional class (WHO-FC) is a powerful predictor of survival especially during follow-up, and worsening FC is known to be a predictor of disease progression.[72]

While the index of suspicion of right ventricular dysfunction increases with physical exam, chest radiography, and electrocardiography, transthoracic echocardiography (TEE) with Doppler are the crucial, noninvasive tests of choice directly revealing hemodynamic signs of PH and right ventricular overload/involvement. Often, the diagnosis, etiology, and pathogenesis of PH are determined clinically with the combined clinical and noninvasive findings listed above. Some patients, however, require additional invasive testing, including RHC to confirm and evaluate the pulmonary system further. Vasoactive testing should be performed in Group 1 patients. This type of testing will identify a subgroup of patients who will benefit from calcium channel blocker therapy. Given the rapid advances of targeted-PAH therapy, patients with echocardiographic findings of PH and suspected PAH should be promptly referred to a specialist center for a baseline evaluation, risk stratification, and assessment of disease progression. Etiology, symptoms, functional class, and RV involvement must be evaluated properly before the initiation of pharmacotherapeutic treatments.

TREATMENT

PH is a complex disease with multiple etiologies and no known cure. The common treatment for all types of PH is symptomatic dependent on the type and severity of the disease. All PH patients should receive a preventive care plan that includes an exercise and pulmonary rehabilitation plan, vaccination schedule against influenza and pneumococcal pneumonia, as well as nutritional and psychosocial support/counseling. Current treatment strategies are divided into two groups, supportive therapy and targeted therapy. Both groups aim to improve the patient's morbidity and mortality risks, clinical symptoms, and functional capacity. Supportive therapies include oxygen, diuretics, and digoxin. PAH therapy includes specific vasodilatory medications classified based on their cellular and molecular mechanisms (Table 4.18). Group 1 (PAH) and Group 4 (CTEPH) are the only two groups with targeted therapies. PAH therapies include endothelin receptor antagonists (ambrisentan, bosentan, macitentan), phosphodiesterase-5 inhibitors (sildenafil, tadalafil, vardenafil), prostacyclin pathway analogs and agonists, the prostanoids (epoprostenol, treprostinil, iloprost, selexipag) and soluble guanylate cyclase stimulator (riociguat). There is recent interest in the limited use of calcium channel blockers (diltiazem and nifedipine and more recently amlodipine) for a small subset of vasoreactive patients diagnosed with Group 1 PAH.[86] Some non randomized controlled clinical trials suggest a potential benefit of calcium channel blockers in a subgroup of people with PAH; however, more randomized clinical trials are needed and there are some concerns about the long-term benefit.[87]

Owing the complexity of the disease, combination therapy to target multiple pathogenic pathways is considered the standard of care in PAH with a phosphodiesterase-5 inhibitor and an endothelin receptor antagonist being the most widely utilized combination.[88] PAH therapy has improved the survival rates. U.S. based REVEAL Registry has reported survival rates at 1, 3, and 5 years of 90.4%, 76.2%, and 65.4%, respectively, compared to 68%, 48%, and 34% before the development of PAH-specific therapy; however, the long-term (5-year) survival rate remains poor despite therapeutic advances.[72] Survival subgroup analysis identified several prognostic indicators associated with survival including

TABLE 4.18 Pulmonary Arterial Hypertension–Specific Drug Therapy

Drug Class	Mechanism of Action	Adverse Drug Reactions
Calcium channel blockers	Inhibition of calcium ions in vascular smooth muscle	Hypotension and peripheral edema Exacerbation of right ventricle failure due to negative inotropic effects
Endothelin receptor antagonists	Competitive antagonist to endothelin-1 receptors	Hepatotoxicity Peripheral edema
Phosphodiesterase inhibitors	Competitive and selective inhibition of phosphodiesterase inhibiting cyclic guanosine monophosphate (cGMP) hydrolysis and elevating cellular cGMP levels	Headache Flushing
Prostacyclin receptor agonists	Binding and activation of the prostacyclin receptor in pulmonary artery smooth muscle resulting in cell hyperpolarization	Headache Jaw pain Nausea Dizziness Flushing Nasopharyngitis Vomiting
Soluble guanylate cyclase (sGC) stimulator	Sensitizes sGC to endogenous nitric oxide and directly stimulates the activity of guanylate cyclase, resulting in vasodilation and antiproliferation of smooth muscle cells	Headache Dyspepsia Nausea Vomiting Peripheral edema Dizziness Anemia Constipation

functional class, baseline 6-minute walk distance (6MWD), mean right atrial pressure (mRAP), and BNP.

Collectively, significant progress has been made in the understanding of the epidemiology, pathobiology, diagnosis, and prognosis of patients with PH, leading to notable improvement in the quality and efficacy of treatments and clinical care.

PATIENT EDUCATION

- PH is a condition with high blood pressure within the vessels in the lungs.
- There are many types and causes of PH.
- PH can occur in isolation or, more commonly, associated with diseases of the heart.
- Some illicit drugs and medications, including diet drugs, have been shown to result in PH and, on the other hand, some cases have no known cause.
- Symptoms include shortness of breath, fatigue, chest pain or pressure, near fainting, palpitations, swelling of the lower legs, and right-sided abdominal pain.
- The diagnosis is made using diagnostic tests including blood work, chest x-ray, and EKG and an ultrasound of the heart. If the suspicion of the disease is high, invasive direct measurement of the pressure in the lungs may be necessary.
- The general treatment is symptomatic and dependent on the underlying cause and severity of the disease.
- In addition to medical therapies, important lifestyle changes are recommended to improve the quality of life. These include smoking cessation, routine exercise, and dietary changes.

4.8C COR PULMONALE

OVERVIEW

Cor pulmonale describes the structural and functional changes of the right ventricle resulting from lung disease. Often viewed as a chronic disease, cor pulmonale also presents as a life-threatening condition in an acute setting.[89–91] Considering their anatomic and physiologic juxtaposition, the impact of pulmonary pathophysiology on cardiac structure and function is not surprising. The degree of cardiovascular involvement, however, is critical because cardiovascular involvement significantly increases the overall mortality risk of the underlying pulmonary disease. The appreciation of the complex and disease-based maladaptive changes of the pulmonary and cardiovascular systems is central to understanding this important cardiopulmonary condition.

EPIDEMIOLOGY

Without hemodynamic and structural measurements of the right side of the heart, the true prevalence of cor pulmonale is difficult to assess and the exact prevalence is unknown. Patients with COPD, the third leading cause of death, are most affected by cor pulmonale and therefore, by association, cor pulmonale has emerged as a common condition. Current estimates are that cor pulmonale accounts for approximately 6% to 7% of all types of heart disease and 10% to 30% of all heart failure admissions in the United States.[92] When cor pulmonale is paired with COPD, the overall mortality rate is much higher than for COPD alone.[90,91] Cor pulmonale is a common incident in patients with venous thromboembolic disease and acute pulmonary embolic event. Approximately 60,000 to 100,000 annual deaths in the United State are due to VTE or PE and about 50% are due to RV failure.[93]

PATHOPHYSIOLOGY

Cor pulmonale is a cardiac complication of parenchymal lung diseases such as COPD. PH often complicates parenchymal lung disease and the increase in pulmonary vascular resistance (PVR) leads to cor pulmonale. The process of increased PVR is likely the result of multiple factors including acidemia, hypercarbia, and increased cardiac output and blood viscosity; however, tissue alveolar hypoxia is considered a major stimulus and critical player. Two distinct mechanisms of action of alveolar hypoxia must be considered: acute hypoxia causing vasoconstriction and chronic hypoxia inducing long-standing structural changes in the pulmonary vasculature.[94,95]

Acute hypoxic vasoconstriction (HVC) is a compensatory response unique to the lung that optimizes ventilation and perfusion ($\dot{V}/\dot{Q}$) matching and blood oxygenation. HVC leads to the diversion of blood from hypoxic lung segment to a better-oxygenated lung segment. Chronic hypoxia (days to weeks) and sustained vasoconstriction result in irreversible pulmonary vascular remodeling.[94] Hypoxic vascular remodeling is characterized by changes in the intima (fibrosis) and media (smooth muscle proliferation and hypertrophy) of the pulmonary arterioles.[94] Remodeling processes result in the narrower and more muscular vessel with less compliance and higher resistance to flow. Several studies show the close association of the severity of cor pulmonale with the degree of alveolar hypoxia and point to the adaptive hypoxic pulmonary vasoconstrictor response as a key contributing factor to the development of the disease.[95,96]

In conditions such as emphysema and a massive pulmonary embolus, the increase in pulmonary vascular resistance is due to the destruction the vasculature or obstruction of blood flow within the pulmonary vascular bed. This destruction/obstruction will lead to an overall decrease in cross-sectional area and increase the total pulmonary vascular resistance.

Pulmonary vascular endothelial dysfunction is an additional factor in the pathogenesis of PH. The endothelium is a dynamic tissue that maintains the balance of constriction and dilation through the production of molecular mediators including nitric oxide (NO) and prostacyclin. An imbalance of these factors is likely involved in the pathogenesis of PH.

Finally, RV systolic dysfunction, hypertrophy, and dilation have also been observed in patients with COPD who did not have PH.[97] This suggests that minor elevations in pulmonary pressures have important negative consequences. It also points to an earlier cardiac involvement in the evolution of the disease than previously thought. This finding also suggests that other additive mechanisms may play an important role in the pathogenesis including inflammation, endothelial dysfunction, and lung hyperinflation.[98]

Normally, the right ventricle is a thin-walled, compliant, low-pressure chamber. Regardless of the mechanism, elevated pulmonary vascular resistance increases the work of the right ventricle. RV function and output are preserved, to a point, due to compensatory mechanisms including RV dilation and hypertrophy. Eventually, however, in the setting of chronic pressure overload, RV systolic and diastolic dysfunction and failure and hemodynamic collapse result.[99,100]

MEDICAL HISTORY AND CLINICAL PRESENTATION

PH and cor pulmonale should be suspected in all patients with primary hypoxic lung disease. The most common symptom is dyspnea on exertion although this is not a specific finding of cor pulmonale. Despite the lack of a specific clinical sign, a careful history of dyspnea is important to differentiate between cardiac, pulmonary, mixed pulmonary and cardiac, and noncardiac and extrapulmonary causes. Critical components include onset and duration, triggers, severity, and the development of additional symptoms including exertional chest pain, fatigue, lethargy, syncope or near-syncope, or any clinical signs of right-sided heart failure. Other factors in the history should include a smoking history, exercise tolerance, allergies, occupational history, history of asthma or coronary artery disease, congestive heart failure, cardiomyopathies, and valvular heart disease (Box 4.3).

SIGNS AND SYMPTOMS

The early diagnosis of cor pulmonale is challenging as the clinical signs are insensitive and the physical finding of RV hypertrophy and failure are late signs. Clinical signs of right-sided heart failure include a widened split of the second heart sound, right ventricular heave, tricuspid regurgitation murmur, and elevated jugular venous pressure, and increased "a" wave, peripheral edema, or ascites should heighten the index of suspicion of cor pulmonale. Additional symptoms of cor pulmonale include:

- Dyspnea on exertion
- Tachycardia and/or palpitations
- Syncope, or near syncopal episodes
- Chest pain
- Lower extremity edema and/or ascites
- Cyanosis

BOX 4.3 Respiratory Diseases Associated With Cor Pulmonale

Obstructive Lung Diseases
COPD
Asthma
Bronchiectasis, bronchiolitis obliterans
Cystic fibrosis
Restrictive Lung Diseases
Idiopathic interstitial pulmonary fibrosis
Connective tissue diseases
Pneumoconiosis
Sarcoidosis
Sequelae of pulmonary tuberculosis
Neuromuscular diseases
Respiratory Insufficiency
Alveolar hypoventilation disorders
Chronic exposure to high altitude
Obesity-hypoventilation syndrome

COPD, chronic obstructive pulmonary disease.

PHYSICAL EXAMINATION

Physical examination findings of advanced disease consistent with right-sided heart failure include:

- Tachypnea
- Jugular venous distention and abnormal wave formation
- Peripheral edema
- Palpable left parasternal lift
- Loud S2 or ejection click, narrow splitting of S2, a holosystolic murmur consistent with tricuspid regurgitation at the left lower sternal border, right-sided S4
- Lung crepitations
- Hepatomegaly and ascites

Physical examination findings associated with COPD including pursed-lip breathing, reduced chest expansion, reduced breath sounds, use of accessory respiratory muscles, and extended (>4 seconds) expiratory time.

DIFFERENTIAL DIAGNOSIS

The differential diagnosis of cor pulmonade is summarized in Table 4.19.

DIAGNOSTIC STUDIES

The diagnosis of cor pulmonale is based on a combination of the evidence of PH with normal cardiac output and the presence of pulmonary disease. Acute cor pulmonale is based on elevated pulmonary artery pressure with clinical signs of right-sided heart failure (Table 4.20).

TABLE 4.19 Differential Diagnosis for Cor Pulmonade

Diagnosis	Description
Atrial myxoma	Sporadic, primary cardiac tumor of primitive mesenchymal cells in subendocardial tissue of the left atrial septum; can lead to mechanical interference of cardiac blood flow and function
Polycythemia	Malignant stem cell disorder of the bone marrow resulting in an increased production of red blood cells and characterized by the elevated absolute red blood cell mass
Left ventricular heart failure	Dysfunction of the left ventricle that reduces the ability of the heart to pump blood to the systemic and coronary circulation
Infiltrative cardiomyopathies	Diseases associated with an infiltrative process of the myocardium characterized by primary decreased ventricular compliance and diastolic dysfunction with preserved systolic function
Pulmonic stenosis	Structural abnormalities in the pulmonic valve leading to obstruction to blood flow from the right ventricle to the pulmonary artery during ventricular systole
Congenital heart disease (left-to-right shunt)	Congenital cardiac malformation in which there is an abnormal connection between the right and left sides of the heart and flow of oxygenated blood to the lungs
Myocardial infarction	Irreversible necrosis of the myocardium resulting from ischemia
Valvular disease and endocarditis	Infection of the endocardium characterized by microbial invasion of the heart valves, which can lead to dysfunction of the blood flow within the heart
Cardiac tamponade	Accumulation of fluid in the pericardial space resulting in diastolic dysfunction, reduced ventricular filling, and possible hemodynamic instability
Acute coronary syndrome	Spectrum of catastrophic clinical presentations resulting from the rupture of an atherosclerotic plaque within the coronary artery leading to partial or complete obstruction of blood flow to the myocardium
Pneumonia	A broadly defined lung infection
Pulmonary embolus	A blood clot in the pulmonary vasculature that occludes the pulmonary arteries and obstructs blood flow to the lungs
Volume overload	Expansion of extracellular volume with the development of hemodynamic and clnical fluid congestion

EVALUATION

History and physical examination findings and diagnostic tests are directed toward evaluating the severity of cor pulmonale and determining the underlying etiology of the primary PH. Diagnostic studies include routine laboratory tests, chest x-ray and EKG. Noninvasive echocardiography provides valuable information about the morphology of the right ventricle and extent of RV involvement and Doppler studies allow for the indirect estimation of pulmonary artery pressure; however, these images may be technically difficult to obtain in COPD patients. RHC is the only direct way to measure the pulmonary pressures and the major determinant of prognosis. Once the diagnosis is made, it should be followed with additional advanced testing directed at determining the underlying etiology. PFTs, ventilation/perfusion scanning, and chest CT may show specific evidence of underlying pulmonary disease.

TABLE 4.20 Diagnostic Studies of Cor Pulmonale

Diagnostic Test	Parameter and Rationale
Lab studies	Complete blood count (CBC) and hematocrit to detect the presence of polycythemia Serum alpha-1 antitrypsin as a cause of chronic obstructive pulmonary disease (COPD) Antinuclear antibody (ANA) Coagulation studies for connective tissue disease Arterial blood gas to evaluate arterial oxygenation, carbon dioxide levels, and pH Brain natriuretic peptide (BNP) to evaluate congestive heart failure and identify significant pulmonary hypertension
Imaging	The sensitivity and specificity of radiologic signs of cor pulmonale is low. Chest x-ray may be used to evaluate size of the right ventricle and right atrium, the pulmonary vasculature, and evidence of vascular congestion, and to suggest primary etiology including emphysema
Electrocardiogram	Evidence for chronic cor pulmonale includes right ventricular hypertrophy or right atrial enlargement, right ventricular strain, or conduction delays associated with right ventricular enlargement: • Right axis deviation • R/S amplitude ratio in V1 >1 • R/S amplitude ratio in V6 <1 • Increase in P wave amplitude in leads 2, 3, and aVF • S1Q3T3 pattern • Incomplete (or complete) right bundle branch block pattern • Low-voltage QRS (peak-to-peak QRS amplitude <5 mm limb leads and <10 mm precordial leads
Transthoracic echocardiography and Doppler ultrasound	To evaluate right ventricular chamber size and wall thickness, right ventricular function, and limited ability to assess pulmonary artery pressure
Right heart catherization	The gold standard for the diagnosis of pulmonary hypertension. Evaluate right ventricular size and function and directly measure pulmonary artery pressure and indirectly measure left atrial pressure

TREATMENT

Treatment of underlying COPD is essential. Specifically, oxygen therapy is the logical treatment of PH since alveolar hypoxia is considered the major determinant of the elevation of pulmonary artery pressure and pulmonary vascular resistance.

Primary treatment consists of the following:

- Long-term oxygen therapy to overcome hypoxemia
- Diuretic to optimize volume status
- Calcium channel blockers to reduce afterload

- Prostacyclin analogs and endothelin-receptor antagonists
- Anticoagulant and thrombolytic therapy for treatment of underlying pulmonary thromboembolic disease

PATIENT EDUCATION

- Cor pulmonale is an impairment of the right ventricle resulting from respiratory disease. Most commonly, cor pulmonale is due to high blood pressure in the lungs. This increase in pressure makes it harder for the right side of the heart to pump blood to the lungs. If it continues, this condition puts a strain on the heart.
- There are many causes of cor pulmonale but COPD is the most frequent cause.
- Symptoms include a fast heart rate, fatigue, lightheadedness or fainting during activities, ankle swelling, cough, chest pain, shortness of breath with exercise, blueish lips and fingers, and right-sided abdominal discomfort.
- A physical exam will be done to make the diagnosis and determine the cause.
- Additional tests including blood work, chest x-ray, EKG, and ultrasound of the heart may be required to help diagnose the condition. Occasionally, more advanced tests including PFTs, a ventilation and perfusion scan, and arterial blood gases may be necessary to identify the underlying lung disease. Rarely, a catheter inserted into the blood vessels will be needed to directly measure the pressure in the lungs.
- Treatment is directed at the reduction of symptoms and improvement in lung function. The treatment selection will be based on the cause of the cor pulmonale.
- Patients who smoke should stop immediately. Patients should avoid strenuous activities, heavy lifting, and travel to high altitudes and keep immunizations up to date including an annual flu vaccine and pneumonia.
- The outlook of the disease will depend on adherence to the treatments and the underlying cause.

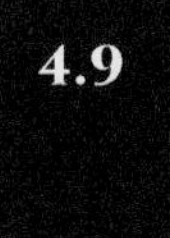

4.9 OCCUPATIONAL LUNG DISEASE: PNEUMOCONIOSIS, PLEURAL LUNG DISEASE

OVERVIEW

Occupational lung disease is a classification of a group of lung diseases that are caused by the chronic inhalation of a variety of mineral or metal dust particles, usually from an occupational exposure, causing damage to the lung parenchyma or the pleural lining. Pneumoconiosis is the general term used to describe a group of ILDs that cause chronic fibrosis, which commonly includes coal worker's pneumoconiosis, silicosis, and asbestosis. Pleural lung disease is the general term used to describe those conditions that cause a diffuse thickening and scarring of the pleural lining, which is common from chronic asbestos exposure. Pleural plaques are the most common manifestation of asbestosis exposure.[101]

EPIDEMIOLOGY

The incidence of pneumoconiosis is directly related to the type and length of exposure time to the dust.[102] As reported in *The Lancet* from a survey of reported deaths in 2013, pneumoconiosis was the cause of 260,001 deaths which increased from 251,000 in 1990.[103] The study was able to further break down the type of pneumoconiosis deaths: 46,000 due to silicosis, 24,000 due to asbestosis, and 25,000 due to coal worker's pneumoconiosis.[103] The number of deaths due to pneumoconiosis has decreased in the United States because of improved working conditions and the governmental regulations.

PATHOPHYSIOLOGY

Pneumoconiosis results when the lungs are not able to efficiently eliminate the dust from the lungs. Normally, the dust is engulfed by alveolar macrophages, moved up the respiratory tree by the mucociliary escalator, and expelled.

The risk of pneumoconiosis is dependent upon the size of the particles and time of exposure. The smaller the particles, the easier it is for them to deposit deeper in the bronchial tree. The longer a patient is exposed to air filled with dust, the more dust that is deposited into the lungs.

When the mucociliary escalator can no longer keep up with the amount of dust in the alveoli, saturation occurs leaving macrophages engulfed with dust filling the alveoli. This stimulates an immune response, entrapping the macrophages and stimulating fibroblasts to produce collagen, eventually leading to fibrosis of the lung parenchyma.

The formation of pleural plaques is common in asbestos exposure. Asbestos is inhaled and accumulates in the lower bronchial tree, causing inflammation, stimulation of the phagocytes, and collagen formation from fibroblasts. It is thought that these hyalinized collagen fibers are transported via the lymphatic system into the pleural space causing pleural plaques. While not cancerous, pleural plaques from asbestos are a marker for high risk of mesothelioma and lung cancer.

MEDICAL HISTORY AND CLINICAL PRESENTATION

Typically, occupational lung disease occurs after years of exposure to the offending agent. Depending on the type of occupational exposure, patients can be asymptomatic or slowly become symptomatic, typically with dyspnea on exertion. Coal worker's pneumoconiosis and silicosis are usually asymptomatic and found incidentally on chest radiographs. Patients with asbestos-related exposure usually develop progressive dyspnea on exertion. There is an acute form of silicosis that occurs with high concentration exposure, in which symptoms occur more rapidly—months to a few years. This condition is rare.

Taking a detailed occupational history is very important. Occupations that place patients at risk for occupational lung disease include coal mining, working with insulation, shipbuilding, railroad locomotive building, asbestos abatement, roofing, construction, pipe fitters, bricklayers, sheet metal workers, and automotive work. Attention should be given to the type of exposure, length of exposure, and use of respiratory safety equipment.

While cigarette smoking does not cause occupational lung disease, it is important to elicit a smoking history because it is common to have concomitant obstructive pulmonary symptoms complicating the clinical picture of occupational lung disease.

SIGNS AND SYMPTOMS

Patients with occupational lung disease may initially present with an abnormal chest x-ray with incidental findings. The chief complaint is dyspnea with exertion that slowly progresses over a long period of time. Cough, sputum production, and wheezing are not typical of occupational lung disease and are more often seen in patients who concomitantly have COPD from cigarette smoking.

TABLE 4.21 Differential Diagnosis for Occupational Lung Disease

Diagnosis	Description
Idiopathic pulmonary fibrosis	Idiopathic slowly progressive pulmonary condition that causes inflammation of the lung parenchyma that leads to pulmonary fibrosis.
Interstitial pulmonary fibrosis	General category of pulmonary disease marked by slow progressive pulmonary fibrosis due to many different triggering agents. It is characterized by inflammation that eventually leads to pulmonary fibrosis.
Tuberculosis	Bacterial infection that can be asymptomatic causing pulmonary cavitary nodules typically in the upper lobes of the lungs. Older infiltrates can have fibrotic scars.
Hypertrophic osteoarthropathy	Orthopedic condition that causes periostitis of the hands and clubbing.
Berylliosis	Chronic pulmonary allergic response to beryllium causing granulomatous pulmonary infiltrates and dyspnea on exertion.
Lung cancer	Early lung cancer can present with minimal symptoms that include dyspnea on exertion and nodular densities on chest radiograph.
Sarcoidosis	Inflammatory granulomatous condition that affects the lungs causing progressive dyspnea on exertion.

PHYSICAL EXAMINATION

The physical examination may be unremarkable. As the disease continues to advance, patients may develop bibasilar inspiratory crackles and clubbing.

The underlying pathophysiology leads to pulmonary fibrosis. If the fibrosis is significant, patients can develop cor pulmonale from increased right-sided heart enlargement and failure leading to peripheral edema, jugular venous distention, hepatomegaly and hepatic congestion, and a right ventricular heave.

DIFFERENTIAL DIAGNOSIS

The differential diagnosis of occupational lung disease is summarized in Table 4.21.

DIAGNOSTIC STUDIES

Pulmonary imaging is the mainstay of occupational lung disease evaluation. Many times, an abnormal chest radiograph is found incidentally. For this reason interpretation should be coupled with a detailed social history including an occupational history and a high index of suspicion for occupational lung disease in the appropriate patient presentation.

Radiologic disease findings can vary by specific occupational lung disease. They are summarized in Table 4.22. The International Labor Organization International Classification of Radiographs of Pneumoconiosis, which is based on size, shape, location, and number of opacities, has developed guidelines for the evaluation of chest radiographs that aid in the classification and assessing severity of occupational lung disease.

While the chest x-ray is the initial screening test for occupational lung disease, high-resolution CT can better define parenchymal involvement, may allow for earlier recognition in symptomatic patients, and can differentiate idiopathic pulmonary fibrosis.[104]

TABLE 4.22 Comparison of Occupational Lung Disease and Radiographic Findings

Occupational Lung Disease	Chest Radiographic Findings
Coal miner's pneumoconiosis	Diffuse small, rounded opacities <1 cm throughout the lungs most prominent in the upper lobes. Over time, they coalesce forming large opacities with pulmonary fibrosis, mainly in the upper lobes.
Silicosis	Innumerable small 1–3 mm rounded opacities usually in the upper lobes. As the disease progresses, the small opacities coalesce forming larger opacities. Calcification of the peripheral hilar lymph nodes is common finding that is suggestive of silicosis.
Asbestosis	Linear reticular streaking in the peripheral lung bases accompanied by bilateral opacities of various shapes and sizes with a ground-glass appearance. Pleural plaques are highly suggestive of asbestosis. Honeycombing in the mid and lower lung fields suggests advanced cases. Hilar lymph nodes are not involved.

While pulmonary imaging is the most helpful in the evaluation of a patient with occupational lung disease, PFTs may be helpful in characterizing pulmonary function over time. Early in the disease process PFTs may not be abnormal. However, over the course of time, patients may show changes in pulmonary function in the following fashion:

- **Coal miner's pneumoconiosis:** Spirometry typically is normal except in very advanced or complicated cases.
- **Silicosis:** Combined obstructive and restrictive pattern on spirometry and a reduction in the diffusion capacity. Initially, there is a reduction in lung volumes and as the disease progresses with fibrosis, a decreased diffusion capacity and obstruction occur.
- **Asbestosis:** Restrictive pattern on spirometry with a reduction in the diffusion capacity.

Laboratory testing is not helpful in the diagnosis of occupational lung disease. However, a CBC, BNP sputum smear and cultures, tuberculin skin testing, and bronchoalveolar lavage may be helpful in excluding other conditions on the differential diagnosis.

EVALUATION

Patients who present with the gradual onset of dyspnea on exertion should undergo a thorough history and physical examination with attention to occupational exposure to mineral or metal dust particles.

TREATMENT

There is no specific treatment for occupational lung disease. However, the following are recommended to improve symptoms and prevent associated complications.

- Smoking cessation
- Avoid further occupational exposure of the offending agent and use respiratory protection
- Pneumococcal and influenza vaccination
- Supplemental oxygen with hypoxia
- Aggressive treatment of concomitant COPD and acute infections

4.10 PLEURAL DISEASES

4.10A PLEURAL EFFUSIONS

OVERVIEW

A pleural effusion is the accumulation of fluid in the pleural space due to the manifestation of underlying disease. In the United States, it is a common clinical problem estimated to affect over 1.5 million patients per year. Pleural effusions are caused by a wide variety of disorders of the lung, pleural diseases, and other extrapulmonary diseases. The fluid accumulation can be harmless; however, if severe enough, it may interfere with lung function and lead to lung compression or collapse. Over the years, significant advances have been made in the understanding of the pleural biology and pathogenesis of pleural effusions. With this understanding, the diagnosis, evaluation, and management of pleural effusions have progressed. Given the wide variety of etiologies and presence of significant comorbidities, expeditious and efficient diagnosis will maximize patient care.

EPIDEMIOLOGY

Fluid accumulation in the pleural space is a common occurrence caused by both benign and serious conditions. In the United States alone, it is estimated that approximately 1.5 million cases of pleural effusions are diagnosed annually, with 16% requiring thoracentesis.[105] Adults account for over 90% of the cases in the United States with the most frequent causes being congestive heart failure, bacterial infections (parapneumonic effusions), and pulmonary emboli.[106–108] Malignancy is the third most common cause of a pleural effusion and is reported in 15% of all cancer patients. In men, lung cancers are the most common malignancy associated with pleural effusion, and for women breast cancers are more common. Combined, these two cancer types account for 50% to 60% of all malignant pleural effusions seen in the United States.[109,110] Viral disease and postcardiac surgery are also common causes of pleural effusions in adults.[111,112] In children, pleural effusions are much more rare and the most predominate etiology is infectious; the incidence of pleural effusions due to congestive heart failure and malignancy in children is a much less frequent cause.[113] A number of less common diseases, such as systemic lupus and pulmonary arterial hypertension (idiopathic and familial), are associated with pleural effusions. Despite the broad etiology of pleural effusions, many are idiopathic and some (30%) have been determined to have multiple causes and underlying pathology.[114]

PATHOPHYSIOLOGY

Both the visceral and parietal pleurae play an important role in fluid homeostasis in the pleural space. Pleural effusions are caused by several physiologic mechanisms including increased pleural membrane permeability, decreased intrapleural pressure, decreased capillary oncotic pressure, obstructed lymphatic flow, or increased pulmonary capillary pressure. Pleural fluid production and movement across the pulmonary capillary is dynamically controlled by the delicate balance of the oncotic and hydrostatic forces within the pulmonary capillaries and pleural space.[115] Governed by Starling's law of fluid exchange, capillaries of the parietal pleura produce an estimated 5 to 10 L of serous fluid per day, most of which is reabsorbed by the lymphatic system. Fluid production from the parietal pleura increases in disease states that result in an imbalance of Starling's forces, an increase capillary hydrostatic pressure, decreased oncotic pressure (transudate) or increased capillary permeability (exudate). In addition, fluid can also enter the pleural space from the interstitial space of the visceral pleura (usually from heart failure), from the peritoneal cavity through a rupture of the diaphragm or the retroperitoneal space. Although the lymphatics have the capacity to reabsorb a significant amount of fluid, an accumulation of pleural fluid may result from not only an increase in production but also a decrease reabsorption such as obstruction of mediastinal lymph nodes. Therefore, the etiology of pleural effusions is quite varied and includes cardiovascular, nephrotic, infectious, and malignant disorders.

Based on the underlying physiologic process, pleural effusions are classified as either transudative or exudative. Transudative effusions are almost always associated with an imbalance of fluid forces (hydrostatic) or protein forces (oncotic) external to the pleural space. This imbalance leads to either an increase in capillary hydrostatic pressure, or a decrease in capillary oncotic pressure, or both, and fluid is pushed through the capillary. As a result, transudative fluid is characterized as extravascular fluid with a low nucleated cell count, low protein count, and low specific gravity.

Exudative effusions primarily result from a disease process, systemic or focal, that disrupts the integrity of the pleural capillary, increasing the permeability. Exudative fluid leaks around the cells of the capillary and, as a result, contains higher concentrations of protein and lactate dehydrogenase (LDH).

The analysis and differential classification of the pleural fluid are pivotal to determining the cause of the effusion.

MEDICAL HISTORY AND CLINICAL PRESENTATION

The clinical presentation is largely determined by the amount of fluid and the underlying disease process. The basic evaluation is directed by the probable causes suggested in the history and physical exam. The initial clinical history should include any recent respiratory infections or fever, especially pneumonia, as these will suggest a parapneumonic process. A history of congestive heart failure or renal or liver impairment suggests a transudative process. A thorough historical review of any pulmonary processes, including PH or PE, is essential. Specific queries about recent, unilateral leg swelling point to deep vein thrombosis and PE, whereas bilateral leg swelling suggests right-sided heart failure. A history of all malignancies (especially lung cancer, breast cancer, or lymphomas), weight loss, or smoking would point toward a neoplastic cause. Pleural effusions may be a symptom of mesothelioma and a thorough occupational history, including dates and amount of exposure to asbestos, should be elicited. Drug-induced lung toxicities also manifest as pleural effusions. There is an increasing list of drugs that may cause exudative effusions including nitrofurantoin, dantrolen, methysergide, amiodarone, inflximab, interleukin-2, procarbazine, methotrexate, clozapine, phenytoin; and therefore, a final important component of the medical history is a drug history, both prescription and illicit drug use.[116,117]

SIGNS AND SYMPTOMS

Signs and symptoms of a pleural effusion vary depending on the etiology. Symptoms and signs may be specific to the respiratory system or nonspecific. A small amount of fluid is usually asymptomatic, and depending on the degree of respiratory reserve, patients are asymptomatic even with a large accumulation of fluid.[118] In light of these variations, the three most common symptoms are dyspnea, cough, and pleuritic chest pain.

The temporal pattern of breathlessness can provide clues to the etiology of the effusion. For example, chronic exertional dyspnea, orthopnea, and nocturnal dyspnea that improve with standing are associated with congestive heart failure. The rapidity with which the exertional dyspnea develops is an important indicator. Rapid onset of dyspnea after exertion is associated with cardiac failure or pulmonary hypertension. The severity of the dyspnea loosely correlates with the effusion size. Breathlessness from pleural effusion, therefore, is likely to be multifactorial and related both to the mechanical distortion of the diaphragm and chest wall as well as to hypoxemia.[119]

Cough is an additional nonspecific symptom, however, cough associated with pleural effusion has been characterized as a mild and nonproductive cough. Conversely, more severe cough and appearance of purulent sputum suggest an infective etiology and would be accompanied by fever, sweating, and fatigue. A bloody sputum suggests an endotracheal lesion.

Pleuritic chest pain is characterized by sudden, sharp, stabbing or burning pain with respiration and implies a degree of inflammation of the parietal pleura. Pleuritic chest pain has many life-threatening causes including PE, myocardial infarction, aortic dissection, pneumothorax, pericarditis, and pneumonia.[120] A thorough evaluation of this pain should be performed to diagnose or exclude these causes.

TABLE 4.23 Differential Diagnosis for Pleural Effusions

Exudative Effusions	Transudative Effusions
Parapneumonic effusion (bacterial, viral, fungal, parasitic infection)	Congestive heart failure
Malignant neoplasm	Cirrhotic liver disease
Pulmonary emboli	Renal failure
Connective tissue disease	Nephrotic syndrome
Pancreatitis	Atelectasis
Postoperative (pulmonary or cardiac)	Hypothyroidism
Chylothorax	Pulmonary emboli
Trauma (esophageal rupture)	Cancer
Occupational exposure (asbestos)	Peritoneal dialysis
Subdiaphragmatic abscess	Hypoalbuminemia
Drug-induced	Superior vena cava obstruction
Ovarian hyperstimulation syndrome	Sarcoidosis
Iatrogenic (drug-induced, radiation therapy, medications)	Pericardial disease
Hemothorax	
Sarcoidosis	

PHYSICAL EXAMINATION

Pleural effusion can be diagnosed on physical examination. For all patients suspected to have a pleural effusion, a thorough exam of the chest should be performed.[121] The physical examination for pleural effusion should include inspection, palpation, percussion, and auscultation of the chest. In patients with a lot of fluid accumulation, chest inspection is notable for trachea shifted toward the opposite side and asymmetric chest expansion. Tachypnea may be present with large effusions as well. Decreased or absent tactile fremitus, dullness to percussion over the fluid area, and uni- or bilaterally diminished or absent breath sounds are also findings consistent with pleural effusion. A pleural friction rub may be heard on auscultation especially if there is an inflammatory process or after thoracentesis. Discontinuous sounds or crackles may also be heard with pleural effusions as distal airways collapse on exhalation and abruptly open during inspiration. Occasionally, egophony is observed at the edge of the effusion.

DIFFERENTIAL DIAGNOSIS

The differential diagnosis for pleural effusions is extensive (Table 4.23). A systematic and expeditious clinical assessment of the etiology of effusion is critical since some causes are associated with poor outcomes.

DIAGNOSTIC STUDIES

Lung imaging is the cornerstone diagnostic study for detecting pleural effusions. While pleural effusions may be diagnosed by physical exam, the chest exam can be challenging in critically ill patients and has a lower sensitivity and specificity than chest ultrasound and chest x-ray.[122] Comparatively, chest ultrasound is more sensitive and specific than chest x-ray. For detecting and determining the volume of fluid, the sensitivity of chest ultrasound is similar to that of CT.[123] CT and ultrasound will provide additional information on pleural thickening and abnormalities of nonpleural structures that will aid in distinguishing etiology.

Thoracentesis and fluid analysis are helpful for determining the physiologic basis of the effusion. The gross appearance of the fluid including the color, character, and odor will provide diagnostic clues. Milky white color is consistent with a high lipid level and suggests chylothorax, while dark green color suggests a biliothorax. Red, blood-stained fluid significantly narrows the differential down to malignancy, trauma and cardiac surgery, pulmonary emboli, and pneumonia. Turbid fluid consistent with cells or cell debris suggests an empyema and viscous fluid points to a mesothelioma. A putrid odor suggests anaerobic empyema and ammonia points to a urinothorax (Table 4.24).

Chemical and biochemical analysis of the fluid provides definitive information to help with the differential. Differentiating between a transudative and exudative process is critical in identifying the underlying cause. Light's criteria rule is a standardized method that compares serum and pleural protein and LDH concentrations to differentiate exudative from transudative effusion effusions.[124] Light's

TABLE 4.24 Diagnoses Established by Pleural Fluid Analysis

Pleural Fluid Analysis	Possible Diagnosis
Turbid to bloody, positive cytology	Malignancy
Turbid to purulent, putrid order and positive culture	Empyema
Ratio of pleural fluid to blood hematocrit >0.5	Hemothorax
Creatinine and pleural fluid creatinine/serum ratio >1 with a pH <7.30	Urinothorax
Milky fluid, presence of chylomicrons, triglycerides >110 mg/dL	Chylothorax
Clear to turbid, white blood cells, mostly polymorphonuclear leukocytes	Parapneumonic effusion
Acid-fast bacillus, adenosine deaminase level, *Mycobacterium tuberculosis* culture	Tuberculosis
Amylase	Pancreatitis, malignancy, esophageal perforation, or tuberculosis
N-terminal pro-brain natriuretic peptide level	Congestive heart failure
Low glucose	Rheumatoid pleurisy Malignant effusion Tuberculous pleurisy Lupus pleuritis Esophageal rupture Complicated parapneumonic effusion or empyema
pH and glucose	pH <7.20 and glucose <60 mg/dL complicated parapneumonic process or empyema
Adenosine deaminase	Malignant vs. tuberculous pleurisy

criteria is 100% sensitive for diagnosing exudative fluid and 93% to 96% sensitive for differentiating between exudative from transudative fluids (Table 4.24).[125] There are times, however, when pleural fluids are misclassified. In congestive heart failure patients on long-term diuretics, for example, the transudate fluid is misclassified as an exudate in 25% of the cases (Box 4.4).[125] Using a modified criterion of serum minus pleural protein concentration level of <3.1 g/dL, rather than a serum/pleural fluid ratio of >0.5, corrects the misidentification.[126] Other factors including local anesthetics, contaminants, and presence of air may confound the pleural fluid values and therefore analysis should always be performed with the clinical context in mind.

Besides protein and LDH, other chemical and biochemical markers of the pleural fluid can provide useful diagnostic information. These measures include total protein concentrations, cholesterol, triglycerides, glucose, creatinine, pH, amylase, adenosine deaminase, NT-pro-BNP, procalcitonin, cancer-related biomarkers, cytology nucleated cells, lymphocytosis, eosinophilia. When an infectious process is suspected, Gram stain and cultures may be used to identify a causative pathogen (Table 4.24).

BOX 4.4 Exudate

At least one of the following criteria is present
Pleural fluid protein/serum protein ratio >0.5
Pleural lactate dehydrogenase (LDH)/serum LDH ratio >0.6
Pleural fluid LDH > two-thirds the upper limits of the laboratory's normal serum LDH

If the results of the fluid analysis are unclear and the pleural effusion remains undiagnosed, percutaneous pleural biopsy or thoracoscopy may be necessary.

EVALUATION

Pleural effusions develop from a variety of systemic, inflammatory, infectious, and malignant conditions. Clinical assessment alone is sometimes capable of identifying transudative effusions but often precise etiologic diagnosis depends on a combination of medical history, physical examination, and imaging test. Pleura effusions are associated with high short-term and long-term mortality rates, and prompt evaluation and management are critical.[127]

History and physical exam findings are suggestive of pleural effusion. If a pleural effusion is suspected, imaging is required to confirm the diagnosis and guide pleural interventions. Standard posteroanterior and lateral chest radiography or more reliable ultrasonography of the thorax are the most important techniques for initial diagnosis. Fluid analysis is always indicated when the cause of the effusion is unclear or in the setting of suspected infection. If imaging and fluid analysis are inconclusive, a pleural biopsy is usually necessary, especially in the diagnosis of malignant effusions. In cancer patients, if the initial cytologic examination is negative, video-assisted thoracoscopy is performed for the direct inspection of the pleural surface and possible pleural abrasion.

TREATMENT

If possible, the initial strategy is to treat the underlying disorder. Treatment depends on the primary condition including antibiotic therapy, diuretics, ultrafiltration, or anticoagulation. In symptomatic patients, a large-volume thoracentesis and/or insertion of a pleural drain may be necessary. Asymptomatic patients and patients with transudative pleural effusions, in general, do not require tube thoracostomy or pleural interventions but are closely followed (every 3 to 6 weeks) for clinical and radiographic changes.[115] In symptomatic patients with persistent recurrent effusions multiple thoracenteses are not recommended. For these patients, chemical pleurodesis or indwelling pleural catheter placement may be required.[128]

PATIENT EDUCATION

- Pleural effusion is sometimes called "water-on-the-lungs" because of an accumulation of fluid in the pleural cavity, which is the space lined by two membranes that enclose the lungs.

- Pleural effusions are common and several diseases can cause a pleural effusion. Heart failure is the most common cause. Pneumonia, cancer, and clots in the lungs are other causes.
- The most common symptoms of pleural effusion are sharp chest pain with breathing, shortness of breath and/or rapid breathing and a dry cough.
- The seriousness of the condition depends on the primary cause.
- X-ray or other imaging modalities such as ultrasound, CT, or MRI are required to evaluate the amount of fluid and make the definitive diagnosis.
- Sometimes, a small sample of the fluid will need to be removed for analysis to determine the cause.
- The treatment is based on the symptoms, the amount of fluid around the lungs, and the underlying cause.
- If there is difficulty breathing, a needle is used to remove the fluid from the chest cavity.
- If the disease is caused by an infection or heart failure then medications such as antibiotics and diuretics can be used to treat the effusion.
- Large volume effusions may require a tube to drain the fluid from the chest over a period of a few days.
- Recurrent effusions occasionally require a drug that stops the fluid formation by scaring the lining of the lung in a procedure called pleural sclerosis or pleurodesis.
- Occasionally, fluid accumulation is ongoing, especially in cases caused by cancer. In these cases, a semipermanent, flexible tube and collection bag, left in place for a longer period, may be required. This will allow patients to manage the fluid removal at home.

4.10B PNEUMOTHORAX

OVERVIEW

Pneumothorax refers to the abnormal collection of gas, usually air, in the pleural space and subsequent collapse of the lung. It may occur in young, apparently healthy adults or in older adults as a result of diffuse lung disease. Accordingly, the clinical presentation varies tremendously depending on the diverse etiology and may be encountered by clinicians in several specialties and a spectrum of severity. This condition can quickly lead to impaired ventilation, oxygenation, and hemodynamic compromise. Early diagnosis and treatment are important to prevent morbidity associated with this potentially fatal complication.

EPIDEMIOLOGY

The two major etiologic forms of pneumothorax are nonspontaneous that occur with known precipitating factors and spontaneous, with no obvious precipitating factors. While each form has varying and unique epidemiologic data and is further subdivided, nonspontaneous pneumothoraces are more common and are considered medical emergencies.

Nonspontaneous pneumothorax can be further divided into traumatic and iatrogenic. In a trauma situation, pneumothorax should not be overlooked as it is the most common life-threatening injury in blunt thoracic trauma and can be seen in approximately 40% to 50% of all penetrating and nonpenetrating chest traumas.[129–131] The cause of the high mortality and morbidity rates in chest traumas is mostly due to delayed pulmonary complications.[132,133]

In the hospital setting, several invasive procedures have been known to cause nonspontaneous iatrogenic pneumothorax including central venous line placement, nasogastric tube placements, pleural aspiration, and biopsy and is more common in mechanically ventilated patients.[134,135] Understandably, most patients with pneumothorax related to mechanical ventilation have more severe underlying lung diseases; however, pneumothorax was found to be an independent predictor of mortality during mechanical ventilation.[136] Not surprisingly, at training hospitals incidence of iatrogenic pneumothorax is proportional to the number of invasive procedures and patients on mechanical ventilation.[137]

Spontaneous pneumothorax is the sudden onset of a collapsed lung without an apparent cause or history of trauma. Spontaneous pneumothorax is further subdivided into primary and secondary, which have varying epidemiologic data. Primary spontaneous pneumothorax occurs in people without underlying respiratory disease, while secondary spontaneous pneumothorax occurs in the presence of respiratory disease.

Primary spontaneous pneumothorax in the absence of clinically apparent lung disease is one of the most common diseases affecting young adults and a significant health burden.[138] Annual incidence rates of 22.7 per 100,000 has been reported with a male-to-female ratio of 3.3:1[139] with the average age of 34 years old for males and 40 for females.[139,140] In addition to age and gender, additional risk factors for primary pneumothorax include tall and thin body habitus and smoking. Some inherited conditions increase the risk of primary pneumothorax including Marfan syndrome, α-1 antitrypsin deficiency, cystic fibrosis, Ehlers-Danlos syndrome, tuberous sclerosis, and homocysteinuria.[141] Readmission and recurrence rates are high (~30%) with a greater percentage occurring within the first year and strong evidence that female sex was a risk factor for recurrence.[142–145]

Secondary pneumothorax is a complication of a preexisting lung disease and more commonly affects the older adult. Similar to primary pneumothorax, secondary pneumothorax is more frequently seen in males; however, the peak incidence occurs later in life (>55 years of age). Secondary pneumothorax is commonly associated with COPD and the severity of COPD correlates with an increase in risk. COPD patients, in general, are at a higher risk of nonspontaneous, iatrogenic pneumothorax. In addition to COPD, the incidence of secondary pneumothorax is high in patients with cystic fibrosis and severe pulmonary disease including pneumonia, connective tissue disease–associated interstitial disease, lymphoma, or other malignancies.[146–148] Because it occurs in patients suffering from diffuse lung disease, secondary spontaneous pneumothorax induces respiratory failure more frequency than primary spontaneous pneumothorax and is a potentially life-threatening condition associated with substantially greater morbidity and mortality rates.[139]

Pneumothorax can occur in neonates and is a life-threatening condition associated with a high morbidity rate. It has an overall neonatal incidence rate of 1% to 2% and increases to >40% in infants with respiratory distress syndrome undergoing intermittent positive pressure ventilation.[149,150]

PATHOPHYSIOLOGY

The pleural space is a negative pressure, fluid-filled space. A pneumothorax is the presence of air or gas in the pleural space due a breach in the visceral or parietal pleura, either by trauma or spontaneous rupture. Normally, throughout the respiratory cycle, the intrapleural pressure remains subatmospheric due to two distinct forces of the inward elastic recoil of the lungs and the outward expansion of the chest wall. These opposing forces provide a slight suction on the lung to keep it expanded throughout the respiratory cycle. Air does not normally exist in the intrapleural space as the net driving pressures direct inspired gases down the pressure gradient from the alveolus through the pulmonary capillary and into the blood. In a pneumothorax, air enters the pleural space from loss of integrity of the chest wall or alveolar sac. When communication avenues develop air flows down the pressure gradient and into the pleural space. The air-flow leak into the pleural space results in an increase in the pleural pressure and compresses the lung tissue. Pneumothorax can occur from air leaks from injuries to the chest and rib fractures or from spontaneous alveolar rupture. The exact pathogenesis of spontaneous alveolar rupture is unclear. It has been proposed that subpleural defects, blebs or bulla, or macroscopically occult pleuropulmonary changes combined with increased shearing forces are predisposing factors that lead to spontaneous alveolar rupture and are the leak source.[151–153]

Tension pneumothorax is a life-threatening rapid accumulation of air in the pleural space and is commonly seen in mechanically ventilated patients. The positive pressure from the mechanical ventilation will increase gas flow through pleura defects. The pleural defects may function as a one-way valve, air enters the pleural space on inspiration but is unable to exit on expiration. This will lead to increasing ipsilateral intrapleural pressure over time and lead to displaced mediastinal structures and contralateral lung compression, chest wall expansion, diaphragmatic depression, and hemodynamic collapse.[130,135,136]

Clinically, the main physiologic change associated with pneumothorax is dependent on the degree of lung collapse. Collapse of the lung results in a decrease in total lung capacity, vital capacity, and oxygenation (PaO_2). Total cross-sectional area of the lung will decrease, which results in a decrease in diffusion capacity.

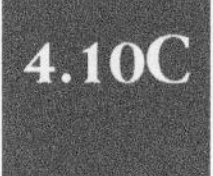

4.10C PRIMARY SPONTANEOUS PNEUMOTHORAX

MEDICAL HISTORY AND CLINICAL PRESENTATION

The clinical presentation and medical history vary depending on the type of pneumothorax. Development of spontaneous pneumothorax is closely correlated with underlying disease, the onset is usually abrupt, and patients often present with acute onset dyspnea and pleuritic chest pain localized to the ipsilateral side. The chest pain typically resolves within 24 hours. Some patients, especially the younger population, may be asymptomatic. The severity of the symptoms depends on the extent of the collapse, the degree of pulmonary reserve, and preexisting lung disease. Symptoms usually occur at rest but may develop during activities including air travel, exercise, scuba diving or after a traumatic event or surgical procedure.

To determine the etiology, a thorough history of significant risk factors including recent accident or trauma, smoking, malignancies, COPD, infection (especially HIV, *Pneumocystis jirovecii*, toxoplasmosis, and Kaposi sarcoma), illicit drug use, air travel should be considered. A history of prior pneumothorax is important as the recurrence rate is high.[142]

SIGNS AND SYMPTOMS

Depending on the degree of involvement, there is a wide range of signs and symptoms of a patient with pneumothorax. Symptoms range from minimal or absent to severe respiratory distress. Chest pain and dyspnea are the most common symptoms.

Chest pain is described as sudden and sharp, unilateral, and pleuritic in nature.

Additional physical signs can be subtle and include reduced lung expansion, hyperresonance, diminished breath sounds, dyspnea, cyanosis, sweating, tachypnea, and tachycardia. Signs of tension pneumothorax are usually more remarkable and consist of chest expansion, hypotension, and hypoxia. Additional signs of hemodynamic instability include jugular venous distention. Patients who progress to this critical state may appear fatigued and anxious.

PHYSICAL EXAMINATION

The physical examination findings will depend on both the degree of lung involvement and preexisting lung disease and therefore do not necessarily correlate with the degree of collapse. Therefore, physical exam findings are variable and range from normal to severe respiratory distress. While small pneumothoraces may not be detectable on physical exam, a large collapse will result in unequal breath sounds, hyperresonance with percussion in the ipsilateral chest wall with asymmetric lung expansion and decreased tactile fremitus. The accuracy and utility of these physical exam findings are limited in a critical setting with a lot of background noise. Cardiovascular findings include tachycardia, pulsus paradoxus, hypotension, and jugular venous distention. Cardiac apical displacement is observed when mediastinal structures are displaced.

DIFFERENTIAL DIAGNOSIS

The differential diagnosis for pneumothorax is summarized in Table 4.25.

DIAGNOSTIC STUDIES

Thoracic imagings the essential procedure in the diagnosis of a pneumothorax (Table 4.26).[154] Although chest CT scanning may be more sensitive in detecting a small pneumothorax, because they are simple, rapid, relatively inexpensive and easy to use, chest radiographs are usually the most common and preferred initial imaging modality in hemodynamically stable patients with a suspected pneumothorax. The initial image should be an upright film and when not definitively observed on an inspiratory film, the pneumothorax may become more visible on expiratory projections. Timely bedside ultrasound testing can also be performed. It has a greater sensitivity compared to the chest radiograph, may be performed within minutes, and is useful in the setting of critically ill, unstable patients. In patients with an uncertain diagnosis following initial imaging, a chest CT may facilitate the diagnosis. If an emergent tube thracostomy is

TABLE 4.25 Differential Diagnosis for Pneumothorax

Diagnosis	Description
Acute aortic dissection	The catastrophic separation of laminal planes of the aortic wall
Acute coronary syndrome	Spectrum of catastrophic clinical presentations resulting from the rupture of an atherosclerotic plaque within the coronary artery leading to partial or complete obstruction of blood flow to the myocardium
Asthma	Chronic disease characterized by variable airflow obstruction that is usually reversible and caused by inflammation and bronchial hyperresponsiveness that is usually reversible
Aspiration pneumonia	Pulmonary complications due to the entry of gastric or oropharyngeal fluids into the lower airways
Chronic obstructive pulmonary disease (COPD), acute exacerbation	Acute resistance to airflow and worsening of respiratory symptoms beyond daily variations
Esophageal perforation	Breach or tear of the esophageal wall
Myocardial infarction	Irreversible necrosis of the myocardium resulting from ischemia
Myocardial ischemia	Reversible imbalance between the coronary blood supply and myocardial oxygen demand
Pericarditis	Inflammation of the pericardium
Pulmonary embolism	A blood clot in the pulmonary vasculature that occludes the pulmonary arteries and obstructs blood flow to the lungs
Pleural empyema and effusion	Inflammatory fluid and debris in the pleural space
Rib fracture	A crack or break in a bone in the thorax
Tuberculosis	A multisystemic infectious disease caused by the bacillus *Mycobacterium tuberculosis*

performed, a rush of air or bubbling in the chest drain after insertion confirms the diagnosis.

EVALUATION

The diagnosis of pneumothorax is based on clinical suspicion and the history and physical examination are key to the diagnosis. Clinical interpretation of the presenting signs and symptoms is crucial for the correct diagnosis. Since the typical signs and symptoms may be minor or absent, a high index of suspicion is required early in the evaluation. Initially, the airway and hemodynamic stability of the patients must be assessed, especially trauma victims. Unstable patients with a clinical high suspicion of a pneumothorax require urgent decompression with needle decompression or tube thoracostomy before imaging. In stable patients, the presence of the pneumothorax should be confirmed by imaging, which will also provide information on the extent and possible cause.

TABLE 4.26 Diagnostic Tests for Pneumothorax

Diagnostic Test	Testing Parameters
Arterial blood gas (ABG)	Evaluate the degree of hypoxemia, acidemia, and hypercarbia
Pulse oximetry	Evaluate the degree of hypoxemia
Chest x-ray	A diagnostic test used in the majority of cases to confirm and localize the pneumothorax
Ultrasound	Sensitive and specific portable and rapid diagnostic test that is useful in an acute, emergent setting
CT	A more sensitive test with greater image resolution; useful in detecting small pneumothoraces, pneumomediastinum, and uncertain or complex cases and calculation of pneumothorax size; also used for detecting occult traumatic pneumothorax

TREATMENT

Treatment of a pneumothorax depends not only on the clinical setting but also on the etiology and associated comorbidities. Importantly, management depends on the clinical status of the patient and the size of the pneumothorax. If the pneumothorax is considered clinically significant (moderate-to-large) treatment consists of an interventional drainage, simple aspiration, and sometimes surgical intervention.[154] Recently, initial drainage in patients with moderate-to-large pneumothorax has been challenged in favor of a more conservative approach, especially in patients without clinically significant symptoms or hemodynamic instability.[155,156] Active intervention is recommended in patients with any size pneumothorax and significant breathlessness.

Observation and supplemental oxygen therapy are recommended for all patients with a pneumothorax. Oxygen therapy accelerates the rate of pleural air absorption. In asymptomatic patients with small pneumothoraces, oxygen administration is usually the only treatment needed.

- Observation
- Supplemental oxygen
- Treatment of the underlying lung disease
- Simple aspiration
- Tube or catheter thoracostomy
- Thoracoscopy
- Mechanical ventilation

PATIENT EDUCATION

- The area surrounding the lungs is a fluid-filled space called the pleural cavity.
- The pleural space is important to normal lung function.
- A pneumothorax occurs when air leaks into this space and causes part or all of the lung to collapse.
- There are several reasons why this occurs including a spontaneous collapse or damage to traumatic damage to the lining or chest wall. In some cases, underlying lung disease can also cause the lung to collapse.
- The symptoms of a pneumothorax include chest pain and shortness of breath or difficulty breathing. Sometimes breathing and heart rate will increase and the patient may have a cough.

- The more severe cases of a pneumothorax result in a decrease in blood pressure, a blue tinge to the lips or skin, and collapse.
- The condition can be diagnosed through physical examination, listening to the lung. Noninvasive imaging studies such as a chest x-ray or ultrasound will also be done to provide more detailed pictures of the lung.
- Depending on the severity of the conditions, the patient may be given supplemental oxygen and observed. In more severe cases the leak will need to be repaired and the lungs inflated. These procedures require more invasive techniques and may require hospitalization.
- The long-term outcome is good, although there may be an increased risk for recurrence.
- Call 9-1-1 if someone is experiencing a sudden, sharp pain in the chest, severe shortness of breath or trouble breathing, a bluish tinge to skin, fainting, or a rapid heart rate.

4.11 SLEEP APNEA

OVERVIEW

Sleep apnea is a serious, common, underdiagnosed sleep disorder that is characterized by disordered breathing resulting in numerous hypoxic episodes throughout sleep preventing the patient from restorative sleep. It is characterized by loud frequent snoring and excessive daytime sleepiness. There are two specific types: obstructive sleep apnea (OSA) resulting from intermittent upper airway obstruction, and central sleep apnea, resulting from intermittent apneas or hypopneas from intermittent disruption of brain signals to the pulmonary muscles. OSA is more common than central sleep apnea. Untreated sleep apnea can lead to high blood pressure, heart disease, stroke, diabetes, and depression.

EPIDEMIOLOGY

OSA is defined by an apnea-hypopnea index (AHI) of ≥5 and is more common in men than women. In the general adult population the incidence was estimated to be 3% to 7% in men and 2% to 5% in women.[157,158] The incidence of OSA increases in certain high-risk groups including patients with obesity and patients with coronary artery disease and diabetes. Men are at higher risk for OSA due to the male habitus, which includes higher incidence of a bull neck and central adiposity. The incidence of OSA rises more quickly in women after menopause so that it is closer to that for men.[159]

In a study by Peppard et al. using data from the Wisconsin Sleep Cohort Study estimated that the incidence of moderate to severe disordered breathing (an apnea-hypopnea index of ≥15) was 10% among 30- to 49-year-old men, 17% among 50- to 70-year-old men, 3% among 30- to 49-year-old women, and 9% among 50- to 70-year-old women.[161] This represents an increased incidence of sleep-disordered breathing of between 14% and 55% depending upon subgroup.[158] The risk of OSA increases with increased age. The prevalence of OSA in persons >65 years of age increases about two to three times compared to that for younger persons for a varied increase from 7% to 40%.[157,160]

There is a definite correlation between obesity and the incidence of OSA. With the rise in obesity rates, OSA, according to the National Healthy Sleep Awareness Project now affects at least 25 million adults in the United States and it continues to increase.[161]

OSA also varies by race. Comparatively, there is a higher incidence of OSA in younger Black individuals compared to Caucasians of the same age, independent of body mass index (BMI).[162]

PATHOPHYSIOLOGY

The physiologic mechanisms of OSA are not fully understood but are multifactorial, including both anatomic and neuromuscular causes. They include upper airway anatomy, the ability of the upper airway dilator muscles to respond to respiratory challenge during sleep, the arousal threshold, and the stability of the respiratory control system.[163]

OSA is caused by either an intermittent partial or complete obstruction of the soft tissue of the pharynx during sleep. The pharynx lacks bony support allowing it to collapse, most notably in the portion from the hard palate to the larynx, especially in a narrower airway anatomy with decreased musculature response to negative pharyngeal pressure.[163] Decreased neuromuscular reflexive response is more pronounced in OSA and is a major component leading to obstruction.[164,165] The obstruction can be exacerbated by a crowded oropharynx from the tongue or enlarged tonsils. The obstruction causes decreased airflow resulting in loud snoring and apneic spells resulting in hypoxia stimulating the sympathetic nervous system. The patient startles, creating a partial arousal, which stimulates the pharyngeal muscle response. This happens in a cyclical pattern throughout the night preventing restorative sleep patterns resulting in daytime drowsiness. The patient constantly vacillates between disordered breathing and wakefulness. Apneas and hypopneas can occur during both REM and non-REM sleep. However, they are increased and more pronounced during REM sleep. More severe events result in longer arousals, which relate to more severe daytime sleepiness.[163]

Central sleep apnea (CSA) is not as common as OSA. Unlike OSA, which is caused by obstructed airflow resulting in apnea and hypopneas, CSA is caused by intermittent periods of absent inspiratory drive creating decreased ventilation and apneas and hypopneas. Just as in OSA, the apneas and hypopneas occur intermittently throughout the night, preventing restorative sleep patterns, with multiple arousals and is associated with daytime somnolence.

Inspiratory drive is regulated by signals from the central chemoreceptors in the brainstem, signals from the peripheral chemoreceptors and the respiratory muscles. Diseases, metabolic derangements, and drugs can affect any one of these levels causing depression of the inspiratory drive and precipitate CSA.[166]

Respiratory drive is regulated with chemoreceptor input centrally responding to changes in CO_2 and peripherally at the carotid body responding to changes in PaO_2 and $PaCO_2$. While chemosensitivity can vary among individuals, highly sensitive chemoresponses place an individual at risk for unstable breathing patterns.[166] Patients who have daytime hypercapnia can experience increased hypercapnia during sleep in turn causing hypoventilation. Physiologically, this can be classified as an "abnormal central pattern generator," impairing the brain from initiating stimulus to breath or an "abnormal respiratory pattern generator" causing impairment of the motor pathways that initiate the act of breathing.[166]

Several things can cause an abnormal central pattern generator. They include insults to the brainstem, including tumor, infarction, congenital malformations, and trauma. Other offenders include congenital central hypoventilation syndrome, drugs that have a respiratory depressant effect, especially opioids, and obesity hypoventilation syndrome.

There are several conditions that can cause an abnormal respiratory pattern generator, impacting peripherally from the upper motor neurons to the respiratory muscles affecting the physical work of breathing. This includes neuromuscular disorders—myasthenia gravis, amyotrophic lateral sclerosis, post-polio syndrome, and Guillain-Barré syndrome. Also, conditions that affect the chest wall and its integrity can impact the work of breathing and cause hypoventilation.

Congestive heart failure is frequently associated with CSA, which often exhibits Cheyne-Stokes respiration. CSA has historically been considered a marker for heart disease.[167] While cardiovascular disease is typically related to OSA, congestive heart failure is more closely linked with CSA.

Sleep apnea results in considerable hypoxia from frequent desaturations. This hypoxia can stimulate an increase in sympathetic tone causing rises in blood pressure, rises in pulmonary arterial pressure from pulmonary vasoconstriction, and arrhythmias.

MEDICAL HISTORY AND CLINICAL PRESENTATION

Patients with OSA are typically male, obese, middle-aged and beyond, who complain of daytime somnolence and nonrestorative sleep despite adequate hours of sleep. Bed partners characteristically complain of loud snoring and frequently observe periods of apnea with partial arousals from sleep and restless sleep with tossing and turning. Because of daytime sleepiness, napping is common, especially when the patient is sitting without stimulation.

Patients with a history of obesity, hypothyroidism, and cigarette smoking are at increased risk of OSA. Postmenopausal women are also at risk. It can be exacerbated by alcohol, sleep medications, and conditions that can cause nasal obstruction. It is also commonly associated with hypertension, type 2 diabetes, stroke, coronary artery disease, and congestive heart failure.

SIGNS AND SYMPTOMS

The most common patient complaint is overwhelming sense of fatigue and exhaustion that manifests as morning sluggishness, daytime sleepiness, and frequent naps despite sleeping many hours at night. Because of the nonrestorative sleep, patients frequently complain of decreased mental sharpness and memory loss, poor judgment, inability to concentrate, personality changes including depression, and headache. Other complaints may include decreased libido and erectile dysfunction, morning dry or sore throat, and dyspepsia.

PHYSICAL EXAMINATION

The physical examination often is normal other than the signs of obesity, which include an elevated BMI of >30 kg/m^2 and an increased neck circumference >17 inches in men and 15 inches in women.

Evaluation should include an assessment of the upper airway. The oropharynx should be inspected for crowding with tonsillar enlargement, excessive soft tissue, and enlarged uvula or tongue. Nasal obstruction from a deviated nasal septum should be evaluated.

Additional assessments in the physical examination should include arterial blood pressure and pulmonary, cardiac, and peripheral vascular examination to look for concomitant conditions including hypertension, pulmonary hypertension and cor pulmonale, coronary artery disease, congestive heart failure, and arterial vascular disease.

DIFFERENTIAL DIAGNOSIS

The differential diagnosis of sleep apnea is summarized in Table 4.27.

DIAGNOSTIC STUDIES

The gold standard test for the diagnosis of sleep apnea is polysomnography (PSG). According to recommendations by the American College of Physicians, patients complaining of daytime sleepiness should undergo a sleep study.[168] PSG can be completed either in a sleep lab or at home depending on comorbidities. The advantage of the sleep lab is that it monitors for conditions other than OSA, including CSA, periodic limb movement, and restless legs syndrome.

The AHI measures the number apneas or hypopneas per hour during sleep. It is used to diagnose OSA. A diagnosis of OSA can be made with an AHI ≥15 or AHI ≥5 with symptoms or cardiovascular comorbidities.[169] Patients with OSA will have apneic episodes on PSG with respiratory muscle effort.

The evaluation of airflow and respiratory muscle activity measured on by PSG is used to evaluate CSA. The diagnosis

TABLE 4.27 Differential Diagnosis for Sleep Apnea

Diagnosis	Description
Narcolepsy	A sleep disorder characterized by daytime tiredness and sudden onset of sleep attacks.
Obesity-hypoventilation syndrome	A condition of hypercapnia caused by failure to breathe deeply from severe obesity. The hypercapnia causes fatigue and somnolence.
Periodic limb movement disorder	A sleep disorder characterized by involuntary periodic limb movements during sleep preventing restorative sleep and causing daytime fatigue.
Chronic hypersomnia	An idiopathic, chronic debilitating neurologic disorder characterized by excessive sleep and daytime somnolence.
Simple snoring	Partial collapse of the soft tissue of the upper airway leads to turbulent airflow that causes snoring.
Hypothyroidism	An endocrine disorder caused by failure of the thyroid gland resulting in low levels of thyroxine and depressed metabolism causing fatigue.
Depression	A psychiatric disorder caused by a disruption of neurotransmitters causing a depressed mood, fatigue, personality changes and trouble concentrating.
Hypersomnia due to substance abuse	Substance abuse can exaggerate the symptoms of hypersomnia leading to daytime drowsiness.

of CSA can be made with the cessation of airflow for 10 seconds with no respiratory muscle effort.[170]

Laboratory studies are not usually helpful with the diagnosis of sleep apnea. Thyroid studies should be ordered to exclude hypothyroidism. Erythrocytosis is a common finding with moderate to severe sleep apnea.

EVALUATION

The evaluation of sleep apnea begins with a high index of clinical suspicion in patients with daytime sleepiness or existing comorbidities. A thorough history and physical exam should be obtained. Patients should be screened for undiagnosed hypothyroidism and depression. Integrating a patient questionnaire, like the Epworth Sleepiness Scale or STOP-BANG, can be helpful in the evaluation of sleep apnea. A consultation with a sleep specialist and a PSG should be obtained to confirm the diagnosis.

TREATMENT

- Weight loss, when necessary, should involve reduction in caloric intake and exercise. Medical or surgical treatment may need to be considered in the severely obese patient who fails to lose weight with conservative treatment.
- Continuous positive airway pressure (CPAP) is the most effective treatment for sleep apnea by keeping the upper airway open with airway pressure.
- Oral appliances can be effective by repositioning the mandible and moving the tongue and soft palate forward.
- Surgical options include uvulopalatopharyngoplasty (UPPP), nasal septoplasty, or tracheostomy for patients who cannot tolerate or fail to respond to nonsurgical treatments.

PATIENT EDUCATION

- Patients should be educated on the serious nature of sleep apnea and the risk of comorbidities from untreated sleep apnea.
- Patients should be apprised of the benefits in weight reduction and its positive impact on better sleep.
- Patients should be educated to avoid alcohol and sedating drugs, which can worsen daytime sleepiness.
- Patients should be encouraged practice good sleep hygiene and avoid sleeping on their back to improve sleep.

SPECIAL CONSIDERATIONS

Sleep apnea is less common in children. However, as the population continues to become more obese, the incidence in children will likely increase. Sleep apnea from enlarged tonsils and adenoids is less common in adults; it is more frequent in children even without being obese. Children with Down syndrome and other craniofacial syndromes are at higher risk for sleep apnea.

KEY POINTS

- Sleep apnea is an underrecognized and underdiagnosed medical condition.
- It is an important disease that can lead to high blood pressure, heart disease, stroke, diabetes, and depression.
- The gold standard test for the diagnosis of sleep apnea is PSG.
- CPAP is the most effective treatment for sleep apnea by keeping the upper airway open with airway pressure.

4.12 RESPIRATORY DISTRESS

OVERVIEW

Acute respiratory distress syndrome (ARDS) was first coined in 1967 by Ashbaugh et al. as "an acute onset of tachypnea, hypoxemia, and loss of compliance after a variety of stimuli."[171] ARDS is an acute inflammatory lung process that leads to pulmonary edema, causing refractory and severe hypoxemia, increasing lung stiffness, and impairs the ability of the lung to eliminate carbon dioxide.[172]

EPIDEMIOLOGY

Studies have demonstrated that up to 5% of hospitalized, mechanically ventilated patients have been diagnosed with ARDS.[173] Additionally, a majority of studies show that of those diagnosed with ARDS, about 25% have been diagnosed with mild ARDS whereas up to 75% have been diagnosed with moderate or severe ARDS.[173] Approximately one-third of patients with mild ARDS will progress to moderate or severe ARDS.[173] Hospital mortality rate associated with ARDS is 40%.[173] The incidence of ARDS varies widely across the globe. Studies have shown substantially lower incidences of ARDS in Australia/New Zealand and Europe as compared with the United States.[173] Reasons for the vast differences in ARDS incidences remains unclear.[173]

PATHOPHYSIOLOGY

There are three overlapping stages in the natural history of ARDS: exudative, proliferative, and fibrotic.[173] The exudative phase represents the acute inflammatory stage of ARDS.[173] Direct or indirect lung insults initiate the exudative phase. These include but are not limited to severe sepsis, multiple blood transfusions, pneumonia, aspiration of gastric contents, lung contusion, toxic inhalation, pancreatitis, or trauma. The exudative phase is characterized by the release of proinflammatory cytokines, influx of neutrophils, and impaired endothelial cell barrier function.[173] Respiratory failure that occurs during this phase is attributed to accumulation of protein-rich fluid in distal airspaces and decreased surfactant production.[173] The fluid accumulation is most prominent in dependent areas of the lung. The proliferative phase develops 2 to 7 days after the initial lung insult and can last up to 21 days.[173] It is characterized by early fibrotic changes and thickening of the alveolar capillaries.[173] In some individuals, the proliferative phase will progress to the fibrotic phase. The fibrotic phase is associated with increased collagen deposition.[173] During this phase, progressive tissue fibrosis occurs and, in some cases, necessitates prolonged mechanical ventilatory support.[173]

Infant respiratory distress syndrome is due to a deficiency of surfactant. The production of surfactant starts at 24 to 25 weeks of gestation and is produced by type 2 pneumocytes.[174] Surfactant reaches adequate levels to support breathing by 36 to 37 weeks of gestation.[174] Therefore, when infants are born at <36 weeks' gestation, the underdeveloped lungs are unable to produce sufficient surfactant to maintain adequate breathing.[174] The deficiency of surfactant leads to poorly compliant lungs due to widespread alveolar collapse.[174]

4.12A ADULT RESPIRATORY DISTRESS SYNDROME

MEDICAL HISTORY AND CLINICAL PRESENTATION

ARDS is marked by the rapid onset of profound dyspnea that usually occurs 12 to 48 hours after onset of the initiating event. Bacterial or viral pneumonia is the most common cause of ARDS.[175]

SIGNS AND SYMPTOMS

Signs and symptoms of ARDS include those of respiratory distress. Tachypnea, labored breathing, and intercostal retractions are present. Respiratory distress progresses to respiratory failure with marked hypoxemia, despite adequate supplemental oxygen support.

PHYSICAL EXAMINATION

On physical examination labored breathing, tachypnea, and intercostal retractions are often noted. Bilateral crackles are heard upon lung auscultation.

DIFFERENTIAL DIAGNOSIS

The diagnosis of ARDS is often clinically challenging and therefore differential diagnosis does not strictly apply. Diagnostic studies should be done to rule out cardiogenic pulmonary edema, bilateral pneumonia, or disseminated malignancy.

DIAGNOSTIC STUDIES

Chest radiography is important and shows diffuse bilateral consolidations of the lung tissue. Arterial blood gas is a useful diagnostic test as it assesses the degree of hypoxemia.

EVALUATION

A thorough history and physical exam should be taken by the clinician. Signs of acute cardiogenic pulmonary edema and pneumonia should be assessed. Comprehensive laboratory studies including CBC, comprehensive metabolic panel (CMP), and arterial blood gas (ABG) should be collected. Chest radiography should be done to assess for pulmonary infiltrates or pulmonary edema. Although CT is not necessary to diagnose ARDS, it can help to rule out other causes of hypoxemia including pneumonia or pancreatitis. Echocardiography should be considered to assess cardiac function and rule out a cardiogenic pulmonary edema.

The Berlin definition recommends the use of three categories of ARDS, based on the degree of hypoxemia determined by the PaO_2/FiO_2 ratio. ABG collection is necessary to calculate this ratio. Mild ARDS is characterized by PaO_2/FiO_2 >200 mm Hg but ≤300 mm Hg. Moderate ARDS is defined as PaO_2/FiO_2 >100 mm Hg, but ≤200 mm Hg and severe ARDS is defined as PaO_2/FiO_2 ≤100 mm Hg.[175]

TREATMENT

- Treatment strategies for ARDS focus on identifying and treating the underlying etiology and secondary conditions and providing supportive care that reduces the progression of lung injury.[173]
- Mechanical ventilation remains the cornerstone of therapy.[176]
- Use of lower tidal volumes per breath, calculated using predicted body weight and lower inspiratory pressures, is recommended for all patients with ARDS.[176]
- For patients with severe ARDS, prone positioning is recommended for at least 12 hours per day.[176]

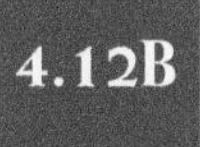

4.12B INFANT RESPIRATORY DISTRESS SYNDROME

MEDICAL HISTORY AND CLINICAL PRESENTATION

Respiratory distress syndrome (RDS) is caused by a deficiency of surfactant and is often called hyaline membrane disease.[174] Newborn infants with RDS typically present during the first 4 to 6 hours of life.[174] It is commonly seen in preterm infants (<36 weeks' gestation) but may also be seen in full-term infants.[174]

SIGNS AND SYMPTOMS

Respiratory distress is recognized as any signs of breathing difficulties in an infant. This includes cyanosis, nasal flaring, grunting, apnea/dyspnea, intercostal muscle retractions, tachypnea (respiratory rate >60 breaths per minute), and tachycardia (heart rate >160 beats per minute).[174]

PHYSICAL EXAMINATION

On physical examination, infants will have evidence of respiratory distress including tachypnea, intercostal muscle retractions, and grunting. There may also be cyanosis if severe hypoxia is present.

DIFFERENTIAL DIAGNOSIS

The differential diagnosis for infant respiratory distress syndrome is summarized in Table 4.28.

DIAGNOSTIC STUDIES

Chest radiography in RDS is an important diagnostic study as it typically shows air bronchograms and reticulonodular shadowing throughout the lung fields. Reticulonodular shadowing is commonly referred to as "ground-glass" appearance.

EVALUATION

The initial evaluation of an infant with RDS should include detailed history taking. Blood tests include CBC, comprehensive metabolic panel, and C-reactive protein.[174] Blood

TABLE 4.28 Differential Diagnosis for Infant Respiratory Distress Syndrome

Diagnosis	Description
Transient tachypnea of the newborn	Usually develops following elective cesarean section Self-limiting, up to 48 hours
Pneumonia	Chest radiography showing patchy infiltrates Blood cultures may be positive for culprit bacteria
Meconium aspiration syndrome	Develops a few hours after birth Secondary to meconium passage in utero Chest radiograph shows bilateral patchy infiltrates

cultures should be drawn to determine if there is infection present. Arterial blood gas is important to determine the degree of hypoxia. Pulse oximetry can also be used to assess the degree of hypoxia.

TREATMENT

- Treatment involves providing appropriate respiratory support, which may range from CPAP to intubation, depending on the work of breathing, degree of respiratory acidosis, FIO_2 requirement.[177]
- There may be consideration given to administering endotracheal surfactant.[177]

COMMON CHIEF COMPLAINTS

APPROACH TO THE PATIENT WITH COUGH

Cough is the most common complaint in primary care, being present in 8% of office visits.[178] Cough can be classified by duration, defined as acute (<3 weeks), subacute or persistent (3 to 8 weeks), and chronic (>8 weeks). Acute cough in both adults and children is most commonly due to viral upper respiratory infection. In this case, associated viral symptoms such as fever, nasal congestion, or sore throat are often present. If the patient presents with a fever and the lung examination reveals signs of consolidation, pneumonia should be suspected. This can be confirmed with a chest x-ray. Patients presenting with acute cough and dyspnea should have further evaluation with pulse oximetry, spirometry, or chest x-ray depending on suspected diagnosis. More severe but less common causes of acute cough include heart failure and occupational exposures. Allergic rhinitis may also present acutely.

The differential diagnosis for subacute and chronic cough includes medication-induced (specifically, ACE inhibitors), postnasal drip [recently renamed upper airway cough syndrome (UACS)], asthma, COPD (specifically chronic bronchitis), or gastroesophageal reflux disease (GERD). In nonsmoking adult patients, not on ACE inhibitors, with normal CXR findings, asthma, nonasthmatic eosinophilic bronchitis, GERD, and UACS account for the majority of cases of chronic cough.[179] Lung cancer should be considered in patients with associated weight loss, hemoptysis, and/or night sweats, especially if there is history of smoking, occupational exposure, or family history. Causes of cough in immunocompromised patients are the same as those in immunocompetent patients, with the addition of tuberculosis, fungal, and atypical infections to the differential diagnosis. Productive and nonproductive cough are generally evaluated the same; however, some causes of cough (i.e., GERD) are more likely to present as a dry cough whereas the presence of sputum points toward causes such as chronic bronchitis or bronchiectasis.[180]

If diagnostic studies are warranted, chest x-ray is typically first line. Indications for radiographic imaging include unexplained chronic cough, cough not responding to empiric therapy, cough with associated dyspnea or suggestion of consolidation on physical examination, or if tuberculosis or lung cancer is suspected. See Figure 4.13 for the approach to the evaluation of the patient with a cough.

APPROACH TO THE PATIENT WITH DYSPNEA

Dyspnea is defined as a subjective perception of shortness of breath. Dyspnea has been associated with increased risk of mortality and is helpful in identifying underlying cardiac or pulmonary disease; thus, a full workup and establishing the underlying cause of dyspnea is important.[181] Dyspnea can generally be classified as respiratory or cardiovascular in origin, though psychogenic causes must not be overlooked. The duration of symptoms can be used to further narrow the differential diagnosis, with the onset of acute dyspnea occurring over hours-days compared to chronic dyspnea, defined as lasting at least 1 month.

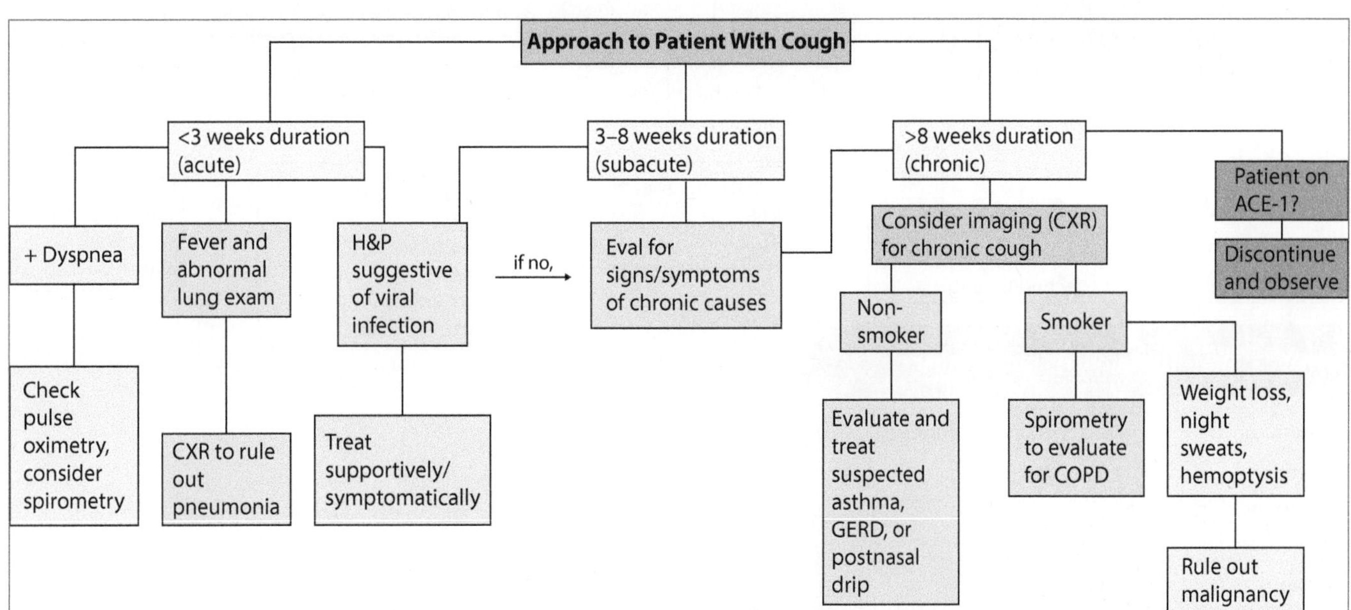

Figure 4.13 Approach to the patient with cough. ACE, angiotensin-converting enzyme; COPD, chronic obstructive pulmonary disease; CXR, chest x-ray; GERD, gastroesophageal reflux disease; H&P, history & physical exam.

The differential diagnosis for acute dyspnea is somewhat narrower than that of chronic dyspnea, and includes myocardial infarction, acute decompensated heart failure, cardiac tamponade, pulmonary embolism, pneumothorax, pneumonia or other pulmonary infection, foreign body aspiration, and anaphylaxis or bronchospasm. Findings of tachycardia, tachypnea, hypoxia, accessory muscle use, cyanosis, or inability to speak in full sentences indicate the need for an urgent/emergent workup. On the other hand, anxiety/panic may present with acute dyspnea in the absence of those red flag findings.

Respiratory causes of chronic dyspnea include hypoxia, hypercapnia, interstitial lung disease, asthma, chronic bronchitis, emphysema, and pulmonary edema. Neuromuscular conditions such as myasthenia gravis and Guillain-Barré syndrome may cause respiratory muscle weakness, and musculoskeletal abnormalities such as kyphoscoliosis may present with restrictive-pattern lung disease. Cardiac causes of chronic dyspnea include heart failure, coronary artery disease, and myocarditis. Differentiating factors can be found in Figure 4.14. Anemia, foreign body aspiration, pregnancy, obesity, and deconditioning are other causes of dyspnea to consider. Finally, clinicians should consider medication-associated conditions. For example, beta blockers may worsen asthma symptoms, NSAIDs lead to fluid retention and bronchoconstriction, and methotrexate may cause interstitial pneumonitis.[181]

APPROACH TO THE WHEEZING PATIENT

Wheezing is defined as the adventitious lung sound produced by turbulent airflow through narrowed airways. The pathophysiologic elements of wheeze include bronchoconstriction or bronchospasm, edema, and excess mucus production.[182] Wheezing is most prevalent in preschool age children (ages 16; Ducharme et al.[183]). In children, viral respiratory infections, bronchiolitis, and asthma are common causes of wheeze. Less common causes include congenital abnormalities, foreign body aspiration, cystic fibrosis, immunodeficiencies, and cardiac or gastrointestinal causes of wheeze.[183] In adults, wheezing is characteristic of asthma, COPD, viral respiratory infections, or heart failure.

The duration and timing of wheeze can provide helpful clues as to the underlying cause. Episodic wheeze associated with other viral symptoms (sore throat, nasal congestion, cough) is indicative of a viral respiratory infection. Intermittent wheezing may indicate allergies or chemical exposure, and may also occur during exercise or as a result

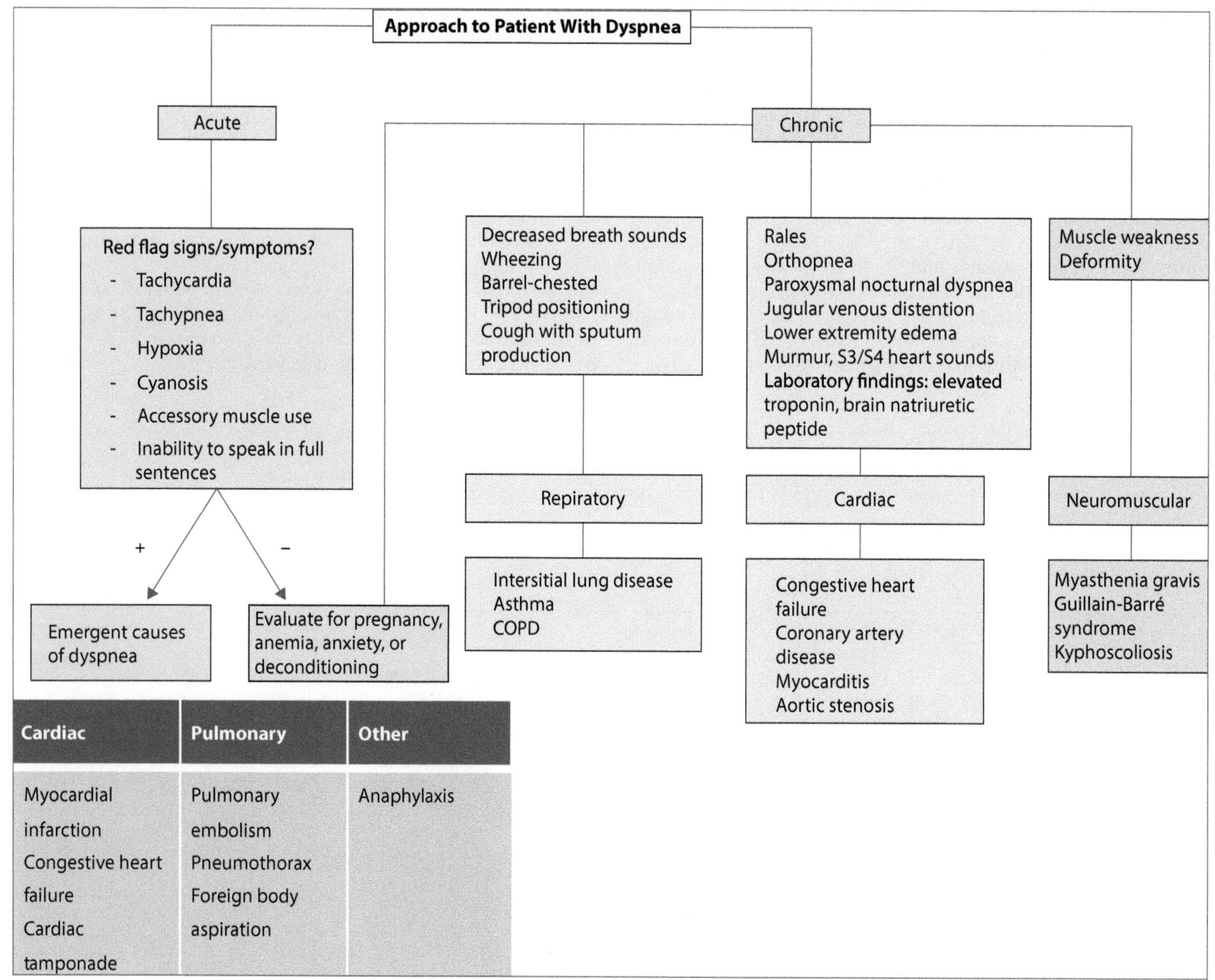

Cardiac	Pulmonary	Other
Myocardial infarction Congestive heart failure Cardiac tamponade	Pulmonary embolism Pneumothorax Foreign body aspiration	Anaphylaxis

Figure 4.14 **Approach to the patient with dyspnea.** COPD, chronic obstructive pulmonary disease

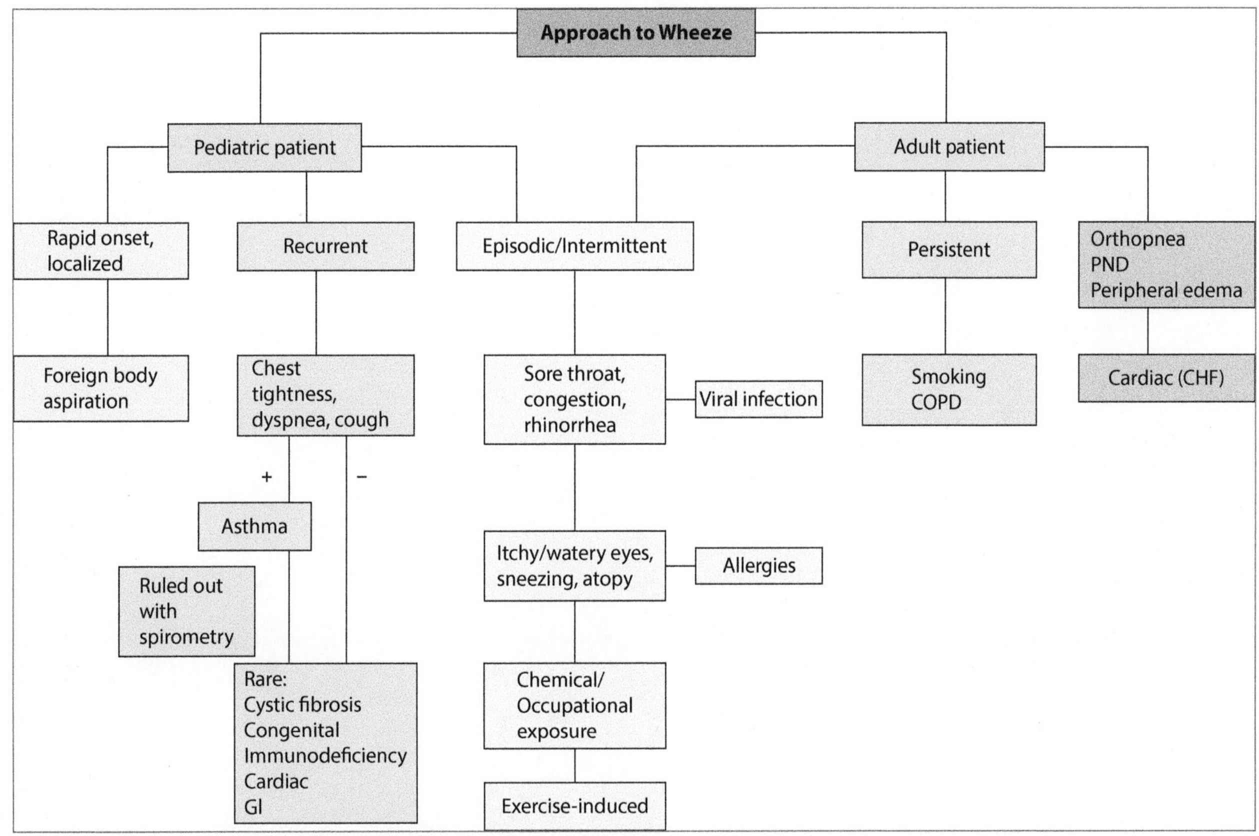

Figure 4.15 Approach to the patient with wheeze. CHF, congestive heart failure; COPD, chronic obstructive pulmonary disease; GI, gastrointestinal; PND, paroxysmal nocturnal dyspnea.

of certain medication use (in particular, beta blockers, aspirin, or NSAIDs). Persistent wheezing in an adult patient suggests smoking and/or COPD. Wheezing associated with peripheral edema, orthopnea, or paroxysmal nocturnal dyspnea should raise suspicion for a cardiac cause of wheeze, most commonly congestive heart failure. See Figure 4.15 for the differential diagnosis for the wheezing patient.

KNOWLEDGE CHECKS

1. Chronic obstructive lung disease and interstitial lung disease present with overlapping symptoms that can sometimes cloud the diagnosis. Compare and contrast the pathophysiology, historical features, physical examination findings, and diagnostic studies of COPD and interstitial lung disease.
2. Interstitial lung disease is a heterogeneous group of disorders. Compare and contrast the findings found on CXR and CT scan with idiopathic pulmonary fibrosis, sarcoidosis, connective tissue interstitial lung disease, and eosinophilic interstitial lung disease.
3. Cor pulmonale is a cardiovascular manifestation of pulmonary disease leading to hypertrophy or dilatation of the right ventricle. List the pulmonary conditions that lead to cor pulmonale.

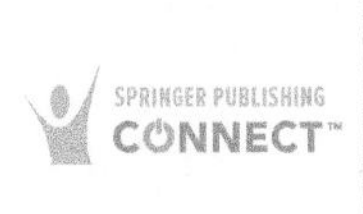

A robust set of instructor resources designed to supplement this text is located at **http://connect.springerpub.com/content/book/978-0-8261-8243-2.** Qualifying instructors may request access by emailing **textbook@springerpub.com.**

REFERENCES

The complete reference list for this chapter appears in the digital version of the chapter, accessible at https://connect.springerpub.com/content/book/978-0-8261-8243-2/chapter/ch04.

CHAPTER 5

CARDIOVASCULAR SYSTEM

CHRISTINE BRUCE

LEARNING OBJECTIVES

- Explain the pathophysiology behind the development of cardiovascular conditions, including hypertension, hypotension, chronic heart failure (HF), coronary artery disease, valvular heart disease (VHD), arrhythmias, pericardial disease, endocarditis, myocarditis, rheumatic heart disease (RHD), peripheral venous disease, and arterial aneurysms.
- Describe the presentation of patients with HF.
- Develop an evaluation and treatment strategy for patients with cardiovascular conditions that include both lifestyle modifications and pharmacotherapy.
- Develop a treatment plan for patients who have resistant hypertension.
- Explain the underlying causes for the various types of shock that are seen in clinical practice.
- Discuss medications used in the management of HF that can improve symptoms versus medications that have a survival benefit.
- Indicate the role of resynchronization pacemaker in the management of HF.
- Distinguish between the three primary conditions seen with acute coronary syndrome (ACS): ST segment elevation myocardial infarction (STEMI), non-ST segment elevation myocardial infarction (NSTEMI), and unstable angina (USA).
- Describe the medical and surgical approaches that are utilized in the management of VHD.
- Assess patients at risk for congenital heart disease.
- Predict appropriate long-term complications for patient with *repaired* coarctation of the aorta and be able to state appropriate management of identified complications.
- Categorize the severity of the patent ductus arteriosus (PDA) by clinical presentation (asymptomatic patient vs. symptomatic patient).
- Compose an appropriate treatment plan based on the clinical presentation of the patient with congenital heart disease.
- Compare the role of ultrasound and arteriography in the evaluation and monitoring of patients with aneurysm.
- Develop a treatment regimen for patients who have aneurysm formation.
- Compare rupture of aneurysm, formation of pseudoaneurysm, and aortic dissection from a clinical standpoint.

INTRODUCTION

Despite the in advances in modern medicine, cardiovascular disease remains the most common mechanism of death for people living in the United States. Atherosclerosis is the primary risk factor for the development of coronary artery disease and patients with diabetes mellitis are considered to have a cardiovascular risk factor equivalent. Women develop cardiovascular disease just as frequently as men but they tend to develop this at a later age and to present with atypical symptoms.

5.1 HYPERTENSION

CHRISTINE BRUCE

5.1A ESSENTIAL HYPERTENSION

OVERVIEW

Essential hypertension constitutes the majority of patients with hypertension and is also known as idiopathic or primary hypertension as no single cause has been identified. Hypertension is a major risk factor for the development of both cardiovascular and renal disease.[1]

Hypertension should only be diagnosed in a patient based on an average blood pressure taken on two or more readings obtained on two or more occasions. It is ideal to have the patient self-monitor blood pressure at home to confirm the diagnosis and self-monitoring can also be used to help to titrate the response to medications.

White coat hypertension can be found by ambulatory blood pressure monitoring that demonstrates normal blood pressure readings when outside the office setting. There is a concern that these patients adversely respond to stressful situations with elevation of their blood pressure. Masked hypertension is the opposite of white coat hypertension as these patients have normal blood pressure readings in the office but elevated blood pressure readings outside the office. Home blood pressure monitoring is reasonable to pursue for these patients. Ambulatory blood pressure measurement is the ideal method of confirming a hypertension diagnosis as well as diagnosing both white coat and masked hypertension.

The goal blood pressure is <140/<90 mm Hg for patients <65 years without other cardiovascular comorbidities and <130/<80 mm Hg for patients who are >65 years. Patients with other cardiovascular conditions such as diabetes or chronic kidney disease also have lower blood pressure goals of <130/<80 mm Hg (Table 5.1).

Essential hypertension is a rise in blood pressure of an unknown cause that increases the risk for cerebral, cardiac, and kidney events.[2] The majority of patients with hypertension do not have symptoms and most patients with hypertension are diagnosed with screening rather than symptoms. It can be difficult to manage patients with hypertension because the medications that are given to treat this asymptomatic condition can produce symptoms that make adherence to treatment more difficult.

Factors that impact blood pressure need to be identified and altered whenever possible. Lifestyle choices impacting blood pressure should also be assessed. These can include use of alcohol, sedentary lifestyle without exercise, smoking, and a high fat and salt intake diet. Because hypertension is a marker for cardiovascular disease, other cardiovascular risk factors should be assessed. It is important to assess for an end organ damage as stricter blood pressure control is needed for patients with end-organ damage.

EPIDEMIOLOGY

In developed countries, the risk of becoming hypertensive during a lifetime exceeds 90%. Risk factors for essential hypertension are the same as other cardiovascular risk factors such as aging, obesity, insulin resistance, diabetes, and hyperlipidemia.[2] One in three U.S. adults has hypertension and hypertension is considered to be the costliest of all cardiovascular diseases. Individuals with hypertension are estimated to face nearly $2,000 higher annual healthcare expenditures compared with their nonhypertensive peers.[3] Despite this high prevalence of hypertension in the U.S. adult population, blood pressure goals are met in fewer than one-half of these patients despite treatment, and about one in six U.S. adults is unaware of their hypertension.[4] Hypertension is higher among people born in the United States when compared to foreigners coming into the United States and the highest risk for the development of hypertension is in native non-Hispanic Black populations.[5]

Hypertension has a disproportional negative effect on the Black population compared to other races.[1] Black patients with hypertension have a more severe cardiovascular course with cardiovascular disease being the most common cause of death in this population.[6] Patients who smoke are also at increased risk of poorer outcomes with hypertension compared to those who have never smoked.[7]

TABLE 5.1 Blood Pressure Classification

Blood Pressure Findings	Criteria
Normal blood pressure (BP)	Systolic BP <120 mm Hg and diastolic BP <80 mm Hg
Stage I hypertension	Systolic BP 130–139 mm Hg and diastolic BP 80–89 mm Hg
Stage II hypertension	Systolic BP of at least 140 mm Hg and diastolic BP of at least 90 mm Hg

PATHOPHYSIOLOGY

Most patients with essential hypertension have normal cardiac output but increased peripheral resistance most pronounced in the small arteriolar walls, which contain smooth muscle cells. Prolonged smooth muscle constriction induces structural changes with thickening of the arteriolar vessel walls, which can be mediated by angiotensin leading to an irreversible rise in peripheral resistance.[8]

Many factors are involved with the development of hypertension including salt intake, obesity and insulin resistance, the renin-angiotensin system (RAS), and the sympathetic nervous system. Other entities contributing to hypertension include genetics, endothelial dysfunction, and neurovascular abnormalities.[8]

The sympathetic nervous system causes an increased cardiac output, which can result in increased peripheral arterial resistance. This increased pressure is transmitted to the capillary bed and affects cell wall homeostasis.[8]

Increased vascular stiffness is fundamental to the development of hypertension and this phenomenon is also associated with the development of atherosclerosis.[9] The kidney plays a significant role in the development of primary hypertension due to its impairment in the renal tubules, which have an impaired ability to secrete sodium leading to increased intravascular volume as salt retention leads to further retention of water.[10]

The RAS is the primary endocrine system affecting control of blood pressure. Renin is secreted from the juxtaglomerular apparatus of the kidney in response to the glomerular underperfusion or due to a recent reduced salt intake. It is also released in response to stimulation from the sympathetic nervous system. Renin converts its angiotensin I, a physiologically active substance, into angiotensin II in the lungs by angiotensin-converting enzyme (ACE). Angiotensin II is a potent vasoconstrictor causing a rise in blood pressure. It also stimulates the release of aldosterone in the adrenal gland causing increased sodium and water retention.[8]

Vascular endothelial cells produce potent local vasoactive agents including the vasodilator molecule nitric oxide and the vasoconstrictor peptide endothelin. Some antihypertensive medications can restore impaired production of nitric oxide, which is one of the main reasons that medications are effective in the management of hypertension.[8] Chronic endothelial injury from metabolic burden and oxidative stress promotes structural and functional vascular alterations in the microvascular network.[11]

The body's inability to produce atrial natriuretic peptide is also involved in the pathophysiology of hypertension as this hormone increases sodium and water excretion from the kidney by acting as a natural diuretic.[8]

Obesity contributes to hypertension due to dietary factors, metabolic endothelial and vascular dysfunction, neuroendocrine imbalances, sodium retention, glomerular hyperfiltration, proteinuria, and maladaptive immune and inflammatory responses. Visceral adipose tissue in particular is resistant to insulin and leptin, causing altered secretion of molecules and hormones including tumor necrosis factor and interleukin 6, which plays a role in the exacerbation of obesity-associated cardiovascular disease.[12]

Aortic wall stiffness is associated with renal organ damage and local carotid artery stiffness is associated with cardiac organ damage.[13] Essential hypertension may largely be a result of maladaption to a high salt diet and hypertension may be an adaptive mechanism to improve salt secretion. Any physiologic state that reduces urinary sodium concentrating ability can increase blood pressure in individuals at risk for salt-induced hypertension. Natriuresis is a crucial element for effective long-term pharmacologic treatment of essential hypertension.[14]

There are genetic influences affecting hypertension and family members tend to follow hypertension patterns already established in their family. The diet may contribute to hypertension, especially diets that have a great deal of salt. Potassium intake is also known to lower blood pressure. Salt leads to hypertension due to the retention of water under the influence of sodium. Volume status influences diastolic blood pressure measurement with the diastolic blood pressure increasing with increased volume in the blood vessel. There is an indirect relationship between levels of blood pressure and physical activity.

MEDICAL HISTORY AND CLINICAL PRESENTATION

The majority of patients with essential hypertension are identified by blood pressure screening rather than having symptoms. The presence of medical conditions such as stroke, myocardial infarction (MI), peripheral arterial disease (PAD), thyroid disease, kidney disease, obstructive sleep apnea, and diabetes should be assessed as these patients have an increased risk for the development of hypertension. Obstructive sleep apnea is a common condition causing secondary hypertension and is the most common secondary cause of resistant hypertension. Patients older than 50 years of age who have a large neck circumference measurement and who snore are most likely to have obstructive sleep apnea.[15]

Family history should be obtained with regard to hypertension along with a premature history of cardiovascular disease as these factors are nonmodifiable but should alert the clinician to early treatment of hypertension.

Review of systems should include questions about palpitations, headaches, sweating, visual changes, hematuria, and claudication. Other psychosocial factors that might impact hypertension and its management include amount of physical activity, use of illicit drugs, smoking and alcohol use, high dietary sodium intake, and emotional stress.

The clinician should perform medication reconciliation; the list should include the use of complementary medication as many of these supplements can increase blood pressure.

SIGNS AND SYMPTOMS

In established hypertension, funduscopic examination will show vasoconstriction and arteriolar narrowing producing arteriovenous nicking and copper wiring. Flame hemorrhages can be seen as a result of retinal hemorrhage. Optic neuropathy can result from ischemia to the optic nerve revealing itself as optic disc pallor or cotton-wool spots.[16]

Uncontrolled long-standing hypertension injures the vascular endothelium especially in patients who also have diabetes, which leads to peripheral vascular disease, claudication, and production of aortic aneurysms.

Brain damage as a result of chronic hypertension can manifest as transient ischemic attacks (TIAs), lacunar infarctions, strokes, and multi-infarct dementia.[17]

Long-standing hypertension that is not controlled leads to hypertensive nephrosclerosis and chronic kidney disease. This is exacerbated in the setting of diabetes, which is one of the microvascular complications seen in this condition. Obesity is also a major risk factor for the development of essential hypertension, diabetes, and chronic kidney disease. Visceral adiposity is especially problematic because of physical compression of the kidneys that occurs. Obesity ultimately leads to glomerular injury that exacerbates hypertension and worsens renal injury.[18]

PHYSICAL EXAMINATION

The physical examination includes measurement of vital signs and measuring the blood pressure in both arms at least 5 minutes after being seated. Clothing covering the arms and antecubital space should be removed so that the stethoscope directly touches the brachial artery. Automated blood pressure cuff measurements can also be taken with the clinician outside the room, which may reduce patient anxiety. The correct size cuff should also be chosen as a cuff that is too small will falsely elevate the blood pressure reading while a cuff that is too large falsely lowers the blood pressure reading. Differences in blood pressure between the arms can suggest aortic coarctation of the aorta or aortic dissection.

The patient's body mass index (BMI) should be calculated as obesity is related to elevated blood pressure. A search for target end-organ damage is pursued in the setting of established or episodic hypertension. Funduscopic examination is performed to assess for retinopathy and papilledema, which signify hypertensive retinal disease. Assessment for elevated jugular venous pressure helps to assess both blood volume and effectiveness of the right side of the heart as a pump. Peripheral edema should be checked to assess for venous insufficiency, heart failure (HF), and chronic kidney disease. Pulses should be palpated and the carotid artery should be auscultated for the presence of bruits, which may be heard in the setting of vascular disease. When compared to the brachial artery palpation, a delayed and weakened femoral pulse suggests aortofemoral blockage (Leriche syndrome).

The heart examination includes measurement of the rate and regularity along with listening for murmurs, rubs, and gallops. The chest should be palpated to assess the location of the point of maximal impulse (PMI), which suggests left ventricular hypertrophy when there is lateral displacement. An S4 may be heard in the setting of hypertension as the atria needs to contract against a hypertrophied and less compliant left ventricle (LV). Long-standing systemic hypertension overloads the LV, which undergoes concentric hypertrophy to overcome systemic vascular resistance. With time, the LV becomes stiffer and requires the atria to contract harder in order to fill this structure.

Secondary causes of hypertension can produce physical examination findings such as buffalo hump, violaceous striae, and abdominal obesity, which is seen with Cushing syndrome. Patients who have episodic palpitations and tachycardia along with sustained blood pressure elevation can be assessed for pheochromocytoma or carcinoid syndrome. Renovascular hypertension may be associated with a renal bruit. Enlargement of the thyroid gland and dry, coarse skin may suggest hypothyroid disease as an underlying cause for hypertension. New-onset atrial fibrillation (AF) and tremor when extending the hands suggest hyperthyroidism as an underlying cause of hypertension.

DIFFERENTIAL DIAGNOSIS

The differential diagnosis for essential hypertension is summarized in Table 5.2.[19,20]

DIAGNOSTIC STUDIES

A baseline EKG can identify left ventricular hypertrophy, which occurs as the heart tries to overcome increased vascular resistance in the systemic circulation. A urinalysis with microscopic examination can identify kidney damage in the setting of diabetes and also chronic kidney disease. Serum creatinine, blood urea nitrogen (BUN), and glomerular filtrate rate (GFR) are important to measure when evaluating a patient for chronic kidney disease as these patients may have lower blood pressure goals. The thyroid-stimulating hormonate (TSH) is the test of choice as the screen for thyroid disease, which increases the risk for hypertension.

If end-organ damage of the heart—particularly left ventricular failure—is suspected, an echocardiogram can be done in order to assess the ejection fraction, concentric versus eccentric ventricular enlargement, and overall wall motion of the LV.

Patient with microalbuminuria in the setting of hypertension have a significantly higher rate of cardiovascular events, both fatal and nonfatal. Evaluation of urinary albumin excretion assessment should be done as part of hypertension

TABLE 5.2 Differential Diagnosis for Essential Hypertension

Diagnosis	Description and Differentiating Features
Medication-induced	The most frequently incriminated drugs are steroids, nonsteroidal anti-inflammatory medications, sympathomimetic agents, central nervous system (CNS) stimulants such as alcohol or amphetamines, and dietary supplements including ginseng and natural licorice. Other implicated agents include sibutramine, antiemetic agents, L-dopa, leflunomide, growth hormone, thyroid hormone, recombinant erythropoietin, antidepressants, and immunosuppressants.
Illicit drug use	Cocaine and methamphetamines predominate.
Coarctation of the aorta	Differential blood pressure between the arms or between the upper extremity and lower extremity, and blood pressure that does not respond to traditional treatment. Patients can have a continuous murmur heard over the back and have delayed or weakened femoral pulses.
Renal disease	Includes both renal parenchymal disease and renal artery stenosis along with fibromuscular dysplasia of the renal artery. Renal bruit may be present. Young women without cardiovascular disease are most likely to have fibromuscular dysplasia as the underlying cause for their secondary hypertension. Renal duplex ultrasound or magnetic resonance angiogram (MRA) confirms diagnosis with the classic finding on MRA demonstrating the string of pearls sign with fibromuscular dysplasia.
Pheochromocytoma	Rare secondary cause of hypertension. Paroxysms of palpitations and elevated blood pressure due to catecholamine release from the adrenal medulla. Serum measurement of metanephrines is the best screen with MRI identifying this chromaffin cell adrenal tumor.
Cushing syndrome/ Cushing disease	State of excessive glucocorticoids in the body. Cushing disease is specific for pituitary adenoma causing increased adrenocorticotropic hormone (ACTH) with increased release of glucocorticoids from the adrenal cortex. Cushing syndrome occurs from any cause of increased glucocorticoid in the body. Screen is with 24-hour urine cortisol measurement, dexamethasone suppression test, or midnight salivary cortisol level with demonstration of increased glucocorticoids in at least two of these three screening tests.
Hyperparathyroidism	Patients will have elevated serum calcium along with low serum phosphate levels. Classic complaints include constipation and abdominal pain, kidney stones, and pathologic fracture. Despite the serum calcium being high, these patients will also have an elevation in their serum parathyroid hormone as these tumors are not subject to negative feedback from the hypothalamus and pituitary glands in the setting of hypercalcemia.
Hyper- and hypothyroidism	Can be identified prior to the onset of symptoms through routine screening that is best done by measurement of serum thyroid-stimulating hormone (TSH). TSH is elevated with hypothyroidism with symptoms including weight gain, cold intolerance, and fatigue. TSH is low in the setting of hyperthyroidism along with demonstration of elevations in T4 and/or T3. Symptoms include heat intolerance, new-onset atrial fibrillation, weight loss, palpitations, anxiety, tremors, and frequent soft bowel movements.
Hyperaldosteronism or Conn syndrome	Unprovoked or unexpected hypokalemia in the setting of hypertension. High levels of the mineralocorticoid aldosterone causes the retention of sodium and therefore water along with the loss of potassium leading to hypertension. Best screen is plasma renin to aldosterone ratio.
Obstructive sleep apnea	Patients with this condition will have disordered sleep with multiple hypopnea or apnea episodes during the night. This condition also leads to lack of nocturnal dip in blood pressure. Patients typically are overweight and bed partners note excessive snoring and apneic breathing. Best test is polysomnography confirming hypoxia, hypopnea, and apnea episodes.
Acromegaly	Increased production of growth hormone that occurs after the onset of puberty. Increased frontal bossing, increased hand and foot size with a doughy handshake and jaw protuberance are noted. Test of choice for evaluation is growth hormone nadir during oral glucose tolerance test.

Source: Data from Dobri G, Niwattisaiwong S, Bena JF, et al. Is GH nadir during OGTT a reliable test for diagnosis of acromegaly in patients with abnormal glucose metabolism? Endocrine. *2019;64:139–146. doi:10.1007/s12020-018-1805-z*

monitoring as urinary microalbuminuria is a risk factor for the development of cardiovascular events.[21]

Specific testing can be done when certain underlying causes are suspected. Obstructive sleep apnea is best assessed with polysomnography. Pheochromocytoma is assessed by measuring plasma metanephrine levels. Primary hyperparathyroidism is suspected when elevated serum calcium levels and elevated hyperparathyroid hormone levels are found on routine and follow-up testing.

Renal vascular disease such as fibromuscular dysplasia is assessed with renal duplex Doppler studies. Other tests include CT or magnetic resonance angiography (MRA) of the renal artery. Coarctation of the aorta is suggested when patients have differential blood pressure between their arms and/or between their arms and legs. In the setting of coarctation, chest x-ray (CXR) can show erosion of the rib and a positive "E" or "three" sign. Evaluation consists of CT or MRA or a transthoracic echocardiogram (TTE).

An electrolyte panel can be done to identify unprovoked hypokalemia, which can be found in the setting of primary hyperaldosteronism. Test of choice in this setting is plasma renin/aldosterone ratio. Cushing syndrome is assessed with two of the following three tests: midnight salivary cortisol level, 24-hour urinary cortisol excretion, or the dexamethasone suppression test.

EVALUATION

Hypertension can present as early as 3 years of age, which is the typical age for screening in the pediatric population. Children who were born prematurely, who have a very low birth weight, or who were patients in the neonatal ICU are at increased risk for the development of hypertension and chronic kidney disease so these patients should have blood pressure screening prior to 3 years of age.[22] Pediatric patients with essential hypertension are older when diagnosed, have a stronger family history of hypertension, and have a lower prevalence of preterm birth than pediatric patients who have secondary hypertension.[23]

For the adult population who are at average risk for the development of hypertension, the U.S. Preventive Services Task Force recommends hypertension screening at age 18 along with treatment for hypertension when elevated blood pressure is found to occur in both clinical and community settings on at least two separate occasions or in those who have signs of end-organ damage as a result of long-standing hypertension.[24]

TREATMENT

Lifestyle modifications are recommended for all patients with hypertension, even those who are only at risk for hypertension. Recommendations include weight reduction and maintenance of a normal BMI, a heart healthy diet, dietary sodium reduction, increasing physical activity, quitting smoking, and moderate alcohol consumption.[25] Utilization of potassium salt substitute is a low-cost effective method for lowering both systolic and diastolic blood pressure.[26] Most hypertensive patients need two or more drugs for blood pressure control along with concomitant statin treatment for cardiovascular risk factor reduction.[2] Despite the availability of effective and safe antihypertensive medications, hypertension goals are not met in most patients.

Reduction in the mean dietary sodium intake in patients with established hypertension reduces systolic blood pressure by 5.5 mm Hg and diastolic blood pressure is lowered by 2.9 mm Hg. Patients without hypertension have no significant effect with sodium reduction with regard to blood pressure lowering.[27]

Management of hypertension after failure of therapeutic lifestyle changes is based upon the underlying patient conditions and demographics. Only when therapeutic lifestyle modifications fail to achieve acceptable blood pressure ranges are medications given. For patients having excessively high blood pressure readings in an established pattern, two medications rather than one should be started. Systolic blood pressure goal for those older than 65 living in the community is <130 mm Hg. Patients who have diabetes also have a lower blood pressure goal, <130/<80 mm Hg, the same blood pressure goals in patients who have chronic kidney disease.

Potassium supplementation can be utilized for treatment without adverse effects in those with normally functioning kidneys. Potassium supplementation has a modest but significant impact on blood pressure and should be considered as an adjuvant antihypertensive agent for patients with essential hypertension.[28]

Lifestyle Modifications

Weight loss leads to 5 to 10 mm Hg reduction in systolic blood pressure. Sodium intake limited to 1,500 to 2,400 mg per day leads to a reduction of 2 to 8 mm Hg of systolic blood pressure. A DASH (dietary approaches to stop hypertension) diet includes fruits, vegetables, low-fat dairy, whole grains, beans, and foods rich in potassium, magnesium, and calcium. Adoption of this type of diet leads to a systolic blood pressure lowering of 8 to 14 mm Hg.[29] Consuming fewer than two alcoholic drinks for a male or one or fewer alcoholic drinks for a female lowers systolic blood pressure by 2 to 4 mm Hg. Exercising at least 30 minutes per day most days of the week leads to long-term reduction of blood pressure of 4 to 9 mm Hg systolically. Patients who participate in an active lifestyle have a 35% reduction in the development of hypertension compared to those with a sedentary lifestyle.[30]

Pharmacologic Therapy

Successful blood pressure management leads to a 28% to 44% reduction in stroke, 20% to 35% reduction in ischemic heart disease, and a significant reduction in HF.[31] Patients with stage 1 hypertension who have clinical cardiovascular disease, those who have a 10-year cardiovascular risk of at least 10%, and patients with stage 2 hypertension should have pharmacologic therapy without delay. Alzheimer disease incidence may be lowered by blood pressure control.[32] Sustained blood pressure reduction in patients with type 2 diabetes also reduces cardiovascular complications.[33] Strict blood pressure control is associated with lower risk of death for patients who develop end-stage kidney disease.[34]

Intensive blood pressure control is associated with a significantly lower rate of cardiovascular disease and all-cause mortality for patients under age 75 without prior cardiovascular or chronic kidney disease and this intensive blood pressure control benefit was also seen in patients older than age 75 with pre existing cardiovascular or chronic kidney disease.[35]

Essential hypertension is associated with large and small vascular remodeling that impacts cardiovascular prognosis. Renin-angiotensin-aldosterone system blockers are the agents that have been shown to affect vascular remodeling to the greatest degree. Lifestyle modifications, including exercise and weight loss, also improve large and small vascular remodeling.[36]

First-line RAS blockers (includes ACE inhibitors [ACEIs], angiotensin receptor blockers [ARBs], and direct renin inhibitors) decrease HF but have a slight increased risk for stroke. When compared to dihydropyridine calcium channel blockers, first-line RAS inhibitors do not differ for all-cause death or total cardiovascular events including MI. Thiazide diuretics are better at decreasing HF and decreasing stroke when compared to RAS inhibitors but there is no difference for all-cause death rates between the two groups and there is no significant difference in blood pressure measurements when RAS inhibitors, dihydropyridine calcium channel blockers, and thiazide diuretics are compared in clinical practice.[37]

Clinical effect of blood pressure control when studied over a 3-year period identified RAS blockers to provide the best blood pressure control and, together with diuretics, the lowest rate of cardiovascular events. Beta blockers were associated with the highest rate of uncontrolled blood pressure and a high cardiovascular event rate.[38]

The ultimate goal of treating hypertension is to lower the blood pressure without causing adverse effects from the medications that are used to lower blood pressure. Many medications promote the lowering of blood pressure. Clinical comorbid conditions may help to determine which agents are chosen. Agents that reduce clinical cardiovascular events include thiazide diuretics, dihydropyridine calcium channel blockers, ACEIs, and ARBs.

The elderly and Black population respond best to thiazide diuretics and dihydropyridine calcium channel blockers. These patients are low renin producers so renin, which results in higher angiotensin II and aldosterone levels, will not be overproduced when intravascular volume drops when diuretics are used. Thiazide diuretics can help to retain calcium in the body, which is helpful in the elderly population concerned about osteopenia but has an adverse effect of increasing serum uric acid levels.[39]

Beta blockers are not considered first-line therapy for hypertension but they may still have a role as part of multiple drug regimens in patients who have underlying HF or previous myocardial damage. Recent updates of blood pressure clinical guidelines have downgraded the use of beta blockers to second- or third-line therapy as these agents are inferior to other agents with regard to lowering cardiovascular risk and overall mortality.[40] Beta blockers behave differently based upon their subtypes. Conventional non vasodilating beta blockers (atenolol and metoprolol) are inferior to first-line recommended antihypertensive agents with regard to cardioprotection because of their inability to decrease central blood pressure along with its adverse effects on glycemic and lipid metabolism. New generation vasodilating beta blockers carvedilol and nebivolol have enhanced hemodynamic and metabolic properties that can result in better prevention of major cardiovascular events in patients with hypertension. These newer generation beta blockers are superior to conventional beta blockers for the prevention of cardiovascular events in patients with essential hypertension. These newer generation beta blockers also possess antioxidant and anti-inflammatory effects, which may be beneficial in the management of hypertension.[41]

Beta blockers may protect the heart through their blocking of the sympathetic nervous system and through their negative chronotropic and inotropic activity. Side effects include fatigue, bronchospasm, erectile dysfunction, and worsening of peripheral vascular disease. These agents should be avoided in HF with reduced ejection fraction (HFrEF) or in decompensated HF as these conditions will temporarily worsen when beta blockers are used in this setting.

The choice of blood pressure medications may depend on comorbidities, contraindications, and medications that could worsen underlying conditions.[42] Table 5.3 summarizes pharmacologic options for blood pressure management.

Indications and adverse effects of antihypertensive agents should be known in order to optimally use these agents. Thiazide diuretics may be used as first-line agents because of their efficacy and known ability to lower morbidity and

TABLE 5.3 Pharmacologic Options for Blood Pressure Management

Comorbidity	Indicated Medications
Heart failure with decreased ejection fraction ACE; postmyocardial infarction (exception is diuretic)	ACE inhibitor or ARB, beta blocker, diuretic, aldosterone antagonist
Chronic kidney disease with proteinuria	ACE inhibitor or ARB
Angina pectoris	Beta blocker, calcium channel blocker
Atrial fibrillation with rapid ventricular response or atrial flutter	Beta blocker, nondihydropyridine calcium channel blocker
Benign prostatic hyperplasia	Alpha blocker
Essential tremor	Noncardioselective beta blocker
Hyperthyroidism	Beta blocker
Migraine prophylaxis	Beta blocker and calcium channel blocker
Osteoporosis	Thiazide diuretic
Raynaud phenomenon	Dihydropyridine calcium channel blocker
Contraindications/Avoid Use Classes	
Angioedema	ACE inhibitor
Bronchospastic disease	Nonselective beta blocker
Pregnancy	ACE inhibitor, ARB, renin inhibitor
Second- to third-degree heart block	Beta blocker, nondihydropyridine calcium channel blocker unless pacemaker is present
Medications Leading to Adverse Actions	
Depression	Beta blockers and central alpha-2 agonists
Gout	Loop and thiazide diuretics
Hyponatremia	Thiazide diuretics
Hyperkalemia	Aldosterone antagonists, ACE inhibitors, ARBs, renin inhibitors
Renovascular disease	ACE inhibitor, ARB, renin inhibitor

ACE, angiotensin-converting enzyme; ARB, angiotensin receptor blocker.

mortality.[41] Side effects of thiazides include hyponatremia, hypokalemia, hyperlipidemia, hyperuricemia, and hyperglycemia. These agents should not be used in a patient with gout due to retention of monosodium urate but they could be considered in patients who are on xanthine oxidase inhibitors such as allopurinol, which prevents the formation of uric acid.

ACEIs are first-line agents for hypertension treatment especially if there is coexisting diabetes, HF, or kidney disease. When used clinically, they also lower the risk for the development of AF.[43] Their primary mechanism of action is vasodilation. They are known to cause hyperkalemia as an adverse action. Cough may be a complication of their use due to the accumulation of bradykinin. They should not be used with ARBs or direct renin inhibitors as there is no additional benefit but there is an increased risk for kidney damage and hyperkalemia since these agents drop the GFR in the kidney. They should not be used in pregnancy as they can result in kidney agenesis in the developing fetus.

ARBs are also first-line agents to treat hypertension and HF when ACEIs cannot be used. They have the same adverse actions as ACEIs with the exception of not causing a cough since there is no accumulation of bradykinin. When ARBs and ACEIs are compared against each other, both groups decrease proteinuria and control blood pressure to the same degree.[44]

The aldosterone receptor blockers are weak potassium-sparing diuretics. These are used as add-on therapy when blood pressure goals are not achieved and are also used as third-line therapy for patients with chronic HF. There is mortality benefit with the use of these agents. Agents in this class include spironolactone and eplerenone. These agents are less effective in the setting of impaired renal function where hyperkalemia may be worsened when using these agents. Spironolactone is also associated with gynecomastia, an adverse effect that is not seen with eplerenone.

Patients who have had previous MI or HF should have ACEIs or ARBs as part of the treatment regimen. Patients with chronic kidney disease who need diuretics are best treated with loop diuretics as these agents will continue to function even with the lowest residual kidney function.

Direct oral inhibitors of renin such as aliskiren can be used to control blood pressure in patients with more severe stages of hypertension and in those with concomitant diseases such as diabetes mellitus and impaired renal function.[45]

Dihydropyridine calcium channel blockers are effective antihypertensive agents. Long-acting dihydropyridine calcium channel blocker, amlodipine, has been shown to have reduced risk for stroke and HF in patients taking this for hypertension.[46] Their use may be limited if peripheral edema occurs as a result of their peripheral arterial vasodilation. They may also be associated with headache and flushing as adverse actions. The nondihydropyridine calcium channel blockers such as diltiazem and verapamil are utilized for rate control than rather than blood pressure control. When calcium channel blockers are utilized in the management of hypertension, long-acting dihydropyridine calcium channel blockers are preferred over intermediate-acting agents due to increased efficacy along with less effect on the autonomic nervous system and heart rate.[47]

Constipation is a side effect with these agents. These medications should be avoided in HFrEF. They should not be used in combination with a beta blocker because of an exaggerated decrease in cardiac function.

Research has shown that patients have improved outcomes treating blood pressure when a nocturnal dip in blood pressure occurs. Administration of amlodipine at bedtime optimizes the antihypertensive effect along with increasing the daytime/nocturnal ratio of blood pressure allowing normalization of the blood pressure pattern and minimizing the morning blood pressure surge.[48]

Vasodilators such as hydralazine and minoxidil work by keeping potassium channels open. Primary side effect is edema. Hydralazine can lead to a lupus-like syndrome. Hydralazine also needs frequent dosing in order to maintain its effect leading to issues with medication adherence. When used in the setting of chronic HF, hydralazine must be paired with isosorbide dinitrate in order to achieve its desired effect. Minoxidil can lead to hair growth. Hydralazine has been used to control hypertension in pregnancy, but its use has been supplanted by nifedipine and labetalol, which have clinical superior effects used in this setting.[49]

Alpha blockers may be used in the setting of hypertension, particularly as add-on therapy. First dose orthostatic hypotension and dizziness can occur. Recommendation is to take this agent at bedtime in order to lessen orthostasis. It is typically not efficacious for use as a single agent antihypertensive, but it can be helpful as additional therapy for men with urinary outlet obstructive symptoms.[50] Medications in this category include prazosin, terazosin and doxazosin. These agents are also utilized as ureteral stone expulsive therapy because of their ability to relax smooth muscles in the genitourinary tract.[51]

Central alpha agonists such as clonidine may be useful as add-on therapy in patients not responding to other agents. These agents are associated with fatigue and depression. Rebound hypertension may occur with the use of these agents. Clonidine can also be given via transdermal patch. Because of its fast onset of action when taken orally, clonidine can be used in the setting of hypertensive urgency/emergency.[52] Clonidine can also be utilized for women with pregnancy-related hypertension as this medication not only lowers blood pressure but also increases formation of the circulating anti-inflammatory cytokine IL-10.[66]

Resistant hypertension can affect up to one in five patients diagnosed and treated for hypertension despite lifestyle and therapeutic treatment.[53] Individualized therapy is needed in order to lower blood pressure as these patients are at increased risk for cardiac and all-cause mortality. Older age and obesity are the primary risk factors for the development of resistant hypertension.[54] Patients should also be assessed for the possibility of secondary causes for this resistant hypertension.

PATIENT EDUCATION

Hypertension is a significant modifiable risk factor for cardiovascular disease, stroke, chronic kidney disease, and death. Systolic blood pressure readings are more impactful in these complications than diastolic blood pressure especially regarding coronary events, HF, stroke, and chronic kidney disease. Isolated systolic hypertension is also associated with an increased risk for the development of AF.[55]

Hypertension is the leading risk factor for death globally. A significant percentage of patients admitted to hospitals have undiagnosed hypertension but despite recognizing elevated blood pressure while in the hospital, there continues to be a lack of postdischarge assessment for elevated blood pressure readings in these hospitalized patients. One explanation for this is the perception that this elevated blood pressure is caused by anxiety, pain, or white coat syndrome and that outside the hospital, the blood pressure will normalize after discharge. This lack of follow-up to elevated blood pressures in hospitalized patients represents a missed public health opportunity for identification of patients with undiagnosed hypertension.[56]

Complications of essential hypertension include left ventricular hypertrophy, microalbuminuria, and cognitive dysfunction.[2]

5.1B URGENT AND EMERGENT HYPERTENSION

OVERVIEW

Hypertensive urgency is defined as acute severe uncontrolled hypertension without end-organ damage while hypertensive emergency includes elevated blood pressure along with signs of end-organ damage with both of these entities failing under the global category of hypertensive crisis.[57]

Hypertensive crisis includes both hypertensive emergency and hypertension urgency with the primary difference being that hypertensive emergency has signs of end-organ damage. Both conditions have a significant elevation in blood pressures, which are typically at least 180 mm Hg systolically and 110 mm Hg diastolically. Hypertensive emergency can be manifested in the eye by papilledema due to damage of the arterioles feeding into the optic disc resulting in optic nerve hemorrhage and swelling. Irrevocable blindness can occur.

Hypertensive emergency can cause aortic wall dissection and rupture of abdominal aortic aneurysm. The brain can be harmed in the setting of both chronic uncontrolled hypertension and acute blood pressure elevations.

Hypertensive emergency can lead to hemorrhagic stroke or subarachnoid hemorrhage from cerebral aneurysm rupture. The LV can be overwhelmed with chronic elevation of systolic blood pressure leading to left ventricular hypertrophy causing HFrEF and problems with relaxation of the LV leading to HFpEF (heart failure with preserved ejection fraction).

Hypertensive emergency can lead to acute MI and chronic kidney disease if not properly identified and treated.

SIGNS AND SYMPTOMS

Patients with hypertensive urgency may present with headache, epistaxis, faintness, and psychomotor agitation. Patients with hypertensive emergencies present with chest pain, dyspnea, and neurologic deficits. End-organ damage seen in the setting of hypertensive emergency includes cerebral infarction, acute pulmonary edema, hypertensive encephalopathy, and cerebral hemorrhage. Cerebral infarction and acute pulmonary edema are the most frequent types of end-organ damage in the setting of hypertensive emergency.[58]

TREATMENT

Hypertensive crisis including hypertensive urgency and hypertensive emergency requires urgent treatment in order to prevent complications and further damage to susceptible organs. Both oral nifedipine and intravenous (IV) labetalol (a combined alpha and beta blocker) are utilized for treatment in this setting.[59] Table 5.4 summarizes pharmacologic options for the management of hypertensive urgencies and emergencies.

5.1C SECONDARY HYPERTENSION

OVERVIEW

Secondary hypertension occurs in 5% to 10% of cases in patients who are diagnosed with hypertension. Parenchymal renal disease, renal artery stenosis, primary hyperaldosteronism secondary to adrenal adenoma, pheochromocytoma, and adenoma of the adrenal or pituitary glands causing Cushing syndrome and Cushing disease are the most common types of secondary hypertension.[60]

Although secondary hypertension is not frequently encountered compared to essential hypertension, there are situations in which a secondary cause of hypertension should be sought. Patients with secondary hypertension have a specific underlying cause responsible for the elevated blood pressure. Secondary hypertension should be suspected in patients with resistant hypertension and secondary hypertension increases with age. If appropriately diagnosed and treated, patients with secondary hypertension can be cured, or at the minimum, show improvement in blood pressure control. As a result, screening for secondary causes of hypertension should be pursued for patients in whom a secondary cause is suspected.[61] Patients presenting with hypertensive crisis should be assessed for secondary hypertension as this may be their presenting symptom.[62]

SPECIAL CONSIDERATIONS

- Hypertension during pregnancy deserves special mention as hypertensive disorders of pregnancy are among the leading preventable contributors of maternal and fetal adverse outcomes. Increased blood pressure has a strong association with unfavorable pregnancy outcomes including stroke and pulmonary edema. A persistent blood pressure measurement ≥160/110 mm Hg that lasts for more than 15 minutes either during pregnancy or in the postpartum state is considered an obstetric emergency requiring appropriate, rapid treatment.[63] Hydralazine, labetalol, and nifedipine are first-line treatment options for the emergent reduction of blood pressure in pregnancy.[63]

TABLE 5.4 Medications Used in the Management of Hypertensive Urgencies/Emergencies

Nitrates (venodilation)	Sodium nitroprusside, nitroglycerin
Calcium channel blockers (dihydropyridines)	Clevidipine—short-acting, intravenous (IV) agent; nicardipine IV
Dopamine-1 agonists	Fenoldopam—able to maintain renal perfusion
Combined alpha and beta blocker	Labetalol
Short-acting beta blocker	Esmolol
Direct arteriolar vasodilator	Hydralazine

5.2 HYPOTENSION

CHRISTINE BRUCE

OVERVIEW

Shock is the clinical expression of circulatory failure resulting in inadequate cellular oxygen utilization. Four pathophysiologic mechanisms are involved with shock: hypovolemic, cardiogenic, obstructive, and distributive factors.[64] Cardiogenic shock can occur with any condition causing direct myocardial damage or anything that inhibits the cardiac contractile mechanism.

Shock may occur as a result of pump failure in the setting of cardiogenic shock, loss of circulating blood volume in the setting of hypovolemia, abnormalities in vasoregulation with distributive shock, or actual obstruction to blood flow known as obstructive shock.

Cardiogenic shock can be preceded by rapid hemodynamic deterioration on a background of preexisting left ventricular systolic dysfunction known as pre-cardiogenic shock. The symptoms include rapid clinical deterioration that precedes overt cardiogenic shock with hypotension, inflammatory response, and end-organ failure. Identification of pre-cardiogenic shock offers an ability to initiate early treatment with the intent to improve clinical outcomes.[65]

Cardiogenic shock is characterized by inadequate cardiac output along with sustained hypotension. Cardiogenic shock often complicates acute MI. Even if the systolic blood pressure is above 90 mm Hg, there can still be peripheral hypoperfusion in these patients who continue to have a substantial risk of in-hospital death despite still having blood pressure that is considered normotensive.[66]

EPIDEMIOLOGY

Patients admitted to the coronary ICU often have shock as part of their overall picture. Two thirds of these patients have their shock caused by cardiogenic shock, 7% have distributive shock, 3% have hypovolemic shock, 20% have a mixed bag picture for shock, and 4% do not fit into any of the categories. For patients having cardiogenic shock, 30% of those patients have acute MI-related cardiogenic shock, 18% have ischemic cardiomyopathy without acute MI, 28% have nonischemic cardiomyopathy, and 17% have a different cardiac cause unrelated to primary myocardial dysfunction.[67]

PATHOPHYSIOLOGY

Cardiogenic shock has also been identified as a result of acute cardiac injury caused by severe acute respiratory syndrome coronavirus. Endomyocardial biopsy of these patients demonstrates low-grade myocardial inflammation and viral particles in the myocardium suggesting either a viremic phase or infected macrophage migration from the lung. This infection can be associated with flulike symptoms rapidly degenerating into respiratory distress, hypotension, and cardiogenic shock.[68]

Hypovolemic shock is caused by a loss of intravascular volume, which can occur from overt bleeding (typically in the gastrointestinal [GI], genitourinary, or pulmonary system) along with trauma, third space losses such as that seen with bowel obstruction, burns, or severe nausea and vomiting.

Distributive shock, caused by loss of vascular regulation, can be caused by sepsis, anaphylaxis, toxins, or neurogenic or endocrine diseases such as that which occurs when there is a disconnection between the brain and spinal cord or adrenal crisis. There is excessive vasodilation with dysfunction noted in the microvascular circulation. This results in blood bypassing the capillary beds, which leads to tissue hypoxia. Even though cardiac output is adequate, it cannot maintain pressure sufficient for normal tissue perfusion.

Obstructive shock is due to actual structural injury, which can be caused by a pulmonary embolism (PE), cardiac tamponade, or tension pneumothorax.

When there is an adequate blood flow, there is interruption of oxygen delivery to the peripheral tissues occurring at the cellular level leading to tissue hypoperfusion and anaerobic metabolism. The body naturally tries to compensate by increasing the force of contraction of the heart and by tachycardia along with tachypnea. Unless there is immediate treatment, the body's compensatory mechanisms cannot meet metabolic demand resulting in irreversible organ damage and ultimately death.

Without treatment, shock precipitates a cascade of pro-inflammatory mediators resulting in cellular damage and end-organ dysfunction.[69] Endothelial activation occurs along with increases in inflammatory markers such as angiopoietin-1 (Ang-1) which promotes vascular quiescence and angiopoietin-2 (Ang-2) that mediates microvascular leak along with various interleukin subsets such as interleukin 6, interleukin 8 and granulocyte colony stimulation factor.[70]

5.2A CARDIOGENIC SHOCK

MEDICAL HISTORY AND CLINICAL PRESENTATION

Patients presenting to the ED with hypotension should be evaluated for cardiogenic etiology as the cause of hypotension in order to plan appropriate therapy. Factors making it more likely to have a cardiogenic etiology for hypotension include shortness of breath as a presenting symptom, electrocardiographic ischemia signs, history of HF, and absence of fever. These patients should have early cardiac interventions employed in order to have the best clinical outcome.[71]

SIGNS AND SYMPTOMS

Clinical features of cardiogenic shock include poor peripheral tissue perfusion, tachycardia, and hypotension, dyspnea, and altered mentation.[64] Specific physical examination signs include elevated jugular venous pressure, peripheral edema, pulmonary rales, cold and mottled extremities, and hypotension.[72] Postural or orthostatic hypotension can be caused by volume depletion, medications, diabetes, alcohol, infection, varicose veins, and problems with the autonomic nervous system. Myocarditis can cause cardiogenic shock. If the right ventricle (RV) is involved with myocarditis, acute right-sided HF along with low cardiac output can be easily missed as these patients will not have the typical HF signs of shortness of breath and pulmonary crackles.[73]

PHYSICAL EXAMINATION

Multiple signs and symptoms are seen with shock with the keynote symptoms being altered mental state and hypotension. As the blood pressure declines, the compensatory mechanisms that are initially involved are tachypnea and tachycardia as the body tries to compensate for poor perfusion by increasing the basal metabolic rate in order to perfuse vital organs. Clinicians assessing these patients will note a prolonged capillary refill time with or without cyanosis, poor production of urine due to decreased blood flow to the kidneys, and rales on lung auscultation if left-sided HF occurs. With progression of HF in this setting, the patient's overwhelmed RV leads to jugular venous distention, hepatojugular reflex, and peripheral edema.

DIFFERENTIAL DIAGNOSIS

The differential diagnosis for cardiogenic shock is summarized in Table 5.5.[74–77]

DIAGNOSTIC STUDIES

Poor perfusion to the tissues leads to the production of lactic acid so elevation of serum lactate levels are consistent with shock and serial assessment of these levels can help to follow the progression of shock and its response to therapy. Venous and arterial blood gases (ABGs) can provide clues to the metabolic state of the patient and can identify whether hypoxia and anaerobic metabolism are occurring. The complete blood count (CBC) can provide clues to the underlying cause for shock with elevation in the white blood cell count being consistent with septic shock and decreases in the hemoglobin and hematocrit occurring in the setting of acute blood loss, but this is only present after fluid resuscitation causes this hemodilution.

Since the kidney is not considered an essential organ by the body during its compensatory mechanism, BUN and creatinine levels should be obtained in order to assess the baseline function of the kidneys. The anion gap is part of the metabolic profile and calculation of this gap in the setting of metabolic acidosis can provide clues to the underlying cause contributing to shock.

EKG is performed to assess for acute coronary syndrome (ACS) as demonstrated by ST segment changes or the development of a new-onset left bundle branch block pattern. Focused ultrasound exam of the abdomen and chest can identify cardiac tamponade, tension pneumothorax, significant spontaneous pneumothorax, free fluid in the abdominal cavity caused by rupture of a hollow viscus, or blood from rupture of abdominal aortic aneurysm or an ectopic pregnancy. A beta-hCG (human chorionic gonadotropin) can confirm pregnancy if ruptured ectopic pregnancy is suspected.

The remainder of diagnostic investigation will depend upon the working differential diagnosis for this patient. If a tension pneumothorax is suspected as the cause of shock, CXR will identify this condition, although immediate treatment is needed, which can be suggested by the identification of tracheal deviation and absence of breath sounds on one side of the chest. CXR demonstrating a widened mediastinum may help to identify aortic dissection as the underlying cause of the patient's shock. Cardiac tamponade can also be suggested by CXR findings showing a globular cardiac silhouette. Echocardiogram can allow the computation of the ejection fraction from the LV and assess for left ventricular wall motion abnormalities.

EVALUATION

The patient is rapidly assessed in the setting of suspected shock as emergent therapy is needed to reduce the risks of

TABLE 5.5 Differential Diagnosis for Cardiogenic Shock

Diagnoses	Description
Takotsubo cardiomyopathy	Can cause acute, nonischemic cardiomyopathy causing apical ballooning in the setting of normal coronary arteries. It is typically related to catecholamine-associated triggers particularly emotional stress but can also occur in the setting of surgical stress or catecholamine-producing tumor such as pheochromocytoma. These patients can present with acute cardiogenic shock.[74]
Acute myocarditis	Can present with cardiovascular collapse but typically these patients will have preceding signs or symptoms of infection, ST segment elevation or depression, elevated troponin levels, localized or diffuse left ventricular wall motion abnormalities, inflammatory cells on biopsy, and evidence of viral infection on laboratory testing.[74]
Exercise-induced left ventricular dysfunction	Can cause apical ballooning along with right ventricular involvement.[74]
Pulmonary embolism	Patients present with syncope, systemic arterial hypotension, cardiogenic shock, cardiac arrest.[75] Patients may have increased risk for prothrombotic states such as postoperative state, prolonged travel, use of high-risk medications such as oral contraceptives, or inherited or acquired coagulopathies.
Basic hypotension	Lower blood pressure with systolic <90 mm Hg does not necessarily result in symptoms or an end-organ dysfunction as patients may normally run blood pressures in this range. Shock is excluded if patients remain asymptomatic over time without signs of organ dysfunction as some patients naturally run a lower blood pressure that is not pathologic.
Obstructive shock	Seen with cardiac tamponade, tension pneumothorax, or massive pulmonary embolism that is interfering with blood being able to be ejected from the heart. Atrial myxomas may also cause obstruction to blood getting into the mitral inflow.[76]
Distributive shock	Anaphylaxis, toxin- or poison-mediated, neurogenic shock (disconnection between the brain and spinal cord with hypotension and bradycardia) and addisonian crisis with loss of glococorticoids, which are needed in order to maintain vascular tone.
Hypovolemic shock	Any loss of blood or intravascular fluid that is not adequately replaced to meet the metabolic demands of the body.
Septic shock	Systemic inflammatory response syndrome (SIRS) with vasodilation, increased permeability, hypovolemia, and ventricular dysfunction or fundamental features.[77]

Source: *Data from Loscalzo J, Roy N, Shah RV, et al. Case 8-2018: a 55-year-old woman with shock and labile blood pressure.* N Engl J Med. *2018;378:1043–1053. doi:10.1056/NEJMcpc1712225; Piazza G, Goldhaber SZ. Fibrinolysis for acute pulmonary embolism.* Vasc Med. *2010;15:419–428. doi:10.1177/1358863X10380304; Lyall A, Ghosh S, Mishra K. Diagnosing obstructive shock: echocardiography is the third eye of a vigilant intensivist.* Indian J Crit Care Med. *2016;20:542–544. doi:10.4103/0972-5229.190376; Joseph MX, Disney PJS, Da Costa R, Hutchison SJ. Transthoracic echocardiography to identify or exclude cardiac cause of shock.* Chest. *2004;126:1592–1597. doi:10.1378/chest.126.5.1592*

morbidity and mortality. The emphasis of this evaluation is on airway, breathing, and circulation. Transesophageal echocardiogram (TEE) is considered the echocardiographic test of choice used to establish the presence or absence of cardiogenic shock. TEE provides better anatomic evaluation than TTE resulting in improved sensitivity and specificity at identifying cardiac dysfunction as the cause of the shock. The performance of TEE as the only image prevents the patient from first having a TTE that is inadequate and having the patient undergo two tests instead of one.[77]

Vital signs are serially measured along with recording of urinary output in the setting of hypovolemic shock. Blood cultures and Gram stain are performed if septic shock is suspected. Neurologic examination is performed for patients who are suspected of having neurogenic shock, which can demonstrate hypotension with bradycardia (an inappropriate response). Patients with addisonian crisis can have hyponatremia, nausea, vomiting, and alterations of consciousness as findings[78] with these patients needing lifesaving glucocorticoid administration to retain vascular tone.

TREATMENT

Treatment of cardiogenic shock consists of methods to improve myocardial oxygenation, peripheral tissue perfusion, and control of tissue congestion, which typically produces an increase in lactic acidosis.[64] Treatments attempt to optimize oxygen delivery and reverse poor perfusion by providing volume resuscitation in the form of crystalloid administration. If this fails, vasopressors are used in order to improve cardiac output and vascular tone along with supporting cardiac function as well as addressing the underlying cause. For all causes of shock, treatment must address the underlying cause in order to reduce the risks of morbidity and mortality.

Patients who are hypotensive who are not fluid overloaded are given intravenous or interosseous access so that fluid resuscitation can be started. For patients who have blood loss contributing to the hypotension, early transfusion of packed red blood cells is provided along with crystalloid fluid as crystalloids are more readily available than packed red blood cells and the patient may not survive the time delay in order to receive the packed red blood cells. Crystalloids alone in this setting are insufficient as they do not improve oxygen delivery to the tissues in the same way the packed red blood cells provide. Packed red blood cell transfusions do not contain clotting factors, so patients receiving multiple units of packed red blood cells should also receive fresh frozen plasma and platelets.[78]

Typically, there is pump failure contributing to cardiogenic shock so dobutamine is indicated if volume resuscitation is not adequate at restoring perfusion to the organs.[77] Heart rate can be lowered in order to allow for enhanced filling of the heart and this can be accomplished with the short-acting beta blocker esmolol or another agent that works to reset the SA node known as ivabradine.[77]

Patients with severe hemorrhage as a result of trauma who are given tranexamic acid within 3 hours of initial injury have improved mortality risk.[80] Transexamic acid acts as an antifibrinolytic agent as it competitively inhibits plasminogen binding sites, which decreases plasmin formation and fibrinolysis.[80]

A known complication of acute MI that designates a very poor prognosis is sustained hypotension, cardiogenic shock, and HF. Application of intra-aortic balloon pump (IABP) counterpulsation as an interventional strategy used in the setting of acute MI treated with fibrinolysis has been shown to be a useful adjunctive therapy in patients with the most severe HF and hypotension when this treatment is continued for at least 48 hours post-MI.[81] IABP counterpulsation therapy simultaneously increases coronary blood flow via augmenting diastolic aorto-coronary pressure gradient and decreases myocardial oxygen demand by reducing afterload.[82]

Extracorporeal membrane oxygenation (ECMO) in veno-arterial configuration provides circulatory support. ECMO in cardiogenic shock provides rapid improvement of circulatory status and a significant increase in tissue perfusion. Its primary use is in the management of patients with severe and rapidly deteriorating cardiogenic shock.[83]

Left ventricular assist device augments cardiac output and reduces left ventricular wall stretch. In a situation of cardiogenic shock, there is improved cardiac power and perfusing augmenting tissue perfusion.[84]

Patients with cardiogenic shock secondary to MI may need to be treated with vasopressors in addition to fluid resuscitation.[85] Norepinephrine may be preferred over epinephrine as it has a lower incidence of refractory shock even though it has a similar effect on arterial pressure and the cardiac index. Heart rate is also most likely to increase significantly with the use of epinephrine while norepinephrine has a neutral effect on heart rate. There is also more lactic acid produced with the use of epinephrine when it is compared to norepinephrine.[85]

Six factors have been identified as independent predictors for 30-day mortality rate in the setting of cardiogenic shock: age older than 73, prior stroke, glucose on admission >191 mg/dL, creatinine >1.5 mg/dL, thrombosis in MI (TIMI) flow grades <3 after percutaneous coronary intervention (PCI), and arterial blood lactate being >5 mmol/L. Higher scores based on these risk factors have an increased mortality risk and these scores can help to risk stratify patients for short-term mortality and help with clinical decision-making.[86]

PATIENT EDUCATION

Despite advances in therapy, shock continues to have a high mortality rate, even when identified early and treated appropriately in an ICU environment. Hospital mortality rate of cardiogenic shock can be as high as 60%.[87]

Patients with shock are continually monitored in an ICU setting. Management of shock is performed in a hospital setting so patient education is done in order to prevent a recurrence of this condition. In a trauma setting leading to massive bleeding and injury, common sense counseling such as seatbelt and helmet use are emphasized. Because cardiogenic shock is a frequent cause of shock overall, aggressive secondary preventive strategies are employed in order to prevent cardiac decline over time. Optimal treatment strategies include the use of hydroxy-methylglutaryl coenzyme A (HMG-CoA) reductase agents (*statins*), ACEIs or ARBs, judicious use of beta blockers, heart healthy diet, control of hypertension and diabetes, and appropriate exercise. If the patient developed shock as a result of anaphylaxis secondary to medication allergy or bee stings, the patient should be counseled to carry and administer epinephrine if recurrence of anaphylaxis occurs.

SPECIAL CONSIDERATIONS

Cardiogenic shock, even properly found and treated, is associated with a much higher morbidity rate and risk for hospitalization than syncope due to vasovagal or postural hypotension.[88] Management of cardiogenic shock includes efforts to unload the heart and to improve blood flow to the coronary artery, which can be best accomplished with PCI or coronary artery bypass grafting.

KEY POINTS

- Despite appropriate identification and management, mortality rate from shock continues to be high.
- Treatment of shock should be directed at trying to reverse the underlying cause.
- Shock is more than just hypotension but also includes signs of poor tissue perfusion, which can include oliguria, confusion, and cold, clammy skin as blood is shunted to the essential organs of heart, lungs, and brain.

5.2B VASOVAGAL SYNCOPE

Jill Cowen and Marie Shaner

OVERVIEW

Vasovagal syncope, also described as a form of reflex syncope, is a transient loss of consciousness due to a sudden drop in heart rate and blood pressure. These episodes are often precipitated by triggers such as prolonged periods of standing, excessive heat, or pain.[89] Once in the supine position, patients will recover heart rate and blood pressure control within minutes. Because of the benign nature of vasovagal syncope, conservative treatment with positional change and improving hydration is often sufficient. Medical management options are available for patients who have symptoms refractory to conservative treatment. Vasovagal mediated response is the most common cause of syncope.[90]

EPIDEMIOLOGY

There is a bimodal distribution in the incidence of vasovagal syncope with peaks during adolescence and senior age groups. Females are twice as likely as males to experience reflex-mediated syncope during adolescence.[91]

PATHOPHYSIOLOGY

Autonomic and cardiovascular compensatory mechanisms are required to perfuse blood to the brain while in the upright position. Cerebral hypoperfusion occurring after several minutes in an upright position causing transient loss of consciousness and loss of postural tone may be attributed to vasovagal syncope once cardiac syncope is ruled out. There may be individual variations in the length of the hemodynamic mechanisms responsible for hypoperfusion and syncope. Gravitational pull in the upright position initially causes decrease in central blood volume, decreased stroke volume, and decreased cardiac output despite increase in heart rate. There is blood pressure variability during this stage but mean systolic pressure may be preserved by an increase in systemic vascular resistance. Circulatory instability occurs after continued decrease in both cardiac output and central blood volume. Ultimately, hypotension and vasovagal loss of consciousness occur with an increase in lower body negative pressure inducing a fall in heart rate and cardiac output.[92]

MEDICAL HISTORY AND CLINICAL PRESENTATION

The clinician's role is to determine if the syncopal event/symptoms described by the patient are consistent with a "vasovagal syncope" or due to another cause.

Vasovagal Syncope

Patients will often describe lightheadedness particularly with positional changes, hot/humid environments, and/or prolonged standing. Visual changes, auditory changes, and palpitations are also common. Patients will also describe either feeling hot or cold. Observers to the patient will often notice the patient to be pale and diaphoretic. If patients do lose consciousness, they are typically unconscious for <1 minute and do not have amnesia of the event but may be confused as to why they are on the ground. Patients typically do not incur injury because they can feel changes building prior to loss of consciousness and are able to subconsciously protect themselves as they fall to the ground. The most common time of presentation is during the adolescent growth spurt. There may be a family history of vasovagal syncope.

Other Faints

Symptoms occurring suddenly resulting in injury, prolonged loss of consciousness, amnesia of the event, bowel/bladder incontinence, symptoms with exercise, or a family history of cardiomyopathy/cardiac dysrhythmia/sudden death, should be worked up more thoroughly to rule out structural heart disease, cardiac dysrhythmia, metabolic disease, or neurologic disorders.

SIGNS AND SYMPTOMS

- Dizziness with positional changes (typically described as lightheadedness not "the room is spinning")
- Palpitations (typically not with sudden onset)
- Paresthesia
- Visual changes (tunnel vision, seeing spots)
- Pallor
- Diaphoresis
- Nausea/vomiting

PHYSICAL EXAMINATION

Orthostatic vital signs should be obtained and are considered positive if the patient experiences symptoms during the testing, the systolic blood pressure drops more than 20 mm Hg, and /or the heart rate increases by 30 beats per minute (bpm) or more. The thyroid should be palpated and assessed for underlying thyroid disease. Respiratory examination should be normal. Cardiac examination should also be normal, but it would not be uncommon to appreciate a marked increase in the patient's heart rate by auscultation with positional changes. Consider further workup for structural heart disease if a murmur is present. Abdominal examination should be normal. Peripheral examination should reveal normally palpable pulses in all extremities with brisk capillary refill. Peripheral edema should not be present.

DIFFERENTIAL DIAGNOSIS

The differential diagnosis for vasovagal syncope is summarized in Table 5.6.

DIAGNOSTIC STUDIES

Diagnostic studies are performed to rule out other disorders. A thorough medical history and physical examination should be able satisfy the diagnosis of benign vasovagal syncope (see above).

- **EKG:** Done as a screening tool for all syncope. The EKG should show normal sinus rhythm with normal QTc interval and no pre-excitation (delta wave) or shortening

TABLE 5.6 Differential Diagnosis for Vasovagal Syncope

Diagnosis	Description
Hypertrophic cardiomyopathy	Left ventricular outflow tract obstruction causing decreased cardiac output and increased risk of ventricular dysrhythmia leading to loss of consciousness and sudden death.
Severe aortic stenosis	Fixed left ventricular outflow tract obstruction leading to decreased cardiac output and loss of conscousness.
Long QT syndrome	Genetic channelopathy increasing the risk of sudden development of ventricular tachycardia/ventricular fibrillation leading to loss of consciousness and sudden death.
Wolff-Parkinson-White (WPW) syndrome	Palpitations due to development of supraventricular tachycardia (SVT). Fast conducting accessory pathway may lead to development of ventricular dysrhythmia and loss of consciousness. If atrial fibrillation develops in these patients, it can be fatal.
Neurologic disorders (seizure)	Loss of consciousness with bowel/bladder incontinence or postictal amnesia.
Metabolic disorders (hypoglycemia/thyroid disease)	Hypoglycemia causing dizziness. Thyroid disease, causing changes in heart rate.

of the QT interval. Any abnormalities in the EKG should raise concern for presence of a cardiac dysrhythmia or structural heart disease.

- **24-hour Holter monitor:** Performed if there is a concern for cardiac dysrhythmia.
- **Echocardiogram:** Performed if the syncopal event or family history raises concerns for structural heart disease.
- **Exercise stress test:** Performed if the syncopal event or family history raises concerns for structural heart disease. Will also be considered if the syncopal event is related to exercise.
- **Tilt table testing (rarely performed):** May be performed by a cardiology electrophysiologist if other testing is inconclusive or there is a suspicion of genetic cardiac dysrhythmia that was not able to be identified by other testing.

TREATMENT

- Initial treatment involves optimizing hydration, increasing salt intake to further improve intravascular volume, and decreasing or eliminating caffeine (a diuretic that decreases intravascular volume). Extensive time should be spent educating patients on potential triggers and avoidance of known triggers if possible. Triggers include hot/humid environments, rapid positional changes, prolonged standing, poor sleep quality, fasting (hypoglycemia), emotional/physical stress/anxiety, pain, or hormonal fluctuations during menstrual cycle.
- Compression stockings may be considered to aid in centralizing intravascular volume during periods of standing.
- Supplemental salt tablets may be utilized to optimize salt intake if patient is unable to adequately obtain salt from dietary means alone.
- If lifestyle modifications are inadequate to control the patient's symptoms, pharmacologic therapy is considered. Typical first-line agent is fludrocortisone 0.1 to 0.4 mg per day. Typical dose is 0.2 mg orally (PO) daily either as a single dose or divided twice daily. Mechanism of action is sodium retention by the kidneys promoting shift of water from the renal tubules back to the vasculature. This medication should be taken with water to increase effectiveness.
- Secondary pharmacologic therapy (if patient fails fludrocortisone) includes beta blockade therapy or vasoconstrictive agents such as midodrine.
  - Consider beta blockade therapy in patients with complaints of palpitations or tachycardia with minimal exertion. Start with a small dose and slowly uptitrate to desired effect. Be mindful that beta blockers may cause hypotension and worsening dizziness.
  - Consider midodrine in patients whose primary complaint is dizziness and hypotension is noted on physical examination. Midodrine is typically dosed three times per day but can be used twice daily as well. Blood pressure should be monitored closely for significant hypertension. Counsel patients to avoid lying supine for at least 30 minutes after receiving a dose of midodrine to avoid sudden elevation in systolic blood pressure.

PATIENT EDUCATION

- Instruct patients to always keep water readily available. Suggest carrying a water bottle.
- Instruct patients to change positions slowly until their symptoms are better managed.
- Avoid potential triggers if possible. Consume even greater amounts of water if a known trigger is unavoidable.
- Discuss diagnosis with teachers, coaches, and supervisors and share with them the plan of action needed if symptoms occur.
- Vasovagal syncope resolves on its own within 1 to 2 years for most patients.
- This diagnosis does not lead to sudden death but may result in injury if patient falls from a significant height. Avoid heights until symptoms are controlled.

5.3 HEART FAILURE

Christine Bruce

OVERVIEW

Chronic HF is one of the most common reasons for hospitalization in the United States. HF, the leading cause of death in the Western world, develops when a cardiac injury or insult impairs the ability of the heart to pump blood and maintain tissue perfusion.[94] It is a clinical syndrome wherein the pumping function of the heart cannot meet the physiologic demands of the body or the heart cannot fill sufficiently in order to meet those demands. With this condition, the heart is either unable to eject enough blood into the systemic circulation (HFrEF) or HFpEF. In the past, these terms were called systolic HF (HFrEF) and diastolic HF (HFpEF). In HFpEF, enough blood is ejected from the ventricles, but the ventricles fail to relax. Left-sided ventricular failure could progress to cause right-sided failure which is the most common underlying cause of the RV to fail. The symptoms of HF include dyspnea, orthopnea, and fatigue due to low perfusion. Signs of HF include rales, jugular venous distention, dependent edema, and an S3 or rarely an S4 heart sound on cardiac auscultation. Treatment includes medications that decrease mortality risk and reduce symptoms, limiting salt and water intake, and elevation of dependent portions of the body.

As the population ages, HF incidence is increasing. While improvements have been made related to cardiovascular mortality relative to ACS, mortality rate related to chronic HF has not improved. The key presenting symptoms of HF are dyspnea upon exertion and dyspnea with recumbency, a condition known as paroxysmal nocturnal dyspnea (PND). Without treatment, the dyspnea with exertion leads to dyspnea at rest. With a heart unable to meet its metabolic demands, patients will also have fatigue and an inability to exercise. If the LV fails, blood will back up in the pulmonary system causing dyspnea and signs of congestion. Increased pulmonary pressure leads to the right side of the heart being overwhelmed with the eventual backup of blood into the jugular venous system, the hepatic system, and peripheral system leading to hepatic congestion and dependent edema.

HF remains the most common diagnosis requiring hospitalization. It is a clinical syndrome but it is typically secondary to another insult. Ischemic heart disease is the most common underlying cause for HF development. Dietary indiscretion with increased sodium intake or fluid overload can exacerbate and precipitate HF with congestion.

HF is characterized by dyspnea, fatigue, and signs of fluid overload leading to peripheral edema and pulmonary rales. HF continues to have high morbidity and mortality rates, especially with aging. HF can be secondary to multiple conditions including coronary artery disease, hypertension, valvular heart disease (VHD), and diabetes. About half of the patients with HF have reduced ejection fraction while the other half have preserved ejection fraction. Mortality rates are similar for both preserved and reduced ejection fraction types of HF.[95]

EPIDEMIOLOGY

Structural heart problems can lead to an inability for the LV to relax, which leads to impairment in ventricular filling. This situation typically will cause an S3 gallop on auscultation of the heart and represents HFpEF. HFrEF occurs when the pumping action of the heart is impaired. Coronary artery disease with ischemia or cardiomyopathy secondary to virus or medications also results in the inability of the heart to sufficiently contract in order to meet its metabolic demands. Underlying cardiovascular disease is commonly present in patients with HF. The most common underlying causes of HF are cardiomyopathy (51%) and coronary ischemia (40%).[96]

PATHOPHYSIOLOGY

HF can occur with any structural problem within the heart. Eccentric ventricular damage leads to a stretching of the cardiac myocytes. Damaged cardiac myocytes lose their ability to contract, and this is a common underlying cause for the development of HFrEF. When the LV has to contract against increased systemic vascular resistance (as is the case with hypertension), the LV develops concentric hypertrophy with an increase in the width and force of contraction, which is part of the Frank-Starling curve.

A complex interaction occurs in the setting of HF between several neurohormones that act to compensate for a failing heart to sustain cardiac output while the heart is decompensating. The adrenergic or sympathetic nervous system is the primary compensatory mechanism in this condition as these levels are elevated in the setting of HF. Acutely, this is a positive effect to restore cardiac function. In the long-term, however, stimulation of the sympathetic nervous system will not be able to maintain cardiac function and the patient develops chronic decompensated HF. The sympathetic nervous system will continue to push the heart to work harder, which is more than the cardiac muscle can handle. This compensatory mechanism in the long run is harmful to the heart, causing further decompensation in cardiac function.[94]

5.3A CHRONIC HEART FAILURE

MEDICAL HISTORY AND CLINICAL PRESENTATION

Comorbidities associated with chronic HF include diabetes, hypertension, chronic obstructive pulmonary disease (COPD), and renal insufficiency. Cardiac ischemia is a frequent cause for beginning HF.[97] It has been demonstrated that patients with systolic blood pressure <89 mm Hg and those with heart rates >76 bpm as a baseline have higher mortality risk in the setting of chronic HF.[98]

Symptoms of HF may be a better predictor for prognosis than even left ventricular ejection fraction.[99] Patients with diabetes have a significantly increased risk for the development of HF. It is well known that the thiazolidinediones adversely affect HF prognosis.

SIGNS AND SYMPTOMS

Fatigue is the most common symptom of HF. Males tend to have less severe HF symptoms including frequency, severity, and distress. Females with HF tend to have more depression-type symptoms.[100] Congestive signs and symptoms include peripheral edema, jugular venous distention, a third heart sound, and pulmonary rales[101] and these signs also have prognostic value when they are present. Peripheral edema is independently associated with increased mortality risk.[102]

Orthopnea occurs with shortness of breath in a recumbent position. When patients recline, dyspnea results as this maneuver moves edema into the intravascular space thereby increasing vascular volume. The supine position increases preload by increasing the left ventricular end-diastolic volume, which results in an increase in pulmonary vascular pressure. This results in fluid leaking into the alveoli and interstitium. Patients with HF may sleep propped up on several pillows or may actually sleep in a recliner because of this orthopnea. PND, the sudden onset of dyspnea with a reclining position, occurs as a result of preload increasing with recumbency. The symptoms occur within minutes to hours with patients getting out of bed and standing in order to repool blood to lessen the symptoms.

Fatigue occurs in the setting of HFrEF due to impairment of the systolic function of the LV. Without adequate perfusion into the systemic circulation, perfusion of vital organs decreases; this is manifested by fatigue, slower mentation, and decreased urinary output. Edema occurs as a result of fluid backing up into the lungs and then into the peripheral circulation. Patients managed at home for HF weigh themselves as increased body weight occurs before the patient becomes overtly symptomatic.

Cough occurring in the setting of HF has been called "cardiac asthma" when it is accompanied by wheezing. This cough related to HF occurs because of the interstitial/alveolar congestion with elevation in the left ventricular end-diastolic pressure. Rales can accompany this increased fluid accumulation. This cough is usually nonproductive. The setting of pulmonary edema or acutely decompensated HF leads to the development of pink, frothy sputum.

PHYSICAL EXAMINATION

The physical examination in a patient with HF focuses on the patient's vital signs, with systolic blood pressure assessing whether there is adequate perfusion to the organs, patient's pulse assessing metabolic demand and catecholamine release, and patient's respiratory rate assessing whether tachypnea is present. Further examination determines whether an S3 is present on heart auscultation along with assessment for the presence of jugular venous distention and the quality of the peripheral pulses.[103]

DIFFERENTIAL DIAGNOSIS

The differential diagnosis of chronic HF is summarized in Table 5.7.[104]

DIAGNOSTIC STUDIES

HF is widely considered to be diagnosed based upon clinical grounds. The primary method of confirming HF as the diagnosis is with N-terminal pro-brain natriuretic peptide (NT-proBNP), which is released into the circulation when cardiac myocytes are stretched.[105] Echocardiogram should be the first diagnostic test performed when the diagnosis has been made as this test has the ability to differentiate between HFrEF and HFpEF.

Because HF can occur in the setting of coronary artery disease, baseline EKG should be done to look for signs of previous myocardial damage or for irregular heart rhythms such as AF, which can lead to the development of HF. Anemia can worsen signs and symptoms of HF so a CBC should also be performed to assess for this condition. If iron deficiency is present, correction should be done in order to improve the number of circulating red blood cells in order to provide oxygen to the tissues. CXR can show dilation of the heart caused by cardiomyopathy and can also show pleural effusion or signs of fluid in the interstitium from backflow of blood from the left side of the heart.

Pump failure in the setting of HF can lead to poor renal perfusion. Acute kidney injury can lead to hyperkalemia due to inefficiency in the body getting rid of potassium and activation of the renin-angiotensin-aldosterone system that leads to salt and fluid retention with more water than salt being retained leading to the development of hyponatremia. Serum electrolytes along with BUN and creatinine and calculation of the GFR. Improving blood flow to the kidneys will prevent activation of the renin-angiotensin-aldosterone system.

Diabetic patients have a higher risk for coronary artery disease and HF so assessment of blood sugar and hemoglobin A1c are also part of this evaluation. Patients with unknown or untreated thyroid disease can also develop HF as an underlying cause. Hypothyroidism leads to hyponatremia from increased fluid retention in the body. Hyperthyroidism can lead to the acute development of AF, which is also a risk factor for the development of HF.

Because of the relationship between coronary disease and HF, full cardiovascular risk factor identification is essential. Patients should have a fasting lipid profile as a baseline prior to treatment in the setting of HF.

Patients can be referred for exercise treadmill test or performance of the "get up and go test" if they are severely

TABLE 5.7 Differential Diagnosis of Chronic Heart Failure

Diagnosis	Description and Differentiating Features
Chronic obstructive pulmonary disease (COPD)	Although the two processes are very different, these conditions may present similarly with dyspnea with or without coughing being present early in these conditions. COPD remains the primary diagnosis that needs to be differentiated from CHF. BNP measurements are the primary means of differentiating between these conditions as it is increased with heart failure and not increased in the setting of COPD.
Pneumonia	Pneumonia causes fever, dyspnea, tachypnea, and signs of consolidation on lung auscultation. Symptoms occur abruptly and are a change from the baseline. Pneumonia is independent of heart disease and depends upon exposure to bacterial or viral pathogens in the environment.
Deconditioning, sedentary lifestyle	Patients who are deconditioned due to physical inactivity are more likely to have dyspnea on exertion, fast heart rates with activity, and fatigue. These conditions are independent of actual cardiac damage (pump failure or inability of the heart to relax and allow adequate filling) and improve when increased activity is undertaken.
Pulmonary embolism (PE)	Because of the high risk for death if PE is not diagnosed and treated, PE should be considered for patients with abrupt chest pain, dyspnea, tachycardia, and tachypnea. Patients with PE typically will have risk factors such as hypercoagulable state, use of estrogen-containing medications, family history of clots/hypercoagulation, long travel, recent surgery or incapacitation, deep venous thrombosis, atrial fibrillation without anticoagulation, or inactivity. PE diagnosis is made with CT angiogram or V̇/Q̇ scanning.
Cardiomyopathy (all-cause)	Cardiomyopathy can occur as a result of alcohol-induced damage to the heart ("holiday heart), postpartum state, viral-induced damage (enteroviruses such as Coxsackie B), tachycardia-induced cardiomyopathy, and damage from previous infarction (ischemic-related cardiomyopathy). When cardiac myocytes are damaged, their ability to function is impaired leading to poor ventricular systolic function.
Liver damage/ cirrhosis	Patients with advanced liver failure will have hepatic congestion (hepatomegaly) along with the development of ascites progressing to esophageal and gastric varices. Abnormal results on serum liver tests can occur. Patients with CHF with hepatomegaly typically will also have abnormalities on lung examination such as rales and irregular heart rhythm (seen with atrial fibrillation) or S3 gallop, findings that are not present in the setting of liver disease/cirrhosis.

BNP, brain natriuretic peptide; CHF, congestive heart failure; V̇/Q̇, ventilation/perfusion.

Source: Data from Güder G, Störk S. COPD and heart failure: differential diagnosis and comorbidity. Herz. *2019;44:502–508. doi:10.1007/s00059-019-4814-7*

deconditioned. Chemical stress testing can be performed for those unable to tolerate the traditional exercise stress test.

EVALUATION

The first and most essential test to order as part of the evaluation for chronic HF is a TTE (transthoracic echocardiogram). This test will allow the calculation of the ejection fraction which will help to separate the underlying cause of HF into that due to HFrEF versus that due to HFpEF. Ventricular wall motion abnormalities can also be found along with identification of a left ventricular mural thrombosis, which would suggest that anticoagulation is needed.

An EKG is performed as a baseline in order to assess for previous STEMI (presence of significant Q waves in anatomically continuous leads) and to assess for potential left bundle branch block due to impaired left ventricular pump function. A lack of R wave progression across the precordium is associated with an age indeterminate anterior wall MI.

CXR can identify cardiomegaly, which can occur in the setting of HF secondary to dilated cardiomyopathy.

A patient who has wheezing without a clear underlying etiology (cardiac asthma versus pulmonary asthma) will have elevation in B-type natriuretic peptide (BNP) and NT-proBNP with cardiac-related dyspnea and these tests are obtained to differentiate between cardiac- and pulmonary-related dyspnea in patients having symptoms. Symptoms are rarely present if the BNP is <400 even though most labs will identify levels of BNP >100 as being abnormal. Obesity may falsely lower the BNP level.

A CBC assesses for anemia, which would further stress the heart by increasing the heart rate to compensate. CBC can identify polycythemia, which increases the risk for a hypercoagulable state and the formation of thrombosis. A complete metabolic panel (CMP) can assess for electrolyte abnormalities, which may occur as a result of HF or from medication-induced electrolyte abnormalities that occur as adverse actions of these medications. The CMP can also identify renal impairment as the kidney can be adversely affected as the body compensates for HF (cardiorenal syndrome). The CMP also identifies liver dysfunction that can occur with hepatic congestion as a result of right-sided HF (cardiohepatic syndrome).

Thyroid function studies are performed to assess for thyroid disease since thyroid dysfunction can precipitate HF or can complicate HF by altering the body's basal metabolic rate.

As part of the assessment for coronary artery risk, a lipid profile is ordered as a baseline but current recommendations base lipid management on cardiovascular risk and not just elevated levels of cholesterol.

If hemochromatosis is suspected as an infiltrative cause of cardiomyopathy leading to HF, a serum ferritin or transferrin saturation level can be obtained to assess for iron overload.

If the patient has cardiomyopathy as the underlying cause for HF, an endomyocardial biopsy may be indicated.

To ascertain the patient's functional cardiac status, a 6-minute walk test can be performed. For patients unable to perform this test, a simple "get up and go" test may be performed. Patients with intermediate risk for coronary disease caused by HF may be referred for an exercise treadmill test. A cardiac MRI and ventriculography can be performed for patients who have cardiomyopathy in order to assess progression or recovery from the cardiomyopathy.

TREATMENT

Medications that decrease mortality risk and slow down the progression of HF include ACEIs, ARBs, aldosterone receptor antagonists, and certain beta blockers specifically carvedilol, bisoprolol, and metoprolol. Beta blockers should be used in a stable patient who does not have decompensated HF since negative inotropic activity of these agents can initially worsen symptoms. Beta blocker therapy may take up to a month until the patient has clinical improvement. Newly introduced neprilysin inhibitors work by inhibiting neprilysin, an enzyme that breaks down endogenous peptides that normally promote urine sodium excretion and vasodilation. Thiazide or loop diuretics may be used to relieve congestive symptoms by reducing the overall fluid buildup in the body. Hydralazine combined with nitrates act as vasodilators, and these have been shown to improve both symptoms and mortality risk in select patients.

The use of a combination medication containing an ARB–neprilysin inhibitor (ARNI) (valsartan/sacubitril) and a sinoatrial node modulator (ivabradine)[106] is used for patients not responding to first-line therapies. Sacubitril/valsartan improved congestion to a greater extent than enalapril alone.[107,108] Improving congestive symptoms by using diuretics and vasodilators improves the quality of life for patients with chronic HF.[107–109]

A fall in BNP following medical treatment has been shown to predict better clinical outcomes.[108] The use of spironolactone as an add-on medication after the use of ACEIs, beta blockers, and diuretics improves congestive symptoms, quality of life, and survival.[107–109]

For patients who have diabetes, there is growing interest of the SGLT2 inhibitors for management of HF with empagliflozin having a positive affect managing HF symptoms and improvement in cardiac function as high as 38% along with demonstrating a mortality benefit.[110]

Elderly patients have improved quality of life scores when home-based therapy for chronic HF is delivered versus the care delivered in specialty heart care clinics.[111] In today's world of remote telemedicine care, chronic HF care delivered over telemedicine was not found to improve survival versus care delivered in the usual manner.[112] Chronic care management of HF improves survival, decreases hospitalization, and improves quality of life when patients are actively treated for this condition.[113]

Management of acute HF exacerbation includes four primary intravenous medications: nitroglycerin, nesiritide, dopamine, and milrinone.[114] Nitroglycerin, a venodilator, is often considered first-line treatment for exacerbations of HF along with diuretics for congestive symptoms. Nesiritide, a natriuretic peptide, and nitroglycerin use were associated with lower mortality rate than the vasopressors dobutamine and milrinone in the setting of acute decompensated HF.[114]

In patients who have HF who also have AF, rhythm control was not superior to rate control when assessed over a 12-month period.[115]

PATIENT EDUCATION

Patients who are closely followed after hospitalization and exacerbation of HF have fewer readmissions and are more likely to follow planned treatments and guidelines.[116] If patients are not adherent to following treatment recommendations, outcomes are clinically worse.[117]

Patients with HF require a great deal of self-care to maintain physical stability, prevent hospitalization, and improve the quality of life. Patients need to monitor and recognize symptoms indicating decompensation in HF early on and take measures to treat this before further decompensation occurs. When self-care occurs, patients have fewer hospitalizations, lower medical cost, and decreased mortality risk. Patients with gradual symptom deterioration have a more difficult time recognizing and correcting the symptoms before exacerbation of HF occurs.[118]

There is a known relationship between HF and deep vein thrombosis (DVT). It is important to educate patients to maintain activity and take steps to prevent DVT in the setting of HF.[119]

5.3B CARDIOMYOPATHIES

OVERVIEW

Cardiomyopathies are a heterogeneous group of heart muscle diseases leading to HF. The major types of cardiomyopathy include dilated cardiomyopathy, hypertrophic cardiomyopathy, and restrictive cardiomyopathy. Dilated cardiomyopathy causes HFrEF and is the most frequent cause of death in spite of improvement in treatment. Dilated cardiomyopathy is also a leading indication for heart transplantation. In hypertrophic cardiomyopathy, outflow obstruction is present and the HF that occurs is most commonly the HFpEF type. Patients with restrictive cardiomyopathy also develop HFpEF early on. HFrEF is found with amyloidosis and hemochromatosis subtypes.[120]

Patients with a diagnosis of restrictive cardiomyopathy need to have constrictive pericarditis ruled out as the underlying cause of restrictive cardiomyopathy as this can be treated surgically. Restrictive cardiomyopathy can be categorized as idiopathic or from amyloid heart disease, endomyocardial fibrosis, or infiltrative disease.[121] Treatment for restrictive cardiomyopathy may include amiodarone for arrhythmias, warfarin for anticoagulation, cardiac support devices, and heart transplant surgery.[121]

Primary cardiomyopathy is confined to the heart muscle with subclassifications listed according to genetic, mixed, and acquired cardiomyopathies. Secondary cardiomyopathies have heart involvement due to systemic or another multiorgan disorder. Subtypes of primary cardiomyopathy include hypertrophic, dilated, and restrictive cardiomyopathies. The subtypes involved both structural and functional disorders of the myocardium.

Dilated cardiomyopathy is defined by the presence of left ventricular dilation along with contractile dysfunction. About 35% of dilated cardiomyopathy is genetically inherited with gene mutations affecting the cytoskeletal, sarcomere, and nuclear envelope proteins. Acquired causes of dilated cardiomyopathy include myocarditis due to exposure to alcohol, drugs and toxins, and metabolic and endocrine disturbances.[122]

Hypertrophic cardiomyopathy is a commonly inherited cardiovascular disease present in 1 in 500 in the general population. There are more than 1,400 mutations over 11 or more genes encoding proteins of the cardiac sarcomeres. It is well known that hypertrophic cardiomyopathy is the most frequent cause of sudden death in young people, but this condition can also lead to functional disability from HF and stroke. Clinical diagnosis is based upon unexplained left ventricular hypertrophy noted on echocardiogram or cardiovascular MRI or upon further investigation of a systolic murmur. Patients having a first-degree relative with hypertrophic cardiomyopathy should have screening performed because of the inherited pattern of this condition.[123]

Restrictive cardiomyopathy is characterized by nondilated LV or RV along with diastolic dysfunction. The three major causes of restrictive cardiomyopathy are cardiac amyloidosis, cardiac sarcoidosis, and cardiac hemochromatosis. Finding the etiology of restrictive cardiomyopathy is challenging, resulting in delay of diagnosis for each of these entities. Early recognition can improve survival in all subtypes of restrictive cardiomyopathy.[124]

EPIDEMIOLOGY

Hypertrophic cardiomyopathy is the development of a hypertrophied, nondilated LV that occurs without another predisposing condition. This is an inherited condition that can have hypertrophy of the LV occurring either in adolescence or later in life. The hypertrophy may be asymmetric and diastolic dysfunction is typically present. The primary concern is obstruction to left ventricular outflow. If the LV cannot empty as a result of this obstruction, the body cannot meet its metabolic demand.

Arrhythmogenic right ventricular cardiomyopathy/dysplasia (ARVC/D) is characterized by progressive replacement of normal myocardium with fibrofatty material. This condition most commonly occurs in the right ventricular inflow and outflow tracts with a small number of patients having left ventricular outflow tract dysfunction. There is a wide variety of muscle function abnormalities leading to a wide variety of symptoms such as arrhythmias, HF, and sudden death.

Restrictive cardiomyopathy consists of a pattern of restrictive ventricular filling. This leads to a reduced diastolic volume in the setting of either normal or reduced systolic volume with normal left ventricular wall thickness. This condition can be idiopathic, inherited, or secondary to hemochromatosis, amyloidosis, sarcoidosis, carcinoid syndrome, or previous radiation therapy.

PATHOPHYSIOLOGY

Dilated cardiomyopathy is characterized by dilated ventricles along with systolic dysfunction. Intrinsic factors leading to dilated cardiomyopathy include genetic variations leading to mutations and disease associated polymorphisms as these genes affect the performance, regulation, and maintenance of cardiac function. These genetic variations contribute to the pathogenesis of hereditary dilated cardiomyopathy. Cardiomyopathy can also occur secondary to other insults occurring in the heart thereby having a nonhereditary cause for the development of dilated cardiomyopathy.[125]

Restrictive cardiomyopathy is a disease of the heart muscle that causes impaired filling of the ventricle along with either normal or reduced ventricular diastolic volume.[129] Restrictive cardiomyopathy histologically has patchy interstitial fibrosis along with myocyte disarray leading to stiffening of the ventricles interfering with diastolic filling of the heart. Restrictive cardiomyopathy patients present with symptoms of dyspnea, peripheral edema, and an inability to exercise because of the symptoms. As the disease progresses, patients can develop hepatomegaly and ascites.

Doxorubicin, a chemotherapeutic agent, is classically a cause of cardiomyopathy as an adverse action of this medication. Chronic alcohol consumption also harms the cardiac myocytes especially if thiamine deficiency is also present.

MEDICAL HISTORY AND CLINICAL PRESENTATION

The most common presenting symptoms of dilated cardiomyopathy are consistent with congestive HF symptoms such as dyspnea upon exertion and PND. Other presenting symptoms can include circulatory collapse, arrhythmias, and thromboembolic events. Neurohormonal changes can occur secondary to myocyte damage and contribute to remodeling of the heart.[122] Patients with restrictive cardiomyopathy typically present with dyspnea upon exertion or palpitations as a result of diastolic dysfunction. Since the symptoms can be consistent with coronary artery disease, cardiac disease should be evaluated to provide early intervention when needed.

SIGNS AND SYMPTOMS

Chest pain, dyspnea upon exertion, palpitations, and syncope can occur in the setting of cardiomyopathy. Patients with restrictive cardiomyopathy have increased jugular venous pressure. An S3 gallop may be present with restrictive cardiomyopathy due to the impaired ability of the LV to relax.

PHYSICAL EXAMINATION

There are no specific signs or symptoms identifying cardiomyopathy because of overlap of signs and symptoms with HF. The PMI can be laterally displaced in the setting of dilated cardiomyopathy. S4 and S3 heart sounds can occur with the volume and pressure overload in the LV in the setting of HFpEF and HFrEF. Patients who have pulmonary fluid backup as a result of HFrEF can have pulmonary rales, jugular venous distention, hepatomegaly, and peripheral edema. Patients with hypertrophic cardiomyopathy may have a systolic murmur that increases with standing after squatting or with Valsalva maneuver.

DIFFERENTIAL DIAGNOSIS

Differential diagnosis of restrictive cardiomyopathy includes radiation therapy to the thorax leading to fibrosis, iron infiltration in the setting of hemochromatosis, and elevated levels of serum ferritin and transferrin saturation (Table 5.8).[126,127] Amyloidosis can cause low voltage QRS complexes on EKG along with increased wall thickness being found on echocardiogram. Amyloidosis diagnosis can be supported by serum protein electrophoresis and urine protein electrophoresis along with analysis of light chains. Technetium cardiac imaging can also identify some subtypes of amyloidosis. Endomyocardial biopsy can definitively diagnose amyloidosis but fat pad biopsy is less invasive and is the preferred diagnostic evaluation strategy.

DIAGNOSTIC STUDIES

Echocardiogram can be utilized to classify the cardiomyopathy according to subtype of dilated, hypertrophic, and

TABLE 5.8 Differential Diagnosis of Restrictive Cardiomyopathy

Diagnosies	Description and Differentiating Features
Takotsubo cardiomyopathy	Mimics acute myocardial infarction/heart failure as a result of emotional or physical stress with apical ballooning of left ventricle in light of normal coronary arteries. This condition causes transient apical ballooning and stress cardiomyopathy. Patients develop chest pain along with ST elevation, T wave inversions, and mild elevations in cardiac markers. After this acute event passes, left ventricular function normalizes.
Brugada syndrome	ST segment elevation in right precordial leads puts the patient at risk for sudden cardiac death due to arrhythmias.
Inflammatory myocarditis	Result of various infections, toxins, and medications. Biopsy reveals inflammatory infiltrates with or without myocyte necrosis. Suspect this condition in a patient with new onset of heart failure following a viral illness with echocardiogram showing dilated left ventricle.
Peripartum cardiomyopathy	Occurs toward the end of pregnancy or within several months following delivery with patients presenting with heart failure secondary to left ventricular systolic function. Can be associated with gestational hypertension or twin pregnancy. Complete recovery ensues some but progressive disease can occur and can even be fatal unless cardiac transplant occurs. Recurrent pregnancy is not recommended as this condition can recur and can be fatal.
Tachycardia-induced cardiomyopathy	Prolonged periods of increased heart rates lead to tachycardia-induced cardiomyopathy. Condition is important to recognize as rate control can prevent the development of this cardiomyopathy.
Amyloidosis	Abnormal starch-like product is deposited in the heart. Patients present with dyspnea or palpitations. Small voltage QRS complexes are noted on EKG. Echocardiogram reveals increased thickening in the atrial septum and left ventricular wall, speckled pattern seen with imaging along with valve thickening as a result of amyloid deposition. Pericardial effusion can also be identified. Despite the larger left ventricular mass, the QRS complex voltage is small.
Hemochromatosis	Can cause dilated or restrictive cardiomyopathy as a result of autosomal recessive disease caused by a mutation of the *HFE* gene leading to iron deposition in the heart and other organs. Cardiac MRI reveals iron deposition.
Sarcoidosis	Systemic granulomatous disorder of unknown etiology. Condition can present with heart failure as a result of cardiomyopathy, rhythm disturbances, and even sudden death. Cardiac MRI can help to identify this invasive condition when the heart is affected.
Acute drug use	Cocaine, sulfonamides, and antiepileptic medications can lead to myocarditis as exemplified by chest pain, dyspnea upon exertion, fatigue, syncope, and palpitations.

Source: Data from Dahlviken RM, Fridlund B, Mathisen L. Women's experiences of Takosubo cardiomyopathy in a short-term perspective: a qualitative content analysis. Scand J Caring Sci. *2015;29:258. doi:10.1111/scs.12158; Probst V, Veltmann C, Eckardt L, et al. Long-term prognosis of patients diagnosed with Brugada syndrome results from the FINGER Brugada Syndrome Registry.* Circulation. *2010;121:635–643. doi:10.1161/CIRCULATIONAHA.109.887026*

restrictive cardiomyopathy. Cardiac MRI and cardiac CT can help to identify the underlying cause of cardiomyopathy along with calculating the end-diastolic volumes and whether an intracardiac thrombus is present. Cardiac catheterization can be performed if echocardiogram is inconclusive.

Echocardiography is the diagnostic modality of choice used to identify hypertrophic cardiomyopathy. Patients with family history of sudden cardiac death or patients who have syncope that is either unexplained or that occurs with exercise should be evaluated for hypertrophic cardiomyopathy. Cardiac MRI provides accurate estimation of the extent of hypertrophy along with the extent of myocardial fibrosis. Coronary angiography can be used to determine if there is coexisting coronary artery disease in patients with hypertrophic cardiomyopathy. Although endomyocardial biopsy will identify this condition, it is rarely needed.

ARVC/D is a difficult diagnosis to make and is evaluated with echocardiogram showing abnormalities in muscle function, MRI, and angiography along with exercise stress testing are used to look for arrhythmias. Histopathologic changes can be seen on endomyocardial biopsy. This condition is inherited primarily in an autosomal dominant pattern so genetic testing can also be used to identify this condition.

Patients with restrictive cardiomyopathy will have biatrial hypertrophy due to the diastolic dysfunction along with nonspecific ST-T wave changes. Echocardiogram confirms the biatrial enlargement along with diastolic dysfunction with normal wall thickness. Cardiac catheterization can be used to distinguish restrictive cardiomyopathy from constrictive pericarditis. Endomyocardial biopsy can also be done to confirm the diagnosis.

A normal EKG is reassuring at ruling out significant cardiomyopathy since these patients tend to have at least a left bundle branch block pattern because of poor systolic function of the LV requiring a long time for the LV contraction to occur. If the patient has coexisting HF as a result of cardiomyopathy, the patient will have an elevation of BNP.

Elevated troponin levels in the blood is strongly associated with poor prognosis in patients who develop cardiomyopathy as a result of contracting a novel coronavirus disease. Myocardial injury in the setting of COVID-19 includes ischemia due to circulatory and respiratory failure, coronary artery thrombotic obstruction due to increased coagulability, and myocarditis caused by systemic inflammation or direct binding of the virus to its receptor, ACE-2, which is abundantly expressed in the heart. Persistent immune activation following viral infection increases the risk of developing dilated cardiomyopathy in COVID-19 patients.[128]

Echocardiogram aids in making the diagnosis of restrictive cardiomyopathy with findings consistent with biatrial enlargement and severe diastolic dysfunction. Echocardiogram will show the ventricles to be of normal size and without wall thickness. Systolic function and wall motion of the LV are typically normal. Pulmonary hypertension is consistent with restrictive cardiomyopathy. Valvular involvement with restrictive cardiomyopathy occurs with tricuspid regurgitation (TR) and mitral valve (MV) regurgitation. Echocardiogram can also help to differentiate constrictive pericarditis from cardiac amyloidosis, which causes restrictive cardiomyopathy.[129]

Amyloidosis is a rare disorder that is characterized by the deposition of amyloid protein aggregates in different organ systems throughout the body causing functional impairment of the affected organs. Because of its nonspecific presentation, it can present with localized or multisystemic amyloid deposits. Echocardiogram and cardiac MRI will show restrictive cardiomyopathy. Congo red staining of biopsy sites can identify amyloid deposition. Patients with amyloidosis can also have elevated serum kappa light chains with the need to differentiate this condition from multiple myeloma, which can also have elevation of light chains in the urine.[130]

Abdominal fat pad biopsy in the identification of amyloidosis allows a less invasive approach than biopsy of the heart or kidneys. Abdominal fat pad excisional biopsy has a high sensitivity for immunoglobulin light chain amyloidosis, but it is less sensitive for the transthyretin type of amyloidosis.[131] Rectal mucosal biopsy can also be performed along with abdominal fat pad biopsy in order to improve the sensitivity of finding light chain amyloidosis.[132]

EVALUATION

Patients suspected of having cardiomyopathy should undergo a baseline EKG along with an echocardiogram, which will aid not only in making the diagnosis but also in identifying the underlying cause. Ejection fraction and end-diastolic pressures are calculated during echocardiography, which can suggest the severity of the cardiomyopathy. Once the diagnosis is made, treatment can be determined. If echocardiography is inconclusive, cardiac MRI or CT angiography (CTA) can be performed. Cardiac catheterization can be done to assess for concomitant coronary artery disease.

Patients should be evaluated for thyroid abnormalities as thyroid disease can lead to cardiomyopathy or can worsen cardiomyopathy if not identified and treated. Genetic testing has a role for patients with hypertrophic cardiomyopathy, hemochromatosis, arrhythmogenic right ventricular outflow obstruction, or amyloidosis, which can be either inherited or acquired.

TREATMENT

Treatment of dilated cardiomyopathy is the same as the treatment of chronic HF, namely ACEIs or ARBs, beta blockers, and diuretics for fluid overload. If arrhythmia is a prominent symptom, implantable cardiac defibrillator can be lifesaving in preventing sudden death. Patients who are refractory to medical therapy may need mechanical circulatory support such as IABP or left ventricular assist device with heart transplant also a consideration.[122]

Treatment for hypertrophic cardiomyopathy includes implantable defibrillators to prevent sudden cardiac death, medications such as beta blockers to decrease chronotropic and inotropic activity of the heart, surgical myectomy or alcohol septal ablation in order to relieve outflow obstruction and symptoms, and radiofrequency ablation to control AF and to prevent embolic stroke.[123]

There is no specific medical therapy for restrictive cardiomyopathy. Loop diuretics are utilized in order to relieve congestive symptoms and this is typically only given late in the course of the disease as patients with restrictive cardiomyopathy require relatively high filling pressures in order to maintain cardiac output. If diuresis is too aggressive, there will be hypoperfusion of the kidneys. Anticoagulation and rate control may be indicated in the setting of AF and restrictive cardiomyopathy. Digoxin is typically not used because it can increase intracellular calcium, which interferes with diastolic relaxation. Cardiovascular mortality in the setting of restrictive cardiomyopathy is related to progressive HF and arrhythmias. Patients who have failed maximal medical therapy may be considered for cardiac transplantation.[133]

PATIENT EDUCATION

Pediatric patients with hypertrophic cardiomyopathy and restrictive physiology may have poor outcomes. Many children with hypertrophic cardiomyopathy develop a restrictive type of cardiomyopathy and these patients have a 3.5-fold increase in hospitalizations and a 5.7-fold increase in death.[134]

SPECIAL CONSIDERATIONS

HF is a syndrome resulting from a process affecting the heart. For this reason, the underlying cause of HF should be identified as its correction is essential in its management. HF can result from an acute MI or could be secondary to dietary or fluid indiscretion. Patient education is key to decreasing recurrence of decompensated HF. Patients with a tendency for decompensated HF should measure their weight daily and take action in response to weight gain. Diuretics are effective in managing fluid overload and in helping to maintain the patient's weight. A consideration for potassium supplementation should occur in patients receiving loop diuretics. Since patients with HF often receive ACEIs or ARBs along with spironolactone as add-on therapy, potassium levels should be serially followed, especially if the patient has impaired renal function.

In the setting of dilated cardiomyopathy, patients with the lowest ejection fractions and those with severe diastolic dysfunction have a worse prognosis.[121]

KEY POINTS

- The incidence of HF is increasing primarily as the population ages and improvements are made in the treatment of coronary artery disease, allowing these patients to survive long enough to develop HF.
- HF occurs secondary to another insult so there should be a search for the provoking factor with treatment addressed at this underlying cause.
- HF is the most common reason for hospitalization in the United States according to the diagnosis related grouping admitting diagnosis.
- Patients need to be active participants in their ongoing care for HF with emphasis on fluid restriction, active lifestyle as much as possible, limiting salt, potassium supplementation to replace sodium in the diet, and medication adherence.

5.4 CORONARY ARTERY DISEASE

CHRISTINE BRUCE

OVERVIEW

More people die from coronary artery disease than any other single condition in the United States. Coronary disease can occur as atherosclerosis progresses slowly over time with buildup of plaque until occlusion interferes with blood supply to the heart. ACS can also occur when a smaller, lipid-laden plaque acutely ruptures resulting in acute occlusion, suggesting that any unstable plaque is at risk for rupture even without a large amount of obstruction.

ACS is made up of three entities: STEMI, NSTEMI, and unstable angina (USA). These conditions are separate from chronic angina pectoris, which has a fixed plaque causing similar complaints but in a predictable fashion. The first time angina occurs or a change occurs in the previously established pattern of angina pectoris, the criteria for USA is met. Three factors are evaluated in order to differentiate each ACS entity: history of the patient, EKG findings, and elevation of cardiac biomarkers such as troponin.

NSTEMI is defined as having elevated cardiac biomarkers signifying cardiac necrosis in the absence of persistent ST segment elevation in patients with chest pain. It carries a poorer long-term prognosis than patients surviving STEMI because of the typical comorbidities of these patients, who tend to be older along with having diverse underlying causes that add complexity to therapeutic decision-making.[135]

Type I NSTEMI is an acute atherothrombotic event and type II NSTEMI occurs as a result of a mismatch of myocardial oxygen supply and demand.

Clopidogrel and aspirin reduce recurrent events when used in ACS. Other agents that may be helpful for ACS include glycoprotein IIb/III inhibitors, thrombolytics used in the setting of STEMI, and PCI used in any ACS patient with ongoing or worsening symptoms.

EPIDEMIOLOGY

NSTEMI has become more common than STEMI in clinical practice. In-hospital mortality rate is significantly lower in NSTEMI patients than in STEMI patients acutely but 1-year mortality rate is similar in both conditions meaning that long-term mortality is higher with NSTEMI. PCI reduces mortality risk in both STEMI and NSTEMI, but PCI is often underutilized in patients with NSTEMI.[136]

ACS occurs more frequently with aging as there is a slow accumulation of lipid-laden plaque surrounded by a thin fibrous cap. Risk factors include age >45 years in men or >55 years in women, family history of coronary artery disease and hyperlipidemia that includes elevated low-density lipoprotein or low high-density lipoprotein levels, hypertension, diabetes mellitus, and smoking. Atherosclerosis is the most common cause for the development of ACS with vasculitis, coronary artery spasm, and aortic stenosis (AS) being other causes. AS interferes with blood flow into the right and left coronary arteries as a result of limitations in getting blood into the systemic circulation. Patients with left ventricular hypertrophy or hypertrophic cardiomyopathy can develop ACS if there is insufficient blood supplying the musculature of the heart.

PATHOPHYSIOLOGY

ACS occurs with plaque rupture, erosion, or ulceration. ACS can occur as a result of a superficial erosion in the coronary artery. Plaques that are complicated by erosion are matrix-rich, lipid poor, and lack prominent macrophage collections. These erosions are unlike plaques that rupture, which typically have thin fibrous caps, large lipid pools, and abundant foam cells. Thrombi that complicate superficial erosions are more platelet rich than the fibrinous clots precipitated by plaque rupture. Multiple processes predispose plaques to superficial erosions including disturbed flow of blood, basement membrane breakdown, endothelial cell death, and detachment potentiated by innate immune activation. ACSs that occur as a result of plaque erosion may not require immediate invasive therapy.[137] Old fibrotic, calcified plaques are less likely to rupture than new lipid-laden plaques.

Following disruption of the plaque, platelet adhesion occurs along with platelet activation leading to platelet aggregation at the site of the rupture. Platelet aggregation forms a white clot and fibrin accumulation forms a red clot. White clot formation results in thrombotic occlusion. Platelet cascade starts thrombus formation. After plaque disruption, there is partial or total occlusion of the artery which may be superimposed on coronary artery spasm. White clot with minimum red clot is typically found with both USA and NSTEMI. Red clots are always part of STEMI. If ACS occurs in patients younger than 50 years of age who are not at risk for coronary disease, consider cocaine use, as this can cause both vasospasm and thrombosis.

When myocardial cells are deprived of blood for 4 hours or longer, irreversible death occurs and these cells are not capable of contracting or conducting an electrical impulse. The area around the infarcted tissue is known as the penumbra and it is this at-risk tissue that can recover if blood is returned to these cells. With ischemia and infarction, the heart becomes irritable and ectopic beats occur along with an increased potential for cardiac arrhythmia. The first hour post-MI is known as the "golden hour" as death can occur as a result of malignant arrhythmia such as ventricular tachycardia (VT) or fibrillation. The majority of cardiac deaths occur from these arrhythmias and not due to massive loss of cardiac tissue. With time, several complications occur over a period of time that is predictable.

RV infarction presents special challenges for management as the RV dilates pushing the interventricular septum into the left ventricular cavity causing decreased left ventricular filling, which results in decreased stroke volume and hypotension. Right and left ventricular failure as a result of infarction can be easily distinguished clinically because right ventricular failure patients have clear lungs on auscultation and there is elevation of jugular venous pressure. Right ventricular infarctions are typically from problems with the right coronary artery (RCA). Treatment of right ventricular MI requires avoidance of venous dilating medications like nitroglycerin as they further decrease the preload and this worsens hypotension.

Although atherosclerosis and plaque rupture is the typical cause of ACS, other causes of acute MI can occur without underlying atherosclerosis, as illustrated in Table 5.9.

TABLE 5.9 Other Causes of Acute Myocardial Infarction

Nonatherogenic Causes	Description
Vasculitis	Causes inflammation of the endothelium. Vasculitis leading to acute myocardial infarction can be due to lupus, polyarteritis nodosa, or Kawasaki syndrome (leads to coronary artery aneurysm).
Cocaine use	Can lead to significant spasm.
Coronary artery embolism	Can occur due to atrial myxoma tumor or atrial or ventricular thrombus.
Hypercoagulable states	Can lead to blockage of a coronary vessel. Hypercoagulable states include polycythemia vera, thrombocytosis, factor V Leiden (activated resistance to protein C), and deficiencies of protein C, protein S, or antithrombin III. The presence of a prothrombin gene or antiphospholipid antibody can also lead to hypercoagulable state and acute myocardial infarction.

5.4A ACUTE MYOCARDIAL INFARCTION

MEDICAL HISTORY AND CLINICAL PRESENTATION

Many patients experiencing chest discomfort initially deny that it is cardiac in nature. Patients may blame this discomfort on indigestion, food intolerance, stress, pneumonia, or anxiety. Denial of symptoms may result in delay of proper evaluation and treatment and lower the chance of successful reperfusion therapy. High-risk factors for coronary events include aging, diabetes, hyperlipidemia, positive family history of coronary disease, hypertension, previous MI, and physical or emotional stress.

SIGNS AND SYMPTOMS

Angina pectoris occurs when there is temporary impaired blood flow to an area of the heart resulting in ischemia rather than myocardial cell death. Patients with angina typically describe a poorly localized, squeezing, or crushing retrosternal pain that may radiate to the arm, jaw, or neck. Patients can also complain of shortness of breath, nausea, epigastric discomfort, diaphoresis, weakness, or dizziness. Anginal patients can predict how much activity will bring about these symptoms and know how long it takes until these symptoms abate (typically <5 minutes). Rest and nitroglycerin bring about the resolution of these symptoms. Because these stable plaques cause interference with blood flow, the body can bypass these narrowed segments of blood vessels in a process known as angiogenesis. If these stable plaques become unstable and rupture, this collateral circulation can supply the blood downstream and prevent infarction since an alternative pathway for circulation exists.

ACS can present as STEMI, NSTEMI, or USA. USA occurs as the first episode of angina or if there is a change in the previously established pattern of stable angina. Patients are suspected of having ACS if chest pressure/discomfort is not relieved after three nitroglycerin doses or if the pain continues despite rest. Diaphoresis is a worrisome sign. Diabetic patients, older adults, and women may have atypical presentation for ACS, which could include weakness, dyspnea, HF, lightheadedness, or pain/pressure in sites other than the chest. Patients with ACS may have a sense of impending doom as a presenting feature.

Patients with actual MI have chest pressure or pain that does not respond to three nitroglycerin doses taken 5 minutes apart. This pain is hard to describe due to its visceral nature. Patients may appear ashen in appearance with diaphoresis. Shortness of breath occurs even if oxygen levels are not decreased. Blood pressure may be lower along with tachycardia. Patients may complain of feeling anxious and be lightheaded.

PHYSICAL EXAMINATION

Patients may have swelling, vomiting, bradycardia, heart block, or tachycardia as signs of acute MI. Tachyarrhythmias can occur due to pain and anxiety increasing the heart rate along with production of ectopic beats due to irritability within the cardiac myocytes. Atypical signs may include shortness of breath as a primary complaint along with palpitations, syncope, weakness, or lightheadedness. Mild or few symptoms can occur in older, diabetic, and female patients. USA may present with rest angina that can last longer than 20 minutes. Patients may also complain of a crescendo pattern of pain with increased intensity, duration, or frequency of chest pain. Some patients with USA may have pain at rest or pain that awakens them. Progressive USA pattern may herald an acute MI.

DIFFERENTIAL DIAGNOSIS

The differential diagnosis for coronary artery disease is summarized in Table 5.10.[138–141]

DIAGNOSTIC STUDIES

Diagnosis of ACS is based upon having a positive finding in at least two of three parameters: patient history, cardiac enzyme biomarkers, and EKG findings. The differentiating feature between USA and NSTEMI is that cardiac biomarkers are elevated only with NSTEMI. EKG findings differentiate STEMI and NSTEMI from each other since both conditions will have positive cardiac biomarkers and similar patient histories that are concerning for cardiac-related chest pain. EKG with STEMI initially shows peaked T waves followed by ST segment elevation. As the STEMI evolves or

TABLE 5.10 Differential Diagnosis for Coronary Artery Disease

Condition	Notable History and Physical Findings	Diagnostic Findings
Angina pectoris	Predictable pattern of chest pain. Responds to nitrates, beta blockers, and rest. Typically lasts 5–15 minutes. Is not typically associated with diaphoresis.	EKG can show ST segment depression in anatomically contiguous leads. Normal troponin levels.
Acute pericarditis and Dressler syndrome	Pleuritic chest pain increasing with deep breathing. Pain lessens with leaning forward and worsens with laying down or inspiration. Pericardial friction rub can be heard on auscultation of the heart. **Dressler syndrome** is postmyocardial pericarditis occurring as an inflammatory condition involving the pleura and pericardium. Dressler syndrome can also occur after PCI and stent placement, pacemaker lead insertion, or blunt cardiac trauma.	EKG shows ST segment elevation in practically all leads with depressed PR segment.
Cocaine-Induced myocardial infarction with coronary vasospasm	Episodes typically occur in patients with normal coronary arteries who use vasospastic drugs such as cocaine and methamphetamines. Suspect in patients with abrupt chest pain who lack cardiovascular risk factors. Treatment for cocaine-induced coronary spasm is with benzodiazepines or nitrates. **Beta blockers need to be avoided in this setting because of unopposed alpha adrenergic stimulation, which would increase heart rate exponentially.**	ST segment elevation in affected leads from areas of the heart affected by impaired blood flow. ST segment depression can also occur as a result of impaired blood flow to a segment of the heart. If infarction occurs, troponin levels will increase.
Pulmonary embolism	Tachypnea, tachycardia, shortness of breath, and anxiety.	Most common EKG finding is sinus tachycardia with a classic S1Q3T3 being often talked about but rarely seen.
Aortic dissection	Complaints of a tearing pain or pain with a ripping quality primarily located between the scapulae in the back.	Chest x-ray shows a widened mediastinum, pulses are decreased and delayed in the lower extremity compared to the pulses proximal to the site of dissection.
Reflux esophagitis	Complaints of indigestion, dyspepsia, burning in the esophagus; possible waterbrash with refluxant entering into the mouth.	Diagnosis of exclusion; EGD in nonacute circumstance can show esophageal irritation. Difficult differentiation at times since both conditions respond to nitroglycerin.
Cholecystitis	Right upper quadrant abdominal pain which remains steady when the pain occurs; patient may have inspiratory arrest on deep inspiration with palpation in the right upper quadrant known as a Murphy sign.	Ultrasound can show cholelithiasis, sludge in gallbladder, thickening of gallbladder wall, or pericholecystic fluid collection.
Tension pneumothorax	Extreme shortness of breath with rapid decline in respiratory system leading to cyanosis and rapid clinical deterioration.	Chest x-ray demonstrates pneumothorax with shifting of the mediastinum due to kinking of the vessels preventing blood return to the heart; tracheal deviation also seen.
Perforated peptic ulcer	Abdominal pain with rigid abdomen on exam and loss of bowel sounds due to peritonitis.	Abdominal upright film will show free air beneath the diaphragm since rupture of an air-filled stomach will cause leakage of air into the peritoneal cavity.
Takotsubo cardiomyopathy	Complaint of chest pain in the setting of emotional turmoil. Clinical presentation is identical to acute MI but no actual myocardial damage occurs.	Identified during heart catheterization or echocardiography showing wall motion abnormalities without significant coronary artery disease. Patients have an elevated brain natriuretic peptide, myoglobulin, and CK-MB levels. Echocardiogram can also identify these wall motion abnormalities that are typically located in the apex.[138]
Cardiac-related syncope	Sudden onset of loss of consciousness with patient having injuries without defensive attempt to prevent injury during syncopal episode.	Can be caused by underlying arrhythmia, which could be due to ACS or reduced left ventricular function, pulmonary embolism, or structural heart disease such as aortic valve stenosis.[139]
Spontaneous pneumothorax	Tall thin patient with acute onset of chest pain that is unilateral in location. Increased risk in those who smoke. In addition to chest pain, there may be dyspnea. Can occur as the result of spontaneous rupture of lung bleb.	Chest film identifies collapse of lung (especially with expiratory phase chest film). Edge of lung may be visualized along with lack of vessel markings in the lung periphery.

TABLE 5.10 Differential Diagnosis for Coronary Artery Disease *(continued)*

Condition	Notable History and Physical Findings	Diagnostic Findings
Hypertrophic cardiomyopathy	Symptoms most common following exercise when there is venous pulling into the extremities. Substernal chest pain. Harsh systolic murmur that lessons with squatting and fist clenching and increases with standing and performing the Valsalva maneuver.	EKG can show with T wave inversions in V2 through the V4. Echocardiogram can show asymmetric hypertrophy of the intraventricular septum with the mitral valve showing increased occlusion of left ventricular output with lower blood volumes.
Costochondritis or Tietze syndrome	Pain reproduced with chest wall pressure; pain increased with inspiration. Tietze syndrome has pain at costochondral, sternoclavicular, or costosternal junctions while costochondritis provides more diffuse pain without focal tenderness.	EKG has nonspecific findings and may have only tachycardia if the patient is experiencing pain.
Myocarditis	Vague chest complaints that can follow viral illness such as Coxsackie B, other echovirus, and even coronavirus infection.[140]	Conduction abnormalities with heart block may occur as evidenced by various heart blocks.
Mitral valve prolapse	Can be associated with midsystolic click or mitral regurgitation. Pain is typically intermittent and may be associated with palpitations. Young females are at increased risk for this condition. Condition is mild but more worrisome if associated with mitral regurgitation. Occurs in 1 in 400 people and is the most common reason for operating on the mitral valve in the United States.[141]	Holter monitor may demonstrate palpitations with this condition. No specific EKG findings and troponin levels remain normal.
Variant or Prinzmetal angina	Chest pain typically occurs at rest. Caused by vasospasm of coronary artery. Vasospasm might be provoked by plaque or endothelial injury. Treated with nitrates or calcium channel blockers. Beta blockers are ineffective.	Cardiac biomarkers remain normal. EKG has ST segment elevation in anatomically contiguous leads that return to baseline when spasm is relieved.

ACS, acute coronary syndrome; EGD, esophagogastroduodenoscopy; MI, myocardial infarction; PCI, percutaneous coronary intervention.

Source: Data from Fröhlich GM, Schoch B, Schmid F, et al. Takotsubo cardiomyopathy has a unique cardiac biomarker profile: NT-proBNP/myoglobin and NT-proBNP/troponin T ratios for the differential diagnosis of acute coronary syndromes and stress induced cardiomyopathy. Int J Cardiol. *2012;154:328–332. doi:10.1016/j.ijcard.2011.09.077; Möckel M. Biomarkers in the diagnosis of cardiovascular emergencies: acute coronary syndrome and differential diagnoses.* Internist. *2019;60(6):564–570. doi:10.1007/s00108-019-0620-9; Kang Y, Chen T, Mui D, et al. Cardiovascular manifestations and treatment considerations in COVID-19.* Heart. *2020;106:1132–1141. doi:10.1136/heartjnl-2020-317056; Levine RA, Jerosch-Herold M, Hajjar RJ. Mitral valve prolapse: a disease of valve and ventricle.* J Am Coll Cardiol. *2018;72:835–837. doi:10.1016/j.jacc.2018.07.006*

if reperfusion occurs, T wave inversion may be seen prior to return of the T waves to the baseline. With STEMI, there is typically reciprocal T wave inversion in other anatomically contiguous leads. Q waves show a completed infarct due to infarcted tissue not being able to conduct electricity. If reperfusion occurs in a timely manner, the patient may never go on to develop Q waves. Once a Q wave develops, it tends to be permanent since dead cardiac tissue does not conduct electricity. If a patient with chest pain has an EKG already showing significant Q waves, this would reflect previous myocardial damage and does not exclude another cardiovascular event.

ACS causes ST segment elevation with typical chest pain pattern in the setting of STEMI. A new-onset left bundle branch block also supports the diagnosis of acute MI and this is treated as a STEMI equivalent. ST segment depression and T wave inversion are less specific for ACS and can be seen with any cardiac conditions including angina pectoris, USA, and NSTEMI. A normal EKG, however, does not rule out an acute MI.

A patient having an acute bout of chest pain who has a positive EKG for STEMI will show ST segment elevation of >1 mm in two anatomic contiguous leads. Flat or downsloping ST segment depression or T wave inversion can be seen in any acute coronary event. Serial EKGs in the setting of ACS may show the initial EKG to be normal or nondiagnostic with subsequent EKGs having a normal appearance despite MI. In the same way that serial enzymes are ordered (typically on presentation and at 2 and 6 hours), EKGs are also performed serially. ST segment monitoring can be done on an ongoing basis and is typically serially followed.

In the setting of Prinzmetal angina, the EKG will show transient ST segment elevation during angina. There is no role for exercise treadmill testing as this condition is not caused by increased physiologic demand on the heart. Ergonovine given intravenously is the most sensitive and specific test that can provoke this spasm. Nitroglycerin can reverse the effects of ergotamine if refractory spasm occurs.[142]

The role of cardiac biomarkers is based on the premise that injured myocardial cells leak enzymes. The initial biomarkers may be normal as it may take 2 hours for them to be seen in the blood. Troponin is both sensitive and specific for myocardial necrosis with the degree of rise mirroring the extent of necrosis. High troponin levels can signify a worse prognosis necessitating early invasive strategy.

Echocardiogram can be used in the setting of ACS since acute MIs have abnormal wall motion abnormalities signified by hypokinesia or dyskinesia that occurs within seconds of coronary artery occlusion. Echocardiogram can detect left ventricular thrombus and aneurysm. Limitation of echocardiogram is that it cannot distinguish new from old MI patterns as wall motion abnormalities can occur acutely or can be permanently seen if there is continued dysfunction of the heart wall motion. In the setting of USA, ischemia is reversible along with wall motion abnormalities. Echocardiogram is most useful in diagnosing MI in the setting of left bundle branch block, if the patient has an abnormal EKG but diagnostic uncertainty, or if pericarditis is suspected in a patient who has an EKG showing ST segment elevation.

Myocardial perfusion imaging (MPI) is useful in identifying reversible wall motion abnormalities as demonstrated by normalization of these abnormalities in the resting phase of the study. A perfusion defect on this study that never normalizes is either a new or old MI. If normalization occurs, this suggests transient ischemia.

EVALUATION

Risk Stratification

Patients are risk stratified according to TIMI (thrombolysis in acute MI) or Grace risk scores that help in both diagnostic and therapeutic decision-making. Points are awarded for the following: age ≥65; ≥3 coronary artery disease risk factors including hypertension, hypercholesterolemia, diabetes, family history of coronary artery disease, or current smoker; known coronary artery disease with stenosis of at least 50%; aspirin used in the past 7 days; severe angina with at least two episodes in 24 hours; ST segment EKG changes of at least 0.5 mm; and positive cardiac markers. TIMI risk index utilizes heart rate, age, and systolic blood pressure in its calculation. Prediction for mortality via TIMI scores is more accurate when applied to male versus female population.[143]

Risk stratification determines whether the patient receives early intervention with cardiac catheterization or whether the patient receives exercise stress testing prior to discharge. The higher the TIMI score, the greater the likelihood of death and the worse the outcome. TIMI scores of 0 to 2 are considered low risk and the patient is given aspirin, beta blockers, nitrates, heparin, statins, and clopidogrel. TIMI scores of 0 or 1, however, do not mean that the patient is not at risk for adverse outcome. Patients with scores of 0 to 2 typically undergo stress testing prior to discharge. Cardiac catheterization is indicated if significant myocardial ischemia is suspected. TIMI scores of 3 to 7 are considered intermediate to high risk. The same treatments are pursued medically with the addition of early cardiac catheterization and PCI, as needed.

Stress testing results can lead to referral for cardiac catheterization if the patient has ST segment depression or elevation, if they cannot achieve appropriate Bruce protocol exercise of 5 mets, if systolic blood pressure does not rise by 10 to 30 mm Hg during exercise, or if the patient is unable to exercise.

An exercise stress test is positive for cardiac ischemia if there are 2 mm ST segment depressions seen in anatomically contiguous leads or if hypotension occurs, as signified as a drop of at least 10 mm Hg in systolic pressure. Exercise stress testing can be used to risk stratify patients regarding further evaluation and prognosis. Patients with ongoing severe symptoms or hypotension are more likely to have triple vessel disease. Stress testing can also assess the effectiveness of therapy. Exercise stress testing is contraindicated in the setting of cardiac instability states such as aortic dissection, acute MI, USA, decompensated HF, uncontrolled ventricular arrhythmias, significant AS (when the patient cannot increase cardiac output when needed), hypertrophic cardiomyopathy, and severe, uncontrolled hypertension.

Exercise stress test interpretation can be difficult in patients who have baseline EKG abnormalities such as left ventricular hypertrophy, bundle branch block pattern, and in those who have a pacemaker. For these patients, nuclear stress imaging in lieu of exercise stress testing can be beneficial in these settings.

The ideal candidate for a patient to undergo exercise stress test is a patient who has intermediate risk for coronary disease as these patients are less likely to have false positive or false negative testing. Exercise stress test should not be performed in low-risk patients who are able to exercise without symptoms or if troponin is normal as findings are more likely to be false positive test results than true cardiac-related problems. Using similar reasoning, normal exercise stress testing in a patient with a high pretest probability for coronary artery disease is more likely to be a false negative test, which would still require additional evaluation.

Chemical stress tests are indicated for patients who are unable to exercise. Dipyridamole (Persantine) or dobutamine can be used to increase myocardial contractility so that a heart can be assessed when placed under stress. When dipyridamole is given to an individual with stable angina, coronary steal syndrome may occur as a result of vasodilation of the coronary arteries without significant obstruction while coronary arteries having obstruction will have the obstructed coronary artery already maximally dilated. In the setting of obstruction, the end result is that blood is diverted or stolen away from the ischemic myocardium to nonischemic areas, which further worsens the ischemia, and this process is demonstrated on the EKG as ST segment depression in the anatomically affected area.

Nuclear stress test involves injection of a radioactive substance (such as thallium) followed by visualization of the perfused heart tissue. Perfusion pictures are done at rest and after exercise to assess for recovery of blood flow patterns. Nuclear stress tests have a higher sensitivity and specificity than exercise treadmill test but are considerably more expensive.

Stress echocardiogram combines exercise stress testing while performing an echocardiogram. Wall motion abnormalities are identified when exercise occurs and clinicians are able to visualize what happens to the heart when stressed.

Cardiac catheterization is indicated in ACS and can also be performed when noninvasive test cannot be done such as patients with morbid obesity or COPD, which limits the interpretation of these noninvasive tests. Results may lead to PCI or coronary artery bypass grafting. Coronary CT can be performed in stable patients who have intermediate risk for coronary artery disease in order to find obstructing lesions.[144]

Patients with ACS will have vital signs immediately taken, chew an 81-mg aspirin, and have pulse oximetry performed with oxygen delivered to the patient if the patient's oxygen level is lower than 94% (the level in which the hemoglobin is fully saturated). EKG is performed urgently and evaluated for acute changes. IV access is obtained in order to deliver medication and fluids.

Troponin levels are normal in the setting of angina pectoris and Prinzmetal angina because there is ischemia but no actual infarction. Patients with Prinzmetal angina can have 24-hour EKG Holter monitor applied, which classically shows a transient elevation of the ST segment but with normal troponin levels. The vasoconstrictive medication ergonovine may be given to provoke vasospasm assessing for coronary artery spasm producing transient ST segment elevation.

Patients with USA and NSTEMI can have an EKG that can be normal or can show ST segment depression or T wave inversions, but troponin levels are normal because there is no myocyte necrosis. If the troponin levels are elevated, NSTEMI is diagnosed, which signifies an infarction beneath the endocardium (sometimes called a subendocardial infarct). This infarct occurs because the coronary vessels run along the epicardium, which is located in the outer one third of the heart, so the endocardium is the farthest area away from the blood supply. NSTEMI causes changes like ST depression or T wave inversion, but it never shows ST segment elevation.

ST elevation in leads V1 and V2 is consistent with anteroseptal MI involving the left anterior descending artery (LAD). Lead V3 and V4 involvement is an anteroapical MI, which means the distal part of the LAD is involved. Lead V5 and V6 involvement signifies an anterolateral MI, which involves the LAD or left circumflex artery. Lateral MI involves leads I and aVL from involvement of the left circumflex artery. Inferior wall MI involves leads II, III, and aVF with blockage of the RCA typically being the culprit. RCA occlusion can also cause right ventricular infarction and right-sided chest leads illustrate these findings. There is ST depression with tall R waves in V1 to V3 in the setting of posterior MI most commonly involving the posterior descending artery and is also demonstrated by obtaining additional EKG in the posterior leads V7 to V9.

TREATMENT

Modern therapy of STEMI includes reperfusion therapy, ideally by primary PCI, antithrombotic therapy, and secondary prevention measures.[145]

Treatment of Unstable Angina/Non-ST Segment Elevation Myocardial Infarction

Aspirin should be administered promptly unless contraindicated. Bolus administration of clopidogrel at 300 to 600 mg or prasugrel 60 mg is given for aspirin-allergic patients. Ticagrelor is also given for patients getting conservative, ischemic-guided medical therapy. Early invasive treatment is recommended for those who have refractory angina or hemodynamic or electrical instability. Patients given early invasive therapy have less postprocedure angina and no difference in mortality compared to those patients given traditional medical therapy of heparin, clopidogrel, and aspirin.[146] Dual platelet aspirin plus clopidogrel is given prior to PCI.[166] Heparin or bivalirudin can be given prior to cardiac catheterization. If the patient is not going for cardiac catheterization, fondaparinux (an indirect factor Xa inhibitor) or low molecular weight heparin is administered. If a history of GI bleeding is noted, a PPI or H2 blocker should be added to the dual antiplatelet therapy. PPI agents can be safely used with clopidogrel such as pantoprazole while avoiding omeprazole and esomeprazole due to impairing the action of clopidogrel due to the cytochrome P450 system.

Patients being given medical therapy are placed on nasal oxygen as indicated for arterial saturation <94% or if respiratory distress is present. Nitroglycerin is indicated for ongoing angina. Beta blockers should be administered within the first 24 hours. ACEI should be given within 24 hours in those with clinical HF or in those with ejection fraction of <40%.[166] Statin therapy is also considered as first-line therapy in ACS with atorvastatin 80 mg being given as soon as possible.

PCI should be considered for revascularization even after thrombolysis has been given; however, PCI should be delayed at least 2 hours after thrombolytics. PCI performed in these settings is now routine and is no longer considered salvage therapy. If conservative treatment was performed, MPI (myocardial perfusion imaging) is indicated prior to discharge of the patient from the healthcare facility.

Postdischarge medications include aspirin, clopidogrel, beta blockers to control heart rate, statins, and ACEI if decreased ejection fraction or HF exists, and in those with diabetes or hypertension.

ST Segment Elevation Myocardial Infarction Treatment

Patients with STEMI and ongoing ischemic symptoms should be treated with PCI.[147] Primary PCI should be done within 90 minutes of contact with the medical system. Emergency transport to PCI-capable hospital is recommended since patients have a better outcome with PCI compared to thrombolytic therapy alone. Although the best results of PCI occur within 12 hours of symptom onset, myocardial salvage of surrounding tissues (known as the penumbra) can occur as late as 72 hours after the initial onset of symptoms.[148]

Fibrinolytic therapy can be considered if PCI cannot be done within the optimal time frame. When fibrinolytic therapy is given, it should be started within 30 minutes of hospital arrival (door to drug therapy). Aspirin should be given before PCI and continued in patients with STEMI who continue to have ischemic symptoms. These patients should be treated with PCI; however, PCI must be delayed at least 2 hours.

Aspirin should be continued indefinitely at 81 mg daily. P2Y12 receptors should be given during primary PCI and continued for 1 year with drug-eluting stent placement and a minimum of 1 month with placement of bare metal stents.[166] Clopidogrel is continued for a longer period of time with drug-eluting stents so that endothelialization of the vessel can occur. Anticoagulation therapy with unfractionated heparin and bivalirudin should be considered as part of this treatment. Urgent PCI of the infarcted artery should be addressed urgently with stent placement. Urgent coronary artery bypass surgery is indicated if the coronary artery anatomy is not anatomically amendable to PCI.

Role of Antiplatelet Therapy

Antiplatelet therapy with aspirin or clopidogrel is recommended in those patients with established coronary artery disease. Dual antiplatelet therapy is recommended after ACS and in patients undergoing PCI either with or without stent placement. Patients who underwent elective PCI without stenting should still receive aspirin or clopidogrel daily for 1 month followed by long-term or lifetime aspirin therapy.

No antiplatelet or oral anticoagulant is required in patients with systolic dysfunction without thrombosis. Risk versus benefit consideration is needed in this setting. LV mural thrombosis patients are recommended to have oral anticoagulant therapy for a minimum of 3 months.[166]

Role for Triple Anticoagulant Therapy

The use of triple anticoagulant therapy includes aspirin, clopidogrel, and warfarin, which is utilized in patients with AF who are at high risk for thromboembolism and who recently had coronary stent placement during PCI.[149] This is considered a matter of clinical judgment balancing the risk of thrombosis against the risk of bleeding. In this setting, bare metal stents are the stents of choice when triple anticoagulant therapy is required. For patients with nonvalvular AF, direct oral anticoagulants can be considered. Triple anticoagulant therapy is the most effective therapy to prevent both coronary stent thrombosis and the occurrence of embolic stroke in high-risk patients. This treatment, however, increases the risk of bleeding 3.7-fold when warfarin is added as part of triple anticoagulant therapy.[150]

Drug-eluting stent should be reserved for high-risk clinical or anatomic situations such as those with diabetes or for coronary lesions that are unusually long, totally obstructed, or in small blood vessels if triple antithrombotic anticoagulant therapy is required.[166]

Thrombolytic Therapy in Acute Coronary Syndromes

Streptokinase and alteplase are given via IV infusion. Reteplase and tenecteplase are given by rapid bolus. Tissue plasminogen activator (tPA) is the most commonly utilized thrombolytic agent and this agent has proven effective results. Streptokinase is less commonly used because of the development of antibodies, which can persist up to a year and is now no longer available in the United States. Patients with diabetes, those with poorly controlled hypertension, and those who are given thrombolytics more than 12 hours after initial onset of chest pain have poorer response to thrombolytic agents.[151]

Absolute contraindications to thrombolytic therapy include active bleeding or known bleeding abnormality, closed head or facial trauma within 3 months, suspected aortic dissection, any prior intracranial hemorrhage, or ischemic stroke within 3 months. Relative contraindications for thrombolytic therapy include recent major surgery within 3 weeks, prolonged cardiopulmonary resuscitation, significant GI bleed within 4 weeks, active peptic ulcer disease, blood pressure that cannot be lowered to predetermined levels (<185/110 mm Hg), or previous ischemic stroke more than 3 months ago.

Antithrombin therapy is given along with PCI as standard practice. Typically, a patient will be given a heparin bolus en route to the catheterization laboratory.

Discharge medications following ACS include "ABCDE": aspirin and antianginal agents, beta blockers and blood pressure control, cholesterol medications and cigarettes stopping, diet therapy and diabetes control, and education and exercise.

Treatment of Prinzmetal angina is with vasodilator drugs including nitrates, which relax vascular smooth muscle and calcium channel blockers. When Prinzmetal angina is associated with coronary atherosclerosis, the prognosis is determined by the severity of the underlying disease. There is no role for beta blockers or large doses of aspirin.[142] Avoiding known triggers precipitating vasospasm is also part of the treatment. Since this condition is seen more commonly in smokers, smoking cessation is advised.

Aspirin

If patient is younger than 50 years, low-dose aspirin should only be used in patients with higher risk for the development of coronary artery disease (CAD). There may be a role for calculation of coronary artery calcium scores risk stratifying patients into low- versus high-risk patients with the lower risk patients not requiring aspirin use.[152]

Considering pooled data sets, coronary calcium scores are able to risk stratify patients for recommending aspirin use for primary prevention against coronary artery disease, which allows comparison of number needed to treat versus number sustaining harm.[153]

Current prevention against coronary artery disease involves exercise, healthy diet, smoking cessation, and statin use rather than aspirin use as a primary prevention strategy since aspirin is associated with GI blood loss.[154] Aspirin for primary prevention reduces nonfatal ischemic events but significantly increases nonfatal bleeding events. The safety and efficacy of aspirin use in primary prevention remain debatable.[155] Aspirin should be used with extreme caution in primary prevention of cardiovascular disease because long-term aspirin use has not been proved to lower cardiovascular mortality risk and in fact, increased cardiovascular mortality rate has been demonstrated in patients who took aspirin twice per day.[156]

Risks of aspirin therapy include hemorrhagic stroke and GI bleeding. Tobacco cessation and control of lipids and blood pressure promote a greater risk reduction than aspirin therapy alone when used as a cardiovascular preventive strategy. Immediate release omeprazole has been shown to decrease GI ulceration in patients taking aspirin and can lessen the occurrence of GI bleeding.[157] On the other hand, patients taking proton pump inhibitors (PPIs) have less platelet activity when taking aspirin, which could lower aspirin's effectiveness.[158] Aspirin has not been shown to affect cardiovascular disease as primary prevention even in patients with diabetes.[159]

Dietary therapy and cardiovascular prevention should be balanced between calories and physical activity in order to achieve or maintain a healthy body weight. Diet recommendations include increasing dietary intake of vegetables and fruits, whole grains, and high fiber foods. Fish, especially oily fish, should be consumed twice every week.[160]

Replacement of saturated fats with polyunsaturated vegetable oils can lower the risk for coronary artery disease by 30% as long as the saturated fats are not replaced with refined carbohydrates and sugars.[161] There should be a minimum intake of partially hydrogenated fats (typically, these fats are solids at room temperature) and beverages and foods with fat and sugars. Foods should be prepared with little or no salt.

Whole grains, fruits/vegetables, nuts/legumes, oils, and tea/coffee are associated with lower cardiovascular risk scores while juices/sweetened beverages, refined grains, potatoes/fries, sweets, and animal foods increase cardiovascular risk.[162]

The Mediterranean and DASH diets are recommended to improve lipid profiles and to decrease cardiovascular disease risk. The Mediterranean diet emphasizes the intake of vegetables, fish, fruit, whole grains, and olive oil and this diet has been shown to be more effective at lowering risk of cardiovascular disease than low-fat diets and approaches the same beneficial effect as statin therapy.[163]

While moderate alcohol intake is associated with a lower risk for coronary artery disease, it is associated with increased risk for the development of other noncardiac disease states such as both ischemic and hemorrhagic stroke.[164]

Statin Therapy

Statins (HMG-CoA reductase agents) remain the drug treatment of choice for managing hyperlipidemia and for coronary artery disease prevention. Statins have much greater benefit when they are utilized in secondary rather than primary prevention against cardiovascular events. Statin use is associated with improved endothelial vasodilator function.[165] Statin therapy should be employed in primary prevention only in high-risk patients such as Framingham risk of at least 20%.[166] Lifetime risk for cardiovascular disease better assesses benefit of statin therapy for low- and intermediate-risk patients.[167] Statins should be utilized for primary prevention of macrovascular complications in patients with type 2 diabetes and other cardiovascular risk factors such as age over 55 years, left ventricular hypertrophy, previous cardiovascular disease, peripheral arterial disease (PAD), smoking, or hypertension.[166]

Statin use has been associated with increased likelihood of diabetes and mild, not clinically relevant elevations in liver transaminase levels but is not associated with cognitive decline, cataract formation, or decline in renal function.[168] Diabetic complications and increased risk for overweight/

obesity has been identified in people taking statins as part of primary prevention.[169]

Blood Pressure Considerations

Control of blood pressure and other cardiovascular risk factors may play a role in the regression of atherosclerotic plaque. Patients whose blood pressure was controlled with amplodipine had fewer cardiovascular events than patients taking atenolol for their blood pressure control.[170] Blood pressure goal is <140/90 mm Hg in patients with stable coronary artery disease and <130/80 mm Hg in patients with previous MI, stroke or TIA, or coronary artery disease risk equivalent condition such as coronary artery disease, PAD, or abdominal aortic aneurysm.[171]

Patients with elevated diastolic pressure should have this pressure lowered slowly and should not decrease the diastolic pressure lower than 60 mm Hg, as this is associated with a higher mortality risk. Patients with diastolic blood pressures in the lowest quartile (40–64 mm Hg) have an increased risk for the development of angina in those with known coronary artery disease.[172]

All patients with coronary disease should be counseled for smoking cessation.

Treatment of Chronic Stable Angina

Patients who have chronic stable angina who have a heart rate >70 bpm should be treated with beta blockers. Beta blockers lower the heart rate and the force of contraction causing a decreased myocardial oxygen demand. Patients with angina need to be classified as stable or unstable. Patients who are unable to tolerate beta blocker therapy or those who continue to have symptoms despite maximum beta blocker therapy should be given ivabradine which inhibits the sinoatrial cells allowing a longer diastolic fill time.[173] Ivabradine slows the heart rate without causing a negative inotropic effect on the heart.

PATIENT EDUCATION

Modifiable Risk Factors for Coronary Artery Disease

Cigarette smoking causes more than twice the number of heart attacks when patients who smoke are compared to patients who are nonsmokers. Patients who quit smoking reduce their risk of MI to that of a nonsmoker within 2 years of stopping smoking.

Hypertension is a well-established risk factor for myocardial ischemia, stroke, kidney failure, and HF. Systolic blood pressure may be more predictive than diastolic blood pressure for cardiovascular risks such as stroke. Systolic blood pressure tends to increase in the elderly population and lower blood pressure goals are now identified in this population.

Inactivity and sedentary lifestyle are risk factors for ischemic heart disease. Moderate exercise provides a protective effect against both ischemic heart disease and cardiovascular events. Vigorous exercise can provide additional benefits from cardiovascular conditioning.

Obesity, especially abdominal obesity, increases the risk for ischemic heart disease and stroke. Increased BMI increases blood pressure, lipid levels, and triglyceride levels while lowering high-density lipoprotein cholesterol. Weight loss as little as 10 to 20 pounds can reduce the risk for cardiovascular disease.

Diabetes causes macrovascular disease and is considered an ischemic heart disease equivalent. Majority of deaths in patients with diabetes are due to cardiovascular disease. Statin medications and aspirin are indicated in the majority of diabetic patients since good blood sugar control alone does not significantly lower the risk for cardiovascular disease.

Overall, mortality rates between patients with STEMI and NSTEMI do not differ over a 30-day window. The cause of death following MI is typically arrhythmia, and arrhythmia is most important in the first hour after MI. Patients who survive 1 month following STEMI treated with PCI have <1.5% annual risk for cardiovascular death.[174]

5.4B ANGINA

Patients with angina have chest tightness, heaviness, or pressure as the description of the pain. Patients may also have abdominal pain if the inferior portion of the heart is involved. Pain can also lead to nausea as an additional complaint. Patients with right-sided damage to the heart may also have hypotension, lightheadedness, or bradycardia that occurs as a result of impairment of the pacemaker system of the heart.

5.4C STABLE ANGINA

Patients with stable angina have a predictable pattern to their chest pain. They also have a predictable pattern to response to nitroglycerin that they take for relief of anginal symptoms. These patterns can persist for years and patients will modify their activity to prevent the onset of chest pain. Precipitants of angina can include exercise, heavy meals, cold, and stressful situations.

5.4D UNSTABLE ANGINA

USA is often referred to as crescendo or preinfarction angina. First episode angina or angina that is a change in the typical pattern of angina fits the criteria for USA meaning that the chest pain has increased severity, frequency, or duration. Patients no longer respond to nitrates as in the past and this angina can also occur at rest. Experts call new-onset angina as unstable. A sudden change in the pattern of angina typically means a physical change within the coronary arteries. which could be occurring in the setting where there is hemorrhage into an atherosclerotic plaque or rupture of a plaque with intermittent thrombus formation.

Some patients with USA already have a coronary thrombosis that is seen during cardiac catheterization. Untreated USA patients can progress to MI in about half of the cases without treatment. Because of the high cardiac risk for USA patients, these patients should be admitted for intensive medical evaluation and treatment.

High-risk features for patients with angina and NSTEMI include repeated or prolonged chest pain lasting at least 10 minutes, elevated troponin levels (with NSTEMI), persistent EKG changes with ST depression or new T wave inversion, hypotension with systolic blood pressure <90 mm Hg, VT, syncope, left ventricular ejection fraction <40%, previous coronary artery bypass grafting or angioplasty, diabetes, and chronic kidney disease.

5.4E PRINZMETAL ANGINA

Patients with Prinzmetal angina (also called variant angina) have coronary artery vasospasm resulting in chest pain. Unlike traditional angina that occurs with activity, Prinzmetal angina usually occurs with rest. Triggers of coronary spasm in the setting of Prinzmetal angina include smoking, cocaine or alcohol use, and the use of triptans in the management of both cluster and migraine headache. EKGs performed during these episodes classically show ST segment elevation in anatomically contiguous leads. There are typically no reciprocal changes seen on the EKG in a patient with Prinzmetal angina. Cardiac biomarkers do not increase with this condition. Historically, this was believed to be a benign condition, but more recent data identify that coronary spasm occurs in an area of plaque, which precipitates the spasm and serious associated adverse outcomes including ACS, arrhythmias, and death.[175]

Prinzmetal angina consists of vasospasm that causes a marked but transient reduction in the luminal diameter. The vasospastic state is focal at a single site and can occur in both normal or diseased vessels. This condition can coexist with Raynaud phenomenon and migraine headaches. Endothelial dysfunction is the primary cause for Prinzmetal angina.[142]

SPECIAL CONSIDERATIONS

COMPLICATIONS

Inflammation from infarction can spread toward pericardium causing postinfarction fibrinous pericarditis; these patients can present with a low-grade fever and sharp pleuritic chest pain that increases with inspiration. This condition is most likely to occur 3 to 14 days after the infarction and results from macrophages cleaning up the necrotic mass with laying down soft granulation tissue. This soft granulation tissue is quite weak so there is a risk of interventricular septum or ventricular free wall rupture, which typically presents 3 to 5 days following MI. Ventricular free wall rupture classically occurs following an anterior wall STEMI and presents at around 5 to 14 days as a result of a large amount of blood leaking into the pericardial cavity causing a pericardial tamponade. Risk for the development of free wall rupture post-MI include inferior wall STEMI, use of oral anticoagulants, and treatment with thrombolytics instead of PCI.[176] The patient may develop pulseless electrical activity with the heart losing its ability to actually pump despite electrical activity being seen on the EKG.

Ventricular septal defect (VSD) is another complication, which presents as a new holosystolic murmur located at the left sternal border.

If a patient has impaired blood flow to the pacemaker of the heart (SA or atrioventricular [AV] node), bradycardia or heart block can occur. In the setting of ACS with myocardial damage, the heart is irritable so dysrhythmias are expected and do not require treatment. Arrhythmias can include tachyarrhythmias originating in both the atria and ventricles. Prolonged tachyarrhythmias can lead to the development of tachycardia-induced cardiomyopathy as another complication.

Ventricular fibrillation (VF) in the immediate MI period is the leading cause of death caused by arrhythmia.

Pump dysfunction can lead to left ventricular aneurysm formation with persistent ST segment elevation that does not return to baseline even several weeks following the acute event. Suspect left ventricular aneurysm formation in the setting of severe anterior wall MI. Echocardiography will show paradoxical movement of the anterior wall of the LV. Mural thrombosis can occur in the setting of left ventricular dysfunction. These patients are at increased risk for systemic embolization. Warfarin is typically prescribed when mural thrombosis is identified.

KEY POINTS

- Cardiovascular disease is the most common cause of death in the United States.
- ACS consists of USA, NSTEMI, and STEMI.
- Risk stratification is important to consider in the evaluation of patients suspected of having ACS.
- Patients with STEMI have improved outcomes with PCI rather than thrombolytic therapy.
- Patients with USA or NSTEMI are not eligible for fibrinolytic therapy as increased obstruction and fatality are associated with these conditions.
- Lifestyle modification including smoking cessation is indicated for both primary and secondary cardiovascular prevention.

5.5 VALVULAR HEART DISEASE

Christine Bruce

OVERVIEW

VHD is demonstrated by either functional or anatomic abnormalities affecting the cardiac valves causing either regurgitation or stenosis when damaged. In developed countries, aortic stenosis (AS) is the most prevalent of all VHDs. As the population ages, this condition develops more frequently. Symptomatic disease is universally fatal if left untreated.[177] Both stenosis and regurgitation will be discussed with regard to the aortic, mitral, tricuspid, and pulmonary valves.

VHD occurs most commonly in the aging population. This condition typically has a slowly progressive course with the earliest symptom typically being exertional dyspnea.

EPIDEMIOLOGY

The prevalence of VHD is 2.5% in developed countries. Both AS and mitral regurgitation (MR) increase dramatically after the age of 65 years due to the degenerative etiologies of these conditions; 75% of VHD is attributed to valve degeneration while 22% of VHD is caused by rheumatic heart disease (RHD). Infective endocarditis (IE) is another major cause of VHD. In developing countries, RHD remains the leading cause of VHD.[178]

PATHOPHYSIOLOGY

VHD can occur as a congenital or acquired condition and the incidence is increasing as patients are living long enough to develop this condition. There is limited understanding of the genetic and molecular etiology of the diseases affecting the heart valves. The most effective therapy option is surgical repair or replacement, but these procedures are not without complications and there is no guarantee of lifelong success.[179]

Aortic VHD and MR most commonly occur from degeneration of the aortic valve (AoV), particularly a bicuspid AoV, followed by the development of MR. Mitral stenosis

(MS) is most commonly caused as a result of rheumatic fever.[180] AS is attributable to traditional cardiovascular risk factors in one-third of cases.[181]

Medications may lead to VHD. Patient using tricyclic antidepressants have a significantly increased risk for the development of VHD. Other antidepressants are associated with a greater risk of VHD but the risk is not as high as that seen with tricyclic antidepressant use.[182] Women who took the combination anorectic agents phentermine and fenfluramine who previously had no history of cardiac disease are at an increased risk for the development of VHD along with pulmonary hypertension.[183]

Regurgitant features of an abnormal valve usually results in volume overload while stenotic lesions affecting heart valves typically lead to pressure overload.

Radiation therapy to the heart can increase the risk for clinically significant VHD as demonstrated in patients given radiation therapy for Hodgkin lymphoma. In this setting, AoVs and MVs are most frequently affected. Patients receiving the highest radiation doses are more likely to develop VHD.[184]

MEDICAL HISTORY AND CLINICAL PRESENTATION

VHD can progress in an indolent manner with the most common symptom initially being exertional dyspnea. Other symptoms include angina, palpitations, syncope, lower extremity edema, and ascites.

SIGNS AND SYMPTOMS

Patients can have chest pain, syncope, palpitations, jugular venous distention and hepatic enlargement, lower extremity edema, and ascites in the setting of VHD.

PHYSICAL EXAMINATION

AS causes a midsystolic, crescendo decrescendo murmur, which is best heard at the right upper sternal border. Murmur can radiate into carotid arteries. In the setting of a bicuspid AoV, soft ejection click can be heard followed by crescendo decrescendo murmur, which presents as a mid to late peaking murmur at the right upper sternal border with diminished A2 and decreased carotid upstroke. A tardus (late) and parvus (slow rise) pulse occurs.

Aortic regurgitation (AR) produces a diastolic decrescendo murmur at the lower left sternal border accentuated with the patient sitting and leaning forward. AR murmur radiates toward the base of the heart. A wide pulse pressure develops with a bounding pulse that rapidly falls. As with other diastolic murmurs, AR murmur is considered to be pathologic. Acute murmur in the setting of AR can occur in the setting of proximal aortic dissection.

MS is a diastolic, low-pitched, decrescendo murmur heard best in the apex of the heart with the patient in the left lateral decubitus position. MS is the only valvular abnormality able to produce an opening snap. These patients can have backup of fluid into the lungs along with right ventricular overload and development of cor pulmonale. Hemoptysis is a late clinical sign of this condition.

MR produces a systolic holosystolic or late systolic murmur heard best at the apex of the heart that radiates to either the axilla or back. No corresponding systolic click occurs if the patient has coexisting MV prolapse (MVP). MR can occur in the setting of acute MI with rupture of the chordae tendon of the MV allowing reflux of blood back into the left atrium (LA) during ventricular contraction.

Tricuspid regurgitation (TR) causes a holosystolic murmur heard best at the lower left sternal border with radiation of the murmur to the left upper sternal border. TR can occur in the setting of illicit IV drug use causing IE preventing the closure of this valve.

Tricuspid stenosis (TS) produces a diastolic murmur heard best at the left lower sternal border. TS occurs most commonly in the setting of IE due to IV drug use.

Pulmonic stenosis (PS) produces a systolic crescendo-decrescendo murmur heard best at the left upper sternal border. PS murmur increases with deep breathing as negative thoracic pressure brings more blood into the right side of the heart.

Pulmonic regurgitation (PR) is a diastolic murmur heard best at the left lower sternal border. It is most likely to occur in the setting of right ventricular volume overload and increased pulmonary pressures.

Innocent flow murmurs are heard best at the right upper sternal border that does not interfere with the natural valve closure sequence. They can be seen in childhood or in situations with increased volume states such as pregnancy, fever, untreated hyperthyroidism, or anemia.

VHD conditions and associated physical examination findings are summarized in Table 5.11.

DIFFERENTIAL DIAGNOSIS

The differential diagnosis for VHD is summarized in Table 5.12.

DIAGNOSTIC STUDIES

Echocardiogram remains the key diagnostic interventional strategy when VHD is suspected. Diagnostic intervention for VHD includes echocardiogram, EKG, and CXR.[185] Echocardiogram visualizes all cardiac valves along with movement of blood within the heart. Congenital and acquired anomalies of the heart can be diagnosed such as ASD, VSD, patent ductus arteriosus (PDA), and pericarditis, and ejection fraction of the LV can be calculated.

EVALUATION

Evaluation for VHD starts with a comprehensive history and physical examination. Historical information of importance includes cyanosis, near or actual syncope, fatigue,

TABLE 5.11 Valvular Heart Disease Conditions and Associated Physical Examination Findings

Cardiac Condition	Associated Findings (ACC/AHA)
Aortic stenosis	Mid to late peaking murmur at the right upper sternal border with diminished A2 and decreased carotid upstroke
Aortic regurgitation	Early, soft decrescendo diastolic murmur at the right upper sternal border best heard leaning forward after expiration
Mitral stenosis	Low-pitched, soft rumbling mid to late diastolic murmur heard at the apex; could be associated with a mitral valve opening snap
Mitral regurgitation	Blowing systolic murmur at the apex radiating to the sternal border, axilla, or back

ACC/AHA, American College of Cardiology/American Heart Association.

TABLE 5.12 Differential Diagnosis for Valvular Heart Disease

Diagnosis	Description
Physiologic flow murmur (innocent murmur)	Murmur grade 1/6 to 2/6 with early to mid-peaking systolic murmur at the upper sternal border that does not change with Valsalva maneuver.
Hypertrophic cardiomyopathy	Mid- to late peaking systolic murmur at the right sternal border that increases with Valsalva maneuver and standing after squatting.
Aortic dissection	Produces a murmur consistent with aortic regurgitation (diastolic decrescendo murmur) with radiation into back producing asymmetric differential in upper extremity blood pressures, asymmetric pulses, or pulsus paradoxus.
Aortic sclerosis	Midsystolic ejection murmur without any associated hemodynamic consequences.
Patent ductus arteriosus (PDA)	Continuous systolic "machinery" flow murmur with the manifestations determined by the degree of left-to-right shunting, which is dependent upon the size and length of the PDA and the difference between pulmonary and systemic vascular resistance.
Ventricular septal defect (VSD)	Infants with small VSDs with a large pressure differential between the left and right ventricle can have a thrill palpated in the third or fourth intercostal space at the left sternal border. Harsh blowing holosystolic murmur is heard best at the left mid to lower sternal border. Large VSDs can produce holosystolic murmur along with diastolic rumble related to the increased flow through the mitral valve.
Atrial septal defect (ASD)	Findings depend on the size of the defect, degree of shunting, and the pulmonary arterial pressure. Midsystolic pulmonary flow or ejection murmur along with a wide, fixed split second heart sound.
Still murmur	Systolic murmur with a vibratory musical quality heard best at the left lower sternal border or between the left lower sternal border and apex. Murmur is louder in the supine position and in hyperdynamic states. Childhood murmur that resolves by adolescence.
Venous hum	Continuous murmur that is loudest when the patient is sitting with extended head. Disappears when the patient is supine or when flexing the head or by applying pressure over the jugular vein when the patient is sitting. Heard best in the left or right upper sternal border or infraclavicular or supraclavicular regions.
Pericarditis	Produces pericardial friction rub when inflamed visceral and parietal pericardial surfaces rub against each other. Rub may not be heard if there is a large amount of pericardial effusion. Scratching quality sound present throughout systole and diastole.
Ebstein anomaly	Congenital malformation of the tricuspid valve and right ventricle with clinical presentation depending on the degree of involvement. Can also occur in infants of mothers taking lithium during pregnancy. Tricuspid regurgitation occurs along with displacement of the valve dividing the right ventricle into two chambers. Considered to atrialize the right ventricle. Results in abnormal right ventricular performance.
Austin Flint murmur	Apical diastolic rumbling murmur associated with aortic regurgitation. Can be misdiagnosed as mitral stenosis.
Mitral valve prolapse	Can be associated with mild, trace, or no mitral regurgitation. There is billowing of any part of the mitral leaflets of at least 2 mm seen on echocardiogram. There is abnormal systolic displacement of one or both leaflets into the left atrium due to a disruption or elongation of the leaflets, chordae, or papillary muscles. Midsystolic click and late systolic murmur can also occur.

inability to keep up with peer activity, palpitations, jugular venous distention with or without edema, and chest pain. Careful auscultation of the heart provides clues to the underlying type of VHD. Special cardiac maneuvers are performed to accentuate these murmurs. Right-sided heart murmurs typically increase with inspiration and squatting due to increased amount of preload. The Valsalva maneuver and standing after squatting decreases the amount of blood entering the heart and would accentuate the murmur associated with hypertrophic cardiomyopathy. An EKG is performed to establish a baseline, and echocardiogram will be the definitive study identifying blood flow within the heart and motion of the cardiac valves.

TREATMENT

Management of VHD should be individualized so that each patient can be treated based on their specific comorbidity while taking into account the patient's needs and preferences.[186] The timing of surgery is dependent upon the type and location of the valvular abnormality. Risk calculators such as the Society of Thoracic Surgery Adult Cardiac Surgery Risk Calculator can be utilized to predict the risk of adverse outcome of surgical intervention.

Medical therapy may alleviate symptoms, but it has not been shown to prevent progression of VHD or to improve long-term survival in this setting.

PATIENT EDUCATION

Aortic Stenosis

Patients who inherit a bicuspid AoV have an increased risk for the development of AS because two leaflets are subject to increased workload leading to sclerosis and calcification compared with the normal three leaflet valve. In addition to degeneration of the AoV over time, other risk factors for the development of this condition include RHD and radiation to the heart. If the AoV damage occurred as a result of RHD, MV disease is invariably present. Patients with diabetes, hypertension, or hyperlipidemia have a 33% increase in the risk for developing severe AS over those without those conditions.[181]

AS causes a pressure overload in the LV causing concentric left ventricular hypertrophy along with fibrosis within the heart. As this condition progresses, diastolic dysfunction occurs and eventually results in systolic HF and pulmonary congestion.

The classic triad of symptoms with AS includes exertional dyspnea, syncope, and chest pain. Survivability dramatically decreases once a patient with AS become symptomatic. In fact, the fourth classic sign associated with AS is sudden death. Patients with AS will have a crescendo decrescendo systolic murmur along with a diminished A2 component of S2.

TTE can determine the cause and severity of AS and calculate both the ejection fraction and the valve aperture. AoV apertures that are 1 cm or less constitute severe AS. Cardiac catheterization measures the gradient across the AoV, which can provide detailed prognostic information regarding cardiac surgery.

The treatment of AS is AoV replacement (AVR) in patients who are symptomatic or who have left ventricular systolic dysfunction with ejection fraction of <50% even if this occurs in an asymptomatic patient. The AoV can also be replaced if the patient is having another open-heart procedure. This procedure can be done through an open technique or through a transcatheter AoV replacement (TAVR). TAVR typically is performed for patients who do not qualify for open-heart surgery as long as there is no coexisting severe AR. There are similar outcomes seen with these procedures with regard to mortality and survival over a 5-year period when TAVR is compared to traditional open AVRs.[187] Balloon valvuloplasty can be used as a bridge to therapy for actual replacement of the AoV.

AVR is indicated when patients become symptomatic. For asymptomatic patients, the risks involved in elective surgery are greater than those of potentially serious complications. Patients with AS are followed with periodic echocardiograms and are encouraged for cardiac risk factor modification. Comorbid conditions are evaluated and treated based upon established guidelines.[188]

Aortic Regurgitation

AR can result from pathology in the aortic root or because of intrinsic valve disease. Underlying chronic causes of AR include ascending aortic dilation, bicuspid AoV, calcific degeneration, radiation to the chest, and previous rheumatic fever. Acute AR can be caused by endocarditis, chest trauma, aortic dissection, and complications of surgical intervention to the AoV.

As in other types of regurgitation, volume overload rather than pressure overload predominates. There is progressive left ventricular dilation with eccentric rather than concentric hypertrophy. This means that there is an increase in the length rather than width of the cardiac myocytes.

Symptoms of AR include shortness of breath with exertion, fatigue, and chest pain. Signs of AR include bounding peripheral pulses, head-bobbing, pistol shot sounds on auscultation over pulses, diastolic decrescendo murmur heard on either side of the sternum, and wide pulse pressures on blood pressure measurement.

TTE is the most important evaluation strategy as this can identify the aortic root along with assessment of left ventricular function. If endocarditis is suspected, TTE is performed. Patients can tolerate this condition for a long period of time so serial assessments are necessary to assess for progression. Once patients become symptomatic, surgical intervention is recommended. Acute AR may need immediate surgery as in the case of proximal aortic dissection or aortic root injury that occurs from blunt cardiac trauma. The procedure of choice is the traditional AVR.

Medical therapy includes medications to control blood pressure with multiple classes of medications being utilized including dihydropyridine calcium channel blockers, ACEIs, and ARBs.

Mitral Stenosis

MS typically results from RHD, which leads to fusion of the mitral commissures with calcification of the valve and abnormalities in the subvalvular structures. There is slow progression of clinical symptoms with gradual enlargement of the LA in the setting of normal left ventricular function. Prominent symptoms include fatigue caused by low cardiac output, dyspnea from pulmonary congestion, and lower extremity edema as a result of right-sided HF due to increased pulmonary pressures. Symptoms initially occur with exertion since there is less diastolic filling time from the tachycardia that occurs with exertion. Enlargement of LA can lead to AF that can be complicated by embolic phenomenon.

MS may cause an opening snap, a loud S1, an increased P2 component of S2, and a diastolic rumble or low-pitched murmur heard at the apex.

Echocardiogram assesses MS severity, pulmonary pressures, and right ventricular function. Treatment of MS is percutaneous balloon mitral commissurotomy (PBMC) in patients who are symptomatic or in asymptomatic patients with an MV aperture <1 cm. Anticoagulation is recommended in patients with MS who develop AF.

Mitral Regurgitation

Acute MR can be caused by IE, angina or MI resulting in papillary muscle ischemia or rupture, or trauma. Chronic MR can be due to MVP, previous radiation therapy, or RHD. MR causes volume overload leading to left ventricular dilation and left atrial dilation and increased pulmonary pressures. As the condition progresses, pulmonary hypertension and right ventricular failure can ensue. MVP is the primary cause for primary MR. Patients with chronic MR due to MVP can develop degeneration of the MV leading to Barlow syndrome resulting in chest pain and palpitations.

MR causes a blowing holosystolic murmur at the apex with possible systolic click if there is associated MVP. Echocardiogram demonstrates this condition along with its blood flow patterns. Treatment for acute MR includes vasodilator therapy to allow easier exit of the blood out of the heart resulting in improved cardiac output. An intra-aortic balloon pump can be used to augment systolic and coronary perfusion pressures. Prompt surgical repair is needed with acute symptomatic MR. Patients with chronic severe MR are best improved with surgery to repair the damaged valve. For patients who are not surgical candidates, MV repair with a clip device delivered percutaneously can be performed.

SPECIAL CONSIDERATIONS

Patients who have VHD should have aggressive management of coronary artery comorbidities. Blood pressure should be controlled to prevent further pressure on the heart. There is a growing need for treatment of adults who have survived congenital heart disease as these patients have normal lifespans. There are fewer indications for antibiotic prophylaxis in the setting of VHD and these decisions are also based upon the type of surgery that is being performed.

KEY POINTS

- Patients with VHD should have serial echocardiograms to assess for progression of the disease as many patients remain asymptomatic while ongoing damage is occurring.
- Most patients who develop symptoms in the setting of VHD benefit from surgery rather than ongoing medical management.
- Patients with known VHD should be counseled regarding the development of symptoms since some symptoms are life-threatening and need to have immediate intervention.
- Although MS is primarily caused by RHD, this condition is more likely to be encountered with immigrants from endemic countries migrating to United States.
- Patients with significant AS should be carefully evaluated prior to an exercise treadmill test being performed as these patients cannot increase cardiac output to the exercising muscles due to their fixed rate of flow across the narrowed AoV aperture.

5.6 CONGENITAL HEART DISEASE

Jill Cowen, Gretchen L. Hackett, Julie Jones, Marnie I. O'Donnell, Catherine Roden, and Aniqa Shahrier

OVERVIEW

Congenital heart disease is a significant cause of morbidity and death in the pediatric population. Congenital heart disease ranges from 6 to 13 per 1,000 live births annually in the United States.[189] These defects can be broken down into two categories: acyanotic heart defects and cyanotic heart defects. An increasing number of children born with congenital heart disease are surviving to adulthood. There are now more adult patients living with congenital heart disease than there are pediatric patients with congenital heart disease. This has necessitated the specialized training of cardiologists to provide care for adult patients with repaired or palliated congenital heart defects.

All newborns are screened with pulse oximetry prior to discharge home from the hospital. If pulse oximetry measures <94%, the patient is evaluated for congenital heart disease. Additionally, patients who have a parent or siblings with congenital heart disease are at higher risk for congenital heart disease themselves and often undergo screening either prior to birth (fetal echocardiogram) or shortly after birth (postnatal TTE). One should have a high index of suspicion for congenital heart disease in all patients under 1 year of age who present with a murmur, show signs of poor weight gain, or have poor oral intake.

PATHOPHYSIOLOGY

The mammalian heart is composed of diverse cell types and structures such as cardiac and smooth muscle cells which contribute to the contractile apparatus and vascular system, the conduction system along with the endothelial, valvular, and interstitial mesenchymal fibroblast cells.[93] As the heart develops during embryogenesis, cardiac cells migrate a considerable distance in an ever-changing environment. Errors in development often lead to the development of congenital heart disease. Many cases of congenital heart disease are idiopathic; however, if a first-degree relative has a congenital heart defect, the risk of congenital heart disease being inherited increases. Additionally, fetal exposure to toxins (prescribed medications or illicit drugs used by the mother) and/or preexisting maternal medical conditions can increase the risk of the fetus developing congenital heart disease.

Syndromic patients have a higher incidence of congenital heart disease as compared to nonsyndromic patients and should always be considered when evaluating a syndromic patient for the first time. Common syndromes associated with congenital heart disease include (but not limited to) trisomy 21 (Down syndrome), trisomy 18 (Edward syndrome), Turner syndrome, Noonan syndrome, Alagille syndrome, and DiGeorge syndrome.

MEDICAL HISTORY AND CLINICAL PRESENTATION

A thorough medical history should be obtained from the patient or patient guardians with focus on feeding difficulties, color changes with feeding or crying, diaphoresis with feeds, or changes in energy level. Assess older children for complaints of chest pain, palpitations, shortness of breath (particularly with activity), presyncope, or overt syncope.

Birth history and complications during pregnancy or delivery should be obtained at the first visit. Medication/drug exposures such as alcohol, cocaine, lithium, and nonsteroidal anti-inflammatory drugs (NSAIDs) should be obtained. Assess for maternal autoimmune disease (e.g., lupus, diabetes/gestational diabetes, preeclampsia, congenital heart disease).

Assess for family history of congenital heart disease, cardiomyopathy, cardiac dysrhythmias, or sudden death.

SIGNS AND SYMPTOMS

Feeding difficulties and failure to thrive are often a sign of congenital heart disease in the newborn period. Sudden onset of chest pain, palpitations, and presyncope or overt syncope during exercise in older children carry a high index of suspicion for congenital heart disease, genetic cardiomyopathy, or genetic tachydysrhythmia that may lead to sudden death.

PHYSICAL EXAMINATION

A full set of vital signs should be obtained. Findings of oxygen desaturation, poor weight gain, blood pressure discrepancies between the upper and lower extremities (coarctation), tachypnea, tachycardia, and/or bradycardia should be further investigated. Complaints of dizziness should be further assessed by performing orthostatic vital signs in the office.

Appearance of pallor, cyanosis, or syndromic features should be noted. Palpation of the fontanelles if open should be performed in addition to auscultation of the fontanelle and temporal region for bruits. Look for findings of increased work of breathing such as intercostal retractions, subcostal retractions, nasal flaring, grunting, or head bobbing.

Auscultation of all lung fields is important, assessing for wheezing, rales, rhonchi, and overall air entry.

Palpation of the anterior chest assessing for PMI, heaves, or lifts is important to assess cardiac placement in the chest (i.e., levocardia versus dextrocardia) and presence or absence of cardiomegaly. The presence of a palpable thrill indicates a pathologic murmur. Auscultate heart sounds in all locations of the anterior chest as well as the axillary region and the midscapular region of the back. Audible murmurs in the axillary regions or back are considered pathologic. Assess the first and second heart sounds (S1 and S2 timing the cardiac cycle with the carotid pulse to identify systole and diastole. Pay attention to the characteristics of S2: physiologically split with inspiration (normal), single and loud (pulmonary hypertension), single (normal result of single ventricle palliation), or fixed split (atrial septal defect [ASD]). Listen for S3 (early diastolic gallop; normal variant if intermittent and in the supine position only; or related to dilated cardiomyopathy if not intermittent) and S4 (late diastolic gallop associated with ventricular diastolic dysfunction/stiff ventricle: never normal). Identify and describe any murmurs present utilizing the following seven characteristics:

1. Intensity of the murmur
   a. **Systolic** I–III (soft to loud; no palpable thrill), IV (loud with diaphragm fully on chest and palpable thrill), V (stethoscope in contact with chest and diaphragm at 45-degree angle off the chest with palpable thrill), VI (diaphragm off chest completely and palpable thrill)
   b. **Diastolic** I–IV (soft to loud)
2. Location in the cardiac cycle (systolic vs. diastolic, continuous, or to and fro: remember to time with carotid pulse)
3. Pitch of the murmur (low and vibratory, high and harsh)
4. Quality of the murmur (crescendo/decrescendo, holosystolic, regurgitant)
5. Location of the murmur on the chest (area it is heard best)
6. Radiation of the murmur (other places heard or isolated)
7. Behavior of the murmur with positional changes or special maneuvers (intensifies, unchanged, or decreases)

Auscultate the abdomen listening for abdominal bruits (descending aorta stenosis, renal artery stenosis). Assess bowel sounds. Palpate liver and spleen for location (different locations if in the presence of heterotaxia) and presence of organomegaly indicating HF.

Palpate peripheral pulses comparing quality of brachial artery to femoral artery and presence or absence of delay (decreased femoral pulses with increased brachial femoral delay is consistent with coarctation of the aorta). Assess temperature of peripheral extremities and capillary refill. Assess nail beds for color and appearance (cyanotic in cyanotic congenital heart disease, clubbing can be seen in older patients with long-standing cyanotic congenital heart disease). Palpate extremities for edema (not typically seen in congenital heart disease but is often noted in the ICU following cardiopulmonary bypass if capillary leak develops).

DIFFERENTIAL DIAGNOSIS

The differential diagnosis for congenital heart disease is summarized in Table 5.13.

TABLE 5.13 Differential Diagnosis for Congenital Heart Disease

Diagnosis	Description
Thyroid disease	Tachycardia or bradycardia with normal heart
Primary respiratory disease	Cyanosis and increased work of breathing with normal heart
Functional murmur	Innocent sound not associated with congenital heart disease
Gastroesophageal reflux and or metabolic disease	Failure to thrive due to feeding difficulties with structurally normal heart
Renal disease	Hypertension without coarcation of the aorta

DIAGNOSTIC STUDIES

Common congenital cardiology diagnostic studies (noninvasive):

1. **Screening:** All newborns should be screened for congenital heart disease prior to discharge home from the hospital after birth/within 72 hours with pulse oximetry. Oxygen saturations <94% should have additional testing completed to rule out congenital heart disease.
2. **EKG:** Inexpensive screening tool to assess for cardiac dysrhythmia, conduction disorders, cardiomegaly, cardiac inflammation, or myocardial ischemia.
3. **24-hour or 48-hour Holter monitor:** Continuous ambulatory cardiac rhythm recording over either 24 or 48 hours. This study is used to assess cardiac rhythm during any symptoms that are reported by the patient during the testing period or screen for any cardiac dysrhythmias that a patient may be prone to as a result of their past medical history. Test provides maximum heart rate, minimum heart rate, and average heart rate and quantification of atrial or ventricular ectopy noted during the study compared to the patient's normal rhythm (i.e., percentage of ectopy during the day). The patient keeps a diary of symptoms during the study but does not need to interact with the recording device. Results of the study are not available until the monitor is returned and downloaded.
4. **30-day cardiac event monitor:** With this outpatient cardiac rhythm monitoring over a longer duration the patient has the ability to actively record their heart rhythm during concerning symptoms.
5. **TTE:** Cardiac ultrasound exam allows for real-time assessment of cardiac anatomy, chamber size, cardiac function, and direction/speed of blood flow. Imaging modalities include two-dimensional echocardiography, three-dimensional echocardiography (3DE), M mode (real-time assessment of chamber size/wall thickness, also used to estimate ejection fraction), color flow Doppler (assesses direction of blood flow), Doppler (assesses speed of blood flow), left ventricular and right ventricular strain (more specific assessment of ventricular function allowing for assessment of specific wall regions in all three axes: longitudinal shortening, horizontal shortening, and radial shortening).
6. **Exercise stress testing:** The patient's hemodynamics are monitored during a standardized exercise protocol (blood pressure, 12-lead EKG, pulse oximetry). This testing may also be combined with TTE to assess wall motion and valve function (pre/post exercise), or nuclear imaging to assess myocardial blood flow (pre-post exercise). Of note, pharmacologic stress testing can be performed in the pediatric population but is rarely indicated.

Advanced Cardiology Diagnostic/Therapeutic Studies

If required, more advanced cardiology imaging options include cardiac MRI/MRA, cardiac CT, TEE, cardiac catheterization, bubble study with echocardiography and transcranial Doppler, and electrophysiology studies. These studies are typically performed by a cardiologist with additional advanced training within the specific testing modality.

If any of these studies are thought to be needed, cardiology consultation is strongly recommended and often required to have these studies performed and interpreted properly.

EVALUATION/TREATMENT

If congenital heart disease is suspected from the history or physical examination, the patient should be referred to a cardiologist for further evaluation and management.

5.6A ATRIAL SEPTAL DEFECTS

An ASD is a hole in the wall separating the right atrium and LA of the heart, is the second most common congenital heart defect, and accounts for approximately 10% to 15% of all congenital heart disease.[190,191] This defect allows oxygenated blood in the LA to cross over and mix with deoxygenated blood flow returning to the right atrium from the body. This is an acyanotic heart lesion that typically does not cause congestive HF, though if significant in size, it may cause right-sided heart enlargement and symptoms such as decreased exercise tolerance and decreased ability to recover from respiratory infections.

EPIDEMIOLOGY

Secundum ASDs comprise approximately 70% of all ASDs and occur twice as often in females compared to males.[192] Patent foramen ovale (PFO) and small secundum ASDs have a high rate of spontaneous closure, whereas larger defects often remain open and may cause right-sided heart enlargement requiring closure.[192] Primum ASDs and sinus venosus defects are rarer and often occur in conjunction with other congenital heart disease.[193] There is no specific genetic association with an isolated ASD; however, ASDs occurring in conjunction with other congenital heart defects often have an underlying genetic cause.[193]

PATHOPHYSIOLOGY

An ASD (see Figure 5.1) is an acyanotic heart lesion allowing oxygenated blood flow from the left side of the heart to mix directly with deoxygenated blood flow returning to the right side of the heart from the body. This is described as a left-to-right shunt. As long as the pulmonary pressures are lower than the systemic pressures (normal physiology), then blood flow moves through the defect from the higher pressure, systemic side, of the heart to the lower pressure, pulmonary side, of the heart. This shunt will cause an increase in blood flow to the lungs. This shunt does not typically cause patients to demonstrate clinical signs of pulmonary overcirculation (i.e., congestive HF); however, if the shunt is significant in size, it may cause right heart enlargement. The first cardiac chamber to become enlarged is typically the right atrium as deoxygenated blood flow from the body returns to the right atrium and mixes with the extra oxygenated flow from the left atrium crossing to the right atrium through the defect.

There are four general types of ASDs: secundum ASD, PFO, sinus venosus ASD, and primum ASD. The most common defects are a secundum ASD and PFO, while the sinus venosus ASDs and primum ASDs are less common.

A secundum ASD (Figure 5.2) is a defect in the middle of the atrial septum that has atrial septal tissue completely surrounding the defect. Specifically, there is tissue above the

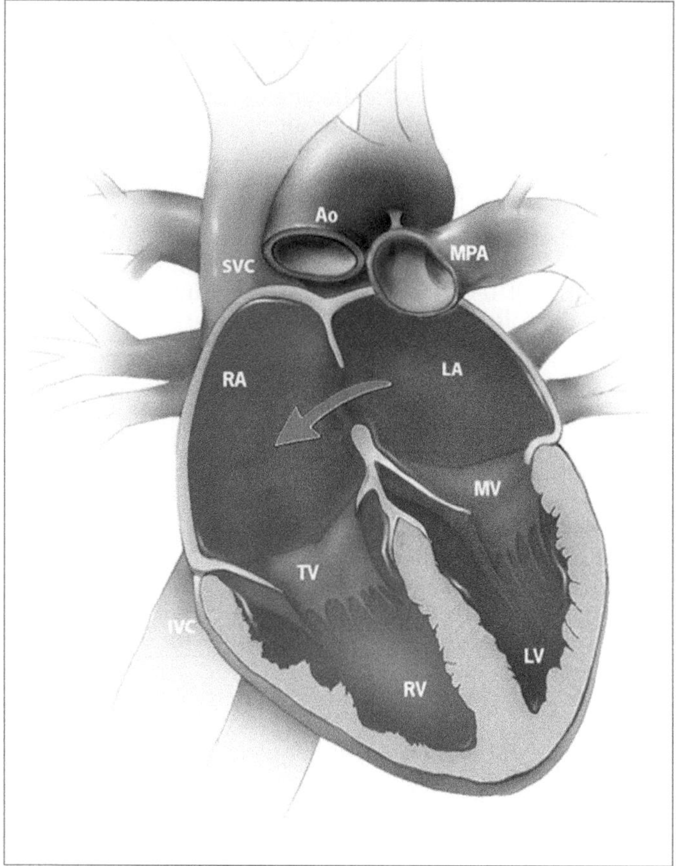

Figure 5.1 Atrial septal defect. Ao, aorta; IVC, inferior vena cava; LA, left atrium; LV, left ventricle; MPA, main pulmonary artery; MV, mitral valve; RA, right atrium; RV, right ventricle; SVC, superior vena cava; TV, tricuspid valve.
(Source: Courtesy of the Centers for Disease Control and Prevention.)

defect and below the defect, but actual absence of tissue at the area of the defect, without overlap of the superior and inferior rims (see Figure 5.2). Trivial (<3 mm) and small (3 mm–<6 mm) secundum ASDs are typically hemodynamically insignificant and have a high probability of undergoing spontaneous closure.[192] Medium-sized defects (6–8 mm) may not spontaneously close but may become small enough to not be hemodynamically significant.[192] Large defects (>8 mm) will not undergo spontaneous closure and typically cause significant right-sided heart enlargement.[192]

A PFO (Latin for "tiny hole") is a specific type of secundum ASD. It also has septal tissue surrounding the defect similar to a secundum atrial; however, there is overlap of the superior and inferior rims (Figure 5.3). The PFO is a normal structure for the fetal heart that allows blood flow from the inferior vena cava (IVC) to bypass the lungs and head straight to the body in the setting of elevated pulmonary vascular resistance in utero. Only a small amount of fetal heart flow goes to the lungs because the lungs are filled with amniotic fluid. Oxygen delivery to fetus is being provided by the placenta. Shortly after birth, the flap should seal over and close as amniotic fluid is cleared from the lungs allowing the lungs to become air filled. However, approximately 20% of the population will still have a PFO as an adult.[190,194]

A sinus venosus ASD (Figure 5.4) is located in the posterior portion of the atrial septum and involves either the superior vena cava (see Figure 5.4; missing superior rim) or the IVC (not shown, missing the inferior rim). These defects

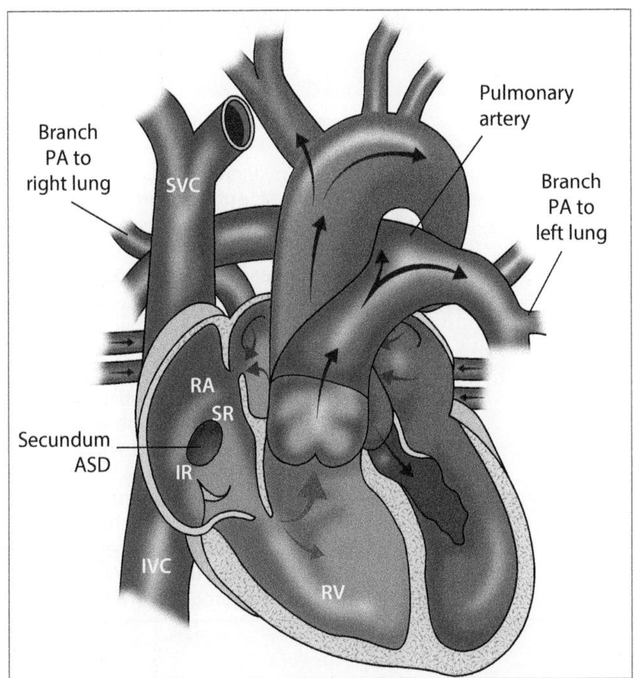

Figure 5.2 **Secundum atrial septal defect. This defect is in the middle of the atrial septum with tissue above and below the defect with an absence of tissue in the area of the defect without overlap of the superior and inferior rims.** ASD, atrial septal defect; IR, inferior rim; IVC, inferior vena cava; PA, pulmonary artery; RA, right atrium; RV, right ventricle; SR, superior rim; SVC, superior vena cava.

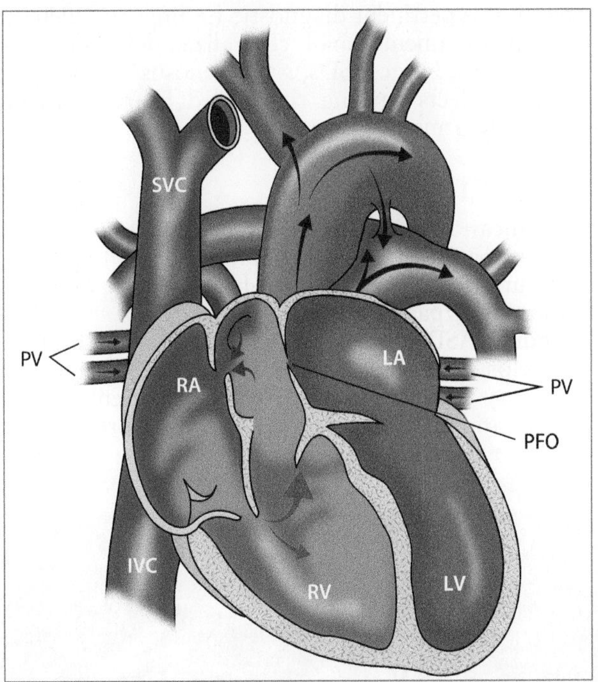

Figure 5.3 **Patent foramen ovale. Septal tissue surrounds the defect, similar to a secundum atrial; however, there is overlap of the superior and inferior rims.** IVC, inferior vena cava; LA, left atrium; LV, left ventricle; PFO, patent foramen ovale; PV, pulmonary vein; RA, right atrium; RV, right ventricle; SVC, superior vena cava.

are hemodynamically significant and will not undergo spontaneous closure. These defects are less common.

A primum ASD (Figure 5.5) involves the atrial septum that is near the AV valves (tricuspid valve [TV] and MV).

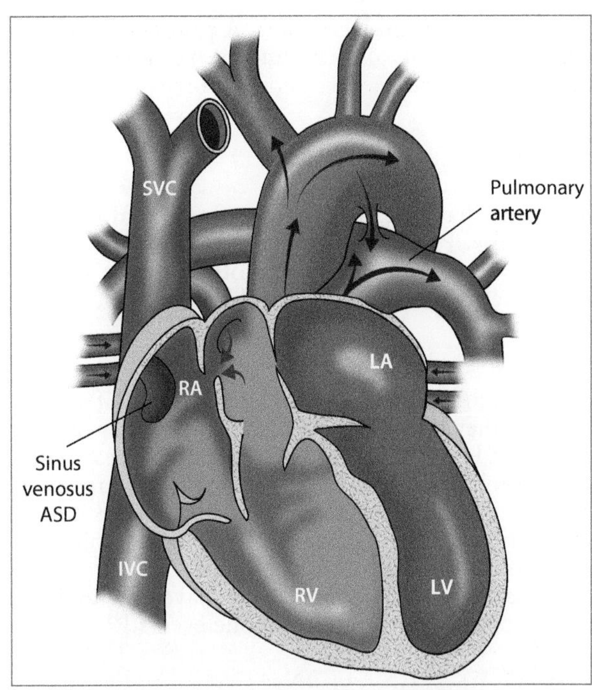

Figure 5.4 **Sinus venosus atrial septal defect. Note absence of superior rim and presence of inferior rim. ASD, atrial septal defect; IVC, inferior vena cava;** LA, left atrium; LV, left ventricle; RA, right atrium; RV, right ventricle; SVC, superior vena cava.

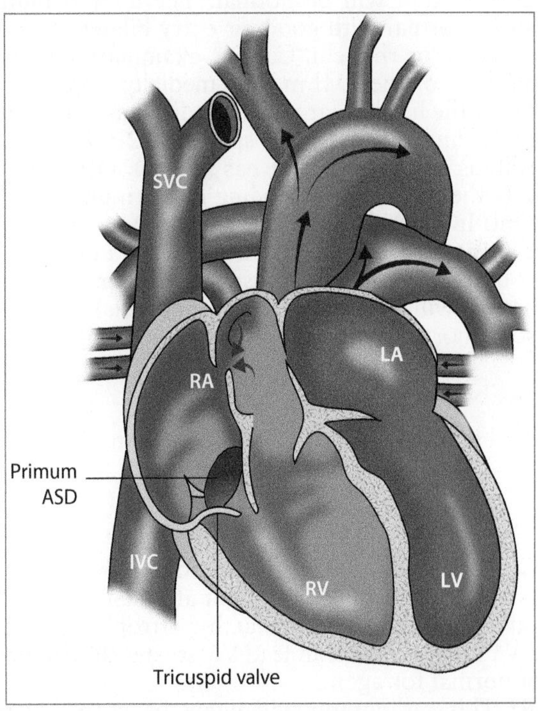

Figure 5.5 **Primum atrial septal defect. Atrial septum is near the atrioventricular valves (tricuspid valve and mitral valve) and lacks the inferior atrial septal rim.** ASD, atrial septal defect; IVC, inferior vena cava; LA, left atrium; LV, left ventricle; RA, right atrium; RV, right ventricle; SVC, superior vena cava.

This defect lacks the inferior atrial septal rim. This defect can occur in isolation or is often associated with another congenital heart defect commonly seen in patients with trisomy 21 called an atrioventricular septal defect/endocardial cushion defect/atrioventricular canal defect (see Section

5.6B Ventricular Septal Defects).[193] A primum ASD will not undergo spontaneous closure and is considered hemodynamically significant.

MEDICAL HISTORY AND CLINICAL PRESENTATION

Most patients have no significant past medical history and appear healthy. Premature infants and newborns are more likely to have a PFO. Patients with other genetic syndromes are more likely to have a congenital heart defect.

SIGNS AND SYMPTOMS

Patients with an ASD are often asymptomatic. If symptoms are present, they will likely be subtle and more generalized. Patients with large ASDs causing right-sided heart enlargement may complain of a decreased exercise capacity, but most patients will not be aware that they had exercise limitations until the ASD is closed. Frequent or prolonged respiratory infections may also be present.

Adult patients with a PFO may have migraine headaches[195] or history of thromboembolic events.[195]

PHYSICAL EXAMINATION

Patients will typically present acyanotic in no acute distress. The patient will show signs of adequate perfusion including brisk capillary refill. Head, ears, eye, nose, and throat exam will be normal unless patients are syndromic (trisomy 21). The thyroid exam will be normal. The lung examination will also be normal with good air entry bilaterally with no wheezes, rales, or rhonchi. Cardiac examination with have a normal PMI or the PMI may be medially displaced if the right side of the heart is large. On cardiac auscultation there will be a normal S1 and fixed split S2 (S2 may be normal if the ASD is small or patient has a PFO). Often the fixed split S2 is the only cardiac finding and a murmur will not be present. In large ASDs, a harsh systolic murmur may be present at the left upper sternal border and a diastolic rumble may be heard along the left sternal border. The vascular examination will be normal. The abdominal examination will also be normal with no hepatosplenomegaly.

DIFFERENTIAL DIAGNOSIS

The differential diagnosis for ASDs is summarized in Table 5.14.

DIAGNOSTIC STUDIES

- **EKG:** This study will likely be normal but may show signs of right axis deviation, right atrial enlargement (tall P waves), or right ventricular hypertrophy (R wave in lead V1 and/or S wave in lead V6 greater than upper limits of normal for age).
- **CXR:** This radiograph will likely be normal with no signs of pulmonary edema (increased pulmonary vascular markings). Cardiomegaly with the right heart shadow being enlarged may be present in large ASDs.
- **TTE (Figure 5.6):** This modality will typically show the location and size of the ASD as well as the direction of the atrial level shunt. The size and function of the right side of the heart can also be assessed. Transthoracic imaging had great resolution in children but may be less ideal in adult patients.
- **TEE:** A sedated imaging study that is obtained by placing a probe in the patient's esophagus to more clearly visualizes the atrial septum. TEE is utilized when transthoracic imaging is suboptimal and there is a clinical suspicion of a heart defect not seen by transthoracic imaging. Cardiology consultation is required to obtain this imaging.

TABLE 5.14 Differential Diagnoses for Atrial Septal Defects

Diagnosis	Description
Anomalus pulmonary venus return/extracardiac shunts	When the pulmonary veins are connected to the right side of the heart or extracardiac connections (arteriovenous malformations) are present, volume overload of the right side of the heart will occur causing right-sided heart enlargement.
Pulmonary stenosis	Physical exam finding is a systolic murmur caused by an abnormality of the pulmonary valve instead of the murmur being caused by extra flow across the pulmonary valve in the setting of an atrial septal defect.
Tricuspid stenosis	Physical exam finding is a diastolic rumble caused by an abnormality in the tricuspid valve instead of the murmur being caused by extra flow across the tricuspid valve in the setting of an atrial septal defect.

EVALUATION

The size of the ASD, location of the defect, and any associated symptoms/pertinent diagnostic findings will determine the need for treatment. Small, centralized defects do not require treatment. Large ASDs, sinus venosus ASDs, primum ASDs, and defects causing right-sided heart enlargement will require treatment.

TREATMENT

- No medication treatment is available.
- Sinus venosus ASDs and primum ASDs will require primary surgical closure via open-heart surgery and cardiopulmonary bypass.
- Secundum ASDs and PFOs can be closed with an atrial septal closure device placed in the cardiac catheterization laboratory under fluoroscopy with the patient sedated. A superior and inferior rim of tissue must be present to hold the device in place.

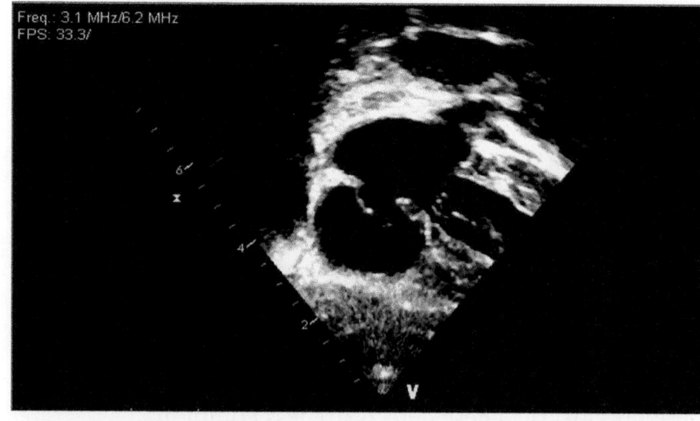

Figure 5.6 Subcostal transthoracic image of a secundum atrial septal defect.

- Primary closure via open-heart surgery is indicated if the ASD is too large to be closed by the atrial septal closure device.

PATIENT EDUCATION

- It may be helpful to utilize a diagram showing the anatomy of the heart and location of the ASD.
- Explain that most patients with a small ASD are asymptomatic and have no changes in their exercise tolerance or their ability to perform tasks (including competitive sports), and will have no limitation to their lifespan as a result of the defect.
- Refer to cardiologist once ASD is identified (if not already established with cardiology)
- Refer patient to cardiologist if surgical closure or device closure is recommended (if not already established with cardiology). Patient will also have an evaluation by the cardiologist or surgeon performing the selected procedure.
- Patient will be followed by a cardiologist until defect undergoes spontaneous closure. Monitoring by cardiologist will continue indefinitely following device or primary closure.
- Instruct patient to report any changes to exercise tolerance and any difficulty recovering from respiratory infections.
- Patient is at risk for endocarditis during the first 6 months following either primary closure or device closure of the ASD. Patient should avoid elective procedures of risk such as dental cleaning/extractions and will require premedication with an antibiotic 1 hour prior to the procedure during this time frame if the procedure is performed.
- Patient is at low risk for atrial dysrhythmias following closure, but instruct patient report any episodes of palpitations, dizziness, or syncope. Then refer to cardiology for cardiac dysrhythmia evaluation.

SPECIAL CONSIDERATIONS

Most premature infants and newborns have a small atrial level shunt (likely a PFO) that can be seen by TTE. Often this is an incidental finding on the echocardiogram that would have been completed for another reason (e.g., presence of a murmur, concerns for other congenital heart disease, or abnormal EKG).

Adults with history of migraine headache not responding to standard medical management may have a hemodynamically significant PFO allowing microemboli to pass from the venous to the arterial side causing headaches.[195] These patients may benefit from device closure of their PFO. Closure of a PFO in patients without history of migraine headaches refractory to standard medical therapy is not recommended.[195]

It is recommended to close a small ASD/PFO in patients with a history of embolic stroke to prevent further stroke.[195] Closure of a small ASD/PFO in patients with no history of stroke is not currently recommended.[195]

The ability to accurately state the presence or absence of a small ASD/PFO in adult patients via TTE is limited due to image quality. Additional image modalities need to be considered if there is a clinical concern (e.g., TEE). Expert consultation is recommended.[195]

KEY POINTS

- ASDs are common acyanotic congenital heart defects.
- ASD patients are often asymptomatic.
- Key physical examination finding with ASDs is a fixed split S2 on cardiac auscultation.
- Diagnostic testing will show right-sided heart enlargement in the setting of large ASDs.

5.6B VENTRICULAR SEPTAL DEFECTS

OVERVIEW

A VSD is a hole in the wall separating the RV and LV of the heart. It is the most common congenital heart defect[196] allowing oxygenated blood in the LV to cross over and mix with deoxygenated blood from the RV. VSD frequently occurs in the setting of other congenital heart disease states. This acyanotic heart defect allows a larger volume of blood than normal to be carried to the lungs, often resulting in pulmonary blood flow more than systemic circulation (resulting in congestive HF). There are a number of anatomic locations where VSDs can be present. Size and location of the defect and symptomatology of the patient play a role in determining the need for surgical intervention.

PATHOPHYSIOLOGY

In the presence of a VSD, oxygenated flow from the LV crosses the ventricular septum and enters the RV. This flow mixes with the deoxygenated blood in the RV and is pumped to the lungs via the pulmonary artery (Figure 5.7). This right-to-left shunt often causes pulmonary overcirculation once the pulmonary vascular resistance decreases. The amount of pulmonary over circulation noted is dependent upon two factors; the size of the defect and the difference between the pressures on the left side of the heart versus the right side of the heart. During fetal life, the pulmonary vascular resistance is elevated and similar to the systemic vascular resistance due to fluid-filled lungs. The lack of a pressure gradient will limit the amount of blood flow that can move through the defect from the left to the right. Over the course of the first 1 to 2 months, the pulmonary vascular resistance will drop, increasing this gradient and allowing more blood flow through the defect and ultimately to the lungs.

In general, VSDs will be described in two ways regarding the magnitude of the ventricular level shunt. A defect that is described as restrictive indicates that the size of the defect is able to restrict the amount of extra blood flow to the lungs in addition to the elevated pulmonary vascular resistance noted in the newborn period. As the pulmonary vascular resistance drops, the size of the defect is the primary limiting factor of extra blood flow. A defect that is described as nonrestrictive indicates that the size of the defect is so large that the only factor that limits extra pulmonary blood flow is the elevated pulmonary vascular resistance initially. As the pulmonary vascular resistance begins to drop, significant pulmonary overcirculation will occur. General rule of thumb: little difference between pulmonary vascular resistance and systemic vascular resistance, less pulmonary overcirculation; larger difference, more pulmonary overcirculation.

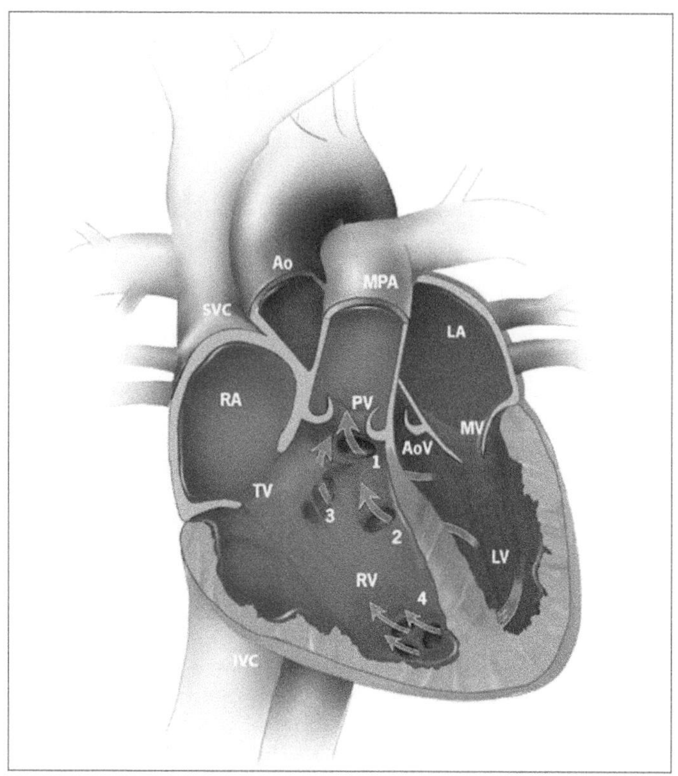

Figure 5.7 **Ventricular septal defect.** Ao, aorta; AoV, aortic valve; IVC, inferior vena cava; LA, left atrium; LV, left ventricle; MPA, main pulmonary artery; MV, mitral valve; PV, pulmonary valve; RA, right atrium; RV, right ventricle; SVC, superior vena cava; TV, tricuspid valve; 1, conoventricular, malaligned; 2, perimembranous; 3, inlet; 4, muscular.
(Source: Centers for Disease Control and Prevention.)

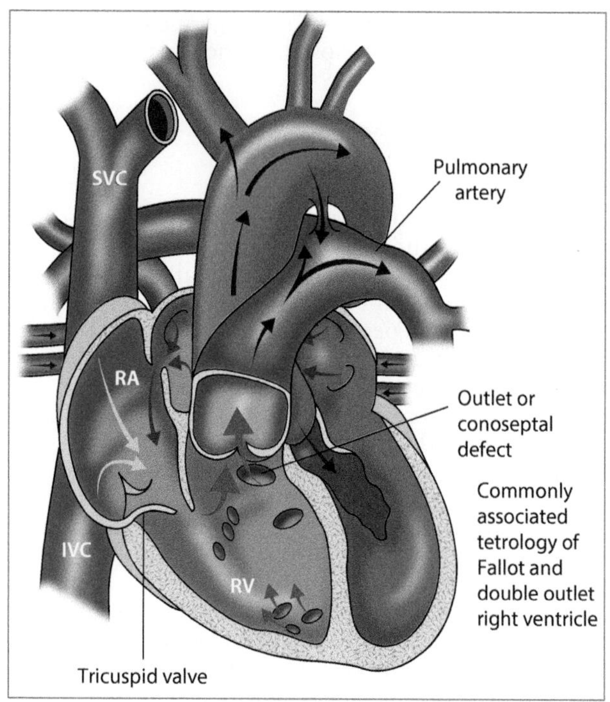

Figure 5.8 **Inlet ventricular septal defect. Commonly associated with atrioventricular canal defect.** IVC, inferior vena cava; RA, right atrium; RV, right ventricle; SVC, superior vena cava.

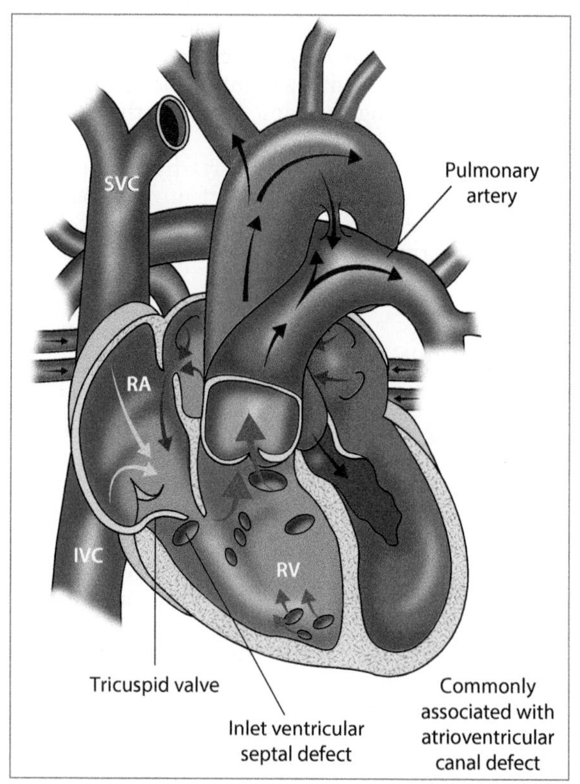

Figure 5.9 **Outlet or conoseptal ventricular septal defect. Commonly associated with tetrology of Fallot and double outlet right ventricle.** IVC, inferior vena cava; RA, right atrium; RV, right ventricle; SVC, superior vena cava.

There are four general locations within the ventricular septum where defects can occur. The ventricular septum can first be broken down into two sections: the noncontractile membranous septum and contractile muscular septum. The membranous septum is further broken down into three sections: the inlet septum (Figure 5.8), the outlet septum (Figure 5.9), and the perimembranous septum (Figure 5.10).

The most common location for a VSD to occur is the perimembranous septum (Figure 5.10). Small defects in this region often undergo spontaneous closure and rarely cause HF. Moderate defects may initially present with clinical signs of HF, but the defect may become smaller over time resulting in resolution of HF symptoms. Large defects will result in HF once the pulmonary vascular resistance decreases and will likely require surgical closure. Occasionally, a small membranous defect is located close enough to the AoV to pull the AoV leaflet into the defect itself. These patients do not present with HF due to pulmonary overcirculation but can develop AoV insufficiency that may lead to volume overload of the LV resulting in pulmonary congestion due to decreased left ventricular function. If AoV insufficiency is noted in the setting of a small membranous VSD, then surgical closure of the VSD is recommended to protect the AoV.

The second most common VSD is located in the muscular portion of the ventricular septum (Figure 5.11). As with the perimembranous VSD, size matters. Small defects have a high likelihood of spontaneous closure and do not cause pulmonary overcirculation. Moderate defects may initially present with clinical signs of HF, but the defect may become smaller over time resulting in resolution of HF symptoms. Large defects will result in HF once the pulmonary vascular resistance decreases and will likely require surgical closure.

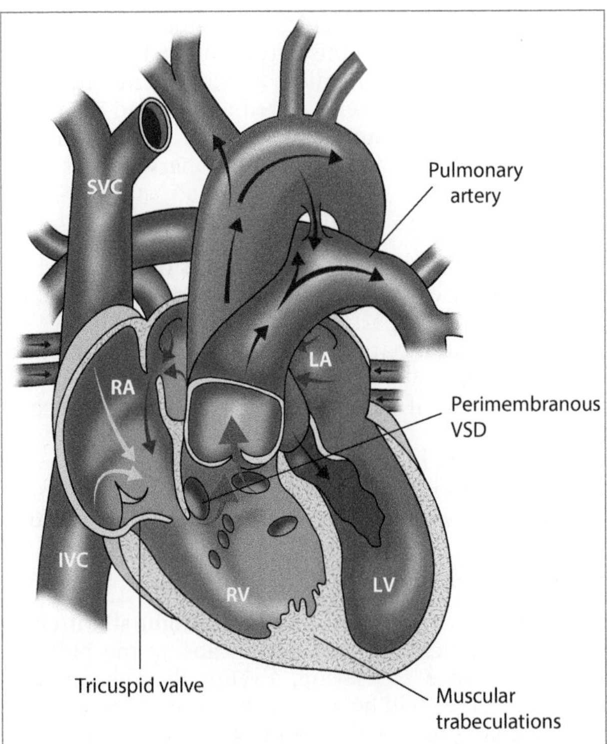

Figure 5.10 **Perimembranous ventricular septal defect. The most common location for a ventricular septal defect. Small defects in this region often undergo spontaneous closure and rarely cause heart failure.** IVC, inferior vena cava; LA, left atrium; LV, left ventricle; RA, right atrium; RV, right ventricle; SVC, superior vena cava; VSD, ventricular septal defect.

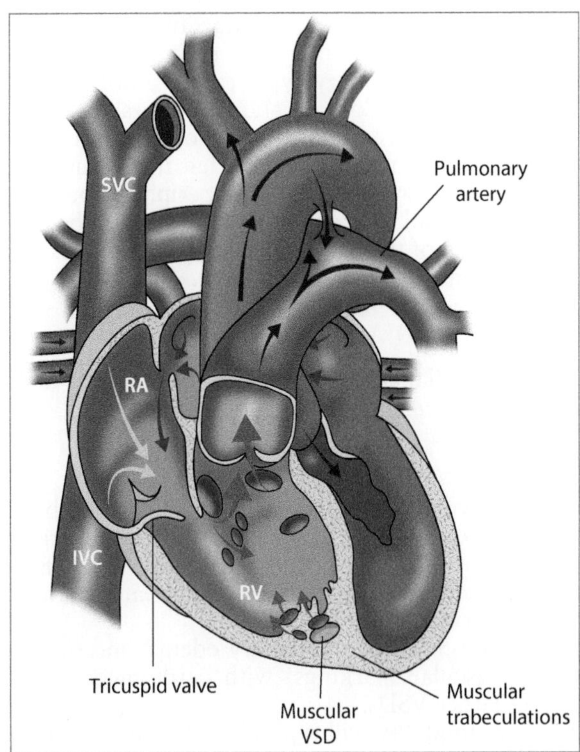

Figure 5.11 **Muscular ventricular septal defect. Small defects have a high likelihood of spontaneous closure and do not cause pulmonary overcirculation. Moderate defects may initially present with clinical signs of heart failure, but the defect may become smaller over time resulting in resolution of heart failure symptoms. Large defects will result in heart failure once the pulmonary vascular resistance decreases and will likely require surgical closure.** IVC, inferior vena cava; RA, right atrium; RV, right ventricle; SVC, superior vena cava; VSD, ventricular septal defect.

The other two membranous defects occur less frequently and are often associated with additional congenital heart defects. Inlet VSDs are commonly associated with AV septal defect/endocardial cushion defect/AV canal defect. Outlet VSDs are commonly associated with tetralogy of Fallot and transposition of the great arteries (TGA). These defects do not close spontaneously and are typically surgically repaired as part of a larger congenital heart surgical repair.

MEDICAL HISTORY AND CLINICAL PRESENTATION

Newborns with a VSD will be asymptomatic at birth but may possess a nonspecific flow murmur on physical examination (if they have a murmur at all). As the pulmonary vascular resistance drops over the course of the next 2 months, the murmur will become a more traditional, harsh, holosystolic murmur.

Additionally, patients with larger VSDs will present with increased work of breathing and failure to thrive (decreased ability to gain weight) as the pulmonary vascular resistance drops. The drop in pulmonary vascular resistance will result in increased blood flow to the lungs and increased volume overload to the left side of the heart. Owing to the pulmonary congestion, patients will become tachypneic. Their metabolic demand will be increased because of the tachypnea and increased burden on the left side of the heart. They will require a higher-than-normal calorie intake per day as a result of this increased metabolic demand but will struggle to take in adequate calories by mouth because of the rate that they are breathing. As a result of the inability to consume enough calories, they often struggle to gain weight. Caloric needs for growth for normal infants is approximately 110–120 kcal/kg/day.[197] Patients with a significant cardiac defect will often require more than 120 kcal/kg/day to gain weight in the face of their defect.[197] The increased respiratory rate also places them at increased risk of aspiration pneumonia.

SIGNS AND SYMPTOMS

Patients with small VSDs will present to clinic asymptomatic with normal weight gain and oral feeding patterns. Patients with larger VSDs will present to clinic with a history of poor weight gain, poor oral feeding, tachypnea, dyspnea with feeding, and diaphoresis with feeding.

PHYSICAL EXAMINATION

Vital signs should be obtained at every visit and will be normal in patients with small defects. Patients with larger defects will show poor weight gain. Height will not be affected. Heart rate may be normal for age or slightly elevated. Heart rhythm will be normal. The blood pressure will be normal. The patient's respiratory rate will be elevated with normal oxygen saturation in room air. The patient will show signs of increased work of breathing, with intercostal/subcostal retractions, but will not have findings of grunting, nasal flaring, or head bobbing. This is called comfortable tachypnea. Auscultation of the lung fields will have good air entry bilaterally and clear lung fields or may have subtle wheezing/rales. Rhonchi will not be auscultated. The cardiac examination will show normal to leftward PMI. A thrill may be palpable on the chest. Cardiac auscultation will reveal a normal S1 and physiologically split S2 (loud single S2 is concerning for pulmonary hypertension and Eisenmenger syndrome; see Special Considerations). A harsh holosystolic murmur will be appreciated at any point on the anterior chest, but most commonly along the left midsternal border. The capillary refill will be brisk. The peripheral pulse exam will be normal in all four extremities. There will be no cyanosis or clubbing of the nail beds. The liver and possibly the spleen will be easily palpable and large.

DIFFERENTIAL DIAGNOSIS

The differential diagnosis for VSDs is summarized in Table 5.15.

DIAGNOSTIC STUDIES

- **EKG:** This will likely be normal with small VSDs but may show signs of left axis deviation, left atrial enlargement (wide P waves), or left ventricular hypertrophy (R wave in lead V6 and or S wave in lead V1 greater than upper limits of normal for age).
- **Chest x-ray:** Signs of pulmonary edema (increased pulmonary vascular markings) with cardiomegaly will be noted in larger VSDs.
- **TTE:** This modality will typically show the location and size of the VSD as well as the direction of the ventricular level shunt. The size and function of the left side of the heart can also be assessed.

TREATMENT

- The patient should be closely monitored by general clinician and pediatric cardiologist for signs of increased work of breathing, poor weight gain, poor PO feeding
- Loop diuretics such as furosemide are considered the first-line therapy to improve work of breathing by decreasing pulmonary edema (ventricular preload)
- ACEIs such as captopril may be added to decrease afterload and help extra blood flow to the lungs.
- Often the feeding regimen will need to be augmented to promote weight gain. The patient may be unable to take in large volumes of formula due to the pulmonary edema and tachypnea. Smaller volumes of formula at higher concentrations are often needed. Placement of a feeding tube may be considered if the patient is unable to safely take in formula by mouth.

TABLE 5.15 Differential Diagnosis for Ventricular Septal Defects

Diagnosis	Description
Viral/bacterial respiratory infection	Tachypnea will be present and likely wheezing. Patient will also likely show signs of respiratory distress such as nasal flaring and head bobbing. Oxygen saturation may be diminished.
Atrioventricular valve insufficiency (mitral or triscuspid valve)	Patient will also have presence of a holosystolic murmur, but will likely not be tachypneic or have poor weight gain.
Atrioventricular septal defect	Patient will present with holosystolic murmur and failure to thrive, but ventricular septal defect is part of a larger congenital heart defect.

- Surgical closure of the defect is considered when the patient continues to demonstrate signs of failure to thrive despite maximizing medical management (maximized preload reduction, afterload reduction, and feeding regimen). Surgical closure can only be accomplished via open-heart surgery and cardiopulmonary bypass.

PATIENT EDUCATION

- Notify clinician if patient shows signs of increased work of breathing, persistent increase in respiratory rate, intercostal retractions (particularly with feeding).
- Notify clinican if patient exhibits findings of diaphoresis with feeding.
- Notify clinician if patient shows signs of struggling with oral feeds.
  - Feeds taking longer than normal.
  - Patient looking more fatigued with feeds.
  - Patient appearing more short of breath with feeding.

SPECIAL CONSIDERATIONS

In the setting of a long-standing left-to-right shunt changes in the lung parenchyma may occur causing the pulmonary vascular resistance to elevate. Eventually, the pulmonary vascular resistance will be greater than the systemic vascular resistance changing the direction of the shunt (now right-to-left). This change in shunt allows deoxygenated flow to mix with the systemic circuit causing cyanosis. This process is called Eisenmenger syndrome. Once present, the defect is no longer fixable. Closing the defect in this situation will decrease cardiac output and can lead to death (the only way flow can get from the right heart to the left heart is through lungs under very high pressure). If the defect is left open, cardiac output is maintained because flow can go through the defect and out to the body (blue flow is better than no flow).

Inability to split the second heart sound on auscultation is concerning for the presence of pulmonary hypertension and possible Eisenmenger syndrome. If identified early, and with aggressive pulmonary hypertension treatment, staged or partial closure of the VSD may be possible.

5.6C COARCTATION OF THE AORTA

OVERVIEW

Coarctation of the aorta is a narrowing of the aortic arch, most commonly at the insertion site of the ductus arteriosus; however, narrowing may occur at any site within the transverse aortic arch. The narrowing can be mild or severe causing hypertension in the upper extremities and hypotension in the lower extremities. Typically, lower extremity pulses are faint or absent. Milder forms of coarctation of the aorta can go undetected in the newborn period but present as hypertension in the older child. Severe coarctation of the aorta can lead to renal ischemia and mesenteric ischemia resulting in septic shock. A common cause of necrotizing enterocolitis in the newborn period is unrecognized coarctation of the aorta. Milder forms of coarctation of the aorta can go undetected in the newborn period but present as hypertension in the older child. Coarctation of the aorta can be easily identified in the primary care office by performing an accurate and thorough history and physical examination and should be strongly suspected in any child who presents with faint or absent lower extremity pulses.

EPIDEMIOLOGY

Coarctation of the aorta accounts for 4% to 6% of all congenital heart defects, occurring in approximately 4 per 10,000 live births.[198] It occurs more commonly in males than females (59%–41%). Most cases occur spontaneously.

PATHOPHYSIOLOGY

The precise cause of coarctation of the aorta is unknown; however, there are two main theories to the development of the disorder: decreased intrauterine flow through the aorta causing underdevelopment of the fetal aortic arch[199] and migration or extension of ductal tissue into the wall of the fetal thoracic aorta.[200]

There is evidence to support increased familial risk of congenital left ventricular outflow tract obstruction (LVOTO).[201] In this setting coarctation of the aorta is often associated with other left ventricular malformations such as bicuspid AoV or Shone's complex and is often seen in patients with Turner syndrome.[202]

5.6D PATENT DUCTUS ARTERIOSUS

OVERVIEW

PDA, failure of the ductus arteriosus to close after birth, is a common acyanotic congenital heart defect often seen in premature infants but can also be found in term infants. Larger defects with lower pulmonary vascular resistance will often lead to increased symptomatology. Symptoms may include pulmonary overcirculation, renal insufficiency, poor weight gain, gut ischemia, and septic shock. The degree of symptomatology seen in the patient is related to the size of the shunt and the patient's pulmonary vascular resistance. Larger defects left untreated may also contribute to chronic lung disease.

EPIDEMIOLOGY

In term infants, narrowing of the ductus arteriosus resulting in functional closure occurs in 50% within 24 hours after birth, 90% within 48 hours, and virtually all within 72 hours. Term infants with persistent PDA typically have abnormal ductal tissue that does not respond to inhibition of prostaglandin synthase (PGE2) and as a result will likely not respond to medical closure methods. The incidence of isolated PDA in term infants is approximately 3 to 8 per 10,000 live births and is more prominent in females than males.[203,204]

Preterm infants often have delayed closure of the ductus arteriosus, often taking weeks to months to close. The length of time to closure is inversely proportional to gestational age.

PATHOPHYSIOLOGY

The ductus arteriosus is a vital structure in the fetal heart allowing blood flow from the right side of the heart to bypass the lungs in utero resulting in a right-to-left shunt across the ductus (fetal lungs filled with amniotic fluid resulting in high pulmonary pressures). This structure typically recedes (closes) within 72 hours after birth resulting in a ligamentous structure (ligamentum arteriosum). Patency of the ductus arteriosus after birth will result in a left-to-right shunt across the ductus as the pulmonary vascular resistance drops (typically within 2–8 weeks; Figure 5.12). Larger left-to-right shunts will lead to left atrial and possibly left ventricular enlargement. Diastolic pressure in the aorta is lowered as a result of continued blood flow from the aorta to the pulmonary artery in diastole as well as systole (Figure 5.13). This drop in diastolic pressure can lead to decreased blood flow to the kidneys and gut, resulting in renal insufficiency or mesenteric ischemia.

MEDICAL HISTORY AND CLINICAL PRESENTATION

A history of prematurity is common; however, a PDA can be seen in term infants as well. Patients will be asymptomatic

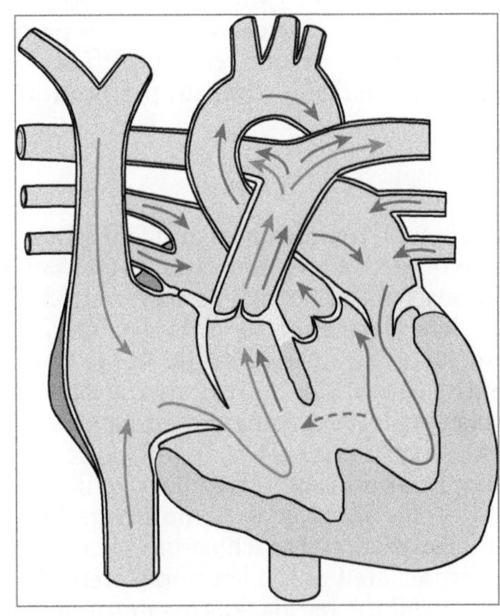

Figure 5.12 Ventricular septal defect with left-to-right shunt.

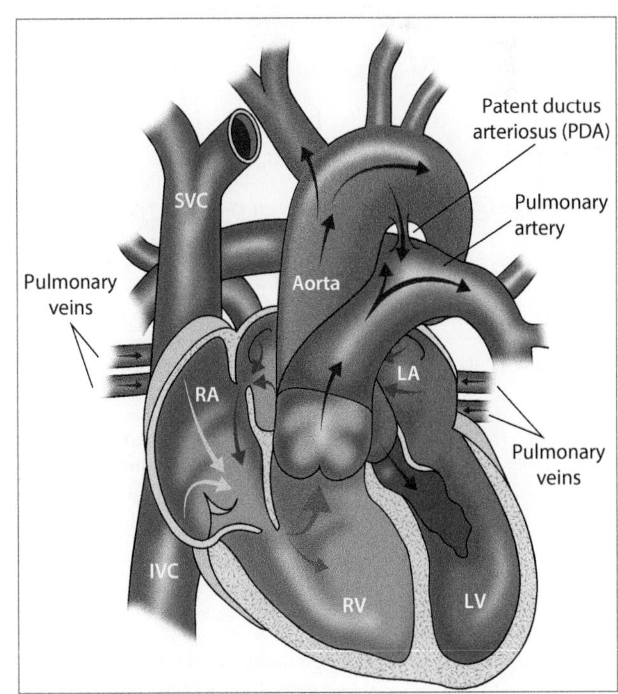

Figure 5.13 Patent ductus arteriosus. Diastolic flow reversal in the distal aorta indicates the patient is at risk for decreased renal/gut perfusion. IVC, inferior vena cava; LA, left atrium; LV, left ventricle; RA, right atrium; RV, right ventricle; SVC, superior vena cava.

with normal growth and development if the PDA is small. Larger PDAs will lead to tachypnea, feeding intolerance, and poor weight gain. Decreased urine output can also be seen due to decreased renal perfusion. Large PDAs can also be a cause of necrotizing enterocolitis secondary to gut ischemia.

SIGNS AND SYMPTOMS

Patients with hemodynamically significant PDAs will present with tachypnea due to pulmonary overcirculation. Patients will be acyanotic. Poor feeding will often be present due to tachypnea but may also be related to abdominal discomfort due to gut ischemia. Increased metabolic demand and decreased ability to feed will result in poor weight gain. Oliguria may be seen due to decreased renal perfusion. Acidosis (often metabolic due to renal insufficiency) may be seen. Septic shock can result from gut perforation (necrotizing enterocolitis).

PHYSICAL EXAMINATION

Patients with hemodynamically significant PDAs will present with tachypnea due to pulmonary overcirculation. Oxygen saturations will be normal as oxygenated blood flow moves from left (systemic) to right (pulmonic). Systolic blood pressure will be normal in the upper and lower extremities, but diastolic blood pressure will be low resulting in a wide pulse pressure causing bounding pulses in the upper and lower extremities. Palmar pulses and/or pulsatile nail beds may be appreciated. Capillary refill will be brisk. Auscultation of the lungs may demonstrate faint rales. A harsh (often described as "machine-like") continuous murmur will be appreciated at the left upper sternal border, left axillary region, and the left back. This murmur will be present with the patient both supine and seated. Abdominal examination will typically be normal (no renal artery bruits) but may demonstrate hepatomegaly secondary to pulmonary overcirculation (i.e., congestive HF).

DIFFERENTIAL DIAGNOSIS

The differential diagnosis for PDA is summarized in Table 5.16.

TABLE 5.16 Differential Diagnosis for Patent Ductus Arteriosus

Diagnosis	Description
Arteriovenous fistula	Continuous murmur without wide pulse pressure.
Venous hum	Innocent, continuous murmur heard in the seated position only (often heard in older children).
Ventricular septal defect	Can also cause acyanotic pulmonary overcirculation. Will have a holosystolic murmur and normal pulse pressure with normal pulses.
Coarctation of the aorta	Systolic murmur heard in the same region as patent ductus arteriosus with bounding upper extremity pulses, diminished lower extremity pulses. Systolic hypertension in the upper extremities and systolic hypotension in the lower extremities.

DIAGNOSTIC STUDIES

EKG will be normal with small ducts but will show left atrial enlargement in larger ducts. CXR will often show pulmonary edema and cardiomegaly in larger, hemodynamically significant PDAs.

Echocardiogram will show the presence of the PDA. The anatomic size of the duct and direction of blood flow through the duct can be determined by color flow Doppler. Continuous Doppler will determine the velocity of blood flow through the duct (high velocities typically indicate more restriction of flow, as in a small duct, and normal pulmonary pressures). An elevated left atrial/aorta diameter ratio is indicative of left atrial enlargement. Diastolic flow reversal in the distal aorta indicates the patient is at risk for decreased renal/gut perfusion.

TREATMENT

- Initial medical management of pulmonary overcirculation is done with fluid restriction and diuresis. Monitor and correct blood gas as indicated. Manage airway (conservative or mechanical ventilation) as needed to maintain oxygen saturation between 90% and 95%.[205]
- Medical closure of the PDA with indomethacin or ibuprofen (nonselective COX inhibitors) is considered after the first week if PDA is still felt to be significant.[205] Use of ibuprofen versus indomethacin is based on availability and institution preference.[205] Ibuprofen can be given IV or orally and is dosed 10 mg/kg for first dose followed by two doses of 5 mg/kg q24h over the course of 72 hours).[205] Indomethacin is administered IV at 0.2 g/kg/dose q12h for a total of three doses. Both agents may require multiple treatment courses.
- Catheter-based closure or surgical ligation of the duct is considered if PDA remains hemodynamically significant and medical closure is unsuccessful.

PATIENT EDUCATION

- Monitor for feeding difficulties, tachypnea during feeds, diaphoresis during feeds.
- Monitor for hoarse/weak cry if surgical ligation was performed (at risk for damage to the recurrent laryngeal nerve resulting in vocal cord paralysis)

KEY POINTS

- PDA is quite common in preterm infants.
- PDA causes left-to-right shunt resulting in pulmonary overcirculation similar to VSD.
- Continuous machinery-like murmur is present.
- Nonselective COX inhibitors are utilized for medical closure of the PDA.

5.6E TETRALOGY OF FALLOT

OVERVIEW

Tetralogy of Fallot is a condition comprising four features: malaligned VSD, overriding aorta, right ventricular outflow tract obstruction with varying degrees of pulmonary valve stenosis or atresia, and right ventricular hypertrophy. The overriding aorta receives blood from both LV and RV through the VSD. Flow through the pulmonary valve and to the lungs is hindered by the RV outflow tract (RVOT) obstruction and pulmonary valve stenosis, causing right ventricular hypertrophy to develop. The clinical presentation of these patients is dependent on the degree of obstruction of blood flow to the lungs and the relative resistance of the pulmonary and systemic vascular systems. It varies from cyanosis to acyanotic at birth with subsequent development of HF symptoms secondary to too much blood flow to the lungs.

EPIDEMIOLOGY

Tetralogy of Fallot occurs in 3 of every 10,000 live births.[206] It accounts for 7% to 10% of all congenital heart lesions and is the most common cyanotic congenital heart disease.[206] If one child in any family is born with tetralogy of Fallot, the risk of having another child with it is 3%.[206] Tetralogy of Fallot is a common occurrence in children with 22q11.2 deletion, also known as DiGeorge syndrome.

PATHOPHYSIOLOGY

The VSD is malaligned, allowing blue blood from the RV and red blood from the LV to both go through the aorta to the body. The direction and degree of shunting depend on the level of RVOT obstruction and pulmonary valve stenosis. If the stenosis is mild, blood shunts from left to right at the VSD. However, if the obstruction is more severe or the pulmonary valve is atretic, there is right-to-left shunting at the VSD. Therefore, the patient's oxygen saturation can vary from normal (>90%) to cyanotic. Because the RV is pumping against a fixed obstruction, it becomes hypertrophied.

Pulmonary Atresia With or Without Major Aortopulmonary Collateral Arteries

In pulmonary atresia, the pulmonary valve does not develop, and a plate of tissue is typically present in that position. Therefore, there is no outflow through the pulmonary valve, and the only outlet for blood in the RV is to go through the VSD to the LV and then the aorta. These patients are ductal dependent as the only way the pulmonary vasculature receives blood is through the PDA.

The main pulmonary artery (MPA) may be hypoplastic or atretic as well. The branch pulmonary arteries are typically hypoplastic but may also have abnormal origins, such as from the aorta or its branches, or may not be present at all. When the pulmonary valve is atretic, sometimes major aortopulmonary collateral arteries (MAPCAs) develop. These are abnormal vessels that directly connect the pulmonary vasculature to the aorta or its branches and act as left-to-right shunts for red blood to travel to the lungs. However, these vessels are frequently too small to ensure adequate blood flow to the lungs or become narrow over time. Also, in some cases the vessels are so large that they steal too much blood from the systemic circulation, leaving the rest of the body with inadequate circulation.

Absent Pulmonary Valve

When the pulmonary valve is absent, only a rudimentary structure may be present. While there is typically at least some degree of outflow obstruction, there is no impedance to retrograde flow back into the RV. This creates a to-and-fro phenomenon in which the majority of the blood that goes out the pulmonary valve travels back into the RV during diastole. The proximal branch pulmonary arteries subsequently become very large and aneurysmal. There is typically not significant cyanosis in these patients as there is an outlet for blood to exit the RV to the pulmonary vascular bed. However, these patients can be very ill at birth as the large branch pulmonary arteries compress the airways and even the aorta.

MEDICAL HISTORY AND CLINICAL PRESENTATION

Tetralogy of Fallot is frequently diagnosed prenatally. Exact detection rates vary by sonographer and institution, but prenatal diagnostic rate can be up to 70%.[207] Clinical presentation varies depending on the amount of RVOT obstruction. If there is a significant degree of RVOT obstruction, blood will shunt right to left at the VSD and the patient will be cyanotic. However, if the RVOT obstruction is less significant, patients will appear acyanotic at birth.

SIGNS AND SYMPTOMS

If there is severe RVOT obstruction at birth, patients will appear cyanotic with adequate systemic perfusion. If there is less significant RVOT obstruction and the VSD is shunting left to right, patients may be acyanotic and asymptomatic at birth. However, pulmonary vascular resistance naturally decreases at 4 to 6 weeks of life, which increases the amount of left-to-right shunting at the VSD and can result in too much blood flow to the lungs, known as pulmonary overcirculation.

PHYSICAL EXAMINATION

The second heart sound (S2) is typically single. A crescendo-decrescendo systolic murmur can be heard at the left upper sternal border due to pulmonary valve stenosis. It can radiate into the back if the degree of stenosis is severe. An AoV ejection click can be heard if there is a significant amount of left-to-right shunting through the VSD. If the degree of RVOT obstruction is mild and there is not significant shunting at the VSD, no murmurs may be auscultated.

Acyanotic patients may have "tet" spells where they become cyanotic abruptly. Blood shunts right to left instead of left to right at the VSD, decreasing the amount of oxygen reaching systemic circulation. Pulmonary blood flow is decreased as less blood flows through the RVOT, further worsening cyanosis as less blood is oxygenated. The murmur of RVOT obstruction and pulmonary valve stenosis is decreased or absent during these episodes as less blood is flowing through the area, decreasing the degree of stenosis. When the spells occur, prompt treatment is necessary (see below).

Physical examination findings of pulmonary overcirculation include tachypnea and increased work of breathing.

DIFFERENTIAL DIAGNOSIS

The differential diagnosis for tetralogy of Fallot is summarized in Table 5.17.

DIAGNOSTIC STUDIES

An echocardiogram is the best study to evaluate these patients. It allows direct visualization of the anatomy, including the RVOT and pulmonary valve, VSD, and aorta. The echocardiogram also allows the ability to measure the degree of obstruction in the RVOT and the direction and intensity of shunting at the VSD.

EKG typically demonstrates right axis deviation and right ventricular hypertrophy.

TABLE 5.17 Differential Diagnosis for Tetralogy of Fallot

Diagnosis	Description
Double outlet right ventricle	The right ventricle supplies blood to both the left and right ventricles. A VSD is always present.
Ventricular septal defect (VSD)	A VSD with significant left-to-right shunting can cause relative pulmonary valve stenosis due to the increased amount of blood flowing across the valve. The aorta is not overriding.
Pulmonary valve atresia	Lack of outflow through the right ventricle mimics tetralogy of Fallot, but the aorta is not overriding.

CXR can demonstrate the classic "boot-shaped" heart due to an upturned cardiac apex secondary to RV hypertrophy, although it is not commonly seen now that patients are diagnosed prenatally or promptly after birth.

While typically not needed for classic cases, CT and MRI, especially angiography, can be useful when evaluating patients with MAPCAs or abnormal pulmonary artery anatomy.

EVALUATION

In addition to the diagnostic studies listed above, the systemic oxygen saturation can indicate the direction of shunting at the VSD. Physical examination allows an estimate of the degree of RVOT obstruction based on the murmur heard (e.g., severe obstruction will cause a loud, short murmur). Blood gases provide further insight into the degree of gas exchange occurring in the lungs and the degree of systemic perfusion and oxygenation. Metabolic acidosis is an indication that systemic perfusion is inadequate. Tetralogy of Fallot patients are at increased risk of cardiac arrhythmias and require telemetry monitoring.

All patients with tetralogy of Fallot should undergo testing for 22q11.2 deletion or DiGeorge syndrome as conotruncal abnormalities are common in these patients.

TREATMENT

- If patients are acyanotic at birth and receive adequate pulmonary blood flow, they may not require any treatment in the acute neonatal period.
- As the heart performs increased work in tetralogy of Fallot, patients require increased caloric intake. This may be provided in the form of calorie fortified formulas or nasogastric feeds if adequate weight gain is not achieved.
- During tet spells, patients assume in the knee-to-chest position to increase systemic vascular resistance and decrease right-to-left shunting at the VSD. Fluid boluses increase preload and cardiac output. They may also be given morphine for pain relief and calming to decrease systemic oxygen consumption. Beta blockers decrease heart rate and therefore cardiac oxygen consumption.
- Patients with pulmonary atresia are given prostaglandin E (PGE) to maintain the PDA until surgical intervention occurs.
- Patients with typical tetralogy of Fallot undergo VSD closure such that the aorta subsequently only receives blood from the LV and transannular patch placement to make the pulmonary valve bigger. They may require resection of RV muscle bundles depending on the degree of RVOT obstruction.
- If patients develop pulmonary overcirculation prior to repair, they may be started on diuretics to decrease the volume of blood going to the lungs. Loop diuretics such as furosemide are typically first-line, but patients may require additional diuretics such as thiazides and spironolactone. If they are having tet spells, patients are placed on beta blockers to slow the heart rate and decrease the amount of RVOT obstruction. However, the best course of action for tet spells is to perform surgical correction.
- Tetralogy of Fallot with pulmonary atresia patients requires surgical intervention acutely, typically within the first week of life. A conduit is placed from the RV to the branch pulmonary arteries and the VSD is closed. If MAPCAs are present, they may be ligated or incorporated into the repair depending on the patient's individual anatomy.

PATIENT EDUCATION

- It is important that patients with tetralogy of Fallot receive evaluation and care by a pediatric cardiologist.
- If patients develop cyanosis, they should be placed in a knee-to-chest position and promptly evaluated in an ED.

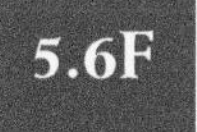

5.6F TRANSPOSITION OF THE GREAT VESSELS

OVERVIEW

TGA refers to discordant ventriculoarterial connections, namely the RV gives rise to the aorta and the LV gives rise to the pulmonary artery. There are two main forms of TGA: D-transposition of the great arteries (D-TGA) and L-transposition of the great arteries (L-TGA). These are determined by the orientation of the aorta in relation to the pulmonary artery. L-TGA is also referred to as "congenitally corrected" transposition. D-TGA is the most common form of cyanotic heart disease to present in the newborn period.[208] If left untreated, this form of congenital heart disease is fatal. Surgical intervention is the standard of care. After intervention, patients require lifelong follow-up with close monitoring.[209]

EPIDEMIOLOGY

D-TGA is most common type of cyanotic heart disease that presents in the newborn period.[208] This congenital heart defect is reported to represent anywhere between 3% to 7% of all congenital heart defects. When assessing only cyanotic congenital heart defects, TGA represents about 20% of congenital heart defects.[210] D-TGA affects males more often than females. Noninheritable risk factors include maternal diabetes, specifically hyperglycemia, vitamin A, ibuprofen, influenza, organic solvents, and pesticides. L-TGA is much less common compared to D-TGA, and is reported to occur in <1% of patients with congenital heart disease.[211]

PATHOPHYSIOLOGY

In typical fetal cardiac development, there is initially a common outflow tract from the ventricles and the aorticopulmonary septum forms in a spiral-like configuration to separate the aorta from the pulmonary artery. In normal development, the subpulmonary conus remains and forms the infundibulum while the subaortic conus regresses. This is thought to result in the typical configuration of the pulmonary artery being anterior and rightward to the aorta. Differential conal development, referring to the subpulmonary conus regressing while the subaortic conus develops, is thought to result in D-TGA.

D-TGA refers to discordant ventriculoarterial connections. Essentially, the RV gives rise to the aorta and the LV gives rise to the pulmonary artery. Typically, the aorta is found anterior and rightward as compared to the pulmonary artery. Associated lesions that can be commonly seen in D-TGA include VSD and LVOTO. The two most common VSD types seen are perimembranous and malalignment. Malalignment VSDs can result in LVOTO. Another important anatomic feature in D-TGA concerns the coronary arteries and impacts surgical planning. Multiple classification systems are used to describe the origins of and anatomy of the coronary arteries in D-TGA.

The anatomy of D-TGA results in two parallel circuits of blood flow. The deoxygenated blood returning from the body to the right atrium via the superior vena cava (SVC) and IVC travels to the RV and exits the aorta to return to the body. The oxygenated blood returns to the LA via the pulmonary veins, travels to the LV, and exits the pulmonary artery to return to the lungs. Without some form of mixing, whether this be at the atrial level, ventricular level, or via the ductus arteriosus, there is no way to get deoxygenated blood to the lungs or oxygenated blood to the body. Thus, some type of communication to allow for mixing is needed for survival. Most infants have both a PFO and PDA at birth, which allows for this mixing. The size of these shunts is what determines the degree of cyanosis present after birth. Ensuring that both the ductus arteriosus remains patent and the forman ovale is of adequate size is the cornerstone of initial management in patients with D-TGA, as noted below. Also of note, infants with D-TGA who also have a VSD will often have higher saturations due to increased mixing.

Another feature seen in D-TGA includes reversed differential cyanosis. This refers to the upper half of the body demonstrating cyanosis while the lower half of the body is pink. This is seen in the immediate newborn period in patients with D-TGA due to oxygenated blood from the pulmonary artery traveling across the ductus arteriosus and going to the descending aorta and lower body. It is due to increased pressures in the pulmonary vascular bed seen normally in the immediate newborn period resulting in shunting of oxygenated blood from the pulmonary artery (higher pressure) to the aorta (lower pressure). Once the pulmonary vascular resistance drops within the first hours to days of life, this finding disappears as the pulmonary vascular pressures become lower than the pressure in the descending aorta.

In normal fetal cardiac development, the primitive heart tube loops toward the right (dextro or d-looped) resulting in the RV being anterior and rightward as compared to the left. In L-TGA, this looping occurs to the left (levo or l-looped), which results in the LV being on the right and the RV being on the left. In other words, there is ventricular inversion or AV discordance. In addition, the aorta typically rises from the left-sided RV and is leftward and anterior as compared to the pulmonary artery, which typically arises from the right-sided LV. By itself, L-TGA results in no abnormality to blood flow through the heart and this is why it is termed "congenitally corrected" transposition. However, most patients with L-TGA have other cardiac lesions including VSDs, LVOTO, and abnormalities of the TV (located on the left), which can result in clinical sequelae dependent upon constellation of defects. Another important consideration for patients with L-TGA is that the conduction system of the heart is often abnormal and can result in arrhythmias, specifically AV block.

MEDICAL HISTORY AND CLINICAL PRESENTATION

Most patients with D-TGA present in the newborn period. In some instances, this form of congenital heart disease can be identified antenatally by fetal echocardiography. In these instances, it is advisable for the infant to be delivered at a medical facility with access to pediatric cardiology and cardiothoracic surgery. For infants without antenatal diagnosis, D-TGA is often identified after echocardiogram is obtained in the setting of cyanosis and tachypnea. For some infants in whom the degree of cyanosis is minimal, mandatory state newborn screening will identify mild hypoxia resulting in echocardiogram and subsequent diagnosis. Presentation in patients with L-TGA is highly variable and often dependent on the presence of associated lesions.

SIGNS AND SYMPTOMS

Cyanosis in varying degrees is a universal feature of neonates with D-TGA. The severity of cyanosis is influenced by the size of the PFO or ASD and resultant mixing of deoxygenated and oxygenated blood in the heart. Other factors that can influence this mixing include the presence or absence of associated defects such as a VSDs and presence of LVOTO. Anatomic variations that allow for more mixing typically result in a lesser degree of cyanosis.

Tachypnea is another symptom often noted in infants with D-TGA. This is typically a "comfortable" tachypnea without other signs of respiratory distress. If D-TGA is not identified early in the newborn period, some infants, specifically those with associated VSDs, can go on to develop HF. In this circumstance one would expect to see tachypnea with other signs of respiratory distress such as retractions or grunting.

As above, signs and symptoms associated with L-TGA are highly dependent on the presence of associated cardiac lesions.

PHYSICAL EXAMINATION

Infants with D-TGA typically present with cyanosis. Some infants will have clinically evident cyanosis prompting further assessment. Other infants may demonstrate no clinical cyanosis with only mild hypoxia detected on routine newborn screening. Tachypnea without other findings of respiratory distress is often present. Signs of decreased perfusion including delayed capillary refill or poor peripheral pulses may be present when there are associated lesions such as coarctation of the aorta. A murmur may be noted on cardiac exam if associated lesions such as VSD or LVOTO are present. The remainder of the physical exam should be within normal limits.

A common feature seen in L-TGA on physical examination is a loud, single second heart sound. This is due to the position of the AoV being anterior in the chest. Other physical exam findings are associated with the presence of other cardiac lesions.

DIFFERENTIAL DIAGNOSIS

The differential diagnosis of TGA should encompass other clinical entities that may result in cyanosis, tachypnea, HF or heart block.

- **Cyanosis:** The potential causes of cyanosis in an infant are numerous. Other forms of cyanotic congenital heart disease should be considered including tetralogy of Fallot, truncus arteriosus, tricuspid atresia, total anomalous pulmonary venous return, pulmonary atresia, and hypoplasic left heart syndrome. Anomalies affecting the airways such as choanal atresia, tracheo-esophageal fistula, and laryngomalacia are of concern. Lung pathology such as pneumonia, pneumothorax, or diaphragmatic hernia are considerations. Numerous metabolic or neurologic disorders can result in apnea leading to cyanosis.
- **Tachypnea/HF:** Other cardiac disorders that can present with tachypnea or overt HF include lesions resulting in significant left-to-right shunting such as a VSD. Certain forms of cardiomyopathy or myocarditis can also lead to this. In an older patient, myocardial ischemia can be a source of HF and resultant tachypnea.
- **Heart block:** Various etiologies including cardiomyopathy, myocarditis, myocardial ischemia, and drugs should be considered when evaluating a patient with heart block.

DIAGNOSTIC STUDIES

The most important tool in the diagnosis of D-TGA is TTE. Other studies that are commonly used include fetal echocardiography, electrocardiography, CXR and cardiac catheterization.

- **Fetal echocardiography:** Fetal echocardiography is indicated in a variety of circumstances related to maternal clinic status or when abnormalities are noted on routine obstetric ultrasound exam. Optimal time for imaging is between 18 and 24 weeks' gestation; however, imaging can be obtained later in gestation as well. Fetal echocardiography can demonstrate D-TGA, identifying the aorta coming from the RV and the pulmonary artery coming from the LV.
- **Transthoracic echocardiography:** TTE is done in the immediate newborn period for infants with positive fetal echocardiogram or those with concerning signs such as cyanosis or failed newborn screen. Again, these images will demonstrate the aorta, typically identified by the presence of coronary arteries, coming from the anterior RV and the pulmonary artery, identified by the branching into the left and right pulmonary arteries, arising from the more posterior LV. TTE also identifies the presence of other lesions such as VSDs or outflow tract obstruction. It is important to note the size of the communication at the atrial level, the presence and size of the ductus arteriosus, and the coronary artery anatomy as well.
- **Electrocardiography:** EKG findings in infants with D-TGA are often normal.
- **Chest radiography:** The classic CXR finding in D-TGA is the "egg on a string" appearance. This is due to the relationship and resultant shape of the abnormally located great vessels. Should an infant develop HF in the setting of D-TGA, one can also see increased pulmonary vascular markings.
- **Cardiac catheterization:** Given the quality of imaging able to be obtained via echocardiogram, cardiac catheterization is typically not required to make the diagnosis of D-TGA. Given that the coronary artery anatomy is important to clarify prior to surgical intervention, however, cardiac catheterization is occasionally used to identify the coronary arteries when echocardiography is inconclusive. In addition, cardiac catheterization is required when a balloon atrial septostomy is required to improve mixing at the atrial level (see Treatment section).

Similar to D-TGA, several tools are used in the diagnosis of L-TGA including TTE and electrocardiography.

- **Transthoracic echocardiography:** In L-TGA, views that allow for characterization of a morphologic LV versus RV are identified to determine the position of the LV versus RV. They include the shape of the ventricle, smooth versus trabeculated endocardial surface, presence of a moderator band (seen in RV), and characteristics of the AV valves.
- **Electrocardiography:** Features include left axis deviation, Q waves in the right precordial leads and also in leads III and aVF. In addition, problems with AV block are also frequently noted due to the abnormal development of the conduction system.

EVALUATION

Evaluation of an infant with suspected TGA should always begin with TTE. Cardiology should also be consulted. Often a CXR and EKG are obtained as part of the initial workup as well. Further testing and intervention will be recommended by cardiology based upon the infant's TTE findings and clinical status.

TREATMENT

Treatment options are different for D-TGA and L-TGA.

D-TGA:

- In D-TGA the goal in the immediate newborn period is to improve oxygen saturation. Three main interventions achieve this goal: (1) supplemental oxygenation, (2) initiation of a prostaglandin E_1 infusion, which opens the ductus arteriosus and allows for shunting of deoxygenated blood across the ductus arteriosus, and (3) a balloon atrial septostomy which is performed in the cardiac catheterization lab. This procedure is indicated for infants in whom the forman ovale is not felt to be of adequate size to allow for mixing. This procedure involves inserting a balloon-tipped catheter into the venous system to the right atrium and subsequently across the PFO into the LA. The balloon is then inflated and the catheter pulled across the PFO into the right atrium creating a larger defect in the atrial septum. This allows for improved mixing of deoxygenated and oxygenated blood in the heart and improves systemic oxygen saturations.

- The preferred procedure for definitive management of D-TGA is the arterial switch operation. This operation is typically performed shortly after birth. Initially, transection of the aorta and pulmonary artery occurs. Button incisions are created around the coronary arteries and are subsequently reimplanted to the pulmonary artery trunk. The aorta is then brought behind the pulmonary arteries and anastomosed to the pulmonary artery trunk to create the "neo-aorta." The repositioning of the pulmonary arteries anterior to the aorta is referred to as the LeCompte maneuver. The defects in the aortic trunk where the coronary arteries were removed are repaired and the pulmonary artery is anastomosed to the aortic trunk to create the "neo-pulmonary artery." This results in anatomic correction of the congenital heart disease with the RV giving rise to the pulmonary artery and the LV giving rise to the aorta.
  - Potential complications that can occur after an arterial switch procedure include obstruction of the coronary arteries, pulmonary stenosis at the site of anastomosis, and regurgitation of the "neo-aortic" valve.
- Prior to the arterial switch procedure, the surgical intervention for D-TGA was an atrial baffle operation. The two forms of this included the Mustard and Senning operation. These procedures involve redirecting blood flow from the SVC and IVC to the LA and blood flow from the pulmonary veins to the right atrium. The Mustard operation achieves this with prosthetic material while the Senning operation uses the patient's atrial septal tissue to redirect blood flow. This results in a physiologic correction of the congenital heart disease.
  - Potential complications that occur after an atrial switch procedure include right ventricular dysfunction, arrhythmia, baffle leaks, and obstruction of the SVC. Given the frequency of these complications, the arterial switch is the preferred operation for patients with D-TGA.
- In the subset of patients with D-TGA associated with VSD and severe pulmonary stenosis, the Rastelli operation is often used. This involves using a patch to close the VSD such that the LV gives rise to the aorta and placing a conduit between the RV and pulmonary artery.

L-TGA:

- Management for patients with L-TGA is largely driven by the presence of associated cardiac lesions and the hemodynamic consequences associated with each. In isolated L-TGA, the major difficulty includes the RV functioning as the systemic ventricle and eventual HF over time.
- The two main categories of repair in L-TGA include physiologic repair and anatomic repair.
  - Physiologic repair refers to surgical interventions that result in the RV remaining the systemic ventricle. This can include interventions such as systemic to pulmonary artery shunts, pulmonary artery bands, VSD closure, and TV repair.
  - Anatomic repair refers to surgical interventions which result in the LV becoming the systemic ventricle. These interventions are typically more complex from a surgical standpoint. The classic intervention is the "double switch," which involves an atrial switch and arterial switch procedure.
- One important feature in the management of L-TGA refers back to the abnormal conduction system and difficulties with AV block. Postoperative AV block is a known risk factor and may require permanent pacing.

PATIENT EDUCATION

- Any neonate with TGA should be under the care of a cardiologist and in a medical facility with available pediatric cardiothoracic surgeons.
- Patients with TGA will be followed by a cardiologist throughout their entire life.
- Always encourage patients to report any changes in respiratory status and exercise tolerance in addition to the presence of palpitations or chest pain to their physician.
- Activity restrictions may be required for patients who have undergone arterial switch or atrial redirection procedures. Refer patients to their cardiologist for sports and activity clearance.

SPECIAL CONSIDERATIONS

Many patients with TGA survive well into adulthood. These patients should be followed by an adult congenital heart disease specialist at least annually. Any patient who underwent an arterial switch operation should have close monitoring of the coronary arteries with various imaging modalities.

KEY POINTS

- The two forms of TGA are D-TGA and L-TGA determined by the relationship of the aorta with respect to the pulmonary artery.
- D-TGA is the most common form of cyanotic congenital heart disease to present in the newborn period.
- Many patients with D-TGA require a balloon atrial septostomy in the newborn period prior to surgical intervention.
- Arterial switch procedure is the standard of care to correct D-TGA.
- Coronary artery anatomy is important for surgical planning in patients with D-TGA.

5.6G EBSTEIN ANOMALY

OVERVIEW

Ebstein anomaly of the TV is a relatively rare congenital cardiac malformation.[212] The defect occurs in <1% of all congenital heart diseases.[213] It is a cyanotic heart defect. Ebstein anomaly can pose serious management challenges from both hemodynamic and electrophysiologic perspectives. It involves a malformation of the TV with adherence of the septal and posterior leaflets to the underlying right ventricular myocardium.[212,214] The anterior leaflet tends to retain mobility but is typically elongated, fenestrated, and tethered. As a consequence, the functional TV orifice becomes distorted and displaced down into the apical portion of the RV, which results in variable degrees of regurgitation and stenosis. This causes right atrial enlargement with expansion of the true right AV groove, as well as dilation of the "atrialized" portion of the RV above the functional TV orifice, where tissue is remarkably thin-walled.

More than one-half of these patients will have some degree of cyanosis from an interatrial communication (either a PFO or ASD), which allows right-to-left shunting. The severity of the TV dysfunction varies widely from patient to patient, such that some are critically ill at birth, whereas others can remain relatively asymptomatic for decades.[212]

These patients contend with an extraordinarily high incidence of tachyarrhythmias. Most can be attributed to accessory pathways (APs) located near the AV node.[212] Atriofasicular fibers and AV nodal reentrant tachycardia are common in Ebstein anomaly.[212,215–217] Other arrhythmias include monomorphic VT.[212,217–219]

EPIDEMIOLOGY

Ebstein anomaly of the TV is a relatively rare congenital cardiac malformation.[212] The defect occurs in <1% of all congenital heart diseases.[213] It is considered a cyanotic heart defect. Ebstein anomaly can pose serious management challenges from both hemodynamic and electrophysiologic perspectives. It is present at birth but the symptoms and signs can occur at any age, with an average life expectancy of the third decade of age as indicated in an earlier report.[213,220]

PATHOPHYSIOLOGY

Ebstein anomaly involves a distinctive malformation of the TV with adherence of the septal and posterior leaflets to the underlying right ventricular myocardium due to failure of embryologic delamination.[212,214] The anterior leaflet tends to retain mobility but is typically elongated, fenestrated, and tethered. As a consequence, the functional TV orifice becomes distorted and displaced down into the apical portion of the RV, which results in variable degrees of regurgitation and stenosis. This causes right atrial enlargement with expansion of the true right AV groove, as well as dilation of the "atrialized" portion of the RV above the functional TV orifice, where tissue is remarkably thin-walled.[212] There is an interatrial communication (either a PFO or ASD), allowing a degree of cyanosis in some patients.

Congenital disorders of all parts of the heart can be associated with Ebstein anomaly, with MVP and left ventricular noncompaction (LVNC) being the two most common ones.[213,221]

The TV deformity and resultant right-sided heart enlargement are the most striking manifestations of this disease. The RA and RV are enlarged to a dramatic degree. There is RA enlargement with expansion of the true right AV groove.[212] However, it is not just a disease of the right side of the heart; in 39% of these patients a myocardial or valvular disorder of the left heart has been also noted.[213,221]

The partial deterioration present in the RV together with the presence of the TV regurgitation will hinder venous return from flowing into the pulmonary circulation. Apart from that, during atrial contraction, the atrialized part of the RV inflates and will behave as a passive reservoir. This will result in a diminished ejection fraction. The ultimate result is RA dilation, therefore increasing the interatrial communication through the ASD resulting in varying degrees of right-to-left shunting.[222,223] The patients with more severe TV disease might experience symptoms of HF to varying degrees.

Ebstein anomaly can pose not only hemodynamic but also serious electrophysiologic challenges. These patients contend with an extraordinarily high incidence of tachyarrhythmias. Most can be attributed to APs located along the posterior and septal border of the TV where the valve leaflets are most abnormal. It is the only congenital heart defect with such a dramatic predisposition toward APs.[212] The APs include both concealed and preexcited Wolff-Parkinson-White pathways. The degree of TV deformity and the area of atrialized RV do not seem to correlate directly with the presence or absence of APs.[212,224] There are patients with only mild forms of Ebstein anomaly who have problematic APs, and others with severe forms of the disease in whom APs are absent.[212] The incidence of APs has been estimated to be between 10% and 38% depending on how the study population was selected and whether manifest and concealed APs were combined.[221,225–231] APs are usually right sided and may even be multiple.[216,232,233]

Atriofasicular fibers and AV nodal reentrant tachycardia are common in Ebstein anomaly.[212,215–217] Exactly why atriofascicular fibers would occur in association with Ebstein anomaly is not understood, but one could speculate that it might represent some sort of electrical compensation for underdevelopment of the right bundle branch.[212]

Other arrhythmias include monomorphic VT arising from the congenitally abnormal muscle in the atrialized portion of the RV.[212,213,217–219,234,235] Atrialized RV is arrhythmogenic probably due to its anatomic characteristics just distal to the His bundle, and with links to the Purkinje fibers, slow conduction is generated and VT is triggered.[213,218,236] As well as a variety of acquired atrial tachycardias and VTs (atrial flutter, AF, polymorphic VT) that develop in response to abnormal hemodynamics and degenerative remodeling.[212]

Histopathologic study of the normal conduction tissues has been performed in Ebstein anomaly hearts.[212,237,238] The compact AV node appears structurally unremarkable and is located as expected in the Koch's triangle, although it is reported to be displaced toward the base, closer than normal to the mouth of the coronary sinus.[212] However, there can be conduction system abnormalities, which are at least partly due to the compression of the AV node by the septal malformation, accessory pathways, and abnormalities of the right bundle branch.[213]

The bundle of His and left bundle branch appear normal, but multiple abnormalities of the right bundle branch have been observed, including atresia, short length, narrow caliber, and fibrosis.[212] In Ebstein anomaly in humans, right bundle branch block is frequent.[213,239,240]

Taussig initially[212,241] observed, "Rhythm concerns were recognized early on as an important feature of Ebstein anomaly. Many patients suffer from repeated attacks of paroxysmal tachycardia"[212] and "sudden death is relatively common."[241]

A conspicuous feature on nearly one-half of Ebstein anomaly hearts is a very prominent ridge along the AV groove. It separates the RA proper from the atrialized portion of the RV. This ridge is found to be more common in autopsy specimens from these patients who had a history of pre-excitation and supraventricular tachycardia (SVT) during life.[212,224] This raises the strong suspicion of a link between the ridge tissue itself and abnormal AV connections.[212]

If the leaflet displacement and valve regurgitation are severe, pulmonary blood flow decreases, the right atrium becomes dilated, and blood is shunted from right to left across an ASD.[222,242] This dysfunction and dilation of the RA and RV lead to progressive patchy myocardial atrophy and fibrosis, which lead to a conduction defect, resulting in an abnormal EKG.[222,243] The abnormally developed TV is also associated with conduction abnormalities, which include delayed intra-atrial conduction, right bundle branch block, and ventricular pre-excitation. This is because the downward displacement of the septal leaflet is related to discontinuity of the central fibrous body and to the septal AV ring leading to direct muscular connection being formed. These create a potential substrate for accessory AV connections.[222,244,245] In addition, although the AV system is situated normally, the AV node may become compressed by the abnormal formation of the central fibrous body. Thus, the right bundle branch may be damaged by marked fibrosis, leading to complete or incomplete right bunch branch blocks.[222,244]

EKG abnormalities of this anomaly include unusually tall and broad P waves due to right atrial enlargement, right bundle branch block caused by abnormalities of the right bundle branch, tachyarrhythmias related to accessory pathways, and pre-excitation of Wolff-Parkinson-White (WPW) syndrome.[213,246] There can be first-degree AV block in the absence of pre-excitation, which is usually a consequence of RA enlargement with long interatrial conduction time rather than true delay at the AV node.[212]

MEDICAL HISTORY AND CLINICAL PRESENTATION

The hemodynamic complications of Ebstein anomaly are directly related to the severity of the leaflet displacement and to the resultant TV regurgitation. In the case of mild displacement and mild valve regurgitation, the patient may be asymptomatic for many years.[222,242] Regular assessments are needed and should include evaluation of the patient's heart rhythm to evaluate any new arrhythmias and exercise testing to quantify the cardiac functional capacity. If the patients develop signs and symptoms of right-sided HF, standard HF treatment is initiated, yet there is little evidence for the actual efficacy of these treatments in patients with Ebstein anomaly.[222,247] Medical management should be individualized and often involves standard HF treatment, such as diuretics, digoxin, beta blocker, and ACEIs to reduce the afterload.[222,235,248] Antibiotic prophylaxis is not usually necessary in those patients who are acyanotic and unoperated. However, it is recommended before dental procedures if there is cyanosis and/or the patient has a prosthetic heart valve.[222,242]

SIGNS AND SYMPTOMS

In the case of mild displacement and mild TV regurgitation, the patient may be asymptomatic for many years. In some cases, children may have cyanosis, arrhythmia, or cardiac failure. In that case ASD closure, valve repair, and valve replacement are performed. But valve reconstruction is preferable to a valve replacement.[222,242] Generally, most develop late rhythm disorders nearly to the same level as patients with a more serious anatomic abnormality.[222,249] These would be felt as symptoms of irregular heartbeats and palpitations.

PHYSICAL EXAMINATION

Physical signs on examination vary markedly, but they are present in the majority of patients.[232]

- Growth, development, and body build of the patient are generally normal, although Kapusta et al. found children with Ebstein anomaly to be slightly shorter than the population average in addition to the mean BMI standard deviation score being slightly decreased.[232,250]
- Older children are often referred for further evaluation of a heart murmur.[232,251,252]
- Cyanosis in all degrees and varying degrees of digital clubbing may be present.[232,250]
- Often a prominent third or even a fourth heart sound is heard.[232,250]
- A patient could have HF symptoms.
- A presentation could be an arrhythmia.

DIFFERENTIAL DIAGNOSIS

The differential diagnosis for Ebstein anomaly is summarized in Table 5.18.[263]

DIAGNOSTIC STUDIES

1. **Echocardiogram:**
   - Two-dimensional echocardiography is the most important diagnostic tool for children with congenital heart disease. It is portable and noninvasive, has no radiation risk, and provides immediate high-resolution anatomic and physiologic information.[232]
   - Three-dimensional echocardiography is a feasible method to evaluate the anatomy and the dynamic function of the abnormal TV. It permits clear differentiation from TV dysplasia. It shows the degree of TV

TABLE 5.18 Differential Diagnosis for Ebstein Anomaly

Diagnosis	Description
Tricuspid valve dysplasia	Leakage of the tricuspid valve causing right atrial enlargement. Patient is acyanotic.
Hypoplastic right heart syndrome	Small right ventricle unable to support pulmonary cardiac output and large right atrium. Patient is cyanotic.
Total anomalous pulmonary venous return	All pulmonary veins draining to right atrium causing right atrial enlargement. Patient is cyanotic.
Partial anomalous pulmonary venous return	One or more of the pulmonary veins, but not all, drain to the right atrium. Patient may be acyanotic or cyanotic.
Uhl anomaly	Congenital malformation of the right ventricle with almost total absence of the right ventricular myocardium.
Right-sided heart failure, cor pulmonale	Ebstein anomaly can be a cause of right-sided heart failure, but not exclusively, symptoms of right-sided heart failure present as dyspnea, palpitations, hepatomegaly, and cyanosis.

regurgitation and adds information regarding septal leaflet insertion and RV volumes. It also visualizes the size, location, and shapes of septal defects.[232]

2. **EKG:**
   - Conduction abnormalities are at least partly due to the compression of the AV node by the septal malformation.[213,221,253] First-degree AV block in the absence of pre-excitation is usually a consequence of RA enlargement with long interatrial conduction time rather than true delay at the AV node.[212]
   - Right bundle branch block is common due to abnormalities of the right bundle.[213,246]
   - Unusually tall and broad P waves due to right atrial enlargement may be present.[213,246,254]
   - Tachyarrythmias related to accessory pathways and WPW syndrome is common.[213,246]
   - VT: Just distal to the His bundle, and with links to the Purkinje fibers, slow conduction is generated and VT is triggered.[213,218,236]
   - Monomorphic VT arises from atrialized RV muscle in Ebstein anomaly.[212,213,217–219,234,235]
3. **Holter monitoring:**
   - This study is needed to assess symptoms and to check for conduction abnormalities, ectopy, and arrhythmia.
4. **Electrophysiology:** This study is used to define conduction and tachyarrhythmias.
5. **CXR:**
   - Pulmonary vascularity may be normal or decreased.[232]
   - If patient is thought to have HF, checking for interstitial edema and pulmonary vascular congestion is needed.[232]
   - The cardiac silhouette may vary from almost normal to typical configuration of a box- or balloon-shaped heart with a narrow waist. This is greatly due to the enlarged right atrium and also the dilated ventricular outflow tract, which can be displaced outward and upward. The aorta cross-section is small, and the pulmonary trunk, which normally appears as a discrete convex bulge, is absent.[232]
   - In a newborn with systemic desaturation and the CXR showing cardiomegaly and decreased pulmonary vascularity, the diagnosis of Ebstein anomaly should be considered.[232]
6. **Exercise testing:**
   - This assists in determining the severity of the disease. Patients may have limited exercise tolerance. Driscoll et al.[232,255] showed that surgical repair improves exercise tolerance mostly because of the elimination of the right-to-left shunt in these patients.[232]
   - It allows for the ability to check for exercise-induced arrhythmia.
7. **Cardiac MRI:**
   - MRI is a powerful tool providing anatomic and hemodynamic information that echocardiography alone cannot provide.[232]

EVALUATION

Ebstein anomaly can pose serious management challenges from both hemodynamic and electrophysiologic perspectives. Patients with this congenital cardiac anomaly need to be monitored with routine cardiology evaluations and cardiac testing as noted previously. If routine testing starts to show abnormalities or if there are concerning symptoms, treatment and close monitoring are necessary. Besides symptoms of right HF the clinician needs to remain vigilant regarding the frequent occurrence of arrhythmia and risk of sudden death.[212,241]

TREATMENT

- Asymptomatic Ebstein anomaly can be kept under close follow-up. Patients with New York Heart Association heart function classes 1 and 2 can be conservatively treated.
- Treatment of right HF involves adjustment of heart rate and preload and exercise restriction. This may include a low-sodium diet, oral diuretics, digoxin, and a low-dose ACEI. Therapeutic control of acute exacerbation of right HF was mainly based on diuretics, vasodilators, cardiotonic, low-sodium diet, and abdominal paracentesis, which can be effective for relieving the congestive HF but is not good for withholding the effusions.[238,254] Yet there is little evidence for the actual efficacy of these treatments in patients with Ebstein anomaly.[213,247]
- Supraventricular arrhythmias are the most common rhythm disturbance in children and tends to be recurrent and drug resistant.[232]
- Radiofrequency ablation is done for life-threatening arrhythmias and drug-refractory tachycardias, although ablations in Ebstein anomaly can be challenging.[216,232] These ablations are more likely to have recurrence compared to other congenital heart diseases.[232,256]
- The surgical approach to Ebstein anomaly has evolved.[212,256] The earliest surgical approach involved shunts, then attempts at improving TV function by valvuloplasty or replacement with excision or plication of redundant tissue of the dilated RA and RV.[212,257] Although right-sided heart hemodynamics usually improved after early types of surgery, later TV dysfunction was common. Only in recent years a more effective technique for TV reconstruction has become available using the cone technique developed by da Silva and colleagues.[258] In this operation, the adherent TV tissue is carefully separated from the underlying RV endocardium, which allows leaflet tissue to be reshaped into a configuration that restores coaptation with a functional annulus that is appropriately located along the true AV groove.[212,259–262]

PATIENT EDUCATION

- Watch for symptoms of heart racing and report occurrences.
- Lifelong cardiac follow-up is essential.
- Antibiotic prophylaxis is not usually necessary in those patients who are acyanotic and unoperated. However, it is recommended before dental procedures if there is cyanosis and/or if the patient has a prosthetic heart valve.[222,247]

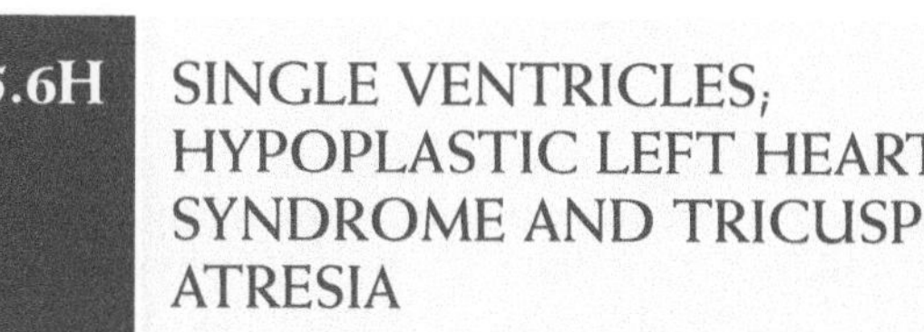

5.6H SINGLE VENTRICLES; HYPOPLASTIC LEFT HEART SYNDROME AND TRICUSPID ATRESIA

OVERVIEW

The single ventricle is among the most complex of all congenital heart diseases. This arises when there is hypoplasia of either the RV or LV resulting in a nonfunctional ventricular chamber, and thereby one single working ventricle. For the purposes of this review, we will focus on hypoplastic left heart syndrome (HLHS) and tricuspid atresia, which results in a hypoplastic RV.

EPIDEMIOLOGY

The incidence of single ventricle is thought to be about 0.08 to 0.4 per 1,000 live births.[264] Prior to 1960s, these children died as infants with little to no surgical or palliation options. Improvements in prenatal screening have potentially decreased live births as some will choose to terminate the pregnancy with such a diagnosis. However, prenatal diagnosis has also been shown to improve patient outcomes in those who choose life for their infants.[265]

Today, the mortality rate for children in the United States with a single ventricle is about 10% within the first year of life. However, the development of the Fontan palliation has resulted in decreased mortality and morbidity rates. There are now many adults, teenagers, and children living with single ventricle physiology. Since this palliation is still relatively new, there is still much to learn about caring for the patient with a single ventricle.

PATHOPHYSIOLOGY

The anatomy of a single ventricle is individualized for each patient. The overall goal of therapy is to get deoxygenated blood flow to the lungs and oxygenated blood flow to the body tissues. There is only one functioning "pump" or ventricle, and therefore, passive flow, blood volume, and adequate hydration become very important.

In HLHS, the systemic pumping chamber (LV) is hypoplastic and nonfunctional. Deoxygenated blood returns to the heart normally via the IVC and SVC. The right atrium is present with a functional TV and functional RV. The RV pumps blood flow to the lungs. The oxygenated blood returns to the LA and crosses an ASD into the right heart again. The RV then pumps the mixed blood back through the pulmonary arteries and via the PDA to the body. In most cases, anatomic structures "downstream" from the hypoplasia are also affected. Therefore, sometimes in HLHS the AoV and aorta are also small and not sufficient. All single ventricle patients must have either an ASD or a VSD in order for complete mixing of oxygen saturated blood and deoxygenated blood for survival. If one is not present, an emergent atrial septostomy will be performed immediately at birth.

In tricuspid atresia, the TV is small and often nonfunctional. The downstream effect results in a small, hypoplastic RV, pulmonary valve, and sometimes small branch pulmonary arteries. In this anatomy, the challenge is to provide adequate blood flow to the lungs for oxygenation. Preoperatively this is achieved through the PDA. Generally, patients with a single LV as their systemic pumping chamber seem to do better than patients with a single RV.

MEDICAL HISTORY AND CLINICAL PRESENTATION

At birth, these infants may appear healthy for the first few hours of life. However, as the PDA closes and the pulmonary vascular resistance falls, these children will become cyanotic, tachypneic, and acidotic and could die if not diagnosed. They are reliant on the PDA to sustain their systemic circulation. As the PDA closes, the oxygen saturation in the peripheral tissues will fall. These infants are very fragile. They are typically cared for in a neonatal ICU in the hospital where the cardiac surgeries will be performed. Prostaglandins (PGE) are used to keep the PDA open until the first stage of surgery can be performed. This usually occurs within a week of life.

Preoperative care consists of maintaining the PDA, providing oxygen and potentially intubation if needed. It is important to note that oxygen saturations of 100% in peripheral tissues is often not a goal in single ventricle physiology because that means that the patient is receiving too much supplemental oxygen, which can be harmful. Typical oxygen saturations should reveal mixing of the oxygenated and deoxygenated blood and are most often targeted at 75% to 85%.

Most infants with single ventricle physiology are diagnosed prenatally. However, recognizing signs and symptoms early may be lifesaving for patients with little to no prenatal care and to those who choose home births.

SIGNS AND SYMPTOMS

Prenatally undiagnosed infants will present in cardiogenic shock with cyanosis, tachypnea, retractions, poor feeding, and decreased level of consciousness.

Prenatally diagnosed infants will be immediately placed on IV prostaglandins to maintain ductal patency. These infants may not have any symptoms. If they develop pulmonary overcirculation, they will have symptoms of tachypnea, retractions, nasal flaring, and head bobbing.

PHYSICAL EXAMINATION

Newborns may present in shock and appear pale and cyanotic, with decreased level of consciousness and decrease in perfusion. Examination of head, eyes, ears, nose, and throat will most likely demonstrate a subtle degree of cyanosis. HLHS does have an association with some syndromes and, therefore, there may be syndromic facial features. The lung exam will be normal. The cardiac exam will reveal a displaced PMI medially. There will be a normal S1 but a single S2 due to the AoV being absent or nonfunctional. A harsh continuous murmur may be heard at the left upper sternal border to left midclavicle indicating the PDA is patent. The abdominal exam will be normal. The perfusion of the extremities may be diminished with decreased capillary refill and decreased lower extremity pulses.

DIFFERENTIAL DIAGNOSIS

The differential diagnosis for HLHS and tricuspid atresia are summarized in Table 5.19. All diagnoses have normal LVs allowing a two-ventricle repair.

TABLE 5.19 Differential Diagnosis for Hypoplastic Left Heart Syndrome and Tricuspid Atresia

Diagnosis	Description
Coarctation of aorta	Obstruction in the aortic arch causing decrease systemic blood flow
Severe aortic stenosis	Obstruction of the aortic valve causing obstruction of systemic blood flow
Interrupted aortic arch	Discontinuation of the aortic arch with the patent ductus arteriosus bridging systemic blood flow

DIAGNOSTIC STUDIES

- **EKG:** 20% of patients with HLHS have a normal EKG. Compared to age-matched controls, patients with HLHS were more likely to exhibit a longer PR interval, a wider QRS complex, decreased left-sided forces, an absence of septal Q waves in the inferior and lateral leads, an abnormal frontal plane QRS axis, and a preexcited appearance.[266]
- **TTE:** The LV is small, muscle bound, and non-apex forming. The LV is echo-bright, indicating endocardial fibroelastosis. The LA is generally small but can be dilated due to a restrictive ASD. There will generally be an ASD. The ascending aorta is hypoplastic with an absent valve or stenotic valve. The MV can be absent or with thickened short leaflets. The right-sided heart structures are generally normal but may have dilated RV.

EVALUATION

Once a newborn is identified as having HLHS, they will be transferred to the ICU to undergo extensive testing which may include ABG, CBC, CMP, continuous telemetry CXR, and TTE.

TREATMENT

- Upon diagnosis, prostaglandin IV must be initiated for ductal patency.
- Surgical palliation is required to sustain life. The first surgery is usually performed in the first week of life. The surgery is a Norwood-Sano or a Norwood-BT shunt (Figure 5.14). The Norwood procedure reconstructs the hypoplastic aortic arch using the pulmonary artery to create one outlet from the RV. The PDA is ligated. Either a Sano shunt (a tube from the RV to the pulmonary artery at the bifurcation) or a BT (Blalock-Taussig) shunt (tube connecting the branch pulmonary artery to the aortic arch; Figure 5.15) is placed.
- Around 4 to 6 months of age the next stage of surgical palliation occurs, the hemi-Fontan or Glenn procedure. During this procedure a cavopulmonary connection is made from the left pulmonary artery to the SVC. The Sano or BT shunt is removed.
- Around 3 to 4 years of life the third stage of surgical palliation occurs, the Fontan completion. Another cavopulmonary connection is made from the left pulmonary artery to the IVC.

PATIENT EDUCATION

These infants are medically fragile. There are often associated feeding difficulties and slow weight gain. We enlist the help of the patient family to provide optimum outcomes. Parents are often asked to weigh their infant daily, record the patient's intake, and monitor the oxygen saturations daily. Parents watch for changes in the baby's oxygen saturations, feeding regimen, weight, and breathing status more closely than normal infants.

SPECIAL CONSIDERATIONS

Single ventricle patients need to maintain adequate hydration since their blood supply to the lungs is largely passive flow. Dehydration can lead to serious health risks. These patients also are often on aspirin or other anticoagulants to ensure patency of the BT, Sano, or cavopulmonary anastomosis. These patients may fatigue sooner than people with

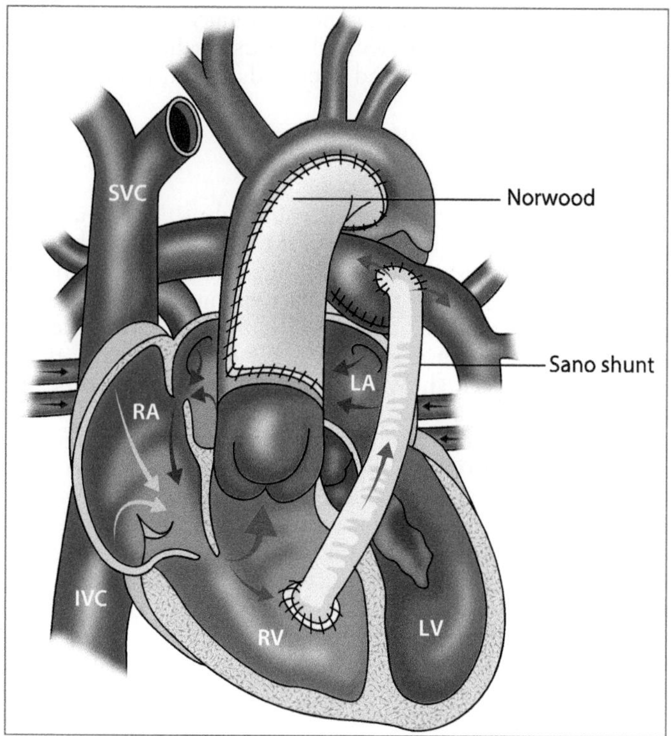

Figure 5.14 Norwood-Sano procedure. IVC, inferior vena cava; LA, left atrium; LV, left ventricle; RA, right atrium; RV, right ventricle; SVC, superior vena cava.

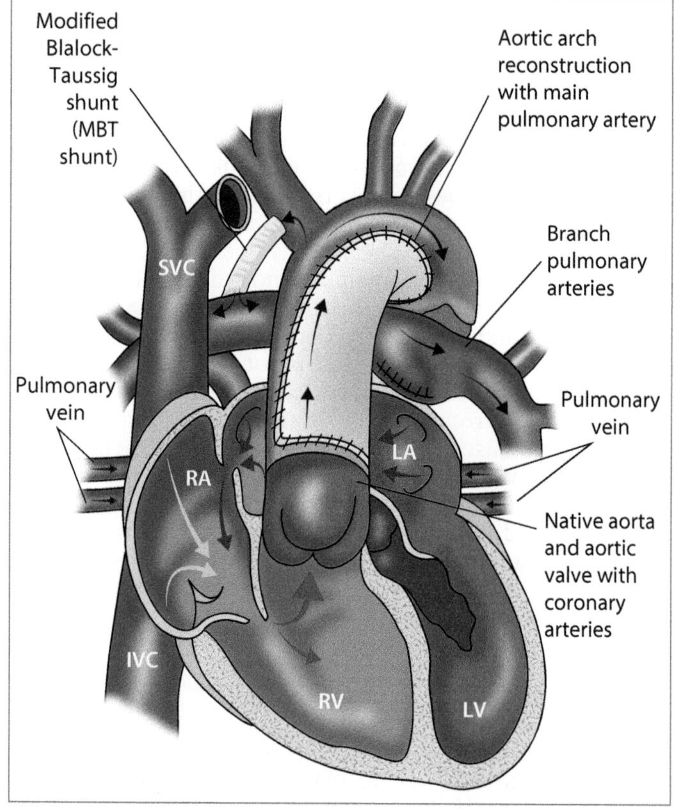

Figure 5.15 Norwood-BT procedure. IVC, inferior vena cava; LA, left atrium; LV, left ventricle; RA, right atrium; RV, right ventricle; SVC, superior vena cava.

normal cardiac anatomy. Complications and adverse outcomes of the Fontan palliation include chylous effusions, abnormal liver enzymes and hepatofibrosis, and protein-losing enteropathy.

KEY POINTS

- Single ventricle patients rely on one good ventricle to sustain life. The pulmonary blood flow is passive.
- Single ventricle patients have a high morbidity and mortality rate in the first year of life.
- Palliation is done in three staged surgeries: The BT shunt or Sano in first week of life, the Norwood or hemi-Fontan at 3 to 5 months of age, and the Fontan completion around age 1 to 2 years.
- Lifelong cardiology care is needed.
- Patients should be on anticoagulation such as aspirin daily and should maintain adequate hydration.

5.7 ARRHYTHMIAS

Christine Bruce

OVERVIEW

The normal heart automatically beats in a regular, coordinated manner due to its automaticity that traditionally starts in the sinoatrial (SA) node. The SA node has the fastest pacemaker, so it dominates the initiation of electrical impulses that trigger a sequence of organized contractions of the atria and ventricles. Both arrhythmias and conduction disorders occur as a result of abnormalities in either the initiation of the electrical impulse, abnormalities in the way that the impulses are conducted, or a combination of both of these processes.

Cardiac conduction abnormalities leading to either arrhythmia or various heart blocks can occur with any heart disorder. Congenital abnormalities of structure such as accessory AV connection or abnormalities in function such as pathology affecting conduction system can lead to cardiac arrhythmias. Systemic conditions such as hyperthyroidism and hypothyroidism; electrolyte abnormalities particularly potassium, magnesium, and calcium abnormalities; medications; and acute intoxication states such as alcohol, cocaine, or excessive caffeine intake can also lead to heart rhythm abnormalities.

EPIDEMIOLOGY

The cardiac conduction system involves specialized cardiac myocytes having automaticity, which allows the intrinsic pacemaker of the heart to start the cardiac conduction. The SA node is located in the superior portion of the right atrium and serves as the pacemaker of the heart as it intrinsically has the fastest setting in its pacemaker. Once the SA node fires, there is an orderly stimulation of other cells from the atria into the AV node, which is located on the right side of the interatrial septum. The AV node delays the conduction and impulse transmission allowing additional filling of the ventricle from the atrium. The bundle of His is a continuation of the AV node and is located at the superior portion of the intraventricular septum where it bifurcates into the left and right bundle branches, which terminate in Purkinje fibers. The right bundle conduction sends impulses to the anterior and apical endocardial regions of the RV. The left bundle is in the anterior portion and posterior portion and stimulates the left side of the intraventricular septum.

The resting sinus heart rate in adult patients typically ranges from 60 to 100 bpm. Bradycardia occurs with cardiovascular toning from aerobic exercise, illness, vagal nerve stimulation, and sometimes with aging. Inspiration causes an increase in heart rate while expiration causes a decrease in heart rate, which leads to a condition called sinus arrhythmia, which is a normal phenomenon. It is for this reason that EKGs are taken with the patient breathing normally without deeply inspiring or expiring.

PATHOPHYSIOLOGY

Pathology producing bradycardia can occur in the sinus node, the AV nodal tissue, and in the specialized His-Purkinje conduction system.[267] Bradycardia is defined as a heart rate of <50 to 60 bpm, which can occur in young athletic individuals and can also be seen in patients as part of normal aging or as an actual disease.[267] Bradycardia can occur in settings that are unrelated to the cardiovascular system. Medical conditions that can induce bradycardia include hypothyroidism, hypothermia, hyperkalemia, and typhoid fever.[268] Bradycardia arrhythmias can occur from abnormalities in the intrinsic pacemaker or with conduction blocks especially within the AV node or the His/Purkinje system. Bradycardia can be caused by Lyme carditis that occurs when bacterial spirochetes infect the pericardium or myocardium triggering an inflammatory response. The most common EKG findings in these patients include AV conduction abnormalities such as first-, second-, and third-degree heart block.[269]

Most tachycardias are due to reentry although some can result from enhanced normal automaticity or from abnormal mechanisms of automaticity.

Reentry is a circular propagation of an impulse around two interconnected pathways that have different conduction characteristics and refractory times. Reentry can be triggered by a premature beat, which starts the continuous circulation pathway leading to tachyarrhythmia. Typically, reentry can be prevented by inducing tissue refractoriness after stimulation. If tissue refractoriness is shortened because of sympathetic stimulation or if the conduction pathway remains stimulated as a result of hypertrophy, reentry can occur. Ischemia can also slow normal impulse conduction causing the reentry circuit to fire.

MEDICAL HISTORY AND CLINICAL PRESENTATION

Patients may have arrhythmia with or without symptoms occurring. If patients are symptomatic, palpitations can be felt as a result of skipped beats, rapid beats, or very forceful beats. If hemodynamic compromise occurs, patients can develop shortness of breath, chest pain, presyncope, or syncope. If hemodynamic compromise is significant, cardiac arrest can occur.

SIGNS AND SYMPTOMS

Assessment of symptoms in a patient with a low heart rate is a critical component in the evaluation and management of bradycardia. Common symptoms of bradycardia include syncope, presyncope, transient dizziness or lightheadedness, fatigue, dyspnea on exertion, or confusion, which results from cerebral hypoperfusion.[267] Significant bradycardia or malignant arrhythmias such as VF, VT, or asystole can cause an abrupt onset of syncope because autoregulation in the cerebral circulation fails to maintain blood flow in the brain. The cerebral cortex initially responds to impaired blood flow by disrupting normal activity in the brain followed by a complete cessation of activity when hypoperfusion deepens.[270] Symptomatic bradycardia requiring pacemaker placement has syncope as a presenting symptom in 33% of patients, dizziness in 22%, overt collapse in 17%, angina in 17%, and HF in 11%.[271] The most common underlying reason for these patients having symptomatic bradycardia is primary disturbance of cardiac automaticity and/or conduction in 49%, adverse drug effect in 21%, acute MI in 14%, pacemaker failure in 6%, intoxication in 6%, and electrolyte disorder in 4%.[271]

Although acute cocaine intoxication is associated with hypertension and tachycardia as a result of catecholamine release, chronic cocaine use can also be associated with sinus bradycardia as there is a sevenfold increase due to cocaine-induced desensitization of the beta-adrenergic receptor secondary to continuous exposure.[272] Bradycardia and hypotension have also been reported in patients using synthetic cannabinoids.[273]

PHYSICAL EXAMINATION

The jugular venous system can identify complete heart block by becoming distended as a result of the atria contracting against a closed AV node. This condition produces a large A wave also known as a cannon wave, which can also occur in the setting of a patient having paroxysmal SVT.

Auscultation of the heart and assessment of the pulse identify whether the patient has a regular or irregular rate. The most common irregularly irregular heart rate is due to atrial fibrillation (AF). AF can be paroxysmal, meaning that it starts and stops spontaneously, or it can be prolonged and can last for decades; it is the most common sustained arrhythmia in clinical practice.

Patients can develop rales heard on lung auscultation if HF occurs as a result of cardiac dysrhythmia. Patients with AF who have a rapid ventricular response do not have enough filling time compromising cardiac output, which leads to poor outflow of blood with dependent edema occurring as a result of lack of forward flow of blood.

DIFFERENTIAL DIAGNOSIS

The differential diagnosis for arrythmias is summarized in Table 5.20.

TABLE 5.20 Differential Diagnosis of Arrythmias

Diagnosis	Description
Focal atrial tachycardia (also called paroxysmal atrial tachycardia)	Abnormal automaticity in the atria with rates between 120 and 250 bpm. P waves are seen before every QRS complex but have a different morphology than the P wave seen in normal sinus rhythm. Underlying causes include cocaine, alcohol, previous cardiac surgery, and digoxin toxicity. Abrupt onset and abrupt stoppage of dysrhythmia.
Atrial flutter	Reentry type of atrial tachycardia with atrial rates 250 to 320 bpm with the ventricular rates 120 to 160 bpm. Typically, pulse is regular with ventricle contracting every two, three, or four P waves. Flutter waves seen in the inferior EKG leads. Transitory rhythm, which will change into another type of rhythm.
Atrial fibrillation	Most common cause of prolonged cardiac dysrhythmia. A type of supraventricular tachyarrhythmia Characterized by uncoordinated atrial activation with variable ventricular response with most common response being rapid. No P waves, no cannon A waves in the jugular venous system, and pulse is irregularly irregular. Can be persistent, paroxysmal, or chronic in nature.
Wolff-Parkinson-White syndrome	Shortened PR interval with slurring on the uptake of the QRS complex, which is known as a delta wave. Most commonly caused by AV reentry tachycardia, atrial flutter, or atrial fibrillation. Congenital heart disease is a known risk factor. Aberrant pathway can be ablated as a method of treatment.
Ventricular tachycardia/ sustained and nonsustained	Often is a sign of a patient with heart disease. Three PVCs in a row meet the criteria for VT. Hard to differentiate from SVT with aberrancy. Electrical axis with a VT is typically extreme right, extreme left. Can be monomorphic or polymorphic dependent on QRS appearance. Sustained VT lasts longer than 30 seconds and can occur with or without a pulse. VT without a pulse is treated the same as ventricular fibrillation. VT is typically associated with ischemic and nonischemic heart disease, Brugada syndrome, and metabolic problems.
Long QT syndrome	Can be inherited or acquired causing the QT interval to be too long compared to the ventricular rate or R-R interval. Electrolyte abnormalities, hypokalemia, and hypomagnesemia can prolong QT interval as can the use of medications such as fluoroquinolones and type III antiarrhythmics such as amiodarone. Increased risk for syncope, torsades de pointes, and sudden cardiac death.
Cardiac arrest	Sudden loss of cardiac output resulting in loss of systemic circulation. Associated with asystole, ventricular fibrillation, pulseless ventricular tachycardia, and pulseless electrical activity. Cardiopulmonary resuscitation immediately needed along with defibrillation when a shockable arrhythmia is present.
Bradycardia	As defined, heart rate <60 bpm, but symptoms do not occur unless heart rate is <50. Treat according to symptoms as this can be a normal variant in hearts that are cardiovascularly conditioned and in those taking beta blockers. If symptomatic, atropine is first-line medication to improve AV nodal conduction. Transplanted hearts do not respond to vagal lytic medications and would instead need beta agonist such as isoproterenol to improve the rate. Pacemaker is definitive treatment for patients not responding to medication. Can be the result of sinus node dysfunction, second- and third-degree heart blocks.
Supraventricular tachycardia	Heart rates typically >150 bpm. Can be paroxysmal with sudden onset and stoppage. Symptoms include palpitations, dizziness, lightheadedness, syncope, and near syncope. Can be caused by reentry circuit which can be treated with radiofrequency ablation. Vagal maneuvers are first-line treatment. Adenosine can be given to stop conduction between the atria and ventricles with the hope that when the heart restarts, the SA node will resume functioning.

AV, atrioventricular; PVCs, premature ventricular contractions; SA, sinoatrial; SVT, supraventricular tachycardia; VT, ventricular tachycardia.

DIAGNOSTIC STUDIES

As part of the initial evaluation, a careful search for reversible causes is conducted with a comprehensive history and physical examination along with review of medications. Additional testing of patients with bradycardia includes performance of a 12-lead EKG, which could suggest structural heart disease, conduction disturbance, or other cardiac conditions that can predispose patients to bradycardia and other arrhythmias. Ambulatory EKG monitoring can be considered to establish a diagnosis or make a symptom-rhythm correlation. Longer term monitoring can result in higher yield for patients who are not having frequent symptoms. Exercise testing can be considered in patients with symptoms temporally related to exercise, asymptomatic second-degree AV block, or suspected chronotropic incompetence. TTE is performed in patients with new left bundle branch block, Mobitz type II AV heart block, or complete AV block. Cardiac CT, cardiac MRI, nuclear imaging, or TEE can be considered in selected patients based upon clinical suspicion and differential diagnosis if more advanced imaging is needed as part of the overall evaluation for cardiac dysrhythmia.[267]

EVALUATION

Twelve-lead EKG is the initial step used in the identification of a cardiac arrhythmia. Sinus bradycardia shows a P wave preceding every QRS complex with a heart rate <60 bpm. If bradycardia arrhythmia occurs without a relationship between the P waves and the QRS complexes, AV heart block is present. If the ventricle is intrinsically beating as an escape rhythm, the QRS complex will be wide, while demonstration of a narrow QRS complex as the escape rhythm typically means that the escape complex is located at or above the AV node.

If the QRS rhythm is irregular and if P waves outnumber the QRS complexes, a second-degree AV heart block is present. If there is gradual prolongation of the PR interval with a subsequent dropped QRS complex, second-degree type I or Wenckebach rhythm is present. A stable QR interval with more P waves than QRS complexes being conducted illustrates a second-degree type II AV heart block.

Tachyarrhythmias identified on EKG can manifest as irregularly narrow QRS complexes, irregularly wide QRS complexes, regular narrow QRS complexes, and irregular wide QRS complexes. Echocardiogram can help to further delineate atrial and ventricular activity in the setting of cardiac arrhythmias and can also enable the calculation of the left ventricular ejection fraction.

Once a patient is diagnosed with a cardiac arrhythmia, the search for and correction of the underlying cause is performed. The CXR can be performed to assess for cardiomegaly or pulmonary abnormalities as many of these patients have coexisting dyspnea.

Patients having intermittent symptoms consistent with arrhythmia can have placement of a Holter monitor to record the heart rhythm on an ongoing basis. Patients having intermittent but serious symptoms can have placement of a loop recorder/event recorder in order to capture the dysrhythmia when symptoms are infrequent.

TREATMENT

Treatment of an arrhythmia depends upon the underlying cause and can include antiarrhythmic medications, implantable cardioverter/defibrillators, and pacemakers including resynchronization pacemaker therapy, which is primarily used in the setting of chronic HF. Radiofrequency ablation therapy can be performed in order to eliminate accessory pathways and circuits when medication is not effective.

There has been a shift in the emphasis of management of bradycardia with the emphasis on the evaluation and management of disease states and not just implanting a pacemaker to treat symptomatic bradycardia.[267] There is a direct correlation between bradycardia and sleep apnea so management of sleep apnea can be an effective treatment for patients with symptomatic nocturnal bradycardia.

Medications that are used to treat bradycardia acutely include atropine, which is a parasympatholytic drug that can affect the SA node conduction and automaticity and enhance conduction through the AV node. Isoproterenol is a pure beta agonist that can be used to treat bradycardia in a transplanted heart since these hearts are denervated and do not respond to the vagolytic medications. The catecholamines dopamine, dobutamine, and epinephrine directly stimulate beta receptors to increase SA node automaticity along with AV conduction. In the setting of overdose of beta blockers or calcium channel blockers, calcium gluconate or calcium chloride can be used along with glucagon as long as the liver is still functional.[267]

Placement of a permanent pacemaker is indicated for patients with symptomatic bradycardia who do not respond to medications or who have second-degree heart block type II or third-degree heart block, which traditionally has the conduction blockage located below the AV node. Patients who have a depressed ejection fraction of <50% respond better to pacemakers placed in the LV instead of the RV in order to ensure a more physiologic ventricular activation.[274]

Antiarrhythmic medications can be given depending on the symptoms and the severity of the underlying arrhythmia (Table 5.21). The Vaughn Williams classification system details the classes of medications of antiarrhythmic medications[275] along with the advice to avoid electrolyte abnormalities and bradycardia in patients taking these medications.

5.7A BRADYCARDIAS

Slow heart rates may be symptomatic for those who have a pathologic underlying cause or can be normal in asymptomatic patients who have excellent cardiovascular conditioning. This can be the result of sinus bradycardia with slow setting of the SA node, either type of second-degree heart block, or third-degree heart block resulting in cardiac rates that are not sufficient to meet metabolic demand. Symptoms may include dizziness, lightheadedness, or palpitations that are felt as a result of ectopic beats that are perceived between the slow cardiac conduction cycles. Treatment can include atropine, which acts as a vagolytic agent to take the brakes off the slow conduction through the AV node, along with pacemaker placement, which is needed in the setting of both sick sinus syndrome and third-degree heart block along with a potential for needing pacemaker in second-degree heart block type II. Bradycardia by itself may not need to be treated unless the patient is having symptoms or has a third-degree heart block.

Sick sinus syndrome refers to a condition in which there is dysfunction of the SA node. This dysfunction comprises inappropriate sinus bradycardia, alternating bradycardia

TABLE 5.21 Antiarrhythmic Medications

Drug Classification	Examples of Medications	Major Mechanism of Action	Therapeutic Effects	Contraindications and Adverse Side Effects
Class IA	Disopyramide, procainamide, quinidine	Sodium channel blockers	Used to suppress atrial and ventricular premature beats, manage SVT, and slow ventricular response in the setting of atrial fibrillation.	Highly anticholinergic with urinary retention, glaucoma, blurred vision, torsades, negative inotropic activity worsening heart failure and hypotension as adverse effects.
Class IB	Lidocaine, mexiletine	Sodium channel blocker without any effect on potassium channels	Primarily used to suppress ventricular arrhythmias.	
Class IC	Flecainide, propafenone	Sodium channel blocker that can slow heart dynamics	Suppression of atrial and ventricular premature beats, SVTs and VTs, atrial fibrillation.	May cause blurred vision paresthesias and GI upset as adverse actions.
Class II: Beta blockers	Atenolol, bisoprolol, esmolol, metoprolol, nadolol, propranolol, timolol	Decrease the rate of automaticity, slow conduction velocity, and prolong refractoriness	Treat SVT, reduce ventricular proarrhythmia effects, block sympathetic effects.	Contraindicated in the setting of asthma, not used for preexisting slow heart rates, can cause depression, interfere with recognition of hypoglycemia, not used with peripheral arterial disease because of interference with blood flow to the extremities.
Class III: Membrane stabilizing medications	Amiodarone, dofetilide, dronedarone, ibutilide, sotalol	Potassium channel blockers, reduce the rate of automaticity and cause QT interval prolongation; block alpha receptors and beta receptors	Treats SVTs and ventricular tachycardia.	May be proarrhythmic especially torsades. Amiodarone contains high-dose iodine affecting the thyroid, pulmonary fibrosis, skin discoloration, hepatic abnormalities, peripheral neuropathy, and lowering of the GFR with long-term use. Can be used for both atrial and ventricular dysrhythmias.
Class IV: Calcium channel blockers (nondihydropyridine type)	Diltiazem, verapamil	Depresses the calcium dependent action potentials and decreases the rate of automaticity, prolongs refractoriness	Treatment of SVTs and slows the ventricular response in the setting of atrial fibrillation or atrial flutter.	Negative inotropic effect can worsen heart failure symptoms.

GI, gastrointestinal; GFR, glomerular filtrate rate; SVT, supraventricular tachycardia; VT, ventricular tachycardia.

and atrial tachycardia, sinus pause or arrest, and SA exit block. This condition predominates in the elderly patient as the conduction system seems not to age well. Sinus pause temporarily causes activity in the SA node to stop and this usually triggers an escape rhythm in other portions of the heart that have automaticity function. Long pauses can cause dizziness and syncope. SA node dysfunction typically has an idiopathic underlying cause as a result of SA node fibrosis. Known causes include increased vagal tone, ischemia, myocarditis, and infiltrative heart disease such as amyloidosis and hemochromatosis. Treatment is with a pacemaker.

5.7B TACHYCARDIAS

Tachycardia is defined as a heart rates >100 bpm and can be caused by conditions that increase the basic metabolic rate (e.g., fever, exercise, or hyperthyroidism). Tachycardias are treated by addressing the underlying cause. Sinus tachycardia typically will have a slow increase in the heart rate with a slow resolution of that fast heart rate. SVT typically has an abrupt onset and cessation of fast heart rates and this classification includes any significant tachycardia that is located above the AV node.

AF is the most common sustained cardiac arrhythmia seen in clinical practice. This condition contributes to mortality and morbidity and is seen more frequently in the elderly population. A serious complication of AF is the development of atrial thromboembolism with resultant systemic embolization and stroke.[276] AF is typically a rapid, irregularly irregular atrial rhythm. Symptoms include palpitations, lightheadedness, and near syncope along with exercise intolerance, dyspnea, and weakness. Atrial thrombi may form increasing the risk of embolic stroke. Patient will have an irregular pulse and diagnosis can be made with EKG or echocardiogram.

Management of AF involves rate control with medications, prevention of thromboembolism by anticoagulation, or rhythm control with attempt to convert AF to sinus rhythm by either medications or electrical cardioversion. Overall management of AF with rate control versus rhythm control remains a contentious strategy. In the setting of AF with HF, there are similar outcomes with regard to mortality, hospitalization, and thromboembolism rates regardless of whether rate control or rhythm control is employed for treatment. Rhythm control has been found to be superior to rate control with regard to improvement in left ventricular ejection fraction, exercise capacity, and quality of life particularly within the group of rhythm control patients, and catheter ablation was found to be superior to the use of antiarrhythmic medications as part of rhythm control.[277]

Conflicting studies have shown no differences in outcome between management of AF with rate control versus rhythm control. Patients having a high risk of arrhythmia recurrence may not benefit with rhythm control strategies as AF frequently recurs for them.[278] Patients without symptoms do not have a clear advantage when given rate control versus rhythm control, and there may be an advantage to ablation therapy in those who undergo this procedure.

Controversy also exists with regard to stroke prevention in the setting of long-standing AF. Antiplatelet therapy in the form of aspirin may be useful in younger patients with lone AF without other risk factors. Data support the use of anticoagulation therapy for patients over 75 years of age in the setting of AF rather than aspirin therapy alone.[279]

Atrial flutter has a rapid, regular atrial rhythm caused by an atrial macroentrant circuit. Patients complain of palpitations, exercise intolerance, dyspnea, lightheadedness, and near syncope. Typically, this dysrhythmia is not long-standing and will transition into another rhythm. Sawtooth waves are seen on EKG and occur as a result of increased atrial contraction but the ventricular response is slower, typically very predictable, occurring every second, third, or fourth atrial contraction. Treatment includes medications to control the rate, anticoagulation to prevent thromboembolism, and cardioversion if the patient needs assistance to return to normal sinus rhythm. This condition may cause hemodynamic compromise and urgent cardioversion is needed in that circumstance. Rate control medications include beta blockers, nondihydropyridine calcium channel blockers, along with electrical therapy in the form of synchronized cardioversion.

Atrial tachycardia is a regular rhythm typically caused by a single atrial focus separate from the SA node. Underlying causes can include atrial automaticity and intra-atrial reentry. This condition often occurs in patients with a structural heart disorder but may also be caused by pericarditis, alcohol intoxication, and medication use such as digoxin. EKG in the setting of atrial tachycardia will show P waves with different morphologies occurring before QRS complexes but if the ventricular rate is too fast, the P wave may be hidden in either the preceding T wave or within the QRS complex itself. Vagal maneuvers can be utilized to slow conduction through the AV node as the first attempt at treatment. Medications used to treat atrial tachycardia include adenosine, beta blockers, and nondihydropyridine calcium channel blockers. Symptomatic patients may need to be treated with synchronized cardioversion. Antiarrhythmic medications such as procainamide, quinidine, and amiodarone may also be used to chemically convert atrial tachycardia back to normal sinus rhythm.

Multifocal atrial tachycardia has an irregularly irregular rhythm caused by random discharge of multiple ectopic atrial foci, which typically occur as a result of COPD. There are at least three different P wave morphologies and the heart rate is above 100 bpm. Treatment is dependent on addressing the underlying pulmonary cause.

Wandering atrial pacemaker is a similar condition to multifocal atrial tachycardia with three or more different P wave morphologies along with an irregular ventricular rate but this rate is <100 bpm.

Junctional tachycardia is caused by abnormal automaticity in either the AV node or tissues adjacent to it. This situation is most likely to occur after open-heart surgery, inferior wall MI, myocarditis, or digoxin toxicity. EKG shows regular narrow QRS complexes either with no P waves or retroconducted P waves. There is a gradual onset of symptoms and if treatment is needed, beta blockers are used to control the faster heart rate along with the correction of the underlying cause.

Long QT syndrome with resultant torsades de pointes, which is a polymorphic type of VT that has an EKG showing rapid, irregular QRS complexes that seem to twist around the baseline. This pleomorphic type of VT can digress into VF. Any medication that prolongs the QT interval such as amiodarone needs to be avoided in this situation. Treatment involves IV magnesium for patients who are magnesium deficient and defibrillation along with discontinuing any medication that prolongs the QT interval. Long QT syndrome can be congenital primarily as an autosomal dominant disorder or can be acquired in the setting of medications such as antiarrhythmics, tricyclic antidepressants, phenothiazines, and antifungals. Electrolyte abnormalities such as hypomagnesemia and hypokalemia can also prolong the QT interval. Patients with long QT syndrome can present with syncope since cardiac output is impaired. Lidocaine shortens the QT interval and may be useful in this setting for drug-induced QT prolongation especially in the setting of tricyclic antidepressant overdose. Patients with congenital QT syndrome are treated with beta blockers, permanent pacing with and without ICD (implantable cardiac defibrillator). These patients also need to avoid any medications that would prolong the QT interval and also keep their electrolytes from being abnormal.

Reentry SVT occurs above the bifurcation of the His bundle. Presenting symptoms include palpitations or chest discomfort. Initial therapy is with a vagal maneuver followed by IV adenosine or nondihydropyridine calcium channel blocker such as verapamil if the QRS complexes are narrow. If the SVT has wide QRS complexes, there is a concern for aberrant conduction, which would necessitate the use of procainamide, amiodarone, or synchronized cardioversion. The underlying pathophysiology for the reentry pathway shows this to be within the AV node, accessory bypass tract, or the pathway existing within the atria or the SA node. AV nodal reentry tachycardia is most commonly triggered by atrial premature beat. Accessory pathway reentry tachycardia has this abnormal tract running from the atria directly to the ventricle and this arrhythmia is triggered by either atrial or ventricular premature beats.

WPW syndrome is a pre-excitation syndrome with a shortened PR interval and a slurring on the upstroke of the QRS caused by an accessory pathway within the bundle of Kent. This condition can be idiopathic or can be seen in the setting of cardiomyopathy. Tachycardias that occur in this condition can lead to AF. Patients typically present with palpitations along with dyspnea, chest discomfort, syncope, or lightheadedness. Treatment is with vagolytic maneuvers, adenosine, nondihydropyridine calcium channel blockers, or radiofrequency ablation of the accessory pathway. Patients with known WPW syndrome and AF should not receive digoxin or nondihydropyridine calcium channel blockers as these agents can cause VF when used in the setting.

VF denotes a quivering, uncoordinated movement in the ventricles without an actual ventricular contraction. Immediate syncope occurs due to lack of cardiac output followed by death without treatment. Since there is still energy within the cardiac conduction system, immediate defibrillation is the most effective treatment. This rhythm frequently occurs in the setting of acute cardiac arrest and is often a terminal rhythm for patients who do not survive. Most patients with this condition have underlying heart disease. Patients who survive cardiac arrest secondary to VF are eligible for ICD placement, which can immediately shock the heart if VF would recur.

VT has at least three consecutive premature ventricular beats occurring at a rate of at least 120 bpm. Patients can be asymptomatic or could have compromised cardiac output in which no pulse is palpable. Patients who develop VT with a pulse who are stable can be treated with antiarrhythmics such as amiodarone or with synchronized cardioversion. VT without a pulse is treated in the same manner as VF with immediate defibrillation. Patients who develop VT typically have significant underlying cardiovascular disease but this could also occur in the setting of electrolyte abnormalities, hypoxemia, or long QT syndrome.

5.7C HEART BLOCK

First-degree AV heart block consists of the SA node dysfunction leading to pulse slowing with resultant prolonged PR interval on the EKG. This condition alone does not warrant treatment. **Type I second-degree heart block or Wenckebach** phenomenon has a progressive lengthening of the PR interval to the point where there is a dropped QRS complex. **Type II second-degree heart block** involves the conduction of impulses being blocked without any slowing or prolongation of the PR interval before the block occurs. When the QRS complex follows the atrial contraction, the PR interval remains the same but there are more P waves than QRS complexes. There is typically a pattern to the dropped beats that occurs such as every second, third, or fourth P wave not being followed by a QRS complex. This leads to an EKG appearance of "group beating." Because the pathology typically occurs below the AV node with this condition, permanent pacemaker is indicated.

Third-degree heart block has independent atrial and ventricular contractions without electrical communication between the atria and ventricles. These patients will have a slow pulse as a result of the ventricular escape pacemaker approximately occurring between 30 and 40 bpm. There is no coordinated conduction between the atria and ventricles in this condition and permanent pacemaker is needed for treatment.

5.7D PREMATURE BEATS

Ventricular premature beats or premature ventricular contractions (PVCs) are single ventricular impulses caused by reentry within the ventricle or by abnormal automaticity within the ventricular cells themselves. They can occur with and without underlying cardiovascular disease and they can be asymptomatic or cause palpitations. These ventricular premature beats are expected after MI due to the irritability of the heart after it is deprived of oxygen. Although it is common to ignore and not treat ventricular premature beats, it is essential that ventricular premature beats are not suppressed by antiarrhythmic medications after MI as there is a higher morbidity associated with their treatment in the setting with the use of these agents.

Premature beats occurring every other beat on a consistent basis is known as ventricular bigeminy and premature beats occurring every third complex is known as ventricular trigeminy. When there are paired ventricular premature beats, couplets are said to occur. Three PVCs in a row meet the criteria for VT. PVCs that have the same appearance on EKGs are known as monomorphic PVCs while PVCs having a different appearance are known as multifocal PVCs.

Known precipitants of PVCs include the use of stimulants such as caffeine, cocaine, alcohol, and sympathomimetic medications along with the patient experiencing anxiety and stress. PVCs occurring on a frequent basis may impact cardiac output as there may not be sufficient time for ventricular filling to occur. Diagnosis of PVCs is on a rhythm strip or EKG. Following a PVC, a compensatory pause typically occurs. The PVC itself also tends to have an opposite polarity than the rest of the QRS complexes. These attributes may help to differentiate PVCs from premature atrial beats with aberrant conduction that typically occur on the same electrical axis and do not have a compensatory pause following the premature atrial contraction.

Treatment of premature beats if needed due to symptoms, is best done with beta blockers, which suppress sympathetic activity. If PVCs increase during exercise in a patient with known coronary artery disease, the patient should be evaluated for potential PCI as this may be a sign of significant progression of the coronary artery disease. Frequent PVCs or continued tachycardic states can lead to the development of cardiomyopathy so there may be some other compelling reasons for treating these conditions.

SPECIAL CONSIDERATIONS

Brugada syndrome is an inherited disorder caused by cardiac electrical abnormalities that results in patients having an increased risk of both syncope and sudden death. The most common inherited gene is *SCN5A* gene which is involved with the voltage dependent cardiac sodium channel.[280] Since this is an electrical disorder, most of these symptomatic patients are young and do not have structural or coronary heart disease when they develop symptoms. The characteristic EKG pattern with Brugada syndrome demonstrates prominent ST segment elevation in V1 and V2 making the QRS complex resemble a right bundle branch block pattern. ST segment is coved leading to the production of an inverted T wave in these leads. Diagnosis may be based upon screening of family members with this condition or as part of an evaluation for patients who have unexplained syncope or cardiac arrest without any underlying structural or coronary artery disease. Precipitants of syncope or cardiac arrest in these patients can be fever or use of class I antiarrhythmic medications, beta blockers, tricyclic antidepressants, and cocaine.

When identified, patients with Brugada syndrome are treated with an implantable cardiac defibrillator.

Patients with inherited primary arrhythmia syndromes may be at increased risk of sudden cardiac death even in the setting of having a normally structured heart. Long QT syndrome and Brugada syndrome along with various cardiomyopathies such as hypertrophic cardiomyopathy may have exercise as a known trigger for ventricular arrhythmia. Many of these patients qualify for placement of an implantable cardiac defibrillator but exercising with this device in place may lead to the delivery of inappropriate shocks and further complications. As a general rule, exercise stressing the heart should generally be avoided in patients with many of these inherited syndromes associated with arrhythmia.[281]

KEY POINTS

- Patients with arrhythmia may be asymptomatic with the arrhythmia being picked up as an incidental finding when an EKG is done for another reason.
- Cardiac arrhythmias involved a range of diagnoses from bradycardia, AV conduction blocks, and tachyarrhythmias.
- Treatment of the underlying cause for the dysrhythmia is most important as part of the treatment regimen.
- Antiarrhythmic medications used to suppress or prevent arrhythmia may have the unexpected adverse action of being proarrhythmic with their use.
- Patients who survive sudden cardiac death second to arrhythmia are typically eligible for placement of an implantable cardiac defibrillator to treat arrhythmias if they recur.

5.8 PERICARDIAL DISEASE

Christine Bruce

5.8A PERICARDITIS

OVERVIEW

Pericarditis is caused by inflammation of the lining of the heart. Fluid can accumulate between the visceral and parietal pericardium leading to pericardial effusion. Patients with acute pericarditis feel better sitting up and leaning forward with pain having a pleuritic component and worsening while taking a deep breath. Treatment is usually medical and is dependent on the underlying etiology if it has been determined since the majority of cases are idiopathic.

Classic triad of acute pericarditis is chest pain, pericardial friction rub, and EKG showing diffuse ST-T wave segment elevation along with depressed PR segment. Pain is pleuritic in nature, retrosternal, and mitigated with sitting up and leaning forward. Acute pericarditis can be caused by severe inflammation, infection, or hemorrhage from either iatrogenic causes such as cardiac surgery or aortic dissection or from direct trauma. Constrictive pericarditis involves scarring and fibrosis that interferes with filling of the heart during diastole.

EPIDEMIOLOGY

About 90% of pericarditis is idiopathic while viral and bacterial infections cause 1% to 2%, tuberculosis 4%, and neoplasms 7%. Autoimmune or inflammatory disease can cause 3% to 5%.[282] Acute pericarditis is the most common cause of all pericardial diseases that are seen in clinical practice. Pericarditis can occur as a result of a STEMI, as a sequela of viral infection, at the time of a dissecting aortic aneurysm from blood leaking into the pericardial space, after blunt or sharp trauma to the chest, from neoplastic invasion of the pericardium, after chest irradiation, as a result of uremia, from autoimmune disorders, and from medication use.[282]

PATHOPHYSIOLOGY

There is usually 15 to 50 mL of straw-colored fluid contained within the visceral and parietal layers of the fibrous pericardium. This fluid can increase in amount and contain markers of inflammation. Both local and systemic conditions can lead to the development of acute pericarditis. Underlying conditions include both idiopathic and viral infections such as coxsackievirus A16 and other enteroviruses. Pericarditis can occur in the setting of chronic kidney disease with resultant uremia, and autoimmune disease such as rheumatoid arthritis (RA), vasculitis, and lupus. Post MI pericardial inflammation or Dressler syndrome occurs following MI up to several weeks following MI. Acute pericarditis can occur as a result of cancer, mostly from local tumor invasion or lymphatic or hematologic spread (Figure 5.16).

MEDICAL HISTORY AND CLINICAL PRESENTATION

Because this condition causes chest pain, patients may be seen in the ED and urgent care centers along with primary care practices. Complications of acute pericarditis include cardiac tamponade, recurrent or chronic pericarditis, and constrictive or constrictive-effusive pericarditis.[283]

Typically, pericarditis is self-limited and treated with nonsteroidal anti-inflammatory medications as first-line therapy for uncomplicated cases.[284] Chest pain is the most common presenting symptom causing sharp and stabbing pain that is pleuritic in nature causing this condition to be confused with MI. Pain is exacerbated by lying down. Pain can occur at rest rather than exertion and does not respond to nitrates. Pericardial friction rub can occur and is described as a scratchy sound best heard with the patient leaning forward.

SIGNS AND SYMPTOMS

Pericarditis typically causes a sudden onset of retrosternal chest pain that is described as sharp and stabbing that is worsened with inspiration or when lying down. Patients are more likely to breathe shallowly and more rapidly. The pain can radiate into the jaw, neck, shoulder, arms, or trapezius and typically lasts hours to days. There is no response of the pain to nitroglycerin. Patients will naturally assume a position of sitting up and leaning forward. Patients avoid exertion because this results in taking a deeper breath which patients avoid at all costs. This pleuritic pain can also cause inspiratory arrest and anxiety.

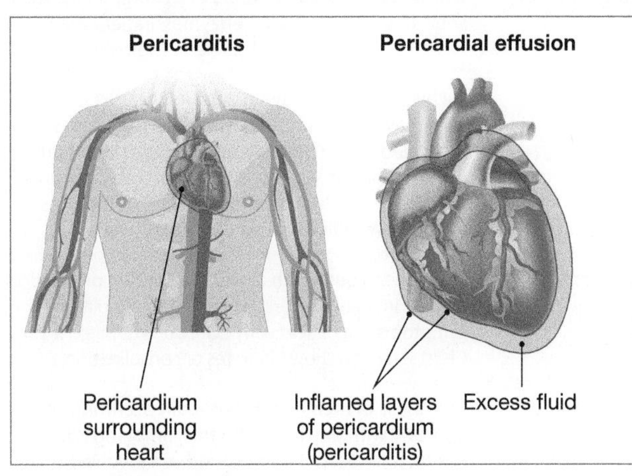

Figure 5.16 Pericarditis.
(*Source: Flamm KL, Granger M, Gawlik K, et al. Evidence-based assessment of the heart and circulatory system. In: Gawlik KS, Melnyk BM, Teall AM, eds.* Evidence-Based Physical Examination: Best Practices for Health and Well-Being Assessment. *Springer Publishing Company; 2021:149, Fig. 6.46.*)

PHYSICAL EXAMINATION

A pericardial friction rub can be present in up to 85% of patients.[282] This pericardial friction rub has a three-phase component on auscultation. This rub is heard best at the lower left lateral sternal border. Fever may be present if infection is part of the etiology. Patients with constrictive pericarditis may have jugular venous distention, hepatomegaly, peripheral edema, and right ventricular heave. Cardiac tamponade can be a life-threatening complication with this condition being diagnosed by finding decreased blood pressure, elevated jugular venous pressure, muffled heart sounds, and pulsus paradoxus.[285]

DIFFERENTIAL DIAGNOSIS

The differential diagnosis for pericardial disease is summarized in Table 5.22.

DIAGNOSTIC STUDIES

Classic EKG findings show ST segment elevation diffusely, occurring in almost all chest leads along with PR segment depression. Echocardiogram will demonstrate the pericardial effusion with a heart otherwise functioning well without wall motion abnormality. Echocardiogram is especially useful in evaluating for possible cardiac tamponade, which can occur in the setting of untreated pericardial effusion. If autoimmune disease or infection is suspected as the cause of the pericarditis, C-reactive protein and erythrocyte sedimentation rate will be elevated. CXR classically shows a water bottle–shaped heart if a pericardial effusion is present. For this feature to be demonstrated, a large pericardial effusion of at least 300 mL needs to be present. If uremia is the underlying cause for the pericarditis, glomerular filtration rate will be low due to an elevation in serum creatinine.

TABLE 5.22 Differential Diagnosis for Pericardial Disease

Condition	Explanation
Myocardial infarction/angina	Pressure-like sensation or a squeezing sensation. Angina responds to nitroglycerin while myocardial infarction continues despite 3 nitroglycerin. EKG, cardiac enzymes, and patient history aid in diagnosis. S4 heart sound may be present.
Costochondritis/ Tietze syndrome	Pain with pressure at the costochondral junction which produces the patient's chief complaint. Heart sounds are normal as are enzymes. Patient may have a history of musculoskeletal overexertion.
Pulmonary embolism	Tachycardia and tachypnea are key features. Chest pain may be pleuritic in nature. EKG will show sinus tachycardia with possible right axis deviation due to increased intrapleural pressure from the pulmonary embolism. V̇/Q̇ lung scan or spiral CT of the chest are positive with negative cardiac enzymes.
Pneumonia	Tachypnea, cough with or without sputum production, change in mental status, exacerbation of pulmonary symptoms in a patient with COPD, unexplained fever. Chest x-ray can show infiltrates or consolidation.
Pneumothorax	Shortness of breath and chest pain occurring abruptly with or without trauma. Smoking is a risk factor. Absent breath sounds on involved side. Simple pneumothorax can occur in young, healthy patients while people with emphysema have an increased risk caused by rupture of a bleb. Expiratory film will highlight the edge of the collapsed lung. Cardiac enzymes are normal.

COPD, chronic obstructive pulmonary disease; V̇/Q̇, ventilation/perfusion.

EVALUATION

A history and laboratory tests, a chest radiograph, and an echocardiogram are used in evaluation.[286] Acute pericarditis is a clinical diagnosis that can be supported by patient's having an elevation in the markers of inflammation such as erythrocyte sedimentation rate or high-sensitivity C-reactive protein, EKG findings to include ST segment elevation diffusely along with PR segment depression, and pleuritic chest pain along with a pericardial friction rub. Serial high-sensitivity C-reactive protein levels can be followed in order to assess response to therapy. CXR can be performed to identify pericardial effusion or other thoracic abnormalities that can result in chest pain.

TREATMENT

Aspirin and NSAIDs are effective treatments for idiopathic and viral causes of acute pericarditis with aspirin being the treatment of choice for post-MI-related pericarditis with NSAIDs and steroids being avoided in this circumstance as NSAIDs increase the risk for further thrombosis formation and steroids increase the risk for recurrent pericarditis. Colchicine added to treatment reduces risk for recurrence by 50%.[287]

Most pericardial effusions related to acute pericarditis can be safely managed with an echocardiogram-guided percutaneous approach. Pericardiectomy remains a definitive treatment for patients with severe symptoms caused by constrictive pericarditis with this procedure typically relieving symptoms.

Subspecialty consultation should be considered if the diagnosis remains uncertain following initial evaluation or based on a failure to respond to treatment. Surgery may be required for recurrent symptomatic effusions or recurrent pericardial tamponade.[283] Typically, pericarditis is self-limited with NSAIDs remaining first-line therapy for uncomplicated cases.[284]

Complications of pericarditis include cardiac tamponade, recurrent pericarditis, and pericardial constriction.[282]

PATIENT EDUCATION

Although acute pericarditis can cause alarming symptoms in patients who have this condition, this condition is typically self-limited and responds to simple treatment with aspirin, glucocorticoids, or colchicine. Because of the abrupt onset of chest pain, cardiovascular evaluation is warranted. Patients are expected to have a full recovery but remain at risk for recurrent pericarditis especially if the underlying cause remains. Acute pericarditis with resultant pericardial effusion may require clinical intervention involving aspiration of the fluid, allowing a pericardial drain to continue drainage of this fluid, or pericardiectomy if significant constrictive pericarditis or cardiac tamponade occurs. Full recovery is expected.

5.8B PERICARDIAL EFFUSION

Pericardial effusion can occur as result of acute pericarditis with an increase in the amount of naturally occurring fluid contained between the visceral and parietal pericardium. This fluid can contain inflammatory markers and proliferate to the point where cardiac tamponade occurs. Pulsus paradoxus, a drop of at least 10 mm Hg of systolic blood pressure during inspiration, can be seen in the setting of pericardial effusion with resultant cardiac tamponade. Patients with large pericardial effusions have the classic CXR finding of a water bottle heart due to the accumulation of this free-flowing fluid, which tends to accumulate mostly in the dependent portions of the heart.

Treatment of pericardial effusion is mostly dependent upon patient's symptoms. Anti-inflammatory medications can calm the inflammatory process, allowing gradual absorption of this additional fluid over time. Patients who are acutely symptomatic may need drainage of this fluid, which can be done during echocardiogram.

KEY POINTS

- The vast majority of cases of acute pericarditis are idiopathic.
- Diagnosis of acute pericarditis is primarily based on clinical grounds with support from patient history and EKG findings.
- Acute pericarditis is self-limited and patients are expected to have complete recovery although recurrence remains a possibility.

5.9 ENDOCARDITIS

Christine Bruce

OVERVIEW

IE refers to infection of the endocardium or simply a focus of infection in the heart.[288] Noninfectious endocarditis occurs when sterile platelets and fibrin thrombi form on cardiac valves along with adjacent structures. This type of noninfectious endocarditis can lead to IE. Complications of this condition include embolization and impairment in cardiac function.

Although the diagnosis of endocarditis can be suggested by echocardiogram, the diagnosis is based upon a constellation of symptoms and signs.

Endocarditis can be a life-threatening disorder. Cardiac valves that may be affected by endocarditis include both native and cardiac valve prosthesis along with other involved structures including permanent pacemakers, implanted cardioverter-defibrillators, or anything that is implanted and sites of previous repair of heart defects.

Risk factors for the development of endocarditis include aging, diabetes, immunosuppressed state, IV drug use, congenital heart disease, and any implanted cardiovascular device. Despite optimal care, mortality rate approaches 30%.[289]

EPIDEMIOLOGY

Endocarditis can occur at any age. Men are typically affected twice as often as women. Patients at highest risk are those who have pathogens inoculated into the body such as that seen with IV drug use. Normal heart valves are fairly resistant to both bacteria and fungi as they do not easily adhere to the endocardial surface. Constant blood flow in the heart also flushes away these pathogens on the endocardial surfaces. Patients with endocarditis who have a predisposing abnormality of the endocardium or who have microorganisms introduced into the systemic circulation are at increased risk for the development of endocarditis.

Endocarditis occurs most often in the MV and AoV while right-sided endocarditis most often occurs on the TV, which is the valve that receives the highest inoculum of pathogens that enter the body from the venous circulation. Major classifications of endocarditis include subacute bacterial endocarditis (SBE), acute bacterial endocarditis (ABE), and prosthetic valve endocarditis (PVE). SBE develops insidiously with slow progression over weeks to months. There may not be an overt source of infection or portal of entry that is identified. This condition may develop on abnormal valves after asymptomatic bacteremia following musculoskeletal, cutaneous, GI, or genitourinary infections. ABE occurs abruptly with rapid progression. Normal valves may be affected. PVE is most likely to occur within 1 year following valve replacement. Both mechanical and bioprosthetic valves may be affected. Infections occurring within 2 months of prosthetic valve placement are typically caused by contamination during surgery with *Staphylococcus epidermidis* being most commonly identified pathogen. Late phase PVE occurs with low virulence organisms and can result from transient asymptomatic bacteremia.

The incidence of IE has increased to 15 cases per 100,000 population.[290] Increased numbers are related to the higher number of permanent cardiovascular devices being implanted, more invasive intravenous catheters being placed in critical care units, increased number of patients undergoing hemodialysis, and increased access to echocardiogram allowing a diagnosis to be made.[288]

Staphylococcus aureus is the predominant pathogen present in about 40% of cases.[290] It can invade and survive within endothelial cells and has a predilection to infecting endovascular tissue.

PATHOPHYSIOLOGY

Endocarditis most commonly affects the heart valves in patients who have congenital heart defects, rheumatic valvular disease, bicuspid valves, MVP, hypertrophic cardiomyopathy, or previous bouts of endocarditis. Prosthetic valves are highest risk. For patients who have noninfected endocarditis, the fibrin-platelet vegetation settles in areas of the endocardium where it releases tissue factors that start the inflammatory cascade.

Microorganisms entering the heart can result from infections of central venous catheters, IV drug use, abscesses, peritonitis, or urinary tract infections. Bacteria can be introduced into the bloodstream during invasive dental and surgical procedures but even a small amount of inoculum can occur during tooth brushing in patients who have gingivitis.

Streptococci and *S. aureus* cause 80% to 90% of cases of IE. Enterococci, gram-negative bacilli, HACEK (*Haemophilus* species, *Aggregatibacter* [formerly *Actinobacillus*] species, *Cardiobacterium hominis, Eikenella corrodens,* and *Kingella* species), and fungi cause the remainder of infections.[291] After colonization with these bacteria, a layer of fibrin and platelets covers these organisms which prevent action by host defenses such as neutrophils, immunoglobulins, and complement.

Once microorganisms adhere to the endocardium, myocardial abscesses develop and destroy tissues and can affect the conductive system if abscesses occur at sites where cardiac automaticity occurs. Valvular incompetence can develop suddenly resulting in HF as vegetations prevent full closure of these valves making them incompetent. Aortitis can result from contiguous spread of infection. Prosthetic valve infections can involve ring abscesses, large vegetations causing obstruction, and mycotic aneurysms leading to dehiscence and conductive disturbances.

Right-sided lesions produce septic pulmonary emboli and left-sided lesions can embolize to any tissue, particularly the kidneys, spleen, and central nervous system (CNS). Mycotic aneurysms can form in any major artery. Cutaneous and retinal emboli may occur. Diffuse glomerulonephritis results from immune complex deposition.

MEDICAL HISTORY AND CLINICAL PRESENTATION

Patients with IE may have a history of IV drug use, implantation of a cardiac device, history of surgery for correction of congenital heart disease, or repair/replacement of a heart valve. Any circumstance in which there is transient bacteremia can result in the development of endocarditis. In the setting of SBE, there may not be any overt clue to the development of bacteremia.

SIGNS AND SYMPTOMS

SBE causes vague constitutional symptoms such as low-grade fever, malaise, and weight loss. Patients may have chills and arthralgias. Patients eventually will develop fever and new-onset murmur or change in previously identified murmur. Regurgitant murmurs can lead to the development of a patient having signs and symptoms consistent with congestive HF. Palatal petechiae may be found.

PHYSICAL EXAMINATION

In the setting of SBE, physical examination can be normal but if signs are present, patients may have pallor, fever, new onset or change in a preexisting murmur, and tachycardia. Roth spots may develop; they are retinal emboli that are described as round or oval hemorrhagic retinal lesions with small white centers. Osler nodes are painful erythematous subcutaneous nodules in the fingers and toes and Janeway lesions are nontender hemorrhagic macules on the palms and soles. Patients may develop splinter hemorrhages under the nails. Patients may present with CNS symptoms such as TIAs, stroke, or subarachnoid hemorrhage if there is rupture of an infected brain aneurysm. Gross hematuria can occur if renal emboli are present. Prolonged infection can result in clubbing of the fingers. Patients with ABE and PVE can have the same type of signs and symptoms but with a much more rapid course.

TABLE 5.23 Differential Diagnosis for Infective Endocarditis

Diagnosis	Description and Differentiating Features
Rheumatic fever	Carditis can occur with rheumatic fever but there is also arthritis, subcutaneous nodules, chorea, and erythema marginatum along with preceding strep infection.
Atrial myxoma	Tumor in the atrium that is gelatinous and may produce emboli. Chest x-ray shows a small atrium with echocardiogram demonstrating the tumor.
Libman-Sachs endocarditis	Seen in the setting of systemic lupus erythematosus with patients having positive antinuclear antibody and antiphospholipid antibody. Blood cultures are negative as this condition is inflammatory and not infectious.
Noninfectious endocarditis	Can be the result of malignancy, systemic lupus erythematosus, tuberculosis, or HIV infection. Valve destruction occurs without bacteremia. Condition results from underlying carcinoma or hypercoagulable state. Evaluation can identify the underlying cause.

DIFFERENTIAL DIAGNOSIS

The differential diagnosis for IE is summarized in Table 5.23.

DIAGNOSTIC STUDIES

Diagnostic studies for IE are summarized in Table 5.24.[292]

EVALUATION

Any patient with bacteremia should be suspected of having IE, especially if the patient has either a newly discovered heart murmur or a change in a previously identified heart murmur. Murmurs that are regurgitant are more concerning for IE than systolic murmurs. Patients develop fever at some

TABLE 5.24 Diagnostic Studies for Infective Endocarditis

Diagnostic Intervention	Rationale/Findings
Blood cultures	A series of three blood cultures are obtained prior to initiation of antibiotic therapy in order to identify the pathogen. Blood cultures should ideally be performed 1 hour apart from each other. All three blood cultures should be positive because bacteremia is continuous.
Echocardiogram	Transthoracic echocardiogram is first-line test to identify vegetations in the heart with transesophageal echocardiogram being reserved for patients with high suspicion of endocarditis who have a negative transthoracic echocardiogram.
Use of clinical criteria	Revised Duke clinical diagnostic criteria include having two or three positive blood cultures, echocardiographic evidence of endocardial involvement showing oscillating intracardiac mass on heart valve, cardiac abscess, dehiscence of prosthetic valve, and new onset of valvular regurgitation as the major criteria.
Additional supporting laboratory studies	Complete blood count showing elevated white blood cell count and possibly a normal chromic, normocytic anemia; erythrocyte sedimentation rate and C-reactive protein being elevated; and increased immunoglobulin levels, and urinalysis showing microscopic hematuria with or without pyuria. EKG should be performed in order to assess for cardiac conduction abnormality.
Testing in the setting of high index of suspicion but negative blood cultures	Serologic studies, histopathology, and polymerase chain reaction assays have distinct roles in the diagnosis of infective endocarditis when blood cultures have tested negative with the highest yield obtained from serologic studies.

Source: Data from Pericart L, Bernard A, Bourguignon T, et al. Comparison of outcome of possible versus definite infective endocarditis involving native heart valves. Am J Cardiol. *2017;119:1854–1861. doi:10.1016/j.amjcard.2017.02.039*

TABLE 5.25 Pathogens and Preferred Antibiotics for Infective Endocarditis

Pathogen	Preferred Antibiotic
Penicillin-susceptible to streptococcus viridans or *Streptococcus gallolyticus* (formerly *S. bovis*)	Penicillin G, ampicillin, ceftriaxone, or amoxicillin plus gentamicin for at least 2 weeks; vancomycin for 4 weeks for those unable to tolerate the preceding therapy
Penicillin-resistant streptococci	Beta-lactam plus gentamicin or vancomycin with or without gentamicin
Methicillin-sensitive staphylococci	Beta-lactam; vancomycin; daptomycin; or trimethoprim/sulfamethoxazole plus clindamycin; 6 weeks of nafcillin for left-sided valvular disease; cefazolin for those with allergies to preceding drugs
Methicillin-resistant staphylococci	Vancomycin; daptomycin; or trimethoprim/ sulfamethoxazole plus clindamycin
Coagulase-negative staphylococci	Vancomycin plus rifampin and gentamicin
Penicillin-sensitive enterococci	Beta-lactam or vancomycin plus aminoglycoside
Penicillin-resistant enterococci (beta-lactamase producing)	Ampicillin/sulbactam or vancomycin plus gentamicin
Penicillin-resistant *Enterococcus faecium*	Linezolid or daptomycin
HACEK organisms	Ceftriaxone; ampicillin/sulbactam with or without gentamicin; ciprofloxacin; ampicillin
IV drug abusers	Nafcillin
Prosthetic valve endocarditis	Similar treatment as native valve treatment based upon most likely pathogen based upon risk
Prophylactic antibiotic regimen for high risk patients for infective endocarditis	Amoxicillin 2 g as a single dose 30 to 60 minutes prior to procedure; ampicillin 2 g IV or IM or penicillin VK 2 g orally or cephalexin 2 g orally, or cefazolin 1 g IV or IM or ceftriaxone 1 g IV/IM or clindamycin 600 mg orally or IV

HACEK, Haemophilus *species,* Aggregatibacter *[formerly Actinobacillus] species,* Cardiobacterium hominis, Eikenella corrodens, *and* Kingella *species; IM, intramuscular; IV, intravenous.*

point in their illness. Blood cultures are mandatory in order to determine the appropriate antimicrobial therapy.

TREATMENT

If vegetations are <1 cm antibiotics will typically resolve this infection. IV antibiotics are the mainstay of therapy with treatment based upon identification of the organism and its susceptibility patterns (Table 5.25)[293]. Antibiotics must be given for a prolonged course. Surgery may be needed for mechanical complications or resistant organisms. Antibiotics are given for 2 to 8 weeks with home IV antibiotic therapy commonly arranged.

Surgical treatment is needed in order to debride necrotic tissue, drain abscesses, or remove foreign material or infected devices. Infected IV catheters need to be removed. Treatment failure may occur because of biofilms adherent to catheters and other devices.

Surgical treatment is indicated for patients with severe MR even in the absence of congestive HF, with mitral annular abscess, uncontrolled sepsis, or multiple embolisms. MV replacement/repair is considered the standard treatment for MV endocarditis that does not respond to antibiotic therapy.

The elderly are most likely to develop IE because of their multiple comorbidities along with the need for valve prosthesis replacement and increased need for placement of cardiac pacemaker.[288]

PATIENT EDUCATION

Antibiotic prophylaxis is now recommended only for patients with underlying cardiac conditions associated with the highest risk of developing IE such as patients with prosthetic valves or previous valve repairs, patients with unrepaired cyanotic congenital heart disease or previously repaired congenital heart disease with residual shunts, or patients with previous cardiac transplant with valvular regurgitation due to a structurally abnormal valve.

Prophylaxis is recommended for dental procedures involving manipulation of gingival tissue or periapical region of teeth or perforation of the oral mucosa. Other procedures requiring prophylaxis include invasive procedures of the respiratory tract and treatment of infected skin or musculoskeletal tissues. Prophylaxis is not recommended for genitourinary or GI tract procedures.

Of all treatment options for prophylaxis, amoxicillin is typically preferred because of higher and more sustained serum concentration arising from increased GI absorption. Clindamycin is the preferred choice for patients allergic to penicillin.

The majority of cases of IE occur independently of medical-surgical procedures and there should be ongoing education to prevent illicit drug use and improve dental hygiene in order to prevent bacteremia.[294]

SPECIAL CONSIDERATIONS

It is more difficult to diagnose IE because of its sometimes subtle presentation. IE should be part of the differential diagnosis for any patient with constitutional symptoms that include fever, which is the most common sign associated with this condition. A new or changing heart murmur should also raise the suspicion for IE. Blood cultures and echocardiography are essential to perform for patients suspected of having this condition.

KEY POINTS

- The incidence of IE continues to increase as patients are living longer and having more invasive procedures along with an escalation in IV drug use.
- Acute IE has rapid progression of symptoms.
- Blood cultures should be given prior to institution of antibiotic therapy in order to prevent false negative blood cultures.

5.10 MYOCARDITIS

Christine Bruce

Myocarditis involves inflammation of the cardiac myocytes that results in acute HF. Myocarditis is underdiagnosed because there are multiple other causes of acute HF, sudden death, and chronic dilated cardiomyopathy. Patients present with nonspecific symptoms including chest pain, dyspnea and palpitations, and complaints consistent with coronary artery disease.[295] Causes of myocarditis include viruses, bacteria, toxins, and various immune syndromes. Viruses are the most common cause of myocarditis that can be manifested as an upper respiratory infection (URI). These URIs are typically caused by adenovirus or echovirus virus. Other viruses leading to myocarditis include parvovirus B19, human herpesvirus 6, and coxsackievirus.[296] Injury to the heart occurs because of early destruction of the myocytes by the virus followed by an immune response causing further destruction.

COVID-19 contributes to cardiovascular complications such as acute myocardial injury as a result of ACS, myocarditis, stress-induced cardiomyopathy, arrhythmias, cardiogenic shock, and cardiac arrest.[140]

Eosinophilic myocarditis (EM) is an acute life-threatening inflammatory disease of the heart. Primary symptom of this condition is dyspnea upon exertion. Peripheral eosinophilia is observed in three-fourths of patients with this condition. This condition leads to an impaired ejection fraction. EM is seen more commonly in the setting of hypersensitivity and eosinophilic granulomatosis with polyangiitis. Corticosteroids are the mainstay of treatment for this condition.[297]

COVID-19-related myocarditis occurs as a result of direct viral injury along with cardiac damage due to the host's immune response. These patients will have a change in the EKG and cardiac biomarkers along with impaired cardiac function. These patients typically may not have significant coronary artery disease to explain the symptoms. Cardiac biomarkers are increased so it is necessary to rule out MI as a cause of the elevation in these markers. The long-term impact of COVID-19 myocarditis remains unknown.[298]

Patients may be asymptomatic prior to the development of myocarditis or could have a viral prodrome. Patients present with acute HF symptoms of dyspnea upon exertion, cough, fatigue, and edema. Cardiac MRI and endomyocardial biopsy can be used to make definitive diagnosis. These studies may be necessary for patients who develop acute HF that remains unexplained. This diagnosis is difficult to make as a result of its heterogeneous presentations and wide variety of pathogens causing myocarditis.[299]

Treatment of myocarditis is the same as management of HF. NSAIDs are of no benefit for treatment of this condition. Prognosis is related to the severity of the HF. Pericarditis may occur in the setting of myocarditis.

Diagnostic approach to myocarditis includes EKG, serum cardiac markers, assessment of markers of inflammation with erythrocyte sedimentation rate or C-reactive protein, and echocardiogram.

5.11 RHEUMATIC HEART DISEASE

Christine Bruce

OVERVIEW

RHD continues to be a major burden in developing countries where it causes most of the cardiovascular morbidity and mortality in young people. This condition results from an abnormal autoimmune response to group A streptococcal infections in a genetically susceptible host.[300]

Acute rheumatic fever is the precursor to RHD and other organs besides the heart can be affected. When the heart is involved with this condition, there may be irreversible valve damage and the development of HF.

Penicillin is an effective prevention against RHD, but it does not prevent group A streptococcal-related glomerulonephritis. Following the development of rheumatic fever, antibiotic prophylaxis is recommended against recurrent episodes of acute rheumatic fever and this is recommended in endemic areas.

RHD is most commonly seen in patients who have limited access to antibiotic therapy for group A beta-hemolytic streptococcal infection; 40% to 60% of patients with acute rheumatic fever develop RHD.[301] Rheumatic carditis is a pericarditis affecting the pericardium, myocardium, and endocardium. Pericarditis is the most characteristic manifestation of acute rheumatic carditis causing precordial or retrosternal chest pain that is relieved when the patient sits or leans forward. RHD may be associated with a pericardial friction rub. Pericarditis and myocarditis patients typically have complete recovery following an acute episode of rheumatic fever.[302]

EPIDEMIOLOGY

RHD leads to about 250,000 deaths per year worldwide.[300] RHD is the leading cause of MS and is seen more commonly in women than men. Patients who are diagnosed with MS should be evaluated for possible RHD as the underlying cause for the development of MS. Rheumatic fever incidence in the Western world had substantially declined over the past five decades but this trend is reversing due to immigration from nonindustrialized countries where the incidence of RHD is higher.[303]

PATHOPHYSIOLOGY

RHD leading to MS causes fusion of the mitral commissures followed by calcification of the valve and structural abnormalities just below the valve.[304] RHD causes the MV leaflets to be thickened with the posterior leaflet being relatively immobile and moving parallel to the anterior leaflet of the MV during systole. There is no associated abnormal formation of the papillary muscle that occurs.[302]

In the setting of RHD, the AoV can have fusion of the commissioners of the AoV making this a distinctive feature of RHD. These patients will also have concentric enlargement of the LV as a result of pressure overload of the LV as the heart attempts to empty blood from a narrowed orifice.[304]

MEDICAL HISTORY AND CLINICAL PRESENTATION

RHD patients with acute myocarditis can present with mild symptoms such as tachycardia or worsening of HF symptoms. Myocarditis can lead to conduction disturbances such as a first-degree AV heart block.[302]

MS caused by RHD causes fatigue from impaired cardiac output, dyspnea from the LA being unable to have forward repulsion of the blood, increased pulmonary pressures with right-sided HF leading to lower extremity edema, hepatomegaly, and jugular venous distention. Symptoms initially occur with exertion because exercise shortens diastolic filling time and increases venous return to the heart in order to have an increase in cardiac output to the exercising muscles.

Patients who have RHD leading to MS may be diagnosed during pregnancy where there is increased blood volume and cardiac output. Other presenting symptoms include new-onset AF with or without systemic embolization or even hemoptysis.

Exertional dyspnea, syncope, and angina are the most common presenting symptoms for AS, but the symptoms will not appear until the stenosis is severe. Once symptoms occur, life expectancy is dramatically altered, and surgical intervention is recommended as soon as symptoms develop.

SIGNS AND SYMPTOMS

Dyspnea that initially occurs with exertion, coughing and wheezing from increased pulmonary pressure, peripheral edema in the dependent regions of the body, hepatomegaly, and increased jugular venous distention are the symptoms seen with RHD. Auscultation of the heart can reveal an opening snap of the MV as the MV is the only valve that can manifest an opening snap.

Because of overload of the LA caused by MS, left atrial enlargement occurs which can lead to AF and development of left atrial thrombus leading to systemic embolization if the thrombus is extracted from the LA.

AS classically causes dyspnea upon exertion, angina, and syncope but these findings occur late in the course of the disease. Chronic AR causes dyspnea, fatigue, and angina.

PHYSICAL EXAMINATION

The physical exam for patients with RHD leading to MS includes a loud S1 when the MV closes, increased impulse felt in the precordium, an opening snap during diastole, increased pulmonic component of S2, and a diastolic rumble with or without murmur that is heard best at the apex of the heart. This murmur can be accentuated by listening to the patient in the left lateral decubitus position. Additionally, there may be signs of pulmonary congestion depending on the severity of the lesion and the volume status of the patient.

Physical exam findings in the setting of severe AS include a late peaking systolic murmur, diminished aortic component of the S2, pulsus tardus (delay in the carotid upstroke), and pulses parvus (decreased amplitude of the pulse caused by low cardiac output). The murmur of AS is best heard in the right upper sternal border. This murmur can radiate into the carotid arteries.

Physical exam findings occurring in the setting of rheumatic-induced AR include bounding peripheral pulses, displacement of the left ventricular apex, and a diastolic decrescendo murmur heard along the right sternal border (aortic root pathology) or left sternal border (valve pathology).

Patients with chronic MR develop a blowing holosystolic murmur heard best at the apex. If the LV is dilated, the apical impulse can be displaced laterally and an S3 may be heard, especially if there is left ventricular dysfunction.

DIFFERENTIAL DIAGNOSIS

The differential diagnosis for RHD is summarized in Table 5.26.

DIAGNOSTIC STUDIES

TTE is the diagnostic study of choice used for patients with MS as this procedure can measure the MV aperture allowing classification of the severity of his condition, pulmonary pressures, and right ventricular function. Severe MS occurs when the MV measures 1.5 cm or less, which corresponds to a mean mitral gradient of more than 5 to 10 mm Hg in the setting of a normal heart rate. Stress echocardiography can be used to assess the response of the mitral gradient and pulmonary pressures when the patient has exertional activity if the diagnosis is in question.

EVALUATION

Patients suspected of having MS caused by RHD need to have a baseline EKG in order to assess for left atrial enlargement, right ventricular hypertrophy caused by cor pulmonale, and AF. Echocardiogram is initially ordered and performed serially every 3 to 5 years to assess the MV aperture and progression of the condition.

TREATMENT

Treatment of rheumatic carditis involves anti-inflammatories with corticosteroids considered to be the treatment of choice with these being given for 4 to 6 weeks or until the inflammatory markers return to normal.[302]

TABLE 5.26 Differential Diagnosis for Rheumatic Heart Disease

Valvular Damage Associated With Rheumatic Heart Disease	Description and Differentiating Features/Findings
Aortic stenosis	Aortic stenosis caused by rheumatic heart disease (RHD) is most likely to occur after or concomitantly with mitral stenosis. This condition is most likely to be secondary to a bicuspid aortic valve rather than RHD as degeneration of the aortic valve occurs in this setting.
Tricuspid stenosis	Nearly always caused by RHD. Since mitral stenosis is virtually always present in this setting, symptoms are more dramatically seen secondary to mitral valve disease. Tricuspid stenosis symptoms include elevated jugular venous pressure, hepatic congestion, and peripheral edema along with a diastolic rumble. If surgery is performed for mitral stenosis, tricuspid stenosis surgery can be addressed at the same time.
Aortic regurgitation	RHD can lead to chronic aortic regurgitation in which volume overload causes progressive left ventricular dilation and eccentric hypertrophy. Symptoms associated with chronic aortic regurgitation include shortness of breath, fatigue, and angina.
Mitral regurgitation	Mitral regurgitation can arise from any part of the complex valve apparatus, which includes the leaflets, annulus, chordae, papillary muscles, and left ventricular free walls. RHD can also cause mitral regurgitation as a result of damage to the mitral valve.

MS caused by RHD is treated in the same manner as MS caused by other conditions. In the setting of AF, warfarin is the currently preferred medication given to prevent thromboembolism. Currently, novel oral anticoagulants (NOACs) have not received formal approval to prevent clot formation in the setting of VHD, but this recommendation may change in the future. Studies to date have evaluated the role of NOACs for anticoagulation with valvular disease but these studies have excluded patients with MS.[305] What has been identified is that patients with AS and MS are at increased risk for both the development of thromboembolism and bleeding when using anticoagulants.[306]

Medical therapy for patients with MS is in the form of medications having negative chronotropic activity such as beta blockers, diuretics, and long-acting nitrates as these agents can improve transvalvular flow across the MV.

Patients with rheumatic-induced MS who need clinical intervention are best treated with PBMC. This procedure is indicated for patients who have a pliable MV but who have ongoing symptoms and in patients who are asymptomatic but have a MV area <1 cm. Patients who have severe stenosis or symptoms in the setting of a nonpliable valve or who are having heart surgery for another reason should undergo MV replacement instead of PBMC.

Indications for AVR include patients who become symptomatic in the setting of AS, those with impaired left ventricular systolic function with ejection fraction <50% in patients who have not yet developed symptoms, or in the setting of a patient having cardiac surgery for another reason. AVR could be considered in patients who have abnormal exercise testing especially if hypotension develops during exercise.

AVR can be done through a traditional open approach or via transcatheter approach with both procedures having similar outcomes. Balloon valvuloplasty could be used as a bridge therapy prior to definitive AVR.

Patients with chronic AR can have medical therapy in the form of dihydropyridine calcium channel blockers, ACEIs, or ARBs if these patients concomitantly have hypertension. Medical therapy is also recommended for symptomatic patients who are not surgical candidates.

In the setting of chronic AR, open AVR is indicated for patients who have symptoms, those who have left ventricular dysfunction, or patients undergoing cardiac surgery for other reasons.

Patients with chronic severe MR have the best outcome with surgery. Surgery is indicated in symptomatic patients with left ventricular ejection fraction >30%, asymptomatic patients with left ventricular dysfunction with ejection fraction of 30% to 60%, and for patients undergoing another type of cardiac surgery. MV repair should be considered in asymptomatic patients who have developed new-onset AF or pulmonary hypertension. Surgical repair is preferred of replacement. Medical therapy with vasodilators is not beneficial in the absence of symptoms or left ventricular dysfunction.

Patients who are not surgical candidates can undergo MV repair with catheter-based clip device delivered percutaneously. This clip helps closure of the MV leaflets reducing regurgitation.

PATIENT EDUCATION

The most common cause of death related to RHD is HF followed by thromboembolism, which occurs most commonly in the setting of AF caused by MS. With an increase in the immigrant population from developing countries into the United States, acute rheumatic fever and its complication of RHD needs to be taken into consideration. Treatment of acute rheumatic fever within 7 days of group A streptococcal pharyngitis prevents rheumatic fever and all of its sequelae except for glomerulonephritis, which occurs as a result of immune complex deposition within nephrogenic strain of group A streptococcal infection. Patients with group A beta-hemolytic streptococcal infection should be treated with penicillin either with a single IM injection or for 10 days orally in order to eradicate this pathogen.

SPECIAL CONSIDERATIONS

In addition to beta-hemolytic group A streptococcal infection, there appears to be a genetic predisposition to the development of acute rheumatic fever. Antibiotics given within 7 days of group A streptococcal pharyngitis prevents the development of rheumatic fever. Antibiotic therapy consists of a single IM dose of benzathine penicillin or 10-day course of penicillin orally.

KEY POINTS

- The incidence of rheumatic fever is increasing in the United States as a result of immigration of patients who have endemic group A beta-hemolytic streptococcal infection without the benefit of antibiotic therapy.
- Rheumatic carditis can be prevented by the appropriate treatment of group A beta-hemolytic streptococcal infection with penicillin as there is no known resistance to penicillin therapy.
- Acute manifestations of RHD is carditis, but due to nonspecific symptoms of carditis, diagnosis is elusive unless clinicians have a high index of suspicion.
- Initial manifestations of acute rheumatic carditis involve MR but patients may only be diagnosed decades later when MS occurs.
- MV repair via balloon commissurotomy is the preferred surgical intervention for patients with symptomatic MS.

5.12 PERIPHERAL ARTERIAL DISEASE

Christine Bruce

OVERVIEW

PAD is characterized by the narrowing of the aortic bifurcation and arteries of the lower extremities or narrowing in the arteries feeding into the upper extremities as these arteries are also peripheral arteries. Lower extremity arterial involvement includes the iliac, femoral, popliteal, and tibial arteries. PAD of the upper extremities primarily involves the origin of the subclavian arteries. The most common cause of PAD is atherosclerosis.

PAD is a coronary artery disease risk equivalent placing patients at risk for MI and stroke. The classic presentation of PAD is calf pain with ambulation but other patients may have atypical symptoms such as peripheral weakness and paresthesia. Patients with nonhealing arterial ulcers are considered to have PAD until proven otherwise.

The initial evaluation for patient suspected of having PAD is by noninvasive screening with ankle-brachial index (ABI), which compares the blood pressure in the ankle is to the blood pressure in the brachial artery. Patient suspected of having PAD affecting the upper extremity should have a comparison of blood pressure between the arms.

PAD serves as a marker for cardiovascular disease. Patients who have ABI of <.90 have a three to six times increase in death from cardiovascular disease.[307] Although intermittent claudication is a well-known presenting symptom for PAD, the majority of patients with PAD are asymptomatic, meaning that a high index of suspicion for PAD is needed to make the diagnosis for early intervention in order to prevent complications from atherosclerosis and coronary disease.[308] Risk factors for the development of PAD are smoking, diabetes, and aging. Patients typically will begin to develop PAD around age 40 with the incidence increasing with aging as a result of the progression of atherosclerosis.

EPIDEMIOLOGY

PAD occurs with atherosclerosis with an increased risk for the development of this condition in patients who smoke, have diabetes, or are hypertensive with smoking constituting the largest risk factor. Women tend to have a greater tendency to develop PAD than men, but this might be the result of women living longer and atherosclerosis becoming more prevalent in the aging population.[309] Asymptomatic PAD is several times more common in the general population than in patients who have intermittent claudication. The incidence of PAD increases to more than 10% among patients in their 60s and 70s. PAD is associated with an increased incidence of both coronary and cerebrovascular disease.[310]

PATHOPHYSIOLOGY

PAD is due to blockage of the artery supplying blood to the upper or lower limbs typically secondary to atherosclerosis. Claudication, the most common symptom that occurs in the setting of PAD is caused by arterial obstruction, inflammation, vascular dysfunction, reduced microvascular blood flow, impaired angiogenesis, and altered skeletal muscle function.[311]

MEDICAL HISTORY AND CLINICAL PRESENTATION

Evaluation of the patient begins with a careful history. Patients with vascular disease often have intermittent symptoms and may not volunteer their symptoms unless directly asked. When questioning the patient about ambulation, the clinician should ask if there are any limitations to walking long distances or walking uphill. Patient should be asked about skin issues and foot ulcers and about the type of footwear that is worn as pressure points on the foot can result in ulceration with difficulty healing.

Patients with atherosclerosis, diabetes, hypertension, or who smoke should be suspected of having PAD since PAD can occur without symptoms. Patient's may admit to limiting activity but may not be clear as to why they are not exercising as much as they had done in the past. Some patients will complain of claudication that occurs with exercise with symptoms abating after stopping exercise. Patients may complain of having thin, shiny skin as a result of arterial insufficiency. Some patients may present with arterial ulcers. Patients with acute arterial occlusion will present with the classic 6 Ps: pain, pallor, paralysis, paresthesias, poikilothermia, and pulselessness. Patient's having nonhealing arterial ulcers are considered to have PAD until proven otherwise.

SIGNS AND SYMPTOMS

Patients may present with classic intermittent claudication in the calf with activity that causes the onset of symptoms sooner with activity as the condition progresses. For asymptomatic patients with PAD, diagnosis is suspected when patients are found to have an abnormal ABI. In addition to exertional claudication, patients may also have exertional leg pain, progressive disease–causing pain at rest, nonhealing arterial wounds, ischemic ulcers, and gangrene. Patients having PAD affecting the upper extremities can present with arm claudication, ischemia in the upper extremity, or dizziness when the upper extremity is exercised in the setting of subclavian steal syndrome.

Patients with PAD may have progressive disease before they are identified. These patients may present with pain at rest, tissue ulceration, nonhealing ulcers, and gangrene. These patients will self-limit their activities due to pain and are at increased risk to undergo amputation. Because PAD is a coronary artery disease equivalent, these patients are at increased risk for cardiovascular mortality.

PHYSICAL EXAMINATION

Physical examination starts with comparison of blood pressure in both arms if upper extremity PAD is suspected. A differential of >15 mm Hg is consistent with subclavian stenosis. Assessment of pulses and bruits is performed. The diameter of the abdominal aorta is assessed to assess for aneurysm. The lower extremities are elevated to assess for pallor followed by placing the lowering of the extremities in dependent position to assess how long it takes for blood to return and for dependent rubor. The feet are carefully examined to assess for skin breakdown, ulceration, fissures, calluses, and tinea.

DIFFERENTIAL DIAGNOSIS

Patients who have intermittent claudication will need to have PAD differentiated from spinal stenosis as this is the primary condition in the differential diagnosis (Table 5.27)[312]. Patients with acute arterial occlusion can develop this condition from progressive atherosclerotic narrowing to the point where blood flow distally is significantly impacted versus embolic blockage from a more central source.

DIAGNOSTIC STUDIES

Clinical evaluation begins with performing an ABI. Blood pressures are checked at the brachial artery and this is compared to the blood pressure obtained in the lower extremity at the dorsalis pedis and posterior tibial arteries. The ABI is calculated using the higher ankle pressure in each leg divided by the higher brachial artery pressure. Normal measurements include the ankle pressures that are the same or slightly higher than the brachial pressure, so normal ABIs are between 1.00 and 1.40. ABI measurements between 0.9 up to 1.0 are considered borderline with mild to moderate PAD being identified at ABIs between 0.41 and 0.90 and severe PAD being <0.40. ABIs >1.40 indicate noncompressible, calcified arteries in the lower extremities making this measurement invalid. For these patients, a toe-brachial index can be used and if this

TABLE 5.27 Differential Diagnosis for Peripheral Arterial Disease

Diagnosis	Description and Differentiating Features
Spinal stenosis	"Pseudoclaudicaton." Patient complains of cramping, tightness, aching, fatigue, weakness or numbness in the calf with activity. Symptoms are typically bilateral. Discomfort can continue with just standing. Symptoms improve with sitting and leaning forward at the waist. Symptoms may continue for up to 30 minutes.
Charcot foot	Diabetic neuropathic osteoarthropathy occurs as a result of recurrent microtrauma to foot with impaired sensation. Neurovascular changes are caused by pathologic innervation of blood vessels as a result of diabetes.[312]
Erysipelas	Redness of the foot due to infection with streptococcus when this infection occurs in the lower extremities. No clear wound edge as margins of wound are indistinct.
Arthritis	Hip arthritis causes groin pain most commonly with symptoms worsening with activity. Knee arthritis with active inflammation can cause a Baker cyst, which can rupture leading to calf pain. ABI measurement in these patients is normal.
Radiculopathy	Lumbar radiculopathy results in pain radiating down the posterior thigh into the calf with symptoms sometimes worsening with activity. Patients may have a history of back pain. Ankle-brachial index is normal.

number is <0.70, it is considered equivalent positive for PAD.

Patient is having borderline measurements can undergo an exercise ABI test that includes ABI measurements at rest and after treadmill walking or performing plantar flexion exercises. If the ankle pressure decreases >30 mm Hg or if the postexercise ABI decreases >20%, PAD is suggested as a diagnosis.

Segmental blood pressure measurements can be performed to localize diseased vessels. Blood pressures are taken at several locations in the lower extremities in order to localize the area of arterial narrowing.

Diagnostic tests used in the evaluation of PAD include arterial duplex ultrasonography, CTA, and MRA. These invasive tests are used preoperatively for planned endovascular or surgical revascularization procedures. Patients with upper extremity PAD undergo similar tests in anticipation of surgical intervention.

EVALUATION

Screening is not recommended for asymptomatic patients. Patients with intermittent claudication or those who have signs of arterial disease including arterial ulcers, thin, shiny atrophic skin, or leg weakness or paresthesias should have ABI performed as the initial test following history taking and physical exam.[313] Diagnostic accuracy is improved with the use of handheld Doppler studies of the peripheral arteries in order to supplement the history and physical examination findings.[314]

TREATMENT

The initial treatment of PAD consists of addressing the risk factors such as smoking cessation, control of diabetes, and statin therapy for atherosclerosis. Walking programs to improve collateral circulation in the lower extremities are encouraged. The ultimate goal of therapy is to improve functional status, symptoms of claudication, and prevention of tissue loss and amputation.

Smoking cessation is of primary importance. Control of blood pressure can also be an effective therapy in the management of PAD. Blood pressure target of <130/80 mm Hg is encouraged. There are no specific classes of blood pressure medications that are recommended over others.

Antiplatelet monotherapy in patients with PAD reduces the risk for MI, stroke, and peripheral arterial events. Aspirin is considered the primary antiplatelet agent in this setting. Clopidogrel can be given for those who cannot take aspirin. There is no evidence for supporting warfarin over aspirin in patients with PAD.

Encouragement of walking or even a supervised exercise program is associated with improved functional performance and is recommended for patients with intermittent claudication.

Patients with symptomatic intermittent claudication can be treated with cilostazol, which is a phosphodiesterase inhibitor that also has antiplatelet and vasodilator activity. Walking distances and symptoms can improve with the use of this agent. Once there is critical limb ischemia, surgical intervention has better outcomes than medical therapy.

Revascularization procedures improve symptoms and functional capacity. Surgery can also improve wound healing in patients with intermittent claudication or critical limb ischemia. Patients who have critical limb ischemia should be referred for surgical intervention. Revascularization can be done with surgical bypass or endovascular revascularization techniques. Endovascular revascularization includes balloon angioplasty, stenting, and atherectomy. Balloon angioplasty combined with stenting has improved long-term success when compared to angioplasty alone.

Patients with complex anatomy may need traditional surgical revascularization rather than endovascular revascularization even though recovery from traditional surgical revascularization is more difficult.

PATIENT EDUCATION

The primary risk factor for the development of PAD is atherosclerosis so patients should have counseling in order to address improvement in diet, physical activity, blood pressure, lipids, and blood sugars in the setting of diabetes. Lifestyle modifications are first-line recommendations. For patients who smoke, smoking cessation is essential because of the damage that smoking does to the arterial vessels.

SPECIAL CONSIDERATIONS

Not all patients with PAD will have symptoms but there can be progression of arterial narrowing with tissue ischemia and ulceration occurring. Exercise can help to develop collateral vessels if atherosclerosis prevents blood flow through native vessels. Patients who present with tissue ischemia will benefit with revascularization.

KEY POINTS

- PAD is one of the manifestations of atherosclerosis making it a cardiovascular equivalent.
- PAD is typically caused by atherosclerosis and it should be noted that these patients have a three- to sixfold increased risk for stroke and MI.
- Acute arterial occlusion needs aggressive treatment to prevent tissue loss.

5.12B ACUTE ARTERIAL OCCLUSION

Acute arterial occlusion occurs as a result of progressive arterial narrowing or acute embolic phenomenon. Risk factors for the development of acute arterial occlusion include aortic atherosclerosis, arterial trauma, recent MI, and AF.[315] COVID-19 infection can be a risk factor for the development of both arterial and venous thromboembolism (VTE) because of excessive inflammation, hypoxia, immobilization, and disseminated intravascular coagulation.[316] Arterial occlusion can occur in the setting of total knee replacement with this risk increasing with longer tourniquet operative times.[317]

Acute arterial occlusion leads to acute leg ischemia, which carries a high risk of amputation and death if left untreated. Catheter-directed thrombolysis can be used to dissolve the clot along with surgical embolectomy to remove the site of obstruction. Surgical or percutaneous revascularization is also part of the management of this condition.[318]

5.13 PERIPHERAL VENOUS DISEASE

Christine Bruce

OVERVIEW

Chronic venous insufficiency is a condition in which the veins or valves of the lower extremities are incompetent with resultant pooling of blood into the legs. Venous hypertension is a primary contributor to this condition in some patients along with this condition being acquired on a congenital basis. Chronic venous insufficiency is twice as prevalent as coronary artery disease in the United States.[319]

Patients with a history of previous DVT are at risk for the development of chronic venous insufficiency because of the dilation of the venous system that occurs with this condition.

Since many risk factors for the development of DVT are known, prevention of this condition is preferred over treatment if DVT develops. Despite these risks being known, thromboprophylaxis has been shown to be underutilized. In the absence of prophylaxis, rates as high as 50% have been reported following orthopedic surgery, and 25% following general surgery.[320]

Chronic venous insufficiency results in impaired venous return resulting in lower extremity discomfort, edema, and skin changes. Post-phlebotic or post-thrombotic syndrome is a symptomatic chronic venous insufficiency state that occurs after the development of DVT. Diagnosis of this condition is by history, physical exam, and duplex ultrasound. Patients with chronic venous insufficiency tend to be older males with history of phlebitis and previous history of significant lower extremity injury while patients with varicose veins tend to be female with a family history of varicose veins.[321]

The most common inherited predisposition for venous clot formation is Leiden factor V, which causes the body to be resistant to activated protein C, while the second most common inherited pattern is prothrombin G20210A gene mutation, which increases circulating prothrombin and enhances thrombin generation. Patients inheriting this pattern are two to three times more likely to develop DVT.[322]

EPIDEMIOLOGY

Chronic venous stasis ulcers of the lower extremity affect up to 5% of the population over 65 years of age and 1.5% of the general population. This condition is caused by chronic venous disease produced by venous hypertension, which typically results from valvular incompetence within the deep venous system or by obstruction of the venous outflow.[323]

Risk factors for the development of chronic venous insufficiency include increasing age with poor venous function, family history of this condition that includes a family history of varicose veins, smoking, occupations requiring long duration of sitting or standing, and previous history of DVT.

Surgery is a known risk factor for the development of DVT with this specific population increasing their risk when patients are older, when they have a high pain index prior to surgery, and if they receive a blood transfusion in the perioperative period.[324] Risk factors for the development of DVT include a deficiency of protein C, protein S, or antithrombin III; resistance to activated protein C; pregnancy or recent childbirth; hyperhomocysteinemia; or oral contraceptive use.[325]

PATHOPHYSIOLOGY

Dilation of the veins in the lower extremity leads to an inability of the valves within these veins to properly close leading to venous hypertension. Sludging of the blood leads to further dilation of these veins producing venous varicosities. Since blood is accumulating in the dependent portions of the body instead of being propelled back into the heart, venous stasis occurs. This venous stasis leads to leakage of hemosiderin, which causes brown pigments to be deposited in the lower extremities.

The most common site for initiation of the thrombus appears to be the valve pocket sinus, due to its tendency to become hypoxic. Activation of endothelial cells by hypoxia or possibly inflammatory stimuli leads to surface expression of adhesion receptors that facilitate the binding of circulating leukocytes and microvesicles. Subsequent activation of the leukocytes induces expression of the potent procoagulant protein tissue factor that triggers thrombosis.[326]

Leiden factor V causes factor Va to be resistant to activated protein C and this is the most prevalent cause of hypercoagulability affecting 5% of the White population. Patients with deficiencies of protein C, protein S, or antithrombin III have an increased risk for venous thrombosis in settings such as using oral contraceptives or having surgery. Cancer increases thrombotic risk by producing tissue factor initiating coagulation, by shedding procoagulant lipid microparticles, and by impairing blood flow. Age is the strongest risk factor for the promotion of thrombosis as a result of fragility of the vessels contributing to stasis, increased coagulation factor levels, impaired function of the venous valves, and decreased amount of natural anticoagulation, along with increased risk of being immobile and increased risk of severe infection.[327]

MEDICAL HISTORY AND CLINICAL PRESENTATION

Venous return from the lower extremity relies on contraction of calf muscles to project the blood from the gastrocnemius veins into and through the deep veins. Venous valve supports this blood flow by directing blood proximally to the heart. Chronic venous insufficiency occurs when venous obstruction, venous valvular insufficiency, or decreased contraction of the muscles surrounding the veins prevents or lowers forward venous flow with resultant increase in venous pressure. Prolonged venous hypertension causes tissue edema, inflammation, and hypoxia which causes the symptoms. DVT is a major risk factor for the development of chronic insufficiency while other factors include trauma, age, and obesity.

Risk factors for the development of post-thrombotic syndrome following DVT include proximal thrombosis, recurrent ipsilateral DVT, and obesity.

SIGNS AND SYMPTOMS

Symptoms of chronic venous insufficiency include aching, itching, restlessness, heaviness in the legs, leg swelling, and pain. These symptoms are worse with prolonged standing or sitting. Ankle swelling due to edema commonly occurs with the edema indenting with the pressure in the affected area. Varicose veins are dilated, palpable, subcutaneous veins more than 3 mm in diameter. Lipodermatosclerosis is localized chronic inflammation and fibrosis affecting both the skin and subcutaneous tissues of the lower leg especially in the medial supramalleolar region. This condition occurs from capillary proliferation, fat necrosis, and fibrosis of the skin and subcutaneous tissues. Dry, scaling hypertrophied skin is seen with venous stasis dermatitis. Venous ulcerations are seen posterior to the medial malleolus and sometimes superior to the lateral malleolus.

Venous stasis dermatitis produces reddish brown hyperpigmentation, induration, and venous stasis ulcers. Venous stasis ulcers may develop spontaneously or following trauma to the skin. These ulcers typically do not penetrate the deep fascia.

Leg edema secondary to chronic venous insufficiency tends to be unilateral and asymmetric. If a patient presents with bilateral edema, a search for a systemic cause is needed. Medications such as dihydropyridine calcium channel blockers or cardiovascular vasodilators such as hydralazine can also result in bilateral edema due to their vasodilating properties.

PHYSICAL EXAMINATION

Physical examination in the setting of chronic venous insufficiency demonstrates edema, dilated veins, thin or hyperpigmented skin, and ulceration. Legs are warm and there may be palpable and visible varicosities noted in the lower extremities.

DIFFERENTIAL DIAGNOSIS

The differential diagnosis for peripheral venous disease is summarized in Table 5.28.[328]

DIAGNOSTIC STUDIES

Chronic venous insufficiency is a clinical diagnosis with venous duplex Doppler ultrasonography being performed in the setting of unclear diagnosis or for those patients who are considering clinical intervention.

EVALUATION

The initial evaluation of patients with peripheral venous disease consists of a duplex ultrasound imaging which combines brightness mode imaging and Doppler investigation. This study can localize the sites of obstruction and demonstrate valvular reflux in both the systemic and deep venous systems. Venous reflux is demonstrated by retrograde or reversed flow and valve closure time of more than 0.5 second.

Phlebography identifies the site and level of obstruction along with any collaterals, although this technique is more commonly used when planning an in situ revascularization procedure. If detailed anatomic information is needed, CT and MR venography can be performed.

Patients with unilateral edema should be evaluated with CT in order to assess for a pelvic or abdominal mass.

Air plethysmography assesses venous function identifying reflux and obstruction. It can be performed in specialized centers if the diagnosis remains obscure after Doppler studies are performed.

TREATMENT

Initial management of chronic venous insufficiency is conservative. Recommendations for treatment include exercise, elevation of the legs, weight loss if needed, and compression stockings with the amount of compression dependent on the stage of the disease. If patients have skin changes or ulceration, at least 30 mm Hg of compression as needed. Knee length stockings are prescribed with professional fitting ideally performed. Topical moisturizers should be used to reduce skin breakdown and prevent infection. Stasis dermatitis may require topical steroids.

Wound care is needed to control drainage from ulcers and prevent maceration of the surrounding skin and consists of hydrocolloids and foam dressings. Patients with spider veins and small varicose veins can undergo injection sclerotherapy, thermocoagulation, or laser therapy. Patients not responding to conservative therapy can be treated with venous ablation, stripping or excision, or even stenting if stenosis and obstruction are present.

Compression stockings used in the setting of DVT is effective at decreasing the risk for the development of post-thrombotic syndrome. Patients using below knee compression stockings have the same benefit than thigh high compression stockings in preventing post-thrombotic syndrome.[329]

Mechanical endovascular ablation is as effective as radiofrequency ablation in the management of great saphenous vein incompetence.[330]

Intermittent pneumatic compression devices have been found to be superior to antiembolic stockings in the prevention of DVT. These devices used a pump to cyclically inflate and deflate hollow plastic leggings providing external compression that squeezes blood and fluid out of the lower legs. It effectively treats severe post-thrombotic syndrome and venous stasis ulcers and can be used in the

TABLE 5.28 Differential Diagnosis for Peripheral Venous Disease

Causes of Lower Extremity Edema	Description and Differentiating Features
Venous insufficiency	Swelling as a result of incompetent valves, dilation of peripheral veins, aging, or gravity from prolonged standing or sitting without elevation of legs.
Venous thrombosis	Acute clot in peripheral vein, which has significance when clot is located in deep venous system of calf, thigh, or pelvic veins with danger being proximal extension or embolism arising from this clot.
Varicose veins	Dilation of superficial veins in the peripheral vascular system results in poor venous return of blood into the central circulation with resultant edema. Varicosities are often inherited versus lifestyle that involves prolonged standing without compressive support on these peripheral veins.
Thrombophlebitis	Inflammation of the peripheral veins as a result of clot being lodged in the veins. Can cause a heavy sensation in the legs, achiness, and swelling. Superficial thrombophlebitis treated with heat application, and elevation with little risk for embolic phenomena to occur unless the deep venous system is affected.
Heart failure	Heart has an inability to appropriately remove blood into the systemic circulation or ventricles have an inability to relax resulting in stiffening of these structures interfering with diastolic filling. As left ventricular failure progresses, there is overloading of the right ventricle resulting in dependent edema, hepatomegaly, and jugular venous distention.
Cirrhosis	Scarring of the functioning liver cells results in ascites along with dependent edema. Majority of cases of cirrhosis occurs in the setting of long-standing alcohol intake or secondary to hepatitis C.
Nephrotic syndrome	Kidney damage to the glomerulus leads to massive proteinuria of at least 3 g/day, hypercoagulability secondary to the loss of anticoagulants in the urine, edema due to the loss of protein, and edema as a result of poor oncotic pressure from this protein loss.
Hypoalbuminemia	Loss of sufficient protein to maintain oncotic pressure in the cell results in leakage of fluid into the interstitium with generalized edema, especially in the lower extremities.
Lymphedema	Dorsal foot buffalo hump present along with loss of the web spaces between the toes (Stemmer sign). Positive findings also include an inability to pinch the skin located on the dorsum of the foot.[328] Duplex ultrasound is normal since this condition is not a problem with venous return.
Diabetic foot ulceration	Patients typically will have long-standing history of diabetes, poor circulation to the feet, and neuropathy that interferes with pain sensation to the legs. Ulcers are most likely on the plantar aspect of the foot or the dorsal aspect of the digits from ongoing trauma to the area. If infected, polymicrobial infection is the rule.
Arterial ulcer	Ulcers are located on the distal margins of the foot where circulation is furthest away from the central blood source. Doppler ankle-brachial index is <0.9, dorsalis pedis and posterior tibialis pulses are decreased, and there may be impaired capillary refill in the toes.
Chronic compartment syndrome	Occurs in muscular athletes who develop chronic calf pain after exercise, which induces significant acute bursts of activity stressing the calf muscles.

operative setting. Stockings alone are insufficient in preventing VTE. Heparin and low molecular weight heparin are efficient chemoprophylactic agents to reduce the incidence of VTE.[331] Prophylaxis does not eliminate the risk for the development of DVT and there is a suggestion that platelets can be a major contributor to hypercoagulability. Aspirin can be an add-on therapy to heparin prophylaxis at further lowering the risk for the development of DVT.[332]

Topical wound care is an important part of the management of venous stasis ulcers. Unna boots consist of zinc oxide impregnated bandages that are applied covered by compression bandages and elevation of the legs. This leads to excellent healing of venous stasis ulcers. Occlusive dressings such as hydrocolloids containing aluminum chloride provide a moist environment allowing wound healing and promoting the growth of new tissue. They are more expensive than Unna boots. Wounds with a lot of drainage may benefit from dressings that are absorptive.

PATIENT EDUCATION

Venous leg ulcers are chronic and are often difficult to heal with only 40% to 70% healing after 6 months of treatment.[333] Post-thrombotic syndrome is a known complication of acute DVT.

Patients with unprovoked DVT are at increased risk for the development of recurrent DVT when compared to patients who developed DVT as a result of known precipitating event such as surgery. Patients with proximal DVT, those diagnosed with cancer, those who were previously given short duration of oral anticoagulation therapy, and those with a history of thromboembolic events had a higher risk of recurrent events.[334] Venous stasis syndrome (VSS) can be a complication of DVT. VSS is most likely to occur due to venous outlet obstruction with or without venous valvular incompetence. VSS is more likely to occur with aging. Presence of varicose veins also increases potential for valvular incompetence and subsequent VSS.[335]

Venous thrombosis, thrombophlebitis, and varicose veins are all part of the clinical expression of venous insufficiency. These entities are discussed in the sections above.

KEY POINTS

- Chronic venous insufficiency is a common disorder with significant morbidity associated with it.
- Patients with chronic venous insufficiency may complain of heaviness, edema, achiness, and paresthesias or may be asymptomatic except for edema.
- The diagnosis of chronic venous insufficiency is based upon the history, physical exam, and Doppler ultrasound findings.
- Conservative treatment is employed for patients with chronic venous insufficiency and includes elevation, compressive stockings, and exercise causing calf contraction to propel blood toward the heart.
- Venous thrombosis can affect any vein but this condition is especially problematic when it affects the deep veins of an extremity in the calf, thigh, or pelvis as these locations have a higher tendency for embolic phenomena to occur.

5.14 ARTERIAL ANEURYSMS AND DISSECTION

Christine Bruce

5.14A ARTERIAL ANEURYSMS

OVERVIEW

Aortic diseases include thoracic and abdominal aortic aneurysms (AAA), aortic atheromas, and aortic dissection and rupture. Patients can present with rupture with a range of symptoms from severe pain to little or no symptoms and aneurysm formation can also be picked up as incidental findings when imaging or echocardiography is done for another reason. Ruptured AAA that is not recognized and treated soon enough can have morbidity and mortality approaching 100% in untreated individuals.[336]

AAA meets the criteria for an aneurysm when the diameter of this vessel is at least 3 cm. Risk factors for AAA formation include being a male, aging, smoking, atherosclerosis, hypertension, and a family history of aneurysm formation.

AAA is most commonly diagnosed incidentally during other screening procedures with the majority of patients being asymptomatic when diagnosed. The U.S. Preventive Services Task Force recommends a one-time screening for AAA for all men age 65 to 75 who have also smoked. AAAs measuring 4 cm or less are serially followed with duplex ultrasonography every 2 to 3 years. Once the AAA reaches 4.1 cm, screening is performed more frequently, every 6 to 12 months.

Once the aneurysm reaches 5.5 cm, CTA or MRA are performed in order to plan the elective surgery and identify whether the aneurysm is suprarenal, juxtarenal, or infrarenal.

By traditional definition, an aneurysm has diameter increase >50% of the normal diameter. Thoracic aneurysms can occur at the aortic root, ascending aorta, aortic arch, and descending aorta. Risk factors for the development of thoracic AAA include connective tissue disease such as Marfan or Ehlers-Danlos syndrome. Increased risk is also seen with bicuspid AoV, trauma, infection, aging, and hypertension. Aneurysms are classified as fusiform, which is circumferential widening of the artery, and saccular, which are localized outpouchings of the arterial wall.

EPIDEMIOLOGY

The average age of patients identified with AAA is 73 years of age with 79% of affected patients being men and 90% of affected patients having a White heritage.[337] Male sex, smoking, and elevated systolic blood pressure readings are associated with a higher prevalence of AAA but there is a paradox in that obesity has a lower incidence of AAA.[338] Areas where smoking has decreased in prevalence have seen a steep decline in AAA mortality. AAAs typically begin below the renal arteries and can extend into the iliacs. Most AAAs are fusiform rather than saccular.

PATHOPHYSIOLOGY

Atherosclerosis is most likely to deposit at the aortic root and ascending aorta making this a common site of aneurysm development. Aneurysms form as a result of cystic medial degeneration and weakening of the aortic wall due to loss of smooth muscle fibers and elastic fiber degeneration. Aneurysms are caused by weakening of the arterial wall, particularly the media, which is a thick layer of elastic fibers arranged in the spiral formation. True aneurysms involve all three layers of the artery: the media, intima, and adventitia. In addition to atherosclerosis, other causes of AAA include trauma, vasculitis, cystic medial necrosis, and postsurgical disruption of previous anastomosis site. Mycotic aneurysms occur as a result of infection with *Salmonella* being the most common bacterial pathogen.

Pseudoaneurysms involve a communication between the arterial lumen and the overlying connective tissue. Typically trauma such as iatrogenic catheter placement of the artery results in damage from arterial rupture creating a blood-filled cavity on the outside of the vessel wall.

AAA is a common degenerative vascular disorder associated with sudden death due to aortic rupture. AAA rupture is a multifaceted biologic process involving biochemical, cellular, and proteolytic influences. AAA rupture occurs when the stress or the force per unit area on the aneurysm wall exceeds wall strength. Aneurysm wall weakening can also occur as a result of proteolytic activities. The most important predisposing factor for aneurysm growth and rupture is aneurysm diameter. Rupture risk also depends on wall stress, aneurysm shape and geometry, intraluminal thrombus, wall thickness, calcification, and metabolic activity.[339]

Complications of AAA include rupture, distal embolization producing pulselessness, coldness, and paralysis distal to the site of the embolization, and disseminated intravascular coagulation as a result of the massive blood loss that occurs as a result of rupture. Embolization can affect the lower extremities, the mesentery, and kidneys depending on the site of aneurysm formation.

MEDICAL HISTORY AND CLINICAL PRESENTATION

Risk factors for the development of aneurysm include prolonged hypertension, dyslipidemia, and smoking. Thoracic aortic aneurysms have additional risk factors of connective tissue disease such as Ehlers-Danlos syndrome or Marfan syndrome. Hematogenous spread of bacteria can produce mycotic thoracic aneurysms. Syphilis can cause aortic root dilation and thoracic aneurysms. Blunt trauma to the chest can injure the aortic wall and produce pseudoaneurysm.

Patients with thoracic aortic aneurysms are typically asymptomatic but can have back pain caused by compression of the vertebral arteries, cough from tracheal irritation, dysphagia from esophageal compression, hoarseness from compression of the recurrent laryngeal or vagus nerve, chest pain due to coronary artery compression, and hemoptysis from erosion of the aneurysm into the lungs themselves.

Patients with ruptured AAA are usually hypotensive and in shock, with complaints of pain in abdomen or back, along with having a palpable pulsatile abdominal mass. Unusual clinical presentations include transient lower limb paralysis, pain under the rib, groin pain, testicular pain, or iliofemoral venous thrombosis.[336] Patients with a ruptured aneurysm may not survive to reach care if the rupture occurs outside a hospital facility.

SIGNS AND SYMPTOMS

The majority of AAAs are asymptomatic. When symptoms occur, they may be due to compression of adjacent structures as the aneurysm expands. Symptoms with ruptured aneurysms include severe back pain, leg weakness, decreased pulse amplitude, and a pulsatile palpable abdominal mass. A bruit may be heard over the abdominal aorta due to the turbulent nature of blood flow.

Because echocardiography is a common procedure, many thoracic aortic aneurysms are discovered incidentally. If patient is symptomatic, hoarseness or dysphasia may be the presenting symptoms caused by compression of the aneurysm on the recurrent laryngeal nerve or the esophagus, respectively.

PHYSICAL EXAMINATION

Physical exam findings consistent with thoracic aortic aneurysm consist of a diastolic heart murmur and a widened pulse pressure that results from AR, which is often seen with thoracic aortic aneurysm. Patients with ruptured thoracic aortic aneurysm present with severe chest pain, back pain, dyspnea, and even sudden cardiac death.

Pulses distal to the site of rupture are decreased in amplitude. AAA may be suspected in asymptomatic patients by hearing an abdominal bruit or feeling a widened abdominal aorta during abdominal palpation, but this is only found in very thin individuals.

DIFFERENTIAL DIAGNOSIS

The differential diagnosis for arterial aneurysms is summarized in Table 5.29.[340]

TABLE 5.29 Differential Diagnosis for Arterial Aneurysms

Conditions Causing Chest and Abdominal Pain	Description and Differentiating Features
Acute myocardial infarction	Can cause abdominal pain especially if the inferior wall of the heart is involved. EKG will show ST segment changes in two or more anatomically contiguous leads along with elevation in cardiac biomarkers such as troponin.
Aortic dissection	Pain is described as a searing or tearing pain starting in the chest or back that migrates into the abdomen as the tear progresses. Other symptoms are related to involvement of the aortic arch producing cerebral embolism or upper extremity ischemia.
Carotid artery dissection	Head or neck pain is the most frequent symptom of carotid artery dissection. Thunderclap headache can also occur with this dissection. Some patients develop Horner syndrome caused by distention of the sympathetic fibers located on the external surface of the internal carotid artery producing ptosis and miosis. Tinnitus, carotid artery bruit, and scalp tenderness can also occur. There may be involvement of cranial nerves IX, X, XI, and XII.
Esophageal spasm	Spasm can result in significant chest pain, which is capable of radiation into the back. Symptoms may be indistinguishable from aortic dissection or rupture along the aortic arch but patients with esophageal spasm will not have hypotension or decreased pulses.
Esophageal rupture	Rupture of the esophagus causes severe chest pain. Since the esophagus contains air, there may be leakage of air into the subcutaneous space, which can be manifested with crepitation palpable in the chest wall. There is not the same extent of hypotension seen with this condition as it is not vascular in nature.
Ulcerated aortic plaque/ erosion	Ulcerated aortic plaque may produce symptoms consistent with ruptured abdominal aortic aneurysm when the ulcerated plaque erodes into the vessel but true perforation of the vessel does not occur. Ultrasound of the abdomen can distinguish between these conditions.
Renal colic	Renal colic produces flank or back pain that can radiate into the anterior abdominal wall and also into the testicle or vulva. Hematuria can occur with both conditions and does not need distinguishing characteristic.
Pancreatitis	Causes pain radiating straight through to the back along with diaphoresis, nausea, and vomiting. Elevation in serum amylase and lipase occurs on diagnostic studies. Abdominal film can show peripancreatic edema and a sentinel loop sign. Chronic pancreatitis is demonstrated by having calcifications within the pancreas.
Mesenteric ischemia	Mesenteric ischemia causes severe abdominal pain from necrosis that develops into the involved bowel wall segments. Arteriography can show embolism or obstruction of the mesenteric vessels.
Cholecystitis	Can cause pain radiating between the scapulae. Pain is steady and progressive but can respond to parenteral ketorolac or opiates. Right upper quadrant ultrasound can demonstrate cholelithiasis, sludge within the gallbladder, and pericholecystic edema. Inspiratory arrest can occur when patients take a deep breath, which is known as a Murphy sign.

Source: Data from English SW, Passe TJ, Lindell EP, Klaas JP. Multiple cranial neuropathies as a presentation of spontaneous internal carotid artery dissection: a case report and literature review. J Clin Neurosci. *2018;50:129–131. doi:10.1016/j.jocn.2018.01.056*

DIAGNOSTIC STUDIES

Screening for thoracic aortic aneurysm may be indicated in patients with a bicuspid AoV, known connective tissue disease, and positive family history. There is no screening recommended for asymptomatic patients. Aneurysms may be picked up incidentally as patients commonly have abdominal imaging for a variety of causes. Diagnosis of aneurysm can be made by imaging tests which include ultrasonography, CTA, or MRA.

After thoracic aortic aneurysm is identified, aortic diameter is carefully measured. This measurement is serially tracked. Once the thoracic aneurysm exceeds 5 cm, there is an increased risk for rupture along with an increased risk of rupture for aneurysms that grow more than 0.1 cm/year. Serial monitoring is typically done on a yearly basis with TTE.

While AAA is a dilation of the abdominal aorta, there are several influences that affect the size of the abdominal aorta and they include age, gender, and body size. Precise measurements of the abdominal aorta also have shortcomings and a true widening of the aorta should be evaluated in relationship to adjacent aortic segments. The best method to demonstrate an expansion of a potential aneurysm is by serial follow-up assessments using the same imaging technique.[341]

If ruptured AAA is suspected an emergency ultrasound exam should be performed.[336] Arrangements should be made for immediate surgical intervention.

EVALUATION

One-time screening is recommended for males between ages 65 and 75, especially if they have ever smoked. Patients identified with AAA as a result of being found as an incidental finding are serially monitored with ultrasound for measuring the diameter of the abdominal aorta. Ultrasound is preferred as a monitoring technique due to low cost and lack of radiation exposure. For preoperative planning, CTA or MRI is performed due to improved anatomic images. For patient suspected of having rupture, immediate ultrasound is performed at the bedside with emergency surgery being indicated for treatment.

TREATMENT

Treatment of aneurysms that are not ruptured involves medical or surgical intervention, depending upon whether the patient has symptoms along with the size and location of the aneurysm. Medical management includes strict blood pressure control, control of lipids to prevent further atherosclerosis, and monitoring through imaging on a regular basis. Patients with known aneurysms should be encouraged to quit smoking. Surgical interventions include open and laparoscopic repair along with endovascular surgery. If an aneurysm is ruptured, emergency surgical treatment is indicated.

Treatment of thoracic aortic aneurysm includes blood pressure control with beta blockers being first-line choices. When the thoracic aneurysm exceeds 5.5 cm in diameter, elective repair is recommended as these patients have an increased risk for aneurysm rupture. If the patient is having coronary artery bypass grafting and has an aneurysm of at least 4.5 cm, aneurysm resection is typically done as part of the coronary artery bypass grafting procedure. Open surgical repair is performed for thoracic aortic aneurysms involving the aortic root, ascending aorta, and aortic arch. Thoracic endovascular aortic repair with stenting can be used to treat a descending aortic aneurysm that is grown to >6 cm.

Endovascular AAA repair has a lower in-hospital mortality rate than open repair at 1% versus 4% for unruptured AAA along with 41% survival with endovascular repair versus 21% survival with open repair of ruptured AAA. Patients with suitable anatomy who undergo endovascular aneurysm repair also have a shorter hospital stay of 2 days versus 7 days.[337]

Medical treatment of AAA involves risk factor reduction to lower the risk for rupture and overall mortality. In addition to having elective repair when the aneurysm reaches 5.5 cm, and aneurysm that grows more than 0.5 cm/year or patients who develop symptoms from AAA such as abdominal or back pain are recommended for elective resection. The decision for performing open versus endovascular aneurysm repair is dependent on the location of the AAA and whether the renal and mesenteric arteries are involved. Endovascular repair has a slightly lower morbidity and mortality in the short term but no differences in long-term mortality. Patients undergoing endovascular aneurysm resection have a higher risk for repeated intervention, endoleak, device failure, and postimplantation syndrome, which is signified by fever, leukocytosis, and elevated C-reactive protein. Following endovascular resection, patients are followed serially with CTA or ultrasound to evaluate the stent graft.[342]

Although women do not develop AAA as frequently as men, they have lower survival after rupture when open repair is undertaken. Women with AAAs tend to be older and have smaller diameter AAA when the repair is performed. Women are also more likely to have perioperative complications due to less favorable vascular anatomy. Patients older than 80 years of age and those who have more comorbidities tend to have worse prognosis.[343]

The shape of the aneurysm also impacts elective repair of an unruptured aneurysm. Saccular AAAs tend to become more symptomatic and more likely to rupture than fusiform AAAs, so early repair of a saccular aneurysm is recommended. Elective treatment of a saccular abdominal aortic aortic aneurysm is approximately 4.5 cm for elective surgery which is smaller than the currently recommended elective repair at 5.5 cm.[344]

Treatment of thoracoabdominal aortic aneurysm is a difficult challenge for vascular surgeons due to the potential for spinal cord injury secondary to ischemia. Two-stage procedures can be done in this situation with the patient having an acute open repair and later, a staged endovascular repair. These aneurysms can also be massively sized, sometimes up to 20 cm in diameter. Because of the massive size of these aneurysms, patients can have symptoms associated with compression, formation of hemothorax, and unstable aneurysm anatomy. For this reason, the initial surgical approach needs to be open rather than endovascular.[345]

Aortoduodenal fistula is a known complication following AAA repair. Patients can present with abdominal pain and melena and bleeding can be massive. Diagnosis can be made with CTA of the aorta. A high index of suspicion is needed for early diagnosis, which ideally is made prior to massive loss of blood.[346]

PATIENT EDUCATION

The best option to avoid AAA rupture is smoking cessation and control of hypertension.[339] Lifestyle modifications in the general measures to avoid atherosclerosis including aggressive blood pressure control are additional factors used in the prevention of aneurysm formation or extension of aneurysm when one has already occurred.

5.14B AORTIC DISSECTION

Aortic dissection occurs as a result of blood escaping through a tear in the aortic intima, which causes a separation between the intima and media creating a false lumen or channel for blood to escape from the systemic circulation. This intimal tear can occur independently or can occur secondary to hemorrhage within the media. This dissection can occur anywhere in the aorta and can extend both proximally or distally into other arteries. Most aortic dissections occur within 5 cm of the AoV or just distal to the origin of the left subclavian artery.

Hypertension ia the biggest risk factor for the development of aortic dissection. Signs and symptoms of aortic dissection include a tearing sensation in the chest or back, wide pulse pressure as a result of AR, and poor blood flow distal to the site of the dissection.

CXR can show widening of the mediastinum which can be used as a screen for patients suspected of having dissection. Echocardiogram and CT aortogram can also identify this condition and can provide additional anatomic information.

Treatment of aortic dissection is highly dependent on the site where dissection occurs. Blood pressure control is performed regardless of other management strategy. Aortic dissection in the proximal aortic arch is treated surgically while dissection distal to origin of the left subclavian artery is primarily managed with blood pressure control without surgery unless patients remain symptomatic. When surgery is performed, a synthetic graft is placed and endovascular stent grafts may be used when dissection occurs in the descending thoracic aorta.

The DeBakey classification system identifies three types of dissection: type I dissection starts in the ascending aorta and extends to at least the aortic arch and perhaps more distally, type II starts in the ascending aorta proximal to the brachiocephalic artery and is confined to the ascending aorta, and type III dissection starts in the descending thoracic aorta distal to the origin of the left subclavian artery. The Stanford classification system has type A which involves the ascending aorta and type B demonstrating the origin of the dissection distal to the left subclavian artery.

Beta blockers are considered to be first-line treatment for management of blood pressure in the setting of aortic dissection. Metoprolol and labetalol are preferred agents and these are administered intravenously. Nitroprusside, an arterial dilator, can also be used for blood pressure control if beta blockers are not effective but this should only be given after beta blocker therapy is instituted.

Patients who survive aortic dissection have aggressive management of blood pressure on a lifetime, long-term basis.

5.14C AORTITIS

Aortitis involves inflammation of the aorta and can lead to aneurysm formation or occlusion of the aorta. This condition can be caused by connective tissue disorders such as Takayasu or giant cell arteritis, ankylosing spondylitis, or infections such as bacterial endocarditis, syphilis, or *Salmonella* or fungal infections. This inflammation typically involves all layers of the aorta and can lead to occlusion of the aorta or its branches. Aortitis can also lead to weakening of the arterial wall and formation of aneurysms. Although this is not a common condition, it may have serious complications including death.

COMMON CHIEF COMPLAINTS

APPROACH TO PATIENT WITH CHEST PAIN

Patients with chest pain or chest discomfort are commonly encountered in outpatient and emergency settings. This chest pain/pressure complaint may be benign or life-threatening. Risk stratification is the first step when encountering this complaint. Typical angina is described as substernal chest pain or pressure that occurs with exertion and pain onset is typically predictable. Anginal chest pain is relieved with rest or nitroglycerin. There is typically no worsening of symptoms over a 2-month period and the symptoms are brought on by either exercise, cold weather, large meals (blood is shunted into the abdomen to digest the food), or stress. Other symptoms include exertional dyspnea, fatigue, and nausea and vomiting.

ACS consists of STEMI, NSTEMI, and USA. The commonality for three processes is disruption of blood flow to a portion of the heart. The diagnosis is made with two positive findings of the following criteria: patient history, cardiac biomarkers, and EKG findings. The difference between NSTEMI and USA is that NSTEMI has an increase in cardiac biomarkers, which is not seen with USA. The distinction between STEMI and NSTEMI is EKG interpretation with STEMI having ST segment elevation in two or more anatomic leads, which is not present with NSTEMI.

USA and NSTEMI involve partial blockage of a coronary artery. Thrombolytics are not used because this therapy could convert a partial to a full occlusion as the disrupted blockage moves downstream. There is a role for PCI with coronary angiography and stent placement

HISTORY

History is vital in helping to determine the underlying cause of chest pain. A patient who is young and otherwise healthy without a congenital or family history of cardiovascular disease most likely does not have an underlying cause. Patients with sickle cell disease can have acute chest wall syndrome presenting with chest pain or dyspnea. Patients in high-risk categories such as elderly, diabetic, male, and those with hyperlipidemia pose a much higher risk for a cardiac-related cause of chest pain.

In the setting of chest pain, the history is typically more valuable than the physical exam with the precipitating event leading to chest pain being important with regard to whether this is new-onset pain or a recurrent episode. The duration, quality, location, radiation, frequency, alleviating factors, and other symptoms such as diaphoresis, palpitations, syncope, presyncope, and lightheadedness should be ascertained. Diaphoresis is especially important, assigning the patient into a higher risk category. Diaphoresis may be the presenting sign of myocardial damage in a patient with a nonspecific complaint such as weakness or fatigue.

Sharp pain and chest wall pain are less likely to be related to ischemia or infarction and more likely to be related to musculoskeletal causes. Ischemia and infarction still need to be ruled out as these complaints are not mutually exclusive from more serious conditions as they can coexist.

Duration of pain is an important discriminating factor. MI typically causes symptoms that last 20 to 30 minutes while angina pain typically resolves within 5 minutes of rest. Both conditions can respond to nitroglycerin, but the response is mitigated with actual MI. Improvement of symptoms can occur as a result of nitroglycerin causing venodilation, pulling blood away from the heart and acting as a coronary artery vasodilator.

Chest pain responding to nitroglycerin can occur with both angina and esophageal spasm. This response does not discriminate between these conditions. Nitroglycerin should cause a headache when it is taken because of its vasodilating properties. Sublingual nitroglycerin is light and heat sensitive so a lack of headache in a patient taking this might signify that the nitroglycerin has lost some of its potency.

Women, elderly, and diabetic patients are more likely to have atypical presentation of chest pain with symptoms such as dyspnea, fatigue, and weakness rather than actual chest pain. Patients may have tachycardia and anxiety, which requires additional evaluation for PE since these symptoms may overlap.

PHYSICAL EXAM

As part of the overall evaluation, blood pressure should be checked in both arms since a difference of systolic pressure of more than 20 mm Hg requires consideration for aortic dissection as the underlying cause of chest pain. Hypotension could suggest a massive PE or cardiogenic shock. Fever might suggest pneumonia or esophageal rupture leading to mediastinitis.

The chest wall is assessed for tenderness, use of accessory muscles of respiration, and respiratory motion. In the setting of trauma, paradoxical movement of the chest wall suggests a flail chest with the need for emergency intervention. Point tenderness of the chest wall may suggest costochondritis.

Right ventricular infarction and right bundle branch block may result in widened splitting of the S2 heart sound as the RV under stress takes even longer to contract. Paradoxical splitting of S2 is associated with left bundle branch block with anterior wall MI. A new-onset left bundle branch block pattern on EKG is treated equivalently as STEMI.

S4 heart sounds occur with both angina and infarction. This occurs due to stiffening of the ventricle requiring the atrium to contract more forcefully. S3 heart sound occurs more frequently with HF. A new diastolic murmur located at the right sternal border could signal aortic dissection (when AR occurs). A new systolic murmur on the left sternal border can signify angina or infarction if this murmur is secondary to MR from papillary muscle rupture of the posterior chordae tendineae which occurs most commonly in inferior and posterior wall MIs.

Lung sounds demonstrating crackles or rales occurs with left ventricular infarction, especially with left anterior wall MI. Spontaneous pneumothorax can lead to asymmetry of breath sounds. Decreased breath sounds at the bases are seen with pleural effusions. Absent breath sounds and shifting of the trachea away from the midline is consistent with tension pneumothorax and immediate intervention with needle decompression of the chest is needed.

Extremities are assessed for pulses, edema, and calf and thigh swelling and tenderness. A normal Homan sign (dorsiflexion of the foot causing calf pain) is not sensitive enough to rule out calf DVT and further evaluation is necessary for these patients since DVT leading to PE is life-threatening. Palpable, tender venous cords are consistent with DVT. Delayed or absent pulses may occur in the setting of aortofemoral occlusion or aortic dissection.

TESTING IN THE SETTING OF CHEST PAIN

The initial test done in the setting of chest pain is a 12-lead EKG. The EKG is performed immediately after patient stabilization and taking vital signs. In an ED setting, the patient has cardiac monitoring and is closely observed. A normal EKG does not rule out a significant myocardial problem. ST segment wave changes in two or more anatomically continuous leads is consistent with damage to that portion of the heart. Most patients with acute chest pain will also have tachycardia unless the blood supply to the SA or AV node is compromised.

It is helpful to compare the current EKG with past EKGs. New-onset left bundle branch block in a patient with chest pain or ST segment elevation in a patient with chest pain is sufficient to lead to emergency reperfusion with thrombolytic or PCI.

Serial cardiac biomarkers play a vital role in risk stratification and diagnosis. Troponin levels are sensitive and specific to a patient having myocardial damage. Troponin I levels are not influenced by patient having underlying kidney disease while troponin T may be elevated in the setting of chronic kidney disease, polymyositis, or dermatomyositis. These biomarkers are obtained at 0, 2, and 6 hours after presentation. Troponin levels may remain elevated for up to 2 weeks after myocardial damage.

Cardiac causes for elevated troponin levels are ACS, coronary spasm or embolism, cocaine or methamphetamine use, stress cardiomyopathy, congestive HF, myocarditis or pericarditis, trauma, infiltrative diseases, and postprocedure (ablation, electric shock, coronary bypass surgery, and post-coronary angioplasty). Noncardiac causes for elevated troponin levels include PE, renal failure, stroke, sepsis, drug toxicity (anthracyclines), and hypoxia.

CXR is performed on patients with chest pain. X-ray findings can identify pneumothorax, pneumomediastinum (esophageal rupture), pleural effusion, and infiltrates consistent with pneumonia. A widened mediastinum suggests aortic dissection. A water bottle appearance to the heart on CXR is consistent with pericardial effusion.

Other tests that are considered include ABGs, BNP hormone levels (increased with HF and cardiac-related asthma symptoms), and spiral CT if PE is considered.

DIAGNOSTIC EVALUATION

For stable patients with chest pain needing further evaluation based on changing symptoms, an exercise treadmill test is considered first-line clinical intervention.[166] The patient who is unable to exercise should undergo either a nuclear MPI study or pharmacologic stress echocardiogram if the pretest probability for coronary disease is more than 10%.[166] Exercise stress testing or other imaging studies should be repeated when there is a change in clinical status.

Coronary CTA is a reasonable alternative in those with intermediate pretest probability of coronary artery disease whose symptoms persist despite normal test results or in those who have had equivocal stress test. CTA is not indicated with known moderate or severe coronary calcification or in those who have had coronary artery stents since interpretation is difficult in these settings.

An echocardiogram is recommended to assess resting left ventricular function and valve disease. This is also useful in patients who have HF or ventricular arrhythmias as wall motion can be seen and an ejection fraction can be calculated.

TREATMENT

Patients with stable chest pain are recommended for lifestyle modifications including diet, weight loss, smoking cessation, and exercise for at least 30 minutes per day most days of the week. Patients should be assessed for chronic kidney disease and psychosocial factors such as depression, anxiety, and poor social support as patients in these circumstances have a worse prognosis.

Medication treatment for patients with stable coronary disease includes aspirin, statins, blood pressure and diabetes control, beta blocker therapy, and, as needed, sublingual nitroglycerin.

Coronary angiography should be considered in patients who survive sudden cardiac death, those with high-risk noninvasive test results, and those whose angina symptoms do not respond to medical management. Coronary artery bypass graft (CABG) is indicated with left main artery disease, proximal LAD disease, and three-vessel disease with left ventricular dysfunction and low ejection fraction. Patients with ischemic LV and ejection fractions <35% have improved outcomes with CABG than with optimal medical therapy.[347] Diabetic patients tend to benefit more from bypass rather than stent placement.

The leading cause of death following PCI is MI and PCI patients have a higher cardiac-related mortality than patients treated with CABG following ACS.[348] There is a need for secondary prevention strategies after coronary disease is identified.

Medical management includes antiplatelet therapy with aspirin with or without clopidogrel as dual antiplatelet therapy. Clopidogrel should be held for 5 days prior to CABG being performed. Heparin is given along with antiplatelet therapy for USA and NSTEMI. Anti-thrombin therapy includes both unfractionated and subcutaneous low molecular weight heparin such as enoxaparin, which should be given until angiography is performed in 2 to 3 days following ACS.

HMG-CoA reductase agents (also known as "statins") are first-line agents used in primary and secondary prevention of coronary artery disease. When plaques are already present, these agents stabilize the plaque reducing the risk for plaque rupture. The highest return on investment with the use of statins is as secondary disease prevention as the number needed to treat in order to prevent recurrence of an acute coronary artery event is much lower than when these agents are used as a primary prevention strategy.

Glycoprotein IIb/IIIa inhibitors work as antiplatelet agents by blocking the receptor involved in platelet aggregation. These agents are only given intravenously and these agents interfere with the final stage of platelet bridging. These agents or clopidogrel are used during PCI with stenting. Patients getting either of these agents at the time of stenting have longer periods of stent patency. Complications of the glycoprotein IIb/IIIa inhibitors include bleeding and thrombocytopenia.

SUMMARY

Chest pain is a complaint that is commonly encountered in clinical practice. A thorough investigation for this complaint should be pursued as some causes of chest pain are life-threatening. Patient education is needed in order to address the underlying cause of chest pain and to prevent recurrent episodes or progression of coronary artery disease, if present. Lifestyle modifications are helpful in addressing coronary artery disease and statin medications can help to lower the risk for both primary and secondary cardiovascular events.

APPROACH TO THE PATIENT WITH HYPERTENSION

Hypertension is found most commonly by screening as the majority of patients with hypertension are asymptomatic. Patients who are found to have significant blood pressure elevation should have emergent treatment and should be assessed for a secondary cause of hypertension. Patients with resistant hypertension should also be assessed for adherence to medication, low-salt diet, alcohol use, and caloric intake as these factors impact blood pressure readings.

Patients with elevated blood pressure who have palpitations and flushing on a recurrent basis can be assessed for pheochromocytoma and carcinoid syndrome. Young females without other risk factors for hypertension can be assessed for fibromuscular dysplasia of the renal artery. Obese patients should be assessed for sleep apnea, which is one of the most common causes of both secondary and resistant hypertension. Patients with unexplained or unprovoked hypokalemia can be assessed for hyperaldosteronism. Patients using corticosteroids or who have a cushingoid appearance with buffalo hump, proximal muscle weakness, and striae can be assessed for Cushing syndrome.

APPROACH TO THE PATIENT WITH ORTHOSTATIC HYPOTENSION

Orthostatic hypotension is a decline in systolic blood pressure of at least 20 mm Hg or diastolic blood pressure decline of 10 mm Hg. When a patient assumes an upright posture, there needs to be rapid cardiovascular adjustments that involve the autonomic nervous system, adequate blood volume, and intact skeletal and respiratory muscle pumps. If the patient does not have sufficient blood volume or has defective sympathetic adrenergic vasoconstriction, orthostatic hypotension develops. Signs and symptoms of this orthostatic intolerance include lightheadedness in the upright position that is relieved by recumbency.[349]

Patients who have both type 2 diabetes and hypertension have an increased incidence of orthostatic hypotension and mortality is increased in these patients if orthostatic hypotension occurs.[350] Orthostatic hypotension is also an independent risk factor for the development of HF.[351]

APPROACH TO THE PATIENT WITH POSTURAL ORTHOSTATIC TACHYCARDIA SYNDROME

Postural orthostatic tachycardia syndrome (POTS) is the most common form of orthostatic intolerance in young people affecting approximately 500,000 people in the United States annually. This condition is most likely to affect young women at the beginning of their working lives. Patients present with heart rate increase of at least 30 bpm standing or during head-up tilt table testing along with the absence of orthostatic hypotension. Patients have a broad range of symptoms in the upright position including palpitations, fatigue, cognitive disturbance, headache, nausea, presyncope, and syncope.[352]

APPROACH TO THE PATIENT WITH DYSPNEA UPON EXERTION

For patients to become symptomatic secondary to HF, the initial symptom is dyspnea upon exertion. If HF is not managed appropriately, this dyspnea will occur with progressively less exertion until dyspnea can occur at rest, which may be a sign of decompensated HF. PND is a fairly specific sign of HF. Orthopnea is frequently seen with HF and this may progress to such a degree that patients sleep in a recliner in order to maintain a more erect position. When the right side of the heart becomes fluid overloaded, patients will have jugular venous distention, which progresses to hepatomegaly and peripheral edema. This edema will be most prevalent in the dependent portions of the body meaning that bed-bound patients will have presacral edema while patients who are ambulatory will develop ankle and pretibial edema. Initial symptoms of fluid overload on the left side of the heart includes wheezing, cough, and rales that are heard on auscultation.

KNOWLEDGE CHECKS

1. Understand the normal relationship between the tricuspid valve and the mitral valve by echocardiogram and be able to describe how this relationship differs in Ebstein anomaly of the tricuspid valve.
2. Understand that Ebstein anomaly is commonly associated tachydysrhythmias. State common dysrhythmias associated with Ebstein anomaly and describe how they would appear on an EKG.

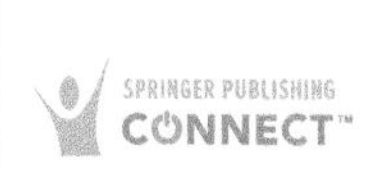

A robust set of instructor resources designed to supplement this text is located at **http://connect.springerpub.com/content/book/978-0-8261-8243-2.** Qualifying instructors may request access by emailing **textbook@springerpub.com.**

REFERENCES

The complete reference list for this chapter appears in the digital version of the chapter, accessible at https://connect.springerpub.com/content/book/978-0-8261-8243-2/chapter/ch05.

To view full list of references, please visit connect.springerpub.com.

CHAPTER 6

HEMATOLOGIC SYSTEM

JAMES VAN RHEE

LEARNING OBJECTIVES

- Describe normal hematopoiesis regarding red blood cell (RBC) production, hemoglobin biosynthesis, hemoglobin structure and function, and RBC metabolism.
- Compare and contrast the various etiologies of the microcytic anemias regarding epidemiology, pathophysiology, clinical presentation, diagnosis, and disease management.
- Compare and contrast the various etiologies of the macrocytic anemias with regard to epidemiology, pathophysiology, clinical presentation, diagnosis, and disease management.
- Compare and contrast the epidemiology, pathophysiology, clinical presentation, diagnosis, and management of various causes of hemolytic anemia.
- Differentiate acute lymphocytic leukemia (ALL) from acute myeloid leukemia (AML) regarding epidemiology, pathophysiology, clinical presentation, diagnosis, and management.
- Differentiate chronic myeloid leukemia (CML) from chronic lymphocytic leukemia (CLL) regarding epidemiology, pathophysiology, clinical presentation, diagnosis, and management.
- Discuss the various myeloproliferative disorders regarding risk factors, epidemiology, pathophysiology, clinical presentation, diagnosis, and management.
- Discuss Hodgkin's lymphoma and non-Hodgkin's lymphoma regarding risk factors, epidemiology, pathophysiology, clinical presentation, diagnosis, and management.
- Compare and contrast monoclonal gammopathies of undetermined significance, plasmacytoma, multiple myeloma (MM), Waldenström's macroglobulinemia, and primary amyloidosis (AL) with regard to epidemiology, pathophysiology, clinical presentation, diagnosis, and management.
- Discuss primary and secondary hemostasis and their role in coagulation.
- Discuss the epidemiology, pathophysiology, clinical presentation, diagnosis, and management of the various clotting factor disorders.
- Discuss the epidemiology, pathophysiology, clinical presentation, diagnosis, and management of von Willebrand disease.
- Compare the various etiologies of thrombocytopenia regarding epidemiology, pathophysiology, clinical presentation, diagnosis, and management.
- Discuss the congenital and acquired conditions resulting in a hypercoagulable state regarding epidemiology, pathophysiology, clinical presentation, diagnosis, and management.

INTRODUCTION

Hematology is the study of the normal and pathologic aspects of blood and the blood elements. The hematopoietic system is made up of RBCs, white blood cells (WBCs), and platelets. The WBCs include neutrophils, lymphocytes, monocytes, eosinophils, and basophils. All cells in the hematopoietic system originate from the pluripotent stem cell.

6.1 ANEMIA

OVERVIEW

Anemia is defined as a reduction in the number of circulating RBCs below the normal limits for age and gender and is among the most common abnormalities encountered in medicine. Anemia is recognized by a low hematocrit, hemoglobin, or RBC count value.

There are many possible causes of anemia: acute or chronic blood loss, drug reactions, autoimmunity, bone marrow suppression via systemic or intrinsic hematopoietic stem cell (HSC) disease processes, and malnutrition. Anemias are classified based on their underlying pathophysiology related to decreased production (i.e., iron deficiency) or increased destruction (i.e., hemolytic anemia) of RBCs.

EPIDEMIOLOGY

Anemia is a common, multifactorial condition among patients. After 50 years of age the prevalence of anemia increases with advancing age and exceeds 20% in those 85 years and older.[1] In nursing home patients, anemia is present in 48% to 63% of residents.[1] Among older adults with anemia, approximately one third have evidence of iron, folate, and/or vitamin B12 deficiency, one third have renal insufficiency and/or chronic inflammation, and the remaining one third have anemia that is unexplained.[2]

PATHOPHYSIOLOGY

The adult erythroid lineage takes its origin from a more complex cell lineage, with HSCs as the earliest precursor cells. HSCs are in the bone marrow and continuously replenish the blood system throughout adult life. To produce adult RBCs, HSCs undergo a relatively long and extensive process of cellular differentiation and proliferation. The primitive cells are characterized by the expression of globin and form a variety of distinguishable hemoglobin tetramers. Once released in the bloodstream, the macrocytic primitive erythrocytes retain proliferative capacity. Beginning early in embryonic life, erythro-myeloid progenitors differentiate in the fetal liver to produce the first definitive erythrocytes. There is an immediate switch to fetal/adult globin when erythropoiesis starts in the fetal liver. Hemoglobin tetramers consisting of α- and γ-globin chains ($\alpha_2\gamma_2$) are known as HbF. These hemoglobins allow the developing fetus to extract oxygen more efficiently from the maternal blood.

Around the time of birth, the site of erythropoiesis switches to the bone marrow and the spleen. The bone marrow is the primary site for adult erythropoiesis, but under erythroid stress conditions, such as low oxygen pressure or anemia, the spleen is used to expand the erythropoietic capacity.

Fetal globin expression is silenced in adult erythropoiesis. Hemoglobin tetramers composed of α- and β-globin ($\alpha_2\beta_2$, HbA1) account for ~97% of all hemoglobin in adult erythrocytes. HbA2 ($\alpha_2\delta_2$) and HbF account, respectively, for ~2% and ~1% of total hemoglobin in most adults.

Immature erythroid-restricted progenitors are identified as the burst forming unit-erythroid (BFU-E). Their growth is dependent on several factors, the most important of which are stem cell factor (SCF), thrombopoietin (TPO), interleukin 3 (IL-3), IL-11, and FLT3-ligand.

More mature erythroid progenitors, colony-forming units-erythroid (CFU-E), consist of small colonies of cells. They are fivefold to eightfold more abundant than BFU-E in bone marrow and under normal circumstances do not appear in the circulation. As progenitors undergo the differentiation process, their numbers increase, with their proliferative potential simultaneously decreasing. Erythrocytes represent the most common cell type in adult blood.

RBCs have an average life span of 120 days (Figure 6.1). New erythrocytes are constantly produced in the bone marrow, which provides a growth environment. This environment supports direct contact and exposure of the developing hematopoietic cells to cell adhesion molecules, growth factors, and cytokines. The earliest erythroid progenitors are responsive to cytokines including TPO, granulocyte-macrophage colony-stimulating factor (GM-CSF), IL-3, and IL-11, and specially to in SCF. At subsequent stages, SCF acts with EPO in the proliferation and expansion of the developing erythroid progenitors. Erythroid cells at the terminal stages of differentiation have shed their nucleus, endoplasmic reticulum, and mitochondria, and, consequently, they are no longer able to proliferate. To maintain the RBC count in the 5 L of blood of an adult individual, 2.4×10^6 new erythrocytes must be produced each second; it takes about 1 week for reticulocytes to

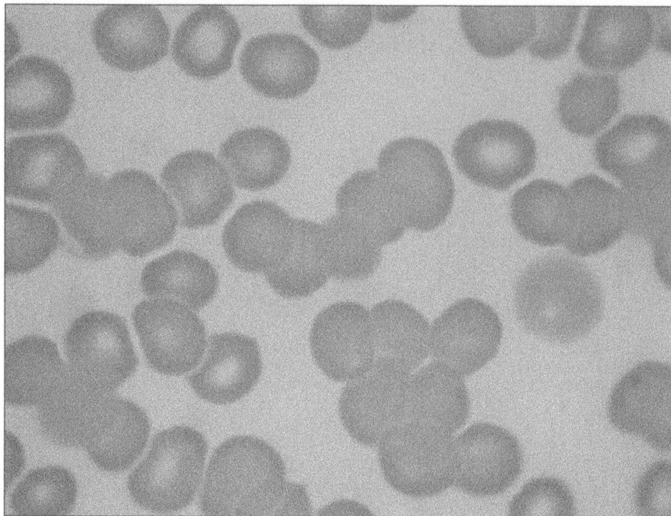

Figure 6.1 Normal red blood cells.
(Source: James Van Rhee and Janie McDaniel.)

complete the maturation process. Mature erythrocytes have a diameter of only about 7 µm. Their small size and biconcave shape create a large surface area for gas exchange and allow the cells to enter the microcapillaries in the tissues.

The iron requirement is based on physiologic needs due to small daily losses in body cells and fluids, losses during menstruation and pregnancy in women, and iron needed for growth in infants, children and adolescents; additional replacement needs are due to pathologic losses, typically from blood loss. In normal healthy men, the daily iron loss is <1.0 mg/day. In healthy menstruating women, the daily iron loss is approximately 1.5 mg/day. The average American diet contains 10 to 15 mg of iron per day.

Dietary iron is consumed and then absorbed in the stomach, duodenum, and upper jejunum; only about 10% of dietary iron is absorbed. The transport across the intestinal lumen is facilitated by ferroportin. Ferroportin is a transmembrane protein that transports iron from inside to outside the cell. This allows iron to be transported from the intestinal cells into the bloodstream. Ferroportin also facilitates the transport of iron in macrophages to apotransferrin for delivery to erythroid cells and the synthesis of hemoglobin.

Under normal conditions, approximately 1% of erythrocytes are removed from circulation every day and replaced by new cells. This rate of erythropoiesis can increase significantly from the baseline level in response to hypoxic stress. Hypoxic stress occurs when there is inadequate oxygen supply to tissues secondary to insufficient numbers of functioning erythrocytes. The increase in erythrocyte production is the primary response to counteract hypoxic stress. Hypoxia stimulates the production of erythropoietin by the cortical interstitial cells in the kidneys.

6.1A IRON DEFICIENCY ANEMIA

MEDICAL HISTORY AND CLINICAL PRESENTATION

Iron deficiency is the most common cause of anemia in the world. With no specific historical or physical examination findings, additional laboratory studies are almost always required to establish the diagnosis of iron deficiency.

BOX 6.1 Causes of Iron Deficiency

Dietary deficiency
Decreased absorption Celiac disease
Increased requirement Pregnancy/lactation
Chronic blood loss Blood donation Gastrointestinal Menstrual
Hemoglobinuria
Iron sequestration
Idiopathic

Iron deficiency develops when there is a decrease in total body iron. The average adult has storage iron reserves of about 200 to 250 mg in females and 750 to 1,000 mg in males.

The most important step in the evaluation of iron deficiency is the identification and treatment of the underlying cause of the decrease in body iron. See Box 6.1 for the common causes of iron deficiency.

In men and postmenopausal women, pathologic blood loss is the most common cause of iron deficiency. In women of child-bearing age, menstrual blood loss adds to iron requirements and each pregnancy leads to iron donation to the fetus. In menstruating patients there must be an increase in the absorption of iron up to 3–4 mg/day and during pregnancy and lactation iron demand goes up 2 to 5 mg/day.

In infants, children, and adolescents, iron deficiency develops when iron requirements for growth surpass the supply from stores and diet. Iron deficiency is infrequently caused by impaired absorption of iron alone and is rarely the result of genetic disorders.

Chronic blood loss is the most common etiology of iron deficiency in adult patients. Gastrointestinal (GI) loss is a major concern and a search must be made for the source of GI blood loss, once other etiologies of blood loss are excluded. Common GI causes include malignancy, ulcers, gastritis, drug-induced lesions (alcohol, salicylates, steroids, and nonsteroidal anti-inflammatory agents), and parasitic infections. Genitourinary blood loss, chronic hemoglobinuria, and hemosiderinuria are less common causes. Repeated blood donation also may lead to iron deficiency. In infants, children, and adolescents, the need for iron for growth may exceed the supply available from diet and stores. In a small percentage of patients, the etiology of the deficiency may not be identified.

SIGNS AND SYMPTOMS

Patients with iron deficiency may have no signs or symptoms or may have features common to all anemias, such as pallor, palpitations, tinnitus, headache, irritability, weakness, dizziness, easy fatigability, and other vague and nonspecific complaints. The presentation is influenced by both the severity of the anemia and the rate of development. As iron deficiency often develops slowly, signs and symptoms may be minimal due to adaptation in the circulatory and respiratory systems. But severe iron deficiency anemia can produce cardiorespiratory failure and may require urgent management.

A relatively specific symptom of iron deficiency is pica. Pica is characterized by the obsessive craving for specific foods, such as ice chips.

Iron deficiency may also produce signs and symptoms independent of anemia, especially in epithelial tissues that have a high iron requirement because of rapid cell turnover. Glossitis, angular stomatitis, esophageal web or stricture, and gastric atrophy may develop. The combination of esophageal web, dysphagia, and severe iron deficiency is called Plummer-Vinson syndrome.

PHYSICAL EXAMINATION

Distinctive physical findings occur in only a small number of patients with iron deficiency but include koilonychia. Koilonychia is thin, brittle fingernails with a concave or "spoon" shape (Figure 6.2); blue sclerae, a bluish hue of the sclerae due to thinning of the sclerae, may also be noted.

DIFFERENTIAL DIAGNOSIS

Other causes of microcytic anemia include anemia of chronic disease, thalassemia, lead poisoning, and sideroblastic anemia (Table 6.1).

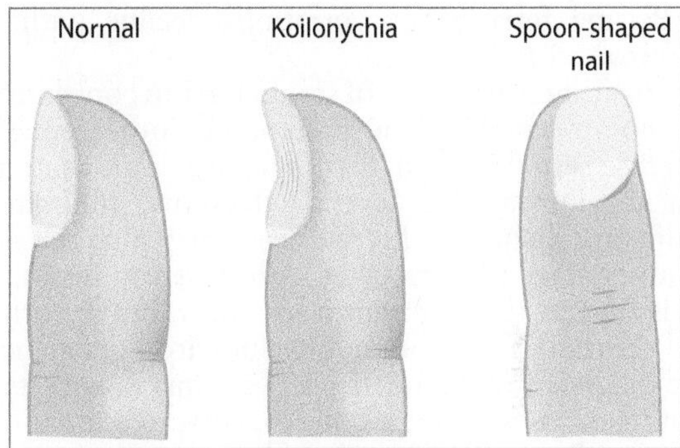

Figure 6.2 Koilonychia (nail spooning) can be noted in iron deficiency and vitamin B12 deficiency.

TABLE 6.1 Differential Diagnosis of Iron Deficiency Anemia

Differential Diagnosis	Description
Thalassemia	Hereditary disorder with reduction in synthesis of globin chains. Abnormal hemoglobin electrophoresis, normal iron studies.
Anemia of chronic disease	Characterized by a history of a chronic systemic disease. Normal ferritin, low serum iron, low total iron-binding capacity.
Sideroblastic anemia	Defect in iron utilization in the porphyrin pathway. Presence of ringed sideroblasts on bone marrow biopsy, elevated serum iron and total iron-binding capacity.
Lead poisoning	Elevated lead levels inhibit enzymes in heme synthesis pathway. Elevated lead levels and increased free erythrocyte protoporphyrin levels.

DIAGNOSTIC STUDIES

Uncomplicated iron deficiency produces a characteristic sequence of changes in laboratory studies. After iron stores are exhausted the plasma iron level falls; the total iron-binding capacity (TIBC), a measure of the plasma transferrin concentration, increases; and the transferrin saturation (the ratio of the plasma iron to TIBC) decreases to <16%. TIBC is an indirect measure the blood's capacity to bind iron to transferrin. Transferrin is a plasma protein that binds iron tightly but reversibly and transports iron via the blood to the liver, spleen, and bone marrow.

With reduction of the amount of iron available for heme synthesis, the erythrocyte zinc protoporphyrin level progressively increases and the reticulocyte count falls. On the peripheral blood smear, the appearance of hypochromic, microcytic erythrocytes will be noted (Figure 6.3). Other RBC abnormalities that may be noted include target cells and pencil-shaped cells. RBC indices, such as mean corpuscular volume (MCV), will decrease. Platelet count is typically elevated, but typically <800,000/μL.

These laboratory measures are not diagnostic of iron deficiency. These characteristic laboratory changes can result not only from iron deficiency but also from many other disorders that impair iron delivery to the erythroid marrow. To detect the absence of storage iron—the defining feature of iron deficiency—measurement of serum ferritin is needed. Ferritin is the principal storage protein for intracellular iron. The amount of ferritin synthesized and secreted into the plasma is proportional to the magnitude of body iron stores. Plasma ferritin concentrations decline with a decrease in iron stores.

Diagnostic interpretation of serum ferritin concentrations is often complicated by the presence of other conditions that increase serum ferritin. Serum ferritin is an acute-phase reactant and increased in several infectious, inflammatory, and malignant disorders. Liver disease may also release ferritin from damaged hepatocytes. A low serum ferritin (<10 mcg/L) is diagnostic of absent iron stores, but a normal or elevated serum ferritin does not exclude iron deficiency.

If the diagnosis of iron deficiency anemia is uncertain after laboratory assessment, a bone marrow examination can be definitive. Prussian blue stain of bone marrow aspiration and biopsy provides information regarding macrophage storage iron by grading of marrow hemosiderin; determination of the proportion of iron supply to sideroblasts; and general morphologic features of hematopoiesis.

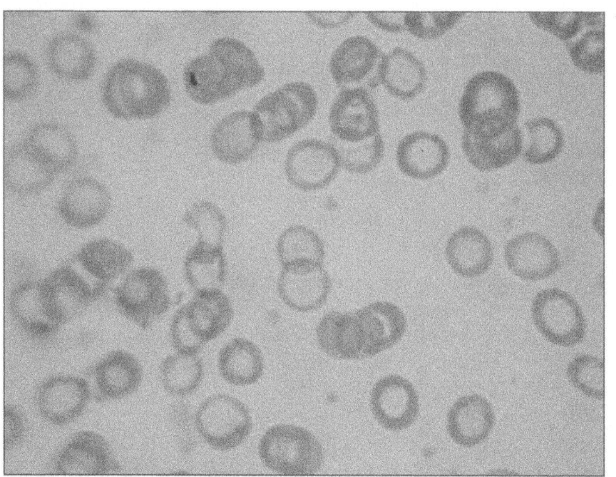

Figure 6.3 Microcytic hypochromic cells noted in iron deficiency anemia (Wright Stain 1,000×).
(Source: James Van Rhee and Jane McDaniel.)

TABLE 6.2 Summary of Laboratory Findings in Iron Deficiency Anemia

Laboratory Test	Iron Deficiency Anemia	Normal Range
Mean corpuscular volume (MCV)	Decreased	80–100 fL
Mean corpuscular hemoglobin (MCH)	Decreased	27–32 pg
Mean corpuscular hemoglobin concentration (MCHC)	Decreased/Normal	30–36 mg/dL
Red blood cell distribution width (RDW)	Increased	10.5%–14.5%
Serum iron	Decreased	30–160 mcg/dL
Total iron-binding capacity (TIBC)	Increased	225–430 mcg/dL
Serum ferritin	Decreased	30–300 ng/mL

See Table 6.2 for a summary of laboratory findings in iron deficiency anemia.

EVALUATION

In some circumstances, a trial of iron is an alternative means of confirming the diagnosis of iron deficiency. Proof that iron deficiency is the cause of an anemia can be diagnosed by a characteristic response to treatment with iron. The definitive diagnostic response consists of both of the following:

- An increase in reticulocytes within 5–10 days of starting adequate iron therapy and then gradually decreasing.
- An increase in hemoglobin and hematocrit, beginning after maximum reticulocytosis and no later than 3 weeks after iron therapy was started, and continuing until the hemoglobin and hematocrit have returned to normal.

Several factors may complicate interpretation of the results of a trial of iron, including poor compliance, malabsorption of iron, continued blood loss, and the effects of coexisting conditions, such as infectious, inflammatory, or malignant disorders. Despite a positive result with iron therapy, the underlying cause of the iron deficiency must be determined.

Rarely, laboratory indicators of iron status are altered by a variety of inherited disorders of iron metabolism. A lifelong history of abnormal iron studies with anemia that is refractory to iron therapy suggests a genetic basis for iron deficiency.

TREATMENT

Iron therapy for iron deficiency can typically be deferred until the underlying etiology has been identified. If concurrent infection or inflammation is present, iron should be withheld until these disorders are resolved or well controlled.

Oral iron is the treatment of choice because of its effectiveness, safety, and cost. Oral iron therapy starts with a ferrous iron salt (ferrous sulfate), taken separately from meals, to maximize absorption, in three to four divided doses, supplying a total of 150 to 200 mg of elemental iron per day in adults or 3 to 6 mg of iron per kilogram per day in children. For milder anemia, a single daily dose of approximately 60 mg of iron may be adequate. After the anemia has been fully corrected, oral iron should be continued to replace storage iron. Most patients can tolerate oral iron therapy without difficulty, but a number may have side effects. The most common side effects are GI, including nausea and constipation, and can be managed by administering iron with food and decreasing the dose.

Parenteral iron therapy, despite the decrease in adverse reactions with newer preparations, should be reserved for the patient who is not able to tolerate oral iron despite repeated modifications in dosage regimen, suffers from iron malabsorption, has iron needs that cannot be met by oral therapy due to prolonged uncontrollable bleeding or other sources of blood loss, or has a coexisting chronic inflammatory state, such as inflammatory bowel disease.

If the expected response to iron therapy does not occur, a complete reevaluation of the patient should begin. An error in diagnosis is common, with the anemia resulting from infection, inflammation, or malignancy being mistaken for iron deficiency anemia. Continued blood loss may also cause an incomplete response. Other nutritional deficiencies, hepatic or renal disease, or infectious, inflammatory, or malignant disorders may delay recovery. If the expected response is not obtained with oral iron therapy, the form and dose of iron used should be reconsidered, compliance with the treatment regimen should be reviewed, and the possibility of malabsorption considered.

In rare cases of severe iron deficiency anemia immediate RBC transfusion may be needed to prevent cardiac or cerebral ischemia. RBC transfusion may also be required to support patients when the chronic rate of iron loss exceeds the rate of replacement.

PATIENT EDUCATION

- The patient and family should be told that the prognosis for iron deficiency is excellent, and that an excellent response to either oral or parenteral iron can be anticipated. The overall prognosis is determined by the underlying cause of the iron deficiency.
- A subjective and clinical response to treatment should be noted in the first few days after treatment is begun. Symptoms may improve before a hematologic response is noted.

6.1B THALASSEMIA

Thalassemia is one of the most common genetic diseases worldwide and is due to unbalanced production of the hemoglobin molecule because of insufficient production of the α- or β-globin chains. The remaining globin chains precipitate in the erythroid precursors and in RBCs, resulting in an anemia from either ineffective production of RBCs, hemolysis of RBCs, or a combination of the two.

MEDICAL HISTORY AND CLINICAL PRESENTATION

In α-thalassemia, there are normally four α-globin genes present, with two located on each copy of chromosome 16. When one α-globin gene is deleted, there is generally no consequence and it is difficult to distinguish between these individuals and those without such deletions.

Patients who have two α-globin genes deleted on the same chromosome or on different chromosomes have microcytic RBC indices and hypochromia along with a mild anemia. These patients are considered to have α-thalassemia trait.

Those with three α-globin genes deleted have a condition known as hemoglobin H disease, which can vary in severity but often involves a moderate to severe anemia that can require regular RBC transfusions.

Deletion of all four α-globin genes is usually incompatible with a viable birth, and fetuses affected by such a condition have a severe form of hydrops fetalis. Fetal β-like globin chain (γ-globin) forms hemoglobin Barts when assembled as a tetramer of four γ-globin chains.

Carriers of β-thalassemia mutations (β-thalassemia trait) have microcytosis, hypochromia, a normal or increased number of RBCs, and often an elevation of the minor adult hemoglobin, along with a mild anemia in some cases. Patients who acquire two β-thalassemia mutations generally have a severe microcytic and hypochromic anemia.

SIGNS AND SYMPTOMS

Thalassemia is genetically transmitted; patients often have a family history of these diseases, and parents of patients will be carriers for these mutations. Patients of Mediterranean, Southeast and South Asian, and Middle Eastern origin are most frequently affected, although these mutations are widespread in many populations around the world. Symptoms vary depending on the severity of the disease and include fatigue, shortness of breath, and jaundice.

PHYSICAL EXAMINATION

Many patients with thalassemia will have hepatosplenomegaly because of extramedullary hematopoiesis. Signs of medullary expansion such as a prominent, protruding forehead can be helpful in assessing the severity of thalassemia. Close examination of growth charts of children with thalassemia is required as this information may affect the decision to transfuse the patient more frequently to support growth.

DIFFERENTIAL DIAGNOSIS

There can be diagnostic confusion between thalassemia trait and iron deficiency anemia as both conditions can have a low MCV and a low mean corpuscular hemoglobin (MCH). Patient with thalassemia trait can have a high RBC count and mild or no anemia. Patients with iron deficiency can have a normal or low RBC count and generally get anemia as a later manifestation.

The Mentzer index (Mentzer index = MCV/RBC count) can be used to separate thalassemia trait and iron deficiency. Patients with a Mentzer index of <13 have thalassemia trait, while those with iron deficiency usually have an index of >13. The Mentzer index should be used in conjunction with other tests, such as iron status and HbA2 levels.[3] Assessment of iron stores is often necessary to distinguish the two (Table 6.3).

TABLE 6.3 Differential Diagnosis of Iron Deficiency Anemia

Differential Diagnosis	Description
Iron deficiency anemia	Due to chronic blood loss or malabsorption. Low serum iron, elevated total iron-binding capacity, and decreased ferritin.
Anemia of chronic disease	Characterized by a history of a chronic systemic disease. Normal ferritin, low serum iron, low total iron-binding capacity.
Sideroblastic anemia	Defect in iron utilization in the porphyrin pathway. Presence of ringed sideroblasts on bone marrow biopsy, elevated serum iron and total iron-binding capacity.
Lead poisoning	Elevated lead levels inhibit enzymes in heme synthesis pathway. Elevated lead levels and increased free erythrocyte protoporphyrin levels.

DIAGNOSTIC STUDIES

A complete blood count (CBC) is used initially to demonstrate the degree of anemia and reveal the presence of hypochromia and microcytosis. The RBC count can be increased in those with thalassemia trait and can be helpful in distinguishing this from iron deficiency. The reticulocyte count will be low due to impaired RBC production.

A blood smear will reveal hypochromic and microcytic RBCs, variation in RBC size (anisocytosis), and unique cells such as target cells. Stains of a smear with brilliant cresyl blue can reveal hemoglobin precipitates that occur in hemoglobin H disease.

Hemoglobin electrophoresis is used to determine whether other hemoglobin types may be present (i.e., hemoglobin E or S) and, if done quantitatively, will indicate whether HbA2 and HbF are elevated, as occurs in β-thalassemia. In hemoglobin H disease, hemoglobin H can be detected and hemoglobin Barts can also be detected in newborn infants.

Once thalassemia has been diagnosed and characterized, genetic testing can often be helpful. Detection of α-thalassemia deletions and β-thalassemia mutations is done by polymerase chain reaction (PCR) testing. Genetic testing to delineate specific mutations may be useful for predicting the clinical course in certain patients.

EVALUATION

At times it may be difficult to differentiate iron deficiency anemia from thalassemia. Both have microcytic hypochromic RBCs. History and physical examination are typically not helpful in the separation of these two disorders. The history may reveal other family members with anemia and the physical examination may reveal splenomegaly. The CBC will reveal anemia with severely microcytic RBCs with an MCV <70 fL. Hemoglobin electrophoresis is needed to confirm the diagnosis. Elevated HbA2 will be noted.

TREATMENT

Depending on the degree of anemia and effects on patient growth and development, transfusion therapy can be utilized in patients with thalassemia. Younger children are typically kept on transfusion regimens to ensure that growth potential is maximized. Thalassemia major patients undergoing chronic transfusions and even thalassemia intermedia patients who may have only rare transfusions have an increased propensity to absorb iron. These patients are at risk for becoming iron overloaded.

To avoid possible complications of iron overload, including cardiac disease, cirrhosis, pancreatic islet cell failure, testicular failure, and joint disease, regular iron chelation needs to be undertaken. Deferoxamine (subcutaneous/intravenous) and deferasirox (oral) are two iron chelators that are available for the treatment of iron overload.

Beyond regular transfusion therapy and iron chelation, few definitive therapies exist. Bone marrow transplantation is potentially curative. There are several other therapies that are currently under investigation, including gene therapy to allow nonmutated forms of the β-globin genes to be introduced into RBC progenitors.

Patients who undergo splenectomy, to decrease hemolysis of RBCs, should be vaccinated against polysaccharide encapsulated organisms including *Streptococcus pneumoniae*, *Haemophilus influenzae* type b, and *Neisseria meningitidis*.

Thalassemia patients may have several endocrine complications including impaired growth and hormone deficiencies. The use of hormone replacement can have a valuable role in treating these patients, but this needs to be done under the guidance of an endocrinologist.

Bone disease seen in thalassemia can also be improved with the use of calcium supplementation, vitamin D, and bisphosphonates.

PATIENT EDUCATION

- With regular transfusion therapies and appropriate iron chelation, patients with thalassemia can live into adulthood. Women with thalassemia can successfully carry pregnancies to term.
- All patients with thalassemia need to be followed by multiple specialists including hematologists, cardiologists, endocrinologists, and psychologists to properly manage the various problems and issues that arise from thalassemia.

6.1C ANEMIA OF CHRONIC DISEASE

The anemia of chronic disease is a common cause of anemia that can develop in patients with malignancy, chronic infection, and rheumatologic conditions; it can also be noted in patients with other chronic diseases such as heart failure and diabetes. There are three different etiologies or pathophysiologic mechanisms of anemia of chronic disease:

- Anemia of inflammation
- Anemia of chronic disease
- Anemia of older adults

The diagnosis of the anemia of chronic disease can be difficult and is mainly one of exclusion.

MEDICAL HISTORY AND CLINICAL PRESENTATION

The presentation of patients with anemia of chronic disease consists of the signs and symptoms of the underlying disease. The symptoms due to anemia are typically mild and consist of fatigue and dyspnea.

SIGNS AND SYMPTOMS

The typical presentation of anemia of chronic disease is that of the underlying condition. Common causes include infectious, inflammatory, or malignant. All share some or all the same features of anemia of chronic disease. Differences will depend on the presentation of the underlying disorder.

PHYSICAL EXAMINATION

A complete physical exam should be performed looking for findings consistent with the underlying chronic disease.

DIFFERENTIAL DIAGNOSIS

Other conditions that can mimic anemia of chronic disease are iron deficiency, erythropoietin deficiency, and myelodysplastic disorders. However, the presence of low serum iron and transferrin levels, and normal or elevated ferritin, should increase the likelihood of anemia of chronic disease.

DIAGNOSTIC STUDIES

There is no single laboratory test that definitively rules in or rules out the diagnosis of anemia of chronic disease. The anemia of chronic disease is typically microcytic or normocytic, and not associated with other abnormalities in the blood. If other abnormalities are noted, such as leukocytosis and thrombocytosis, these changes are typically secondary to the underlying cause (i.e., inflammation).

Iron studies typically show low serum iron, low TIBC, an elevated percentage saturation, and elevated ferritin (Table 6.4).

TABLE 6.4 Comparison of the Laboratory Findings in Anemia of Chronic Disease and Iron Deficiency Anemia

Laboratory Test	Anemia of Chronic Disease	Iron Deficiency Anemia	Normal Range
Mean corpuscular volume (MCV)	Normal/ decreased	Decreased	80–100 fL
Mean corpuscular hemoglobin (MCH)	Normal/ decreased	Decreased	27–32 pg
Mean corpuscular hemoglobin concentration (MCHC)	Normal/ decreased	Decreased/ normal	30–36 mg/dL
Red blood cell distribution width (RDW)	Normal	Increased	10.5%–14.5%
Serum iron	Decreased	Decreased	30–160 mcg/dL
Total iron-binding capacity (TIBC)	Decreased	Increased	225–430 mcg/dL
Serum ferritin	Elevated	Decreased	30–300 ng/mL

Bone marrow exam should not be necessary but may be required to exclude other causes of anemia or to diagnose an underlying condition.

Serum erythropoietin may be elevated, but often not as elevated as in those with other forms of anemia (i.e., iron deficiency).

Erythrocyte sedimentation rate (ESR) is often elevated, secondary to underlying etiology.

Imaging studies are typically not helpful but may be necessary to uncover the underlying condition that is causing the anemia and may be helpful to rule out other causes of anemia.

EVALUATION

Clinical signs and symptoms in anemia of chronic disease are usually those of the underlying disorder (infection, inflammation, or malignancy). Anemia of chronic disease should be suspected in patients with microcytic or normocytic anemia who also have chronic illness, infection, inflammation, or cancer. If anemia of chronic disease is suspected a serum iron, TIBC, reticulocyte count, and serum ferritin should be obtained. Hemoglobin is usually >8 g/dL unless an additional mechanism contributes to anemia, such as iron deficiency.

A serum ferritin level of <100 ng/mL in a patient with inflammation (<200 ng/mL in patients with chronic kidney disease) suggests that iron deficiency may be superimposed on anemia of chronic disease. However, since serum ferritin is an acute-phase reactant it may be falsely elevated.

TREATMENT

The most effective therapy is to reverse the underlying cause. While rare, transfusions may be needed if the anemia is severe enough to cause symptoms. Erythropoietin has been shown to be effective in improving quality of life in patients with anemia in the setting of chronic kidney disease. With the use of erythropoietin, the target hemoglobin should not be above 10 g/dL.

PATIENT EDUCATION

- Typically, the anemia of chronic disease is mild. Anemia of chronic disease may be a poor prognostic indicator for some conditions (e.g., heart failure), but the anemia typically is not directly related to morbidity or mortality.

6.1D SIDEROBLASTIC ANEMIA

Sideroblastic anemias are characterized by the presence of ringed sideroblasts. Ringed sideroblasts are erythroblasts containing a perinuclear distribution of iron-laden siderotic granules surrounding the nucleus. These granules, deposited in mitochondria, form a ring around the nucleus. In sideroblastic anemias, both the erythroblasts and circulating erythrocytes also tend to contain iron-laden granules called Pappenheimer bodies. Pappenheimer bodies appear as basophilic granules on a routine peripheral blood smear.

Sideroblastic anemia arises from defects in the production of heme. Heme is a non-covalent molecular complex of reduced iron with protoporphyrin IX. Defects in the production of heme can be due to the following:

- Inadequate biosynthesis of protoporphyrin IX
- Failure of iron to couple with protoporphyrin IX

- Disruption of the transport of protoporphyrin IX precursors and iron in and out of the mitochondria

With any of these mechanisms there is a defect in iron utilization and inadequate production of intact hemoglobin molecules causing hypochromic RBCs.

MEDICAL HISTORY AND CLINICAL PRESENTATION

Sideroblastic anemias can be inherited or acquired. The most common form of acquired sideroblastic anemia is idiopathic refractory sideroblastic anemia (IRSA), or refractory anemia with ringed sideroblasts. This is a form of myelodysplastic syndrome and has been shown to be associated with mutations in RNA splicing. Other acquired forms of sideroblastic anemia are due to medications, radiation, or myeloproliferative diseases. Medications most commonly causing sideroblastic anemia are alcohol, isoniazid (INH), and chloramphenicol. Anemia associated with these drugs is rarely severe.

The major hereditary form of sideroblastic anemia is X-linked sideroblastic anemia, a defect in heme synthesis, due to mutations in the gene coding for the enzyme (delta-aminolevulinic acid synthetase-2 [ALAS-2]) that is the rate-limiting catalyst of the first step in heme biosynthesis. Family history in younger patients is needed if there is a suspicion of an inherited form.

SIGNS AND SYMPTOMS

In cases of sideroblastic anemia that have gone undetected for prolonged periods of time, signs and symptoms of iron overload may be apparent, including bronzing of the skin, arthropathies, glucose intolerance, or even myocardial dysfunction. Most adults present with acquired sideroblastic anemia and may present with signs and symptoms of the underlying etiology. A detailed medication and alcohol history should be obtained.

PHYSICAL EXAMINATION

There are no physical examination findings typical of sideroblastic anemia. Findings of possible underlying etiologies may be noted.

DIFFERENTIAL DIAGNOSIS

Ringed sideroblasts, with or without anemia, have been documented in other genetic disorders:

- Erythropoietic porphyria (anemia can occur)
- Zinc overload or copper deficiency
- Thiamine-responsive megaloblastic anemia

While all these conditions can present with ringed sideroblasts, most patients will have either IRSA; a myelodysplastic syndrome which occurs in the latter decades of life; or X-linked sideroblastic anemia, which often presents in childhood or early adolescence.

DIAGNOSTIC STUDIES

Sideroblastic anemia will present with anemia and a low reticulocyte count with no nutritional deficiencies or underlying systemic conditions that could be another cause of the anemia. Examination of the peripheral blood will frequently reveal a dimorphic population of RBCs, or anisocytosis with basophilic granules in the RBC. An elevated RBC distribution width (RDW) value and the presence of siderotic granules (Pappenheimer bodies) are noted. Ringed sideroblasts and Pappenheimer bodies are both best appreciated by seeing the bone marrow aspirate for peripheral blood smear with Prussian blue stain.

Considering a possible diagnosis of sideroblastic anemia should prompt a Prussian blue staining of the peripheral smear and a bone marrow examination. Patients with sideroblastic anemia often exhibit some indication of iron overload such as:

- Elevated ferritin
- High saturation of transferrin
- Elevation in serum iron

Ringed sideroblasts seen in patients with acute alcohol toxicity are rarely the cause of anemia and will resolve when blood alcohol levels fall. Anemia in this setting is most often due to GI bleeding or folate deficiency.

Myelodysplastic syndrome associated with IRSA should be considered if there is an abnormal neutrophil count or platelet count on peripheral blood smear.

EVALUATION

The gold standard for diagnosis of sideroblastic anemia is examination of the bone marrow aspirate and biopsy with Prussian blue stain for the presence of ring sideroblasts.

In adults, IRSA is most frequently diagnosed because a myelodysplastic syndrome is suspected based on a refractory anemia with no other likely cause.

Patients suspected of sideroblastic anemia should have studies of iron stores (ferritin, iron/TIBC) performed.

Sideroblastic anemias are often dimorphic. The MCV may be normal or microcytic but a broad distribution of large and small cells is seen on the peripheral smear. This is noted by an elevated RDW value on the CBC.

Bone marrow examination is required to confirm the diagnosis of sideroblastic anemia.

TREATMENT

Sideroblastic anemia never presents as a hematologic emergency. Initial therapy should be provided with pyridoxine (vitamin B6). Pyridoxine is a co-factor that stimulates steps in the heme biosynthetic pathway. A 3-month trial is needed to determine if the therapy will be effective. Pyridoxine is useful in many patients with inherited forms of sideroblastic anemia but is less effective in acquired disease.

With drug-induced disease the medication should be stopped if that is an option.

Transfusion support for patients is indicated if the anemia is producing significant symptoms.

The myelodysplastic syndrome associated with acquired sideroblastic anemia can be treated successfully with immunosuppressive agents, such as steroids or cyclosporine. These therapies are frequently not effective and should be maintained for only a short trial.

Allogeneic stem cell transplantation has been attempted for inherited forms of sideroblastic anemia, but long-term outcomes have yet to be determined.[4]

PATIENT EDUCATION

- The prognosis of idiopathic sideroblastic anemias is related to the severity of the anemia and the risk of developing iron overload. With aggressive management of iron overload, blood transfusion support, and pyridoxine patients should live into adulthood.

- IRSA has a favorable prognosis among the myelodysplastic syndromes (MDS) but is still a life-threatening illness. Survival varies depending on the severity of the anemia, the success in managing iron overload, and the presence of abnormalities in neutrophils or platelets.
- A normal karyotype carries the most favorable prognosis. Monosomy 7 or deletions of the long arms of chromosome 7 are associated with a worse prognosis.

6.1E VITAMIN B12 DEFICIENCY

Vitamin B12 (cobalamin) plays an important role in the enzymatic reactions responsible for RBC formation and myelination of the nervous system. Deficiency in vitamin B12 may lead to megaloblastic anemia and numerous neurologic dysfunctions. Deficiency may be caused by malabsorption, malnutrition, or an increased demand. The most common underlying cause of vitamin B12 deficiency is pernicious anemia, an autoimmune disease characterized by the absence of intrinsic factor (IF). IF is a protein that is crucial for vitamin B12 absorption in the terminal ileum. Since the daily allowance for vitamin B12 is quite small compared with the large body stores, vitamin B12 deficiency develops over 7 to 10 years in adults. Etiologies are noted in Table 6.5.

MEDICAL HISTORY AND CLINICAL PRESENTATION

A detailed past medical history should be obtained as there are several conditions that should raise suspicion for either subclinical or clinical vitamin B12 deficiency.The following historical information should be investigated:

- Malabsorptive GI diseases, such as sprue, celiac disease, partial gastrectomy, short bowel syndrome, inflammatory bowel disease, and bariatric surgery, carry an increased risk of vitamin B12 deficiency.
- Strict vegetarians and chronic alcoholics should also be considered at risk of developing vitamin B12 deficiency.
- Young adults with a history of nitrous oxide abuse by inhalation should be considered at risk of developing vitamin B12 deficiency.
- Pancreatic insufficiency patients are at risk of developing vitamin B12 deficiency because of the associated malabsorption of vitamin B12 that cannot be released from dietary protein and is unable to bind to IF.
- Chronic therapy with either metformin or omeprazole has shown an increased risk of development of vitamin B12 deficiency.
- Infections with *Helicobacter pylori* have been associated with vitamin B12 and folate deficiencies and should be considered in the presence of upper GI symptoms.

TABLE 6.5 Etiologies of Vitamin B12 Deficiency

Mechanism	Etiology
Malabsorption	
Decreased intrinsic factor (IF)	Pernicious anemia Atrophic gastritis Gastrectomy
Decreased uptake of IF-vitamin B12 complex	Crohn's disease Celiac disease Pancreatic insufficiency Surgical resection of ileum
Malnutrition	Chronic alcoholism Anorexia nervosa Strict vegan diet
Increased demand	Pregnancy Breastfeeding *Diphyllobothrium latum* infection Leukemia

SIGNS AND SYMPTOMS

The signs and symptoms of vitamin B12 deficiency include fatigue due to anemia, neurologic symptoms, and glossitis. Pernicious anemia is typically associated with a positive family history for pernicious anemia or with other autoimmune diseases. In many cases, the classic manifestations may be absent.

PHYSICAL EXAMINATION

Vitamin B12 deficiency presents with nonhematologic manifestations that include a beefy, red, smooth tongue. Patients present with signs of anemia (e.g., fatigue) and/or neurologic manifestations including paresthesia, spasticity, ataxia, and neuropsychiatric disorders. See Table 6.6 for the clinical signs of vitamin B12 deficiency.

DIFFERENTIAL DIAGNOSIS

Causes of macrocytosis other than vitamin B12 deficiency include folate deficiency, azidothymidine (AZT) therapy, chemotherapy, elevated alcohol intake and/or liver dysfunction, hypothyroidism, myelodysplastic syndrome, and MM. Macrocytosis may be hidden or absent in the presence of concomitant iron deficiency or thalassemia, although these cases tend to have an increased RDW.

Severe megaloblastic anemia can be misdiagnosed as erythroleukemia and in rare cases AML.

DIAGNOSTIC STUDIES

Laboratory evaluation of vitamin B12 deficiency is straightforward and manifests with anemia, macrocytosis (MCV

TABLE 6.6 Clinical Manifestations of Vitamin B12 Deficiency

Hematologic	Megaloblastic anemia Pancytopenia
Neurologic	Paresthesia Peripheral neuropathy Demyelination of dorsal columns and corticospinal tract
Psychiatric	Irritability/personality change Memory impairment/dementia Depression Psychosis
Cardiovascular	Possible increased risk of myocardial infarction and stroke

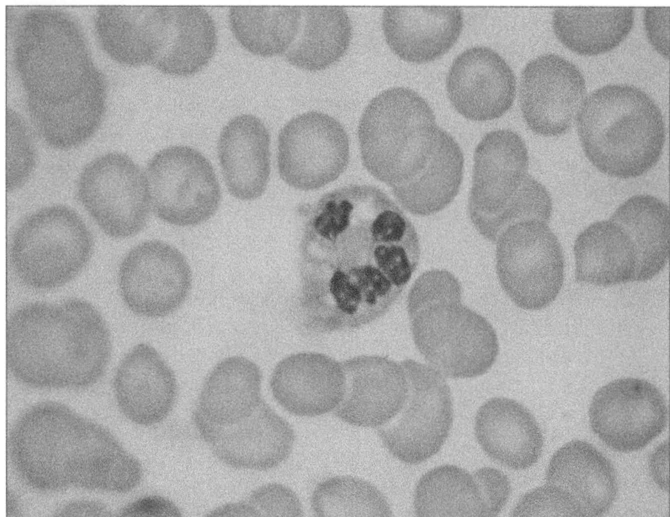

Figure 6.4 **Hypersegmented neutrophil.**
(Source: James Van Rhee and Janie McDaniel.)

>100 fL with ovalocytosis), with possible thrombocytopenia and neutropenia, and neutrophil hypersegmentation (at least 5% of neutrophils with five lobes or at least 1% with six lobes) (Figure 6.4). Hypersegmentation of neutrophils is a useful diagnostic sign and can be present with neurologic findings and in the absence of anemia. RBC morphology reveals the presence of macrocytes and ovalocytes. Reticulocyte count is typically reduced but may be normal.

Serum or plasma vitamin B12 levels or of metabolites are required to confirm a diagnosis of vitamin B12 deficiency. Final confirmation of the diagnosis may require noting normal vitamin B12 levels after treatment.

Serum or plasma vitamin B12 levels <200 pg/mL may be indicative of vitamin B12 deficiency but may not be indicative of true B12 deficiency, which must be demonstrated by both clinical and laboratory findings. Vitamin B12 deficiency is highly unlikely when vitamin B12 values are >300 pg/mL.

Vitamin B12 plays an important role in homocysteine and methylmalonic acid metabolism. Vitamin B12 is required for the conversion of homocysteine to methionine and the conversion of L-methylmalonyl-coenzyme A to succinyl-coenzyme A. With vitamin B12 deficiency the levels of homocysteine and methylmalonic acid will increase. These levels will increase before the drop in serum vitamin B12 levels.

The diagnosis of pernicious anemia is primarily based on the presence of antibodies directed against IF in conjunction with increased serum levels of gastrin and pepsinogen. An increase in serum gastrin and pepsinogen above the normal range is very sensitive for diagnosing pernicious anemia, but not very specific, since these values increase in a variety of other conditions.

Increased lactic dehydrogenase (LDH) and bilirubin confirm the presence of ineffective erythropoiesis due to vitamin B12 deficiency, which results in altered maturation of erythroid precursors.

EVALUATION

Diagnosis of vitamin B12 deficiency is relatively straightforward. The presence of anemia, macrocytosis, ovalocytosis, neutrophil hypersegmentation, and neurologic manifestations, along with low vitamin B12 levels, strongly supports the diagnosis.

Examination of the bone marrow does not distinguish vitamin B12 from folate deficiency and should be reserved for cases in which there is a suspicion of an underlying hematologic malignancy. In vitamin B12 deficiency the marrow is hypercellular with characteristic features of megaloblastic erythropoiesis and presence of large metamyelocytes.

Intestinal malabsorption of vitamin B12 should be investigated. While the presence of anti-IF antibodies and serum gastrin and pepsinogen levels aids in diagnosing pernicious anemia, upper endoscopy and small bowel studies should be considered in selected cases. Small-bowel study with biopsy should be considered when celiac disease is suspected along with anti-endomysial antibodies and anti–tissue-transglutaminase antibodies.

TREATMENT

Standard treatment is vitamin B12 replacement. High-dose oral vitamin B12 is as effective as intramuscular (IM) for correcting the anemia and neurologic symptoms.[5] More rapid improvement is noted with IM therapy and should be used in severe vitamin B12 deficiency or in patients with severe neurologic symptoms.

Patients who have had bariatric surgery should receive 1 mg of oral vitamin B12 per day indefinitely.

Normalization of serum homocysteine and methylmalonic acid following vitamin B12 supplementation is a strong additional confirmation of the diagnosis of B12 deficiency.

The reticulocyte count will increase after treatment, peaking at 1 week following vitamin B12 administration. If reticulocyte response is inadequate it may indicate concurrent iron deficiency.

PATIENT EDUCATION

- Patients with pernicious anemia require regular screening for thyroid disease and iron deficiency. These patients are also at higher risk of developing GI malignancies, such as carcinoids and gastric cancer.
- Use of vitamin B12 in patients with elevated serum homocysteine levels and cardiovascular disease does not reduce the risk of myocardial infarction or stroke or alter cognitive decline.

6.1F FOLATE DEFICIENCY

Folate, absorbed in the small intestine, plays an important role in homocysteine metabolism; folate is required for the conversion of homocysteine to methionine. With folate deficiency the levels of homocysteine will increase. The level of homocysteine will increase before a drop in the serum folate level.

Folate deficiency should be considered in patients with reduced dietary intake and alcoholism. Reduced dietary intake may be noted in patients with chronic diseases, institutionalization in nursing homes, and advanced old age. Folate deficiency may also be a consequence of intestinal malabsorption, noted in celiac disease and inflammatory bowel disease. Folate deficiency can be drug-induced and should be considered in patients treated with metformin, cholestyramine, methotrexate, phenytoin, trimethoprim, and pyrimethamine.

MEDICAL HISTORY AND CLINICAL PRESENTATION

Evaluation of the patient should include a complete medical history. Increase risk of folate deficiency is noted in patients with poor nutritional intake, malabsorption disorders, hepatobiliary dysfunction, and possible increased folate catabolism. A detailed medication history should be obtained. Drugs that affect folate metabolism include methotrexate, 5-fluorouracil, hydroxyurea, pyrimethamine, pentamidine, phenytoin, and trimethoprim/sulfamethoxazole. Drugs that affect folate absorption include metformin and cholestyramine.

SIGNS AND SYMPTOMS

The signs and symptoms noted in folate deficiency are those of anemia. General symptoms include fatigue, pallor, jaundice, and cognitive decline. Chest pain and shortness of breath are noted if tissue hypoxia and organ ischemia have developed as a result of the anemia.

PHYSICAL EXAMINATION

Folate deficiency presents with nonhematologic manifestations that includes a beefy, red, smooth tongue and angular cheilitis. There are no neurologic findings noted with folate deficiency.

DIFFERENTIAL DIAGNOSIS

Macrocytosis is a common finding in adult patients, with an estimated incidence around 2–3%, but most cases do not have anemia.[6] Causes of macrocytosis other than folate deficiency include vitamin B12 deficiency, azathioprine therapy, chemotherapy, elevated alcohol intake and/or liver dysfunction, hypothyroidism, myelodysplastic syndrome, and MM. Macrocytosis may be hidden or absent in the presence of iron deficiency or thalassemia.

Severe folate deficiency can be misdiagnosed as erythroleukemia and AML. Infections with *Helicobacter pylori* have been associated with vitamin B12 and folate deficiencies and should be considered in the presence of upper GI symptoms.

DIAGNOSTIC STUDIES

Serum folate values below 3.0 ng/mL may indicate folate deficiency and values above 4 ng/mL rule out folate deficiency. Serum folate levels are influenced by dietary intake of folate.

The RBC folate assay is recommended, over serum folate assay, because it is not affected by recent intake of folate-containing food and better represents true tissue folate levels. Values below 140 ng/mL have been interpreted as diagnostic of folate deficiency. RBC folate can also decrease in the presence of vitamin B12 deficiency.

Metabolic intermediates assays can be useful in cases with indeterminant folate levels. Serum homocysteine is elevated in folate deficiency, while serum/urine methylmalonic acid levels are normal. These assays are helpful in the differential diagnosis with vitamin B12 deficiency, which is associated with increases in both serum homocysteine and methylmalonic acid.

Increased LDH and bilirubin are noted and confirm the presence of ineffective erythropoiesis due to folate deficiency.

Bone marrow aspirate and biopsy are rarely needed to make the diagnosis of folate deficiency. In folate deficiency the marrow is hypercellular with characteristic features of megaloblastic erythropoiesis and presence of large metamyelocytes. The bone marrow does not aid in distinguishing folate deficiency from vitamin B12 deficiency and should be reserved for cases in which there is a suspicion of an underlying hematologic malignancy.

EVALUATION

The possible diagnosis of folate deficiency should be considered if on the CBC there is the presence of anemia, macrocytosis (MCV >100 fL with ovalocytosis) and hypersegmented neutrophils (defined as 5% of neutrophils with five lobes or 1% with six lobes). The reticulocyte count will be decreased. Direct measurement of folate levels in RBCs or serum/plasma and of metabolites is required to confirm a diagnosis of folate deficiency. Final confirmation of the diagnosis may require showing a normalization of the biochemical markers of folate deficiency following folate therapy.

A serum folate sample should be taken before any meal, as serum folate may transiently normalize following a folate-containing meal. A similar effect can also be noted following blood/plasma transfusions. Folate levels may be below the normal range due to low intake in the preceding few days, during pregnancy, because of increased alcohol intake, or during therapy with anticonvulsant drugs such as carbamazepine, phenobarbital, and phenytoin.

Folate and vitamin B12 deficiency may both be present in the same patient, so in the workup of a possible folate deficiency, vitamin B12 metabolism should always be assessed.

TREATMENT

Oral folic acid (1–5 mg daily) is typically adequate to treat folate deficiency. Normalization of homocysteine following folate supplementation is an additional confirmation of the diagnosis of folate deficiency. Incomplete therapeutic response is associated with only transient normalization of these parameters. Incomplete response should trigger further investigation of other diagnoses.

The reticulocyte count promptly increases after treatment, peaking at 1 week following folate administration. A blunted response may be indicative of the presence of iron deficiency.

PATIENT EDUCATION

- Folic acid supplements decrease homocysteine levels. Patients with increased cardiovascular disease risk secondary to elevated homocysteine levels should be treated with folic acid.

6.1G HEMOLYTIC ANEMIA

Hemolytic anemia is the premature destruction of RBCs. It can be acute or chronic, and can be life-threatening, and it should be considered in all patients with an unexplained normocytic or macrocytic anemia. Hemolytic anemias present with laboratory evidence of increased RBC destruction, including elevated LDH, elevated indirect bilirubin, decreased haptoglobin, and increase in reticulocytes.

Premature destruction of RBCs can occur and can be intravascular or extravascular in the monocyte-macrophage

TABLE 6.7 Etiologies of Hemolytic Anemia

Etiology	Example	Mechanism	Vascular Location
Autoimmune hemolytic anemia	Warm or cold autoantibodies	Splenic trapping, phagocytosis, complement activation	Extravascular or intravascular
Drug induced	Drug-induced thrombotic microangiopathy, drug-induced immune hemolytic anemia	Direct, toxin, phagocytosis, fragmentation	Extravascular or intravascular
Enzymopathy	G6PD or PK deficiencies	Oxidative lysis	Intravascular
Hemoglobinopathy	Sickle cell disease, hemoglobin C disease	Splenic trapping	Extravascular
Infection	Infection with *Plasmodium* (malaria), *Babesia*, or *Clostridium perfringens*	Direct, toxin, phagocytosis, fragmentation	Extravascular or intravascular
Membrane structural abnormalities	HS, HE, PNH	Splenic trapping	Extravascular
Extrinsic nonimmune disorders	TTP, HUS, DIC, HELLP syndrome, MAHA, drug-induced thrombotic microangiopathy	Fragmentation	Intravascular
Systemic disease	Hypertensive emergencies, systemic lupus erythematosus, scleroderma, liver disease, hypersplenism	Splenic trapping, fragmentation	Extravascular or intravascular
Trauma	Endovascular devices, aortic stenosis, extracorporeal membrane oxygenation, arteriovenous malformation, burns	Fragmentation, direct trauma	Intravascular

DIC, disseminated intravascular coagulation; G6PD, glucose-6-phosphate dehydrogenase; HE, hereditary elliptocytosis; HELLP, hemolysis, elevated liver enzymes, and low platelet count; HS, hereditary spherocytosis; HUS, hemolytic uremic syndrome; MAHA, microangiopathic hemolytic anemia; PK, pyruvate kinase; PNH, paroxysmal nocturnal hemoglobinuria; TTP, thrombotic thrombocytopenic purpura.

system of the spleen and liver; extravascular destruction is more common. The etiologies of hemolysis are numerous, and mechanisms include (see Table 6.7):

- Hemoglobinopathies, such as sickle cell disease, leading to splenic destruction via multiple mechanisms
- Membrane disorders, such as hereditary spherocytosis (HS), due to inherited protein deficits, leading to increased RBC destruction
- Enzyme deficiencies, such as glucose-6-phosphate dehydrogenase (G6PD) deficiency, secondary to hemolysis due to oxidative stress or decreased energy production in the cell
- Immune-mediated hemolytic anemia, in which antibodies bind with the RBCs resulting in phagocytosis or complement-mediated destruction
- Extrinsic nonimmune causes, such as microangiopathic hemolytic anemia (MAHA), infections, direct trauma, and drug-induced hemolysis, resulting in fragmentation of the RBCs

MEDICAL HISTORY AND CLINICAL PRESENTATION

The clinical presentation of hemolytic anemias is variable and nonspecific. Acute hemolytic anemia should be considered in the patient who presents with acute jaundice or hematuria in the presence of anemia. The clinical presentation of patients with chronic hemolytic anemia include lymphadenopathy, hepatosplenomegaly, cholestasis, and choledocholithiasis. Other nonspecific symptoms include fatigue, dyspnea, hypotension, chest pain, and tachycardia.

SIGNS AND SYMPTOMS

Table 6.8 summarizes history and physical examination findings in hemolytic anemia.

PHYSICAL EXAMINATION

Physical examination findings are nonspecific. Rapid onset of findings with no history of bleeding is consistent with a hemolytic anemia. Jaundice and dark urine may be noted with hemolysis. Splenomegaly may indicate an overwhelming of the reticuloendothelial system. Laboratory confirmation is key.

DIAGNOSTIC STUDIES

The initial laboratory workup of the patient with possible hemolytic anemia should begin with a CBC. Evaluate for anemia and then classify the anemia as normocytic or macrocytic. Once an anemia is identified, other tests that should be obtained include evaluation of the peripheral blood smear, reticulocyte count, LDH level, haptoglobin, unconjugated bilirubin levels, and a urinalysis (see Table 6.9).

- LDH is intracellular and increased levels are noted in hemolysis of RBCs.
- Haptoglobin is a protein that binds to free hemoglobin in the circulation, and levels are decreased in RBC hemolysis.
- Unconjugated bilirubin levels rise as its production exceeds elimination capability.
- Increase in reticulocytes is noted in RBC hemolysis leading to macrocytic RBCs, unless another etiology for the anemia such as iron deficiency or bone marrow suppression is present.
- Urinalysis may be positive for hemoglobinuria in hemolytic anemia despite no visible RBCs on microscopic examination of the urine.

The presence of increased reticulocytes, elevated LDH, elevated unconjugated bilirubin, and decreased haptoglobin levels confirms the presence of hemolysis. The absence of

TABLE 6.8 History and Physical Examination Findings in Hemolytic Anemia

History and Physical Examination Findings	Types of Hemolytic Anemia
Acute-onset jaundice	All hemolytic anemias
Diarrhea	HUS (*Escherichia coli* 0157:H7)
Fever, chills	AIHA, DIC, HUS, infection (malaria, *Babesia* infection)
Hematuria	PNH, intravascular hemolysis
History of malignancy	Warm autoantibody hemolytic anemia
Medications	Drug-induced thrombotic microangiopathic anemia, drug-induced immune hemolytic anemia, G6PD deficiency
Positive family history of hemolytic anemia	Sickle cell disease, HS, HE, G6PD deficiency, PK deficiency
Recent infection with Epstein-Barr virus or *Mycoplasma pneumoniae*	Cold autoantibody hemolytic anemia

AIHA, autoimmune hemolytic anemia; DIC, disseminated intravascular coagulation; G6PD, glucose-6-phosphate dehydrogenase; HE, hereditary elliptocytosis; HS, hereditary spherocytosis; HUS, hemolytic uremic syndrome; PK, pyruvate kinase; PNH, paroxysmal nocturnal hemoglobinuria.

these findings should lead to the evaluation of other possible causes of the anemia.

Examining the peripheral blood smear is important in identifying the specific etiology of various hemolytic anemias. The peripheral blood should be examined for the presence of spherocytes, schistocytes, sickle cells, bite cells, or blister cells.

- **Spherocytes (Figure 6.5):** Caused by membrane deficits or repeated small membrane removals by macrophages
- **Schistocytes (Figure 6.6):** Fragmented cells that result from intravascular destruction
- **Sickle cells (Figure 6.7):** Elongated cells that occur when hypoxia leads to the development of rigid protein strands in the RBCs causing a change in cell shape
- **Bite and blister cells:** Cells that result from partial phagocytosis and occur in oxidative causes of anemia

The direct antiglobulin test (DAT), or direct Coombs test, further differentiates immune hemolytic anemia from nonimmune causes. In the patient with an acquired hemolytic anemia the DAT is used to determine whether the RBCs

TABLE 6.9 Initial Laboratory Tests for Hemolysis

Test	Finding in Hemolysis	Cause
Haptoglobin	Decreased	Binds free hemoglobin
LDH	Elevated	Released from lysis of RBCs
Peripheral blood smear	Abnormal RBCs	Based on cause of anemia
Reticulocyte count	Increased	Marrow response to anemia
Unconjugated bilirubin	Increased	Increased hemoglobin breakdown
Urinalysis	Presence of urobilinogen and blood	Free hemoglobin and its metabolites

LDH, lactate dehydrogenase; RBCs, red blood cells.

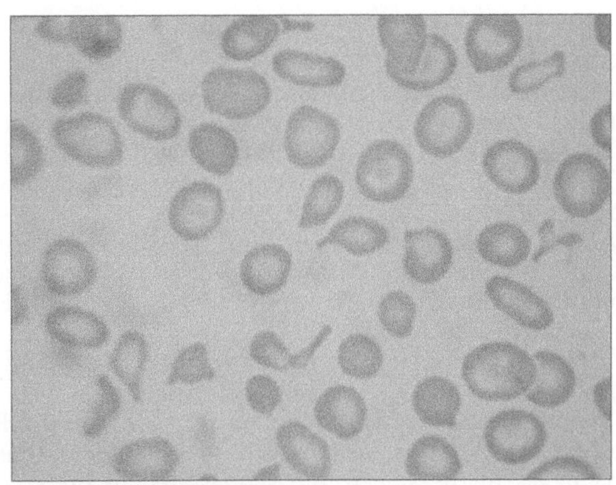

Figure 6.5 **Spherocytes.**
(Source: James Van Rhee and Janie McDaniel.)

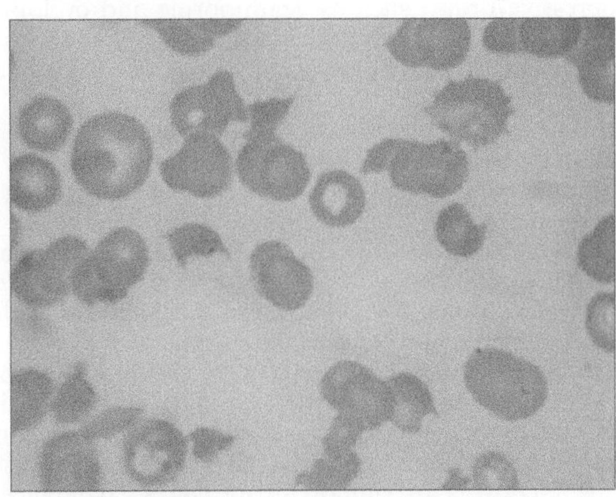

Figure 6.6 **Schistocytes.**
(Source: James Van Rhee and Janie McDaniel.)

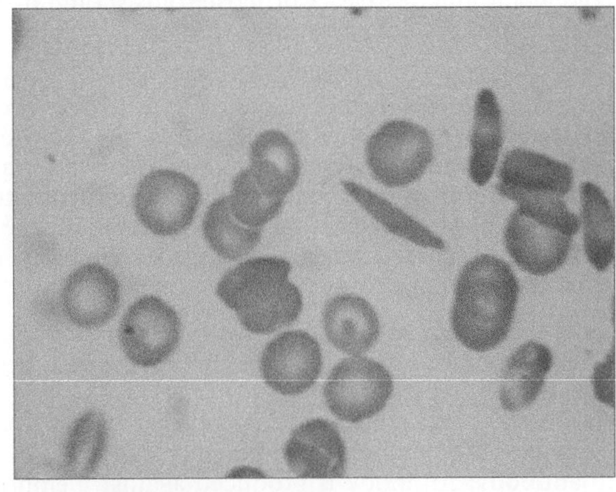

Figure 6.7 **Sickle cells.**
(Source: James Van Rhee and Janie McDaniel.)

have surface bound immunoglobulin G (IgG) and/or complement. The main use of the DAT is to determine if the hemolysis is immune dependent or immune independent. The underlying mechanism of the DAT is that anti-human globulin (AHG) agglutinates antibody-coated cells.

EVALUATION

Immune Hemolytic Anemia

AUTOIMMUNE HEMOLYTIC ANEMIA

Autoimmune hemolytic anemia (AIHA) is caused by autoantibody-mediated destruction. The classic laboratory finding is a positive DAT. AIHA is organized into two subgroups based on the binding temperatures of the autoantibody, either cold and warm agglutinins. Many cases of AIHA are idiopathic; however, viral and bacterial infections, autoimmune conditions, connective tissue disorder, lymphoproliferative malignancies, and blood transfusions are associated with AIHA.

Warm autoantibodies are more common than cold autoantibodies and involve IgG antibodies that react with the RBC membrane at normal body temperatures. These RBCs coated with IgG, are then removed by reticuloendothelial macrophages in the spleen and sequestered in the spleen, which can lead to splenomegaly. First-line treatment of warm autoantibodies is glucocorticoids. Second lines of therapy include splenectomy, rituximab, and other immunosuppressive drugs, such as azathioprine and cyclophosphamide. Management should also include treatment of the underlying condition, blood transfusions as needed, and supportive care.

Cold autoantibodies involve IgM antibodies. These autoantibodies react at low temperatures with antigens on the RBC surface leading to RBC cell lysis on rewarming via complement fixation causing intravascular hemolysis. Primary chronic cold agglutinin disease accounts for a small percentage of all cases and should be suspected in elderly patients with chronic hemolytic anemia, symptoms such as Raynaud phenomenon, and agglutination of RBCs on peripheral blood smear. Development of these cold autoantibodies is also associated with secondary cold agglutinin disease due to infections, such as *Mycoplasma* pneumonia and infectious mononucleosis, or malignant processes. Treatment consists of supportive measures, avoidance of triggers, and management of the underlying disease. Studies have shown that the combination of fludarabine and rituximab or rituximab alone can be effective in treating patients with cold agglutinin disease.[7] Corticosteroids should not be used to treat primary cold agglutinin disease.

DRUG-INDUCED IMMUNE HEMOLYTIC ANEMIA

Drug-induced immune hemolytic anemia is a rare occurrence that results from druginduced antibodies. The most common drug groups causing an immune hemolytic anemia include antimicrobials, nonsteroidal anti-inflammatory drugs, antineoplastic medications, and antihypertensives. There are three common mechanisms of drug-induced immune hemolytic anemia (Table 6.10).

- **Hapten-induced:** The drug, which is the hapten, binds to the RBC membrane and antibodies are now made directed against the hapten.
- **Immune complex:** Antibody is produced against part-drug, part-RBC membrane components.
- **Autoantibody:** Antibody is produced against membrane components producing a reaction similar to that of autoimmune disease.

TABLE 6.10 Drug-Induced Immune Hemolytic Anemia

Mechanism	Hapten	Immune Complex	Autoantibody
DAT	Positive	Positive	Positive
Anti-IgG	Positive	Rarely positive	Positive
Anti-C3d	Rarely positive	Positive	Negative
Examples	Cephalothin Ampicillin	HCTZ Antihistamines Rifampin/INH Sulfonamides Quinidine	L-Dopa Ibuprofen α-Interferon Methyldopa

DAT, direct antiglobulin test; HCTZ, hydrochlorothiazide; IgG, immunoglobulin G; INH, isoniazid.

The DAT is positive in patients with drug-induced immune hemolytic anemia. Currently, cefotetan, ceftriaxone, piperacillin/tazobactam, and nonsteroidal anti-inflammatory drugs predominate. The progression of this condition is typically gradual, and treatment involves removal of the offending agent and RBC transfusion as needed.

Nonimmune Hemolytic Anemia—Acquired

MICROANGIOPATHIC HEMOLYTIC ANEMIA

MAHA is hemolytic anemia that occurs when RBCs fragment, and results in schistocytes on the peripheral blood smear. This can be caused by trauma from an endovascular device or microthrombi. Thrombotic microangiopathies (TMAs) are a group of disorders that share MAHA as a key feature. Two of the major TMAs are thrombotic thrombocytopenic purpura (TTP) and hemolytic uremic syndrome (HUS).

THROMBOTIC THROMBOCYTOPENIC PURPURA

TTP is characterized by thrombocytopenia, fever, renal injury, presence of schistocytes, and neurologic dysfunction. This presentation has significant overlap with the presentation of HUS, but HUS typically has more renal injury and less neurologic dysfunction. TTP can be diagnosed by noting a significantly reduced ADAMTS13 enzyme activity. The ADAMTS13 enzyme cleaves von Willebrand factor (vWF) aggregations and, when this ADAMTS13 enzyme is lacking or nonfunctional, large vWF multimers form. These multimers trap platelets, leading to the development of microthrombi and RBC destruction by shearing the RBCs, creating schistocytes.

TTP is life-threatening and requires timely diagnosis and treatment. Additional laboratory findings include a negative DAT result and normal coagulation testing. Assessment of ADAMTS13 enzyme activity is diagnostic for TTP, but making a presumptive diagnosis based on clinical presentation and basic labs is important. Once a presumptive diagnosis is made, immediate treatment with plasma exchange and glucocorticoids should be started. Plasma exchange removes affected platelets and autoantibodies while replenishing ADAMTS13 enzyme levels.

HEMOLYTIC UREMIC SYNDROME

HUS is characterized by MAHA, acute kidney injury, thrombocytopenia, and neurologic dysfunction. HUS can be separated from TTP based on ADAMTS13 enzyme activity. HUS is most commonly caused by a Shiga toxin producing

Escherichia coli HUS (STEC-HUS) but is also caused by STEC organisms such as *Escherichia coli* O157:H7 and *Shigella dysenteriae*. The primary source of STEC infection is inadequately cooked ground beef; but fruits, vegetables, poultry, and contaminated drinking water have also been implicated. It most commonly affects children and presents with abdominal pain with diarrhea, following 5–10 days later with MAHA, acute kidney injury, and thrombocytopenia. *Streptococcus pneumoniae* infection, HIV infection, and influenza have also been associated with HUS in rare cases, and present without the classic prodrome. Treatment of STEC-HUS is supportive care and continued evaluation of renal function. Antibiotics are not recommended for GI STEC because they may increase the risk of HUS. Eculizumab has been shown to be effective in the treatment of HUS.[8]

OTHER MICROANGIOPATHIC HEMOLYTIC ANEMIA SYNDROMES

Other clinical entities that cause MAHA include HELLP syndrome (hemolysis, elevated liver enzymes, and low platelet count) and disseminated intravascular coagulation (DIC). HELLP syndrome is related to pregnancy and shares many of the same characteristics of TTP and HUS. TTP and HUS do not usually induce liver enzyme elevations as in HELLP syndrome. A low LDH–to–aspartate transaminase ratio can aid in distinguishing HELLP syndrome because the rate of hemolysis is higher in the other TMAs and hepatic involvement is higher in HELLP syndrome. DIC also can result in MAHA due to fibrin-rich microthrombi. DIC causes thrombocytopenia, prolonged coagulation studies, positive D-dimer test results, decreased fibrinogen levels, and elevated fibrinogen degradation products.

DRUG-INDUCED THROMBOTIC MICROANGIOPATHY

Drug-induced TMA occurs when a medication causes the formation of platelet microthrombi, resulting in MAHA through induced antibodies or direct toxicity. These antibodies interact only in the presence of the drug. The clinical features are like those of other MAHA syndromes. In a 2015 review, the overall incidence of drug-induced TMA was 5% of all MAHA cases.[9] Quinine, cyclosporine, and tacrolimus made up over half of all drug-induced TMA cases. The management of drug-induced TMA includes discontinuing the offending agent and providing supportive care; plasma exchange is not beneficial, except in the cases involving ticlopidine.

Other etiologies include hypersplenism and physical and infectious etiologies. Hypersplenism is the increased pooling and/or destruction of RBCs by the enlarged spleen. Splenomegaly is noted in hypersplenism and is characterized by a reduction in one or more of the blood's cellular elements in the presence of normocellular or hypercellular bone marrow. Most cases of anemia secondary to hypersplenism are asymptomatic. Physical etiologies include burns, snake venom, and toxic chemicals.

Infectious etiologies include *Plasmodium, Babesia,* and *Clostridium perfringens*. Malaria, caused by various species of *Plasmodium*, is the most common etiology of hemolytic anemia in the world. Symptoms include fever, splenomegaly, hemolytic anemia, and thrombocytopenia. The anemia is typically normocytic, normochromic and increased reticulocytes may not be noted secondary to suppression of erythropoietic precursors. Diagnosis is made by observation of the parasite in the RBCs on blood films. *Babesia* intraerythrocytic protozoa are transmitted by ticks. Diagnosis is made by examination of blood smear and serologic testing.

Nonimmune Hemolytic Anemia—Congenital

The congenital hemolytic anemias typically present in infancy or early childhood. The family history may be positive for hemolytic anemia and infants may have significant hyperbilirubinemia. Patients present with pallor, jaundice, and possibly splenomegaly. Laboratory studies reveal a reticulocytosis, elevated indirect bilirubin, and abnormalities on peripheral blood smear, and are DAT negative.

MEMBRANE DISORDERS

HS is due to protein mutations involved in the interactions between the lipid bilayer and spectrin-based cytoskeleton on the RBC membrane. This mutation leads to a loss of RBC surface area and the formation of a spherocyte. HS is an autosomal dominant disorder and is most commonly noted in people of northern European ancestry; 1 in 2,000 people in northern Europe and North America are affected.[10] Patients present with pallor, splenomegaly, and jaundice; laboratory testing reveals spherocytes on peripheral blood smear, increased reticulocytes, and a negative DAT. The osmotic fragility test is considered the gold standard for diagnosing HS but is falsely negative in about 25% of patients.[10] Recent studies note eosin-5-maleimide (EMA) binding test as the appropriate screening test. EMA binding is deficient in HS.[11] Treatment includes splenectomy, which reduces hemolysis; splenectomy is indicated in moderate to severe disease. Cholecystectomy should be considered at the time of splenectomy as gallstone development is common in patients with chronic hemolysis.

Hereditary elliptocytosis (HE) is the second most common membrane disorder, behind HS. In HE the RBCs are elliptical or oval, which results from defects in the protein connection in the RBC membrane. HE is an autosomal dominant disorder, with a prevalence of 1 in 2,000–4,000 worldwide, and is most common in individuals of African, Mediterranean, or Southeast Asian descent. Most patients are asymptomatic, but neonates can present with jaundice, hemolysis, and hydrops fetalis. Patients with severe disease should be considered for splenectomy.

HEMOGLOBIN DISORDERS

Sickle cell anemia is an inherited disorder caused by a point mutation leading to a substitution of valine for glutamic acid in position six of the beta chain of hemoglobin. Membrane abnormalities from sickling and oxidative damage caused by hemoglobin S, along with impaired deformability of sickle cells, leads to splenic trapping and removal of cells. Some degree of intravascular hemolysis occurs as well. Sickle cell disease is more common in People of African descent, including African Americans, Hispanic Americans from Central and South America, and people of Middle Eastern, Asian, Indian, and Mediterranean descent. Sickle cell disease symptoms typically appear by 4 months of age. Symptoms include pallor, jaundice, bone pain, edema, and recurrent painful episodes and chronic organ disease secondary to vasoocclusion. Laboratory testing reveals sickle cells on peripheral blood smear, and hemoglobin electrophoresis reveals a predominance of hemoglobin S. Treatment is mostly supportive. Hydration and pain medications are used to treat acute painful crisis. Transfusions are used as needed. Hydroxyurea, inhibitor of ribonucleotide reductase, has been shown to increase HbF, which inhibits hemoglobin S polymerization, and is approved for treatment in patients with frequent painful crisis. All patients should be up to date on immunizations for *Streptococcus pneumoniae*, *Haemophilus influenzae*, hepatitis B, and influenza.

Hemoglobin C (HbC) disease is one-fourth as frequent among African Americans as sickle cell disease. Laboratory testing reveals mild anemia and mild reticulocytosis. The predominant RBC abnormality on the peripheral smear is an abundance of target cells, and crystal-containing cells may also be seen. Splenomegaly may be the only physical finding. The frequency of acute painful episodes is approximately half that found in sickle cell disease, with life expectancy two decades longer. However, significant morbidity can occur. The incidence of fatal bacterial infection is less than in sickle cell anemia, but there is an increased risk of *S. pneumoniae* and *H. influenzae* infection.

ENZYME DISORDERS

Oxidative hemolysis occurs when normal processes are unable to reduce ferric iron, also known as methemoglobin, to ferrous iron, which carries oxygen. This results in the denaturing of ferric hemoglobin into multimers, called Heinz bodies, and leads to premature RBC destruction by phagocytosis. G6PD is an integral part of the protective systems, and when it is deficient, oxidative insults may cause hemolysis. G6PD deficiency is an X-linked disorder and is common in individuals of Mediterranean and African descent. Classically, fava beans, sulfa drugs, and primaquine were the primary triggers of oxidative hemolysis, but the list of medications to avoid in persons with G6PD deficiency is extensive and noted in Table 6.11. The diagnosis is made by G6PD activity testing. Treatment is discontinuation of the drug and supportive care. Methylene blue is indicated for the treatment of severe methemoglobinemia from a non-G6PD cause, but it is possibly harmful and contraindicated in persons with G6PD deficiency.

Pyruvate kinase (PK) deficiency, an autosomal recessive disorder, is the most common enzyme deficiency causing hemolysis. The enzyme PK is important in energy generation in the cell. Although it is the second most common enzyme disorder to G6PD deficiency, most patients with G6PD deficiency never suffer a hemolytic episode. PK deficiency is noted worldwide but is more common among people of northern European descent. Splenomegaly is often present and patients with severe hemolysis may be chronically jaundiced and may develop gallstones, transient aplastic anemia (AA) crises, and folate deficiency. Since the hemolysis is extravascular with a variable intravascular hemolysis, an increased LDH, hyperbilirubinemia, and low haptoglobin levels may be present. The reticulocyte count increases after splenectomy. RBC morphology is nonspecific in PK deficiency. Laboratories perform quantitative PK enzyme analysis and analyze the mutant enzyme by comprehensive kinetic studies. Many patients do not require therapy. Some require RBC transfusions and splenectomy has documented benefit in severe cases.

TABLE 6.11 Drugs to Avoid in G6PD Deficiency

Class	Drug
Analgesics	Acetylsalicylic acid Acetaminophen
Antibiotics	Nitrofurans Quinolones Chloramphenicol Sulfonamides
Anthelmintic	Beta-naphthol Niridazole Stibophen
Antimalarial	Mepacrine Pamaquine Pentaquine Primaquine
Antimycobacterial	Dapsone Para-aminosalicylic acid Sulfones
Antineoplastic	Doxorubicin Rasburicase
Cardiovascular drugs	Dopamine Procainamide Quinidine Hydralazine Methyldopa
Genitourinary analgesics	Phenazopyridine
Gout preparations	Colchicine Probenecid
Other	Fava beans Naphthalene

G6PD, glucose-6-phosphate dehydrogenase.

PATIENT EDUCATION

- The presentation of hemolytic anemia varies and is nonspecific. There is no single specific diagnostic test for hemolytic anemia.
- RBC morphology can be helpful in identifying the type of hemolytic anemia.

6.1H APLASTIC ANEMIA

AA can be inherited or acquired. Inherited forms usually present during the first decade of life, but in rare cases may manifest in adulthood. Inherited forms may result from DNA repair defects (Fanconi anemia), abnormally short telomeres, or abnormalities of ribosomal biogenesis. Acquired forms of AA are most commonly due to autoimmune attack directed at HSCs. This immune attack is primarily directed by cytotoxic T-cells that target HSCs and cause apoptosis leading to hematopoietic failure.

Acquired AA is extremely rare. The estimated incidence is 2 per 1 million persons in the United States.[12] The disease is most common between the ages of 15 and 30 years, but a second peak occurs after age 60.[12] Environmental toxins such as insecticides and benzene may slightly increase the risk for developing bone marrow failure, and certain medications (i.e., antiseizure medications) may rarely lead to AA.

Acquired AA is potentially fatal bone marrow failure disorder and is characterized by pancytopenia and a hypocellular bone marrow. AA is characterized as nonsevere (nSAA), severe (SAA), or very severe (vSAA) depending on the depth of pancytopenia. SAA and vSAA have a high mortality rate if they are not treated appropriately. nSAA is not usually life-threatening and may not require treatment.

MEDICAL HISTORY AND CLINICAL PRESENTATION

The following historical questions should be asked:

- History of exposures and thorough review of medication history

- Family history of cytopenia, physical anomalies, or pulmonary fibrosis
- Family history of other blood dyscrasias or pulmonary fibrosis, which is suggestive of inherited bone marrow failure
- History of previous blood counts to determine how long the patient may have had this disorder

SIGNS AND SYMPTOMS

AA may present with the following signs and symptoms:

- Fatigue
- Dyspnea on exertion
- Easy bruising and bleeding
- Petechiae most commonly in the mouth or lower extremity
- Pallor
- Headache
- Fever secondary to infection

PHYSICAL EXAMINATION

The following physical examination findings may be noted.

- Pallor in the conjunctivae and nail beds
- Petechiae in the oral cavity and lower extremities
- Splenomegaly (unusual)
- Weight loss, lymphadenopathy, fevers, or other systemic complaints (rare)
- Signs of inherited bone marrow failure disorders, which include short stature, skin and nail abnormalities, early graying of the hair, and missing or abnormal digits

DIFFERENTIAL DIAGNOSIS

The differential diagnosis of pancytopenia is broad; however, the differential diagnosis of pancytopenia with a hypocellular marrow is more restricted, as noted below in Table 6.12.

DIAGNOSTIC STUDIES

The laboratory tests listed in Table 6.13 are used in the evaluation of the patient with possible AA.

TABLE 6.12 Differential Diagnosis for Aplastic Anemia

Differential Diagnosis	Description
Myelodysplastic syndromes (MDS)	Hypercellular bone marrow is common. MDS are more common in older patients (median age 60 years) but may occur at any age.
Large granular lymphocyte leukemia	This disorder of clonal T-cells presents with pancytopenia, and bone marrow is often involved with interstitial lymphocytic infiltrates. Diagnosed by flow cytometry from the peripheral blood. Splenic involvement is common.
Paroxysmal nocturnal hemoglobinuria (PNH)	This clonal hematopoietic stem cell disease may present with pancytopenia.
Inherited bone marrow failure syndromes (e.g., Fanconi anemia, dyskeratosis congenita, and Shwachman-Diamond syndrome)	Typically present in the first decade of life. Specific testing is available to rule out these disorders.

EVALUATION

Evaluation of AA aids in the specific diagnosis of the various types of AA. Criteria are noted in Table 6.14.

TREATMENT

- Allogeneic HSC transplantation (HSCT) from a matched sibling donor is the treatment of choice for children and young adults with SAA and vSAA. Immunosuppressive therapy (IST) is the treatment of choice for individuals over age 40 and those who do not have a matched sibling donor.
- Alternative donor transplants are usually reserved for SAA and vSAA patients who have not responded to IST.
- Patients with SAA will require support with blood products. Goal of therapy is to minimize symptoms such as cardiac complications and bleeding. Blood products should be irradiated to prevent transfusion-associated graft-versus-host disease (GVHD) in patients who could proceed to transplantation. Blood products should also be filtered to reduce the incidence of viral infections and prevent alloimmunization.
- IST with antithymocyte globulin and cyclosporine (ATG/CsA) is first-line therapy for patients with SAA who are

TABLE 6.13 Laboratory Testing Results Noted in Patients With Aplastic Anemia

Laboratory Test	Results
CBC with leukocyte differential	Pancytopenia with the ratio of neutrophils to lymphocytes (normally 3–4:1) inverted. The presence of nucleated RBCs, blasts, or dysplastic appearing neutrophils is atypical and should raise suspicion for MDS or leukemia.
Reticulocyte count	Absolute or corrected reticulocyte count is always low in AA.
Complete metabolic profile	Hepatitis/aplasia syndrome presents with severely elevated bilirubin and transaminases. Mild elevations in LDH may be suggestive of a paroxysmal nocturnal hemoglobinuria (PNH) clone.
Peripheral blood flow cytometry	Detection of cells missing glycosylphosphatidylinositol anchored protein (GPI-AP) is a hallmark of PNH. A small to moderate population of GPI-AP deficient cells (usually 0.1% to 15%) can be found at diagnosis in up to 70% of patients with acquired AA.
Fanconi anemia screen on peripheral blood	Increased chromosomal breakage in response to diepoxybutane or mitomycin C is diagnostic of Fanconi anemia. Patients with acquired AA do not show an increase in chromosomal breaks.
Bone marrow aspirate, biopsy, iron stain, and flow cytometry	A hypocellular bone marrow biopsy is required for the diagnosis of AA. A rough estimate of what constitutes normal cellularity can be calculated by subtracting the patient's age from 100.
Bone marrow karyotyping and fluorescence in situ hybridization	Abnormal cytogenetic studies in the setting of a hypocellular bone marrow suggest a diagnosis of MDS. The most common and worst prognostic cytogenetic abnormality to evolve from AA is monosomy 7. Trisomy 8 and 13q abnormalities have a more favorable prognosis and sometimes respond to immunosuppressive therapy.

AA, aplastic anemia; CBC, complete blood count; LDH, lactate dehydrogenase; MDS, myelodysplastic syndromes; RBCs, red blood cells.

TABLE 6.14 Diagnostic Criteria for Aplastic Anemia[13]

Aplastic Anemia Classification	Diagnostic Criteria
Severe aplastic anemia (SAA)	Hypocellular bone marrow (<25% cellularity) and at least two of the following: • Absolute neutrophil count <0.5 × 10⁹/L • Absolute reticulocyte count <60 k/mm³ • Platelet count <20k × 10⁹/L
Very severe aplastic anemia (vSAA)	Same as SAA except absolute neutrophil count <0.2 × 10⁹/L.
Nonsevere aplastic anemia (nSAA)	Hypocellular bone marrow and peripheral blood cytopenia that do not meet criteria for SAA

Source: Data from Guinan EC. Diagnosis and management of aplastic anemia. Hematology Am Soc Hematol Educ Program. 2011;2011:76-81. doi: 10.1182/asheducation-2011.1.76. PMID: 22160015.

over age 30 years, lack human leukocyte antigen (HLA)-matched sibling donors, or are not HSCT candidates for other reasons.
- High-dose cyclophosphamide can be used to treat AA, but its use is limited because of its high rate of toxicity.
- Eltrombopag, a colony-stimulating factor, is the standard of care in AA.

PATIENT EDUCATION

- The mortality risk from AA correlates with the peripheral blood counts. Patients with SAA and vSAA are at greatest risk if not treated promptly. The mortality rate in these patients can approach 50% in the first year without therapy.
- nSAA is rarely life-threatening and may not require therapy. Patients could anticipate that one-third of patients with nSAA improve spontaneously, one-third continue with cytopenia in the nSAA range, and one-third progress to SAA over time.

SPECIAL CONSIDERATIONS

- Iron deficiency anemia is the most common cause of anemia in childhood and typically is seen between 6 and 24 months of age. Deficiency typically develops when rapid growth and expanding blood volume put a demand on iron stores. Dietary risk factors include extended exclusive breast feeding more than 6 months without iron supplementation, consuming low iron formulas, and excessive whole milk intake.
- Symptoms and laboratory findings are those typically noted in adults. Children may develop tachycardia and a systolic ejection murmur. With severe anemia congestive heart failure may develop. Treatment consists of 3 to 6 mg/kg/day of elemental iron.
- Infants exclusively fed by breast-feeding or born to strict vegetarian mothers are at increased risk of developing vitamin B12 deficiency. In infants it manifests primarily with neurologic symptoms and failure to thrive.
- Pregnancy and lactation will increase folate requirements, doubling the daily requirement needs.
- Patients with chronic RBC hemolysis and skin diseases characterized by massive exfoliation also have increased folate demands.
- Inadequate folate levels are also associated with increased birth defects; this can be prevented if the daily folate intake is 400 mcg or greater.

KEY POINTS

- Iron deficiency is the most common anemia in the world and the most common etiology is blood loss. Diagnostic testing includes decreased serum iron, elevated TIBC, and decreased ferritin; treatment is elemental iron.
- Anemia of chronic disease is due to infection, inflammation, or malignancy. Hemoglobin is typically >8 g/dL.
- AA involves hypoplasia of the bone marrow affecting RBCs, WBCs, and platelets.
- The long-term complications of sickle cell anemia include pulmonary hypertension, chronic kidney disease, stroke, aseptic necrosis, and infection.

6.2 LEUKEMIA

OVERVIEW

Leukemia is a progressive, malignant disease of the WBCs. It is characterized by abnormal proliferation and development of leukocytes and their precursors in the blood and bone marrow. Leukemia is classified as acute or chronic, according to the degree of cell differentiation; and as myeloid or lymphocytic, according to the predominant type of cell involved. The exact cause of leukemia is unknown, but genetic and environmental risk factors have been identified. Typical signs and symptoms might include fatigue, weight loss, fever, pallor, ecchymoses, petechiae, dyspnea, bleeding, and recurrent infections. Definitive diagnoses often require bone marrow biopsy and/or blood analysis.

EPIDEMIOLOGY

In 2018, there were about 60,300 new cases of leukemia with about 24,300 deaths.[14] The prevalence of leukemia is generally higher in Caucasians and in males and increases with age. Approximately 1.5% of persons will be diagnosed with leukemia in their lifetime.[14]

PATHOPHYSIOLOGY

Several genetic syndromes, including Down syndrome and neurofibromatosis, are associated with an increased risk of childhood acute lymphocytic leukemia (ALL) and AML. Persons exposed to ionizing radiation, such as those receiving radiation treatment, have an increased risk of developing ALL, AML, and CML.

Occupational and environmental exposure to benzene is an established risk factor for leukemia in adults, most commonly AML. Household pesticide exposure in utero and in the first 3 years of life has been associated with an increased risk of childhood ALL. Obesity may also increase the risk. A history of hematologic malignancy is also a risk factor for developing a different subtype of leukemia later in life.

Normal WBC maturation sequence begins with the blast form, derived from HSCs. In the myelocytic series the cell matures from a blast to a mature neutrophil through a series of steps.

6.2A ACUTE LYMPHOCYTIC LEUKEMIA

ALL is a neoplasm involving lymphoblasts of either the B-cell or T-cell type. ALL is primarily a disease of children, with most of cases occurring in patients under 6 years of age. The incidence of ALL is about 1.8 per 100,000 persons per year, with 5,930 new cases diagnosed each year in the United States.[13] Approximately 85% are precursor B-cell phenotype, with precursor T-cell disease accounting for the remainder.

Treatment of childhood ALL has been very successful over the past decades. Current treatment for pediatric ALL has a reported complete remission rate of 95% to 99%, with estimated 5-year event-free survival rates of 80% to 85%. Results for adults with ALL have not kept pace with those of children, with a disease-free survival rate of 41%, and overall survival rate of 43%.[15]

ALL is typically associated with a proliferation of small to medium-size blasts with scant agranular cytoplasm involving primarily the bone marrow and the peripheral blood.

When the primary location of lymphoblasts is in the bone marrow or peripheral blood it is termed ALL; when the primary location of the lymphoblasts is in the lymph nodes or extranodal tissues it is termed lymphoblastic lymphoma (LBL). In patients who have both bone marrow and nodal involvement the distinction between ALL and LBL is arbitrary. There is no agreed upon number of lymphoblasts that is required for a diagnosis of ALL.

MEDICAL HISTORY AND CLINICAL PRESENTATION

The clinical presentation of patients with ALL is often insidious. Symptoms include fatigue, lethargy, or the presence of constitutional symptoms such as fevers, night sweats, and weight loss. Patients can present with symptoms resulting from anemia, such as dyspnea or lightheadedness, infections due to neutropenia, or easy bruising or bleeding from thrombocytopenia.

Children often have a more aggressive and dramatic presentation that includes extreme pain in the extremities and joints. Lymphadenopathy, splenomegaly, and hepatomegaly are seen in about 20% of patients with ALL. Symptoms from central nervous system (CNS) involvement at presentation is rare, and if present often manifest as symptoms from cranial nerve involvement, due to leptomeningeal leukemic deposits.

SIGNS AND SYMPTOMS

The clinical presentation of patients with ALL is vague and includes fatigue, lethargy, fevers, night sweats, or weight loss. Patients may also present with dyspnea, lightheadedness, infections, or easy bruising and bleeding. A full review of systems is needed and symptoms related to possible infections such as low-grade fevers or night sweats should be investigated.

PHYSICAL EXAMINATION

Lymphadenopathy, splenomegaly, and hepatomegaly are seen in about 20% of patients with ALL.

A complete neurologic examination is required in all patients with ALL. With T-cell ALL, radiographic imaging is performed to establish extramedullary sites of disease, and in male patients, a testicular exam should be performed.

DIFFERENTIAL DIAGNOSIS

The differential diagnosis for patients with ALL, with pancytopenia, and with no circulating lymphoblasts includes AML and marrow failure syndromes such as myelodysplastic syndrome or AA.

Children and young adults who present with severe back, joint, or extremity pain should be evaluated for Still disease and other rheumatologic disorders.

With the presence of circulating blasts, ALL must be distinguished from other leukemic disorders including Burkitt leukemia, AML, CLL, and the leukemic phase of several lymphomas.

DIAGNOSTIC STUDIES

ALL is diagnosed by the presence of lymphoblasts in the peripheral blood or bone marrow. Lymphoblasts in ALL are typically small to intermediate size, and have scant cytoplasm, with a high nuclear-to-cytoplasmic ratio. The nucleolus is often indistinct, and the cytoplasm varies from blue to blue-grey in color with occasional vacuoles. Lymphoblasts can be distinguished from their normal B-cell precursors, which have a higher nuclear-to-cytoplasmic ratio, homogeneous chromatin, and no obvious nucleoli.

Cytochemistry has been used to distinguish ALL from myeloid leukemia. Both B- and T-cell lymphoblasts are negative for myeloperoxidase. B-cell lymphoblasts are often positive for PAS (periodic acid-Schiff) stain, a marker for intracellular glycogen, in a coarse "block-like" pattern.

Immunophenotyping by flow cytometry of peripheral blood or bone marrow is now the method of choice to diagnose ALL. B-ALL/LBL lymphoblasts are almost always positive for CD19, cytoplasmic CD22, and CD79a.

T-ALL/LBL lymphoblasts will variably express CD1a, CD2, CD3, CD4, CD5, CD7, and CD8.

Cytogenetic analysis should be performed on the bone marrow or peripheral blood of all patients with ALL. Cytogenetic and immunophenotypic analysis serves to define several genetic subsets of the disease. One subtype of B-ALL/LBL is Philadelphia chromosome positive (Ph+) ALL. This arises from a reciprocal translocation involving chromosomes 9 and 22, t(9;22)(q34;q11.2). The frequency of Ph+ ALL increases with age as it is noted in approximately 3% of children but found in about 25–30% of adult patients.[16,17] Ph+ ALL has a poor prognosis since Ph+ stem cell is thought to be more primitive than other B-ALL initiating cells. Patients with Ph+ ALL are treated with combination chemotherapy, including a tyrosine kinase inhibitor (TKI).

EVALUATION

A CBC is the first step in the evaluation of the patient with possible leukemia. A WBC count over 20,000/µL is noted in about one-third of patients with ALL. Acute leukemia can also present with pancytopenia. The next step in evaluation involves the evaluation of the peripheral blood smear for the presence of immature WBCs, followed by a bone marrow aspirate or core biopsy (Figure 6.8). Flow cytometry and cytogenetic analysis play an important role in the diagnosis and evaluation of the patient with ALL. A lumbar puncture should be performed to evaluate for presence of disease in the CNS.

TREATMENT

Once a diagnosis of ALL is made, it is important to start therapy immediately.

The main treatment for ALL in adults is long-term chemotherapy. Treatment involves three phases: induction, consolidation, and maintenance therapy. Treatment typically lasts 2 years.

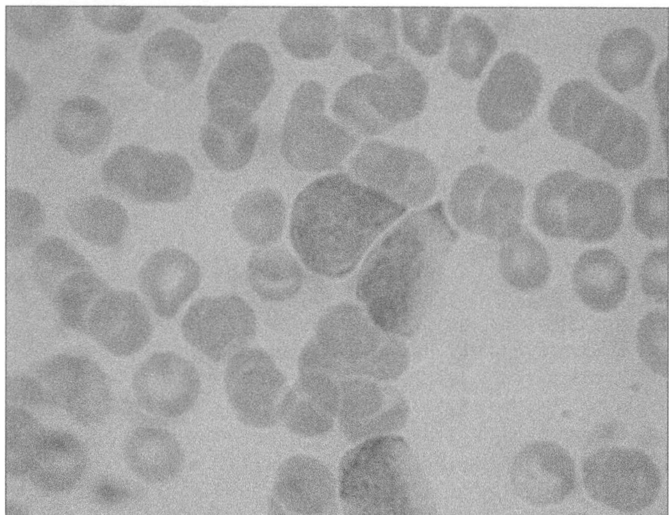

Figure 6.8 **Acute lymphocytic leukemia with blasts in the peripheral blood.**

During induction the goal is remission. Combinations of chemotherapy are utilized including vincristine, prednisone, and doxorubicin. Some protocols may also add cyclophosphamide, L-asparaginase, and possible high-dose methotrexate or cytarabine. If the patient is positive for Philadelphia chromosome imatinib or dasatinib is added.

Because of the possible spread of disease to the CNS, or if leukemia cells are noted in the CNS at the time of diagnosis, treatment of the CNS is needed. Treatment of the CNS is typically started during induction therapy and continued throughout treatment. Treatment of the CNS consists of intrathecal chemotherapy, often with methotrexate, but occasionally cytarabine or prednisone is used as well. Radiation therapy to the brain and spinal cord can also be utilized. If the patient goes into remission, consolidation therapy is the next step. Consolidation therapy typically lasts a few months and consists of the same chemotherapy agents used in induction, but in higher doses.

After consolidation, the patient is put on a maintenance chemotherapy program of methotrexate and 6-mercaptopurine (6-MP). In some cases, this may be combined with other drugs such as vincristine and prednisone. Maintenance typically lasts for about 2 years.

Allogeneic stem cell transplant should be considered in certain subtypes of ALL or in patients with the poor prognostic factors.

Children with standard-risk ALL receive three drugs for the first month of treatment: L-asparaginase,vincristine, and dexamethasone. In high-risk groups, a fourth drug, such as daunorubicin, is added. Children with Ph+ ALL may also be started on imatinib.

Intrathecal chemotherapy should be given to all children. The chemotherapy agent used is typically methotrexate. Hydrocortisone and cytarabine may be added in high-risk children. Side effects to intrathecal chemotherapy include seizures. Radiation therapy to the brain can be used with some high-risk patients, such as those with T-cell ALL. Recently it has been found that many children, even with high-risk ALL, may not need radiation therapy if given more intensive chemo therapy. Side effects of brain radiation include slowing of growth and development.

Because the treatment for ALL is complicated and of such long duration, complications are common. The use of corticosteroid long durations can lead to immune suppression and an increased risk of infection, including fungal infections. Corticosteroids can also cause significant mood alterations, hyperglycemia, and loss of bone density. In pediatric patients, corticosteroids can lead to growth plate fractures and potential growth stunting. In older adolescents and young adult patients, the use of high-dose corticosteroids is associated with avascular necrosis.

Hepatotoxicity may also develop as a result of the use of anthracyclines, vinca alkaloids, asparaginase, or antimetabolites. The risk of hepatotoxicity may increase with the use of other hepatically cleared agents, such as antibiotics and antifungal therapies.

PATIENT EDUCATION

- The prognosis of ALL is highly variable and dependent on factors such as age, immunophenotype, and the presence of the Philadelphia chromosome or other cytogenetic or molecular abnormalities.
- The leading cause of death is infection.
- Complication of chemotherapy may include tumor lysis syndrome. To avoid this the patient should be started on intravenous fluids and allopurinol prior to starting chemotherapy.

6.2B ACUTE MYELOID LEUKEMIA

AML is a cancer of blood-forming cells. AML occurs when abnormal blood cell formation is favored at the expense of normal maturation. An accumulation of malignant hematopoietic cells called blasts fills the marrow space and often appears in the peripheral blood. Many patients with leukemia present with high WBC counts in which the blood cells are replaced by these immature myeloid blasts.

Leukemic cells are characterized by a high nuclear-to-cytoplasmic ratio and a very immature appearing chromatin pattern. This uncontrolled proliferation and accumulation of immature hematopoietic cells and bone marrow failure lead to anemia, thrombocytopenia, and neutropenia/leukopenia. If the blast count in the blood is very high, these cells can cause microthrombi/microhemorrhage leading to deteriorating mental status and/or respiratory failure.

AML may also present in a more chronic way with progressive fatigue, especially in older adults. AML is a disease of older adults with a median age of approximately 65 years.

The World Health Organization (WHO) classification requires 20% blasts in the bone marrow or blood to make the diagnosis of AML.[18] They further divide AML into various groups based on genetic abnormalities.

MEDICAL HISTORY AND CLINICAL PRESENTATION

The diagnosis of AML is straightforward, although some patients may be asymptomatic when a CBC check is ordered for other reasons. Patients present with signs or symptoms associated with bone marrow failure. Fatigue or dyspnea, due to anemia and cytokine release from the malignant myeloblasts, is frequently noted; abnormal bleeding is noted due to thrombocytopenia, specifically in mucosal surfaces such as the nose and gums and/or fine punctate bleeding in the skin, noted as petechiae, mainly on the lower extremities.

Patients may present with an infection, particularly pneumonia or soft tissue infection, due to the neutropenia. Occasionally, patients can present with extramedullary leukemia; leukemic cells are noted in nonmarrow sites. Particularly in AML-monocytic subtypes, deposits of leukemic cells may be noted in the skin, meninges, and gums.

DIC may be the clinical presentation with AML. This activation of the clotting system is due to the release of tissue factor (TF) from leukemic blasts during cell turnover. Patients with DIC and thrombocytopenia, typically noted in acute promyelocytic leukemia (APL), may present with devastating bleeding complications such as major intracranial hemorrhage (ICH).

The most important risk factor for AML is age. Most patients with AML have no predisposing factors; however, chemotherapy for other cancers, particularly alkylating agents or topoisomerase II inhibiting drugs can lead to the development of leukemia.

Other risk factors for AML include exposure to ionizing radiation from military, industrial, or therapeutic sources and exposure to certain industrial solvents such as benzene.

SIGNS AND SYMPTOMS

Gingival hypertrophy may be noted on oral examination. Cranial neuropathies caused by basilar skull infiltration or headache and vomiting due to increased intracranial pressure from decreased cerebrospinal fluid flow can be signs of leukemic meningitis. The most common extramedullary manifestation of AML is leukemia cutis, leukemic infiltration of the skin, which presents as pearly or opalescent nodules.

PHYSICAL EXAMINATION

On physical examination, lymphadenopathy and splenomegaly are commonly noted, particularly in the monocytic subtypes of AML. The monocytic subtypes of AML may also present with gingival hypertrophy, leukemic infiltration of the skin, and meningeal signs from leukemic meningitis. Petechiae or microhemorrhages in the skin may be noted.

DIFFERENTIAL DIAGNOSIS

Patients with abnormal blood counts can have several conditions other than AML, an elevated WBC count with >20% peripheral blasts, anemia, and thrombocytopenia is a typical presentation for acute leukemia and is rarely confused with other conditions.

ALL most closely resembles AML. ALL can present like AML, but the blasts are lymphoid rather than myeloid in origin. Lymphoid blasts tend to have less cytoplasm, fewer or no granules, as well as fewer nucleoli than in myeloblasts. Auer rods are not seen in ALL, but the absence of Auer rods, present in only half of AML cases, does not exclude AML.

In the absence of Auer rods on Wright-stained smears, another level of testing is required to differentiate between lymphoblasts and myeloblasts. Immunophenotypic analysis is the main technique used to delineate lymphoid antigens versus myeloid antigens.

Other conditions in which the WBC count can be high include leukemoid reactions, CML, or indolent lymphoproliferative neoplasms (e.g., CLL or hairy cell leukemia). In chronic phase of CML and in leukemoid reaction there should be few or no blasts and a preponderance of midrange myeloid cells such as bands, myelocytes, metamyelocytes, and promyelocytes.

Two important related entities to AML in which peripheral myeloblasts can be seen include MDS and myeloproliferative neoplasms. Patients with MDS, mainly those with increased blasts, frequently convert to AML after months to years.

The myeloproliferative neoplasms, particularly myelofibrosis (MF), can present with elevated WBC counts, some degree of peripheral blasts, and abnormal platelet. Bone marrow examination in MF will show a small number of myeloblasts and infiltration with fibroblasts.

DIAGNOSTIC STUDIES

Patients generally have a normocytic anemia and thrombocytopenia. The WBC count, generally elevated, may be low, particularly in most patients with the subtype APL or in older adults.

Peripheral blood smear typically reveals the presence of blasts. About half of patients with AML will have blasts that display Auer rods, a concretion of peroxidase/lysozyme-containing granules that appear as rod-like structures singly or in clusters in the cytoplasm of myeloblasts and are commonly noted in APL (Figure 6.9).

Several other laboratory findings may be noted. Serum potassium may be elevated due to tumor lysis, or depressed due to myeloblast-induced renal tubular electrolyte losses. The serum phosphate and uric acid may be high in tumor lysis syndrome, with hyperphosphatemia leading to hypocalcemia.

Elevated hepatic transaminases may be elevated secondary to infection or leukemic infiltration of the liver. Serum alkaline phosphatase is elevated. Elevated direct bilirubin may occur secondary to presence of biliary stones or infections. Low serum albumin may indicate a more chronic presentation with evidence of malnutrition.

Serum creatinine and blood urine nitrogen should be obtained to evaluate the patient's hydration status and evaluation of possible renal failure. Presence of renal failure may indicate underlying renal dysfunction or may indicate renal damage from uric acid released related to tumor lysis syndrome.

Some patients with AML, especially APL, may present with DIC. Evaluation of possible DIC includes obtaining prothrombin time (PT)/INR, partial thromboplastin time (PTT), and fibrinogen.

The most important laboratory study in a patient with known or suspected AML is a bone marrow aspirate and

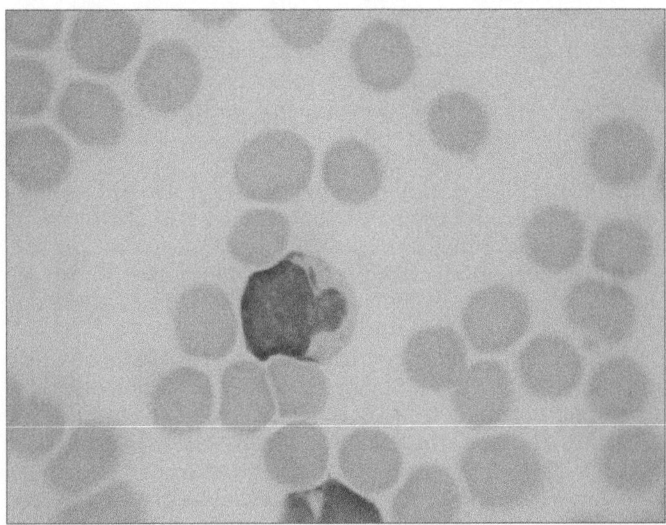

Figure 6.9 Acute myeloid leukemia blast with the presence of Auer rods.

biopsy. Cytochemistry may be performed on the bone marrow aspirate smear including tests for peroxidase, nonspecific esterase, and PAS. Bone marrow aspirate should be sent for flow cytometric analysis to definitively diagnose AML. Definitive diagnosis is made with the detection of myeloid antigens such as CD33 (present in 90% of patients with AML), CD13, CD15, CD11, CD14, and CD117. Bone marrow should be sent for cytogenetic analysis. Cytogenetic testing is used to determine prognosis and guide therapy. Two cytogenetic abnormalities, inversion of chromosome 16 and translocation t(8;21), are characteristic of a favorable prognosis. In some cases, with APL, if cytogenetic analysis is not available, other diagnostic studies may be obtained. FISH (fluorescence in situ hybridization) is used to detect the characteristic t(15;17) translocation of APL, and PCR is used to detect the fusion gene product, which is pathognomonic for APL.

EVALUATION

The following studies should be obtained in the evaluation of patients with possible AML:

- CBC with differential
- Chemistry panel, including uric acid
- Bone marrow aspirate and biopsy with cytogenetic and genetic testing
- Chest radiograph
- PT, PTT (partial thromboplastin time), fibrinogen
- HLA type

A definitive diagnosis of AML made on a blood smear would only be possible if >20% of the WBCs were blasts and if at least some of these cells contained Auer rods; otherwise, examination of the bone marrow or peripheral blasts using cytochemical and/or immunophenotypic analysis would need to be undertaken.

TREATMENT

Many patients require intravenous hydration. Intravenous saline should be given to patients who are dehydrated due to renal losses, vomiting, or lack of oral intake. Transfusion of blood products may be needed as well. Platelet transfusion should be given to patients who are bleeding and thrombocytopenic; prophylactic transfusions are indicated if the platelet count is <10,000/μL.

AML patients are at risk of developing tumor lysis syndrome. If serum uric acid is elevated and/or there are other signs of tumor lysis, alkalization of the urine should be considered to prevent uric acid deposition. Prior to starting chemotherapy prophylactic allopurinol, a xanthine oxidase inhibitor, should be administered.

Leukostasis is a common complication of AML. Leukostasis can lead to the development of microthrombi in the cerebral or pulmonary vasculature. Saline hydration and a rapid acting ribonucleotide reductase inhibitor, hydroxyurea, can lower the WBC count over a few days, while definitive therapy is being initiated.

The definitive therapeutic approach to AML depends on specific disease-and patient-related features. The treatment protocol for AML is divided into two stages: induction therapy followed postremission consolidating therapy. In the induction phase, chemotherapy is given to reduce the tumor burden to a low level so that a complete remission is achieved. Complete remission is defined as no leukemic cells detected in the bone marrow, peripheral blood, or extramedullary sites. Relapse is inevitable if no additional therapy is provided in the postremission setting.

Induction therapy for non-APL AML consists of an anthracycline-like agent for 3 days, with cytarabine for 7 days. A mid-cycle bone marrow examination should be done, and if this bone marrow is adequately cellular and contains >10% blasts, then a reinduction strategy consisting of another 3+7 days of chemotherapy, or 2 days of daunorubicin plus 5 days of cytarabine, should be administered. The overall complete remission rate for younger adults with AML is approximately 60% to 80%.[18]

For those who fail to achieve remission after 1 or 2 cycles of induction chemotherapy, the prognosis is poor. These refractory patients are then treated with a high-dose cytosine arabinoside based regimen. If this treatment is successful, the patient should have an allogeneic stem cell transplant using the best available donor.

If remission is achieved, a high-dose chemotherapy (high-dose cytosine arabinoside) approach with autologous stem cell rescue or allogeneic stem cell transplantation is used postremission.

Patients with APL are treated as soon as possible with all trans retinoic acid (ATRA). ATRA will ablate the DIC and restore hemostasis to a normal state. APL is the most curable subtype of AML. Chemotherapy for APL consists of idarubicin plus ATRA induction, along with three courses of anthracycline/ATRA consolidation, followed by maintenance therapy with ATRA plus 6-MP and methotrexate. If AML relapses after a period of remission, the outcome is poor.

PATIENT EDUCATION

- The prognosis of patients with AML depends largely on age and cytogenetics. Age is a critical prognostic factor, since patients older than age 55 to 60 are rarely cured of this disease, yet patients under age 40 can expect a 40% cure rate.
- The prognosis in APL is related to WBC count and platelet count at time of diagnosis. A WBC count <10,000/μL and a platelet count >40,000/μL have the best prognosis.

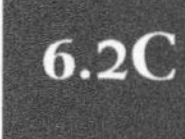

6.2C CHRONIC LYMPHOCYTIC LEUKEMIA

CLL is the most common leukemia in the Western world and is a disease of older adults, with median age at diagnosis of around 70.

CLL is a lymphoproliferative disorder that arises from mature B-cells and leads to the development of functionally incompetent, clonal malignant cells. Accumulation of large numbers of CLL cells leads to the characteristic clinical findings of the disease: lymphocytosis, lymphadenopathy, and hepatosplenomegaly in early stage disease, and cytopenia due to crowding out the bone marrow in advanced disease.

CLL is staged using the Rai staging system (Table 6.15), which is based on lymphocytosis; patients must have at least 5,000/μL monoclonal lymphocytes. Rai staging is used to determine risk groups when determining treatment options. Stage 0 is low risk; stages I and II are intermediate risk; and stages III and IV are high risk.

TABLE 6.15 Rai Staging System for Chronic Lymphocytic Leukemia

Rai Stage	Description
Stage 0	Lymphocytosis; no enlargement of the lymph nodes, spleen, or liver; RBC and platelet counts are near normal.
Stage I	Lymphocytosis; enlarged lymph nodes; spleen and liver are not enlarged; RBC and platelet counts are near normal.
Stage II	Lymphocytosis; enlarged spleen and possibly enlarged liver; lymph nodes may or may not be enlarged; RBC and platelet counts are near normal.
Stage III	Lymphocytosis; lymph nodes, spleen, or liver may or may not be enlarged; anemia; platelet counts are near normal.
Stage IV	Lymphocytosis; enlarged lymph nodes, spleen, or liver; anemia; thrombocytopenia.

RBC, red blood cell.

MEDICAL HISTORY AND CLINICAL PRESENTATION

Most cases of CLL are spontaneous and do not have clearly identifiable risk factors.

Caucasians are at higher risk for CLL, with Asians at the lowest risk. There is also a male predominance, and the risk of developing CLL increases with age.

SIGNS AND SYMPTOMS

Many people with CLL have no early symptoms. Those who develop signs and symptoms may experience painless lymphadenopathy, fever, fatigue, upper left quadrant discomfort secondary to splenomegaly, night sweats, weight loss, and frequent infections.

PHYSICAL EXAMINATION

A fourth of all patients with CLL are asymptomatic at diagnosis; those who present with symptoms exhibit a wide range of symptoms. New lymphadenopathy is frequently the first presenting physical examination finding. At times patients may present with "B symptoms," including fever, night sweats, and weight loss. In patients with more advanced disease pallor due to anemia or easy bleeding/bruising due to thrombocytopenia may be noted.

As CLL can impair the normal immune system response, findings of frequent infections may be noted.

DIFFERENTIAL DIAGNOSIS

Table 6.16 summarizes the differential diagnosis for CLL.

DIAGNOSTIC STUDIES

A CBC and differential will reveal an elevated WBC count with an absolute lymphocytosis. Examination of the peripheral blood smear will show many small lymphocytes and the presence of smudge cells (Figure 6.10). Peripheral blood should also be sent for cytogenetics to evaluate for common cytogenetic abnormalities, as results can affect both prognosis and treatment selection.

Bone marrow biopsy is not required at the time of initial presentation, as the diagnosis can be made from peripheral blood flow cytometry. Bone marrow biopsy should be performed prior to starting treatment to establish a baseline, after completing treatment to evaluate response, and if the disease should relapse.

Peripheral blood flow cytometry is the most sensitive and specific test to establish the diagnosis of CLL. To make the diagnosis the absolute B-lymphocyte count should be ≥5,000/µL, with mainly mature-appearing lymphocytes; and demonstrate clonality.

Other tests that may be beneficial include testing for beta-2 microglobulin and LDH, which serve as markers of disease burden. Serum protein electrophoresis should be evaluated to rule out monoclonal gammopathy; and HIV and hepatitis B and C testing are performed because of the risk of reactivation with treatment.

TABLE 6.16 Differential Diagnosis for Chronic Lymphocytic Leukemia

Differential Diagnosis	Description
Lymphocytic lymphoma	Lymph node-only involvement by malignant CLL cells, with fewer than 5,000/µL circulating clonal B-cells. May develop disease consistent with CLL.
Mantle cell lymphoma	B-cell malignancy that can be mistaken for CLL. Cyclin D1 expression and FISH for the t(11;14) (IgG/CCND1) are both positive in MCL and negative in CLL.
Follicular lymphoma	Distinguished by the cleaved nuclei with irregular contours characteristic of centrocytes in follicular lymphoma and by immunophenotype.
T-cell prolymphocytic leukemia	Separated by a different immunophenotype.
Hairy cell leukemia	Hairy cell leukemia can also have circulating disease, but with a different phenotype. Cells also have hair-like projections.
Lymphoplasmacytic lymphoma	Plasmacytoid-appearing cells and associated with significant paraproteinemia.

CLL, chronic lymphocytic leukemia; FISH, fluorescent in situ hybridization; IgG, immunoglobulin G; MCL, mantle cell lymphoma.

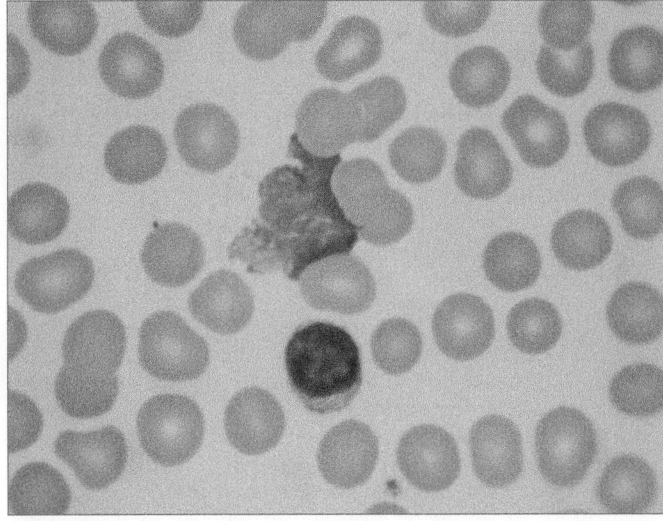

Figure 6.10 **Small lymphocyte and smudge cell noted in chronic lymphocytic leukemia.**

TREATMENT

It is not necessary to initiate emergent therapy for CLL. Even with extreme lymphocytosis a definitive diagnosis should be made prior to starting treatment. If acute onset of anemia or thrombocytopenia is present, steroids should be started and will typically lead to correction of the anemia or thrombocytopenia.

Tumor lysis syndrome may be seen in patients following initial treatment or with transformed disease, and should be treated with intravenous hydration, allopurinol and/or rasburicase, and electrolyte management.

The choice of definitive therapy for patients with CLL depends on their physical condition, prognostic risk factors, and stage. Early stage patients without symptoms can be followed with close observation. CBC should be checked at least every 3 months, and if counts remain stable the interval can be increased to every 6 months. Those with more advanced disease or symptoms should undergo treatment.

Although long-term remissions can be achieved, conventional treatment for CLL is not curative. First-line therapy is a combination of fludarabine, cyclophosphamide, and rituximab.

For patients with low-risk disease or serious comorbidities, first-line treatment consists bendamustine and rituximab followed by fludarabine and rituximab or fludarabine as single therapy or with cyclophosphamide or the oral alkylating agent chlorambucil.

Because of treatment intensity complications can develop. Myelosuppression is common in patients on chemoimmunotherapy or alemtuzumab, and transfusion support may be required. Growth factor support with pegfilgrastim should be provided when the absolute neutrophil count is <1,000/μL.

There is a high risk of opportunistic infections, and prophylactic antibiotics may be required. Prophylactic medications should be continued for at least 6 months after completing therapy, and indefinitely in the relapsed setting.

Patients receiving alemtuzumab should be monitored for *Cytomegalovirus* infection and if present antiviral therapy should be started.

PATIENT EDUCATION

- CLL is typically an indolent lymphoproliferative disorder. Long-term remissions are possible, but no conventional therapy is curative. The goal of therapy is to prevent complications and optimize quality of life.
- With treatment median survival has improved significantly at all stages of disease, particularly in those with advanced disease. Cytogenic abnormalities indicate a poor prognosis.

6.2D CHRONIC MYELOID LEUKEMIA

CML is a malignant disease arising from a primitive HSC in the bone marrow that involves all three myeloid lineages: granulocytes, erythroid cells, and megakaryocytes. Patients typically present with an elevated WBC count consisting of mature neutrophils; a smaller number of immature granulocytes are often present in the blood. CML is defined by the presence of the *BCR/ABL1* fusion gene, which results from the reciprocal translocation t(9;22)(q34;q11.2). This abnormal chromosome 22 is the Philadelphia chromosome.

The Philadelphia chromosome, which results from the reciprocal translocation, t(9;22)(q34;q11.2), is the hallmark of CML. This mutation results in dysregulation of myeloproliferation.

At the time of diagnosis most patients are still in the chronic phase, and the differentiation and maturation of granulocytes proceed relatively normally. Over time, CML can progress to a more advanced disease.

MEDICAL HISTORY AND CLINICAL PRESENTATION

CML is classified into three phases. These phases are based on the number of immature WBCs in the peripheral blood or bone marrow. The chronic phase is defined as having <10% blasts in the peripheral blood or bone marrow. Symptoms are usually mild.

The accelerated phase is defined as peripheral blood with >15% but <30% blasts; or 20% or more of basophils in the blood; or 30% or more blasts and promyelocytes in the blood; or platelet count <100,000/mm^3, not due to treatment; or new chromosome changes in the leukemia cells with Philadelphia chromosome. In this phase symptoms may include fever, decreased appetite, and weight loss.

The blast phase, or acute phase, is defined as >20% blasts in the blood or bone marrow with large clusters of blasts noted in the bone marrow. Blasts may spread to other tissues and organs. Symptoms often include fever, decreased appetite, and weight loss. This phase presents like an acute leukemia.

The median age for CML is 60 years old and is very uncommon in children. CML occurs in both males and females and is not familial. Risk factors for CML include radiation exposure, benzene exposure, and prior chemotherapy for another disorder.

SIGNS AND SYMPTOMS

About one-third of newly diagnosed patients with CML in chronic phase present with no symptoms, and the diagnosis is made on a routine blood count. The most common presenting symptoms are fatigue, related anemia, and modest weight loss, due to early satiety from splenomegaly. Fever and bleeding are relatively uncommon. Other symptoms may include weakness, night sweats, and bone pain caused by leukemia cells infiltrating the bone and joint.

The accelerated phase is characterized by increasing symptoms related to the anemia or thrombocytopenia, increasing spleen size, and constitutional symptoms of fever, sweats, and weight loss.

PHYSICAL EXAMINATION

Physical exam findings are limited and related to the anemia and thrombocytopenia. Splenomegaly is common.

DIFFERENTIAL DIAGNOSIS

The differential diagnosis of CML is noted in Table 6.17.

DIAGNOSTIC STUDIES

CBC and differential are the first step in the evaluation of the patient with CML. The WBC count and platelet count are elevated. The platelet count is rarely >1 million/μL. Most of the WBCs are mature neutrophils and bands, but the entire spectrum of granulocytic differentiation is present.

TABLE 6.17 Differential Diagnosis of Chronic Myeloid Leukemia

Differential Diagnosis	Description
Myeloproliferative disorders	Varies depending on type.
Leukemoid reaction	Secondary to infection or stress, elevated white blood cell count, normal absolute count of basophils, and elevated leukocyte alkaline phosphatase level.
Chronic myelomonocytic leukemia	Monocytosis, normal absolute count of basophils, and lack of Philadelphia chromosome.

A high percentage of blasts or basophils could indicate more advanced disease.

Genetic testing should be completed to document the *BCR/ABL1* fusion, which is always present. The Philadelphia chromosome, which results from the reciprocal translocation, t(9;22)(q34;q11.2), gene should also be documented.

Serum LDH level will be elevated, and the elevation is proportional to the mass of leukemia cells that are turning over.

Bone marrow biopsy and aspiration for cytologic and histologic evaluation will reveal a markedly elevated ratio of myeloid to erythroid (M:E) cells, often to >20:1. Increased numbers of blasts or promyelocytes, or increased reticulin fibrosis in the marrow, may indicate more advanced disease.

EVALUATION

The most definitive diagnostic test is a molecular genetic test to document the presence of the *BCR/ABL1* fusion gene. This can be done with a FISH assay or by RT-PCR (reverse transcriptase polymerase chain reaction). Both tests can be done on granulocytes in the peripheral blood, as they do not require dividing cells. Also, a bone marrow exam provides a sample of dividing marrow cells by aspiration that will demonstrate the t(9;22) by cytogenetic analysis of metaphase cells.

TREATMENT

In patients with CML in the chronic phase, most of the circulating cells are mature neutrophils. Those with WBC count >100,000/µL often have no symptoms, and asymptomatic patients rarely require emergency interventions.

Patients with more advanced disease and large numbers of blasts and promyelocytes in the blood may develop symptoms from leukostasis. Treatment is leukapheresis and starting hydroxyurea to lower the WBC count.

The definitive treatment for patients with CML in the chronic phase involves an oral TKI, such as imatinib, dasatinib, or nilotinib. These drugs are well tolerated and effective with a majority of patients achieving a complete cytogenetic response within 3–6 months. Remissions are long lasting and may persist for more than 10 years. If resistance develops switching to another TKI or an allogeneic HSC transplant should be considered.

Other treatment options include interferon, alone or in combination with low-dose cytarabine or imatinib can produce a complete cytogenetic response in chronic phase CML. Busulfan, an alkylating agent, has been used to suppress myeloproliferation in CML.

Allopurinol is used when starting treatment with a TKI to reduce the risk of hyperuricemia and urate nephropathy.

RBC transfusions are useful to treat the anemia that may be present.

Neutropenia may develop with treatment with TKIs. Supportive care with prophylactic antibiotics or filgrastim is recommended.

PATIENT EDUCATION

- Most deaths follow a blast or accelerated phase of the disease.
- TKIs are the treatment of choice.

SPECIAL CONSIDERATIONS

- Safety during pregnancy is not established for the TKIs for the treatment of CML. This should be discontinued when pregnancy occurs. Depending upon disease status, interferon can be substituted.

KEY POINTS

- ALL is most common in children. CNS involvement is common, and most patients receive intrathecal chemotherapy and corticosteroids. In children response is excellent.
- AML is most common in adults. Several subtypes involve immature myeloid cells. Chromosomal and molecular genetic abnormalities are common.
- CLL is an indolent lymphoproliferative disease involving mature lymphocytes and noted in older patients.
- CML involves the Philadelphia chromosome. Peripheral blood smear aids in the diagnosis. TKIs are the treatment of choice.

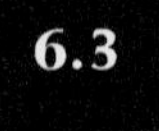

6.3 MYELOPROLIFERATIVE NEOPLASMS

OVERVIEW

Myeloproliferative disorders are a group of slow-growing blood cancers in which the bone marrow produces too many abnormal RBCs, WBCs, and platelets. The type of myeloproliferative disorder is based on which cell is being produced in abnormal numbers. There are six types of myeloproliferative disorders: CML, polycythemia vera, primary myelofibrosis (PMF), essential thrombocytosis (ET), chronic neutrophilic leukemia, and chronic eosinophilic leukemia.

EPIDEMIOLOGY

Risk factors for myeloproliferative neoplasms include intense radiation and petrochemicals, such as benzene or toluene. Many people with myeloproliferative disease have an acquired mutation in the *JAK2* gene.

6.3A POLYCYTHEMIA VERA

Polycythemia vera is a clonal HSC disorder due to unregulated production of RBCs, WBCs, and platelets; thrombotic and hemorrhagic events; pruritus; erythromelalgia;

splenomegaly; and MF. The disease is influenced by genetics related to *JAK2* V617F allele.

The elevated WBC count is associated with extramedullary hematopoiesis, which may manifest as splenomegaly; the liver may also be involved and present with an elevated alkaline phosphatase. Splenomegaly can lead to portal hypertension and varices development due to increased blood flow to the liver.

Pulmonary hypertension and pulmonary fibrosis are significant complications in patients with an aggressive form of polycythemia vera.

MEDICAL HISTORY AND CLINICAL PRESENTATION

Polycythemia vera is most common in women, the elderly, individuals of Ashkenazi extraction, and family members of patients with other myeloproliferative neoplasm such as polycythemia vera, essential thrombocytosis, or primary MF.

SIGNS AND SYMPTOMS

The symptoms associated with polycythemia vera are nonspecific and due to increased blood viscosity, hypercoagulability, inappropriate release of inflammatory cytokines, and organomegaly. The most common symptoms include headache, itching, impaired cognition, weakness, dizziness, extremity and abdominal pain, and easy bruising.

PHYSICAL EXAMINATION

Pruritus and erythromelalgia are early symptoms associated with polycythemia vera, but their absence does not mitigate against the diagnosis. In women, there is an increased predilection for hepatic vein thrombosis and this is often the first manifestation of the disorder.

DIFFERENTIAL DIAGNOSIS

The differential diagnosis of polycythemia includes any cause of erythrocytosis, such as the following:

- Hypoxia secondary to carbon monoxide exposure, high altitude, and chronic pulmonary disease
- Renal disease, including renal artery stenosis and glomerulonephritis
- Tumors, including hypernephroma and hepatoma
- Drugs, such as anabolic steroids and erythropoietin

Conditions that promote plasma volume contraction and pseudoerythrocytosis, including hypertension, diuretics, tobacco use, and androgenic steroids can mimic erythrocytosis.

DIAGNOSTIC STUDIES

Laboratory results are the most important finding in making the diagnosis of polycythemia vera. The WHO has developed diagnostic criteria. The diagnosis of polycythemia vera requires the presence of all three major criteria or the first two major criteria and the one minor criterion.[19,20] See Table 6.18 for these criteria.

EVALUATION

Polycythemia vera is difficult to diagnose based on clinical grounds. The diagnosis is made with an elevation in RBCs, WBCs, and platelets, with or without splenomegaly. If there is an isolated erythrocytosis, even with isolated erythrocytosis and the *JAK2* mutation, another cause of erythrocytosis is more likely. If the hematocrit is <50% or the hemoglobin <16.0 g/dL, the presence of an absolute erythrocytosis is not assured and a RBC mass and plasma volume determination should be performed to avoid confusion with pseudoerythrocytosis due to plasma volume contraction.

Elevation in RBC mass is only noted in polycythemia vera, so a RBC mass measurement is needed to distinguish this disorder from other myeloproliferative disorders.

TABLE 6.18 WHO Diagnostic Criteria for Polycythemia Vera

Major criteria	1) Hb >16.5 g/dL (men)/>16.0 g/dL (women) or Hct >49% (men)/48% (women) or increased red blood cell mass
	2) Bone marrow biopsy showing hypercellularity for age with trilineage growth including prominent erythroid, granulocytic, and megakaryocytic proliferation with pleomorphic, mature megakaryocytes
	3) Presence of *JAK2* V617F or *JAK2* exon 12 mutation
Minor criteria	1) Subnormal serum erythropoietin level

Hb, hemoglobin; Hct, hematocrit; WHO, World Health Organization.

TREATMENT

Because of hyperviscosity, thrombosis is an risk to the patient with polycythemia vera. Once the diagnosis is established, therapeutic phlebotomy should be started to reduce the RBC mass and decrease blood viscosity. Phlebotomy is the quickest and most direct method for reducing the RBC mass, provoking a rapid increase in the plasma volume, and an improvement in platelet function, reducing the risk of thrombosis.

The therapeutic goal of phlebotomy is a hematocrit of 45% or less in a man and 42% or less in a woman.

If there is marked elevation of the leukocyte count or the uric acid is 10 mg/dL or greater, allopurinol should be started. If there is ocular migraine or erythromelalgia not relieved by phlebotomy, low-dose aspirin should be given.

Thrombocytosis causing transient ischemic attacks, unresponsive to aspirin, will require platelet count reduction with hydroxyurea.

Irradiation and chemotherapy are not effective in controlling the complications of polycythemia vera. Pegylated interferon alpha is the only therapy that has produced complete remissions in polycythemia vera.

Pruritus can be a significant symptom. Therapy should begin with a long-acting antihistamine. If pruritus is not controlled hydroxyurea or photochemotherapy or pegylated interferon alpha should be considered.

Massive splenomegaly in polycythemia vera is difficult to manage. It is usually refractory to chemotherapy and with no long-lasting response to irradiation. Splenectomy is associated with a high morbidity rate secondary to splanchnic vein thrombosis, intra-abdominal hemorrhage, extreme leukocytosis or thrombocytosis, hepatomegaly due to extramedullary hematopoiesis, and abdominal wall weakness or herniation.

PATIENT EDUCATION

- Polycythemia vera has a slow clinical course and progressive increase in the blood counts and spleen size.
- Treatment often requires no more than periodic phlebotomy and attention to specific symptoms.

6.3B ESSENTIAL THROMBOCYTOSIS

ET is a clonal disorder of the pluripotent HSC in the bone marrow. It is related to the other chronic myeloproliferative neoplasms, including polycythemia vera, myeloid metaplasia and MF, and CML. On CBC there is an elevated platelet count (thrombocytosis).

TPO is the key hormone that regulates megakaryocyte differentiation and proliferation in the marrow. TPO stimulates platelet production. Disease states associated with secondary or reactive thrombocytosis are due to either direct or indirect increases in TPO production. The thrombocytosis in ET is caused by increased sensitivity of the megakaryocytic cell line to TPO.

MEDICAL HISTORY AND CLINICAL PRESENTATION

Most patients with ET are asymptomatic at presentation and are diagnosed incidentally by finding thrombocytosis on routine blood tests. Patients with ET may present with a history of unexplained bleeding tendency, venous or arterial thrombosis, and vascular ischemic manifestations.

Bleeding tends to occur at superficial sites with easy bruising, including exaggerated bruising with the use of aspirin and nonsteroidal anti-inflammatory drugs. Other bleeding manifestations include mucosal hemorrhage, such as epistaxis, hemoptysis, gingival bleeding, or bleeding from the GI or genitourinary tracts. A history of thrombosis may take the form of venous thromboembolism (VTE), most commonly deep vein thrombosis or pulmonary embolism. Other thrombosis locations include portal, hepatic (Budd-Chiari syndrome), splenic vein, and mesenteric thrombosis.

Peripheral vascular disease manifests as microvascular ischemia, including the syndrome of erythromelalgia. Erythromelalgia is characterized by intense burning or throbbing pain over the plantar aspects of the feet or palmar aspects of the hands. The pain may be associated with the areas of warmth and erythema, but palpable peripheral pulses of large peripheral arteries are still present. Erythromelalgia is quickly responsive to aspirin therapy.

SIGNS AND SYMPTOMS

ET is most frequently diagnosed in older individuals, median age of about 60 years of age, and the gender distribution is equal. ET is rarely seen in children. Most patients are asymptomatic. No environmental risk factors have been identified.

PHYSICAL EXAMINATION

The physical exam in most patients is normal. Splenomegaly is found in about 40% but is not diagnostic. Hepatomegaly is seen in about 20% of cases. Lymphadenopathy is not noted. Physical examination will reveal signs consistent with bleeding and easy bruising. Other bleeding manifestations include mucosal hemorrhage.

DIFFERENTIAL DIAGNOSIS

Thrombocytosis is much more commonly due to secondary causes. See Table 6.19 for causes of secondary (reactive) thrombocytosis.

Most worrisome in the differential diagnosis of thrombocytosis is the possibility of an occult malignancy.

TABLE 6.19 Causes of Secondary Thrombocytosis

Transient	Sustained
Acute blood loss	Cancer
Acute infection or inflammation	Chronic infection or inflammation
Response to vigorous exercise	Drug reactions
Rebound from thrombocytopenia	Iron deficiency
	Hemolytic anemia
	Asplenia

DIAGNOSTIC STUDIES

Thrombocytosis must be first confirmed by repeat blood counts. If repeat platelet count is normal, no further evaluation is needed.

If thrombocytosis is confirmed and there are elevations in hemoglobin and hematocrit and WBC count, another cause of myeloproliferative neoplasm should be considered. In those with isolated thrombocytosis, secondary causes should be sought.

Peripheral blood smear should be examined to check for possible giant platelets, and a bone marrow aspiration and biopsy should be obtained. The bone marrow may reveal giant megakaryocytes.

TREATMENT

Not all patients require treatment. Urgent therapy is needed in patients with active cerebrovascular, coronary, or digital ischemia. A rapid lowering of platelets is obtained with oral hydroxyurea, and antiplatelet therapy with aspirin can be started immediately unless there is an absolute contraindication.

The long-term treatment of patients is dictated by stratification of thrombotic risk. High risk is defined as age over 60 and previous history of thrombosis or vascular events. Low-risk patients have none of these characteristics and can be followed without therapy, even without aspirin. Low-dose aspirin can be given to ET patients with lower risk, unless there is a history of significant bleeding complications.

High-risk patients should be treated to reduce the platelet count and maintain it within normal range. The treatment of choice is hydroxyurea. Blood counts should be monitored so that platelet count is kept low without suppressing hemoglobin and WBC count.

Anagrelide is second-line platelet-reducing therapy for high-risk patients. Many patients cannot tolerate this drug because of its vasodilatory and positive inotropic properties that can cause fluid retention, palpitations, arrhythmias, heart failure, and headaches. Anagrelide is also associated with reversible bone marrow fibrosis.

An alternative second-line drug is pegylated interferon alfa; its use is limited by severe side effects that make it intolerable for about 20% of patients.

PATIENT EDUCATION

- Prognosis in ET is variable. Thrombotic and vascular complications are the major causes of death in ET.
- A small group of patients have transformation to acute leukemia, myelodysplasia, or MF.

6.3C PRIMARY MYELOFIBROSIS

PMF is a chronic malignant hematologic disorder that is a myeloproliferative neoplasm. It is characterized by splenomegaly, a leukoerythroblastic picture on peripheral smear, bone marrow fibrosis, cytopenia, and systemic symptoms.

Annual incidence is 1.5 cases per 100,000 persons.[21] There is a link between excessive radiation exposure and chronic exposure to several industrial solvents such as benzene and toluene and the development of MF.

The exact pathogenesis of PMF is unknown but it is thought to be due to a mutation in a pluripotent HSC, resulting in clonal proliferation. Bone marrow fibrosis is thought to be secondary to the abnormal deposition of collagen derived from normal fibroblasts. Fibroblasts in PMF are induced to proliferate and produce excessive collagen by growth factors and cytokines secreted by megakaryocytes. Bone marrow fibrosis is not an irreversible process in PMF.

MEDICAL HISTORY AND CLINICAL PRESENTATION

PMF is rare and is mostly a disease of the elderly. The average age at diagnosis is 65 years with most patients between the ages of 50 and 69. Approximately 5% of patients are diagnosed before the age of 40. While rare, a higher incidence has been reported in Ashkenazi Jews.[22]

SIGNS AND SYMPTOMS

The most common presenting complaint is fatigue. While often the result of anemia, fatigue can be a significant burden, even in patients who are not anemic. Patients also present with splenomegaly. Splenomegaly can result in left upper quadrant abdominal pain, left shoulder pain, early satiety, and diarrhea. Patients with more advanced disease may have systemic symptoms such as weight loss, bone pain, night sweats, and fevers.

PHYSICAL EXAMINATION

Extramedullary hematopoiesis, a hallmark finding, can present as splenomegaly, hepatomegaly, lymphadenopathy, or pericardial or pleural effusion.

DIFFERENTIAL DIAGNOSIS

Acute MF is characterized by acute presentation of bone marrow fibrosis, fever, pancytopenia and teardrop poikilocytosis, and no splenomegaly. The bone marrow is characterized by the appearance of immature myeloid cells and blast cells. Acute MF is treated with aggressive chemotherapy followed by stem cell transplantation, and prognosis is poor.

Other disorders can cause bone marrow fibrosis and have a similar clinical presentation of PMF. They include nonmalignant conditions such as tuberculosis, hypoparathyroidism, systemic lupus erythematosus, scleroderma, and Gaucher disease as well as malignant conditions such as AML, MM, Hodgkin and non-Hodgkin lymphoma, and hairy cell leukemia.

DIAGNOSTIC STUDIES

The following laboratory studies are indicated for the diagnosis and prognostication of PMF:

- CBC is important. Anemia with a hemoglobin <10 g/dL is seen in 60% of patients, leukopenia is noted in 15% to 25% of patients, and leukocytosis is noted in 33% of patients. As the disease progresses thrombocytopenia becomes more common. Platelets may be abnormally large.
- Examination of the peripheral blood smear and bone marrow are essential for the diagnosis. Leukoerythroblastosis with teardrop RBCs strongly suggests the diagnosis (Figure 6.11). Leukoerythroblastosis is also characterized by the presence of nucleated RBCs and immature myeloid elements in a majority of cases.
- Bone marrow biopsy and successful bone marrow aspiration is unusual, with a dry tap occurring in most cases. Bone marrow cytogenetic studies are used to assist in determining prognosis.

EVALUATION

Diagnosis of PMF requires meeting all three major and at least two minor criteria in the list in Table 6.20.

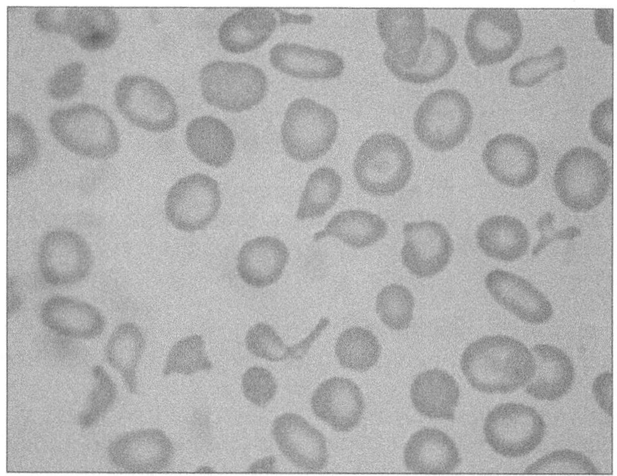

Figure 6.11 Teardrop red blood cells noted in primary myelofibrosis.

TABLE 6.20 Diagnostic Criteria for Primary Myelofibrosis

Major Criteria	Minor Criteria
Presence of megakaryocyte proliferation and atypia	Leukoerythroblastosis
Not meeting WHO criteria for other myeloproliferative neoplasm	Increase in serum LDH level
Demonstration of *JAK2, CALR,* or *MPL* mutations	Anemia
	Palpable splenomegaly
	Leukocytosis >11 × 10^9/L

LDH, lactate dehydrogenase; WHO, World Health Organization.
Source: Data from Arber DA, Orazi A, Hasserjian R, et al. The 2016 revision to the World Health Organization classification of myeloid neoplasms and acute leukemia. Blood. *2016;127:2391. doi:10.1182/ blood-2016-06-721662*

TREATMENT

Active therapy is indicated for the following conditions: symptomatic anemia, symptomatic splenomegaly, portal hypertension, significant thrombocytopenia, and systemic symptoms such as bone pain, fevers, night sweats, and weight loss. Allogeneic stem cell transplantation is currently the only curative option.

Ruxolitinib is indicated for patients with intermediate or high-risk MF and is an excellent palliative agent. It has been shown to reduce the degree of splenomegaly, improve systemic symptoms, and improve quality of life.[23] Side effects include anemia and thrombocytopenia

Other therapeutic options include androgen preparations and combinations of thalidomide or lenalidomide and prednisone for anemia; hydroxyurea is used for reduction of splenomegaly and systemic symptoms. Melphalan and busulfan can be used in patients in a hyperproliferative phase and can stabilize the leukocytosis and reduce splenomegaly.

Splenectomy is a possible treatment for patients with massive splenomegaly that is unresponsive or intolerant to medical treatments, or in patients with severe life-threatening thrombocytopenia and anemia.

PATIENT EDUCATION

- PMF is a disease with a highly variability outcome based on how advanced the disease is at the time of diagnosis.
- The patient and their family should be informed that PMF is a hematologic malignancy.
- Clinical course varies: Some patients can have stable disease for many years without developing any complications or can rapidly decompensate due to the development of systemic symptoms, progression to AML, or thrombotic or hemorrhagic complications.
- Median overall survival period from the time of diagnosis is approximately 6–7 years.

6.3D MYELODYSPLASTIC SYNDROMES

The MDS are a heterogeneous group of clonal bone marrow failure syndromes characterized by cytopenia, clonally restricted hematopoiesis, and a risk of progression to AML. About a fourth of patients will progress to AML.

Most MDS cases are idiopathic and only a small percentage are secondary to prior exposure to a DNA damaging agent such as alkylating agent/topoisomerase inhibitor chemotherapy or ionizing radiation.

MDS can be diagnosed at any age but is most commonly noted in older patients with an average of 71 years. Allogeneic HSCT is the only curative therapy for MDS, and all other treatments for MDS are palliative in nature, although some therapies can extend survival and improve quality of life. MDS are a collection of related diseases of the bone marrow. While they are heterogeneous in their presentation, they share many pathophysiologic features:

- They are clonal disorders in that they arise from an abnormal hematopoietic precursor and have clonally expanded and evolved.
- Ineffective hematopoiesis is present with dysplasia and increased apoptosis of differentiating cells leading to both quantitative and qualitative defects of mature cells in the peripheral blood.
- They have an increased risk of progression to AML.

The current classification of MDS includes six major categories.

- MDS with multilineage dysplasia (MDS-MLD): dysplasia noted in at least 10% of early cells of two or three of the cell types (RBCs, WBCs, or platelets) in the bone marrow, decreased number of cells in at least one cell line, and <5% blasts in the bone marrow and rare blasts in the peripheral blood. This is the most common type of MDS.
- MDS with single lineage dysplasia (MDS-SLD): dysplasia noted in at least 10% of early cells of one cell type (RBCs, WBCs, or platelets) in the bone marrow, decreased number of cells in one or two cell lines and normal in the others, and <5% blasts in the bone marrow and rare blasts in the peripheral blood. This type of MDS is rare and progression to AML is rare.
- MDS with ring sideroblasts (MDS-RS): at least 15% of the early RBCs are ring sideroblasts or 5% of the cells have a mutation in the *SF3B1* gene. This type of MDS is rare and rarely converts to AML. This is further divided into two subtypes:
  - MDS-RS with single lineage dysplasia (MDS-RS-SLD): dysplasia in only one cell line
  - MDS-RS with multilineage dysplasia (MS-RS-MLD): dysplasia in more than one cell type
- MDS with excess blasts (MDS-EB): more blasts are noted in the bone marrow than normal, at least one cell type is low in number, and there may or may not be severe dysplasia in the bone marrow. This type makes up 25% of cases of MDS and is most likely to convert to AML. There are two subtypes:
  - MDS-EB1: blasts in 5% to 9% of the cells in the bone marrow or 2% to 4% of the cells in the peripheral blood.
  - MDS-EB2: blasts in 10% to 19% of the cells in the bone marrow or 5% to 19% of the cells in the peripheral blood.
- MDS with isolated del(5q): missing a part of chromosome 5, have low numbers of one or two cell lines, and dysplasia in at least one cell type in the bone marrow. This type of MDS is rare, occurs most often in older females, are rarely develops into AML.
- MDS, unclassified (MDS-U): this type does not fit any of the other type criteria and is rare.

MEDICAL HISTORY AND CLINICAL PRESENTATION

MDS are diseases of older patients; the median age at diagnosis in the United States is about 71 years.

Exposures to ionizing radiation, alkylating agents (e.g., melphalan, chlorambucil), and topoisomerase inhibitors (e.g., etoposide, topotecan, anthracyclines) are known risk factors for developing MDS.

There is a moderate male predominance (<1.5:1), probably related to occupational exposures. Work in agriculture and the petroleum industries and cigarette smoking may slightly increase risk.

The 5q syndrome, an uncommon type of MDS with a relatively indolent natural history, has a female predominance.

Patients diagnosed with MDS under age 50 who do not have a history of exposure to a DNA damaging agent might have a germline disorder predisposing to MDS, such as Fanconi anemia. MDS may arise in patients with AA or paroxysmal nocturnal hemoglobinuria (PNH).

SIGNS AND SYMPTOMS

Signs and symptoms vary depending on the cell type affected. They may present with signs of anemia (fatigue, dizziness, weakness), leukopenia (frequent infections), and thrombocytopenia (bruising and bleeding). Other symptoms include weight loss, fever, bone pain, and loss of appetite.

PHYSICAL EXAMINATION

Physical examination findings vary depending on the cell types affected. Patients may present with signs of anemia (pallor, cardiac murmur) and thrombocytopenia (bruising and petechiae).

DIFFERENTIAL DIAGNOSIS

The differential diagnosis includes the following:

- Vitamin B12 (cyanocobalamin) or folate deficiency
- Copper deficiency
- Medication effect (especially methotrexate, azathioprine, or chemotherapeutics)
- Alcohol abuse
- HIV infection
- Autoimmune disorders (e.g., immune thrombocytopenia (ITP), Felty syndrome)
- Congenital syndromes (e.g., congenital or cyclic neutropenia, Fanconi anemia)

MDS can be difficult to distinguish from other hematologic disorders, including AA, myeloproliferative neoplasms, PNH, or AML.

DIAGNOSTIC STUDIES

Almost all patients present with anemia that is typically macrocytic or normocytic. Up to half of patients are also neutropenic and thrombocytopenic. Isolated thrombocytopenia is rare without anemia in MDS; if noted, other causes (such as ITP or medications) should be ruled out. The bone marrow in MDS is usually hypercellular.

The peripheral smear will reveal cytopenia with neutrophil hypogranularity or hypolobated, giant or hypogranular platelets, or oval macrocytic erythrocytes.

Bone marrow aspirate and trephine core biopsy will reveal dysplasia in >10% of cells, and may show an increase in myeloid blasts, monocyte precursors, or the presence of pathologic ring sideroblasts.

Other tests such as flow cytometry, MDS FISH panels, and molecular genetic tests may aid in the diagnosis.

EVALUATION

The diagnosis of MDS is based on the presence of three main features:

- Unexplained decreases in one or more of the cell lines, including hemoglobin <10 g/dL, absolute neutrophil count <1,800/μL, and platelet count <100 × 10^9/L.
- Morphologic evidence of significant dysplasia, >10% erythroid precursors, granulocytes, or megakaryocytes in the peripheral blood or bone marrow.
- Blast forms account for <20% of total nucleated cells in the bone marrow and peripheral blood. Values >20% are considered AML.

Initial diagnostic evaluation should include the following:

- CBC with differential and evaluation of the peripheral smear
- Bone marrow aspirate, biopsy, and cytogenetic analysis
- Serum vitamin B12 levels and folate levels
- Serum ferritin level
- Serum LDH
- Serum creatinine and liver function tests
- Serum copper level
- HLA typing if possible allogeneic transplant
- PT and activated partial thromboplastin time (aPTT)
- Type and crossmatch for possible transfusion

TREATMENT

MDS are typically subacute diseases and most cases do not require emergent management. Exceptions are cases in which abnormalities in the peripheral blood can lead to life-threatening conditions. These include:

- Severe bleeding with thrombocytopenia or hypofunctioning platelets
- Severe thrombocytopenia
- Fever and neutropenia
- Severe or symptomatic anemia

Goals of MDS therapy depend in part on the stage of disease, and include symptom control, reduction of transfusion needs, delay of disease progression, improvement in quality of life, and extension of survival.

Except for allogeneic HSCT there are no curative therapeutic options. Three medications have been approval for MDS: azacitidine, decitabine, and lenalidomide. For higher-risk patients and if the patient is a transplant candidate, allogeneic stem cell transplant is the treatment of choice. Azacitidine or decitabine may be used as a bridge to transplant. If the patient does not wish a transplant or is not a candidate, a hypomethylating agent (i.e., azacitidine or decitabine) is the most appropriate initial therapy.

PATIENT EDUCATION

- The prognosis of patients with MDS is highly variable.
- Poor prognostic criteria include:
  - Age over 60 years
  - Increased blast cells in the bone marrow
  - Chromosomal abnormalities such as abnormalities of chromosome 7 or complex karyotypes with more than two abnormalities
  - Cytopenia in more than one cell line instead of just a single cytopenia
  - Transfusion dependence
  - Comorbidities and impaired functional status

SPECIAL CONSIDERATIONS

- Polycythemia vera is most common in women, particularly in the reproductive age range; management should include avoidance of mutagenic drugs, such as hydroxyurea and other chemotherapeutic agents, and anagrelide.
- In polycythemia vera phlebotomy is safe and important therapeutically, because in pregnancy there is normally plasma volume expansion, making it even more difficult

to assess the size of the RBC mass. This will not harm the fetus and will provide protection from thrombosis for the mother.

- In women with high-risk ET who are considering pregnancy, interferon alfa is the treatment of choice. Hydroxyurea is teratogenic.

KEY POINTS

- ET is a clonal abnormality resulting in thrombocytosis. Patients are at risk of thrombosis.
- MF is excessive bone marrow fibrosis with loss of hematopoietic cells and extramedullary hematopoiesis. The treatment of choice is ruxolitinib.
- Polycythemia vera is a chronic myeloproliferative disorder with increased production of all cell lines. Treatment is phlebotomy.

6.4 LYMPHOMA

OVERVIEW

Lymphoma is a group of blood malignancies that start in the lymphatic system or the lymph nodes. There are two main types of lymphomas:

- **Hodgkin lymphoma (HL):** There are five types of HL and all involve the presence of Reed-Sternberg cells. Any lymphoma that does not involve Reed-Sternberg cells is a non-Hodgkin lymphoma (NHL). See Table 6.21 for the types of HL.
- **NHL:** There are many different types of NHL. They are divided into aggressive and indolent types. See Table 6.21 for the types of NHL.

EPIDEMIOLOGY

There are approximately 8,500 new cases of HL per year in the United States.[24] It is most common in young adults, and the majority are cured. NHL is a very common malignancy.

TABLE 6.21 Types of Hodgkin and Non-Hodgkin Lymphomas

Hodgkin Lymphoma (HL)	Non-Hodgkin Lymphoma	
	Aggressive	Indolent
Nodular lymphocyte-predominant HL	Diffuse large B-cell lymphoma	Follicular lymphoma
Classical HL	Anaplastic large cell lymphoma	Cutaneous T-cell lymphoma
Nodular sclerosis classical HL	Burkitt lymphoma	Lymphoplasmacytic lymphoma
Lymphocyte-rich classical HL	Lymphoblastic lymphoma	Marginal zone B-cell lymphoma
Mixed cellularity classical HL	Mantle cell lymphoma	MALT lymphoma
Lymphocyte-depleted classical HL	Peripheral T-cell lymphoma	Small-cell lymphocytic lymphoma

MALT, mucosa-associated lymphoid tissue.

In the United States, there are approximately 90,390 new cases per year, with approximately 21,680 deaths.[24]

PATHOPHYSIOLOGY

A major function of the immune system is to protect against disease and invasion by antigens. These antigens include bacteria, fungi, viruses, toxins, or foreign body. An antigen is any substance that can spark an immune response. There are two types of immune systems, the innate immune system and the adaptive immune system.

The innate immune system includes physical barriers that overlay the epithelium in the respiratory, GI, and genitourinary tracts; complement proteins; cytokines; and membrane bound receptors and cytoplasmic proteins that bind to molecules expressed on the surfaces of invading microbes.

The adaptive immune system is based on antigen-specific receptors expressed on the surfaces of T- and B-lymphocytes. The adaptive immune system is highly specific in its ability to recognize and defend against specific foreign agents using both the cellular and humoral immune systems.

Various cells are involved in the immune response, including B-lymphocytes and T-lymphocytes.

The B-lymphocytes respond to a specific antigen and secrete antibodies that react to the specific antigen. B-lymphocytes produce one specific antibody. These antibodies are called immunoglobulins and there are five major types of immunoglobulins (IgG, IgM, IgA, IgD, and IgE). Antibodies lock onto the antigen and mark the antigen for death via phagocytosis. When a B-lymphocyte comes across its triggering antigen it produces cells called plasma cells. Each plasma cell produces a specific antibody. Whenever the antibody and antigen interlock, the antibody marks the antigen for destruction. B-lymphocytes are not able to penetrate the cell, so it is left to T-lymphocytes to attack the target cells.

T-lymphocytes are cells that are programmed to recognize, respond to, and remember antigens. T-lymphocytes contribute to the immune defenses in two ways. Helper T-cells coordinate the immune response. They communicate with other cells and stimulate B-cells to produce more antibodies. Others attract more T-cells or phagocytes. The killer T-cells attack other cells. Killer T-cells are useful for fighting viruses as they recognize small parts of the virus on the infected cells and destroy the infected cells.

6.4A HODGKIN LYMPHOMA

HL, a monoclonal B-cell disorder, is divided into two subgroups: classical Hodgkin lymphoma (CHL) and nodular lymphocyte predominant Hodgkin lymphoma (NLPHL). CHL is divided into four distinct entities: nodular sclerosis, mixed cellularity, lymphocyte-rich, and lymphocyte-depleted; the subtypes have little prognostic significance with current therapies. Differentiating between CHL and NLPHL is important, as they have distinct natural histories and treatment options are different. Staging is based on the Ann Arbor system (Table 6.22).[25]

Approximately 8,500 cases of HL are diagnosed annually in the United States.[24] Patients with NLPHL are frequently male and in the 30- to 50-year age group. There is a bimodal age distribution with the first peak in the third decade of life

TABLE 6.22 Ann Arbor Staging System

Stage	Description
I	Involvement of a single lymph node region (I) or a single extra-lymphatic organ or site (IE)
II	Involvement of two or more lymph node regions on the same side of the diaphragm (II) or localized involvement of an extra-lymphatic organ or site (IIE)
III	Involvement of lymph node regions on both sides of the diaphragm (III) or localized involvement of an extra-lymphatic organ or site (IIIE) or spleen (IIIS) or both (IIISE)
IV	Diffuse or disseminated involvement of one or more extra-lymphatic organs, with or without associated lymph node involvement

and the second after the age of 50. The highest rates in the United States occur among Caucasians, followed by African Americans, Hispanics, and Asians.

A history of infectious mononucleosis increases the risk of HL two- to threefold, and points toward Epstein-Barr virus (EBV) as an etiologic agent. There is a 10-fold higher risk of HL among HIV-infected persons compared with HIV-negative persons.

MEDICAL HISTORY AND CLINICAL PRESENTATION

CHL presents with painless cervical and/or supraclavicular lymphadenopathy. Lymph node involvement is frequently contiguous. Systemic symptoms, or B symptoms, including fever (temperatures >38° C), night sweats, or weight loss (>10% baseline body weight) are present more commonly in advanced disease than early disease. Chest pain, cough, dyspnea, and superior vena cava (SVC) syndrome are rare.

SIGNS AND SYMPTOMS

Disease localized to the mediastinum will develop chest pain and cough. Disease located in the retroperitoneum present with abdominal or back pain. B symptoms are common and are present more frequently in older patients and in those with HIV. Pruritus occurs infrequently. Alcohol-related pain in the sites of involvement is rare, with an incidence of <2%.[26]

PHYSICAL EXAMINATION

The most common presentation for CHL is painless cervical and/or supraclavicular lymphadenopathy. B symptoms may be noted. Patients with extensive disease may have multiple nodal chains involved, along with splenomegaly. A small percentage of patients will present with an excoriated rash secondary to pruritus. Rarely patients will present with complications such as SVC syndrome, pericardial tamponade, neurologic complaints due to spinal cord compression, or symptoms associated with paraneoplastic syndromes.

NLPHL presents with solitary cervical, axillary, or inguinal lymphadenopathy with no consistent pattern of spread. Presence of any other symptoms related to the disease, including B symptoms, is unusual. Most patients present with early stage disease, and mediastinal involvement is rare.

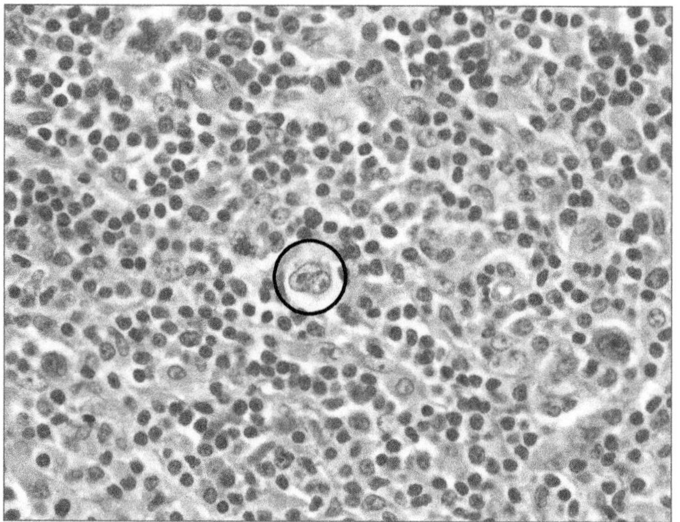

Figure 6.12 **Reed-Sternberg cell noted in Hodgkin lymphoma (at center).**

DIFFERENTIAL DIAGNOSIS

Other lymphoma subtypes, such as those noted in NHL, can mimic CHL. Nonmalignant conditions are in the differential diagnosis as well, including rheumatologic and infectious diseases, such as fever of unknown origin (FUO), acute HIV infection, infectious mononucleosis, and sarcoidosis.

DIAGNOSTIC STUDIES

An excisional lymph node biopsy is typically required to diagnose HL. A needle biopsy should not be used as the sole means of diagnosis. The presence of Hodgkin/Reed-Sternberg cells (HRS) (Figure 6.12) in a background of inflammatory cells is required for a diagnosis of CHL.

CHL causes mass lesions in the centriaxial lymph nodes and usually spreads in a contiguous pattern. When extranodal involvement occurs, it commonly involves the liver, bone, lungs, and bone marrow. If extensive mediastinal involvement is present, direct extension to the chest wall, pericardium, or pleura may occur. Spread to distant organs is preceded by splenic involvement.

Once the diagnosis of HL has been made, imaging studies are essential for disease staging. CT has been replaced by PET/CT for staging patients, though CT is the first test obtained in the workup of a patient. A baseline PET/CT is useful in monitoring response to therapy.

EVALUATION

Necessary laboratory tests include a CBC with differential; comprehensive metabolic panel with alkaline phosphatase, albumin, and calcium levels; and an ESR. The WBC count, absolute lymphocyte count, hemoglobin, albumin, and ESR should be obtained prior to starting therapy as they aid in predicting response to therapy. Elevated alkaline phosphatase does not necessarily predict liver or bone involvement. Testing for HIV is indicated in patients with known risk factors and in patients with unusual disease presentations.

TREATMENT

For patients who present with complications therapy should be started immediately. In most cases the optimal treatment is chemotherapy, rather than radiotherapy. Treatment of HL is largely dictated by the patient's stage and risk factors at the time of presentation.

Current treatment strategies for early stage HL consists of 4 cycles of Adriamycin, bleomycin, vinblastine, and dacarbazine (ABVD) and radiotherapy.

Unfavorable HL is defined by the presence of bulky disease. Three-fourths of patients with early stage unfavorable HL are cured with combined modality therapy with 4 to 6 cycles of ABVD followed by radiation therapy.

The current standard of care for advanced stage HL is with 6 cycles of ABVD. Other options include escalated BEACOPP (bleomycin, etoposide, doxorubicin, cyclophosphamide, vincristine, procarbazine, and prednisone). Cure is based on the number of international prognostic score factors and ranges from 42% to 82%.[27]

Brentuximab vedotin (BV), an antibody-drug conjugate targeting CD30, is used in patients who have failed either two prior regimens or an autologous stem cell transplant.

The standard therapy for relapsed HL is with high-dose chemotherapy, followed by autologous stem cell transplant.

Complications with chemotherapy are common.

- ABVD is a moderate to highly emetogenic regimen and patients should be premedicated with a serotonin (5-HT_3) antagonist and a steroid.
- Treatment with vinblastine can lead to autonomic and peripheral neuropathy. The neuropathy is typically transient and neuropathic pain can be effectively treated with gabapentin or pregabalin.
- Constipation is a common side effect from vinblastine and can be prevented with an aggressive bowel regimen.
- Bleomycin pulmonary toxicity is noted in patients treated with ABVD. It presents as a pneumonitis and may progress to a fibrosis. Treatment consists of stopping the bleomycin and administration of corticosteroids. Patients should be assessed for pulmonary symptoms prior to every cycle of bleomycin and withholding until a chest radiograph is obtained to evaluate for bilateral interstitial infiltrates if symptoms develop.

Patients with HL have impaired immunity and should receive annual influenza vaccinations. Women treated with chest radiation before the age of 25 have an increased risk of developing breast cancer by age 55. Annual mammography and breast MRI are recommended starting 8 to 10 years following mediastinal radiation in women treated between 10 and 30 years of age. Patients with HL are at increased risk for lung cancer, particularly in patients over 40 years of age and smokers, who were treated with alkylating agents or chest radiation. Screening for lung cancer with low-dose spiral CT should be considered.

PATIENT EDUCATION

- Nearly 80% of patients will be cured of HL. The goal of therapy is curative, even for patients with advanced stage disease and poor prognostic features. The response rates and mortality rates are largely influenced by stage, the number of favorable or unfavorable features that a patient has at the time of diagnosis, and response to the initial treatment.
- Prognosis varies depending on the number of risk factors present. See Table 6.23 for freedom from progression and overall survival rates in patients with advanced disease. Most relapses occur within the first 2 years after diagnosis.

TABLE 6.23 The International Prognostic Score for Hodgkin Lymphoma

Score	5-Year Freedom From Progression Rate (%)	5-Year Overall Survival Rate (%)
0	84	89
1	77	90
2	67	81
3	60	78
4	51	61
5 or more	42	56

One point given for each of the following: *Serum albumin <4 g/dL, hemoglobin <10.5 g/dL, male gender, age >45 years, stage IV disease, white blood cell (WBC) count ≥15,000/μ, absolute lymphocyte count <600/μ, and/or <8% of the total WBC count.*

Source: Data from Hasenclever D, Diehl V. A prognostic score for advanced Hodgkin's disease. International Prognostic Factors Project on Advanced Hodgkin's Disease. N Engl J Med. *1998;339(21):1506. doi:10.1056/NEJM199811193392104*

6.4B NON-HODGKIN LYMPHOMA

NHL consists of a diverse group of malignant neoplasms derived from B-cell progenitors, T-cell progenitors, mature B-cells, mature T-cells, or natural killer cells. See Table 6.21 for the various types on NHLs. The Ann Arbor staging used in HL is also used in NHL.

MEDICAL HISTORY AND CLINICAL PRESENTATION

The clinical presentation of NHL varies depending on the type of lymphoma and the areas of involvement. Some NHLs behave indolently with waxing and waning lymphadenopathy for years, while others are highly aggressive, resulting in death within weeks if left untreated.

Several diseases, infectious agents, and drugs or toxins have been associated with the development of NHL. These include:

- A personal or family history of lymphoma or prior hematopoietic malignancy, past radiation or chemotherapy treatment, use of immunosuppressive agents, or organ transplantation.
- Exposure to certain agricultural pesticides, hair dyes, and dioxins.
- Infections associated with NHL include HIV, human T lymphotropic virus type I (HTLV-I), EBV, and hepatitis B and C.
- Other associated disorders linked to NHL include autoimmune diseases, immunodeficiency disorders, mixed cryoglobulinemia, inflammatory GI diseases, and obesity.

SIGNS AND SYMPTOMS

Aggressive lymphomas commonly present acutely or subacutely with a rapidly growing mass, systemic B symptoms, and/or elevated levels of serum LDH and uric acid. These types of lymphomas include diffuse large B-cell lymphoma, Burkitt lymphoma, precursor B- and T-lymphoblastic leukemia/lymphoma, and adult T-cell leukemia-lymphoma.

Indolentlymphomasareinsidious,presentingonlywithslow growing lymphadenopathy, hepatomegaly, splenomegaly, or cytopenia. These types of lymphomas include follicular lymphoma, CLL/small lymphocytic lymphoma, and splenic marginal zone lymphoma.

The natural history of NHL shows significant patient-to-patient variability. Less common presentations include skin rash, pruritus, exaggerated reactions to insect stings or bites, fatigue, malaise, FUO, ascites, and effusions.

PHYSICAL EXAMINATION

The physical examination should be directed to all potentially involved lymphoid sites evaluating for lymphadenopathy. Approximately 20% of patients with NHL present with mediastinal adenopathy on clinical examination or chest radiograph. Mediastinal involvement presents with persistent cough, chest discomfort, or without clinical symptomatology but with an abnormal chest radiograph. Pleural disease may also be noted.

If the liver is involved diffuse hepatosplenomegaly may be noted. Ascites may also be present.

Extranodal disease may be noted in the following areas: GI tract, skin, testis, bone, and kidney. Symptoms due to extralymphatic disease are associated with aggressive NHL and are uncommon in the indolent lymphomas.

DIFFERENTIAL DIAGNOSIS

The differential diagnosis includes CHL. Nonmalignant conditions in the differential diagnosis include rheumatologic and infectious diseases, such as FUO, acute HIV infection, infectious mononucleosis, and sarcoidosis.

DIAGNOSTIC STUDIES

Several laboratory abnormalities may be noted in NHL. CBC, WBC differential, platelet count, and examination of the peripheral smear may reveal the presence of atypical cells; the presence of malignant cells in the peripheral blood is generally indicative of extensive marrow involvement. Unexplained anemia, thrombocytopenia, or leukopenia may be due to bone marrow infiltration, hypersplenism from splenic involvement, or immune destruction.

Several blood chemistry abnormalities may be present. Hypercalcemia and hyperuricemia may develop during the disease but are rare at the time of presentation. Hyperuricemia and tumor lysis syndrome are noted in Burkitt lymphoma and are more frequent in patients with underlying renal failure. Serum LDH elevation associated with NHL may be due to high tumor burden, extensive infiltration of the liver, coincident hemolytic anemia secondary to immune-mediated RBC destruction, or particularly rapidly growing forms of NHL. An elevated LDH greater than two to three times normal is associated with a poorer prognosis.

EVALUATION

Imaging studies are a major component in the staging evaluation of patients with NHL and may help in the selection of a biopsy site for diagnosis. The preferred imaging modality is integrated PET/CT or CT scan alone.

Lymph node biopsy is essential to the diagnosis of NHL. If other diagnostic tests do not support another diagnosis, a lymph node should be considered for biopsy if one or more of the following lymph node characteristics is present: significant lymph node enlargement, persistence of lymphadenopathy for more than 4 to 6 weeks, or progressive increase in size.

Bone marrow involvement occurs in up to half of all patients with NHL. Bone marrow involvement with NHL is usually focal, but on occasion patients may have extensive disease and present with pancytopenia and systemic symptoms. All patients with NHL should undergo a bone marrow aspiration and biopsy prior to the initiation of treatment as part of their staging evaluation.

After the initial tissue biopsy provides a diagnosis of NHL, the following baseline laboratory tests should be obtained:

- CBC, WBC differential, platelet count, and examination of the peripheral smear
- Complete chemistry profile including blood urea nitrogen, creatinine, alkaline phosphatase, aspartate aminotransferase, alanine aminotransferase, LDH, calcium, uric acid, albumin, and electrolytes
- Serum protein electrophoresis
- HIV, hepatitis B and C serology
- Beta-2 microglobulin levels

These tests may contribute to staging and assistance with guiding therapy.

TREATMENT

There are multiple treatment options for patients with NHL. Chemotherapy is commonly used and drugs from different groups are combined. One combination is called CHOP, which consists of the drugs cyclophosphamide, doxorubicin (hydroxydaunorubicin), vincristine (Oncovin), and prednisone. Another common combination leaves out doxorubicin and is called CVP. Chemotherapy is often combined with an immunotherapy medication, such as rituximab (Rituxan). Immunotherapy is used to boost the patient's own immune system or used to kill lymphoma cells or slow their growth.

Monoclonal antibodies are designed to attack a specific target on the surface of lymphocytes. Several monoclonal antibodies are now used to treat NHL. Antibodies that target the CD20 antigen on B-lymphocytes include:

- **Rituximab (Rituxan):** Often used with chemotherapy or by itself
- **Obinutuzumab (Gazyva):** Often used with chemotherapy to treat small lymphocytic lymphoma/CLL; also used along with chemotherapy in treating follicular lymphoma
- **Ofatumumab (Arzerra):** Used mainly in patients with SLL/CLL who are not responding to other treatments
- **Ibritumomab tiuxetan (Zevalin):** A monoclonal antibody attached to a radioactive molecule that brings radiation directly to the lymphoma cells

Side effects are common, but mild and include itching, chills, fever, nausea, rashes, fatigue, and headaches. More serious reactions include chest pain, palpitations, swelling of the face and tongue, cough, dyspnea, and dizziness or lightheadedness. All monoclonal antibodies can cause inactive infections to become active again.

Other monoclonal antibodies targeting CD52 include alemtuzumab (Campath); side effects include fever, chills, nausea, rashes, and neutropenia. Monoclonal antibodies that target CD30 include BV (Adcetris); common side effects can include neuropathy, pancytopenia, fatigue, fever, nausea and vomiting, infections, diarrhea, and cough. Monoclonal antibodies that target CD79b include polatuzumab vedotin-piiq (Polivy); common side effects can include peripheral neuropathy, pancytopenia, fatigue, fever, decreased appetite, diarrhea, and pneumonia.

Other drugs used in the treatment of NHL are noted in Table 6.24.

TABLE 6.24 Treatment Options for Non-Hodgkin Lymphoma

Drug Group	Drug Names	Side Effects	Other
Immunomodulating drugs	Thalidomide (Thalomid) Lenalidomide (Revlimid)	Neutropenia Neuropathy Thrombosis	Birth defects if taken in pregnancy
Chimeric antigen receptor (CAR) T-cell therapy	Axicabtagene ciloleucel (Yescarta) Tisagenlecleucel (Kymriah)	High fever Chills Flu-like symptoms Neurologic changes Pancytopenia Palpitations	Side effects can be life threatening
Proteasome inhibitors	Bortezomib (Velcade)	Pancytopenia Nausea Loss of appetite Neuropathy	Often used to treat multiple myeloma
Histone deacetylase (HDAC) inhibitors	Romidepsin (Istodax) Belinostat (Beleodaq)	Pancytopenia Arrhythmias Nausea and vomiting	
Kinase inhibitors	Ibrutinib (Imbruvica) Acalabrutinib (Calquence)	Diarrhea Pancytopenia Headache	Serious side effects include hemorrhage, infections, and atrial fibrillation
PI3K inhibitors	Idelalisib (Zydelig) Copanlisib (Aliqopa)	Diarrhea Fever Fatigue Nausea Pancytopenia	

Radiation is used to treat NHL in the following situations:

- NHL stage I or II
- Advanced lymphomas along with chemotherapy
- Stem cell transplant patients may receive whole body radiation with high-dose chemotherapy
- Radiation therapy can be used as palliative care when disease has spread to brain or spinal cord

Stem cell transplant procedures, including autologous stem cell transplant and allogenic stem cell transplant, are also possible treatment options.

PATIENT EDUCATION

- Prognosis varies by type and stage of lymphoma and individual patient factors.

6.5 MULTIPLE MYELOMA

OVERVIEW

MM is a B-cell neoplasm characterized by expansion of plasma cells within the bone marrow and extramedullary sites. The classic clinical manifestations include lytic bone lesions, hypercalcemia, anemia, cytopenia, and renal dysfunction.

The most important predictors of prognosis are the International Staging System (ISS) stage and cytogenetic findings. Other findings associated with high-risk disease include extensive extramedullary disease, significant renal impairment or failure, plasmablastic features, and plasma cell leukemia.

The mainstays of therapy include the immunomodulatory drugs thalidomide, lenalidomide, and pomalidomide, as well as the proteasome inhibitors bortezomib and carfilzomib. A majority of patients respond to initial therapy, with at least a partial response.

High-dose melphalan and autologous stem cell transplantation (ASCT) remain a cornerstone of therapy in appropriately selected patients.

EPIDEMIOLOGY

MM is a relatively uncommon cancer. In the United States, there are approximately 34,900 new cases of MM per year and MM accounts for 12,400 deaths per year.[24] The incidence of disease is equal in males and females. A higher incidence is noted in African Americans and with exposure to certain toxics, such as agent orange, benzene, radiation, and pesticides.[28]

PATHOPHYSIOLOGY

Normal B-cell differentiation results in the production of plasma cells and memory B-cells. After exposure to an antigen with specificity for the immunoglobulin receptor, B-cells aggregate in germinal centers and undergo somatic hypermutation and immunoglobulin class switch, producing high affinity IgG or IgA antibodies. Mutations occurring during somatic hypermutation and class switch are likely involved in the pathogenesis of MM. Chromosomal abnormalities are detected in up to 90% of MM patients.

MEDICAL HISTORY AND CLINICAL PRESENTATION

Some patients with MM have no symptoms at all. Others have symptoms related the extent of the disease at the time of presentation. Skeletal system complaints include bone pain, most often in the back, the hips, and skull; bone weakness, either diffuse osteoporosis, or where there is a plasmacytoma; and broken bones secondary to minor stress or injury.

Pancytopenia can present with signs of anemia, including weakness, dyspnea, and dizziness; signs of leukopenia, including recurrent infections; and thrombocytopenia, including bleeding and bruising. If hypercalcemia is present polydipsia, polyuria, dehydration, constipation, abdominal pain, and decreased appetite may be noted. Neurologic complaints can be noted including peripheral neuropathy and signs of spinal cord compression, including severe back pain and lower extremity numbness and weakness.

SIGNS AND SYMPTOMS

General symptoms in MM include several unspecific findings such as fatigue and generalized weakness, bone pain, weight loss, night sweats, recurrent infections with encapsulated organisms, and paresthesia. A careful review of musculoskeletal symptoms is important, and sites of potential involvement of plasmacytoma or pathologic fracture should be imaged.

Cardiopulmonary symptoms such as shortness of breath, exertional dyspnea, orthopnea, and dependent edema should raise concern of cardiac involvement.

Table 6.25 Diagnostic Criteria for Plasma Cell Disorders

Disease	Definition
MGUS	Serum monoclonal protein level <3 g/dL <10% bone marrow clonal plasma cells No evidence of other B-cell lymphoproliferative disorder
Smoldering multiple myeloma	Serum monoclonal protein ≥3 g/dL (IgG or IgA) and/or bone marrow clonal plasma cells ≥10% Absence of myeloma defining event or amyloidosis
Multiple myeloma	Evidence of end organ damage secondary to a plasma cell disorder defined by: • Hypercalcemia (serum calcium >11.5 mg/dL) • Renal insufficiency (serum creatinine >2 mg/dl or an estimated glomerular filtration rate <40 mL/min • Anemia (hemoglobin <10 g/dL or >2 g/dL below the normal reference value) • Lytic bone lesions, pathologic fractures, or severe osteopenia Any one or more of the following biomarkers of malignancy: • Clonal bone marrow plasma cell >60% • Involved:uninvolved serum free light chain ratio ≥100 • >1 focal lesion on MRI studies

IgA, immunoglobulin A; IgG, immunoglobulin G; MGUS, monoclonal gammopathy of undetermined significance.

Dizziness, visual symptoms, headache, and other neurologic abnormalities should raise concern for hyperviscosity.

PHYSICAL EXAMINATION

Physical examination findings are dependent on the extent of the disease. Common symptoms include conjunctival pallor, lower extremity edema, bony protuberances, and pain on palpation of the spine or long bones.

DIFFERENTIAL DIAGNOSIS

Differential diagnosis includes monoclonal gammopathy of undetermined significance (MGUS), smoldering MM, lymphoplasmacytic lymphoma, Waldenström macroglobulinemia, plasmablastic lymphoma, and prostate cancer. It is important to distinguish MGUS from other plasma cell disorders to determine prognosis, and disease management. The International Myeloma Working Group (IMWG) established the guidelines of diagnostic criteria for plasma cell disorders.[29] See Table 6.25 for diagnostic criteria.

The annual rate of transformation from MGUS to MM, or another related disorder such as B-cell lymphoma, Waldenström macroglobulinemia and immunoglobulin light chain amyloidosis, is approximately 1%.[30]

DIAGNOSTIC STUDIES

Several laboratory abnormalities are noted in MM. The CBC will reveal anemia, most likely normocytic normochromic. Chemistry profile reveal low serum albumin and possible elevations in serum creatinine and calcium levels. Lactic dehydrogenase levels may be elevated and is a useful indicator of a patient's prognosis; elevated levels mean advanced disease and poor prognosis.

A 24-hour urine sample should be obtained for urine protein electrophoresis and urine immunofixation to evaluate for the presence of myeloma protein.

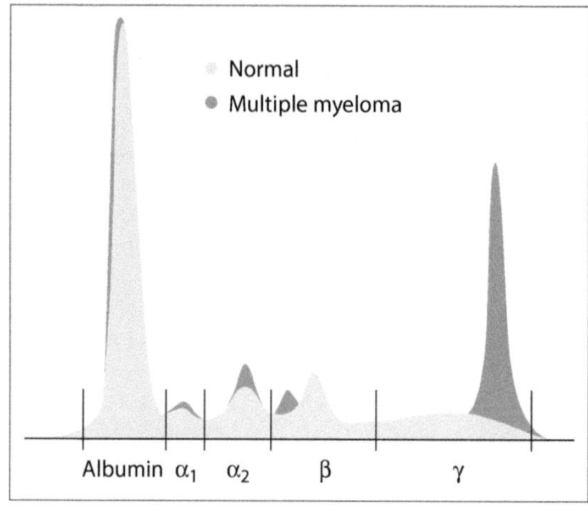

Figure 6.13 Serum protein electrophoresis, comparing normal and multiple myeloma.

Serum electrophoresis will reveal the presence of monoclonal antibodies produced by the myeloma cells. Immunofixation or immunoelectrophoresis is used to determine the exact type of abnormal antibody (IgA, IgD, IgE, IgG, and IgM). Finding of a monoclonal antibody in the blood may be the first step in diagnosing MM (Figure 6.13).

These immunoglobulins or antibodies are made up of protein chains: two heavy chains and two light chains. Light chains can be filtered through the kidney into the urine; these urine proteins are known as Bence Jones protein. Urine protein electrophoresis and urine immunofixation are used to identify these monoclonal antibodies in urine.

Beta-2 microglobulin is a protein produced by the myeloma cells. Levels of beta-2 microglobulin is a useful indicator of a patient's prognosis with high levels indicating advanced disease and worse prognosis.

Bone marrow biopsy and aspiration will detect the presence of increased number of plasma cells in the bone marrow. Other tests performed on the bone marrow aspirate include immunohistochemistry to identify myeloma cells; flow cytometry to identify specific markers to identify myeloma cells, lymphoma cells, or cancer cells; and chromosome analyses, including karyotype and FISH, to identify chromosomal abnormalities that may be present in myeloma.

A skeletal survey is performed as part of the diagnostic evaluation to assess for MM-related bone abnormalities. CT and MRI are more sensitive and should be utilized in the initial diagnostic evaluation of patients with significant musculoskeletal symptoms. Fluorodeoxyglucose (FDG) PET imaging can be highly informative as well, particularly in patients with suspected extramedullary involvement.

The diagnosis of MM requires a plasma cell tumor (proven by biopsy) OR at least 10% plasma cells in the bone marrow AND at least one of the following:

- High blood calcium level >11 mg/dL
- Poor kidney function creatinine clearance <40 mL/min or serum creatinine >2 mg/dL
- Anemia: hemoglobin <10 g/dL
- Bone lesions >5 mm noted on imaging studies (CT, MRI, PET scan)
- 60% or more plasma cells in the bone marrow

Smoldering myeloma is used to define early myeloma that is not causing any symptoms. People with smoldering myeloma have some signs of MM, such as:

- Plasma cells in the bone marrow between 10% and 60%
- High level of monoclonal immunoglobulin (M protein) in the blood
- High level of light chains in the urine (also called Bence Jones protein)

But they have normal blood counts, normal calcium levels, normal kidney function, no bone or organ damage, and no signs of amyloidosis.

EVALUATION

The initial laboratory evaluation of suspected MM should include a comprehensive metabolic panel, CBC with differential, serum protein electrophoresis with immunofixation, 24-hour urine for both total protein and urine protein electrophoresis, quantitative immunoglobulins, serum-free light chain analysis, and beta-2-microglobulin.

Bone marrow evaluation is an essential part of the diagnostic evaluation. The marrow may reveal diffuse or focal plasma cell involvement. The plasma cells are often dysplastic, with prominent nucleoli and an increase in the nuclear-to cytoplasmic ratio.

Cytogenetic analysis is performed for common MM-related mutations such as trisomy, deletion (del) 13, del 17, t(4;14), t(11;14), chromosome 1 amplification, and t(14;16).

A full evaluation that includes skeletal bone survey should be undertaken at time of diagnosis. It is important to identify sites of bone disease, particularly plasmacytomas or impending fracture.

A 24-hour urine sample should be obtained at diagnosis for both total protein quantification and urinary protein electrophoresis.

The IMWGs *Revised International Staging System for Multiple Myeloma* is used to stage MM.[31] Criteria for MM staging is noted in Table 6.26.

TREATMENT

Therapy for MM does not need to be initiated emergently, but there are several important exceptions, which follow:

- Hypercalcemia with mental status changes is treated with intravenous fluid hydration, intravenous bisphosphonates or calcitonin, and starting chemotherapy.
- Hyperviscosity with associated neurologic or cardiopulmonary manifestations is treated with plasmapheresis and chemotherapy.
- Renal failure is treated with chemotherapy or the proteasome inhibitor bortezomib.
- Spinal compression fracture or plasmacytoma, with existing or impending spinal cord compression, is treated with oral or intravenous corticosteroid in combination with local therapy targeting the lesions, either a decompressive procedure or radiation therapy.

Treatment options vary on disease risk and transplant eligibility.[32] Transplant-eligible patients with standard risk disease are treated with either two-drug regimens, such as lenalidomide-dexamethasone or bortezomib-dexamethasone, or with three-drug regimens such as lenalidomide-bortezomib-dexamethasone, bortezomib-thalidomide-dexamethasone, or cyclophosphamide-bortezomib-dexamethasone.

Patients with high-risk disease should be treated with lenalidomide-bortezomib-dexamethasone as an induction regimen based on the high-level of response and favorable toxicity profile associated with this combination. Cyclophosphamide-bortezomib-dexamethasone is also a highly active three-drug regimen.

In newly diagnosed transplant-ineligible patients, the long-time standard of care melphalan-prednisone, has been replaced by regimens such as lenalidomide-dexamethasone, bortezomib-dexamethasone, bortezomib plus melphalan-prednisone, cyclophosphamide-bortezomib-dexamethasone, and lenalidomide-bortezomib-dexamethasone.

Patients with standard-risk disease are typically treated with two-drug regimens such as lenalidomide-dexamethasone or bortezomib-dexamethasone. Bortezomib-dexamethasone may be preferred in patients with renal impairment, although lenalidomide-dexamethasone can be used in the setting of renal impairment with dose modification.

Transplant-ineligible patients with high-risk disease should receive three-drug therapy with regimens such as bortezomib-thalidomide-dexamethasone, lenalidomide-bortezomib-dexamethasone, or cyclophosphamide-bortezomib-dexamethasone.

Prophylactic antibiotics are used in the management of MM as well. Antiviral agent such as acyclovir or valacyclovir is given to patients receiving bortezomib, due to the increased incidence of herpes zoster reactivation among patients. Patients receiving high-dose or prolonged treatment with corticosteroids are considered for *Pneumocystis jirovecii* prophylaxis, most often with Bactrim; and patients who receive either thalidomide, lenalidomide, or pomalidomide should receive aspirin to reduce the likelihood of thrombotic event.

TABLE 6.26 Staging of Multiple Myeloma

Stage	Description	Median Progression-Free Survival (Months)
Stage I	• Beta-2 microglobulin ≤3.5 g/dL and albumin ≥3.5 g/dL • Standard risk for CA • Normal LDH	62
Stage II	• Does not meet criteria for stage I or stage III	44
Stage III	• Beta-2 microglobulin of 5.5 g/dL or more, and *either* • High risk for CA or high LDH	29

CA, chromosomal abnormalities; LDH, lactate dehydrogenase.
Source: Data from Palumbo A, Avet-Loiseau H, Oliva S, et al. Revised International Staging System for multiple myeloma: a report from International Myeloma Working Group. J Clin Oncol. 2015;33(26): 2863–2869. doi:10.1200/JCO.2015.61.2267

PATIENT EDUCATION

- With the currently available induction regimens, the overall response rate in patients with newly diagnosed disease is >90%.
- In patients who undergo stem cell transplant following induction therapy, the mean duration of response is approximately 2 years.

6.6 BLOOD TRANSFUSIONS

OVERVIEW

Transfusion reactions are defined as adverse events associated with the transfusion of whole blood or one of its components. These range in severity from minor to life-threatening. Reactions can occur during the transfusion, defined as acute transfusion reactions, or days to weeks later, defined as delayed transfusion reactions, and may be immunologic or nonimmunologic. The most common presentation includes fever, chills, urticaria, and itching. Respiratory distress, high fever, hypotension, and hemoglobinuria can indicate a more serious reaction.

Types of transfusion reactions include the following: acute hemolytic, delayed hemolytic, febrile nonhemolytic, anaphylactic, simple allergic, septic (bacterial contamination), transfusion-related acute lung injury (TRALI), and transfusion-associated circulatory overload (TACO). With all suspected transfusion reactions, the transfusion should be stopped immediately, and the blood bank notified.

EPIDEMIOLOGY

Transfusion reactions range in frequency from relatively common (mild allergic and febrile nonhemolytic reactions) to rare (anaphylaxis, acute hemolytic, and sepsis). Fatal adverse events may occur most commonly with TRALI.

As a result of advances in blood screening and data systems, the risks and deaths associated with the transfusion of blood products have decreased greatly.

PATHOPHYSIOLOGY

Acute hemolytic transfusion reactions occur when the patient's plasma contains antibodies directed against the antigens on the transfused RBCs. Preformed IgM or IgG antibodies bind to RBCs and fix complement, leading to assembly of a membrane attack complex and intravascular hemolysis. Activation of the complement cascade leads to release of C3a and C5a. C3a and C5a promote release of serotonin and histamine from mast cells and this promotes bronchial and intestinal smooth muscle contraction.

Hemolysis associated with delayed hemolytic transfusion reactions is due to coating of RBCs with immunoglobulin and C3b. RBCs then undergo extravascular hemolysis being cleared by the reticuloendothelial system. Intravascular hemolysis can also occur with delayed hemolytic transfusion reactions.

Allergic transfusion reactions are due to preformed antibodies to plasma proteins in the transfused blood component.

Febrile transfusion reactions are due to cytokines released from leukocytes and platelets during storage or that are released when transfused. These preformed antibodies react with transfused leukocytes or platelets causing release of cytokines and a febrile reaction.

TRALI is due to transfusion of antibodies to HLA or neutrophil antigens, and transfusion of biologic modifiers that activate pulmonary endothelial cells and prime neutrophils, leading to pulmonary edema.

TACO is due to the sudden infusion of fluid with high oncotic pressure that occurs during a transfusion. This occurs in patients who cannot respond to the sudden change in volume.

Septic reactions are most likely associated with platelet transfusions. Plasma and cryoprecipitate transfusions rarely cause septic reactions because they are stored frozen and they rarely cause hemolytic reactions. Presenting signs for septic reactions include fever, chills, rigors, or shock.

Infectious or immunologic adverse effects can be seen with transfusion of blood products. Many of these infectious risks are addressed during the donor screening process and blood units are screened for various pathogens. See Table 6.27 for the infectious risk of blood transfusions.[33]

TABLE 6.27 Infectious Risks of Blood Transfusion

Infection	Risk
HIV	1 in 1,467,000
Hepatitis C	1 in 1,149,000
Hepatitis B	1 in 292,000
West Nile virus	Uncommon
Cytomegalovirus	50–85% of donors are carriers. Leukocyte reduction is protective.
Bacterial infection	1 in 2–3,000 (mostly platelets)
Parasitic infection	Relatively uncommon

Source: Data from Zou S, Stramer SL, Dodd RY. Donor testing and risk: current prevalence, incidence, and residual risk of transfusion-transmissible agents in US allogeneic donations. Transfus Med Rev. *2012;26:119. doi:10.1016/j.tmrv.2011.07.007*

DIAGNOSTIC STUDIES

If an acute transfusion reaction or a delayed hemolytic transfusion reaction is suspected the following steps should be taken:

- Confirm that the correct blood component unit was transfused. All paperwork, tags, labels, and patient identifiers should be reviewed and matched. A clerical error is a very common cause of a hemolytic transfusion reaction.
- Tests should be performed to detect possible hemolysis. These tests include urine for hemoglobin and inspecting the serum for visible hemolysis.
- Check ABO typing and DAT to confirm the patient's blood type and to determine if antibodies are coating the patient's RBCs. This would suggest an immune mechanism for the hemolysis.
- Antibody screen should be completed on a new blood sample from the patient to determine whether anti-RBC antibodies are present that were not detected prior to the transfusion.
- Repeat crossmatch between the patient's serum and a sample from the transfused RBC unit to determine whether the unit was fully compatible with the patient.

Additional tests for a suspected nonhemolytic acute transfusion reaction depend on the presenting signs and symptoms. If the reaction is associated with rigors and/or significant fever, a Gram stain and culture should be performed on a sample from the blood component and the patient's blood. If the reaction is associated with significant dyspnea, then test for brain natriuretic peptide (BNP) to determine if circulatory overload is likely.

TREATMENT

The following treatment options should be considered in suspected transfusion reactions:

- Supportive fluids should be provided to maintain blood pressure and adequate renal perfusion, unless TACO is suspected.
- Antipyretics can be given to treat fevers; if the fever is high and rigors present broad-spectrum antibiotics should be given.
- Antihistamines can be used to treat mild-moderate allergic reactions, corticosteroids are used to treat severe allergic reactions, and epinephrine is used for anaphylactic reactions.

- Oxygen should be given if hypoxia or dyspnea is present or TRALI is suspected.
- If TACO is suspected diuretics should be given and intravenous (IV) fluids limited.
- If hypotension is present vasopressors should be considered.

Further transfusion with RBCs should not be given until the workup has ruled out a hemolytic reaction or determined the etiology of a hemolytic reaction. If a RBC transfusion is emergently needed, emergency release O Rh(D) units may be the safest.

Suspected delayed hemolytic transfusion reactions rarely need immediate therapy, but the same immediate therapies for acute hemolytic transfusion reactions may be indicated for delayed hemolytic transfusion reactions.

BLOOD COMPONENTS

The primary use of a RBC transfusion is to increase the oxygen-carrying capacity of the blood. RBC transfusion is indicated in patients with anemia who have evidence of impaired oxygen delivery. With acute blood loss, volume replacement is often required along with plasma and platelets.

The decision to transfuse patients should be made in each individual case. There is no uniform hemoglobin value below which transfusion should occur. Many studies and guidelines support the use of a restrictive transfusion strategy, including in the ICU setting and with postoperative anemia.

RBCs should not be given for volume replacement or for any reason other than correction of acute or chronic anemia when nontransfusion alternatives are not an option. The decision to transfuse should not be based on a single hemoglobin value without considering all physiologic factors affecting oxygenation and clinical status in a patient.

One unit of RBCs usually increases the hemoglobin concentration by approximately 1.0 g/dL in an average-size, nonbleeding adult. For pediatric or neonatal patients, as well as for adult patients who cannot tolerate a transfusion of the total volume within 4 hours, splitting of the units should be considered.

The transfusion of platelets is indicated in the treatment of patients with bleeding due to severely decreased or dysfunctional platelets. Platelet transfusion may also be used prophylactically in patients with rapidly falling or low platelet counts secondary to bone marrow disorders or chemotherapy. Platelet transfusions are not recommended for patients with rapid platelet destruction (e.g., ITP, heparin-induced thrombocytopenia [HIT], TTP) except when there is clinically significant and/or life-threatening bleeding.

The two types of platelet transfusions are apheresis and pooled. Apheresis platelets may be selected based on similar HLA typing to the recipient's when a recipient fails to respond to platelet transfusion because of the presence of anti-HLA antibodies.

The donor plasma in the platelet unit should be ABO compatible, but not necessarily group-specific, with the recipient's RBCs. The same compatibility guidelines are used for platelets and plasma products.

One random donor platelet concentrate should increase the platelet count by 5,000 to 10,000/µL in an average-size patient who is not refractory. Generally, a pool of 6 to 8 platelet concentrates or a single apheresis unit is sufficient to correct or prevent bleeding in a normal-size adult.[34] Transfusion of apheresis platelets should result in increments like those achieved by transfusion of pooled platelets. If the post-transfusion platelet count does not rise to the expected level, this could be due to sepsis, alloimmunization, fever, ITP, or DIC.

Plasma products include frozen plasma citrate phosphate dextrose (CPD), apheresis fresh frozen plasma (AFFP), and cryosupernatant plasma CPD, also called cryo-poor plasma. Plasma products must be ABO compatible with the recipient's blood type but not necessarily group specific.

Frozen plasma CPD (FP) is made up of 280 mL of plasma separated from an individual unit of whole blood collected in CPD anticoagulant and frozen within 24 hours. FP contains all coagulation factors but with slightly reduced amounts of clotting factors V and VIII.

AFFP is collected by apheresis and frozen within 8 hours. It contains both labile clotting factors V and VIII, plus nonlabile coagulation factors. Sodium citrate anticoagulated AFFP units have a volume of 490 mL while ACD-A anticoagulated AFFP units have a volume of 250 mL.

Cryosupernatant plasma CPD (CSP) or cryo-poor plasma has a volume of 270 mL of plasma separated from an individual unit of whole blood prepared following cryoprecipitate production. It contains all coagulation factors but has reduced levels of the high molecular weight vWF multimers.

AFFP/FP is used in the treatment or prevention of clinically significant bleeding due to a deficiency of one or more plasma coagulation factors. This includes treatment of:

- Bleeding patients or patients undergoing invasive procedures who require replacement of multiple coagulation factors (e.g., patients with severe liver disease or DIC)
- Patients receiving massive transfusions with clinically significant coagulation abnormalities
- Patients on warfarin anticoagulation who are bleeding or need to undergo an invasive procedure before vitamin K can reverse the warfarin effect
- Patients being treated for TTP and adult HUS by plasma exchange
- Patients being treated by plasma exchange when the exchange fluid must include coagulation factors

Plasma transfusion is not indicated for volume replacement alone, or for a single coagulation factor deficiency if specific recombinant products or plasma-derived virally inactivated products are available. Plasma transfusion is not indicated or effective in reversal of an international normalized ratio (INR) below 1.8.

Hypovolemia without coagulation factor deficiencies should be treated with other plasma volume expanders such as 0.9% sodium chloride, Ringer lactate solution, albumin, or hydroxyethyl starches.

Plasma is not indicated when specific therapy such as vitamin K, prothrombin complex concentrates (PCCs), cryoprecipitate, or specific coagulation factor replacement can be used.

The plasma volume used should be able to achieve a minimum of 30% of plasma clotting factor concentration, which is typically 10 to 15 mL/kg of body weight; for the treatment of warfarin reversal the dose is 5 to 8 mL/kg body weight.

Cryoprecipitate is used for fibrinogen replacement in acquired hypofibrinogenemia or as empiric therapy in a bleeding patient. If the plasma fibrinogen level is <100 mg/dL cryoprecipitate should be given. Cryoprecipitate is used as a factor VIII concentrate for hemophilia, von Willebrand disease (vWD), and hypofibrinogenemia. With fibrinogen deficiency it should only be used if there is active bleeding or a planned surgical procedure.

One unit of cryoprecipitate contains approximately 285 mg of fibrinogen. The amount of cryoprecipitat required for transfusion will depend on the severity of the bleeding condition.

6.7 HEMOSTATIC DISORDERS

OVERVIEW

The goal of this overview is to briefly summarize the two main pathways of hemostasis (primary hemostasis and secondary hemostasis) as well as anticoagulant mechanisms and fibrinolysis. In addition, this section will discuss disorders of hemostasis and the mechanisms of the various drugs that are available to impact these pathways to prevent either thrombosis or bleeding. While many of the main drugs that are used to treat disorders of hemostasis have been used for decades, greater understanding of hemostasis has led to development of various new drugs that have come onto the market recently or are close to coming onto the market. Thus, improved understanding of hemostasis continues to lead to benefits for patients.

Hemostasis is the physiologic process that stops bleeding at the site of an injury while maintaining normal blood flow elsewhere in the circulation. There are two main components of hemostasis. Primary hemostasis consists of platelet aggregation and platelet plug formation. Platelets are activated in a multistep process that results in their adherence to the site of injury and to each other, creating a platelet plug. Secondary hemostasis involves the coagulation cascade and results in the deposition of fibrin into and around the platelet plug. The fibrin forms a mesh that strengthens and stabilizes the clot. Primary and secondary hemostasis occur simultaneously and are intertwined. The fibrinolytic pathway also plays a significant role in limiting hemostasis. Thrombus formation or bleeding can occur whenever this process is disrupted.

Platelets are small fragments produced from megakaryocytes. The normal platelet count ranges from 150 to 450 million per milliliter of blood and they circulate for about 7 to 10 days. In a healthy blood vessel with normal blood flow, platelets do not adhere to surfaces or aggregate with each other. If the vessel is injured platelets are exposed to subendothelial matrix, and adhesion and activation of platelets begin.

When the endothelium is injured, the subendothelial matrix is exposed and immediately initiates primary hemostasis. Primary hemostasis consists of three main events.

- **Platelet adhesion:** With endothelial injury, platelets bind to exposed subendothelial matrix proteins with the aid of adhesion molecules or the receptors transmembrane glycoproteins (GP) and either integrins or non-integrin. Abnormalities in either GPIb-IX-V complex or vWF can result in inherited hemorrhagic disorders such as Bernard-Soulier syndrome (GPIb deficiency) or vWD (abnormality or deficiency in vWF).
- **Platelet activation:** Once platelets adhere they become activated, degranulate and release the content of the alpha granules (contain vWF and coagulation factors) and dense granules (Wcontain adenosine diphosphate [ADP] and serotonin), and recruit additional platelets to the site. Thrombin, which is generated by the coagulation cascade, is another platelet activator.
- **Platelet plug formation:** Fibrinogen forms links between activated platelets to form a stable platelet plug. Further stabilization is accomplished through secondary hemostasis.

Secondary hemostasis consists of the cascade of coagulation serine proteases that results in the cleavage of soluble fibrinogen by thrombin. Thrombin cleavage generates insoluble fibrin that forms a crosslinked fibrin mesh at the site of an injury. Fibrin generation occurs simultaneously to platelet aggregation. In intact and healthy blood vessels this cascade is not activated and several anticoagulants, including thrombomodulin and heparin sulfate proteoglycans, prevent its activation.

When the vascular system is injured, blood is exposed to TF. The complex of TF and factor VIIa activates factor X and factor IX. This activation pathway is called the extrinsic pathway. Factor IXa also activates factor X, in the presence of factor VIIIa. Factor Xa, with its cofactor Va, then activates the conversion of prothrombin to thrombin. Thrombin cleaves fibrinogen to generate fibrin. Thrombin is responsible for positive feedback activation of coagulation; this leads to clot propagation. Thrombin activates factor XI, which then activates factor IX and thrombin activates cofactors VIII and V. This is the intrinsic pathway of coagulation, a positive feedback loop. Thrombin also has an important role in limiting the coagulation cascade by binding to thrombomodulin on endothelial cells and activating protein C. Activated protein C (APC), in the presence of protein S, will downregulate the coagulation cascade as it cleaves and inactivates the procoagulant cofactors VIIIa and Va.

The function of the fibrinolytic system is to dissolve blood clots during the process of wound healing and to prevent blood clots in healthy blood vessels. The fibrinolytic system is composed of plasmin, which cleaves and breaks down fibrin. Plasmin is generated from plasminogen by the proteases tissue plasminogen activator (tPA) and urokinase plasminogen activator (uPA).

EPIDEMIOLOGY

The prevalence of the various bleeding disorders varies greatly. See Table 6.28 for the prevalence of the various bleeding disorders.

6.7A PLATELET DISORDERS

Bleeding that develops spontaneously, without associated surgery or injury, is considered pathological. Bleeding associated with a local pathologic process may be exacerbated by disorders of the hemostatic process, or spontaneous bleeding can develop in their presence. Platelet disorders may be due to thrombocytopenia or platelet dysfunction.

Thrombocytopenia can be due to decreased production, increased destruction, or sequestration in the spleen. Spontaneous bleeding is rare outside of severe thrombocytopenia (<20,000 cells/μL), which is seen in immune or drug-induced thrombocytopenia, in acute leukemia, or following cytotoxic chemotherapy. Mild thrombocytopenia (<50,000–75,000 cells/μL) can contribute to excessive bleeding provoked by trauma or menses.

Platelet numbers may be normal but their function impaired. Platelet dysfunction is typically an acquired problem, related to drugs, uremia or liver disease. Platelet inhibition is the goal with treatment with aspirin, clopidogrel, and the GPIIb/IIa (GPIIb/IIIa) receptor antagonists; increased bleeding risk has been noted with all these medications.

TABLE 6.28 Prevalence of Bleeding Disorders

Bleeding Disorder	Prevalence	Bleeding Disorder	Prevalence
Factor V deficiency	<1 in 1 million	von Willebrand disease	1 in 100
Factor VII deficiency	1 in 500,000	Glanzmann thrombasthenia	1 in 1 million
Factor VIII deficiency (hemophilia A)	1 in 500 male births	Bernard-Soulier syndrome	<1 in 1 million
Factor IX deficiency (hemophilia B)	1 in 30,000 male births	Wiskott-Aldrich syndrome	1 in 1 million
Factor X deficiency	1 in 500,000	Immune thrombocytopenia purpura	3.3 in 100,000 new cases per year
Factor XI deficiency	4% in Ashkenazi Jews	Thrombotic thrombocytopenia purpura	3.7 in 1 million new cases per year
Factor XIII deficiency	>200 cases reported		

MEDICAL HISTORY AND CLINICAL PRESENTATION

History and physical examination are the most important elements of the diagnostic evaluation. With the history the diagnosis will be readily evident, and laboratory testing can then be used to confirm initial diagnosis.

SIGNS AND SYMPTOMS

Platelet disorders present with cutaneous and mucosal bleeding, while bleeding in the setting of coagulation defects most often takes the form of larger ecchymoses that spread to deeper tissues, such as hemarthrosis.

Spontaneous bleeding suggests a more severe underlying defect. Multisystem illness should prompt consideration of DIC or TTP/HUS. A past medical history of liver disease or uremia may lead to platelet disorders. Liver disease reduces clotting factor production and increased consumption, both thrombocytopenia and platelet dysfunction, and increased fibrinolysis. Uremia will cause platelet dysfunction.

In pregnant women who hemorrhage, consider HELLP syndrome, fatty liver of pregnancy with accompanying liver failure, or TTP/HUS.

Drugs can induce severe thrombocytopenia, AA, and vascular purpura. Antiplatelet and anticoagulant medications contribute to the development of bleeding events.

PHYSICAL EXAMINATION

Physical examination can assist in determining if bleeding is due to a platelet disorder. Vital signs, including orthostatic measurements, are used to estimate the acuity and significance of blood/volume loss. Skin examination may reveal the presence of petechiae. The presence of petechiae suggests a platelet disorder or vasculitis. Petechiae are typically be found in dependent areas, such as the lower extremities with sparing of the soles of the feet. Petechiae secondary to thrombocytopenia will not be palpable, while petechiae secondary to vasculitis will be. Ecchymoses will be multiple, blue-purple areas, without spread to deeper soft tissues in the case of a platelet disorder. The presence of bleeding, petechiae and purpura on the nasal or oral mucosa suggests a platelet disorder. Splenomegaly may be present as the spleen can sequester up to 90% of platelets leading to mild to moderate thrombocytopenia.

DIFFERENTIAL DIAGNOSIS

The differential diagnosis for platelet disorders is noted in Table 6.29.

DIAGNOSTIC STUDIES

Platelet count value below 50,000 cells/μL is highly suggestive of thrombocytopenia as a cause of or contributor

TABLE 6.29 Differential Diagnosis of Platelet Disorders

Thrombocytopenia	Description
Acute leukemia	Presents with thrombocytopenia, leukopenia, and anemia. Constitutional symptoms, such as fever and weight loss are noted. Blasts are noted on the blood smear.
Disseminated intravascular coagulation (DIC)	DIC occurs in association with a secondary condition and associated with serious bleeding or clotting complications.
Thrombotic thrombocytopenic purpura (TTP)	Characterized by schistocytes on the blood smear and neurologic findings.
Immune thrombocytopenic purpura (ITP)	Immune mediated, present with bleeding and no splenomegaly
Drug-induced thrombocytopenia	Immune-mediated thrombocytopenia due to side effect of drugs. Heparin-induced thrombocytopenia is a thrombocytopenic reaction characterized by predisposition to thrombosis.
Platelet Dysfunction	**Description**
von Willebrand disease (vWD)	Genetic defect with absent or defective vWF.
Bernard-Soulier syndrome	Inherited disorder of blood clotting, thrombocytopenia, megakaryocytes, prolonged bleeding time
Wiskott-Aldrich syndrome	Abnormal immune system function with microthrombocytopenia, eczema and bleeding
Glanzmann thrombasthenia	Genetic disorder with impaired platelet function due to a defect in GPIIb/IIIa
Gray platelet syndrome	Platelet alpha granule deficiency with myelofibrosis and large agranular platelets

TABLE 6.30 Bleeding Risk Related to Platelet Level

Platelet Count	Risk Level
<150,000/μL	Less than 150,000/μL is the definition of thrombocytopenia but platelet counts between 100,000–150,000/μL are unimportant for bleeding risk, even with surgery or trauma.
50,000–100,000/μL	Between 50,000 and 100,000/μL may indicate a risk for bleeding with certain types of surgery or trauma, but not associated with spontaneous bleeding, and are safe in patients taking drugs such as aspirin and clopidogrel.
30,000–50,000/μL	Between 30,000 and 50,000/μL suggest a possible risk for bleeding with surgery or trauma, but rarely associated with petechiae, purpura, or spontaneous bleeding.
10,000–30,000/μL	Between 10,000 and 30,000/μL are associated with petechiae, purpura, and spontaneous bleeding; and excessive bleeding with surgery or trauma.
<10,000/μL	Less than 10,000/μL are associated with spontaneous bleeding; spontaneous, severe, and life-threatening bleeding is uncommon unless other disorders are present.

to bleeding. Peripheral smear should be reviewed to ensure there is no evidence of pseudothrombocytopenia. See Table 6.30 for the risk of bleeding with various platelet counts.

The peripheral blood smear should be examined to exclude pseudothrombocytopenia and evaluate platelet morphology or clumping pattern abnormalities that may suggest the presence of a congenital platelet function disorder.

The bleeding time (BT) is a diagnostic test for platelet function disorders. It will be prolonged in the setting of thrombocytopenia or platelet dysfunction, including vWD. The test is nonspecific, poorly reproducible, and insensitive. Because of these limitations the test is used infrequently.

Platelet function analyzer test (PFA-100) measures the formation of the hemostatic plug. An abnormal closure time suggests platelet dysfunction, including vWD. It is a more sensitive test for vWD than the BT. The PFA-100 is affected by anemia and thrombocytopenia but is normal in coagulopathies or vascular dysfunction.

Platelet aggregometry uses several different methods to measure platelet aggregation with the addition of agonists to the patient's sample. This test detects platelet defects and is used to monitor platelet inhibition by drugs such as aspirin, clopidogrel and GPIIb/IIIa receptor antagonists.

EVALUATION

If the patient with bleeding has a normal PT, INR, and aPTT this may indicate a platelet disorder. These possible disorders include vWD and disorders of fibrinolysis or vascular integrity.

Low platelets will confirm thrombocytopenia. If the platelet count is >50,000/μL, this is unlikely to cause bleeding, and other causes should be sought.

If the platelet count is normal, PFA-100 testing can be used to assess for platelet dysfunction or vWD. A history of antiplatelet medication use or symptoms of uremia suggests a source of platelet dysfunction. If there is a concern about vWD, a vWF antigen immunoassay, ristocetin cofactor (RCoF) activity, and factor VIII level testing should be obtained. Abnormal platelet morphology suggests the possibility of an inherited disorder of platelet function.

TREATMENT

General approach to the treatment of significant active bleeding includes local control of the bleeding and maintaining hemodynamic stability and airway control. Further treatment is directed by the patient's status and laboratory testing results.

When appropriate, blood products should be transfused. Packed RBCs should be given when there is ongoing severe bleeding, regardless of hemoglobin level. If platelets are <50,000 cells/μL, give 1 unit of single donor platelet pheresis product or 5–6 units of pooled platelet concentrates; this will increase platelets by approximately 30,000 cells/μL. Platelets may not be fully functional until 4 hours after transfusion and alloimmunization should be considered if at 15 minutes post-transfusion the platelet count has not increased by at least 10,000 platelets/μL. If the platelet count responds initially but declines at 24 hours, this suggests consumption from sepsis, DIC, or drug effect. In TTP platelet transfusion may worsen the disease.

If there is concurrent decrease in coagulation factors the transfusing of fresh frozen plasma (FFP) should be considered. FFP contains all the coagulation factors and should be considered in patients with factor deficiency, with DIC, currently taking warfarin with an elevated INR, or with massive transfusions.

6.7AA THROMBOCYTOPENIA

Two major causes of thrombocytopenia include ITP and TTP.

Immune Thrombocytopenic Purpura

ITP is a heterogeneous group of disorders characterized by autoimmune-mediated platelet destruction and impairment of platelet production. In ITP the platelets life span is reduced as a result of an antibody-mediated clearance of platelets by tissue macrophages. Platelet production may be impaired in ITP by antibody- and cell-mediated suppression of megakaryopoiesis. ITP refers to all forms of immune-mediated thrombocytopenia, whether occurring in the absence of an evident predisposing etiology (primary) or as a sequela of an associated condition (secondary). A platelet count of $<100 \times 10^9/L$ is recommended as the cutoff for diagnosis. ITP is classified by duration of disease. ITP diagnosed within the last 3 months is newly diagnosed, 3 to 12 months ago is persistent, and >12 months ago is chronic. The incidence of ITP in adults is estimated to be 1.6 to 3.9 per 100,000 persons per year. Adult-onset ITP incidence has a bimodal distribution, with peaks during young adulthood and among the elderly. Among young adults, ITP is approximately twice as common in females as in males; in the elderly, it affects males and females equally.[35]

Thrombotic Thrombocytopenic Purpura

TTP is a life-threatening disorder caused by systemic platelet adhesion and aggregation. TTP is a TMA and is characterized by organ ischemia, profound thrombocytopenia, presence of schistocytes, and severe deficiency of the plasma vWF-cleaving protease, ADAMTS13.

ADAMTS13 deficiency may be familial, due to defective enzyme production, or acquired via an autoantibody.

Familial TTP typically appears in infancy or childhood and is recurrent. Patients with familial TTP have <5% to 10% of normal plasma ADAMTS13, both during and between episodes.

The absent or severely reduced plasma ADAMTS13 activity in familial TTP is a consequence of homozygous (or double heterozygous) mutations in both *ADAMTS13* alleles located on chromosome 9.

MEDICAL HISTORY AND CLINICAL PRESENTATION

Immune Thrombocytopenic Purpura

The major clinical manifestation of ITP is an increased risk of bleeding. Nonhemorrhagic manifestations include fatigue and reduced quality of life. Bleeding in ITP is primarily mucocutaneous, but petechiae, purpura, ecchymoses, epistaxis, gingival bleeding, and menorrhagia are common. Major GI hemorrhage and hematuria occur less frequently. ICH is rare. A history of recent use of prescription, over-the-counter, and recreational drugs as well as herbal supplements should be obtained to rule out drug-induced thrombocytopenia.

Thrombotic Thrombocytopenic Purpura

The major clinical manifestations of TTP are secondary to severe thrombocytopenia and ischemia. Bruising or purpura and rarely bleeding of the nose and gums may be noted. Large ecchymoses may occur. The classic presentation of TTP includes the following five findings:

- Fever
- Change in mental status
- Thrombocytopenia
- Renal insufficiency
- MAHA

TTP may occur late in pregnancy or immediately after delivery, in HIV/AIDS patients, and in the first few weeks of taking clopidogrel or ticlopidine. TMAs are at times noted during the immunosuppression, due to cyclosporine or tacrolimus, associated with HSC or solid organ transplantation.

SIGNS AND SYMPTOMS

Immune Thrombocytopenic Purpura

The presentation of primary ITP is a healthy individual with isolated thrombocytopenia and an unremarkable peripheral blood smear, and on physical examination the only finding may be bleeding secondary to thrombocytopenia. Some patients with ITP suffer from disabling fatigue, apprehension of bleeding, withdrawal from important professional and recreational activities, and poor quality of life. Adults with chronic ITP have a mildly increased risk of thromboembolism, hematologic malignancy, and other autoimmune disorders such as systemic lupus erythematosus.

Thrombotic Thrombocytopenic Purpura

The signs and symptoms of TTP may be subtle and nonspecific. Patients may experience influenza-like or diarrheal illness before developing TTP. Neurologic symptoms are common and vary greatly in severity. Other symptoms include fatigue, confusion, headaches, seizures, and stroke-like symptoms.

PHYSICAL EXAMINATION

Immune Thrombocytopenic Purpura

Physical examination may only present with evidence of bleeding. Bleeding may be noted in the oral and nasal cavity and the skin examination may reveal petechiae, purpura, or ecchymoses.

Thrombotic Thrombocytopenic Purpura

Physical examination will present with signs of bleeding and the microangiopathic anemia. Patients may also have jaundice, skin pallor, tachycardia, dyspnea, and petechiae.

DIFFERENTIAL DIAGNOSIS

Immune Thrombocytopenic Purpura

When evaluating a patient for primary ITP all possible etiologies for a secondary ITP should be excluded.

After non-autoimmune causes of thrombocytopenia have been excluded, a thorough history and physical examination should be conducted to evaluate for a predisposing infection, malignancy, autoimmune disorder, or immune deficiency. Separating primary ITP from secondary etiologies is critical in respect to treatment and prognosis. See Table 6.31 for a list of secondary causes of ITP.

Thrombotic Thrombocytopenic Purpura

Several other disorders can present like TTP. See Table 6.32 for a list of secondary causes of TTP. Plasma ADAMTS13 levels are usually within a broad normal range in the above disorders.

DIAGNOSTIC STUDIES

Immune Thrombocytopenic Purpura

Diagnosis of ITP is a diagnosis of exclusion. CBC will reveal thrombocytopenia with normal-appearing platelets. Review of the peripheral blood smear should be done to rule out artifact or platelet clumping as a cause of thrombocytopenia. Testing for hepatitis C and HIV should be obtained as they both can present with thrombocytopenia. Other tests to rule out other possible etiologies include coagulation studies, *Helicobacter pylori* testing, thyroid function tests, anti-nuclear antibody (ANA) test, assessment of vitamin B12 and folate, and bone marrow biopsy.

TABLE 6.31 Etiologies of Secondary Immune Thrombocytopenic Purpura

Category	Examples
Autoimmune disorders	Systemic lupus erythematosus Antiphospholipid syndrome Evans syndrome
Infections	Human immunodeficiency virus Hepatitis C virus *Helicobacter pylori*
Lymphoproliferative disorders	Chronic lymphocytic leukemia
Congenital immune deficiencies	Common variable immune deficiency Autoimmune lymphoproliferative syndrome
Drugs	Alemtuzumab Purine analogs

TABLE 6.32 Differential Diagnosis of Thrombotic Thrombocytopenic Purpura

Differential Diagnosis	Description
Hemolytic uremic syndrome (HUS)	Caused by Shiga toxin-producing bacteria (e.g., *Escherichia coli* O157:H7) or defective control or hyperactivity of the alternative complement pathway. Acute renal failure is prominent.
Disseminated intravascular coagulation (DIC)	Plasma D-dimers are elevated. Venous thromboembolism is common.
Malignant hypertension	Elevated blood pressure with end-organ damage.
Collagen vascular disease/severe vasculitis	Positive ANA and elevated erythrocyte sedimentation rate.
Evans syndrome	Autoimmune thrombocytopenia and AIHA.
Preeclampsia/eclampsia/HELLP syndrome	Pregnant with elevated blood pressure and urine positive for protein, for HELLP have hemolysis with elevated liver function tests and low platelets.
Antiphospholipid syndrome	Autoimmune hypercoagulable state. Detection of specific antibodies.
Heparin-induced thrombocytopenia (HIT)	History of heparin usage.

AIHA, autoimmune hemolytic anemia; ANA, anti-nuclear antibody; HELLP, hemolysis, elevated liver function tests, low platelets.

Thrombotic Thrombocytopenic Purpura

Before beginning treatment, the patient should be tested for ADAMTS13 activity, to determine if the enzyme is absent, reduced, or within normal range. If ADAMTS13 is <5% to 10%, then it should be determined if an ADAMTS13 autoantibody is present. Elevated serum LDH is noted due to release from fragmenting RBCs and ischemic tissue cells. Patients with familial TTP always present with absent or severely reduced plasma levels of ADAMTS13.

Normal levels of ADAMTS13 indicate that TTP is not present.

ADAMTS13 can be reduced below the normal range in liver disease, disseminated malignancies, sepsis, pregnancy, and in newborns. The ADAMTS13 level in these conditions is not reduced to the extremely low values (<5 to 10%) found in patients with familial or autoantibody-mediated TTP.

EVALUATION

Immune Thrombocytopenic Purpura

There is no gold standard laboratory test for ITP. Most compelling is the presence of a response to ITP-specific therapy. The initial evaluation of suspected primary ITP involves excluding non-autoimmune causes of thrombocytopenia and exclusion of secondary causes. A careful history, physical examination, CBC, and review of peripheral blood smear are the first steps in the evaluation.

Thrombotic Thrombocytopenic Purpura

TTP is characterized by a MAHA and thrombocytopenia. These characteristics are also noted in HUS. Other symptoms for TTP include fever, change in mental status, and mild renal insufficiency. TPP can be confirmed by showing decreased levels of ADAMTS13.

TREATMENT

Immune Thrombocytopenic Purpura

The goal of therapy is to provide a hemostatic platelet count, typically a platelet count of 20 to 30 × 10^9/L or greater, while minimizing treatment-related morbidity. Treatment is rarely indicated for patients with platelet counts >20–30 × 10^9/L. Patients with extensive bleeding symptoms, comorbidities, or lifestyles that predispose them to bleeding and those who require an invasive procedure may benefit from a higher platelet count. A platelet count of 50 × 10^9/L or higher in patients who require antithrombotic therapy is indicated.

First-line therapy consists of corticosteroids, supplemented with intravenous immunoglobulin (IVIG) or immunoglobulin anti-D as needed. This will stop any bleeding and raise the platelet count acutely in patients with newly diagnosed or newly relapsed disease.

Thrombotic Thrombocytopenic Purpura

In familial ADAMTS13-deficient TTP, FFP or cryoprecipitate-poor plasma infusion is sufficient to reverse episodes of familial TTP within a few days. To treat acquired ADAMTS13 autoantibody-mediated TTP, FFP or cryoprecipitate-poor plasma infusion is used initially until daily plasma exchange can be started. FFP or cryoprecipitate-poor plasma infusion alone is not as effective as plasma exchange and may lead to volume overload. In acquired TMA not associated with ADAMTS13 deficiency, any medication that may induce the disorder should be stopped. Common medications include clopidogrel, ticlopidine, bevacizumab, mitomycin, gemcitabine, quinine, total body irradiation, chemotherapeutic agents, cyclosporine, and tacrolimus. Familial ADAMTS13-deficient TTP is treated with periodic infusion of FFP or cryoprecipitate-poor plasma in patients who lack effective ADAMTS13 synthesis.

PATIENT EDUCATION

Immune Thrombocytopenic Purpura

- Primary ITP in adults is a chronic disease. Approximately 80% to 90% of patients respond to standard first-line treatments, but many will relapse and require additional therapy.
- The chance of long-term survival with proper treatment and follow-up is excellent.
- The likelihood of achieving a sustained remission lessens as the duration of disease increases.
- It is estimated that 5% to 10% of patients presenting with primary ITP will eventually develop systemic lupus erythematosus or another autoimmune disorder.

Thrombotic Thrombocytopenic Purpura

- Familial ADAMTS13-deficient TTP
  - Episodes are usually recurrent and can be treated successfully with infusions of FFP or cryoprecipitate-poor plasma.
- Acquired ADAMTS13 autoantibody-mediated TTP
  - 80% of patients with acquired anti-ADAMTS13 autoantibody-mediated TTP enter clinical remission after 10 or more plasma exchange procedures using FFP or cryoprecipitate-poor plasma.
  - Cognitive impairment may be noted after treatment in some patients.
  - Relapses occur in about one third of patients, often within the first year after the initial episode.

6.7AB PLATELET FUNCTION DISORDERS

Inherited platelet function disorders are a heterogeneous group of bleeding disorders of varying severity due to defects in platelet adhesion, GP expression, receptor function, signaling pathways, aggregation, and granular contents and abnormalities in procoagulant activity. These disorders are typically associated with normal platelet counts and characterized by bleeding symptoms, which include epistaxis, extensive bruising, menorrhagia in women, and the possibility of life-threatening excessive bleeding with surgery, injury, or childbirth.

Bernard-Soulier Syndrome

Bernard-Soulier syndrome (BSS) is a rare autosomal recessive bleeding disorder, on a rare occasion acquired with myelodysplasia/AML. Prevalence is 1 in 1 million births. It typically presents in early childhood.

Mutations in genes lead to a defective GPIb/IX/V complex. This complex is the principal receptor for vWF and is crucial to platelet adhesion to an injured endothelium.

MEDICAL HISTORY AND CLINICAL PRESENTATION

Common bleeding symptoms reported include menorrhagia, ecchymosis without trauma, GI hemorrhage, dental bleeding, epistaxis, and petechiae.

SIGNS AND SYMPTOMS

BSS is characterized by moderate to severe mucocutaneous bleeding and surgical bleeding, large granular platelets, thrombocytopenia, and abnormal platelet aggregation in the presence of ristocetin. Other symptoms include bleeding gums, bruising, epistaxis, and abnormal menstrual periods.

PHYSICAL EXAMINATION

Physical examination reveals bleeding of mucous membranes, such as oral mucosa and nasal mucosa.

DIFFERENTIAL DIAGNOSIS

Because of variable thrombocytopenia, BSS is confused with chronic ITP.

Because of the large platelet size, the macrothrombocytopenia syndromes should be considered. The macrothrombocytopenia syndromes present with sensorineural hearing loss, cataracts, nephritis, and inclusion bodies in the WBCs.

Type 2B vWD is due to a mutation that leads to an increased affinity of the abnormal vWF for blood platelets. Patients with type 2B vWD present with variable thrombocytopenia and excessive bleeding symptoms. In type 2B vWD, there is platelet aggregation to very low doses of ristocetin.

DIAGNOSTIC STUDIES

Evaluation begins with a CBC, manual peripheral blood smear review, and a PFA-100. On peripheral blood smear there is variable thrombocytopenia with large platelets. With PFA-100 testing the closure time is prolonged. A complete drug history is needed prior to performing a PFA-100 or other platelet studies, since recent nonsteroidal anti-inflammatory drug or aspirin use can lead to false positive results. Also, herbal medications and certain foods (garlic and fatty foods) can prolong the closure time in the collagen/epinephrine cartridge.

To verify the diagnosis, light transmission platelet aggregometry should be done to demonstrate the significantly reduced or absent platelet aggregation in the presence of ristocetin and thrombin. Verification of the molecular defect and definitive confirmation of this diagnosis requires flow cytometry.

TREATMENT

Bleeding events in BSS are controlled by platelet transfusion. If mucosal bleeding is present tranexamic acid can be given. Affected patients should avoid contact sports and medications such as aspirin, which can increase bleeding.

Glanzmann Thrombasthenia

Glanzmann thrombasthenia (GT) is a rare, inherited (autosomal recessive disorder), moderate to severe bleeding disorder, rarely acquired with APL.

GT is seen with increased prevalence in populations with high consanguineous marriage rates (i.e., South Indian Hindus, Iraqi Jews, French Gypsies, Jordanian nomadic tribes) and most cases are noted outside the United States.

GT is due to a qualitative or quantitative defect in GPIIb/IIIa leading to an inability to aggregate platelets despite normal adhesion. There are three subtypes of GT:

- **Type 1 disease:** Absent platelet aggregation and clot retraction
- **Type 2 disease:** Absent platelet aggregation and normal clot retraction
- **Variant disease:** No common feature

MEDICAL HISTORY AND CLINICAL PRESENTATION

Patients present in early childhood with moderate to severe mucocutaneous bleeding, including menorrhagia, epistaxis, gingival bleeding, GI hemorrhage, and ecchymosis.

SIGNS AND SYMPTOMS

The symptoms of this disease are usually apparent at birth or during infancy. Symptoms vary from mild to life-threatening bleeding. Symptoms include easy bruising, epistaxis, bleeding gums, menorrhagia, abnormal bleeding after surgery, and rarely hematemesis, hematuria, or hematochezia.

PHYSICAL EXAMINATION

Physical examination reveals bleeding of mucous membranes, such as oral and nasal mucosa.

DIFFERENTIAL DIAGNOSIS

Several conditions present with features that are similar to GT. Hemophilia, a rare inherited blood clotting disorder caused by an inactive or deficient factor VIII or IX, presents with joint bleeding and elevated PTT.

Bernard-Soulier syndrome, a rare inherited blood clotting disorder, is characterized by platelet abnormalities due to abnormal GPIb/IX/V complex. Symptoms include profuse bleeding, such as nosebleeds and heavy menstrual bleeding. Petechiae and purpura are noted on physical exam.

May-Hegglin syndrome is a rare inherited disorder of blood platelets and certain WBCs characterized by reduced numbers of giant platelets. Patients do not have excessive bleeding unless platelet count is very low.

Storage pool disease (SPD) is a rare inherited disorder of blood platelets characterized by clotting dysfunction due to the platelets' inability to store and release certain clotting factors. Symptoms include mild bleeding, nosebleeds, and heavier than normal menstrual periods. Some patients with SPD may have thrombocytopenia.

DIAGNOSTIC STUDIES

If there is clinical suspicion of GT other causes of mucocutaneous bleeding should be ruled out with a PT, PTT, CBC, fibrinogen activity, and vWD panel including RCoF assay, vWF antigen, and factor VIII activity, all of which will be normal in GT. Platelet morphology and quantity will be normal with GT. PFA-100 will reveal a significantly prolonged closure time in both collagen/ADP and collagen/epinephrine tests.

To verify the diagnosis light transmission platelet aggregometry should be completed to demonstrate the absent response to all platelet agonists, including arachidonic acid, ADP, collagen, and epinephrine.

Definitive diagnosis can be made by defective or absent GP expression of IIb/IIIa by flow cytometry and gene sequencing.

TREATMENT

Simple bleeding can be controlled with local pressure. Some individuals with GT may require blood platelet transfusions. If transfusions are needed HLA matched transfusion is best as some patients develop antibodies to transfused platelets.

A recombinant factor VIIa (rFVIIa) product can be used to treat GT. This medication is used to treat bleeding episodes and perioperative management when platelet transfusions are not effective.

PATIENT EDUCATION

- Failure to make a timely diagnosis of GT can lead to excessive and/or fatal bleeding, especially following surgical procedures.
- Platelet alloimmunization is common; utilizing HLA matched platelets is key to prevention of alloantibodies.
- Genetic counseling is recommended for people with GT and their families.

von Willebrand Disease

vWF is a multimeric protein that has a critical role in hemostasis. vWF is produced and secreted by endothelial cells and platelets and, after binding to platelet GPI receptors, causes platelets to adhere to injured endothelial cells.

Another function of vWF is to bind to coagulation factor VIII and protect it from proteolysis. vWF-bound factor VIII can circulate longer than would be possible in the absence of vWF.

Deficiency or defective vWF results in vWD, which is a common mild congenital bleeding disorder. The gene encoding the vWF monomer is on chromosome 12. There are several types of congenital vWD. Type 1 is a quantitative disorder in vWF production or release and accounts for a majority of all cases of vWD. Type 2 is a qualitative or functional defect in vWF and makes up a fourth of all cases of vWD. Type 3 is a quantitative deficiency in vWF production or release and is very rare.

MEDICAL HISTORY AND CLINICAL PRESENTATION

vWD is typically an inherited bleeding disorder, only rarely acquired. A family history of bleeding affecting both males and females is suggestive of vWD. The bleeding is mild and patients typically present for evaluation of easy bruising, excessive bleeding with dental extractions or surgery, recurrent epistaxis, or excessive menstrual bleeding.

Mucocutaneous bleeding is the most common symptom of most patients with vWD. vWD type 3 and type 2N present like severe hemophilia A in males in that joint and muscle bleeding can occur.

vWD can be acquired in association with MM, lymphoproliferative or myeloproliferative disorders, hypothyroidism, and cardiac disorders such as aortic stenosis and use of left ventricular assist devices.

SIGNS AND SYMPTOMS

The specific symptoms and severity of vWD can vary greatly. Some patients may be asymptomatic or have only mild symptoms and others will have moderate to severe bleeding. Patients may develop symptoms in infancy, and others do not develop symptoms until adulthood. Mild symptoms include mild bleeding from the mucous membranes and the skin including chronic epistaxis and bleeding from the gums. Easy bruising and prolonged bleeding from minor cuts may occur. Women may experience menorrhagia or heavy bleeding during and following childbirth. Iron deficiency anemia can develop if the bleeding is left untreated.

PHYSICAL EXAMINATION

The most common sites of hemorrhage include mucous membranes, skin, and the uterus. Muscle and joint bleeding occur with more severe disease. Menorrhagia is common in women with vWD and presents with severe menorrhagia with blood clots >1 inch in diameter, bleeding that requires a pad or tampon change more than hourly, and low serum ferritin levels.

The physical examination should be directed at detecting signs of bleeding, including size, location, and distribution of ecchymoses, hematomas, and petechiae; signs of anemia; and other causes of bleeding, including liver disease, splenomegaly, and gynecologic lesions.

DIFFERENTIAL DIAGNOSIS

Hemophilia A and platelet disorders can resemble vWD clinically. Hemophilia A is an X-linked deficiency of factor III that primarily affects males.

DIAGNOSTIC STUDIES

The standard laboratory assessment of vWD includes tests for vWF antigen, RCoF and factor VIII coagulant activity. A follow-up test that evaluates the distribution of vWF multimers may be useful in some patients.

The vWD panel consists of the following:

- vWF antigen (vWF:Ag) is an enzyme-linked immunosorbent assay (ELISA) that is used to quantify the plasma vWF:Ag level. The mean value for plasma vWF:Ag varies with blood type as patients with type O blood have a mean level of 74%; type A 103%; type B 110%; and type AB 126%.
- RCoF assay measures vWF functional activity in plasma. Ristocetin promotes the binding of large vWF multimers from plasma onto formalin-fixed normal platelets that retain exposed GPIb. There is considerable variability in the RCoF assay.
- Factor VIII activity level is decreased to varying degrees when vWF is quantitatively or qualitatively deficient/defective. In vWD the decrease in factor VIII is often not below a level that prolongs the PTT.

The BT test and PFA-100 are screening tests that give variable results and are not reliable indicators of effective versus ineffective hemostasis.

The typical vWD panel results for the various types of vWD are noted in Table 6.33.

vWF may be elevated during an acute phase reaction. Patients with a significant deficiency of vWF may have values that increase considerably during infection or injury. vWF also increases during pregnancy and during estrogen/oral contraceptive use. If testing is done during an acute phase reaction, concurrent measurement of a plasma marker of inflammation, such as C-reactive protein, should be obtained to aid in the interpretation of the panel results.

TREATMENT

The goals of treatment are cessation and subsequent prevention of bleeding. This can be achieved with DDAVP (1-desamino-8-D-arginine vasopressin) and/or concentrates containing both vWF and factor VIII.

DDAVP or desmopressin induces the secretion into circulation of vWF multimers stored in the endothelial cells. This raises the plasma level of both vWF multimers and factor VIII. DDAVP is most effective in type 1 vWD. Complications with DDAVP treatment include dilutional hyponatremia and seizures. DDAVP should not be given to people with type 2B vWD because of possible worsening thrombocytopenia.

Another treatment option is Humate-P, which is a concentrate that contains all vWF multimers and factor VIII; it is given by either rapid IV infusion or continuous infusion.

Bleeding in vWD types other than type 1 will likely require vWF-containing concentrate. This is also the case with type 1 vWD that is inadequately responsive to DDAVP.

TABLE 6.33 von Willebrand Disease Panel Results

Type	vWF Antigen (%)	Ristocetin Cofactor Assay (%)	Factor VIII Activity Level (%)	Ratio of Ristocetin Cofactor to vWF Antigen
Normal	***52–214***	***51–215***	***56–191***	***>0.5–0.7***
Type 1	<30	<30	Decreased or normal	>0.5–0.7
Type 2A	30–200	<30	Decreased or normal	<0.5–0.7
Type 2B	30–200	<30	Decreased or normal	<0.5–0.7
Type 2M	30–200	<30	Decreased or normal	<0.5–0.7
Type 2N	30–200	30–200	Markedly decreased	>0.5–0.7
Type 3	<10	<10	Markedly decreased	N/A

vWF, von Willebrand factor.

PATIENT EDUCATION

- Most patients with vWD have a favorable prognosis if bleeding is treated and prevented appropriately.
- Individuals with vWD should be discouraged from participating in high-impact sports/activities, such as football, boxing, rugby, wrestling. Helmets should be worn in sports with possible head injury.
- Patients on vWF prophylaxis should treat themselves whenever they can foresee potentially threatening activity.

6.7AC THROMBOCYTOSIS

Thrombocytosis is defined as a platelet count above 450,000/µL. There are several causes of temporary increases in platelet count, including inflammation and certain infections, but generally they have little or no long-term consequence. If two platelet counts, 3 months apart, are elevated the cause of the thrombocytosis should be determined.

There are many etiologies of thrombocytosis: Distributive thrombocytosis can be seen when an asplenic patient redistributes up to half of their platelets from the spleen to the peripheral bloodstream. This type of thrombocytosis is rarely of any consequence to the patient. Consistent thrombocytosis is usually due to a primary marrow disease of excess myeloproliferation, typically polycythemia vera or ET; or is reactive in nature, usually due to iron deficiency or chronic inflammation.

The pathophysiology of reactive thrombocytosis in patients with inflammation is secondary to IL-6, released from leukocytes stimulated with bacterial or tissue breakdown products and in malignancies due to the direct tumor production of IL-6. IL-6 acts on hepatocytes to stimulate the production and release of TPO, the primary regulator of platelet production.

MEDICAL HISTORY AND CLINICAL PRESENTATION

Iron deficiency is the most common cause for reactive thrombocytosis. The symptoms of anemia are fatigue, lethargy, exertional dyspnea, and palpitations.

The second major cause of reactive thrombocytosis is inflammation; patients will show the signs and symptoms of the underlying inflammatory disease, such as rheumatoid arthritis, inflammatory bowel disease, and cancer.

The presentation of a myeloproliferative neoplasm is subtle or found upon routine blood testing. Occasionally, an acute thrombosis of the coronary arteries, cerebral arteries, or deep venous or hepatic vein thrombosis is the presenting feature of a myeloproliferative neoplasm such as polycythemia vera or ET.

SIGNS AND SYMPTOMS

Iron deficiency presents like most other causes of anemia, but with additional symptoms such as pica, perioral cheilitis, and glossitis. Inflammatory disorders will present with the examination findings of the underlying inflammatory disease. Myeloproliferative neoplasms present with a ruddy complexion and splenomegaly.

DIAGNOSTIC STUDIES

The first step in the evaluation of possible thrombocytosis is to obtain a CBC and differential. The platelet count is elevated in everyone with thrombocytosis, but the presence of abnormalities in other blood cells may lead to the correct diagnosis. An elevated leukocyte count (neutrophils) could indicate inflammation, or if basophilia and/or eosinophilia is noted, then a myeloproliferative neoplasm should be considered.

An elevated RBC count could indicate polycythemia vera, as inflammation and iron deficiency both cause anemia, and an examination of the RBC MCV is important, as a patient with polycythemia vera who is also iron deficient may present with normal or low RBC counts, and only with thrombocytosis.

Laboratory tests that may assist in determining the etiology include the C-reactive protein if inflammation is suspected. If elevated, then more specific tests for the evaluation for rheumatoid arthritis, systemic lupus erythematosis, and inflammatory bowel disease should be obtained.

If iron deficiency is suspected because of an appropriate patient history and low MCV, serum iron, iron-binding capacity, and ferritin levels will establish the diagnosis.

If a primary marrow disorder is suspected, the Jak2 V617F test will establish a myeloproliferative neoplasm as the cause; the test is positive in nearly every person with polycythemia vera, but only positive in about half of patients with ET.

TREATMENT

In most patients with thrombocytosis, emergent treatment is rare.

The only indication for emergent therapy of thrombocytosis is impending or ongoing thrombosis, arterial or venous. This is typically found in the setting of a myeloproliferative neoplasm such as polycythemia vera or ET. The platelet count should be reduced immediately by daily apheresis, and if a myeloproliferative neoplasm is confirmed, therapy with a cytoreduction agent (hydroxyurea) and, unless contraindicated (because of bleeding), an anti-platelet function agent should be started.

In the chronic setting, treatment is usually indicated only for thrombocytosis due to a myeloproliferative neoplasm.

Recently Jak2 inhibitors have become available for the treatment of Jak2 mutation-positive primary MF. This treatment is usually reserved for patients who have failed other modalities.

PATIENT EDUCATION

- For most patients with thrombocytosis, the elevated platelet count is inconsequential, and the patient's prognosis is dependent entirely on the underlying cause of marrow reactivity.
- In patients with myeloproliferative neoplasms prognosis is usually good, with minimal impact on long-term survival.

6.7B COAGULATION DISORDERS

Coagulation factor deficiencies can be due to underproduction, consumption, or direct inhibition by autoantibodies or medications.

Hemophilia A and B, X-linked inherited bleeding disorders, result from genetic mutations leading to underproduction of factors VIII and IX, respectively. Acquired clotting factor deficiencies are due to consumptive processes such as DIC or autoantibody formation, directed at factors V or VIII.

MEDICAL HISTORY AND CLINICAL PRESENTATION

The medical history is important in the evaluation of the bleeding patient and will assist in separating the platelet disorders from the coagulation factor disorders. In the patient with a coagulation factor disorder, bleeding often takes the form of larger ecchymoses that spread to deeper tissues. Hemarthrosis suggests hemophilia or other severe inherited coagulation defect. Delayed bleeding after injury or procedure indicates a coagulation disorder.

History of multisystem disease should prompt the consideration of DIC, TTP, or HUS. A history of previous excessive bleeding with injury or procedures indicates a possible inherited disorder. A past medical history of liver disease can be associated with decreased clotting factor production and bleeding and malabsorption can lead to vitamin K deficiency and associated coagulopathy.

Obtaining a medication history is important. The risk of bleeding increases greatly in the setting of dual or triple antithrombotic therapy, often used in the treatment of cardiovascular disease. Many drugs interact with warfarin and potentiate its effect. The following medications can increase the effects of warfarin: antibiotics (fluoroquinolones, macrolides, metronidazole, tetracyclines, trimethoprim-sulfamethoxazole, cephalosporins), azole antifungal agents, antiarrhythmics (amiodarone, propafenone), cholesterol-lowering agents, glucocorticoids, omeprazole, cimetidine, and selective serotonin reuptake inhibitors.

SIGNS AND SYMPTOMS

Signs and symptoms of the coagulation factor disorders include delayed oozing of blood from deep lacerations or wounds, prolonged bleeding after circumcision or dental extraction, IM or intra-articular hematomas, CNS bleeding, or hematuria.

In hemophilia the factor activity level can assist in predicting the patient's symptoms (see Table 6.34).

TABLE 6.34 Predictive Value of Factor Levels in Hemophilia

Factor Level (%)	Severity of Hemophilia	Specific Symptoms
<1	Severe	Spontaneous intraarticular and intramuscular bleeding
1–5	Moderate	Predominantly soft tissue bleeding
5–30	Mild	Risk of bleeding after trauma or surgery, spontaneous bleeding rare

PHYSICAL EXAMINATION

Physical examination findings in patients with coagulation disorders are consistent with any underlying disorder and bleeding. Vital signs may be abnormal if there has been significant blood loss, skin may reveal deep hematomas, and joints may reveal hemarthrosis.

DIAGNOSTIC STUDIES

The evaluation of the patient with a possible coagulation disorder consists of several standard tests.

- **PT and INR:** Used to evaluate the extrinsic and common coagulation pathways.
- **aPTT:** Used to evaluate the intrinsic and common coagulation pathways.
- **Fibrinogen:** Measures fibrinogen levels, which will be decreased in fibrinogen deficiency and normal in dysfibrinogenemia.
- **Thrombin time (TT) and reptilase time (RT):** Measure the rate of fibrin clot formation; levels will be prolonged in fibrinogen disorders and TT will be elevated in the presence of heparin and dabigatran.
- Other tests: Include platelet count, individual factor activity levels, fibrinogen degradation products, and euglobulin clot lysis test.

EVALUATION

The evaluation of the patient with possible coagulation factor disorders begins with a detailed history and physical examination combined with targeted laboratory evaluation. Laboratory test result interpretation is noted below.

- Normal PT and INR and prolonged aPTT
  - These results suggest a disorder of the intrinsic pathway, most often hemophilia, vWD, or exposure to heparin, dabigatran, or edoxaban. Acquired inhibitors to factors VIII, IX, XI, or XII can also present in this way, as can a lupus inhibitor, but the latter does not present with bleeding.
  - Early onset of bleeding problems or a family history of bleeding can provide a clue to congenital coagulation factor deficiencies such as hemophilia, and individual factor assays can confirm the diagnosis of inherited or acquired specific factor deficiencies.
  - vWD is often accompanied by factor VIII deficiency, so additional vWD testing (as described above) may be indicated in patients with isolated aPTT prolongation.
  - A prolonged TT supports measurable heparin or dabigatran levels.
- Prolonged PT and INR and normal aPTT
  - Results suggest a disorder of the extrinsic pathway, often from liver disease, vitamin K deficiency, warfarin or rivaroxaban exposure, or factor VII deficiency.
  - Correction of PT/INR on repeat testing following vitamin K administration can diagnose vitamin K deficiency.
  - Factor VII deficiency can be confirmed with a factor VII assay.
  - A 50:50 mixing study can help to assess for an inhibitor.
- Prolonged PT, INR, and aPTT
  - Results suggest a common pathway disorder, including deficiency or inhibitors of prothrombin, fibrinogen, or factors V or X; advanced liver disease; DIC; supratherapeutic warfarin or heparin dosing; or combined factor deficiencies/inhibitors.
  - Fibrinogen concentration and TT or RT can be checked to assess for fibrinogen or fibrinolytic disorders. Fibrinogen levels will be low in hypofibrinogenemia and hyperfibrinolytic states, but not in dysfibrinogenemia.
  - Since factor VIII is not vitamin K dependent, a normal or elevated factor VIII assay suggests liver disease. A low level of factor VIII is suggestive of DIC.
  - Low platelets and low or low-normal fibrinogen plus elevated fibrin degradation products will often be found in DIC.
  - Specific factor assays are available to evaluate for deficient prothrombin or factor V or X.

6.7BA FACTOR DEFICIENCIES

Hemophilia A and B are X-linked inherited bleeding disorders. Hemophilia A and B are seen in all racial and ethnic groups. There are approximately 24.6 cases per 100,000 males of hemophilia A and 5.0 cases per 100,000 males of hemophilia B; 1 in 5,000 live male births result in a boy with hemophilia A.[36]

Factor VIII normally circulates with its carrier protein, vWF. Factor VIII serves as a cofactor that enhances the activation of factor X by factor IX.

The presence of factors VIII and IX results in a dramatic increase in the rate of thrombin generation. Because factors VIII and IX form a complex to activate factor X, the absence of either results in an elevated aPTT and a normal PT. The bleeding presentation of these two factor deficiencies is similar.

Hemophilia A, factor VIII deficiency, is common, accounting for approximately 80–85% of all factor deficiency cases.

Since both hemophilia A and B are X-linked recessive mutations, most affected individuals are male. Females, who are heterozygous, have approximately 50% of normal physiologic levels of factor VIII or IX. Typically, carriers of the disease have sufficient levels of factors to have no bleeding concerns; however, some carriers have factor VIII or IX levels in the mild hemophilia range and manifest bleeding symptoms such as heavy menstrual bleeding or postpartum hemorrhage.

MEDICAL HISTORY AND CLINICAL PRESENTATION

Hemophilia should be suspected if there is a positive family history in a female whose father or brother are diagnosed with hemophilia gives birth to a male child or in unexpected or unexplained bleeding in a newborn male infant, particularly following circumcision, cephalohematoma, ICH with minimal birth trauma, or large ecchymoses in neonates with a normal platelet count.

Hemophilia should also be suspected if there is spontaneous or traumatic hemarthrosis following minimal injury in a male of any age. Patients with hemophilia A or B can bleed into virtually any organ or tissue; except for joints and superficial mucous membranes, most bleeding episodes occur following trauma. Other clinical features include continued bleeding, hematoma expansion, and progression of secondary inflammation beyond what is expected for the injury.

Soft tissue purpura over the trunk or extremities, without accompanying systemic signs such as fever should lead to a consideration of a possible diagnosis of hemophilia. Patients who present with only petechiae are much more likely to have a platelet defect.

SIGNS AND SYMPTOMS

Prolonged bleeding with minimal trauma is an early sign of hemophilia. Bleeding can occur anywhere in the body, with prolonged superficial bleeding from minor abrasions or lacerations. Joint bleeding is common in hemophilia.

PHYSICAL EXAMINATION

Patients with hemophilia typically appear normal when no active bleeding. With recent or active bleeding, the patient may present with hypotension, tachycardia, pallor, bruising, abdominal pain and distention, and joint or muscle swelling and pain.

DIFFERENTIAL DIAGNOSIS

The differential diagnosis for hemophilia A and B includes vWD, factor XI deficiency, and acquired hemophilia A. Each of these disorders can present with a prolonged aPTT, normal PT, normal platelet count, and normal functional fibrinogen level.

vWD is an autosomal inherited bleeding disorder that results from abnormal vWF. vWF is produced in vascular endothelial cells and platelets. vWD presents with abnormal levels of factor VIII, plus abnormal vWF-mediated platelet agglutination in response to the reagent ristocetin. The exception is type 2N vWD which results in a low factor VIII level but normal qualitative vWF function.

Factor XI deficiency requires differentiation from hemophilia A and B. Factor XI assay should be obtained when both factor VIII and IX assays are normal in an individual with bleeding or when there is a family history of factor XI deficiency.

Acquired hemophilia A may present as acute unexplained bleeding in an individual with no prior history of abnormal bleeding. Acquired hemophilia A occurs most commonly after age 50 and affects both genders equally. Bleeding symptoms typically include mucocutaneous bleeding, deep soft tissue hemorrhage and large ecchymosis; and hemarthrosis is uncommon. On laboratory evaluation, the prolonged aPTT does not correct in a 1:1 ratio mixing study with normal plasma as it does in both vWD and inherited hemophilia A.

DIAGNOSTIC STUDIES

The following coagulation screening test results are noted in both hemophilia A and B:

- Normal PT
- Abnormal PTT
- Normal platelet count
- Normal fibrinogen level or thrombin clotting time

With these results a factor VIII assay should be obtained. If the factor VIII assay is low, then hemophilia A is the most likely diagnosis in a male patient. vWD must be excluded if there is no supportive family history. If the factor VIII assay is normal, a factor IX level should be obtained. A low level of factor IX indicates hemophilia B.

TREATMENT

Acute

Severe bleeding requires immediate infusion of factor VIII concentrate for hemophilia A or factor IX concentrate for hemophilia B. Treatment dosing of factor VIII or IX concentrate is based on achieving and maintaining adequate hemostasis in the bleeding patient. Delay in therapy leads to worse clinical outcome, regardless of the type or severity of the hemophilic bleed.

For major or life-threatening bleeding initial replacement therapy with clotting factor concentrate should be dosed to achieve a plasma level of at least 100% of the normal physiologic level. This is defined as 1 unit of factor VIII or IX per milliliter of plasma. Not all types of bleeding require replacement of the deficient clotting factor to 100% of normal.

If a factor VIII or factor IX inhibitor is present, alternative therapy such as rFVIIa or activated prothrombin complex concentrate (aPCC, containing some activated factors II, VII, IX, or X) may be required. If an inhibitor is present, consultation with experts is required as dosing requires expertise in treating inhibitors.

For mild dental bleeding or epistaxis, the oral antifibrinolytic agents, epsilon-aminocaproic acid or tranexamic acid, alone may suffice in achieving and maintaining hemostasis. These agents are more likely to be effective in patients with mild hemophilia A or B.

For patients with mild hemophilia A, desmopressin or DDAVP offers another option when the bleeding is mild. DDAVP induces release of factor VIII-binding vWF from endothelial cells. A single dose of DDAVP results in a threefold or greater increase in the baseline factor VIII level.

PATIENT EDUCATION

- For young children with severe hemophilia A or B who have normal joints, significant joint morbidity can be pre-empted by institution of a primary prophylaxis regimen.
- Children with hemophilia can expect a normal lifespan and can participate in all but the most physically violent activities and sports.
- Any head injury can become life-threatening in an individual with hemophilia, especially those with severe phenotypes. Such an injury requires prompt infusion of a "high dose" of the patient's prescribed factor and evaluation quickly in an emergency center with CT imaging capability.

There are several other rare inherited coagulation factor deficiencies. Table 6.35 summarizes these disorders.[36]

TABLE 6.35 Other Inherited Coagulation Factor Deficiencies

Factor Deficiency	Prevalence	Bleeding	Laboratory Findings	Half-life	Treatment
Fibrinogen	1 in 1 million	None to severe	↑PT, PTT, TT, BT	2–4 days	Fibrinogen concentrate, cryoprecipitate
Prothrombin	1 in 1 million	Mild to moderate	↑PT, PTT	3 days	PCC, FFP
Factor V	1 in 1 million	Moderate	↑PT, PTT, BT	36 hours	FFP
Factor VII	1 in 500,000	Mild to severe	↑PT	4–6 hours	Factor VIIa
Factor X	1 in 500,000	Mild to severe	↑PT, PTT	40 hours	PCC, FFP
Factor XI	1 in 1 million	Mild to moderate	↑PTT	40–70 hours	Factor XI concentrate, factor VIIa, FFP
Factor XII	1 in 1 million	No bleeding	↑PTT	60 hours	Not needed
Factor XIII	1 in 2 million	Moderate to severe	All normal	10–14 days	Factor XIII concentrate, FFP, cryoprecipitate

BT, bleeding time; FFP, fresh frozen plasma; PCC, prothrombin complex concentrate; PT, prothrombin time; PTT, partial thromboplastin time; TT, thrombin time.
Source: Data from Ruiz-Saez A. Occurrence of thrombosis in rare bleeding disorders. Semin Thromb Hemost. *2013;39(6):684–692. doi:10.1055/s-0033-1353391*

TABLE 6.36 Acquired Risk Factors and Risk of Venous Thromboembolism

Clinical Condition	Venous Thromboembolism Risk (Odds Ratio)
Major general surgery	>10
Cancer	2–9
Major trauma	>10
Immobilization	<2
Arthroscopic knee surgery	2–9
Chemotherapy	2–9
Oral contraceptives	2–9
Pregnancy	2–9
Congestive heart failure or respiratory failure	2–9
Hormone replacement	2–9
Increasing age	<2
Obesity	<2

Source: Data from Anderson FA, Spencer FA. Risk factors for venous thromboembolism. Circulation. *2003;107(suppl 1):23. doi:10.1161/01.CIR.0000078469.07362.E6*

TABLE 6.37 Inherited Hypercoagulable States

Disease	Prevalence (%)	
	General Population	Patients with Venous Thromboembolism
Deficiency of Coagulation Inhibitors		
Antithrombin deficiency	0.02–0.2	1
Protein S deficiency	0.03–0.1	2
Protein C deficiency	0.2–0.4	3
Dysfunction of Coagulation Factors		
Factor V Leiden (heterozygous)	5	20
Prothrombin gene mutation (heterogeneous)	2	6
Dysfibrinogenemia		0.8

6.7BB HYPERCOAGULABLE STATES

A hypercoagulable state is any acquired or inherited condition that increases the risk of thromboembolism. Inherited hypercoagulable states are usually the result of heterozygous mutations.

Acquired causes of hypercoagulability are more common than inherited hypercoagulable states. Acquired causes of hypercoagulability and the risk of thromboembolism are noted in Table 6.36.[37]

Except for antiphospholipid syndrome and HIT, there are no laboratory diagnostic tests to identify which patients with acquired disorders are at risk for VTE.

There are a variety of inherited hypercoagulable states. See Table 6.37 for a summary of the inherited hypercoagulable states.

Antithrombin III Deficiency

Antithrombin binds and inactivates activated factor Xa and factor IIa (thrombin). Its activity is accelerated by the presence of heparin. Antithrombin deficiency can result from mutations that affect protein production leading to type I antithrombin deficiency or synthesis of a dysfunctional protein leading to type II antithrombin deficiency. Type I antithrombin deficiency is the most common inherited form among patients with thrombosis, while type II deficiency is the most common form in the general population.

Acquired causes of antithrombin deficiency include acute thrombosis, DIC, heparin therapy, nephrotic syndrome, and liver disease.

Protein C Deficiency

Protein C circulates in an inactive form that is activated by thrombin bound to the endothelial membrane proteins thrombomodulin and endothelial protein C receptor. APC functions as an anticoagulant by cleaving and inactivating factors Va and VIIIa. These reactions are accelerated in the presence of free protein S. Protein C is a vitamin K dependent coagulation protein. Acquired protein C deficiency can result from vitamin K deficiency, vitamin K antagonist therapy, acute thrombosis, DIC, or liver disease.

Protein S Deficiency

Protein S serves as a cofactor for protein C, assisting protein C with inactivation of factors Va and VIIIa. Protein S exists in the plasma in two forms, free and bound to C4b-binding protein, a complement protein. Reductions in free protein S are associated with reduced protein S activity. Free protein S also serves as a cofactor for the inactivation of factor Xa.

Acquired protein S deficiency can result from vitamin K deficiency, vitamin K antagonist therapy, acute thrombosis, DIC, and liver disease, as well as pregnancy, estrogen therapy, and inflammatory disorders, which increase the concentration of C4b-binding protein

Factor V Leiden

Factor V Leiden is a mutation that disrupts the first APC cleavage site in factor Va. Factor V Leiden mutation slows the inactivation of factor Va, a critical cofactor for factor Xa activation of prothrombin and factor VIIIa.

Prothrombin Gene *G20210A* Mutation

The prothrombin *G20210A* gene mutation increases the efficiency of prothrombin mRNA resulting in an increase in prothrombin protein levels.

Hyperhomocysteinemia

Homocysteine is an amino acid that converts to methionine by methionine synthase with vitamin B12 as a cofactor. Homocysteine is converted to cysteine via cystathionine by cystathionine beta synthase with vitamin B6 as a cofactor. Patients with homocystinuria have cystathionine beta synthase mutations. High concentrations of homocysteine have been associated with vascular damage and an increased risk of venous and arterial thromboembolism.

Dysfibrinogenemia

Mutations in the chains of fibrinogen can result in fibrinogen molecules that are resistant to fibrinolysis.

MEDICAL HISTORY AND CLINICAL PRESENTATION

The presence of thrombophilia has been weakly associated with recurrent VTE. Clinical features associated with a greater chance of underlying thrombophilia include:

- **Unprovoked thromboembolism:** The presence of a provoking risk factor, such as surgery, suggests that an underlying hypercoagulable state is less likely.
- **VTE at young age (younger than 50 years):** Hypercoagulable states often precipitate VTE early in life.
- **Recurrent VTE:** Thrombophilia may be present, particularly in the setting of recurrent unprovoked VTE.
- **Unusual location:** Mesenteric vein thrombosis and cerebral venous sinus thrombosis are often associated with thrombophilia in the absence of other risk factors.
- **Autoimmune disorder:** Presence of an autoimmune disorder indicates that antiphospholipid syndrome could be present.
- **Thrombosis during treatment:** Thrombosis during treatment with unfractionated or low molecular weight heparin (LMWH) should prompt consideration of HIT.

Testing for hypercoagulable states should be obtained in the following situations:

- Idiopathic or recurrent VTE
- VTE at age <40 years
- VTE with strong family history
- VTE in unusual vascular sites
- Warfarin-induced skin necrosis
- Recurrent pregnancy loss

SIGNS AND SYMPTOMS

The most common signs and symptoms are those associated with deep venous thrombosis and pulmonary embolism. Deep venous thrombosis presents with pain, swelling and redness at the site of the thrombosis. Pulmonary embolism presents with chest pain, dyspnea, and palpitations.

Venous thrombosis may occur in unusual places such as veins in the brain, liver, mesenteric, kidney, and upper extremity.

PHYSICAL EXAMINATION

Physical examination findings are consistent with deep venous thrombosis or pulmonary embolism. Protein C deficiency can cause purpura fulminans that leads to tissue death and bleeding into the skin and other organs. Protein C and protein S deficiency has also been linked to skin necrosis in patients taking warfarin.

DIAGNOSTIC STUDIES

Factor V Leiden diagnosis relies upon the APC resistance assay and factor V Leiden DNA-based assays. The APC resistance assay is the screening test for factor V Leiden.

The APC resistance assay can be done in the presence of heparin, warfarin, or acute thrombosis. Positive results are confirmed with the factor V Leiden PCR test.

Prothrombin gene *G20210A* mutation diagnosis relies upon DNA-based assays. These assays can be done in the presence of anticoagulation or acute thrombosis.

Antithrombin deficiency diagnosis relies upon antithrombin activity assays. These assess the functional level of antithrombin in patient plasma by determining residual thrombin activity after addition of heparin and an excess of thrombin.

Protein C deficiency diagnosis depends on the protein C activity level and is the appropriate screening test for protein C deficiency. Protein C antigen assays can be performed if the protein C activity is low to determine the patient's deficiency type.

Protein S deficiency is diagnosed by checking protein S activity. Total and free protein S antigen assays can be ordered if protein S activity levels are low. Protein S activity assays have a high false positive rate, so all abnormal tests should be repeated to confirm the diagnosis.

Antiphospholipid syndrome diagnosis is made based on the presence of clinical events and positive laboratory assays. Laboratory abnormalities must be present on at least two assays performed at least 12 weeks apart. Antiphospholipid syndrome is associated with one or more confirmed episodes of arterial, venous, or small vessel thrombosis. Pregnancy losses are also considered objective manifestations. Laboratory tests include a positive lupus anticoagulant test, IgG and IgM cardiolipin antibody, and anti-beta-2 GPI IgG or IgM antibody.

Hyperhomocysteinemia diagnosis is based upon fasting homocysteine levels. Homocysteine levels are affected by folate, vitamin B12, and pyridoxine deficiencies, renal failure, smoking, and advancing age.

EVALUATION

The laboratory workup should begin with the following tests: PT, PTT, fibrinogen level, anti-cardiolipin antibody assay, antithrombin level, C-reactive protein, and homocysteine level.

TREATMENT

Treatment recommendation for antithrombin deficiency is antithrombin concentrate in VTE patients with antithrombin deficiency in high-risk clinical situations such as surgery or delivery. Therapy should keep the antithrombin level at 80% to 120%.

Homozygous protein C deficiency causes the thrombotic syndrome known as purpura fulminans. Protein C concentrate should be administered to control this prothrombotic state until effective anticoagulation can be achieved. Protein C concentrate can be used to prevent thrombosis in patients with protein C deficiency during risk periods when anticoagulation must be interrupted such as during major surgery or delivery.

All patients with known thrombophilia should receive adequate VTE prophylaxis during risk periods such as major surgery, trauma, medical illness, or postpartum period.

The presence of antithrombin deficiency, protein S deficiency, protein C deficiency, or antiphospholipid syndrome is considered an indication for long-term anticoagulation in patients with VTE and arterial thromboembolism.

Presence of the prothrombin gene mutation alone is not considered a justification for long-term anticoagulation.

SPECIAL CONSIDERATIONS

- Patients known to have thrombophilic disorders with or without previous thrombosis should avoid hormonal contraceptives.
- In pregnancy:
  - Patients with factor V Leiden or prothrombin gene mutation homozygosity and no previous VTE but a positive family history of VTE should be considered for antepartum and postpartum prophylactic or intermediate dose LMWH or postpartum vitamin K antagonists (INR2-3).
  - For pregnant women with factor V Leiden or prothrombin gene mutation heterozygosity or protein C or protein S or antithrombin deficiency and no previous VTE but a positive family history of VTE, antepartum surveillance and postpartum prophylactic or intermediate dose LMWH or vitamin K antagonists (INR 2-3) are suggested.
  - For patients with no personal or family history of VTE and factor V Leiden or prothrombin gene mutation heterozygosity, antepartum surveillance and postpartum prophylactic or intermediate dose LMWH or vitamin K antagonists (INR 2-3) for at least 6 weeks are recommended.
  - Antepartum and postpartum surveillance is suggested for women with other hypercoagulable states and no personal or family history of VTE.
  - Patients with a pregnancy associated or hormonal therapy associated episode of VTE should consider antepartum and postpartum (prophylactic or intermediate dose) prophylaxis.

KEY POINTS

- Hypercoagulable state should be considered in patients with recurrent episodes of thromboembolism and no risk factors for embolism.

Long-term anticoagulation should be considered.

6.7BC DISSEMINATED INTRAVASCULAR COAGULATION

DIC is a serious, life-threatening condition that is secondary to a wide variety of conditions. This complex syndrome involves excessive intravascular coagulation leading to microthrombosis and organ failure and with bleeding due to inactivation and excessive consumption of platelets and clotting factors.

Normal hemostasis depends on thrombin generation via activation of the coagulation cascade. The chief activator of coagulation is TF. TF is present in most cells of the body; if the cells are stimulated, damaged, or injured, proinflammatory cytokines are released and induce TF release into the local environment. This results in the generation of thrombin via the TF/factor VIIa pathway to promote hemostasis. Any TF or thrombin that escapes the area of injury is neutralized.

DIC is a result of overproduction of TF and thrombin. Excessive thrombin leads to micro- and macrovascular clotting that causes impaired organ perfusion, organ ischemia, and end-organ damage. With excessive clotting there is development of thrombocytopenia and consumption of clotting factors. Excessive thrombin converts plasminogen to plasmin, which leads to fibrinolysis, excess fibrin degradation products, and excessive bleeding. The excessive bleeding leads to increased vascular permeability, hypotension, and shock. See Figure 6.14 for the pathophysiology of DIC.

MEDICAL HISTORY AND CLINICAL PRESENTATION

Systemic infections and sepsis are the most common causes of DIC. Purpura fulminans, commonly noted in meningococcemia, is a severe form of DIC characterized by diffuse microthrombi of the skin leading to hemorrhagic necrosis. Extensive acute tissue damage and hemorrhagic shock are triggers of DIC. Many obstetric causes of DIC occur because of TF leakage from the damaged placenta or uterus. Malignancies such as solid tumors and APL are associated with DIC. See Table 6.38 for triggers of DIC.

SIGNS AND SYMPTOMS

Signs and symptoms of DIC are those of the underlying triggering event and several nonspecific signs such as bleeding from many body sites, blood clots, bruising, hypotension, dyspnea, change in mental status, and fever.

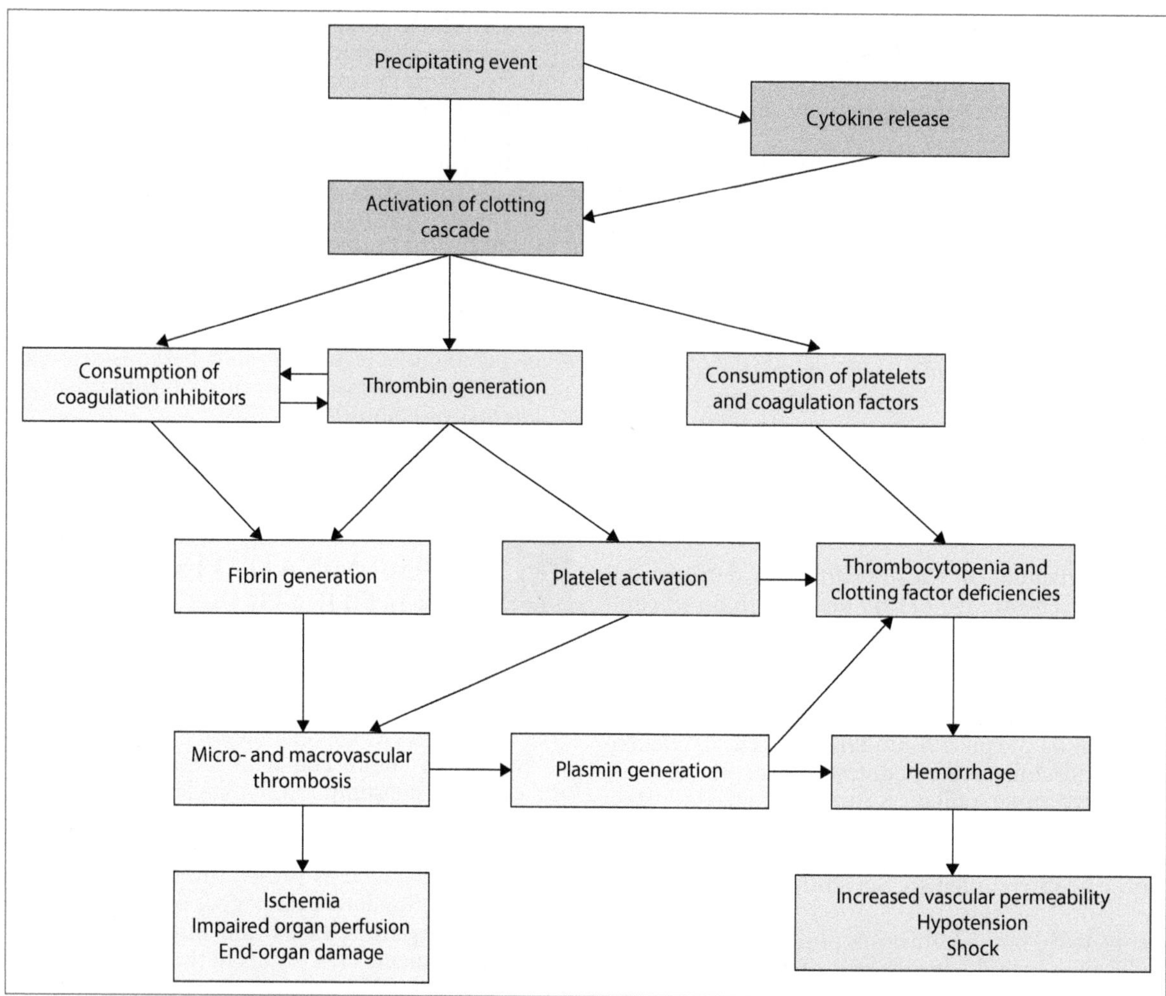

Figure 6.14 Pathophysiology of disseminated intravascular coagulation.

TABLE 6.38 Etiologies of Disseminated Intravascular Coagulation

Infections	Neoplasia	Tissue Damage	Obstetric Causes
Gram-positive bacteria	Malignant solid tumors	Crush injuries	Abruptio placentae
Gram-negative bacteria	Acute promyelocytic leukemia	CNS injuries	Placenta previa
Spirochetes	Cancer chemotherapy	Burns	Retained products of conception
Rickettsias	Tumor lysis syndrome	Heatstroke	Amniotic fluid embolism
Protozoa		Hemolytic transfusion reaction	Uterine atony
Fungi		Acute transplant rejection	Therapeutic abortion
Viruses		Shock	Toxemia of pregnancy

CNS, central nervous system.

PHYSICAL EXAMINATION

The key feature in DIC is bleeding at multiple sites. In the postoperative patient, there is bleeding from all incisions, from wounds, and at insertion sites of intravascular devices. Hemorrhage from the nose, gums, and skin petechiae and ecchymoses may be noted. Thrombosis associated with DIC can occur in venous or arterial, small or mid-size/large vessels. Thrombosis often leads to multiorgan failure and organ failure is the leading cause of death.

DIFFERENTIAL DIAGNOSIS

For any patient with a risk factor for DIC who presents with hemorrhage, thrombosis, or both, the diagnosis of DIC is almost certain. No single laboratory test can be used to diagnose DIC. With any acute thrombohemorrhagic emergency, the following should be considered within the differential diagnosis: TTP, HIT, and HELLP syndrome in pregnant patients. See Table 6.39 for differential diagnosis of DIC.

DIAGNOSTIC STUDIES

In acute DIC the classic laboratory findings include prolongation of the PTT, PT, and TT; production of FDP or D-dimer; and thrombocytopenia. PT and PTT prolongations are secondary to consumption of coagulation factors, while a prolonged TT is due to elevated fibrin split products

TABLE 6.39 Differential Diagnosis of Disseminated Intravascular Coagulation

Features	Acute DIC	HELLP	TTP	HIT
Pathophysiology	Increased thrombin and plasmin	Ischemia of placenta	ADAMTS13 deficiency	Antiplatelet antibodies secondary to heparin
Physical examination	Bleeding and thrombosis	No bleeding, may have preeclampsia	No bleeding, microvascular thrombosis	No bleeding, microvascular thrombosis
PT/PTT	Increased	Normal	Normal	Normal
Platelets	Low	Low	Low	Low
FDP/D-dimer	Elevated	Slight elevation	Slight elevation	Slight elevation
Clinical findings	Always an underlying cause	Pregnant and increasing liver function tests	Schistocytes present, increased creatinine and LDH, change in mental status	Exposure to heparin, heparin associated platelet antibodies
Therapy	Treat underlying cause	Uterine evacuation	Plasma exchange	Stop heparin

DIC, disseminated intravascular coagulation; FDP, fibrin degradation products; HELLP, hemolysis, elevated liver function tests, low platelets; HIT, heparin-induced thrombocytopenia; LDH, lactate dehydrogenase; PT, prothrombin time; PTT, partial thromboplastin time; TTP, thrombotic thrombocytopenic purpura.

and decreased fibrinogen levels. The production of large amounts of FDP/D-dimer is the result of plasminogen being rapidly converted to plasmin, with resultant lysis of fibrin into FDP. None of the above abnormalities are specific for DIC, which remains a clinical diagnosis.

EVALUATION

The initial evaluation includes a complete history to identify triggering events and physical examination to identify the presence of thrombosis and/or bleeding. The initial laboratory assessment includes platelet count, fibrinogen level, PT, PTT, TT, and FDP/D-dimer. Examination of the blood smear can detect thrombocytopenia and schistocytes, but neither are specific for DIC.

TREATMENT

The primary focus is to identify and treat the underlying cause. If it is infectious, appropriate antibiotics need to be initiated. If it is a complication of pregnancy, prompt evacuation of the uterus is needed. If the etiology is trauma, efforts should be made to aggressively repair injuries, and to minimize the DIC-provoking acidosis, hypothermia, and hypotension. If the etiology is malignancy, all measures to treat the underlying malignancy should be undertaken.

The survival rate in DIC is determined by the ability to identify and reverse the underlying pathophysiologic mechanism. Coagulation tests will not improve until the underlying etiology.

Transfusion of blood products, such as packed RBCs, FFP, cryoprecipitate or platelet concentrates, are typically not sufficient to overcome the process. Some post-transfusion patients do improve, but this is due to the etiology being self-limited.

Patients with active bleeding or high risk for bleeding requiring invasive procedures/surgeries should be considered for transfusion of blood products. Goal should be to maintain a platelet count of 50,000–75,000/mm^3 and hematocrit level of 25%–35%. The fibrinogen level should be maintained at 50–100 mg/dL, with cryoprecipitate transfusion being the preferred product.

Improvement in the patient's status will be evident by improvement in the clinical situation, with correction of hypotension and acidosis. Serial monitoring of PT, PTT, TT, D-dimer, and platelet count should be done and observed for improvement.

PATIENT EDUCATION

- Acute DIC has a mortality rate of about 65–85%. Survivors are typically young and healthy. Obstetric etiologies show low mortality and morbidity rates with prompt delivery.
- Mortality rate is high in cases related to sepsis and neoplastic disease.
- Progressive end-organ failure is the most common cause of death.

COMMON CHIEF COMPLAINTS

APPROACH TO ANEMIA

There are various ways of classifying anemia. Utilizing the reticulocyte count can assist in dividing the anemias into the decreased production and increased destruction groups. If the corrected reticulocyte count is low, then the patient has a decreased production anemia. The decreased production anemias are then divided into the microcytic, normocytic, and macrocytic subtypes, based on MCV. The microcytic anemias include iron deficiency, thalassemia, sideroblastic, and anemia of chronic disease. They can be separated out with iron studies and hemoglobin electrophoresis. The normocytic anemias include anemia of chronic disease and blood loss. The macrocytic anemias include vitamin B12 and folate deficiency; diagnosis is made by testing the vitamin B12 and folate levels.

If the reticulocyte count is elevated, then the patient has an increased destruction or hemolytic anemia. The hemolytic anemias are either congenital or acquired. A positive family history points toward a congenital hemolytic anemia. The congenital hemolytic anemias include membrane abnormalities, hemoglobin abnormalities, or enzyme abnormalities.

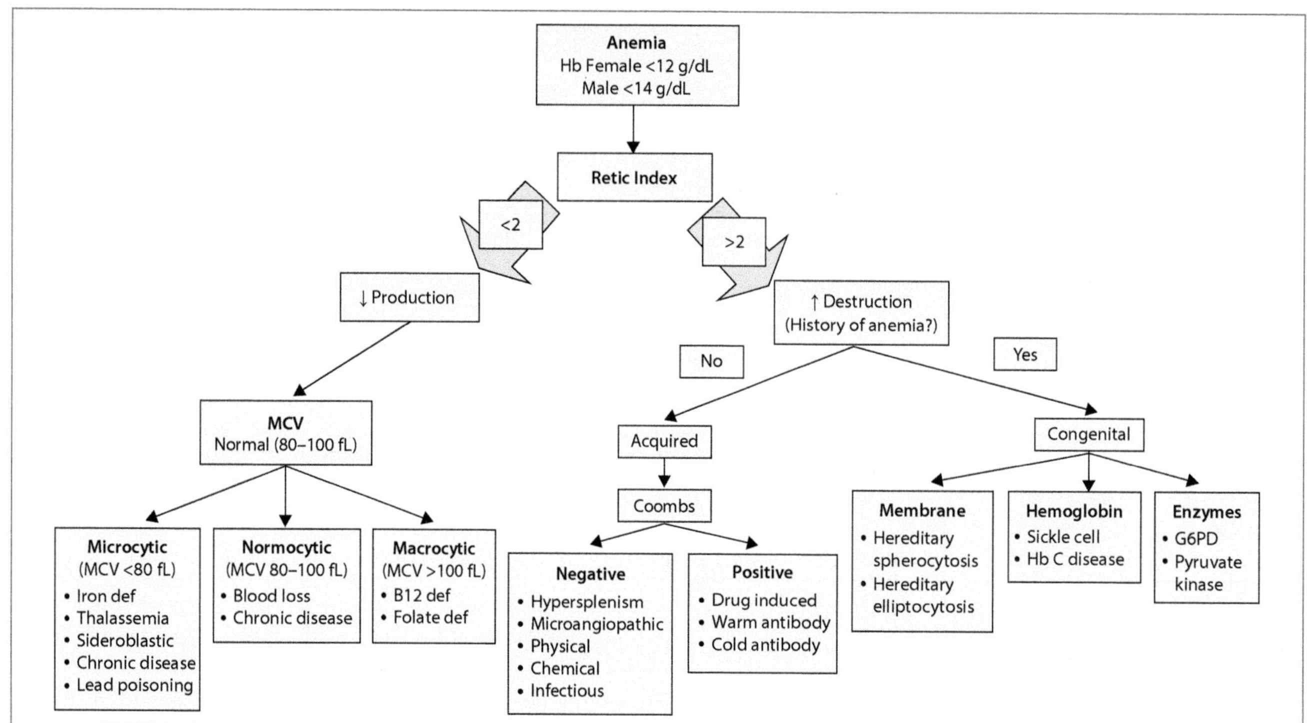

Figure 6.15 Approach to anemia flowchart. def, deficiency; G6PD, glucose-6-phosphate dehydrogenase; Hb, hemoglobin; MCV, mean corpuscular volume.

If the hemolytic anemia is acquired a direct Coombs test should be ordered. If the direct Coombs is negative the possible etiologies include hypersplenism, microangiopathic, physical etiologies, and infections. If the direct Coombs is positive the anemia could be drug induced, warm autoantibody, or cold autoantibody. Figure 6.15 summarizes the approach to the evaluation of the patient with anemia.

KNOWLEDGE CHECKS

1. Iron deficiency anemia and anemia of chronic disease often present with similar signs and symptoms. Compare and contrast iron deficiency anemia with anemia of chronic disease.
2. The hemolytic anemias consist of several complex disorders. Develop a focused approach based on an understanding of the pathophysiology of the various diseases.
3. The hematologic malignancies are due to abnormal proliferation of progenitor cells. Create a table outlining the various leukemias and lymphomas.
4. Compare and contrast the presentation, laboratory findings, and treatment of the platelet and coagulation factor disorders.

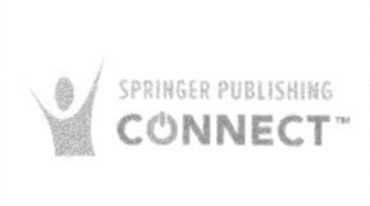

A robust set of instructor resources designed to supplement this text is located at **http://connect.springerpub.com/content/book/978-0-8261-8243-2.** Qualifying instructors may request access by emailing **textbook@springerpub.com.**

REFERENCES

The complete reference list for this chapter appears in the digital version of the chapter, accessible at https://connect.springerpub.com/content/book/978-0-8261-8243-2/chapter/ch06.

CHAPTER 7

ONCOLOGY

JAMES VAN RHEE

LEARNING OBJECTIVES

- Develop a basic understanding of genetics as it relates to the development of various malignancies.
- Discuss the risk factors, pathophysiology, presentation, diagnosis, and management of common malignancies.
- Describe the risk factors, pathophysiology, clinical presentation, diagnosis, and management of the common oncologic emergencies.
- Describe the approach to weight loss in the outpatient setting.

INTRODUCTION

Cancer is a heterogeneous group of conditions characterized by the abnormal division and proliferation of cells. The etiology is often multifactorial, but cancer may be related to upregulation of oncogenes, downregulation of tumor suppressor genes, or epigenetic phenomena that lead to unregulated cell division and growth. Cancers can present in a variety of ways depending on the cell type affected; they can be solid tumors such as breast, lung, or colon cancer or liquid tumors such as lymphoma and leukemia. In 2018, over 1,735,000 new cases of cancer were diagnosed in the United States and over 609,600 people died from the disease.[1] The most common cancers, in descending order, are breast cancer, lung and bronchus cancer, prostate cancer, colon and rectum cancer, melanoma of the skin, bladder cancer, non-Hodgkin lymphoma, kidney and renal pelvis cancer, endometrial cancer, leukemia, pancreatic cancer, thyroid cancer, and liver cancer. In 2016, the incidence of new cancer cases was 436 per 100,000 men and women per year (Figure 7.1) and there were 156 deaths per 100,000 per year (Figure 7.2).[2]

7.1 ONCOLOGY GENETICS

Several factors influence the various etiologies of cancer, including genetic, environmental, medical, and lifestyle factors, all of which interact to produce a given malignancy. Knowledge of cancer genetics is improving our understanding of cancer biology, assisting in the identification of at-risk individuals, enhancing our ability to characterize malignancies, establishing treatment that best matches the molecular components of the malignancy, and leading to the development of new therapeutic options. This expanding knowledge has implications for all aspects of cancer management, prevention, screening, and treatment.

Genetic information provides a means of identifying individuals who have an increased risk of cancer. Sources of genetic information include the following:

- Patient DNA sample: can be obtained and analyzed at any time
- Patient family history: can identify people with an increased risk of cancer or serve as a step in the identification of an inherited cancer predisposition
- Physical examination findings
- Medical records

Penetrance is defined as the proportion of individuals carrying a pathogenic variant who will manifest the disease. For example, common genetic variants that are associated with cancer susceptibility have a lower penetrance than rare genetic variants. In adults, penetrance is usually described by the individual's age and sex. For example, the penetrance for breast cancer in female carriers of *BRCA1/BRCA2* pathogenic variants is often quoted by age 50 and by age 70. There are many methods for estimating penetrance but determining an individual's risk of cancer involves some level of imprecision.

7.2 CANCER STAGING AND EVALUATION

The stage of cancer at the time of diagnosis is one of the key factors that defines prognosis and is critical in determining the appropriate treatment.

OVERVIEW

The TNM Classification of Malignant Tumors (TNM) is the standard for classifying the extent of disease. It is a classification system of the anatomic extent of disease. This classification system is used for solid tumors but is not used for leukemia or cancer of the central nervous system (CNS). Many of the common cancers have their own specific TNM classification.

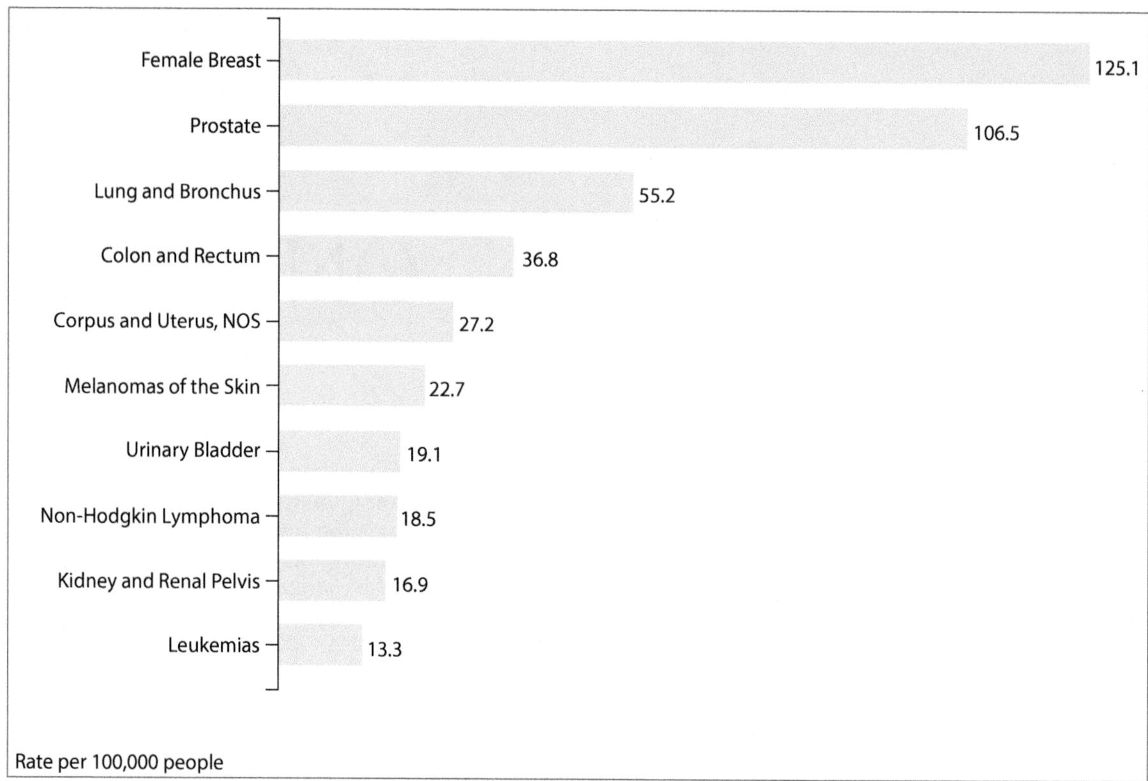

Figure 7.1 Top 10 cancers by rate of new cancer cases in the United States, 2017. NOS, not otherwise specified. *(Data source: U.S. Cancer Statistics Working Group. U.S. Cancer Statistics Data Visualizations Tool, based on November 2019 submission data [1999–2017]. U.S. Department of Health and Human Services, Centers for Disease Control and Prevention, and National Cancer Institute; June 2020. https://www.cdc.gov/cancer/dataviz)*

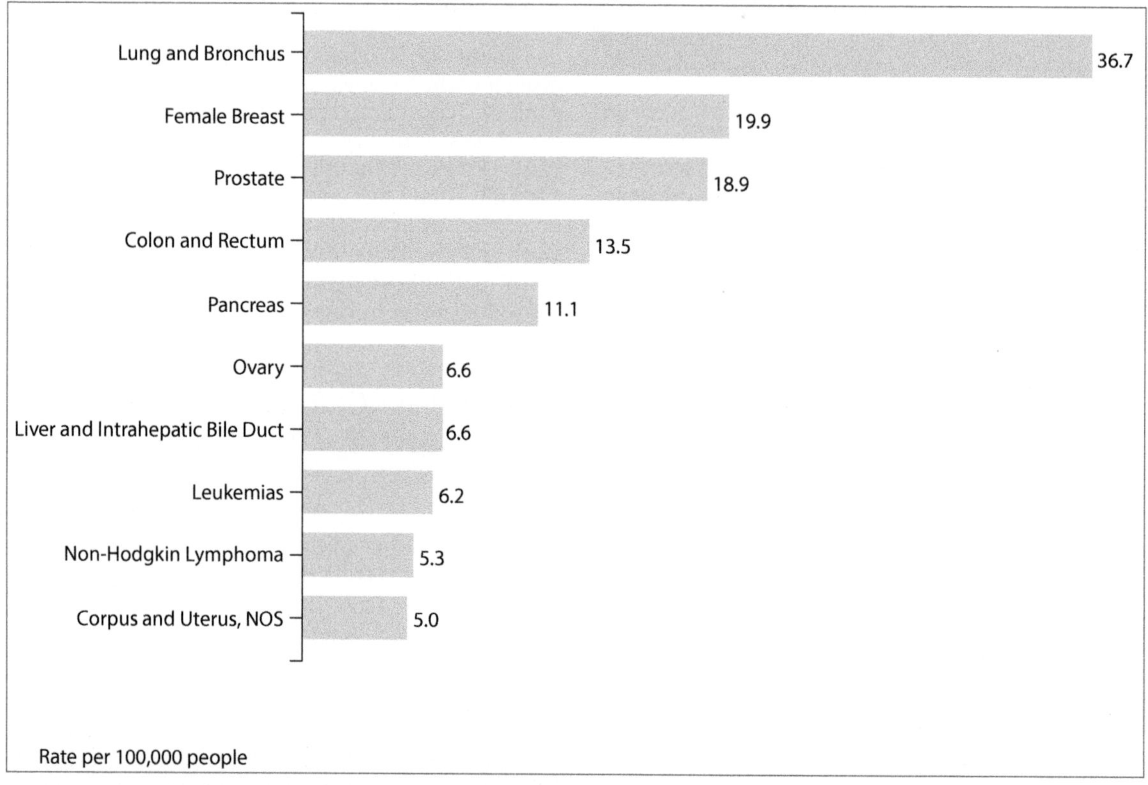

Figure 7.2 Top 10 cancers by rates of cancer deaths in the United States, 2017. NOS, not otherwise specified. *(Data source: U.S. Cancer Statistics Working Group. U.S. Cancer Statistics Data Visualizations Tool, based on November 2019 submission data [1999–2017]. U.S. Department of Health and Human Services, Centers for Disease Control and Prevention, and National Cancer Institute; June 2010. https://www.cdc.gov/cancer/dataviz)*

TABLE 7.1 TNM Classification

Level	Description
T	**The size or local extent of the primary tumor**
Tx	Tumor cannot be assessed
Tis	Carcinoma in situ
T0	No evidence of tumor
T1, T2, T3, T4	Size or extension of primary tumor
N	**Spread to regional lymph nodes**
Nx	Lymph nodes cannot be assessed
N0	No regional lymph node spread
N1	Regional lymph node involvement
N2	Spread that is between N1 and N3
N3	Spread to distant or numerous regional lymph nodes
M	**Presence of distant metastasis**
M0	No distant metastasis
M1	Metastasis to distant organs
Other modifiers	
G	Grade of cancer cell and ranges from low grade or highly differentiated to high grade or poorly or undifferentiated, scored as 1 to 4
S	Presence of elevated serum tumor markers, scored as 0 to 3
R	Surgical resection completeness, borders free of cancer or not, scored 0 to 2
L	Invasion of lymphatic vessels, scored 0 to 1
V	Invasion into a vein, scored 0 to 2

The TNM classification system describes the stage of a cancer using specific codes:

- T describes the size of the primary tumor and if it has invaded local tissue; definition is specific for each cancer location.
- N describes if nearby lymph nodes are involved; the number of positive nodes or involvement of specific regional nodes is noted.
- M describes the presence or absence of distant metastasis.

The TNM classification includes staging algorithms for almost all cancers, with the exception of pediatric cancers. See Table 7.1 for a general outline of the TNM classification system. The values shown may not be used for all cancers.

7.3 LUNG CANCER

OVERVIEW

There are two major types of lung cancer: non-small cell lung cancer (NSCLC) and small cell lung cancer (SCLC). NSCLC accounts for 85% of all lung cancers and includes adenocarcinoma, squamous cell carcinoma, and large cell carcinoma.[3] SCLC accounts for the remaining 15% of all lung cancers.[3] SCLCs grow more rapidly than NSCLCs and are more responsive to chemotherapy.

EPIDEMIOLOGY

Lung cancer is the second most common type of cancer, behind prostate cancer in men and breast cancer in women. In 2018, approximately 234,000 new cases of lung cancer were diagnosed, composing 13% of all cancers diagnosed. Deaths from lung cancer totaled approximately 154,000 in 2018, or 25% of all cancer deaths.[1] The average age at diagnosis is 70 years.

Age-adjusted lung cancer incidence rates in the United States for men have declined since 1982. This decrease is due to changes in risk behaviors, mainly smoking. The incidence rate in men has decreased at twice the rate as women due to difference in smoking uptake and cessation rates.

In the United States, the decline in lung cancer deaths is most likely due to tobacco control initiatives. There was a 45% decrease in male lung cancer deaths between 1990 and 2015 and lung cancer deaths in women declined 19% from 2002 to 2015.[1] Estimates of mortality in 2018 are 83,550 deaths for men and 70,500 for women, around 25% of annual cancer fatalities.[1]

Lung cancer, along with liver and pancreatic cancer, has one of the lowest survival rates with a 5-year relative survival rate for all stages combined at 18% for new cancer diagnoses between 2003 and 2009.[1] Lung cancer is often not diagnosed until advanced stage disease is present, even more so in Black Americans in comparison to White Americans. Advanced lung cancer has an extremely poor prognosis, with a 5-year survival rate of only 5%.[1]

PATHOPHYSIOLOGY

The most important risk factor for the development of lung cancer is tobacco smoking. Almost 80% of all lung cancers in the United States are smoking related.[1] Exposure to secondhand smoke also increases the risk. Nonsmokers exposed to secondhand smoke increased the risk of developing lung cancer by 20% to 30%.[4] Cancer risk declines after smoking cessation, but it never returns to baseline. About 10% to 20% of people who develop lung cancer have never smoked or have smoked minimally.[5]

Several other environmental exposures may increase the risk of developing lung cancer:

- **Asbestos:** This natural mineral was used as fireproofing in building materials and some manufacturing processes. When inhaled, the fibers can irritate the lung and cause lung disease.
- **Radon:** This odorless gas is released by some soil and rocks that contain uranium. Some homes may have high levels of radon, which may increase the risk of developing lung cancer.
- **Industrial substances:** Exposure to arsenic, uranium, beryllium, vinyl chloride, nickel chromates, coal products, mustard gas, chloromethyl ethers, gasoline, and diesel exhaust increase the risk of lung cancer.
- **Radiation exposure:** X-rays to the chest and other radiation exposure can increase the risk of lung cancer, especially in people who smoke.

- **Air pollution:** Trace amounts of diesel exhaust, coal products, and other industrial substances in air pollution can increase the risk of lung cancer.
- **Tuberculosis:** Tuberculosis causes scarring of lung tissue, which can be a risk factor for developing lung cancer.
- **Genetics:** The development of lung cancer can occur via inherited or environmentally acquired gene mutations.
- **Military service:** Both past and current military personnel may have had exposure to industrial substances and asbestos-bearing materials, as well as exposure to tactical chemicals, such as Agent Orange.

Chronic obstructive pulmonary disease (COPD), alpha-1 antitrypsin deficiency, and pulmonary fibrosis increase susceptibility to lung cancer.

There are several genetic factors linked to the development of lung cancer. Respiratory epithelial cells require prolonged exposure to cancer-promoting agents and accumulation of multiple genetic mutations before becoming neoplastic.

Although oncogenic driver mutations can cause or contribute to lung cancer among smokers, these mutations are more likely to be a cause of lung cancer among nonsmokers.

7.3A SMALL CELL LUNG CANCER

SCLC is an aggressive epithelial tumor with neuroendocrine characteristics, and it accounts for 15% of all lung cancer diagnoses.[3] SCLC has a rapid doubling time and metastasizes early; approximately two-thirds of patients present with metastatic disease.[6]

The prognosis for SCLC is poor; the average survival of patients diagnosed with localized disease is <2 years, while that of patients with metastatic disease is <1 year.

Genetically, SCLC is hallmarked by abnormalities of several tumor suppressor genes. *TP53* is mutated in 70% to 90% of SCLC cases.[7] Deletion of the short arm of chromosome 3 (3p) is common in SCLC; three tumor suppressor genes are in this chromosomal region.

MEDICAL HISTORY AND CLINICAL PRESENTATION

Common presenting symptoms include cough, hemoptysis, weight loss, and dyspnea. Due to the development of paraneoplastic syndromes, noted in up to 10% of patients, patients with SCLS can present with several other syndromes, including[8]:

- **Syndrome of inappropriate secretion of antidiuretic hormone (SIADH):** This is observed in 7% to 16% of SCLC patients and is a euvolemic, hypoosmotic, hyponatremia due to inadequate suppression of antidiuretic hormone secretion.[8] Most patients are asymptomatic or have mild symptoms that include headache, fatigue, weakness, and mild cognitive changes. If the sodium drop is rapid, severe symptoms such as seizures and coma may present.
- **Cushing syndrome:** This syndrome is seen in 1.6% to 4.5% of SCLC patients and is associated with the symptoms secondary to glucocorticoid excess.[8] It presents with hypertension, hypokalemia, weakness, or edema.
- **Lambert-Eaton syndrome:** Rarely, SCLC patients will develop a Lambert-Eaton syndrome. Patients present with progressive symmetric lower extremity proximal muscle weakness without atrophy. Ptosis may also be observed.

SIGNS AND SYMPTOMS

Most lung cancers do not cause symptoms until they have spread. The most common symptoms of lung cancer include:

- Persistent cough
- Hemoptysis
- Chest pain that is often worse with deep breathing or coughing
- Hoarseness
- Weight loss
- Shortness of breath
- Fatigue
- Recurrent pulmonary infections
- New onset of wheezing

Other symptoms may develop with metastasis. These include bone pain, headache, extremity weakness, seizures, jaundice, and lymphadenopathy.

PHYSICAL EXAMINATION

Physical examination findings include decreased or absent breath sounds on lung examination, tachypnea, and pallor. Other nonspecific findings include fever, decreased oxygen saturations, lymphadenopathy, hepatomegaly, and clubbing of the fingers.

DIFFERENTIAL DIAGNOSIS

Differential diagnosis includes tumors such as those that may be mistaken for SCLC: primitive neuroectodermal tumor, atypical carcinoid, and large cell neuroendocrine carcinoma. Small cell carcinoma may also arise from extrapulmonary sites including the cervix, prostate, pancreas, and small intestine.

DIAGNOSTIC STUDIES

The diagnostic test of choice is biopsy of the primary tumor or a metastatic site, including pleural or pericardial effusion.

Radiographic studies are also recommended including chest x-ray; CT scan of the chest, abdomen, and pelvis; PET scan or bone scan to evaluate for bone metastases; MRI of the brain with gadolinium, the preferred test, or CT scan with contrast of the head to evaluate for brain metastases.

Laboratory studies include complete metabolic profile and complete blood count (CBC) with differential; pulmonary function tests for patients who may need radiation or surgery; and bone marrow biopsy and aspirate.

EVALUATION

The U.S. Preventive Services Task Force (USPSTF) recommends annual screening for lung cancer with low-dose CT scan in adults age 55 to 80 years who have a 30 pack-year smoking history and currently smoke or have quit within the past 15 years. Screening can be discontinued once a person has not smoked for 15 years or develops a health problem that substantially limits life expectancy or the ability or willingness to have curative lung surgery.[9]

TREATMENT

- Treatment of the specific paraneoplastic syndromes is indicated. For SIADH, management consists of treatment of the underlying tumor and acute management includes fluid restriction, intravenous (IV) saline, and possible oral salt tablets. Cushing syndrome is treated with an adrenal enzyme inhibitor, such as ketoconazole or metyrapone should be started to suppress cortisol levels. Lambert-Eaton syndrome treatment begins with treatment of the underlying cancer along with pyridostigmine, intravenous immunoglobulin (IVIG), or prednisolone. For the patient with symptomatic brain metastases, whole brain radiotherapy should be started and if significant edema is present, steroids should be considered.
- SCLC doubles rapidly and metastasizes early. Patients should be started on therapy immediately, within 1 to 2 weeks of diagnosis. If the patient presents with symptomatic disease, treatment should be initiated emergently.
- Almost all patients diagnosed with SCLC should receive chemotherapy; those with early stage disease should also receive local therapy, either radiation or surgery. Even patients with poor performance status—if this status is secondary to newly diagnosed SCLC—should be offered therapy, as the disease is highly responsive.
- Patients with limited disease SCLC should receive four cycles of platinum-based chemotherapy. Cisplatin or carboplatin should be given, in combination with etoposide. Hyperfractionated radiotherapy should be started during the first two cycles of chemotherapy. With combined treatment, approximately 14.3% of limited disease SCLC patients will be disease free at 3 years.[10]
- Patients with extensive disease SCLC (TNM stage IV) should receive systemic chemotherapy only with palliative intent. Etoposide plus a platinum agent is considered the standard of care.
- Patients with stage I (parenchymal only) SCLC may be candidates for surgical resection, lobectomy with thoracic lymphadenectomy, followed by chemotherapy. All patients with resected SCLC should receive adjuvant platinum-based chemotherapy.
- Over 50% of SCLC patients will develop intracranial metastases. Prophylactic cranial irradiation (PCI) decreases the incidence of brain metastases. Overall prognosis after relapse is poor.

7.3B NON-SMALL CELL LUNG CANCER

NSCLC accounts for about 85% of lung cancer cases and includes the following histologic subtypes: adenocarcinoma, squamous cell carcinoma, large cell carcinoma, and undifferentiated. Adenocarcinoma tumors and large cell tumors are peripheral lesions and tend to metastasize early in the clinical course, while squamous cell tumors are central, often cavitate, and metastasize late.

Specific mutations have been found in non-squamous cell NSCLC tumors and should be considered when selecting therapy. About 50% of NSCLC have molecular aberrations in activating kinases.[11] Several treatment agents that specifically target some of these alterations have been developed and are being used in the treatment of NSCLC. These include epidermal growth factor receptor (EGFR) inhibitors erlotinib and afatinib, and the anaplastic lymphoma kinase (ALK) inhibitors crizotinib and ceritinib. Immunotherapy in the form of immune checkpoint inhibitors are used as second-line therapy.

MEDICAL HISTORY AND CLINICAL PRESENTATION

Common presenting symptoms include chronic cough, hemoptysis, and weight loss. History may be significant for smoking, asbestos exposure, tuberculosis infection, or a high-risk occupation. Symptoms will vary depending on the size and location of the tumor. Other common symptoms may include fatigue, dyspnea, and chest pain.

Smoking is associated with about 90% of lung cancer cases.[12] The risk of developing lung cancer increases with increased duration and intensity of smoking. A person who smokes one pack of cigarettes daily has a 20-fold increased risk of lung cancer compared with a never smoker.[13] The risk of lung cancer declines after smoking cessation, but even after stopping for 10 to 20 years the risk is still five times higher than in a person who never smoked.[13] Persons who live in a household with a smoker have a 30% increase in the risk of lung cancer compared to never smokers who do not live in such an environment.[13]

Asbestos exposure increases the risk of lung cancer fivefold, but smokers who are exposed have a >50-fold increase in risk of lung cancer.[13] Other exposures such as radon, uranium, arsenic, nickel-cadmium, chromium, and chloromethyl ether increase the risk of cancer.

SIGNS AND SYMPTOMS

NSCLC may present with signs or symptoms related to the primary tumor, local growth, local invasion, distant metastases, or paraneoplastic syndromes.

Thoracic signs and symptoms include the following:

- **Bronchial obstruction:** Cough, dyspnea, hypoxia, hemoptysis, wheezing, postobstructive pneumonia, or pneumonitis
- **Chest wall invasion:** Pain or palpable mass
- **Tumor compression of local structures:** Superior vena cava syndrome (SVCS), dysphagia due to esophageal compression, or cardiac symptoms
- **Pleural or pericardial effusion:** Pain, dyspnea, tamponade, or arrhythmias
- **Horner syndrome:** Due to invasion of sympathetic chain, diaphragmatic paralysis due to phrenic nerve palsy, hoarseness due to involvement of recurrent laryngeal nerve, ulnar pain, and vasomotor changes from involvement of eighth cervical and first thoracic nerves

Metastatic disease symptoms include:

- **Bone:** Pain, fracture, spinal cord, or nerve root compression
- **Brain:** Headache, dizziness, nausea/emesis, seizures, or focal neurologic deficits
- **Liver:** Anorexia, right upper quadrant (RUQ) pain, jaundice, or weight loss
- **Bone marrow:** Pancytopenia

Paraneoplastic syndromes are common with lung cancer and are more commonly seen in SCLC than in NSCLC. See Section 7.3A Small Cell Lung Cancer for symptoms related to paraneoplastic syndromes.

PHYSICAL EXAMINATION

Physical examination findings of NSCLC depend on the tumor location. NSCLC with a central location may cause crackles, wheezing, hoarseness of the voice, and tachypnea. If located in a peripheral location it may present with pleurisy and reduced chest expansion.

DIFFERENTIAL DIAGNOSIS

The solitary pulmonary nodule is defined as a single density, with well-circumscribed margins, surrounded by normal lung parenchyma, and measuring 1 to 6 cm in greatest diameter. The differential diagnosis of a pulmonary nodule is noted in Table 7.2.

The probability that a single pulmonary nodule is cancer is based on several characteristics of the nodule, including size, growth over time, patient's age, and smoking history. See Table 7.3 for the probability of solitary nodule being malignant or benign.

The first step in the evaluation is to obtain prior radiographs for comparison. This would allow a determination of whether the nodule is new and allow an estimation of its growth. If using high-resolution CT scans, follow-up imaging should be considered at 3 months after the nodule is initially detected and then every 3 to 6 months to assess the growth pattern of the lesion.

For large lesions, a PET scan may be helpful. A nodule may be positive on PET scan in patients with infections or granulomatous disease, so all positive PET scans should be biopsied.

DIAGNOSTIC STUDIES

A biopsy is needed to confirm a diagnosis in all patients with suspected lung cancer. Central lung lesions may be sampled during bronchoscopy, endobronchial ultrasound, or blind biopsy. Lymph nodes may be sampled via blind biopsy, endobronchial ultrasound, or transesophageal ultrasound. Palpable lymph nodes can be sampled by fine needle aspiration.

If a minimally invasive approach is not feasible, a thoracotomy or video–assisted thoracic surgery may be required for sampling of lung nodules, and a mediastinoscopy may be required to biopsy any lymph nodes. Biopsy of distant sites of disease is often performed as it may accomplish tissue diagnosis and staging at the same time.

Imaging studies play an important role in the evaluation of the patient with NSCLC. Chest x-ray and chest CT scan are important to identify location and extent of disease and are the first step in the evaluation of the patient with possible lung cancer. Once the diagnosis has been made a PET-CT is used to evaluate for nodal and distant disease. If PET-CT is not available, CT of chest/abdomen/pelvis plus nuclear bone scan may be used. PET-CT has a sensitivity of approximately 90% and a specificity of 80%.[14]

If distant disease is suspected based on PET-CT, a confirmatory biopsy should be considered prior to deeming a person to have stage IV disease (Figure 7.3).

To determine the presence of brain metastases a brain MRI is indicated. CT scan can be used if an MRI is contraindicated.

If a pleural effusion is present a thoracentesis should be performed to determine if the effusion is malignant; this would be considered stage IVA disease. Since cytology analysis of the fluid typically has low yield for malignant cells, effusions are considered malignant if they have positive cytology, are hemorrhagic, or are exudative. Exception to this would be if there is another clear explanation for an exudative effusion, such as pneumonia.

TABLE 7.2 Differential Diagnosis for Solitary Pulmonary Nodule

Malignant	Benign
Primary lung cancer	Infectious
Bronchial carcinoid	Granulomatous disease
Metastatic disease—breast, colon, renal, germ cell, and melanoma	Abscess
	Vascular
	Hamartoma

TABLE 7.3 Probability of Malignancy Based on the Appearance of a Single Pulmonary Nodule

Characteristic	Increased Probability of Malignant	Decreased Probability of Malignant
General appearance	Spiculated	Smooth
Calcification	Absent	Present
Nodule size	>2.3 cm	<1.5 cm
Growth rate		Stable >2 years

EVALUATION

Clinical outcome for a patient diagnosed with NSLC is related to the stage at the time of diagnosis. Two-thirds of patients diagnosed with lung cancer present with locally advanced or metastatic disease and it is presumed that early detection would lead to improved patient outcomes.

The USPSTF recommends annual screening for lung cancer with low-dose CT scan in adults age 55 to 80 years who have a 30 pack-year smoking history and currently smoke or have quit within the past 15 years. Screening can be discontinued once a person has not smoked for 15 years or develops a health problem that substantially limits life expectancy or the ability or willingness to have curative lung surgery.[15]

TREATMENT

Most cases of NSCLC do not require urgent treatment, but several disease-related complications may need to be treated urgently. These complications may occur at any time during the disease.

- **Hypercalcemia:** Treat with IV fluids and bisphosphonates; use of diuretics is generally discouraged, particularly in the setting of dehydration.
- **Spinal cord compression:** Initiate corticosteroids immediately and treat with radiation therapy and/or surgery.
- **Cardiac tamponade:** Treat with pericardiocentesis with or without a pericardiotomy.
- **SVCS:** Consider steroids, radiation therapy, and possible stent.

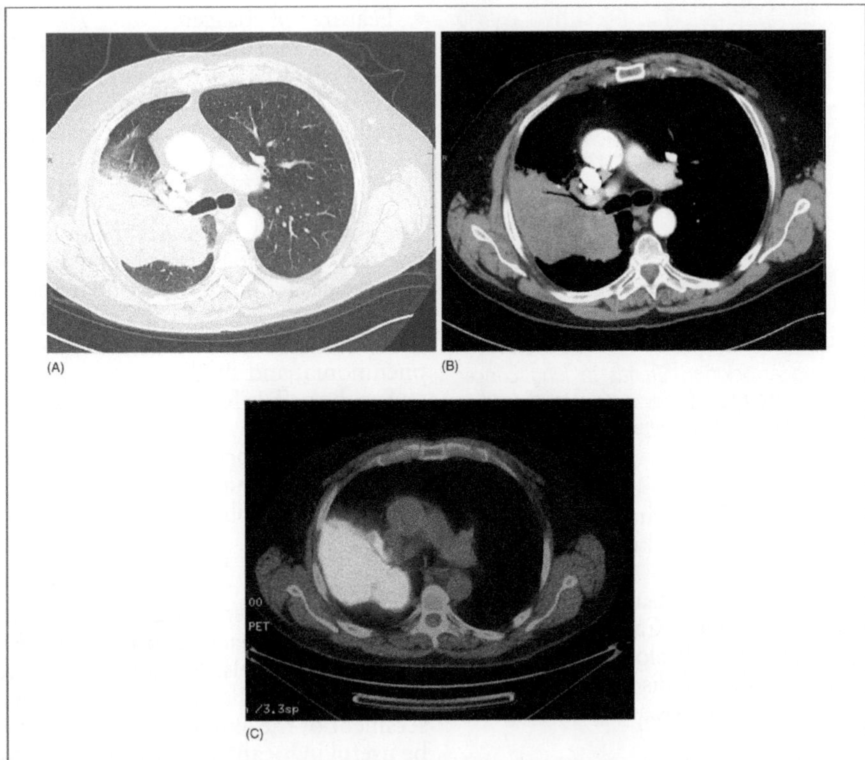

Figure 7.3 Lung carcinoma, 66-year-old male with lung cancer. Patient had shortness of breath and chronic cough. (A) CT axial lung window shows large consolidative opacity in the right upper lung. (B) CT axial mediastinal window shows the same mass, with better assessment of the mediastinum. Small right paratracheal node is present (arrow). (C) PET-CT axial image shows FDG-avid mass with SUV max 14.7. No metabolic activity was seen in the adjacent nodes. FDG, fluorodeoxyglucose; SUV, standardized uptake value.

(Source: Viswanathan C, Duran C. Principles of body imaging in cancer. In: Stubblefield MD, ed. Cancer Rehabilitation. *2nd ed. Springer Publishing Company; 2018)*

- **Hemoptysis:** Treat with radiation therapy or endobronchial ablative techniques.
- **Brain metastases:** Initiate steroids and treat with whole-brain radiation therapy, stereotactic radiation, surgical resection, or a combination of these modalities.

The treatment of NSCLC depends on the stage of the malignancy. Surgical resection is the main therapy for these stages of NSCLC. A lobectomy with hilar and mediastinal lymph node biopsy is procedure of choice. If the lesions are proximal, surgical options include pneumonectomy and sleeve resection. If the surgical margins are positive for malignant cells, resection or radiation therapy should be considered. If surgery is contraindicated, conventional fractionated radiation therapy or stereotactic body radiation therapy should be started. Postoperative chemotherapy is recommended 6 to 12 weeks after resection of stage II and III NSCLC. Cisplatin-based chemotherapy is recommended.

Pancoast tumors adjoin the brachial plexus and are associated with Horner syndrome or shoulder/arm pain. Pancoast tumors are treated with a combination of concurrent chemotherapy and radiation therapy, followed by surgery and additional chemotherapy.

Stage III disease includes mediastinal nodal involvement or direct mediastinal invasion. Treatment consists of local treatment including surgery, radiation therapy, or both; and systemic cisplatin-based chemotherapy.

Stage IV NSCLC includes patients with distant disease, bilateral lung involvement, or malignant effusions. Treatment consists of chemotherapy, cisplatin based, or molecular targeted therapies alone. Biologic agents like the anti-vascular endothelial growth factor monoclonal antibody bevacizumab or the anti-EGFR monoclonal antibodies cetuximab or necitumumab can be used in addition to chemotherapy. Certain tumors, those with *EGFR* mutations, can be treated with tyrosine kinase inhibitors.

PATIENT EDUCATION

- Lung cancer survival rates vary depending on the type of cancer and the stage at diagnosis. See Table 7.4 for 5-year survival rates.
- Patients diagnosed with early stage disease and treated with definitive therapy should be monitored for recurrence of disease and second primary development. The monitoring frequency for stages I–III is clinical and radiographic surveillance chest CT every 4 to 6 months for 2 years, then every 12 months for years 2 through 5.

7.3C CARCINOID TUMOR

Typical carcinoid tumor is a rare primary, neuroendocrine, malignant tumor. The incidence of carcinoid tumors is estimated at 4.7 per 100,000.[16] About 45% of patients with small bowel carcinoid tumors develop carcinoid syndrome, while the tumors of other origins, such as bronchi, pancreas, biliary, and thymus, are much less likely to cause carcinoid syndrome.[17] The syndrome normally presents between the

TABLE 7.4 5-Year Survival Rates for Lung Cancer

Stage	Survival (%)
All stages	16.8
Localized	54
Regional	26.5
Distant	4
Unstaged	7.4

Source: Data from American Lung Association. Trends in lung cancer morbidity and mortality. November 2014. https://www.lung.org/getmedia/ee16997d-52d9-4d05-a967-ddf90d209922/lc-trend-report.pdf.pdf

ages of 40 and 60 years. Bronchial carcinoid tumors are more common in women, and there is no known genetic or environmental predisposing factor.

Most carcinoid tumors are discovered incidentally with few demonstrating hormonal activity. Carcinoid tumors causing carcinoid syndrome are typically slow growing with vague symptoms including abdominal discomfort present for >9 years, on average, before a diagnosis is made.

MEDICAL HISTORY AND CLINICAL PRESENTATION

Bronchial carcinoid and adenoid cystic carcinoma have a propensity for the trachea or major bronchi and may present with wheeze, cough, or hemoptysis. Endobronchial metastases, common with renal cell carcinoma, melanoma, and lymphomas, also have the same symptoms. Endobronchial obstruction may present with symptoms of pneumonia, including fever, sweats, and pleurisy.

Ectopic hormone secretion is rare with these primary or metastatic tumors, but Cushing syndrome and acromegaly have been reported with bronchial carcinoid tumors. Flushing and diarrhea, the carcinoid syndrome, has been reported with patients with bronchial carcinoid tumors with hepatic metastases.

SIGNS AND SYMPTOMS

Symptomatic tumors cause the carcinoid syndrome through release of bioactive substances including serotonin and histamine. The carcinoid syndrome is characterized by symptoms such as intermittent flushing, diarrhea, abdominal pain, right-sided heart disease, and wheezing. Episodic flushing is the key symptom, although bronchial carcinoids typically present with wheezing and dyspnea. Flushing is usually confined to the face, neck, and upper trunk. The classic carcinoid flush is best described as cyanotic and lasts 30 seconds to 30 minutes. The flush may be spontaneous, but there are precipitating factors such as anesthesia, defecation, eating, medications, and palpation of the liver. The bronchial flush may be much more severe and prolonged, associated with hypotension, tachycardia, periorbital edema, and salivation along with diarrhea and severe bronchoconstriction.

PHYSICAL EXAMINATION

Findings that increase the likelihood of carcinoid syndrome include the following:

- Observation of the typical face, neck, and upper trunk flush
- Features of rosacea
- Systolic murmur along the lower left sternal border suggestive of tricuspid regurgitation
- Pellagra, due to increased use of tryptophan by the carcinoid tumor that results in niacin deficiency

DIFFERENTIAL DIAGNOSIS

The differential diagnosis includes the granulomatous lung diseases, including histoplasmosis, blastomycosis, coccidioidomycosis, actinomycosis, and tuberculosis. Other conditions that may be confused with carcinoid tumor include nodular sarcoidosis, Wegener granulomatosis, cryptogenic organizing pneumonia, and single or multiple pulmonary nodules.

See Box 7.1 for the differential diagnosis for episodic flushing.

A careful history should help exclude drugs or medications as a cause of recurrent flushing. Observation of the flush itself is key to eliminating the other diagnoses on the list.

DIAGNOSTIC STUDIES

Confirmatory tests for carcinoid syndrome include urinary 5-hydroxyindoleacetic acid (5-HIAA) and/or plasma chromogranin A levels. Radiolabeled octreotide imaging allows localization of the responsible carcinoid tumor and an assessment of the extent of disease. CT scan or MRI scans may be useful in localization of carcinoid tumors and in detection of metastases, but the octreoscan is the imaging of choice.

Most bronchial carcinoid tumors do not secrete hormones, but if flushing and/or diarrhea (carcinoid syndrome) is present, a 24-hour urine 5-HIAA level may be elevated.

Carcinoid tumors may also produce adrenocorticotropic hormone (ACTH) or corticotropin releasing hormone (CRH) resulting in Cushing syndrome, growth hormone causing acromegaly, or human chorionic gonadotropin (hCG) and/or alpha-fetoprotein in patients with germ cell tumors.

For bronchial carcinoid tumors, blood or urine tests for corticotropin or 5-HIAA will be elevated and may suggest the diagnosis in the patient with the appropriate clinical syndrome. See Table 7.5 for summary of the 5-HIAA and plasma chromogranin A tests. Octreotide scan provides localization of suspected carcinoid tumor but should not be done unless 5-HIAA or chromogranin A is elevated.

TREATMENT

- Management includes surgery for localized disease, hepatic artery embolization for control of liver metastases, and administration of octreotide for symptom control.

Box 7.1 Differential Diagnosis of Episodic Flushing

Drugs: levodopa, bromocriptine, diltiazem	Alcohol	Nicotinic acid
Anaphylaxis	Pheochromocytoma	Medullary thyroid cancer
Systemic mastocytosis	Menopause	Emotional distress
VIPoma		

TABLE 7.5 Characteristics of Tests Used in Carcinoid Syndrome

Characteristic	5-HIAA	Plasma chromogranin A
Normal range	2–8 mg/day	Varies with assay
Sensitivity, specificity	35%–75%, 88%–100%	53%–68%, 84%–94%
Elevated levels	Carcinoid tumor Foods: avocado, banana, eggplant, walnuts, pecans, kiwi, pineapple, plums Medications: acetaminophen, caffeine, guaifenesin, phenobarbital, ephedrine, nicotine, methamphetamine, melphalan, mesalamine	Carcinoid tumor chronic atrophic gastritis, liver cirrhosis, chronic hepatitis, pancreatitis, inflammatory bowel disease, heart failure, renal failure, hyperthyroidism, chronic obstructive pulmonary disease, and rheumatoid arthritis Drugs: proton pump inhibitors
Decreased levels	Ethanol, corticotropin, MAO inhibitors, imipramine, levodopa, aspirin, heparin, isoniazid	
Notes	Unreliable in diagnosing gastric or bronchial carcinoids. Serotonin levels should be checked in its place.	Correlates with burden of disease and recurrence.

5-HIAA, 5-hydroxyindoleacetic acid; MAO, monoamine oxidase.
Source: Data from Corcuff J, Chardon L, El Hajji Ridah I, Brossaud J. Urinary sampling for 5HIAA and metanephrines determination: revisiting the recommendations. Endocr Connect. *2017;6:R87.*

- Octreotide should be started with a short-acting agent and then transition to a long-acting agent. Long-acting agents include sandostatin and lanreotide. Side effects include nausea, abdominal discomfort, bloating, loose stools, and malabsorption, all of which tend to diminish with time.

PATIENT EDUCATION

- Carcinoid tumors that are discovered incidentally confer a prognosis that is dependent on the origin and evidence of metastasis. Long-term consequences of the carcinoid syndrome include fibrosis with right-side cardiac valve abnormalities and fibrosis may also affect the small bowel or the lungs.
- Patients should consider taking a multivitamin containing niacin in addition to the management of carcinoid syndrome.

7.3D MESOTHELIOMA

Pleural mesothelioma is a rare locally invasive, lethal malignancy associated with asbestosis as most cases are linked to asbestos exposure. Approximately 3,000 cases are diagnosed annually in the United States.[18] The life expectancy without treatment is <12 months.[19,20] Asbestos is a group of hydrated magnesium silicate fibrous materials and is used with restrictions in cement, ceiling tiles, brake linings, and shipbuilding. Pleural mesothelioma is more prevalent in men secondary to the occupational association.

Pleural mesothelioma is subdivided into three histologic subtypes: epithelioid, biphasic/mixed, and sarcomatoid. The subtypes are an important prognostic factor and dictate therapy. The typical presentation is a pleural effusion of unknown etiology. Epithelioid tumors are the most common mesothelioma subtypes. Epithelioid tumors have the best prognosis and are most likely to respond to chemotherapy. Sarcomatoid tumors are classified as stage IV, considered nonoperable and have the worst prognosis.

MEDICAL HISTORY AND CLINICAL PRESENTATION

Asbestos exposure is the major risk factor for pleural mesothelioma. The lifetime risk in people with asbestos exposure is up to 10%.[21] Insulation workers are at greatest risk and other occupational risk groups include carpenters, electricians, mining/milling, general shipyard, heating, and construction workers. Patients with pleural mesothelioma present with dyspnea, nonpleuritic chest pain, cough, chest wall pain, weight loss, fever, night sweats, and fatigue.

SIGNS AND SYMPTOMS

There is a 20- to 60-year latency period from exposure to asbestos to development of disease. Clinical signs and symptoms include dyspnea, nonpleuritic chest pain, and cough due to pleural effusion. Nonspecific symptoms include fevers, night sweats, fatigue, and weight loss.

Patients may also be asymptomatic and present with a chest wall mass, pleural effusion, or other pleural pathology on imaging.

PHYSICAL EXAMINATION

Physical examination findings are related to the presence of pleural effusions. Findings include decreased breath sounds, dullness to percussion, egophony, and palpable chest wall masses.

DIFFERENTIAL DIAGNOSIS

Diagnosing pleural mesothelioma and separating benign from malignant pleural disease are difficult. The differential diagnosis includes metastatic adenocarcinoma with pleural effusion. Diagnosis is based on histology and immunohistochemical (IHC) staining.

DIAGNOSTIC STUDIES

Tissue diagnosis is required. Initial evaluation consists of a CT chest/abdomen with contrast and PET-CT for staging. If the patient is being considered for surgical resection, the fluid should be drained and then pulmonary function tests should be performed, along with an echocardiogram to evaluate heart function, and ventilation/perfusion study. Staging studies should also be performed to determine treatment options.

EVALUATION

Tissue diagnosis is required, and surgical biopsy offers the highest yield. Other diagnostic studies include CT of the thorax with contrast and thoracentesis with cytology and pleural biopsy.

TREATMENT

- Clinical stage I–III that are epithelial or have mixed histologic features are evaluated for possible surgical intervention.
- Clinical stage IV or sarcomatoid history are considered unresectable and are treated with chemotherapy. First-line chemotherapy is the combination of cisplatin and pemetrexed. Thoracentesis is indicated in cases of severe dyspnea and large pleural effusions for symptom control. If surgery is indicated, the procedures of choice are extrapleural pneumonectomy or pleurectomy/decortication.

PATIENT EDUCATION

- Pleural mesothelioma is a very difficult to treat, mostly fatal, and rarely curable with a median overall survival of 9 to 17 months.[21] Surgical resection is only possible in a small group of patients, so the goal of therapy is typically palliative.

KEY POINTS

- The main factor contributing to lung cancer is smoking, but about 15% of all lung cancer patients have never smoked cigarettes and have suspected driver mutations.
- Lung cancer can be SCLC or NSCLC.
- Manifestations can include cough, fever, hoarseness, pleural effusion, pneumonia, and metastases to the brain, liver, and bone.
- Consider yearly screening with low-dose helical CT for current or former smokers age ≥55 years at high risk.
- Treat early-stage NSCLC with resection when pulmonary reserve is adequate, followed by chemotherapy.
- Treat advanced stage SCLC and NSCLC with chemotherapy and/or immunotherapy.

7.4 GASTROINTESTINAL CANCER

OVERVIEW

Gastrointestinal (GI) cancers refer to malignant conditions of the GI tract and accessory organs of digestion, including the esophagus, stomach, biliary system, pancreas, small intestine, large intestine, rectum, and anus. The symptoms are related to the organ affected and can include obstruction, bleeding, or other associated problems. The diagnosis often requires endoscopic examination with biopsy. The prognosis and treatment depend on tumor location, cancer type, and whether it has invaded other tissues or metastasized.

Overall, the GI tract and the accessory organs of digestion are responsible for more cancers and more deaths from cancer than any other system in the body.

EPIDEMIOLOGY

According to the American Cancer Society, GI cancers have the overall highest incidence and are the second leading cause of death in the United States.[1] See Table 7.6 for a summary of GI cancer statistics.

PATHOPHYSIOLOGY

The pathogenesis varies with each of the various GI cancers. Esophageal cancer is due to chronic inflammation, metaplasia, and dysplasia due to gastroesophageal reflux (GERD) leading to Barrett esophagus or long-term exposure to irritants. For gastric cancer, the most important environmental risk factor is infection with *Helicobacter pylori*—as well as dietary factors and lifestyle effects such as smoking or alcohol. Cancer of the small intestine is linked to familial adenomatous polyposis (FAP) and Crohn disease. Colon cancer can develop via genetic or environmental causes. Genetic etiologies include FAP and hereditary nonpolyposis colorectal cancer (CRC). Hepatocellular carcinoma (HCC) is linked to infection with hepatitis B and hepatitis C. Pancreatic cancer is due to inherited and acquired mutations; *K-ras* mutation is the most common.

TABLE 7.6 Gastrointestinal Cancer Facts

	Esophageal Cancer	Gastric Cancer	Pancreatic Cancer	Hepatic Cancer	Small Intestine Cancer	Colorectal Cancer
Estimated new cases in 2019	17,290	26,240	55,400	42,220	10,470	142,500
% of all new cancer cases	1.0	1.5	3.2	2.4	0.6	8.2
Estimated deaths in 2019	15,850	10,800	44,330	30,200	1,450	50,630
% of all cancer deaths	2.6	1.8	7.3	5.0	0.2	8.3
5-year survival rate (2007–2013)	19%	31%	8%	18%	68%	64%
Lifetime risk (%)	0.5	0.9	1.6	1.0	0.3	4.2

Source: Data from American Cancer Society. Cancer Facts & Figures 2018. *American Cancer Society; 2018. https://www.cancer.org/content/dam/cancer-org/research/ cancer-facts-and-statistics/annual-cancer-facts-and-figures/2018*

7.4A ESOPHAGEAL CANCER

Esophageal cancer has two main histologic types: squamous cell carcinoma and adenocarcinoma. The incidence of esophageal cancer is increasing. Although the incidence of squamous cell carcinoma has been stabilized, the incidence of adenocarcinoma is increasing rapidly in the United States. Several environmental exposures play a role in the development of esophageal cancer, and genetics also play a role with a molecular mutation related to the p53 tumor suppressor gene *TP53*, which is linked to many cancers, including esophageal.

Despite improvements in both diagnosis and treatment, esophageal cancer continues to have a poor prognosis, with 5-year survival rates <19%.[1]

MEDICAL HISTORY AND CLINICAL PRESENTATION

In squamous cell carcinoma the two major risk factors are tobacco use and alcohol. The use of tobacco increases the risk of esophageal cancer in alcoholics compared with rates for the general population. Other risk factors include hot food and beverages, low fruit and vegetable consumption, and male sex.

For adenocarcinoma, obesity increases the risk of GERD, which in turn increases the risk of Barrett esophagus. Barrett esophagus increases the risk of progression to cancer depending on the degree of dysplasia. Other risk factors include tobacco use and male sex.

SIGNS AND SYMPTOMS

Signs and symptoms of esophageal cancer depend on the stage of the disease. Many patients are unaware of the presence of precancerous disease or early stage cancer such as Barrett's esophagus for esophageal adenocarcinoma. As the cancer grows, symptoms gradually appear.

Early symptoms include gastric reflux, dysphagia, chest pain, back pain, and weight loss. Symptoms of advanced disease include hoarseness due to recurrent laryngeal nerve involvement, Horner syndrome due to invasion of sympathetic nerve, recurrent pneumonia, cough due to fistula development, hiccups due to phrenic nerve involvement, and dyspnea due to tracheal stricture from tumor invasion.

PHYSICAL EXAMINATION

Patients with esophageal cancer typically have normal physical examinations unless the disease has metastasized. Once metastasized, the physical examination findings will be consistent with the location of the metastases; for example, jaundice may appear with liver metastases.

DIFFERENTIAL DIAGNOSIS

See Table 7.7 for the differential diagnosis for esophageal cancer.

TABLE 7.7 Differential Diagnosis for Esophageal Cancer

Diagnosis	Description
Esophageal varices	Dilated submucosal veins secondary to portal hypertension and seen in cirrhosis.
Achalasia	Risk factor for squamous cell carcinoma. Esophageal motility disorder with dysphagia to solids and liquids, progressive.
Benign tumors	Show signs of dysphagia and differentiate based on biopsy.
Gastroesophageal reflux disease	Due to decreased lower esophageal sphincter tone; presents with regurgitation, heartburn, and dysphagia.
Esophagitis	Inflammation due to infections, pill-induced, or reflux. Presents with dysphagia and odynophagia.
Booerhaave syndrome	Spontaneous esophageal perforation that is thought to arise from a rapid increase in intraluminal esophageal pressure.
Esophageal diverticulum	Noted over the age of 70 and presents with dysphagia, regurgitation, halitosis, and odynophagia.

DIAGNOSTIC STUDIES

Esophageal cancer is best diagnosed by upper endoscopic examination of the esophageal lesion with biopsy to confirm the diagnosis. Improper movement of vocal cord may suggest recurrent laryngeal nerve paresis. Staging of esophageal cancer is based on the depth of tumor into or through the esophageal wall (T category), the presence of metastatic regional lymph nodes (N category), and distant metastases (M category).

Other diagnostic studies include barium esophagram, which can provide information on tumor location, size, and shape; endoscopic ultrasound is used to evaluate depth of tumor and regional lymph node involvement. The major role of CT scan is to detect local tumor invasion into adjacent structures and detection of distant metastatic disease such as lung and hepatic metastases.

PET imaging is useful in detecting regional lymph nodes that are not near the primary tumor. PET is the most important modality for distant metastatic disease detection.

EVALUATION

Initial evaluation consists of upper endoscopy with biopsy. Once the diagnosis has been made, testing for proper staging should be completed. This includes CT and PET scans. Staging is very important in determining prognosis and treatment options.

TREATMENT

- A tissue diagnosis is necessary to confirm the presence of a malignancy before the initiation of therapy unless there are acute airway emergencies or progressive life-threatening conditions. These emergent life-threatening conditions include tracheoesophageal or bronchoesophageal fistula. Fistula development is a very poor prognostic factor and patients usually die within 1 to 2 months. Therapy should be supportive to maintain quality of life and may include stenting of the esophagus and airways.
- Perforation of esophageal cancer can occur, and the patient should be started on antibiotics and acid suppression therapy, and operative management should be undertaken.

- GI bleeding can occur from the tumor and should be treated with fluid resuscitation and blood transfusion to stabilize the patient and endoscopic hemostasis such as electrocoagulation to control bleeding.
- Treatment of esophageal carcinoma (stage 0, MI, M2, and M3 with lymphatic invasion) is esophagectomy. If stage IB, stage II and III preoperative chemoradiotherapy following esophagectomy is recommended. Chemotherapy consists of various combinations of carboplatin, cisplatin, paclitaxel, and fluoropyrimidine. Chemoradiotherapy is a reasonable approach for patients who are not surgical candidates. Radiation therapy with or without chemotherapy and/or intraluminal brachytherapy are useful alternatives to esophagectomy for patients with esophageal cancer. Brachytherapy should be considered an alternative to stent placement palliation of dysphagia.

PATIENT EDUCATION

- Primary prevention includes treatment of GERD and Barrett esophagus, weight loss, avoiding tobacco and alcohol, and a diet with increased fruits and vegetables.

7.4B GASTRIC CANCER

Gastric adenocarcinoma makes up 95% of all gastric malignancies, occurs in approximately 26,000 patients, and is estimated to result in approximately 11,000 deaths annually.[1] It is most common in older persons with a median age of diagnosis of 60 years. Gastric carcinoma is frequently associated with *Helicobacter pylori* infection of the stomach. *H. pylori* gastritis is widespread and more common in poorly developed countries, and gastric cancer is more common in these populations. There are several dietary risk factors for gastric cancer. Gastric cancer is more common in people who eat smoked and preserved foods, and less common in those who consume fresh meats and vegetables.

Genetic risk for gastric adenocarcinoma is rare.

MEDICAL HISTORY AND CLINICAL PRESENTATION

History of unexplained weight loss, early satiety, and dysphagia is common. Lymphadenopathy may be noted in the left axilla or around the umbilicus. The skin rash of acanthosis nigricans, particularly in the axillary areas, is noted with gastric cancer. There may be a history of iron deficiency anemia.

SIGNS AND SYMPTOMS

Symptoms of gastric cancer include diffuse abdominal pain, bloating, weight loss, hematemesis, weight loss, melena, and dysphagia. Other symptoms include those related to iron deficiency anemia. Many patients with the intestinal form of gastric cancer will have *H. pylori* present in the stomach and chronic gastritis.

PHYSICAL EXAMINATION

Patients with gastric cancer typically appear weak. Common physical examination findings include abdominal distention, abdominal mass, and pallor. Lymphadenopathy may be noted in the left axilla and periumbilical area; this would indicate intraperitoneal carcinomatosis.

Rectal examination may reveal a firm anterior mass on palpation. This is known as Blumer's shelf and is due to metastases from the primary tumor.

DIAGNOSTIC STUDIES

The diagnostic test of choice is an upper endoscopy with biopsy of areas of the stomach suspicious for malignancy.

Endoscopic ultrasound is useful in defining the depth of tumor penetration of the stomach wall; it is less specific for defining lymph node metastases but can demonstrate enlargement of perigastric lymph nodes suggesting tumor involvement.

Metastatic carcinoma to the stomach is rare, though occasionally melanoma will metastasize to the stomach mucosa.

Gastric cancers may overexpress the human epidermal growth factor receptor 2 (HER2). Some patients with overexpression of HER2 may respond to treatment with anti-HER2 monoclonal antibody trastuzumab.

CT scanning is useful in staging, as it can detect liver and lung metastases and enlarged lymph nodes. PET/CT is useful in detecting metastases in some cases.

EVALUATION

In a patient suspected of having a gastric neoplasm, the primary means of diagnosis is upper endoscopy with biopsy. Patients with dysphagia as a significant symptom should be evaluated by endoscopy for distal esophageal, gastroesophageal junction, and proximal gastric masses.

TREATMENT

- The primary therapy of gastric cancer is gastrectomy if indicated. Contraindications to gastrectomy include presence of metastatic disease where resection of the primary tumor could not be done for cure, locally advanced stomach tumor making gastrectomy technically impossible, and inability to tolerate surgery.
- When a diagnosis is made at the time of surgery, postoperative chemoradiation is indicated.
- Pre- or postoperative chemotherapy consists of epirubicin, cisplatin, and fluorouracil (5-FU). Adjunctive therapy with either peri-operative chemotherapy or postoperative chemoradiation has been convincingly demonstrated to improve survival.

PATIENT EDUCATION

- Untreated gastric cancer has a 5-year survival rate of almost 0% in patients with disseminated disease and about half survive 5 years with localized disease.
- Prognosis is poor secondary to complications such as ascites, GI bleeding, distant metastasis, weight loss, recurrence of disease, and complications due to treatment.

7.4C COLORECTAL CANCER

Colorectal adenocarcinoma is the fourth most common malignancy in the United States. Incidence of new CRC in 2018 was estimated to be approximately 140,250 with total number of deaths 50,630.[1] Incidence rates have been decreasing by approximately 3.5% each year since 2005 in patients over age 55 due to improvements in screening, risk factor modification, and improved treatments.[1]

The lifetime risk of CRC is 5%.[22] The median age of diagnosis is 72 years, with a clear majority of new CRCs occurring in individuals over the age of 50. It is estimated that it takes 10 years for the development of frank carcinoma from the earliest precursor lesions. Current screening guidelines recommend colonoscopy every 10 years after the age of 50 years in average risk individuals.

Autosomal dominant familial syndromes with increased risk and early onset of CRC include FAP in 1% of all cases and hereditary nonpolyposis CRC in 3% of cases.

MEDICAL HISTORY AND CLINICAL PRESENTATION

Hereditary CRC syndromes, personal or familial history of CRC or polyps, history of ulcerative colitis (UC), and acromegaly cause the greatest increase in risk for CRC.

Hereditary colorectal syndromes include FAP, hereditary nonpolyposis coli, Peutz-Jeghers syndrome, and MUTYH-associated polyposis. Family history of CRC in one first-degree relative increases the risk about twofold. Patients with adenomatous polyps >1 cm are at three to six times higher risk of CRC.[23] The risk of CRC is increased in patients with UC and varies depending on the duration and extent of involvement. The annual incidence is estimated at about 0.5% between 10 to 20 years after diagnosis, increasing to 1% annually thereafter.[24]

The incidence and mortality of CRC appear to be higher in African Americans and mortality appears to be higher in men. Other risk factors include history of diabetes mellitus, androgen deprivation, and acromegaly.

Alcohol consumption, especially more than two to three drinks a day, may increase risk of CRC, smoking has been associated with increased risk of developing polyps, and dietary factors, such as long-term consumption of red or processed meats and caffeine, have inconsistently been shown to be associated with an increased risk.[25]

SIGNS AND SYMPTOMS

GI signs and symptoms include abdominal pain and/or discomfort, which may be associated with nausea and vomiting; altered bowel movements or even bowel obstruction, more commonly with left-sided tumors; and GI bleeding ranging from occult blood loss to melena and/or hematochezia. Metastatic disease symptoms vary depending on location; liver metastases may cause anorexia; RUQ pain and jaundice and nonspecific symptoms include weight loss, fatigue, anemia and occasionally fever of unknown origin.

PHYSICAL EXAMINATION

The most common physical examination findings include emaciation, lethargy, and pallor. Other findings include fever, abdominal pain or discomfort, ascites, rectal bleeding, and jaundice. Patients with Peutz-Jeghers syndrome present with characteristic freckling of the mouth, lips, fingers, and toes (Figure 7.4).

DIFFERENTIAL DIAGNOSIS

See Table 7.8 for the differential diagnosis for CRC.

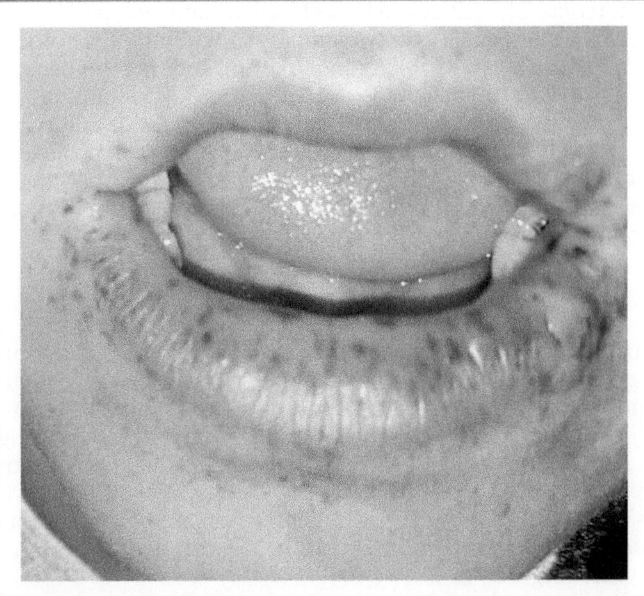

FIGURE 7.4 Peutz-Jeghers syndrome.
(Source: Courtesy of Massryy)

TABLE 7.8 Differential Diagnosis for Colorectal Cancer

Diagnosis	Description
Irritable bowel syndrome	Presents with abdominal pain and alteration of bowel habits
Diverticulitis	Left lower guardant abdominal pain, fever, and rebound tenderness
Inflammatory bowel disease	Presents with persistent diarrhea, abdominal pain, rectal bleeding, weight loss, and fatigue
Gastrointestinal infections	Present with fever, diarrhea, and abdominal pain
Hemorrhoids	Present with pain with defecation, hematochezia, and anal discharge

The presence of CRC must be ruled out in any patient with persistent symptoms, especially in those older than 40 years.

DIAGNOSTIC STUDIES

The diagnosis of symptomatic patients is via colonoscopy with biopsy. CT scan and PET scan are used in staging CRC. Staging is used to determine prognosis and treatment options. Screening for CRC is the centerpiece in the care of asymptomatic patients and reduces the incidence, morbidity, and mortality of CRC.

All patients with CRC should also be evaluated with a CBC, blood chemistries, and liver function tests. Carcinoembryonic antigen (CEA) is associated with CRC but has low diagnostic ability due to overlap with several benign conditions. This marker is not recommended for screening but should be obtained in patients with known CRC to aid in staging, treatment planning, and assessment.

Carriers of FAP and MUTYH-associated polyposis gene mutations or at-risk family members should undergo colonic surveillance with flexible sigmoidoscopy and/or colonoscopy every year starting at the age of 10 years, and continuing until age 35 to 40 years, if negative.[26] Patients diagnosed with, or strongly suspected to have, hereditary nonpolyposis coli should be offered colonoscopy starting at the age of 20 to 25 years or 2 to 5 years prior to the earliest age of colon cancer diagnosis in the family.[27]

EVALUATION

Current guidelines, by the American Cancer Society, recommend CRC risk assessment by age 40 in patients without known family history to determine the age to initiate screening. Patients with average risk are advised to start screening at age 50, using one of several options including colonoscopy every 10 years, annual fecal-based tests, flexible sigmoidoscopy every 5 years, a combination of annual fecal tests and sigmoidoscopy every 5 years or CT colonography every 5 years (Figure 7.5).[28]

Patients with a family history of early CRC or advanced adenoma in a first-degree relative below 60 years or with more than one first-degree relative at any age should be offered screening colonoscopies at the age of 40 years, or 10 years younger than the earliest diagnosis in the family.[28]

Screening options include:

- Colonoscopy is the preferred screening test, since polyps can be removed at the time of the procedure, and the full colon is examined.
- Flexible sigmoidoscopy requires no sedation and less bowel preparation but is limited to the lower half of the colon. If a lesion is noted larger than 1 cm the patient should be referred to colonoscopy.
- Double-contrast barium enema is no longer widely used and is typically reserved for patients who cannot undergo colonoscopy.
- CT colonography requires a colonoscopy if positive findings are noted.
- Fecal occult blood test (FOBT) is the most common stool test used but is not recommended for screening on a single specimen due to low sensitivity. FOBT should be performed on three successive specimens while on a prescribed diet.
- Stool DNA test is a noninvasive test and identifies DNA changes in cells of a stool sample. If positive, a colonoscopy is indicated.

The USPSTF recommends low-dose aspirin use for the primary prevention of colorectal cancer in adults ages 50 to 59 years who have a 10% or greater 10-year CVD risk, who are not at increased risk of bleeding, have a life expectancy of at least the next 10 years, and are willing to

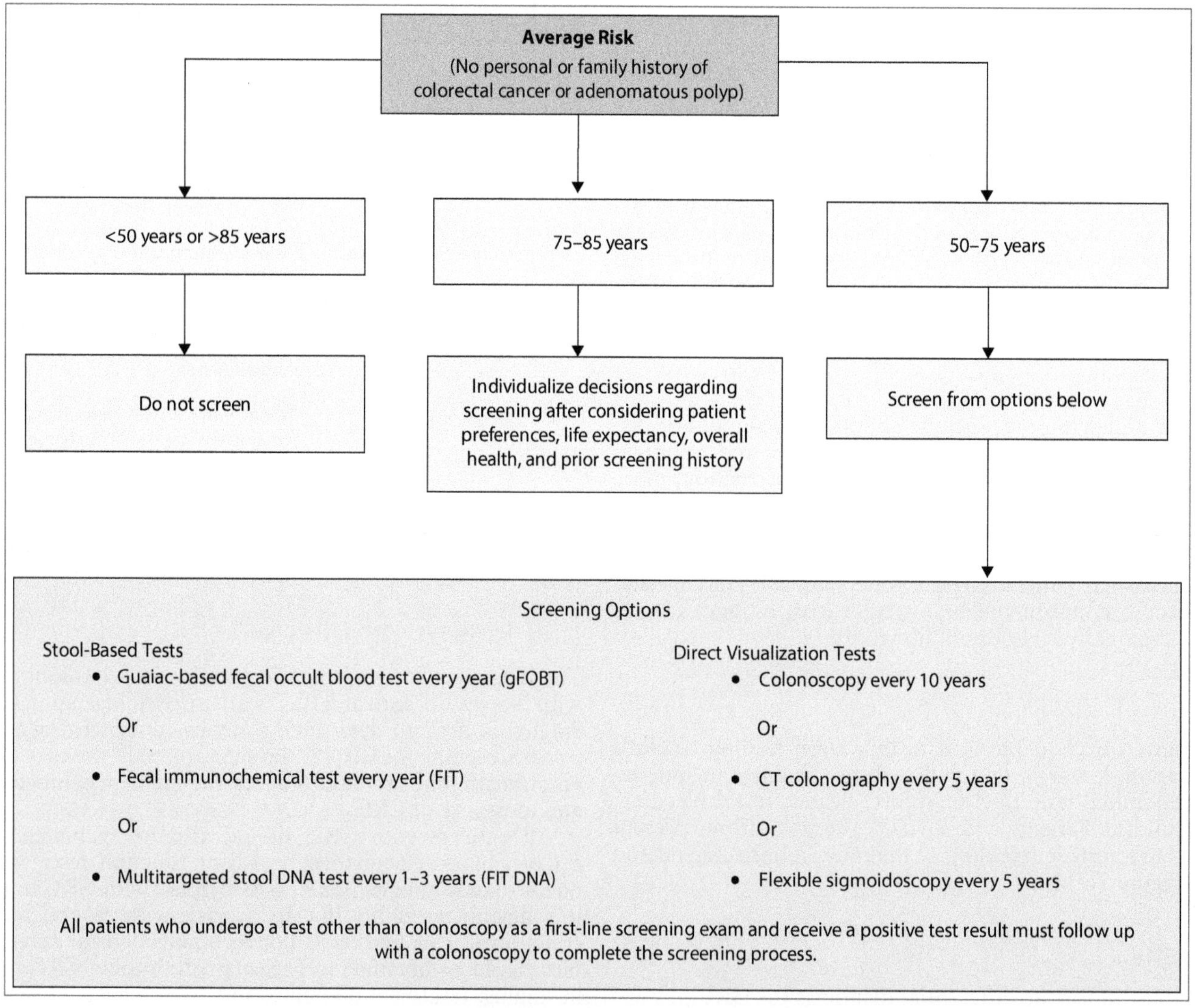

Figure 7.5 American Cancer Society recommendations for colorectal cancer screening.

take low-dose aspirin daily for at least 10 years.[29] Celecoxib (selective cyclooxygenase 2, COX-2 inhibitor) is used to reduce polyp burden in patients with FAP as an adjunct to endoscopy and surgery.

TREATMENT

- Most cases of colorectal cancer do not require urgent initiation of treatment. There are several complications that may require emergent treatment.
- Bowel obstruction and/or perforation are uncommon but may be seen with cecal or sigmoid carcinomas.
- Emergent surgery may be needed. Melena is more often seen with colon cancer and hematochezia with rectal cancer. While this is rarely life threatening, it may require emergent management including surgery or transfusions. Extensive liver metastases may cause liver failure due to infiltration and/or biliary obstruction. Biliary stenting and urgent initiation of chemotherapy may be indicated.
- Brain metastasis is uncommon. Treatment options include steroids, whole-brain radiation therapy, stereotactic radiation, surgical resection, or a combination.
- Treatment of colorectal cancer varies depending on the disease stage. Stage I tumors encompass TNM stages T1 and T2 N0M0. These are small tumors with no lymph node involvement. Surgical resection is the standard treatment.
- Surgical resection is the mainstay of treatment for stage II colon cancer. To decrease the risk of distant recurrences, adjuvant chemotherapy, with fluoropyrimidine-based adjuvant therapy, for 6 months should be considered for stage II colon cancer patients with high-risk features.
- Surgical resection is the mainstay of treatment for stage III colon cancer, with adjuvant chemotherapy following surgery. Stage III rectal cancer patients are routinely treated with preoperative therapy.
- Stage IV includes metastases. Patients with potentially resectable metastatic disease should be reevaluated every 2 months to see if resection is possible. Most stage IV patients are treated with palliative care to prolong survival by stopping tumor progression, minimize tumor-related symptoms, and maintain quality of life.

PATIENT EDUCATION

- The most important predictor of outcome is the stage of disease at diagnosis. Surgical resection is the only potentially curative modality and is employed in patients with stages I–III and select stage IV patients.
- The 5-year relative survival rate is 64% for colon cancer and 67% for rectal cancer. Only 39% of colorectal cancer patients are diagnosed with localized disease, for which the 5-year survival rate is 90%.[1]

7.4D PANCREATIC CANCER

Pancreatic adenocarcinoma is the most common cancer of the pancreas and is currently the fourth leading cause of cancer death in the United States.[1] The disease presents clinically late in its course so most patients with this disease are not candidates for surgical resection.

Patients for whom a resection is feasible will undergo either a partial or total pancreatectomy with curative intent, followed by adjuvant therapy. Patients without distant metastases but with unresectable primary disease, referred to as locally advanced pancreatic adenocarcinoma, are treated with chemotherapy, which is at times followed by chemoradiation.

For patients with distant metastases, chemotherapy for symptom management and extension of life is standard treatment.

Pancreatic adenocarcinoma is characterized by activating mutations in the *KRAS* gene. Although *KRAS* mutations are common in many malignancies, it has >90% prevalence in pancreatic adenocarcinoma.[30] Mutations in, or loss of, the *CDKN2A* and *TP53* tumor suppressors are also very frequent (90% and 75%, respectively).[30]

MEDICAL HISTORY AND CLINICAL PRESENTATION

Several factors are linked to the increased incidence of pancreatic cancer. Heritable factors are linked to 10% of cases.[31] The occurrence of three first-degree relatives with pancreatic cancer formally defines familial pancreatic cancer; additionally, having two or more affected first-degree relatives increases risk and justifies screening. Several lifestyle and environmental factors may contribute to risk of pancreatic ductal adenocarcinoma (PDA). These include tobacco use, high-fat diet, diabetes, exposure to wood pulp or petroleum products, and chronic pancreatitis.

SIGNS AND SYMPTOMS

The most common symptoms of pancreatic cancer include mid epigastric pain, jaundice, sudden unexplained weight loss, and dark urine and light-colored or greasy stools.

PHYSICAL EXAMINATION

Patients with pancreatic cancer are usually in their 50s and appear cachectic, with signs of malnutrition. Patients mostly present with palpable abdominal mass, epigastric tenderness radiating to the back, hepatosplenomegaly, and signs of metastasis in advanced stages. Jaundice with or without a palpable gallbladder (Courvoisier sign) is noted in pancreatic head tumors. The signs of metastasis include left supraclavicular lymphadenopathy, palpable periumbilical mass, metastatic palpable mass in the rectal pouch, and the involvement of other nodes in the cervical area.

DIFFERENTIAL DIAGNOSIS

Pancreatic cancer must be differentiated from other pancreatic disorders including chronic pancreatitis, autoimmune pancreatitis, pancreatic pseudocyst, choledocholithiasis, and neuroendocrine tumors of the pancreas. Pathologies of the bile duct and duodenum such as choledocholithiasis, cholelithiasis, choledochal cysts, cholangiocarcinoma, bile duct strictures and ampullary cancer should be differentiated from pancreatic cancer based on imaging and biopsy findings.

DIAGNOSTIC STUDIES

Diagnosing patients with pancreatic cancer can be difficult. Early manifestations are subtle. History and physical examination are the beginning of any diagnostic workup and staging.

Laboratory studies include the CBC, metabolic profile including liver function tests, and the tumor marker CA 19-9. The CBC will reveal a mild, normocytic anemia, fasting glucose tolerance is often impaired, and liver function tests may be elevated if liver metastases have occurred. CA 19-9 is a tumor marker in metastatic disease and in assessing response to therapy. CA 19-9 levels >1,000 U/mL are associated with unresectable disease. CA 19-9 is not a screening or a diagnostic test but should be evaluated preoperatively in resectable patients. Postoperative CA 19-9 levels in the normal range are a favorable prognostic feature. Decreases in high CA 19-9 levels during treatment are predictive of improved survival.

A triphasic multidetector CT scan with thin cuts through the pancreas is the cornerstone of establishing diagnosis and assessing surgical options.

Endoscopic ultrasound can be useful in the evaluation of PDA, particularly for characterizing potentially resectable patients' nodal involvement more closely.

A chest x-ray or CT scan of the chest is recommended in patients prior to surgery to complete staging.

EVALUATION

Screening for pancreatic adenocarcinoma is not cost-effective except for high-risk families. In this case endoscopic ultrasound and magnetic resonance cholangiopancreatography can be used to screen.

When a pancreatic malignancy is suspected, an abdominal CT scan with contrast should be obtained. CT scan can identify a lesion in the pancreas with 89% to 97% sensitivity and can often discriminate between ductal adenocarcinoma and neuroendocrine tumors.[32] A CT should also be used to evaluate vascular involvement and for determining surgical options (Figure 7.6).

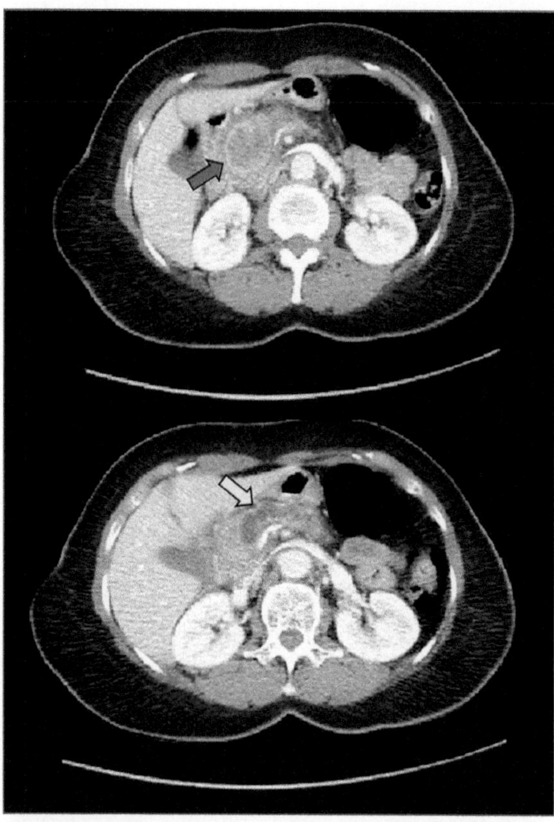

Figure 7.6 **Abdominal CT with intravenous contrast demonstrating pancreatic adenocarcinoma in the head region (red arrow) with upstream pancreatic ductal dilation (yellow arrow).**

(Source: Mulki R, Mekaroonkamol P, Lopez-Aguilar AG, et al. Diagnosis and staging of pancreatic cancer. In: Bekaii-Saab T, El-Rayes BF, Pawlik TM, eds. Handbook of Gastrointestinal Cancers: Evidence-Based Treatment and Multidisciplinary Patient Care. *Springer Publishing Company; 2019, Figure 20.1.)*

Benign lesions such as intraductal papillary mucinous neoplasms or mucinous cystic neoplasms may be difficult to discriminate from their malignant counterparts. Biopsy of a mass in the pancreas is not necessarily required prior to resection. False negative biopsies are common and should not delay surgical resection in most cases.

TREATMENT

- Surgery is the initial treatment of choice in cases that appear to be surgically resectable. Metastases to lymph nodes beyond the field of resection should be considered unresectable, as should distant metastases, superior mesenteric artery (SMA) or celiac encasement >180 degrees, aortic invasion, or an unreconstructible superior mesenteric vein/portal occlusion.
- Four surgical procedures are deployed for pancreatic cancer resection and include pancreatoduodenectomy, total pancreatectomy, regional or extended pancreatectomy, or distal pancreatectomy with or without splenectomy.
- Adjuvant chemotherapy treatment for 6 months should be considered for all resected patients suitable for therapy. Commonly used regimens include gemcitabine or 5-FU and leucovorin. Adjuvant therapy has been shown to double the long-term survival compared to observation alone.
- Patients with unresectable locally advanced disease are managed with chemotherapy, with or without chemoradiation.
- Metastatic disease is common at the time of presentation. The most common sites of metastases are the liver and peritoneum. Systemic chemotherapy, coupled with symptom management, is the mainstay of treatment for patients with metastatic disease. Gemcitabine and FOLFIRINOX (oxaliplatin, irinotecan, leucovorin, followed by a 5-FU bolus) are the chemotherapy protocols of choice. The addition of the EGFR inhibitor erlotinib or nab-paclitaxel to gemcitabine provides additional survival benefit.

PATIENT EDUCATION

- The prognosis of pancreatic cancer is determined to a large extent by the stage at which the disease is diagnosed. Resectable patients who receive adjuvant therapy have a median survival of 24 months and up to one in four will be alive 5 years after resection.[33]
- Those with metastatic disease at diagnosis have a median survival of 6 months with gemcitabine or longer with combination regimens, although survival past 2 years is rare.[34]
- Decline in CA 19-9 levels in response to therapy is an encouraging prognostic sign.

7.4E HEPATOCELLULAR CANCER

HCC is the most common primary malignant tumor of the liver and the fifth most common cause of cancer-related death in the United States.[1] Incidence in the United States has increased threefold in the past two decades, secondary to increases in chronic hepatitis C virus (HCV) and nonalcoholic steatohepatitis (NASH).

Although surgical resection and liver transplantation are potential cures, a clear majority of patients present with advanced disease and curative treatment modalities are not an option.

Most cases of HCC are due to chronic liver disease resulting from chronic HCV or hepatitis B virus (HBV) infection alone or exacerbated by comorbid conditions such as chronic alcohol use, metabolic syndrome, and infectious diseases.

In the United States, chronic HCV infection with associated cirrhosis is the major risk factor of developing HCC. Patients with chronic HCV infection and cirrhosis have a 2% to 6% per year incidence of developing HCC and the incidence is made worse by comorbid conditions, mainly chronic alcohol use.[35] Complete eradication of the HCV reduces the risk of developing HCC, but these patients still have some risk for cancer and should continue to be monitored.

Hepatitis B virus (HBV) is a risk factor for HCC, but this risk is decreasing in the United States due to the hepatitis B vaccine. Patients with chronic HBV infection without cirrhosis have a 0.3% to 0.6% per year incidence of HCC.[36] Patients with concomitant cirrhosis have a 3–8% per year incidence of HCC.[36]

Other risk factors include cirrhosis from any cause of liver disease, including alcoholic liver disease, NASH, hereditary hemochromatosis, alpha-1 antitrypsin deficiency, and Wilson disease, also predisposes to HCC.

MEDICAL HISTORY AND CLINICAL PRESENTATION

In a patient with known cirrhosis, a decline in hepatic function should heighten clinical suspicion for the development of HCC. However, a lack of known chronic liver disease at presentation does not preclude the possibility of HCC. Many patients with HCC have cirrhosis as their initial presentation.

The history obtained should ask about past events concerning for hepatic decompensation, including prior variceal bleeding, hepatic encephalopathy, or increased abdominal girth associated with ascites. Social history should evaluate the use of alcohol and/or tobacco products, with emphasis on quantity and duration of use. A family history of HCC should also be documented.

SIGNS AND SYMPTOMS

The clinical presentation of HCC varies considerably and is often dependent on the degree of hepatic reserve. Many patients are asymptomatic at the time of diagnosis or have their tumors incidentally discovered on imaging done for unrelated reasons. Given that most patients with HCC have concomitant cirrhosis, the first manifestation of HCC can be hepatic decompensation, such as jaundice, hepatic encephalopathy, or ascites.

The most common symptoms on initial presentation include abdominal pain, weight loss, weakness, ascites, and jaundice.

PHYSICAL EXAMINATION

On physical examination the stigmata of cirrhosis or portal hypertension should be noted, such as ascites, hepatomegaly, splenomegaly, or periumbilical varices. The sclerae and oral cavity should be examined for jaundice.

Paraneoplastic syndromes are rare in HCC. Hypoglycemia may be noted early in the disease from a defect in processing of preinsulin-like growth factor by the hepatocytes and polycythemia may be noted due to synthesis of erythropoietin by the hepatocytes.

DIFFERENTIAL DIAGNOSIS

In patients with known cirrhosis, chronic HBV, or chronic HCV infection who present with a new liver mass on imaging, HCC is the diagnosis of choice until proved otherwise. Other primary malignant and benign tumors of the liver can mimic the radiologic findings of HCC and include intrahepatic cholangiocarcinoma, hepatic adenoma, hepatic hemangioma, and focal nodular hyperplasia of the liver.

DIAGNOSTIC STUDIES

HCC can be diagnosed in most cases without the need for a biopsy if characteristic radiologic features are present in the appropriate imaging studies. These imaging studies consist of either contrast-enhanced CT or MRI, consisting of unenhanced, arterial, venous, and delayed phase images.

Lesions <1 cm are thought to have a higher likelihood of being dysplastic nodules rather than HCC and repeat imaging should be done in 3 to 6 months to monitor growth or change.

There is currently no role for PET imaging to either aid in the diagnosis or staging of HCC; if concerned about metastatic disease, a bone scan, chest CT, and/or MRI of the head is indicated.

In the past alpha fetoprotein (AFP) level >200 ng/mL and a mass on cross-sectional imaging was sufficient for the diagnosis of HCC. AFP can be elevated in patients with intrahepatic cholangiocarcinoma and/or hepatic metastases from other malignancies such as gastric cancer.

EVALUATION

The initial evaluation of a patient with possible HCC should include a CBC, liver function tests, basic metabolic profile, coagulation panel, hepatitis serologies, and AFP. AFP is obtained at baseline as prognostic marker and can be used to assess response to treatment.

Imaging studies consisting of either contrast-enhanced CT or MRI should also be obtained.

TREATMENT

- The initial therapy for HCC is based on tumor characteristics, underlying liver function, and the overall performance status of the patient.
- Patients with a single focus of HCC, preserved liver function, and a good overall performance status should undergo surgical resection of the lesion consisting of a partial hepatectomy.
- Liver transplant should be considered in patients with multifocal disease consisting of three or fewer lesions <3 cm, or a solitary lesion <5 cm.
- Percutaneous ablation techniques are indicated in patients with either a single focus of HCC or three or fewer nodules anatomically eligible for liver transplantation, but with comorbidities excluding them for surgical resection or transplantation.
- Patients with advanced stage HCC with a good performance score and preserved liver function are treated with systemic chemotherapy, which includes sorafenib, a multikinase inhibitor. Common adverse effects of sorafenib include fatigue, diarrhea, and hand-foot syndrome.
- Many patients present with end -stage HCC, for which no treatment options are available. In these cases, supportive care, including pain management and palliative care service, is indicated.

- The recurrence rate following surgical resection for early stage HCC approaches 70% over a 5-year period. Recurrences in the first 2 years following resection are most likely secondary to metastases via vascular transit from the original tumor location, while recurrences following 2 years are secondary to new lesions that occur due to a defect in the liver parenchyma due to cirrhosis.

PATIENT EDUCATION

- Surveillance for HCC should be offered to patients who have >1.5% risk per year of developing HCC.[37] At-risk groups should be screened with abdominal ultrasound every 6 to 12 months.
- Survival and recurrence are linked to treatment and disease stage.

KEY POINTS

- Alcohol, tobacco, and human papillomavirus infection are risk factors for squamous cell carcinoma of the esophagus; Barrett esophagus due to chronic reflux is a risk factor for adenocarcinoma of the esophagus.
- *Helicobacter pylori* infection is a risk factor for some stomach cancers, the initial symptoms of gastric cancer are nonspecific and often resemble those of peptic ulcer disease.
- Colorectal cancer is one of the most common cancers. Right-sided lesions usually manifest with bleeding and anemia; left-sided lesions usually manifest with obstructive symptoms.
- Routine screening for colon cancer should begin at age 50 for patients with average risk; typical methods involve colonoscopy or annual FOBT and/or flexible sigmoidoscopy.
- Pancreatic cancer is highly lethal.
- Pancreatic cancer is treated with a Whipple procedure when surgery is feasible and adjuvant chemotherapy and radiation therapy.
- HCC is usually a complication of cirrhosis and is most common where hepatitis B is prevalent.
- Diagnosis of HCC is based on the AFP level and liver imaging results.
- Prevention of HCC involves use of the hepatitis B vaccine and management of disorders that can cause cirrhosis.

7.5 BREAST CANCER

Breast cancer is the most common cancer in women in the developed world. In 2018, there were about 266,000 new cases of breast cancer and over 40,000 deaths.[1] In women breast cancer is the second leading cause of cancer deaths. There has been a slight decrease in the incidence of breast cancer which is in line with the decrease in use of hormone replacement therapy and improved screening of the disease.

OVERVIEW

Most breast malignancies arise from epithelial elements and are categorized as carcinomas. Breast carcinomas are a diverse group of lesions that differ in microscopic appearance and biologic behavior, although these disorders are often discussed as a single disease. There are several types of breast cancer.

The noninvasive breast cancers include ductal carcinoma in situ (DCIS) and lobular carcinoma in situ (LCIS). This distinction is primarily based upon the growth pattern and cytologic features of the lesions.

The invasive breast carcinomas consist of several histologic subtypes, listed below, along with their incidence.[38]

- Infiltrating ductal: 76%
- Invasive lobular: 8%
- Ductal/lobular: 7%
- Mucinous (colloid): 2.4%
- Tubular: 1.5%
- Medullary: 1.2%
- Papillary: 1%

Other subtypes include metaplastic breast cancer and invasive micropapillary breast cancer, which account for <5% of cases.

EPIDEMIOLOGY

The lifetime risk for breast cancer in the United States is 1 in 8 (12%) with a 1 in 35 (3%) chance of dying from breast cancer.[39] The United States has the highest annual incidence rates of breast cancer in the world. It is the most common cancer and the second-most common cause of cancer death, after lung cancer, in women.[1]

PATHOPHYSIOLOGY

DCIS refers to malignant ductal cells that are confined in the ducts of the breast and have broken through the basement membrane to become invasive. These lesions do not have metastatic potential, but they do have the potential to become invasive. DCIS lesions also have the common tumor markers associated with invasive breast cancers, estrogen, and progesterone receptors. If DCIS is not surgically treated, there is significant risk of developing an invasive cancer in the area.

LCIS arises in the terminal duct lobular unit and may spread into the ducts; the basement membrane is intact, and the cells fill more than half of the lumen.

Breast cancer is not one disease but includes several types of cancer. In the past, classification was based on histologic features, but more recently molecular or genetic factors have replaced older definitions.

Breast cancers are commonly sensitive to hormones. Approximately 80% of breast cancers are found to have estrogen and/or progesterone receptors.[40] HER2 was initially described in the 1980s and was shown to be associated with a more aggressive form of breast cancer. Approximately 13% of breast cancers do not express estrogen or progesterone receptors and are HER2 normal.[40]

MEDICAL HISTORY AND CLINICAL PRESENTATION

The risk of getting breast cancer appears to be linked to both inherited and environmental factors with the latter having the greater impact for many women.

The Gail Model is used to assess the risk of getting breast cancer. The Gail Model uses the following features: age of menarche, age of first childbirth, family history, history of prior breast biopsies, and age.

For women with an increased risk (Gail Model score >1.67% 5-year risk) of getting breast cancer are often recommended to undergo risk reduction strategies, including chemoprevention.[41] Studies of tamoxifen, raloxifene, and the aromatase inhibitor exemestane have all shown that the incidence of breast

TABLE 7.9 Risk Factors for Breast Cancer

Strong Risk Factor (Risk >4X normal)	Moderate Risk Factor (Risk 2–4X normal)	Weak Risk Factor (Risk 1–2X normal)
Advancing age	Over 30 years old at birth of first child	Early menarche (before age 12)
Female gender	Past breast biopsy with any signs of cell abnormality or hyperplasia	Late menopause (after age 54)
Previous breast cancer diagnosis	Postmenopausal obesity (high BMI)	Alcohol: moderate to heavy alcohol consumption
Increased bone density	Chest wall radiation (strong risk factor if in last 10 years)	Prolonged hormone replacement therapy, particularly with both estrogen and progesterone
BRCA mutations or family history with premenopausal or bilateral breast cancer		Family history of breast cancer if affected relatives were older or postmenopausal and not *BRCA* mutation carrier

BMI, body mass index.

cancer can safely be reduced in women with an increased risk of developing breast cancer.[42]

Other risk factors are listed in Table 7.9.

SIGNS AND SYMPTOMS

DCIS is usually asymptomatic and identified first with an abnormal mammogram. It will rarely present as a palpable mass, but spontaneous nipple discharge that is bloody, pink tinged, clear, or serous in nature may be a presenting symptom. LCIS is usually asymptomatic and will be found as an incidental finding on biopsy of the breast for other findings.

Breast cancer may present with signs and symptoms or may present asymptomatically as an abnormal imaging finding. Approximately half of all breast cancers in the United States present as palpable masses. Most patients with early breast cancer are asymptomatic other than a possible mass.

Other findings include new thickening, redness, swelling, heat, or a rash. Any change in the breast should be considered as suspicious. If the patient is premenopausal there may be breast changes related to her menstrual cycle and a re-examination at a different time in her cycle may be indicated. Nodal areas should be examined, and this should include the axillae as well as the supra- and infraclavicular areas.

PHYSICAL EXAMINATION

Patients with breast cancer usually are generally well appearing. Physical examination of patients with breast cancer is usually remarkable for a lump in the breast, peau d'orange, an inverted nipple. Nipple discharge may be noted, and lymphadenopathy may be noted in the axilla and supra- and infraclavicular areas.

DIFFERENTIAL DIAGNOSIS

Breast cancer must be differentiated from other diseases such as cysts and inflammatory and noninflammatory solid lumps. Breast symptoms such as nipple discharge and mastalgia should be investigated as well. Nipple discharge can be due to papilloma, duct ectasia, and infection.

DIAGNOSTIC STUDIES

Mammography is the first step in the screening and evaluation of breast mass. On mammography a cancer often

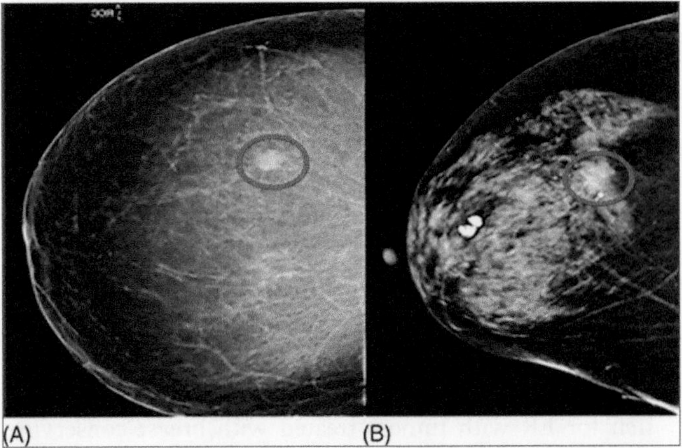

Figure 7.7 A breast cancer lesion (circle), note the calcification. *(Source: Campassi C, Ho L, Galandak J, et al. Breast imaging: breast cancer screening, diagnosis, staging, and surveillance. In: Tkaczuk KHR, Kesmodel SB, Feigenberg SJ, eds.* Handbok of Breast Cancer and Related Breast Disease. *Springer Publishing Company; 2016, Fig. 1.3.)*

appears as a cluster of calcifications or as structural abnormalities. With mammographic screening, about 84% of breast cancers in women over the age of 50 and 75% of cancers in women age 46 to 50 will be diagnosed by mammography.[43] If the screening mammogram suggests changes that may be malignant, diagnostic mammograms are done to provide further views of the breast (Figure 7.7).

Ultrasound may be used to assess if a mass or abnormality is cystic or solid. Lesions that look like simple cysts are rarely malignant. Complex cysts or solid lesions require further diagnosis.

MRI is recommended in women with a high risk of breast cancer such as *BRCA* mutation carriers and when other imaging such as mammogram and ultrasound are not conclusive.

An abnormality noted on mammography, MRI, or ultrasound that is suspicious of cancer should be biopsied with a core biopsy, which can establish the diagnosis and give further information that is necessary for treatment planning.

For patients presenting with nipple discharge, a ductogram can be performed to identify the area of tumor, which is seen as a filling defect in the duct or a cutoff filling of the duct with contrast, or a narrowing of the duct.

Because needle biopsy provides only a sample of the mammographic abnormality, excision of the lesion will provide the final confirmation of the lesion. The pathology examination will characterize the histology, nuclear grade, and evidence of necrosis as well as the size of the involved area and margin width on resected specimens.

EVALUATION

Regardless of whether the cancer is diagnosed by mammogram or physical examination, a tissue diagnosis is necessary. This is done via a radiologically guided biopsy done by ultrasound, mammogram, or MRI.

Estrogen receptor (ER) status should be obtained on all in situ and invasive cancers. Progesterone and HER2 status are done on invasive cancers.

A single standard for the clinical staging of breast cancer is not available. MRI can be used in staging as it will identify multifocal cancers and the extent of the local disease, enabling better surgical planning.

Although PET scans may be helpful in staging high-grade cancers, its role in lower grade breast cancers and lobular cancers is questioned. Currently PET scans are not recommended for staging in most cases.

Bone scans should be considered in patients with stages II and III cancer as the bones are the most common site of advanced disease.

TREATMENT

- DCIS may be treated with breast conserving surgery or mastectomy with or without immediate reconstruction. For DCIS treated with breast conserving surgery, radiation is indicated in most circumstances to reduce risk of local recurrence. Current guidelines recommend tamoxifen for ER with tumors treated with breast conserving surgery. The benefit of tamoxifen for ER negative tumors is uncertain.
- LCIS confers risk for breast cancer in both breasts. Local resection after a core needle biopsy showing LCIS is warranted to confirm the diagnosis of LCIS only and to rule out DCIS or invasive cancer. Radiation post excision is not indicated. Tamoxifen and raloxifene, selective ER modulators, block the effects of endogenous estrogen and are used as chemoprevention. Both are approved for breast cancer prevention in premenopausal women.
- Surgery remains the primary treatment of breast cancer. The primary surgery is removal of the tumor and surrounding tissue to ensure clear margins. This may be done by breast conserving surgery such as a lumpectomy or partial mastectomy, or by removal of the entire breast with a mastectomy.
- All invasive cancers should be assessed for ER and progesterone receptor status. Patients with endocrine sensitive tumors should be considered for hormone treatment.
- Because of the differences in the endocrine axis, hormonal therapy recommendations depend on the menopausal status of the woman. In premenopausal women, tamoxifen is the mainstay of treatment. In postmenopausal women tamoxifen along with aromatase inhibitors are used as hormonal therapy. Chemotherapy is used for the treatment of breast cancer in the adjuvant setting and along with endocrine therapy has improved survival. Chemotherapy agents used include taxanes and anthracyclines.
- Radiation is given to further decrease the risk of the cancer recurring locally but has also been shown to improve survival. Radiation may be given to the breast only, or to breast and regional lymph nodes. Postmastectomy radiation is indicated if the tumor is >5 cm, margins are positive, or there are involved lymph nodes.

PATIENT EDUCATION

- DCIS is curable and the prognosis is excellent. Because it is noninvasive, the tumor does not have the capacity to spread distantly.
- For patients with DCIS treated with breast conserving surgery with or without radiation, follow-up consists of breast exam every 6 months and mammogram of the ipsilateral breast every 6 months for 3 years to assess changes from surgical scarring and radiation; when changes are stable the frequency can be decreased to yearly.
- LCIS is a risk factor for the development of subsequent breast cancer in either breast. This risk can be reduced by endocrine systemic therapy, with tamoxifen for premenopausal women, and tamoxifen, raloxifene, or exemestane for postmenopausal women.
- For patients who elect observation with or without chemoprevention, enhanced surveillance is planned. This includes physical exam and breast imaging at 6-month intervals. Bilateral mammograms should be performed annually.
- The survival of patients with early breast cancer has improved greatly. The 5-year survival rate for early localized breast cancer is 99% and 90% for invasive disease.

KEY POINTS

- Breast cancer is the second leading cause of cancer death in women.
- Screen women by doing clinical breast examination, mammography (beginning at age 50 and often at age 40), and, for women at high risk, MRI.
- For most women, treatment requires surgical removal, lymph node sampling, hormone therapy or chemotherapy, and radiation therapy.
- Hormone therapy, such as tamoxifen, is recommended if tumors have hormone receptors.

7.6 GYNECOLOGIC CANCER

OVERVIEW

The gynecologic cancers include cervical, ovarian, uterine (endometrial), and vaginal/vulvar malignancies. The three major malignancies—cervical, ovarian, endometrial—are generally asymptomatic early in the disease process and only develop signs and symptoms as the disease progresses. These three may spread by direct extension to surrounding organs or via the lymphatic system.

There are over 110,000 new gynecologic cancers per year in the United States and over 32,000 deaths.[1] The gynecologic cancer with the highest incidence is uterine cancer, ovarian cancer is a distant second, and cervical cancer is third. Vaginal cancer and vulvar cancer are uncommon.

EPIDEMIOLOGY

Cervical cancer occurs most often in women over 30 years of age. Over the past 40 years, the number of deaths from cervical cancer has decreased by 65% because of regular

Pap tests, but over 13,000 women are diagnosed with cervical cancer annually.[1] Women age 40 to 44 years have the highest incidence of cervical cancer.

Ovarian cancer, which affects 20,000 individuals annually, is the tenth most common type of cancer and the fifth leading cause of cancer death among women.[1] All women are at risk for ovarian cancer, 90% of cases occur in women age >40 years, but the greatest incidence is in those over age 60.[1] The lifetime risk of ovarian cancer is as high as 60% in women who carry the *BRCA* gene.[1]

Cancer of the uterus usually occurs in women who are going through menopause or are postmenopausal. Endometrial cancer is the fourth most common gynecologic cancer and each year, 63,230 U.S. women are diagnosed with uterine cancer.[1] Women age 65 to 69 years have the highest incidence of this type of cancer.

PATHOPHYSIOLOGY

Gynecologic cancers spread via direct extension to surrounding organs, metastasis through the lymphatic system, typically via the pelvic or para-aortic lymph nodes, or via the hematogenous route. Ovarian cancer may spread through the peritoneum through the peritoneal fluid.

Endometrial cancer is associated with a positive family history or factors that increase the patient's exposure to estrogen. Obesity, polycystic ovary syndrome, hereditary nonpolyposis colorectal cancer, and exposure to tamoxifen are risk factors related to increased estrogen exposure.

Cervical cancer is the most preventable and secondary to unfavorable behaviors including smoking, multiple sexual partners, and unprotected sexual activity. Human papilloma virus (HPV) is linked to almost all cases of cervical cancer. HPV invades the epithelial cells via microtrauma and replicates in a nonlytic manner. This nonlytic manner does not cause the release of proinflammatory agents and allows for persistent infection and the development of precancerous lesions. Smoking leads to metaplasia of the cervical cells; nicotine has been found on cervical cells, and has caused damage to the cellular DNA, producing instability of the cervical epithelium.

The etiology of most cases of ovarian cancer remains unclear. One theory is based on the idea that an increasing number of ovulations or proliferations of the ovary epithelium leads to increased abnormal cell repair and mutations, which lead to the formation of cancer cells. Chronic inflammation from exposure to talc or asbestos has been linked to cancer development. The tumor suppressor genes *BRAC1* and *BRCA2* are linked to the development of ovarian carcinoma.

7.6A CERVICAL CANCER

Cervical cancer is highly preventable, is an uncommon cancer in the United States, and makes up 4.8% of all cancer deaths in females.[1] Persistent HPV infection is responsible for most cervical cancer cases, and cervical cancer typically follows the development of preinvasive cervical lesions. Cervical screening programs have resulted in the detection and treatment of preinvasive lesions, which has led to a dramatic decrease in the incidence of invasive cervical cancer.

HPV is a group of >200 viruses, of which 40 are spread through direct sexual contact. Several HPV types cause genital warts and a dozen HPV types cause certain types of cancer—cervical, anal, oropharyngeal, penile, vulvar, and vaginal.

The currently used vaccine is Gardasilt 9. Gardasil 9 prevents infection with HPV types 16 and 18, which cause 70% of cervical cancers.[44] Gardasil also prevents infection with HPV types 6 and 11, which cause most genital warts. Gardasil also prevents infection cancer-causing types (31, 33, 45, 52, and 58).

Current immunization recommendations include[45]:

- All children 9 to 14 years of age should get two HPV vaccine shots 6 to 12 months apart. If the two shots are given <5 months apart, a third shot will be needed.
- HPV vaccine is recommended for young women through age 26, and young men through age 21.
- Adolescents who get their first dose at age 15 or older need three doses of vaccine given at 0, 1–2 months, and 6 months.
- Persons who have completed a valid series with any HPV vaccine do not need any additional doses.

The vaccines do not prevent other sexually transmitted diseases, nor do they treat existing HPV infections or HPV-caused disease.

Cervical cancer generally has a favorable prognosis as it is often detected at an early stage and is effectively treated with surgery or chemoradiation. Advanced stage disease is highly treatable with chemotherapy and radiation, with a 5-year survival rate of about 50% in stage III disease.[46]

HPV DNA is detected in nearly all cervical cancers of both squamous and adenocarcinoma histology. While there are hundreds of HPV strains, HPV-16 and HPV-18 have been most commonly associated with squamous cell carcinoma and adenocarcinoma, respectively. HPV carcinogenesis is mediated through its oncogenes E6 and E7.

Most cervical cancer is squamous cell, followed by adenocarcinoma, which is increasing in incidence. This may be related to the decreased ability of Pap smears to detect adenocarcinomas and upper cervical lesions. Clear cell carcinoma, a rare form of cervical adenocarcinomas, has been linked with prenatal exposure to diethylstilbestrol (DES), a drug that was used to prevent miscarriages in the 1940s and 1950s.

MEDICAL HISTORY AND CLINICAL PRESENTATION

Most cervical cancers are a result of persistent HPV infection. Risk factors for increased exposure to HPV include first coitus at a young age, multiple sexual partners, history of other sexually transmitted diseases, contraceptive use, and high parity.

SIGNS AND SYMPTOMS

Most early stage cervical cancer is asymptomatic and is typically diagnosed following an abnormal Pap smear. Women with early stage cancer sometimes complain of watery vaginal discharge or postcoital spotting. Advanced cervical cancer almost always has some form of abnormal vaginal bleeding and may present with symptoms related to the local spread of disease. This includes unilateral or bilateral ureteral obstruction and lower extremity swelling from deep venous thrombosis. The classic triad of findings with advanced cervical cancer is sciatic pain, leg swelling, and hydronephrosis. Patients sometimes present with malodorous vaginal discharge from large necrotic cervical tumors or fistulas.

PHYSICAL EXAMINATION

Most women with cervical cancer are asymptomatic at the early stage of disease. Patients in advance stage of cancer may have such symptoms as abnormal vaginal bleeding, vaginal discharge, abdominal and pelvic pain, and urinary hesitancy. Physical examination in late cervical cancer is usually remarkable for cervical mass, pallor, and pedal edema.

DIFFERENTIAL DIAGNOSIS

Cervical cancer must be differentiated from other diseases that cause abnormal vaginal bleeding, such as cervical polyps, cervical leiomyoma, and invasion from endometrial cancer, vaginal cancer, cervical lymphoma, or cervical ectopic pregnancy.

DIAGNOSTIC STUDIES

Diagnosis is typically made during routine screening with Pap smear. Stage I cancers are confined to the cervix and if not clinically visible are stage IA and only detected microscopically by colposcopy or cervical biopsy. Any tumor confined to the cervix that is clinically visible is considered stage IB.

Stage II lesions are those that extend beyond the cervix (excluding the uterus) but not to the pelvic sidewall or lower third of the vagina. Parametrium may be involved and is assessed by a rectovaginal examination.

Tumors involving the lower third of the vagina without extension to the sidewall are considered stage IIIA while tumors that extend to the pelvic sidewall or result in hydronephrosis or a nonfunctioning kidney are considered stage IIIB. Extension to the pelvic sidewall is determined by pelvic and rectovaginal exam.

Tumor that extends beyond the pelvis into adjacent mucosa of the bowel or bladder is considered stage IVA disease. Biopsy by cystoscopy or proctoscopy is required for confirmation of diagnosis. Patients may present with hematuria. Disease spread to other distant organs is considered stage IVB.

Patients with stage IB or greater disease should be evaluated with additional imaging. Chest x-ray should be obtained if extrapelvic disease is confirmed.

A combined PET-CT is the most sensitive way of identifying suspicious lymph nodes. PET-CT is more sensitive for the detection of positive nodes and is preferred over CT alone if it is available. MRI is indicated for tumors high in the endocervix. MRI aids in the differentiation between uterine and cervical primary lesions, which may be managed differently.

EVALUATION

Cervical cancer is definitively diagnosed by cervical biopsy and the imaging studies noted above are used for staging of disease.

TREATMENT

- Treatment recommendations for cervical cancer are primarily based on clinical stage and assessment of nodal involvement.
- Surgery, abdominal or vaginal hysterectomy, is generally reserved for women with lower stage disease and smaller lesions (IA, IB, and selected IIA). Oophorectomy is not routinely indicated unless there is an adenocarcinoma, in which case removal of the ovaries should be considered. Women who wish to maintain fertility or who are poor surgical candidates could be treated with cone biopsy and careful surveillance.
- Chemoradiation is the preferred treatment for women with stage IB–IVB disease.
- Radiation therapy may be administered as intracavitary brachytherapy and/or external beam radiation therapy (EBRT). EBRT is often combined with chemotherapy. Systemic chemotherapy is used as primary treatment for women with stage IVB or recurrent disease. Systemic chemotherapy consists of cisplatin (with gemcitabine, topotecan, or paclitaxel).

PATIENT EDUCATION

- Radiation and surgery yield cure rates of 92% for patients with early stage disease.[46]
- Radiation therapy plus concurrent chemotherapy is the treatment of choice for patients with locally advanced disease.
- Overall 5-year survival is based on various stages[46]:
  - Localized: 92%
  - Regional: 56%
  - Distant: 17%
  - All stages: 66%

7.6B OVARIAN CANCER

Ovarian cancer is less common than cervical and endometrial cancer but causes more deaths in the United States than cervical and endometrial malignancies combined. There are no known effective screening tests for ovarian cancer, symptoms are nonspecific, and many patients present with advanced disease.

Epithelial cancers of the ovaries, including serous, mucinous, endometrioid, and clear cell adenocarcinoma, account for about 90% of ovarian cancers.[1] The rest are stromal, including granulosa and Sertoli-Leydig tumors; and germ-cell, including dysgerminoma, endodermal sinus tumors, malignant teratoma, and embryonal carcinoma tumors.

The major risk factors for the development of ovarian cancer are a positive family history of ovarian cancer and genetic predisposition. Most women with a genetic basis for ovarian cancer have either *BRCA1* or *BRCA2* genetic abnormalities.

The definitive pathophysiology associated with the development of ovarian cancer remains to be identified.

MEDICAL HISTORY AND CLINICAL PRESENTATION

Ovarian cancer should be considered in any woman presenting with at least moderately severe, but nonspecific abdominal/pelvic pain or bloating lasting several weeks.

Other possible risk factors include a personal history of infertility, breast cancer, and prolonged use of post-menopausal hormone replacement. Multiple pregnancies, premenopausal use of oral contraceptives, undergoing a bilateral tubal ligation, or prophylactic oophorectomies in the postmenopausal period have been shown to decrease the risk of ovarian cancer.

SIGNS AND SYMPTOMS

Ovarian cancer is called the silent killer because symptoms do not develop until the end-stage disease is present. Patients with advanced disease present with acute symptoms such as dyspnea secondary to pleural effusion, nausea and vomiting secondary to bowel obstruction, pain and swelling in the lower extremities secondary to venous thromboembolism. Patients with early, late, or advanced disease present with subacute symptoms such as abdominal pain, abdominal bloating and distention, early satiety, increased urinary urgency and frequency, pelvic pain and pressure, abdominal or pelvic mass, fatigue, weight loss, abnormal vaginal bleeding, and painful intercourse.

PHYSICAL EXAMINATION

Physical examination findings vary but may include a palpable adnexal mass, fluid wave due to ascites, decreased breath sounds due to the presence of a pleural effusion, and high-pitched bowel sounds due to a bowel obstruction.

DIFFERENTIAL DIAGNOSIS

The differential diagnosis for ovarian cancer includes tubo-ovarian abscess, ectopic pregnancy, salpingitis, fallopian tube carcinoma, leiomyoma, pregnancy, diverticular abscess, colorectal cancer, and bladder cancer.

DIAGNOSTIC STUDIES

The standard workup for a woman suspected of having ovarian cancer includes the performance of a CT scan of the abdomen and pelvis to document the presence of a pelvic mass and reveal the extent of intraperitoneal and extraperitoneal tumor spread.

The serum CA-125 antigen level is often obtained but is not specific for ovarian cancer. However, because most patients with advanced ovarian cancer will have an elevated serum level of this tumor antigen, the finding of a normal serum value would suggest the possibility of a nonovarian site in a patient with radiographic findings highly suggestive of malignant disease.

EVALUATION

The evaluation includes laboratory studies; imaging studies such as CT scan, MRI, or ultrasound; and surgical exploration to make the definite diagnosis. Routine lab work includes a CBC, metabolic profile, and tumor markers. Tumor markers include CA-125 for epithelial ovarian cancer and alpha-fetoprotein and hCG for germ cell ovarian cancer.

TREATMENT

- Surgical exploration is essential for staging and selection of best treatment options. Even in the setting of regionally advanced disease, standard initial treatment for epithelial ovarian cancer includes an attempt at maximal surgical cytoreduction. Platinum-based combination chemotherapy, carboplatin and paclitaxel or docetaxel, is administered after surgical cytoreduction.
- While a large majority of patients with advanced ovarian cancer will respond to platinum-based chemotherapy, recurrence of the disease process is common. For recurrence >6 to 12 months following the completion of platinum-based therapy, reintroduction of a platinum regimen is the accepted treatment.

PATIENT EDUCATION

- Ovarian cancer is a highly chemotherapy-sensitive malignancy. Patients with advanced intra-abdominal disease or spread outside the abdominal cavity will achieve symptomatic benefit and long-term disease-free survival.
- With disease recurrence or disease that has not achieved a clinically defined complete response to primary chemotherapy, there is no second-line strategy that has legitimate curative intent. The 5-year stage-specific survival rates for invasive epithelial ovarian cancer are localized disease 92%, regional 76%, distant 30%, and all stages 47%.[47]

7.6C ENDOMETRIAL CANCER

Endometrial carcinoma is the most common gynecologic malignancy of the female reproductive tract. Endometrial cancer usually occurs in postmenopausal women with a median age at the time of diagnosis of 61 years. Women have a 2.5% lifetime risk of developing endometrial cancer, which accounts for 7% of all cancers in women.[1] Mortality is almost twofold higher in the African American population. There are two clinical-pathologic types of endometrial cancer. Type I is an estrogen-dependent endometrial carcinoma that is associated with excess estrogen stimulation, and includes obesity, polycystic ovary syndrome, diabetes mellitus, unopposed estrogen replacement therapy, and the use of tamoxifen. Type II is an estrogen-independent carcinoma that is aggressive and has an overall poor prognosis.

MEDICAL HISTORY AND CLINICAL PRESENTATION

Vaginal bleeding in postmenopausal women is the most common symptom of uterine cancer. Patients may present with a watery blood-tinged discharge. Other symptoms include dyspareunia, dysuria, pelvic pain, abdominal bloating, and constipation.

SIGNS AND SYMPTOMS

Most patients with endometrial cancer present with abnormal vaginal bleeding. Asymptomatic women with endometrial carcinoma are identified during cervical cancer screening when atypical endometrial cells are noted. Early symptoms include abnormal menstrual periods, metrorrhagia in premenopausal women, most menopausal bleeding, and postcoital bleeding. Advanced symptoms include polyuria and dysuria, pelvic pain and dyspareunia, and fatigue and weight loss.

PHYSICAL EXAMINATION

Physical examination in endometrial cancer reveals vaginal bleeding, pallor, and possibly pedal edema. Early in disease physical examination may be normal. In advanced stages of the disease the patient may appear lethargic, pale, and confused. Regional lymphadenopathy may be present. On abdominal examination the uterus may be enlarged, and ascites may be present.

DIFFERENTIAL DIAGNOSIS

Several other conditions can present with abnormal bleeding. They include menorrhagia, anovulation in a premenopausal or a perimenopausal patient, polycystic ovary syndrome or endocrinopathies that affect ovulation such as hypothyroidism or hyperthyroidism, hyperprolactinemia, and Cushing syndrome.

There are also several anatomic causes of vaginal bleeding that can mimic endometrial cancer. These include uterine polyps, leiomyomas, arteriovenous malformations, endometritis, and pelvic inflammatory disease.

DIAGNOSTIC STUDIES

Endometrial biopsy will establish the diagnosis of endometrial cancer. Surgical staging must be done to aid in determining prognosis and treatment. The standard surgical approach includes a total abdominal hysterectomy, bilateral salpingo-oophorectomy with or without lymph node dissection, and peritoneal washings. Laparoscopy and robotic-assisted surgery are alternatives to the traditional procedure. Endometrial carcinoma is staged according to the International Federation of Gynecology and Obstetrics (FIGO) system.

CT, MRI, and PET are used in the staging of endometrial carcinoma, as imaging studies help differentiate between organ-confined or locally advanced disease. Imaging studies are not a substitute for surgical staging.

EVALUATION

A complete history and physical examination should be obtained and the presence of hereditary or acquired coagulopathies should be noted. A review of current medications should be completed and document the use of anticoagulant, antiplatelet, and nonsteroidal anti-inflammatory medications.

Initial laboratory tests include a CBC plus differential, chemistry profile, coagulation profile including prothrombin time/international normalized ratio (PT/INR), partial thromboplastin time (PTT), thrombin time, serum D-dimers, and fibrinogen level. Endometrial biopsy is the test of choice, and staging of the carcinoma is completed during surgical procedures.

TREATMENT

- Treatment of uterine bleeding should be undertaken to stabilize the patient. Various methods to treat bleeding include intrauterine tamponade, uterine curettage, high-dose IV estrogen, uterine artery embolization, high-dose oral estrogen, high-dose oral contraceptives, high-dose progestins, tranexamic acid, and endometrial ablation.
- Surgery, radiation therapy, hormone therapy, and chemotherapy are used either alone or sequentially to treat endometrial carcinoma depending on disease stage and histologic grade.
- The standard surgical approach includes a total abdominal hysterectomy, bilateral salpingo-oophorectomy with or without lymph node dissection, and peritoneal washings.
- Radiation therapy consists of EBRT and intravaginal irradiation.
- Chemotherapy, cisplatin with platinum and taxanes, is often used in conjunction with radiation therapy for first-line treatment of women with advanced disease (stage III) after initial surgery. In patients who have distant or visceral disease chemotherapy alone is often used.
- The stage of the malignancy directs the treatment.
    - Stage I is typically observation or vaginal brachytherapy with or without external radiation.
    - Stage II is treated with vaginal brachytherapy and/or pelvic radiation therapy.
    - Stage III treatment consists of chemotherapy with or without radiation therapy or tumor directed radiation therapy.
    - Stage IV is chemotherapy, hormonal therapy, and radiation therapy.

PATIENT EDUCATION

- The most important prognostic factors at diagnosis are stage, grade, depth of invasive disease, and histologic subtype. The 5-year survival rate is stage dependent[48]:
    - Localized: 95%
    - Regional: 69%
    - Distant: 17%
    - All stages: 81%
- Caucasian women have a higher survival rate than non-White patients at each disease stage.

KEY POINTS

- Ovarian cancer affects mostly postmenopausal and perimenopausal women; nulliparity, delayed childbearing, early menarche, and delayed menopause increase risk.
- If cervical cancer is suspected, ultrasound is done first, then measure tumor markers (CA-125), and surgically stage tumors.
- Screen all women for cervical cancer by doing Pap and HPV tests at regular intervals.
- HPV vaccination is recommended for girls and boys.
- Endometrial cancer is one of the most common cancers among women.
- Endometrial sampling is recommended for women with abnormal bleeding, particularly those >40 years.
- Treatment of endometrial cancer is usually total hysterectomy, bilateral salpingo-oophorectomy, lymphadenectomy, and sometimes radiation therapy and/or chemotherapy.

7.7 BONE CANCER

OVERVIEW

Fewer than 0.2% of all cancers are primary bone cancer.[1] It is much more common for bones to be the site of metastasis from other cancers.

There are many different types of bone cancer. The two most common are Ewing sarcoma and osteosarcoma. These occur mainly in children and young adults. Ewing sarcoma can occur in the bone or the soft tissue. Chondrosarcoma is cancer of the cartilage and is more common in adults.

Benign bone tumors do not spread to other tissues and organs and are not usually life threatening and can often be cured with surgery. Types of benign bone tumors include osteoid osteoma, osteoblastoma, enchondroma, and chondromyxoid fibroma.

Bone metastasis is common and noted with breast cancer, prostate cancer, and lung cancer.

EPIDEMIOLOGY

Bone cancer estimates for 2018 are approximately 3,450 new cases and 1,590 deaths from bone cancer.[1] In adults, over 40% of primary bone cancers are chondrosarcomas, followed by osteosarcomas (28%), chordomas (10%), Ewing tumors (8%), and malignant fibrous histiocytoma/fibrosarcoma (4%).[49] In children and teenagers, osteosarcoma (56%) and Ewing sarcoma (34%) are much more common than chondrosarcoma (6%).[49]

PATHOPHYSIOLOGY

Macrophages play a role in tumor growth, dissemination of cancer cells, and metastasis development.

Macrophages can promote inflammation and cytotoxic immune response or downregulate T-cell activity and promote tissue vascularization; both are beneficial to the development of cancer.

The clinical features of conventional osteosarcoma point to an origin in a mesenchymal cell or osteoblasts involved in a metaphyseal endochondral ossification. No unifying genetic alteration has been identified.

7.7A OSTEOSARCOMA

Osteosarcoma is the most common malignant bone tumor in children and adolescents. About 900 new cases of osteosarcoma are diagnosed in the United States each year, with >400 being diagnosed in the pediatric population.[50] Osteosarcoma makes up <1% of all cancers diagnosed in the United States each year.[1]

The most common primary tumor site of origin is the femur, followed by the tibia, humerus, fibula, pelvis, scapula, and jaw.

Between 10% and 20% of patients will have metastatic disease at presentation, most commonly to the lung. The presence of metastatic disease at presentation is a poor prognostic sign decreasing overall survival from 70% to below 20%.[51]

Spontaneous development is the most common clinical scenario for the development of osteosarcoma. Other risk factors include exposure to ionizing radiation and alkylator and/or anthracycline based regimens of chemotherapy.

Multiple genetic factors have been associated with osteosarcoma. Osteosarcoma has been shown to be associated with mutations at loci on chromosomes 13q and 18p.

Secondary osteosarcoma can develop following malignant transformation of Paget disease of bone or other benign bone lesions.

MEDICAL HISTORY AND CLINICAL PRESENTATION

Osteosarcoma most commonly presents with pain at the involved primary tumor site that may have been present for 3 or more months prior to the diagnosis. Localized swelling in the involved area can develop. The pain is often worse with activity and is precipitated by minor trauma. Pathologic fracture is an infrequent presenting sign. Pain is reproducible upon palpation.

SIGNS AND SYMPTOMS

Signs and symptoms of the osteosarcoma include pain at site and pain that presents at night or rest. Patient may not have localized swelling and a pathologic fracture may be noted at presentation. If metastatic disease to the lung is present, cough or chest pain may be noted.

PHYSICAL EXAMINATION

Patients present with pain or localized swelling at the primary tumor site, most commonly the femur followed by the tibia and humerus. Pulmonary metastases are found in approximately 10% to 20% of cases at diagnosis.[51] Symptoms of pulmonary metastases include cough, chest pain, and/or hemoptysis in patients with widespread pulmonary disease.

DIFFERENTIAL DIAGNOSIS

Several diseases and conditions can present like osteosarcoma, including osteomyelitis, Ewing sarcoma, chondrosarcoma, benign bone tumors, and soft tissue sarcomas.

DIAGNOSTIC STUDIES

Diagnosis is made by biopsy. Radiograph of the affected area is often sufficient in making the diagnosis of osteosarcoma. The tumor has a characteristic appearance, and the lesion will have a mixed lytic and sclerotic appearance. Osteosarcoma more commonly develops in the metaphysis of long bones, unlike Ewing sarcoma, which more commonly develops in the diaphysis. Periosteal new bone formation with the lifting of the bone cortex is common as is the classic "sunburst" appearance, which refers to radiating calcification at the site of disease (Figure 7.8).

Lactic dehydrogenase (LDH) and serum alkaline phosphatase can be elevated.

A CT scan of the chest is needed to evaluate for pulmonary metastases, a bone scan to evaluate for skeletal metastases, or a PET scan to identify metastatic disease. MRI of the site is essential for evaluating extent of local disease.

TREATMENT

- Treatment is multimodal and includes surgical resection and intensive chemotherapy.
- After diagnosis, patients receive preoperative chemotherapy prior to surgical resection of the primary tumor and metastatic sites. Limb-sparing procedures, surgical

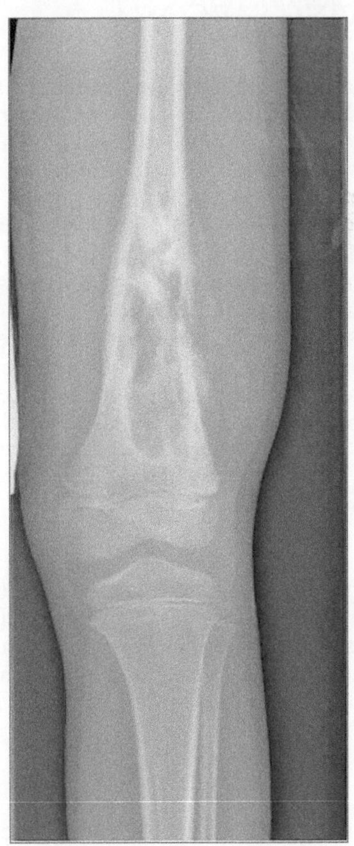

Figure 7.8 Classic x-ray appearance of an osteosarcoma of the distal femur of a skeletally immature patient showing a permeative lesion with a wide zone of transition, cortical destruction with soft tissue extension, and periosteal elevation.

techniques that achieve full tumor resection with negative margins but allow for continued function of the involved limb, is the treatment of choice.

- Preoperative systemic chemotherapy shows a clear benefit in addition to surgery. Patients treated with surgery alone will develop metastatic recurrence in >80% of cases.
  - Chemotherapeutic agents include doxorubicin, cisplatin, and high-dose methotrexate. After surgery, maintenance chemotherapy includes doxorubicin, cisplatin, and high-dose methotrexate.
  - Effective surgical control is essential for cure of osteosarcoma.
- Osteosarcoma is not radiosensitive, and radiation is usually not indicated.
- Metastatic disease at presentation is similarly treated with aggressive chemotherapy and surgical control.

PATIENT EDUCATION

- Patients with a new diagnosis of nonmetastatic osteosarcoma have an overall survival rate of approximately 65% to 70% with conventional therapy.[52]
- Patients with metastatic disease have an overall survival rate between 10% and 20%.[52]
- The most important predictor of overall survival at diagnosis is the presence of metastatic disease at presentation.
- Recurrent osteosarcoma after conventional treatment has a grim prognosis.

7.7B EWING SARCOMA

Ewing sarcoma and primitive neuroectodermal tumors are known as the Ewing sarcoma family of tumors. A majority of the tumors originate in the axial and appendicular skeleton, with a minority of cases arising in the soft tissue.

Almost all the bone and soft tissue tumors of the Ewing sarcoma family of tumors share a translocation, and in 85% to 90% the translocation is t(11:22)(q24;q12).

Most patients are between 14 and 30 years of age at diagnosis but may present at any age.

Ewing sarcoma family of tumors is more common in males (60%) than females (40%) and is rare in people of African or Asian descent compared to Caucasians. The overall incidence for Ewing sarcoma is 0.128 per 100,000 population.[53]

MEDICAL HISTORY AND CLINICAL PRESENTATION

Most commonly there is bone pain, and there may be a mass. The most common site is the pelvis. Typically, pelvic lesions present with pain as the mass would have to be extremely large to be visible or palpable in most patients. Patients with pelvic lesions may also present with symptoms of sciatic nerve pain.

SIGNS AND SYMPTOMS

The most common presentation of Ewing sarcoma includes localized bone pain, swelling, fever, decreased appetite, and weight loss. The patient may present with a fracture from minor trauma, called a pathologic fracture. Diagnosis cannot be certain without a biopsy of the lesion.

PHYSICAL EXAMINATION

Most commonly there is bone pain, and possibly a mass. Sciatic nerve pain may be noted and is described as a burning or searing pain radiating from the back or from and down the back of the leg. Ewing sarcoma and primitive neuroectodermal tumors of the spine or paraspinal soft tissue may present with back pain and possibly neurologic symptoms related to the level of the lesion. Chest wall Ewing sarcoma and primitive neuroectodermal tumors may present as chest wall pain and pleural effusion and most often have an associated rib lesion. Extremity lesions present with pain, and there may be a visible mass or asymmetry between the involved and normal extremity. Patients present with metastatic disease in approximately one-fourth of cases. The most common site of metastasis is the lung, followed by bone and bone marrow.

DIFFERENTIAL DIAGNOSIS

Other tumors in the same site may present with similar symptoms. For example, osteosarcoma may present with bone pain and a mass. Unlike Ewing sarcoma, osteosarcoma almost never presents with systemic symptoms such as fever. Chest wall Ewing sarcoma and primitive neuroectodermal tumors may be mistaken for a pulmonary infection.

Pelvic, vertebral, and extremity lesions may present like osteomyelitis; although osteomyelitis may cause pain, a mass would be uncommon.

DIAGNOSTIC STUDIES

Lab tests are nonspecific and variable and include mild anemia, elevated erythrocyte sedimentation rate (ESR), and elevated LDH.

Imaging is the most important first step toward diagnosis. The first step is a plain x-ray of the site. Periosteal destruction will be noted if there is a bone lesion. In long bones the typical lesion is in the diaphysis. Periosteal reaction, bone destruction, and an associated soft tissue mass are common findings (Figure 7.9). If the plain film is positive, then MRI

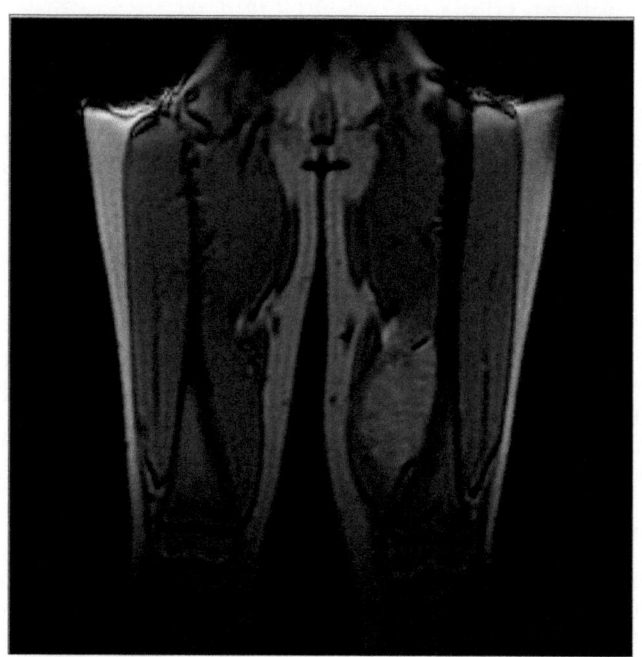

Figure 7.9 MRI of Ewing sarcoma in soft tissue of left thigh in a young female.
(Source: Courtesy of Jim Van Rhee.)

should be obtained. If MRI is not possible, CT with contrast is indicated. If there is no bone lesion on plain film, the next step would also be MRI.

An evaluation for metastasis should include CT of the chest with contrast and a whole-body bone scan and a bone marrow examination. A PET scan should be considered.

The diagnosis must be made by tissue biopsy. Although a diagnosis may be established by a fine needle biopsy, open biopsy is recommended to obtain sufficient tissue.

TREATMENT

- Treatment for Ewing sarcoma and primitive neuroectodermal tumors is several cycles of multiagent chemotherapy, followed by restaging, then local control (either surgery, radiation, or both) and then continuing chemotherapy for up to a year.
- Chemotherapy consists of vincristine, cyclophosphamide, doxorubicin alternating with ifosfamide and etoposide. For metastatic disease treatment consists of the same agents every 2 weeks.
- Although most of the Ewing sarcoma family of tumors are sensitive to radiation, radiation is avoided if complete resection is possible. Radiation can disturb growth, and second malignancies such as osteosarcoma may develop. Radiation is generally reserved for patients with unresectable tumors or those with positive margins after surgery.

PATIENT EDUCATION

- Young patients with localized Ewing sarcoma family of tumors who receive chemotherapy have a 5-year overall survival rate of 88%.[54] Overall relapse rate has been reported to be 80% to 90%.
- For patients with pulmonary metastases from only the Ewing sarcoma family of tumors the survival rate at 5 years is 54%.[54]

KEY POINTS

- Osteosarcoma is the second most common primary bone tumor.
- X-ray of osteosarcoma presents with sclerotic or lytic features and diagnosis is by biopsy.
- Treatment of osteosarcoma includes chemotherapy and surgery.
- Ewing sarcoma diagnosed by biopsy and x-ray reveals multiple layers of subperiosteal reaction (onion-skin appearance).
- Treatment of Ewing sarcoma consists of surgery, chemotherapy, and radiation therapy.

7.8 RENAL CANCER

OVERVIEW

Malignancies of the urinary tract system consist of renal cell carcinoma (RCC), bladder carcinoma, Wilms tumor (WT), and lymphoma. RCC develops in the proximal renal tubules that make up the kidney's filtration system. Transitional cell carcinomas are the most common type of bladder cancer. These cancers start in the transitional cells that line the inside of the bladder. WT is rare but most common in children and is treated with radiation therapy and chemotherapy, while other types of urinary tract malignancies are treated with chemotherapy, radiation therapy, and surgery. Lymphoma is rare and is associated with lymphadenopathy throughout the body. Lymphoma is treated with chemotherapy.

EPIDEMIOLOGY

In 2018, there were approximately 150,000 new cases of urinary tract carcinomas and approximately 33,000 deaths.[1]

7.8A WILMS TUMOR

WT is the most common childhood renal tumor, accounting for about 6% of all childhood malignant disease with approximately 500 new cases diagnosed in the United States each year.[55] Over 66% of cases are diagnosed in children <5 years of age, with equal distribution between males and females.[56]

WT arises from clusters of embryonal kidney cells that persist into childhood. Certain genetic conditions, such as WAGR syndrome and Beckwith-Wiedemann syndrome, are associated with WT.

The clear majority of WT occur sporadically. Approximately 10% of patients have congenital anomalies that may suggest a genetic predisposition to cancer, and approximately 1% to 2% of patients have another family member with WT.[57]

MEDICAL HISTORY AND CLINICAL PRESENTATION

The most common clinical presentation is abdominal distention or an abdominal mass. Abdominal pain is also noted, usually resulting from local distention or hemorrhage. Patients may present with hematuria and hypertension. Some patients may present with fever.

Approximately 10% of patients with WT show signs of an associated syndrome. One of the most common is syndromes is WAGR syndrome, which includes WT, iris absence, genitourinary malformations, and mental retardation.

SIGNS AND SYMPTOMS

Signs and symptoms of WT include asymptomatic abdominal mass, abdominal pain, and urinary tract infections. Common symptoms of WT include abdominal tenderness and hematuria. Other symptoms include hypertension, fever, anemia, and varicocele.

PHYSICAL EXAMINATION

Physical examination findings of patients with WT include high blood pressure, fever, pallor, absent iris, and a palpable abdominal mass. The abdominal mass rarely crosses the midline. Genitourinary malformations may be present.

DIFFERENTIAL DIAGNOSIS

The differential diagnosis for WT includes the following:

- Neuroblastoma or hepatoblastoma
- RCC, clear cell sarcoma of the kidney
- Benign processes involving the kidney such as polycystic dysplastic kidneys or hematomas

In neonates and very young infants, most renal tumors are congenital mesoblastic nephroma rather than WT.

DIAGNOSTIC STUDIES

The diagnosis of WT is confirmed histologically. Most children with renal tumors have favorable histology for WT.

The main approach is immediate nephrectomy, if feasible without excessive morbidity. This procedure allows for histologic confirmation and accurate staging and lymph node assessment.

The staging system includes:

- **Stage I:** Tumor is confined to the kidney with no penetration of the renal capsule, and no invasion of veins or lymphatics of the renal sinus, and the tumor is resected completely.
- **Stage II:** Tumor penetrates the renal capsule or extends into local blood vessels but is completely resected with negative surgical margins.
- **Stage III:** Tumor is not resected completely.
- **Stage IV:** Tumors have disseminated outside the abdomen.
- **Stage V:** Bilateral disease affects both kidneys.

EVALUATION

The presurgical evaluation includes an abdominal ultrasound for assessment of blood vessels for flow and tumor thrombus, an abdominal/pelvis CT or MRI scan, and a CT scan of the lungs.

For patients with clear cell sarcoma and rhabdoid tumor of the kidney, an MRI of the brain and a bone scan are required.

TREATMENT

- The treatment of WT includes three modalities: surgery, chemotherapy, and radiation therapy. The three main chemotherapeutic agents that are used are vincristine, dactinomycin, and doxorubicin. Radiotherapy is given for patients with distant metastatic disease and patients with local stage III disease that was incompletely resected.
- Although most patients with WT do well, approximately 10% to 15% experience relapse and most will relapse within 2 years.[58] Treatment of recurrent WT includes chemotherapeutic agents that were not part of the initial chemotherapy protocol.

7.8B BLADDER CANCER

In 2018, an estimated 81,190 new cases of bladder cancer were diagnosed in the United States and 17,240 patients died from bladder cancer.[1] In the United States, bladder cancer is the fourth most common malignancy in men and is three times more common in males than females.[1] The median age at diagnosis is 70 years. Bladder cancer is strongly associated with cigarette smoking, which increases the risk of bladder cancer two- to four fold. Other risk factors include occupational exposure to aromatic amines in occupations such as painters, leather workers, dry cleaners, and petroleum workers; prolonged treatment with cyclophosphamide; chronic inflammation from indwelling catheters or bladder stones; chronic infection with *Schistosoma haematobium*; and prior irradiation to the pelvis. Bladder cancer is one of the extracolonic malignancies that may be seen in patients with Lynch syndrome.

In the United States, 90% of bladder cancers are urothelial (transitional cell) carcinomas and there are three major groups: nonmuscle invasive disease, muscle invasive disease, and metastatic bladder cancer.

Nonmuscle invasive disease is the most common type of bladder cancer and is characterized by high local recurrence rates and prolonged survival. Tumors with muscle invasion into the lamina propria of the bladder have a higher rate of recurrence and almost half will progress to higher stages of disease.

MEDICAL HISTORY AND CLINICAL PRESENTATION

Hematuria, macroscopic or microscopic, is a common presenting symptom with intermittent painless gross hematuria as the most common presentation. Irritative voiding symptoms, such as dysuria, frequency, nocturia, and urgency, are also noted at the time of diagnosis.

SIGNS AND SYMPTOMS

While hematuria is the most common presenting symptom in a newly diagnosed cancer patient, patients with metastatic bladder cancer may present with constitutional symptoms including fatigue, fever, anorexia, weight loss, and night sweats. Other manifestations include dyspnea on exertion due to anemia; cough, hemoptysis, or chest pain due to lung metastases; flank pain due to hydronephrosis; abdominal pain due to liver metastases; and severe back pain due to vertebral metastases.

PHYSICAL EXAMINATION

Early in the disease the physical examination may be normal. An abdominal mass may be noted in patients with extensive disease, hepatomegaly and lymphadenopathy in metastatic disease, and lymphedema in localized advanced disease.

DIFFERENTIAL DIAGNOSIS

Several nonmalignant disorders of the urinary system and kidneys can present with isolated microscopic hematuria or gross hematuria. These include:

- Nephrolithiasis
- Urinary tract infections
- Chronic irritation of the bladder mucosa due to indwelling Foley catheter
- Benign prostatic hyperplasia
- Primary kidney disease, such as nephritic syndrome and IgA nephropathy
- Radiation cystitis in patients with history of radiotherapy to the pelvis

Isolated microscopic hematuria or gross hematuria with or without lower urinary tract symptoms can be noted in other pelvic malignancies:

- Transitional cell carcinoma of the urethra
- Advanced prostate cancer with invasion into the bladder
- Advanced adenocarcinoma of the rectum with invasion into the bladder
- Transitional cell carcinoma of the upper urinary tract: ureter, renal pelvis
- RCC

DIAGNOSTIC STUDIES

Imaging or cystoscopy studies are the first step in the evaluation. Imaging studies may show a thickened bladder wall, bladder mass, perivesical stranding changes, hydronephrosis, regional lymphadenopathy, and visceral or skeletal metastases. Cystoscopy findings may include papillary masses, sessile masses, or erythematous patches. Urine cytology has a high specificity and moderate sensitivity for the detection of high-grade tumors.

If imaging and cystoscopy, or cytologic findings are abnormal, the next step is a transurethral resection of bladder tumor. A definitive tissue diagnosis of bladder cancer is established at the time of transurethral resection. The pathologic specimen must include the muscularis propria layer of the bladder to identify any muscle wall invasion.

A normocytic, normochromic anemia of chronic disease is not uncommon in patients with bladder cancer. Leukocytosis can be caused by urinary tract infection. Serum creatinine and estimated glomerular filtration rate (GFR) help establish the patient's baseline renal function. Elevations of the serum alkaline phosphatase can be seen in patients with liver or bone metastases; if elevated, patients should have a bone scan.

EVALUATION

Intermittent painless gross hematuria in an adult may be a manifestation for bladder cancer and mandates urologic evaluation. The initial evaluation of a patient with painless gross hematuria includes a complete history and physical examination, urinalysis, urine cytology, CBC with differential, serum metabolic profile, coagulation profile, and office cystoscopy.

A complete history and physical examination should be obtained. A history of hereditary or acquired coagulopathies should be noted and current medications should be thoroughly reviewed. The use of anticoagulant, antiplatelet, and nonsteroidal anti-inflammatory medications should be noted.

Initial laboratory tests include a CBC, complete metabolic profile, and coagulation studies. A urologic consultation is required.

Cystoscopy should be performed to identify the source of bleeding, look for clot formation and retention, and to initiate a three-way Foley catheter irrigation. Emergent fulguration of a bleeding bladder tumor may be required.

TREATMENT

- Patients with locally advanced bladder cancer may present with tumor-related obstructive uropathy and concomitant renal insufficiency. This can be caused by tumor invasion of ureteral orifices or by extrinsic compression of the ureter by metastatic lymph nodes.
  - Placement of a percutaneous nephrostomy or insertion of a ureteral stent should be considered in patients with bladder cancer-related obstructive uropathy.
- Treatment for nonmuscle invasive urothelial carcinoma of the bladder includes transurethral resection of bladder tumor to remove all visible tumors, adjuvant intravesical chemotherapy with mitomycin C, valrubicin, gemcitabine, or intravesical immunotherapy with bacillus Calmette-Guérin (BCG) to reduce tumor recurrence.
- High-grade nonmuscle invasive bladder cancer has a high risk of local recurrence and progression to higher stages of disease. After complete endoscopic resection of high-grade nonmuscle invasive tumors, adjuvant intravesical therapy with BCG should be considered.

Radical cystectomy, bilateral pelvic lymphadenectomy, and urinary diversion are the standard treatment of muscle invasive bladder cancer. Some patients with muscle invasive disease have micrometastases at the time of radical cystectomy. Induction chemotherapy with methotrexate, vinblastine, doxorubicin, and cisplatin is a standard induction cisplatin-based combination chemotherapy regimen.

PATIENT EDUCATION

- The 5-year survival rate varies little with the age of the patient and ranges from 78% to 97% for localized disease and 8% to 12% for distant disease.[59]
- Many patients with metastatic or unresectable transitional cell carcinoma of the bladder have incurable disease. The most common sites of metastatic spread include the lymphatic system, liver, lungs, and bones and most are diagnosed during the first 2 to 3 years after radical cystectomy.
- The median overall survival for patients with metastatic transitional cell carcinoma of the bladder treated with cisplatin-based combination chemotherapy is 15 months.[60]

7.8C RENAL CELL CANCER

RCC accounts for 3% of malignant tumors and is the tenth leading cause of cancer deaths in the United States.[1] An estimated 65,300 new renal cell cancers were diagnosed in 2018 with over 17,000 deaths.[1] It is most common in patients in their 60s, and there is a male-female predominance of 2:1.

The majority of RCC tumors are sporadic. In patients with bilateral renal tumors or who are young, under 40 years of age, a genetic cause of RCC should be considered.

Patients with tuberous sclerosis are at risk to develop bilateral renal tumors. These patients may have cutaneous lesions, CNS hamartomas, and pulmonary cysts. Renal tumors in these patients are generally benign.

The major environmental risk factor associated with RCC development is cigarette smoking, with a relative risk of approximately two- to three fold.

Obesity is a recognized risk factor. Autosomal dominant polycystic kidney disease is not considered a risk factor for RCC.

MEDICAL HISTORY AND CLINICAL PRESENTATION

Most patients present with gross or microscopic hematuria, flank pain, and an abdominal mass. The classic triad of flank pain, hematuria, and mass are found in only 10% to 15% of patients and are usually a sign of advanced disease. Symptoms of metastatic disease occur in about 25% of patients at the time of presentation. Because of widespread use of CT scans and ultrasound, renal tumors are frequently identified in patients with no symptoms.

SIGNS AND SYMPTOMS

Signs and symptoms include hematuria, flank pain, and abdominal mass. Patients can present with no symptoms, and the discovery of the tumor is incidental.

Symptoms of metastases or paraneoplastic syndromes, when present, have a negative prognostic sign. These signs and symptoms include hypercalcemia, unexplained fever, and wasting syndrome.

There are several RCC subtypes, based on the cell type involved. These include clear cell, which is the most common; papillary RCC; and other rare types including chromophobe, collecting duct, unclassified, and medullary.

PHYSICAL EXAMINATION

Early in the disease the physical examination may be normal. An abdominal or flank mass may be noted in patients with extensive disease.

DIFFERENTIAL DIAGNOSIS

Solid lesions of the kidney are considered RCC until proved otherwise. Other causes of solid masses in the kidney include renal angiomyolipoma, renal pelvis urothelial cancer, renal abscesses, or adrenal tumors.

DIAGNOSTIC STUDIES

On urinalysis hematuria will be noted. CBC may reveal anemia, but erythrocytosis secondary to increased erythropoietin production may be noted. Hypercalcemia may be noted. Elevated alkaline phosphatase may indicate the presence of bone metastases.

CT and MRI scanning are the most important imaging tests for RCC and can confirm the presence of a mass and assist with staging the lesion. RCC on imaging presents as a small mass lesion with a peripheral location with contrast enhancement and calcification.

EVALUATION

Most renal tumors are discovered incidentally during an imaging procedure, and patients are asymptomatic. The classic presentation that includes the triad of hematuria, flank pain, and a palpable mass are seldom noted. Past medical history and smoking history are important, as well as an occupational and environmental exposure history. There are no biomarkers that are helpful during the initial evaluation.

TREATMENT

- Surgery is the primary treatment for RCC. Partial nephrectomy should be considered first line, unless the tumor is over 7 cm, and then a radical nephrectomy should be done.
- No effective chemotherapy is available for metastatic disease. Vinblastine, interferon-alpha and interleukin-2 may bring about a partial response and bevacizumab can slow progression of disease.
- Some new targeted medications, such as vascular endothelial growth factor (VEGF), Raf-kinase, and mTOR inhibitors are effective in advanced disease.

PATIENT EDUCATION

- The 5-year survival rates are[61]:
  - Localized: 93%
  - Regional: 70%
  - Distant: 12%
  - All stages: 75%
- Since treatment of metastatic RCC rarely produces complete responses, and cure is unlikely, current therapy is focused on control of disease progression.

KEY POINTS

- WT is most common in children under 5 years of age and presents with a painless, palpable abdominal mass.
- WT is diagnosed by biopsy and treated with surgery and chemotherapy.
- Risk of bladder cancer increases with smoking, cyclophosphamide use, chronic irritation, or exposure to certain chemicals.
- Over 90% of bladder cancers are transitional cell carcinoma.
- For suspect bladder cancer in patients with unexplained hematuria, diagnosis is made with cystoscopy biopsy.
- RCC is an adenocarcinoma and accounts for 90% to 95% of primary malignant renal tumors.
- Symptoms of RCC do not develop until the tumor is large or metastatic, so incidental discovery is common.
- Treat localized RCC with radical nephrectomy.

7.9 TESTICULAR CANCER

Testicular cancer is the most common cancer among males between 20 and 40 years of age. The major risk factors are a personal history of cryptorchidism and a family history of testicular cancer in a brother or father.

Testicular cancers are typically aggressive and rapidly progressive cancers that require rapid workup and treatment. Testicular cancers are almost always first discovered by the patient as either a tender or nontender mass and must be considered as a possible diagnosis in a man with testicular pain or tenderness.

OVERVIEW

Testicular cancer should be suspected when a patient discovers a painless testicular mass, either unintentionally or by self-examination, or when a testicular mass is discovered by routine physical examination.

The primary risk factors for a testicular germ cell tumor is a history of cryptorchidism, testis cancer in the other testicle, or a family history of testis cancer, particularly in a man's brother or father. Testicular cancer is not known to be associated with any behaviors, such as smoking.

Testis cancer is most commonly diagnosed between the ages of 15 and 40, with nonseminomas predominating in younger men, and seminomas in middle-aged men. Testis cancer is most common in White males and is exceedingly rare in men of African ancestry. Men with Klinefelter syndrome are at increased risk of developing mediastinal germ cell tumors.

EPIDEMIOLOGY

Testicular cancer is the most common malignancy in men 15 to 35 years of age and it accounts for approximately 1% of all cancers in men.[1] About 95% of testicular tumors are malignant and derived from germ cells, whereas the remaining 5% are non-germ cell or stromal tumors derived from Leydig and Sertoli cells of the gonadal stroma. Malignant tumors include five basic cell types: seminoma, embryonal carcinoma, yolk sac tumor, choriocarcinoma, and teratoma.

PATHOPHYSIOLOGY

The pathophysiology of germ cell tumors is poorly understood. They appear to develop from a precursor lesion called intratubular germ cell neoplasia (ITGCN).

The precursor for ITGCN appears to be an arrested primordial germ cell or gonocyte. In a normal boy these primitive germ cells no longer exist at the time of birth, so the changes to these cells occur in utero. These premalignant cells then lay quiet until stimulated by testosterone after puberty.

There are no specific exposures or behaviors that have been clearly linked to an increased risk of germ cell tumors. The only modifiable risk factor for testis cancer is cryptorchidism.

MEDICAL HISTORY AND CLINICAL PRESENTATION

The most common symptom is a painless lump in the testicle, which is pathognomonic for testicular cancer, and swelling in the testicle. The patient may also note a heaviness in the scrotum, inguinal lymphadenopathy, and weight loss. The patient may have no signs or symptoms. A history of cryptorchidism should be investigated.

SIGNS AND SYMPTOMS

Testicular cancer should be considered, and a testis exam performed for any adolescent, young adult, or middle-aged male who complains of the following:

- Back pain
- Gynecomastia
- Lower extremity edema
- Unexplained dyspnea
- Infertility
- Testicular or pelvic pain
- Abdominal mass

Testicular cancer can result in gynecomastia, back pain (from retroperitoneal adenopathy), infertility, thromboembolisms, hemoptysis, and testicular pain.

PHYSICAL EXAMINATION

Testicular cancer may be detected on self-examination or during routine physical examination. The testicle examination may reveal an enlarged, indurated, painful, or tender testicle. Testicular cancer can also result in testicular atrophy, gynecomastia, back pain, or palpable supraclavicular adenopathy.

The key physical examination elements include palpation of the testes, palpation of the breasts, complete lymph node examination, and abdominal examination.

DIFFERENTIAL DIAGNOSIS

The differential diagnosis for a testicular mass and/or tenderness includes hydrocele, spermatocele, orchitis, epididymitis, germ cell tumors, and non-germ cell cancers. Tumors can be distinguished from other abnormalities with a transscrotal ultrasound. Although most painful lesions of the testis are not malignant, testis cancers can be painful and/or tender, so the presence of pain or tenderness does not exclude cancer.

DIAGNOSTIC STUDIES

Biopsy is needed to diagnose and divide testicular germ cell tumor into the two major histologic types: seminomas and nonseminomas, which include embryonal carcinomas, teratomas, yolk-sac tumors, and choriocarcinomas.

The tumor markers hCG and alpha-fetoprotein, and LDH levels should be obtained. The results will assist with diagnosis, staging and risk assessment, evaluation of response to therapy, and early detection of relapse. If the tumor markers are elevated prior to orchiectomy, they should be repeated after surgery to see if they are returning to normal.

Alpha-fetoprotein is normally secreted during gestation and declines to low levels at 1 year of age. Elevated levels are found in most patients with embryonal and teratocarcinomas of the testis, as well as in patients with extragonadal germ cell tumors. Pure seminomas do not secrete alpha-fetoprotein. Alpha-fetoprotein can also be elevated in HCC, GI cancers, benign liver disease, particularly hepatitis, and chemotherapy-induced liver damage.

hCG is a glycoprotein hormone normally secreted by the placenta. The beta subunit is normally present during pregnancy so high levels in males and nonpregnant females is indicative of cancer. hCG is secreted by choriocarcinomas, embryonal cell carcinomas, teratomas, and pure seminomas.

LDH is a useful marker, especially for staging seminoma and nonseminoma germ cell tumor.

Transscrotal ultrasound can confirm the presence of a hypoechoic, heterogeneous mass. CT scans are used to identify metastatic disease in the retroperitoneal lymph nodes, lungs, posterior mediastinal lymph nodes, liver, and pelvic lymph nodes.

EVALUATION

Scrotal/testicular nodules and masses are a common complaint of male patients. If an emergent intervention is needed, a timely referral should be made. If nonemergent, a testicular ultrasound should be obtained. If the mass is heterogeneous it should be regarded as neoplasm until proved otherwise. Most testicular tumors are derived from the germ cells, and the most common is a seminoma. The other tumors are stromal in origin, such as Leydig cell, Sertoli cell, or granulosa cell. The most common bilateral testis tumor and most common metastatic tumor of the testicles is lymphoma. All require prompt radical orchiectomy for tissue diagnosis and staging. Tumor markers should also be obtained.

TREATMENT

- Germ cell tumors are aggressive and rapid growing cancers. Inguinal orchiectomy is the treatment of choice and should be done as soon as possible. Chemotherapy is indicated for metastatic disease and should be started as soon as possible.
- Following orchiectomy if there is persistent elevation of serum tumor markers this typically represents metastatic disease, regardless of staging studies.
- Regardless of the treatment used, the long-term disease-specific survival of germ cell testicular cancer is over 95%.
- For stage I seminomas and nonseminomas in which the postorchiectomy serum tumor markers are normal, most are cured by orchiectomy alone and need no additional treatment. The relapse risk is high for seminomas and nonseminomas. Close surveillance is mandatory for men who do not undergo postorchiectomy treatment so that relapses can be promptly treated. For stage I seminomas, there are two alternatives to surveillance: single agent chemotherapy with carboplatin or subdiaphragmatic radiation. Clinical stage I seminoma that relapses during surveillance almost always relapses to the retroperitoneum and can usually be salvaged with radiation therapy.
- Postorchiectomy chemotherapy is also an effective treatment strategy for stage I nonseminomas with normal serum tumor markers and the standard treatment consists of bleomycin, etoposide, and cisplatin.

- Stage II seminomas are uncommon and there are two standard treatments: either radiation therapy or chemotherapy. Chemotherapy consists of bleomycin, etoposide and cisplatin, or etoposide plus cisplatin.
- Stage III germ cell tumors are treated with multiagent cisplatin-based chemotherapy. The most common combination includes bleomycin, etoposide, and cisplatin.

PATIENT EDUCATION

- The goal of treatment for testis cancer is cure, regardless of stage. The overall 5-year survival rate is 95%; it is 99% for local disease and 73% for distant disease.[1]
- The USPSTF has reaffirmed its 2004 recommendation against screening for testicular cancer in adolescent and adult males without any symptoms.
- Surveillance of patients with testicular cancer consists of regularly scheduled physical examination, tumor marker monitoring, chest x-ray, and CT of the chest and abdomen.

KEY POINTS

- Testicular cancer is the most common solid cancer in males age 15 to 35 and is often curable.
- Assess scrotal masses with ultrasonography and obtain alpha-fetoprotein and beta-hCG levels.
- Treatment includes radical inguinal orchiectomy, usually with radiation therapy (for seminomas) and retroperitoneal lymph node dissection (for nonseminomas).

7.10 PROSTATE CANCER

OVERVIEW

Prostate adenocarcinoma is the most common cancer and the second leading cause of cancer death in men in the United States, with 164,690 new cases and 29,430 deaths in 2018.[1] One in nine men will be diagnosed with prostate cancer during their lifetime. While a common diagnosis, most men who have prostate cancer will not die from it; the survival rate for all stages of prostate cancer is 99%.[1]

Screening for prostate cancer with digital rectal examination and prostate specific antigen (PSA) is controversial. Localized prostate cancer is curable with appropriate local therapy. Patients are classified as low-risk, intermediate-risk, and high-risk localized prostate cancer based on clinical stage, Gleason score, and the serum PSA level.

In men with metastatic prostate cancer, androgen deprivation therapy (ADT) is the most effective initial treatment.

EPIDEMIOLOGY

There are several risk factors for the development of prostate cancer. African Americans are affected more than Caucasians. The risk of developing prostate cancer increases with increasing age. Clinically diagnosed prostate cancer is rare before age 40. The incidence of prostate cancer in men age 35 to 44 is 0.5%; the incidence in men age 45 to 54 is 8.7%; the incidence in men age 55 to 64 is 32.7%; the incidence in men age 65 to 75 is 39.3%; and the incidence in men over age 75 is 18.9%.[62]

Family History

Men with a first-degree relative with prostate cancer have a twofold increased risk of developing prostate cancer in their lifetime. Patients with two first-degree relatives with prostate cancer have a five fold increased risk of developing prostate cancer.

Dietary factors for prostate cancer are controversial. Low consumption of products containing lycopene, such as tomatoes, and high consumption of alpha-linolenic acid, found in vegetable oils, soybeans, and walnuts, have been associated with higher incidence of prostate cancer.

Increased sexual activity, >21 ejaculations per month, has been shown to decrease the risk of prostate cancer. Chronic prostatic inflammation has been linked with high-grade disease.

Screening guidelines vary with specific organizations. See Table 7.10 for the various guidelines.

PATHOPHYSIOLOGY

Development of prostate cancer is thought to occur through a multistep carcinogenesis process by which normal prostatic epithelium progresses through proliferative inflammatory

TABLE 7.10 Prostate Cancer Screening Guidelines by Organization

Organization	Guidelines
American Urological Association	Under the age of 40 should not be screened. Those 40–54 years of age and at average risk should not be routinely screened; those at higher risk (e.g., positive family history or African American race) should have an individualized screening decision. Those 55–69 years of age should consider PSA screening based on values and preferences. Over the age of 70 years or those with <10–15-year life expectancy should not have PSA screening.
American Cancer Society	Recommends a discussion of the pros and cons of PSA testing based on individual risk.
U.S. Preventive Services Task Force	Recommends that the decision to undergo PSA-based screening for prostate cancer should be an individual one for men aged 55 to 69 years and recommends against PSA-based screening in men over age 70.

PSA, prostate-specific antigen.

Source: Data from American Urological Association. Early detection of prostate cancer. https://www.auanet.org/guidelines/prostate-cancer-early-detection-guideline; Wolf AM, Wender RC, Etzioni RB, et al. American Cancer Society guideline for the early detection of prostate cancer: update 2010. CA Cancer J Clin. 2010;60(2):70–98; U.S. Preventive Services Task Force. Prostate cancer screening. https://www.uspreventiveservicestaskforce.org/Page/Document/UpdateSummaryFinal/prostate-cancer-screening

atrophy to prostatic intraepithelial neoplasia, and finally to prostatic adenocarcinoma.

MEDICAL HISTORY AND CLINICAL PRESENTATION

Prostate cancer is a slow growing, potentially lethal disease usually found in men over the age of 50. Although the disease has been reported in all age groups, almost 60% of all prostate cancers occur in men over the age of 65.[62] While many patients present with no symptoms, common symptoms of prostate cancer include changes in bladder habits, hematuria, hematospermia, and painful ejaculation.

SIGNS AND SYMPTOMS

Most men with localized prostate cancer do not have any symptoms and are often diagnosed from an abnormal digital rectal examination or elevated serum PSA level.

Other presenting symptoms in patients with localized prostate cancer can be similar to those associated with benign prostatic hypertrophy and include urinary urgency, urinary frequency, weak urinary stream, urinary outflow obstruction, hematuria, dysuria, irritative voiding symptoms, urinary tract infections, or pelvic pain.

Men with more advanced disease who have bulky pelvic lymph node metastases may present with hydroureter/hydronephrosis or lower extremity edema.

Men with bony metastases often present with bone pain or may present with signs and symptoms of spinal cord compression, including lower extremity weakness, sensory loss, and paralysis.

PHYSICAL EXAMINATION

Digital rectal examination may reveal an asymmetric boggy mass palpated in the anterior wall of the rectum or hard nodular prostate. Common physical examination findings of prostate cancer include cachexia, pallor, lower extremity lymphedema, and bone tenderness.

DIFFERENTIAL DIAGNOSIS

Prostate cancer must be differentiated from benign prostatic hypertrophy, prostatitis, renal carcinoma, renal stones, bladder cancer, and cystitis. See Table 7.11 for the differential diagnosis of prostate cancer.

DIAGNOSTIC STUDIES

The diagnosis of prostate cancer is confirmed with a biopsy, using a transrectal approach with ultrasound guidance. Determining the initial treatment approach for prostate cancer depends on accurate classification into different risk-groups based on three diagnostic parameters: PSA level, clinical stage, and Gleason score. Combinations of these three parameters allow classification of patients into high-risk, intermediate-risk, and low-risk groups. Risk stratification indicates the likelihood of disease recurrence or persistence after appropriate local therapy. See Table 7.12 for risk classification criteria.

A serum PSA should be performed in all patients and compared to previous PSA values, if available.

The Gleason score, which is determined by examining biopsy tissue, is a measure of the tumor grade or degree of differentiation. Each biopsy core is evaluated for the presence of cancer, and if cancer is present is assigned a primary and secondary Gleason score.

The primary Gleason score, ranging from 1–5, reflects the tumor grade/differentiation that is the most prevalent in that biopsy specimen. The secondary Gleason score, ranging from 1–5, reflects the tumor grade/differentiation that is the second most prevalent pattern. The Gleason sum score, ranging from 2–10 with higher scores meaning a more aggressive tumor, guides prognosis and treatment.

Imaging studies include a bone scan to evaluate bone metastases. CT scan of the chest/abdomen/pelvis with IV contrast agent should be considered to evaluate for diffuse metastases.

An MRI evaluation may be useful in confirming extraprostatic tumor extension, demonstrating presence or absence of seminal vesicle invasion, and evaluating pelvic lymph nodes for tumor involvement. The use of PET imaging for the staging or monitoring of prostate cancer is not recommended.

TREATMENT

- Treatment options are based on the risk category. For very low risk patients, active surveillance is a popular approach to treatment. Since the morbidity and mortality risks are very low, active monitoring may be all that is needed.
  - This involves actively monitoring the course of the disease with the expectation to intervene if the cancer progresses. Active surveillance is especially attractive for men who have a limited overall life expectancy. This approach includes PSA test every 6 months, digital rectal examination every 12 months, and repeat prostate

TABLE 7.11 Differential Diagnosis for Prostate Cancer

Diagnosis	Description
Benign prostatic hypertrophy	Signs of urinary obstruction including urinary hesitancy, frequency, and possible urinary retention. Digital rectal exam reveals a rubbery enlarged prostate.
Prostatitis	Presents with frequency, urgency, dysuria, and perineal pain. May also note fever, nausea, and vomiting. Digital rectal exam reveals a very tender prostate.
Renal carcinoma	Presents with hematuria, flank pain, and abdominal mass. CT scan of abdomen will reveal renal mass.
Renal stones	Symptoms include flank pain, hematuria, nausea and vomiting, urinary frequency, and urgency. Stone present on x-ray or CT scan.
Bladder cancer	Presents with hematuria, urinary frequency and urgency, and dysuria. Diagnosed with cystoscopy revealing a mass.
Cystitis	Presents with suprapubic tenderness, urgency, frequency, and dysuria. Urinalysis positive for bacteria and white blood cells.

TABLE 7.12 Risk Stratification in Prostate Cancer

Risk Group	Risk (%)	PSA (ng/mL)	Stage	Gleason Sum Score
Very low risk	1–2	≤10	T1	≤6
Low risk	5–10	≤10	Stage T1–T2a	≤6
Intermediate risk	15–20	10–20	Stage T2b–T2c	7
High risk	30–40	≥20	Stage T3a	8–10

PSA, prostate specific antigen.
Source: Data from National Comprehensive Cancer Network. NCCN clinical practice guidelines in oncology. Prostate cancer: version 4.2018. https://www2.tri-kobe.org/nccn/guideline/urological/english/prostate.pdf

biopsy every 1 to 2 years. With the increased risk of aggressive disease in African Americans with very low risk prostate cancer, active surveillance may not be an option.

- In low-risk patients, radical prostatectomy and radiation therapy are initial treatment options, and the choice of primary therapy may depend on patient age, medical comorbidities, complications of each treatment, and patient preferences.
  - The main complications of radical prostatectomy include urinary incontinence and erectile dysfunction.
  - Complications with radiation therapy include urinary incontinence, rectal irritation, and erectile dysfunction.
- In the intermediate-risk patient the most appropriate treatment options include radical prostatectomy with or without pelvic lymph node dissection, or radiation therapy combined with short-term ADT.
  - The ADT uses a form of luteinizing hormone releasing hormone (LHRH) agonist/antagonist, which may be combined with an oral antiandrogen. Commonly used LHRH agonists include leuprolide or goserelin with the antiandrogen drug bicalutamide.
- In high-risk patients, prostatectomy is generally not done because of the low chance of complete surgical resection. Most patients receive radiation therapy combined with long-term ADT.
- Locally advanced prostate cancer treatment options include EBRT with or without brachytherapy combined with long-term ADT; radical prostatectomy plus pelvic lymphadenectomy in selected patients without fixation to adjacent organs; or ADT alone.
- Surveillance should be started in patients after primary therapy for localized or locally advanced disease. A surveillance plan includes PSA measurements and rectal examinations every 3 months for the first year, PSA measurements and rectal examinations every 6 months for the second year, and PSA measurements and rectal examinations every 12 months thereafter.
- With metastatic prostate cancer, ADT should be initiated immediately in all patients even in the absence of symptoms. Androgen suppression is achieved with the use of LHRH agonists or antagonists. Chemotherapy can also be used for metastatic prostate cancer. Most protocols include mitoxantrone and docetaxel.

PATIENT EDUCATION

- The prognosis for localized prostate cancer is excellent.
- In patients with metastatic prostate cancer, the goals of therapy are palliative and focus on treatment or prevention of pain and other skeletal-related complications.

KEY POINTS

- Prostate cancer development increases with advancing age.
- Complications due to bone metastases are common.
- Diagnose prostate cancer by transrectal ultrasound-guided needle biopsy.
- Localized prostate cancer is treated with prostatectomy and radiation therapy.

7.11 BRAIN CANCER

OVERVIEW

Brain tumors account for 85% to 90% of all primary CNS tumors.[63] These vary in aggressiveness from oligodendrogliomas, which can be associated with prolonged survival, to glioblastomas, with a median survival of <2 years.

All varieties of diffuse glioma share several common characteristics. Patients typically present with seizure, headaches, or focal neurologic deficits. The natural history of untreated diffuse glioma is progressive invasion of normal brain tissue. Diffuse gliomas are not surgically curable tumors. After surgery, further treatment options depend on tumor grade, and range from observation alone to treatment with radiation and chemotherapy. In addition to primary brain tumors, there is also brain metastases. The most common cancers that spread to the brain are bladder, breast, lung, kidney, leukemia, lymphoma, and melanoma.

EPIDEMIOLOGY

This year an estimated 23,800 adults and 3,700 children in the United States will be diagnosed with a primary tumor of the brain.[2] Diffuse gliomas are mostly noted in adults.[63] The incidence rates of glioblastoma range from a low of 0.16 per 100,000 person-years in children age 0 to 19 years to a high of 15.24 per 100,000 person-years in adults age 75 to 84 years.[63] Brain and other nervous system cancer is the ninth leading cause of death for men and women.[1] It is estimated that 16,800 adults died from primary cancerous brain and CNS tumors in 2018.[1] Diffuse gliomas are more common in males and Caucasians.

PATHOPHYSIOLOGY

The only risk factor for glioblastoma is exposure to ionizing radiation, most frequently in the form of therapeutic radiation. This is an infrequent cause of glioma; most cases have no recognized cause.

Genetic predisposition to infiltrating gliomas appears to be relatively uncommon, although gliomas may be inherited as a part of several familial diseases, such as type 1 neurofibromatosis, Turcot syndrome, and Li-Fraumeni syndrome.

Gliomas are graded based on microscopic features and these grades are described in Table 7.13.

SIGNS AND SYMPTOMS

The most common symptoms of brain tumors are headache, seizures, visual changes, and changes in personality. The

TABLE 7.13 Glioma Grading System

Grade	Description
I	Slow growing tumors that are unlikely to spread, cured by surgery
II	Slow growing and unlikely to spread, but recurrence is common
III	Present with rapidly growing cells but no necrotic cells, grow rapidly
IV	Actively dividing with development of new blood vessels and areas of necrotic tissue, grow rapidly and spread

headaches tend to be worse when the patient awakens in the morning and resolve in a few hours, worsen with coughing and exercise, occur during sleep, and have associated vomiting, double vision, weakness, and numbness. General symptoms include nausea, loss of appetite, and vomiting.

Other symptoms may include changes in alertness and memory loss; changes in hearing, smell, and taste; clumsiness; dizziness or vertigo; muscle weakness and numbness; and problems with eyesight, such as decreased vision, diplopia, or blindness.

PHYSICAL EXAMINATION

Physical examination findings will vary depending on the location of the tumor. Common physical examination findings include altered level of consciousness, anisocoria, papilledema, and focal neurologic deficits.

Neurologic deficits can include cognitive and behavioral impairment, such as impaired judgment, memory loss, lack of recognition, and spatial orientation disorders; personality or emotional changes; focal deficits such as hemiparesis, hypoesthesia, visual impairment, aphasia, ataxia, and facial paralysis; and sensory impairments involving sense of smell, impaired hearing, and double vision.

DIFFERENTIAL DIAGNOSIS

In glioma patients who present with symptoms there are several conditions in the differential diagnosis. Nonmalignant conditions include demyelinating disease, subacute stroke, infection/abscess, congenital malformations, leukoencephalopathies, and sarcoidosis. Other malignant conditions include metastatic disease, primary CNS lymphoma, and hemangioblastoma.

DIAGNOSTIC STUDIES

Brain cancer is a pathologic diagnosis, and tissue confirmation is needed prior to treatment. Biopsy is most often chosen when gross total resection cannot be safely performed and no debulking surgery is necessary. Biopsy has the advantage of low morbidity and mortality. Imaging studies include an MRI, which has a higher specificity and sensitivity than CT scan. Typical MRI findings include solitary ring-enhanced lesions on T1 postcontrast imaging; patchy or indistinct enhancement is noted in diffuse gliomas.

Basic laboratory studies after diagnosis of glioma should be performed to assess the patient's ability to tolerate chemotherapy or monitor the effects of concurrent medications.

TREATMENT

- Antiepileptic therapy is indicated in patients who present with seizure activity. Phenytoin is used as a first-line antiepileptic drug. Levetiracetam has become widely used in patients with intracranial tumors.
  - There is no proven role for long-term prophylactic antiepileptic therapy in patients with a brain tumor who have not experienced a seizure. Prophylactic antiepileptic drugs may be used for a limited period after surgery but should be discontinued as soon as appropriate.
- Asymptomatic edema seen on imaging does not require steroid treatment, except in rare circumstance in which there is significant midline shift, or the patient is at risk for herniation.
  - In patients with significant symptoms, dexamethasone is started and tapered over time. Cerebral edema may worsen during radiation therapy and increased steroid requirements may be needed.
- The current therapy for newly diagnosed glioblastoma involves surgery, radiation therapy, and temozolomide chemotherapy.
- Definitive therapy for glioma is surgery. Infiltrating glioma is not surgically curable, owing to the extension of microscopic disease. Resection may not be possible if the tumor is in brain areas such as motor strip or Broca's area. A repeat contrast-enhanced MRI should be completed within 48 hours after surgery to establish extent of resection.
- Involved-field radiation is the centerpiece of postsurgical treatment of high-grade glioma. Stereotactic radiosurgery systems, such as Gamma Knife, deliver large doses of radiation to well-defined targets, with little radiation to surrounding structures.
- Temozolomide chemotherapy is part of the standard-of-care treatment of glioblastoma. Temozolomide is an oral alkylating agent used in combination with radiation therapy for patients with newly diagnosed glioblastoma.

PATIENT EDUCATION

- The median survival time associated with glioblastoma has improved with the use of temozolomide.
- Patients treated with radiation and temozolomide have a median survival of around 12 to 16 months.
- Gliomas are primary tumors that originate in the brain parenchyma.
- Signs and symptoms, treatment, and prognosis vary with location of the glioma.

7.12 THYROID CANCER

OVERVIEW

Thyroid cancer refers to four kinds of tumors involving the thyroid gland: papillary, follicular, medullary, and anaplastic. Papillary and follicular tumors are the most common and typically benign. Medullary and anaplastic tumors are malignant. Medullary tumors have a good prognosis if they are restricted to the thyroid gland and a poor prognosis if metastases have occurred. Anaplastic tumors are rapid growers and respond poorly to treatment.

Thyroid nodules are diagnosed by ultrasound-guided fine needle aspiration or thyroidectomy. Treatment includes surgery and radioactive iodine.

EPIDEMIOLOGY

In 2018, an estimated 53,900 adults in the United States were diagnosed with thyroid cancer.[1] Thyroid cancer is the fifth most common cancer in women and is the most common cancer in women 20 to 34 years of age.[1]

Women are three times more likely to have thyroid cancer than men, but women and men die at similar rates.

Localized thyroid cancer is most common at the time of diagnosis and the 5-year survival rate is greatest for localized papillary, follicular, and medullary thyroid cancers. For localized anaplastic thyroid cancer, the 5-year survival rate is much lower.

Regional thyroid cancer, cancer that has spread to nearby tissues, organs, or lymph nodes, has a very high 5-year survival rate with papillary, follicular, and medullary cancer. For regional anaplastic thyroid cancer, the rate is much lower.

Medullary and anaplastic thyroid cancers are a rare type of thyroid cancers and are more likely to metastasize.

PATHOPHYSIOLOGY

Two types of cells are located within the thyroid parenchyma: the follicular cells and the supporting cells. Thyroid cancer begins in the follicular cell of the thyroid gland. Cancers derived from follicular cells are generally differentiated thyroid carcinomas.

Thyroid irradiation is the only modifiable cause of thyroid cancer. External radiation of the thyroid and exposure to ionizing radiation from nuclear fallout, especially during childhood and whole-body radiation for bone marrow transplantation, are associated with a significantly increased risk of papillary thyroid carcinoma.

Thyroid cancer can be found in about 10% of first-degree relatives of patients with papillary thyroid carcinoma.

MEDICAL HISTORY AND CLINICAL PRESENTATION

History should be focused on family history of thyroid cancer and the presence of risk factors. Risk factors include a primary relative with thyroid cancer, head and neck radiation during childhood, and the extremes of age (<30 or >60 years of age).

Rapid growth of a thyroid mass over several weeks or months is of concern for cancer. Tracheal compression or invasion by thyroid cancer can result in dyspnea, cough, or hemoptysis. Posterior invasion may result in recurrent laryngeal nerve damage, vocal cord dysfunction, and hoarseness.

SIGNS AND SYMPTOMS

It is common for people with thyroid cancer to have few or no symptoms. Thyroid cancers are often diagnosed by routine examination of the neck during a physical exam. They are also unintentionally found by x-rays or other imaging scans. People with thyroid cancer may experience the following: neck mass, hoarseness, lymphadenopathy, dysphagia, dyspnea, or cough.

PHYSICAL EXAMINATION

On thyroid examination the presence of a thyroid nodule >1 cm should be evaluated. The nodule may be soft to palpation and may not be easily identified or may appear more firm or hard.

Pemberton's maneuver if positive, development of facial flushing and/or distended jugular veins when both arms are raised at the side of the head for 1 minute, indicates the presence of significant obstruction in venous flow from a retrosternal goiter.

Invasion of tumor beyond the thyroid gland can be detected on exam when a nodule does not move up and down with swallowing. Careful examination for adenopathy of the paratracheal area and along the jugular chain lateral neck should be performed, especially ipsilateral to the thyroid nodule.

DIAGNOSTIC STUDIES

Once a thyroid nodule is identified the following should be performed:

- Thyroid-stimulating hormone level
- Thyroid ultrasound

If the thyroid-stimulating hormone level is low, radioiodine imaging should be performed. If the nodule is hot the patient should be evaluated and treated for thyrotoxicosis; hot nodules are rarely malignant and should not be biopsied. If the nodule is cold or warm a fine needle aspiration should be considered. If the thyroid-stimulating hormone level is normal or elevated a fine needle aspiration should be done.

A fine needle aspiration of the thyroid should be considered if the ultrasound of the thyroid reveals a mass that is hypoechoic, shows micro- or macrocalcifications, infiltrative margins, increased central vascularity, or unilateral adenopathy.

TREATMENT

- Near-total or total thyroidectomy is the recommended procedure for all patients with differentiated thyroid cancer. Complete thyroidectomy is suggested for all patients with a thyroid cancer tumor >1 cm found after lobectomy, especially if there are additional nodules seen in the contralateral lobe by ultrasound, metastatic lymph nodes, a family history of thyroid cancer, or a history of head and neck radiation.
- Long-term follow-up of thyroid cancer includes thyroid-stimulating hormone suppression, monitoring serum thyroglobulin levels, and periodic ultrasound exams of the neck. Because thyroid-stimulating hormone is a growth factor for thyroid cells, the thyroid hormone (levothyroxine) dose is adjusted until the thyroid-stimulating hormone is suppressed below the normal range. Serum thyroglobulin level generally falls over time, but patients with persistent or progressive disease will show thyroglobulin levels that rise.
- Radioiodine ablation therapy, with radioactive iodine, is indicated in patients with distant metastases, extrathyroidal extension of the tumor, or primary tumor size >4 cm.
- EBRT is used in thyroid cancer as a palliative treatment for locally advanced or otherwise unresectable disease in patients older than 45 years.

PATIENT EDUCATION

- Thyroid malignancies usually are slow growing and have a cause-specific 5-year survival of 98% but it varies by stage, with distant disease 5-year survival rate of 56%.[1]
- These cancers may demonstrate local invasion into the trachea, esophagus, and recurrent laryngeal nerve causing respiratory symptoms, cough, hemoptysis, dysphagia, and hoarseness.
- Distant metastatic disease typically travels via the blood to the lungs and bone.
- There are four types of thyroid cancer: papillary, follicular, medullary, and anaplastic.
- Most tumors present as asymptomatic nodules.
- Diagnosis is typically by fine needle aspiration.
- Treatment is surgical removal followed by ablation.

7.13 ONCOLOGIC EMERGENCIES

OVERVIEW

Oncologic emergencies are classified as metabolic, hematologic, structural, or treatment-related. Tumor lysis syndrome is a metabolic emergency that presents as severe electrolyte abnormalities. Treatment focuses on rehydration, maintaining urine output, and lowering uric acid levels. Hypercalcemia of malignancy is treated with aggressive rehydration and IV bisphosphonates. Febrile neutropenia is one of the most common complications related to cancer treatment, particularly chemotherapy. It is treated with empiric antibiotics. Structural oncologic emergencies are caused by direct compression of nontumor structures by metastatic disease. SVCS presents as facial edema with development of collateral venous circulation. Intravascular stenting plus chemotherapy and radiation therapy lead to superior outcomes. Malignant spinal cord compression is managed with steroids and/or surgery and radiation therapy.

EPIDEMIOLOGY

Complications can occur from the effects of cancer or from cancer treatment. Some oncologic emergencies take months to develop, while others develop over hours, causing devastating outcomes such as paralysis and death. In many patients, cancer is not diagnosed until a related condition emerges.

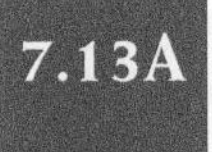

7.13A SUPERIOR VENA CAVA SYNDROME

SVCS is defined by the obstruction of blood flow through the superior vena cava because of intraluminal thrombus, invasion, or external compression. The obstruction can be due to processes involving the lung, regional lymph nodes, and other mediastinal structures. This leads to thrombosis due to inflammatory processes, as noted with neoplastic or infectious disorders or foreign bodies, mainly central venous catheters or pacemaker leads. Because of the obstruction the venous pressure in the upper body is increased and venous collaterals form, establishing alternate routes for the return of venous blood to the right atrium.

MEDICAL HISTORY AND CLINICAL PRESENTATION

SVCS is a complication of malignancy, with nonmalignant etiologies increasing due to the use of intravascular devices. Most cases of malignant SVCS are due to NSCLC (50%), SCLC (25%–35%), and non-Hodgkin lymphoma (NHL) (10%–15%).[64] Other malignancies, such as thymoma, primary mediastinal germ cell neoplasms, mesotheliomas, and solid tumors with mediastinal lymph node metastases, account for the remaining causes. Nonmalignant causes include intravascular devices, infections, and postradiation.

SIGNS AND SYMPTOMS

Symptoms that should raise the suspicion of SVCS include headache, dizziness, stupor, syncope, and visual disturbances, which suggest cerebral edema; facial or upper extremity swelling, dilated anterior chest or collateral veins, epistaxis, and hemoptysis suggest increased venous pressure. Findings suggestive of severe or life-threatening disease include syncope after bending, hypotension, confusion, and significant laryngeal edema. These symptoms can get better over time after several weeks of progression due to development of collaterals.

PHYSICAL EXAMINATION

Physical examination findings include edema and possibly cyanosis of face, neck, and arms; dilated neck veins and increased number of collateral veins covering the anterior chest wall; tongue swelling, and in severe cases, proptosis, obtundation, laryngeal edema, and stridor.

DIAGNOSTIC STUDIES

A high clinical index of suspicion is necessary and once the diagnosis is suspected, a contrast-enhanced chest CT should be used to confirm the diagnosis by defining the level and extent of venous blockage and identify collaterals. Venography is the gold standard and can be slightly superior to CT to define the level and extent of obstruction, but it does not provide any etiologic information; it is rarely used except for patients who are undergoing stent placement or other endovascular procedures. Magnetic resonance venography can be used in patients with contrast dye allergy or other contraindications to iodine contrast dye. Laboratory tests are mostly used for etiologic diagnosis and for evaluation of comorbidities, rather than for the diagnosis of SVCS.

EVALUATION

The diagnosis requires confirmation with imaging, but the clinical suspicion is raised by signs and symptoms of central vein obstruction. Symptoms are more severe if the superior vena cava obstruction is distal to the azygos vein and are usually exacerbated by bending forward or lying down.

TREATMENT

- Once diagnosed, the severity of the symptoms will dictate the management. An etiologic diagnosis should be established before treatment is instituted.
- SVCS usually has a relatively chronic onset, on average 45 days of symptoms before presentation. If the patient is known to have a malignancy that likely explains the SVCS, then treatment should be immediately initiated.

- The patient with proven intravascular thrombosis and no malignancy that is secondary to intravascular devices can be treated immediately after diagnosis with thrombolysis and possibly device removal and/or stent placement.
- The only truly emergent situation is the patient who presents with signs of severe airway compromise or the patient with cerebral edema or hemodynamic compromise. These patients require immediate treatment.
  - Immediate management consists of airway stabilization, endovascular stenting, and radiation therapy. In stable patients the major treatments include endovascular stents and thrombolytic therapy.
- In cases of intravascular thrombosis due to intravascular device, removal of the device is recommended; anticoagulation, treatment of the malignancy, and stenting may be indicated.

PATIENT EDUCATION

- SVCS is frequently caused by malignancy and every effort should be made to diagnose the underlying etiology.
- Deferring treatment until a full diagnostic workup is completed does not impact outcomes for stable patients.
- For patients with NSCLC, SVCS is a poor prognostic sign, with a median survival around 5 months.

7.13B NEUTROPENIC FEVER

Neutropenic fever is a common complication of chemotherapy for people with cancer. Neutropenic fever is very concerning for patients treated for hematologic malignancies, given the myelosuppressive nature of their treatment. These infections can progress rapidly, so immediate medical therapy is warranted.

Neutropenia is defined by the absolute neutrophil count (ANC), which is the sum of circulating segmented and band neutrophils. Neutropenia is defined by an ANC $<1.0 \times 10^9$/L. Severe neutropenia is a count of <500 cells/microliter or a count that is expected to decrease to less than this level within 48 hours. Profound neutropenia is an ANC <100 cells/microliter. As the severity and duration of neutropenia increases, so does the risk of infection.

MEDICAL HISTORY AND CLINICAL PRESENTATION

The Infectious Diseases Society of America defines fever in neutropenic patients as a single temperature measurement by oral or tympanic membrane of ≥38.3 °C (101 °F) or a temperature of >38 °C (100.4 °F) for >1 hour.[65] A history should include a complete review of systems, use of any prophylactic antimicrobial agents, recent use of therapeutic antimicrobial agents, previous infections, and comorbidities.

SIGNS AND SYMPTOMS

All patients should have a detailed history taken and physical examination performed. Fever may be the only presenting sign of infection in neutropenic patients, as they may not be able to mount a typical inflammatory response. Signs of infection may be absent or subtle.

PHYSICAL EXAMINATION

Physical examination should be complete and sites most likely to be a source of infection should be investigated. Common sites of infection include the skin, catheter insertion sites, the oral mucosa, sinuses, lungs, abdomen, genitals, and perianal areas. A digital rectal examination should be avoided, as infection can be introduced by the manipulation of the fragile mucosa of the anus.

DIAGNOSTIC STUDIES

Diagnostic studies should include a CBC with differential, complete metabolic profile, coagulation panel, and urinalysis. Microbiology testing should include blood and urine cultures, and any other possible sources of infection as determined by the history and physical examination. Chest x-ray or CT of the chest may be warranted depending on respiratory symptoms or signs on physical examination.

TREATMENT

- The infectious agent will be identified occasionally. Gram-positive organisms are most commonly isolated, but gram-negative rods, including *Pseudomonas* should be considered.
- Empiric broad-spectrum antibiotics should be administered within 1 hour of fever documentation. Dose adjustments should be made due to hepatic or kidney dysfunction. Antibiotic therapy should cover both gram-positive and gram-negative organisms and ensure coverage for *P. aeruginosa*. The Infectious Diseases Society of America recommends empiric monotherapy with an antipseudomonal beta-lactam agent, such as cefepime, ceftazidime, imipenem-cilastatin, meropenem, or piperacillin-tazobactam. Vancomycin is typically not recommended as part of first-line therapy but can be added for skin and soft tissue infections, sepsis or hemodynamic instability, pneumonia, or if an indwelling line is suspected as a source of infection.

PATIENT EDUCATION

- The initial antimicrobial regimen should be continued until the fever subsides and then for a minimum of 2 to 3 days afterward.
- If vancomycin or other specific gram-positive coverage was started empirically, it can be discontinued after 48 hours if there is no evidence of gram-positive infection.
- If a causative organism is identified the antibiotics should be continued for the minimum time frame of the infection and until the ANC recovers to >500 cells/microliter.
- If fever persists without a causative organism identified, then empiric antifungal coverage should be added after 5 to 7 days of broad-spectrum empiric antibiotics.

7.13C SPINAL CORD COMPRESSION

Spinal cord compression is caused more commonly by lesions outside the spinal cord than by lesions within it. Compression may be acute, subacute, or chronic.

Acute compression develops within minutes to hours. It is often due to trauma or metastatic tumor. It is occasionally due to abscess and rarely due to spontaneous epidural hematoma. Acute compression may follow subacute and chronic compression, especially if the cause is abscess or tumor.

Subacute compression develops over days to weeks. It is usually caused by metastatic extramedullary tumor, subdural or epidural abscess or hematoma, or cervical or, rarely, thoracic herniated disk. Chronic compression develops over months to years. It is commonly caused by spinal stenosis.

Lesions that compress the spinal cord may also compress nerve roots or, rarely, occlude the spinal cord's blood supply, causing spinal cord infarction.

SIGNS AND SYMPTOMS

Acute or advanced spinal cord compression causes segmental deficits, paraparesis or quadriparesis, hyporeflexia followed by hyperreflexia, extensor plantar responses, loss of bowel and bladder sphincter tone, and sensory deficits. Subacute or chronic compression may begin with local back pain that radiates down the distribution of a nerve root and sometimes hyperreflexia and loss of sensation are noted. Sensory loss may begin in the sacral segments. Complete loss of function may follow suddenly and unpredictably, possibly resulting from secondary spinal cord infarction.

PHYSICAL EXAMINATION

Spinal percussion tenderness is prominent if the cause is metastatic carcinoma, abscess, or hematoma.

Intramedullary lesions tend to cause poorly localized burning pain rather than radicular pain and to spare sensation in sacral dermatomes and usually result in spastic paresis. Spinal cord compression is suggested by spinal or radicular pain with reflex, motor, or sensory deficits, particularly at a segmental level.

DIFFERENTIAL DIAGNOSIS

Acute spinal cord compression must be differentiated from other diseases with similar presentation such as transverse myelitis, Guillain-Barré syndrome, diabetic neuropathy, multiple sclerosis, amyotrophic lateral sclerosis, and peripheral neuropathy.

DIAGNOSTIC STUDIES

MRI should be done immediately if available, and if not available a CT myelography should be obtained. MRI is diagnostic for spinal cord compression.

TREATMENT

Treatment of spinal cord compression centers on relieving the pressure on the cord. Incomplete loss of function may be reversible, but complete loss of function is rarely reversible. If spinal cord compression is due to a tumor, IV dexamethasone should be started immediately, followed by immediate surgery or radiation therapy. Surgery is indicated when neurologic deficits worsen despite nonsurgical treatment, the spine is unstable, tumors recur after radiation therapy, or an abscess or a compressive subdural or epidural hematoma is suspected.

7.13D TUMOR LYSIS SYNDROME

Tumor lysis syndrome is characterized by metabolic abnormalities including hyperuricemia, hyperkalemia, hyperphosphatemia, and hypocalcemia due to the rapid release of intracellular contents into the peripheral circulation. These metabolites can cause acute renal failure and a wide range of symptoms. Tumor lysis syndrome is observed after the initiation of cancer therapy for acute lymphoblastic leukemia and Burkitt lymphoma.

When tumor cells lyse, electrolytes, proteins, and nucleic acids are released into the bloodstream. This sudden influx can result in hyperuricemia, hyperkalemia, and hyperphosphatemia with subsequent hypocalcemia and have detrimental effects on the kidneys, myocardium, and CNS.

The release and catabolism of nucleic acids, specifically purine nucleic acids that are metabolized by xanthine oxidase into uric acid, can lead to hyperuricemia. The level of phosphorus in cancer cells is four times the levels found in normal cells, so the rapid release of intracellular phosphorus can lead to hyperphosphatemia. The kidneys initially act to remedy this by increasing excretion and decreasing tubular resorption; the kidneys can become overwhelmed and acute kidney injury can develop.

Hypocalcemia is a consequence of hyperphosphatemia and is included in the metabolic derangements that constitute tumor lysis syndrome. Hyperkalemia results from the rapid release of intracellular potassium into the bloodstream.

MEDICAL HISTORY AND CLINICAL PRESENTATION

Clinical tumor lysis syndrome is defined as the presence of laboratory tumor lysis syndrome with the addition of one of the following complications: renal insufficiency, cardiac arrhythmias, or seizures.

SIGNS AND SYMPTOMS

Signs and symptoms in tumor lysis syndrome are due to the electrolyte abnormalities. Other signs and symptoms include nausea, seizures, arrhythmias, and tetany. Hyperkalemia can cause GI distress, such as nausea, vomiting, diarrhea, and anorexia. Severe hyperphosphatemia may lead to nausea, vomiting, diarrhea, lethargy, and seizures. Severe hypocalcemia is associated with muscular effects, muscle cramps, paresthesia, tetany; cardiac abnormalities such as arrhythmias, heart block, hypotension; and neurologic consequences such as confusion, delirium, seizures.

PHYSICAL EXAMINATION

The physical examination findings are due to the electrolyte abnormalities. Other findings include fever, tachycardia, edema, arrhythmia, and tetany.

Acute obstructive uropathy can cause hematuria, flank pain, hypertension, azotemia, acidosis, edema, oliguria, anuria, lethargy, and somnolence.

DIAGNOSTIC STUDIES

Tumor lysis syndrome is diagnosed based on laboratory abnormalities. Laboratory findings include:

- Uric acid ≥8 mg/dL
- Potassium ≥6 mEq/L
- Phosphorus ≥4.5 mg/dL
- Calcium ≤7 mg/dL

Clinical tumor lysis syndrome is defined as laboratory tumor lysis syndrome plus at least one of the following:

- Creatinine ≥1.5 × upper limit of normal
- Cardiac arrhythmia
- Seizure

EKG abnormalities may be noted secondary to the development of hyperkalemia; this includes peaked T waves or widening of the QRS complex, arrhythmias, or asystole.

EVALUATION

Tumor lysis syndrome is diagnosed based on both laboratory and clinical findings. Definitions of clinical tumor lysis syndrome and laboratory tumor lysis syndrome were standardized by Cairo and Bishop in 2004.[66] Based on their classification, laboratory tumor lysis syndrome occurs when two or more metabolic values are abnormal or if they change by 25% within 3 days before or 7 days after initiation of therapy.

TREATMENT

- Prevention is key in the management of tumor lysis syndrome; those at risk should be proactively treated. The centerpiece to preventive care is aggressive IV hydration along with close electrolyte monitoring before and during treatment. Hydration should be started 24 hours before chemotherapy is started. IV hydration promotes increased urine flow, which leads to improved intravascular volume, renal perfusion, and glomerular filtration, which all promote excretion of uric acid and phosphate. Loop diuretics may also be used to maintain brisk urine flow but are contraindicated in patients with hypovolemia or obstructive uropathy. Urinary alkalization is no longer recommended.
- The standard of care for hyperuricemia is aggressive hydration and the use of a hypouricemic agent, such as allopurinol or rasburicase. Allopurinol is a xanthine oxidase inhibitor and blocks the conversion of xanthine and hypoxanthine to uric acid. Allopurinol should be used as prophylaxis, initiated 1 to 2 days before chemotherapy, and continued for 3 to 7 days. Rasburicase is a recombinant urate oxidase that converts uric acid into water-soluble allantoin. It is used as the initial management of hyperuricemia in pediatric and adult patients undergoing therapy for leukemia, lymphoma, or solid tumors who are at risk of tumor lysis syndrome and subsequent hyperuricemia. Rasburicase is contraindicated for use in pregnant and lactating women and in those with glucose-6-phosphate dehydrogenase deficiency.
- Elevated serum potassium may be acutely reduced by the administration of regular insulin, immediately followed by 50% dextrose, and then an hour-long infusion of 10% dextrose to prevent hypoglycemia; inhaled β-agonists; and use of loop diuretics.
- Hyperphosphatemia is managed with a low-phosphorus diet and short-term use of oral phosphate binders like aluminum hydroxide or aluminum carbonate. Calcium carbonate should be avoided in patients with hypercalcemia.

KEY POINTS

- Neutropenia is defined as a neutrophil count <500/µL.
- Neutropenic fever should be treated with broad-spectrum antibiotics.
- Tumor lysis syndrome is treated with hydration and allopurinol. Electrolytes should be monitored closely.
- Spinal cord compression presents with back or radicular pain with sensory or motor deficits.
- Spinal cord compression is diagnosed by MRI or CT myelogram; treatment is corticosteroids as soon as possible and surgery.
- SVCS presents with headache, facial swelling, and dilated veins in the neck, face, and upper chest.

7.14 CHEMOTHERAPY

Chemotherapeutic agents are used to directly or indirectly inhibit the proliferation of rapidly growing cells.

In general, chemotherapeutic agents cause the same general side effects because of the damage they cause to rapidly growing cells but can also cause neurotoxicity. These general side effects include:

- Mucositis and stomatitis, esophagitis, and enteritis associated with diarrhea
- Myelosuppression with neutropenia and lymphocytopenia, increasing the risk of infection
- Thrombocytopenia, increased bleeding risk
- Fatigue due to anemia
- Hair loss
- Chemotherapy-induced peripheral neuropathy in a "stocking-glove pattern"
- Centrally induced vomiting
- Gonadal damage

See Table 7.14 for a list of common chemotherapy agents including drug class, indications, and side effects.

SPECIAL CONSIDERATIONS

Cancer during pregnancy is uncommon. Cancer rarely directly affects the fetus.

Breast cancer is the most common cancer diagnosed during pregnancy, affecting about 1 in 3,000 women who are pregnant. Due to the changes to the breast that occur during pregnancy, it may be more difficult to detect and may be diagnosed later. Other cancers that occur in pregnancy include cervical cancer, thyroid cancer, lymphoma, melanoma, and gestational trophoblastic tumor.

Diagnosis of cancer in pregnancy is challenging as many of the common symptoms of cancer, such as bloating, headaches, and breast changes, are also noted as a normal part of pregnancy.

Diagnostic tests for cancer may or may not be safe to the pregnant woman and fetus. Some limitations are:

- **X-ray:** The radiation level in diagnostic x-rays is too low to harm the fetus. When possible, women should use a lead shield to cover the abdomen during x-rays.
- **CT scans:** CT scans are used to diagnose and determine if metastases are present. CT scans of the head or chest are usually safe during pregnancy. When possible, a lead shield should be used to protect the abdomen from radiation. CT scans of the abdomen or pelvis should be done only if necessary.
- MRI, ultrasound, and biopsy are generally safe during pregnancy.

Cancer treatment during pregnancy requires a multidisciplinary approach. Several factors should be considered when determining treatment option: pregnancy stage; type, location, size, and stage of the cancer; and personal wishes of the patient and her family.

Considerations for delaying treatment include:

- Treatment during the first 3 months of pregnancy is more likely to cause fetal harm. Treatment should be delayed until the second or third trimester.
- If cancer is diagnosed late in pregnancy, treatment can be delayed until after the child is born.
- Some treatments can harm the fetus at any time during the pregnancy. Radiation therapy can cause damage to fetal cells depending on the radiation dose and area of the body being treated.

TABLE 7.14 Review of Chemotherapeutic Agents

Drug Class	Subgroup	Drug	Mechanism of Action	Side Effects	Indications
Alkylating agents	**Oxazaphosphorines**	Cyclophosphamide Ifosfamide	Alkylation of DNA/RNA → cross-links DNA at guanine N-7 → impaired DNA synthesis Cyclophosphamide and ifosfamide require activation in liver	**Hemorrhagic cystitis:** prophylactic administration of **mesna** (sodium 2-mercaptoethane sulfonate) and fluids, or N-acetylcysteine Myelosuppression Bladder carcinoma (cyclophosphamide)	Leukemia Multiple myeloma Gynecologic tumors Lung cancer
	Nitrogen mustards	Busulfan Chlorambucil Melphalan		In rare cases, pulmonary fibrosis	Multiple myeloma CLL, CML
	Hydrazine	Temozolomide		Emetogenic Myelotoxic	Glioblastoma
	Platinum-based agents	Cisplatin Carboplatin Oxaliplatin	Cross-links between DNA strands → ↓ DNA replication	Emetogenic Nephrotoxic Ototoxic Neurotoxic (central and peripheral neuropathies)	Bladder cancer Lung cancer Testicular cancer Ovarian cancer
Topoisomerase inhibitors	**Topoisomerase I inhibitors**	Irinotecan Topotecan	Inhibition of topoisomerase I → ↓ DNA replication	Myelotoxic	Ovarian cancer Colorectal cancer Small cell lung cancer
	Topoisomerase II inhibitors	Etoposide Teniposide	Inhibition of topoisomerase II → ↑ DNA degradation and ↓ DNA replication	Myelotoxic	Many solid tumors Leukemias Lymphomas
		Anthracyclines Doxorubicin Daunorubicin Idarubicin		Cardiotoxic: can cause dilated cardiomyopathy with systolic CHF	
Mitotic inhibitors	**Vinca alkaloids**	Vincristine Vinblastine	Binding and destruction of tubulin in microtubules → mitotic arrest in metaphase	**Neurotoxic** (especially vincristine leads to peripheral neuropathy) Paralytic ileus, constipation (especially vincristine) Myelotoxic (vinblastine decreases blasts) Increased risk of opportunistic infections	Many solid tumors Leukemia Lymphomas Hodgkin lymphoma: vinblastine NHL: vincristine
	Taxanes	Docetaxel Paclitaxel	Stabilization of microtubules → ↓ mitotic spindles → mitotic arrest in metaphase	Myelotoxic Pulmonary fibrosis	Breast cancer Ovarian cancer Prostate cancer Gastric cancer

(continued)

TABLE 7.14 Review of Chemotherapeutic Agents *(continued)*

Drug Class	Subgroup	Drug	Mechanism of Action	Side Effects	Indications
Antimetabolites	**Antifolates**	Methotrexate	Inhibition of dihydrofolate reductase by displacing dihydrofolate → ↓ formation of purine nucleotides	Myelotoxic Hepatoxic Mucositis	Sarcomas Choriocarcinoma ALL Lymphomas
		Pemetrexed			Pleural mesothelioma Non-small cell lung cancer
	Pyrimidine antagonists	Cytarabine 5-Fluorouracil (5-FU) Gemcitabine Capecitabine	Incorporation of false pyrimidine analogs into DNA → ↓ DNA replication	Myelotoxic	Breast cancer Transitional cell cancer Colorectal cancer Pancreatic cancer
	Purine analogs	6-Mercaptopurine (6-MP) Azathioprine (prodrug for 6-MP)	Incorporation of false purine analogs into DNA → ↓ DNA replication	Myelosuppression Nephrotoxicity Neurotoxicity	Acute leukemias
		Cladribine			Hairy cell leukemia
	Purine antagonists	Fludarabine	Inhibition of DNA polymerase → DNA strands break	Myelotoxic	CLL
	Ribonucleotide reductase inhibitors	Hydroxyurea	Inhibition of ribonucleotide reductase → ↓ DNA replication → massive cytoreduction	Myelotoxic Hyperuricemia	CML
Other	**Antibiotics**	Bleomycin	Induces formation of free radicals → DNA strand breaks, arrests the cell cycle in G phase	Pulmonary fibrosis	Testicular cancer Hodgkin lymphoma
		Actinomycin D	DNA intercalation → interference with DNA transcription → ↓ RNA synthesis	Nephrotoxic Interstitial pneumonia	Wilms tumor Ewing sarcoma Rhabdomyosarcoma
		Mitomycin			Urinary bladder carcinoma
		Anthracyclines Doxorubicin Daunorubicin Idarubicin	Induces formation of free radicals → DNA strand breaks DNA intercalation → DNA strand breaks and ↓ DNA replication Topoisomerase II inhibitor	Cardiotoxic, can cause dilated cardiomyopathy with systolic CHF	
	Enzymes	l-Asparaginase	Cleavage of the amino acid l-asparagine by l-Asparaginase	Allergic reactions	Acute leukemias
	Proteasome inhibitors	Bortezomib	Inhibit degradation of ubiquitinated apoptotic proteins such as p53 → programmed cell death	Cytopenia Peripheral neuropathy	Multiple myeloma
	Tyrosine kinase inhibitors	Imatinib Erlotinib	Prevents phosphorylation and activation of multiple proteins by tyrosine kinases → cell dysfunction and death	Cytopenia Edema	CML GI stromal tumors

ALL, acute lymphoblastic leukemia; CHF, congestive heart failure; CLL, chronic lymphocytic leukemia; CML, chronic myelogenous leukemia; NHL, non-Hodgkin lymphoma.

Several treatment options are available during pregnancy:

- Surgery poses little risk to the fetus and is safe during all trimesters.
- Chemotherapy can be used, but only during certain times in pregnancy:
  - During the first 3 months of pregnancy, chemotherapy increases the risk of birth defects or pregnancy loss.
  - During the second and third trimesters the placenta acts as a barrier between the woman and the fetus. Recent studies suggest that fetuses exposed to chemotherapy while in utero do not show abnormalities immediately after delivery or during growth and development compared with babies not exposed to chemotherapy.
  - Chemotherapy in the last trimester may cause side effects in the woman and these side effects may indirectly harm the fetus.
  - Women who are receiving chemotherapy after a pregnancy should not breastfeed, as chemotherapy can transfer to the infant through breast milk.

KEY POINTS

- In the United States, cancer is the second most common cause of disease behind cardiac disease.[1]
- There are numerous risk factors for cancer including tobacco, radiation, sunlight, obesity, diet, alcohol, age, and infectious agents.
- Key clinical manifestations include weight loss, persistent cough, change in bowels, unexplained anemia, and development of a new lump.
- Early detection of cancer is key to long-term survival.
- Cancer staging is important in determining treatment options and prognosis.

COMMON CHIEF COMPLAINTS

APPROACH TO WEIGHT LOSS

Weight loss is classified as voluntary or involuntary. Serious medical or psychiatric disorders are often the etiology of progressive involuntary weight loss. Weight loss that is clinically significant is defined as a loss of >5% of usual body weight over 6 months.

The strongest independent predictor of involuntary weight loss is patient age, smoking history, and poor self-reported health. Mortality rates increase when weight loss is involuntary.

Common etiologies for involuntary weight loss are noted in Table 7.15.

Malignancy was noted to be the cause of involuntary weight loss in up to one-third of weight loss patients. Weight loss and anorexia are noted in over half of cancer patients at the time of diagnosis. Cancer cachexia is due to a decrease in muscle mass and seems to be due to tumor necrosis factor and interleukins 1 and 6. Cancer can also lead to weight loss due to the presence of pain, abdominal distention, nausea and vomiting, infections, dysphagia, obstruction, and the adverse effects of chemotherapy and radiation therapy.

Evaluation of the patient with involuntary weight loss starts with a complete history and physical examination. The history should include a complete review of systems. The Nine Ds (Box 7.2) will assist in the evaluation of weight loss.

TABLE 7.15 Etiologies of Involuntary Weight Loss in Adults

Conditions	Medications
Endocrine disorders Hyperthyroidism Diabetes mellitus Chronic primary adrenal insufficiency	Anticonvulsants
Gastrointestinal disorders Malabsorption disorders Inflammatory bowel disease	Antidepressants
Malignancy	Levodopa
HIV infection	Digoxin
Chronic heart disease	Metformin
Severe chronic lung disease	Exenatide
Chronic kidney disease	Liraglutide
Depression	Thyroid medication

BOX 7.2 The Historical Nine Ds for the Evaluation of the Weight Loss Patient

- Dentition
- Dysgeusia
- Dysphagia
- Diarrhea
- Depression
- Dementia
- Disease
- Dysfunction
- Drugs

The physical examination should be complete, and the findings of the various chronic diseases assessed. For example, spider angiomas may be noted in patients with chronic liver disease. Abnormal physical examination findings are most commonly noted in patients with underlying malignancy.

Laboratory studies should include a CBC with differential, complete metabolic profile, hemoglobin A1c, urinalysis, stool hemoccult, sedimentation rate, and C-reactive protein. Imaging studies should start with a chest x-ray. See Table 7.16 for the laboratory abnormalities noted in patients with unexplained involuntary weight loss due to underlying malignancy.

The management of the patient with unexplained weight loss depends on the specific underlying cause.

TABLE 7.16 Laboratory Test Predictors of Unexplained Weight Loss in Cancer Patients

Test	Value	Odds Ratio (95% CI)
White blood cell count	>12,000/mm³	3.6 (1.3–10.1)
Albumin	<3.5 g/dL	6.7 (3.3–14.3)
Alkaline phosphatase	>300 U/L	11.9 (3.9–36.3)
Lactate dehydrogenase	>500 U/L	12.5 (3.9–39.8)

Source: Data from Hernandez JL, Matorras P, Riancho JA, Gonzalez-Macias J. Involuntary weight loss without specific symptoms: a clinical prediction score for malignant neoplasm. Q J Med. *2003;96:649. doi:101093/qjmed/hcg107*

KNOWLEDGE CHECKS

1. Presentation of the various types of malignancies is nonspecific. Describe a general approach to the evaluation of the patient with a possible malignancy.
2. Screening for various malignancies can improve prognosis. Create a table of the various malignances and their screening methods, including frequency, sensitivity, and specificity.
3. Oncologic emergencies can develop with a number of malignancies. Describe the common oncologic emergencies including their presentation and treatment.

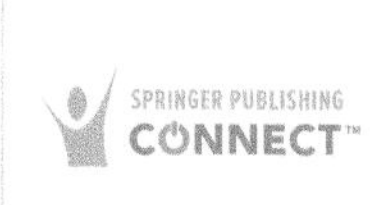

A robust set of instructor resources designed to supplement this text is located at **http://connect.springerpub.com/content/book/978-0-8261-8243-2.** Qualifying instructors may request access by emailing **textbook@springerpub.com.**

REFERENCES

The complete reference list for this chapter appears in the digital version of the chapter, accessible at https://connect.springerpub.com/content/book/978-0-8261-8243-2/chapter/ch07.

CHAPTER 8

GASTROINTESTINAL SYSTEM

ELIZABETH THOMPSON, NANA BERNASKO, JESSICA DAHMUS, AND BRANDON HEADLEE

LEARNING OBJECTIVES

- Distinguish between oropharyngeal and esophageal dysphagia.
- Develop the workup for gastrointestinal (GI) motility disorders.
- Describe the treatment for common GI disorders, including gastroesophageal reflux disease (GERD), irritable bowel syndrome (IBS), nausea and vomiting, diarrhea, and constipation.
- Describe the evaluation and workup of abdominal pain.
- Develop the evaluation of inflammatory bowel disease.
- Evaluate acute and chronic GI bleeding.
- Describe the workup for elevated liver enzymes and differentiate cholestatic versus hepatocellular enzyme abnormalities.
- Diagnosically evaluate viral hepatitis A, B, and C.
- Detail the implications of cirrhosis of the liver.
- Describe the evaluation and implications of pancreatitis.
- Develop a colon cancer screening protocol.

INTRODUCTION

Gastroenterology includes several subspecialties such as general gastroenterology, motility, hepatology, and inflammatory bowel disease (IBD), which frequently overlap. This chapter organizes disorders into those of the esophagus, stomach/duodenum, small intestine, large intestine, and rectum; GI bleeding; peritoneal disorders; liver diseases; pancreatic diseases; and common GI complaints.

Altered anatomy from surgery or congenital defects can result in motility disorders and/or malabsorptive syndromes, which can impair any portion of the GI tract, and will be discussed under the topic of small intestine disorders. IBD can occur in any portion of the GI tract, from the mouth to the anus, but will be addressed under the topic of large bowel disorders.

The enteric nervous system and brain–gut axis encompass many GI motility disorders including esophageal motility disorders, functional GI disorders, and IBS.

Pathologic conditions secondary to chronic GI disease can progress to esophagitis, esophageal stricturing disease, Barrett esophagus, and pancreatitis, which frequently involve therapeutic intervention.

The hepatology subspecialty is often considered a separate entity from gastroenterology. This topic will detail the evaluation of elevated liver enzymes, chronic hepatitis, metabolic liver diseases, liver tumors, and hepatocellular carcinoma.

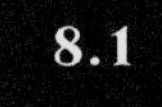

8.1 DISORDERS OF THE ESOPHAGUS

OVERVIEW

The esophagus is a muscular tube that allows transfer of material from the mouth through the upper esophageal sphincter, and propulsion of a bolus through the esophagus through the lower esophageal sphincter (LES) and into the stomach. The upper third of the esophagus is composed of striated muscle and the lower third is composed of smooth muscle. The midesophagus is composed of both striated and smooth muscle. Disruption of the passage of foodstuffs can present with a spectrum of symptoms and pathology, ranging from nonerosive reflux disease (NERD) to malignancy.

PATHOPHYSIOLOGY

The process of swallowing has three phases, which are the oral, pharyngeal, and esophageal phases. Digestion itself begins in the oral cavity. Good oral health is necessary to begin the oral phase of swallowing and the process of digestion. Saliva contains amylase to aid in the digestion of starch. Saliva also contains bicarbonate to neutralize refluxed gastric acid and provides protection from microbes. Salivary glands supply mucus and saliva for mastication to aid in the transport of food around the oral cavity to the teeth to form a bolus. The food bolus is pressed against the hard palate toward the pharynx by the tongue through muscular contraction. The hypoglossal nerve (cranial nerve [CN] XII) is responsible for muscular contraction of the tongue. The facial nerve (CN VII) innervates the mandibular muscles.[1]

The pharynx connects the nose and mouth to both the trachea and esophagus. It can be divided into the nasopharynx, oropharynx, and hypopharynx. It has two separate functions, which include respiration and ingestion of food and liquids. The muscles of the nasopharynx prevent the food bolus from entering the nasal passages. The oropharynx works to propel the food bolus backward into the esophagus. The hypopharynx contains the upper esophageal sphincter.[2]

During the process of swallowing, the soft palate elevates to seal the nasopharynx, preventing reflux of contents into the nasal cavity. For swallowing to occur, the pharynx is activated by a sequence of contraction and relaxation of the pharyngeal muscles to force the bolus to the upper esophageal sphincter. The upper esophageal sphincter is kept closed in the nonswallowing state by the tonic constriction of the cricopharyngeus. Once the process of swallowing begins, the thus upper esophageal sphincter relaxes until the bolus reaches the esophagus. The hypoglossal nerve (CN XII), facial nerve (CN VII), and vagus nerve (CN X) innervate the pharyngeal musculature. The vagus nerve innervates the upper esophageal sphincter and cricopharyngeus.[1]

The esophageal phase of swallowing begins after the passage of the bolus through the upper esophageal sphincter. The contractile function of the upper third of the esophagus is controlled by somatic nerves from the brain. They innervate the motor end plates that terminate on the striated muscle fibers through the release of acetylcholine via nicotinic receptors.[2] The bolus is transported through the esophageal lumen in conjunction with the swallowing reflex, as this transitions to smooth muscle in the lower third of the esophagus.

Autonomic regulation of swallowing in the lower two-thirds of the esophagus involves the vagus nerve and enteric nervous system. The vagus nerve innervates the smooth muscle of the esophagus through *vagal efferents*, which synapse with myenteric neurons through acetylcholine and the smooth muscle through muscarinic receptors and substance P. The esophagus contains *sensory afferents* that communicate to the vagus region of the brain in the dorsal vagal complex. The esophagus also contains enteric neurons that sense esophageal contents and contribute to the coordination of local reflexes that control swallowing and esophageal peristalsis. Normal esophageal peristalsis and sphincter relaxation occur through the activity of the vagus nerve and enteric nervous system. This is mediated by nitric oxide release from inhibitory nerves in the myenteric plexus. The solid food bolus is propelled along the esophagus by coordinated muscular contraction and relaxation through primary peristalsis. Gravity helps to assist in movement of liquid. Distention of the esophagus creates secondary peristalsis, which clears any remaining material refluxed from the stomach.[2]

In the smooth muscle esophagus, inhibitory (relaxatory) and excitatory (contractile) motor neurons in the myenteric plexus are activated by preganglionic fibers that originate in the dorsal motor nucleus of the vagus. Inhibitory neurons release nitric oxide, which relaxes the muscle allowing bolus passage. This is known as deglutitive relaxation, which increases in duration from proximal to distal, producing peristaltic contractions. Postganglionic excitatory neurons release acetylcholine and other neurotransmitters including serotonin, which promote contraction of the muscle wall. This sequence of events requires central coordination, in conjunction with local reflexes. This is activated by mechanical stimulation to produce an esophageal contraction that clears the esophageal lumen of the swallowed bolus.[3]

Hormonal and neurogenic factors along with the diaphragm work to prevent backflow of gastric contents into the esophageal lumen by maintaining a lower esophageal pressure and a functional LES. The LES is the antireflux mechanism. It is a segment of smooth muscle that is normally chronically contracted and maintains a pressure approximately 15 mm Hg above the intragastric pressure. Relaxation of the LES permits the bolus to be transported into the stomach.

The sphincter pressure can be influenced by meal composition and medications. Inappropriate relaxation of the LES can also be exacerbated by obesity and other diseases. Dysfunction of the LES can result in the reflux of gastric contents into the lower esophageal lumen, causing GERD. Prolonged exposure to acid and pepsin from backflow of gastric contents can cause injury to the esophageal squamous epithelium, resulting in esophagitis.

8.1A GASTROESOPHAGEAL REFLUX DISEASE

MEDICAL HISTORY AND CLINICAL PRESENTATION

GERD is a common disease in the United States, affecting up to 20% of the Western population. It results from the backflow of gastroduodenal contents into the esophageal lumen, which may produce injury to the esophageal mucosa. For most patients with GERD, the predominant mechanism of reflux is transient LES relaxations.[4]

Severe reflux is common in patients with scleroderma or connective tissue disease causing chronically low LES pressure and a hypotensive LES. Other risk factors for GERD include hiatal hernia (see Section 8.16 Hiatal Hernia and Abdominal Wall Hernias), increased gastric volume, obesity, alcohol, tobacco, and pregnancy. The obesity epidemic contributes to the increased incidence of GERD. Obesity causes increased pressure on the diaphragm, which can result in reflux of gastric contents into the esophagus.

Heartburn or pyrosis is defined as retrosternal burning discomfort in the epigastric area that may radiate upward toward the neck, occurring after meals. Dysphagia is defined as difficulty in swallowing and odynophagia is pain with swallowing.

Uncontrolled reflux can result in esophagitis and can cause esophageal stenosis, webs, and stricturing disease. A Schatzki ring can cause a benign stricture in the lower esophagus and often requires serial dilations to achieve symptomatic improvement in dysphagia.

Benign peptic strictures are usually due to acid reflux and result from esophageal injury. Radiation therapy for head and neck cancer or esophageal cancer or mediastinal radiation for other malignancies can result in esophageal strictures, even many years after treatment.

Patients who present with symptoms occurring at least twice a week for 8 weeks or more can be considered to have GERD. Alarm signs that necessitate a prompt workup with an upper endoscopy or imaging study to rule out malignancy include dysphagia, odynophagia, unexplained weight loss, family history of esophageal cancer, anemia, and new onset of symptoms in patients over the age of 50.

SIGNS AND SYMPTOMS

The more common manifestations of GERD that patients present with include heartburn, regurgitation, and dysphagia. Other symptoms include globus (sense of a lump in the throat), noncardiac chest pain, and bilious vomiting. Extraintestinal manifestations can include cough, hoarseness, laryngitis, dental disease, sinusitis, and pulmonary fibrosis.

PHYSICAL EXAMINATION

The physical examination is often normal in a patient presenting with GERD. Obesity should be documented.

DIFFERENTIAL DIAGNOSIS

The differential diagnosis for GERD includes cardiac etiology in any patient presenting with a complaints of chest pain. Differential diagnosis includes chronic esophagitis, Barrett esophagus, functional dyspepsia, esophageal motility disorder, and gastroparesis.

A diagnosis of GERD can be suggested by presenting symptoms and whether there is a response to a trial of a proton pump inhibitor (PPI) medication.

DIAGNOSTIC STUDIES

A barium swallow x-ray or an upper GI series can evaluate the esophageal anatomy for strictures, rings, or webs. Findings suggestive of a stricture or mass would necessitate an urgent endoscopy.

Patients who continue to be symptomatic or require chronic PPI medication to control symptoms of reflux should undergo an upper endoscopy study to evaluate for chronic esophagitis. An esophagogastroduodenoscopy (EGD) is performed under sedation. A flexible endoscope with a camera is passed orally down the length of the esophagus, through the gastroesophageal junction into the stomach, through the pylorus, and into the first portion of the duodenum. Esophageal biopsies are obtained if there are abnormalities noted such as salmon-colored mucosa (consistent with Barrett esophagus), ulcer, or rings.

Twenty-four-hour pH impedance testing can further evaluate for extraintestinal manifestations of GERD and nonacid reflux. Impedance pH monitoring is performed with insertion of a transnasal catheter that is worn by the patient for 24 hours. This detects movement of fluid and gas into the esophagus and measures pH, enabling detection of acid and nonacid reflux episodes. Information is transmitted to a monitor worn on the waist of the patient and the patient is instructed to record events on a diary.

A wireless capsule or "bravo" study is a wireless pH capsule that is placed endoscopically and allows recording of acid reflux for 48 hours. This device measures acid reflux by detecting drops in esophageal pH to <4.0. The patient records events on a diary during that time period.

An esophageal manometry study defines the integrity of the LES and can determine if there is a hypotensive LES as a cause for reflux (see Section 8.1D Esophageal Motility Disorders for further information on esophageal manometry).

EVALUATION

A patient with GERD who undergoes an upper endoscopy and has a normal examination, without evidence of inflammation, is classified as having NERD. A patient with NERD can be treated symptomatically with as-needed (PRN) PPI therapy.[5] Esophageal biopsies will rule out chronic reflux esophagitis, eosinophilic esophagitis, or Barrett esophagus.

TREATMENT

The goal of treatment in a patient with GERD is to prevent complications from the disease. Lifestyle modifications are the cornerstone of managing and treating GERD. It is reasonable to consider a short-term trial of a daily PPI for symptom management if lifestyle changes and H2 blockers do not provide relief.

For symptomatic treatment of GERD, over-the-counter (OTC) antacids or histamine antagonists (H2 blockers) can be used. OTC antacids include calcium carbonate, sodium bicarbonate, magnesium hydroxide, and aluminum hydroxide. H2 blockers include ranitidine, cimetidine, and famotidine. These agents provide quick relief and are appropriate for short-term management of symptoms.

A patient with a peptic stricture from GERD requires repeated dilation of the stricture. A PPI is indicated for long-term acid suppression. PPI medications include omeprazole, esomeprazole, lansoprazole, pantoprazole, and rabeprazole.

Risks versus benefits need to be considered in long-term use of PPI medication. The use of PPIs over many years has been controversially implicated in osteoporosis, kidney disease, and dementia. PPI therapy and safety outcomes including dementia, bone fracture, chronic kidney disease, and pneumonia have shown no association with PPI therapy on 3-year follow-up. There is, however, a significant association with enteric infections, specifically with *Clostridium difficile*.[6]

Potential side effects of PPI therapy include diarrhea and drug–drug interactions. Long-term use of PPI medication can potentially affect iron and vitamin B12 absorption, and this should be periodically monitored in patients who remain on PPIs for >5 years.[7]

Surgery for reflux is controversial. Before this is performed, a patient should undergo further evaluation of reflux. Abnormal 24-hour pH scores are a significant predictor of successful outcome following fundoplication surgery for reflux.[8] Patients with typical GERD symptoms with normal pH testing are less likely to have a successful outcome following surgery for reflux.[9]

PATIENT EDUCATION

- Classic complaints of heartburn can often be managed with lifestyle changes.
- For overweight or obese patients, counseling on weight reduction is essential. Weight reduction can provide benefit in controlling not only reflux disease but many other diseases.
- Smoking is a risk factor for which patients should be counseled.
- Dietary triggers can reduce LES pressure and can cause reflux. Examples include caffeine, spicy foods, chocolate, peppermint, pepper, alcohol, and fatty foods.
- Patients should be told to avoid late time meals and to raise the head of the bed at night to control nocturnal symptoms.
- If pharmacotherapy is required, patient should be educated on proper dosing. A PPI should be dosed approximately 30 minutes before eating to ensure maximum effectiveness. Antacids and H2 blockers should be dosed 2 or more hours away from the PPI.

8.1B ESOPHAGITIS

MEDICAL HISTORY AND CLINICAL PRESENTATION

Esophagitis is an inflammatory process of the esophagus and is an endoscopic diagnosis. It can result from GERD and can be a cause of unexplained chest pain. Medications and bacterial or viral infections can also be a cause of esophagitis (Table 8.1).[10]

Eosinophilic esophagitis (EoE) is a condition that may require endoscopic retrieval of a food bolus. EoE typically presents with recurrent dysphagia often associated with food impaction. After removal of the food bolus, high-dose PPI therapy (twice daily dosing) is prescribed. An EGD should then be performed 12 weeks later with biopsies of the proximal and distal esophagus.

DIAGNOSTIC STUDIES

The classic endoscopic findings in EoE include a ringed appearance of the esophagus. Untreated disease can result in narrowing of the esophagus and strictures. The diagnosis is based on pathology findings showing eosinophilic infiltration of 15 or more eosinophils per high-power field. The disease is incompletely understood. Evidence suggests that this is an allergic disorder mediated by antigen sensitization either through foods or aeroallergens. Disorders associated with eosinophilic infiltration include Crohn disease, infectious esophagitis such as *Candida* or herpesvirus infection, GERD, drug induced, and cardiovascular disease (CVD).[11]

TREATMENT

- Approximately 25% to 40% of patients with suspected EoE respond to PPI therapy and eosinophils are no longer seen on esophageal biopsies when endoscopy is repeated. These patients are considered to have PPI responsive esophageal eosinophilia.
- If histologic findings of eosinophilia persist despite PPI therapy, then treatment with topical corticosteroids is added. Topical fluticasone is prescribed in doses ranging from 220 to 440 mcg twice daily whereby the inhaled steroid is swallowed for 6 to 12 weeks and during this interval most patients will respond symptomatically and histologically.

TABLE 8.1 Los Angeles Grade System of Esophagitis

Grade	Description
0	No esophagitis
A	One or more mucosal breaks <5 mm long without extending between mucosal folds
B	One of more mucosal breaks >5 mm long not extending between mucosal folds
C	One or more mucosal breaks continuous between the tops of more than two mucosal folds, involving <75% of the circumference
D	One mucosal break involving ≥75% of the circumference

Source: Data from Lundell LR, Dent J, Bennett JR, et al. Endoscopic assessment of esophagitis: clinical and functional correlates and further validation of the Los Angeles classification. Gut. *1999;45(2):172–180. doi:10.1136/gut.45.2.172*[10]

- Depending upon the response, the steroid therapy can be reduced to 1 week out of each month. Symptoms are more likely to recur within 18 months in half of patients who discontinue therapy.
- An alternative to a swallowed fluticasone inhaler is a liquid-based formulation of budesonide containing .5 mg of budesonide mixed in a 10–15 mL slurry that can be taken twice a day.[11]

PATIENT EDUCATION

- A referral to an allergist is usually recommended in patients with histologic findings of persistent esophageal eosinophilia. The most common allergenic foods are dairy, eggs, wheat, soy, peanuts, and fish/shellfish.[12]
- Elemental or amino based formula diets have also been shown to be effective in alleviating symptoms, but they are not well tolerated in an oral form.

8.1C BARRETT ESOPHAGUS

MEDICAL HISTORY AND CLINICAL PRESENTATION

In patients with chronic esophageal injury from reflux, Barrett metaplasia can develop when mucus-secreting columnar cells replace reflux-damaged esophageal squamous cells. Barrett esophagus is defined by pathology as either intestinal metaplasia, low-grade dysplasia or high-grade dysplasia. *Metaplasia,* in which one cell type replaces another, results from chronic tissue injury. *Dysplasia* is defined has having neoplastic epithelium that remains confined within the basement membrane. Carcinomas are preceded by dysplasia and they can also coexist with dysplasia. Treatment of dysplasia lowers the incidence of carcinoma. High-grade dysplasia is usually confirmed by two expert GI pathologists.

The annual risk of esophageal adenocarcinoma is approximately .25% for patients without dysplasia and 6% for patients with high-grade dysplasia.[13] Risk factors for progression to adenocarcinoma in Barrett esophagus include long segment of Barrett esophagus, erosive esophagitis, presence of a large hiatal hernia, advanced age, age <30 years at onset of GERD symptoms, male sex, White race, family history, tobacco use, and obesity. Protective factors for Barrett esophagus and esophageal adenocarcinoma include the use of nonsteroidal anti-inflammatory drugs (NSAIDs), use of statins, *Helicobacter pylori* infection, and a diet high in fruits and vegetables.[14]

SIGNS AND SYMPTOMS

There are no specific signs and symptoms for Barrett esophagitis. Findings on endoscopy show columnar mucosa extending above the gastroesophageal junction and lining the distal esophagus.

DIAGNOSTIC STUDIES

A diagnosis of Barrett esophagus is defined by pathology from esophageal biopsies showing intestinal metaplasia with goblet cells. The extent of esophageal columnar metaplasia defines whether there is long segment (greater than ≥3 cm of columnar metaplasia) or short segment (<3 cm) Barrett esophagus.

TREATMENT

- Long-term PPI therapy is indicated in a patient with Barrett esophagus. A surveillance endoscopy is generally recommended in 1 year for intestinal metaplasia and if stable, EGDs are performed at intervals of 3 to 5 years.
- Low-grade dysplasia is surveyed by a repeat EGD in 3 to 6 months with extensive surveillance biopsies to confirm that this is the highest lesion. An EGD is then performed annually or endoscopic ablative therapy can be considered.[14]
- High-grade dysplasia warrants endoscopic intervention. An endoscopic ultrasound (EUS) should be performed prior to considering endoscopic techniques to confirm that the stage of the lesion is superficial and appropriate for endoscopic resection.
- *Endoscopic mucosal resection* or *endoscopic ablation* is performed by an advanced therapeutic gastroenterologist.
- Surveillance endoscopy is performed every 3 months for the first year after treating high-grade dysplasia, then every 6 months for the next year, and then annually thereafter.[14–16]

SPECIAL CONSIDERATIONS

- *Adenocarcinoma of the esophagus* is the most common cause of esophageal cancer in the United States. It is usually discovered at a very late stage and the prognosis is poor. There are no specific guidelines for screening for this and usually a patient is not symptomatic until a very late stage. Approximately 40% of patients report no symptoms of GERD at the time of presentation. Risk factors include Barrett esophagus, tobacco use, and obesity. A diet rich in fruits and vegetables is thought to be protective. Patients with chronic GERD are at an increased risk for Barrett esophagus, however, it is unrealistic to screen based on the presence of GERD symptoms given that 20% of the U.S. population experiences weekly acid reflux. The role of screening for Barrett esophagus with upper endoscopy remains unclear. The American College of Gastroenterology guidelines suggest that the highest yield in screening should be reserved for patients over the age of 50 with chronic GERD symptoms.[17]
- *Squamous cell cancer of the esophagus* is the most common form of esophageal cancer worldwide. There is a high incidence found in Turkey, northeastern Iran, Kazakhstan, northern and Central China, and southern and eastern Africa. It occurs more commonly in the midesophagus, while adenocarcinoma usually occurs in the lower esophagus. While tobacco use is a risk factor for both adenocarcinoma and squamous cell cancers of the esophagus, alcohol consumption is a risk factor only for squamous cell cancer of the esophagus. Other risk factors for squamous cell esophageal cancer include achalasia, caustic injury, human papillomavirus (HPV), history of thoracic radiation, low socioeconomic status, poor oral hygiene, and nutritional deficiencies.[18]

8.1D ESOPHAGEAL MOTILITY DISORDERS

MEDICAL HISTORY AND CLINICAL PRESENTATION

Motility disorders of the esophagus can involve both the striated and smooth muscle. These disorders frequently present with dysphagia (refer to Section 8.11 Dysphagia and Table 8.35). Oropharyngeal dysphagia can present with upper esophageal symptoms or aspiration. A patient with oropharyngeal dysphagia will often complain of increased difficulty swallowing liquids compared to solids. A patient will often have difficulty initiating a swallow and transferring a food bolus from the mouth into the esophagus. Regurgitation of food or fluid may occur from the upper esophagus, immediately with swallowing. Nasal regurgitation can also occur. Risk factors for this condition include neurologic or muscular diseases. Previous radiation therapy to the head or neck can also cause upper esophageal symptoms. A Zenker diverticulum arises just above the cricopharyngeus muscle in the posterior wall of the hypopharynx. The diverticulum can retain food and material and can be a cause of delayed regurgitation, halitosis, and aspiration. Dysphagia is usually due to compression of the diverticulum into the esophagus.

A patient with esophageal dysphagia will have complaints of dysphagia mainly with solid food and a sensation of food sticking or getting "hung up" in the esophagus. This can occur from a mechanical process impairing movement such as a Schatzki ring or stricture, malignancy, or an esophageal motility disorder. Disease of the smooth muscle or excitatory nerves include weak muscle contractions or decreased LES tone, which can be seen in scleroderma or collagen vascular disease, myotonic dystrophy or neuromuscular disorders. Disorders of inhibitory innervation include achalasia and diffuse esophageal spasm.

Diffuse esophageal spasm is characterized by multiple simultaneous nonperistaltic contractions and abnormal esophageal peristalsis due to loss of deglutitive inhibition and impairment of inhibitory nerve function of the smooth muscle esophagus. Some patients will progress to achalasia. Achalasia is an esophageal motility disorder that is characterized by failed esophageal peristalsis and failure of the LES to relax with swallowing. It results from degeneration of postganglionic inhibitory neurons. In the United States, there is usually no known cause and it is considered idiopathic. It is an uncommon disorder, affecting approximately 1 in 100,000 people and usually manifests between the ages of 25 and 50.[19]

Hypercontractile esophageal motility disorders include jackhammer esophagus and distal esophageal spasm. These disorders typically present with chest pain. The causes are unknown but thought to be related to disturbed neuromuscular function. There are no established associations between these esophageal motility disorders and clinical disease. Jackhammer esophagus occurs more commonly in younger populations, while distal esophageal spasm is more common in older patients.[3]

SIGNS AND SYMPTOMS

Common presentations of an esophageal motility disorder include dysphagia, noncardiac chest pain, globus sensation, gagging, and vomiting. Dysphagia to liquids and solids is slowly progressive in achalasia and symptoms include regurgitation of undigested food, liquid, foam, and/or mucus. There may be a history of significant weight loss as the disease progresses due to inability to tolerate oral feedings.

PHYSICAL EXAMINATION

Physical examination may be normal. Evaluate body mass index (BMI). Evaluate neck and chest for abnormalities suggesting external compression.

DIFFERENTIAL DIAGNOSIS

CVD must first be excluded in any patient presenting with chest pain. Noncardiac chest pain differential diagnosis includes esophageal motility disorder, gallbladder disease, pancreatitis, chest wall pain, pericarditis, or mediastinal pain from inflammation or tumor.

The differential diagnosis for dysphagia includes oropharyngeal dysphagia, esophageal motility disorder, reflux, chronic esophagitis, EoE, stricture, and malignancy.

DIAGNOSTIC STUDIES

A barium swallow x-ray is a helpful imaging tool for evaluating the esophageal anatomy. Structural abnormalities in the upper esophagus such as a cricopharyngeal bar or Zenker diverticulum can be identified by barium swallow or videofluoroscopic swallowing study. An upper endoscopy study is indicated for a patient presenting with dysphagia or odynophagia to ultimately rule out malignancy.

If a patient has risk factors for pharyngeal dysphagia or has upper esophageal symptoms, a videofluoroscopy swallowing study with speech therapy is indicated. This is performed in conjunction with a speech therapist, whereby the patient under supervision is given soft food items to eat while the swallowing study is performed.

An esophageal manometry study is the gold standard for diagnosing an esophageal motility disorder. This is performed while the patient is awake. A transnasal catheter with pressure sensors is passed into the esophagus through the LES and into the stomach. The patient is then given sips of water. Esophageal manometry measures the strength or amplitude, duration, and nature of contractions (peristalsis) in the esophageal body. The lower esophageal resting pressure and LES pressure are also measured.

EVALUATION

The classic radiologic finding of achalasia on a barium swallow study is a "bird beak" sign, which shows a dilated esophagus with narrowing and tapering at the LES. It is essential that an upper endoscopy be performed to rule out pseudoachalasia or malignancy.

A transient cricopharyngeal bar can be an incidental finding on an x-ray in up to 5% of individuals without dysphagia and can be reproduced during a Valsalva maneuver.

A cervical esophageal web can be an incidental finding or may be a cause of intermittent solid food dysphagia. Plummer-Vinson syndrome is a condition seen more commonly in females with dysphagia who are found to have an esophageal web and iron deficiency anemia.

An esophageal manometry study consistent with achalasia will show 100% failed peristalsis and impaired relaxation of the LES.

In distal esophageal spasm, abnormal simultaneous or spastic contractions occur in the mid- to distal esophagus. Jackhammer esophagus, formerly called nutcracker esophagus, is characterized by high pressure esophageal contractions.

Ineffective esophageal motility is defined has having esophageal aperistalsis with a normal or low LES pressure. It is also known as scleroderma esophagus. A connective tissue disorder should be included in the differential diagnosis in a patient diagnosed with ineffective esophageal motility.

Esophagogastric junction (EGJ) outflow obstruction is defined as having normal peristalsis with a high LES pressure. CT of the chest should be obtained to rule out extrinsic compression. An upper endoscopy is essential to rule out malignancy in a patient found to have EGJ outflow obstruction.

TREATMENT

- Table 8.2 lists treatment for esophageal motility disorders.
- Treatment for symptomatic Zenker diverticulum is diverticulectomy with criocopharyngeal myotomy. This is performed endoscopically with an advanced therapeutic gastroenterologist or referred to an otolaryngologist.[19]
- Achalasia
  - Treatment is directed toward relaxing or disrupting the LES.
  - Treatment of achalasia does not restore peristalsis.
  - Mild symptoms can be treated empirically with medications that help relax the LES such as sublingual nitroglycerin, calcium channel blockers, anticholinergic drugs, or phosphodiesterase inhibitors.
  - Temporary relief can be achieved by endoscopic botulinum toxin injections to the LES. Pneumatic dilation can also be performed. This involves successive dilation with a pneumatic balloon, designed to tear the muscles of the LES. This incurs a small risk (<4%) of esophageal rupture.
  - A Heller myotomy is a minimally invasive surgical procedure that can be performed laparoscopically.
  - Peroral endoscopic myotomy (POEM) is performed endoscopically by making a mucosal incision 10–15 cm proximal to the LES and creating a submucosal tunnel 2–4 cm onto the gastric cardia. A circular muscle myotomy is performed with the tunnel, dividing the circular layer of the LES.
    - The advantages of POEM over laparoscopic Heller myotomy include no abdominal incisions, more rapid recovery, avoidance of vagal nerve injury, and avoidance of intra-abdominal incisions.
    - POEM is becoming a more favorable approach due to low risk and good outcomes. However, there is a high rate of gastroesophageal reflux following this and many patients may require lifelong PPI therapy for symptomatic reflux or erosive esophagitis.[20]

PATIENT EDUCATION

- There is no cure for an esophageal motility disorder and treatment is directed toward improving symptoms.

TABLE 8.2 Esophageal Motility Disorders and Treatment

Esophageal Motility Disorder	Treatment
Aperistalsis/absent contractility Ineffective esophageal motility	Target GERD therapy; treatment cannot restore peristalsis nor can it improve smooth muscle contractility
Esophageal spasm Hypercontractile esophagus/ jackhammer esophagus	Anticholinergic, calcium channel blocker (nifedipine 20 mg), nitrate, trazodone, or phosphodiesterase-5 inhibitor (sildenafil)
Achalasia EGJ outflow obstruction	Botox, pneumatic dilation, myotomy (POEM or surgical myotomy)

EGJ, esophagogastric junction; GERD, gastroesophageal reflux disease; POEM, peroral endoscopic myotomy.

- There are treatments for reducing LES pressure, but there are no treatments for improving esophageal peristalsis.
- Patients should be advised on modifying eating behavior to eat slowly, chew food well, and separate solids from liquids.

SPECIAL CONSIDERATIONS

- Caustic injury can cause esophageal stricture. In children caustic injuries are typically accidental; however, in adults the majority are due to suicide attempts.[21] Ingestion of alkali (e.g., drain cleaners, household cleaning products, and disc batteries) will typically cause more damage to the esophagus compared to the stomach or duodenum. Acid ingestion tends to cause more severe gastric injury. Aspiration of either acid or alkali can cause laryngeal and tracheobronchial injury. There is a higher risk of perforation and complications in caustic injury; therefore, an EGD is recommended within 12 hours and no longer than 24 hours after ingestion to classify the mucosal injury, specifically in suicide cases to help predict outcomes.[22] There is also a significant risk of squamous cell esophageal cancer following such injury. Surveillance endoscopy is recommended every 2 to 3 years beginning 10 to 20 years after caustic ingestion.[16]
- Infectious esophagitis usually presents with odynophagia and is more common in the immunosuppressed and elderly. Immunosuppressed patients can develop herpes simplex virus (HSV) and cytomegalovirus (CMV) infections from reactivation of latent viruses. *Candida* infection can result from colonization due to stricture or obstruction and can also be associated with HSV and CMV infections. Diagnosis is by endoscopy and biopsy.

KEY POINTS

- Neurologic diseases including cerebrovascular accident, central nervous system (CNS) disease, reduced level of consciousness, trauma, dementia, and CNS tumors can impact the oropharyngeal phase of swallowing and lead to aspiration.
- Neuromuscular disease such as myasthenia gravis is a risk factor for aspiration from oropharyngeal dysfunction.
- Dysphagia is an "alarm" symptom, necessitating a prompt upper endoscopy.
- PPIs should be used at the lowest effective dose and the need for their continued use should be periodically reassessed.
- Manifestations of chest pain from an esophageal motility disorder or GERD can mimic cardiac disease, which must first be ruled out.

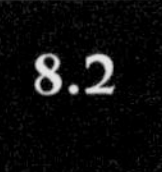

8.2 DISORDERS OF THE STOMACH/DUODENUM

OVERVIEW

The stomach functions to break down an ingested food bolus into smaller particles. This is accomplished through a complex process of endocrine and exocrine secretions. Coordinated activity between the CNS and the stomach is also necessary for the process of digestion from the stomach through the pylorus and into the first portion of the small intestine, the duodenum.

The stomach is divided into the fundus and corpus (body) which are considered oxyntic mucosa, and the pyloric or antrum region, which is antral mucosa. The proximal stomach consists of the cardia, fundus, and proximal portion of the corpus. The distal portion of the stomach is called the antrum. The proximal stomach serves as a reservoir to move gastric contents to the distal stomach where grinding and mixing of the meal is accomplished to produce chyme that eventually gets absorbed into the small intestine.

Phasic contractions in the distal stomach contract and relax, while tonic contractions in the proximal stomach are sustained contractions. Specific motility patterns, known as the migrating motor complex (MMC), help to move food and particles beginning in the stomach.[23] The proximal stomach relaxes to accommodate the meal. Phasic contractions of the distal part of the stomach propel food against the pylorus. The pylorus separates the stomach from the duodenum and acts as a sphincter that controls the material that leaves the stomach and empties into the duodenum. The function of the pylorus is independent of the distal stomach and proximal small bowel segments. Nitric oxide from both vagal and intrinsic pathways works to relax the pylorus. The presence of nutrients, hypertonicity, and duodenal acid contribute to feedback reflexes from the duodenum that result in closure of the pylorus.[24]

PATHOPHYSIOLOGY

Gastric motility is also controlled by the enteric nervous system and smooth muscle cells. Serotonin (5-hydroxytryptamine, or 5-HT) is localized in the enterochromaffin cells of the GI mucosa and within neurons of the enteric nervous system and effects neuromodulation of the gut smooth muscle function. Myenteric neurons of the stomach provide coordination of gastric motility during fasting periods. The enteric nervous system includes the interstitial cells of Cajal, which are considered the "pacemaker" of the stomach and are located within the deep muscular plexus of the stomach and duodenum.[23] Diseases of connective tissue and neurologic or paraneoplastic disorders can interfere with the function at any of these levels, resulting in abnormal gastric emptying.

The oxyntic mucosa in the gastric fundus contains parietal cells, chief cells, enterochromaffin-like (ECL) cells, D cells, and ghrelin. G cells in the antral mucosa secrete gastrin and also contain D cells that secrete somatostatin. The parietal cells in the fundus secrete hydrochloric acid which helps to sterilize the stomach. The parietal cells also secrete intrinsic factor, which is necessary for vitamin B12 absorption. Chief cells secrete pepsinogen, an inactive precursor to pepsin, which is involved in protein digestion. Histamine is a paracrine agent, secreted by ECL cells, to help regulate gastric secretion.[25]

Once food is propelled into the stomach, gastrin is released and binds to cholecystokinin-2 receptors on the ECL cells causing histamine secretion. Histamine binds to the histamine 2 receptors on the parietal cells and is coupled to hydrochloric acid secretion through activation of hydrogen potassium adenosine triphosphatase (H^+-K^+-ATPase), also known as the proton pump. PPI medications inhibit the function of the parietal cell H^+-K^+-ATPase, and greatly reduce acid secretion, decrease somatostatin secretin, and subsequently stimulate gastrin secretion.[25] Gastrin is a trophic hormone, which results in the growth of fundic gland polyps, commonly seen with chronic use of PPI, which are considered benign.

Gastric acid facilitates the digestion of protein and absorption of iron, magnesium, and calcium. The parietal cells in the stomach release intrinsic factor, which is needed for vitamin B12 absorption. By lowering the pH, gastric acid also limits bacterial growth in the stomach, which potentially helps in preventing infections such as *Helicobacter pylori* and *Clostridium difficile* and may have a role in preventing spontaneous bacterial peritonitis (SBP).[26,27]

8.2A GASTRITIS

MEDICAL HISTORY AND CLINICAL PRESENTATION

Acute gastritis is a common mucosal acute inflammatory process and is usually transient. It is often triggered by NSAIDs and can resolve if the stimulus is removed.

Helicobacter pylori (*H. pylori*) infection is another cause of gastritis. *H. pylori* is endemic in certain areas of the world and can be associated with household contacts. It can be transmitted by the fecal-oral route, usually in childhood. *H. pylori* is a motile, flagellated, gram-negative bacterium that survives in an acid environment in the antrum of the stomach. It produces urease, which converts urea to ammonia, generating areas of acid neutralization in the stomach.

Risk factors for GI toxicity from NSAIDs include older age, chronic use of high-dose NSAIDs, and history of an ulcer. The damaging effects of NSAIDs are due to cyclooxygenase, the enzyme involved in prostaglandin synthesis. Prostaglandins are mediators of defensive mechanisms that stimulate secretion of mucus and bicarbonate to protect gastric mucosa, resist acid penetration, and promote healing and angiogenesis. Cyclooxygenase-2 (COX-2) specific inhibitors are NSAIDs that do not significantly affect the upper GI prostaglandin levels. A COX-2 selective inhibitor is an alternative drug to an NSAID that can relieve pain and inflammation without causing damage to the upper GI tract by sparing mucosal prostaglandin production.

H. pylori is considered a carcinogen and if left untreated is a risk factor for gastric adenocarcinoma and gastric mucosa associated lymphoid tissue (MALT) lymphoma. *H. pylori* gastritis results in a reduction in hydrochloric acid production. The extent of acid loss is directly related to the development of gastric cancer. The chronic inflammation caused by this infection, in addition to genetic susceptibility, can cause gastric intestinal metaplasia. Treatment of *H. pylori* gastritis reduces this risk.[28]

SIGNS AND SYMPTOMS

Gastritis often presents with upper abdominal pain. Pain may be described as burning or dull. Symptoms may include bloating and indigestion.

PHYSICAL EXAMINATION

The physical examination may be normal in uncomplicated acute gastritis. The abdomen should be examined for guarding or rebound. A rectal examination is performed to evaluate for blood.

DIFFERENTIAL DIAGNOSIS

The differential diagnosis for gastritis includes peptic ulcer disease, NSAID-induced gastritis, *H. pylori* infection, GERD, or functional dyspepsia.

DIAGNOSTIC STUDIES

Laboratory studies include complete blood count (CBC) with differential.

A fecal *H. pylori* antigen or a urea breath test are noninvasive ways to screen for *H. pylori* and are appropriate for younger patients without alarm features.

Upper endoscopy is indicated if the patient has hemoccult positive stools or persistent unexplained pain.

EVALUATION

If the physical examination and labs are normal and if the patient's history is suggestive of NSAID use as a potential cause of abdominal pain, it is reasonable to prescribe a PPI to assess for symptomatic improvement. Discontinuation of the NSAID and treatment with a PPI for 12 weeks is a recommended.

If the urea breath test or fecal antigen test is positive for *H. pylori*, the patient should be treated accordingly. Follow-up testing after completion of therapy should be performed to ensure eradication.

The presence of atrophic gastritis and intestinal metaplasia on endoscopy may be a potential precursor for stomach cancer; however, there currently are no U.S. guidelines for management. The European guidelines suggest endoscopic surveillance every 1 to 2 years.[29]

TREATMENT

- Positive testing for *H. pylori* requires a 10- to 14-day regimen of twice daily PPI and antibiotics (Table 8.3).[30]
  - At least 4 weeks or more following completion of therapy, a repeat urea breath test or an *H. pylori* stool antigen test should be ordered to document clearance.
- For patients negative for *H. pylori*, treatments used to help protect the GI mucosa include misoprostol, a prostaglandin analog, histamine H2 receptor agonist, or PPI.
- NSAIDs are appropriate in patients at low risk of GI complications. Co-therapy with a PPI or misoprostol is preferred for patients with GI risk factors. For patients at high risk, a COX-2 inhibitor should be considered in place of a traditional NSAID.[31]

PATIENT EDUCATION

- Patients should be counseled on smoking cessation if indicated and avoidance of NSAIDs to reduce the risk of developing ulcer disease.
- If *H. pylori* positive, patients should be counseled on the necessity to ensure this is eradicated due to the risk of gastric cancer.
- Prior to stool or breath testing, the patient needs to be off PPIs or H2 blockers for 2 weeks and off bismuth/antibiotics for 4 weeks to ensure accurate results.

8.2B PEPTIC ULCER DISEASE

OVERVIEW

An ulcer is a loss of surface epithelium that extends into the muscularis mucosa. It develops from a defect in the gastric duodenal wall and extends through the muscularis

TABLE 8.3 *Helicobacter pylori* **Treatment Regimens**

Therapy	Dosage
First-Line Therapy	
Triple therapy, 14 days	Standard dose PPI BID Clarithromycin 500 mg BID Amoxicillin 1 g BID *or* metronidazole 500 mg TID
Second-Line Therapy	
Bismuth quadruple therapy, 10–14 days	Standard dose PPI BID Bismuth subsalicylate 525 mg QID Metronidazole 250 mg QID Tetracycline 500 mg QID
Levofloxacin-based, 10 days	Standard dose PPI BID Levofloxacin 250–500 mg BID Amoxicillin 1 g BID
Clarithromycin sequential, 10–14 days total	Standard dose PPI BID Amoxicillin 1 g BID for the first 5 days Clarithromycin 500 mg BID *and* tinidazole 500 mg bid for the next 5 days
Additional Regimens	
Levofloxacin sequential, 10–14 days total (for clarithromycin-resistant strains)	Standard dose PPI BID Amoxicillin 1 g BID for the first 5 days Levofloxacin 500–1,000 mg BID and metronidazole 500 mg BID (or tinidazole 500 mg BID) for the next 5 days
Quadruple non-bismuth therapy, 10–14 days (clarithromycin/ metronidazole dual resistance)	Standard dose PPI BID Amoxicillin 1 g BID Clarithromycin 500 mg BID Nitroimidazole 500 mg BID
Hybrid therapy, 14 days total (may have higher cure than sequential)	Standard dose PPI BID Amoxicillin 1 g BID for 14 days Clarithromycin 500 mg BID *and* nitroimidazole 500 mg BID for the last 7 days

BID, twice daily; PPI, proton pump inhibitor; QID, four times daily ; TID, three times daily.

mucosa into the deeper layers of the wall. It is >5 mm and is visible by endoscopy or radiographic imaging. Erosions are superficial mucosal lesions that are <5 mm. Unlike ulcers, erosions are unlikely to cause bleeding or perforation.

Peptic ulcer disease includes ulcerations in the stomach and duodenum, caused by an imbalance of protective and aggressive factors including impaired GI mucosal defense mechanisms. Complications of peptic ulcer disease include hemorrhage, perforation, and gastric outlet obstruction. Hemorrhage is the most frequent complication. Peptic ulcer disease is the most common cause of upper GI bleeding. Perforation can lead to peritonitis and release of contents into the peritoneal cavity (see Section 8.7A Peritonitis). Perforation of an ulcer is unusual with the advent of PPIs. Prior to this, surgery for ulcer complications included vagotomy with partial gastric resection or drainage procedures, which caused marked alterations in normal gastric physiology.[32]

MEDICAL HISTORY AND CLINICAL PRESENTATION

NSAIDs and *H. pylori* infection are the most common causes of peptic ulcer disease. The risk is higher with both conditions together. Less common causes of peptic ulcer disease include physiologic stress, acid hypersecretory states, and malignancy.

NSAIDs are a common cause of gastric ulcers, while *H. pylori* infection is the most common cause of duodenal ulcers in developed countries. Older patients are less likely to experience pain compared to younger patients. Risk factors for peptic ulcer disease with NSAID use include older age, frailty, smoking, significant comorbidities, alcohol abuse, and use of antiplatelet or anticoagulant medications.

SIGNS AND SYMPTOMS

Peptic ulcer disease is associated with epigastric pain that can be described as an ache, gnawing sensation, or hunger-like sensation often occurring at night. Eating can exacerbate pain with gastric ulcers. Eating and antacids may temporarily relieve the pain of a duodenal ulcer.

H. pylori infection may or may not present with upper abdominal pain. Severe disease can be associated with anemia, hematemesis, melena, anorexia, or weight loss.

PHYSICAL EXAMINATION

Physical examination is usually normal in uncomplicated peptic ulcer disease. Evaluate for orthostasis or hemodynamic compromise in complicated disease. Evaluate the abdomen for signs of peritonitis or palpable mass. A rectal examination should be performed to assess for occult blood or melena.

DIFFERENTIAL DIAGNOSIS

The differential diagnosis for peptic ulcer disease includes *H. pylori*, NSAID-induced ulcer disease, functional dyspepsia, gastroparesis, GERD, Zollinger-Ellison syndrome (ZES), gastroduodenal Crohn disease, biliary tract disease, pancreatitis, mesenteric ischemia, cardiac ischemia, abdominal aortic aneurysm, and malignancy.

DIAGNOSTIC STUDIES

- Laboratory studies include CBC with differential, liver enzyme tests, and lipase. Consider abdominal ultrasound and EKG.
- Urea breath test and *H. pylori* stool antigen test both identify current infection.
- Endoscopy with biopsy is the standard procedure for diagnosis of peptic ulcer disease.

EVALUATION AND TREATMENT

- Refer to Section 8.6A Upper Gastrointestinal Bleeding for treatment of ulcer disease for patients on clopidogrel or aspirin.
- Positive *H. pylori* testing requires treatment (see Table 8.3).[30] It is essential that eradication of *H. pylori* be documented, with either a follow-up *H. pylori* stool antigen test or a urea breath test 4 to 6 weeks after treatment is completed.

PATIENT EDUCATION

- Smoking cessation is recommended if indicated. The patient is counseled to avoid NSAIDs. In place of NSAIDS, acetaminophen as directed can be recommended for pain.

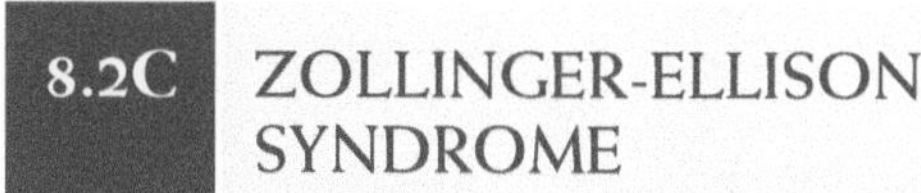

8.2C ZOLLINGER-ELLISON SYNDROME

MEDICAL HISTORY AND CLINICAL PRESENTATION

ZES is an uncommon condition associated with gastric acid hypersecretion. It is caused by hypersecretion of gastrin by gastrinomas and results in refractory peptic ulcers and diarrhea.

Gastrinomas are neuroendocrine tumors which can arise from the duodenum or pancreas. These usually occur sporadically; however, up to 25% are associated with multiple endocrine neoplasia type 1 (MEN1). MEN1 is an autosomal-dominant inherited syndrome characterized by pancreatic neuroendocrine tumors, pituitary tumor, and hyperparathyroidism.[33]

The unregulated gastrin production from the gastrinoma binds to cholecystokinin (CCK-2) receptors on the ECL cells, resulting in histamine release. Histamine binds to the H2 receptors on the parietal cells to stimulate acid release. Gastrin has trophic effects on gastric epithelial and ECL cells. Parietal cell mass also increases due to chronic hypergastrinemia. Diarrhea results from inactivation of pancreatic enzymes from gastric hypersecretion, leading to steatorrhea and malabsorption.[33]

A patient with ZES often will present with symptoms of peptic ulcers due to excessive gastric secretion and complications such as perforation and stricture and will likely be refractory to standard PPI therapy.

SIGNS AND SYMPTOMS

Signs and symptoms of ZES include diarrhea, weight loss, abdominal pain, reflux, nausea, vomiting, and history of peptic ulcers.

PHYSICAL EXAMINATION

The physical examination findings may be normal in ZES. Evaluate BMI and weight trend. Evaluate for pallor, abdominal tenderness, jaundice (if liver involvement), or dental erosion (from excessive acid).

DIFFERENTIAL DIAGNOSIS

The differential diagnosis for hypergastrinemia includes chronic atrophic gastritis, *H. pylori* infection, chronic PPI use, and hypochlorhydria.

DIAGNOSTIC STUDIES

Upper endoscopy is indicated to evaluate for ulcers or gastrinoma.

A fasting gastrin level off PPI should be obtained in a patient suspected with ZES. It is recommended that gastric pH also be measured to rule out secondary causes of hypergastrinemia. A serum gastrin level greater than 10 times the upper limit of normal (ULN) in the setting of a gastric pH <2 is diagnostic of ZES.[34]

A secretin stimulation test can differentiate a patient with gastrinomas from other causes of hypergastrinemia. Secretin stimulates the release of gastrin by gastrinoma cells. Normally gastric G cells are inhibited by secretin. A patient with ZES will have a dramatic rise in gastrin level with administration of intravenous (IV) secretin; serum gastrin level falls or remains unchanged in other disorders.

EVALUATION

Most gastrinomas occur in the first and second portion of the duodenum and tend to be small and multiple. Pancreatic gastrinomas are often larger than 1 cm. Since gastrinomas express somatostatin receptors, this can be used for tumor imaging with PET scanning.

TREATMENT

- The treatment goals of ZES are to control gastric acid hypersecretion in an effort to reduce symptoms and complications. Long-term use of high dose of oral PPI at three to four times above the normal dosing is utilized.
- Somatostatin analogs such as octreotide alone or in combination with alfa-interferon are indicated for initial antitumor therapy for metastatic disease.
- Surgery is recommended in patients with ZES without MEN1 syndrome who do not have metastatic disease. Surgery is controversial in ZES patients with MEN1 due to gastrinomas being multifocal and surgery is rarely curative. In patients with MEN1, resection is recommended after surgery for primary hyperparathyroidism and only for tumors >2 cm.[33]

8.2D GASTROPARESIS

MEDICAL HISTORY AND CLINICAL PRESENTATION

Gastroparesis is defined as a delay in gastric emptying in the absence of an obstructing lesion in the stomach or distal GI tract. Disorders that interfere with the neuromuscular coordination of the stomach can result in gastroparesis. The most common causes are diabetic, idiopathic, and postsurgical. Hypothyroidism, scleroderma, Parkinson disease, and trauma from head injury or spinal cord injury are also risk factors for gastroparesis.

The patient may have a history of chronic reflux not controlled with PPI or H2 blockers. There is often an overlap of functional dyspepsia. Symptoms of nausea, vomiting, and postprandial pain may have coincided following a viral illness.

Medications such as opiates, tricyclic antidepressants (TCAs), dopamine, and calcium channel blockers can also delay gastric emptying and cause symptoms.

SIGNS AND SYMPTOMS

The signs and symptoms of gastroparesis include epigastric fullness, nausea, reflux, weight loss, early satiety, and vomiting of ingested food hours to days from previous consumption. Symptoms of dumping syndrome or rapid gastric emptying can mimic those of gastroparesis and can be seen in Roux-en-Y gastric bypass patients.

PHYSICAL EXAMINATION

Evaluate for orthostasis, pallor, skin turgor, or temporal wasting. Evaluate the oral cavity for glossitis, cheilosis, and dentition. The abdominal examination includes inspection for surgical scars or abdominal distention and evaluation for bowel sounds. Assess for Carnett sign and Murphy sign and palpate for tenderness or mass.

DIFFERENTIAL DIAGNOSIS

The differential diagnosis for gastroparesis includes dumping syndrome, gastric outlet obstruction, peptic ulcer disease, cholecystitis, choledocholithiasis, extrinsic abdominal mass, stomach cancer, and biliary tract cancer.

DIAGNOSTIC STUDIES

- Thyroid-stimulating hormone (TSH), comprehensive metabolic panel (CMP), HbA1c (if the patient is diabetic)
- Abdominal CT scan to rule out extrinsic compression
- An upper endoscopy to exclude a mechanical obstruction
- If a mechanical obstruction is ruled out, a 4-hour gastric emptying scintigraphy using radionuclide technetium-99m–labeled food, such as oatmeal or eggs, can characterize gastric emptying. Alternatively, a wireless motility capsule can be used to measure not only gastric but also small and large bowel motility.

EVALUATION

A 4-hour solid emptying study consistent with gastroparesis will show >10% retention at 4 hours.

TREATMENT

- Gastroparesis is treated with a gastroparesis diet, composed of small, frequent meals that are low in fat and low in fiber. A referral to a nutritionist should be considered, especially if the patient has diabetes or if unable to consume enough by mouth to maintain nutritional status.
- Vitamin/mineral supplementation is usually necessary due to a restricted diet.
- Antiemetic is given to control nausea.
- A pro-kinetic drug such a metoclopramide can be considered for short-term treatment, but long-term use is contraindicated due to the risk of extrapyramidal side effects.
- Erythromycin has prokinetic effects, but its use is limited due to tachyphylaxis.
- Referral to a center with an IRB/IND license for prokinetic drug treatment with motilium.
- Consider supplemental small bowel enteral feedings if nutritional status cannot be maintained on an oral diet.
- Treament for rapid gastric emptying includes small frequent meals, low in carbohydrate, rich in fat and protein. Medication treatment includes guar gum, psyllium, pectin, acarbose, or an anticholinergic such as dicyclomine or hyoscyamine. A somatostatin analog such as octreotide can be given for diarrhea. The patient should be instructed to lie down for 30 minutes after eating.

PATIENT EDUCATION

- Patients with gastroparesis should be counseled to follow a diet low in fat, low in fiber, divided into six small meals. Supplementation with an oral liquid nutrition supplement may be needed. Patients should be educated that symptoms of gastroparesis can vary and can flare with a viral illness.
- Patients with dumping syndrome need less carbohydrate and higher fat, protein, and fiber content to help slow the emptying.

8.2E PYLORIC STENOSIS

OVERVIEW

Hypertrophic pyloric stenosis causes gastric outlet obstruction due to hypertrophy of the circular muscle that surrounds the pyloric channel. Correction of this in infants is the most common abdominal surgical procedure during the first 6 months of life. The incidence in the United States of infantile hypertrophic pyloric stenosis is approximately 3 in 1,000 live births, is highest among northern European ancestry, and occurs in approximately 50% of identical twins.[35]

MEDICAL HISTORY AND CLINICAL PRESENTATION

The infant usually presents at 3 to 4 weeks of age with projectile vomiting following feedings. This may begin with mild spitting up but progresses to the point of forceful vomiting that may be expelled through mouth and the nostrils.

SIGNS AND SYMPTOMS

- Nonbilious emesis
- Loss of interest in feeding

PHYSICAL EXAMINATION

- Assess volume status
- Assess for wasting
- Abdominal examination for a palpable "olive-like" pyloric mass

DIFFERENTIAL DIAGNOSIS

The differential diagnosis of infantile hypertrophic pyloric stenosis includes GERD.

DIAGNOSTIC STUDIES

- Noncontrast x-ray of the abdomen
- Ultrasound of the pylorus

EVALUATION

X-ray will show a distended stomach and a paucity of gas beyond the stomach.

TREATMENT

- Treatment is a surgical pyloromyotomy.

8.2F DUODENAL ATRESIA

MEDICAL HISTORY AND CLINICAL PRESENTATION

An atresia is a congenital defect of a hollow viscus that can result in obstruction of the lumen, occurring most commonly near the ampulla of Vater. Duodenal atresia represents approximately 60% of small intestinal atresias. Approximately 50% of infants with duodenal atresia have an associated chromosomal anomaly, usually trisomy 21. It is an isolated finding in up to half of the cases. Other associated congenital defects include intestinal malrotation, esophageal atresia, imperforate anus, Meckel diverticulum, pancreatic defects, congenital heart disease, CNS lesions, and renal anomalies.[35]

An infant with duodenal atresia is often a preterm infant who has early intolerance to feeding with vomiting and upper abdominal distention. The vomiting may be intermittent and variable in severity, so this can remain undiagnosed for years.

SIGNS AND SYMPTOMS

- An infant with duodenal atresia will usually have gastric distention and bilious vomiting
- If the obstruction is more proximal, nonbilious emesis occurs
- There may be poor weight gain or history of aspiration

PHYSICAL EXAMINATION

- Evaluate growth

DIFFERENTIAL DIAGNOSIS

Duodenal stenosis, duodenal web, intestinal malrotation, mid-gut volvulus.

DIAGNOSTIC STUDIES

- Noncontrast x-ray

EVALUATION

A plain radiograph of an infant with duodenal obstruction will show a "double bubble" sign of air in the stomach and in the first portion of the duodenum with an absence of air beyond the second bubble.

TREATMENT

- Nasogastric (NG) tube placement for decompression, correction of fluid and electrolyte abnormalities. Definitive treatment is surgical correction with duodenojejunostomy or duodenoduodenostomy.
- Approximately 12% of patients may require revision or another surgery over the years.

SPECIAL CONSIDERATIONS

- *Autoimmune gastritis* is a chronic atrophic gastritis associated with serum antiparietal cell and anti-intrinsic factor antibodies, usually affecting the fundus of the stomach and seen more commonly in adults over the age of 50. During the course of the disease, there is loss of parietal cells, which can lead to vitamin B12 malabsorption. Advanced disease results in achlorhydria and intrinsic factor deficiency. Owing to loss of regulatory inhibition there is a rise in serum gastrin. Lack of intrinsic factor causes pernicious anemia, which is the vitamin B12 deficiency associated with chronic atrophic autoimmune gastritis. Pernicious anemia also occurs in conjunction with other autoimmune diseases including Graves disease and thyroiditis.
- Hypertrophic pyloric stenosis rarely occurs in adults. Thickening of the pylorus in adults is usually associated with peptic ulcer disease; however, malignancy needs to be ruled out with an upper endoscopy.

KEY POINTS

- Patients older than 55 and those with alarm symptoms such as heme positive stool or unexplained anemia should undergo an upper endoscopy.
- Following treatment for *H. pylori* gastritis, it is essential that eradication of this be documented due to the increased risk of stomach cancer.
- Consider gastrinoma or ZES in a patient with refractory peptic ulcers and diarrhea.

8.3 DISORDERS OF THE SMALL INTESTINE

OVERVIEW

The small intestine is where most digestion and absorption of nutrients occur. The average length of the small bowel in adults is approximately 22 feet or 7 m. Fluid absorption is an important function of the small intestine. In healthy adults, the GI tract secretes about 4 L of fluid, which includes 2 L of gastric acid and 1.5 L of pancreatic-biliary secretions in response to the 2 to 3 L of consumption daily.

The small intestine is divided into three parts: the duodenum, the jejunum, and the ileum. The duodenum is located in the upper small bowel. Chyme from the stomach enters the duodenum where bile salts, enzymes, and bicarbonate further aid in digestion. Bile is produced in the liver, stored in the gallbladder, and is released into the duodenum to aid in the digestion of fats and fat-soluble vitamins. Pancreatic enzymes released from the pancreas are needed to digest carbohydrate and fats. Bicarbonate is released from the pancreas to neutralize acid from the stomach. The jejunum is the second portion of the small bowel and occupies the proximal two-fifths of the small bowel.

Most nutrient absorption involving proteins, carbohydrates, vitamins, and minerals occurs in the first half of the jejunum; however, iron absorption occurs mainly in the duodenum. The ileum occupies the distal three-fifths of the small intestine and mainly absorbs water, bile salts, and vitamin B12. The ileocecal valve is a one-way valve that is located between the ileum and the cecum. This helps control the passage of contents into the colon. The ileocecal valve increases the contact time of nutrients and electrolytes with the small bowel and also minimizes movement of bacteria from the large bowel into the small bowel by preventing reflux or backflow.

The proximal small bowel of heathy individuals has a predominance of gram-positive aerobic bacteria that usually do not exceed more than 10^4 colony forming units per milliliter. The distal small bowel is a transition zone with the microbiota consisting of dense populations of anaerobes, usually $>10^{12}$ CFU/mL. The upper gut is less populated with microbes due to the gastric acid barrier and are dominated by those that can resist gastric acid such as *H. pylori* and *lactobacilli*. The gut microbiota serves as a barrier effect preventing invasion by pathogenic organisms, regulating immune function and motility, digestion of food, and production of short-chain fatty acids. It also serves to regulate colonic water and electrolyte transport, production of vitamins, metabolism of drugs, and maintenance of overall homeostasis in the GI tract.[36]

PATHOPHYSIOLOGY

Surgically altered anatomy after intestinal resection is described in terms of location of the anastomosis, which has implications for nutritional management and prognosis.

The three categories are (a) jejunoileal anastomosis following resection of a portion of the jejunum and ileum with retention of the ileocecal valve and the entire colon; (b) jejunocolic anastomosis following resection of the ileum, ileocecal valve, part of the colon, and parts of the jejunum; and (c) end-jejunostomy following resection of the entire ileum and colon, or the colon is present but disconnected. A stoma in the abdomen is connected to the remnant jejunum (Figure 8.1).

In adults, the duodenum and proximal jejunum are uncommon sites of resection. However, resection of these areas of the intestine results in gastric hypersecretion and micronutrient deficiencies. The jejunum has a large absorptive surface. The proximal 100–150 cm of the jejunum is the primary site of carbohydrate, protein, and water-soluble vitamin absorption. When the jejunum is resected, there is a temporary reduction in absorption of most nutrients.[37]

Resection of the terminal ileum is associated with vitamin B12 malabsorption. The distal terminal ileum also is the site for absorption of bile acids. In adults with resection of >100 cm of the terminal ileum, there is decreased reabsorption of bile acids into the enterohepatic circulation, resulting in a reduction in the bile salt pool. The liver is unable to compensate and bile acid losses exceed the compensatory increase in hepatic bile acid production causing fat malabsorption.[38]

Steatorrhea can occur as a result of deconjugation of bile acids by intraluminal bacteria resulting in a deficiency of intraluminal bile acids necessary for micelle formation. Bacteria-derived deconjugated bile acids, such as lithocholic acid, can injure enterocytes that can affect carbohydrate and protein absorption.

Fat malabsorption resulting in steatorrhea can cause fat-soluble vitamin deficiencies. The increased passage of bile acids into the colon can induce bile acid diarrhea or a choleretic enteropathy. Given the diminished bile acid pool, bile acid sequestrants may worsen steatorrhea and should be avoided in patients who have >100 cm of the terminal ileum resected.

The colon helps to slow intestinal transit and stimulate intestinal adaptation. (Refer to Section 8.4 Disorders of the Large Intestine, overview.) Patients with extensive small bowel with <100 cm of remnant bowel and without a colon, such as an end-jejunostomy, are at high risk for dehydration and electrolyte losses and require long-term parenteral nutrition.[39]

In short bowel syndrome with a colon in continuity, calcium preferentially binds to unabsorbed fatty acids in the lumen. Oxalate then passes freely into the colon and is absorbed into the circulatory system and filtered by the kidney, resulting in oxalate nephrolithiasis and risk for progressive obstructive nephropathy.[40]

Physiologic changes and adaptations that occur following small bowel surgery are divided into three phases: the acute phase, the adaptation phase, and the maintenance phase. During the acute phase, which lasts 3 to 4 weeks immediately after resection, there is high intestinal fluid losses—up to 6 to 8 L/day—and electrolyte abnormalities. This phase is associated with malnutrition and requires enteral and parenteral nutrition support. Gastric hypersecretion occurs because of loss of cholecystokinin and secretin feedback inhibition that normally regulates gastrin and gastric acid secretion. This is usually transient, lasting a few months.[41] The increase in acid load results in an increased stool volume contributing to diarrhea and electrolyte losses. The reduction in pH results in deactivation of pancreatic enzymes and fat malabsorption occurs.

The adaptation phase begins within 2 to 4 days of bowel resection and lasts for 12 to 24 months. The intestinal villi will grow in length and thickness, which then leads to an increase in surface area. Patients with jejunoileal anastomoses have the remnant ileum and intact colon that can compensate and usually are not at risk to develop electrolyte imbalances or major nutrient deficiencies.[42] Following jejunal resection, intestinal transit may remain normal due to the "ileal brake" for unabsorbed lipids, which cause a delay in gastric emptying when they reach the ileum. Preserving the colon exerts a braking effect on the rate of early gastric emptying of liquids. This helps to facilitate absorption of nutrients within the small intestine.[43]

During the adaptation phase over the course of 1 to 2 years, there are structural and functional changes to the remaining small bowel and colon that increase nutrient absorption and slow the GI tract. Glucagon-like peptide 2 (GLP-2) appears to be an important mediator of intestinal adaptation. It is an intestinal growth factor produced by the enteroendocrine L cells of the ileum and colon and works to promote crypt cell growth, reduce enterocyte apoptosis, and stimulate blood flow.[44] The maintenance phase following bowel resection is where the absorptive capacity of the remaining bowel will be maximized.

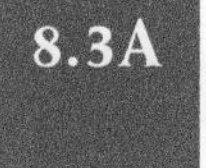

8.3A MALABSORPTION DISORDERS: SHORT BOWEL SYNDROME

MEDICAL HISTORY AND CLINICAL PRESENTATION

Defects in intestinal luminal and brush border processing, or injury to any portion of the small intestine, can result in malabsorption and nutrient deficiencies. Gut stasis,

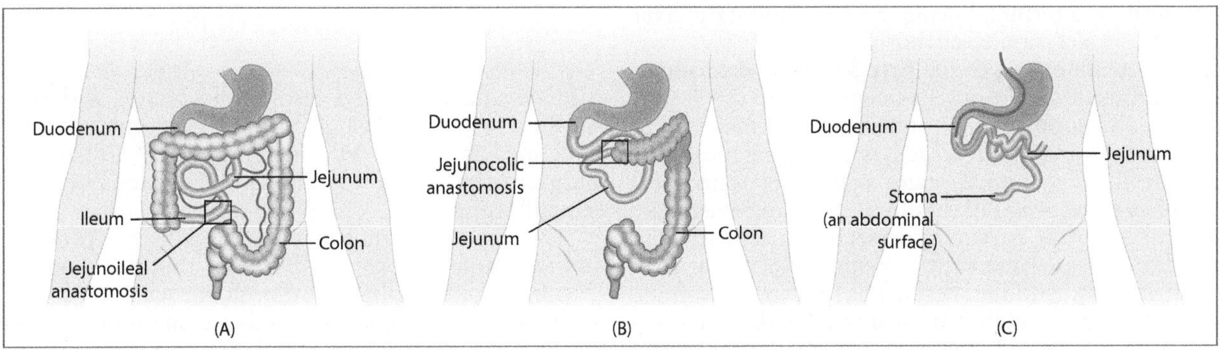

Figure 8.1 **(A) Jejunoileal anastomosis; (B) jejunocolic anastomosis; and (C) jejunostomy.**

dysmotility, and altered anatomy can cause changes in the gut microbiome, resulting in malabsorption.

Short bowel syndrome is the most common cause of intestinal failure and can result from surgical resection for Crohn disease, trauma, malignancy, radiation, or mesenteric ischemia. In children and infants, short bowel syndrome can occur from necrotizing enterocolitis or congenital intestinal abnormalities such as midgut volvulus, atresias, or gastroschisis.

The clinical presentation of short bowel syndrome and eventual need for parenteral nutrition are dependent on the remaining small bowel following intestinal resection. An intact and healthy duodenum, proximal jejunum, and distal 100 cm of the ileum will have a good prognosis for long-term adaptation of the small bowel. The loss of the terminal ileum or resection of >70% of the small bowel will have long-term consequences from severe malabsorption.[45]

SIGNS AND SYMPTOMS

Steatorrhea can present with pale, greasy, foul-smelling stools. This leads to diarrhea, electrolyte imbalances, kidney stones, dehydration, weight loss, and vitamin and mineral deficiencies.

PHYSICAL EXAMINATION

Assess BMI. Assess skin turgor and mucus membranes for hydration status. Assess for signs of malnutrition such as temporal wasting. Assess for indwelling central lines or feeding tubes. Examine the abdomen for surgical scars.

DIFFERENTIAL DIAGNOSIS

The differential diagnosis for malabsorption that occurs because of short bowel syndrome includes gastric hypersecretion, small intestinal bacterial overgrowth (SIBO), bile salt diarrhea, steatorrhea, and exocrine pancreatic insufficiency.

DIAGNOSTIC STUDIES

- CBC with differential, electrolytes, calcium, kidney panel, ferritin, iron profile, hepatic function, prealbumin, vitamin B12, folate, vitamin D, and vitamin A levels
- Kidney, ureter, and bladder (KUB) x-ray or kidney ultrasound to assess for kidney stones

EVALUATION AND TREATMENT

- The need for long-term total parenteral nutrition (TPN) will depend upon the length of small bowel resected, the site of resection, and the presence of colon in continuity with the small bowel. The long-term risks of TPN in a patient without a terminal ileum include cholestatic liver disease and progression to cirrhosis.
- During the acute phase, or the first 3 to 4 weeks following bowel resection, IV fluid replacement with 0.9% normal saline and supplemental potassium and magnesium are required. Stoma and fecal losses should be measured and replaced every 1 to 2 hours with a separate solution. An H2 blocker or PPI should be given intravenously initially to suppress gastric hypersecretion and to help reduce fluid losses. Pancreatic enzyme replacement may also be necessary. Antidiarrheal drugs such as loperamide or tincture of opium will be needed to treat diarrhea.
- Parenteral and/or enteral nutrition should be introduced once the patient is hemodynamically stable. There is a risk for development of cholelithiasis due to interruption of the enterohepatic bile salt circulation in a patient on TPN; therefore, prophylactic ursodeoxycholate can be considered.
- A patient with a limited terminal ileum resection of <100 cm should be prescribed a bile acid sequestrant for diarrhea, such as colestipol 1 to 2 g with meals, or cholestyramine, 2–4 g with meals.
- If >100 cm of the terminal ileum has been resected, a patient will require a low-fat diet and should not be given a bile acid sequestrant.
- Medium chain triglycerides do not require micellar solubilization and are absorbed directly into the portal circulation, thereby providing additional calorie supplementation in a patient with an intact colon. Correction of dehydration, a low oxalate diet, and calcium citrate supplementation are necessary to reduce the development of kidney stones in a patient with an intact colon.[40]
- There is a risk for fat-soluble vitamin deficiency due to malabsorption and supplementation is necessary. If the proximal small bowel has been resected, additional iron, folate, and calcium supplementation is needed. Resection of >60 cm of the terminal ileum requires lifelong vitamin B12 replacement, either daily sublingually or intramuscular injection given monthly.
- Teduglutide is a recombinant analog of human glucagon-like peptide 2, approved by the U.S. Food and Drug Administration (FDA) in 2012 for the treatment of adults with short bowel syndrome who are dependent on TPN.
  - This drug works by regeneration of cells in the intestinal lining and promotes intestinal adaptation by improving absorption of fluids and nutrients. It may have modest benefits in weaning of parenteral nutrition in patients with short bowel syndrome.
  - The trophic effects of teduglutide can increase the risk of accelerated neoplastic growth. A colonoscopy needs to be performed to rule out colon polyps prior to initiating treatment.[46]

PATIENT EDUCATION

- A patient who has persistent intestinal failure after a period of intestinal adaptation and cannot be weaned from TPN may need to be considered for a small bowel transplant.

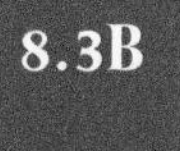

8.3B MALABSORPTION DISORDERS: SMALL INTESTINAL BACTERIAL OVERGROWTH

MEDICAL HISTORY AND CLINICAL PRESENTATION

SIBO is a malabsorptive disorder associated with significant gut stasis resulting in a change in the gut microbiome. SIBO is defined as overgrowth of bacteria $\geq 10^6$ CFU/mL of aerobic gram-negative or strict anaerobic bacteria obtained from jejunal aspirate.[36]

The sequelae from the underlying disease process results in the manifestations of SIBO. The vascular damage, nerve dysfunction, atrophy of smooth muscles, and fibrosis in systemic sclerosis results in reduced small bowel clearance, causing SIBO. Resulting malabsorption can lead to malnutrition and can also interfere with drug absorption.[47]

Reduced gastric acid production or failure of the gastric barrier such as atrophic gastritis, gastric bypass surgery, or the use of PPIs are risk factors for SIBO. Altered small bowel anatomy and adhesions from intestinal surgeries cause small bowel stasis. Immunodeficiency syndromes such as IgA deficiency, combined variable immune deficiency, and T cell deficiency are also risk factors for SIBO.[45]

SIGNS AND SYMPTOMS

Signs and symptoms of SIBO can include weight loss, diarrhea, flatulence, bloating, steatorrhea, abdominal distention, abdominal discomfort, or constipation.

PHYSICAL EXAMINATION

Physical examination can be normal. Assess BMI. Assess skin turgor and assess for signs of fat-soluble vitamin deficiencies. Assess neurologic status for signs of vitamin B12 deficiency. Inspect the abdomen for surgical scars and signs of abdominal distention.

DIFFERENTIAL DIAGNOSIS

The differential diagnosis for SIBO includes fat malabsorption, exocrine pancreatic insufficiency, celiac disease, IBS, pseudo-obstruction, and IgA deficiency.

DIAGNOSTIC STUDIES

Lab studies include IgA, tissue transglutaminase antibody, CBC with differential, calcium, magnesium, electrolytes, vitamin B12, and vitamin D.

Small bowel aspiration and culture are considered the gold standard for diagnosing SIBO; however, this is invasive and costly. There are also limitations with using this method to diagnose SIBO because of the possibility of patchy locations of organisms in the mid or distal small bowel.

Hydrogen breath testing is an inexpensive and noninvasive alternative for diagnosis of SIBO. An increase of breath hydrogen after oral administration of the substrate is diagnostic of SIBO. Although diarrhea is more common in SIBO, methane-predominant SIBO seems to be associated with constipation. There are several limitations in breath testing including proper test preparation and wide variation in interpretation and diagnostic criteria.[36]

EVALUATION

When fat malabsorption is present, there is a risk for deficiencies of the fat-soluble vitamins; however, vitamin K usually remains normal due to bacterial synthesis of menaquinones. There is a risk for vitamin B12 deficiency due to inhibition of absorption by anaerobic organisms and by consumption of vitamin B12 by enteric microbes within the intestinal lumen before it can be absorbed. Folate levels may be elevated in SIBO due to bacterial synthesis.[36]

TREATMENT

- Treatment of SIBO consists of oral antibiotics for 7 to 14 days (Table 8.4).[47] Clinical response is used as a guide of successful therapy.
    - Relapse is common and problematic for those with stasis syndromes associated with SIBO. A cyclical regimen of rotating antibiotics for 1 to 2 weeks each month can be considered, depending upon the rapidity of return of symptoms and their severity.

TABLE 8.4 Small Intestinal Bacterial Overgrowth Adult Treatment Regimens

Antibiotic	Dosage (Treat 7–10 Days)
Amoxicillin-clavulanate	500 mg TID or 875 mg BID
Rifaximin	400 mg TID
Metronidazole	250 mg TID
Trimethoprim-sulfamethoxazole double-strength	160/800 mg BID
Ciprofloxacin	250 mg BID
Neomycin	500 mg QID

BID, twice a day; QID, four times a day; TID, three times a day.

- For methane producers in constipation-associated with SIBO, a combination of rifaximin and neomycin can be considered.

PATIENT EDUCATION

- Multivitamin and mineral supplementation. A separate vitamin D supplement may be recommended.

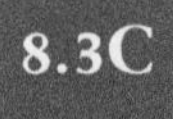

8.3C MALABSORPTION DISORDERS: CELIAC DISEASE

MEDICAL HISTORY AND CLINICAL PRESENTATION

Celiac disease, also called celiac sprue, is a mucosal disorder of the small intestine. It is immune-mediated and can occur in genetically susceptible people. Gluten exposure from products containing wheat, barley, rye, and/or triticale causes injury to the small intestine, resulting in malabsorption.

The disease is rare in patients of Asian or African descent but occurs in approximately 1% of European Caucasians.[45] The prevalence of this disease is increased in patients with type 1 diabetes, Down syndrome, Sjögren syndrome, autoimmune thyroiditis, and autoimmune liver disease.

Malabsorption from small bowel injury can cause weight loss, anemia, and osteoporosis. There is also an increased risk of small bowel lymphoma.

SIGNS AND SYMPTOMS

A patient with celiac disease can be asymptomatic. Signs and symptoms can vary and include diarrhea, abdominal cramps, or constipation. Extraintestinal manifestation include anemia, arthralgias, and fatigue.

PHYSICAL EXAMINATION

The physical examination in celiac disease is often normal. The presence of dermatitis herpetiformis is associated with a 90% prevalence of celiac disease; however, few patients present with this. This rash is characterized by papulovesicular lesions on the extensor surfaces of the extremities, trunk, buttocks, neck, or scalp with a worsening of rash after consumption of gluten-containing food.

DIFFERENTIAL DIAGNOSIS

The differential diagnosis includes IBS, microscopic colitis, lactase deficiency, common variable immune deficiency (CVID), autoimmune enteropathy, SIBO, lymphoma, refractory sprue, Crohn disease, and drug-induced enteropathy, such as that from the angiotensin receptor blocker olmesartan.

DIAGNOSTIC STUDIES

A patient presenting with diarrhea, unexplained anemia, or a family history of celiac disease should be screened with serologic testing including immunoglobulin A (IgA) and tissue transglutaminase antibody (tTgAb). A deficiency of IgA can result in a false negative tTgAb test, and therefore, a low IgA would be an indication for an upper endoscopy and duodenal biopsies to rule out celiac disease.

A gluten-free diet can normalize both serologic studies and pathology findings; therefore, it is imperative that a patient be consuming gluten for several months prior to being tested for celiac disease in order to obtain accurate results. Genetic testing for human leukocyte antigen (HLA) DQ2 and DQ8 can be considered to ultimately rule out celiac disease if both markers are negative. However, one or both markers are positive in 50% of the population; thus genetic testing does not confirm celiac disease and can only rule it out.

Celiac disease is confirmed in a patient with positive serologic testing by an upper endoscopy and biopsies of the duodenum. Pathology can show varying degrees of villous atrophy, crypt hypertrophy, and an increase in intraepithelial lymphocytes.

EVALUATION

Endoscopy findings show flattening of villi in the small bowel; biopsies show villous atrophy and lymphocytic infiltration.

TREATMENT

- The treatment for celiac disease is a lifelong gluten-free diet, which should result in symptomatic and histologic improvement. There is an increased risk for folate, calcium, and iron malabsorption from small intestinal injury, so supplementation may be needed until the small bowel heals.
- After following a gluten-free diet for several months, compliance can be assessed by repeating a tTgAb test with the goal of normalization of this level. This test should then be performed annually.
- Consider periodic bone density screening.
- Aside from clinical judgment, there are no specific screening guidelines for small bowel lymphoma in such patients.

PATIENT EDUCATION

- A patient diagnosed with celiac disease should be referred to a nutritionist for instruction on a gluten-free diet and should be counseled on adequate nutrient intake.
- The patient should also be counseled on weight-bearing exercise for bone health.

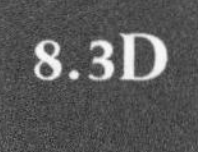

8.3D MALABSORPTION DISORDERS: LACTOSE INTOLERANCE

MEDICAL HISTORY AND CLINICAL PRESENTATION

Lactose is a disaccharide consisting of galactose bound to glucose and requires hydrolysis at the intestinal brush border by the enzyme lactase. Lactose intolerance is a clinical syndrome due to deficiency of lactase in the brush border of the small intestine. Lactose malabsorption occurs when there is failure to digest and/or absorb lactose in the small intestine. Lactose passes into the large intestine due to lactase deficiency. The undigested lactose within the intestinal microbiota results in bacterial fermentation of lactose and production of gases including hydrogen, carbon dioxide, methane, and short-chain fatty acids.

The activity of lactase in the small intestine is highest in infancy and is reduced in most populations during childhood.

Lactase deficiency refers to having a lower level of intestinal brush border lactase enzyme activity compared to that of normal individuals. Genetic risk factors include African or Asian descent. The likelihood of lactose intolerance depends on the amount of lactose consumed, lactase expression on the intestinal brush border, and the microbiome in the small intestine.[48]

SIGNS AND SYMPTOMS

In children, stool may be watery and frothy. Adults may complain of borborygmi, abdominal cramps, abdominal pain, bloating, flatulence, and diarrhea.

PHYSICAL EXAMINATION

The physical examination is usually normal in a patient with lactose intolerance.

DIFFERENTIAL DIAGNOSIS

The differential diagnosis for lactose intolerance includes celiac disease, SIBO, IBS, IBD, and drug- or radiation-induced injury.

DIAGNOSTIC STUDIES

A presumptive diagnosis of lactose intolerance can be made in a patient with mild symptoms that occur following ingestion of lactose and resolve within 5 to 7 days after avoiding foods containing lactose.

A lactose hydrogen breath test is the test of choice to assess lactose malabsorption and symptoms of lactose intolerance. An oral challenge with a standard dose of lactose is given and the excretion of hydrogen in expiratory air is then measured. However, non-hydrogen-producing microbiota can result in a false negative hydrogen breath test and false positive tests can result from SIBO, rapid transit, and altered bowel anatomy.

TREATMENT

- Most patients with lactose intolerance can tolerate up to 12 g of lactose, or the equivalent of 250 mL of milk, without symptoms.[49]

- Lactase supplementation is recommended in patients with lactose intolerance to improve lactose digestion and symptoms.
- Patients who avoid dairy products may require calcium supplementation and should periodically have vitamin D levels monitored.

8.3E MALABSORPTION DISORDERS: WHIPPLE DISEASE

MEDICAL HISTORY AND CLINICAL PRESENTATION

Whipple disease is an uncommon multisystemic process that can be potentially unmasked by immunosuppressive therapy.[50] It is caused by *Tropheryma whipplei*, which is ubiquitous in the environment. It more often affects White, middle-aged men of European ancestry who may have an underlying genetic predisposition leading to colonization of *T. whipplei* throughout the intestinal tract. It can be a mimicker of many different illnesses.

SIGNS AND SYMPTOMS

Classic Whipple disease presents over time and is characterized by migratory arthralgias, chronic diarrhea, weight loss, and malabsorption. Neurologic involvement can occur in the setting of classic Whipple disease or as a manifestation of relapse after treatment.

PHYSICAL EXAMINATION

Assess BMI over time. Perform skin examination assessing for hyperpigmentation, abdominal examination for tenderness, and cardiac examination to assess for murmur. Assess for lymphadenopathy.

DIFFERENTIAL DIAGNOSIS

The differential diagnosis includes IBD, infectious causes of chronic diarrhea, connective tissue disease, HIV infection, tuberculosis, and hyperthyroidism.

DIAGNOSTIC STUDIES

An upper endoscopy with biopsies of the small intestine for *T. whipplei* testing is recommended in a patient suspected for Whipple disease. Histologic testing is done with periodic acid-Schiff staining, polymerase chain reaction (PCR) testing, and immunohistochemistry.

EVALUATION

Whipple disease should be considered in a patient presenting with arthralgias, diarrhea, abdominal pain, and weight loss when all other conditions have been ruled out.

TREATMENT

- Treatment of Whipple disease without CNS involvement includes an initial phase of an IV antibiotic such as ceftriaxone or penicillin for 2 weeks, followed by trimethoprim/sulfamethoxazole twice daily for 1 year.
- For patients with CNS involvement, parenteral treatment can be extended for 4 weeks.
- Most extraintestinal manifestations resolve within a year. Long-term antibiotic suppressive therapy is usually needed.

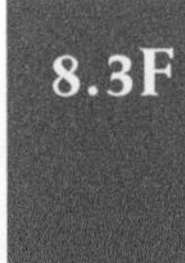

8.3F SMALL BOWEL MOTILITY DISORDERS: CHRONIC INTESTINAL PSEUDO-OBSTRUCTION

MEDICAL HISTORY AND CLINICAL PRESENTATION

An *ileus* is the absence of intestinal peristalsis without mechanical obstruction. Postoperative ileus refers to obstipation and intolerance of oral intake due to nonmechanical factors that disrupt the normal coordinated propulsive motor activity of the GI tract. Postoperative ileus can affect the stomach, small intestine, or colon. Small bowel function normally resumes activity within several hours postsurgery. Within 24 to 48 hours the stomach usually starts functioning and within 3–5 days after surgery the colon should resume normal activity.

As opposed to an ileus, chronic intestinal pseudo-obstruction (CIPO) is a rare disorder, with unknown prevalence and incidence. It is primarily a disorder of small bowel motility characterized by recurrent symptoms of intestinal obstruction associated with radiologic findings of small bowel dilation, but in the absence of mechanical obstruction.

Primary causes of CIPO are uncommon and usually present in childhood. They include familial visceral myopathies, mitochondrial dysfunction, or sporadic visceral neuropathies such as Hirschsprung disease. CIPO is usually characterized by occlusive symptoms at birth. Urologic involvement is common. There is a high risk of colonic and small bowel volvulus from severe gut dilation, dysmotility, and/or malrotation.[51]

Secondary forms of CIPO are more common in adults and usually occur in older age. These can arise from systemic disorders that affect GI motility characterized by chronic abdominal pain and distention with superimposed acute episodes of pseudo-obstruction. Secondary or acquired causes of CIPO include connective tissue disorders such as scleroderma, neuromuscular disorders, paraneoplastic syndrome, amyloidosis, and myasthenia gravis. Viral etiologies include CMV, Epstein-Barr virus, and varicella zoster. Other risk factors include Ehlers-Danlos syndrome, jejunal diverticulosis, and radiation enteritis.[52]

Infections from *Trypanosoma cruzi* (Chagas disease) can also be a cause of secondary CIPO. Chagas disease is common in Latin America. It is also associated with dysphagia and cardiomyopathy.[51] Drugs such as opioids, TCAs, anticholinergic agents, phenothiazines, and antiparkinsonian medications can also be a secondary cause of CIPO.[53]

SIGNS AND SYMPTOMS

Intermittent abdominal pain, nausea, vomiting, bloating, constipation, and intestinal dilation are seen with SIBO. Diarrhea can be present due to SIBO.[52]

PHYSICAL EXAMINATION

Overall assessment for orthostasis, pallor, and skin turgor. Abdominal examination to assess for distention or surgical scars. Auscultation for bowel sounds.

DIFFERENTIAL DIAGNOSIS

Acute colonic pseudo-obstruction (Ogilvie syndrome), polypharmacy, electrolyte imbalance, connective tissue disease, Chagas disease, enteric neuropathy, amyloidosis, paraneoplastic syndrome.

DIAGNOSTIC STUDIES

- Abdominal x-ray is performed to rule out obstruction.
- Laboratory testing to identify secondary causes of CIPO should include testing to screen for diabetes, celiac disease, connective tissue and skeletal muscle disorders (antinuclear antibody, anti-double-stranded DNA and SCL-70, creatine phosphokinase, aldolase), and hypothyroidism.
- Others tests include serology for Chagas disease, urinary catecholamines for pheochromocytoma, and enteric neuronal autoantibodies (anti-Hu or type 1 antineuronal nuclear antibodies) in patients with suspected paraneoplastic syndrome. If paraneoplastic syndrome is suspected, then occult malignancy of the lung, ovary, and/or breast should be ruled out.
- Urinary porphyrins should be assayed in patients with severe, otherwise unexplained abdominal pain. Other studies that should be ordered include a CBC with differential, electrolytes, hepatic function panel, albumin, vitamin B12, fasting cortisol, C-reactive protein (CRP), and erythrocyte sedimentary rate.[51]
- An upper enteroscopy should be performed to the level of the proximal jejunum in patients suspected of having CIPO to identify intraluminal or extraluminal occlusion.

EVALUATION

Acute intestinal pseudo-obstruction in scleroderma is considered a gastroenterologic emergency and chronic CIPO can lead to sepsis in such patients. Most patients have spontaneous resolution with bowel rest, NG decompression, IV hydration, and correction of electrolyte abnormalities.[47]

Malnutrition from poor oral intake can occur and supplemental small bowel enteral tube feedings may be needed. Alternatively, some patients require TPN if there is whole gut dysmotility.

In children, venting ostomies may be helpful as a bridge to transplantation in selective cases, but they are characterized by high complications rates. In adults, venting ostomies can also be helpful. Surgical resection may be an option for selected patients with proven segmental gut dysfunction. A multidisciplinary team approach is the best management strategy for such patients.[51]

TREATMENT

- The treatment goals of CIPO include appropriate nutritional support, promotion of GI motility, and treatment of complications. Erythromycin is a macrolide antibiotic that has been shown to accelerate gastric emptying and improve symptoms of CIPO.[51] Its use is limited due to the development of tachyphylaxis. Subcutaneous octreotide has shown to have beneficial effects in scleroderma related CIPO by improving bacterial overgrowth in these patients.[54]
- For treatment of an ileus, early postoperative enteral feeding may be advantageous for recovery. Gum chewing has also been proposed to help stimulate bowel recovery after surgery through the parasympathetic/vagal cholinergic stimulation of the GI tract. Medication efficacy varies, depending upon the target organ, with greater success in the stomach and colon, as opposed to the small bowel.[55]
- Erythromycin is a macrolide antibiotic and is also a motilin receptor agonist and may be effective in the short term to help accelerate gastric emptying.

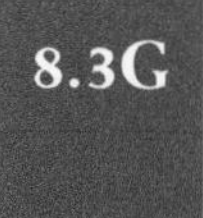

8.3G SMALL BOWEL MOTILITY DISORDERS: BOWEL OBSTRUCTION

MEDICAL HISTORY AND CLINICAL PRESENTATION

A bowel obstruction occurs when there is disruption to the normal flow of intraluminal contents. An obstruction leads to progressive dilation of the intestine proximal to the blockage. The bowel will decompress distally as luminal contents pass. Early diagnosis is essential in preventing complications of perforation or ischemia.

Obstruction of the small intestine can be partial or complete. In a low-grade or incomplete intestinal obstruction, some gas or fluid can pass beyond the point of obstruction. In a high-grade or complete obstruction, nothing passes beyond it. The intestinal tract dilates proximal to the point of obstruction and fills with GI secretions and swallowed air, and the luminal pressures increase. When the intraluminal pressure exceeds the venous pressures, there is a loss of venous drainage, which can compromise arterial flow and lead to ischemia, necrosis, and perforation.

A closed loop obstruction is a type of complete obstruction occurring when the intestine is obstructed at two locations. This is a surgical emergency and can progress to bowel strangulation or perforation. Intestinal volvulus is an example of a closed loop obstruction that results in torsion of arterial inflow and venous drainage.[56]

Adhesions from prior abdominal surgery are the main cause of small bowel obstruction, accounting for 60% to 85% of cases. Other causes of small bowel obstruction include Crohn disease, neoplasm, abdominal wall or groin hernia, prior irradiation, gallstone ileus, volvulus, and Meckel diverticulum.[56]

SIGNS AND SYMPTOMS

Symptoms associated with an acute small bowel obstruction include nausea, vomiting, cramping abdominal pain, and obstipation (inability to pass flatus or stool).

PHYSICAL EXAMINATION

Evaluate for signs of dehydration such as tachycardia, orthostatic hypotension, decreased urine output and dry mucous membranes. Examine the abdomen for distention. Acute obstruction is characterized by high-pitched bowel sounds; however, it may be hypoactive with increased abdominal distention. Distention of the bowel can result in tympany to percussion; this can indicate free intra-abdominal air. Tenderness to light percussion can be indicative of peritonitis.

DIFFERENTIAL DIAGNOSIS

The differential diagnosis for a small bowel obstruction is broad. Diagnoses to consider include gastroenteritis, intussusception, pancreatitis, esophageal rupture, IBD, mesenteric ischemia, large bowel obstruction, acute appendicitis, diabetic ketoacidosis, and pelvic inflammatory disease.

DIAGNOSTIC STUDIES

A plain x-ray can confirm a bowel obstruction in most patients. Findings on x-ray include dilated loops of bowel with air-fluid levels. The cause of a bowel obstruction is usually not apparent on x-ray, as it is difficult to establish a transition point between the dilated proximal and nondilated distal small bowel. X-rays are less useful for differentiating small from large bowel obstruction and partial obstruction from ileus.[56]

An abdominal CT can identify a specific transition point and severity of obstruction, either partial or complete. An acute intestinal obstruction will show GI tract dilation proximal to the site of obstruction, with decompression distally. A CT scan can aid in determining the etiology by identifying hernias, masses, or inflammatory changes. Complications of ischemia or perforation can also be identified.[56]

TREATMENT

- Initial management of a small bowel obstruction includes placing the patient NPO (nothing by mouth), fluid resuscitation, and electrolyte repletion. Significant distention, nausea, or vomiting, may require NG tube decompression.
- Surgical consult is needed for possible surgical intervention to clear the obstruction when necessary.

8.3H INTESTINAL INTUSSUSCEPTION

MEDICAL HISTORY AND CLINICAL PRESENTATION

An intussusception occurs from invagination of one segment of the bowel into an immediately adjacent segment. This can occur in the small or large bowel and results from alteration of normal peristalsis by a lesion in the bowel that creates the invagination.

Intussusception is a common abdominal emergency in children and the second most common cause of intestinal obstruction next to pyloric stenosis. It can occur from either anatomic or infectious etiologies, and often can be managed nonoperatively. The most common type of intussusception in children is ilecolic. This can be seen in patients with cystic fibrosis, foreign body ingestion, intestinal parasites, or feces that result in a lead point in the ileum. Infections that result in mesenteric lymphadenopathy, or hypertrophy of Peyer patches from adenovirus or rotavirus can also cause an intussusception.[57]

Noninfectious etiologies in both children and adults include celiac and Crohn disease.

Most adult intussusceptions occur in the small intestine. Benign causes of intussusception include Meckel diverticulum, adhesions, or lipomas. Malignant tumors in the small bowel such as adenocarcinoma, GI stromal tumor, carcinoid tumor, neuroendocrine tumors, leiomyosarcoma, and lymphoma can cause intussusception.

Approximately 25% of adult intussusceptions occur in the colon. Intussusception is rare in adults, and bowel resection is usually indicated due to obstruction. Adenocarcinoma is the most common malignant cause and colonic lipoma is the most common benign cause of intussusception in the colon.[57]

SIGNS AND SYMPTOMS

The classic presentation in young children includes an acute onset of colicky abdominal pain. Vomiting may occur shortly after the onset of pain. There can be passage of blood and mucus in the stool, described as a "currant jelly" (brick red) appearance.

Adult patients will usually present with symptoms of obstruction including intermittent cramping abdominal pain, nausea, vomiting, obstipation, bleeding, and change in bowel habits.

PHYSICAL EXAMINATION

In children a "sausage-shaped" mass can often be palpated in the right upper quadrant (RUQ).

Physical examination in an adult may show a distended abdomen, decreased bowel sounds, abdominal tenderness, or palpable abdominal mass. Pain out of proportion to physical exam findings can indicate peritonitis or ischemia, especially if the patient presents late in the course of the disease.

DIFFERENTIAL DIAGNOSIS

The differential diagnosis for intussusception in an adult includes abdominal hernia, appendicitis, gastric volvulus, and cyclic vomiting syndrome.

DIAGNOSTIC STUDIES

A plain x-ray may show signs of obstruction including distended loops of bowel and the absence of gas. Other radiographic findings include an obscured liver margin, lack of air in the cecum precluding visualization, or a target sign. The sensitivity and specificity of diagnosing intussusception by a trained sonographer are close to 100%. The classic feature is a target or donut sign caused by edema forming a ring around the intussusception.[57]

Because of the nonspecific clinical presentation, an abdominal CT scan is recommended for a timely diagnosis.

A barium or water-soluble enema may reveal a "cup-shaped" filling defect and may potentially have a therapeutic effect in a patient with colonic or ileocolic intussusception.

EVALUATION

Findings on imaging that warrant surgery include signs of obstruction, intussusception with a lead point mass, and ileocolic intussusception due to the high association with malignancy.

TREATMENT

- Treatment in children depends upon the type of intussusception. Ileocolonic intussusception requires reduction by ultrasound-guided fluoroscopic enema. Small bowel intussusception in children is uncommon and can be monitored; this usually reduces spontaneously without surgery.[57]
- A colonoscopy can be considered in adults and allows for biopsy; however, there is an increased risk of perforation. Caution must be taken when proceeding with this.[57]

8.3I MESENTERIC ISCHEMIA

MEDICAL HISTORY AND CLINICAL PRESENTATION

A reduction in blood flow to the small intestine can be classified as either acute, with a sudden onset of hypoperfusion, or chronic. Acute mesenteric arterial occlusion can result from superior mesenteric arterial embolism (50%), superior mesenteric arterial thrombosis (15% to 20%), nonocclusive mesenteric ischemia (20% to 25%), and mesenteric venous thrombosis (5% to 10%). Acute mesenteric ischemia is considered a medical and surgical emergency, with a mortality rate of over 50%.[58]

Chronic mesenteric ischemia is also known as "intestinal angina" and results from reduced blood flow due to atherosclerosis causing narrowing of at least two of the three major vessels, which are the celiac axis, superior mesenteric artery (SMA), and inferior mesenteric artery (IMA). Collateral vessels usually compensate for the reduced blood flow, so most patients are asymptomatic.

Acute mesenteric ischemia can occur as a result of an acute thrombosis from chronic intestinal ischemia. Pain presents with sudden onset lasting several hours.

SIGNS AND SYMPTOMS

Postprandial pain, weight loss, and an abdominal bruit are considered the classic diagnostic presentation of chronic mesenteric ischemia.

PHYSICAL EXAMINATION

Physical examination findings usually show minimal tenderness or may be normal. An epigastric bruit can be found in about 50% of patients.

DIFFERENTIAL DIAGNOSIS

The differential diagnosis for acute mesenteric ischemia includes acute myocardial infarction, acute pancreatitis, aortic dissection, peptic ulcer disease, and gastritis.

DIAGNOSTIC STUDIES

- Lab studies include CBC with differential, electrolytes, hepatic function, lipase, amylase, cardiac enzymes, lipase. Initial laboratory studies are usually normal in mesenteric ischemia.
- Plain films of the abdomen will exclude a perforation or obstruction.
- The gold standard in the diagnosis of acute mesenteric ischemia is mesenteric angiography.

EVALUATION

A high index of clinical suspicion should prompt a mesenteric angiography study.

TREATMENT

- Treatment goal of acute mesenteric ischemia is to restore intestinal blood flow after the cause of the event is corrected. Aggressive hemodynamic support and monitoring are required. Emergent laparotomy is required if there are peritoneal signs or suspicion of perforation.[58]
- When chronic mesenteric ischemia is diagnosed based on symptoms and stenosis of two or more mesenteric arteries, the treatment is to restore the mesenteric arterial blood flow. The patient should be referred to a vascular specialist for endovascular therapy.

KEY POINTS

- Many diseases are associated with intestinal malabsorption, including celiac disease, chronic pancreatitis, scleroderma, amyloidosis, systemic mastocytosis, lymphoma, Crohn disease, cystic fibrosis, radiation enteropathy, tropical sprue, and intestinal failure.
- Short bowel syndrome presents with a spectrum of malabsorption challenges and is a complicated condition.
- SIBO can also be a cause of unexplained diarrhea in older adults.
- Early diagnosis of small bowel obstruction is necessary to prevent complications of perforation and ischemia.
- Acute mesenteric ischemia is a medical and surgical emergency and should be suspected in any patient over the age of 50 who presents with abdominal pain out of proportion to physical findings.

SPECIAL CONSIDERATIONS

- *Tropical sprue* occurs in selected countries among natives and tourists from the Caribbean or tropical Asia. Symptoms are nonspecific and include diarrhea, weight loss, anorexia, and steatorrhea. Megaloblastic anemia from folate and/or vitamin B12 deficiency can occur. Biopsy and histology cannot distinguish between celiac and tropical sprue. Other diseases of malabsorption should be ruled out. Treatment with tetracycline or poorly absorbed sulfonamide is recommended for 1 to 2 months and nutritional deficiencies such as vitamin B12, folic acid, vitamin D, and calcium should be corrected.[45]
- Whipple disease can mimic *Mycobacterium avium* infection in immunocompromised patients and is differentiated with Ziehl-Neelsen staining. *M. avium* is acid fast and *T. whipplei* is not. If there is CNS involvement, PCR and cytologic testing of cerebrospinal fluid is diagnostic.[45]

8.4 DISORDERS OF THE LARGE INTESTINE

OVERVIEW

The large intestine begins at the terminal ileum where contents open into the cecum, through the ileocecal valve. The large intestine includes the cecum, appendix, colon, rectum, and anal canal. The colon is divided into the right, transverse, left, and sigmoid segments. The right colon is fixed in the retroperitoneum; however, the position of the cecum and appendix are variable, which has clinical importance. Up to 60% of people have a retrocecal position of the appendix, which can cause an atypical presentation in appendicitis.[59]

The vascular supply to the intestines includes the celiac artery, SMA, and IMA. SMA supplies blood to the small and large bowel. Most of the colon's blood supply comes from branches of the SMA and IMA. Branches of the internal iliac artery supply the rectum and there are numerous collaterals between these vascular systems. When a major vessel becomes occluded, collateral pathways develop in order to supply blood. The two watershed regions in the large bowel that have fewer collaterals and are more susceptible to ischemia are the splenic flexure (SMA and IMA) and the rectosigmoid (IMA and internal iliac artery).[60]

The colon is responsible for receiving 1 to 1.5 L each day from the small intestine, which is composed of salt water and undigested material such as fiber and incompletely absorbed carbohydrates. The colon absorbs water, nutrients, and vitamins; compacts feces; secretes potassium and chloride; and propels waste material toward the rectum. Material is retained in the sigmoid colon until the gastrocolonic response stimulates emptying into the rectum. The rectoanal inhibitory reflex is activated when the rectum is distended, which causes relaxation of the internal anal sphincter. Contraction of the puborectalis muscle and external anal sphincter blocks defecation long enough for rectal accommodation to occur.

Poorly absorbed substances cause osmotic retention of water in the lumen, limiting water absorption and potentially causing diarrhea. Large organic polymers, such as fiber, absorb water. The water-holding capacity of solids is a factor in regulating stool consistency. Fat does not bind water as well as carbohydrates, making fatty stool looser in consistency.

The microbiome within the colon also modulates colon physiology. Bacterial fermentation produces short-chain fatty acids that are absorbed by the colon, increasing sodium and fluid absorption and impacting colon motility. Fermentation results in the production of carbon dioxide, hydrogen, and methane, which can contribute to gas and bloating. These gases also affect colon motility.[61]

8.4A IRRITABLE BOWEL SYNDROME

MEDICAL HISTORY AND CLINICAL PRESENTATION

IBS is a functional bowel disorder. It is a symptom-based condition defined by altered bowel habits associated with abdominal pain in the absence of underlying pathology causing these symptoms. Defecation provides relief of pain. IBS can also be defined as a disorder of brain–gut interactions associated with changes in GI motility, visceral perception, mucosal and immune function, gut microbiome, and/or CNS processing.[62]

Other GI disorders associated with IBS include GERD and functional dyspepsia. Somatic pain syndromes associated with this disorder include fibromyalgia, chronic fatigue syndrome, and chronic pelvic pain. Psychiatric disorders associated with IBS include depression, anxiety, and somatization.

IBS is a complex disorder and the pathophysiology is not completely understood. Risk factors include genetic predisposition, exposure to environmental factors, and psychosocial factors. An abnormal stress response, in combination with psychological distress and an infectious or inflammatory response, may alter intestinal permeability. This can then trigger a physiologic response of inflammatory cells, edema, and release of cytokines or chemokines, resulting in IBS symptoms. Coexisting depression or somatization may also affect gut permeability, the immune system, and the microbiome, leading to IBS symptoms. IBS symptoms may further exacerbate underlying anxiety, depression, or somatization.[63] Approximately half of patients with IBS develop GI symptoms first, and then subsequently develop mood disorders.[64]

The Rome IV criteria represent the current standard for diagnosing IBS. The previous Rome III criteria were updated in 2016 by a group of international experts.[63,65] Subtypes of IBS are categorized by predominant stool pattern as constipation predominant (IBS-C), diarrhea predominant (IBS-D), or mixed type vacillating between constipation and diarrhea (IBS-M). Individuals who meet the criteria for IBS, but cannot be classified as IBS-D, IBS-C, or IBS-M, are considered to have unclassified IBS (IBS-U).[65] Recurrent abdominal pain or discomfort occurs at least 3 days per month over the prior 3 months with at least two out of three characteristics that include (1) improvement with defecation, (2) onset associated with a change in frequency of stool, and (3) onset associated with a change in form of stool. IBS-C is defined as hard or lumpy stool ≥25% and loose or watery stool with <25% of bowel movements. IBS-D is characterized by having loose or watery stool ≥25% of the time and hard or lumpy stool with <25% of bowel movements. Mixed IBS is defined as hard or lumpy stool ≥25% and loose or water stool with ≥25% of bowel movements. The established criterion is fulfilled for the last 3 months with symptom onset at least 6 months before the diagnosis.[65]

SIGNS AND SYMPTOMS

Patients with IBS present with abdominal pain associated with a variety of GI complaints, which can include diarrhea, constipation, bloating, gas, and nausea.

Identifying the patient's predominant bowel pattern is necessary for diagnostic testing and treatment. The Bristol Stool Form Scale is a validated tool assessing stool appearance, ranging from a score of 1 (hard and lumpy stool) to a score of 7 (liquid stool).[66]

PHYSICAL EXAMINATION

A history and physical examination should be performed in every patient evaluated for IBS. The presence of a mass, ascites, hepatomegaly, or splenomegaly necessitates further workup. An anorectal examination should be performed to evaluate sphincter tone and squeeze pressure, which can help identify defecatory dyssynergia.

DIFFERENTIAL DIAGNOSIS

The differential diagnosis for IBS associated with diarrhea includes carbohydrate intolerance, bile acid malabsorption, exocrine pancreatic insufficiency, infection, celiac disease, tropical sprue, SIBO, IBD, and microscopic colitis.

In patients presenting with constipation, the differential diagnosis includes defecatory dyssynergia and slow transit constipation. Defecatory dyssynergia is a common clinical problem in patients with chronic constipation and can overlap with IBS. Slow transit constipation can occur with defecatory dyssynergia and IBS (see Section 8.14 Constipation).

DIAGNOSTIC STUDIES

Concerning features or "red flags" that warrant further workup before diagnosing IBS include symptom onset over the age of 50, severe or progressively worsening symptoms, unexplained weight loss, nocturnal diarrhea, family history of colon cancer, rectal bleeding or melena, and unexplained iron deficiency anemia. A patient presenting with red flag features should undergo a colonoscopy to rule out malignancy of the large bowel. In patients with diarrhea, biopsies of the colon and terminal ileum are necessary to rule out microscopic colitis or IBD.

Laboratory studies include TSH, CBC with differential, hepatic function studies, and electrolytes. For diarrhea predominant symptoms other labs include erythrocyte sedimentation rate (ESR), CRP, IgA, and tTgAb. For diarrhea predominant symptoms, stool studies include *Clostridium difficile*, enteric pathogens, and parasites. Further studies can include fecal fat and pancreatic elastase to evaluate for bile acid malabsorption or pancreatic insufficiency.

EVALUATION

Many conditions can overlap with IBS, including the conditions listed under the differential diagnosis. A negative workup is reassuring for IBS. A patient who has tested negative for celiac while consuming a regular diet, and then eliminates gluten and has subsequent symptom improvement, can be considered to have nonceliac gluten sensitivity. Food allergies are uncommon, but food intolerances are common in IBS.

TREATMENT

- In general, a low-fat diet is recommended for all IBS patients, as fat is known to exacerbate the gastrocolic reflex and can trigger diarrhea.
- Short-chain poorly absorbed carbohydrates, such as FODMAPs (fermentable, oligosaccharides, disaccharides, monosaccharides, and polyols), can lead to increased small intestinal and colonic water secretion and fermentation, causing an increase in short-chain fatty acids and gas.[67] A low FODMAP diet has been shown to have more efficacy in improving IBS symptoms in IBS-D compared to IBS-C.
- There is moderate quality of evidence to support nonpharmacologic interventions for IBS such as soluble fiber and peppermint oil.[63] Soluble fiber supplementation in includes psyllium, wheat dextrin, or methycellulose powder.
- Peppermint oil also has anti-spasmodic effects by relaxing smooth muscle through blockade of calcium channels.[68]
- Probiotics are live microorganisms that, when given in adequate amounts, may confer a health benefit to the host and may represent an option for diseases characterized by dysbiosis, such as IBS. The mechanisms by which they provide benefit in IBS remains unknown. Meta-analyses have shown significant but small benefit can be obtained with probiotics in IBS. Treatment of IBS is complicated by a high placebo response and the pathophysiologic and clinical heterogeneity of the IBS population.[69]
- Anticholinergic drugs such as hyoscyamine and dicyclomine may provide short-term symptomatic relief of abdominal spasms and cramps in all subtypes of IBS. They reduce pain by decreasing smooth muscle contraction.[63]
- Two classes of antidepressants can be used as adjuvant treatment of IBS: TCAs and selective serotonin reuptake inhibitors (SSRIs). The doses used to treat IBS are lower than those used to treat depression.[70]
- SSRIs have less visceral analgesic effects compared to TCAs but may be more effective for improving well-being and anxiety-specific GI symptoms.[71] Side effects of SSRIs include nausea, diarrhea, and sexual dysfunction.
- IBS-C
  - Table 8.5 summarizes treatment options available for IBS-C; many of these overlap with the treatment of idiopathic constipation.
  - An intestinal secretagogue can be added to a bowel regimen or used alone to treat IBS-C.

TABLE 8.5 Treatment Options for Constipation-Predominant Irritable Bowel Syndrome

Treatment	Mechanism	Special Considerations
High-fiber diet	Increase colonic transit, normal bowel pattern	Caution in slow transit constipation
Stool softener (docusate)	Stool surfactant, soften stools	Not effective by itself to treat opiate-related constipation
Osmotic laxative (polyethylene glycol, lactulose, magnesium)	Works in the colon to draw water into the stool	Caution in renal disease with magnesium-containing drugs
Stimulant laxative (Dulcolax, senna)	Works in the colon to stimulate peristalsis	Avoid chronic use due to dependence of bowel peristalsis. Melanosis coli seen during colonoscopy
Lubiprostone 8 mcg BID* or 24 mcg BID†	Chloride channel-2 activator in small bowel	Dose with food (to help minimize nausea side effect)
Linaclotide 72 mcg, 145 mcg, or 290 mcg once daily	Guanylate cyclase c agonist in the entire small bowel	Take on empty stomach (to help minimize diarrhea side effect)
Plecanatide 3 mg once daily	Guanylate cyclase c agonist in the proximal small bowel	May have less diarrhea compared to linaclotide
Prucalopride 2 mg or 1 mg once daily	5-HT4 agonist, enhances peristalsis in the gut	Approved for **constipation**; caution for suicidal ideation; reduce dose in renal disease
Tegaserod 6 mg BID	5-HT4 agonist	Approved in **IBS-C for women** <65 years old with no more than 1 cardiovascular risk factor
SSRI (citalopram, fluoxetine)	Decrease abdominal discomfort	Adjuvant treatment in **IBS-C**

**Dose approved for IBS-C.*
†Dose approved for chronic idiopathic constipation and opioid-induced constipation not caused by cancer.
BID, twice daily; IBS-C, constipation-predominant irritable bowel syndrome; 5-HT4, 5-hydroxytryptamine type 4; SSRI, selective serotonin reuptake inhibitor.

- Prucalopride is a prokinetic drug that was approved by the FDA in January 2019 for treatment of constipation. It is a serotonergic agent and activates 5-HT4 receptors, promoting acetylcholine release, colonic smooth muscle contractions, and peristaslsis. There is a warning on the drug because of an association with suicidal ideation and behavior due to the potential serotonergic effects.
- In 2019, the FDA approved reintroduction of tegaserod, a 5-HT4 agonist, for the treatment of IBS-C in women under 65 years of age and with no more than one risk factor for CVD.
- Adjuvant treatment with an SSRI may be a better choice in treating IBS-C due to the potential side effect of diarrhea.

- IBS-D
  - Other treatment options for IBS-D, some of which overlap with the treatment of diarrhea, are shown in Table 8.6.
  - Alosetron is a 5-HT3 antagonist approved by the FDA for management of IBS-D in women. Patients need to be counseled on the side effects of constipation and risk for obstruction and, in rare cases, ischemic colitis.
  - Eluxadoline is not recommended in patients with alcohol dependence or preexisting pancreaticobiliary disease. It is contraindicated in patients without a gallbladder due to the significantly increased risk of pancreatitis.
  - The TCAs used more commonly as adjuvant therapy in IBS-D include desipramine, nortriptyline, and amitriptyline. Adverse side effects include dry mouth, drowsiness, and weight gain.

PATIENT EDUCATION

- Treatment of IBS begins with educating the patient about the condition and explaining that a negative workup is a positive finding and helps support the diagnosis. Structured exercise intervention has been shown to lead to greater improvement in overall IBS symptoms.[72]
- High FODMAP food items include, but are not limited to, cow's milk, soy milk, apples, cherries, peaches, watermelon, onions, garlic, mushrooms, wheat, high fructose corn syrup, and some sugar substitutes. Refer to website www.eatright.org.
- For further information on IBS, refer to www.niddk.nih.gov.

8.4B *CLOSTRIDIUM DIFFICILE* INFECTION

MEDICAL HISTORY AND CLINICAL PRESENTATION

Clostridioides difficile is a spore-forming gram-positive rod that causes *C. difficile* infection. It is the major infectious cause of antibiotic-induced diarrhea and is the most commonly recognized cause of infectious diarrhea in healthcare settings. *C. difficile* infection is defined as having diarrhea and a stool test positive for either *C. difficile* toxin or colonoscopy pathology findings showing pseudomembranous colitis.[73] *C. difficile* infections have increased in prevalence since 2000 in the community, even among healthy people previously at low risk, and has become less responsive to treatment. Almost any antibiotic has been associated with *C. difficile*; however, the highest risk appears to be associated with third- and fourth-generation cephalosporins, fluoroquinolones, carbapenems, and clindamycin.[73,74]

Patients with IBD are at risk for primary *C. difficile* infection and recurrent disease. They also have an increased risk of morbidity and mortality.[73] *C. difficile* infection requires

TABLE 8.6 Treatment Options for Diarrhea-Predominant Irritable Bowel Syndrome

Treatment	Mechanism	Special Considerations
Bulk fiber daily (psyllium, methylcellulose, or wheat dextrin)	Bulk stool, normalize stool consistency	
Low FODMAP diet (fermentable, oligosaccharides, disaccharides, monosaccharides, and polyols)	Reduce absorption of osmotically active short chain carbohydrates	Consider referral to nutritionist
Low-fat diet	Reduce gastrocolic reflex	
Antidiarrheal drugs PRN (loperamide, atropine/diphenoxylate)	Slows intestinal motility by affecting water and electrolyte absorption through the bowel	Risk for megacolon and ileus; discontinue if distention or constipation develop
Anticholinergic drugs PRN (hyoscyamine, dicyclomine)	Antispasmodic, relax intestinal smooth muscle	Side effects include dizziness, dry mouth, constipation
Eluxadoline 75 mg BID or 100 mg BID; approved for IBS-D	Mu-opioid receptor antagonist	Contraindicated if gallbladder removed; pancreatitis risk
Alosetron .5 mg BID or 1 mg BID	5-HT3 receptor antagonist	Caution for ischemic colitis, severe constipation Approved for women only with IBS-D
TCA (nortriptyline 10 mg HS or amitriptyline 10 mg HS)	Slow GI transit via anticholinergic and noradrenergic effects	Adjuvant therapy for pain associated with IBS
Ondansetron (antiemetic)	5-HT3 receptor antagonist	Adjuvant to treat nausea associated with IBS-D
Rifaximin 550 mg TID × 2 weeks	Antibiotic for flare of IBS-D	Very expensive

BID, twice daily; GI, gastrointestinal; HS, at night; 5-HT3, 5-hydroxytryptamine type 3; IBS, irritable bowel syndrome; IBS-D, diarrhea-predominant irritable bowel syndrome; PRN, as needed; TCA, tricyclic antidepressant.

prompt diagnosis and treatment in patients with IBD to avoid inappropriate treatment with glucocorticoids or immunosuppressive therapy. Other risk factors for *C. difficile* infection include age >65, recent hospitalization, and use of PPIs. There is an epidemiologic association between PPI use and *C. dfficile* infection; therefore, it is recommended that unnecessary PPIs be discontinued.[73]

SIGNS AND SYMPTOMS

Watery diarrhea (≥3 loose stools in 24 hours) is the major symptom of *C. difficile* infection. Other manifestations include lower abdominal pain and cramping, low-grade fever, and nausea. Symptoms range from mild diarrhea to potentially life-threatening pseudomembranous colitis. Diarrhea may occur during or after antibiotic therapy. The risk is highest in the first month following antibiotic therapy, but it can also occur up to 3 months following antibiotic therapy.[73,74]

PHYSICAL EXAMINATION

Physical examination findings may be normal. Severe and complicated *C. difficile* infection is associated with systemic signs including hypotension, ileus, or megacolon. Abdominal examination revealing decreased bowel sounds, abdominal rigidity, guarding, and rebound tenderness may suggest bowel perforation from megacolon. A prompt surgical evaluation should be obtained for such patients.

DIFFERENTIAL DIAGNOSIS

The differential diagnosis for *C. difficile* infection includes ulcerative colitis (UC), microscopic colitis, postinfectious IBS, celiac disease, and noninfectious antibiotic–associated diarrhea.

DIAGNOSTIC STUDIES

Diagnostic studies include stool testing for *C. difficile*, CBC with differential, and CMP.

A patient presenting with severe colitis symptoms should undergo x-ray imaging to rule out megacolon.[74]

EVALUATION

C. difficile infection can be classified based on disease severity. Mild to moderate disease includes diarrhea without systemic signs of infection, a white blood cell (WBC) count of <15,000 cells/mL, and a serum creatinine <1.5 times baseline. Severe disease is associated with systemic signs of infection which includes a WBC count >15,000 cells/mL or serum creatinine ≥1.5 times the premorbid level.[73,74]

TREATMENT

- Metronidazole is no longer recommended as first-line treatment for *C. difficile* infection unless disease is mild or if vancomycin or fidaxomicin are unavailable (Table 8.7).[73]
- Asymptomatic patients should not be retested for *C. diffcle* and it is recommended that repeat testing not be performed within 7 days during the same episode of diarrhea.[73]
- Recurrent *C. difficile* is defined by having resolution of *C. difficile* infection symptoms while on appropriate therapy followed by recurrence of symptoms within 2 to 8 weeks after treatment has stopped.

TABLE 8.7 Treatment Regimens for *Clostridium difficile*

Infection Grade	Treatment Regimen
Initial infection: nonsevere disease and severe disease	Vancomycin 125 mg QID × 10 days *or* Fidaxomicin 200 mg BID × 10 days
Initial infection: fulminant disease	Vancomycin 500 mg PO or via NG tube QID *and* Metronidazole 500 mg IV q8h *or* Rectal vancomycin given as retention enema 500 mg/100 mL normal saline PR q6h
First recurrence for non-severe and severe disease	If vancomycin used for first episode, then pulsed and tapered vancomycin regimen* *or* Fidaxomicin 200 mg BID × 10 days If fidaxomicin or metronidazole used initially, then vancomycin 125 mg QID × 10 days
Second or subsequent recurrence for nonsevere and severe disease	Vancomycin pulsed and tapered regimen* *or* Fidaxomicin 200 mg BID × 10 days *or* Vancomycin 125 mg QID × 10 days, then rifaximin 400 mg TID × 20 days *or* Fecal microbiota transplant

**Pulsed and tapered vancomycin regimen: 125 mg PO QID × 10–14 days, then 125 mg PO BID × 7 days, then 125 mg PO once daily × 7 days, then 125 mg q2–3 days for 2–8 weeks.*

BID, twice daily; IV, intravenously; NG, nasogastric; PO, orally; PR, per rectum; q8h, every 8 hours; QID, four times daily; TID, three times daily.

- Persistent diarrhea without resolution during initial therapy should prompt an evaluation for other causes of diarrhea. Specifically, a colonoscopy should be considered to rule out IBD.
- Fecal microbiota transplantation (FMT) restores gut microbiota diversity through instillation of donor stool into the GI tract of a patient with *C. difficile* infection. FMT is recommended for patients with multiple recurrences of *C. difficile* infection who have failed appropriate antibiotic treatments.[73]

PATIENT EDUCATION

- Patients with *C. difficile* infection should avoid PPIs. (See Section 8.1A Gastroesophogeal Reflux Disease, Treatment.)
- Before PPI therapy is reinstituted, risks and benefits should be assessed.
- Future use of antibiotics should be particularly judicious in patients with a history of *C. difficile* infection.

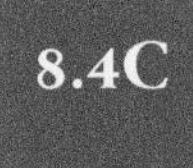

8.4C COLONIC ISCHEMIA (ISCHEMIC COLITIS)

MEDICAL HISTORY AND CLINICAL PRESENTATION

Intestinal ischemia can affect the small or large intestine and can be triggered by any process that reduces intestinal blood flow. *Colonic ischemia*, also called ischemic colitis, is the most common type of mesenteric ischemia. It is more common in the older adult and is the cause of up to 15% of patients who are hospitalized with acute lower GI (LGI) bleeding.[75] *Acute mesenteric ischemia* affects the small bowel and should be suspected in patients with abdominal pain out of proportion to physical findings. (See Section 8.3I Mesenteric Ischemia.)

Colonic ischemia is caused by hypoperfusion from vascular disease or by hematologic conditions associated with increased blood viscosity such as polycythemia vera. The ischemic involvement is usually segmental due to collateral circulation. Areas of the colon with less collateral circulation such as the splenic flexure and rectosigmoid junction are most commonly affected. Large vessels are not involved.

The etiologies of colonic ischemia include nonocclusive colonic ischemia, embolic and thrombotic arterial occlusion, and mesenteric venous thrombosis. Nonocclusive colonic ischemia due to hypoperfusion of the mesenteric microvasculature is the most common cause, occurring most prominently at the splenic flexure and rectosigmoid.[60]

Patients with vascular risk factors such as diabetes, coronary artery disease, and peripheral vascular disease are at higher risk for colonic ischemia. Other risk factors include a history of IBS, constipation, and aortic aneurysm repair.[76]

Constipation and constipation-inducing drugs may be a risk due to increased colonic pressure and reduced blood flow as a result of fecal impaction. Illicit drugs, including amphetamines and cocaine, can increase the risk of ischemia because of vasoconstriction, hypercoagulation, and direct endothelial injury.[60]

SIGNS AND SYMPTOMS

The clinical presentation depends upon the extent and duration of ischemia. Patients typically present with abrupt cramping abdominal pain that usually affects the left side of the abdomen, associated stool urgency, and development of bloody diarrhea within 24 hours. Patients usually do not appear acutely ill at presentation. Compared to small intestinal ischemia, the pain that accompanies colonic ischemia is less severe and tends to occur laterally, rather than periumbically.[60]

PHYSICAL EXAMINATION

Physical examination may be normal in mild cases. Assess vital signs to evaluate for orthostatic hypotension. On abdominal exam, assess for abnormal bowel sounds, signs of distention, rebound tenderness, or guarding.

DIFFERENTIAL DIAGNOSIS

The differential diagnosis for colonic ischemia (ischemic colitis) includes IBD, infectious colitis, C. *difficile* colitis, and colon cancer.

DIAGNOSTIC STUDIES

Initial lab studies include CBC, CMP, serum lactate level, lactate dehydrogenase (LDH) level, creatinine kinase level, and amylase level. Stool studies should be ordered for C. *difficile* toxin, stool cultures, and ova and parasite testing.

An abdominal plain film is usually nonrevealing; however, findings of "thumbprinting" suggest submucosal hemorrhage and edema. A CT scan with IV and oral contrast agent is recommended as the imaging modality for patients suspected of colonic ischemia to assess the distribution and phase of colitis.

EVALUATION

Colonic ischemia is often segmental, involving the left colon; however, isolated right colon ischemia has a different clinical presentation and worse outcome than that affecting any other region of the colon.[60] Imaging findings of edema, bowel wall thickening, and thumbprinting are suggestive of ischemia. Nonspecific findings of segmental wall thickening may be seen, which is also seen in both infectious colitis and Crohn colitis.

Abnormal imaging findings such as nonspecific colonic wall thickening should prompt a colonoscopy for diagnosis; however, in severe disease biopsies should be limited.

A colonoscopy should not be performed in patients who have signs of acute peritonitis or findings of irreversible ischemic damage on imaging. Surgical intervention may be indicated in patients with the presence of colonic ischemia accompanied by peritonitis, hemodynamic instability, pancolonic colonic ischemia, or gangrene.

The underlying medical condition contributing to ischemia should be corrected. A repeat colonoscopy can be performed several months afterward to confirm healing and to rule out other underlying pathology.

TREATMENT

- Symptoms usually resolve within 24 to 48 hours and specific therapy is not indicated for mild disease.
- Treatment for a patient with colonic ischemia is conservative management with bowel rest, IV hydration, antibiotics if indicated, and serial abdominal examinations.
- Marked colonic distention may require decompression with a rectal or NG tube.
- Vasoconstrictive medications such as digitalis, glycosides, vasopressin, and diuretics should be held. Close monitoring is needed should surgical intervention be warranted.

PATIENT EDUCATION

- Ensure adequate blood pressure control for optimal colonic perfusion. Educate patients on maintaining hydration. Avoid potential drug triggers.

8.4D DIVERTICULAR DISEASE

MEDICAL HISTORY AND CLINICAL PRESENTATION

Diverticulosis refers to the presence of diverticula in an asymptomatic individual. It is often an anatomic finding on screening colonoscopy and is the most common structural abnormality of the colon. The presence of diverticulosis increases with age. It is estimated that this affects 30% of people by age 60, and up to 65% by age 80. The prevalence of diverticulosis is much lower in vegetarians, presumably due to a higher fiber diet.[77] The majority of people who have diverticulosis will remain asymptomatic. Asymptomatic disease does not require treatment.

A diverticulum is a sac-like protrusion of the colonic wall. Diverticulosis is the presence of diverticula. Diverticulitis is defined as having inflammation of a diverticulum. Diverticular bleeding occurs from segmental weakness of the vasa recta associated with a diverticulum and is characterized by painless hematochezia.

Diverticular disease occurs in the presence of diverticula associated with symptoms and includes complications of infection or GI bleeding. It is more common in Western countries and in people who have adopted a Western lifestyle. It usually affects the left side of the colon; however, individuals from Asia generally have right-sided disease.[77]

The major causes and risk factors for the development of diverticulosis in Western countries are linked to low dietary fiber intake and age. Other environmental factors include high red meat intake, obesity, smoking, sedentary lifestyle, alcohol, and NSAIDs.

Acute diverticulitis occurs primarily in the sigmoid colon. Cecal diverticulitis or right-sided diverticulitis is uncommon in the United States. It usually presents in young people or in Asian populations and can present similarly to acute appendicitis. Meckel diverticulitis can also present similarly to acute appendicitis. This occurs as a diverticulum in the distal small intestine and can migrate into the right lower quadrant (RLQ) area, mimicking appendicitis.

SIGNS AND SYMPTOMS

A gradual onset of left lower quadrant (LLQ) pain is the most common complaint in patients presenting with acute diverticulitis. Pain can be constant with intermittent spasms and loose bowel movements. Other complaints include nausea and vomiting, constipation, diarrhea, and urinary symptoms.

PHYSICAL EXAMINATION

Physical examination will reveal LLQ pain and tenderness. Findings of rigidity, rebound tenderness, or guarding may be indicative of peritonitis.

DIFFERENTIAL DIAGNOSIS

The differential diagnosis for acute diverticulitis includes ischemic colitis, IBD, appendicitis, colorectal cancer, pyelonephritis, pelvic inflammatory disease, ovarian torsion, and ectopic pregnancy.

DIAGNOSTIC STUDIES

- Lab studies include a CBC with differential.
- Contrast–enhanced abdominal CT scan is needed to distinguish complicated from uncomplicated disease

EVALUATION

Complicated diverticulitis includes the development of an intra-abdominal, pelvic, or retroperitoneal abscess, peritonitis, or perforation and requires inpatient treatment and surgical consultation. Other complications from diverticulitis include fistula development between the colon and bladder, vagina, uterus, other bowel segments, or abdominal wall. Resection of the affected bowel segment is usually required.[78,79]

TREATMENT

- Treatment of acute diverticulitis includes bowel rest and antibiotics. A clear liquid diet is recommended, with gradual advancement as the patient clinically improves.
- Uncomplicated diverticulitis is treated in the outpatient setting with at least a 7-day course of antibiotics that will cover gram-negative rods and anaerobes (Table 8.8).
- IV antibiotics and hospitalization are recommended in geriatric patients and those with severe comorbidities, oral intolerance, or immunosuppression.[77]
- Treatment for complicated diverticulitis includes IV antibiotics, fluids, and pain control (Table 8.9).[77]
- An abscess may be amenable to CT-guided percutaneous drainage or may require surgery. If there is an obstruction, surgical resection is necessary to rule out cancer.
- Recurrent episodes of diverticulitis tend to be uncomplicated. It is estimated that one-fifth of patients treated medically for acute uncomplicated diverticulitis may have recurrence. The risk is slightly higher in patients under the age of 45. Surgery does not eliminate the risk of recurrence, as there can be residual or newly formed diverticula.
- Surgical resection may not resolve chronic abdominal symptoms and can also increase the risk of defecatory dysfunction. The effect of surgery on the recurrence of

TABLE 8.8 Oral (Outpatient) Antibiotic Regimens for Acute Diverticulitis

Antibiotic(s)	Dose
Metronidazole *plus*	500 mg q8h
Ciprofloxacin *or*	500 mg q12h
Trimethoprim-sulfamethoxazole *or*	160 mg/800 mg q12h
Levofloxacin	750 mg daily
Amoxicillin-clavulanate	875 mg/125 mg q12h

q8h, every 8 hours; q12h, every 12 hours.

TABLE 8.9 Intravenous (Inpatient) Antibiotic Regimens for Acute Diverticulitis

Antibiotic(s)	Dose
Metronidazole *plus*	500 mg q8h *plus*
Ciprofloxacin *or*	400 mg q12h *or*
Levofloxacin *or*	500 mg daily *or*
Ceftriaxone *or*	1–2 g daily *or*
Cefotaxime	1–2 g q6h
Ampicillin-sulbactam	3 g q6h
Piperacillin-tazobactam	3.75 or 4.5 g q6h
Ticarcillin-clavulanate	3.1 g q8h
Imipenem	500 mg q6h
Meropenem	1 g q8h

q6h, every 6 hours; q8h, every 8 hours; q12h, every 12 hours.

divericulitis is unknown. Approximately 10% of patients who undergo elective resection may experience a short-term complication related to surgery. The present data are limited, but patient-centered outcomes after sigmoid resection suggest improved to stable quality of life.[79] When considering surgical intervention for prevention of recurrence, the potential impact of surgery on quality of life needs to be considered.

- Aspirin and NSAIDs may perpetuate the development of diverticulitis by both direct topical injury to the colon and through disruption of the mucosal integrity by impairing prostaglandin synthesis. Presently, no studies have evaluated the effect of aspirin on patients with a history of acute diverticulitis, but regular use of aspirin suggests an increased risk of diverticulitis. There is also a positive association with NSAID use and perforated diverticulitis. The potential risks of aspirin therapy in a patient with a history of diverticulitis needs to be weighed against both the risk of GI bleeding and increased risk of diverticulitis. This is especially important in those patients with a risk of CVD, in whom secondary prevention with aspirin reduces the risk of myocardial infection and death.
- The use of non-NSAID options should be considered for pain control and should be weighed against the potential for recurrent diverticulitis and its complications.[79]

PATIENT EDUCATION

- During an episode and treatment phase of diverticulitis, a low-residue diet is recommended.
- A higher fiber intake is associated with a reduced risk of recurrence, so in general, a high-fiber diet is recommended following treatment of diverticulitis.[77] Foods such as nuts may confer beneficial effects in diseases such as diabetes and CVD, and therefore, the potential broader health benefits of these foods should be weighed against potential risk in the setting of diverticulosis.[79]

8.4E APPENDICITIS

MEDICAL HISTORY AND CLINICAL PRESENTATION

The vermiform appendix is located at the base of the cecum, near the ileocecal valve, and is a true diverticulum of the cecum. The appendiceal orifice opens into the cecum. As opposed to diverticular disease, which consists of a protuberance of a subset of enteric wall layers, the appendiceal wall contains all the layers of the colonic wall: mucosa, submucosa, muscularis, and the serosal covering.[59]

Appendicitis is one of the most common causes of acute abdomen. Obstruction of the appendiceal lumen is believed to lead to the development of appendicitis. Appendicitis remains the most common surgical emergency in every decade of life. Diagnosis of appendicitis is more often delayed, and perforation occurs more often in patients <3 years of age, in those >64 years of age, and in pregnancy where displacement of the cecum by the developing fetus makes the diagnosis more challenging.[80]

Appendicitis can present as either an uncomplicated acute appendicitis or complicated disease such as perforation, intra-abdominal abscess, or with appendicoliths. Severe complications of appendicitis are diffuse peritonitis from a perforated appendicitis and intra-abdominal abscess.

SIGNS AND SYMPTOMS

Early symptoms include nausea and anorexia. The symptoms of appendicitis can vary, depending upon the location of the tip of the appendix. RLQ pain, abdominal rigidity, and periumbilical pain radiating to the RLQ characterize appendicitis. An inflamed anterior appendix produces RLQ pain, whereas a retrocecal appendix can cause a dull abdominal ache.

PHYSICAL EXAMINATION

Physical signs include McBurney point tenderness, which is described as maximal tenderness approximately 2 inches from the anterior superior iliac spine on a straight line from the anterior superior iliac spine to the umbilicus. Rovsing sign is described as having pain in the RLQ with palpation of the LLQ. This can be indicative of right-sided local peritoneal irritation. A psoas sign refers to having RLQ pain with passive extension of the right hip and is associated with a retrocecal appendix.[59,81] Obturator sign produces RLQ pain with internal rotation of the hip with a flexed thigh.

DIFFERENTIAL DIAGNOSIS

The GI differential diagnosis to consider includes perforated appendix, cecal diverticulitis, Meckel diverticulitis, ileitis, or Crohn disease. Gynecologic conditions that can present with similar symptoms include pelvic inflammatory disease, tubo-ovarian abscess, ruptured ovarian cyst, mittelschmerz, ovarian and fallopian tube torsion, ectopic pregnancy, and endometriosis.

DIAGNOSTIC STUDIES

The initial recommended imaging study, especially in children and pregnant women, is ultrasonography. Ultrasound is often nondiagnostic in overweight and obese patients; therefore, a CT scan is more helpful in evaluating appendicitis in these groups. The use of clinical decision-making tools in conjunction with ultrasound may reduce the use of CT in evaluating suspected appendicitis.[81]

EVALULATION

The Alvarado score is one of several diagnostic tools that has been validated to stratify patients into low-, moderate-, and high-risk categories in clinical decision-making in children and adults. It is an eight-item, 10-point tool that is a validated as a clinical decision rule in children and adults. Signs and symptoms of migration of pain, anorexia, nausea/vomiting, rebound pain, temperature ≥37.3 °C (99.1 °F), and polymorphonuclear leukocytes (PMN) ≥75% each equate to 1 point. Two points are given to RLQ tenderness and leukocytosis ≥10,000/µL. An Alvarado score ≥7 is considered high risk. Moderate risk is a score of 4–6 and low risk is a score <4.[81,82]

TREATMENT

- Appendectomy, either open laparotomy or laparoscopy, is the standard of treatment for acute appendicitis and is performed after correction of volume depletion and electrolyte imbalances. IV antibiotics are given to decrease wound infection rates.[59]
- Some suggest that IV antibiotic therapy alone can treat appendicitis; however, this carries a risk for treatment failure and recurrent appendicitis.

8.4F LARGE BOWEL OBSTRUCTION

MEDICAL HISTORY AND CLINICAL PRESENTATION

When a blockage of the colon occurs, fluid and gas cannot be decompressed distally. If the ileocecal valve is competent, the colon cannot decompress contents proximally into the small bowel. This can result in a closed loop obstruction, which can potentially result in colonic ischemia and perforation. The cecum is the segment of the colon with the largest diameter and has the highest risk of ischemia. An obstruction can cause an increase in intraluminal pressure and an increased colon diameter, which then results in higher wall tension in the cecum. When the wall tension exceeds capillary perfusion pressure, ischemia occurs. Acute dilation of the cecum to 10 cm is suggestive of ischemia. A diameter >13 cm can result in perforation.[56]

The most common cause of large bowel obstruction in adults is colorectal cancer, which accounts for over half of all cases. Obstruction usually occurs distal to the splenic flexure where the colon diameter is smaller. Right-sided cancer can also cause obstruction if the tumor size occludes the lumen or by a lead point of an intussusception.[56]

A colonic volvulus is the twisting of the colon, which can result in partial or complete obstruction of the bowel lumen. This can potentially lead to ischemia and gangrene. Colonic volvulus is the most common benign form of colonic obstruction and accounts for approximately 15% of large bowel obstructions in the United States. Other benign causes include postoperative adhesions, strictures secondary to recurrent diverticulitis, and incarceration from hernia.

The sigmoid colon is the most common site of volvulus, accounting for about 60% of cases, followed by the cecum in approximately 35% of cases. Sigmoid volvulus is more commonly seen between the ages of 40 to 60 or in the elderly or debilitated who suffer from chronic constipation. In young people, sigmoid volvulus is associated with megacolon, most commonly from Hirschsprung disease or Chagas disease.[83]

Colonic pseudo-obstruction can be acute or chronic. It is characterized by the presence of dilation of the bowel on imaging.[84] Ogilvie syndrome is characterized by acute dilation of the colon in the absence of an obstruction. This is a rare diagnosis but is more common than once thought.[85] It can occur at any age, but most commonly in patients over the age of 60.[84]

SIGNS AND SYMPTOMS

The majority of patients with a colonic obstruction will have a diffusely distended abdomen and present with periumbilical or hypogastric pain. Pain may vary from vague discomfort to extreme pain. Diarrhea may result from passage of liquid stool around an obstruction. Other symptoms may include nausea, vomiting, and obstipation. If the ileocecal valve is incompetent, vomiting can occur.

PHYSICAL EXAMINATION

Assess for abdominal distention. Bowel sounds may be hyperactive or absent. Abdominal tenderness may suggest perforation or ischemia.

DIFFERENTIAL DIAGNOSIS

Differential diagnosis to consider for large bowel obstruction includes malignancy, megacolon, adhesions, acute gastric dilation, fecal impaction, volvulus, and ischemia. Other diagnoses to consider include ileus due to recent surgery, peritonitis, and electrolyte imbalance.

DIAGNOSTIC STUDIES

A supine or erect (or left lateral decubitus) x-ray with two views is the initial imaging study of choice. An acute mechanical obstruction usually shows colonic air-fluid levels. The absence of rectal gas can also indicate a colonic ileus, so this is not a specific finding for a large bowel obstruction. If additional studies are necessary for diagnosis, CT or barium enema is recommended.

EVALUATION

A sigmoid volvulus will show a "bent inner-tube" or U-shaped appearance or "coffee-bean" sign from a markedly distended sigmoid loop with fluid levels extending toward the diaphragm on erect films.[83] If the ileceal valve is incompetent, there will also be distention of the small bowel.

A cecal volvulus will show radiologic features of a massively dilated cecum in the left upper quadrant (LUQ) or epigastrum. It involves the terminal ileum, cecum, and proximal right colon.[83]

Colonic pseudo-obstruction on abdominal x-ray shows distal obstruction with segmental proximal colonic dilation.

TREATMENT

- NG aspiration and fluid and electrolyte resuscitation are the initial management of a colonic obstruction.
- If there is no evidence of peritonitis, urgent endoscopic decompression should be performed for sigmoid volvulus. This allows for restoration of colonic perfusion and provides an assessment of colonic mucosa. Complete colonoscopy should be avoided due to the risk of perforation in a distended and unprepped bowel. There is an increased risk for recurrence after endoscopic reduction; therefore, placement of a rectal tube after detorsion can reduce this risk.
- Elective sigmoid resection can prevent subsequent recurrence. A colonoscopy is recommended prior to elective sigmoid resection to evaluate for concurrent neoplasm.[83]
- Surgery is indicated for the management of cecal volvulus. A delay in diagnosis and treatment can result in mortality risk of up to 60% from complications of ischemia, infarction, peritonitis and sepsis.[83]
- Colonic obstruction due to adenocarcinoma requires referral to surgery, medical oncology, and/or surgical oncology. This is generally treated with partial colectomy and ileocolic anastomosis or end-ileostomy. Obstruction from a proximal cancer can be managed with endoscopic placement of a colonic stent.
- Patients with acute colonic pseudo-obstruction should be monitored with early abdominal x-rays and physical examination every 12 to 24 hours to evaluate the colonic diameter. Medical management of Ogilvie syndrome includes the use of an acetylcholinesterase inhibitor such as neostigmine to stimulate colonic parasympathetic tone and to facilitate decompression if the cecal diameter exceeds 10 cm. If this fails or if the patient is not

a candidate for neostigmine or cholinergic therapy, then early decompressive colonoscopy can be performed.[85] If the cecal diameter exceeds 12 cm, endoscopic or surgical decompression is indicated.[84]

8.4G COLON CANCER SCREENING AND COLON POLYPS

Colorectal cancer accounts for 9% of new cancers in men and 11% in women each year. Cancer of the large intestine involves a malignant transformation of the glandular epithelium. Almost all colorectal cancers are *adenocarcinoma.* A *polyp* is any proliferation that protrudes above the surface of the lumen of the bowel and can be identified by colonoscopy. A polyp can be non-neoplastic (such as a benign hyperplastic polyp) or neoplastic (such as adenomatous polyp, which has a malignancy potential). An isolated hyperplastic hamartoma or inflammatory polyp is considered benign. *Hyperplastic polyps* are the most common polyps in the colorectum and have no malignancy potential. *Adenomatous polyps* are neoplastic and considered premalignant. *Serrated polyps* are also considered precursor lesions to colorectal cancer. Advanced adenomas include those with the following features: ≥1 cm, villous histology, high-grade dysplasia, and ≥3 in number.[86]

The U.S. Multi-Society Task Force (MSTF) on Colorectal Cancer is a panel of expert gastroenterologists representing the American College of Gastroenterology, the American Gastroenterological Association, and the American Society for Gastrointestinal Endoscopy. The MSTF recommends that clinicians offer colorectal cancer screening beginning at age 50. Screening should begin at age 50 years in average risk persons, except in African Americans, for which limited evidence supports screening beginning at 45 years. Discontinuation of screening should be considered when persons up to date with screening who have prior negative screening coloscopy reach age 75 or have <10 years of life expectancy. Persons without prior sceening should be considered for screening up to age 85, depending upon age and comorbidities. It is suggested that persons with one first-degree relative with colorectal cancer or a documented advanced adenoma at age <60 years or with two first-degree relatives with colorectal cancer and/or documented advanced adenomas undergo colonoscopy every 5 years beginning 10 years younger than the age at which the youngest first-degree relative was diagnosed or age 40, whichever is earlier. It is recommended that persons with one or more first-degree relatives with colorectal cancer or documented advanced adenomas be offered annual fecal immunochemical test (FIT) if they decline colonoscopy. The MSTF considers FIT an essential element for colorectal cancer screening options that clinicians should offer to patients. The advantages of colonoscopy include high sensitivity for cancer and all classes of precancerous lesions and 10-year interval between normal examinations. The disadvantages of colonoscopy include the need for thorough bowel cleansing, and slight risk of complications such as bleeding, aspiration, and perforation compared to other screening methods. The advantages of FIT include lower cost and being a noninvasive screening method. Disadvantages include the need for yearly testing and poor or no sensitivity for serrated lesions.[87]

The newest noninvasive test approved by the FDA for colorectal cancer screening is a combination of a FIT and markers for abnormal DNA, FIT-DNA (also called Cologuard, Exact Sciences, Boston, MA).[88] The Center for Medicaid and Medicare Services has approved this for reimbursement and recommends this be performed at 3-year intervals for colon cancer screening purposes. However, it has been suggested that annual FIT is more effective and less costly than FIT-DNA every 3 years for large organized screening programs.[89] The FIT-DNA has better specificity in the 50- to 65-year age group and may be appropriate to offer for those who seek a noninvasive test with very high sensitivity for cancer. The current evidence suggests that asymptomatic patients with a positive FIT-DNA test and a negative high-quality colonoscopy do not need to have the colonoscopy repeated.[87]

CT colonography has replaced the double contrast barium enema as another alternative for colon cancer screening. The advantages of the CT colonography include a lower risk of perforation compared to colonoscopy and high sensitivity for adenomas ≥1 cm. The disadvantages include the need for a bowel preparation at most centers. CT colonography has less sensitivity for polyps <1 cm compared to colonoscopy and cannot detect flat and serrated lesions. In addition, radiation exposure and cost are disadvantages of CT colonography. However, this can be an appropriate option to consider in patients who have had a failed colonoscopy due to anatomic reasons.

A flexible sigmoidoscopy can screen for distal colon or rectosigmoid cancers, but has the disadvantage of not viewing the right side of the colon. The cost and risks of this procedure are much less compared to colonoscopy, which includes a limited bowel prep and no need for sedation. It has been suggested that a combination of flexible sigmoidoscopy every 5 years plus yearly FIT screening can be used as a lower risk, cost-effective method of colon cancer screening.[90]

Most colon cancers are sporadic, but approximately 25% of colorectal cancer patients have a family history. Approximately 3% to 5% of colorectal cancers are due to germline mutations. There are two autosomal dominant inherited colorectal cancer predisposition syndromes: (1) familial adenomatous polyposis (FAP) and (2) hereditary nonpolyposis colorectal cancer (HNPCC), also called Lynch syndrome. FAP is the second most common inherited colorectal cancer syndrome. It is characterized by having hundreds to thousands of adenomas, which progress to colorectal cancer in all affected persons. Once the diagnosis is made, a prophylactic colectomy or proctocolectomy is recommended. Patients with FAP are also at increased risk for other malignancies, including periampullary duodenal cancer, thyroid cancer, pancreatic cancer, and desmoid tumors.[91]

In contrast to FAP, only a few adenomatous polyps may characterize Lynch syndrome. Lynch syndrome is the most common cause of inherited colorectal cancer. Patients with newly diagnosed colon cancer can be screened for Lynch syndrome using microsatellite instability testing or immunohistochemistry staining for the mismatch repair proteins. Persons affected with Lynch Syndrome are at risk for many other cancers including uterine, ovarian, gastric, urothelial, sebaceous, and biliary cancers. Diagnosis of an autosomal dominant cancer-susceptibility syndrome in patients with cancer may provide important information about prognosis, treatment, and future cancer risks. This also allows for relatives to undergo genetic counseling and testing to help identify if they are at risk and whether or not they would benefit from intensive cancer surveillance. Management of Lynch syndrome includes intensive endoscopic surveillance and possible prophylactic colon and gynecologic surgery.[91]

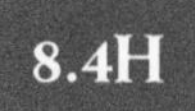

8.4H INFLAMMATORY BOWEL DISEASE

OVERVIEW

IBD is a group of chronic complex and remitting inflammatory conditions of the GI tract that leads to symptoms that can severely diminish a patient's quality of life and are expensive to treat. IBD includes Crohn disease (CD) and ulcerative colitis (UC) and is characterized by the abnormal response of the body's immune system. Whereas CD involves transmural discontinuous inflammation and can affect anywhere from the mouth to the anus, UC is characterized by diffuse mucosal continuous inflammation and is limited to the colon. Sometimes, a definite diagnosis of CD or UC cannot be made; this is known as indeterminate colitis. The cause of IBD is unknown, but it is theorized that environmental, genetic, and immunologic factors may be involved.[92]

EPIDEMIOLOGY

In 2015, the Centers for Disease Control and Prevention (CDC) estimated that IBD affects 3 million (1.3%) U.S. adults.[93] A systematic review by Molodecky et al. reported that the highest annual incidence of UC in North America was 19.2 per 100,000 person-years and prevalence was 505 per 100,000 persons. The highest reported incidence for CD was 20.2 per 100,000 person-years in North America, and prevalence was 322 per 100,000 persons.[94] Although IBD is most prevalent among individuals of European descent living in wealthy Western countries, newly industrialized countries in Asia, the Middle East, Africa, and South America have reported rapid increases in incidence.[94] The prevalence of IBD has been increasing globally, due to being diagnosed predominantly in young individuals, being chronic and incurable, and having low mortality rate.[93] As the incidence of IBD outpaces death, the number of patients diagnosed with IBD will likely continue to increase over time.[95] The average onset of IBD is frequently in the late teens and twenties; however, it may occur at any age and affects men and women equally.[92]

PATHOPHYSIOLOGY

The pathogenesis of IBD is not well understood but it is believed to be the result of the dysregulation of the immune system that results in chronic inflammation of the bowel. It is theorized that genetic, environmental, and immunologic factors may be involved in the dysregulation of the immune system.[92] According to the Crohn's and Colitis Foundation, between 5% and 20% of people with IBD have a first-degree relative who has IBD. The genetic risk is greater with CD than UC.[96] Genetic risk for IBD varies among different populations.[97] For instance, the lifetime risk of IBD in first-degree relatives is at least twofold higher in Ashkenazi Jews than in non-Jews.[98] Some environmental factors that play a role in the development of IBD include cigarette smoking, antibiotic use during childhood, and low levels of vitamin D, although these are not universal in all populations, disease states, or even geographically.[99] Mucosal immunity has also been studied in IBD pathogenesis. Dysfunctions of adaptive immune and innate pathways may contribute to intestinal inflammatory response in patients with IBD.[100]

MEDICAL HISTORY AND CLINICAL PRESENTATION

Crohn Disease

The inflammatory process involves transmural discontinuous inflammation and can affect anywhere from the mouth to the anus. Inflammation tends to commonly develop in the small and large intestine and the perianal region. The behavior of CD is divided into inflammatory, stricturing, or perforating disease. It is important to determine the disease behavior to choose appropriate treatments.[101] Complications of CD can include intestinal obstruction due to strictures, abscesses, and fistulas.

Ulcerative Colitis

Unlike CD, UC is characterized by diffuse continuous mucosal inflammation and is limited to the colon. The rectum is usually always involved, with the inflammation process extending proximally to varying degrees. Complications of UC can include rupture of the bowel and severe bleeding.

SIGNS AND SYMPTOMS

With both CD and UC, symptoms depend on the severity of the extent of disease. Symptoms and signs of IBD include diarrhea, abdominal pain, weight loss, anemia, malnutrition and, at times, rectal bleeding. The onset of symptoms in CD tends to be insidious whereas in UC onset is frequently acute or subacute.

DIFFERENTIAL DIAGNOSIS

Table 8.10 summarizes the differential diagnosis for IBD.

DIAGNOSTIC STUDIES

No single laboratory test is specific or diagnostic of IBD. CBC may show elevated WBC count, decreased hemoglobin secondary to GI bleeding, and increased platelets as an acute phase reactant. CMP can show liver enzyme abnormalities for those at risk of primary sclerosing cholangitis (PSC), and albumin which is not only an indication of malnutrition but also an index of severity of IBD.[102] ESR and CRP are both nonspecific markers that may be elevated in the setting of inflammation. Vitamin B12, folate, vitamin D, iron, ferritin, and total iron binding capacity (TIBC) may be abnormal. The prevalence of iron deficiency anemia in North America was estimated at 2.9%.[103] Stool studies such as fecal calprotectin can help differentiate between IBS and IBD. Infectious enterocolitis should be excluded by bacteriologic and parasitologic examinations.

Magnetic resonance enterography (MRE) is the preferred study due to lack of radiation as well as precision. A CT enterography (CTE) can also be performed. A capsule endoscopy allows for diagnostic imaging, but no intervention. A patency capsule should be done beforehand if stricturing disease is being considered. Abdominal x-ray may show colonic dilation or air-fluid levels if there is an obstruction. Colonoscopy with terminal ileal intubation remains the mainstay in the assessment of IBD, as it allows for direct visualization of the bowel mucosa and sampling of tissue. Obtain biopsies in each segment of the bowel to determine extent and histologic degree of inflammation.

TABLE 8.10 Differential Diagnosis for Inflammatory Bowel Disease

Diagnosis	Description
Infectious gastroenteritis	Acute onset, typically short duration, presentation tends to vary depending on pathogen.
Colorectal cancer	Presentation depends on location. Symptoms may include ill-defined abdominal pain, weight loss, occult bleeding, altered bowel pattern.
Irritable bowel syndrome	Diarrhea, constipation or alternating between constipation and diarrhea. Abdominal pain relieved with bowel movements.
Ischemic colitis	Acute abdominal pain, urgency, hematochezia.
Diverticulitis	Fever, abdominal pain and tenderness, may be recurrent, typically short duration.
Radiation to the bowel	Presentation depends on the location of radiation; symptoms can include hematochezia, weight loss, and abdominal pain.

TREATMENT

Treatment of IBD is aimed at achieving and maintaining remission. The overarching goal for treatment of IBD is mucosal healing, which is defined as resolution of endoscopic inflammatory changes.[104] Assessment of healing occurs with noninvasive metrics such as ESR, CRP, and fecal calprotectin as well as with endoscopy with biopsies to evaluate histology.

Medications used in treatment include aminosalicylates, corticosteroids, immunomodulators (IMMs), antibiotics, and biologics. Treatment of IBD is based on the disease phenotype (CD vs. UC), severity of disease (mild, moderate, severe, fulminant), disease distribution (ileal, ileocolonic, colonic, perianal, small bowel, upper tract), and risk of progression (low, moderate/high). Therefore, staging the disease prior to determining best course of action is paramount.[105] Patient gender, childbearing plans, and potential adherence to treatments also are important in the choice of therapy. Finally, treatment of IBD is best carried out in the outpatient setting. However, at times when the disease is flaring, this care can initially take place in the hospital, which may affect treatment options. Generally speaking, care has transitioned from a step-up format, to a top-down format, implying the use of the more potent, though potentially more risky medications initially and then deescalating over time once in remission.

Mesalamine (5-ASA) preparations have been shown to be effective in all types of UC. Selecting the appropriate formulation depends on the location of disease. If pancolitis, at least 2 g/day of an oral agent targeted to colonic release (Lialda) would be preferred, as opposed to limited rectal disease, in which case nighttime use of at least 1 g/day of a suppository (Canasa) or enema (Rowasa) preparation would be more appropriate. Mesalamines are not indicated as monotherapy in CD. However, in cases of colonic CD, they may be useful adjuncts. Sulfasalazine, in combination with folic acid, has been shown to be effective for the extraintestinal joint pain complaints in IBD patients.

If a patient presents with anything more than mild disease, consideration for advanced therapies would be appropriate and would include use of a biologic, an IMM, or combination therapy with both. This discussion should include possible side effects (pancreatitis: IMM) and risks such as increased risk of infection (hepatitis B, reactivation of latent tuberculosis, herpetic infections), and increased risk of nonmelanomatous skin cancers and lymphomas.

In an acute setting for at least moderate to severe disease, after ruling out common infections such as *C. difficile* infection, early use of IV steroids can result in rapid improvement in symptoms. Depending on a patient's oral status, either methylprednisolone (Solu-Medrol) 15–20 mg IV q8 h or prednisone 40 mg orally (PO) daily (best given in the morning to avoid sleep disruption).[106] However, steroids are not a long-term treatment plan. Guidelines support their use for a maximum of 4 months, usually in the context of a scheduled taper, and generally the nonsystemic variations are preferred over the systemically active ones. If the opportunity to avoid steroids entirely presents itself in favor of early use of biologics, that is preferred. Biologic agents, first FDA approved in 1998 for the treatment of CD, are indicated either alone or in combination with an IMM.

Biologics are grouped broadly into anti-tumor necrosis factors (anti-TNFs; infliximab, adalimumab, certolizumab, golimumab), anti-integrins (vedolizumab), anti-interleukin 12/23 (ustekinumab), and small molecules/Janus kinase (JAK) inhibitors (tofacitinib). Dosing regimen for induction and maintenance is shown in Table 8.11.

Therapeutic drug monitoring in combination with biologic use allows for optimization of dosing while also checking for development of antidrug antibodies, which can weaken or even completely neutralize the active agent and lead to loss of response. When using IMM such as azathioprine (AZA), 6-mercaptopurine (6MP), or methotrexate (MTX), various forms of monitoring and supplementation are recommended. Initial AZA dosing should be based on evaluation of thiopurine methyltransferase (TPMT) enzyme activity to determine the relative metabolism potential for each patient. Appropriate starting dose of 1.5–2.5 mg/kg/day for AZA;

TABLE 8.11 Dosing Regimen for Induction and Maintenance of Pharmacotherapy for Inflammatory Bowel Disease

Medication	Induction	Maintenance
Infliximab, IV	5 mg/kg at week 0, 2, 6	5 mg/kg q 8 weeks
Adalimumab, SC	160/80/40 mg at week 0, 2, 4	40 mg SC q 2 weeks
Certolizumab (CD), SC	400 mg at week 0, 2, 4	400 mg SC q 4 weeks
Golimumab (UC), SC	200 mg at week 0, 100 mg at week 2	100 mg SC q 4 weeks
Vedolizumab, IV	300 mg at week 0, 2, 6	300 mg q 8 weeks
Ustekinumab	260–520 mg IV × 1 (weight based*)	90 mg SC q 8 weeks
Tofacitinib	10 mg PO BID	5–10 mg PO BID

<55 kg: 260 mg; 55–85 kg: 390 mg; >85 kg: 520 mg.

BID, twice daily; CD, Crohn disease; IV, intravenously; PO; orally; q, every; SC, subcutaneously; UC, ulcerative colitis.

0.75–1.5 mg/kg/day for 6MP, and 15–25 mg MTX weekly either PO or IV. MTX does not require chronic monitoring, but it should be taken with 1 mg of folic acid daily. At times, patient tolerance can be improved with the use of antiemetic such as Zofran 20 minutes prior. In patients with UC not responding to maximal medical therapy, consultation with a colorectal surgeon with specialization in IBD should be recommended for consideration of proctocolectomy.

At times when local infectious complications develop, such as perianal abscesses or microperforations, antibiotic therapy is indicated, providing coverage for anaerobes using ciprofloxacin/metronidazole, for example. It is also important to eliminate or at least minimize use of NSAIDs, which have been shown to exacerbate IBD.

Given the increased risk of thromboembolic events, it is important to utilize deep vein thrombosis (DVT) prophylaxis in hospitalized IBD patients. Ambulation is insufficient, even in young, otherwise healthy patients. If a patient has recently been exposed to steroids and flares unexpectedly or without obvious trigger, performing even limited endoscopic evaluation and biopsy for CMV infection is prudent, as this would require treatment with IV ganciclovir 5–7.5 mg/kg twice a day (BID) for 2–3 weeks.[107] Additionally, inquiring about recent NSAID use can provide clues to possible etiology of disease worsening. If a patient with IBD is found to have concomitant *C. difficile* infection, preference is for use of vancomycin over metronidazole.[106] Fecal transplantation can also be used for *C. difficile* treatment, though it is not yet approved for noninfectious therapy of IBD. Postoperatively, high-risk CD patients should be started within 4 weeks on biologic therapy or combination therapy with IMM to prevent disease recurrence.[106] When treating IBD patients, it is important to have a contact at a nearby academic center for curbside consultation regarding treatment options and consideration for clinical trials if possible. This may open up additional therapeutic options for patients.

KEY POINTS

- IBS is a symptom-based disorder; therefore, treatments address the symptom of abdominal pain and the bowel issues of diarrhea and constipation. Individuals with IBS have lower quality of life and higher levels of anxiety.
- Risk factors for severe *C. difficile* infection include age >65, renal failure, immunosuppression, and WBC counts >24,000 cells/mL.
- *Colonic ischemia* should be considered in a patient presenting with LLQ abdominal pain and bloody diarrhea. Most patients have self-limiting symptoms that resolve spontaneously, but up to 10% of patients develop life-threatening colonic necrosis and gangrene.
- Radiographic features of diverticulitis can resemble those of colon cancer; therefore, patients who are symptom free who are at least 6 to 8 weeks following treatment from an initial episode of diverticulitis confirmed by CT scan should undergo a colonoscopy.
- CT has a high accuracy in diagnosing appendicitis and can often diagnose alternative mimickers of appendicitis, potentially decreasing the rate of negative appendectomies.
- IBS can overlap with IBD. There is no increased risk of colon cancer in IBS. The risk of colon cancer increases in IBD 8 to 10 years after the onset of disease if more than one-third of the colon is involved.

SPECIAL CONSIDERATIONS

- *Segmental colitis associated with diverticula (SCAD)*, also referred to as diverticular colitis, is a newly recognized entity of diverticular disease. It is uncommon and estimated to occur in approximately 1% of patients with diverticulosis. It is defined as having segmental chronic inflammation of the colon and can be difficult to distinguish from IBD endoscopically. Biopsies of the rectum and colon are necessary to rule out IBD. Unlike IBD, long-term medication treatment is unnecessary in SCAD. Treatment with mesalamine has been suggested for SCAD; however, it does not reduce the risk of developing diverticulitis.[78]
- *Symptomatic uncomplicated diverticular disease* (SUDD) is characterized by nonspecific attacks of abdominal pain from a diverticular source in the absence of inflammation or altered bowel habits. Pain is described as colicky but can be constant. Defecation or passing flatus provides relief of pain. SUDD shares similar features as IBS; however, the overlap between IBS and SUDD affects mostly people over the age of 65.[79] A high-fiber diet with a combination of both soluble and insoluble fibers and cyclical treatment with a nonabsorbable antibiotic, such a cylical rifaximin for 1 week a month, may be effective in reducing symptoms.[78,81]
- *Pregnancy and IBD:* Very few agents are prohibited in pregnancy, with the exception of MTX, which is a known abortifacient. The biologics (including those other than certolizumab, which was developed with pregnancy in mind) can be safely continued through pregnancy, though some dose adjustment around the estimated date of delivery is recommended. However, if disease is severe enough, doses should not be withheld. Vaccination considerations for children: no live virus vaccines for 6 months, meaning that this should only delay the rotavirus vaccine. Breastfeeding is safe. Steroids are acceptable after 12 weeks.[108]

8.5 RECTAL DISORDERS

OVERVIEW AND PATHOPHYSIOLOGY

Material entering the rectum is dependent upon mucosal absorption, motility, luminal contents, and the microbiome of the colon. Defecation depends upon the capacity of the rectum, the ability of the rectum to expel stool, the ability of the pelvic floor and sphincter muscles to maintain continence and prevent stool leakage, and the ability of these muscles to relax in order to defecate. Luminal contents are retained in the sigmoid until enough water is absorbed to change the contents from a viscous liquid to a soft stool. The gastrocolic response stimulates emptying from the sigmoid into the rectum. The rectal-anal inhibitory reflex (RAIR) is activated when the rectum is distended, which causes relaxation of the internal anal sphincter.[61]

The pelvic floor contains superficial and deep muscles that support the rectum, bladder, and uterus. The internal anal sphincter and external anal sphincter are located within the superficial layers along with the perineal body and transverse perineal muscles. The levator ani are the deeper muscles within the pelvic floor and are composed of the pubococcygeus, iliococcygeus, and puborectalis.[109] The puborectalis muscle is composed of skeletal muscle and maintains the anorectal angle, which controls stool evacuation and supports the integrity of the pelvic floor.[61]

The junction of the colorectal mucosa and anal mucosa forms the dentate line, which is where the anatomic anal canal starts. It ends at the junction of the anal mucosa and perianal skin, or the anal verge. The anal canal is 3 to 4 cm long and is supported by the anal sphincters. The internal anal sphincter is composed of smooth muscle and is involuntary. It is innervated by sympathetic and parasympathetic fibers. It contributes to approximately 85% of the resting tone and is in a constant state of contraction. The tonic contraction of the internal anal sphincter is reflexively inhibited by the RAIR, in response to distention of the rectum, allowing defecation to occur. The external sphincter is striated muscle innervated by the pudendal nerve with fibers originating from S2–S4. It maintains approximately 15% of the resting sphincter tone and 100% of voluntary squeeze pressures. The pudendal nerve innervates the puborectalis muscle, which is the middle layer of the pelvic floor muscle. The branches from the sacral nerve roots of S3 and S4 innervate the deeper muscles, which include the pubococcygeus, iliococcygeus, and coccygeus.

The voluntary effort of bearing down by a Valsalva maneuver during normal defecation with contraction of the rectum and perineal muscles results in an increase in intra-abdominal pressure. At the same time, the puborectalis and anal sphincters relax, allowing the anorectal angle to widen and the perineum to descend. Stool evacuation results from coordination of these muscles, facilitating the movement of stool from the rectum. The pelvic floor and external anal sphincter muscles are responsible for continence by contracting to prevent evacuation and relaxing in order to allow for defecation (Figure 8.2).[110]

Anorectal disorders can range from benign conditions such as hemorrhoids to potentially life-threatening conditions of malignancy.

8.5A FECAL INCONTINENCE

MEDICAL HISTORY AND CLINICAL PRESENTATION

Fecal incontinence, or the inability to hold stool in the rectum, is an embarrassing and debilitating condition. All patients with rectal complaints should be questioned about this. A detailed history including bowel habit history, history of physical and/or sexual abuse, and obstetric history are essential to this evaluation. Symptoms can range from minor soiling to involuntary passage of bowel movements.

There are several subtypes of fecal incontinence. Passive incontinence from a hyposensitive rectum results in involuntary passage of stool without awareness. Afferent nerve injury can result in an inability to detect rectal filling and can occur in a patient with diabetic neuropathy, spinal cord injury, or multiple sclerosis. Urge-related incontinence resulting in discharge of fecal matter despite attempts to retain content occurs in a hypersensitive rectum. This is caused by a noncompliant rectum leading to irresistible urgency and can be seen in patients with UC, history of radiation injury, or previous rectal resection. Fecal seepage is the passive leaking of stool associated with normal evacuation, caused by obstructive sphincter closure, and can be seen in a patient with rectal prolapse or prolapsed hemorrhoids. Sphincter weakness can occur from tears of the internal or external anal sphincter from trauma; pudendal nerve injury related to obstetric injury, diabetes, or multiple sclerosis; and CNS injury such as spina bifida, spinal injury, stroke, or multiple sclerosis.

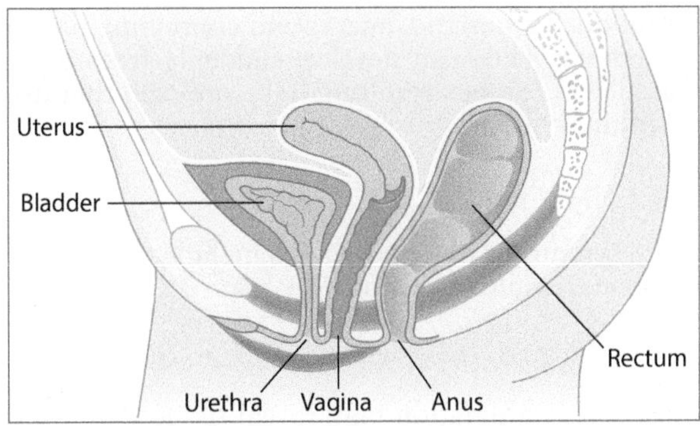

Figure 8.2 **Anatomy of the anal canal and rectum.**

Functional causes of fecal incontinence include fecal impaction with overflow, which can be seen in defecatory dyssynergia and/or spinal cord injury. Diarrhea with rapid transit and loose or watery stools can occur in IBS or infectious diarrhea. Social indifference from dementia, special needs, or mental illness can also be a cause of functional fecal incontinence.[111,112]

SIGNS AND SYMPTOMS

A patient with fecal incontinence may complain of not reaching the bathroom on time, occasional accidental leakage of stool, or passage of feces when believing that one is passing gas.

PHYSICAL EXAMINATION

- Abdominal examination to palpate for mass. Rectal examination to inspect for hemorrhoids, skin tags or rash. Rectal digital exam to palpate for mass or stool retention. Rectal digital examination to assess baseline sphincter tone, whether there is an increase in pressure associated with squeezing, and assessment of the anal sphincter and the puborectalis muscle.

DIFFERENTIAL DIAGNOSIS

The differential diagnosis for fecal incontinence includes overflow diarrhea from constipation, fecal impaction, rectal cancer, proctitis, colitis, infectious diarrhea, and malabsorption.

DIAGNOSTIC STUDIES

The diagnostic studies for fecal incontinence are summarized in Table 8.12.

EVALUATION

A **rectocele** is an abnormal sac-like protrusion of the rectal wall that can protrude anteriorly toward the vagina, or posteriorly toward the sacrum. This is often an incidental finding. Rectoceles that are >3 cm and those that retain barium or stool are considered clinically significant. The first-line

TABLE 8.12 Diagnostic Studies for Fecal Incontinence

Diagnostic Test	Rationale
Stool studies	Infection, parasites, and/or malabsorption
Abdominal x-ray	Constipation
Flexible sigmoidoscopy/ colonoscopy	Biopsies for cancer, microscopic colitis
Barium or magnetic resonance defecography	Rectum and pelvic floor evaluation; rectocele, enterocele, intussusception, rectal prolapse, and megarectum
An anorectal manometry study (ARM) with balloon expulsion	Defecatory dyssynergia

management is treating the underlying dyssynergia; otherwise surgical treatment without treating the dyssynergia carries a high risk of recurrence.[109]

An electromyographic (EMG) study of the anal canal involves the placement of a probe to evaluate the EMG activity of the striated muscles surrounding the anal canal. This provides information concerning the innervation of the pelvic floor muscles, but does not measure sensory thresholds or compliance, and therefore, EMG does not replace anorectal manometry (ARM). EMG can complement the ARM by differentiating neurologic causes of low squeeze pressure.[112]

Endoanal ultrasonography and MRI can identify and characterize sphincter injury of the internal and external anal sphincter. These can be considered if medical management, pelvic floor therapy, and biofeedback fail and if a sphincter defect is suspected.

TREATMENT

- Management of functional fecal incontinence and urge continence relies on conservative measures including pelvic floor retraining, biofeedback, and a consistent bowel regimen.
- An injectable bulking agent dextranomer, in stabilized hyaluronic acid, is approved for treating fecal incontinence. It is injected into the submucosal space surrounding the anal canal.
- If a patient is refractory to conservative management, a referral for a sacral nerve stimulator (SNS) to a urogynecologist who specializes in such can be considered.[113]

PATIENT EDUCATION

- Educate that constipation can result in overflow fecal incontinence
- Antidiarrheal agents should be avoided
- Fiber and laxatives can improve condition
- Physical therapy with biofeedback training may be recommended

8.5B FECAL IMPACTION

MEDICAL HISTORY AND CLINICAL PRESENTATION

Fecal impaction results from an abnormal accumulation of hard and compacted stool in the rectum, which can occur over several days to weeks, with a failure to evacuate. Risk factors and conditions that predispose to fecal impaction include neurologic diseases, diabetes, dementia, dehydration, and immobility.

SIGNS AND SYMPTOMS

Sign and symptoms of fecal impaction may include vague abdominal pain, constipation, and passage of watery stool from overflow. Solitary rectal ulcers can occur with fecal impaction.

PHYSICAL EXAMINATION

Physical examination findings can reveal a palpable firm mass.

DIFFERENTIAL DIAGNOSIS

The differential diagnosis for fecal impaction includes polypharmacy, chronic constipation, defecatory dyssynergia, megarectum, rectal cancer, and colon cancer.

DIAGNOSTIC STUDIES

- Laboratory studies include CBC, metabolic profile, calcium level, and thyroid function testing.
- Plain abdominal x-ray can be performed to evaluate for megarectum or megacolon.
- Abdominal CT may be required to evaluate for extrinsic compression that might be obstructing the colon.

EVALUATION

- Further workup with a colonic transit study can be considered to evaluate for slow transit constipation. An ARM and balloon expulsion testing can identify defecatory dyssynergia.
- Solitary rectal ulcer syndrome is often associated with evacuation disorders. It is characterized by erythema and a single or a few ulcers and a patient may not be symptomatic from the ulcer. Anal cancer can also present as a painless ulcer. Nonhealing ulcers should be biopsied to rule out malignancy, infection, and IBD.

TREATMENT

- Enemas and/or digital disruption should relieve the impaction. Following this, a flexible sigmoidoscopy or colonoscopy should be performed to rule out a secondary cause.
- Long-term management includes a bowel regimen of stool softeners, laxatives, and/or enemas as needed to maintain soft stools and regular bowel movements.

8.5C HEMORRHOIDS

MEDICAL HISTORY AND CLINICAL PRESENTATION

Hemorrhoids are dilated vascular channels between the anal mucosa and underlying internal anal sphincter. Internal hemorrhoids are located above the dentate line and arise from the superior hemorrhoidal plexus. They are usually painless due to visceral innervation with overlying rectal mucosa. Internal hemorrhoids typically do not cause pain, but can present with bright red bleeding per rectum, mucus discharge, and a sense of rectal fullness. Bleeding from internal hemorrhoids presents with bright red blood on the toilet paper, dripping of blood into the toilet bowel, or blood coating the surface of stool. Ongoing blood loss can lead to iron deficiency anemia. Internal hemorrhoids can prolapse into the anal canal and cause pain.

External hemorrhoids are located below the dentate line and arise from the inferior hemorrhoidal plexus. They can be painful due to somatic innervation containing numerous pain receptors. They can develop suddenly from an acute intravascular thrombus resulting in severe pain that usually peaks within 48 hours.

SIGNS AND SYMPTOMS

Signs and symptoms of hemorrhoids include rectal pruritus, burning, pain, and/or bleeding.

PHYSICAL EXAMINATION

An anoscopic examination may reveal tissue with evidence of chronic vascular dilatation and friability.

DIFFERENTIAL DIAGNOSIS

The differential diagnosis includes anal fissure, abscess, IBD, proctitis, colon cancer, rectal cancer, and anal cancer.

EVALUATION

Hemorrhoids are graded from 1 to 4. Grade 1 hemorrhoids bulge into the lumen, but do not extend past the dentate line. Grade 2 hemorrhoids prolapse out of the anal canal with straining and can be reduced spontaneously. Grade 3 hemorrhoids prolapse out of the anal canal with straining and require manual reduction. Grade 4 hemorrhoids are not able to be reduced and are at risk for strangulation.[114]

TREATMENT

- Acute symptoms can be conservatively managed with sitz baths and topical analgesia. Excision with clot evacuation performed within 48 hours after onset of symptoms can significantly decrease the incidence of recurrence. After 48 hours from the onset of symptoms, the thrombus will start to organize, and evacuation likely will not be successful, so the hemorrhoids should be managed conservatively.[115]
- Patients with symptomatic hemorrhoids should avoid straining. The first-line treatment of constipation includes fiber supplementation, stool softeners and/or osmotic laxatives. A steroid suppository can be prescribed to reduce pain and inflammation. Topical preparations containing hydrocortisone and/or lidocaine can be prescribed to reduce symptoms of burning and pruritus.
- Patients who do not respond to medical management and/or who have grade 4 hemorrhoids should be referred for surgical intervention. In-office surgical procedures include rubber band ligation, sclerotherapy, and coagulation.
- Failure of medical and office treatment and/or grade 4 hemorrhoids may need a surgical hemorrhoidectomy. Hemorrhoidopexy fixes the anal cushions in place with a circular stapler. In a hemorrhoidectomy, the hemorrhoid cushions are surgically dissected away from the sphincter muscles and are resected. Complications of hemorrhoidectomy include severe pain, urinary retention, bleeding, and fecal impaction.[114]

8.5D PRURITUS ANI

MEDICAL HISTORY AND CLINICAL PRESENTATION

Pruritus ani is an idiopathic condition that is characterized by severe perianal itching or burning. Poor hygiene of the perineum or seepage can irritate the anoderm, leading to pruritus. Other causes include topical irritants from soap or laundry detergent. Fecal soiling or hemorrhoids can also cause pruritus ani. Pinworms (*Enterobius vermicularis*) are the most common cause of this in children in whom perianal inching is most severe at night.

The patient history should include history of diabetes, psoriasis, eczema, recent antibiotic use, vaginal discharge, and anal intercourse.

SIGNS AND SYMPTOMS

Signs and symptoms of pruritus include an uncomfortable perianal sensation, itchiness, or burning.

PHYSICAL EXAMINATION

- Skin examination for rash.
- Rectal exam to evaluate for erythema, excoriations, or tenderness.

DIFFERENTIAL DIAGNOSIS

Differential diagnosis includes hemorrhoids, fecal incontinence, or dermatologic conditions such as lichen planus, eczema, and seborrheic dermatitis. Infectious etiologies include candidiasis, dermatophytosis, parasites, and superimposed bacterial infection.

DIAGNOSTIC STUDIES

- Pinworms are diagnosed by applying cellophane tape to the perianal skin to collect eggs and view under a microscope.
- Stool study will reveal ova and parasites.
- Refractory pruritus may require a biopsy to rule out a cutaneous malignancy.[114]

TREATMENT

- Treatment of pruritus ani is directed at treating the underlying cause.
- Topical capsaicin .006% or topical hydrocortisone can be effective, but hydrocortisone should not be applied for >2 weeks due to risk of perianal skin thinning.

PATIENT EDUCATION

- Patient education on proper perineal care includes avoiding excessive cleaning or scrubbing. The use of lanolin wipes can help facilitate cleaning following bowel movements. Soaps and topical ointment are generally not recommended.The perineum should be kept dry and the use of a blow dryer on the perineum following bathing may be helpful. Food items including coffee, tea, cola, beer, chocolate, and citrus products should be avoided for a few weeks, and after resolution of the symptom each item can be added back sequentially to identify a trigger.

8.5E ANAL FISSURE

MEDICAL HISTORY AND CLINICAL PRESENTATION

An anal fissure is a split in the anoderm distal to the dentate line. Patients present with severe perianal pain during and after the passage of stool. The etiology of anal fissure may include trauma, ischemia, and elevated anal pressure. Blood flow is poor in the posterior midline, which slows healing. The elevated anal canal pressure is thought to be due to increased internal anal sphincter tone and spasm of the muscle underneath the tear.

SIGNS AND SYMPTOMS

The pain from an anal fissure is often described as passing knives or shards of glass. Blood may be noted on the tissue. Constipation may develop secondarily due to fear of pain with passing stool.

PHYSICAL EXAMINATION

With gentle traction on the buttocks to evert the anus, physical examination will reveal a linear tear at the anoderm midline, which may appear as a fresh laceration on a white ulcerated base. Chronic anal fissures may reveal an external hemorrhoid or "sentinel pile." A limited digital exam may cause severe pain, but sphincter spasm may be felt.

DIFFERENTIAL DIAGNOSIS

The differential diagnosis for an atypical fissure, such as lateral fissure or ulcer occurring off the midline includes CD, malignancy, syphilis, tuberculosis, or HIV infection.

DIAGNOSTIC STUDIES

A full anoscopic examination should be deferred until this has healed. Most fissures occur in the posterior midline.

TREATMENT

- The goal of treatment of an anal fissure is to relax the anal sphincter and to stop the cycle of sphincter spasm and tearing.
  - Stool softeners and regular bowel movements are necessary to minimize trauma to the area. Sitz baths can provide relief.
  - A very small amount of topical .2% nitroglycerin ointment applied to the fissure can help healing.
  - Injection of botulinum toxin into the internal anal sphincter is effective at relieving spasm.
- A chronic refractory anal fissure may require surgery. The gold standard surgical treatment is a lateral internal sphincterotomy. Fecal incontinence is a known complication. There is also a higher cost associated with this, which is why medical management remains the cornerstone of treatment.[114]

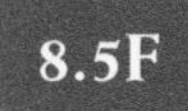

8.5F ANAL ABSCESS AND FISTULAE

MEDICAL HISTORY AND CLINICAL PRESENTATION

Anorectal abscesses and fistulae represent different stages of the same anorectal disorder spectrum. *Abscess* defines the acute phase of infection and can present with pain, swelling, and fever. An anorectal abscess usually arises from an infected anorectal gland. A perianal fistula is a track that can form from the infection through the perianal tissues, creating a connection between the infected anal crypt gland and the perineum.[116]

Fistulae can either be intersphincteric, transsphincteric, suprasphincteric, or extrasphincteric and an MRI can differentiate the anatomy of such.

Pilonidal disease can be an acute or chronic abscess or draining sinus that occurs over the sacrococcygeal or perianal area. This can occur from an infected hair follicle that becomes obstructed and ruptures into the subcutaneous tissues forming an abscess.

A rectovaginal fistula usually presents with passage of stool and flatus through the vagina. There may be varying degrees of incontinence. Rectovaginal fistulae can result from obstetric injury, CD, diverticulitis, radiation, undrained cryptoglandular disease, tumor, and malignancies of the rectum, cervix, or vagina.

SIGNS AND SYMPTOMS

Perianal fistula may present with drainage of blood, purulence, or stool from an external opening in the perianal area. An abscess usually causes a constant throbbing pain, while a fistula can be intermittently painful and associated with pruritus.

PHYSICAL EXAMINATION

An area of persistent pain and swelling can be visualized and palpated in a patient presenting with an anorectal abscess; however, if the abscess is in the intersphincteric space, this may not be visible. Upon palpation with a digital rectal examination, a boggy area of tenderness and fluctuance may be palpated.[117]

Physical examination in pilonidal disease may show small midline pits, or abscesses can be seen near the midline of the coccyx or sacrum. Acute suppuration can be seen in an undrained abscess. Chronic draining sinuses may have multiple mature tracts with hairs protruding from the openings.

A rectovaginal fistula may show an opening in the vagina or rectum that can be visualized or palpated. The fistulae are classified as low, middle, or high depending on location.

DIFFERENTIAL DIAGNOSIS

The most common cause of a perianal fistula is an anorectal abscess. The differential diagnosis for a perianal fistula includes Crohn disease, hidradenitis suppurativa, radiation proctitis, foreign body, HIV infection, tuberculosis, actinomycosis, and malignancy.

Differential diagnosis for pilonidal disease includes hidradenitis suppurativa, furuncle, actinomycosis, and Crohn disease.

DIAGNOSTIC STUDIES

The majority of anorectal abscess or fistula-in-ano do not require imaging, although in complex tract or recurrent disease imaging studies are necessary. Endoanal ultrasound can delineate fistula tracts and identify horseshoe tract extensions. In patients with complex suppurative anorectal conditions or supralevator abscess, a CT scan provides details that otherwise would not be obtained without anesthesia. In patients with Crohn disease, a CT scan is necessary to differentiate isolated rectal inflammation from fistulae and abscesses.[117] A barium enema can identify a rectovaginal fistula.

EVALUATION

Complications of an undrained anorectal abscess can be severe. Without prompt drainage, infection can spread rapidly, resulting in extensive tissue loss, sphincter injury, sepsis, and ultimately death.

TREATMENT

- The treatment of an anorectal abscess requires surgical incision and drainage. Antibiotics are not routinely required in the management of an uncomplicated anorectal abscess, except in cases of immunosuppression, extensive cellulitis, or prosthetic devices.[117] Drainage in the operating room with anesthesia allows for full evaluation and extent of the disease. If the internal opening of a fistula is identified and external sphincter involvement is minimal, a fistulotomy may be performed at the time of abscess drainage.

- Simple anal fistula can be treated with a fistulotomy or with debridement and fibrin glue injection. Treatment options for a complex anal fistula includes anal fistula plug, endoanal advancement flaps, and seton and/or staged fistulotomy. Ligation of the intersphincteric fistula tract (LIFT) procedure involves placement of a seton for 8 or more weeks to allow fibrosis of the tract. The tract can then be identified, ligated, and divided with possible closure of the internal opening and widening of the external opening for drainage, using an intersphincteric approach. With this approach, the sphincter muscle is not divided in an effort to preserve continence.[117]
- In a patient with Crohn disease, asymptomatic fistulae do not require surgical treatment. For complex fistulae associated with Crohn disease, palliation can be provided with long-term drainage setons to allow healing of inflammation. Endorectal and anodermal advancement flaps can be used to treat complex Crohn fistulae in selected patients with normal rectal mucosa who do not have active proctitis. Permanent diversion or proctectomy may be required in complex Crohn fistulae in a patient with uncontrollable symptoms to prevent sepsis.[117]
- Pilonidal abscesses can be drained under local anesthesia by inserting a probe into the primary opening and unroofing the abscess. Skin care, perineal hygiene, and drainage of abscesses may reduce the need for surgery. Definitive surgical treatment is recommended for cysts that fail to heal after 3 months.

8.5G PROCTITIS

MEDICAL HISTORY AND CLINICAL PRESENTATION

Proctitus is a nonspecific term that refers to inflammation of the anus or rectum. Inflammatory proctitis is usually self-limiting and confined to the rectum. It is a mild form of UC and only 10% of patients will progress to colonic UC.

Radiation proctitis can occur following radiation therapy for prostate, bladder, testicular, and gynecologic cancers. Radiation therapy is believed to cause damage to the vascular endothelium. Acute radiation injury is characterized by diarrhea, tenesmus, pain, hematochezia, and incontinence and resolves with discontinuation of therapy.

Proctitis can also occur from sexually transmitted diseases. *Neisseria gonorrhoeae* accounts for approximately 30% of infectious proctitis in the United States, *Chlamydia trachomatis* 19%, *herpes simplex* virus 16%, and *treponema pallidum* causing syphilis 2%.[118] Approximately 80% or more of all anal cancers are associated with human papilloma virus (HPV). The most common subtypes are HPV16, HPV18, and HPV33.[118]

SIGNS AND SYMPTOMS

Signs and symptoms of proctitis include rectal bleeding, diarrhea, pain, and tenesmus.

PHYSICAL EXAMINATION

Herpes proctitis is characterized by painful perianal vesicles and ulcers and diagnosed by viral culture of the vesicle or biopsy of the ulcer.

Anorectal syphilis is characterized by an asymptomatic perianal or anal ulcer.

An anoscopic examination will show friable and edematous mucosa with pus occurring with gonococcal proctitis.

DIFFERENTIAL DIAGNOSIS

The differential diagnosis for proctitis includes UC, infectious proctitis, and inflammatory proctitis.

DIAGNOSTIC STUDIES

The diagnostic studies for proctitis are summarized in Table 8.13.

EVALUATION

Colonoscopy or flexible sigmoidoscopy will reveal friability, granularity, and erosions, but the colon proximal to the rectum is normal appearing in inflammatory proctitis.

TREATMENT

The treatments for inflammatory, radiation, and infectious proctitis are summarized in Table 8.14.

KEY POINTS

- Overflow diarrhea from constipation can present with complaints of fecal incontinence. Consider abdominal x-ray in a patient with a complaint of fecal incontinence.
- Rectal cancer and anal cancer can coexist with hemorrhoids; sigmoidoscopy or colonoscopy should be considered following treatment of hemorrhoids.
- *Condylomata acuminata* or HPV can also infect the anus and is a risk factor for anal cancer.

SPECIAL CONSIDERATIONS

- Proctalgia fugax is defined as having recurrent episodes of pain localized to the anus or lower rectum. It is a functional GI disorder characterized by attacks of spasm or pain. Treatment of proctalgia fugax is often unnecessary due to the infrequent nature of symptoms. Topical treatments with nitroglycerin or diltiazem, TCAs, botulinum toxin injection, and nerve blocks can be offered if treatment is indicated.[114]
- *Condylomata acuminata* are characterized by cauliflower appearing warts in the perianal region. A patient may be asymptomatic or may present with pruritus, discharge,

TABLE 8.13 Diagnostic Studies for Proctitis

Diagnostic Test	Rationale
Colonoscopy/flexible sigmoidoscopy	Confirm infectious etiology or inflammatory bowel disease
Darkfield microscopy	Syphilis
Thayer-Martin agar plating	Gonorrhea

TABLE 8.14 Treatment for Proctitis

Condition	Treatment
Inflammatory proctitis	Steroid foams/hydrocortisone retention enemas; mesalamine orally, suppository, or enema
Radiation proctitis	Argon plasma coagulation/laser; topical steroids; mesalamine orally, suppository, or enema
Infectious proctitis	Same as methods for eradication of other sites from sexually transmitted infections

bleeding, or anal pain. HPV is the cause of condylomata acuminata. In the United States, it is the most common sexually transmitted virus and is the most common anorectal infection in homosexual men, especially in HIV-positive patients. This is diagnosed by anoscopy as warts often extend internally. Differential diagnosis includes condylomata lata from secondary syphilis and anal squamous cell carcinoma. Condylomata are usually painless and nonulcerated, while anal squamous cell cancer is usually painful and may be ulcerated. The extent of the disease and risk of malignancy determine treatment. Minimal disease can be treated in the office setting with topical agents such a 25% podophyllin in tincture of benzoin or bichloracetic acid.

8.6 GASTROINTESTINAL BLEEDING

OVERVIEW

The ligament of Treitz is the anatomic landmark that separates upper GI (UGI) and LGI bleeds. It is a ligament of the duodenum that suspends the duodenojejunal flexure from the retroperitoneum. Bleeding that occurs proximal to the ligament of Treitz is considered an UGI bleed. Acute LGI bleeding occurs most commonly in the colon but can occur anywhere distal to the duodenum. Bleeding that occurs distal to the duodenum and between the ileocecal valve can also be considered small bowel bleeding and is often obscure.

Hematochezia is defined as bright red blood passed per rectum and is the most common presentation of LGI bleeding. Approximately 15% of patients hospitalized with severe hematochezia have an UGI source of bleeding.[119] Acute overt LGI bleeding accounts for approximately 20% of all cases of GI bleeding and most stop spontaneously and have a good outcome. However, older patients with comorbidities have an increased risk of morbidity and mortality.[120]

UGI bleeding can present with hematemesis (vomiting of fresh blood), "coffee ground" emesis, and/or melena. Melena is defined black, tarry stools with a distinctive strong odor. This occurs due to hemoglobin being converted to hematin by bacterial degradation. Melena usually indicates an UGI source of bleeding and can originate from the oropharynx, nasopharynx, esophagus, stomach, small bowel, or the right side of the colon.[121]

Maroon stools are defined as maroon-colored blood mixed with melena and may be indicative of bleeding from the right colon, although UGI bleeding or small bowel bleeding with rapid transit can also produce maroon-colored stools.

UGI and LGI bleeding can both present with hemodynamic instability. General supportive measures include supplemental oxygen by nasal cannula. The patient should be kept NPO to prepare for an urgent endoscopy. Two large-caliber (18 gauge or larger) peripheral IV catheters should be inserted for IV access. Placement of a pulmonary artery catheter should be considered in patients with hemodynamic instability or if close monitoring during resuscitation is needed. If the blood pressure fails to respond to initial resuscitation, the rate of fluid administration should be increased and urgent intervention such as angiography considered. Patients with active bleeding should receive 500 mL of normal saline over 30 minutes while being typed and cross-matched for a blood transfusion. Packed red blood cells (RBCs) should be transfused to maintain the hemoglobin above 7 g/dL. Endoscopic hemostasis may be considered in patients with an international normalized ratio (INR) of 1.5–2.5 prior to or concomitant with the administration of reversal agents. Platelet transfusions should be considered to maintain a platelet count of 50×10^9/L in patients with severe bleeding requiring endoscopic homeostasis. In patients on anticoagulation, a multidisciplinary approach should be used when deciding whether to discontinue medications or use reversal agent to balance the risk of ongoing bleeding with the risk of thromboembolic events.[120,122]

8.6A UPPER GASTROINTESTINAL BLEEDING

MEDICAL HISTORY AND CLINICAL PRESENTATION

Hematemesis or melena suggests a bleed in the upper GI tract, or proximal to the ligament of Treitz. Risk factors for UGI bleeding include alcohol abuse, liver disease, coagulopathy, and history of previous GI bleeding. Medications such as NSAIDs, aspirin, anticoagulants, and/or antiplatelet agents also increase the risk of GI bleeding. The most common causes of UGI bleeding are peptic ulcer disease, esophageal varices, and erosive esophagitis.[123]

Aortoenteric fisula is a rare, but life-threatening cause of UGI bleeding and can manifest with an episode of hematemesis or hematochezia. This occurs most commonly in the duodenum and is known as a "herald bleed." It can stop for several days, but subsequent massive bleeding and death can occur from this. A patient with a history of abdominal aortic aneurysm or aortic graft needs to have an aortoenteric fistula ruled out.[123]

An UGI bleed commonly presents as a medical emergency. Age, comorbidities, and severity of bleed are factors to consider for the need of an urgent endoscopy. A patient judged to be high risk with a major bleed requires active resuscitation with fluid replacement of crystalloid and blood.[121] An upper endoscopy should be performed within 24 hours of presentation once the patient is hemodynamically stable. If the patient is hemodynamically unstable, urgent endoscopy should be performed after resuscitation.[124]

An increased ratio of blood urea nitrogen (BUN) to creatinine is seen in UGI bleeding due to absorption of blood by the small intestine. Clinical features identified to predict the risk of complications can categorize patients as either low or high risk.[125] Depending upon the risk score, patients can be stratified to be managed in an ICU setting to receive urgent endoscopy versus low-risk patients who can be managed as an outpatient.[125] Patients with a risk score >0 are considered high risk (Table 8.15).[126]

SIGNS AND SYMPTOMS

Upper abdominal pain may suggest a peptic ulcer. Dysphagia, unexplained weight loss, and early satiety are symptoms suspicious for malignancy. Odynophagia or dysphagia associated with hematemesis suggests an esophageal ulcer. Pill esophagitis from a retained pill in the esophagus can cause bleeding if it erodes at the site of a vessel. A patient with a variceal hemorrhage may present with ascites or jaundice, suggestive of end-stage liver disease. Symptoms suggesting

TABLE 8.15 Glasgow Blatchford Score*

Variable	Score
Blood urea (mmol/L)	
6.5–7.9	2
8.0–9.9	3
10.0–24.9	4
Hemoglobin (g/dL)	1
Male 12–12.9	3
10–11.9	6
<10	1
Female 10–11.9	6
<10	
Systolic blood pressure (mm Hg)	
100–109	1
90–99	2
<90	3
Pulse >100 bpm	1
Melena	1
Syncope	2
Hepatic disease	2
Cardiac failure	2

**Score >0 considered high risk.*

TABLE 8.16 Diagnostic Studies for Upper Gastrointestinal Bleeding

Diagnostic Test	Rationale
CT scan/CT angiogram	After repair of abdominal aortic aneurysm, loss of tissue plane between aorta and duodenum or gas demonstrating graft infection[124]
Esophagostrostomy (EGD)	Bleeding site for upper GI bleed
No additional testing	Mallory-Weiss tear from repeated vomiting/retching is clinical diagnosis alone
EGD with electrocautery, epinephrine injection, thermal coagulation	Dieulafoy lesion: dilated aberrant submucosal vessel, usually located along the proximal stomach, near the esophagogastric junction, that erodes the overlying epithelium
EGD with laser therapy, heater probe, or multipolar electrocoagulation	Gastric antral vascular ectasia or "watermelon stomach" appears endoscopically as longitudinal rows of erythematous mucosa that radiate from the pylorus into the antrum; chronic upper GI bleeding mostly

EGD, esophagogastroduodenoscopy; GI, gastrointestinal.

significant bleeding include dizziness, palpitations, confusion, and clammy skin.

PHYSICAL EXAMINATION

Signs of mild to moderate hypovolemia include resting tachycardia and normal to borderline low blood pressure. Orthostatic hypotension can be observed with a blood volume loss of at least 15% and supine hypotension can be seen with a blood volume loss of at least 40%. Petechiae or ecchymoses can be signs of coagulopathy. Hypoactive bowel sounds can indicate an ileus or obstruction. Hyperactive bowel sounds might suggest a UGI bleed due to stimulation of peristalsis by blood in the upper GI tract, while normoactive bowel sounds are suggestive of an LGI bleed.[121] Significant abdominal tenderness accompanied by peritoneal irritation such as involuntary guarding suggests perforation. A rectal examination is performed to assess stool for melena, hematochezia, or occult blood.

DIFFERENTIAL DIAGNOSIS

Causes of UGI bleeding are either variceal or nonvariceal. A patient with advanced liver disease and portal hypertension can present with life-threatening hematemesis due to variceal bleeding from esophageal and/or gastric varices. (See Section 8.8D Liver Disease, Cirrhosis, and Its Complications, Variceal Hemorrhage.) The differential diagnosis for non-variceal GI bleeding sources include peptic ulcer, Mallory-Weiss tear, malignancy, hemorrhagic gastritis, esophagitis, anastomotic ulcers, angiodysplasia, or Dieulafoy lesion.

DIAGNOSTIC STUDIES

The diagnostic studies for UGI bleeding are summarized in Table 8.16.

EVALUATION

The goal of endoscopic therapy is to eliminate persistent bleeding and prevent rebleeding. Pre-endoscopic therapy with a PPI can decrease the need for endoscopic therapy.[127] Patients with cirrhosis should receive vasoactive drugs and antibiotics. An upper endoscopy can localize and identify the source of UGI bleeding and therapy can be given to stop the bleeding or to prevent recurrence. An ulcer with active bleeding or nonbleeding visible vessels should receive endoscopic therapy. This can include injection therapy such as epinephrine, thermal probes, or clips. Epinephrine injection therapy should be followed by a second modality such as thermocoagulation.[124]

TREATMENT

- Recurrent bleeding should be treated with endoscopic therapy, but with subsequent bleeding transarterial embolization or surgery should be considered.
- A patient with high-risk stigmata such as active bleeding, visible vessels, and/or clots generally should be hospitalized for 3 days after endoscopic therapy if there is no rebleeding and no other reason to be hospitalized. They should be given clear liquids orally soon after endoscopy. A patient with clean based ulcers can be given a regular diet and discharged after endoscopy if they are hemodynamically stable.[127]
- After securing hemostasis, a high-dose IV PPI by continuous infusion for 72 hours is recommended in a patient with a high-risk endoscopic lesion followed by twice daily oral PPI on days 4 to 14 to reduce the risk of rebleeding.[128] When used for secondary prevention, aspirin should be continued or reintroduced soon after hemostasis is achieved. Early reintroduction of other antithrombotic drugs is also recommended after hemostasis is achieved to reduce thrombotic events and death.[124,129]

- Patients with peptic ulcer disease generally receive 4–8 weeks of once daily oral PPI therapy. The FDA recommends avoiding the use of omeprazole or esomeprazole in patients who are taking clopidogrel due to cytochrome metabolic incompatibility.[130] Patients with *H. pylori* associated bleeding ulcers should receive *H. pylori* therapy (see Table 8.3). Maintenance antisecretory therapy is not needed after it is documented that *H. pylori* has been eradicated unless the patient also requires NSAIDs or antithrombotics. In patients with idiopathic ulcers, long-term antiulcer therapy with a daily PPI is recommended.[127]

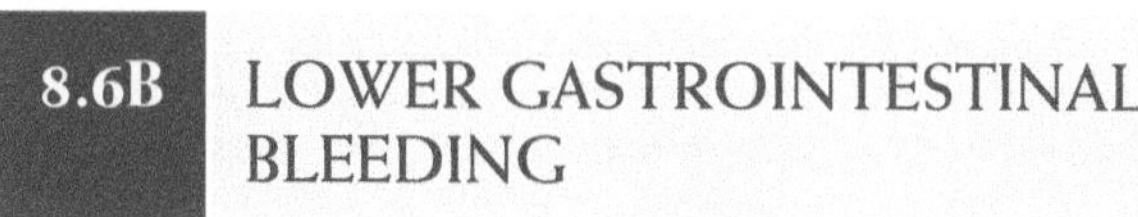

8.6B LOWER GASTROINTESTINAL BLEEDING

MEDICAL HISTORY AND CLINICAL PRESENTATION

The most common cause of LGI bleeding is *diverticulosis*. Most patients with diverticulosis are asymptomatic, but 3% to 20% will experience bleeding, with massive bleeding occurring in 3% to 5% of patients.[131]

Patients with severe hematochezia require urgent attention. High-risk features in LGI bleeding include hemodynamic instability, persistent bleeding, significant comorbid illness, advanced age, hospitalization for another reason, prior history of bleeding from diverticulosis or angiodysplasia, current aspirin use, prolonged prothrombin time, hypoalbuminemia, nontender abdomen, no diarrhea, anemia, elevated BUN level, or abnormal WBC count.[132]

For patients with LGI tract bleeding and hemodynamic instability, exclusion of an upper GI tract source of bleeding is first recommended.[120] Once the patient is hemodynamically stable, a colonoscopy should be performed after adequate colon cleansing for most patients presenting with an acute LGI bleed. If the patient is intolerant to oral intake and is at low risk of aspiration, an NG tube can be considered to facilitate the colon prep. Four to 6L of polyethylene glycol or the equivalent should be administered over 3 to 4 hours until the rectal effluent is clear of blood and stool. The terminal ileum should be intubated by the endoscopist to rule out a proximal bleed suggestive of a small bowel etiology.

SIGNS AND SYMPTOMS

See Section 8.6A Upper Gastrointestinal Bleeding.

PHYSICAL EXAMINATION

See Section 8.6A Upper Gastrointestinal Bleeding.

DIFFERENTIAL DIAGNOSIS

The most common colonic cause of severe hematochezia is diverticulosis. Other causes of LGI bleeding include internal hemorrhoids, ischemic colitis, rectal ulcers, IBD, delayed postpolypectomy bleeding, colonic polyps, colorectal cancer, colonic angiodysplasia, or radiation telangiectasia.

DIAGNOSTIC STUDIES

A colonoscopy can be both diagnostic and therapeutic for patients presenting with acute LGI bleeding; however, ischemic colitis is generally not amenable to endoscopic therapy (see Section 8.4C: Colonic Ischemia [Ischemic Colitis]).

In many ambulatory patients with hematochezia, the bleeding stops spontaneously, allowing for an elective diagnostic evaluation. (See Sections 8.5C Hemorrhoids, 8.5E Anal Fissure, and 8.5G Proctitis.)

EVALUATION

A surgical consult should be considered for patients with high-risk clinical features and ongoing bleeding. Generally, surgery for an acute LGI bleed should be considered after other therapeutic options have failed. The extent and success of prior bleeding control measures, severity and source of bleeding, and level of comorbid disease should be considered. Radiographic interventions can be considered in patients with high-risk clinical features and ongoing bleeding who have a negative upper endoscopy and who do not respond adequately to hemodynamic resuscitation efforts, if unlikely able to tolerate a bowel preparation for an urgent colonoscopy.[120]

TREATMENT

- Postpolypectomy bleeding can occur immediately or up to days or weeks following polyp removal. Risk factors include large polyp size (>2 cm), location on the right side of the colon, and resumption of antithrombotic therapy. This can be treated mechanically with a clip, band ligation, or contact thermal endotherapy, with or without use of a diluted epinephrine injection.[120]
- Diverticulosis most commonly involves the sigmoid and descending colon; however, approximately 50% of diverticular bleeding originates proximal to the splenic flexure. Bleeding is usually self-limiting and stops spontaneously with bowel rest. Diverticular hemorrhage is treated endoscopically with epinephrine injection, coagulation, and clipping of the site of active bleeding, visible vessel, or adherent clot.
- Medical therapy for hemorrhoids is covered under Section 8.5C Hemorrhoids. Occasionally, hemorrhoids may bleed profusely and require emergency hemostasis with banding.
- Rectal varices are vascular structures located proximally to internal hemorrhoids that can cause painless hematochezia. They can be treated with either sclerotherapy or portosystemic shunts.
- Solitary or multiple rectal ulcers can be a cause of LGI bleeding, especially in elderly or debilitated patients. Treatment for active bleeding is treated endoscopically with epinephrine injection and bipolar coagulation.
- Radiation proctitis usually is associated with mild, chronic rectal bleeding. This tends to develop 6 to 18 months after radiation treatment for prostate, gynecologic, or bladder tumors. Damage is caused by altered vascularity and mucosal ischemia. Endoscopically this is identified by rectal telangiectasia and friability and is treated with argon plasma coagulation.
- IBD can present with painless, bloody diarrhea. (See Section 8.4H Inflammatory Bowel Disease.) Endoscopic findings reveal friable, ulcerated, and edematous mucosa. Biopsies can help differentiate this from ischemic colitis. For refractory UC, surgical colectomy is curative.
- Infectious colitis is characterized by an acute onset of bloody diarrhea associated with abdominal pain and/or fever and a stool culture positive for an organism. *Campylobacter jejuni*, *Salmonella*, *Shigella*, invasive

Escherichia coli, E coli 0157:H7, and *C. difficile* are common infectious causes of LGI bleeding. Treatment is directed toward the causative organism. Severe pseudomembranous colitis that risks perforation may require a surgical colectomy.

- GI angiodysplastic lesions (GIADs) can be found in different parts of the GI tract but have a higher prevalence in the right side of the colon and cecum.[133] They can also occur in the small bowel and upper GI tract, specifically in patients with left ventricular assist devices (LVADs).[134] Endoscopic therapy for short-term and initial therapy for actively bleeding lesions with contact thermal therapy using argon plasma coagulation is recommended. This should be followed by medical therapy to induce remission in patients at high risk of recurrence.[133]

PATIENT EDUCATION

- In patients with established high-risk CVD and a history of LGI bleeding, aspirin used for secondary prevention should be continued. Aspirin for primary prevention of cardiovascular events should be avoided in most patients with LGI bleeding. Nonaspirin NSAID use should be avoided in patients with a history of acute LGI bleeding, especially if secondary to diverticulosis or angioectasia.[120]
- In patients on dual antiplatelet therapy or monotherapy, with nonaspirin antiplatelet agents such as thienopyridine, nonaspirin antiplatelet therapy should be resumed as soon as possible and at least within 7 days based on multidisciplinary assessment of cardiovascular and GI risks. Dual antiplatelet therapy should not be discontinued in patients with an acute coronary syndrome within the past 90 days or coronary stenting with the past 30 days.[120]

8.6C SMALL BOWEL AND OBSCURE GASTROINTESTINAL BLEEDING

MEDICAL HISTORY AND CLINICAL PRESENTATION

Obscure GI bleeding is bleeding of unknown origin that persists or recurs following an initial workup of nonrevealing colonoscopy and upper endoscopy. Obscure overt GI bleeding presents with evidence of bleeding such as hematemesis, melena, or hematochezia. Obscure occult GI bleeding refers to bleeding that is not visible in the stool and occurs when minute amounts of blood pass through the GI tract. Obscure occult bleeding is detected by guaiac testing and patients develop iron deficiency.

Patients with LVADs are at an increased risk of obscure occult GI bleeding, primarily from *gastrointestinal angiodysplastic lesions* (GIADs). GIADs are dilated communications between veins and capillaries. The increased risk of bleeding is thought to be from several factors. Patient with continuous low flow LVADs have a decrease in activity of von Willebrand factor, possibly leading to an acquired von Willebrand syndrome. There is also some degree of gut hypoperfusion from a low pulse pressure system with continuous low flow devices. Increased sympathetic tone may potentially result in smooth muscle relaxation and GIAD formation. Continuous flow devices also require the patient to be anticoagulated to prevent pump thrombosis. When combined with aspirin or other antiplatelet agents, the risk for GI bleeding is significantly increased.[134]

For the initial evaluation of a suspected upper GI source of bleeding, an EGD is indicated. A repeat examination is performed that may yield a cause, even if the initial EGD is negative. However, for a second look for a suspected upper GI source of bleeding, a push enteroscopy is appropriate to consider. Similar to an upper endoscopy, a push enteroscopy is performed orally under sedation with a longer endoscope and is passed into the jejunum. The distal duodenum and proximal jejunum can be examined. A repeat colonoscopy should also be considered if there is suspicion for a LGI tract source of bleeding with special attention to intubate the terminal ileum to evaluate the mucosa and to inspect for blood that may be potentially coming from the small intestine. If the second look examinations of the upper and lower GI tract are negative, then further small bowel evaluation is needed. This usually includes a combination of imaging and endoscopy studies.[135]

SIGNS AND SYMPTOMS

See Section 8.6A Upper Gastrointestinal Bleeding.

PHYSICAL EXAMINATION

See Section 8.6A Upper Gastrointestinal Bleeding.

DIFFERENTIAL DIAGNOSIS

Differential diagnosis for small bowel bleeding includes small bowel tumors, Crohn disease, angioectasia, NSAID enteropathy, Meckel diverticula, and small bowel varices.

DIAGNOSTIC STUDIES

The diagnostic studies for small bowel and obscure GI bleeding are summarized in Table 8.17.[136]

EVALUATION

Patients with a positive RBC scan should be referred immediately to angiography for treatment.

There is no capability for therapeutic intervention with video capsule endoscopy, but if significant lesions are found, the patient can be referred for specific management and treatment.[135]

CT enterography allows detection of inflammatory lesions, neoplasms, and vascular lesions.

TREATMENT

Deep enteroscopy has the advantage of diagnostic and therapeutic capabilities including biopsy, dilation, polypectomy, hemostasis, and foreign body removal.

KEY POINTS

- Diverticular bleeding is the most common form of hematochezia in patients over the age of 60.
- A high index of suspicion is needed with a "herald" bleed in a patient with an aortoenteric fistula from a prosthestic aortic graft and is a surgical emergency with a 100% mortality rate if not recognized.
- Risk factors for GIADs include advanced age, chronic renal insufficiency, cirrhosis, valvular heart disease, von Willebrand disease, and connective tissue disease. Bleeding from these is usually mild and intermittent and is a cause of chronic iron deficiency anemia.

TABLE 8.17 Diagnostic Studies for Small Bowel and Obscure Gastrointestinal Bleeding

Diagnostic Test	Rationale
CT angiography	Ability to perform selective mesenteric embolization, detects site of active bleeding[136]
Radioisotope bleeding scans	Detects overt small bowel bleeding in the general area of bleeding
Capsule endoscopy/deep enteroscopy	Detects slower rates of bleeding. Evaluates the entire small bowel for occult bleeding, once the upper GI tract and colon have been excluded.[136] CT enterography should be considered before video capsule endoscopy in patients with a history of IBD, prior radiation, history of small bowel surgery, and/or suspected small bowel stenosis to prevent capsule retention. The limitations of double-balloon enteroscopy include invasiveness, prolonged procedure time, and manpower required. There is also a higher risk of pancreatitis in the peroral approach.
Tagged red blood cell scintigraphy	Localizes site of bleeding to guide angiography treatment in setting of ongoing bleeding[137]
Multiphasic CT enterography or MR enterography	Preferred imaging studies of choice for investigating obscure small bowel bleeding.[136] CT enterography best for suspected small bowel bleeding, but MR can be considered in patients with contraindications for CT or to avoid radiation exposure.[137]

IBD, inflammatory bowel disease; GI, gastrointestinal; MR, magnetic resonance

SPECIAL CONSIDERATIONS

- The most common cause of GI bleeding in children is from a *Meckel diverticulum*. It is characterized by painless melena or bright red blood per rectum, often referred to as "currant jelly." It is a congenital anomaly in the GI tract causing an ileal diverticulum. This can be diagnosed with technetium scanning and is treated by surgical resection of the diverticulum.

8.7 PERITONEAL DISORDERS

OVERVIEW

The peritoneum is a membrane covered by a layer of mesothelial cells. It is composed of the parietal and visceral peritoneum. The parietal peritoneum covers the abdominal wall, the inferior surface of the diaphragm and the pelvis. The visceral peritoneum covers most of the intraperitoneal organs including the stomach, jejunum, ileum, transverse colon, liver, and spleen. It also covers the anterior aspect of the duodenum, left and right colon, pancreas, kidneys, and adrenal glands.[137]

The accumulation of fluid within the peritoneal cavity results in *ascites*. A patient with ascites will often have complaints of fullness, shortness of breath, unexplained weight gain, and abdominal distention. Causes of ascites include portal hypertension, heart failure, tuberculosis, dialysis, and malignancy. Cirrhosis is the most common cause of ascites due to portal hypertension (see Section 8.8D Liver Disease, Cirrhosis, and Its Complications).

Ascitic fluid analysis bold ascitic fluid analysis with a diagnostic paracentesis is necessary to determine the serum ascites albumin gradient (see Section 8.8D Liver Disease, Evaluation).

8.7A PERITONITIS

OVERVIEW

Inflammation of the visceral and parietal peritoneum is usually caused by infection, which can result in perforation of a hollow viscus and is considered secondary peritonitis. Secondary peritonitis is also called "surgical peritonitis" because surgical intervention is usually required to treat this.

In primary or spontaneous bacterial peritonitis (SBP), a specific intra-abdominal source cannot be identified. Most patients with SBP have portal hypertension (see Section 8.8D Liver Disease, Cirrhosis and Its Complications). Primary peritonitis can also occur with ascites associated with nephrotic syndrome. Primary peritonitis is treated with IV antibiotics directed against the triggering organism, which is classically the gram-negative rods with *E. Coli* being most common.[138]

MEDICAL HISTORY AND CLINICAL PRESENTATION

Peritonitis is characterized by abdominal pain. Inflammation of the peritoneum can be associated with an ileus, resulting in nausea and vomiting.

Patients on immunosuppressive drugs may have minimal signs of peritoneal pain. Patients with cirrhosis and ascites may also not complain of pain unless the peritoneum is involved.

Continuous ambulatory peritoneal dialysis is a risk factor for peritonitis. A patient on this type of dialysis can present with pain and/or a cloudy effluent.

Extrapulmonary infection from *M. tuberculosis* can result in tuberculous peritonitis. Risk factors for this infection include HIV infection, cirrhosis, diabetes, and underlying malignancy.

SIGNS AND SYMPTOMS

Signs and symptoms include abdominal pain, nausea, vomiting, and fever.

PHYSICAL EXAMINATION

Assess vitals signs and appearance of the patient. Peritonitis usually manifests with abdominal tenderness, guarding, rigidity, and rebound tenderness.

A patient with surgical peritonitis may be immobile due to pain with movement. Free air in the peritoneal cavity will cause exquisite tenderness with light percussion. Assess for peritoneal signs including rebound tenderness, involuntary guarding, and severe tenderness with palpation. Iliopsoas and obturator signs can suggest retroperitoneal or pelvic inflammation and abscess.

DIFFERENTIAL DIAGNOSIS

The more common causes of secondary peritonitis include perforated peptic ulcer disease, appendicitis, diverticulitis, cholecystitis, pancreatitis, and complications from surgery.

Peritonitis can also occur from rupture of an ectopic pregnancy, ovarian cyst, or a ruptured aneurysm.[137]

DIAGNOSTIC STUDIES

- Lab studies include CBC with differential, electrolytes, renal panel, and hepatic function panel.
- Chest x-ray or upright or decubitus x-ray may show free air.
- Ultrasound can evaluate abscess, bile duct dilation, or large fluid collections.
- CT scan of the abdomen and pelvis with oral and IV contrast is the most sensitive imaging study for evaluating acute abdominal pain.

EVALUATION

Laboratory and imaging studies in addition to laparotomy or laparoscopy confirm the diagnosis of surgical peritonitis.

TREATMENT

- Most cases of surgical peritonitis require fluid resuscitation, antibiotic therapy, and urgent laparotomy or laparoscopy.
- Not all patients with peritonitis require surgery. A localized peritonitis in the LLQ from acute sigmoid diverticulitis can be treated with IV antibiotics and bowel rest. An abscess can be treated with antibiotics and percutaneous drainage.

KEY POINTS

- Peritonitis is considered a medical and possible surgical emergency and requires prompt attention

8.8 DISEASES OF THE LIVER AND BILIARY TRACT

8.8A APPROACH TO ABNORMAL LIVER ENZYMES

OVERVIEW

Liver enzymes, including alanine aminotransferase (ALT), aspartate aminotransferase (AST), alkaline phosphatase (ALP), and bilirubin, are important laboratory values that clinicians encounter on a daily basis. Their abnormality patterns play a key role in forming a differential diagnosis and spurn further evaluation. Understanding the metabolism of these enzymes is important in guiding further management. Of note, the term "liver function enzymes" will not be used to describe the above terms as labs representing true liver synthetic function are albumin and prothrombin time. AST, ALT, ALP, and bilirubin reflect liver injury, rather than function. The proposed evaluation of abnormal liver enzymes is highly influenced by the 2017 American College of Gastroenterology clinical guideline on the evaluation of abnormal liver chemistries.[139]

Hepatitis, or the inflammation of the liver, is characterized by hepatocyte injury due to multiple possible mechanisms or diseases. Acute hepatitis is a disease process that develops and occurs within a 6-month period, while chronic hepatitis involves the persistence of hepatic inflammation past the 6-month window. Cirrhosis is a result of continued hepatocyte injury and eventual tissue fibrosis and scarring, leading to organ architectural distortion and altered physiology.

PATHOPHYSIOLOGY

Serum aminotransferases (transaminases), ALT and AST, are markers of hepatocellular injury. ALT is present primarily in the liver in its cytoplasm, making it a more specific marker of hepatocellular injury.[139,140,141] Elevations in these values can occur in a number of conditions, and evaluating the degree of elevation (number of times above the ULN), the ALT:AST ratio, and the time course of the elevation are important factors to consider when determining the diagnosis. Table 8.18 and Box 8.1 highlight the causes of elevated AST and ALT. Certain conditions may produce a greater rise in one transaminase over the

TABLE 8.18 Hepatic Causes of Elevated Aspartate Aminotransferase and Alanine Transaminase

Generally AST > ALT	Generally ALT > AST
Alcohol-associated liver disease	NAFLD
Cirrhosis	Acute and chronic viral hepatitis
Ischemic hepatitis	Drug-induced liver injury
Congestive hepatopathy	Toxic hepatitis (Amanita exposure)
Acute Budd-Chiari syndrome	Hemochromatosis
Hepatic artery damage/ thrombosis/occlusion	Autoimmune hepatitis
	Wilson disease
TPN	Alpha-1 antitrypsin deficiency
	Celiac disease
	Acute bile duct obstruction
	Liver trauma
	Post-liver surgery
	Veno-occlusive disease/sinusoidal obstructive syndrome
	Diffuse malignancy infiltration
	HELLP syndrome
	Acute fatty liver of pregnancy
	Sepsis
	Hyperemesis gravidarum
	Hemophagocytic lymphohistiocytosis

ALT, alanine aminotransferase; AST, aspartate aminotransferase; HELLP, hemolysis, elevated liver tests, low platelets; NAFLD, nonalcoholic fatty liver disease; TPN, total parenteral nutrition.

Source: Data from Kwo PY, Cohen SM, Lim JK. ACG clinical guideline: evaluation of abnormal liver chemistries. Am J Gastroenterol. 2017;112(1):18–35. doi:10.1038/ajg.2016.517

BOX 8.1 Nonhepatic Causes of Elevated Aspartate Aminotransferase and Alanine Transaminase

- Skeletal muscle damage/rhabdomyolysis
- Cardiac muscle damage
- Thyroid disease
- Heat stroke
- Hemolysis
- Adrenal insufficiency

Source: Data from Kwo PY, Cohen SM, Lim JK. ACG clinical guideline: evaluation of abnormal liver chemistries. Am J Gastroenterol. 2017;112(1):18–35. doi:10.1038/ajg.2016.517

other due to multiple factors such as pyridoxine deficiency (alcohol-associated liver disease [ALD]) and mitochondrial injury.

ALP is a zinc metalloproteinase.[142] Its half-life in serum is approximately 7 days. It is found on the canalicular membrane of hepatocytes and is also present in bone (marker of bone growth or turnover), placenta, small intestine, and kidney. Additionally, patients with blood type O or B may have transiently elevated ALP after a fatty meal.[143] An elevated ALP can occur in the setting of biliary obstruction due to increased canalicular synthesis of the enzyme.[144] Unlike bilirubin, ALP may be elevated in instances of minor biliary obstruction. Table 8.19 lists the typical causes of abnormal ALP.

Serum gamma-glutamyl transferase (GGT) is an enzyme synthesized by hepatic canalicular cells as well as in the kidney, pancreas, spleen, heart, brain, and seminal vesicles. It can be used to determine if the ALP rise is of hepatic or bone origin. GGT can also be elevated in patients who drink alcohol, although it possesses a low sensitivity, making its use in clinical practice questionable.[145] ALP can also be fractionated into bone, intestinal, and hepatic origins to better determine the exact cause of ALP rise.

Bilirubin results from the breakdown of old RBCs. It primarily circulates in the serum unconjugated and bound to albumin. Conjugation via uridine 5'-diphospho (UDP)-glucuronosyltransferase allows bilirubin to become water-soluble, thereby enabling it to be excreted into bile. Bacteria in the colon then convert it to urobilinogen, allowing it to be excreted in urine and stool. By understanding the life cycle of bilirubin, one may then appreciate the potential etiologies of why this value could be elevated (Figure 8.3). Box 8.2 demonstrates causes of elevated unconjugated bilirubin, while Box 8.3 lists causes of elevated conjugated bilirubin.

The total bilirubin (TB) is a marker of both conjugated (direct) and unconjugated (indirect) bilirubin. It is usually <1.1 mg/dL. Fractionating bilirubin into direct and indirect components can be helpful in determining the cause of the total elevation as an elevated direct bilirubin may be a marker of cholestasis or hepatocellular injury, rather than hemolysis. Bilirubin has a longer half-life compared to ALT, AST, and ALP at almost 3 weeks, thereby explaining why jaundice can take longer to resolve after a patient is recovering from hepatitis or obstruction.

TABLE 8.19 Causes of Abnormal Alkaline Phosphate

Hepatobiliary	Nonhepatic
Bile duct obstruction, stricture, or cholestasis	Bone disease (osteomalacia, Paget disease)
Ductopenia	Primary bony malignancy
AIDS cholangiopathy	Bony metastasis
Cholestatic liver disease (PBC, PSC)	Hyperthyroidism
Drug-induced liver injury	Hyperparathyroidism
Infiltrative diseases of the liver*	Pregnancy (third trimester)
Hepatic abscess	Chronic renal failure
Hepatocellular carcinoma	Lymphoma
Viral hepatitis	Extrahepatic malignancy
Cirrhosis	Congestive heart failure
Vanishing bile duct syndrome	Childhood growth
Ischemic cholangiopathy	Infection
Alcohol-associated liver disease	Inflammation
Intrahepatic cholestasis of pregnancy	Influx of ALP after a fatty meal
Benign postoperative jaundice	Blood types O and B
ICU jaundice	Myeloid metaplasia
TPN	Peritonitis
Liver allograft rejection	Diabetes mellitus
Acute alcoholic hepatitis	Gastric ulcer
Sickle cell liver crisis	Increasing age, especially women
Sepsis	
Congestive heart failure	
Hemophagocytic lymphohistiocytosis	

Infiltrative diseases of the liver include sarcoid, granulomatous hepatitis, tuberculosis, amyloid, metastatic cancer, and lymphoma.

ALP, alkaline phosphatase; PBC, primary biliary cholangitis; PSC, primary sclerosing cholangitis; TPN, total parenteral nutrition.

Source: Data from Kwo PY, Cohen SM, Lim JK. ACG clinical guideline: evaluation of abnormal liver chemistries. Am J Gastroenterol. *2017;112(1):18–35. doi:10.1038/ajg.2016.517*

EVALUATION

History should not only include assessment for risk factors of liver disease such as evaluating for other medical conditions, travel, food, and alcohol exposures, but also devote a large portion of time to discussing medication exposures, not forgetting to emphasize over-the counter, herbal, supplemental, and vitamin use.

Physical exam may assess for stigmata of chronic liver disease such as telangiectasias, spider angiomas, jaundice and scleral icterus, asterixis, ascites, and splenomegaly.

When evaluating abnormal liver enzymes, it is important to determine the type of injury, after the abnormalities have been confirmed with an additional serum test. This can be determined by comparing the elevations in transaminases

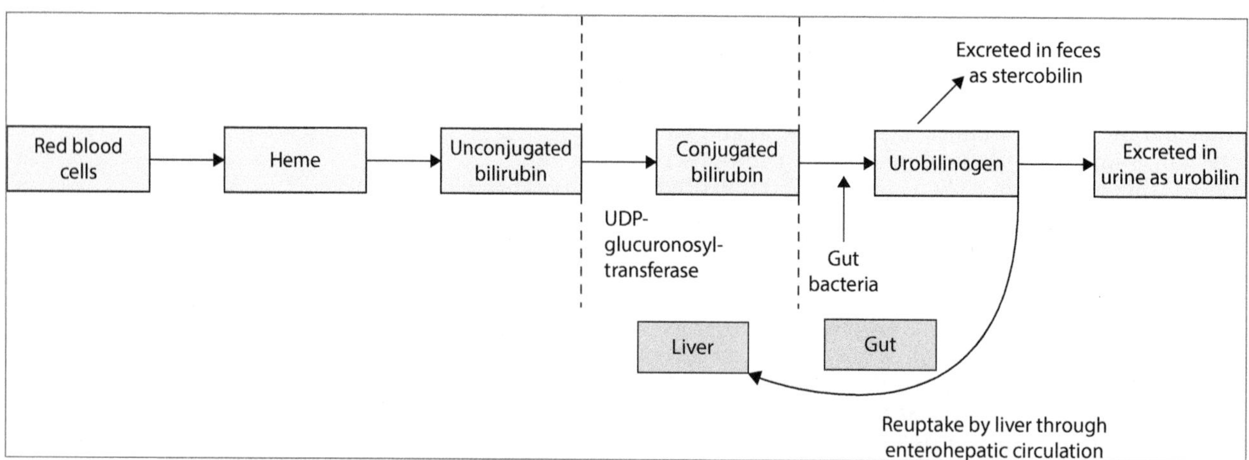

Figure 8.3 Bilirubin metabolism. UDP, uridine 5'-diphospho.

BOX 8.2 Causes of Elevated Unconjugated Bilirubin

Gilbert syndrome
Crigler-Najjar syndrome
Hemolysis
Ineffective erythropoiesis
Resorption of large hematomas
Neonatal jaundice
Hyperthyroidism
Medications
Post-blood transfusion

Source: Data from Kwo PY, Cohen SM, Lim JK. ACG clinical guideline: evaluation of abnormal liver chemistries. Am J Gastroenterol. *2017;112(1): 18–35. doi:10.1038/ajg.2016.517*

BOX 8.3 Causes of Elevated Conjugated Bilirubin

Bile duct obstruction, stricture, or cholestasis
AIDS cholangiopathy
Cholestatic liver disease (PBC, PSC)
Drug-induced liver injury
Infiltrative diseases of the liver*
Hepatocellular carcinoma
Viral hepatitis
Cirrhosis
Ischemic hepatitis
Wilson disease
Autoimmune hepatitis
Vanishing bile duct syndrome
Intrahepatic cholestasis of pregnancy
Benign postoperative jaundice
ICU jaundice
TPN
Acute alcoholic hepatitis
Sickle cell liver crisis
Sepsis
Congestive heart failure
Hemophagocytic lymphohistiocytosis
Ductopenia
Dubin-Johnson syndrome
Rotor syndrome

**Infiltrative diseases of the liver include sarcoid, granulomatous hepatitis, tuberculosis, amyloid, metastatic cancer, and lymphoma.*

PBC, primary biliary cholangitis; PSC, primary sclerosing cholangitis; TPN, total parenteral nutrition.

Source: Data from Kwo PY, Cohen SM, Lim JK. ACG clinical guideline: evaluation of abnormal liver chemistries. Am J Gastroenterol. *2017; 112(1):18–35. doi:10.1038/ajg.2016.517*

(ALT and AST) and ALP compared to their ULN. A situation in which the rise in ALT and AST are greater than the ALP is defined as a hepatocellular injury, while a greater rise in the ALP compared to ALT and AST is a marker of a cholestatic injury. A mixed pattern of injury occurs when both the ALP and AST/ALT elevations are similar.

Hepatocellular injury can be further broken down based on the degree of AST/ALT elevation (Table 8.20). This may aid in narrowing a differential diagnosis.

It is also important to assess for signs of acute liver failure (ALF; changes in INR and altered mental status [encephalopathy], see Section 8.8C Acute Liver Failure for further discussion), and consider referral to a liver transplant center if this occurs.

Cholestatic hepatitis should prompt a different differential diagnosis. Isolated ALP elevations without rise in bilirubin should lead to further evaluation with serum GGT. If the GGT is abnormal, a RUQ ultrasound should be obtained to evaluate for liver parenchymal abnormalities. Additionally, medications should be evaluated, and an antinuclear antibody, antimitochondrial antibody (AMA), and anti-smooth muscle antibody (anti-SMA) should be checked to evaluate for primary biliary cholangitis (PBC) and PSC. A liver biopsy may need to be performed.

Ductal dilation on initial ultrasound or the addition of elevated bilirubin with an elevated ALP warrants further evaluation with magnetic resonance cholangiopancreatography (MRCP) or endoscopic retrograde cholangiopancreatography (ERCP) to evaluate for gallstone disease or PSC. If workup is unremarkable, a liver biopsy may need to be pursued.

Isolated elevations in bilirubin should prompt evaluation for an unconjugated or conjugated cause by assessing the direct and indirect bilirubin. Direct bilirubin is elevated in conjugated hyperbilirubinemia and may be a result of sepsis, TPN, cirrhosis, or biliary obstruction. A RUQ ultrasound should be performed to assess liver parenchyma (nodular or smooth contour) and to look for evidence of gallstone disease (biliary ductal dilation, a visualized gallstone). Further evaluation may be done with MRCP or ERCP if suspicion for choledocholithiasis is high. Unconjugated hyperbilirubinemia should lead to an evaluation for Gilbert disease and hemolysis.

8.8B GALLSTONES AND GALLSTONE DISEASE

OVERVIEW AND EPIDEMIOLOGY

Gallstones, or cholelithiasis, is a widely prevalent disease in Western countries, being found in about 6% of men and 9% of women in the United States.[146] The majority of gallstones are asymptomatic but gallstone disease, or when gallstones cause symptoms, is the most common GI cause of hospitalization and is a significant source of both inpatient and outpatient resource utilization.[147,148]

Gallstone prevalence varies by geographic region but appears most prevalent in Western Caucasian, Hispanic, and Native American populations. There is a higher prevalence in women compared to men. The prevalence of gallstones and gallstone disease appears to be rising due to the obesity epidemic. Risk factors for gallstones and gallstone disease due to cholesterol stones are listed in Box 8.4.

PATHOPHYSIOLOGY

Gallstones are composed of a mixture of cholesterol, calcium salts, proteins, and mucin. They are classified as cholesterol, black pigment, or brown pigment stones based on the

TABLE 8.20 Laboratory Assessment of Different Degrees of Aspartate Aminotransferase and Alanine Aminotransferase Elevation

Elevation Amount	Differential Diagnosis	Initial Laboratory Assessment	Follow-up
Borderline (<2 × ULN) or Mild (2–5 × ULN)	NAFLD, chronic viral hepatitis, hemochromatosis May consider PSC, PBC, Wilson disease, AAT deficiency, celiac sprue, thyroid or muscle disease, or tick-borne illness if initial assessment unrevealing	CBC, AST/ALT, ALP, TB, albumin, INR, HBsAg, HBsAb, HBcAb, HCV Ab, iron panel, abdominal US	Consider repeat liver enzymes in 3–6 months if no abnormalities If persistently elevated, continue evaluation and broaden differential and lab assessment
Moderate (5–15 × ULN)	NAFLD, acute and chronic viral hepatitis, hemochromatosis, PBC, PSC, Wilson disease, AAT, AIH	Same as above plus: HAV IgG and IgM, ceruloplasmin, ANA, SMA, immunoglobulins	Consider liver consultation if work-up unrevealing or patient shows signs of acute liver failure
Severe (>15 × ULN)	Acute viral hepatitis, shock liver, vascular disorders of the liver, DILI, AIH, acute biliary obstruction, diffuse infiltration of the liver, liver trauma/surgery, veno-occlusive disease/sinusoidal obstruction syndrome, HELLP syndrome, and Wilson disease	CBC, AST/ALT, ALP, TB, albumin, INR, HBsAg, HBsAb, HBcAb, HCV Ab, HAV IgG and IgM, ceruloplasmin, ANA, SMA, immunoglobulins, HSV, EBV, CMV, Anti-LKM, IgG4, serum drug panel, urine toxicology Abdominal US with Doppler	Consider N-acetylcysteine if there is concern for acetaminophen overdose Consider intravenous acyclovir if HSV is a concern Urgent hepatology consultation or transfer to a transplant center if patient shows signs of acute liver failure
Massive (ALT >10,000 U/L)	Shock liver/ischemic hepatopathy, DILI, rhabdomyolysis; may also have underlying additional liver disease	Same workup as in severe elevations	Same as in severe elevations

AAT, alpha-1 antitrypsin; Ab, antibody; AIH, autoimmune hepatitis; ALP, alkaline phosphatase; ALT, alanine aminotransferase; ANA, antinuclear antibody; anti-LKM, anti-liver kidney microsomal antibody; AST, aspartate aminotransferase; CBC, complete blood count; CMV, cytomegalovirus; DILI, drug-induced liver injury; EBV, Epstein-Barr virus; HAV, hepatitis A virus; HBcAb, hepatitis B core antibody; HBsAb, hepatitis B surface antibody; HBsAg, hepatitis B surface antigen; HCV, hepatitis C virus, HELLP, hemolysis, elevated liver tests, low platelets; HSV, herpes simplex virus; IgG, immunoglobulin G; IgG4, immunoglobulin G4; IgM, immunoglobulin M; INR, international normalized ratio; NAFLD, nonalcoholic fatty liver disease; PBC, primary biliary cirrhosis; PSC, primary sclerosing cholangitis; SMA, smooth muscle antibody; TB, total bilirubin; ULN, upper limit of normal; US, ultrasound.

BOX 8.4 Risk Factors for Cholesterol Gallstones and Gallstone Disease

Female sex
Age <50
Family history of gallstones
Pregnancy and states of increased estrogen
Diabetes mellitus
Dyslipidemia
Obesity
Rapid weight loss
Medications*
Conditions that promote gallbladder stasis†
Diseases of the ileum such as Crohn disease

**Fibrates, ceftriaxone, somatostatin analogues, oral contraceptive pills.*
†Prolonged fasting and parenteral nutrition, spinal cord injury.

predominant constituent. The majority of gallstones in the Western world are cholesterol stones.[149] Cholesterol stones are formed as a result of hepatic secretion of bile supersaturated with cholesterol, stasis of bile within the gallbladder, and nucleation of cholesterol molecules to form crystals.

Black pigment stones form as a result of calcium salts crystallizing in the gallbladder, typically in settings of older age, chronic hemolytic stages like sickle cell disease, TPN, and Crohn disease. Brown pigment stones can form anywhere in the biliary tract and result from bile stasis and infection due to bacterial enzymes deconjugating bilirubin.

The most common forms of symptomatic gallstone disease can be organized into four categories: biliary pain or colic, acute cholecystitis, choledocholithiasis, and cholangitis. Other conditions such as chronic cholecystitis, Mirizzi syndrome (external compression of the common hepatic duct by a stone in the cystic duct), gallbladder carcinoma, cholecystoenteric fistula, and Bouveret syndrome (gastric outlet obstruction due to a gallstone) are rare complications of gallstone disease. Figure 8.4 shows the possible complications and locations of the most common complications of gallstone disease.

Biliary colic pain is a result of intermittent obstruction of the cystic duct with either a gallstone or biliary sludge. It does not cause inflammation of the gallbladder, but the brief obstruction of the gallbladder neck can lead to pain due to gallbladder contraction.

Acute cholecystitis results from an impacted stone in the cystic duct, resulting in bile stasis causing inflammation of the gallbladder mucosa. Because of the acute inflammation, patients may develop fever. There is risk of secondary gallbladder infection due to ongoing inflammation and inability of bile to escape. If a gallstone is large enough, it may cause external compression of the bile duct, known as Mirizzi syndrome.

Choledocholithiasis, or a stone obstructing the biliary duct, occurs when a gallstone or sludge passes from the gallbladder but becomes lodged somewhere along the biliary tree. Stones may be able to pass through the ampulla of Vater, leading to resolution of the obstruction, but they may also become impacted. Gallstone pancreatitis may result if a stone is lodged at the ampulla due to the inability of pancreatic enzymes to be excreted. Patients who have had a previous cholecystectomy are still at risk of developing

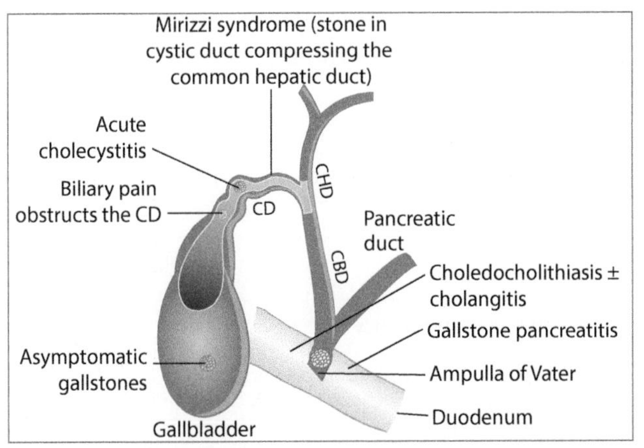

Figure 8.4 Location of some of the consequences of gallstone disease. CBD, common bile duct; CD, cystic duct; CHD, common hepatic duct.

choledocholithiasis, although at a lower rate than those with an intact gallbladder.

Cholangitis results from bile stasis due to choledocholithiasis. Because of stasis, the bile becomes superinfected and can result in bacteremia and an ascending infection along the entirety of the biliary tree. Patients may have ensuing septic shock and coagulopathy as a result of the infection.

MEDICAL HISTORY, CLINICAL PRESENTATION, AND PHYSICAL EXAM

Presentation is dependent upon the type and location of gallstone disease. Many individuals who possess gallstones are asymptomatic, but gallstones or sludge that intermittently or fully obstructs the cystic duct (biliary colic or cholecystitis), obstructs the biliary tree (choledocholithiasis), or obstructs and causes infection within the biliary system (cholangitis) may cause symptoms such as RUQ abdominal pain, nausea, vomiting, diaphoresis, or fever.

Patients with biliary colic or acute cholecystitis typically will have dull, colicky, RUQ or epigastric pain that starts after ingestion of a fatty meal. There may be radiation of the pain into the right shoulder. Pain is steady rather than intermittent when it occurs. Pain is responsive to ketorolac, a parenteral nonsteroidal anti-inflammatory medication. There should be no association of the pain with movement or bowel habits.

Patients with acute cholecystitis, choledocholithiasis, or cholangitis will typically have exquisite RUQ tenderness to palpation due to stimulation of the gallbladder (Murphy sign).[150]

Acute cholangitis is characterized by fever, jaundice, and abdominal pain (Charcot triad). Addition of hypotension and encephalopathy is concerning for more complicated disease (Reynold pentad). Patients may become bacteremic as a result of gram-negative bacterial translocation from the biliary tree into the circulation.

DIFFERENTIAL DIAGNOSIS

Differential diagnosis of episodic RUQ pain in addition to gallstone disease includes peptic ulcer disease, diverticulitis, reflux esophagitis, pancreatitis, renal colic, colon cancer, IBS, radiculopathy, costochondritis, and angina pectoris.

Laboratory abnormalities of acute cholecystitis, choledocholithiasis, and cholangitis include leukocytosis, abnormal liver enzymes, and, occasionally, abnormal pancreatic enzymes. The pattern of liver enzyme elevations may be helpful in differentiating the location of the patient's obstruction. Typically, acute cholecystitis will not have bilirubin abnormalities, but choledocholithiasis will elevate bilirubin due to the prevention of bile flowing freely into the small intestine. There are typically no laboratory abnormalities with biliary colic.

DIAGNOSTIC STUDIES

The diagnostic studies for gallstones and gallstone disease are summarized in Table 8.21.[151,152]

TREATMENT

- Patients with asymptomatic gallstones typically do not require treatment due to low risk of developing symptoms over time (only 15–25% of patients will become symptomatic after 10–15 years).[153]
  - Only those with risk factors for gallbladder cancer (gallbladder adenomas, porcelain gallbladder, gallstones >3 cm) should discuss the risk versus benefits of elective cholecystectomy with a specialist.

TABLE 8.21 Diagnostic Studies for Gallstones and Gallstone Disease

Diagnostic Test	Rationale
Ultrasound	First test in assessment of gallbladder and biliary abnormalities, >95% sensitivity in detecting gallstones.[152] Sludge and ductal dilation detected. Dilated cystic duct consistent with downstream obstruction. Patients with previous cholecystectomy may also have a slightly dilated bile duct due to previous surgery.[153]
Hepatobiliary scintigraphy (HIDA scan)	Follow-up test for acute cholecystitis in symptomatic patient with normal ultrasound. Lack of radioactive tracer into the gallbladder diagnoses acute cholecystitis.
MRCP (magnetic resonance cholangiopancreatography)	Choledocholithiasis is suspected, but not fully appreciated, on ultrasound.
Endoscopic ultrasound (EUS)	Used when there is an intermediate risk of choledocholithiasis when ultrasound is unrevealing. The procedure requires the patient to be placed under anesthesia and undergo internal ultrasound to evaluate the bile ducts for evidence of stone, sludge, or biliary ductal dilation. If that is found, endoscopic retrograde cholangiopancreatography (ERCP) can be performed immediately after while the patient is still under anesthesia. ERCP does have the potential to cause acute pancreatitis, something that MRCP does not cause.
CT of abdomen	Less useful in evaluating gallbladder disease; helpful in assessing for complications of gallstone disease such as abscess, perforation, or pancreatitis.
Cholecystokinin challenge (CCK)	Assesses functional activity of gallblader by calculating ejection fraction (EF) after stimulation with CCK. Poor EF <35% consistent with gallbladder inertia and qualifies patient for cholecystectomy.

HIDA, hepatobiliary iminodiacetic acid.

- Patients with biliary colic have a risk of developing acute cholecystitis or other complications at a rate of 2% to 3% per year.[154] Because of this elevated risk, it is recommended that patients with biliary pain undergo elective laparoscopic cholecystectomy.
- Cholecystectomy is the gold standard of treatment for acute calculous cholecystitis. Additional care for acute cholecystitis includes supportive care with IV fluids and pain management.
- Patients with choledocholithiasis benefit from ERCP, an endoscopic procedure that involves inserting a wire into the common bile duct, injecting contrast agent to evaluate for biliary defects, cutting the biliary sphincter (biliary sphincterotomy), and using tools within the endoscope to remove stones and sludge from the bile due to relieve the obstruction. Patients should ideally then undergo laparoscopic cholecystectomy during the same hospital admission in order to avoid future complications of gallstone disease.[155]
- Acute cholangitis requires emergent ERCP for stone removal and biliary decompression to prevent complications of sepsis. Patients with signs of cholangitis should also be given IV antibiotics to cover gram-negative and anaerobic organisms and have close inpatient monitoring if septic shock develops. Like patients with choledocholithiasis, patients with acute cholangitis should undergo cholecystectomy after the initial obstruction is relieved. Untreated cholangitis has a high mortality rate from septic shock.
- Gallstone dissolution therapy with ursodeoxycholic acid (UDCA) may be considered in special circumstances of patients with symptomatic gallstones who are not able to undergo surgery. If this treatment is discontinued, the stones will return.

8.8C ACUTE LIVER FAILURE

OVERVIEW AND EPIDEMIOLOGY

ALF is defined by severe acute liver injury and is characterized by hepatic encephalopathy (HE; mental status changes) and impaired synthetic function (elevated prothrombin time/INR) in a patient without preexisting liver disease.[156] Other names include fulminant hepatic failure or fulminant hepatitis. It can be differentiated from acute hepatitis due to the presence of encephalopathy. Twenty-six weeks is the cutoff to designate acute versus chronic liver failure.

Acetaminophen toxicity, viral hepatitis, and drug-induced hepatitis are the most common causes of ALF in adults. Acetaminophen toxicity is the most common cause in the United States, comprising up to 46% of cases.[157] Up to 15% of cases do not have a discernable cause.[158] The disease carries increased morbidity and mortality.

Box 8.5 lists the typical conditions that may cause ALF. Alcohol may cause an alcoholic hepatitis, which is typically an acute-on-chronic liver failure since most people with this condition have been actively drinking for long periods of time and likely already have a component of a chronic liver injury before this severe injury.

PATHOPHYSIOLOGY

The pathophysiology of ALF is dependent upon the etiology of the liver failure. Further description of the pathology of the most common causes of liver failure are discussed below.

BOX 8.5 Etiology of Acute Liver Failure

Acetaminophen toxicity
Viral hepatitis (hepatitis A, B, D, E; CMV, EBV, HSV, VZV, adenovirus)
Other drugs or toxins
Autoimmune hepatitis
Acute fatty liver of pregnancy
Amanita phalloides (mushroom poisoning)
Budd-Chiari syndrome
Wilson disease
Cryptogenic/idiopathic
Tumor infiltration (typically breast cancer, small cell lung cancer, lymphoma, melanoma, and myeloma)
Other: ischemic hepatitis, sinusoidal obstructive syndrome, sepsis, HELLP syndrome, heat stroke, hepatectomy, hemaphagocytic lymphohistiocytosis

CMV, cytomegalovirus; EBV, Epstein-Barr virus; HELLP, hemolysis, elevated liver enzymes, low platelets; HSV, herpes simplex virus; VZV, varicella zoster virus.

MEDICAL HISTORY AND CLINICAL PRESENTATION

Medical history helps to determine the etiology of liver failure. By definition, patients with ALF will present with encephalopathy. Symptoms may also include fatigue, lethargy, poor appetite, nausea, vomiting, RUQ pain, pruritus, and abdominal distention.

PHYSICAL EXAMINATION

Physical examination findings may include sceral icterus, jaundice, hepatomegaly, RUQ tenderness with palpation, asterixis, and altered mental status. Encephalopathy findings can range from mild confusion and sleep disturbances to a comatose state. Severe encephalopathy may be accompanied by cerebral edema and intracranial hypertension, which can lead to clinical signs such as hypertension, bradycardia, respiratory depression, abnormal pupillary reflexes, and seizures.

DIAGNOSTIC STUDIES

The hallmark features of ALF are prolonged prothrombin time and encephalopathy in the setting of elevated transaminases AST and ALT. Patients may have severe derangements in their hepatic transaminases, but they may only be mildly elevated, especially in cases of early injury. Initial laboratory evaluation is used to assess the underlying etiology and severity of the liver failure. Box 8.6 lists the initial laboratory analysis that should be pursued when ALF is suspected.

Transjugular approach liver biopsy may be needed if the etiology of ALF cannot be determined. It is helpful in diagnosing conditions such as malignant infiltration, autoimmune hepatitis (AIH), certain viral infections, and Wilson disease.[157]

BOX 8.6 Initial Laboratory Analysis in Acute Liver Failure

Prothrombin time/INR
Serum chemistries: sodium, potassium, chloride, bicarbonate, BUN, creatinine, glucose, calcium, magnesium, phosphate, LDH
Liver chemistries: AST, ALT, alkaline phosphatase, GGT, total bilirubin, albumin
Complete blood count
Arterial blood gas (to evaluate pH for acidosis)
Lactate
Acetaminophen level
Toxicology screen (urine or serum)
Viral hepatitis serologies (anti-hepatitis A IgM, hepatitis B surface antigen, anti-hepatitis B core IgM, anti-hepatitis C virus Ab, hepatitis C RNA, anti-herpes simplex virus Ab, anti-varicella zoster antibodies, anti-hepatitis E IgM)
Autoimmune markers (antinuclear antibody, antismooth muscle antibody, immunoglobulin levels)
Ceruloplasmin level (Wilson disease)
Pregnancy test
Blood type and screen
HIV-1 and HIV-2
Amylase and lipase
Arterial ammonia

Ab, antibodies; ALT, alanine aminotransferase; AST, aspartate aminotransferase; BUN, blood urea nitrogen; GGT, gamma glutamine transferase; IgM, immunoglobulin M; INR, international normalized ratio; LDH, lactate dehydrogenase.

Source: Data from Lee WM, Stravitz RT, Larson AM. Introduction to the revised American Association for the Study of Liver Diseases Position Paper on acute liver failure 2011. Hepatology. *2012;55(3):965–967. doi:10.1002/hep.25551*

TREATMENT

- Patients with ALF should be admitted to the hospital and, at least initially, have close monitoring in an intensive care setting due to the risk of rapid clinical deterioration and development of cerebral edema.[159] The nearest transplant center should also be contacted to determine if the patient would require tertiary care including liver transplantation.
  - Neurologic monitoring every 1–2 hours along with frequent laboratory assessment of liver synthetic function and enzymes is paramount.
  - Patients may require endotracheal intubation if their mental status deteriorates due to worsening HE. Intracranial pressure monitoring may be required in this situation due to the high risk of cerebral edema and subsequent brainstem herniation. Routine treatment of cerebral edema should commence if it is identified.
- N-acetylcysteine (NAC) is an IV antidote used for acetaminophen toxicity.[160] It should be given early in the disease course and, due to its low side effect profile, may be given empirically when the etiology of ALF is still under investigation. Penicillin G and silibinin (milk thistle) are antidotes used for mushroom poisoning with *Amanita phalloides* species.[161] Patients with suspected HSV or varicella-zoster virus infection should be empirically treated with IV acyclovir.[162]
- Conditions such as acute fatty liver of pregnancy and HELLP (hemolysis, hepatic enzyme elevation, and low platelets) syndrome require expeditious delivery of the infant. Typically, liver failure will resolve after delivery, although some patients may require liver transplantation.
- Aside from antidotes that are effective for a small number of conditions, supportive care and workup for potential transplantation remain the hallmarks of ALF treatment. Because of the liver's inability to carry out its normal functions and gluconeogenesis, patients will develop hypoglycemia, hypophosphatemia, hypomagnesemia, and hypokalemia. These electrolytes need to be monitored closely (at least every 4 hours) and replaced as necessary, especially in the early stages of disease.
- Secondary complications of ALF are due to critical illness and include, but are not limited to, acute renal failure, sepsis, coagulopathy, and cardiovascular collapse. Close monitoring and treatment for these are needed. Blood products for thrombocytopenia or prolonged prothrombin time should only be given in the setting of active bleeding or before invasive procedures at risk for bleeding.[157] Patients should receive stress-ulcer prophylaxis with H_2 blockers or PPIs.
- The overall prognosis for survival of ALF without requiring a liver transplant is 55%.[163] There are multiple prognostic models to determine when a patient should be listed for transplantation; however, they do not reliably predict outcome and candidacy for liver transplantation. Urgent transplantation is indicated in ALF when there appears to be a poor prognosis based on laboratory values and clinical course. Patients with ALF due to Wilson disease or mushroom toxicity have overall very poor prognosis and should be considered for liver transplant expeditiously.[164]

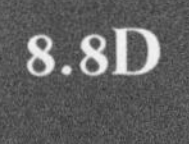

8.8D LIVER DISEASE, CIRRHOSIS, AND ITS COMPLICATIONS

OVERVIEW

Cirrhosis is a multifaceted disease with multiple potential etiologies. Physiologic alterations, potential complications, and etiologies of cirrhosis are discussed in this section

Cirrhosis is an end-stage complication of progressive hepatic fibrosis leading to alterations in the liver's architecture and the formation of regenerative nodules along with alterations in liver physiology. When patients develop cirrhosis, their condition is typically irreversible; however there have been instances of improvement with treatment of the inciting factor. Patients with cirrhosis are susceptible to multiple complications due to portal hypertension and distortion of the liver's architecture from hepatic scarring. Complications include ascites, variceal bleeding, abdominal infection (especially SBP), encephalopathy, hepatic hydrothorax, hepatopulmonary syndrome, portopulmonary hypertension, and renal failure, including hepatorenal syndrome. Life expectancy is severely reduced.

Cirrhosis is termed "compensated" or "decompensated" depending if clinical complications of portal hypertension have manifested with patients having decompensated cirrhosis having an overall worse prognosis. Conditions that would lead to an individual being called a "decompensated cirrhotic" would include bleeding esophageal varices, HE, persistent ascites, and hepatocellular carcinoma (HCC).

EPIDEMIOLOGY

Many causes of chronic liver disease can lead to the development of fibrosis and, eventually, cirrhosis. Potential etiologies of cirrhosis are listed in Box 8.7. Descriptions of the most common chronic liver diseases will be discussed in upcoming sections. Additional, but much less common, causes of cirrhosis include celiac disease, medications such as MTX and isoniazid, idiopathic adulthood ductopenia, granulomatous liver disease, idiopathic portal fibrosis, polycystic liver disease, infection, veno-occlusive disease, and hereditary hemorrhagic telangiectasia.

BOX 8.7 Common Causes of Cirrhosis

- Alcoholic liver disease
- Chronic hepatitis B
- Chronic hepatitis C
- Primary biliary cholangitis
- Primary sclerosing cholangitis
- Autoimmune hepatitis
- Hereditary hemochromatosis
- Wilson disease
- Alpha-1 antitrypsin deficiency
- Nonalcoholic fatty liver disease
- Congestive hepatopathy

In the United States, the most common causes of cirrhosis and indications for liver transplantation are chronic hepatitis C, alcoholic liver disease, and nonalcoholic fatty liver disease (NAFLD).[165] NAFLD currently ranks as the second-most common indication for liver transplant but will likely overtake viral hepatitis as the number one cause in the future since hepatitis C is now highly curable.

PATHOPHYSIOLOGY

The physiologic alterations in cirrhosis are a result of fibrosis, or scarring, which leads to alterations in hepatic blood flow and hepatocyte function and efficiency. Hepatic fibrosis leads to liver architecture distortion through the formation of regenerative nodules. This scarring leads to alterations in blood flow through the liver and enlargement of splanchnic vasculature. Because blood is unable to flow through the liver as it previously did, it finds alternative routes. This process is known as portal hypertension, which is defined as a portal pressure gradient (the difference between the pressure of the portal vein and hepatic veins) being >5 mm Hg (a normal portal pressure gradient is between 3 and 5 mm Hg). Blood is not filtered optimally, which leads to increased splanchnic vasodilators and abnormalities in renal salt and water homeostasis and activation of the renin-angiotensin-aldosterone system (RAAS) and sympathetic nervous system (SNS). Although a patient may be clinically volume-overloaded, their renal system perceives a low sodium state due to decreased flow through the renal vasculature due to splanchnic and renal vasodilation. This in turn results in the body becoming sodium-avid, leading to further free water accumulation. Portal hypertension leads to the risk of developing complications of cirrhosis. The two most common complications of portal hypertension are esophageal varices and ascites. Figure 8.5 illustrates this process.

Portal hypertension may also develop in a setting other than cirrhosis, termed noncirrhotic portal hypertension. Etiologies include extrahepatic portal vein obstruction (portal vein thrombosis), splenic vein obstruction, schistosomiasis,

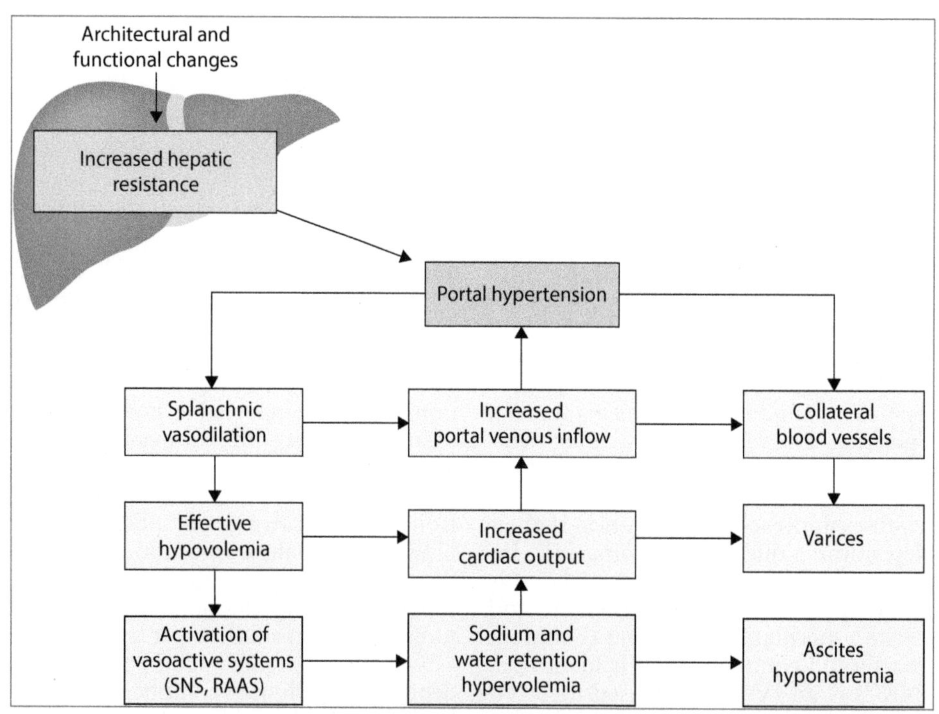

Figure 8.5 Pathophysiology of portal hypertension. RAAS, renin-angiotensin-aldosterone system; SNS, sympathetic nervous system.

nodular regenerative hyperplasia, and arterial-portal vein fistula. Patients with noncirrhotic portal hypertension can develop similar complications that patients with cirrhosis face related to portal hypertension, including bleeding esophageal varices, splenomegaly, and ascites.

MEDICAL HISTORY AND CLINICAL PRESENTATION

Cirrhosis may be the result of a number of diseases and conditions. Thorough history taking is important to assess for any risk factors of any of the possible etiologies.

SIGNS AND SYMPTOMS

Table 8.22 lists possible associated signs and symptoms of patients with chronic liver disease. Additional symptoms in more advanced liver disease can include jaundice, dark urine, pruritus, hematemesis, melena, hematochezia, worsening abdominal distention, and asterixis.

DIAGNOSTIC STUDIES

Abnormal laboratory values indicating a possible underlying liver disease include thrombocytopenia, prolonged prothrombin time/elevated INR, and decreased albumin. Thrombocytopenia is a result of portal hypotension and congestive splenomegaly in advanced liver disease. The liver also helps synthesize thrombopoeitin, vitamin K–dependent clotting factors, and albumin; therefore, scarring and dysfunction of this organ will result in abnormal laboratory values. Liver transaminases (AST and ALT) are typically elevated but can be normal in cases of more progressive disease with poorer functioning liver producing these transaminases. Patients frequently also have hyponatremia, hyperbilirubinemia, anemia, and leukopenia in advanced liver disease.

EVALUATION

Patients with cirrhosis will typically possess a nodular liver contour due to the "lumpiness" of the regenerative hepatic nodules. Asymptomatic patients may also be incidentally found to have imaging findings of abnormal liver contour, prompting further clinical evaluation.

TABLE 8.22 Symptoms and Signs of Chronic Liver Disease and Cirrhosis

Symptoms	Signs
Fatigue	Skin: Spider angiomata, palmar erythema, ecchymoses
Abdominal pain	Eyes: Scleral icterus
Day/night reversal	Musculoskeletal: Loss of proximal muscle mass, temporal wasting, Dupuytren contracture
Peripheral neuropathy	Cardiovascular: Hypotension
Muscle cramps	Abdominal: Ascites, hepatomegaly, splenomegaly, liver nodularity, caput medusa
Weight gain (due to ascites)	Reproductive: Gynecomastia, gonadal atrophy
Weight loss (due to sarcopenia)	Neurologic: Asterixis, altered consciousness, sleep disturbances
Confusion (related to toxinaccumulation or hepatic encephalopathy)	Mouth: Foul odor on the breath (*fetor hepaticus*)
Low libido	
Amenorrhea or irregular menstrual bleeding	

Although imaging is helpful in determining presence of a structural abnormality, it can rarely determine the underlying etiology of cirrhosis. Further investigation should be made into *what* led to the abnormal imaging findings in the first place. A specific etiology of cirrhosis can be made in 85–90% of cases.[30] It is imperative to obtain a thorough clinical history and physical examination in order to evaluate a time course of symptoms and any risk factors for the most common conditions. Special focus should include alcohol history, illicit drug use, weight history (any periods of obesity), and risk factors for metabolic syndrome, travel, medications, occupational exposures, tattoos, and family history. Laboratory assessment is also helpful in determining the etiology of the liver disease.

Liver biopsy may also be used to make a diagnosis of cirrhosis; however, it may not be necessary if imaging and laboratory evaluation strongly suggest a diagnosis and definitive etiology. Transjugular approach liver biopsy may determine a hepatic venous pressure gradient to determine the risk of developing complications of cirrhosis due to elevated portal pressures. Referral to a hepatologist should be considered when the diagnosis remains unclear or if liver biopsy is considered. Specialty care may also be beneficial for further cirrhosis and underlying liver disease management.

Ascites, the accumulation of fluid within the abdomen, is the most common complication of cirrhosis, and cirrhosis is the most common cause of ascites. Other etiologies of ascites include alcoholic hepatitis, heart failure, cancer (peritoneal carcinomatosis and massive liver metastases), pancreatitis, tuberculosis, Budd-Chiari syndrome (BCS), sinusoidal obstructive syndrome, lymphatic leak, myxedema, and nephrotic syndrome.

Physical examination findings in ascites include bulging flanks, abdominal distention, and umbilical hernia. Shifting dullness, the ability to percuss fluid in the abdomen, and fluid-wave elicitation are exam maneuvers, although they are not fully diagnostic due to operator error. Ultrasound may be used to identify ascites and assist with paracentesis.

To determine the etiology of ascitic fluid, a diagnostic paracentesis must be performed. A diagnostic paracentesis is a bedside procedure where by a small amount of ascitic fluid is removed under aseptic conditions from the abdomen and sent for analysis. No blood products need be given before the procedure as complication rates are typically low. Large-volume paracenteses have been performed in cirrhotic patients with platelet counts as low as 19,000 cells/mm^3 and INR as high as 8.7.[166]

Key ascitic fluid analysis parameters include fluid cell count, total protein, and albumin. A serum albumin-ascites gradient (SAAG) may then be calculated by subtracting the ascitic fluid albumin from the serum albumin. A cutoff value of 1.1 g/dL is used to differentiate the type of ascites. A patient with ascites due to portal hypertension will have a SAAG ≥1.1 g/dL. Figure 8.6 displays a flowchart of ascitic fluid analysis using SAAG and total protein. It also lists potential other tests to perform to determine the etiology of the ascites.

Complications of ascites include SBP, hepatorenal syndrome, umbilical hernia, and hepatic hydrothorax. SBP is a result of gut bacterial translocation into the ascitic fluid, causing systemic infection. Patients may present with abdominal pain, fever, nausea, and vomiting, or may be asymptomatic with the only indication of disease being renal failure or relative leukocytosis. SBP is diagnosed by assessing an ascitic fluid sample. Patients with SBP will have an ascitic fluid neutrophil count ≥250 cells/mm^3 or a positive ascitic fluid culture.

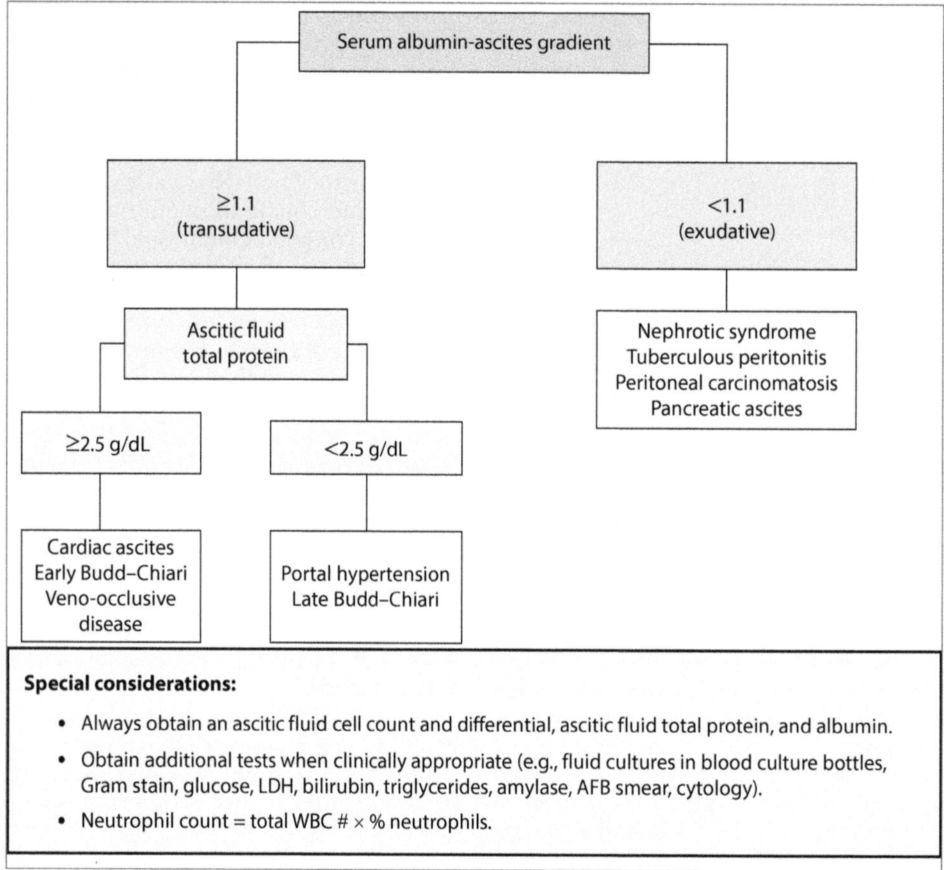

Figure 8.6 Evaluation of ascites. AFB, acid-fast bacilli; LDH, lactate dehydrogenase; WBC, white blood cell.

If SBP is suspected, there should be no delay in performing a diagnostic paracentesis and starting empiric antibiotics, typically with cefotaxime or another third-generation cephalosporin. If an organism is identified on culture, antibiotics may be narrowed to the culprit organism. Antibiotics should be continued for 5 days. If SBP is present, patients should also receive IV albumin (1.5 g/kg body weight within 6 hours and 1.0 g/kg body weight on day 3) to decrease risk of mortality related to renal failure.[167] Patients who have survived an episode of SBP should receive lifelong prophylaxis with daily norfloxacin or trimethoprim/sulfamethoxazole.[168]

Treatment of large-volume ascites includes alcohol cessation, a 2,000 mg sodium-restricted diet, and dual diuretic therapy with spironolactone (an aldosterone antagonist) and furosemide in a 100 mg:40 mg ratio. Large-volume paracenteses may also be considered in patients who do not respond to dual diuretic therapy. If patients require more than 5 L of ascitic fluid removal at a time, albumin should be given to the patient in the amount of 6 to 8 g/L of fluid removed to avoid development of renal failure and hepatorenal syndrome.

Refractory ascites, or fluid overload that is not responsive to a sodium-restricted diet and high-dose diuretic therapy, can be potentially treated with the placement of a transjugular intrahepatic portosystemic shunt (TIPS) to divert blood flow from the splanchnic circulation to the liver (Figure 8.7). Owing to changes in blood flow and unloading of the liver's ability to remove toxins after the procedure, patients are at a higher risk of developing HE and this potential complication should be considered prior to TIPS deployment in already encephalopathic patients.

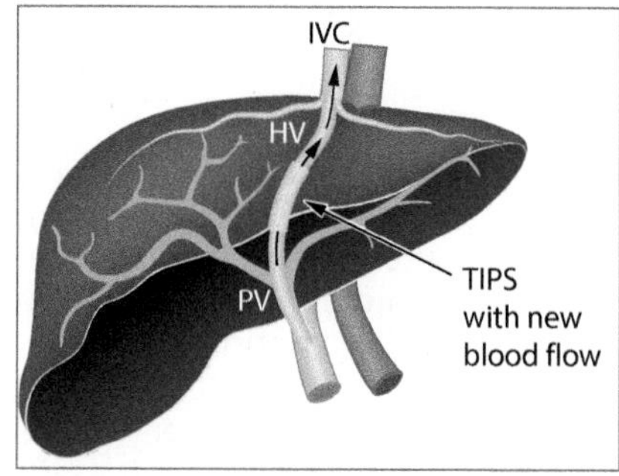

Figure 8.7 Transjugular intrahepatic portosystemic shunt (TIPS). HV, hepatic vein; IVC, inferior vena cava; PV, portal vein.

Variceal Hemorrhage

Esophageal and gastric varices are a complication of rising portal pressures and the formation of portosystemic collaterals in the setting of portal hypertension. These collaterals become engorged with blood, leading to the enlargement of veins that are at risk of oozing or rupture. These bleeding episodes can be massive, with patients losing large amounts of their blood volume and requiring a large volume of blood transfusions. Patients may also develop portal hypertensive gastropathy or gastric antral vascular ectasias (GAVE) as a result of portal hypertension. Although these do not bleed as severely as varices, they are a potential source of continued blood loss leading to iron deficiency anemia in cirrhotic patients.

The goal of treatment is to avoid complications such as variceal hemorrhage. If the endoscopist finds varices that are concerning for future bleeding events (medium to large varices, small varices with red wale signs, decompensated cirrhotics with small varices), they may prophylactically place bands on the varix to decompress it *or* start the patient on a nonselective beta blocker (NSBB) such as propranolol, nadolol, or carvedilol. The choice of therapy is influenced by patient preference, local resources and expertise, and patient underlying contraindications.[169,170]

NSBBs work in portal hypertension by inhibiting beta-adrenergic receptors in the circulation, which allows for unopposed alpha-adrenergic activity and leads to generalized vasoconstriction. Additionally, they decrease portal flow through decreased cardiac output via beta-1 adrenergic blockade. NSBBs are not tolerated well due to hypotension, bradycardia, and fatigue. Carvedilol, a combined alpha and beta blocker, is slightly better tolerated, but it can cause greater decreases in mean arterial pressure due to its anti-alpha-1 adrenergic activity, leading to peripheral vasodilation.[171] NSBBs are not helpful in patients who do not have varices or clinically significant portal hypertension. Table 8.23 outlines these medications.

Variceal bleeding is not a subtle event. Patients will typically present with hematemesis, tachycardia, hypotension, and pallor. Melena may or may not be present. The treatment of bleeding varices involves endoscopic banding or cyanoacrylate injection, after the patient has been hemodynamically stabilized with a secured airway. Additionally, patients should receive blood transfusions conservatively, so portal pressures are not raised too high. A hemoglobin goal of 7–9 g/dL is appropriate. In instances of GI hemorrhage, patients with cirrhosis should be empirically placed on IV ceftriaxone for a 7-day course to avoid SBP because of increased risk of bacterial translocation in the setting of active oozing. IV vasoactive drugs such as octreotide, somatostatin, or vasopressin should be considered to decrease portal pressures during active hemorrhage. After initial stabilitzation, patients should be followed as an outpatient for further variceal banding and should be placed on a NSBB.

Like refractory ascites, TIPS may be considered for the treatment of severe variceal hemorrhage or recurrent variceal hemorrhage despite endoscopic variceal ligation and NSBB. Patients typically do not require NSBB or endoscopic surveillance after TIPS has been performed.

Hepatic Encephalopathy

HE is a type of cognitive impairment associated with cirrhosis. The pathogenesis of this condition is not fully understood. Its presentation ranges from subtle behavioral and attention changes to coma (see Table 8.24). Personality changes may include apathy and irritability. Additionally, early-stage HE is frequently accompanied by sleep-wake cycle disturbances and significant daytime sleepiness.[172] Physical examination findings may include hypertonia or diminished deep tendon reflexes.[173] Asterixis, or "flapping tremor," is frequently present in the early grades of the disorder. This can be observed in actions that require postural tone (hyperextension of the wrists or squeezing of the fingers) and appears as a "flap" and is known as asterixis.

HE may occur due to a number of reasons and its occurrence should prompt investigation of the precipitating factor. Potential causes of HE include infection, GI bleeding, medications, constipation, or new hepatocellular cancer. Medication issues could include lactulose or rifaximin noncompliance or underdosing, or diuretic overdose (intentionally or as a result of renal failure from hypovolemia). Additional causes of encephalopathy that should be investigated include hypoglycemia, substance intoxication, medication or drug side effects, intracranial bleeding, and epilepsy. Blood ammonia may be elevated or normal in HE but has no bearing on the diagnosis of HE.[174] Diagnosis of HE is made through the exclusion of other causes of brain dysfunction and mental status changes.[175]

HE treatment is reserved for patients with overt HE (grades II–IV) or as prophylaxis after an episode of overt HE.[176] Medical treatment includes lactulose and rifaximin.

Lactulose is a nonabsorbable disaccharide that works through multiple mechanisms. It is degraded by gut bacteria resulting in an acidic lumen pH, thereby preventing the diffusion of ammonia into the blood so it is excreted in stool. It acts as an osmotic laxative, promoting gut peristalsis, which leads to decreased time for ammonia absorption in the gut. It also promotes the growth of beneficial bacteria in the intestines. Medication dosing is titrated so that patients may have three bowel movements per day. If patients are not having that many bowel movements or they are showing signs of worsening HE, the dose may be increased. Lactulose may also be given as a retention enema in cases of high-grade HE when oral administration of medications via NG tube is not possible.

Rifaximin is an antibiotic that inhibits bacterial RNA synthesis, thereby altering the composition of gut bacteria. It is given as an add-on therapy with lactulose in the instances when lactulose does not fully improve HE despite escalating doses. It is given orally, in doses of 550 mg twice daily or 400 mg three times daily.

TABLE 8.23 Medications for Guideline-Appropriate Management of Esophageal Varices

Medication	Mechanism of Action	Recommended Dose	Treatment Goals
Propranolol	Competitively blocks beta-1 and beta-2 adrenergic receptors	20–40 mg twice a day Maximal dose of 320 mg/day in patients without ascites, 160 mg/day in patients with ascites	Resting heart rate 55–60 bpm Systolic blood pressure should not drop below 90 mm Hg
Nadolol	Competitively blocks beta-1 and beta-2 adrenergic receptors	20–40 mg once daily Maximal dose of 160 mg/day in patients without ascites and 80 mg/day in patients with ascites	Resting heart rate 55–60 bpm Systolic blood pressure should not drop below 90 mm Hg
Carvedilol	Nonselectively blocks beta- and alpha-adrenergic receptors	Start with 6.25 mg once daily and increase to twice per day after 3 days Maximal dose of 12.5 mg/day	Systolic blood pressure should not drop below 90 mm Hg

TABLE 8.24 Grading of Hepatic Encephalopathy Severity

Grade	Features
I	Behavioral changes, sleep disturbances
II	Disorientation, lethargy, inappropriate behavior
III	Marked confusion, severe lethargy but arousable to verbal stimuli
IV	Comatose, unresponsive to pain, decorticate or decerebrate posturing

Hepatocellular Carcinoma

HCC can be a result of cirrhosis but may also develop in a number of conditions. Cirrhosis is typically the main cause of HCC, with over 80% of cases of HCC being due to cirrhosis.[177] Additional risk factors include hepatitis B virus (HBV) infection, chronic hepatitis C virus (HCV) infection, hereditary hemochromatosis (HH), NAFLD, and aflatoxin exposure.

All patients with cirrhosis should undergo HCC surveillance via liver ultrasound (or equivalent imaging) every 6 months. If HCC is identified, multidisciplinary evaluation should occur to determine the optimal treatment strategy for the patient. Lesions should not be biopsied due to risk of tumor seeding.

Treatment options of HCC depend upon multiple factors including patient's functional status, whether they are listed for transplant and, if so, the size of the lesion. Options may include tumor resection, radiofrequency ablation, alcohol ablation, transarterial chemoembolization, sorafenib, or routine surveillance.

ADDITIONAL TREATMENT AND SURVEILLANCE IN CIRRHOSIS

The treatment strategies and screening guidelines for the main complications of cirrhosis are listed above. Additional general management strategies include vaccination against hepatitis A and B, nutritional and functional status optimization, and risk mitigation. Routine evaluation is important in identifying patients at risk for decompensation, further decompensation, or liver transplant candidacy.

All patients with chronic liver disease should be immunized against hepatitis A virus (HAV) and HBV if they aren't already immune. Patients with cirrhosis have a greater risk of malnutrition and sarcopenia, which are both negative prognostic factors.[178] Continued or increased physical activity along with frequent high-calorie high-protein small meals should be encouraged. Daily protein intake should be 1.2–1.5 g/kg/day.[179]

Patients should avoid things that may worsen disease such as alcohol use, NSAID therapy, hepatotoxins, obesity, and shellfish (risk of *Vibrio vulnificus* infection). Patients may also benefit from treatment of the underlying cause of cirrhosis (treatment of hepatitis C, phlebotomy) under the guidance of a cirrhosis specialist. Patients may safety take up to 2 g of acetaminophen daily with cirrhosis but should avoid NSAIDs due to altered renal function in the setting of portal hypertension.

PATIENT EDUCATION

- Patients should be counseled extensively about the risks of worsening liver disease in the setting of continued alcohol consumption. Patients with other underlying liver disorders, especially NAFLD, nonalcoholic steatohepatitis (NASH), viral hepatitis, and hemochromatosis, are at higher risk of worsening liver fibrosis or HCC with continued alcohol ingestion.[180] Therefore, there is no safe level of alcohol intake with these diseases.[181]
- Liver transplant is a potential treatment strategy for patients with decompensated cirrhosis. Referral to a transplant center for evaluation is recommended as multiple factors comprise a patient's transplant candidacy.

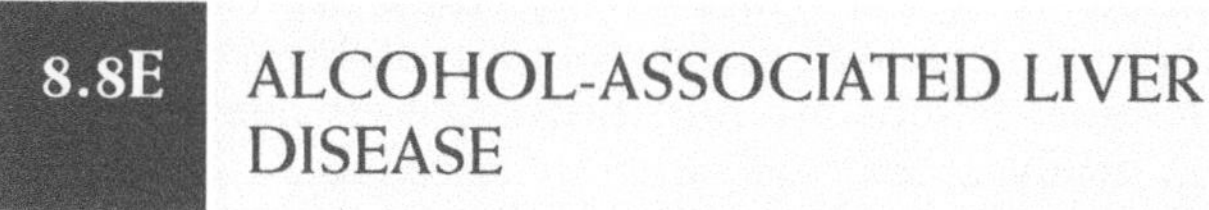

8.8E ALCOHOL-ASSOCIATED LIVER DISEASE

OVERVIEW AND EPIDEMIOLOGY

ALD encompasses a broad range of clinical and histopathological findings. It may range from alcohol use disorder (AUD) to hepatic steatosis to alcohol-associated hepatitis to cirrhosis. The disease has a high mortality rate. In 2012, it was estimated that 5.5 per 100,000 U.S. deaths were due to ALD.[148] It competes with chronic hepatitis C as the leading indication for liver transplantation in the United States.[182]

PATHOPHYSIOLOGY

The pathogenesis of liver disease related to alcohol consumption is incompletely understood since not all patients develop clinically significant liver disease despite high levels of alcohol ingestion. Normally, ethanol is primarily metabolized in the liver via multiple pathways. It is first metabolized to acetaldehyde by the enzyme alcohol dehydrogenase, followed by further conversion to acetate in the hepatocyte mitochondria.[183] Alcoholic hepatic injury typically first manifests as hepatocyte steatosis (Figure 8.8). It appears to be a result of a disruption of multiple metabolism pathways due to altered oxidation of hepatic fatty acids and increased lipogenesis.[184] With abstinence from alcohol, continued hepatocyte injury may be avoided and steatosis is able to resolve, thus returning to normal liver parenchyma. However, with continued liver injury, steatosis may progress to steatohepatitis, or even fibrosis, through multiple proposed mechanisms, including inflammatory cytokines, oxidative

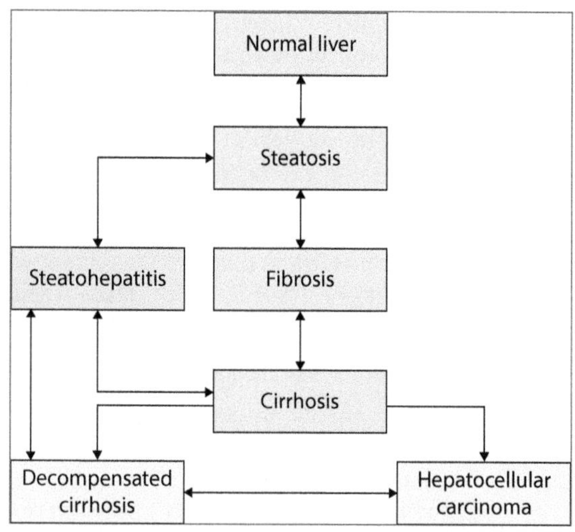

Figure 8.8 Natural history of alcohol-associated liver disease.

stress, and toxic metabolic products of alcohol. With abstinence from alcohol, there is a chance of recovery at each stage, but continued drinking prevents improvement.

PREDISPOSING FACTORS

Risk factors for liver injury and progressive liver disease include female sex, daily drinking, smoking, binge drinking, and the presence of other underlying liver diseases.[185–188] Some research has shown that coffee consumption may be protective against cirrhosis and alcohol-induced cirrhosis.[189]

MEDICAL HISTORY AND CLINICAL PRESENTATION

Owing to the social stigma associated with alcohol misuse, patients may not be forthcoming with their true amount of alcohol consumption. Additionally, patients frequently underestimate serving sizes of beverages and may unintentionally believe they are drinking less than the tolerated amount. A standard drink contains 14 g of alcohol, which is the equivalent of 12 oz. of beer (5% alcohol), 8–9 oz. of malt liquor, 5 oz. of table wine, or 1.5 oz. of distilled spirits. Per the U.S. Department of Health and Human Services, the upper limit of safe drinking is 1 standard drink per day for women and 2 standard drinks per day for men.[190] Binge drinking is defined as 5 drinks in men and 4 drinks in women over a period of 2 hours.

PHYSICAL EXAMINATION

Other than signs of acute alcohol withdrawal syndrome (tachycardia, tremor, psychomotor agitation, hallucinations) or the odor of alcohol on the breath, there are no specific signs or physical examination findings specific to ALD. Many of the signs and symptoms of chronic liver disease from other etiologies are shared with ALD (see Table 8.22). Patients may also be asymptomatic. Clinicians should have a high index of suspicion but should remember to rule out other causes of chronic liver disease along the way.

DIAGNOSTIC STUDIES

Liver-related enzymes, bilirubin, GGT, and certain immunoglobulins may be elevated in a setting of prolonged alcohol use but are not specific to alcohol use and may be elevated as a result of other conditions. GGT and AST may also be elevated after recent excessive alcohol use.[191] Additionally, patients may show evidence of a macrocytic anemia.

Hepatic steatosis may be appreciated on multiple imaging modalities including ultrasound, CT, or MRI. Transient elastography may be used to evaluate for fibrosis and is a less invasive method of detecting this compared to liver biopsy.

Alcohol-associated steatohepatitis (AH) is a clinical syndrome with specific histopathologic findings of neutrophilic lobular inflammation, degenerative changes in hepatocytes (ballooning and Mallory-Denk bodies), steatosis, and pericellular fibrosis. Frequently, however, liver biopsy is not necessary in making a diagnosis if a clinical diagnosis can be made. The clinical presentation is broad, ranging from lack of symptoms to liver failure. The syndrome is typically accompanied by jaundice, anorexia, fever, and tender hepatomegaly. A clinical diagnosis is made based on the findings: acute jaundice, ongoing alcohol consumption without >60 days of abstinence from alcohol, AST >50 IU/L, AST/ALT ratio >1.5 (typically a 2:1 ratio), both AST and ALT <400 IU/L, and serum TB >3.0 mg/dL.[192] Additionally, one must rule out other causes of acute jaundice and hepatitis including ischemic hepatitis, metabolic liver disease, drug-induced liver disease, and acute AIH. An individual can have both AH and concomitant cirrhosis.

A diagnosis of alcoholic cirrhosis may be made through a thorough clinical history, by a careful evaluation of a patient's past and current drinking history, and by excluding other causes of liver disease.

TREATMENT

- The mainstay of treatment in any ALD is cessation of alcohol use. Referral to a drug and alcohol rehabilitation program, an addiction counselor, or support group such as Alcoholics Anonymous are important additional components of therapy.
- In cases of AH, the Maddrey discriminant function (MDF), a lab-based prognostic score, is used to calculate the severity of AH and short-term (28-day) mortality outcomes in order to determine if a patient would benefit from corticosteroids.[193] A score >32 corresponds to severe disease and prednisolone 40 mg/day should be initiated if there are no clinical contraindications such as uncontrolled infection. Additionally, optimal nutrition (>21 kcal/kg/day) and supportive care are the mainstays of treatment of AH. Pentoxifylline was previously used to treat AH in patients who could not take corticosteroids but is now no longer recommended as a treatment in the 2020 AASLD (American Association for the Study of Liver Diseases) guidelines.[181,194]

8.8F VIRAL HEPATITIS

MEDICAL HISTORY AND CLINICAL PRESENTATION

The hepatitis viruses can cause both acute and chronic hepatitis. Generally, hepatic injury is a result of the body's immune response to the virus. Each of the viruses (hepatitis A through E, CMV, Epstein-Barr virus [EBV], HSV, and adenovirus) may present similarly but require different treatment. Laboratory assessment is imperative in identifying and the virus and treating the infection. Table 8.25 outlines key characteristics of hepatitis A through E. More in-depth discussion of these will be presented in subsections below.

Typical presentations of acute viral hepatitis include malaise, anorexia, nausea, vomiting, and abdominal pain. Dark urine, acholic stools, jaundice, and pruritus may also be seen. Physical examination findings may include jaundice, scleral icterus, hepatomegaly, and RUQ tenderness to palpation.[195] Laboratory abnormalities typically include significant elevations in serum transaminases, serum bilirubin, and ALP.

Prevention is key in viral hepatitides. Good handwashing and cooking practices are key in avoiding hepatitis A and E. Vaccinations are available for HAV before travel to endemic countries as well as HBV. Infants who are born to mothers who are HBV surface antigen (HBsAg) positive receive hepatitis B immune globulin within 12 hours after birth and are started on hepatitis B vaccination to attempt to prevent vertical transmission and start to develop protection against future exposure to hepatitis B. Mothers with high HBV viral loads or who are HBV e antigen (HBeAg) positive should receive antiviral therapy to reduce risk of transmission.[196]

TABLE 8.25 Characteristics of Hepatitis A, B, C, and E

Virus	Type of Hepatitis	Source	Diagnosis	Treatment	Complications
HAV	Acute	Fecal-oral	Anti-HAV IgM, anti-HAV IgG indicates previous infection	Supportive care	Rare cases of acute liver failure, cholestatic hepatitis, relapsing hepatitis, autoimmune hepatitis
HBV	Acute and chronic	Perinatal, percutaneous, and sexual exposure (bloodborne)	Please see Table 8.26 on interpretation of HBV serologic patterns	Supportive care in acute phase, antiviral drugs in chronic phase in certain circumstances	Fulminant hepatitis, HCC, cirrhosis, extrahepatic manifestations
HCV	Acute and chronic	Bloodborne, body fluids	Anti-HCV	8–12 weeks of oral therapy, depending on genotype	HCC, cirrhosis
HEV	Acute, rarely chronic	Fecal-oral, blood-borne, mother-to-child transmission	Anti-HEV IgM	Supportive care, potential liver transplant in acute liver failure	Acute liver failure, cholestatic hepatitis

HAV, hepatitis A virus; HBV, hepatitis B virus; HCC, hepatocellular carcinoma; HCV, hepatitis C virus; HEV, hepatitis E virus; IgG, immunoglobulin G; IgM, immunoglobulin M.

Hepatitis A

HAV is an RNA virus that is transmitted via the fecal-oral route through person-to-person contact or consumption of contaminated food or water. It typically causes an acute, self-limited hepatitis that resolves and incurs lifelong immunity to the individual. There is no chronic HAV infection. Symptoms of acute HAV infection are similar to symptoms with any acute hepatitis. Acute infection rarely progresses to ALF. Treatment relies on supportive care. Hepatitis A immunoglobulin can be given after known exposure to HAV and there is a vaccination which can prevent this infection.

Hepatitis B

It is estimated that worldwide, approximately 2 billion people have evidence of past or present HBV infection.[197,198] Prevalence varies based on global geographic area with a <2% population prevalence in the United States. A large percentage of individuals who have chronic HBV infection in higher-prevalence areas is due to vertical transmission perinatally.[196] The virus is transmitted via blood with the majority of transmission occurring through mother-to-child contact during birth (vertical transmission) or through unprotected sexual intercourse, through injection drug use, or during early childhood (horizontal transmission).

The HBV is a DNA virus with a complex, multiparticle structure. Three of its proteins are utilized in serum diagnosis and are helpful in determining what phase of infection a person may have. The HBsAg is an envelope protein on the outer surface of the virion. It indicates the virus is "preSSSent" in the body. Anti-HBs is the antibody to HBsAg and indicates clearance or immunity to the virus. Hepatitis B core antigen (HBcAg) is an antigen expressed in infected hepatocytes. Its antibody, anti-HBc, is expressed in serum. It indicates if a patient has been in "CCContact" with the virus at one time or another but cannot differentiate between a current infection or previous exposure, unlike HBsAg and anti-HBsAg. The HBeAg is a secretory protein of the virus. It is a marker of HBV "EEEnfectivity," as the presence of this antigen is typically associated with high levels of HBV DNA and higher rates of HBV transmission/infectivity.

HBV infection is a more complex condition to diagnose as its serologies allude to different disease presentations. The following list describes HBV infection terms, while Table 8.26 explains what different serology combinations mean.

- **Window period:** Period in acute infection when HBsAg has become negative but anti-HBs is not yet positive, signaling recovery. Only the anti-HBc IgM will be positive at this time.
- **Immune tolerant phase:** Active viral replication is occurring (HBeAg and HBV DNA are positive), but little damage is occurring to the liver (ALT normal) because the body has not mounted an immune response to the virus.
- **Immune active/clearance phase:** The body is trying to eliminate infection so damage is occurring to hepatocytes (ALT is elevated). HBeAg may transition to anti-HBe (seroconversion). There is a higher risk of cirrhosis and HCC development in this phase.
- **Inactive chronic hepatitis B infection:** Liver abnormalities improve after the immune active state and seroconversion to anti-HBe with reduced HBV DNA levels.

In acute HBV infection, about 70% of patients will have a subclinical course without jaundice, while 30% will have a more appreciable illness.[199] Although less common, ALF may occur in 0.1% to 0.5% of patients.[200] In adults who have acute HBV hepatitis, the rate of progression to chronic HBV hepatitis is <5%.[201] However, if infection is acquired perinatally or during early childhood, the rates of progression are significantly higher. Perinatal progression to chronic hepatitis is around 90% while progression between the ages of 1 to 5 is at 20–50%.[196,202] Chronic HBV infection is defined by the persistence of HBsAg for >6 months.

Most patients with chronic HBV are asymptomatic but may experience symptoms during flares. Between 10% and 20% of patients have extrahepatic manifestations, which are a result of circulating immune complexes and may include fever, skin rashes, arthralgia, and arthritis. Polyarteritis nodosa and glomerular disease are more specific extrahepatic complications of chronic HBV infection.[203] Patients may also develop cirrhosis as a result of chronic infection and the signs and symptoms are similar to any patient with cirrhosis described above.

Just as serologic assessment may be confusing in HBV, decisions on who should receive treatment can be complex and nuanced. The 2018 AASLD Hepatitis B Guidelines help to organize and define the correct treatment plans and timing to initiate treatment for HBV individuals.[204] Antiviral treatment is rarely needed in acute HBV infection, since

TABLE 8.26 Serologic Patterns and Interpretations in Hepatitis B

HBsAg	Anti-HBs	Anti-HBc	HBeAg	Anti-HBe	HBV DNA	ALT	Interpretation
+	–	IgM	+	–	+++	Elevated	Acute hepatitis B
–	–	IgM	–	–	+	Elevated	Window period
–	+	IgG	–	+ or –	+ or –	Normal	Recovery from acute hepatitis B (immunity)
+	–	IgG	+	–	+++	Normal or mildly elevated	Chronic hepatitis B, immune tolerant phase
+	–	IgG	+ or –	+ or –	+++	Elevated	Chronic hepatitis B, immune active phase
+	–	IgG	–	+	– to ++	Normal or mildly elevated	Inactive chronic hepatitis B
–	+	–	–	–	–	Normal	Vaccination (immunity)
–	–	–	–	–	–	Normal	Susceptible to infection, never vaccinated

ALT, alanine aminotransferase; anti-HBc, hepatitis B core antibody; anti-HBe, hepatitis B e antibody; anti-HBs, hepatitis B surface antibody; HBeAg, hepatitis B e antigen; HBsAg, hepatitis B surface antigen; IgG, immunoglobulin G; IgM, immunoglobulin M.

such a large proportion of patients recover and develop immunity. Additionally, patients who are anti-HBc positive should be considered for treatment if they are set to start immunosuppressive therapy, due to the risk of HBV reactivation. Those who do not meet the parameters for treatment should have close monitoring of ALT, HBV DNA, and HBeAg according to guideline parameters in the event of needing to start therapy. Treatment options include pegylated interferon, tenofovir, or entecavir.

HBV infection increases an individual's risk for developing HCC, even in the absence of cirrhosis. Patients with HBV infection plus active hepatitis, family history of HCC, Asian ethnicity (males over the age of 40 and females over the age of 50), or African ethnicity should undergo routine ultrasound evaluation every 6 months to assess for the development of HCC.[205] HBV DNA level is an independent predictor of cirrhosis and HCC.[206]

Hepatitis C

Hepatitis C is a bloodborne viral illness with growing prominence and increased treatment options. The World Health Organization estimated in 2015 that 71 million people had chronic HCV infection.[207]

Injection drug use remains the most important risk factor for HCV acquisition in the United States.[208] People born between the years 1945–1965, those who received a blood transfusion before 1992, and those who currently or previously injected drugs should be screened for HCV infection by testing for anti-HCV in serum. Because of the advances in treatment of hepatitis C, current guidelines suggest a one-time hepatitis C screen for all adults over age 18 in the United States. HCV currently remains the most common cause of chronic liver disease and most common indication for liver transplantation, although NAFLD may take its place in the coming decades.

Unlike hepatitis B, the majority of patients infected with HCV do not spontaneously clear the virus. Chronic HCV infection typically occurs in 50–85% of cases.[209] Patients typically have a slow, indolent, and asymptomatic course, not being diagnosed until routine clinical screening or with a diagnosis of cirrhosis many years later. Symptoms, if present, are nonspecific. Extrahepatic manifestations such as essential mixed cryoglobulinemia, membranoproliferative glomerulonephritis, thyroiditis, or porphyria cutanea tarda are possible. Serum transaminases can be normal or elevated.

Diagnosis can be initiated after finding a positive HCV antibody (anti-HCV). If positive, further evaluation should include assessing total HCV RNA load and HCV genotype in order to determine optimal treatment modality.

Newer, significantly more effective treatments of chronic HCV infection have emerged in the past few years, compared to previous interferon-based therapy. Direct-acting antiviral therapy has proved to be >95% effective at curing the disease.[210] Treatment duration ranges from 8 to 12 weeks, depending on the regimen (either glecaprevir/pibrentasvir or sofosbuvir/velpatasvir). Treatment algorithms through the AASLD have been developed to recommend the appropriate pretreatment workup, medication regimens and monitoring, and post-treatment assessment of cure, known as sustained viral response (SVR).[211] The patient should have a quantitative HCV RNA and hepatic function panel checked 12 weeks after completing therapy. Algorithms are available for treatment-naïve noncirrhotics and treatment-naïve compensated cirrhotics. Caution is advised regarding treating decompensated HCV cirrhotics or patients who had previously received HCV treatment. These patients should be seen in expert consultation with a hepatologist for further treatment recommendations. Full treatment recommendations and continuously updated guidelines are available at www.hcvguidelines.org.

Hepatitis D

Hepatitis D virus (HDV) is a defective virus that requires HBV to be present for virion assembly and secretion. Acute HBV and HDV coinfection is typically more severe than acute HBV and is more likely to cause ALF.[212]

Hepatitis E

Hepatitis E virus (HEV) is an RNA virus transmitted via mainly the fecal-oral route, although it can be transmitted via blood transfusion or perinatal transmission. Acute HEV infections are typically asymptomatic, although patients may show the symptoms of acute hepatitis mentioned above. Occasionally, patients may develop extrahepatic manifestations of disease such as thrombocytopenia, acute thyroiditis, membranous glomerulonephritis, and neurologic disease, to name a few.[213] ALF is a rare complication but can be seen, especially in those who are pregnant, are malnourished, or have preexisting liver disease. Chronic HEV infection is rare but can be seen in immunocompromised patients.

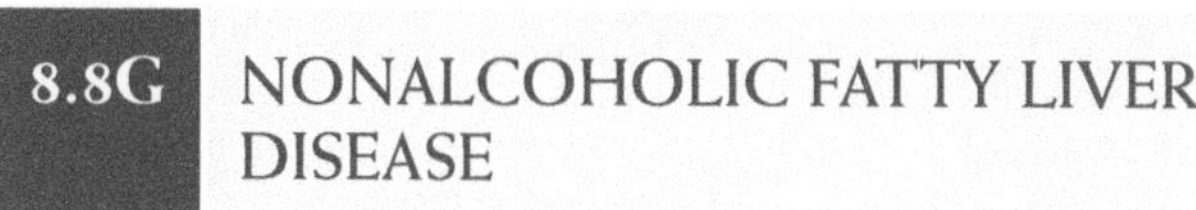

8.8G NONALCOHOLIC FATTY LIVER DISEASE

OVERVIEW AND EPIDEMIOLOGY

NAFLD is the presence of hepatic steatosis on imaging or histology with no other secondary causes of fat accumulation (e.g., heavy alcohol use, medications, genetics). It is characterized histologically as nonalcoholic fatty liver (NAFL) versus NASH if there is inflammation with hepatic injury (seen in NASH). NASH biopsies may have fibrosis present due to hepatocyte injury. Patients with this condition are at risk for developing cirrhosis. "Burned-out" NAFLD is believed to be a major course of cryptogenic cirrhosis (cirrhosis without an identifiable etiology).[214]

The estimated global prevalence of NAFLD based on imaging is around 25.24%.[215] The highest prevalence is reported in the Middle East, followed by South America, while the lowest prevalence is seen in Africa. It is more difficult to determine the prevalence of NASH due to the need for a liver biopsy to confirm this diagnosis. Studies estimate the prevalence of NASH in the general population is between 1.5% and 6.45%.

The most significant risk factor for the development of NAFLD is the presence of the metabolic syndrome (elevated waist circumference, triglyceride level, blood pressure, fasting glucose, and/or decreased high-density lipoproteins [HDLs]). Additional risk factors associated with NAFLD include obesity, type 2 diabetes, dyslipidemia, and polycystic ovary syndrome.[216,217]

PATHOPHYSIOLOGY

While the pathogenesis of NAFLD is not fully understood, it is thought to be due to a combination of excessive lipid accumulation in the liver, insulin resistance inducing hepatic steatosis, along with further oxidative injury leading to hepatocellular injury and steatohepatitis.[218,219] Additional likely components of disease development include genetic factors, hepatic iron accumulation, antioxidant deficiencies, and an abnormal gut microbiome.[220–222]

MEDICAL HISTORY, CLINICAL PRESENTATION, AND PHYSICAL EXAMINATION

Frequently, patients may present to a specialty clinic for further workup of hepatic steatosis appreciated on imaging. They may be asymptomatic, with or without findings of liver enzyme abnormalities. More progressive disease may present with physical exam findings appreciable in cirrhosis and chronic liver disease (see Section 8.8D Liver Disease, Cirrhosis, and Its Complications).

Patients should be evaluated for possible comorbid conditions such as type 2 diabetes, hyperlipidemia, hypertension, obstructive sleep apnea, and any of the treatments for these conditions and the metabolic syndrome. Patients may have a history of previous obesity and have current weight loss due to bariatric surgery, chronic liver disease, or intentional weight loss through diet and exercise. Careful history taking should also focus on alternative explanations for hepatic steatosis such as alcohol use or misuse, medications, or risk factors for other liver diseases such as hepatitis C or Wilson disease. Table 8.27 lists the common causes of secondary hepatic steatosis.

Patients with clinically significant liver disease may not be overweight or obese at the time of evaluation. They may have "burned-out" NAFLD and care should be taken to assess their past peak weights to assess for previous obesity.

DIAGNOSTIC STUDIES

A diagnosis of NAFLD is made when there is evidence of steatosis on imaging and no other source of hepatic steatosis or liver disease such as elevated alcohol consumption, medications, or chronic liver disease. However, it is possible to have hepatic steatosis as a result of metabolic syndrome *and* have other underlying liver diseases.

Although liver biopsy is not necessary to make a diagnosis of NAFLD, it may be helpful when an etiology is uncertain, to make a diagnosis of NASH, or to assess for fibrosis.

Clinical decision aids can be useful in determining if patients are at higher risk of possessing fibrosis in NAFLD. Calculators include the fibrosis-4 index (FIB-4) or NAFLD Fibrosis Score (NFS). Vibration-controlled transient elastography may also be of benefit.

TREATMENT AND SURVEILLANCE

The most common cause of death in patients with NAFLD is not chronic liver disease, but rather CVD.[222] Because of the increased risk of cardiovascular complications, treatment strategies should focus on addressing CVD risk factors and any manifestations of the metabolic syndrome. Patients with NAFL or NASH are not at higher risk for serious liver injury with statin use and are recommended to be placed on this medication if a high enough CVD risk is present.[224,225]

Cancer-related and liver-related death are the second- and third-leading causes of death in this disease.[226] NAFLD is considered the third most common cause of HCC, even in the absence of cirrhosis.[227] Patients with NASH, especially those with evidence of fibrosis, have an increased risk of developing cirrhosis and increased liver-related mortality rate compared to those with only NAFL.[228] Because patients with NASH, rather than NAFL, have higher risk of liver-

TABLE 8.27 Causes of Secondary Hepatic Steatosis

Macrovesicular Steatosis	Microvesicular Steatosis
Excessive alcohol	Reye syndrome
Hepatitic C, genotype 3	Medications (valproate, antiretroviral medications)
Wilson disease	Acute fatty liver of pregnancy
Lipodystrophy	HELLP syndrome
Starvation	Inborn errors of metabolism
Parenteral nutrition	
Abetalipoproteinemia	
Medications (amiodarone, methotrexate, tamoxifen, corticosteroids)	

HELLP, hemolysis, elevated liver enzymes, low platelets.

related mortality, pharmacologic therapy aimed at improving liver disease should be limited to those with NASH only.

The key treatment strategy for NAFLD is weight loss. Adults who are able to lose at least 5% of their body weight had improvement in hepatic steatosis, with further histologic improvements with larger amounts of weight loss.[229,230] Bariatric surgery may also be considered in patients with NAFL or NASH.

Potential pharmacologic therapies for NASH include pioglitazone and vitamin E. Pioglitazone may be used in NASH patients without type 2 diabetes but side effects such as weight gain and bone loss limit its use. Vitamin E is still under investigation but may also be used in nondiabetic NASH patients and is associated with a modest increased risk of prostate cancer.[231]

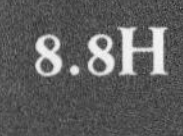

8.8H PRIMARY SCLEROSING CHOLANGITIS (PSC)

OVERVIEW AND EPIDEMIOLOGY

PSC is an idiopathic, chronic, cholestatic liver disease that involves inflammation and fibrosis of both the intrahepatic and extrahepatic bile ducts that cannot be attributed to another disease.[232] This inflammatory response leads to multiple biliary strictures; if another cause of stricturing disease can be determined, it is called secondary sclerosing cholangitis (see Box 8.8). It is a progressive disorder that can develop into cirrhosis, portal hypertension, hepatic decompensation, or cholangiocarcinoma in a majority of patients.[233]

The population prevalence of PSC varies based on geographic region. In the United States, the estimated prevalence is 1 to 16 per 100,000 people.[234] A diagnosis of PSC is frequently accompanied by a diagnosis of IBD, most commonly UC, although the converse is not true. The prevalence of PSC in IBD is around 5%, while the prevalence of IBD in PSC is around 60% to 80%.[235,236]

PATHOPHYSIOLOGY

The cause of PSC is not fully known. Because of its association with IBD, it is hypothesized that there is a role for autoimmunity in the pathogenesis of the disease.

MEDICAL HISTORY, CLINICAL PRESENTATION, AND PHYSICAL EXAMINATION

The presentation of the disease varies widely, from persistently abnormal liver enzymes to sudden onset pruritus to findings of advanced liver disease and to, rarely, cholangitis. Patients may develop nonspecific symptoms such as fatigue. RUQ pain is not a frequent symptom in this condition. Because it is a cholestatic liver disease, the ALP level will typically be elevated, although it can be normal. Serum aminotransferase levels may also be modestly elevated (two to three times above the ULN).[237]

DIAGNOSTIC STUDIES

Serum liver enzymes may be abnormal as a result of this condition. Additionally, immunoglobulin G (IgG) levels may be elevated in up to 60% of patients.[238] IgG4 levels have been found to be elevated in a subset of PSC patients (about 10%). Patients with this finding typically have a more rapidly progressive disease in the absence of treatment, but typically respond to corticosteroids (unlike typical PSC patients).[239,240] Because of this, an IgG4 level should be checked at least once in the initial workup.[241,242] An AMA could be checked in order to rule out PBC.

Imaging of the biliary tract is the most important diagnostic step. Ultrasound is rarely helpful in obtaining a diagnosis but is, an important test for PSC care maintenance. ERCP was previously held as the gold standard for diagnosing this disease. However, because of the risk of complications such as cholangitis and pancreatitis, it has been replaced by MRCP as the diagnostic test of choice, with a diagnostic sensitivity and specificity of ≥80% and ≥87%, respectively.[240,243–245] Diagnosis may be missed with MRCP in cases of early or small duct PSC (a variant of the disease) where the ductal changes are too small to fully appreciate.[246] The characteristic cholangiogram findings are multiple short strictures alternating with normal or dilated biliary segments, producing a "beading" pattern on imaging.[245] There may also be longer strictures, termed a dominant stricture, increasing concern for an underlying cholangiocarcinoma.[247]

Liver biopsy is typically not necessary in diagnosing PSC if imaging findings confirm a diagnosis. However, if imaging findings are unrevealing, a biopsy may be performed to evaluate for small duct PSC or for PSC-AIH overlap syndrome.[246,248]

Causes of secondary sclerosing cholangitis must be excluded before a diagnosis of PSC can be made (Box 8.8).

BOX 8.8 Secondary Causes of Sclerosing Cholangitis

- AIDS cholangiopathy
- Cholangiocarcinoma
- Choledocholithiasis
- Autoimmune hepatitis
- Diffuse intrahepatic metastasis
- Eosinophilic cholangitis
- Hepatic inflammatory pseudotumor
- Histocytosis X
- IgG4-associated cholangitis
- Intra-arterial chemotherapy
- Ischemic cholangitis
- Mast cell cholangiopathy
- Portal hypertensive biliopathy
- Recurrent pancreatitis
- Recurrent pyogenic cholangitis
- Surgical biliary trauma

IgG4, immunoglobulin G4.
Source: Data from Chapman R, Fevery J, Kalloo A, et al. Diagnosis and management of primary sclerosing cholangitis. Hepatology. *2010;51(2):660–678. doi:10.1002/hep.23294*

TREATMENT AND SURVEILLANCE

There is no effective medical treatment for PSC. Endoscopic therapy with ERCP may be used in cases of rising serum bilirubin or pruritus, prompting concern for biliary obstruction, or findings of a dominant stricture on imaging. A dominant stricture is a stenosis or narrowing in the biliary ductal system ≤1.5 mm in the common bile duct or ≤1 mm in the hepatic duct.[249] This is an important finding to look out for due to the concern for the development of cholangiocarcinoma. Endoscopic brushing can help obtain cells from this area to evaluate for disease, although it has low sensitivity for diagnosis. The area can then be endoscopically dilated. There is a risk of developing cholangitis with injection of contrast agent during this procedure, so it should be performed only when absolutely necessary. Additionally, because of this risk, perioperative antibiotics during ERCP should be given.

Owing to the high association of IBD with PSC, colonoscopy with biopsies should be performed soon after PSC diagnosis to rule out concurrent asymptomatic IBD. If IBD is appreciated, PSC patients should undergo colonoscopy every 1 to 2 years.

PSC patients frequently have gallbladder abnormalities, including gallbladder polyps. These polyps run the risk of developing into gallbladder adenocarcinoma. Patients should have annual ultrasound exams performed to screen for mass lesions in the gallbladder. Cholecystectomy should be performed if any mass lesion is identified, no matter the size, due to risk of malignancy.[250]

There is an increased risk of developing cholangiocarcinoma in patients with PSC.[251] Cholangiocarcinoma is a cancer of the epithelial cells of the intra- and extrahepatic bile ducts. It is a rare malignancy but has high mortality rate due to its advanced presentation at diagnosis. For PSC patients in the United States, there is about a 1.5% risk per year of developing cholangiocarcinoma after diagnosis.[252] Additional risk factors for development of cholangiocarcinoma include smoking, alcohol use, older age, liver fluke infection, Caroli disease, choledochal cyst, bile duct adenoma, chronic intrahepatic stones, chemical agents such as vinyl chloride, and cirrhosis.[253] Cholangiocarcinoma should be suspected if PSC patients have a change in their clinical status or liver enzymes. Imaging with CT or MRCP should be utilized if cholangiocarcinoma is suspected, and ERCP should be performed to obtain brushings if a dominant stricture is appreciated. There is currently no medical therapy for cholangiocarcinoma.[254] Surgical resection is a possible option for patients with local, early disease without cirrhosis, although 3-year survival rates are still <20%.[255]

Owing to the progressive nature of this disease, there is a risk of developing portal hypertension and/or cirrhosis and its complications. Patients with advanced liver disease should be monitored for fat-soluble vitamin deficiencies.[256] Other than cirrhosis as its main indication, liver transplantation may be considered in PSC patients with intractable pruritus, recurrent bacterial cholangitis, or early stage cholangiocarcinoma.[257] Five-year survival rates for PSC patients who undergo liver transplant are approximately 85%.[258]

8.8I PRIMARY BILIARY CHOLANGITIS

OVERVIEW AND EPIDEMIOLOGY

PBC (formerly known as primary biliary cirrhosis) is a chronic, cholestatic, autoimmune disease characterized by T-lymphocyte-mediated attacks on small intralobular bile ducts, leading to their destruction and disappearance. Like PSC, it is a chronic, progressive condition that runs the risk of developing into advanced liver disease with cirrhosis and liver failure. Globally, about 1 in 1,000 women over the age of 40 have PBC.[259] It is a female-predominant disease, although men can develop this condition and the male clinical presentation is typically more severe.

PATHOPHYSIOLOGY

The exact cause of PBC is unknown but multiple mechanisms appear to contribute, including environmental, immunogenetic, and epigenetic risks.[260,261] Suggested risk factors, based on several case-control cohort studies include urinary tract infections (UTIs), reproductive hormone replacement, nail polish, and previous cigarette smoking.[262,263] T-lymphocytes attack the small intralobular bile ducts of the liver, leading to their destruction and disappearance.

MEDICAL HISTORY AND CLINICAL PRESENTATION

Like PSC, the clinical presentation of PBC ranges from an asymptomatic state with abnormal liver enzymes to portal hypertension and cirrhosis to intractable pruritus. Symptoms vary but can include fatigue, pruritus, RUQ discomfort, and jaundice.[264] Fatigue and pruritus are two major symptoms of this disorder that significantly negatively impact patient quality of life. Because of elevated lipids in this condition, patients may have xanthoma or xanthelasma on examination. Patients may have scratch marks on their body as a result of the continuous scratching. Pruritus has been reported to decline in advanced liver disease.[265]

Sjögren syndrome, CREST syndrome, scleroderma, and Raynaud disease occur more often in PBC than the general population.[266] Compared to AMA-positive PBC patients, AMA-negative PBC patients have been found to have more nonhepatic autoimmune conditions.[267]

DIAGNOSIS STUDIES

Patients will typically have an elevated ALP, signifying cholestasis. Aminotransferases may also be slightly elevated. AST/ALT elevations greater than five times the ULN may be a clue to a concurrent AIH (termed PBC/AIH overlap syndrome). AMA positivity is a key diagnostic feature of this disease; 95% of patients with PBC will have a positive AMA.[268] In 5% of cases, termed seronegative PBC, patients will not possess the antibody. A liver biopsy is not always needed for diagnosing PBC, but may be helpful in AMA-negative patients or when multiple diagnoses are suspected, such as AIH or NASH.[269] Histology from liver biopsy will typically show evidence of chronic nonsuppurative, granulomatous, lymphocytic small bile duct cholangitis.

To make a diagnosis of PBC, a patient must have two out of three features[263]:

1. Serologic evidence of cholestasis with ALP elevation
2. Presence of AMA or other PBC-specific autoantibodies (sp100 or gp210)
3. Histologic evidence of nonsuppurative cholangitis affecting the interlobular and septal bile ducts

Additional serologic features of the disease include elevated immunoglobulins (specifically IgM), elevated GGT, and elevated cholesterol levels.[270] Although this is a cholestatic condition, bilirubin may not be elevated initially. It may, however, climb in advanced liver disease and is a major predictor of poor outcomes.[271]

TREATMENT

UDCA is first-line therapy for PBC at a dose of 13 to 15 mg/kg/day once a day or in divided doses. It is used in all stages of PBC when liver enzymes are abnormal. Asymptomatic AMA-positive patients without liver enzyme abnormalities do not need UDCA. Treatment response is measured by following liver enzymes. The medication does not improve fatigue, pruritus, bone disease, or other autoimmune features seen in PBC.[263] If patients do not respond to UDCA, obeticholic acid may be considered as second-line treatment, but not in decompensated liver disease.

Cholestyramine, colestipol, and colesevelam (anion-exchange resins) may be used as first-line therapy for pruritus. If utilized, special consideration must be taken in administration times as it interferes with the absorption of UDCA. Rifampicin and opiate antagonists are second- and third-line agents for the treatment of pruritus.

Patients need to be followed lifelong for this disease. Routine monitoring of liver tests should occur every 3 to 6 months, indefinitely. Thyroid status should be assessed annually. A summary of routine PBC follow-up can be seen in Box 8.9. Men have a higher risk of developing HCC in PBC. Because of this, they should undergo routine ultrasound screening, in addition to those with cirrhosis.[272]

Like PSC, and any chronic cholestatic disease for that matter, patients should undergo routine bone mineral density testing, typically every 2 to 3 years, due to the risk of hepatic osteodystrophy. They should be given vitamin D and calcium supplementation, as necessary.

Patients may develop sicca syndrome with dry eye and mouth and may use lubricating drops and saliva substitutes, respectively. For more severe dry eye, patients should be referred to an ophthalmologist. Cyclosporine drops may have beneficial effects in dry eyes. Patients with dry mouth should follow up with a dentist due to higher risk of dental caries due to lack of lubricating saliva.

Because of the progressive nature of this disease, there is a risk of developing precirrhotic portal hypertension due to nodular regenerative hyperplasia or biliary cirrhosis and its complications.[273] Transient elastography can be utilized in evaluation of fibrosis and cirrhosis and used for disease prognosis. Cirrhosis complication management should be employed with these patients (see Section 8.8D Liver Disease, Cirrhosis, and Its Complications). Patients with advanced liver disease should be monitored for fat-soluble vitamin deficiencies.[256] Along with cirrhosis with an elevated MELD score, liver transplantation may be considered in PBC patients with intractable pruritus. Chronic fatigue does not improve after transplantation.

BOX 8.9 Routine Clinical Surveillance in Primary Biliary Cholangitis

Liver enzymes every 3–6 months
Bone mineral density assessment every 2–3 years
Fat-soluble vitamin evaluation annually if bilirubin >2.0 mg/dL
Upper endoscopy every 1–3 years if cirrhotic, Mayo risk score >4.1, or transient elastography score ≥17 kPa
Ultrasound in men, or those with known or suspected cirrhosis, every 6 months

Source: Data from Lindor KD, Bowlus CL, Boyer J, Levy C, Mayo M. Primary biliary cholangitis: 2018 practice guidance from the American Association for the Study of Liver Diseases. Hepatology. *2019;69(1):394–419.doi:10.1002/hep.30145*

8.8J AUTOIMMUNE HEPATITIS

OVERVIEW AND EPIDEMIOLOGY

AIH is a chronic, inflammatory liver disease in which circulating autoantibodies stimulate a T-cell-mediated attack upon the liver, leading to progressive inflammation and, later, fibrosis. Because there is no key feature of this disease, but rather, a constellation of variable findings, diagnosis can be difficult.

The disease may occur but present differently across all ethnic groups. There is an overall female predominance of this disease. In adults, 71% to 95% of AIH patients are women.[274]

PATHOPHYSIOLOGY

Although the pathology is not fully known, hepatic inflammation is hypothesized to be a result of environmental triggers, upregulated immune mechanisms, and a genetic predisposition that trigger immune and autoimmune processes.

MEDICAL HISTORY AND CLINICAL PRESENTATION

Patient presentation may vary from an asymptomatic individual with incidentally noted abnormal liver enzymes to a patient presenting with ALF to a patient with cirrhosis of unknown etiology. Patients may be asymptomatic in up to 34% of cases.[275] From 25% to 75% of patients may have an acute presentation, with ALF occurring in 3% to 6% of North American and European patients.[276,277]

Frequently, patients may have concurrent autoimmune diseases such as autoimmune thyroid disease, celiac disease, or autoimmune skin disease (vitiligo, leukocytoclastic vasculitis, alopecia areata).[278] Additionally, there may be clinical overlap with other autoimmune hepatic diseases such as PBC and PSC based on cholestatic liver abnormalities or histologic findings concerning for either disease in addition to AIH. Drug-induced liver injury (DILI) may also mimic AIH, with the most common drugs implicated being minocycline, nitrofurantoin, and infliximab.[279]

PHYSICAL EXAMINATION

Patients may initially have nonspecific symptoms such as fatigue, nausea, jaundice, abdominal pain, or arthralgias.[280] Physical examination is typically unhelpful, unless there are signs of advanced chronic liver disease (e.g., telangiectasias, splenomegaly, ascites).

DIAGNOSTIC STUDIES

Diagnosis of AIH requires the presence of multiple clinical, laboratory, and histologic features and the exclusion of other causes of liver disease. Laboratory abnormalities include elevated aminotransferases, elevated serum immunoglobulins (typically IgG), and the presence of characteristic autoantibodies.[281] Patients may show IgG4 positivity.[282] Histologic findings may include interface hepatitis, or a lymphoplasmacytic infiltration surrounding the portal triad spreading into the surrounding lobule, plasma cell infiltration, lobular hepatitis, and centrilobular necrosis.[283] Autoantibodies that may be elevated include antinuclear antibodies (ANA), smooth muscle antibodies (anti-actin antibodies), or liver kidney microsome type 1 (anti-LKM1), although up to 20% of cases will be negative for all three autoantibodies (seronegative AIH).[284] Because of the nonspecific presentation and high proportion of seronegative AIH, liver biopsy is necessary to make a full diagnosis of AIH. Histologic assessment is also helpful in identifying or excluding other diagnoses, grading the inflammation severity, and assessing for signs of and severity of fibrosis. Scoring systems may be helpful in making a diagnosis in complex cases.[285]

Because of its association with other autoimmune diseases, patients with AIH should be screened for celiac and thyroid disease at the time of diagnosis. Additionally, if the patient shows signs or symptoms of other autoimmune diseases such as IBD, diabetes, or rheumatoid arthritis, further investigation should be performed.[286]

TREATMENT

Treatment of AIH involves immunosuppressive therapy. First-line induction therapy includes prednisone with azathioprine (AZA). The goal of therapy is for normalization of liver enzymes and IgG levels, termed biochemical remission.[287] If remission is achieved, prednisone may be gradually reduced, with close monitoring of biochemical tests. AZA is continued indefinitely. Thiopurine methyltransferase (TPMT) enzyme activity should be evaluated prior to initiation of AZA therapy due to risk of toxic metabolite buildup if the enzyme activity is low. Toxicity of AZA therapy include leukopenia or thrombocytopenia. Therapy is typically lifelong due to risk of relapse.

Glucocorticoid therapy alone should be considered in patients who present with acute severe AIH or ALF.[286] Patients with ALF should be immediately evaluated for liver transplant. Patients with acute severe AIH who do not respond to glucocorticoids should also be evaluated for transplant.

Because AIH treatment involves immunosuppressive therapy, patients should receive routine vaccinations prior to initiation of therapy, especially live, attenuated vaccinations. This includes hepatitis A and hepatitis B vaccination if patients are not already immune.[288] HBsAg-negative/anti-HBc-positive patients should undergo periodic serologic monitoring of HBsAg and HBV DNA during immunosuppressive therapy to detect HBV reactivation and the need for antiviral therapy, since they are at moderate risk of hepatitis B reactivation.[204]

Patients with risk factors for osteoporosis should undergo routine bone mineral density testing, typically every 2 to 3 years. They should be given vitamin D and calcium supplementation, if necessary. Bisphosphonates may be used in patients with osteoporosis and osteopenia.

Routine care and monitoring should occur for patients with concomitant cirrhosis (see Section 8.8D Liver Disease, Cirrhosis, and Its Complications).

8.8K DRUG-INDUCED LIVER INJURY

OVERVIEW AND EPIDEMIOLOGY

DILI is a common but difficult-to-diagnose condition. It accounts for about 10% of all cases of acute hepatitis.[289] It is the most common cause of ALF in the United States, with acetaminophen being the most common culprit medication.[158,290] Medications, herbal therapies, vitamins, and supplements are all potential injurious sources. Drugs may either cause an intrinsic (dose-based, such as with acetaminophen) or idiosyncratic (unpredictable) reaction. After acetaminophen, the next most common medications to cause DILI in the United States are antibiotics and antiepileptics.[291] Female sex, age, malnutrition, and alcohol abuse may increase a person's risk for developing DILI, although data are not robust.

MEDICAL HISTORY AND CLINICAL PRESENTATION

DILI will typically present within the first 6 months of starting a new medication, although some medications may have a longer latency period. Patient presentations range from asymptomatic with abnormal liver enzymes to jaundice and pruritus, to ALF.

SIGNS AND SYMPTOMS

Typical symptoms include fatigue, anorexia, nausea, vomiting, low-grade fever, RUQ abdominal pain, jaundice, dark urine, and pruritus. Patients may have hepatomegaly on exam. Patients with coagulopathy as a result of abnormal liver synthetic dysfunction may show signs of easy bruising or bleeding. Patients with ALF will develop encephalopathy.

DIAGNOSTIC STUDIES

DILI remains a diagnosis of exclusion. Clinicians must take into account other etiologies of liver disease that could be the cause or additive to the patient's presentation. It is paramount to obtain a full medication, vitamin, supplement, and herbal history from a patient, even with drugs that were taken on an as-needed basis or only once. Please refer to Section 8.8A Approach to Abnormal Liver Enzymes for recommended laboratory and imaging evaluations.

Evaluating the latency, type of injury (hepatocellular versus cholestatic), and outcome of the injury can be helpful in determining if the drug is the culprit in the liver injury. An R-value is a measurement to assess the type of injury pattern. Table 8.28 displays the calculation and categorization of injury. Table 8.29 organizes the most common drugs implicated in DILI and their typical hepatic injury patterns. This is not an exhaustive list of all the causes of DILI and many potential drugs or herbal therapies are not included. The National Library of Medicine's *LiverTox* website (www.livertox.nih.gov) is a helpful, free resource that allows one to search a concerning medication and receive detailed information about the possibility of injury and pattern of injury.[292]

In asymptomatic cases, avoidance of the proposed offending agent is a possible test of determining if the medication

TABLE 8.28 Calculation of R-Value in Assessment of Drug-Induced Liver Injury

R = ALT/ULN ALT ÷ ALP/ULN ALP	Type of Injury
R >5	Hepatocellular
R = 2–5	Mixed injury pattern
R <2	Cholestatic

ALP, alkaline phosphatase; ALT, alanine aminotransferase; ULN, upper limit of normal.

TABLE 8.29 Common Medications and Herbal Supplements Implicated in Drug-Induced Liver Injury, Organized Based on Hepatic Injury Pattern

Hepatocellular	Mixed	Cholestatic
Isoniazid	Fluoroquinolones	Amoxicillin/clavulanic acid
Macrolides	Phenytoin	Trimethoprim/sulfamethoxazole
Nitrofurantoin	Carbamazepine	Anabolic steroids
Minocycline	Azathioprine	Amiodarone
Lamotrigine		Azathioprine
Valproate		Erythromycin
NSAIDs		
Allopurinol		
Green tea extract (catechin)		
Kava kava		

NSAIDs, nonsteroidal anti-inflammatory drugs.

was the culprit. By following liver chemistries and allowing a "washout" period, one may be able to determine that the removed drug was the offending agent. Cholestatic injuries typically take longer to resolve than hepatocellular injuries.

Liver biopsy may be considered when diagnosis remains uncertain or when multiple competing diagnoses are present. Typically, if liver enzymes have not fallen by 50% within 60 or 180 days of stopping the hypothesized offending drug, one should consider liver biopsy.[293] Rechallenging a patient with the suspected offending drug is not advised because of the risk of rapid and severe recurrence of liver injury.[294]

TREATMENT

Withdrawal of the offending agent is the treatment of choice for DILI. NAC infusion is specifically used in acetaminophen toxicity and L-carnitine may be used in cases of valproic acid overdose. Liver enzymes should be followed periodically until they return to normal. Up to 13.6% of patients may develop chronic DILI, especially patients with a cholestatic injury pattern.[295] Hepatology consult may be considered if the cause is not clear, there is concern for chronic DILI or chronic liver disease, or the patient is developing ALF. Patients with signs of ALF (coagulopathy and encephalopathy) should be transferred to a tertiary care center that has the ability to perform liver transplantation, if necessary.

8.9 METABOLIC LIVER DISEASES

8.9A HEMOCHROMATOSIS

OVERVIEW AND EPIDEMIOLOGY

Hemochromatosis, a disease of iron overload, is a condition with primary and secondary causes (Table 8.30).[296] HH is a genetic disorder due to iron overload through increased iron absorption. It is the most common genetic disorder in Caucasians, particularly in patients of northern European descent. Estimated prevalence is 1 per 250 individuals.[297] HH-related iron overload can be primarily broken down into *HFE*-related and non-*HFE*-related forms.

TABLE 8.30 Causes of Iron Overload

Type of Iron Overload	Cause
Hereditary hemochromatosis	*HFE*-related
	C282Y/C282Y
	C282Y/H63D
	Other *HFE* mutations
	Non-*HFE*-related
	Hemojuvelin (*HJV*)
	Transferrin receptor-2 (*TfR2*)
	Ferroportin (*SLC40A1*)
	Hepcidin (*HAMP*)
	African iron overload
Secondary iron overload	Iron-loading anemias/ineffective erythropoeisis
	Thalassemia major
	Sideroblastic anemic
	hemolytic anemia
	Aplastic anemia
	Pyruvate kinase deficiency
	Pyridoxine-responsive anemia
	Parenteral iron overload (iatrogenic)
	Red blood cell transfusions
	Iron-dextran injections
	Long-term hemodialysis
	Chronic liver disease
	Porphyria cutanea tarda
	Hepatitis C
	Hepatitis B
	Alcoholic liver disease
	Nonalcoholic fatty liver disease
	Portacaval shunt
	Dysmetabolic iron overload syndrome
Miscellaneous	Neonatal iron overload
	Aceruloplasminemia
	Congenital atransferrinemia

Source: Data from Phatak PD, Bonkovsky HL, Kowdley KV. Hereditary hemochromatosis: time for targeted screening. Ann Intern Med. *2008;149(4):270–272. doi:10.7326/0003-4819-149-4-200808190-00009*

The *HFE* gene defect on chromosome 6 affects protein product C282Y.[298] *HFE*-related HH is an autosomal recessive disorder with C282Y mutation homozygotes (C282Y/C282Y) accounting for 85% to 90% of patients presenting with HH. A small proportion of *HFE*-related iron overload patients are compound heterozygotes (C282Y/H63D).[299] The remaining 10% to 15% of patients with HH related iron-overload (non-*HFE*-related) have mutations in other genes involved in iron homeostasis.[300]

Currently, screening of family members or of individuals with abnormal liver tests has led to increased identification of this disorder. Prior to screening becoming more widely used, patients were typically identified through symptoms and physical exam findings of this disease, with women, on average, being identified approximately 10 years later due to the proposed "protective" effect of blood and iron loss through menstruation.

Because of its higher prevalence compared to other forms of iron overload, *HFE*-related HH will be the main focus in this subsection with consideration of alternative causes being done when evaluating a patient with iron overload.

PATHOPHYSIOLOGY

The development of iron overload and subsequent liver damage in HH is multifaceted. The four main mechanisms of iron overload development include (1) increased intestinal dietary iron absorption, (2) decreased expression of hepcidin, (3) altered function of the HFE protein, and (4) iron-induced tissue injury.

Iron is primarily absorbed in the duodenum.[301] It is first absorbed along the apical membrane of the enterocyte and transferred across the basolateral membrane. Iron that is absorbed is either stored as ferritin in the enterocyte or transferred across the basolateral membrane to the plasma via the transporter ferroportin. Patients with *HFE*-related HH have increased basolateral transfer of iron from the enterocytes to the plasma.[302]

Hepcidin is an iron-regulatory hormone. Normally, hepcidin is secreted by hepatocytes into the circulation. In states of iron excess or in inflammation, hepcidin will bind to ferroportin, a molecule found in macrophages and on the basolateral surface of enterocytes. By binding to ferroportin, the molecule is then internalized and degraded, preventing the ferroportin from binding intestinal iron and its subsequent release of iron into the enterocyte and macrophage which is then exported into the circulation.[303,304,305]

MEDICAL HISTORY AND CLINICAL PRESENTATION

As mentioned previously, C282Y homozygosity significantly increases one's chance to develop symptomatic HH. The prevalence of C282Y homozygosity is approximately 1 in 250 Caucasians. However, fully expressed disease (phenotypic expression) with end-organ manifestations is seen in <10% of these individuals (incomplete clinical penetrance).[306,307] Symptomatic *HFE*-related HH typically presents around age 40 to 50 but may be appreciated later in women due to menses and childbirth.

SIGNS AND SYMPTOMS

Potential symptoms of this disorder are not specific but may include fatigue, RUQ abdominal pain, arthralgias (typically the second and third metacarpophalangeal joints), chondrocalcinosis, impotence, decreased libido, and symptoms of heart failure or diabetes. Physical examination findings may include enlarged liver, extrahepatic manifestations of chronic liver disease (see Table 8.22), testicular atrophy, congestive heart failure, skin hyperpigmentation ("bronze diabetes"), or arthritis.

DIAGNOSTIC STUDIES

Diagnosis of hemochromatosis is made based on increased iron stores, manifested by increased serum ferritin or transferrin saturation (TS) levels. Further evaluation for HH can be made through *HFE* gene testing to evaluate C282Y status (C282Y homozygosity or C282Y/H63D heterozygosity). The initial approach evaluates indirect markers of iron storage: TS and serum ferritin. TS is the ratio of serum iron to total iron-binding capacity. A TS value of 45% or greater should prompt further evaluation for a syndrome of iron overload. Serum ferritin is also elevated in this condition but is a less specific laboratory value as it can be elevated in conditions that cause inflammation. However, if either TS or ferritin is abnormal, it should prompt performing *HFE* gene mutation analysis. Family screening is also recommended for all first-degree relatives of patients with HH (*HFE* mutation analysis, ferritin, and TS).

Liver biopsy is currently rarely used in the diagnosis of HH but can be used to evaluate for the presence of fibrosis or cirrhosis to aid in disease prognostication, especially in patients without identified genetic susceptibility. Biopsy may also aid in determining hepatic iron concentration and location of iron deposition to better determine the cause of iron overload. A serum ferritin level >1,000 mcg/L is associated with an increased risk of cirrhosis or advanced fibrosis. The AASLD recommends liver biopsy for disease staging in C282Y homozygotes or compound heterozygotes if ferritin is >1,000 mcg/L or if liver enzymes are abnormal.[296]

TREATMENT

Phlebotomy is the mainstay of treatment of hemochromatosis, and has shown improvement in morbidity and mortality in those who have not yet developed cirrhosis and/or diabetes.[308] It should be performed in any person with labs or symptoms consistent with iron overload. A summary of treatment of hemochromatosis, adapted from the AASLD 2011 guidelines, can be appreciated in Box 8.10.

One unit of blood contains 200–250 mg of iron. Typically, patients will have a unit of blood removed once or twice per week, as hemoglobin allows. Serum ferritin is followed during the initial stages of phlebotomy with a goal level between 50 and 100 mcg/L. Iron deficiency should be avoided. Depending on the level of iron overload, therapeutic phlebotomy may take up to 2 to 3 years to adequately reduce iron stores. After ferritin and TS levels are appropriate, patients may undergo routine serum monitoring to determine when maintenance phlebotomy may be helpful. Blood acquired from therapeutic phlebotomy has been deemed safe for donation and transfusion by the American Red Cross and FDA.[309]

Symptoms such as malaise, fatigue, skin pigmentation, insulin requirement in diabetics, and abdominal pain may

BOX 8.10 Treatment of Hemochromatosis

Hereditary hemochromatosis
One phlebotomy (removal of 500 mL of blood) weekly or biweekly
Check Hct/Hb prior to each phlebotomy
Allow Hct/Hb to fall by no more than 20% of prior level
Check serum ferritin level every 10–12 phlebotomies
Stop frequent phlebotomy when serum ferritin reaches 50–100 mcg/L
Continue phlebotomy at intervals to keep serum ferritin between 50 and 100 mcg/L
Avoid vitamin C supplements
Secondary iron overload due to disorders of erythropoiesis
Deferoxamine at doses of 20–40 mg/kg body weight per day
Deferasirox given orally
Consider follow-up liver biopsy to ascertain adequacy of iron removal
Avoid vitamin C supplements

Hb, hemoglobin; Hct, hematocrit.

Source: Data from Phatak PD, Bonkovsky HL, Kowdley KV. Hereditary hemochromatosis: time for targeted screening. Ann Intern Med. *2008;149(4):270–272. doi:10.7326/0003-4819-149-4-200808190-00009*

improve with phlebotomy. Hepatic fibrosis and cirrhosis may regress with phlebotomy, although this is not universal.[310] Advanced cirrhosis is not reversed with iron removal. Patients who develop decompensated cirrhosis should potentially be referred for liver transplantation. Unfortunately, arthropathy, hypogonadism, and advanced cirrhosis typically do not respond if they had developed prior to treatment initiation.

Iron chelation therapy with parenteral deferoxamine is the treatment of choice for secondary iron overload syndromes that involve ineffective erythropoiesis. This therapy can be challenging due to the high cost of the drug, the need to use it as an infusion, and its neurotoxicity. Deferasirox, an oral iron-chelating drug, has recently been approved in the United States as well but has multiple potentially serious side effects including hepatic failure, GI bleeding, and renal injury.

Patients with HH and advanced fibrosis or cirrhosis are at increased risks of developing HCC, even after successful phlebotomy.[311] They should be screened regularly for HCC per AASLD guidelines.[272]

8.9B WILSON DISEASE

OVERVIEW, EPIDEMIOLOGY, AND PATHOPHYSIOLOGY

Copper is an essential metal that is a cofactor for many proteins. It is absorbed in the enterocytes in the duodenum and proximal small intestine and is transported to the liver via the portal circulation by binding to albumin and the amino acid histidine. The liver uses copper for its own function but also creates and secretes the copper-containing protein, ceruloplasmin. Unused copper is excreted into bile. A small amount of copper is excreted in urine.

Wilson disease is an autosomal recessive disorder that leads to absent or reduced function of the ATP7B protein due to an abnormal *ATP7B* gene on chromosome 13.[312] This causes impaired hepatocellular excretion of copper into bile, leading to hepatic copper accumulation and injury and eventual copper deposition into other body tissues via copper release into the bloodstream. Additionally, copper is not incorporated into ceruloplasmin correctly.

The prevalence of disease is approximately 30 affected individuals per 1 million people.[313]

MEDICAL HISTORY, CLINICAL PRESENTATION AND PHYSICAL EXAMINATION

The consequences of Wilson disease can be explained based on where copper primarily deposits in the body, typically the liver, cornea, and brain. This is no one clinical picture of a Wilson disease patient as patients frequently do not have all organ systems affected. A list of the possible clinical features of Wilson disease can be seen in Table 8.31. Typically, patients will manifest liver disease at a younger age (as young as 1 year old) than those typically diagnosed with chronic liver disease, but the disease can present at any age. Liver disease manifestations can be variable, ranging from only mild liver enzyme abnormalities to fulminant hepatic failure.

Wilson disease may present with fulminant hepatic failure, with severe coagulopathy or encephalopathy. A key laboratory feature of wilsonian fulminant hepatic failure may include an incongruency between the serum TB (typically higher than expected due to hemolysis) and ALP (typically low or normal range for patient's age). Additionally, the AST may be significantly higher than the ALT due to hepatic mitochondrial injury.

TABLE 8.31 Possible Clinical Features of Wilson Disease

Organ System	Clinical Features
Hepatic	Hepatomegaly Splenomegaly Elevated serum aminotransferases Fatty liver Acute hepatitis Labs similar to autoimmune hepatitis Cirrhosis Acute liver failure
Neurologic	Movement disorders (tremor, involuntary movements) Rigid dystonia Drooling Dysarthria Pseudobulbar palsy Dysautonomia Migraine Insomnia Seizures (rare)
Psychiatric	Depression Personality changes Neurosis Psychosis
Other systems	Ocular: Kayser-Fleischer rings, sunflower cataracts Renal: Aminoaciduria and nephrolithiasis Skeletal: Osteoporosis and arthritis Cutaneous: Lunulae ceruleae Hematologic: Hemolytic anemia Cardiac: Cardiomyopathy, dysrhythmias Gastrointestinal: Pancreatitis Endocrine: Hypoparathyroidism, menstrual irregularities, infertility, repeated miscarriages

Kayser-Fleischer (KF) rings are an ocular manifestation of this condition, although not specific to this disease. KF rings may also be seen in some chronic cholestatic liver diseases like PBC, PSC, or familial cholestatic syndromes. They are not necessary for making the diagnosis of Wilson disease. Slit-lamp examination will reveal the presence of these copper deposits within the Descemet membrane of the cornea.

DIAGNOSTIC STUDIES

Because of the wide range of presentations and severity, thinking about and making a diagnosis of Wilson disease can be difficult and, at times, frustrating. Multiple tests can aid in diagnosis, but few can make a diagnosis alone. Important factors that can help contribute to a diagnosis include the presence of KF rings, ceruloplasmin <20 mg/dL, or 24-hour urinary copper excretion >40 mcg.

A low serum ceruloplasmin can aid in diagnosis of this disorder but, by itself, is insufficient to make a certain diagnosis as it can be decreased due to multiple other conditions such as intestinal malabsorption, nephrotic syndrome, and malnutrition. Additionally, patients with Wilson disease can have normal to elevated serum ceruloplasmin levels due to hepatic inflammation. Urinary cooper excretion can be elevated in Wilson disease, making 24-hour urinary copper analysis helpful in making a diagnosis. Performing a provocative test with D-penicillamine administration followed by 24-hour urinary copper collection can further aid in diagnosis. A level of 25 μmol or greater in 24 hours is diagnostic for Wilson disease, although it lacks sensitivity.[314]

Liver biopsy may be necessary when all three diagnostic criteria aren't present at once. Hepatic tissue copper concentration, obtained via liver biopsy, may also aid in diagnosis. Classic liver biopsy specimens show interface hepatitis.

TREATMENT

- There are three main lifelong therapies for Wilson disease: chelation with D-penicillamine, trientine, and zinc. Outcomes are best when patients are identified and treated early, prior to the onset of symptoms. Table 8.32 lists the medications, mechanism of action, doses, and side effects for treatment of Wilson disease.[315]
- Medication efficacy monitoring using any of these therapies involves measuring 24-hour urinary copper. Urine copper excretion values <200 mcg/day may indicate noncompliance with therapy or overtreatment. A confirmatory test involves measuring non-ceruloplasmin-bound copper. Elevated values (>15 mcg/dL) are consistent with nonadherence and low values (<5 mcg/dL) are consistent with overtreatment.
- Dietary elimination of copper-rich foods such as organ meats, shellfish, nuts, chocolate, and mushrooms can further aid in management of this disease, but should not be the mainstay of treatment. These foods should be avoided for at least the first year of treatment.
- Routine clinical monitoring should occur at least twice per year after copper levels have been initially stabilized to monitor treatment side effects and for signs of hepatic, psychiatric, or neurologic worsening. Patients may require more frequent monitoring at the initiation of chelation therapy.
- Patients require lifelong chelation treatment to prevent further copper deposition and typically do very well if therapy is continued and tolerated. Frequently, hepatic disease may improve but neurologic Wilson disease may not entirely improve. Therapy should never be interrupted or discontinued (even in pregnancy) as this could lead to the development of intractable liver failure.[316] Liver transplant plays a limited role in disease treatment but is the treatment of choice in fulminant hepatic failure. Patients with neurologic or psychiatric Wilson disease have poorer liver transplant outcomes.[317]

8.9C HEPATIC VENOUS OUTFLOW TRACT OBSTRUCTION

OVERVIEW AND EPIDEMIOLOGY

Hepatic venous outflow tract obstruction, or BCS, is an obstruction of flow through the hepatic veins. Primary BCS involves occlusion of the hepatic vein by thrombus or phlebitis, while secondary hepatic venous obstruction may be due to other factors such as external vein compression or invasion by malignancy. Hepatic venous outflow may also be caused or influenced by cardiac disease, pericardial disease, or sinusoidal obstruction syndrome.[318]

This condition is more common in women in their third or fourth decade of life in non-Asian countries, while Asian countries show a male predominance occurring in the fifth decade of life.[319,320]

PATHOPHYSIOLOGY

Obstruction may occur at one or multiple areas of the hepatic venous system including small hepatic veins, large hepatic veins, or the inferior vena cava (IVC).[321] The disease may be categorized further based on timing and severity. Presentations may range from ALF to subacute to chronic disease. ALF is seen in about 5% of cases, while an additional 20% are acute, nonfulminant cases.[318] Typically, an underlying risk factor for thrombosis is found in up to 87% of patients, usually from a myeloproliferative disorder or hypercoagulable state.[322]

TABLE 8.32 Overview of Available Treatments for Wilson Disease

Drug	Mechanism of Action	Dose	Potential Side Effects
D-penicillamine	Increases urinary excretion of copper; inhibits collagen cross-linking	Initial: 1–1.5 g/day (adults) or 20 mg/kg/day (children) divided into 2–3 doses Maintenance: 0.75–1 g/day as needed to maintain appropriate copper levels *Note:* Consider dose reduction during pregnancy and surgery to promote wound healing	May have worsened neurologic symptoms with initiation of treatment,[316] risk of immunosuppression, rash, pemphigus, elastosis perforans serpiginosa, hypothyroidism, loss of taste, gastrointestinal upset, aplastic anemia, leukopenia, lupus-like syndrome, thrombocytopenia, hepatotoxicity, proteinuria *Note:* Excreted in breast mild; women should not breast-feed while taking this medication
Trientine	Increases urinary copper excretion; may interfere with intestinal copper absorption	Initial and maintenance: 1–1.2 g/day divided into 2–3 doses Consider dose reduction during pregnancy and surgery to promote wound healing	Less significant toxicity, gastritis, iron deficiency, bone marrow suppression
Zinc	Interferes with absorption of copper from the GI tract; increases copper excretion in stool	Initial: 150 mg elemental zinc in 3 divided doses (adults) Maintenance: Titrate dose based on urinary copper levels	Risk of neurologic deterioration during initial treatment, gastritis, possible immunosuppression, clinically insignificant elevations in serum lipase

MEDICAL HISTORY, CLINICAL PRESENTATION, AND PHYSICAL EXAMINATION

Symptoms vary depending on the acuity of the obstruction. Patients with an acute presentation may have fever, abdominal pain, abdominal distention due to ascites, lower extremity edema, GI bleeding as a result of portal hypertension, or HE as a result of altered blood flow to the brain.[320] Those with a subacute or chronic presentation may be asymptomatic or have nonspecific symptoms, since the slow, progressive process of obstruction may have allowed the body to generate collateral blood flow. Multiple subcutaneous veins may be prominent on examination in patients with IVC obstruction.

DIAGNOSTIC STUDIES

Diagnosis is made by hepatic venous imaging, typically by Doppler ultrasound demonstrating decreased or absent flow in the large hepatic vein, or even retrograde or turbulent flow. Collateral vessels may be appreciated on imaging. The portal and splenic veins should also be evaluated to exclude additional thrombi as well as for signs of malignancy.

TREATMENT

- Indefinite anticoagulation therapy is recommended in cases of idiopathic DVT, especially if the underlying hypercoagulable disorder is not identified or curable.[323] There is minimal data regarding anticoagulation in patients with BCS, so the recommendation of indefinite anticoagulation is generalized to this group as well.
  - If a myeloproliferative disorder is found, attempts should be made to treat the disorder.
  - The AASLD recommended in their 2009 guidelines to initiate permanent anticoagulation therapy in patients with BCS and attempt to correct underlying risk factors for venous thrombosis, if possible.[318]
- Some patients' findings may be amenable to more invasive treatment strategies such as angioplasty, stenting, or portosystemic shunting. However, decision for undergoing these procedures should be made by a multidisciplinary team.
- Oral contraceptives are contraindicated in patients with primary BCS. Pregnancy may be considered in the setting of anticoagulation during gestation, although robust data on successful pregnancies are not available other than a few case reports.
- Complications of thrombosis and portal hypertension should utilize a treatment strategy similar to portal hypertension treatment in cirrhosis. Patients with thrombosis who do not improve over time may require TIPS or even liver transplantation.

8.9D LIVER LESIONS

OVERVIEW

There are many potential causes of lesions in the liver. Lesions can be solid, cystic, or a combination of the two. The differential diagnosis is broad for both types with different management based on the diagnosis. In addition to a thorough history and physical exam, imaging modality and radiographic interpretation are key components of identification and management. Because of such a broad differential diagnosis, only brief descriptions of the most common lesions will be mentioned below.

A cystic lesion is a predominately fluid-containing lesion. It can be further categorized into simple and complex cystic lesions. Simple cysts have no evidence of features such as septations or surface irregularity, while complex cysts do. Simple and complex cysts can be singular or multifocal. Table 8.33 displays the differential diagnosis for cystic lesions.

Solid lesions appreciated on radiographic imaging have a different differential diagnosis, which is listed in Table 8.34.

Hepatic hemangiomas, the most common cause of benign solid hepatic lesions, are benign vascular lesions of unknown etiology, thought to arise from congenital hamartomas. They are typically discovered incidentally during imaging for other purposes or during surgery, as most patients are asymptomatic. Ultrasound studies indicated a frequency of this finding in about 0.7% to 1.5% of the population.[325] They occur more frequently in women than men, with a 3:1 female-male ratio.[326] These lesions typically are asymptomatic and usually do not expand over time. They do not require follow-up imaging unless the patient were to become symptomatic.

Focal nodular hyperplasia (FNH), the second most common etiology of solid hepatic lesions, occurs most commonly in women ages 30 to 50.[327] They are caused by injury to the portal tract leading to the formation of arteriovenous shunts. This thereby leads to hyperperfusion of local arteries causing

TABLE 8.33 Differential Diagnosis for Cystic Liver Lesions

Type of Cystic Liver Lesion*	Differential Diagnosis	
Simple	Benign developmental hepatic cyst Biliary hamartoma (von Meyenburg complex) Caroli disease Adult polycystic liver disease	
Complex	Neoplasm	Biliary cystadenoma or cystadenocarcinoma Cystic metastases Hepatocellular carcinoma Cavernous hemangioma Embryonal sarcoma
	Infectious or inflammatory	Abscess Pyogenic Amebic Echinococcal cyst
	Posttraumatic and miscellaneous	Pseudocyst Hematoma Biloma Infected or hemorrhagic cysts

Cystic lesions are first categorized as "simple" or "cystic" and further categorized by etiologic class.

Source: Vachha B, Sun MR, Siewert B, Eisenberg RL. Cystic lesions of the liver. AJR Am J Roentgenol. 2011;196(4):W355–W366. doi:10.2214/AJR.10.5292

TABLE 8.34 Differential Diagnosis for Solid Liver Lesions

Type of Solid Liver Lesion*	Diagnosis
Benign	Hepatic hemangioma Focal nodular hyperplasia Hepatic adenoma Idiopathic noncirrhotic portal hypertension and nodular regenerative hyperplasia Regenerative nodules Inflammatory pseudotumor (rare)
Malignant	Hepatocellular carcinoma Cholangiocarcinoma Metastatic disease Soft tissue sarcomas (rare) Fibrolamellar carcinoma (rare) Hepatoblastoma (rare) Non-Hodgkin lymphoma (rare)

**Lesions are organized by "benign" or "malignant" etiologies. More common causes are listed first.*

local tissue injury and hepatic stellate cell activation.[328] A central scar on imaging is highly suggestive of this condition. Like hepatic hemangiomas, management should be conservative after diagnosis of FNH has been made in asymptomatic patients. Surgical resection, embolization, and radiofrequency ablation are possible options for treatment of symptomatic lesions. The American College of Gastroenterology recommends follow-up with annual abdominal ultrasound for 2 to 3 years in women diagnosed with FNH on oral contraceptive pills (OCPs) but not in women off OCPs.[329]

Hepatocellular adenomas are benign hepatic neoplasms. These lesions are more likely than hemangiomas and FNH to present symptomatically.[330] These lesions have a risk of rupturing and bleeding. Because there is a hormonal association, these lesions may grow in size during pregnancy, although it is not a contraindication to pregnancy if the lesions are <5 cm.[328] Although benign, there is a small risk of these lesions transforming into HCC. Resection should be considered when adenomas are ≥5 cm, while those <5 cm may be managed conservatively. They should be reimaged with CT or MRI every 6 months for at least 2 years to evaluate growth patterns and radiographic findings concerning for cancer. OCPs, anabolic steroids, and hormone-containing intrauterine devices should be avoided in patients with this type of lesion.

Simple cysts are fluid-containing lesions with smooth, thin walls and no findings of complex internal features such as septation, calcification, or nodularity.[324] They have well-defined margins and smooth walls on imaging and do not require further workup or treatment.

Hepatic abscesses are localized collections of pus in the liver. They can be pyogenic, amebic, or fungal. Pyogenic abscesses are typically a result of complications of direct spread from biliary tract disease such as ascending cholangitis or indirect spread via the circulation to the portal vein (portal phlebitis), such as from peritonitis or hematogenous seeding. Typically, the pathogens are polymicrobial, from gram-positive or gram-negative organisms or anaerobes, especially if the abscess is a result of peritonitis from a ruptured colonic diverticulum. Typical symptoms include RUQ pain and fever, but other symptoms include nausea or vomiting. Liver enzymes may be abnormal as a result of the disruption in the liver parenchyma.[331] Patients may also have a leukocytosis or anemia as a result of the infection. Imaging of the area, typically an ultrasound or CT scan with IV contrast is indicated as part of the evaluation for this condition. Blood cultures should also be checked, as they are positive in up to 50% of cases of pyogenic liver abscess.[332] Treatment involves CT or ultrasound-guided aspiration and drainage of the lesion in order to identify the pathogen and control the infection. Aspirate should be sent for Gram stain and culture. Antibiotic therapy is driven by the specific organism and resistance patterns gained by culture. The initial empiric antibiotic coverage should take into account the likely source of the abscess but also be broad-spectrum and parenteral. Typical regimens include a third-generation cephalosporin plus metronidazole, a beta-lactam/beta-lactamase inhibitor combination (e.g., piperacillin-tazobactam) with or without metronidazole for *Entameba histolytica* (amebic abscess) coverage, or ampicillin plus gentamicin plus metronidazole. Clinicians should consider adding vancomycin to the regimen if *Staphylococcus aureus* is a concern. The antibiotic regimen can then be tailored based on blood and aspirate culture results. Antibiotics should be continued for 4 to 6 weeks based on the patient's clinical response.[333]

Echinococcal cysts, or hydatid cysts, are caused by *Echinococcus granulosis* or *E. multilocularis*. Patients may present with abdominal pain or jaundice. History may be notable for travel to an endemic area such as the Mediterranean or contact with sheep. Laboratory findings may show eosinophilia, positive serology. These cysts have risk of rupture, producing biliary colic, obstructive jaundice, cholangitis, pancreatitis, peritonitis, or acute hypersensitivity reaction, including anaphylaxis. Diagnosis can be made with a combination of imaging and serology.[334] Treatment involves medical therapy with albendazole, but surgical resection or liver transplantation may be considered in complicated cases such as in rupture or complicated cysts.[335]

MEDICAL HISTORY, CLINICAL PRESENTATION, AND PHYSICAL EXAMINATION

Many solid lesions are found incidentally during imaging for other reasons. Frequently, they are also asymptomatic but can potentially lead to symptoms such as pain, pruritus, palpable mass, fever, weight loss, or early satiety.

DIAGNOSTIC STUDIES

Most liver lesions can be identified through thorough history, physical exam, laboratory assessment, and imaging. Imaging findings of multiple solid lesions concerning for metastatic disease may prompt further body imaging or laboratory assessment to determine the primary source of the metastatic lesion.

Contrast-enhanced multiphased CT or MRI may be helpful in better identifying the characteristics, size, and relative location of the lesion. Ultrasound can also be used to evaluate lesions, although image quality may not be adequate to fully determine the etiology of the lesion. Contrast enhancement during ultrasound can be a helpful tool in better evaluating lesions.

The size of a solid lesion is an important factor to consider in helping determine the etiology and follow-up plan. Lesions <1 cm are typically benign findings and may be harder to characterize radiographically.[336]

If initial workup cannot secure a diagnosis, lesion biopsy can be considered provided that this would change the patient's management.

TREATMENT

Treatment and surveillance of lesions depend on each individual etiology of the lesion. The typical treatment recommendations are outlined above.

KEY POINTS

- A patient's history and physical examination are the most important tools to utilize when assessing liver enzyme abnormalities. A thorough history and exam should be obtained prior to testing and to guide further testing.
- Cirrhosis is a multifaceted disease with multiple causes and complications. Careful attention should assess for the presence of more severe, or decompensating, complications such as ascites, encephalopathy, varices, and HCC.
- Many patients with conditions that increase their risk of developing cirrhosis may slow or prevent progression with proper treatment and surveillance.
- The differential diagnosis of liver lesions is broad, and accurate diagnosis, treatment, and surveillance of the lesion are dependent on the patient's history and imaging characteristics.

8.10 DISEASES OF THE PANCREAS

OVERVIEW

Pancreatitis refers to inflammation of the pancreas. Episodes can be either acute or chronic, presenting as either sudden onset but generally short-lived symptoms in the acute phase or more insidious in chronic pancreatitis resulting in organ damage and ensuing organ dysfunction.

8.10A ACUTE PANCREATITIS

EPIDEMIOLOGY

Data regarding the incidence of acute pancreatitis vary, but estimates range from 13 to 45/100,000 persons and the inflammation accounts for over 330,000 hospital admissions per year.[337] This number is felt to be increasing due to the association between the increase in obesity rates and gallstone pancreatitis as the most common etiology for the disease, particularly in the United States. Gallstones and alcohol are felt to account for 70% to 80% of all cases of acute pancreatitis.[337] It may also be caused by hypertriglyceridemia, can be drug induced, may follow ERCP, can be influenced by hereditary factors, or may be idiopathic.

It is estimated that 15% of patients who suffer from acute pancreatitis will experience recurrent episodes. These recurrent episodes can then progress to chronic pancreatitis.

PATHOPHYSIOLOGY

The inflammation that develops in acute pancreatitis is caused by the premature activation of intracellular trypsinogen through prolonged Ca^{2+} signals. This is turn causes acinar cell injury and the release of chemokines.[338] This results in the recruitment of neutrophils and macrophages leading to cell death and inflammation. Mutations in *SPINK1* and *PRSSI*, which are associated with hereditary pancreatitis, are thought to lead to inappropriate activation of this inflammatory cascade.

The exact mechanism as to the development of pancreatitis in alcoholic pancreatitis and biliary pancreatitis is unclear. In biliary pancreatitis, the passage of stones from the gallbladder into the common bile duct is thought to cause either obstruction of the pancreatic duct or reflux of bile into the pancreatic duct (Box 8.11).

SIGNS AND SYMPTOMS

The primary symptom in patients suffering from acute pancreatitis is abdominal pain. This typically presents as epigastric pain that can radiate to the back and can be associated with nausea and vomiting. When the pancreatitis is severe it can lead to systemic inflammatory response syndrome (SIRS) and organ dysfunction. A patient can exhibit fever, tachycardia, and tachypnea. Additional clinical findings in this scenario include temperature >30 °C, respiratory rate >24 breaths per minute, heart rate >90 bpm, WBC count >12,000 cells/mL, or >10% bands. Cullen sign (periumbilical ecchymosis), Grey Turner sign (flank ecchymosis), and Fox sign (bilateral bruising in inguinal areas) can be seen in cases of hemorrhagic pancreatitis.

PHYSICAL EXAMINATION

If the patient is exhibiting signs of organ dysfunction or SIRS, they will be tachycardic and tachypneic and may be febrile. The most obvious findings on physical exam will be tenderness in the epigastric region.

DIFFERENTIAL DIAGNOSIS

Perforated viscus, cholecystitis, bowel obstruction, vascular disease, renal colic, inferior myocardial infarction, pneumonia, diabetic ketoacidosis, and duodenal ulcer are included in the differential diagnosis.

EVALUATION

Elevations in serum amylase and lipase are classically used to diagnose acute pancreatitis. An elevation of three times the ULN is used to confirm the diagnosis. Lipase is more specific to pancreas inflammation but there are other disease states for which lipase can be elevated such as inflammation

BOX 8.11 Causes of Acute Pancreatitis

Autoimmune
Biliary (gallstones, gallbladder sludge, microlithiasis)
Drug reactions
Genetic (*CFTR, PRSS1, SPINK1*)
Iatrogenic (e.g., post-ERCP)
Infection
Metabolic (e.g., hypercalcemia, hypertriglyceridemia)
Malignancy (e.g., pancreatic adenocarcinoma, ampullary tumors)
Structural (e.g., pancreatic divisum)
Toxic (e.g., scorpion venom)
Traumatic
Vascular

ERCP, endoscopic retrograde cholangiopancreatography.

in the salivary glands and ovaries. Additionally, if a biliary source such as choledocholithiasis is suspected, liver studies will often also be elevated. A metabolic panel along with lipid panel should be obtained to assess for hypertriglyceridemia and hypercalcemia.

Abdominal ultrasound is key in the diagnosis of acute pancreatitis, particularly as it pertains to evaluating the biliary system. A CT is not always necessary when the clinical presentation and labs results support the diagnosis; however, CT with contrast can be helpful to assess for complications such as pancreatic necrosis or acute pancreatic fluid collections, pseudocysts, and abscesses. It is common to see enlargement of the pancreas on CT due to edema as well as peripancreatic fat stranding in uncomplicated pancreatitis. In complicated pancreatitis such as pancreatic necrosis, the affected areas of the pancreas do not enhance with findings being focal or diffuse. MRCP can be helpful to further evaluate for choledocholithiasis or if pancreatic divisum (a genetic, anatomic variant in the pancreatic ducts) is suspected.

If the etiology of the pancreatitis remains unclear after the above noted workup, EUS and genetic testing can be considered.

TREATMENT

- In uncomplicated pancreatitis the treatment is centered on supportive measures including adequate fluid resuscitation, pain control, and bowel rest. Once patients are pain free, they can be started on a clear liquid diet. If unable to tolerate oral intake, enteral nutrition, either through NG or nasojejunal feeds, should be initiated. Because of complications that can arise with TPN, this should be avoided unless the patient fails enteral nutrition.
- For patients whose pancreatitis is due to gallstones, cholecystectomy should be pursued so as to reduce the risk of recurrent pancreatitis. If the patient is not a surgical candidate, an ERCP with biliary sphincterotomy and stone removal can be considered.
- Acute pancreatitis can be severe when complicated by organ failure, pancreatic necrosis, and pancreatic pseudocysts that can cause gastric outlet obstructions. Depending on the expertise at the treating facility, either percutaneous or endoscopic drainage can be performed in these instances. Conservative management is favored when the necrotic collections are sterile, especially in the acute phase (<2–4 weeks).[339] Surgical approach to pancreatic necrosis was previously the treatment strategy of choice; however, advancements in endoscopic necrosectomy have made it the preferred choice in patients requiring intervention due to either infection or symptoms.

PATIENT EDUCATION

- After developing pancreatitis, patients should be mindful of avoiding alcohol and smoking and should follow a low-fat diet.

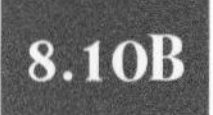

8.10B CHRONIC PANCREATITIS

EPIDEMIOLOGY

Chronic pancreatitis affects 42 to 73 per 100,000 adults in the United States.[340] It is estimated that 10% of patients who suffer from acute pancreatitis will go on to have chronic pancreatitis. The majority of chronic pancreatitis is seen in patients with a history of alcohol abuse. Other risk factors include smoking, genetic factors, hypercalcemia, hypertriglyceridemia, and autoimmune disorders. All age groups are affected by chronic pancreatitis. The variability is due to the underlying cause. Those individuals whose chronic pancreatitis is from alcohol abuse tend to be older, between ages 40 and 60, whereas patients with genetic mutations usually present between ages 10 and 40.

PATHOPHYSIOLOGY

Chronic pancreatitis is thought to develop over time beginning with cell injury and progressing to inflammation and, with prolonged inflammation, fibrosis. It is thought that an acute event occurs and subsequently causes acinar cell injury thus leading to acute pancreatitis. Repeated insults through recurrent and chronic inflammation activation leads to fibrosis of pancreatic parenchyma.[340] When fibrosis affects the pancreatic duct, strictures can develop that then lead to ductal obstruction. This leads to tissue loss and atrophy. Calcifications form due to stagnant secretions. Other theories involve the idea that hypersecretion leads to plug formation in the pancreatic duct, thus leading to calcification, obstruction, and acinar cell dysfunction and atrophy. This theory is specifically thought to be associated with the cystic fibrosis transmembrane regulator (*CFTR*) gene dysfunction.

MEDICAL HISTORY AND CLINICAL PRESENTATION

Abdominal pain is the primary presenting symptom in chronic pancreatitis. As tissue damage progresses, exocrine pancreatic insufficiency, weight loss, and endocrine insufficiency occur. The pattern of pain in chronic pancreatitis can vary between no pain, mild to moderate intermittent pain, severe intermittent pain, and constant pain of varying degrees. Nausea and vomiting can also be present, particularly during episodes of acute pain. Patients with exocrine pancreatic insufficiency report symptoms of maldigestion and steatorrhea or oily, greasy stool. They may also suffer from weight loss and fat-soluble vitamin deficiencies.

SIGNS AND SYMPTOMS

Abdominal pain, primarily in the epigastric region, is the most common symptom. A portion of patients have no pain, but exhibit signs of pancreatic insufficiency such as malabsorption, which can present as oily, greasy bowel movements, diarrhea, weight loss, and subsequent nutritional deficiencies.

PHYSICAL EXAMINATION

Pain is usually present with palpation in the epigastric region, as is seen in acute pancreatitis. If the disease has progressed to include malnutrition, patients may exhibit decreased subcutaneous fat stores, temporal wasting, muscle atrophy, and other signs of malnutrition.

DIFFERENTIAL DIAGNOSIS

Differential diagnosis includes cholangitis, cholecystitis, gastritis, Crohn disease, intestinal perforation, mesenteric artery ischemia, myocardial infarction, pancreatic cancer, and peptic ulcer disease.

EVALUATION

CT with contrast is a valuable first step in the evaluation of suspected chronic pancreatitis. Amylase and lipase are less helpful in the chronic stage of pancreatitis as these patients are often unable to mount serologic response with elevated lipase levels. Calcifications, morphologic changes in the pancreatic duct, or both are indicators of chronic pancreatitis. Further imaging can be obtained with MRI with MRCP. Abnormalities within the ductal system such as dilation or irregularity can be identified on this imaging technique. MRI also allows for evaluation of the pancreatic exocrine function by adding secretin infusion. After infusion, the radiologists evaluate duodenal filling to assess this function. Secretin infusion can also improve visualization of the side branches, which helps identify more subtle changes of chronic pancreatitis. In centers where it is available, EUS can be a valuable tool in diagnosing chronic pancreatitis.

In addition to imaging studies, assessment for nutritional deficiencies should be undertaken, particularly assessment of the fat-soluble vitamins. Reports of steatorrhea should be assessed by 72-hour fecal fat collection or fecal elastase test.

TREATMENT

- Treatment focuses on pain control and correction of nutritional deficiencies either through appropriate dietary guidance or replacement of pancreatic enzymes. Tylenol and NSAIDs should be used as first-line agents when addressing pain. In patients who report severe pain, strong opioids can be considered; however, careful monitoring and a pain management plan must be in place given the risk of opioid dependence. As there is a strong component of neuropathic pain present in chronic pancreatitis, pregabalin is an option to address this neuropathic pain. The use of pancreatic enzymes has been shown to help reduce pain, even when pancreatic insufficiency is not present. Patients must be counseled against alcohol consumption and smoking.
- Endoscopic therapy, primarily ERCP, is used when main duct abnormalities are present. This can include mechanical lithotripsy and extraction of stones that are causing pancreatic duct obstruction and pancreatic duct stenting of strictures. By alleviating any obstruction in the pancreatic duct, ductal hypertension is alleviated, which results in reduced pain. When medical and endoscopic therapy is exhausted, surgical treatment is considered the last line in therapeutic management. Surgical options include partial resection such as Whipple procedure or distal pancreatectomy. Other options are geared toward addressing drainage issues such as in the Peustow procedure. In the subset of patients whose underlying etiology is a genetic mutation or idiopathic who do not respond to medical or endoscopic therapy, complete pancreatectomy with islet autotransplantion is also an option.
- Patients diagnosed with chronic pancreatitis should be regularly assessed for complications such as exocrine insufficiency and vitamin D deficiency. While there are currently no set guidelines for monitoring for the development of pancreatic cancer, these individuals would benefit from a surveillance program given that they are at higher risk for the development of this disease.

PATIENT EDUCATION

- As with acute pancreatitis, patients with chronic pancreatitis should avoid alcohol and smoking and ensure that their nutritional needs are adequately met.

SPECIAL CONSIDERATIONS

- Autoimmune pancreatitis is a rare cause of pancreatitis but one that can lead to chronic pancreatitis. There are two types that have similar but also distinct characteristics.
- Type 1 autoimmune pancreatitis is the more common type and patients present with symptoms of obstructive jaundice and weight loss. On laboratory investigations, serum IgG levels will often be high and IgG subclass 4 will be positive. On imaging, the pancreas will often appear uniformly enlarged, often described as sausage-shaped or with the presence of a pseudocapsule.
- Type 2 autoimmune pancreatitis is less common and is not associated with IgG serum abnormalities but is associated with the presence of IBD, specifically UC.
- Type 2 also presents with obstructive jaundice and can present as a focal mass of the pancreas, often in the head of the pancreas. Additionally, abdominal pain, weight loss, acute pancreatitis, and inflammation are present more often in type 2.
- In both types, it is imperative that pancreatic adenocarcinoma be ruled out as the etiology for the patient's symptoms. Type 1 can usually be diagnosed by serologic and imaging characteristics, whereas in type 2, a core needle biopsy is needed for staining and histologic confirmation. In both instances, corticosteroids, and in rarer instances, an IMM such as azathioprine, is the treatment of choice. Relapses can occur but are more common in type 1 autoimmune pancreatitis.[341]

KEY POINTS

- Alcohol and gallstones are two of the most common causes of acute pancreatitis.
- Suspect pancreatic cancer in a patient with new onset type 2 diabetes and unexplained weight loss.

8.11 DYSPHAGIA

MEDICAL HISTORY AND CLINICAL PRESENTATION

Dysphagia, or difficulty swallowing, is a subjective symptom that can present with a spectrum of complaints. It can be described at a sensation of food "sticking" in the esophagus or chest, a lump in the throat, or chest pain. Odynophagia is pain with swallowing. Globus is a sensation characterized by a lump or tightness in the pharyngeal or cervical area, not caused by an underlying motility or anatomic disorder.

The patient history is necessary to help distinguish between oropharyngeal dysphagia and esophageal dysphagia (see Section 8.1D Esophageal Motility Disorders).

Oropharyngeal dysphagia, also called transfer dysphagia, can present with complaints of initiating a swallow and is associated with coughing, choking, or nasal regurgitation. This results from abnormalities in the oral and pharyngeal phases of swallowing (see Section 8.1 Disorders of the Esophagus). Symptoms are usually localized to the upper esophagus. Disorders associated with oropharyngeal dysphagia and esophageal dysphagia are listed in Table 8.35.

Esophageal dysphagia is usually described as a sensation of food taking longer to swallow, a sensation of food sticking in the throat, retrosternal pain, and/or regurgitation after swallowing. The history should elicit types of foods

TABLE 8.35 Causes of Dysphagia

Oropharyngeal Dysphagia	Esophageal Dysphagia
Parkinson or extrapyramidal lesion	Esophageal cancer
Cerebrovascular accident	Esophageal stricture/benign peptic stricture
Amyotrophic lateral sclerosis	Schatzki ring
Brain tumor	Extrinsic compression
Myasthenia gravis	Foreign body
Polymyositis/dermatomyositis	Eosinophilic esophagitis
Plummer-Vinson syndrome	Infectious esophagitis (*Candida*, cytomegalovirus)
Neoplasm	Achalasia
Radiation therapy (acute or chronic)	Scleroderma esophagus
Cricopharyngeal bar/Zenker diverticulum	Esophageal spasm or lower esophageal sphincter dysfunction
Proximal malignancy	Chagas disease

that trigger symptoms, and the timing course and associated symptoms. Dysphagia to both solids and liquids can suggest an esophageal motility disorder (see Section 8.1D Esophageal Motility Disorders). Dysphagia to solids only may be indicative of an esophageal stricture. Odynophagia may suggest an infectious etiology.

The Rome IV criteria classify functional dysphagia as a functional esophageal disorder. Functional dysphagia is defined as a sensation of abnormal bolus transit through the esophagus. This diagnosis requires excluding oropharyngeal dysphagia, lesions in the esophagus, GERD, EoE, and major motility disorders of the esophagus.[342] In addition to functional dysphagia, the other functional esophageal disorders are functional chest pain, functional heartburn, reflux hypersensitivity, and globus sensation.

PHYSICAL EXAMINATION

Physical examination should include inspection of the oropharynx, assessment of dentition, assessment of motor functions of the tongue and lips, and neck exam for mass or asymmetry.

DIFFERENTIAL DIAGNOSIS

The differential diagnosis of dysphagia includes esophageal cancer, GERD, esophageal motility disorder, EoE, infectious esophagitis, hiatal hernia, esophageal stricture, and oropharyngeal dysphagia.

DIAGNOSTIC STUDIES

Dysphagia is considered an "alarm" symptom and necessitates direct visualization with an upper endoscopy to exclude malignancy and stricture.

An x-ray barium swallow is a noninvasive way to evaluate the esophageal anatomy and to help determine the urgency of an upper endoscopy.

Esophageal manometry is the gold standard for identifying an esophageal motility disorder (see Section 8.1D Esophageal Motility Disorders).

EVALUATION

See Section 8.1D Esophageal Motility Disorders.

Biopsies of the esophagus are obtained to rule out Barrett esophagus, EoE, and infectious esophagitis.

An ENT consult may also be necessary for a laryngoscopy study to exclude a proximal lesion such as laryngeal or pharyngeal cancer.

TREATMENT

- Refer to Section 8.1A Gastroesophageal Reflux Disease for a discussion of treatment. No treatment can improve peristalsis in esophageal motility disorders. Treatment is aimed at controlling GERD if this is associated with these disorders.
- A patient with oropharyngeal dysphagia should undergo a speech therapy evaluation and modified barium swallow or videofluoroscopy study, which allows assessment of the oropharyngeal swallow mechanism.
- Functional dysphagia may improve over time and treatment is not always necessary. A trial of a TCA medications can be considered. Symptomatic improvement is sometimes seen with empiric dilation.

PATIENT EDUCATION

- Lifestyle recommendations such as eating in the upright position, chewing food carefully, weight reduction if indicated, and avoiding food triggers are the general instructions given to patients for management of functional dysphagia.

8.12 DYSPEPSIA

OVERVIEW

The Rome committee is a multinational group of experts in the field that first formed in 1990 and meet regularly to review and revise diagnostic criteria for all functional GI disorders. The most recent Rome IV criteria consider functional dyspepsia a gastroduodenal disorder. Functional dyspepsia has two distinct syndromes: postprandial distress syndrome and epigastric pain syndrome.[343] The other gastroduodenal disorders within this category include belching disorders, nausea and vomiting disorders, and rumination syndrome.

MEDICAL HISTORY AND CLINICAL PRESENTATION

Dyspepsia is a symptom that is defined as difficult digestion. It is called "functional" when there is no organic cause for the symptoms. There is frequently an overlap of GERD, IBS, and the other gastroduodenal disorders.

The prevalence of uninvestigated dyspepsia is approximately 20%. There is an increased risk in females, those with *Helicobacter pylori* infection, smokers, and NSAID users. Over 75% of patients presenting with dyspepsia have a normal upper endoscopy with no structural abnormality and are considered to have functional dyspepsia.[344]

The underlying pathophysiology in functional dyspepsia is not well understood and multifactorial, which may include impaired gastric accommodation, hypersensitivity to gastric distention, delayed gastric emptying, altered duodenal sensitivity, and altered CNS processing.[345]

SIGNS AND SYMPTOMS

Symptoms of dyspepsia include bothersome postprandial fullness, early satiety, abdominal bloating, epigastric pain, epigastric burning, belching, nausea, and vomiting.

PHYSICAL EXAMINATION

The physical examination may be normal or abdominal exam may show nonspecific epigastric tenderness. Focal tenderness that increases with abdominal wall contraction and palpation is considered a positive Carnett sign and suggests musculoskeletal or abdominal wall pain.

DIFFERENTIAL DIAGNOSIS

The history, including symptom characteristics, onset, and chronicity, is necessary to help differentiate between GERD, gastroparesis, biliary disease, and obstruction. Other possibilities include *H. pylori*, celiac disease, Barrett esophagus, peptic ulcer, and gastric or esophageal cancer.

DIAGNOSTIC STUDIES

Patients without alarm symptoms should be tested for *H. pylori* with either a urea breath test or stool antigen assay.

EVALUATION

Functional dyspepsia is a diagnosis of exclusion. Alarm symptoms that necessitate an urgent upper endoscopy include new onset of symptoms in those over the age of 55, overt GI bleeding such as melena or hematemesis, dysphagia, persistent vomiting, unintentional weight loss, family history of gastric or esophageal cancer, palpable abdominal mass, epigastric mass of abnormal adenopathy, and/or iron deficiency anemia.

TREATMENT

- Eradication of *H. pylori* infection if present. Symptom impact is often limited and delayed.
- PPIs are the preferred initial treatment for epigastric pain syndrome. A prokinetic may provide symptom benefit for postprandial distress syndrome.
- An antidepressant can be considered for refractory symptoms, especially with epigastric pain syndrome. Psychological therapy should be offered when dyspepsia is refractory to medical therapy.[346]

8.13 NAUSEA AND VOMITING

OVERVIEW

Nausea and vomiting are common chief complaints that patients present with to primary care and gastroenterology practices. A careful history is necessary to further define and clarify these complaints and to distinguish between acute (lasting <1 week) and chronic vomiting, lasting >1 month. Nausea and vomiting can reflect many diseases and conditions affecting the GI tract, CNS, or endocrine system. Lifestyle and polypharmacy are also factors.

Nausea is a subjective sensation in the throat or epigastrium causing an impending urge to vomit. Vomiting, or emesis, is a partial voluntary act resulting in the expulsion of gastric or intestinal contents by mouth. Retching can be associated with nausea and consists of spasmodic movements, but the glottis stays closed. It may or may not result in vomiting.

Regurgitation involves the retrograde flow of esophageal contents into the mouth and is a common complaint in GERD. Rumination is the regurgitation of undigested food from the stomach back into the mouth. There is usually not a bitterness associated with rumination, and the contents are swallowed again.

The vomiting or emetic center is located in the medulla and is the point of initiating emesis. Afferent neural pathways from the GI tract activate the emetic center. The emetic reflex involves multiple receptors, including stimulation of brain 5-hydroxytryptamine-3 (5-HT3) serotonin receptors that trigger release of dopamine, which then stimulates dopamine 2 receptors in the emetic center. Histamine H1 and muscarinic M1 receptors inhibit motion sickness, vestibular nausea, and pregnancy-related symptoms. Cannabinoid receptors in the dorsal vagal complex inhibit the emetic reflex. Neurokinin 1 (NK1) receptors bind to substance P and are part of the terminal emetic pathways. Activation of the NK1 receptors by substance P is thought to trigger chemotherapy-induced emesis.[347]

Nausea develops through activation of the cerebral cortex and at the same time the stomach relaxes and antral and intestinal peristalsis is inhibited. Efferent pathways initiate the act of vomiting, which include the phrenic nerves to the diaphragm, the spinal nerves to the abdominal muscles, and visceral efferent vagal fibers to the larynx, pharynx, esophagus, and stomach. Contraction of the diaphragm and abdominal muscles and relaxation of the LES together with a strong retrograde peristaltic contraction in the small bowel, pushes the enteric contents into the stomach and toward the mouth. Protective reflexes are activated to prevent pulmonary aspiration.

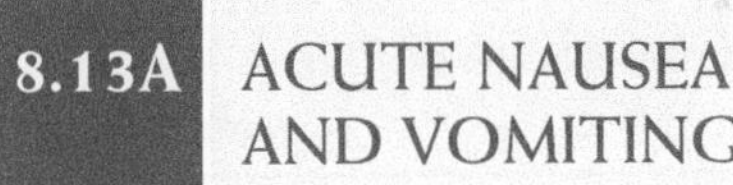

8.13A ACUTE NAUSEA AND VOMITING

MEDICAL HISTORY AND CLINICAL PRESENTATION

Acute vomiting can be secondary to infection, medications, toxins, or metabolic conditions such as uremia or diabetic ketoacidosis. In the acute presentation of nausea and vomiting, the patient needs to be assessed for emergent care such as shock, electrolyte imbalance, viscus perforation, poisoning, cerebral edema, and if appropriate, pregnancy.

SIGNS AND SYMPTOMS

Orthostatic hypotension and sinus tachycardia require immediate correction with IV fluids. Fever and/or abdominal pain suggest sepsis from intra-abdominal infection. Dizziness suggests a CNS etiology. Early morning nausea and vomiting in a female of childbearing age suggest pregnancy.

PHYSICAL EXAMINATION

Physical exam may be normal if due to a self-limiting viral etiology. Tachycardia, fever, and/or periumbilical pain can be present in emergent illness requiring immediate attention.

DIFFERENTIAL DIAGNOSIS

The differential diagnosis for acute nausea and vomiting includes acute gastroenteritis, acute drug toxicity, and metabolic, endocrine, or CNS etiologies (Table 8.36).

DIAGNOSTIC STUDIES

Diagnostic laboratory studies for evaluation of acute nausea and vomiting include electrolytes, renal panel, glucose, CBC with differential, thyroid function studies, hepatic function, amylase, lipase, and if indicated, pregnancy screen. Arterial blood gases in the appropriate setting should be considered to assess acid-base status as prolonged vomiting results in hypokalemic, hypochloremic metabolic alkalosis.

Plain x-ray should be obtained to evaluate for obstruction or stool impaction.

CT scan is indicated if intra-abdominal process such as pancreatitis, appendicitis, or peritonitis is suspected.

MRI of the head is indicated if CNS etiology is suspected to rule out hydrocephalus, tumor, or inflammatory, vascular, or ischemic lesion.

EVALUATION

GI and/or surgical consult(s) will be indicated for pancreatitis and/or biliary stones. Surgical consult is indicated for cholecystitis, appendicitis, obstruction, and/or peritonitis.

TREATMENT

- For self-limiting acute nausea and vomiting, hydration is essential. A low-residue diet is recommended until symptoms dissipate. Treatment with an antiemetic such as ondansetron, a serotonin 5-HT3 receptor antagonist, or a dopamine receptor antagonist such a prochlorperazine can be considered.
- For labyrinthitis or vertigo, an antihistamine to block H1 receptors such as meclizine or hydroxyzine can be considered, but they are very sedating. Scopolamine blocks muscarinic M1 receptors but can be associated with visual disturbances. Anticholinergic side effects need to be considered in patients with glaucoma, benign prostatic hyperplasia, and asthma.
- NK1 receptor antagonists such as oral aprepitant or parenteral fosaprepitant are FDA approved for use in preventing vomiting in patients undergoing chemotherapy. Nausea and vomiting during pregnancy correlates with the level of human chorionic gonadotropin (hCG) and most cases resolve by the end of the first trimester. Hyperemesis gravidarum occurs in 0.3–1% of pregnancies and results in dehydration and electrolyte abnormalities from severe vomiting and begins in the first trimester. It is more common with multiple gestations. It can also be associated with hypothyroidism, eclampsia, HELLP syndrome, and acute fatty liver of pregnancy. Oral and IV hydration, correction of electrolyte imbalance, and thiamine should be given prior to dextrose to avoid Wernicke encephalopathy. Ondansetron or metoclopramide can be prescribed for nausea.[348]

8.13B CHRONIC NAUSEA AND VOMITING

MEDICAL HISTORY AND CLINICAL PRESENTATION

A detailed history is essential to evaluate and treat chronic nausea and vomiting. Underlying pathology needs to be ruled out with abdominal radiographic imaging, small bowel studies, and endoscopy studies. Polypharmacy also needs to be ruled out (see Table 8.36).

The nausea and vomiting disorders, per the Rome IV criteria, include chronic nausea and vomiting syndrome,

TABLE 8.36 Differential Diagnosis for Nausea and Vomiting

Abdominal	Drugs	Metabolic	Central Nervous System	Other
Mechanical obstruction	Levodopa/dopamine agonists/ropinirole	Pregnancy	Dysautonomia	Collagen vascular disease
Peptic ulcer disease	Opiates	Hyperemesis gravidarum	Labyrinthine disease	Cardiac ischemia/infarction
Crohn disease	NSAIDs/aspirin	Parathyroid disease	Intracerebral lesion	Cannabis hyperemesis
Appendicitis	Anticonvulsants	Addison disease	Hydrocephalus	Cyclic vomiting
Acute cholecystitis	GLP1 agonists	Uremia	Pseudotumor cerebri	Rumination syndrome
Acute hepatitis	Cancer chemotherapy	Ketoacidosis	Migraine headaches	Fatty liver of pregnancy
Pancreatitis	Antidepressants	Hyponatremia	Visceral neuropathy	Paraneoplastic syndrome
Mesenteric ischemia	Lubiprostone	Porphyria	Demyelinating disease	Post vagotomy
Peritonitis	Sulfasalazine	Hypercalcemia	Meningitis	Eating disorder
GI dysmotility	Azathioprine			Alcohol abuse
GI malignancy	Antiarrhythmics/ antihypertensives			Mitochondrial disease
	Theophylline			

GI, gastrointestinal; GLP-1, glucagon-like peptide-1; NSAIDs, nonsteroidal anti-inflammatory drugs.
Source: Data from Malagelada JR, Malagelada C. Nausea and vomiting. In: Feldman M, Friedman LS, Brandt LJ, eds. Sleisenger and Fordtran's Gastrointestinal and Liver Disease. *10th ed. Elsevier; 2016:207–220.*

cyclic vomiting syndrome, and cannabinoid hyperemesis syndrome.[349]

Cyclic vomiting syndrome is defined as having stereotypical episodes of acute vomiting, lasting up to a week and having an absence of vomiting between episodes. A patient will have a history of presenting to the ED on numerous occasions with intractable nausea and vomiting and will feel well for many months between episodes. Cyclic vomiting syndrome is more common in children and young adults. There is also a strong association with a history or family history of migraine headaches.

Cannabis hyperemesis syndrome, similar to cyclic vomiting syndrome, also presents with stereotypical episodic vomiting, but the history includes prolonged excessive cannabis use. It may be associated with pathologic bathing behavior, such as prolonged hot baths or showers in an effort to relieve symptoms. Vomiting episodes are relieved by cessation of marijuana use.

A patient who presents with significant weight loss in the setting of nausea and vomiting, with a normal GI workup, should be evaluated for an underlying motility disorder. Risk factors for GI motility disorders include diabetes, thyroid disease, connective tissue disease, benign joint hypermobility/Ehlers-Danlos syndrome, and neurologic disease including Parkinson disease.

Achalasia can present with gradual weight loss and spontaneous vomiting of fluid or food (see Section 8.1D Esophageal Motility Disorders).

A patient with chronic nausea, vomiting, abdominal pain, and/or diarrhea may have dumping syndrome. Risk factors for this include history of Nissen fundoplication, bariatric surgery, esophagectomy, antrectomy, and pyloromyotomy.

PHYSICAL EXAMINATION

Physical examination may be normal, or the patient may exhibit signs of malnutrition including temporal wasting, poor skin turgor, cheilosis, poor dentition, and poor wound healing.

DIFFERENTIAL DIAGNOSIS

The differential diagnosis for chronic nausea and vomiting includes a GI motility disorder such as achalasia, gastroparesis, CIPO, and whole gut dysmotility (see Sections 8.1D Esophageal Motility Disorders, 8.2D Gastroparesis, and 8.3F Chronic Intestinal Pseudo-Obstruction).

Other possibilities to consider in the differential diagnosis are listed in Table 8.36.

DIAGNOSTIC STUDIES

An upper endoscopy study is indicated to rule out gastric outlet obstruction if this has not already been done.

The diagnosis of cyclic vomiting syndrome is clinically based as there are no specific tests or biomarkers.

Workup for non-GI causes include CT of the brain and lab studies to evaluate for metabolic etiology.

TREATMENT

- Treatment of nausea and vomiting from a GI motility disorder is directed toward treating the underlying motility disorder.
- Treatment for cyclic vomiting syndrome includes IV hydration with 10% dextrose replacement with potassium replenishment and possible sedation with an IV benzodiazepine as the treatment for acute attacks. Prophylactic therapies for cyclic vomiting syndrome include a low-dose TCA at bedtime such as amitriptyline or nortriptyline, which can be titrated to 80–100 mg/day. Supplemental coenzyme Q10 200 mg bid or L-carnitine 100 mg/kg/day in two divided doses can be added. A biopsychosocial approach is also needed to successfully treat cyclic vomiting syndrome.[350]
- Treatment of cannabis hyperemesis syndrome is cessation of marijuana.

PATIENT EDUCATION

- Patients with cyclic vomiting syndrome should be counseled on remaining on a prophylactic regimen.
- For abortive therapy, immediate treatment at the onset of symptoms can be done similar to treatment with a migraine headache. This includes taking a sublingual antiemetic such as promethazine immediately with the onset of nausea.
- The patient should lie down in a dark room to "sleep it off."
- Avoidance of marijuana is essential to control nausea and vomiting from cyclic vomiting or cannabis hyperemesis syndrome.

KEY POINTS

- A careful medication history can often reveal a cause of nausea.
- Cessation of marijuana is necessary for treating chronic nausesa and vomiting.
- An image study of the brain should be considered to rule out CNS etiology for nausea and vomiting.
- Consider autonomic testing if GI etiology is ruled out in a patient with chronic nausea.

8.14 CONSTIPATION

MEDICAL HISTORY AND CLINICAL PRESENTATION

Constipation is defined by bowel symptoms of difficult or infrequent passage of stool, hard stool, or a feeling of incomplete evacuation. Functional constipation differs from IBS-constipation predominant (IBS-C) because pain is not included in the definition of this order. The history should include assessment of medications and medical diseases that might be factors associated with constipation (Table 8.37). A detailed history should be obtained including duration of symptoms, history of bowel movements, stool consistency, and associated symptoms such as abdominal pain. Social history should document any history of sexual abuse or rectal trauma.

The Rome IV criteria classify functional constipation as a bowel disorder. The diagnostic criteria for this include two of the following symptoms: (1) straining during more than 25% of defecations, (2) lumpy or hard stools (Bristol scale 1–2) with more than 25% of defecations, (3) sensation of incomplete evacuation with more than 25% of defecations, (4) sensation of anorectal obstruction or blockage in more than 25% of defecations, (5) manual maneuvers (digital evacuation, support of the pelvic floor) to facilitate more than 25% of defections, and (6) fewer than three spontaneous bowel movements per week. Within these diagnostic criteria, loose stools are rarely present without the use of laxatives and there is insufficient criteria for IBS. Symptom onset time includes onset of symptoms at least 6 months prior to diagnosis and fulfilling criteria for the last 3 months.[65]

TABLE 8.37 Risk Factors for Constipation

Conditions	Medications
Pregnancy	Opioids
Diabetes	NSAIDs
Thyroid disease	Calcium channel blockers
Heavy metal poisoning (arsenic, lead, mercury)	Diuretics
Autonomic neuropathy	Ondansetron
Amyloidosis	Alosetron
Intestinal pseudo-obstruction	Anticholinergic agents
Neurologic disease (Parkinson disease, multiple sclerosis, spinal cord injury)	Calcium, iron supplements
Chagas disease	Aluminum-containing antacids

NSAIDs, nonsteroidal anti-inflammatory drugs.

Defecatory dyssynergia can overlap with constipation with similar complaints, however, a patient may also have fecal incontinence (see Section 8.5 Rectal Disorders). Dyssynergia is characterized by a paradoxical anal contraction during defecation, inadequate anal sphincter relaxation, and/or poor push effort due to impaired coordination of abdominal, rectal, and anal muscles (see Figure 8.2). This results in the inability to have a complete bowel movement. Digital maneuvers are often required in order to evacuate. Risk factors for defecatory dyssynergia include older age, postmenopausal state, multiple childbirths, history of sexual abuse, and chronic constipation. Defecatory dyssynergia affects up to 33% of patients with chronic constipation.[351]

Slow transit constipation is characterized by a delay in stool transit and is often refractory to treatment. It is characterized by very infrequent bowel movements (<1 bowel movement per week).

SIGNS AND SYMPTOMS

Signs and symptoms of constipation include straining with bowel movement, hard stools, sensation of incomplete evacuation, sensation of anorectal obstruction or blockage, manual maneuvers needed to evacuate, or fewer than three bowel movements per week.

PHYSICAL EXAMINATION

Physical examination includes abdominal examination for inspection of scars, auscultation for bowel sounds, percussion for mass, and palpation for mass or tenderness. Physical examination findings on a digital rectal examination may include poor sphincter tone, poor push effort, or inability to relax the external anal sphincter.[352]

DIFFERENTIAL DIAGNOSIS

Differential diagnosis for constipation includes functional constipation, IBS, defecatory dyssynergia, slow transit constipation, fecal impaction, Hirschsprung disease, megacolon, colon cancer, or opioid-induced constipation if a patient is on chronic narcotic medications.

DIAGNOSTIC STUDIES

Laboratory studies for the initial evaluation of constipation include basic metabolic panel, glucose, calcium, TSH, and CBC.

An x-ray of the abdomen can assess the severity of constipation and rules out obstruction or megacolon.

A colonoscopy is indicated if the patient has "red flags" such as unexplained anemia, unexplained weight loss, severe abdominal pain, hemoccult positivity, and/or a rectal mass on physical examination.

ARM testing with balloon expulsion is the test of choice to evaluate for defecatory dyssynergia. It can screen for Hirschsprung disease by assessing for the presence of a rectal-anal inhibitory reflex. An ARM study measures the resting rectal and anal pressures. During attempted defecation, rectal sensation, rectal-anal reflexes, and rectal compliance are measured. The rectal-anal inhibitory reflex (RAIR) triggers the anal sphincter to relax. The RAIR is mediated by the myenteric plexus and in Hirschsprung disease, this reflex is absent.

A balloon expulsion test uses a 50-mL balloon filled with water that is placed into the rectum. The patient is given a stopwatch and left alone on a commode and stops the watch when the balloon is expelled. A patient with normal defecation will be able to expel the balloon within 1 minute.

Defecatory dyssynergia should be excluded or identified and treated before pursing colonic transit time. A Sitz marker study measures colonic transit time. An x-ray is taken on day 1 following the administration of 24 radiopaque markers. Another x-ray is taken on day 5. Slow transit constipation is diagnosed if >20% of the markers remain in the colon on day 5.

EVALUATION

If megacolon is shown on an x-ray, the patient should be referred to colorectal surgery.

The diagnosis of slow transit constipation is made with physiologic studies that include radiopaque marker transit study, scintigraphy, or wireless motility capsule.[353]

If an ARM study indicates the absence of a RAIR, a referral to a colorectal surgeon may be indicated to consider a full thickness biopsy to rule out Hirschsprung disease.

TREATMENT

- There are many medication options for treating constipation; however, diet and lifestyle should be the first step in management.
- Psyllium, cellulose, and methylcellulose are bulk fiber sources, but will not be effective for slow transit constipation and may worsen symptoms.
- Constipating medications should be avoided (Table 8.37). Polyethylene glycol is an osmotic laxative that should also be started as a first-line medication to treat constipation. If needed, treatment for constipation can also include the addition of other medications such as a stimulant laxative, secretagogue, or prokinetic (see Table 8.5).
- If a patient is on opioid medication, the goal is to eventually wean from this if possible. Naloxegol is a peripheral opioid receptor antagonist that can treat opioid-induced constipation in a patient who requires chronic opioids.
- Treatment for defecatory dyssynergia includes medical treatment for constipation and physical therapy and biofeedback with a trained therapist who specializes in such. The goals of biofeedback are to correct the dyssynergia

by improving the coordination of the abdominal, rectal, and anal sphincter muscles and to improve rectal sensory perception if the patient has difficulty with sensation in the rectum.[109] Treatment for slow transit constipation requires stimulant laxatives and multiple other categories of laxatives. Physical therapy and biofeedback to treat dyssynergia are also needed. A patient with slow transit constipation that remains refractory to these measures may require referral to a colorectal surgeon.
- Repeated forceful straining, defecatory dyssynergia, and/or trauma from digital maneuvers are often the cause of solitary rectal ulcer syndrome. A sigmoidoscopy or colonoscopy may reveal a small shallow ulcer with white slough or hyperemic mucosa on the wall of the rectum. The cornerstone of management of solitary rectal ulcer is behavioral therapy to include avoiding excessive straining and discontinuing the use of digital maneuvers. Physical therapy and biofeedback may be effective.[109]

PATIENT EDUCATION

- Patient education on diet, exercise, and lifestyle is the first step in managing functional constipation. A high-fiber diet consisting of 20 to 25 g of fiber per day is recommended, along with increasing fluid intake. Dietary sources of fiber include high-fiber grain and cereals, wheat bran, nuts, seeds, and skins of fruit and vegetables.
- A "squatty potty" may be helpful for a patient suspected of having dyssynergia. Counsel on avoiding straining.

KEY POINTS

- A careful medication history may reveal a cause of constipation.
- A history of sexual abuse can be a factor in refractory constipation and evacuation disorders and all patients should be questioned about this.
- A physical therapist trained in treating defecatory disorders is essential for treatment.

8.15 DIARRHEA

OVERVIEW

Diarrhea is a symptom that includes bowel pattern changes of an increase in stool frequency and loose or watery consistency. It can be defined has an increase in stool weight or volume of more than 200 g or 200 mL per 24 hours in a person consuming a Western diet.

The average adult consumes approximately 2 L of fluid per day under normal conditions. There is an additional 7 L from salivary, gastric, pancreatic, biliary, and small intestinal sources, which totals approximately 9 L over 24 hours. Approximately 7.5 L (85–90%) of fluids are absorbed by the small intestine. The colon absorbs another 1.3 L (approximately 10%). The unabsorbed solutes, 200 mL (approximately 2%), account for the average stool mass. The small intestine has a maximum absorptive capacity of approximately 12 L and the colon has a capacity of up to 6 L, for a total of 18 L.[354]

The evaluation of diarrhea begins with a thorough history and physical exam. Diarrhea should be characterized as acute (lasting <1 month) or chronic (lasting >1 month). Diarrhea can be further characterized into secretory, osmotic, malabsorptive, inflammatory, or functional etiologies.

Osmotic diarrhea is a watery diarrhea that results from large amounts of poorly absorbed sugars or sugar alcohol. Acquired deficiencies such as lactase and intolerances to fermentable oligosaccharides, disaccharides, monosaccharides, and polyols are triggers for osmotic diarrhea. With osmotic diarrhea, the stool osmotic ion gap is abnormally elevated. The stool osmotic ion gap is calculated by measuring the stool sodium and potassium with the equation: $290 - 2\ (Na + K)$. Osmotic diarrhea resolves with fasting and subsides when the offending substance is removed.

Secretory diarrhea results in large amounts of watery diarrhea and is caused by either increased intestinal secretion or decreased absorption. Infection is the most common cause of secretory diarrhea. Other causes include endocrine tumors, gastric hypersecretion, enterotoxins, bile salt malabsorption, and laxative abuse. Unlike osmotic diarrhea, secretory diarrhea does not resolve with fasting.

Inflammatory or bloody diarrhea results from disruption of the intestinal mucosal integrity (see Section 8.4H Inflammatory Bowel Disease). Stools may have mucus, blood, or pus associated with ulcers in the mucosa. This can occur from a self-limiting infectious colitis, neoplasia, radiation, or chronic infectious etiology.

Functional diarrhea occurs from altered intestinal motility. In IBS, the diarrhea tends to be variable and may alternate with periods of constipation. Pain distinguishes IBS from functional diarrhea.

8.15A ACUTE DIARRHEA

MEDICAL HISTORY AND CLINICAL PRESENTATION

The most common cause of acute diarrhea is infection. Recent travel to an endemic area can suggest traveler's diarrhea or parasitic infection. Traveler's diarrhea is defined as having the passage of three or more loose to diarrheal stools within 24 hours. Depending upon the cause, this can be associated with nausea, vomiting, abdominal discomfort, hematochezia, or fever. The symptoms can last for 2–10 days after arrival to a new location or at any time during foreign exposure.[354]

Giardia, Entamoeba, Cryptosporidium, and *Cyclospora* are types of parasitic causes of diarrhea. *Entamoeba* can cause a chronic intestinal infection and can result in liver abscess. *Cryptosporidium* can cause chronic infection in immunocompromised patients.[355]

A recent history of antibiotic use is a risk factor for *C. difficile* diarrhea (see Section 8.4B *Clostridioides difficile* infection).

Enteropathogenic *E. coli* can cause a bacterial diarrhea that can be seen in daycare outbreaks and can lead to death in infants.[355]

Other bacterial causes of diarrhea come from foodborne illness (Table 8.38). *Salmonella* and *Campylobacter* account for the majority of laboratory-confirmed causes of foodborne illnesses. Foodborne illnesses due to *Salmonella, Shigella,* and *S. aureus* tend to be more common during the summer months. *Campylobacter jejuni* is more common in the spring and fall. Norovirus and *Bacillus cereus* infections occur year-round.[356]

TABLE 8.38 Bacterial Causes of Foodborn Illnesses

Pathogen	Sources	Mean Incubation Time	Symptoms
Bacillus cereus	Fried rice, cream, meatballs	2–9 hours	Diarrhea, cramps, vomiting
Campylobacter jejuni	Milk, chicken, beef	48 hours	Diarrhea (+/– bloody), fever, cramps, n/v, headache, myalgias
Clostridium perfringens	Beef, turkey, chicken, especially when reheated	12 hours	Diarrhea, cramps
Escherichia coli spp.	Salads, beef	24–96 hours	Diarrhea, cramps, nausea, fever, myalgias bloody diarrhea (HUS)
Listeria monocytogenes	Dairy, raw vegetables, beef, poultry, coleslaw	Unknown	Diarrhea (+/– bloody), fever, cramps, n/v
Salmonella spp.	Eggs, meat, poultry	24 hours	Diarrhea (+/– bloody), n/v, fever, cramps, fever
Shigella spp.	Milk, salads (potato, tuna, or turkey)	24 hours	Cramps, fever, headache, diarrhea (+/– bloody), n/v
Staphylococcus aureus	Ham, pork, canned beef	3 hours	Diarrhea, n/v, cramps
Vibrio parahaemolyticus	Seafood, salted vegetables	12 hours	Diarrhea, cramps, n/v, headache, fever
Yersinia enterocolitica	Chocolate or raw milk, pork	72 hours	Fever, cramps, diarrhea, vomiting, pharyngitis, rash, arthritis, mesenteric adenitis

HUS, hemolytic uremic syndrome; n/v, nausea and vomiting.
Source: Data from Kew MC, Varma RR, Dos Santos HA, Scheuer PJ, Sherlock S. Portal hypertension in primary biliary cirrhosis. Gut. *1971;12(10):830–834. doi:10.1136/gut.12.10.830*

SIGNS AND SYMPTOMS

Acute diarrhea from an infectious cause can be accompanied by fever, nausea and vomiting, abdominal pain, headache, or myalgias.

PHYSICAL EXAMINATION

Evaluate for orthostatic changes and skin turgor. Perform an abdominal examination for tenderness to evaluate for peritonitis.

DIFFERENTIAL DIAGNOSIS

The differential diagnosis for acute infectious diarrhea includes self-limiting viral gastroenteritis and bacterial diarrhea.

DIAGNOSTIC STUDIES

If the patient is ill-appearing, lab studies to obtain include CBC with differential, serum electrolytes, BUN, and creatinine. Abdominal x-ray should be obtained to assess for megacolon.

Stool tests include fecal leukocytes and if positive, stool cultures. Other studies include stool for *Clostridium difficile* toxin A and B, and stool tests for ova and parasites.

EVALUATION

Acute diarrhea in developed countries is often self-limiting and treated with supportive care, including a low-residue diet and oral fluid hydration. Patients presenting with fever, bloody diarrhea, or abdominal pain need further evaluation and possible hospitalization. Profuse diarrhea in older adults or immunocompromised patients should prompt an extensive workup including flexible sigmoidoscopy or colonoscopy.

TREATMENT

- Fluid and electrolyte replacement are of utmost importance in the acute setting. Infants and elderly are a higher risk for dehydration and may require IV fluid and electrolyte replacement.
- Antimotility agents such as Imodium should be avoided if the cause is not known.
- Treatment of traveler's diarrhea is usually empiric. Ciprofloxacin 500 mg daily × 3 days is used for empiric treatment; however, antibiotic resistance is a growing concern. Rifaximin 200 mg BID is the treatment of choice for nondysenteric traveler's diarrhea. Azithromycin is the recommended treatment if travel includes areas such as Southern Asia, Central and South America, and Northern Africa where there is an increase in quinolone-resistant organisms.[354]

PATIENT EDUCATION

- When traveling out of the country, patients should be instructed not to consume unfiltered water or water that has not been treated with bleach or tincture of iodine. Avoid fruit skins and raw vegetables and consume only food that is thoroughly cooked.
- Patients should check with the CDC or contact the local hospital travel clinic for updates on prophylactic measures if traveling to endemic parts of the world.

8.15B CHRONIC DIARRHEA

MEDICAL HISTORY AND CLINICAL PRESENTATION

Chronic diarrhea, defined as diarrhea lasting >1 month, tends to be noninfectious; however, reevaluating for infectious etiology should be considered. Parasites are the most common infectious cause of persistent diarrhea.

Up to 10% of patients who have had infectious diarrhea may develop a postinfectious IBS.

Medications can also be a cause of chronic diarrhea resulting in microscopic colitis. This presents as watery diarrhea and—in some cases—nocturnal diarrhea can occur. Advanced age is also a risk factor for microscopic colitis. Common medication triggers for microscopic colitis include NSAIDs, PPIs, ranitidine, and sertraline.

Diarrhea can also occur following bowel resection and loss of intestinal surface area (see Section 8.3A Short Bowel Syndrome).

SIGNS AND SYMPTOMS

There is a wide spectrum of diarrheal symptoms related to malabsorption and maldigestion (see Section 8.3A Short Bowel Syndrome). The more common complaints of maldigestion are nonspecific and similar to that of IBS and can include flatulence, abdominal distention, and borborygmi.

PHYSICAL EXAMINATION

Physical examination findings may be normal in chronic diarrhea. Rectal examination can assess for fecal impaction or rectal mass. Other uncommon disease conditions can present with distinct physical exam findings (Table 8.39).

DIFFERENTIAL DIAGNOSIS

Chronic diarrhea from malabsorption can occur from celiac disease, Whipple disease, mesenteric ischemia, short bowel syndrome and SIBO, bile acid diarrhea, or pancreatic exocrine insufficiency.

Chronic inflammatory diarrhea can result from IBD, infectious disease (tuberculosis, yersiniosis, *C. difficile* infection strongyloidiasis, CMV infection, and HSV infection), radiation colitis, ischemic colitis, colon cancer, and lymphoma.

Chronic watery diarrhea can occur from osmotic and/or secretory diarrhea. Endocrine disorders resulting in secretory diarrhea include hyperthyroidism, Addison disease, villous adenoma, carcinoid, ZES, neuropathy, postvagotomy diarrhea, and post–gastric surgery dumping syndrome.

DIAGNOSTIC STUDIES

Diagnostic studies include a 24- to 72-hour stool analysis for fecal fat. Consider a pancreatic elastase stool study to evaluate for pancreatic insufficiency. Consider repeating *C. difficile* and ova and parasite studies.

TABLE 8.39 Chronic Diarrhea and Physical Examination Findings

Disease	Physical Examination Findings
Amyloidosis	Macroglossia and hepatomegaly
Addison disease	Hyperpigmentation
Medullary thyroid carcinoma	Thyroid nodule, lymphadenopathy
Mastocytosis	Flushing, urticaria
Carcinoid	Flushing

CT or MRI of the abdomen and pelvis can be performed to exclude structural disease.

Biopsies can provide additional information during sigmoidoscopy, colonoscopy, and esophagogastrostomy.

The incidence of chronic diarrhea caused by peptide-secreting hormones is very low; therefore, screening is not recommended unless there are signs and symptoms consistent with a tumor syndrome (Table 8.39).[357] If history is suggestive of carcinoid tumor syndrome, urinary 5-hydroxyindoleacetic acid (5-HIAA), metanephrine, and histamine should be obtained. Plasma peptides are measured for gastrin, calcitonin, vasoactive intestinal peptide (VIP), somatostatin, and chromogranin A. Scintigraphy with radiolabeled octreotide combined with PET or CT can help identify peptide-secreting tumors.

EVALUATION

Identifying and eliminating the causative agent will improve osmotic diarrhea.

Endoscopy biopsies can guide treatment of chronic colitis. Microscopic colitis shows a normal-appearing colon on direct observation during colonoscopy. The diagnosis is based on colon biopsies showing lymphocytes and/or collagen bands on pathology.

TREATMENT

- Treatment may include an empiric trial of a bile acid sequestrant for bile acid diarrhea or pancreatic enzyme supplementation for pancreatic insufficiency.
- Treatment options for microscopic colitis include Pepto-Bismol, mesalamine, cholestyramine, or budesonide. The diarrhea usually resolves after discontinuing the offending medication and following 3–6 months of treatment, although relapses can occur.
- For treatment of IBS-D, see Section 8.4A Irritable Bowel Syndrome.
- For treatment of underlying IBD, see Section 8.4H Inflammatory Bowel Disease.
- For treatment of malabsorptive diarrhea, refer to the discussion of treatment under Section 8.3 Disorders of the Small Intestine.

PATIENT EDUCATION

- The patient should be educated on avoiding any identified triggers of diarrhea.

SPECIAL CONSIDERATIONS

- Immunocompromised patients have higher chronicity and increased morbidity and mortality due to impaired immune function that can lead to less common presentations and the development of opportunistic infections.
- CMV infection can lead to necrotizing colitis or perforation. Prompt recognition and management of symptoms are essential in such patients.

KEY POINTS

- Microscopic colitis can recur. Avoid medication triggers including NSAIDs, PPI, sertraline, and rantidine.
- If initial GI workup is negative, consider an abdominal flat plate x-ray to rule out overflow diarrhea.

8.16 HIATAL HERNIA AND ABDOMINAL WALL HERNIAS

The crural diaphragm wraps around the esophagus to help maintain the LES pressure. The crural diaphragm is composed of striated muscles and forms the esophageal hiatus and also works as an antireflux barrier at the gastroesophageal junction. A hiatal hernia occurs when the EGJ and a portion of the gastric fundus protrude through the hiatus in the crural diaphragm into the chest (Figure 8.9).

A diaphragmatic hernia is often an incidental finding on endoscopy or x-ray. A type I "sliding" hiatal hernia results in the gastroesophageal junction displaced above the diaphragmatic hiatus with a portion of the gastric cardia. Types II–IV are considered paraesophageal hernias and are due to defects in the phrenoesophageal membrane. A type II hernia occurs when a portion of the gastric fundus migrates through the phrenoesophageal membrane into the mediastinum, but the gastroesophageal junction remains at the level of the diaphragm. A type III paraesophageal hernia is considered a "mixed-type" resulting in the gastroesophageal junction being displaced cranially and a defect in the phrenoesophageal membrane causing the fundus to be displaced adjacent to the LES. When nongastric structures such as the spleen, colon, small bowel, or pancreas herniate through the phrenoesophageal membrane, this is considered a type IV paraesophageal hernia.[358]

A small hiatal hernia does not warrant intervention in asymptomatic patients. Hiatal hernias can result in GERD symptoms of heartburn, dysphagia and regurgitation and can be a risk for esophagitis and Barrett esophagus by disrupting the normal gastroesophageal reflux barrier. A symptomatic paraesophageal hernia can cause chest pain or shortness of breath. It can also result in iron deficiency anemia due to Cameron lesions and ulceration resulting from the fundus moving in and out of the diaphragm. A potential complication of a paraesophageal hernia includes strangulation leading to volvulus, ischemia, or gangrene.

Surgical consult with minimally invasive surgery is indicated for a symptomatic paraesophageal hernia. If a hiatal hernia is thought to be a factor in persistent reflux symptoms despite PPI therapy, prior to referring to surgery, it is recommended that further workup be done to evaluate for an esophageal motility disorder and to document reflux. See Sections 8.1A Gastroesophageal Reflux Disease and 8.1D Esophageal Motility Disorders. A significant esophageal motility disorder may preclude surgery.

A gastric volvulus occurs when the stomach twists on itself. It rarely occurs unless associated with a diaphragmatic hernia. Up to 20% of cases occur in children under the age of 1, usually associated with a congenital diaphragmatic defect. Most cases in adults occur in the fifth decade of life. Acute gastric volvulus is considered a surgical emergency. It presents with severe pain in the lower chest or upper abdomen. Persistent retching is common. Borchardt triad includes pain, unproductive retching, and inability to pass an NG tube. A gastric volvulus on CT scan imaging will show findings of the stomach in the chest. Endoscopy is not recommended due to the risk of perforation.[359]

Chronic gastric volvulus can occur from a paraesophageal hernia and can cause mild intermittent symptoms of dysphagia, postprandial fullness, bloating, and heartburn. An upper GI x-ray or CT scan may show a large diaphragmatic hernia. Treatment is surgical.

An abdominal wall hernia protrudes through the retaining walls of the abdomen. It is considered external if the hernia sac protrudes through the abdominal wall. Internal hernias are contained within the abdominal cavity and may not necessarily have a sac. A hernia is considered reducible if the protruding contents can be returned to the abdomen. It is considered incarcerated when the contents cannot be replaced. When the blood supply of the protruding organ is compromised then the hernia is considered to be strangulated, which can result in ischemia or necrosis of the organ. It is difficult to determine whether a hernia is incarcerated or strangulated; therefore, all incarcerated hernias are considered urgent and require surgical intervention.[359]

Groin hernias include femoral and inguinal hernias. Umbilical, epigastric, spigelian, lumbar, and incisional hernias are considered ventral hernias.

Large inguinal hernias may cause difficulty with sigmoidoscopy and colonoscopy; therefore, surgical repair may be indicated prior to undergoing either of these procedures.

Incisional hernias occur after a prior operation. Conditions that increase intra-abdominal pressure such as obesity, collagen vascular disorders, surgical repair of the aorta, and ascites can increase the risk of postoperative occurrence. Parastomal hernias occur in up to 50% of cases after stoma placement. A dilated bowel prior to stoma placement can result in bowel shrinkage after stoma placement, which can increase the space between the bowel wall and fascia, resulting in hernia formation.[359]

Epigastric hernias occur through midline defects of the rectus sheath between the umbilicus and xiphoid process. It

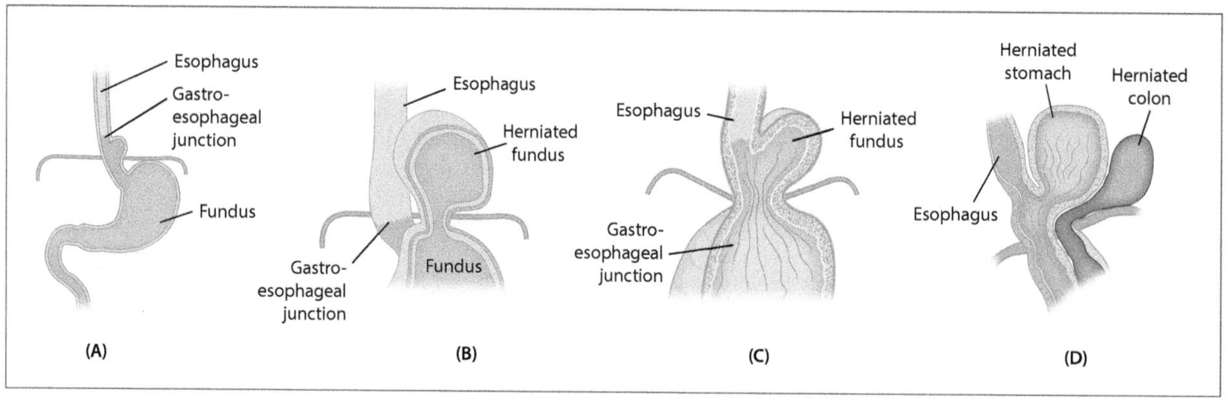

Figure 8.9 **Types of hernias. (A) Type I, sliding hiatal hernia; (B) type II, paraesophageal hernia; (C) type III, mixed; (D) type IV, paraesophageal hernia.**

is unusual for bowel to become incarcerated in an epigastric hernia due to the location in the upper part of the abdominal wall. A patient with an epigastric hernia can present with pain, which can be mistaken for peptic ulcer or biliary disease. An ultrasound or CT scan image can aid in the diagnosis.

Congenital umbilical hernias in infants usually close spontaneously. They occur in approximately 30% of African American infants. Repair of an umbilical hernia is recommended in an adult who is symptomatic or if difficult to reduce.

Spigelian hernias are very rare and usually occur in older patients, around the age of 60. They occur through defects in the fused transversus abdominis muscle and internal oblique muscle, located lateral to the rectus sheath and more commonly below the level of the umbilicus. They are difficult to diagnose due to the anatomic location. Patients with a spigelian hernia usually have abdominal wall pain. This condition can be mistaken for appendicitis or diverticulitis. Ultrasound and CT scan can help to confirm the diagnosis.[359]

TABLE 8.40 Location and Differential Diagnosis of Abdominal Pain

Location	Differential Diagnosis
Epigastric	Pancreatitis, esophagitis, cardiac, aneurysm
Umbilical	Early appendicitis, small bowel obstruction, mesenteric ischemia, aneurysm
Hypogastric	IBD, diverticulitis, IBS, UTI, gynecologic
RUQ	Cholecystitis, pyelonephritis, referred pain from pleurisy or pneumonia
RLQ	Appendicitis, IBD, cholecystitis, hernia, pyelonephritis, gynecologic
LUQ	Peptic ulcer, splenic infarct, pancreatitis, IBS, pyelonephritis, pneumonia
LLQ	Diverticulitis, IBD, IBS, hernia, pyelonephritis

IBD, inflammatory bowel disease; IBS, irritable bowel syndrome; LLQ, left lower quadrant; LUQ, left upper quadrant; RLQ, right lower quadrant; RUQ, right upper quadrant; UTI, urinary tract infection.

COMMON CHIEF COMPLAINTS

APPROACH TO ABDOMINAL PAIN

Abdominal pain is a very common GI complaint and remains the number one complaint in U.S. ED visits. A careful history and physical examination are essential to establish and organize a differential diagnosis. Symptom pattern, timing, and duration can suggest specific etiologies. The evaluation for acute abdominal pain more commonly occurs in the hospital or emergency room setting, while chronic abdominal pain is usually evaluated in the outpatient office setting. Many patients undergo a negative workup for acute abdominal pain and are discharged from the ED or hospital to follow up with their primary care clinician or a gastroenterologist.

The two mechanisms of pain are somatic and visceral pain. Somatic pain occurs from irritation of the parietal peritoneum, abdominal wall, or diaphragm. Pain is usually constant and worse with movement of the peritoneum. Visceral pain results from stretching of the abdominal viscera, such as an obstructed lumen, or from inflammation. Visceral pain can be intermittent or constant and is often associated with autonomic symptoms of nausea, vomiting, diaphoresis, or pallor. Other mechanisms of pain include ischemia, musculoskeletal, metabolic, neuropathic, and functional.[360]

The location of pain can help guide the initial workup and differential diagnosis (Table 8.40). Severe pain of sudden occurrence is often a medical emergency, such as a perforated viscus, obstruction, or acute ischemia.

Laboratory studies include CBC, urinalysis, liver function tests, serum lipase, electrolytes, and pregnancy test. However, lab studies may be normal in older patients and immunocompromised patients and care must be taken to not to be falsely reassured with the finding of normal studies. Calcium binding protein, calprotectin, and leucine-rich alpha-2-glycoprotein (LRG) are new biomarkers of inflammation and have excellent sensitivity and negative predictive value in identifying acute appendicitis and colitis.[361]

Diagnostic imaging will depend upon the likely diagnosis, pregnancy status, and clinical condition. The choice of image should also consider the potential cumulative radiation dose.

Functional GI disorders and disorders of brain–gut interaction are classified by the Rome Foundation primarily on symptoms, as opposed to physiologic criteria. Chronic abdominal pain is often referred to as "functional" when there are no structural or metabolic disorders using currently available diagnostic methods that can explain symptoms.

The Rome IV classification for functional GI disorders that can be a component of chronic abdominal pain includes bowel disorders/IBS (see Section 8.4A Irritable Bowel Syndrome), gallbladder and sphincter of Oddi disorders, and centrally mediated disorders of GI pain.[343]

Centrally mediated disorders of GI pain include centrally mediated abdominal pain syndrome (formerly known as functional abdominal pain syndrome) and narcotic bowel syndrome/opioid-induced GI hyperalgesia.

Centrally mediated abdominal pain syndromes have diagnostic criteria that must be present for at least 6 months before diagnosis. These include (1) continuous abdominal pain, (2) infrequent relationship of pain with physiologic events (e.g., eating, defecation, or menses), (3) pain limiting daily functioning, (4) pain is not intentionally produced, and (5) pain that isn't explained by other structural or functional GI disorders or other medical conditions.

The diagnostic criteria for narcotic bowel syndrome/opiate-induced GI hyperalgesia must be present for at least 6 months prior and includes (1) chronic recurring abdominal pain treated with narcotics, (2) pain not explained by a current or previous GI diagnosis, and (3) two or more of the following: pain worsens or doesn't resolve with escalating dosages of narcotics, worsening of pain when narcotic dose wanes, and/or progression of the frequency, duration, and intensity of pain episodes. Treatment requires an understanding of the patient, sound patient-clinician relationship, and educating the patient about treatment. Treatment may include either a TCA, SSRI, or serotonin-norepinephrine

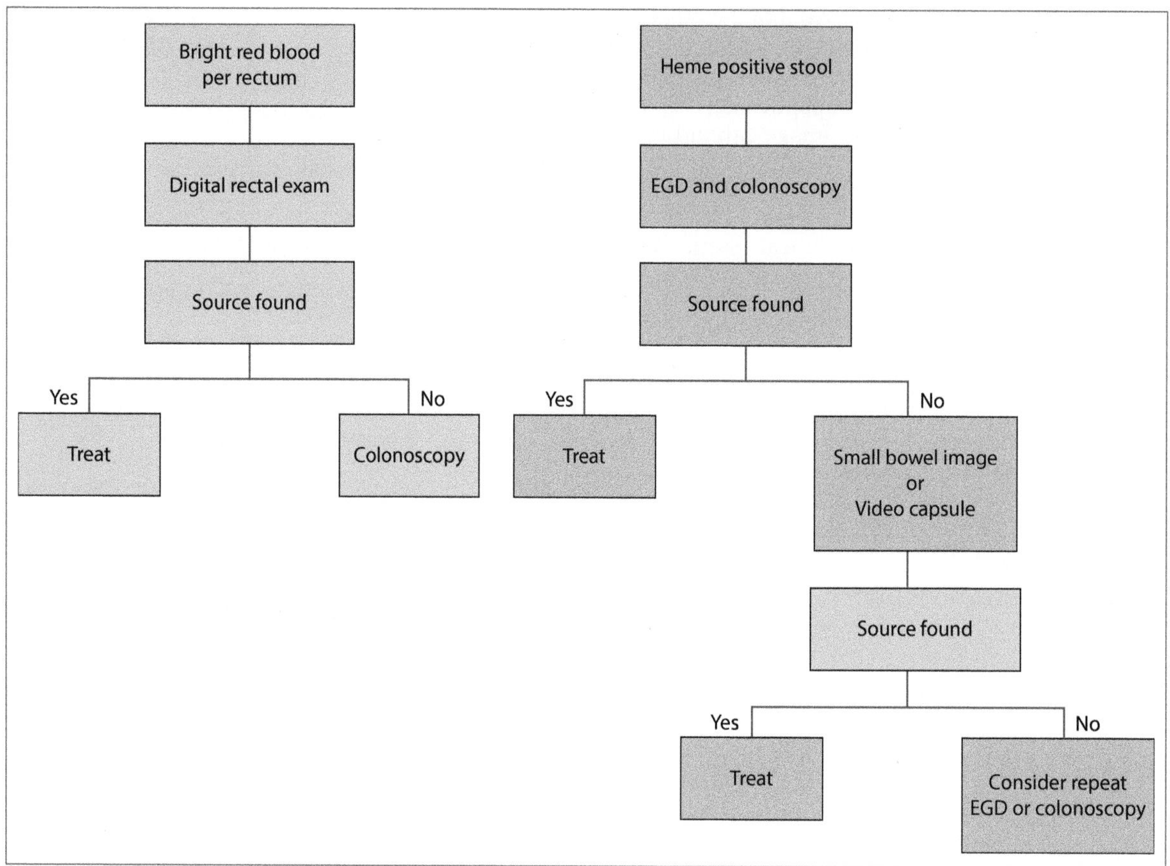

Figure 8.10 **Outpatient approach to gastrointestinal bleeding.** BRBPR, bright red blood per rectum; EGD, esophagogastroduodenoscopy.

reuptake inhibitor. Opiate detoxification is the goal and requires mental health professional, primary care clinician, and family support.[361]

Treatment of chronic abdominal pain requires an effective patient-clinician relationship and knowing when to refer to a mental health professional or a multidisciplinary functional GI or pain treatment center. Opioid treatment should be avoided and is contraindicated due to the risk for narcotic bowel syndrome. Pharmacologic treatment includes tricyclic antidepressants (receptor sites of action are norepinephrine, 5-hydroxytryptamine, histamine and acetylcholine), SSRIs (5-hydroxytryptamine receptor site of action), or serotonin-norepinephrine reuptake inhibitors (norepinephrine and 5-hydroxytryptamine receptor sites of action).[361]

APPROACH TO GI BLEEDING

The approach to GI bleeding depends on whether it is an acute overt GI bleed, obscure GI bleed or chronic occult bleed (see Section 8.6 Gastrointestinal Bleeding).

There are multiple diagnostic procedures available for investigating the GI tract in a patient who presents in the outpatient setting with iron deficiency anemia or a positive hemoccult test result. A complaint of black stool needs to be confirmed by a guaiac test for the presence of hemoglobin degradation products because items such as bismuth, licorice, and iron preparations can turn stools black. Fecal immunochemical testing (FIT) is more specific for human blood and results are not impacted by food intake or medication. A suggested algrithim for a presentation of GI bleeding in hemodynamically stable patients is shown in Figure 8.10.

KNOWLEDGE CHECKS

1. Obesity is a major risk factor for many chronic diseases and several overlapping GI conditions. How does obesity contribute to reflux? What are the potential implications of persistent reflux in the setting of obesity?
2. How is an asymptomatic patient with incidental findings of elevated liver enzymes appropriately evaluated?
3. What effects do neurologic deficits have on swallowing and gastric motility?
4. What additional workup is considered in a 30-year-old patient with a history of irritable bowel syndrome who continues to have abdominal pain?
5. How is a new-onset diarrhea and fecal incontinence evaluated in a 40-year-old female?

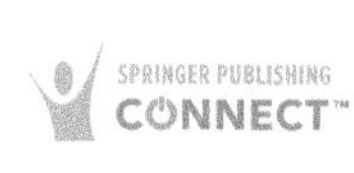

REFERENCES

The complete reference list for this chapter appears in the digital version of the chapter, accessible at https://connect.springerpub.com/content/book/978-0-8261-8243-2/chapter/ch08.

CHAPTER 9

NUTRITION

ANNE WILDERMUTH

LEARNING OBJECTIVES

- Identify types and degrees of malnutrition and discuss treatment and long-term management of each type.
- Identify the epidemiology and pathophysiology, discuss appropriate evaluation, and analyze treatment options and patient education recommendations for obesity.
- Recognize, describe, and differentiate the risk factors, etiology, pathophysiology, clinical findings, assessment, differential diagnosis, prognosis, complications, prevention, and management of the following disorders: anorexia nervosa (AN), bulimia nervosa, binge-eating disorder, and refeeding syndrome.
- Identify the role in metabolism, physiology, and clinical importance for health and nutrition of the following vitamins and minerals: thiamine (B1), riboflavin (B2), niacin (B3), pyridoxine (B6), folate (B9), cyanocobalamin (B12), vitamin A, vitamin C, vitamin D, vitamin E, vitamin K, copper, and calcium.
- Recognize, describe and differentiate the risk factors, etiology, pathophysiology, clinical findings, assessment, differential diagnosis, prognosis, complications, prevention, and management of the following vitamin and mineral deficiencies and toxicities: thiamine (B1), riboflavin (B2), niacin (B3), pyridoxine (B6), folate (B9), cyanocobalamin (B12), vitamin A, vitamin C, vitamin D, vitamin E, vitamin K, copper, and calcium.
- Recognize, describe and differentiate the risk factors, etiology, pathophysiology, clinical findings, assessment, differential diagnosis, prognosis, complications, screening, prevention, and management of the following inborn errors of metabolism: galactosemia, maple syrup urine disease (MSUD), and phenylketonuria (PKU).
- Identify the different macronutrients and discuss their role in human nutrition, including recommended macronutrient distribution per the U.S. Dietary Guidelines for Americans and determination of energy and water requirements.
- Discuss recommended nutrition therapy and provide appropriate patient education for cardiovascular disease, renal disease, and diabetes mellitus.
- Define altered consistency diets and mechanically altered diets and discuss indications, potential complications, and necessary monitoring for each.
- Define nutrition support, enteral nutrition (EN), and parenteral nutrition (PN) and discuss indications for use, types of access for delivery, potential complications, and role of the healthcare team in providing and monitoring this type of nutrition.

INTRODUCTION

Understanding nutrition is of vital importance for clinicians, as diet has a significant impact in prevention of disease and disease treatment. Nutrition plays a role in many phases of healthcare, from optimizing pediatric growth and development to prescribing a diet during a hospitalization to recognizing and treating vitamin deficiencies. PAs will frequently encounter nutrition-related diagnoses, manage these conditions, and provide initial dietary counseling.

Every 5 years the U.S. Department of Agriculture and the U.S. Department of Health and Human Services publish updated Dietary Guidelines for Americans to help health professionals understand and educate patients on eating a healthy diet.[1] Patient education handouts reflecting the current Dietary Guidelines for Americans are available in 21 different languages and for specific age groups from preschool to adult at www.ChooseMyPlate.gov; these are excellent resources to help support clinicians' nutrition education efforts.[1]

Registered dietitians (RDs) are highly trained nutrition professionals who complete extensive didactic and clinical training, sit for a national board examination, and complete continuing education; they play a critical role on the healthcare team. RDs practice in a wide variety of settings, including private practice, as part of the patient-centered medical home, in specialty clinics, and in hospitals. It is helpful and appropriate to refer patients to an RD when nutrition counseling is needed and to consult a dietitian in the hospital for patient nutrition education, diet therapy, and nutrition support.

9.1 MALNUTRITION

Jannelle Reynolds

OVERVIEW

Malnutrition is a broad term defined as any nutritional imbalance, encompassing undernutrition states and deficiencies of micronutrients (see Sections 9.4–9.6).[2,3] The World Health Organization (WHO) considers both kwashiorkor and marasmus, both typically found in resource-limited settings, to be indicators of severe acute malnutrition (SAM).[4] The American Society of Parenteral and Enteral Nutrition (ASPEN) has defined adult malnutrition by etiology and presence of inflammation (see Table 9.1).[3] ASPEN further characterizes adult malnutrition by severity, both moderate (nonsevere) and severe; these determinations are made considering adequacy of energy intake, duration of weight loss, loss of subcutaneous fat, muscle wasting, fluid accumulation, and grip strength.[3] Malnutrition also encompasses overnutrition, or an overabundance of macronutrients or other substances, which will be discussed elsewhere (see Section 9.2 Obesity).[5]

EPIDEMIOLOGY

Prevalence rates are impacted by age, marital status, healthcare setting, and the tools used to assess malnutrition risk.[6] According to a UNICEF estimate, approximately 198 million children worldwide are affected by malnutrition.[7] Protein-energy malnutrition occurs in about 50% of hospitalized older patients.[2] Risk factors for malnutrition include low socioeconomic status, food scarcity, lack of quality healthcare, lack of education on nutrition and a healthy diet, chronic infections, neglect, cultural and religious food customs, inadequate breastfeeding, and incomplete immunizations.[2]

TABLE 9.1 Types of Malnutrition

Malnutrition Term	Definition
Protein-energy malnutrition	Broad term that encompasses all types of malnutrition caused by lack of adequate protein and calories.
Kwashiorkor	Edematous malnutrition caused by inadequate intake of protein; typically seen in developing nations, particularly when weaning from breast milk.
Marasmus	Muscle and fat wasting syndrome characterized by inadequate protein and energy intake; typically develops over months in areas of famine.
Starvation-related malnutrition	Pure chronic starvation, including anorexia nervosa; not associated with systemic inflammation.
Chronic disease-related malnutrition	Associated with chronic disease, including cancer, chronic organ failure, and autoimmune disease; associated with mild to moderate systemic inflammation.
Acute disease-or injury-related malnutrition	Associated with major infection, burns, trauma, or other acute conditions associated with a marked inflammatory response.

PATHOPHYSIOLOGY

Protein-energy malnutrition affects every organ system.[5] Causes consist of impaired intake, increased metabolic requirements, increased losses from impaired digestion and/or absorption, and excessive nutrient losses.[5,8] In infants, protein-energy malnutrition results in growth retardation and alters brain development by reducing synapses and delaying myelination.[2] In older populations, protein-energy malnutrition is either primary, from a decrease in nutrient intake, or secondary, from an increase in catabolic stress such as cancer, chronic obstructive pulmonary disease (COPD), or sepsis.[2] Malnutrition causes an increase in protein breakdown and disrupts protein synthesis.[5] Protein requirements can increase by more than 20% in those with infection due to the rise in acute-phase proteins.[9] Protein loss occurs from the breakdown of skeletal muscle and organ tissue breakdown, including the liver, kidneys, heart, and gastrointestinal (GI) tract. Patients show a low concentration of glutamine, glutamic acid, urea cycle amino acids, and alanine, which are critical for several metabolic pathways like gluconeogenesis.[2,5] Severe protein-energy malnutrition can lead to renal insufficiency, impaired wound healing, cognitive impairment, muscle weakness, immune deficiency, hypothermia, decreased metabolic rate, and death.[2,5]

Children who present with protein-energy malnutrition are deficient in total protein, with lower total serum protein and albumin in kwashiorkor than in marasmus.[2] In the acute phase of protein-energy malnutrition, serum insulin levels are decreased and growth hormone levels elevated.[2] Severe protein-energy malnutrition significantly affects the heart, causing decreased stroke volume and oxidative damage to the cell membranes leading to a reduction in sodium-potassium pumps.[2] The remaining pumps work more slowly, which causes a buildup of intracellular sodium and potassium leakage leading to electrolyte and fluid imbalance.[2,5] Protein deficiency and the subsequent lack of immune mediators leads to immune deficiency and an increased risk of infection.[2,5] Decreased protein also leads to an increase risk of drug toxicity and worsening of existing conditions.[2]

MEDICAL HISTORY AND CLINICAL PRESENTATION

Patients will have a history of limited dietary intake from food insecurity or scarcity or from lack of access or intake of a varied diet, including adequate protein and micronutrients.[4,7] Patients with secondary malnutrition often have a history of chronic illness.[5] Patients may present with complaints of hunger, but this sensation may diminish over time.[4,7] Limited dietary protein may result in significant peripheral edema and anasarca.[5]

SIGNS AND SYMPTOMS

Signs and symptoms vary widely, from increased infection incidence to skin breakdown, as malnutrition can affect nearly every organ system.[2,5] Edema is indicative of a lack of dietary protein.

PHYSICAL EXAMINATION

Clinical features of protein-energy malnutrition can vary based on severity, chronicity, and other nutrient deficiencies. Marasmus clinical features include the following:

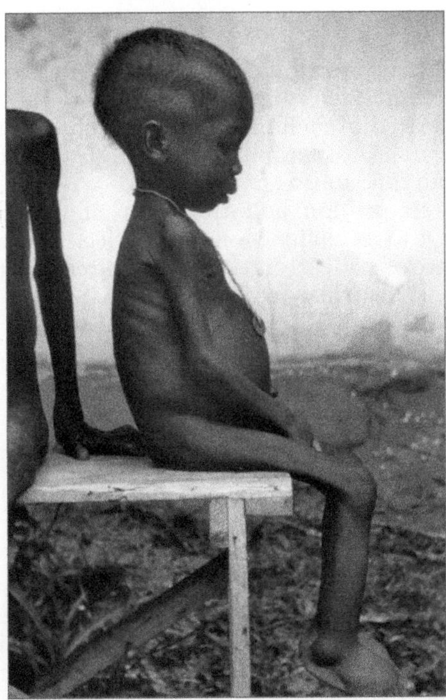

Figure 9.1 **Kwashiorkor in a pediatric patient; note the protuberant abdomen, presumably from hepatosplenomegaly, muscle wasting, and pedal edema.**

(Source: Centers for Disease Control and Prevention/Dr. Lyle Conrad, Public Health Image Library. https://phil.cdc.gov/Details.aspx?pid=6901)

growth retardation, wasting of subcutaneous fat and muscle, increased appetite, irritability, sunken eyes, and mild skin and hair changes.[2,5] Children with marasmus fail to thrive and are emaciated, are cachectic, lack subcutaneous fat, have muscle wasting, and may have chronic infections.[2,5] Kwashiorkor clinical features include the following: growth retardation, muscle wasting, preservation of subcutaneous fat, edema, hepatomegaly, psychomotor retardation, loss of appetite, fatigue, apathy, and severe skin and hair changes.[2,5] Pediatric patients with kwashiorkor, in addition to the above features, often have a protuberant abdomen (Figure 9.1). Skin and hair have a high cellular turnover rate and have high protein requirements, which is why they are significantly affected by protein deficiency.[5] Skin changes can include lanugo, ulcerations, depigmentation, and hyperpigmentation; hair changes can include depigmentation, straightening, different colored bands (flag sign), straightening of hair at bottom and curly at top (forest sign), and sparse, thin, easily pluckable hair.[5] Pavement dermatosis, in which skin is cracked with pale areas in between the cracks, is seen in kwashiorkor is due to the inelasticity of skin.[5]

DIFFERENTIAL DIAGNOSIS

Table 9.2 summarizes the differential diagnosis for malnutrition. Other diagnoses to consider include celiac disease or other malabsorptive GI disease, anorexia nervosa (AN), cancer, congestive heart failure, and AIDS.

DIAGNOSTIC STUDIES

Malnutrition is a clinical diagnosis; however, diagnostic studies are important to assess for degree of malnutrition, electrolyte disturbances, dehydration, and organ damage.[5]

TABLE 9.2 Differential Diagnosis to Consider in the Evaluation of Malnutrition

Diagnosis	Description
Chronic kidney disease	Fatigue, malaise, anorexia, nausea, vomiting, impaired mentation, weight loss, cachexia, muscle wasting, edema, electrolyte abnormalities
Cirrhosis	Weakness, fatigue, weight loss, nausea, vomiting, anorexia, peripheral edema, electrolyte abnormalities, anemia
Depression	Decreased food intake, weight loss, memory impairment, anhedonia
Inflammatory bowel disease	Electrolyte abnormalities, weight loss, diarrhea, malaise, fever, erythema nodosum, anemia and fatigue
Hypothyroidism	Lethargy, failure to thrive, eczema skin changes, fatigue, hair changes

EVALUATION

A detailed diet history with food availability, preferences, and medication history is critical to diagnosing and assessing malnutrition. No solitary parameter diagnosis defines malnutrition. As such, ASPEN guidelines suggest a diagnosis of malnutrition when two or more of the following six characteristics are present: insufficient energy intake, weight loss, loss of muscle mass, loss of subcutaneous fat, localized or generalized fluid accumulation, and diminished functional status measured by hand grip strength. Screening tools may be helpful to identify adolescents and adults at risk; many are available, including the Malnutrition Screening Tool or the Mini Nutritional Assessment.[6] The WHO recommends screening children using a mid-upper arm circumference (MUAC) and assessing for pitting edema.[4] A complete social history and depression screening are critical to assess the environmental and psychological factors contributing to and occurring because of malnutrition. A physical examination covering all body systems should be performed. Anthropometric assessments, including use of growth charts for pediatric patients, MUAC, and body mass index (BMI) are critical for both the initial assessment and monitoring; presence of significant edema may artificially alter true dry patient weight.[4,5,8] Laboratory assessment should include a complete blood count (CBC), complete metabolic profile (CMP) for renal and liver function and albumin, prealbumin, erythrocyte sedimentation rate (ESR), and thyroid-stimulating hormone (TSH).[4,5] Additional serum laboratory studies that may be beneficial include the following: zinc, iron, vitamin D, cortisol, growth hormone, and insulin.[4,5] Additionally, a urinalysis for urine urea, skin biopsy, and hair pull analysis may be beneficial.[2,5]

Laboratory tests results vary but can show increased levels of aspartate aminotransferase (AST) and alanine aminotransferase (ALT), iron deficiency anemia, reduced reticulocytes and leukopenia, hypoalbuminemia, low prealbumin, hypoglycemia, high levels of cortisol and growth hormone, hypokalemia, hypomagnesemia, reduced urine urea, and low blood pH (metabolic acidosis).[2] Potassium levels are low in kwashiorkor and marasmus, but usually much lower in kwashiorkor when corrected for acidosis.[2] This leads to increased sodium and water retention in cells and rise in sodium pumps and therefore edema.[2] No single laboratory test can indicate nutritional status; diagnostic studies should be reviewed in the context of the patient's history and physical exam to accurately diagnose malnutrition.

TREATMENT

- The first priority is to stabilize the patient by correcting fluid and electrolyte imbalances, treating infections, correcting specific nutrient deficiencies, and managing acute complications. Complications can include diarrhea, dehydration, shock, hypoglycemia, hypothermia, and sepsis.[9] Intravenous fluids and medications should be avoided whenever possible; oral rehydration is preferred.[4]
- Patients with an appetite, who are clinically well and alert, may be treated as outpatients. If medical complications, edema, or a poor appetite are present, patients should be hospitalized for treatment.[4]
- Children with SAM should be provided with 5,000 IU of vitamin A daily either in a micronutrient formulation or as part of a meal.[4] High-dose vitamin A should be given to all children with SAM during initial treatment (see Section 9.4 Fat-Soluble Vitamin Disorders).[4]
- In resource-limited countries, ready-to-use therapeutic food (RUTF) in specific nutrient formulations for each treatment stage, available through UNICEF, is the preferred initial nutrition for children with SAM. Refeeding syndrome is a concern; additional thiamine supplementation may help prevent refeeding syndrome.[10] It is preferable to begin feeding as soon as possible and to slow nutrition and correct electrolytes should refeeding syndrome develop (see Section 9.3B Refeeding Syndrome).[4] Initial treatment is with high carbohydrate and low fat, protein, and sodium meals, as absorption of the latter is significantly impaired in SAM.[4] It is critical to initially feed in frequent, small amounts as internal organs recover.[4]
- Once the patient is medically stable, nutritional rehabilitation should provide high energy and protein. A reasonable target for pediatric patients is 175 kcal/kg and 4 g/kg of protein; a reasonable target for adults is 60 kcal/kg and 2 g/kg of protein.[9]
- Patients may benefit from a multivitamin with minerals supplement.[4]
- Milk-based diets are often utilized in nutritional rehabilitation, as they are rich in high-quality protein.[9] Vegetable-based proteins, such as legumes, are inferior to milk-based diets in terms of clearance of edema and rise in serum albumin; however, mixed-protein diets are reasonable and effective.[9]
- Adults with malnutrition should be referred to an RD whenever possible; if a patient with malnutrition is hospitalized, consult dietetic services.

PATIENT EDUCATION

- With appropriate treatment, there is a high recovery rate, and skin and hair changes are typically reversible with treatment. Growth potential may be permanently altered, and some physical and intellectual disabilities may persist.
- Optimizing the diet as much as possible is important to prevent recurrence. Seeing an RD may be helpful to make dietary changes.

KEY POINTS

- Protein-energy malnutrition is common in both resource-limited settings and in hospitalized patients, particularly those who are older and chronically ill.
- Malnutrition affects immune function, wound healing, and organ function.
- Prompt recognition and treatment of malnutrition is imperative to regain function of any affected organ systems and improve patient outcomes. If untreated and severe, malnutrition can lead to death.

9.2 OBESITY

MIA J. HYDE

OVERVIEW

Obesity, one of the most common disorders in medical practice, is currently an epidemic in the United States. This condition of excessive accumulation of adipose tissue puts patients at a higher risk for more serious chronic diseases, such as type 2 diabetes, cardiovascular diseases, sleep apnea, orthopedic problems, cancers, psychosocial issues, and others. Not only do these chronic, and often preventable, conditions contribute to increased patient morbidity and mortality, but they also contribute to inflated health-care costs.

The prevalence of obesity has risen dramatically over the past several decades, to the point that it is now widely recognized as one of our nation's primary health issues. Current predictions project that obesity will soon surpass smoking as the leading cause of preventable death in the United States. According to the Centers for Disease Control and Prevention National Center for Health Statistics, the prevalence of obesity was 39.8% and affected about 93.3 million U.S. adults in 2015–2016.[11] Experts anticipate that 85% of adults will be overweight or obese by 2030.[12]

EPIDEMIOLOGY

Figure 9.2 depicts the overall prevalence of self-reported obesity by state among U.S. adults with statistics gathered through 2011.

Throughout the last 50 years, the prevalence of obesity in the United States has steadily climbed, jumping from 13% in 1960–1994 to 35% in the last 10-year period of data collection.[12] Certain subpopulations are affected more than others, with Hispanics (43%) and non-Hispanic Blacks (48%) having disproportionately higher rates.[12] Gender also plays a role, with women exhibiting more extreme obesity than men, regardless of race or ethnicity.[12] Socioeconomic status also displays trends within subpopulations, but differs by gender, race, and ethnicity. Most prevalent trends include lower obesity rates in persons with higher education levels and either high-end or low-end income levels. Middle-income groups tend to have the highest obesity rates.

PATHOPHYSIOLOGY

Obesity has a multifactorial base of origin. It is considered the direct result of an imbalance between the intake of

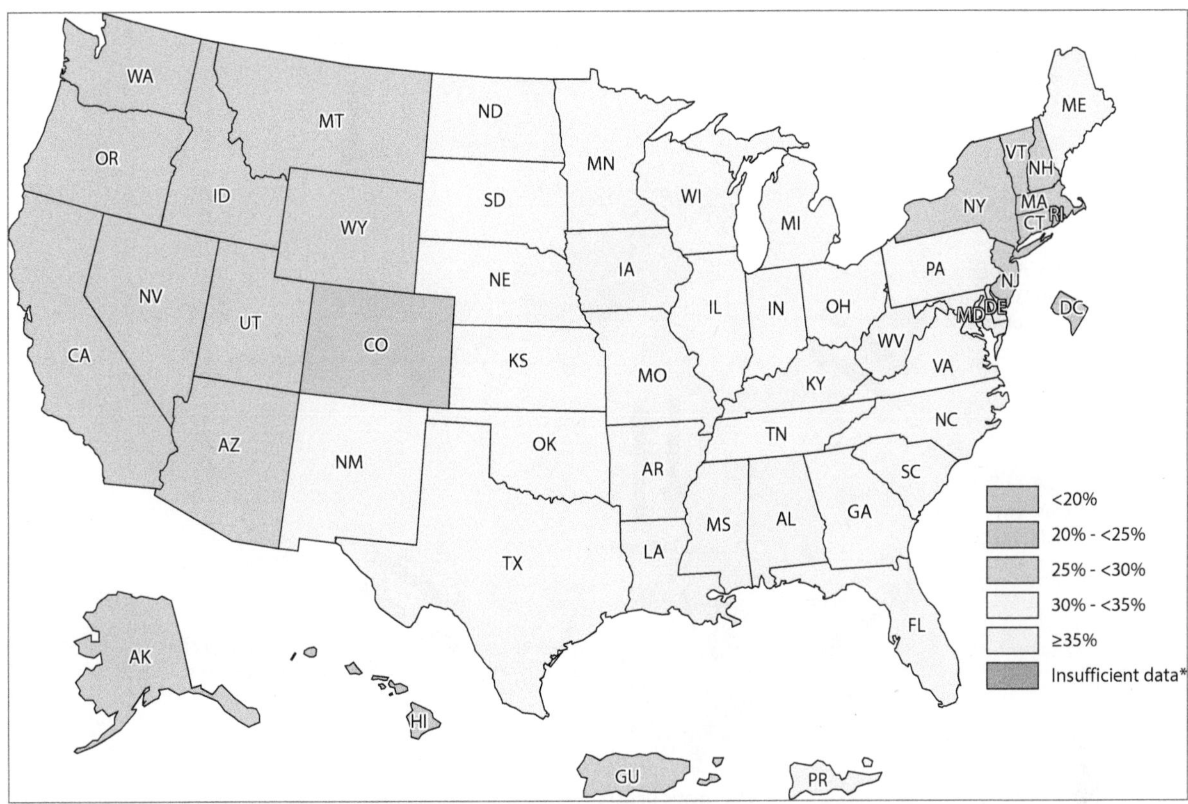

Figure 9.2 Prevalence of self-reported obesity among U.S. adults by state and territory, 2018.
(Source: From Centers for Disease Control and Prevention. Behavioral Risk Factor Surveillance System Survey Data. U.S. Department of Health and Human Services, Centers for Disease Control and Prevention; 2018.)

TABLE 9.3 Factors Influencing Obesity

Dietary	Neuroendocrine	Social/Behavioral	Environmental/Lifestyle	Genetic
Infant feeding practices	Cushing syndrome	Socioeconomic status	Sedentary/limited activity	Autosomal recessive traits
Frequency of eating	Polycystic ovary syndrome	Ethnicity	Sleep deprivation	Autosomal dominant traits
High-fat diets	Hypogonadism	Psychological factors	Aging restrictions	X-linked traits
Overeating	Growth hormone deficiency	Night eating syndrome	Medications (antipsychotics, antidepressants, glucocorticoids)	Chromosomal abnormalities
	Hypothyroidism	Binge-eating		Prader-Willi syndrome
	Hypothalamic obesity			

excess calories and the decreased expenditure of energy. Yet, genetics, aging, environmental, behavioral, and lifestyle influences play an important role as well. Five genes affecting appetite control have been identified in mice, each with a human homolog. Mutations of these genes have been shown to result in obesity in mice. Although these findings are interesting, only a small percentage of human obesity is believed to be due to genetic mutation. The overwhelming majority of human obesity is due to interactions of multiple genes, environmental factors, and behavior (Table 9.3).

The brain is the key modulator of body weight. There are various negative feedback loops originating in the arcuate nucleus of the hypothalamus and the nucleus tractus solitarius that contribute to the development of obesity.[13–15] These feedback processes are needed for energy expenditure, digestion, absorption, transport, and storage of nutrients and utilization of substances for fuel. The brain, responding to the information delivered by these processes, initiates metabolic and cognitive responses accordingly regarding need for food or satiety.

Afferent signals from adipose tissue and the GI tract carry messages about surplus or deficit of nutrients. Circulating hormones, such as insulin, leptin, and ghrelin, are primary players in this circuit of feeding and hunger (Figure 9.3).[13] Insulin is produced in the pancreas in response to increased glucose levels and incretin stimulus.[13] The increase in insulin occurs to normalize glucose levels, unless there is a defect

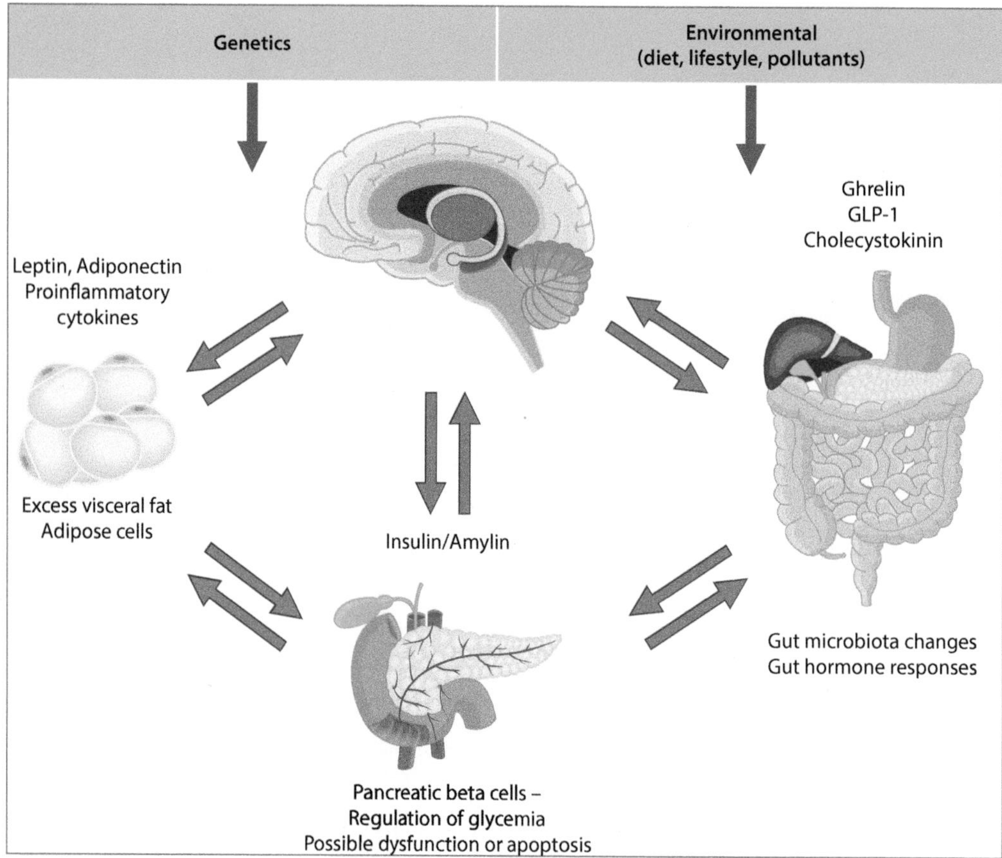

Figure 9.3 **Pathophysiology of obesity, involving various genetic and environmental factors that interfere with target organs linked by neurohormonal pathways.** GLP-1, glucagon-like peptide-1.

present in the pancreatic beta cells. Destruction of the beta cells can occur over time in obese patients due to chronic fuel excess, resulting in metabolic stress and damage of target organs. Leptin is produced in adipose cells and is closely correlated with body fat mass. Leptin can be anorexigenic, meaning appetite is decreased. Yet, most obese individuals have elevated plasma leptin concentrations from increased fat stores, which they fail to respond to, known as leptin resistance. Other gut hormones that act as inhibitors of food intake include adiponectin, glucagon-like peptide-1 (GLP-1), cholecystokinin, pancreatic polypeptide, and peptide YY3-36.[15] Ghrelin, a peptide hormone produced in the gut, is an orexigenic, meaning appetite is increased.[15] Serum concentrations increase in anticipation of a meal and decrease following food ingestion. Other food intake stimulators include melanocyte-stimulating hormone, growth hormone-releasing hormone, and neuropeptide Y.[15]

MEDICAL HISTORY AND CLINICAL PRESENTATION

Historical information is a key component to the evaluation of a patient regarding obesity. Many cases of obesity can be diagnosed based on the history findings. The patient may admit to an increase in food intake, lack of exercise, or sedentary lifestyle and have no other symptoms or risk factors. If this is not the case, clinicians must rule out a secondary cause of obesity. Obese patients rarely have an identifiable secondary cause, but it must be considered in all.[13,14]

The background gathered from a patient will assist in the determination of the cause of obesity and development of a management plan individualized to the patient's specific needs. Patients may present with the following complaints, or may be diagnosed in conjunction with comorbid conditions:

- Decreased exercise tolerance
- Fatigue
- Shortness of breath
- Sleep apnea
- Heartburn
- Skin conditions, including acanthosis nigricans
- Inability to succeed in weight loss
- Comorbid conditions, including diabetes mellitus, metabolic syndrome, polycystic ovary syndrome, coronary disease, dyslipidemia, venous problems, and reproductive difficulty

The medical history should include the following:

- Age of onset
- Recent or significant weight changes or life events that may have triggered weight change
- Previous weight loss attempts, including timing and duration of weight loss attempt, method of attempt (diet change, activity increase, prescription medication, and/or over-the-counter medications or supplements), and outcome of attempt
- Weight status as a child, highest/lowest weight as an adult, and highest/lowest weight in last 5 years
- Past medical history, including chronic disease, surgeries, obstetric and menstrual history for females, and medication reconciliation, including supplements and over-the-counter medications
- Family history of obesity and/or other comorbid conditions
- Social history including occupation; alcohol, tobacco, or drug use; sleep habits; nutritional history including a detailed food diary; and exercise history

SIGNS AND SYMPTOMS

Patients with obesity may present with various signs and symptoms, ranging in degree from obvious to very subtle. Clinical presentations will also vary based on the degree of obesity, mild to morbid. It is important in patients with subtle findings, or signs of secondary comorbid conditions, to screen for and consider obesity in the differential diagnosis. Often management of obesity is an important factor in treating the secondary cause or condition.

Some common presenting signs and symptoms may include breathlessness, fatigue, high blood pressure, snoring, joint pain, insomnia, depression, heartburn, urinary frequency, anovulation, and skin rash. Other symptoms may be specific to obesity-related conditions such as heart disease, diabetes, gallbladder disease, colon cancer, osteoarthritis, and others.

EXHIBIT 9.1 Obesity Classifications by Body Mass Index

BMI is calculated by weight (kg)/height (m^2)
BMI >25 = overweight (grade I)
BMI >30 = obese (grade II)
- 30–34.9 = class 1 obesity
- 35–39.9 = class 2 obesity

BMI ≥40 = morbid obesity (grade III)

BMI, body mass index.

PHYSICAL EXAMINATION

A comprehensive physical exam to rule out secondary causes of obesity is recommended for patients presenting for initial evaluation.[14] Generally, obesity can be defined by an abnormally elevated BMI (Exhibit 9.1).[13]

Table 9.4 outlines additional physical examination components to assess in addition to BMI screening.

DIFFERENTIAL DIAGNOSIS

Table 9.5 summarizes the differential diagnosis for obesity.

DIAGNOSTIC STUDIES

Initial diagnostic studies are utilized to assess for secondary causes of the patient's obesity as well as to assess for medical consequences of the condition and include the following:

- **Lipid panel:** At a minimum, this should include a fasting cholesterol level, triglycerides, and high-density lipoprotein cholesterol (HDL-C).[13] If findings reveal reduced HDL-C and elevated triglyceride, this would suggest a typical dyslipidemia seen with metabolic syndrome. A low-density lipoprotein cholesterol (LDL-C) may also be included and is often found to be elevated in obese individuals.
- **Liver and thyroid function tests:** Results of these tests will likely be normal in obese patients, but elevated transaminase levels may indicate nonalcoholic steatohepatitis (NASH) or fatty liver disease. If TSH levels are elevated, it would be beneficial to screen further for hypothyroidism to evaluate it as a secondary cause of obesity.

TABLE 9.4 Physical Examination Components in the Evaluation of Obesity

Physical Examination Category	Assessment
Vital signs	Blood pressure, pulse, respirations, temperature, pulse oximetry
General assessment	Level of distress Appearance—type of obesity (gynecoid, android, cushingoid)
Head/neck	Facial appearance, thyroid assessment, neck diameter
Skin/integument	Rash, skin turgor, skin dryness, hair or nail changes, hair distribution
Eyes	Vision changes, corneal abnormalities Intraocular vascular or retinal changes
Ear/nose/throat	Oral examination for mucosal or gingival changes
Respiratory	Anteroposterior/transverse diameter, observation of respiratory effort, auscultation of lung fields
Cardiovascular	Assessment for rhythm, regularity, murmurs, S3/S4 heart sounds, lifts, or thrills Assessment of peripheral vessels, carotids, bruits
Abdomen	Waist circumference (>35 inches female, >40 inches male), inspect for striae/scars, auscultate, palpate for liver/spleen enlargement or masses
Genitourinary	Male: Genitourinary/rectal examination exam if indicated Female: Pelvic examination to assess uterus and ovaries; may include bladder if indicated based on symptoms and patient presentation
Musculoskeletal	Inspect and evaluate joints for any signs of osteoarthritic or rheumatic changes, muscle wasting, weakness; may need more in-depth assessment based on patient symptoms
Neurologic	Assess for neuropathy in extremities, coordination, possibly memory if patient presentation indicates
Psychological	Assess mood, emotional status, screen for depression or anxiety

Source: Data from Tsai AG, Bessesen DH. Obesity. Ann Intern Med. *2019;170(5):ITC33–ITC48. doi:10.7326/AITC201903050*

TABLE 9.5 Differential Diagnosis to Consider When Evaluating a Patient for Obesity

Diagnosis	Description
Depression	Feelings of sadness, loss of interest or pleasure, changes in appetite, trouble sleeping, loss of energy, fatigue, feeling of worthlessness or guilt, difficulty concentrating, suicidal thoughts
Type 2 diabetes mellitus	Polydipsia, polyphagia, dry mouth, frequent urination, changes in weight, fatigue, blurred vision, tingling in hands or feet, slow healing wounds, headaches, skin rashes
Metabolic syndrome	Increased waist circumference, polydipsia, polyphagia, frequent urination, fatigue, blurred vision, weight gain, high blood pressure, headaches, high cholesterol
Fatty liver disease	Abdominal pain, feeling of fullness in upper abdomen, loss of appetite, nausea, weakness, jaundice, edema of abdomen or legs, mental confusion
Gastroesophageal reflux disease	Burning sensation in chest (usually after eating and worse at night), chest pain, difficulty swallowing, sore throat, sensation of lump in throat, regurgitation of food or sour liquid
Hirsutism	Oily skin, deepening voice, loss of hair, acne, decreased breast size, increased muscle mass, enlargement of clitoris
Insulinoma	Blurring or double vision, mental confusion, anxiety, irritability, dizziness, mood swings, weakness, sweating, hunger
Kallmann syndrome and idiopathic hypogonadotropic hypogonadism	Undescended testicles, small penile size, facial defects (cleft palate or lip), short fingers or toes, development of only one kidney, hearing loss, color blindness, abnormal eye movements
Lipodystrophy, generalized	Abnormal distribution of body fat, symptoms consistent with diabetes and fatty liver disease
Polycystic ovariy syndrome	Irregular periods or anovulatory, difficulty conceiving, excessive hair growth, weight gain, thinning hair or hair loss, oily skin or acne
Cushing syndrome	Weight gain, thin arms/legs, rounded "moon" face, increased fat around base of neck, fatty hump between shoulders, easy bruising, striae, muscle weakness
Medication-induced obesity	Weight gain due to offending medication, especially antipsychotics, antidepressants, antiepileptics, corticosteroids
Growth hormone deficiency	Anxiety or depression, hair loss (men), decreased sexual interest and function, decreased muscle mass and strength, difficulty concentrating and memory loss, dry skin, elevated triglyceride levels, fatigue
Binge-eating disorder	Fatigue, weight gain, anxiety/depression or mood swings, hunger, weight change, dental caries, compulsive behavior

- *Glucose and insulin studies.* All patients with obesity should be screened for diabetes. The preferred diagnostic study by the American Diabetes Association is a fasting blood glucose and a hemoglobin A1c (HbA1c).[13] Type 2 diabetes is diagnosed when the fasting glucose is 126 mg/dL or greater or the HbA1c is 6.5% or higher.

If the history and/or physical exam findings indicate the need for additional studies to rule out neuroendocrine causes, these can be considered on a case-by-case basis. For example, one may consider a 24-hour urine cortisol level if Cushing syndrome is suspected, a sleep study if sleep apnea is suspected, or a hormone panel including follicle-stimulating hormone and luteinizing hormone if polycystic ovary syndrome is suspected.

TREATMENT

Individuals diagnosed with obesity require an individualized care plan based on their comorbidities, risk factors, and individual current health status and psychosocial circumstances.

- It is crucial that realistic goals are established by and with the patient. Weight loss should be gradual over a long term, approximately 2 pounds per week to promote adherence and prevent return of weight. Patients should expect to lose 8% to 10% of their weight over a 3- to 6- month period.[13,14]
- First-line management is a conservative approach addressing nutritional needs, physical activity levels, and behavioral support.
- Patients should be encouraged to follow a healthful meal pattern and decrease daily caloric intake. The assistance of a dietitian is beneficial if available for consultation. A good guideline is to decrease caloric intake by 500 to 1,000 kcal/day. To promote accountability, encourage the use of a food diary and avoidance of processed foods and eating take-out meals.[14]
- Physical activity should be increased with limitations placed on sedentary time. Encourage patients to strive for 30 to 60 minutes of activity most days of the week. They may start slowly and progress to a goal of exercising 5 days per week.[13,14]
- For behavioral support, offer community resources for support groups or healthy lifestyle groups. Institute a bidirectional plan of care and support, where by the clinician has frequent contact with the patient regarding their progress and questions.
- Second-line management may incorporate pharmacotherapeutic treatment as an adjunct to lifestyle interventions and first-line management approach. The addition of medication should be considered only in patients with a BMI >30 or a BMI 27 to 29.9 with a comorbid condition.[13,14]
- Medications available to treat obesity consist of centrally acting drugs that impair dietary intake, peripherally acting drugs that impair dietary absorption, and drugs that increase energy expenditure. The choice of which drug to employ should be based on the individual patient's comorbidities and contraindications (Table 9.6).[13,14]

TABLE 9.6 Pharmacotherapeutic Options Approved for Long-Term Management of Obesity

Generic Name	Mechanism of Action	Usual Dosing (Adult)	Precautions
Orlistat 60, 120 mg	Pancreatic lipase inhibitor	120 mg three times daily with fat-containing meal	Fecal incontinence, GI side effects Contraindicated in pregnancy
Lorcaserin 10 mg (Controlled Class C-IV)	Serotonin-2C receptor agonist	10 mg twice daily	Decreased liver/kidney function Contraindicated in pregnancy Not for use with other serotoninergic meds
Phentermine-topiramate (Controlled Class C-IV)	Combination med	Initial: 3.75 mg phentermine/23 mg topiramate once daily × 14 days; then titrate based on response. Max: 15 mg phentermine/92 mg topiramate daily	Abuse potential Topiramate is teratogenic Contraindicated in pregnancy, glaucoma, hyperthyroidism Must taper off dose over at least 1 week Decreased liver/kidney function
Bupropion 8 mg-naltrexone 90 mg	Combination med	Week 1: 1 tab once daily Week 2: 1 tab twice daily Week 3: 2 tabs in a.m. and 1 tab in evening Week 4: 2 tabs twice daily Max: 4 tabs daily	Contraindicated in patients with hypertension, seizures, eating disorder, pregnancy or breastfeeding Do not use with or within 14 days of MAO inhibitors
Liraglutide	GLP-1 agonist	Initial: 0.6 mg subcutaneously daily Increase at weekly intervals (1.2, 1.8, 2.4 mg) until recommended dose of 3 mg daily	Gastrointestinal side effects, possibly hypoglycemia Decreased liver/kidney function Contraindicated in pregnancy Possible increased risk for thyroid cancer

GI, gastrointestinal; GLP-1, glucagon-like peptide-1; MAO, monoamine oxidase.

- Bariatric surgery is an increasingly prevalent treatment option for patients with more severe grades of obesity. Roux-en-Y gastric bypass (RYGB) and sleeve gastrectomy are the most common bariatric procedures in the United States.[14] RYGB can be done laparoscopically and typically results in a reduction of over 30% of an individual's initial body weight.[14] Complications are relatively frequent in patients who undergo RYGB and include peritonitis, wound infection, thromboembolic disease, and nutritional deficiencies (iron, vitamin B12, folate, calcium, and vitamin D); however, it is very effective for maintaining weight loss.[13,14] Another surgical option is adjustable gastric banding. Although the surgical time is shorter, the hospital stay is shorter, and there are fewer complications, gastric banding patients frequently experience weight regain.[13,14]

PATIENT EDUCATION

PAs must advocate for their patients with obesity by providing current and comprehensive information that is individualized to patient needs and circumstances.

- Present the details of diagnosis to the patient in a nonjudgmental manner and ask for their input on establishing a management plan that will be agreeable; this increases the likelihood of compliance and success.
- Explain the medical process leading to obesity and any underlying comorbidities as well as the risk to their overall health.
- Help patients establish realistic goals for weight loss and lifestyle modifications that are achievable and not overwhelming.
- Ensure patients are supported by instituting frequent follow-up, whether by phone, return visits, and/or family or support groups. When patients do follow-up, continue to encourage them in their efforts and point out the positive health improvements, such as lower blood pressure or cholesterol levels.
- Discuss setbacks and advise them on ways to meet these challenges. Goals can always be adjusted to promote continued efforts toward success.
- Patient handouts are a great resource to ensure that accurate medical information is being shared. Other community resources to consider are nutritional consultants, physical activity or gym facilities, and behavioral support groups.

KEY POINTS

- Obesity is extremely prevalent in the United States and may present as the primary concern or in association with a comorbid condition.
- Excess calorie intake and insufficient energy expenditure are the primary cause, in combination with genetics and patient lifestyle.
- Compassionate, patient-centered, individualized treatment is essential. Initial treatment is with lifestyle modification. Referral to a dietitian for nutrition counseling may be beneficial.

9.3 EATING DISORDERS

MARK AKSAMIT

9.3A ANOREXIA NERVOSA

OVERVIEW

AN has the highest fatality rate of all eating disorders with a mortality rate of 0.51% per year, 25% of which is due to suicide.[16] The American Psychiatric Association's *Diagnostic and Statistical Manual of Mental Disorders,* Fifth Edition

EXHIBIT 9.2 Anorexia Nervosa Severity Classification by Body Mass Index in Adults

Mild: BMI 17–18.49 kg/m^2
Moderate: BMI 16–16.99 kg/m^2
Severe: BMI 15–15.99 kg/m^2
Extreme: BMI ≤15 kg/m^2

BMI, body mass index.

(*DSM-V*) provides three main diagnostic criteria: a restriction of energy intake relative to requirements leading to a very low body weight, intense fear of weight gain or persistent behavior preventing weight gain despite a low weight, and disturbance in the way one's body weight is experienced or undue influence of body weight on self-esteem.[17] Disease severity in AN is characterized by BMI in adults and by BMI for age percentile in children and adolescents (Exhibit 9.2).[17] AN has subclassifications of binge-eating/purging type, in which the individual engages in binge-eating or purging behaviors, such as self-induced vomiting or laxative misuse, or restricting type, in which the individual does not engage in these behaviors.[17] These subclassifications are based on behaviors during the last 3 months and may fluctuate throughout the disease course.[17]

EPIDEMIOLOGY

In the United States, AN has a lifetime prevalence of 0.9% in adult females and 0.3% in adult males; however, actual prevalence may be higher, as concealment of the disease is common in eating disorders.[18] In adolescents age 13 to 18 years, AN has a lifetime prevalence of 0.3% of females and 0.3% of males, with a median age of onset of 12.3 years of age, or sixth and seventh grades in the United States.[19] AN, which is thought to be most prevalent in industrialized, high-income countries, commonly develops during adolescence or young adulthood and rarely begins after age 40.[17]

PATHOPHYSIOLOGY

Development of AN is multifactorial, having biologic, social, and behavioral components. Significant data suggest a genetic component contributes to the development of AN, potentially linked to specific serotonergic, dopaminergic, opioidergic, or appetite regulation genes, though genetic heritability estimates for AN are broad, ranging from 28% to 74%.[20] First-degree relatives of individuals with AN are 11 times more likely to develop AN than relatives of control subjects.[20] Social and environmental factors, such as living in a culture that values thinness, weight-centric sports participation, and model envy, are also associated with increased risk of AN development.[17] Patients with AN frequently have comorbid mood or anxiety disorders, though mood disorders may improve as weight is restored.[17,21] Individuals with anxiety disorders or who demonstrate obsessive behavior in early life are at higher risk for development of the disease.[17]

MEDICAL HISTORY AND CLINICAL PRESENTATION

Concealment and fear of disease discovery is common in AN, so patients may not readily admit to restrictive eating; wearing baggy clothing, social withdrawal, and concerns about eating in public are common.[17,22] Patients will appear thin and/or malnourished, and may present with mood-related complaints, like depressed mood, insomnia, and anxiety.[17] Patients will often express intense fear of weight gain or describe a pattern of activity to prevent weight gain despite their thinness.[17] Body dysmorphia, when the patient has a disturbed view of their actual weight or appearance, such as describing themselves as fat when actually emaciated, is common; patients may also experience inappropriate influence of their weight on self-esteem.[17,22] Patients with AN frequently obsess about food, which can take many forms: hoarding recipes, memorizing caloric values of foods, obsessive meal planning, weighing food, overusing artificially sweetened products, and overestimating calories consumed.[17,22] Limiting the diet to a few "safe" foods and eliminating consumption of calorically dense foods are common behaviors.[22] Inflexible thinking and a strong desire to control one's environment are common in AN.[17]

The SCOFF questionnaire can be a useful screening tool in the primary care setting for eating disorders, particularly AN and bulimia nervosa.[23] A positive SCOFF screen of two or more "yes" responses has a sensitivity of 100% for AN; specificity is reported at 89.6%.[23]

SIGNS AND SYMPTOMS

Presenting symptoms are highly variable depending on illness severity and duration and the patient's transparency about food restriction. Symptoms may include complaints of feeling cold, amenorrhea, dizziness, chest pain, hair loss, hyperpigmented skin, lower extremity edema, depressed mood, anxiety, and/or insomnia.[17] Amenorrhea, which was a diagnostic criterion in the *DSM-IV* but was dropped in the *DSM-V*, is common, especially at very low BMI; menarche may be delayed in prepubertal females.[17]

PHYSICAL EXAMINATION

Physical examination abnormalities in AN are related to starvation. Anthropometric measurements will reveal a low BMI or dropping off an established growth curve in children and adolescents.[17] Abnormal vital signs are common and include hypotension, bradycardia, and hypothermia.[17] Development of lanugo, or diffuse fine, downy body hair, may occur; other dermatologic changes include hair loss or thinning, brittle nails, and hyperpigmented skin (Figure 9.4).[17,24] Peripheral edema may develop as serum albumin lowers in starvation, during weight restoration, or if diuretic or laxative abuse is stopped.[17] Russell sign, or knuckle callouses, in addition to dental erosions or dental fractures may be present in self-induced vomiting (see Figure 9.6).[24] The cardiac exam may reveal midsystolic clicks and a late systolic murmur from mitral valve prolapse.[25]

DIFFERENTIAL DIAGNOSIS

Table 9.7 summarizes the differential diagnosis for AN.

DIAGNOSTIC STUDIES

Diagnostic studies in AN are completed to assess for starvation-related abnormalities that contribute to morbidity and mortality (Table 9.8).

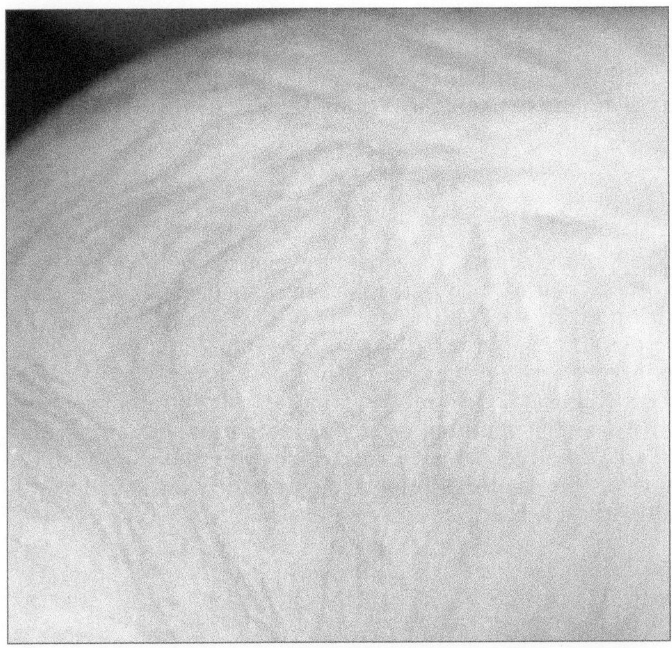

Figure 9.4 Lanugo. Diffuse, downy, fine body hair associated with anorexia nervosa.

EVALUATION

Evaluation of AN is best accomplished with a multidisciplinary team of clinicians, psychiatrists or psychologists, and RDs experienced in treating this disease. Patients with AN who are medically unstable, which may be indicated by severe bradycardia, hypotension, orthostatic hypotension, cardiac dysrhythmias, evidence of organ compromise, severe dehydration, electrolyte imbalance, or extremely low body weight should be admitted for inpatient medical stabilization.[22] Additionally, patients with AN should undergo suicide risk assessment.[17]

TREATMENT

- Patients with AN who are medically unstable or at risk for suicide should be admitted for stabilization.[22] If a patient cannot control binge-eating/purging, amount of exercise, or consuming adequate calories independently and/or lack familial support, inpatient hospitalization in an eating disorder unit or an intensive outpatient program should be considered.[22]
- Medically stable patients with AN who are capable of compliance regarding calorie intake, limiting exercise, and purging and who have good support can be treated

TABLE 9.8 Diagnostic Studies in Anorexia Nervosa

Laboratory Study	Potential Findings
Complete blood count with differential	• Leukopenia with lymphocytosis • Anemia
Chemistries: Complete metabolic profile, serum phosphorus, serum magnesium, and prealbumin	• Elevated blood urea nitrogen (BUN), suggesting dehydration • Hypoglycemia • Hypokalemia, hypomagnesemia, hypophosphatemia • Elevated serum bicarbonate and hypochloremia (metabolic acidosis from self-induced vomiting or laxative abuse) • Decreased albumin and prealbumin
Thyroid panel	• Low thyroid-stimulating hormone (TSH) • Low T3 • Low reverse T3 • Low-normal T4
Electrocardiography	• Bradycardia • Prolonged QTc interval
Echocardiography	• Decreased cardiac mass • Mitral valve prolapse • Myocardial fibrosis • Pericardial effusion
DEXA for bone density	• Low bone density, osteopenia, or osteoporosis
Urinalysis	• High specific gravity (dehydration) • Ketones (starvation)

These laboratory studies assess for biochemical abnormality and organ dysfunction as a result of starvation or binge-eating/purging compensatory behaviors. Values typically normalize with nutritional rehabilitation and cessation of compensatory behaviors.

DEXA, dual-energy x-ray absorptiometry; QTc interval, corrected QT interval; T3, triiodothyronine; T4, thyroxine.

TABLE 9.7 Differential Diagnosis to Consider in the Evaluation of Anorexia Nervosa

Diagnosis	Description
Medical conditions that cause weight loss, including cancer, AIDS, hyperthyroidism, or malabsorptive GI disease	Patients typically have other clinical features of their disease in addition to weight loss. Patients with these conditions rarely experience body dysmorphia or participate in behaviors that prevent weight gain.
Schizophrenia	Chronic or recurrent psychosis may manifest in unusual eating patterns. Patients with schizophrenia rarely have fear of weight gain or body dysmorphia.
Substance use disorders (SUDs)	Patients with SUD may lack adequate nutritional intake, leading to low body weight, but rarely have fear of weight gain or body dysmorphia. SUD may be comorbid condition of AN, so a patient should be screened for an eating disorder if they express fear of weight gain or body dysmorphia.
Bulimia nervosa	Bulimia nervosa has significant clinical overlap with AN, including episodes of binge-eating and purging and body dysmorphia, but body weight is at or above a normal BMI.
Avoidant/restrictive food intake disorder	Individuals with this disorder will have low body weight from lack of interest in eating or avoidance of eating. They do not have a fear of weight gain or body dysmorphia.

AN, anorexia nervosa; BMI, body mass index; GI, gastrointestinal.

as outpatients with close supervision, such as with weekly weigh-in visits with the primary care clinician.[22] Care should be coordinated to keep the interdisciplinary team apprised of the patient's condition.

- The initial priority of treatment is nutritional rehabilitation and weight restoration; however, psychotherapy is critical to successfully treating AN.[22,26] Research suggests family-based treatment (the Maudsley method) is best for adolescents with AN; adults with AN benefit the most from individual cognitive-based therapy.[22,26] It is essential that treating clinicians be experienced in managing AN.
- Weighing should occur on a set schedule of days at a consistent time of day; weighing first thing in the morning after the patient has voided is optimal.[27] Patients should be weighed in a hospital gown and underwear only.[27]
- Optimal rate of initiating nutritional rehabilitation is unclear; starting at 1,500 to 1,800 daily calories in AN in a hospitalized patient who can be closely monitored is likely reasonable, with subsequent increases of 200 to 300 calories per day.[22,27,28] Goal weight gain in hospitalized patients is 2 to 3 pounds per week until ideal body weight is achieved; lower goals for weekly weight gain in an outpatient setting with medically stable patients are reasonable to facilitate treatment alliance.[28] The diet should be well balanced with macronutrients distributed according to the standard diet regimen in the United States: carbohydrates 45% to 65% of calories, fat 20% to 35% of calories, and protein 10% to 35% of calories.[1] A daily multivitamin is indicated during nutritional rehabilitation.[22]
- Pharmacologic agents have not been consistently proved to aid in weight restoration or prevent relapse of AN; however, selective serotonin reuptake inhibitors (SSRIs) may help treat comorbid depression and/or suicidal ideation.[22]
- Relapse is very common, and approximately half of patients never fully recover.[22] Regular psychotherapy, high variety in foods consumed, and the degree to which the ideal body weight is achieved are positive predictors of lasting recovery.[22]

PATIENT EDUCATION

- Treatment with a multidisciplinary team experienced in treating AN is important to achieving recovery.
- Recovered patients will have higher daily caloric requirements than control subjects for at least 6 months following weight restoration.

9.3B REFEEDING SYNDROME

OVERVIEW

Refeeding syndrome, characterized by fluid and electrolyte shifts during nutritional rehabilitation of any malnourished patient, is an important complication to consider in patients with AN as nutrition is reintroduced.[10]

EPIDEMIOLOGY

The precise incidence of refeeding syndrome is unknown, with high variability reported in the literature partly due to a lack of consensus on diagnostic criteria, but risk is highest in the first 2 weeks of active weight restoration.[10,29] Presence of hypophosphatemia is included as a diagnostic criterion in most definitions of refeeding syndrome.[10]

PATHOPHYSIOLOGY

The pathogenicity of refeeding syndrome primarily revolves around hypophosphatemia, triggered by a transition from catabolism to anabolism when nutrition is reintroduced, which also triggers hypokalemia and hypomagnesemia, thiamine deficiency, and volume overload (Figure 9.5).[30] Severe complications can ensue from this chain of metabolic events, including sudden cardiac death, congestive heart failure, rhabdomyolysis, respiratory failure, acute tubular necrosis, and Wernicke encephalopathy (WE).[30]

MEDICAL HISTORY AND CLINICAL PRESENTATION

Clinicians should be concerned about the possibility of refeeding syndrome in any malnourished patient who will be fed by any route, including oral, enteral, and parenteral.[28] The National Institute for Health and Clinical Excellence (NICE) has developed guidelines for identifying patients at high risk of developing refeeding syndrome (Exhibit 9.3).[28] More recent weight loss, larger amount of weight loss, and rapidity of weight restoration directly increase risk of developing refeeding syndrome.[10,28]

SIGNS AND SYMPTOMS

Presenting symptoms in early refeeding syndrome may be difficult to detect, but as the condition progresses, signs of volume overload including lower extremity edema and dyspnea become evident.[10,28] If rhabdomyolysis occurs, patients may experience muscle weakness or swelling.[10] Seizures can also occur.[10]

PHYSICAL EXAMINATION

Vital signs should be obtained several times a day in the first few days of nutritional rehabilitation and daily for the first several weeks.[28] Tachycardia and presence of pretibial edema may signify impending refeeding syndrome, though peripheral edema is common during nutritional rehabilitation and may be transient and uncomplicated.[28] Physical examination findings in refeeding syndrome due to volume overload include tachypnea, respiratory distress, diffuse coarse lung sounds, and peripheral edema.[10] Large muscle swelling or weakness may be present in rhabdomyolysis.[10] A lack of phosphorus and phosphorus-dependent molecules, like adenosine triphosphate (ATP), can result in myocardial dysfunction and a lack of diaphragmatic contraction causing respiratory failure, hypoxia, and seizures.[30]

DIFFERENTIAL DIAGNOSIS

Table 9.9 summarizes the differential diagnosis for refeeding syndrome.

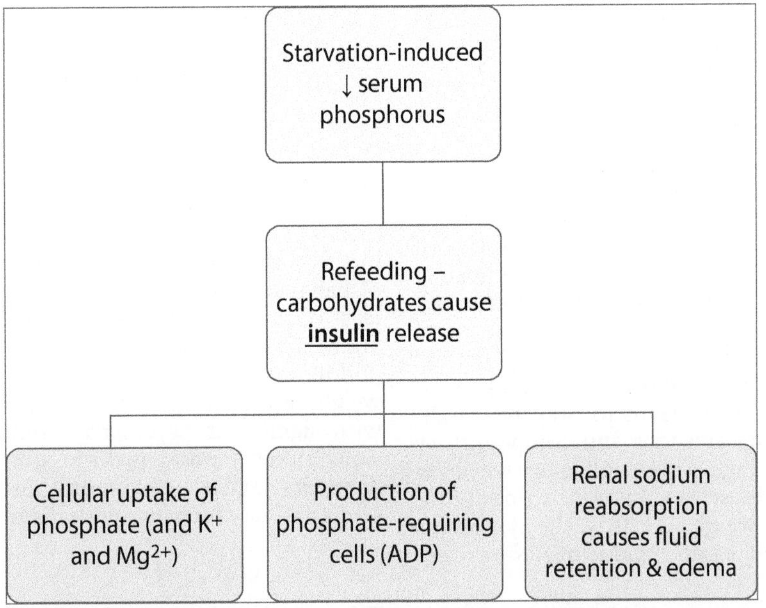

Figure 9.5 **Pathogenicity of hypophosphatemia in refeeding syndrome.** ADP, adenosine diphosphate.

EXHIBIT 9.3 NICE Criteria for Identifying Patients at High Risk of Developing Refeeding Syndrome

Patients are considered at risk if they fall into either set of criteria.

Patient has one or more of:

- BMI ≤16 kg/m^2
- Unintentional weight loss of >15% in the previous 3–6 months
- Little or no nutritional intake for >10 days
- Low levels of potassium, phosphorus, or magnesium before refeeding

Patient has two or more of:

- BMI ≤18.5 kg/m^2
- Unintentional weight loss of >10% in the previous 3–6 months
- Little or no nutritional intake for >5 days
- History of alcohol misuse or drugs, including insulin, chemotherapy, antacids, or diuretics

BMI, body mass index; NICE, National Institute for Health and Clinical Excellence.

Source: With permission from Mehler PS, Winkelman AB, Andersen DM, Gaudiani JL. Nutritional rehabilitation: practical guidelines for refeeding the anorectic patient. *J Nutr Metab.* 2010;2010:625782. doi:10.1155/2010/625782

DIAGNOSTIC STUDIES

Diagnostic evaluation in refeeding syndrome is indicated to assess serum electrolytes, including potassium, as part of a basic or complete metabolic panel and serum magnesium and phosphorus. These laboratory studies should be obtained prior to initiating nutritional rehabilitation and regularly during the first 2 weeks of refeeding; consider obtaining these labs daily if abnormalities are present and every other day if electrolytes are within normal limits.[28]

TABLE 9.9 Differential Diagnosis for Refeeding Syndrome

Diagnosis	Description
Hungry bone syndrome	Hypocalcemia and hypophosphatemia in the postoperative period following parathyroidectomy.
Medications impairing intestinal phosphorus absorption	Antacids, especially those containing aluminum and magnesium, phosphate binders, and niacin may result in hypophosphatemia.
Hyperparathyroidism	Excessive parathyroid hormone can cause hypophosphatemia.
Vitamin D deficiency	Causes decreased gastrointestinal phosphate absorption and increased urinary phosphate excretion, due to secondary hyperparathyroidism.

Source: Adapted from Boateng AA, Sriram K, Meguid MM, Crook M. Refeeding syndrome: treatment considerations based on collective analysis of literature case reports. Nutrition. *2010;26(2):156–167. doi:10.1016/j.nut.2009.11.017*

Hypophosphatemia, hypomagnesemia, and/or hypokalemia suggest refeeding syndrome.

TREATMENT

- Preventing refeeding syndrome is preferable to treatment of refeeding syndrome. Normalizing serum phosphorus, magnesium, and potassium as much as possible, while avoiding significant delay in providing nutrition, is optimal. Nutrition is often started slowly and gradually increased to goal caloric intake, which also helps prevent refeeding syndrome.[10,28,30]
- Should refeeding syndrome occur, patients should be hospitalized and undergo cardiac monitoring. Nutritional rehabilitation should be slowed, and electrolytes should be aggressively corrected.[10,28,30]

9.3C BULIMIA NERVOSA

OVERVIEW

According to the *DSM-V,* bulimia nervosa is characterized by recurrent episodes of binge-eating with subsequent compensatory behaviors utilized as a means to control weight.[17] Binge-eating is defined as consuming a larger quantity of food than what most individuals would eat in a similar period of time (within 2 hours) under similar circumstances.[17] A binge-eating episode must be accompanied by a sense of a lack of control over eating.[17] As a result of binge-eating episodes, an individual may engage in recurrent, inappropriate, compensatory behaviors as a means to prevent weight gain. Further, the binge-eating episodes and compensatory behaviors must occur, on average, at least once per week for 3 months and the individuals' self-evaluation is unduly influenced by body shape and weight.[17] Lastly, the symptoms should not be better explained by an episode of AN or other psychiatric condition.[17]

EPIDEMIOLOGY

Bulimia nervosa has become increasingly prevalent over the years as improved diagnostic criteria and awareness have led to more formal diagnosis. A shift from the more restrictive diagnostic criteria in the *DSM-IV* to the more inclusive *DSM-V* criteria has led to a greater proportion of the population meeting criteria for bulimia nervosa.[17] Further, the Epidemiological Catchment Area Study, which was the largest survey of psychiatric disorders in the United States to date, was carried out prior to the establishment of formal criteria for bulimia nervosa. With these caveats in mind and the tendency for patients to underreport binge-eating episodes and compensatory behaviors, the prevalence rate of bulimia nervosa in the United States is likely between 1% to 3% in the female population, but may be as high as 19% in college-age women.[31] Bulimia nervosa has a median age of onset of 18 years old and is overwhelmingly a disorder of young, White, middle- to upper-class females. In the United States, bulimia nervosa is more common in females than males at a ratio of 3:1.[31] Individuals with bulimia nervosa are typically of normal weight, rarely underweight, but growing research suggest there is a large population of overweight to significantly overweight patients with bulimia nervosa.[17,31]

PATHOPHYSIOLOGY

Bulimia nervosa is a biopsychosocial condition and it is likely that all these domains play a role in the proposed psychopathology. Disruptions in the neuronal processes of body image, taste rewarding, and self-regulation are thought to be implicated in bulimia nervosa, yet the structural basis for these functional and behavioral deficits remains largely unknown.[32,33] Monoamine imbalances, particularly a deficiency of serotonin in certain areas of the brain, are thought to be crucial to the manifestation of bulimia nervosa as well.[32] However, it remains uncertain if the deficiency of serotonin is a direct cause or consequence of bulimia nervosa at this time. Further, significant societal/cultural pressures exist that idealize the concept of thinness alongside the prejudice that exists against obesity could further reinforce these proposed pathways.[32]

MEDICAL HISTORY AND CLINICAL PRESENTATION

Patients with bulimia nervosa typically present with a history of recurrent binge-eating episodes and resultant compensatory behaviors such as self-induced vomiting, use of diuretics, use of laxatives, fasting, and/or excessive exercise as a means to prevent weight gain.[17,32] Vomiting is the most prevalent means of compensatory behavior utilized to control weight in this population.[17] It is important to establish the pattern of behaviors, that is, binging/purging episodes, occurring at least once per week over the course of at least 3 months to attain an accurate diagnosis.[17] Further, self-esteem may be unduly influenced by concern surrounding body image and weight in this population. Patients will frequently present with significant psychiatric comorbidity including depression, anxiety, posttraumatic stress disorder, substance use disorders (SUDs), personality disorders, and body dysmorphia that may interfere with diagnostic clarity.[17]

SIGNS AND SYMPTOMS

The majority of signs and symptoms can be elicited by attaining an exhaustive history and physical examination. Binge episodes occur and are typically followed by compensatory behaviors of purging, excessive exercise, misuse of diuretics, or fasting, which leads to caloric restriction.[17] This cycle typically follows the classic sequence of caloric restriction, binging, and subsequent compensatory behaviors.[17] Triggers for binges include, but are not limited to, psychosocial stressors, depressed mood, dietary restriction, and negative self-image in context of body shape or size. Self-esteem is heavily influenced by body weight and shape, but not to the same degree as observed in patients with AN. The most common medical symptoms of bulimia nervosa are constipation, bloating, abdominal pain, irregular menses, and lethargy.[17,34]

PHYSICAL EXAMINATION

Physical examination of the individual with bulimia nervosa should follow the same principles as the general population. Every individual should receive a complete physical examination guided by the medical status of the patient. Clinicians should pay close attention to the potential body systems impacted by the complications and comorbidity of bulimia nervosa. Common physical examination findings of bulimia nervosa include dry skin, tachycardia, parotid gland swelling, erosion of dental enamel, and hypotension.[17,34] Other exam findings could include scarring of the dorsum of the hand from self-induced vomiting, known as Russell sign, hair loss, and edema (Figure 9.6).[17,34]

DIFFERENTIAL DIAGNOSIS

Table 9.10 summarizes the differential diagnosis for bulimia nervosa.

DIAGNOSTIC STUDIES

Laboratory tests indicated for patients with bulimia nervosa include serum electrolytes, serum creatinine, blood urea nitrogen (BUN), CBC with differential, liver function test, and urinalysis.[17,32] Electrolyte imbalances are common and consist of possible hypochloremia and secondary hypokalemia related to emesis.[17] Metabolic alkalosis is also common with elevations in serum bicarbonate.[17] Severely ill individuals with bulimia nervosa should have an EKG along with serum magnesium, phosphorus, and calcium.[17,32]

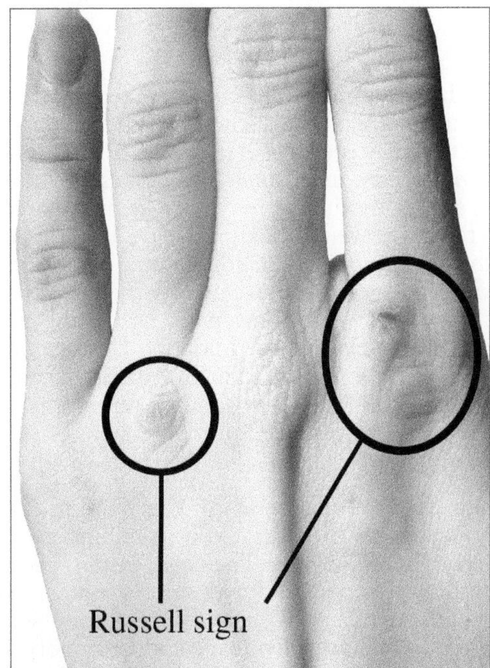

Figure 9.6 **Russell sign, associated with self-induced vomiting. Note the scarring, callouses, and erythema to the dorsal hand.**

All females of childbearing age should have a pregnancy test. Indicated laboratory tests should always be guided by symptoms and examination findings including evaluation of any suspected medical complications/comorbidity.

EVALUATION

It is important to establish a good rapport with the patient initially as they may not willingly disclose vital information about their condition. A full physical examination, ordering of appropriate laboratory studies, and an exhaustive psychiatric assessment are essential.[22] The psychiatric assessment should include an extensive psychiatric history and mental status examination.[17,22] A thorough psychiatric assessment is usually best accomplished by a referral to a clinician who specializes in psychiatry. Ideally, patients with bulimia nervosa should be managed with an integrative care team that, if feasible, includes a primary care clinician, psychotherapist, and psychiatric clinician.[22,32] The coordination of care between this team will allow for more extensive, appropriate, and exhaustive interventions to ensure the best possible outcomes longitudinally for the patient. Ongoing management should include evaluation and targeted treatment of any of the medical or psychiatric comorbidities or complications that may arise because of bulimia nervosa.

TREATMENT

- Medical stabilization is the initial priority, and patients may require hospitalization to achieve physiologic stability.[22,32] Consider treatment in an inpatient eating disorder facility or in a partial hospitalization program for patients who cannot control compensatory behaviors or who lack adequate outpatient support. Suicidal patients should be admitted until stabilized.
- Psychotherapy potentially includes individual, group, family, and behavioral modalities.[32,35] Cognitive behavioral therapy has the most evidence of efficacy in bulimia nervosa.[32]

TABLE 9.10 Differential Diagnosis to Consider in the Evaluation of Bulimia Nervosa

Diagnosis	Description
Anorexia nervosa (AN)	In contrast to bulimia nervosa, patients with AN have abnormally low body weight, as indicated by a body mass index (BMI) of <18.5 kg/m^2. Characteristic physiologic and anatomic sequelae occur in AN that are not seen in bulimia nervosa because of the weight loss/low BMI associated with AN.
Binge-eating disorder (BED)	Binge episodes only, no compensatory behaviors or purging. No restriction of diet between episodes of binging in BED as there is in bulimia nervosa.
Unipolar major depression	Overeating and suicidal ideation can occur in both, but compensatory behaviors (purging) and preoccupations with weight in bulimia nervosa help distinguish these two conditions.
Borderline personality disorder (BPD)	Distinguished by inappropriate compensatory behaviors to control weight in bulimia nervosa that is not present in BPD. Both conditions can have suicidality, identity disturbance, and impulsivity.
Prader-Willi syndrome	Genetic disorder consisting of obesity, obsession with food, hyperphagia, cognitive impairment (typically mental retardation), and hypogonadism. May have behavioral problems as well. No inappropriate compensatory behaviors as a means to control weight.
Klein-Levin syndrome	Self-limited condition that typically affects adolescent males. Symptoms consist of hyperphagia, hypersomnia, and behavioral disturbances. No inappropriate compensatory behaviors as a means to control weight.

- Pharmacotherapy may include antidepressants, such as an SSRI.[32] Antidepressants may be beneficial even if the patient with bulimia nervosa is not clinically depressed.[32] Bupropion should not be utilized in the treatment of bulimia nervosa because of an increased risk of seizures.[32]

PATIENT EDUCATION

- Bulimia nervosa is an eating disorder that consists of binge-eating episodes and purging behaviors. Episodes of excessive overeating are called "binges."
- Unhealthy measures used to prevent weight gain are "purges" and can include self-induced vomiting, excessive exercise, misuse of medications, and fasting.
- There is no specific test for bulimia nervosa.
- Bulimia nervosa can cause numerous medical and mental health complications.
- Bulimia nervosa is treated with psychotherapy and/or medications and/or lifestyle/behavioral modifications.
- Individuals with bulimia nervosa can get better with treatment, but it is often a chronic condition that requires ongoing treatment to prevent recurrence of functionally impairing symptoms.

9.3D BINGE-EATING DISORDER

OVERVIEW

The diagnosis of binge-eating disorder (BED) is relatively new and remains somewhat controversial. Over the years since diagnostic criteria were created, it has become the most common eating disorder.[36] The diagnosis of BED did not exist in the *DSM-IV* but was added to the *DSM-V*, which was released in May 2013.[31] BED is characterized by episodes of binge-eating that are nearly identical to episodes of binge-eating in bulimia nervosa. According to the *DSM-V*, binge-eating episodes characteristic of BED are accompanied by at least three of the following five symptoms: eating more rapidly than normal, eating until feeling uncomfortably full, eating large amounts of food when not feeling physically hungry, eating alone because of embarrassment about how much one is eating, feeling disgusted with oneself or feeling depressed or very guilty afterward.[17] Episodes must occur, on average, once per week for at least 3 months.[17] In contrast to bulimia nervosa, no regular use of inappropriate, compensatory weight loss behaviors such as purging or excessive exercise occur.[17] Lastly, binge-eating episodes must not occur solely during the course of bulimia nervosa or AN and severity of the condition is graded by the number of episodes of binge-eating per week.

EPIDEMIOLOGY

Minimal data exist outside the United States regarding the prevalence of BED. However, one such community survey of 24,124 respondents from 14 different countries found that the median age of onset of BED is late teens to early 20s with a median age of 24 years.[31] The lifetime risk of BED is significantly higher for women than for men, and this population is far more likely to be obese. Even still, <50% of this population seeks treatment for BED. The survey also found that the lifetime prevalence rates ranged from 0.8% to 1.9% with a median of 1.4%, and in the United States this rate was higher at 2.6%.[31] BED seems to aggregate in families as heritability estimates range from 41% to 57%.[37] BED carries significant medical and psychiatric comorbidity, including an increased risk for metabolic syndrome and its components, anxiety (namely phobias), depression, attention deficit/hyperactivity disorder, personality disorders, and substance misuse.[17,38]

PATHOPHYSIOLOGY

The neuropathophysiology of BED remains largely unknown, but several hypotheses have been developed. BED closely resembles a compulsive/impulsive disorder. There are minimal human neuroimaging studies in BED to date, but these limited studies suggest there are several cognitive alterations that occur because of the condition.[37] These alterations seemingly affect impulsivity, compulsivity, executive functioning, attention, and decision-making.[37] Further, these alterations imply that the striatum and cortex play a key role in BED, as the altered functioning of corticostriatal pathways is similar to those seen in substance misuse.[37] Lastly, animal and human genetic studies also suggest that there are distinct changes in opioidergic and dopaminergic pathways associated with binge-eating behaviors.[37]

MEDICAL HISTORY AND CLINICAL PRESENTATION

Patients with BED can be difficult to detect as there is frequently significant shame associated with the condition and its sequelae that may prevent presentation or conversation.[17,38] These individuals are more likely to be obese, may have specific psychiatric comorbidity, may have greater than expected dissatisfaction with weight, and may have larger weight fluctuations than the general obese population.[17,38] As a result, this patient population tends to have greater medical comorbidity including hypertension, chronic pain, and diabetes mellitus that may be key indicators for initiating conversation about BED.[17,38] All of these factors can lead to significant impairment in psychosocial functioning and perceived quality of life.

SIGNS AND SYMPTOMS

Binge-eating episodes in the *DSM-V* are defined as nearly identical to the episodes associated with bulimia nervosa, but key differences in BED exist.[17] The binge-eating episodes associated with BED tend to be of lower caloric content than those associated with bulimia nervosa, and some research has shown that the criterion that an individual eat more rapidly than usual is not always fulfilled.[17,37] Individuals with BED tend to have more severe obesity and earlier onset of obesity than the general obese population.[36] Further, these individuals tend to have more significant medical and psychopathology than what is seen in the general obese population.[36]

PHYSICAL EXAMINATION

Much like bulimia nervosa, physical examination of the individual with BED should follow the same principles as the general population of patients with obesity. This should include careful examination of the patient's nutritional status both currently and historically. Further, every patient should receive a complete physical and psychiatric examination guided by the medical status of the individual. Clinicians should pay close attention to the potential body systems impacted by the complications and comorbidity of BED. This should include careful examination of waist circumference and BMI. In general, a BMI of ≥25 is considered overweight and ≥30 is considered obese.[13,14,39] Waist circumference cutoffs for overweight is >35 inches in females and >40 inches in males.[14]

DIFFERENTIAL DIAGNOSIS

Table 9.11 summarizes the differential diagnosis for BED.

DIAGNOSTIC STUDIES

There are no definitive laboratory tests indicated for the individual with BED. However, it is recommended that diagnostic studies follow the same basic principles as the general population with significant attention to the medical and psychiatric comorbidities that frequently accompany BED.

EVALUATION

Initial evaluation of the individual with BED should owe careful attention to the patient's psychiatric, medical, and nutritional status. Ongoing evaluation should closely monitor for the complications and comorbidities of the condition. Individuals with BED are far more likely to have significant medical and psychiatric comorbidity than the general population, and if these conditions emerge, they warrant prompt attention by the clinician. In busy primary care settings,

TABLE 9.11 Differential Diagnosis to Consider for Binge-Eating Disorder

Diagnosis	Description
Bulimia nervosa	This disorder will have characteristic binge-eating episodes but is separated from binge-eating disorder (BED) by inappropriate, compensatory behaviors to prevent weight loss only seen in bulimia nervosa and not BED.
Night eating syndrome	Defined by recurrent episodes of nighttime eating or evening hyperphagia not better explained by medications, changes in the sleep-wake cycle, medical disorders, medications, substance use, or BED.

the BED Screener or BEDS-7 may be useful as a screening tool to prompt further investigation as it is highly sensitive (100%) but has minimal specificity (38.7%).[40]

TREATMENT

- Psychotherapy potentially includes cognitive behavioral, interpersonal, and dialectical behavioral therapies.[36]
- Medication management includes consideration of SSRI, serotonin and norepinephrine reuptake inhibitors (SNRIs), lisdexamfetamine, and topiramate.[36] Pharmacotherapeutic agents typically help to reduce binge-eating episodes, but there is limited evidence that shows these medications help substantially with weight loss.[36]
- Behavioral weight loss programs may be helpful in symptom management.

PATIENT EDUCATION

- BED is an eating disorder that consists of recurrent binge-eating episodes. A binge-eating episode consists of consuming an amount of food, in a discrete period of time, that is larger than what most people would consume in the same amount of time under similar circumstances.
- Binge-eating episodes may affect mood and perceived self-worth, and often include eating until uncomfortably full, eating more rapidly than normal, and eating when not feeling physically hungry. These episodes occur, on average, at least once per week for 3 months or more.
- There is no specific test for BED.
- BED can cause numerous medical and mental health complications.
- BED is treated with psychotherapy and/or medications and/or lifestyle/behavioral modifications, such as weight loss programs. Individuals with BED can get better with treatment, but it is often a chronic condition that requires ongoing treatment to prevent recurrence of functionally impairing symptoms.

KEY POINTS

- AN has the highest mortality rate of all psychiatric conditions, and most commonly begins in adolescence or early adulthood. Illness severity is determined by BMI.
- Treatment of AN is best accomplished by an experienced multidisciplinary team, including medical clinicians, RDs, and mental health clinicians. The initial treatment priority is nutritional rehabilitation.
- Patients with AN who are medically unstable require hospital admission. Subsequent treatment of AN can be completed in inpatient eating disorder units, partial hospitalization/day programs, or on an outpatient basis, depending on access to resources, available support system, and patient compliance with treatment.
- Relapse is common in AN and patients typically require lifelong awareness and management of eating behaviors.
- Refeeding syndrome is a serious, sometimes fatal, condition that occurs when nutrition is provided to malnourished patients, causing severe fluid and electrolyte shifts. Hypophosphatemia is the primary electrolyte abnormality that contributes to disease manifestations.
- Prevention of refeeding syndrome is preferable to treatment; correct electrolyte abnormalities as much as possible without significant delay of providing lifesaving nutrition. Begin feeding slowly, and advance to caloric goal over several days.
- If refeeding syndrome occurs, noted by hypophosphatemia, hypokalemia, and edema, reduce caloric intake and aggressively correct electrolyte imbalance.
- Bulemia nervosa is characterized by binge-eating and subsequent purging episodes in an effort to control weight. Patients with bulemia nervosa may be of normal body weight, but are frequently overweight or obese.
- Comorbid mood disorders are common with bulemia nervosa.
- Treatment of bulemia nervosa is best achieved with both psychotherapy and pharmacotherapy.
- BED is a relatively new inclusion in the *DSM-V* and is characterized by eating large quantities of food, even when not hungry, without the presence of compensatory behaviors to control weight.
- Patients with BED are often overweight or obese, and medical complications of BED are often related to body weight.
- Treatment of BED includes psychotherapy and potentially pharmacotherapy; medical complications associated with obesity should be screened for and treated.

9.4 FAT-SOLUBLE VITAMIN DISORDERS

Mariah K. Jackson and Shaun Grammer

OVERVIEW

The fat-soluble vitamins are vitamins A, D, E, and K. These four vitamins have unique and crucial roles within the body (Table 9.12). As described by their name, fat-soluble vitamins are soluble in fats and are absorbed similarly to triglycerides, being packaged into micelles and entering the enterocyte to be repackaged into chylomicrons for transportation through the lymphatic system to the liver. Because of this nature, fat-soluble vitamin deficiencies are often seen within disease states that can cause fat malabsorption, such as short bowel syndrome, chronic pancreatitis, cystic fibrosis, and other GI diseases.[41,42] Fat-soluble vitamins can be stored in the body, which increases vitamin toxicity risk, compared to water-soluble vitamins, which in general are not stored.

9.4A VITAMIN A

METABOLISM AND FUNCTION OVERVIEW

Vitamin A refers to a group of compounds called retinoids and carotenoids, with the active form being retinol.[41,43]

TABLE 9.12 Fat-Soluble Vitamins and a Summary of Their Sources, Deficiency, and Toxicity Patterns

Vitamin Name	Alternate Names	Recommended Intake or Biomarker Level (>19 Years Old, Male/Female)	Sources	Risk Factors for Deficiency	Manifestations of Deficiency	Manifestations of Toxicity
Vitamin A	Retinol	900 mcg/700 mcg RAE	Liver, dairy, orange fruits and vegetables	Fat malabsorption, poor diet	Night blindness, Bitot spots, xerophthalmia	Hepatotoxicity, nausea/vomiting, birth defects
Vitamin D	Cholecalciferol	Serum 25(OH)D ≥30 ng/mL	Sun-derived, fortified foods, eggs, fatty fish	Fat malabsorption, poor sun exposure	Children: Rickets Adults: Osteomalacia Other: Secondary hyperparathyroidism	Hypercalcemia, nausea/vomiting, renal failure
Vitamin E	α-Tocopherol	15 mg	Vegetable oils, avocado, nuts	Fat malabsorption	Neuropathy, hemolytic anemia	Interference with anticoagulants
Vitamin K	Phylloquinone, menadione	120 mcg/90 mcg	Dark green leafy vegetables, gut bacteria	Fat malabsorption, no infant supplementation, antibiotic use	Bleeding/bruising, increased PTT	Hemolytic anemia

25(OH)D, 25-hydroxyvitamin D; PTT, partial thromboplastin time; RAE, retinol activity equivalent.

Dietary sources of vitamin A come from both plants (carotenoids) and animals (retinoids). They include liver, dairy products, fish oils, eggs, and primarily yellow-orange fruits and vegetables like carrots, cantaloupe, sweet potatoes, and winter squash. Animal and plant sources of vitamin A are absorbed differently, as plant sources from carotenoids, like β-carotene, have poorer absorption rates. Vitamin A has many biologic roles within the body, which can be generalized into vision, growth and reproduction, immune function, epithelial cell maintenance, and gene expression.[42,43] Vitamin A is integral to the visual cycle, helping the eye transduce light creating signals for the brain to interpret what is being seen. Vitamin A is also highly important to normal cellular proliferation and differentiation, such as maintaining conjunctival membranes and cornea, as well as gene expression for structural proteins, like keratin.[42,43]

REQUIREMENTS, DEFICIENCY, AND TOXICITY

Because of absorption rate differences, the retinol activity equivalent (RAE) was created. The Recommended Dietary Allowance (RDA) of vitamin A is 900 mcg RAE for males and 700 mcg RAE for females, 19 years or older.[43] Vitamin A deficiency and toxicity impact its core functions. A primary outcome of vitamin A deficiency is progressive stages of blindness, including night-blindness, or compromised low-light adaptation, xerophthalmia, Bitot spots, and keratomalacia (Figure 9.7). Additional deficiency responses include impaired immunity function, compromised bone growth, and follicular hyperkeratosis.[41,43] As vitamin A is readily stored, it has the potential to accumulate to toxic levels, known as hypervitaminosis A. Acute hypervitaminosis A causes nausea, vomiting, and malaise symptoms and may result from single or short-term dose of >150,000 mcg of retinol, while chronic high levels of vitamin A result in hepatotoxicity, usually from intake of retinol of >30,000 mcg/day for months, up to years.[43] During pregnancy, excess vitamin A is teratogenic and can lead to birth defects. The potential for negative consequences of vitamin A is usually from excess supplementation over dietary intake. Excessive consumption of β-carotene does not produce the same consequences as described, but can lead to a nontoxic, reversible, yellow-orange coloration of the skin known as carotenoderma, as β-carotene is stored in subcutaneous fat.[42]

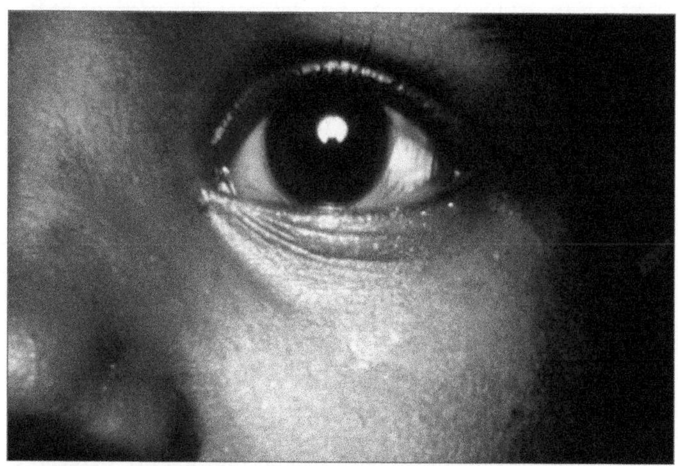

Figure 9.7 Bitot spot. The white plaque seen on the eye is caused by excessive drying of the eye from vitamin A deficiency.
(Source: Public Health Image Library, Centers for Disease Control and Prevention, Dr. J Justin Older. https://phil.cdc.gov/Details.aspx?pid=18894)

9.4B VITAMIN D

METABOLISM AND FUNCTION OVERVIEW

Vitamin D is needed throughout the body, not just for bone maintenance, but also for several other physiologic and immune functions, cell proliferation and apoptosis, insulin secretion, and beta-oxidation.[41,44] Vitamin D is known as the sunshine vitamin, as production starts in the skin through a photolytic process with a derivative of cholesterol (7-dehydrocholesterol) in order to turn into vitamin D3. Vitamin D3 is then converted to 25-hydroxyvitamin D (25(OH)D) by the liver. 25(OH)D is the major circulating form of vitamin D and correlates best with calcium absorption in adults. When required, 25(OH)D is converted by the kidney and other cells to the active form of vitamin D, 1,25-dihydroxyvitamin D (1,25-$(OH)_2D$). Once

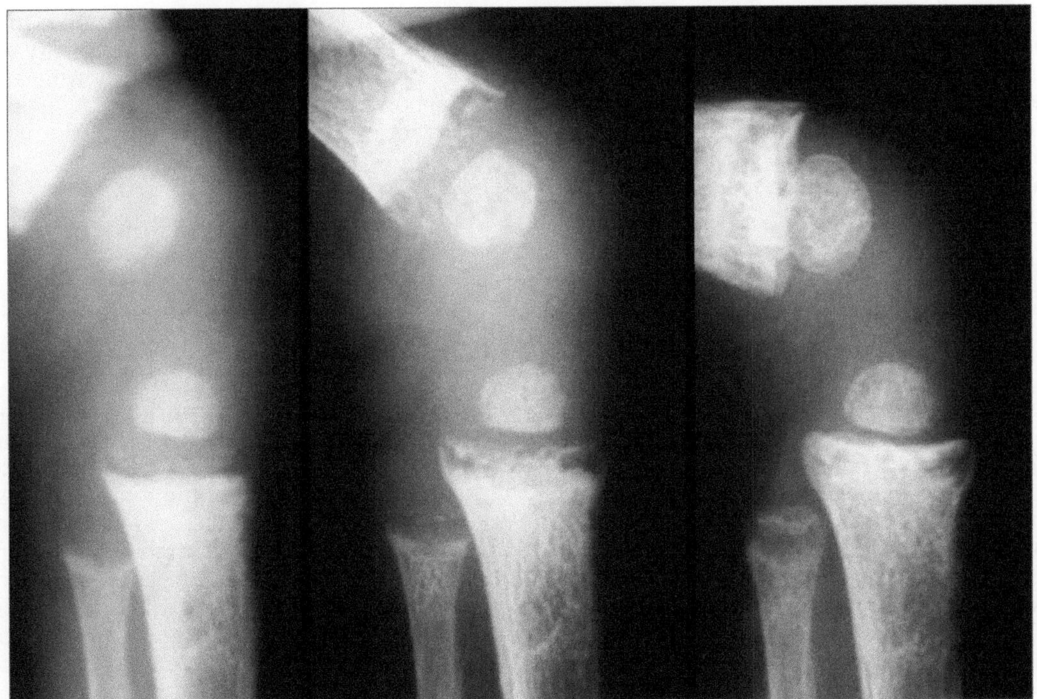

Figure 9.8 Rickets. Serial x-rays of the knee in a patient being treated for rickets. Note the severe osteomalacia near the joint space in the leftmost x-ray and subsequent improvement in calcium deposition on the right, noted by the increased radiodensity.

(Source: Public Health Image Library, Centers for Disease Control and Prevention. https://phil.cdc.gov/Details.aspx?pid=21274)

activated, it can work to enhance intestinal calcium absorption, kidney calcium reabsorption, and promote osteoclast formation.[44] 1,25-$(OH)_2$D is physiologically regulated and serum measurements do not reflect vitamin D status, unlike serum 25(OH)D, which is the biomarker used to define vitamin D deficiency.[45] Endogenous production of vitamin D3 is the primary source of vitamin D, as very few food sources contain vitamin D. However, foods such as fatty fish, eggs, and fortified dairy and cereals are important sources of vitamin D.

REQUIREMENTS, DEFICIENCY, AND TOXICITY

In 2011, the recommendations for vitamin D intake increased to 600–800 IU daily for adequacy, which differs from needs for optimal health, including bone and calcium metabolism, which is based on maintaining a minimum serum 25(OH)D level of 30 ng/mL (75 nmol/L).[45–48] Factors that contribute to vitamin D deficiency include living at more northern latitudes, darker skin tones, and overweight or obese status.[48,49] These lifestyle and innate factors impact the endogenous formation of vitamin D and may require further reliance on additional sources of vitamin D to prevent deficiency. Vitamin D deficiency can lead to rickets (children), osteomalacia (adults), and secondary hyperparathyroidism (Figure 9.8).[41,43] Vitamin D supplementation to combat deficiency needs to be individualized per surrounding factors, as individuals may require between 1,000 and 10,000 IU/day, to a 50,000 IU weekly dose for 12 weeks, followed by 1,000 IU daily in order to return to and maintain individuals at the minimum level of 30 ng/mL of 25(OH)D.[50] While fat soluble, there is a wide margin for vitamin D toxicity, with toxicity reports showing toxicity at doses of 50,000 IU to 2 million IU daily or 25(OH)D levels >150 ng/mL, manifesting with hypercalcemia, nausea/vomiting, and renal failure.[51]

9.4C VITAMIN E

METABOLISM AND FUNCTION OVERVIEW

Like vitamin A, several forms are encompassed under the term vitamin E. Vitamin E refers to eight compounds, divided into two classes: tocopherols (α-, β-, γ-, and δ-tocopherol) and tocotrienols (α-, β-, γ-, and δ-tocotrienols). Of these, α-tocopherol is the primary form consumed and utilized by the body and thus is what the intake recommendation is based upon.[43,52] The primary sources of vitamin E include plant oils, or foods with high amounts of unsaturated fats, like nuts, seeds, and avocados. Vitamin E is primarily an antioxidant, working against free radicals in the body that cause oxidative stress in highly susceptible targets, like polyunsaturated fats within cell membranes.[41,43,52] To prevent lipid peroxidation, vitamin E works as the reducing agent, donating electrons to the free radical, sparing other biologic structures like cell membranes from being oxidized. Once vitamin E is oxidized, it relies on other reducing agents like vitamin C or glutathione to reacquire electrons to continue scavenging for free radicals.[41,43] Besides antioxidant functions, vitamin E plays a role in cell proliferation and differentiation and it impacts cell signaling and cardiovascular disease prevention.[52]

REQUIREMENTS, DEFICIENCY, AND TOXICITY

Vitamin E requirements were determined based on the amount needed to prevent red blood cell peroxide-induced hemolysis, creating an RDA of 15 mg α-tocopherol for men and women ≥19 years old.[43,52] Deficiency of vitamin E may lead to hemolytic anemia secondary to erythrocyte membrane fragility, and nervous system issues like axonal degeneration, peripheral neuropathy, and ataxia.[41] Vitamin E can be stored, so there is potential for toxicity, but the risk of vitamin E toxicity appears to be low, with high tolerable upper limit (UL) of 1,000 mg/day.[43] Despite the low risk of vitamin E toxicity on its own, large doses of vitamin E are known to interfere with vitamin K and therefore those who are deficient in vitamin K or on anticoagulants should be monitored for increased hemorrhagic risk.

9.4D VITAMIN K

METABOLISM AND FUNCTION OVERVIEW

There are three major forms of vitamin K. The vitamin K available from plant foods (K_1, phylloquinone) is found mostly in leafy dark green vegetables, such as spinach, broccoli, and kale. Vegetable oils can also contain significant amounts of vitamin K. Vitamin K_2 menaquinone, is primarily produced by the bacteria that line the GI tract, but can also be found in some fermented foods.[53] Finally, vitamin K is also available in a synthetic form as a supplement as K_3 or menadione. Vitamin K is best known for its role as a cofactor in blood clotting, as it is needed by several vitamin K–dependent coagulation proteins. These proteins include factors II (prothrombin), VII, IX, and X, as well as proteins C and S.[41,43,53] Besides coagulation, vitamin K plays a role in bone health, needed by the proteins osteocalcin and matrix Gla protein. When vitamin K is low or insufficient these proteins will be impaired, impacting bone metabolism. Although vitamin K can be stored, there is a rapid turnover rate of use by the body; therefore, reserves are minimal.

REQUIREMENTS, DEFICIENCY, AND TOXICITY

Adequate intake (AI) of vitamin K was set at 90 mcg for females and 120 mcg for males, 19 years old and older and no tolerable UL has been established, with little risk of toxicity from daily oral intake.[43] Vitamin K deficiency may manifest as increased prothrombin time, bleeding or bruising, and potentially osteoporosis.[53] Deficiency of vitamin K can be seen with malabsorption conditions, poor bacterial vitamin K production secondary to chronic antibiotic use, and poor placental transfer and sterile gut in newborns.[43,53] Newborns in the United States are often routinely given vitamin K to counteract their innate deficiency at birth. Vitamin K toxicity is rare, but cases of supplement abuse have been shown to cause hemolytic anemia and hyperbilirubinemia.[41] Because of vitamin K's effects on clotting, people taking certain anticoagulation medications, such as warfarin, are often advised to maintain a diet with consistent levels of vitamin K intake, avoiding very high doses of vitamin K that can negate the effects of the medication. Patients taking warfarin should consult healthcare clinicians to make sure they have adequate nutrient intake.

KEY POINTS

- Fat-soluble vitamins are absorbed best when eaten with fat-containing foods, are absorbed like fats, and can be stored mainly in the liver or adipose tissue.
- Vitamin A is needed for vision, growth, cell maintenance, and gene expression and has the highest risk for fat-soluble vitamin toxicity. Pregnant women with excessive vitamin A intake are at risk for teratogenic effects on fetal development.
- Vitamin D is needed for bone and calcium homeostasis, immune system, and other biologic functions. Vitamin D deficiency is highly prevalent in the northern hemisphere.
- Vitamin E is an antioxidant found in polyunsaturated fats. Effects from deficiency and toxicity are rarely seen.
- Vitamin K is a cofactor in blood clotting and bone health. Newborns and persons on anticoagulant medications warrant special consideration with this vitamin.

9.5 WATER-SOLUBLE VITAMIN DISORDERS

Jonathan Kilstrom, Richard D. Bennett

The water-soluble vitamins include the following: vitamin B1 (thiamine), vitamin B2 (riboflavin), vitamin B3 (niacin), vitamin B6 (pyridoxine), vitamin B12 (cyanocobalamin), folate, biotin, pantothenate, and vitamin C (ascorbate). Water-soluble vitamins are not stored in significant quantities in the body; they are readily excreted in the urine, typically in response to serum levels. As such, they need to be consumed on a regular basis to ensure nutritional requirements are met.

Toxicity of water-soluble vitamins is rare or nonexistent. Treatment of water-soluble vitamin deficiency is with supplementation of the missing vitamin or vitamins.

9.5A VITAMIN B1 (THIAMINE) DEFICIENCY: BERIBERI AND WERNICKE-KORSAKOFF SYNDROME

OVERVIEW

Vitamin B1, also known as thiamine, is a water-soluble vitamin that plays important roles in carbohydrate metabolism, branched-chain amino acid (BCAA) metabolism, and ultimately neurologic and cardiac function.[54] Dietary sources include many types of grains, legumes, pork, and yeast; additionally, many breads and cereals are fortified with thiamine. Fruits, vegetables, and dairy products are poor sources, and thiamine is also denatured at high pH and high heat, so food processing can limit thiamine availability.[55] Most thiamine in the body is in the form of thiamine diphosphate, also known as thiamine pyrophosphate, which is the primary active form of the vitamin.[56,57]

EPIDEMIOLOGY

Healthy children and adults with an intact small intestine who consume a broad range of foods generally maintain adequate levels of thiamine without supplementation; the 2003–2006 National Health and Nutrition Examination Survey (NHANES) indicated <6% of Americans ingested less than the estimated average requirement (EAR) of thiamine.[58] Thiamine supplementation may be beneficial in specific populations at high-risk for deficiency, however, such as those with alcohol use disorder, AIDS, malnutrition, bariatric surgery recipients, or excessive water-soluble vitamin loss.[56]

Toxicity is extremely rare, as is typically the case with water-soluble vitamins; only trace amounts are stored in the liver, and thiamine is readily excreted in the urine in response to elevated serum values.[54] Thiamine has two well-defined deficiency states, *beriberi* and *Wernicke-Korsakoff syndrome*.

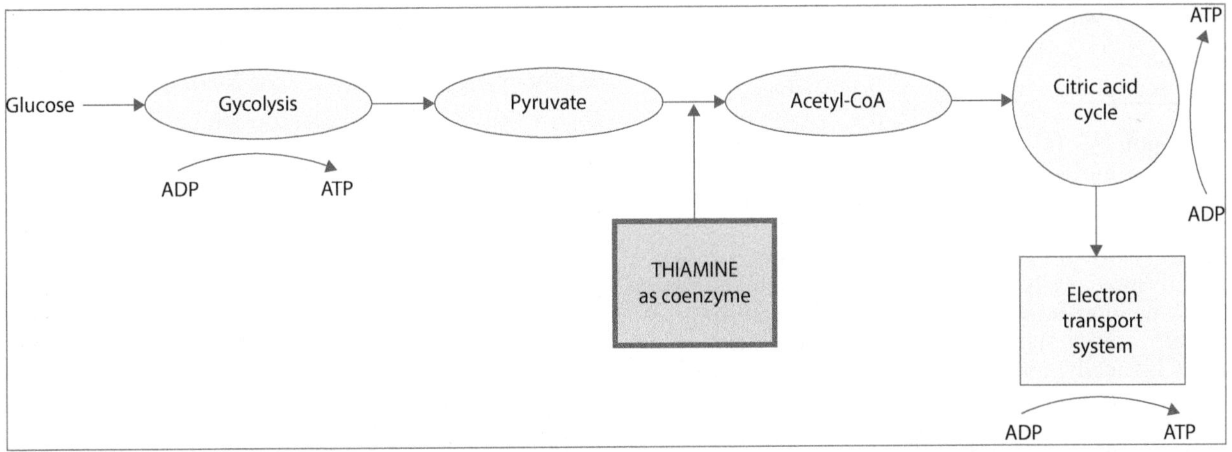

Figure 9.9 Role of thiamine in glucose metabolism. ADP, adenosine diphosphate; ATP, adenosine triphosphate; CoA, coenzyme A.

In its early stages, thiamine deficiency presents with nonspecific symptoms like anorexia, muscle weakness, and mental changes such as irritability and confusion.[54] Beriberi is relatively rare in developed countries, unless restricted or absent in a sole energy source like infant formula or total PN, but it is still seen in populations that consume primarily white polished rice or white cereals.[56] Wernicke-Korsakoff syndrome is a more commonly seen phenotype of thiamine deficiency in the United States, most commonly in patients with alcohol use disorder, but also in non-alcohol- related etiologies due to inadequate consumption, impaired absorption, or increased losses.[56,57] Prevalence of *Wernicke encephalopathy* (WE), the acute phase of the syndrome, was identified in 0.4% to 2.8% in autopsies in the Western world; however, clinically diagnosed cases have lower prevalence, potentially indicating WE is an underrecognized process.[57,59]

PATHOPHYSIOLOGY

Thiamine is absorbed, in small percentages, primarily in the jejunum and has a short half-life, so it must be continually ingested.[55,56]

Thiamine plays a critical role in glucose metabolism; in anaerobic glycolysis, it ultimately facilitates glucose's conversion to ATP, a usable form of energy by cells (Figure 9.9).[60] Thiamine is a critical coenzyme for bridging anaerobic glycolysis and the citric acid cycle by functioning as a coenzyme for the decarboxylation of pyruvate to acetyl coenzyme A (CoA).[54,60] When there is an absence of adequate thiamine, inhibition of the citric acid cycle and electron transport chain ensues and ultimately inhibits glucose from being converted to ATP.[60] As the central nervous system relies on glucose as its primary fuel source, a lack of thiamine, resulting in a lack of ATP production, can cause significant deleterious cellular effects during times when little glucose is available.[54,60] Because the body can store small amounts, approximately 30–50 mg, of thiamine, thiamine deficiency typically takes between 4 and 12 weeks to develop.[57,61]

A long-held belief, based on the role of thiamine in glucose metabolism, is that thiamine must be administered before dextrose in hypoglycemic patients to prevent rapid onset of WE due to limited thiamine stores inhibiting glycolysis.[60] Hypoglycemia is common in alcoholic ketoacidosis, which makes this scenario a somewhat common occurrence. Research is limited regarding this scenario but suggests that prolonged dextrose administration prior to thiamine administration may induce WE, but short-term dextrose administration for hypoglycemia with intravenous or intramuscular thiamine given as soon as possible thereafter is likely safe.[60]

Thiamine deficiency can occur due to low ingestion, poor absorption, increased losses, and increased utilization.[56] Examples of low ingestion include alcohol use disorder, particularly when alcohol intake leads to reduced food intake, PN without thiamine supplementation, and AN.[56,62] Poor absorption can result from any malnourished state or gastric bypass.[56,62] Increased losses can occur with diuretic use, renal replacement therapy, and hyperemesis gravidarum.[62] Pregnancy and lactation are known to require increased thiamine utilization, which can rapidly amplify thiamine deficiency.[61,62]

MEDICAL HISTORY AND CLINICAL PRESENTATION

Beriberi can occur in all ages, and a careful nutritional history will reveal malnutrition, undernutrition, or a very limited diet. Worldwide, outbreaks of beriberi have been observed in Thailand, West Africa, and refugee camps in Guinea, Djibouti, and Nepal.[61] Infantile beriberi mainly affects infants breastfed by women with thiamine deficiency, and symptom onset is rapid with death frequently occurring within days.[61] Adult beriberi has two primary phenotypes, wet and dry. Dry beriberi is defined by nervous system complications, including neuropathy and motor weakness. Wet beriberi gets its name from the presence of edema, typically peripheral but at times systemic, and heart failure in addition to neuropathy. Additionally, wet beriberi can result in dilated cardiomyopathy, which may present with arrhythmias and sudden cardiac death.

Wernicke-Korsakoff syndrome is a neuropsychiatric disease continuum comprising two clinical patterns of thiamine deficiency, WE acutely and Korsakoff syndrome (KS) chronically.[57] Patients often have a history of alcohol use disorder, as patients with Wernicke-Korsakoff syndrome are 8–10 times more likely to have this condition than the general population.[56,57] WE, if untreated, can lead to permanent brain damage, KS, and death.[57,63] KS is characterized by irreversible global amnesia after an incomplete recovery from WE, where recurrent short-term memories cannot be assimilated into long-term memory, and generally, patients are unaware of their illness.[57,63] Patients with KS have limited capability to function outside of regimented, normal habits and may be unable to safely live independently.[57,63]

SIGNS AND SYMPTOMS

Bilateral, symmetric peripheral neuropathy, especially of the legs, is the predominant symptom of dry beriberi.[54,61] Motor weakness and muscle wasting in the distal extremities are also common.[54,61] In wet beriberi, patients present with signs of dyspnea and edema in addition to neuropathy.[54,61] GI symptoms, like anorexia, constipation, and mild cramping, are common in both forms.[61]

Infantile beriberi can take several forms, from cyanosis, edema, and dyspnea early in infancy to symptoms mimicking bacterial meningitis, often accompanied by vomiting, in older infants.[61] Initial symptoms may be constipation and fussiness.[61] Classically, infants with beriberi present with a piercingly loud, high-pitched cry.

WE has a classic triad of symptoms—encephalopathy, oculomotor dysfunction, and gait ataxia—however, the occurrence of all three symptoms concurrently in patients occurs only 17% of the time, making diagnosis challenging, especially when patients concurrently present with alcohol intoxication.[57,63] Encephalopathy, manifesting in a range of symptoms from disorientation to altered level of consciousness, is the most commonly seen symptom in the WE triad.[57,63] KS is characterized by irreversible memory deficits in the presence of an intact sensorium; confabulation is frequently a feature.[57,63]

PHYSICAL EXAMINATION

On physical examination, adults with dry beriberi initially present with diminished sensation in the distal extremities; loss of tactile sensation and peripheral vibratory sensation occur early.[63] Neurologic impairment can progress to reduced deep tendon reflexes, muscle wasting, significant muscle weakness, and foot or wrist drop.[63] In wet beriberi, the same neurologic symptoms are present, but cardiac symptoms predominate. Patients often present with tachycardia, lower extremity peripheral edema or anasarca, and other signs of congestive heart failure, like pulmonary congestion, manifesting as diffuse crackles on auscultation. If a pleural effusion is present, egophony, dullness to percussion of the affected region, or diminished breath sounds to the affected region may be present.

Infantile beriberi can present with cyanosis and fluid overload, both of which are poor prognostic indicators if not immediately treated; this is most common in infants 1 to 3 months of age. A meningitis-like presentation with meningismus, vomiting, and sweating is more common in older infants, especially between 7 and 9 months of age. Neurologic manifestations in infants can also include aphonia due to paralysis of the vocal cords.

DIFFERENTIAL DIAGNOSIS

Table 9.13 summarizes the differential diagnosis for thiamine deficiency.

As thiamine deficiency frequently initially presents with nonspecific symptoms, the differential diagnosis is extensive and requires consideration of many neurologic and cardiac conditions.

DIAGNOSTIC STUDIES

There is not a single, reliable diagnostic study for thiamine deficiency, nor is there a specific threshold under which all patients develop disease, and as such beriberi, WE, and KS are largely clinical diagnoses, made by careful history taking that matches clinical manifestations of the disease.[54,56,57]

TABLE 9.13 Differential Diagnosis to Consider in the Evaluation of Thiamine Deficiency

Diagnosis	Description
Delirium	Waxing and waning disturbance in attention throughout the course of a day in addition to a change in cognition, both of which are not better explained by another diagnosis.[18]
Dilated cardiomyopathy from other conditions, such as viral myocarditis, ischemic heart disease, HIV infection, or substance use disorders	Dilation and compromised contraction of one or both ventricles, potentially resulting in heart failure, arrhythmias, or sudden cardiac death. Symptoms include dyspnea and edema.
Diabetic polyneuropathy	Symmetric polyneuropathy of the distal upper and lower extremities while results in impairment of vibratory sensation, reduced deep tendon reflexes, and loss of pain and light touch sensation.
Guillain-Barré syndrome (GBS)	Progressive, symmetric, typically ascending muscle weakness and diminished deep tendon reflexes, which can lead to respiratory muscle paralysis. GBS is thought to be caused by an immune response to infection.
Charcot-Marie-Tooth disease	Inherited disorder affecting sensory and motor nerves, often appearing in childhood, presenting with distal extremity weakness, muscle atrophy, and foot drop.

Serum thiamine levels can be measured, but are not particularly sensitive or specific indicators of thiamine status in acute illness; erythrocyte thiamine transketolase activity, which is dependent on thiamine, can be a useful laboratory study, particularly in combination with other laboratory studies like measurement of urinary thiamine excretion.[54,56]

Ancillary tests are useful to evaluate cardiac function in wet beriberi. An EKG is useful assess for arrhythmias. Chest x-ray is useful in evaluating wet beriberi and may reveal cardiomegaly, pulmonary congestion, and/or pleural effusions. Echocardiography is important in wet beriberi to evaluate the size of the ventricles, which are enlarged in dilated cardiomyopathy, and to assess ejection fraction; heart failure is generally high-output in beriberi.[61,62]

Neuroimaging does not have a central role in the diagnosis of WE or KS, though brain MRI frequently reveals mammillary body atrophy in WE and KS.[57,63] Neuroimaging and laboratory studies are frequently ordered in the case of altered mental status to assess for other possible diagnoses.[57]

TREATMENT

- The U.S. RDA is 0.5 mg to 0.9 mg daily for children, 1.2 mg daily for adult men, and 1.1 mg daily for adult women, which is generally easily obtained through a typical Western diet.[54] Prophylactic thiamine supplementation can be considered for at-risk populations.[57]
- Thiamine dosages for deficiency states and recommended duration of supplementation are variable in the literature, with the least being required for mild thiamine deficiency and the highest doses being recommended for Wernicke-Korsakoff syndrome. Large doses are tolerated safely and well, given rapid urinary excretion of excess amounts.[57,60,64]

- Hypoglycemic patients at risk for thiamine deficiency should be given dextrose to restore normoglycemia as quickly as possible, followed by thiamine administration intravenously or intramuscularly as soon as possible.[60]
- Mild thiamine deficiency, such as limited neuropathy, can be treated with oral thiamine for 2 weeks.[64]
- Beriberi should be treated with IV thiamine for several days followed by a transition to oral thiamine daily for at least 6 weeks.[56,64]
- Wernicke-Korsakoff syndrome should be treated with high-dose thiamine intravenously for several days followed by a transition to oral thiamine daily for at least 1–3 months.[57,64]

PATIENT EDUCATION

- Encourage a diet that includes a wide variety of fruits, vegetables, protein sources, and whole grains.[1]
- If alcohol is consumed, it should be in moderation and not more than one drink per day for women and two drinks per day for men of legal drinking age.[1]

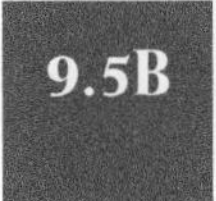

9.5B VITAMIN B2 (RIBOFLAVIN) DEFICIENCY

OVERVIEW

Vitamin B2, also known as riboflavin, is a water-soluble vitamin that plays a key role as a coenzyme in multiple oxidation-reduction biochemical reactions in the body.

EPIDEMIOLOGY

Cases of true riboflavin deficiency, known as ariboflavinosis, are rare as the vitamin is in many common foods such as dairy products, fish, green vegetables, meats, and fortified breads and cereals. Developing countries and areas where starvation is prevalent are more likely to experience riboflavin deficiency. Patients with a history of endocrine disorders, AN, malabsorptive syndrome, and long-term use of barbiturates have increased risk of deficiency.[65]

PATHOPHYSIOLOGY

Flavin adenine dinucleotide (FAD) and flavin mononucleotide (FMN) are hydrolyzed by gastric acids and proteolytic enzymes into free riboflavin. The proximal intestine is the primary absorption site. Rates of absorption increase with intake of other foods and in the presence of bile salts. Riboflavin has also been noted to circulate in the enterohepatic system in small amounts.[54]

MEDICAL HISTORY AND CLINICAL PRESENTATION

Riboflavin deficiency can go undetected due to its vague and nonspecific symptoms. Often, other vitamin deficiencies are present due to poor nutrition and/or absorption. Patients may have a history of a malabsorptive syndrome, endocrine disorder, AN, or long-term use of barbiturates. Patients who are vegetarians or vegans are also at increased risk, especially if they are athletes, due to the lack of dairy and meat in their diet.

SIGNS AND SYMPTOMS

Patients may present with pharyngitis, hyperemia of pharyngeal mucous membranes, chelitis, stomatitis, glossitis, seborrheic dermatitis, and normochromic-normocytic anemia.[54]

PHYSICAL EXAMINATION

Patients with riboflavin deficiency may show signs including hyperemia of the mouth and throat, glossitis, angular stomatitis, chelitis, seborrheic dermatitis, hair loss, and conjunctival erythema. Cataracts may develop with severe and long-standing deficiency.

DIFFERENTIAL DIAGNOSIS

Most patients with riboflavin deficiency are also deficient in other water-soluble vitamins and show signs and symptoms of their deficiencies.[54]

DIAGNOSTIC STUDIES

Routine testing of riboflavin is not indicated in otherwise healthy individuals. Measurement of erythrocyte glutathione reductase (EGR) activity can be used to assess riboflavin levels. Results are expressed as an activity coefficient of EGR (EGRAC). Levels between 1.2 and 1.4 are considered low and >1.4 are deficient.[54] EGRAC is not reliable in patients with glucose-6-phosphate dehydrogenase deficiency.[66]

Less commonly, erythrocyte flavin can be measured to determine the cellular concentration of riboflavin, and urinary flavin can be measured to estimate the amount of urinary excretion over 24 hours.[66]

EVALUATION

Patients presenting with signs and symptoms of riboflavin deficiency and those with a known history of malnutrition or malabsorptive disorders should be evaluated for riboflavin and other water-soluble vitamin deficiencies.

TREATMENT

- Riboflavin deficiency should be treated with oral riboflavin 5–10 mg taken once daily with food.[66]
- The RDA for riboflavin is[66]:
  - Children: 0.5–0.9 mg daily
  - 1.3 mg daily for adult men
  - 1.1 mg daily for nonpregnant women
  - 1.4 mg daily for pregnant women
  - 1.6 mg daily for lactating women

PATIENT EDUCATION

- Those at risk for riboflavin deficiency should be educated on receiving the RDA of riboflavin either in supplement form or by adding foods to their diet with naturally occurring or fortified riboflavin.
- Riboflavin supplements should be taken with food to increase rates of absorption.
- There are no known adverse effects from excessive intake of riboflavin.

9.5C VITAMIN B3 (NIACIN) DEFICIENCY

OVERVIEW

Vitamin B3, also termed niacin, plays a key role in the synthesis and metabolism of proteins, carbohydrates, and fatty acids and plays an important role in the oxidation of all living cells.[67] The term "niacin" refers to nicotinamide and nicotinic acid. Niacin is found in plant and animal foods.

EPIDEMIOLOGY

Niacin deficiency, also termed pellagra, was first documented over 250 years ago. It was prevalent throughout Africa, Asia, Europe, and the United States due to the introduction of diets high in nonalkalized maize. Today, outbreaks continue to occur among refugee populations due to a lack of well-balanced diets.[67]

Those with underlying vitamin B6 (pyridoxine), zinc, and/or copper deficiencies are likely to also experience niacin deficiency due to their roles as key enzyme cofactors in the conversion of tryptophan, an amino acid found in high-protein foods, to niacin in the liver.[67]

PATHOPHYSIOLOGY

Niacin is naturally found in meats, seeds, grains, legumes, and corn products treated with alkali.[68] In the body tissues, nicotinamide adenine dinucleotide (NAD) and nicotinamide dinucleotide phosphate (NADP) are synthesized from nicotinic acid, nicotinamide, and tryptophan and are the two metabolically active forms of niacin.[67]

Niacin is absorbed equally with or without the presence of concurrent food intake. Dietary NAD and NADP are converted to nicotinamide and nicotinic acid in the intestine and are then converted back into NAD and NADP for cellular function. Niacin is absorbed through a passive process by the kidneys, liver, and erythrocytes.[69] The drugs rifampin and isoniazid are known to inhibit the absorption of niacin.[67]

MEDICAL HISTORY AND CLINICAL PRESENTATION

Patients with niacin deficiency often have a history of poor nutrition due to poverty. Those at highest risk may have a high intake of maize-based products and a diet lacking in meat, eggs, grains, and legumes. Patients with an underlying deficiency in vitamin B6, zinc, and/or copper are also at increased risk.[67]

Patients with niacin deficiency present with pellagra, a disorder characterized by photosensitive dermatitis, diarrhea, dementia, and if left untreated, death.

SIGNS AND SYMPTOMS

Pellagra is the hallmark of severe niacin deficiency. It is a condition comprising the "four Ds": photosensitive dermatitis, diarrhea, dementia, and possibly death.

Patients may experience a symmetric hyperpigmented rash to sun-exposed areas that will resemble a sunburn. This most often occurs around the neck. Patients may also present with a bright red tongue, diarrhea, vomiting, insomnia, anxiety, headache, disorientation, delusions, dementia, and encephalopathy. If left untreated, death may result.[54,70]

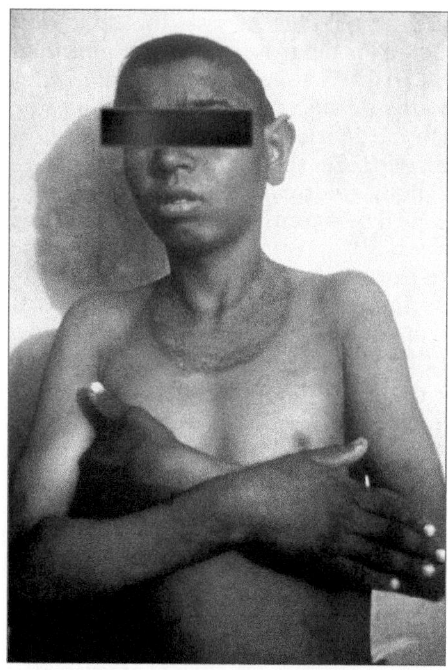

Figure 9.10 **Pellagra, with the classic scaly skin and sores on sun-exposed areas, commonly including the neck and hands. Pellagra is caused by vitamin B3 (niacin) deficiency.**

(Source: Public Health Image Library, Centers for Disease Control and Prevention. https://phil.cdc.gov/Details.aspx?pid=3757)

PHYSICAL EXAMINATION

A symmetric, hyperpigmented rash resembling a sunburn on the neck, hands, and other sun-exposed areas is the most characteristic finding of pellagra (Figure 9.10). Patients may also have a bright red tongue on physical exam and show signs of memory loss and depression.[70]

DIFFERENTIAL DIAGNOSIS

Table 9.14 summarizes the differential diagnosis for niacin deficiency.

DIAGNOSTIC STUDIES

Testing for niacin levels is not widely available. Urinary N-methylnicotinamide is the most reliable and sensitive measure of niacin status. A 24-hour excretion rate <5.8 μmol/day is considered niacin deficient and a rate between 5.8 and 17.5 μmol/day is considered low intake.[54]

Urinary N-methyl-2-pyridone-5-carboxamide, urinary 2-pyridone/N-methylnicotinamide ratio, and erythrocyte NAD/NADP can also provide an assessment of niacin status.[54,71]

CBC, serum albumin, serum protein, liver function, and gamma-glutamyl transferase laboratory tests should also be considered to assess the patient's overall nutritional status and possible hepatic involvement if the patient has a history of chronic alcohol abuse.

EVALUATION

Patients presenting with signs and symptoms of niacin deficiency and those with a known history of malnutrition or malabsorptive disorders should be evaluated for niacin and other water-soluble vitamin deficiencies.[70] Evaluation of overall nutrition status and possible organ involvement

TABLE 9.14 Differential Diagnosis to Consider in the Evaluation of Niacin Deficiency

Diagnosis	Description
Dermatitis	Can be caused by multiple conditions and substances. In niacin deficiency, the rash tends to be symmetric, bilateral, and well defined in areas exposed to the sun.
Diarrhea	Frequent loose stools, but no cutaneous involvement.
Dementia	Memory loss due to chronic and progressive degenerative brain diseases. There should not be cutaneous involvement.
Riboflavin (vitamin B2) deficiency	Similar symptoms to niacin deficiency and often co-occurs with niacin deficiency. Patients are more likely to have symptoms of oral edema and erythema with pain, cheilosis and angular stomatitis, glossitis, seborrheic dermatitis.
Pyridoxine (vitamin B6) deficiency	Similar symptoms to niacin deficiency. Patient are more likely to present with weakness, cheilosis, glossitis, stomatitis, and peripheral neuropathy.
Peripheral neuropathy	Numbness and paresthesias, most commonly affecting the lower extremities. May also have balance difficulties. May be difficult to distinguish from other types of polyneuropathy in niacin deficiency.
Depression	Anhedonia, decreased libido, weight changes, sleep problems, low energy, depressed mood, excessive guilt, suicidal ideations, and poor concentration for >2 weeks. There should be no cutaneous involvement in cases not caused by niacin deficiency.

secondary to chronic conditions such as alcoholism should also be considered. If pellagra is present, prompt niacin supplementation should be initiated.

TREATMENT

- Niacin is dosed as a "niacin equivalent" (NE). One NE is equal to 1 mg of niacin or 60 mg of dietary tryptophan.[72] Nicotinamide is typically the preferred formulation of supplementation or replacement as large doses of niacin can cause nausea, vomiting, paresthesias, and skin flushing.
- Marginal deficiency
  - Nicotinamide 15–20 mg daily
- Severe deficiency (pellagra)
  - Nicotinamide 100–250 mg three times daily for 5 days, followed by 50–300 mg/day[73]
  - Multivitamin once daily
- The U.S. RDA for niacin is[54]:
  - **Adult males:** 16 mg daily
  - **Nonpregnant females:** 14 mg daily
  - **Pregnant females:** 18 mg daily
  - **Children:** 6–12 mg daily

PATIENT EDUCATION

- Patients at risk for niacin deficiency should be educated on appropriate food sources of niacin and supplementation if needed.
- Cutaneous and most neurologic symptoms of niacin deficiency should improve within 48 hours of treatment.[54]
- Niacin deficiency should be treated with a multivitamin supplement to ensure other potential vitamin deficiencies are also treated.
- Moderate to high doses of niacin (1,000 to 3,000 mg daily) can decrease total and LDL-C, but is more likely to result in side effects.[54]
- Nicotinamide is generally better tolerated than niacin, but does not have lipid-lowering properties.[54]

9.5D VITAMIN B6 (PYRIDOXINE)

OVERVIEW

Vitamin B6 is a water-soluble compound that has six different chemical structures that include pyridoxine, pyridoxal, pyridoxamine, and each of their phosphorylated compounds. The most common active form is pyridoxal 5,-phosphate (PLP).[76] The human body cannot synthesize vitamin B6, so it must be obtained from an outside source, such as a food source or supplementation. The typical American diet supplies sufficient vitamin B6 for the human body. Vitamin B6 is heat-stable during cooking and is most commonly found in fish, potatoes, poultry, bananas, nuts, and legumes. Vitamin B6 found in plant-based food is less stable than other sources. Therefore, some strict vegetarian diets may require additional supplementation.[74,75] Vitamin B6 is currently being investigated in a variety of areas for disease prevention (Table 9.15).[74]

PATHOPHYSIOLOGY

Vitamin B6 is involved as a cofactor in several metabolic reactions, most commonly associated with protein metabolism. Vitamin B6 has also been demonstrated to have a role

TABLE 9.15 Vitamin B6 and Disease Prevention

Disease Prevention	Current Evidence
Immune system function	Immune system support has been demonstrated at recommended daily intake and may be more important in the older population.[74]
Coronary artery disease	Studies have found a correlation between vitamin B6 levels and cardiovascular events. However, prospective, controlled studies have failed to demonstrate a direct effect from vitamin B supplementation.[76–78]
Homocysteine	Studies have demonstrated the effect of B vitamins at significantly reducing homocysteine levels. However, the effect was not demonstrated in vitamin B6 alone. Vitamin B9 (folate) appeared to have the greatest effect. The reduction of homocysteine levels from B vitamins has not been shown to improve cardiovascular outcomes.[79–84]
Alzheimer disease	Observational studies have correlated B vitamin intake and cognitive function. However, prospective, controlled studies have failed to demonstrate a direct effect from B vitamin supplementation.[85,86]
Depression	Multiple studies have found a decreased risk of developing depressive symptoms in patients using B vitamin supplementation.[87,88]
Nausea/vomiting of pregnancy	Vitamin B6 has been demonstrated to be effective for nausea and vomiting during the first trimester of pregnancy.[89,90]

in the formation of hemoglobin, serotonin, dopamine, and epinephrine.[74,91] Additionally, a role in the release of glucose through the release of stored glycogen and gluconeogenesis has been demonstrated. Finally, vitamin B6 is critical in the regulation of homocysteine levels in the body.

DEFICIENCY AND TOXICITY

Deficiency of vitamin B6 is uncommon but more prevalent in alcoholism due to decreased dietary intake and improper metabolism.[75,92] Deficiency may also be seen with malabsorption syndromes and associated with common medications, including estrogen-based contraceptives, nonsteroidal anti-inflammatory drugs (NSAIDs), and medications used to treat tuberculosis (isoniazid) and Parkinson disease.[75,93,94] Signs and symptoms of deficiency may include dermatitis, irritability, and electroencephalographic abnormalities.[75] Rarer symptoms include depression, confusion, immune system dysfunction, and seizures.[95,96]

Toxicity of vitamin B6 is extremely rare and only associated with excessive dietary supplement intake. In the rare occurrence of toxicity, patients may present with painful sensory neuropathy. Excessive dietary supplementation may interfere with the effectiveness of some medications, including phenobarbital, phenytoin, and antiparkinsonian medications.[74,97]

9.5E VITAMIN B9 (FOLATE)

OVERVIEW

Vitamin B9 is a water-soluble compound that has different chemical structures depending on the source. Natural dietary sources and metabolically active forms in the body are folates. Supplements and fortified dietary sources contain synthetic forms: folic acid, folinic acid, or levomefolic acid (5-methyltetrahydrofolate).[98]

Vitamin B9 is most commonly found in green leafy vegetables, citrus fruit, legumes, and fortified foods.[98] Prior to the U.S. requirement of fortification of food with folic acid, the estimated occurrence of low serum folate levels in the population was 24% compared to <1% currently.[99]

PATHOPHYSIOLOGY

Folic acid is the most commonly used synthetic form but is inactive until converted by the body. The conversion of folic acid to the active 5-methyltetrahydrofolate is a one-step process using the enzyme methylenetetrahydrofolate reductase (MTHFR). Natural sources of folates are less bioavailable due to an additional step requiring conversion to folic acid before absorption by the intestines.[98] Vitamin B9 is involved as a cofactor in several metabolic reactions, most commonly associated with protein and nucleic acid metabolism and regulation of homocysteine levels in the body.[79–84,98] Vitamin B9 is currently being investigated in a variety of areas for disease prevention (Table 9.15). Additionally, vitamin B9 is critical in the development of the fetus during pregnancy, specifically related to prevention of neural tube defects and congenital cardiac anomalies.[98,100–104] However, 76% of women of childbearing age in the United States are not consuming the recommended dietary intake (RDI) of the vitamin for pregnancy.[105]

DEFICIENCY AND TOXICITY

Deficiency in vitamin B9 most commonly is due to insufficient dietary intake.[98] However, several other factors may cause a significant deficiency (Table 9.16).[98,106,107] Patients with deficiencies of vitamin B9 may present with signs and symptoms of megaloblastic anemia and elevated homocysteine levels. Deficiencies are often treated with folic acid supplementation. Treatment of megaloblastic anemia with folic acid should only occur with monitoring of serum vitamin B12 levels; folic acid may correct the megaloblastic anemia while leaving a vitamin B12 deficiency leading to permanent neurologic damage.[98]

TABLE 9.16 Cause of Vitamin B9 Deficiency

Deficiency Cause	Details
Dietary	Most common cause
Lifestyle	Alcoholism[32] Insufficient dietary intake Decreased intestinal absorption Smoking[33]
Conditions of increased requirement	Pregnancy Cancer Chronic inflammatory diseases
Malabsorption	Crohn disease Ulcerative colitis Celiac disease
Medication	Chronic, high-dose nonsteroidal anti-inflammatory drugs (NSAIDs) Anticonvulsants Phenytoin, phenobarbital, and primidone Cholesterol-lowering agents Cholestyramine and colestipol Antifolate activity Methotrexate, trimethoprim, pyrimethamine, triamterene, and sulfasalazine
Genetic	Influences absorption, transport, or metabolism

A common genetic deficiency involves a decreased availability of MTHFR preventing the conversion of folic acid to the active 5-methyltetrahydrofolate. Patients with this deficiency may exhibit a variety of psychiatric conditions, including depression and anxiety, due to a decreased production of the neurotransmitters norepinephrine, dopamine, and serotonin.[108] Toxicity of vitamin B9 is extremely rare and only associated with excessive dietary supplements.[98]

9.5F VITAMIN B12 (CYANOCOBALAMIN)

OVERVIEW

Vitamin B12 is a water-soluble compound that has two chemical structures metabolically active in the body: methylcobalamin and 5-deoxyadenosylcobalamin. Supplements and fortified dietary sources most commonly use the synthetic form of cyanocobalamin, which can be converted to the active forms in the body.[109] Vitamin B12 is most commonly found in meat, poultry, fish, eggs, and some dairy products.[110] Therefore, strict vegan diets often require supplementation. However, some evidence has indicated that certain plant-based foods have adequate vitamin B12.[111]

PATHOPHYSIOLOGY

Vitamin B12 is involved as a cofactor with two enzymes. Methylcobalamin is a cofactor for the enzyme methionine synthase involved in the conversion of homocysteine to the amino acid methionine; methionine leads to additional reactions that result in adequate functioning of DNA, RNA, and proteins. 5-Deoxyadenosylcobalamin is a cofactor for the enzyme l-methylmalonyl-CoA mutase involved in the conversion of l-methylmalonyl-CoA to succinyl-CoA; succinyl-CoA enters the citric acid cycle and is involved with energy production.[109] Vitamin B12 is currently being investigated in a variety of areas for disease prevention (Table 9.15).

Vitamin B12 absorption is dependent on a functioning GI system. Gastric acid and enzymes are required for the release of vitamin B12 from natural dietary food sources; the synthetic form of cyanocobalamin does not require gastric acid since it is already free. Once released, vitamin B12 will bind to a carrier protein in the stomach while being transported to the duodenum. In the duodenum, vitamin B12 will be released from the carrier protein through actions of pancreatic enzymes and will bind to intrinsic factor from gastric parietal cells, which will be absorbed in the presence of calcium from the pancreas.[110,112]

DEFICIENCY AND TOXICITY

Deficiency in vitamin B12 is rare in healthy adults due to the body's ability to store adequate amounts of the vitamin, requiring very minimal daily intake. Deficiency most commonly occurs in older patients due to insufficient GI absorption. The two most common causes of deficiency are pernicious anemia and food-bound vitamin B12 malabsorption (Box 9.1).

Pernicious anemia is a megaloblastic anemia due to autoimmune disorder decreasing available intrinsic factor resulting in decreased vitamin B12 absorption. Treatment consists of parenteral vitamin B12 administration. However, sufficient daily oral vitamin B12 will passively absorb without the presence of intrinsic factor to maintain adequate vitamin levels.[113]

Food-bound vitamin B12 malabsorption is associated with atrophic gastritis and *Helicobacter pylori* infection resulting in a GI environment that prevents the release of vitamin B12 from natural dietary food sources. Treatment consists of oral supplementation of vitamin B12 since cyanocobalamin does not require release for absorption. Additionally, treating the *Helicobacter pylori* infection has been shown to improve vitamin B12 absorption.[110,112,114]

Patients with deficiencies of vitamin B12 may present with signs and symptoms of megaloblastic anemia and elevated homocysteine levels. Additionally, vitamin B12 deficiency may cause permanent neurologic damage through damage of the myelin sheath resulting in paresthesia, decreased vibration and position sense, and memory disturbance. Finally, changes in mucosal cells may occur causing glossitis.[113]

Deficiency of vitamin B12 can be confirmed through laboratory studies. Vitamin B12 levels can be measured and may return as decreased or low-normal. In the case of low-normal, deficiency can be confirmed through measuring methylmalonic acid (elevated) and homocysteine (elevated) levels. Additionally, parietal cell antibodies may be elevated in pernicious anemia.[113] Toxicity of vitamin B12 is extremely rare and has not been documented in healthy individuals.

BOX 9.1 Causes of Vitamin B12 Deficiency

Pernicious anemia (autoimmune)
Food-bound vitamin B12 malabsorption (atrophic gastritis and *Helicobacter pylori* infection)
Gastrointestinal surgical resection
Malabsorption syndromes (celiac disease)
Pancreatic insufficiency
Strict vegetarian diet
Alcoholism
Drugs (proton-pump inhibitors, cholestyramine, chloramphenicol, neomycin, and colchicine)

Source: With permission from Linardon J, Wade T, de la Piedad Garcia X, Brennan L. Psychotherapy for bulimia nervosa on symptoms of depression: a meta-analysis of randomized controlled trials. Int J Eat Disord. *2017;50(10):1124–1136. doi:10.1002/eat.22763*

9.5G VITAMIN C

INTRODUCTION

Vitamin C, also known as l-ascorbic acid or ascorbate, is a water-soluble and an essential component for maintaining connective tissue networks throughout the body. Dietary intake of vitamin C is required as humans lack the ability to produce vitamin C.[115]

Vitamin C is found in fruits and vegetables. Tomatoes, citrus fruits, and potatoes are the major sources of vitamin C in the American diet. Vitamin C can be given as an oral supplement or as an injection. As a water-soluble vitamin, there is virtually no storage in the body, and plasma concentrations are directly related to dietary intake.[115]

PATHOPHYSIOLOGY

It functions as a cofactor, reducing agent, and antioxidant in a number of biochemical reactions. These reactions are crucial for the correct formation and stabilization of collagen (a major component of connective tissue) and the formation of the neurotransmitters dopamine, epinephrine, and norepinephrine. Vitamin C has a role in production of carnitine (used in fatty acid metabolism), folic acid metabolism, and the metabolism of prostaglandins and cyclic nucleotides (used in cell signaling). Vitamin C enhances iron absorption and may play a role in antioxidant regeneration. Vitamin C is thought to play a role in immune function though studies on the effect of vitamin C in various disease states and the common cold remain inconclusive.[116–118]

TOXICITY AND DEFICIENCY

Vitamin C deficiency is rare in the industrialized world where fruits and vegetables are readily available as well as foods fortified with vitamin C. However, vitamin C deficiency results in scurvy. In the United States scurvy is seen primarily in those living in poverty, older adults, and alcoholics.[115,119] Scurvy is the oldest recognized nutritional deficiency characterized by irritability, appetite loss, low-grade fever, bleeding into the skin and from the gums, changes in hair, and easy bruising.[119] In pediatric populations bone and teeth formation may be disrupted by vitamin C deficiency.[119] Iron deficiency can also occur through blood loss as well as impaired iron absorption. High doses of vitamin C can cause diarrhea, nausea, and generalized GI distress.

TABLE 9.17 Recommended Dietary Allowances of Vitamin C at Various Life Stages

Age	Recommended Amount
Birth to 6 months	40 mg
Infants 7–12 months	50 mg
Children 9–13 years	45 mg
Males 14–18	75 mg
Females 14–18	65 mg
Adult males	90 mg
Adult females	75 mg
Pregnant teens	80 mg
Pregnant women	85 mg
Breastfeeding teens	115 mg
Breastfeeding women	120 mg

TABLE 9.18 Upper Limits for Vitamin C Intake During Various Life Stages

Age	Upper Limit
Birth to 12 months	Not established
Children 1–3 years	400 mg
Children 4–8 years	650 mg
Children 9–13 years	1,200 mg
Teens 14–18	1,800 mg
Adults	2,000 mg

TREATMENT

- Effective treatment of deficiency is accomplished with vitamin C supplementation.[115,120]
- The RDA of vitamin C can typically be obtained through the diet (Table 9.17).[115]
- ULs for vitamin C intake should not be exceeded (Table 9.18).[115]

KEY POINTS

- Thiamine deficiency is common in patients with alcohol use disorders.
- Consider WE in patients who present with oculomotor disturbance, gait ataxia, and encephalopathy.

9.6 MINERAL DISORDERS

9.6A CALCIUM DEFICIENCY

OVERVIEW

Calcium plays a critical role in normal cellular function. The diverse roles of calcium in physiologic processes such as cardiac and muscular contraction, vasodilation, vascular contraction, neuromuscular signaling, intracellular signaling, hormone secretion, skeletal structural integrity, and blood coagulation make it the most abundant mineral in the body and key for normal physiologic functioning.[121–123]

Dairy products including milk, yogurt, and cheese are rich in calcium and are the major source of calcium in the American diet. Other sources include vegetables such as kale, broccoli, varieties of cabbage, and spinach. Fortified grain products, juices, drinks, and cereal may provide a source of calcium in the diet.[121] Supplements typically are available as calcium carbonate and calcium citrate. Calcium carbonate is best absorbed when taken with food, while calcium citrate can be taken with or without food.[121]

PHYSIOLOGY

Extracellular calcium concentrations are tightly regulated through the feedback mechanisms of parathyroid hormone and vitamin D signaling pathways between kidney, bone, intestine, and parathyroid glands.[122,124] Serum calcium does not change with changes in dietary intake.[124] The skeletal system serves as the reservoir for calcium in the body and is used to maintain constant concentrations of calcium in blood, intercellular fluid, and muscle tissue.[123]

DEFICIENCY

Daily variations in calcium intake have little effect. Calcium levels are so tightly regulated, and the reservoir of calcium is so large, that effects of calcium deficiency are seen only with chronic reductions in calcium intake over years. Hypocalcemia is generally the result of an underlying medical condition and may result in numbness, tingling, cramping, lethargy, convulsions, and heart arrhythmias.[121] Long-term dietary deficiency leads to osteopenia and can lead to osteoporosis. Risks of bone fractures increase, especially in the older adult.

Hypercalcemia can result in kidney damage, soft tissue calcification, vascular calcification, hypercalciuria, and kidney stones.[124] High levels of calcium in the blood are usually caused by an underlying malignancy or primary hyperparathyroidism.

Calcium deficiency is covered in detail elsewhere in discussions on osteoporosis, parathyroid disease, and renal disease.

TREATMENT

- RDI of calcium varies by age (Table 9.19).[121] Calcium supplementation should be provided if dietary intake is inadequate.

9.6B WILSON DISEASE

OVERVIEW

Wilson disease (WD) is the classic disorder of copper metabolism. It is a rare autosomal recessive genetic disorder involving mutations of the P-type ATPase copper transporter *ATP7B*.[125,126] It was first identified by Samuel Alexander Wilson over a century ago as a familial nervous disease associated with liver cirrhosis.[125] It was noted to be inherited and associated with extrapyramidal neurologic signs and symptoms. It was later discovered that patients with WD had elevated liver and brain copper levels leading to the development of chelation therapies as the mainstay for

TABLE 9.19 Calcium Recommended Dietary Intake by Life Stage

Age	Male	Female	Pregnant	Lactating
0–6 months	200 mg (adequate intake [AI])	200 mg (AI)		
7–12 months	260 mg (AI)	260 mg (AI)		
1–3 years	700 mg	700 mg		
4–8 years	1,000 mg	1,000 mg		
9–13 years	1,300 mg	1,300 mg		
14–18 years	1,300 mg	1,300 mg	1,300 mg	1,300 mg
19–50 years	1,000 mg	1,000 mg	1,000 mg	1,000 mg
51–70 years	1,000 mg	1,200 mg		
71+ years	1,200 mg	1,200 mg		

Source: From Office of Dietary Supplements. Calcium: fact sheet for health professionals. National Institutes of Health. Updated August 17, 2021. https://ods.od.nih.gov/factsheets/Calcium-HealthProfessional

treatment.[125] Chelation and nonchelation treatments now exist for effective lifelong treatment of WD patients.[125,127,128]

WD is characterized by neurologic disease, hepatic disease, and copper deposition in tissues. Patients exhibit neurologic deficits and symptoms of liver disease, sometimes confusing the diagnosis with other hepatic encephalopathies.

EPIDEMIOLOGY

As a single gene, autosomal recessive condition, WD exhibits "hot spots" in its global distribution but varies considerably among different populations.[128] This may be due in large part to the more than 500 *ATP7B* mutations now identified and the variable penetrance of mutations.[128] Studies identifying genotype-phenotype have largely been unsuccessful. It has been suggested that modifier genes may be responsible for the variability of copper tolerance in individuals with *ATP7B* mutations.[128]

Recent genetic analysis studies predict a disease prevalence of 1:7,000–1:9,000 in certain populations, which is significantly higher than the originally predicted 1:30,000 prevalence figure and is based on genetic analysis of patients in the United Kingdom.[125,126,128] The clinical prevalence is much lower than the predicted prevalence, which again suggests variable penetrance of mutations and other modifying genes that may regulate the patient's ability to handle elevated copper levels without symptoms of WD.[125,126,128]

PATHOPHYSIOLOGY

Copper is an essential micronutrient and essential cofactor for various enzymes within the cell. Copper-containing transcription factors are part of the machinery needed for the cell to maintain its integrity, produce energy, divide, signal, and respond to various cell stresses.[125] However, the cell requires copper levels to be tightly controlled. Aberrant copper levels lead to inappropriate cell signaling in the brain leading to various brain disease forms. Elevated copper levels in the liver result in cellular damage and progressive liver disease. Morbidity and fatality in WD arise predominantly from late detection with signs and symptoms being attributed to other more common neurodegenerative and cirrhotic diseases.[125,128]

MEDICAL HISTORY AND CLINICAL PRESENTATION

WD is most often diagnosed in teenagers; however, late-onset WD is also seen in older adults.[125,128] Signs and symptoms in the pediatric patient include asymptomatic hepatomegaly, elevated liver enzymes, changes in behavior, movement disorders, or school failure.[125] Older patients may present with symptoms of liver failure, movement disorders, memory changes, and behavioral changes.[128] As copper is deposited in tissues, it can appear as Kayser-Fleischer rings of brown or rust coloring around the iris.[125]

SIGNS AND SYMPTOMS

Signs and symptoms include symptoms associated with acute or chronic liver failure including jaundice, abdominal pain, and skin sensitivity and irritation. Changes in behavior, mood, and cognitive function are also seen in WD. Changes in executive function are seen with preservation of verbal and short-term memory. Extrapyramidal symptoms including "wing-beating tremor" or "flapping tremor" as well as various parkinsonian symptoms such as shuffling gait, fine motor tremor, and foot tapping may be seen.[128] Rest, action, or intention tremors may be present as well as involuntary facial grimacing, helping to differentiate from parkinsonism.[128] Dystonic tremor is commonly seen in WD patients.[128]

PHYSICAL EXAMINATION

For clinical evaluation, observation of manifestations of liver damage and neurologic symptoms are suggestive of WD. Observation of the classic visible corneal-pigmented rings (Kayser-Fleischer rings), which may require slit-lamp evaluation, helps to establish the diagnosis. In general, clinical manifestations of liver damage, neurologic symptoms, and Kayser-Fleischer rings are the triad to make a clinical diagnosis (Figure 9.11).

DIFFERENTIAL DIAGNOSIS

Differential diagnosis includes any cirrhotic liver disease and cause of hepatic encephalopathy. Other causes of movement disorders including Parkinson disease, drug-related dystonic movement disorders, and other neurodegenerative diseases should be considered. As these are more commonly

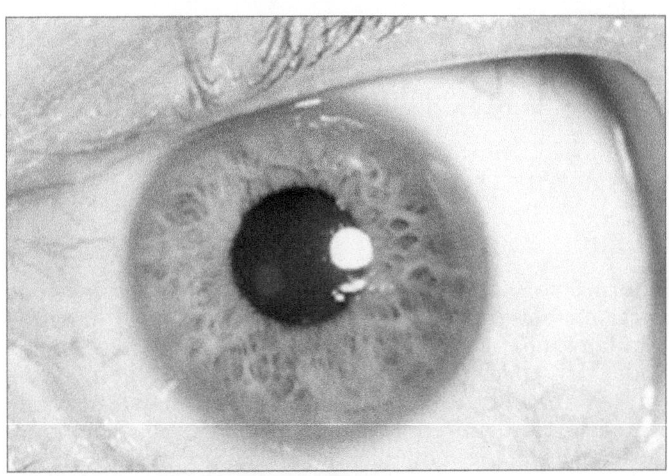

Figure 9.11 Kayser-Fleischer ring associated with Wilson disease. Note the copper-colored circumcorneal deposition, which can also sometimes appear greenish or red-brown.
(Source: Herbert L. Fred, MD, Hendrik A. van Dijk.)

encountered diseases, it can make the time to reach a definitive diagnosis and initiate treatment excessively long for WD patients.

DIAGNOSTIC STUDIES

Diagnostic studies are helpful in the diagnosis of WD. Liver function studies showing elevated liver enzymes in either an acute or a chronic pattern are frequently observed. Ceruloplasmin levels <0.2 g/L are seen; 24-hour urinary copper values >100 mcg in adults are common.[128] Visible corneal-pigmented ring under slit-lamp exam is indicative of improper copper metabolism. Genetic studies can be performed to identify the exact mutation in the *ATP7B* gene.[128]

TREATMENT

- The mainstay of WD treatment is lifelong copper chelation. Chelating agents bind copper from the various tissues and allow copper to be excreted into the stool and/or eliminated by urine excretion.
- D-penicillamine is commonly used and causes the excretion of large amounts of urine copper but is slow in removing copper from the brain.[125,128] Trientine is a multiamine metal chelating agent and is recommended for patients with neurologic involvement.[128] Zinc preparations interfere with GI copper absorption.[125,128] Tetrathiomolybdate interferes with copper absorption or binds with copper in the plasma.[128]
- Vitamin E levels may be reduced in WD patients; therefore, supplementation may help alleviate some symptoms.

PATIENT EDUCATION

- Patients should be counseled concerning the need for lifelong treatment to reduce morbidity and mortality from WD. Drug side effects should be discussed and the correct drug should be used according the needs of the patient and the side effect profile.
- Monitoring every 6 months is suggested to ensure clinical and biochemical response to medication.
- Patients should be routinely screened for hepatocellular carcinoma, and any newly developed hepatic or neurologic symptoms should be investigated and suggest and uncontrolled copper levels.

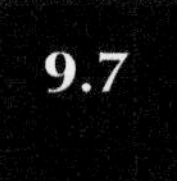

9.7 METABOLIC DISORDERS—INBORN ERRORS OF METABOLISM

CAREY A. WHEELHOUSE

OVERVIEW

Inborn errors of metabolism are genetic conditions that affect metabolism of nutrients. Inborn errors of metabolism may inhibit the breakdown of carbohydrates, amino acids, fatty acids, urea, or other types of metabolic pathways.[129] Inability to breakdown nutrients may lead to elevated levels of intermediate metabolites, which in turn cause neurologic complications, developmental delay, and, in some cases, death.[129] Early identification and treatment are often vital to the prognosis of affected children, and newborn screening for inborn errors of metabolism is recommended.[129]

9.7A GALACTOSEMIA

OVERVIEW

Galactosemia is an inborn error of carbohydrate metabolism. Galactosemia is inherited through an autosomal recessive pattern, and results in diminished ability to break down galactose. Classic galactosemia presents in the newborn period and requires prompt identification and treatment. Untreated, galactosemia leads to life-threatening complications including jaundice, hepatomegaly, and neonatal sepsis.[130,131]

EPIDEMIOLOGY

Galactosemia is a rare disorder, occurring in approximately 1 in every 14,000 to 80,000 live births worldwide.[132] Incidence may vary among populations. Higher prevalence of galactosemia has been reported in South Africa, Ireland, and Argentina.[130,132] In the United States, galactosemia occurrence has been reported at 1 in every 30,000 to 60,000 live births.[131]

PATHOPHYSIOLOGY

Galactosemia is genetic disorder of carbohydrate catabolism resulting from decreased activity of the galactose-1-phosphate uridyltransferase (GALT) enzyme.[130–132] Typically, the GALT enzyme aids in galactose catabolism by converting galactose 1-phosphate and uridine diphosphate glucose to uridine diphosphate galactose and glucose 1-phosphate (Figure 9.12).[130,131] However, in individuals with galactosemia, diminished GALT enzymatic activity leads to potentially life-threatening elevations in total galactose and galactose 1-phosphate.[130,132]

MEDICAL HISTORY AND CLINICAL PRESENTATION

Classic galactosemia is an autosomal recessive disorder present at birth, resulting in complete or near complete deficiency of the GALT enzyme. Affected newborns may not present with symptoms of classic galactosemia until they have begun feeding. Upon consumption of galactose in breast milk or cow's milk formula, affected individuals have acute symptoms development.[131] Symptoms progress rapidly in the first few days of life.[131] If left untreated, affected newborns have a poor prognosis and often die from complications of classic galactosemia.[130,131]

Variant forms of galactosemia also exist, with most variant forms having partial deficiency of the GALT enzyme. Duarte variant galactosemia is the most common variant

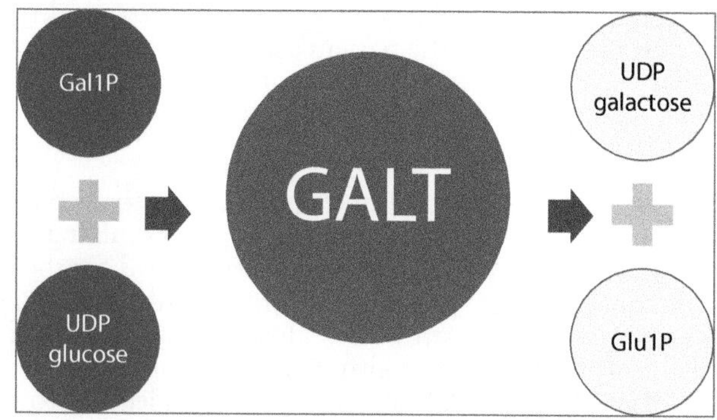

Figure 9.12 GALT enzyme activity. The GALT enzyme breaks down galactose 1-phosphate (Gal1P) and UDP glucose, converting them into UDP galactose and glucose 1-phosphate (Glu1P). GALT, galactose-1-phosphate uridyltransferase; UDP, uridine diphosphate.

form, and is associated with 25% residual GALT activity.[131] Newborn screening may identify some variant forms of galactosemia; however, follow-up testing is recommended to assess the severity of GALT deficiency.[131]

SIGNS AND SYMPTOMS

Clinical symptoms of galactosemia present after consumption of galactose, which is found in both breast milk and milk-based infant formula.[130,131] Early symptoms include poor feeding, jaundice, vomiting, and diarrhea.[131] Within the first few days of life, untreated classic galactosemia results in failure to thrive, hepatomegaly, sepsis, and subsequent death.[130] Affected individuals who are treated appropriately may still have long-term complications, including speech and learning deficits, cataracts, growth delay, reduced bone mineral density, neurologic disorders, and ovarian dysfunction.[130,133]

PHYSICAL EXAMINATION

All newborns should undergo a thorough newborn exam with newborn screening. Children who develop symptoms of lethargy, poor feeding, vomiting, diarrhea, or jaundice after beginning feeding should be assessed for galactosemia with physical examination and follow-up diagnostic testing. Assessment for hepatomegaly may be an indicator of galactosemia. All children should undergo routine well-child examinations to evaluate for age-appropriate cognitive, motor, language, and socioemotional development.

DIFFERENTIAL DIAGNOSIS

Liver dysfunction may cause secondary hypergalactosemia. Causes of liver dysfunction in the newborn period may include congenital hepatitis, congenital hepatic arteriovenous malformations, patent ductus venosus, tyrosinemia, or Fanconi-Bickel syndrome.[130] Additionally, newborn screening for children with galactosemia may show elevated levels of phenylalanine suggesting a diagnosis of PKU. However, children with galactosemia have elevated levels of tyrosine, whereas children with PKU will have low levels of tyrosine.[132]

DIAGNOSTIC STUDIES

Newborn screening is the first step in identifying galactosemia. Follow-up diagnostic tests for both Duarte variant and classic galactosemia include low or absent hemolysate GALT activity, elevated hemolysate galactose 1-phosphate levels, and elevated urinary galacticol levels.[131]

EVALUATION

Children diagnosed with galactosemia should be treated with dietary restriction of galactose immediately.[132] Affected children should be followed closely in the days following diagnosis, monitoring for symptom development. Asymptomatic children should be monitored every 3 to 4 months in the first 2 years of life, progressing to annual follow-up thereafter.[132] Follow-up should include assessment of hepatic function, growth and development and ophthalmologic evaluation, and may include laboratory assessment of urine galactitol or total blood galactose.[132] As affected females reach puberty, assessment of ovarian function should be performed through evaluation of luteinizing hormone, FSH, and estradiol levels.[132]

TREATMENT

Early treatment with dietary restriction of galactose is necessary to reduce the risk of morbidity and mortality in the neonate.[130,132] In infancy, dietary restriction is met through use of soy-based infant formulas.[132] As the child ages, they are weaned to solid foods, maintaining a lifelong dietary restriction of galactose. Dietary restrictions include avoidance of dairy products and high-galactose-containing fruits and vegetables, such as watermelon and figs.[132] Some legumes with high levels of galactose, such as garbanzo beans, are not recommended.[133] Even with lifelong dietary restriction of galactose, patients with galactosemia may go on to develop cognitive, neurologic, and developmental complications.[130,133]

PATIENT EDUCATION

Patients and their parents should be educated on the importance of early identification and lifelong dietary restriction of galactose. Patients and parents should also be educated on the adverse outcomes associated with the diagnosis. Medical clinicians should discuss the importance of routine monitoring of the patient throughout childhood. Female patients with galactosemia should be educated on the possibility of ovarian dysfunction.

9.7B MAPLE SYRUP URINE DISEASE

OVERVIEW

MSUD is an autosomal recessive disorder affecting amino acid metabolism.[134] MSUD is characterized by elevated levels of BCAAs in the blood and urine, as well as a maple syrup odor to the urine. There are five types of MSUD. Classic MSUD is present at birth, and is often identified on newborn screening.[134] The mainstay of treatment is dietary restriction of BCAAs. Failure to diagnose and treat MSUD promptly may result in feeding difficulties, developmental delay, and potentially life-threatening neurologic complications.[134,135]

EPIDEMIOLOGY

MSUD is a rare genetic disorder, with incidence occurring around 1 in every 185,000 live births worldwide, though incidence varies among populations.[134,136] Mennonite populations in the midwestern and northeastern parts of the United States have the highest rates of MSUD, reporting about one case of MSUD for every 200 live births.[134,136]

PATHOPHYSIOLOGY

Patients with MSUD have dysfunctional metabolism of three BCAAs: leucine, isoleucine, and valine.[134] Leucine, isoleucine, and valine are vital to cellular function, protein synthesis, and glucose metabolism.[134] Typically, metabolism of these BCAAs occurs through a multistep process within the liver or, more commonly, skeletal muscle mitochondria.[134] First, leucine, isoleucine, and valine are broken down into α-ketoacids by the branched-chain aminotransferase enzyme. Next, an enzyme complex called the branched-chain α-ketoacid dehydrogenase (BCKAD) converts the α-ketoacids into acetoacetate, acetyl-CoA, and succinyl-CoA.[134,135] However, in individuals with MSUD, the BCKAD complex does not function fully, resulting in elevated levels of BCAAs in the blood and urine (Figure 9.13).[134,135] Elevated levels of these BCAAs subsequently lead to irreversible neurologic dysfunction, developmental delay, and decreased cognitive function.[134,136] In particular, elevated levels of leucine may cause severe illness and neurotoxicity.[134,135]

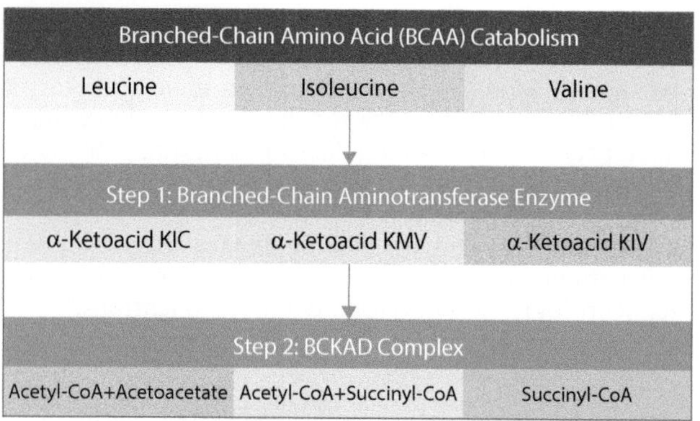

Figure 9.13 **Summary of BCAA catabolism. The BCAAs leucine, isoleucine, and valine are initially broken down into α-ketoacids by the branched-chain aminotransferase enzyme, most commonly occurring within skeletal muscle mitochondria. Next, the α-ketoacids undergo oxidative carboxylation in the BCKAD complex, eventually breaking down into acetyl-CoA, succinyl-CoA, and acetoacetate. In MSUD, step 2 of this pathway is affected.** BCKAD, branched-chain α-ketoacid dehydrogenase; CoA, coenzyme A; KIC, ketoisocaproic; KIV, ketoisovaleric; KMV, keto methylvaleric; MSUD, maple syrup urine disease.

MEDICAL HISTORY AND CLINICAL PRESENTATION

There are five phenotypical presentations of MSUD: classic, intermittent, intermediate, thiamine-responsive, and E3-deficient. Approximately 80% of MSUD cases are classic MSUD.[136] Classic MSUD presents in the newborn phase, with affected individuals having BCKAD function of 2% or less.[134,136] Clinical presentations of classic MSUD include a characteristic maple syrup odor to the urine, poor feeding, and irritability in the newborn phase.[134,136] As the child ages, cognitive impairment, hyperactivity, and neurologic dysfunction develop. Blood levels of BCAAs and urine levels of branched-chain ketoacids are elevated in classic MSUD.[134,136]

Less commonly, a variant form of MSUD may occur. Variant forms of MSUD are associated with BCKAD functioning between 3% and 40%, and symptoms present at variable periods ranging from the newborn phase to later in infancy.[134,136] Individuals with higher levels of BCKAD functioning may have typical growth and development trajectories but present with ketoacidosis in times of stress or acute illness.[134,136]

SIGNS AND SYMPTOMS

Symptoms of classic MSUD often present shortly after birth.[134] Children with MSUD have a characteristic odor of maple syrup in their cerumen, as well as in their urine.[134,136] Typically, characteristic odor of cerumen is the first sign to present in children with MSUD.[135] Initially, newborns may present with poor feeding and irritability.[134,136] Symptoms may quickly progress to dystonia or bicycling-like movements, seizures, altered levels of consciousness, and ketoacidosis.[134,136]

Elevated levels of leucine in the blood, even if only minimal elevations may be neurotoxin.[135] Leucine toxicity may occur with fasting, exercise, and times of physiologic stress, such as an acute illness, injury, or surgical procedure.[135] Leucine toxicity leads to encephalopathy, brain edema, and possibly death.[137]

PHYSICAL EXAMINATION

A thorough newborn exam with newborn screening should be performed, with particular attention paid to odor of the cerumen. While classic and E3-deficient forms of MSUD typically present in the neonatal period, variant forms of MSUD may not.[136] All children should undergo routine well-child examinations to evaluate for age-appropriate cognitive, motor, language, and socioemotional development. Additionally, a diagnosis of MSUD should be considered in infants and children who present with symptoms of encephalopathy and ketoacidosis sporadically, when acutely ill, or when associated with fasting.

DIFFERENTIAL DIAGNOSIS

MSUD should be differentiated from other inborn errors of metabolism resulting in cognitive delay and neurologic complications. Positive newborn screening for MSUD, elevated plasma BCAA levels, and presence of branched-chain ketoacids in the urine differentiate MSUD from other inborn errors of metabolism. Additionally, characteristic maple syrup odor to cerumen and urine may differentiate MSUD from other inborn errors of metabolism.

DIAGNOSTIC STUDIES

Because of the importance of early identification and treatment in patient prognosis, newborn screening for MSUD is recommended.[134,136] However, variant forms of MSUD may not be identified on newborn screening, and false positives may occur in the presence of benign hydroxyprolinemia.[134,136] Additional diagnostic testing may be performed through blood and urine analysis. Plasma leucine, isoleucine, and valine levels are typically elevated in MSUD, but may occasionally present in the normal range.[136] When this occurs, elevated ratios of these BCAAs to other amino acids in the blood, such as the leucine: alanine molar ratio, aid in the diagnosis of MSUD.[135] Additionally, alloisoleucine presence in plasma indicates MSUD, and further diagnostic testing is not needed. Urine testing may performed to aid in the diagnosis of MSUD and includes screening for α-ketoacids in the urine through the urine DNPH (2,4-dinitrophenylhydrazine) test, or through urine organic acid analysis.[134,136] Presence of branched-chain ketoacid in urine organic acid analysis points toward a diagnosis of MSUD, and is usually detected within the first 3 days of life.[136]

EVALUATION

Patients with MSUD should be monitored weekly in their first year of life, and monthly thereafter for appropriate development, presence of neurologic signs and symptoms, and plasma BCAA levels.[135,137] Patients with MSUD must consider the impact of illness and injury on their prognosis, and should be monitored closely in times of acute illness, injury, trauma, or surgery.[135] The urine DNPH test may be used to screen for α-ketoacids presence in the urine on an outpatient basis, aiding patients in appropriate "sick day" treatment during times of physiologic stress.[134,137]

TREATMENT

- Treatment of MSUD targets prevention of neurologic and cognitive complications, as well as promotion of normal growth and development.[137] Treatment is best initiated within 72 hours of birth, and early treatment is associated with lower morbidity and mortality rates, as well as less medical cost for the family.[135]
- Treatment for MSUD includes both maintenance of lifelong dietary restriction of BCAAs, as well as "sick day" medical management during times of acute physiologic

stress.[134,135] Dietary management should include metabolic specialists. Children with MSUD may require special formula that restricts BCAAs while also providing appropriate nutrients for optimal brain development.[137] Additionally, formula may include sodium chloride to control brain edema.[137] Children may be weaned to table foods between 1 and 2 years of age, and continue to supplement their diet with BCAA-free amino acid foods.[134,137] Plasma leucine levels are targeted at 100–300 µmol/L in the neonatal period, 75–100 µmol/L in children <5 years old, and 75–300 µmol/L in children over the age of 5.[137,138]

- In episodes of physiologic stress, such as acute illness or injury, treatment is targeted at both the infection or injury, as well as preventing neurologic complications and cerebral edema.[137] In acute management, patients with MSUD should stop all protein intake for a duration of 1 to 3 days, monitoring plasma BCAA levels at least daily.[134,137] Adequate caloric intake and hydration should be provided through IV dextrose 10% to 12.5% at a rate of 2–3 L/day for adults.[134] Fluid rates for children are calculated by weight.[1] Serum sodium levels should be monitored closely.[135] Mannitol and furosemide may be used for prevention of cerebral edema.[135] As the patient improves, protein may gradually be introduced back into the diet.
- Classic MSUD patients with hepatic BCKAD dysfunction may also be candidates for liver transplantation. As BCKAD dysfunction more commonly occurs in skeletal muscle, liver transplant is not recommended for all patients with classic MSUD. Most patients treated with liver transplant have an unrestricted diet after transplantation.[134]

PATIENT EDUCATION

- Children treated with appropriate dietary restriction of BCAAs can have age-appropriate development. Patients and their parents should be educated on the importance of lifelong dietary restriction of BCAAs, as well as the adverse outcomes associated with elevated levels of BCAAs.
- Patients and parents should also be educated about the impact that illness, injury, surgery, and fasting may have on their BCAA blood levels, as well as the neurologic complications that may arise.
- Clinicians should discuss the importance of routine BCAA plasma monitoring and stress the importance of medical evaluation and management during times of physiologic stress.

9.7C PHENYLKETONURIA

OVERVIEW

PKU is a genetic disorder that affects amino acid metabolism. PKU is characterized by elevated levels of phenylalanine. If left untreated, elevated levels of phenylalanine may cause lasting cognitive and intellectual impairments, as well as neurologic and behavioral complications.[139–141] PKU is often identified during newborn screening, but PKU may also be diagnosed after the newborn period. Individuals with PKU respond well to restrictive dietary treatment.

EPIDEMIOLOGY

Incidence of PKU is rare, with approximately 1 in 10,000 new diagnoses reported per year in European populations.[142] African American populations have a lower incidence of PKU, reporting only one new diagnosis per 50,000 people per year.[142]

PATHOPHYSIOLOGY

PKU is an autosomal recessive disorder.[139,140] Individuals with classic PKU have a deficiency in phenylalanine hydroxylase, a liver enzyme involved in amino acid metabolism.[139–141] Typically, phenylalanine hydroxylase converts phenylalanine into tyrosine, ridding the body of nearly three-fourths of its dietary phenylalanine intake in the process.[140] However, in an individual with PKU, phenylalanine hydroxylase enzyme deficiency leads to inability to break down phenylalanine, causing subsequent elevated levels of phenylalanine.[139–141] PKU may range from mild to severe, depending on the amount of phenylalanine in the individual's blood.[141]

MEDICAL HISTORY AND CLINICAL PRESENTATION

As an autosomal recessive genetic disorder, PKU is present at the time of birth in affected individuals. Parents of children with PKU are carriers and may not be aware of their carrier status prior to birth. Identification of PKU is often found on newborn screening.[140] Children with PKU who are not identified through newborn screening may present with neurologic, cognitive, and/or behavioral symptoms in the early developmental stages.[140]

SIGNS AND SYMPTOMS

Untreated PKU is associated with irreversible neurologic manifestations, which may include headaches, seizures, encephalopathy, abnormalities of gait, upper extremity tremor, hyperactive reflexes, loss of vision, and/or alterations in sensation.[140] Cognitive manifestations, such as low IQ and difficulties with memory, are also common. Psychiatric symptoms, including hyperactivity, anxiety, social isolation, and low self-esteem, may also be present.[139,140]

PHYSICAL EXAMINATION

A thorough newborn exam with newborn screening should be performed on all neonates. Additionally, all children should undergo routine well-child examinations to evaluate development, including age-appropriate cognitive, motor, language, and socioemotional development. Close attention should be paid to neurologic and psychiatric assessment in suspected individuals.

DIFFERENTIAL DIAGNOSIS

Other disorders resulting in abnormalities of phenylalanine levels in neonates include tetrahydrobiopterin (BH4) deficiency, maternal PKU, and tyrosinemia of the newborn.

DIAGNOSTIC STUDIES

Classic PKU is diagnosed when blood phenylalanine levels are >1,200 µmol/L.[141] However, mild cases of PKU have been reported with phenylalanine levels of 600 to 900 µmol/L, and moderate PKU has been reported with blood phenylalanine levels of 900 to 1,200 µmol/L.[141] Brain MRI of adults with symptomatic PKU, either due to late diagnosis or dietary treatment noncompliance, have demonstrated nonspecific changes in white matter.[140]

EVALUATION

Evaluation for PKU should occur as part of routine newborn screening. In individuals diagnosed with PKU, weekly monitoring of blood phenylalanine levels should occur until 12 months of age. From ages 1 to 12, blood phenylalanine levels should be monitored two times per month. After 12 years of age, blood phenylalanine levels may be measured monthly.[143]

TREATMENT

- Treatment of PKU is done through lifelong restriction of dietary phenylalanine consumption, targeting intake of dietary phenylalanine to <10 g/day.[139,141] Dietary restriction is recommended for PKU patients with blood phenylalanine levels >360 µmol/L. Dietary restriction is not recommend for blood phenylalanine levels <360 µmol/L.[141] Dietary restriction is ideally started within the first week of life.[144]
- In infancy, children with PKU consume breast milk or standard infant formula at an individualized level of tolerance, with phenylalanine-free l-amino acid infant formula supplementation to meet nutritional needs of the child.[145] Children are then weaned into a low-phenylalanine diet, typically starting with vegetables, with dietitian directed weaning occurring between 17 and 26 weeks of age.[145]
- A low-phenylalanine diet includes avoidance of high-phenylalanine foods, including proteins such as fish, meat, eggs, and nuts, as well as breads and pasta.[139] Recommended foods include those low in phenylalanine, such as fruit, vegetables, and oils. Protein substitutes and low protein foods are also recommended to prevent growth and protein deficiencies.[139] Adjunctive pharmacologic treatment with sapropterin or pegvaliase may also be considered in some patients with PKU.[146]

PATIENT EDUCATION

- Children treated with appropriate dietary restriction of phenylalanine often have age-appropriate cognitive development that is similar to that of children without PKU.[139] However, dietary noncompliance at any time may result in neurologic and/or psychiatric symptom development, as well as changes in the white matter of the brain.[139]
- Parents should be educated on the pathophysiology of PKU, the importance of lifelong compliance with dietary phenylalanine restriction, and the positive developmental prognosis for children with appropriate dietary treatment.[140]
- In addition to dietary treatment, it is important to consider psychosocial impacts of PKU on affected children and their families. Children may have difficulty understanding or accepting a diet that differs from their siblings, parents, or peers.
- Parents of children with dietary restrictions due to PKU have higher levels of depression and lower levels of social support when compared to parents who do not have children with dietary restrictions.[141] Additionally, parents have reported difficulty in managing dietary needs for children with and their siblings without PKU simultaneously.
- Parents should not only be educated on the pathophysiology, treatment, and prognosis for PKU, but also be provided education and recommendations for familial psychosocial support.[141]

9.8 NUTRITIONAL SUPPORT

9.8A NUTRITIONAL REQUIREMENTS

Megan Timmerman

INTRODUCTION

Established in 1941 by the National Academy of Sciences and Institute of Medicine, Food and Nutrition Board, the RDA was established as a set of guidelines to prevent nutritional deficiencies. The RDA initially sought to define sufficient intake for protein, energy, and eight vitamins and minerals; this was later expanded to include 25. The goal of the RDA is to define sufficient nutritional intake to meet the needs of the majority of Americans, based on age and gender. These guidelines have served as the foundation for nearly all state and federal food and nutrition programs, as well as policy development in the United States since their creation in 1941.

In 1989, research was beginning to show the effect diet had on disease states, specifically nutrient deficiencies and chronic disease. Created in 1994, the Dietary Reference Intakes (DRIs) were established to define a minimum or lowest level of intake to maintain health. The DRI seek to define a relationship between indicators of adequacy, prevention of chronic illness, and nutrient intake. The DRI serve as a foundation to assess and plan nutrient intakes of healthy individuals in both America and Canada, and values are categorically divided by age and gender. The DRIs are based on four nutrient-based values that serve as a reference: EAR, RDA, Tolerable Upper Intake Level (UL), and AI. Expanding upon the initial values set by the RDA, the DRIs have now been established for 51 nutrients: macronutrients, energy, vitamins, and minerals.

The Dietary Guidelines for Americans were established in 1980 by the U.S. Department of Agriculture and the U.S. Department of Health and Human Services to serve as a guide to identify a nutritionally adequate diet to promote health and reduce chronic disease. The Institute of Medicine's DRIs serve as a source for the development of the Dietary Guidelines for Americans.

ASSESSING ENERGY AND MACRONUTRIENT REQUIREMENTS

Calories

Energy is needed by the human body to maintain function of organs and their physiologic properties. Macronutrients are energy-supplying nutrients and are split into four categories: protein, fat, carbohydrates, and alcohol. Each macronutrient source provides its own energy amount, kilocalories (kcal) per gram (Table 9.20).

TABLE 9.20 Kilocalories Provided per Gram by Energy Source

Macronutrient Source	Kcal Provided per Gram
Carbohydrate	4 kcal/g
Protein	4 kcal/g
Fat	9 kcal/g
Alcohol	7 kcal/g

Energy requirements are established based on age, gender, height, weight and level of daily physical activity. Estimated Energy Requirements (EERs) are calculated based on BMI, age, and gender and are multiplied by an activity factor. EER is not an exact recommendation, but rather a range of energy needed to maintain caloric balance. There is no current RDA established for energy consumption, and guidelines established are intended to maintain weight. Excess calories cannot be excreted by the body and are stored as fat by the body for future use.

EXHIBIT 9.4 Harris-Benedict Equations

BMR calculation for men (metric)
BMR = 66.47 + (13.75 × weight in kg) + (5.003 × height in cm) – (6.755 × age in years)

BMR calculation for women (metric)
BMR = 655.1 + (9.563 × weight in kg) + (1.850 × height in cm) – (4.676 × age in years)

BMR, basal metabolic rate.

TABLE 9.21 Harris-Benedict Activity Factors

Level of Activity	Multiplier Factor
Sedentary: little to no exercise	BMR × 1.2
Mild activity: light exercise, 1–3 days/week, 20 minutes	BMR × 1.3
Moderate activity: 30–60 minutes, 3–4 days/week	BMR × 1.5
High intensity: 60+ minutes of high intensity, 5–7 days/week	BMR × 1.7–1.9

BMR, basal metabolic rate.

One of the most widely used methods of estimating caloric needs of Americans is the Harris-Benedict Equation (Exhibit 9.4). This equation seeks to define an individual's basal energy requirement (basal metabolic rate, BMR). This equation factors in gender, age, height, and weight to calculate the resting metabolic rate. The calculated BMR is then multiplied by an activity factor to determine an individual's daily estimated caloric needs (Table 9.21). Once calculated, this equation serves as a framework to identify caloric needs of individuals.

Equations, such as the Harris-Benedict Equation, serve as reliable tools to estimate caloric needs in patients using anthropometric equations easily obtained during clinic visits. The accuracy of this tool decreases with increasing BMI, especially in women, but can still serve as a reference point to assess estimated needs.[147]

A pound of body weight equates to roughly 3,500 calories; to lose 1 pound per week, a person needs to reduce intake by approximately 500 calories each day. The Harris-Benedict Equation and other similar tools allow for a starting place to determine estimated needs for weight loss. The Dietary Guidelines for Americans serve as a guide to assist patients with making dietary changes to influence overall health and wellness (Table 9.22).

Protein

Protein is an important component of each cell in the human body, playing both structural and functional roles. Sources of dietary protein include animal sources, such as meat, fish,

TABLE 9.22 Daily Nutritional Goals for Age-Sex Groups Based on Dietary Reference Intakes & *Dietary Guidelines* Recommendations

	Source of Goal	Child 1–3	Female 4–8	Male 4–8	Female 9–13	Male 9–13	Female 14–18	Male 14–18
Calorie level(s) assessed		1,000	1,200	1,400, 1,600	1,600	1,800	1,800	2,200, 2,800, 3,200
Macronutrients								
Protein, g	RDA	13	19	19	34	34	46	52
Protein, % kcal	AMDR	5–20	10–30	10–30	10–30	10–30	10–30	10–30
Carbohydrate, g	RDA	130	130	130	130	130	130	130
Carbohydrate, % kcal	AMDR	45–65	45–65	45–65	45–65	45–65	45–65	4–65
Dietary fiber, g	14g/1,000 kcal	14	16.8	19.6	22.4	25.2	25.2	30.8
Added sugars, % kcal	DGA	<10%	<10%	<10%	<10%	<10%	<10%	<10%
Total fat, % kcal	AMDR	30–40	25–35	25–35	25–35	25–35	25–35	25–35
Saturated fat, % kcal	DGA	<10%	<10%	<10%	<10%	<10%	<10%	<10%
Linoleic acid, g	AI	7	10	10	10	12	11	16
Linolenic acid, g	AI	0.7	0.9	0.9	1	1.2	1.1	1.6

AI, adequate intake; AMDR, acceptable macronutrient distribution range; DGA, Dietary Guidelines for Americans; RDA, recommended dietary allowance.
Source: U.S. Department of Health and Human Services and U.S. Department of Agriculture. 2015–2020 Dietary Guidelines for Americans. 8th ed. U.S. Department of Health and Human Services; 2015. *https://health.gov/dietaryguidelines/2015/guidelines*

poultry, eggs, and dairy. Animal proteins are often referred to as complete protein sources, as they contain all nine essential amino acids. Nonanimal sources, which include nuts, seeds, vegetables, legumes, plants, and grains, are incomplete protein sources, lacking one or more of the nine essential amino acids; however, if they are eaten in various combinations they can become complete proteins. The nine essential amino acids are leucine, isoleucine, lysine, methionine, phenylalanine, threonine, tryptophan, valine, and histidine.

Protein deficiency affects all organs of the body and all organ systems. AI of protein, as well as nonprotein energy sources, are necessary to prevent the development of protein-energy malnutrition. The RDA for protein remains 0.8 g/kg/day. The Acceptable Macronutrient Distribution Range (AMDR) recommendations for adults are 10–35% of total energy from protein and 5–20% for children.

Carbohydrates

Carbohydrates serve as the primary energy source to all cells in the body. Main carbohydrate sources in the diet include grains, dairy products, fruits, and vegetables, as well as added sugar and sweets. Carbohydrate requirements are established to define to minimum amount of carbohydrate essential for brain function. Long-term effects of inadequate consumption of carbohydrate intake can lead to ketosis. The AMDR recommendation for adults is 45–65% of total calories from carbohydrates.

Dietary Fiber

Dietary fiber refers to the nondigestible portion of carbohydrates consumed as a natural component of plant foods. Other fiber sources in the diet include synthetic fiber sources, also known as functional fiber. Fiber can be categorized as soluble or insoluble. Soluble fiber dissolves in water and can help lower blood cholesterol and glucose levels; types of soluble fiber include oat bran, barley, nuts, seeds, beans, lentils, and peas. Insoluble fiber does not dissolve in water and can be helpful to increase stool bulk and treat constipation; sources include fruits, vegetables, and oat bran. Fiber is considered a nonessential nutrient; therefore, RDA, UL, and lower limits have not been determined, but recommendations for AI have been established. For men and women under the age of 50 years, recommended amounts are 38 g/day and 25 g/day respectively. This reduces to 30 g/day and 21 g/day for those over the age of 50 years.

Fat

Dietary fat serves as a main energy source for the body and is the most calorically concentrated macronutrient. Dietary fat aids in the absorption of fat-soluble vitamins and other food components. Fatty acids are the building blocks of fats, and as fat is digested, it is broken down into fatty acids. Fatty acids serve vital roles in the human body, including energy storage. Fatty acids are divided into four categories: saturated, monounsaturated, polyunsaturated, and trans fats.

Saturated and *trans fat* sources are associated with an increased risk of heart disease and should be limited in the diet. No RDA has been established for these fat sources, and general nutrition recommendations are that intake of these fats should be limited to reduce risk of heart disease. Saturated fat sources are naturally occurring and are solid at room temperature. Sources of saturated fat include meat, full-fat dairy, and palm and coconut oil. Increased consumption of saturated fats has been shown to increase risk of coronary vascular disease.

Trans fats are chemically altered fat sources and are common in commercially processed foods, which allow for increased shelf life of these products. Research has shown that increased consumption of trans fats increases risk of heart disease by increasing LDL levels and decreasing HDL levels. Trans fats are a required inclusion on nutrition labels.

When consumed in moderation, *monounsaturated* and *polyunsaturated* fatty acids are associated with a decreased risk of heart disease. Unsaturated fats come from both animal and plant-based sources, including vegetable oils. These oils are often liquid at room temperature. Foods that are high in polyunsaturated fats are plant-based oils, including sunflower, soybean, and corn oil, and nuts and seeds, including walnuts, flaxseed, and soy products. Monounsaturated food sources include oils such as olive, canola, peanut, sesame, and sunflower oil, as well as avocado and other nuts and seeds.

Essential fatty acids are fatty acids that cannot be made by the body and therefore must be consumed in the diet. Humans require two essential fatty acids, linoleic acid, also known as omega-6, and alpha-linoleic acid, also known as omega-3. Linoleic acid is an essential component of the membrane of cells; it can be found in nuts, seeds, and vegetable oils, including safflower, corn, and soybean oils. Dietary sources of alpha-linoleic acid include vegetable oils, including canola, flaxseed, and soybean, as well as fatty fish and fish oils. A RDA has been established for linoleic acid and alpha-linoleic acid.

There is no established UL or RDA for total fat. The AMDR for fat is set at 20–35% of total calories. Inadequate intake of fat in the diet can lead to increased risk of chronic disease and slowed growth in infants and children.

Water

A large percentage of the human body is composed of water; this percentage decreases with age. Water is essential to maintain homeostasis, vascular volume, transport, and removal of nutrients and waste from the body. Sources of water in the diet include food, beverages, and tap water. Approximately 80% of water in the diet comes through beverages and tap water with 20% coming from moisture from food products. General recommendations for adults include approximately 90 ounces of water daily for women and 125 ounces of water daily for men. No RDA is set for water, but an AI exists (Table 9.23). Deficiencies of water in the diet, excessive exercise, or prolonged exposure to heat can increase losses and may cause dehydration. Severe dehydration can lead to death. Excessive consumption of water is rare but can lead to hyponatremia.

Alcohol

Alcohol is a calorie source when consumed as part of the diet. The Dietary Guidelines for Americans recommends no more than moderate consumption of alcohol, if alcohol is consumed. Moderation is defined as 1 drink per day for women and 2 per day for men for individuals 21 years and over. Examples of 1 serving size of alcohol include 12 ounces of regular beer, 5 ounces of wine, and 1.5 ounces of distilled alcohol. When examining the diet for overall caloric consumption, a detailed review of calories consumed from liquid calorie sources, including alcohol, should be examined. Both alcoholic beverages and sweetened beverages can substantially increase daily caloric intake.

TABLE 9.23 Dietary Reference Intakes for Water

Life Stage Group	AI of Water (L/day)
Infants:	
0–6 months	0.7
7–12 months	0.8
Children:	
1–3 years	1.3
4–8 years	1.7
Males:	
9–13 years	2.4
14–18 years	3.3
>19 years	3.7
Females:	
9–13 years	2.1
14–18 years	2.3
>19 years	2.7
Pregnancy:	
>14 years	3.0
Lactation:	
>14 years	3.7

These recommendations are based on median intakes from healthy individuals.
Source: Institute of Medicine. Water. In: Otten JJ, Hellwig JP, Meyers LD, eds. Dietary Reference Intakes: The Essential Guide to Nutrient Requirements. Institute of Medicine; 2006.

Summary

The DRI and Dietary Guidelines for Americans serve as a framework to assess and guide patients in maintaining a healthy diet and making dietary changes. Using equations such as Harris-Benedict enables basic anthropometric measurements to provide meaningful insight into energy needs, allowing clinicians to counsel patients on weight maintenance, gain, or loss. Counseling patients about their diet should take cultural and religious needs and food preferences into serious consideration, as this will improve compliance with recommendations and improve quality of life. It is critical to inquire about these needs early on when providing dietary counseling and patient education. Completing a 24-hour recall, where patients are interviewed about what they ate and drank, quantities of each, timing of each, and where they consumed the meal on a typical eating day, may be very helpful to gain a complete picture of a patient's eating patterns and preferences.

9.8B DIET THERAPY

Ryan Mullane and Heidi Webb

INTRODUCTION

Therapeutic diets may be beneficial to treat or manage different medical conditions. Consulting an RD or referring a patient to one may be helpful when prescribing a therapeutic diet, implementing the diet, and helping the patient manage the dietary change. Diets can be altered both in consistency and in macronutrients, micronutrients, or fluids that are added or removed. Additionally, therapeutic diets may be prescribed by disease state, such as for cardiovascular disease, diabetes, or renal disease. Consideration of the goals of care, practicability of patients implementing the dietary change, and patient compliance should all be considered when prescribing a therapeutic diet. Liberalizing very restrictive diets to improve adequacy of nutritional intake should be considered when feasible based on the patient's condition and goals of care.

ALTERED CONSISTENCY DIETS

Clear Liquid Diet

Clear liquid diets are composed of transparent liquids; they typically provide <1,000 calories per day, most of which comes from carbohydrate.[148] A clear liquid diet may be beneficial when preparing for endoscopy or colonoscopy. Often clear liquid diets are prescribed as the first oral diet following GI surgery. Adequate water can be contained in this diet, as long as patient intake is sufficient. Because a clear liquid diet lacks in adequate calories, protein, fat, and many micronutrients, it should not be continued for more than 24 hours in most circumstances.[148]

Full Liquid Diet

Full liquid diets include all liquids and food that would be liquid at room temperature, such as ice cream or sorbet.[148] Adequate fluid intake can be achieved with a full liquid diet; if a patient requires a fluid restriction, it is important to include solid food that is liquid at room temperature in the fluid calculation.[148] As full liquid diets also include dairy, which is a good protein source, and fats and oils like melted butter and olive oil, adequate nutritional intake is possible on a full liquid diet.[148] It may, however, be difficult to get adequate micronutrients and fiber. Full liquid diets are often prescribed for diet advancement in patients who have been on clear liquids or in patients who have difficulty consuming solid foods. Diarrhea is possible given the potentially high fat content of this diet. Unless working with an RD to ensure nutritional adequacy of a prolonged full liquid diet, this diet should be prescribed temporarily.

Mechanically Altered Diets

Both solid foods and liquids can be mechanically altered to change the consistency. This is frequently done for patients with dysphagia, as thickened fluids and texture modifications make the swallowing process slower and safer for patients at risk of aspiration.[149] Other potential indications for altering food consistency include poor dentition and esophageal strictures. Patients with acute stroke are at high risk for dysphagia and should undergo dysphagia screening as soon as feasible before oral intake is allowed.[149] It may also be beneficial to screen nonstroke patients, including those with witnessed gagging, coughing, or choking episodes and those with aspiration pneumonia. If a dysphagia screen is failed, a formal swallow evaluation using videofluoroscopy or fiberoptic endoscopic evaluation can follow for diagnosis.[149] Formal swallow evaluations will help discern what texture and consistency of foods can be safely consumed.[149] Solid food can be chopped, minced, pureed, or liquidized, and drinks can have thickener added to the desired consistency (Figure 9.14). Mechanically altered diets can be designed to meet all nutritional needs, and RDs, occupational therapists, and speech therapists can help counsel patients on diet implementation at home.[148]

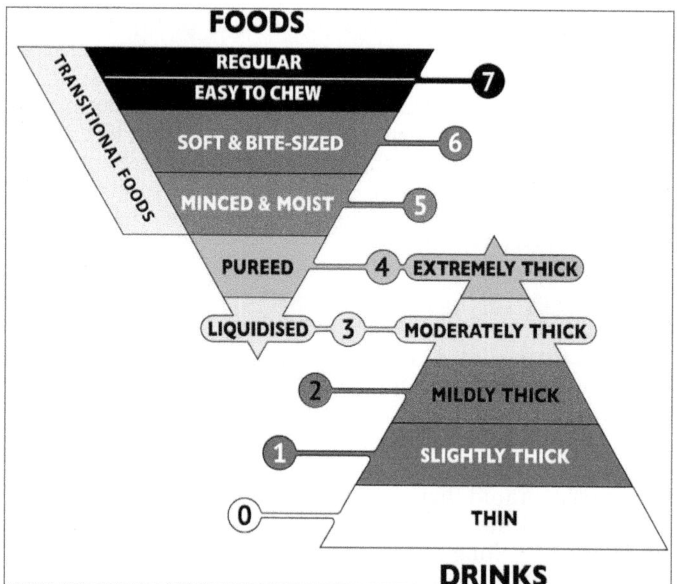

Figure 9.14 **Schematic from the International Dysphagia Diet Standardisation Initiative indicating levels of mechanical alteration of foods. The green and yellow portions are the most restrictive, utilized when the risk of dysphagia is the highest.**

(Source: International Dysphagia Diet Standardisation Initiative. The IDDSI framework. https://iddsi.org/framework)

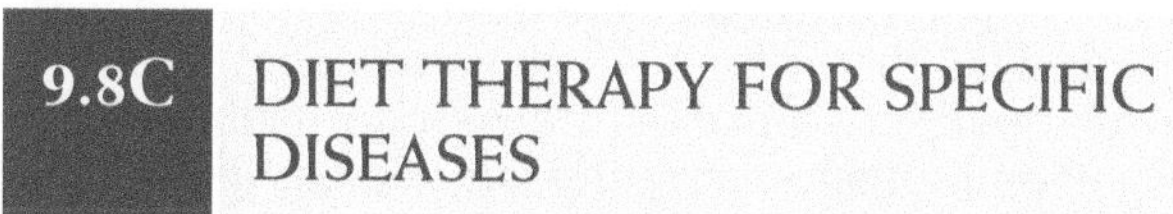

9.8C DIET THERAPY FOR SPECIFIC DISEASES

Ryan Mullane and Heidi Webb

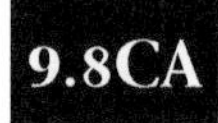

9.8CA CARDIOVASCULAR DISEASE

OVERVIEW

Diet and exercise remain key measures not only for management of cardiovascular disease, but also for prevention of cardiovascular disease. A healthy diet and lifestyle are key tools to fight cardiovascular disease. Caloric intake at its fundamental level is eating or drinking to maintain weight versus lose weight versus gain weight. Caloric requirements vary and are dependent upon age, gender, level of physical activity, and sometimes medical comorbidities. Individuals with cardiovascular disease should aim to consume a variety of nutritious foods from all food groups, especially nutrient-dense foods. The mainstay of dietary intake should focus on a variety of fruits and vegetables, fiber-rich whole grains, low-fat diary, skinless poultry and nonfried fish, nuts and legumes, and vegetable oils.[150] Caution should be taken to limit saturated fats, trans fats, sodium, red meat, sweets, and sugar-sweetened beverages, which are all nutrient-poor foods.[150]

EPIDEMIOLOGY

Heart disease remains the leading cause of death for both men and women in the United States, and is the leading global cause of death.[151]

PATHOPHYSIOLOGY

Detailed pathophysiology of coronary artery disease and other types of cardiovascular disease are discussed elsewhere (see Chapter 5, "Cardiovascular System"). Cardiovascular disease is complex and multifaceted, and genetics, lifestyle, and comorbid conditions are significant factors in disease development.

PHYSICAL EXAMINATION AND DIAGNOSTIC STUDIES

Cardiovascular disease can affect virtually all organ systems, depending on type, severity, and degree of control of the illness. Specific physical examination findings associated with cardiovascular diseases are discussed elsewhere (see Chapter 5, "Cardiovascular System"). Diagnostic evaluation and expected findings vary by disease; however, regular monitoring of lipid panels and electrolytes is advised.

TREATMENT

Carbohydrates, protein, and fat are all sources of macronutrients that can be part of a healthy diet; however, macronutrient intake must be balanced with the calories burned on a daily basis to maintain, gain, or lose weight.

Carbohydrates come in the form of sugar, starches, and fiber, and they are classified as either simple or complex, depending on the chemical structure and how quickly the sugar is digested and absorbed.[150] To simplify, simple sugars are digested quickly and give the body a quick surge of glucose to the bloodstream. Complex carbohydrates are digested more slowly and supply a steadier release of glucose into the blood-stream. In the setting of cardiovascular disease, patients should aim to limit foods that are higher in refined, processed, simple sugars and consume more complex carbohydrates, such as legumes and starchy vegetables, focusing on whole-grain choices.

Protein comes from both plant and animal sources. Protein intake should consist of lower fat options that are higher in minerals and fiber; plant-based protein sources, lean meats, fish, and poultry are advisable sources.[153] Protein should be limited to 2–3 ounces per serving and be incorporated into meals that combine meat and vegetables. The American Heart Association (AHA) recommends eating two servings of fish weekly, especially fatty fish like salmon, lake trout, sardines, and albacore tuna, all of which are high in omega-3 fatty acids.

Dietary guidelines regarding type and source of fat intake have been dynamic for several years. In 2017, the AHA issued a Presidential Advisory entitled "Dietary Fats and Cardiovascular Disease" with purpose of examining clinical trials in a more systematic fashion regarding the type, content, and amount of dietary fat to better establish dietary guidelines.[153] This report advised decreasing saturated fat intake and replacing it with polyunsaturated fats and monounsaturated fats.[153] There is evidence to suggest that omega-3 fatty acid supplementation is reasonable and safe for patients with existing coronary heart disease and heart failure with reduced ejection fraction; evidence is unclear on the role of omega-3 fatty acid supplementation for prevention of heart disease and recommendations are not currently in place.

Patients with cardiovascular disease have been found to benefit from both the Mediterranean diet and also the Dietary Approaches to Stop Hypertension (DASH) diet. The Mediterranean diet is very close to AHA guidelines but does not mimic them exactly. The Mediterranean diet is based heavily on dairy products, fish and poultry, fruits, nuts, vegetables, bread and other cereals, potatoes, beans, seeds, use of olive oil, and wine in low to moderate amounts. The Mediterranean diet has been shown to reduce adverse events, or even prevent the development, of cardiovascular disease and other disease states including breast cancer, depression, colorectal cancer, diabetes, obesity, asthma, erectile dysfunction, and cognitive decline.[154] The Mediterranean diet has been shown in randomized controlled studies to reduce waist-to-hip ratio, improve the lipid panel, and improve markers of inflammation; it has also been shown to reduce cardiovascular death and nonfatal cardiac events.[154]

The DASH diet is rich in fruits, vegetables, legumes, and low-fat dairy and is low in snacks, sweets, meats, and saturated and total fats. The structure of the DASH diet consists of 4–5 servings of fruit, 4–5 servings of vegetables, 2–3 servings of low-fat dairy, and <25% fat. The DASH diet was found to significantly lower blood pressure independent of sodium intake with significantly lower systolic and diastolic blood pressure compared to a control diet. However, further studies have shown an even bigger benefit of combining the DASH diet with a low-sodium diet; it is recommended to limit sodium to 2.3 g daily in the traditional DASH diet, though limiting sodium to 1.5 g daily lowers blood pressure even more.[150] The DASH diet has also been associated with decreased risk of coronary artery disease and stroke death.[150,155]

Alcohol should be used in moderation if at all. The AHA defines moderation as no more than one drink per day in women and no more than two per day in men.[156] Excessive alcohol use can lead to higher triglyceride levels, hypertension, heart failure, cardiomyopathy, and increased caloric intake.[156] Low to moderate intake of alcohol is allowed in the Mediterranean diet.[154] One potential benefit to alcohol is a slight rise in HDL cholesterol. Caffeine use in moderation, 1–2 cups per day, does not seem to be harmful in regard to increased risk of cardiovascular disease and may offer some degree of benefit. However, in patients with cardiac arrhythmia, caffeine should be consumed with caution and only after discussion with a clinician.

PATIENT EDUCATION

- Heart disease remains a significant comorbid condition for patients in the United States and worldwide.
- Nutrition therapy is critical for both primary and secondary prevention of cardiovascular disease and cardiac events.
- Dietary guidelines support nutrition-rich foods from a variety of food groups.
- The Mediterranean diet and the DASH diet both have positive effects in the management of cardiovascular disease.

9.8CB DIABETES

OVERVIEW

Diabetes, including type 1, type 2, and prediabetes, are multifaceted chronic conditions that can be difficult to manage, especially long term. Nutrition therapy and dietary guidelines can be one of the most challenging aspects of patient self-management because of lack of knowledge and understanding, adherence, and/or cost. However, lifestyle modification and dietary changes remain cornerstones of diabetes management, often in conjunction with pharmacologic management.

PATHOPHYSIOLOGY

Type 1 diabetes is a condition of absolute insulin deficiency due to destruction of pancreatic beta cells; in type 2 diabetes and prediabetes, there is insulin resistance and relative insulin deficiency.[157]

PHYSICAL EXAMINATION AND DIAGNOSTIC STUDIES

Diabetes can affect virtually all organ systems, depending on type, severity, and degree of control of the illness. Specific physical examination findings associated with diabetes and diagnostic criteria are discussed elsewhere (see Chapter 16, "Endocrine System"). Regular monitoring of hemoglobin A1c and lipid panels is advised.

TREATMENT

The American Diabetes Association Standards of Care recognizes the goals of nutrition therapy are to be individualized to the patient and to (1) achieve and maintain body weight goals; (2) attain target glycemic, blood pressure, and lipid goals; and (3) delay or prevent complications of diabetes.[158] Nutrition therapy should take into account these goals as well as additional medical comorbidities and patient beliefs including culture, religion, and tradition. Acknowledgment and incorporation of these beliefs can help guide improvement in medical nutrition therapy.[157] Emphasis should be on developing healthy eating patterns that will withstand a lifetime. Patients should have frequent, intensive follow-up to assure adherence to lifestyle modifications. Health-care professionals should take care to not reprimand or shame eating patterns. In patients with prediabetes, active and effective nutrition therapy may prevent the onset of diabetes and its complications.[157] Since the standard of care for nutrition in diabetes and prediabetes focuses on individualizing goals of nutrition therapy, there is no specific recommendation for macronutrient distribution. Macronutrient requirements and distribution will vary by patient population in regard to several factors. Nutritional therapy for patients with diabetes should focus on nutrient-dense food choices and portion control. The Mediterranean diet, the DASH diet, and plant-based diet have all been shown to have significant benefit in patients with type 2 diabetes (see Section 9.8C Diet Therapy for Specific Diseases for a description of the Mediterranean and DASH diets).[154] A plant-based diet tends to fall somewhere in between the Mediterranean diet and the DASH diet in terms of foods included, but excludes animal products. There is no evidence to support any one diet over another in patients with type 1 diabetes.[158] Weight management and portion control are cornerstones for treatment of type 1, type 2, and prediabetes.[158] In general, sodium intake should also be limited to <2.3 g daily.[159]

Patients should not be counseled to maintain strict low carbohydrate diets. In fact, strict low carbohydrate diets should be avoided in women who are pregnant or breastfeeding, in patients with a history of disordered eating, in patients with renal disease, and in those with type 2 diabetes maintained on a sodium-glucose cotransporter 2 (SGLT-2) inhibitor due to potential increased risk for ketoacidosis.[158] Studies investigating the ideal amount of carbohydrates for patients with diabetes remain inconclusive.[158,160] All people with diabetes, regardless of age, should minimize carbohydrate intake from refined carbohydrates and other added simple sugars. Carbohydrate intake should be obtained from vegetables, fruits, legumes, dairy, and whole grains.[158]

For patients with type 1 diabetes and patients with type 2 diabetes who take prandial insulin, focus should be on education to allow the patient to understand the relationship between carbohydrate intake and insulin needs. For patients on fixed insulin doses, meal planning is imperative and should ideally mimic a fixed schedule in regard to type and amount of carbohydrate.[157] Education on use of insulin-to-carbohydrate ratios for meal planning is imperative, especially for patients with type 1 diabetes to improve glycemic control. Patients with type 2 diabetes on prandial insulin could potentially benefit from use of insulin-to-carbohydrate ratios as well, though this is less commonly counseled on in clinical practice.

Research also remains inconclusive regarding the ideal amount of protein intake in individuals with diabetes or prediabetes. Protein intake should be individualized to the patient and consider their current eating habits, additional health maintenance goals, and comorbid conditions. There is, however, some evidence that supports better management of type 2 diabetes with diets slightly higher in protein content, which is theorized to be related to increased satiety seen in higher protein diets.[158] Patients with diabetic kidney disease should avoid a diet with higher protein content; this patient population is advised to maintain the current RDA of 0.8 g of protein/kg/day.[158]

There is no standard of care regarding fat intake for patients with diabetes and prediabetes. As with most patient populations, the type of fat is held in higher regard than the amount of total fat consumed. In general, patients should focus on a diet higher in polyunsaturated and monounsaturated fats. Patients with diabetes and prediabetes are recommended to follow general population guidelines for the intake of saturated fat, trans fat, and dietary cholesterol, as this should constitute a minimal part of a patient's diet. Saturated fats should be limited whenever possible, and patients should be counseled to replace saturated fats with unsaturated fats to avoid replacing them with refined carbohydrates.[158]

Moderate alcohol use has not been found to be significantly detrimental to long-term glycemic control; however, it should be noted that alcohol use can increase risk of hypoglycemia, especially in patients using sulfonylureas or insulin, can lead to weight gain, and with heavy use can lead to hyperglycemia.[158]

PATIENT EDUCATION

- Nutrition therapy and diet guidelines remain a pillar for management of type 1 diabetes, type 2 diabetes, and prediabetes. the current standard of care focuses on individualizing macronutrient distribution to meet each patient's unique nutritional needs and eating preferences.
- Patients should focus on eating nutrient-rich foods and should specifically minimize intake of refined carbohydrates, added sugars, and saturated and trans fats.
- Weight management and portion control are the cornerstones for nutrition therapy.

9.8CC RENAL DISEASE

OVERVIEW

The kidneys serve a vital role in nutrition by maintaining appropriate electrolyte concentrations and serving as an endocrine organ. With declining glomerular filtration rate (GFR) in kidney disease, patients experience alterations in electrolyte levels as well as changes in protein requirements and fluid balance.[161] Malnutrition and protein-calorie wasting are very common in patients with a variety of kidney diseases. Nutritional assessment and education are critical components in the management of patients with kidney diseases. This section will cover how changes in kidney function lead to changes in the sodium, potassium, and phosphorus requirements for patients and will delve into the nutritional recommendations for patients with kidney disease.

EPIDEMIOLOGY

About 15% of adults in the United States (37 million people) are estimated to have chronic kidney disease.[162] Nutrition is a vital part of managing patients with chronic kidney disease as malnutrition is common; roughly 40% of patients on hemodialysis will have protein-energy wasting.[163] Electrolyte disturbances, including hyperkalemia, hyponatremia, and hyperphosphatemia, are frequently encountered, with hyperkalemia being observed in around 50% of patients.[164]

PATHOPHYSIOLOGY

Declining kidney function leads to abnormalities in the regulation of sodium, potassium, and phosphorus homeostasis. The kidneys are the primary organ regulating sodium, potassium, and phosphorus; the kidneys excrete about 90% of the daily potassium intake while working to expel the approximate daily phosphorus that is ingested.[165,166] Sodium handling by the kidneys is a complex process, involving transporters, the renin-angiotensin-aldosterone system, and the sympathetic nervous system. Progressive kidney dysfunction causes the accumulation of each of these electrolytes, leading to hypertension (from sodium retention), cardiac arrhythmias (from hyperkalemia), and bone disease (from hyperphosphatemia).

Beyond electrolyte abnormalities, protein-calorie wasting can occur. Protein-calorie wasting is a body state in which there is a loss of protein in patients with kidney disease. It is due to anorexia and chronic inflammation with dialysis patients having further protein losses in their dialysate.[167]

MEDICAL HISTORY AND CLINICAL PRESENTATION

Patients with kidney disease will often have hypertension related to the retention of sodium and water. Muscle wasting can be seen in patients with protein-calorie wasting.

DIAGNOSTIC STUDIES

Electrolytes in patients with kidney disease should be monitored every 3–12 months, depending on the degree of the patient's kidney dysfunction. Low serum albumin levels are frequently used as a marker of protein-calorie wasting and malnutrition in patients with kidney disease.

EVALUATION

Assessment of nutritional status can involve food diaries and calorie counters. Once patients have begun treatment and undergone education, repeating laboratory tests, such as serum phosphorus and serum albumin, and monitoring vital signs, especially blood pressure and weight, can be useful to determine compliance with therapies.

TREATMENT

The initial treatment for hypertension or fluid retention associated with kidney disease is a sodium restriction. Recommended daily sodium intake is usually less than about 2.5 g/day, which is effective in lowering blood pressure.[168,169]

BOX 9.2 Foods With High Potassium Content

Avocado	Bananas
Beans	Chocolate
Milk	Peanut butter
Tomatoes	Yogurt

BOX 9.3 Foods With High Phosphorus Content

Beer	Cheese
Chocolate	Dark-colored sodas
Milk	Processed meats

Fluid restrictions are useful in patients with hyponatremia due to kidney disease or who are dialysis-dependent. Typical fluid restrictions range from 1 L to 2 L of fluid intake per day.

Patients with hyperkalemia due to kidney disease should avoid foods with high potassium content, while patients with hyperphosphatemia should focus on foods with low phosphorus content (Boxes 9.2 and 9.3).

Healthy diets with plenty of fruits and vegetables are associated with a lower mortality rate in patients with kidney disease.[170,171] Higher consumption of sugar-sweetened beverages has been associated with an elevated risk of developing chronic kidney disease, and patients with chronic kidney disease should be advised to instead drink water, coffee, or other beverages.[172]

Malnutrition is managed best with a multidisciplinary approach to define an individualized nutritional plan. Patients with end-stage renal disease often require increased protein intake of 1.0–1.2 g/kg/day.[161]

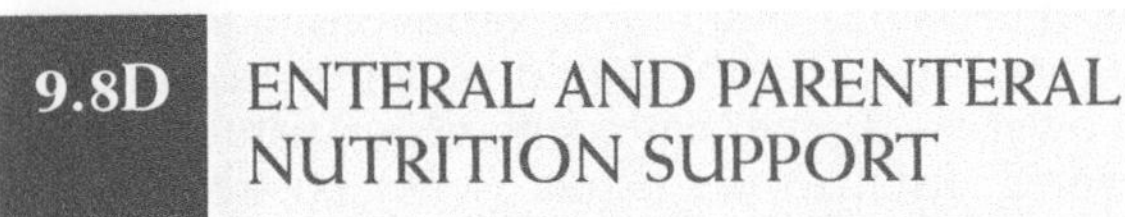

9.8D ENTERAL AND PARENTERAL NUTRITION SUPPORT

Laura Beerman

OVERVIEW

EN and PN are important clinical therapies; both fall under an umbrella category of *nutrition support*. The purpose of EN and PN is to provide the body with all the essential nutrients to preserve lean body mass and maintain immune function when unable to achieve this balance via an oral diet.

NUTRITION ASSESSMENT

Nutrition assessment determines the nutrition goal based on weight history, comorbidities, history of oral intake, and current clinical condition. Energy needs can be calculated by indirect calorimetry, formulas predicting BMR, and predictive equations. Indirect calorimetry is the gold standard for calculating energy expenditure of critically ill patients; however, the equipment is expensive to purchase and warrants a high level of clinical expertise. There are many formulas available to estimate BMR where activity factors or illness-associated stress factors are applied, including Harris-Benedict, Mifflin-St. Jeor, and Ireton-Jones.[173] Predictive weight-based equations are the most straightforward; this type of calculation is often used as it is convenient and widely accepted by clinicians.[174] Additionally, clinical research supports its use when indirect calorimetry is not available or feasible. The American Society of Parental and Enteral Nutrition (ASPEN) is a multidisciplinary international organization for medical professionals who practice in the area of nutrition support. ASPEN guidelines suggest a range of 20 to 35 kcal/kg/day for adults. It is generally accepted to start with 25 kcal/kg of the appropriate reference weight, either actual body weight or adjusted body weight, with adjustment made to clinical response; critically ill patients with high nutritional needs may benefit from starting with a higher weight-based target. Patients with a BMI <25 should generally have needs calculated initially based on their actual body weight, patients with a BMI ≥25 should have needs calculated based on adjusted body weight (Exhibit 9.5). Adjusted body weight is a useful equation in other clinical situations also, as some medications and intravenous fluids are dosed based on adjusted weight.

PROTEIN REQUIREMENTS

Protein requirements in critical illness are calculated using grams per kilogram of body weight within the range of 1.1 to 1.5 g/kg/day with underweight patients requiring up to 1.9 g/kg/day.[175] For burn patients, particularly those with extensive injury, requirements may reach 2.0 g/kg/day.[176] Feeding too much protein can result in acute kidney injury and kidney stones.

FLUID REQUIREMENTS

Fluid requirements are most essential to estimate and incorporate into the nutrition support prescription. Total body water makes up 50% to 60% of body weight. Fluid balance, with total intake and output measured over several days, is helpful to assess these needs; on average, a healthy adult will require 30–40 mL/kg/day. High GI losses require much higher volumes. Insensible losses from the lungs and skin can add up to 1 L/day and should be accounted for to maintain healthy fluid balance.[177]

EXHIBIT 9.5 Formula to Calculate Adjusted Body Weight and Ideal Body Weight in Adults

Adjusted body weight = ideal body weight + 0.25 (adjusted body weight – ideal body weight)

Ideal body weight:
Men: 110 pounds for the first 5 feet of height + 5 pounds for each additional inch
Women: 100 pounds for the first 5 feet of height + 5 pounds for each additional inch

ENTERAL NUTRITION SUPPORT

EN, colloquially known as tube feeding, is a method of providing a complex blend of nutrients, which contain protein, carbohydrate, and fat along with vitamins and minerals, when unable to ingest adequate nutrients by mouth. EN mandates that a functional GI tract is available, as this type of feeding utilizes a tube to deliver nutrients to the gut and relies on effective gut absorption. Patients can be fed exclusively by EN or use EN to meet some of their needs when they cannot meet all needs by oral intake. Nutrition assessment determines patients' nutrient needs for enteral feedings; ASPEN guidelines aid in this process.[178] Initiation of EN is an ASPEN-indicated therapy in the hospitalized patient with inadequate oral intake for 7 days. In cases of trauma and burns, feeding on hospital day 1 if metabolically stable supports the normal pathways of nutrient utilization. Patients with moderate to severe malnutrition need frequent reassessment of oral intake and may benefit from starting feedings sooner than 7 days. Short-term enteral feedings used during the hospital stay, either as the sole source of nutrition or as a supplement to the oral diet, are indicated according to the above guidelines and hospital policy. When oral intake improves based on established nutrition goals, feedings are slowly weaned down and stopped. When the patient cannot eat or the oral diet is suboptimal, EN is continued on hospital discharge until nutritional goals can be met orally.

The length of need for EN determines the type of feeding tube to place. A nasogastric, nasoduodenal, or nasojejunal tube can be used for feedings lasting up to 4 to 6 weeks. These tubes carry less risk than more permanent tubes, and are typically placed at the bedside, intraoperatively, or by interventional radiology.[179] The malnourished patient who is unable to tolerate the surgical procedure for a more permanent EN tube placement uses the nasoenteric tube until more permanent access can be safely placed. Surgical gastrostomies or jejunostmy tubes, percutaneous endoscopic gastrostomy (PEG) tubes, percutaneous endoscopic jejunostomy (PEJ) tubes, and low-profile gastrostomies are placed for long-term feedings estimated at 6 weeks or longer.

After the tube is in place and ready for use, the next step is to determine the method of feeding delivery. Bolus feedings are given intermittently with a syringe multiple times per day, typically consisting of about an 8-ounce volume. Bolus feedings are only appropriate if feeding into the stomach, as the stomach acts as a reservoir to hold the formula during the early process of digestion and then empties into the small bowel over time. Regulated feedings given with a programmed pump deliver a prescribed volume of formula per hour over a designated time. Tubes that feed into the duodenum or jejunum require a regulated pump method, as there is no reservoir to hold the food. Pump feeding can be run continuously or intermittently over a predetermined number of hours.

Assessment of disease state and the ability of the small bowel to absorb the feeding helps to determine product selection.[181] Standard formulas contain intact nutrient sources and require intact gut absorption; elemental and semi-elemental formulas contain "predigested" nutrient sources, which may be preferable for patients with impaired absorption (Table 9.24). Disease-specific products are available but are significantly more expensive and may have limited clinical benefit. Generally, the type of protein contained determines the category, and the medical condition guides specific product selection. There are many formulas on the market and they

TABLE 9.24 Descriptions of the Primary Types of Enteral Nutrition Formulas, Including Standard, Elemental, and Disease-Specific

Standard Product	Elemental or Semi-Elemental Product	Disease-Specific Product
Intact whole proteins made from casein, whey, soy	Short chain peptides, the building blocks of protein or free amino acids, proteins in their most basic form.	Various types of proteins
With and without fiber	Do not contain fiber	No fiber; designed for renal or liver disease
Most economical	Cost more than standard products	Most expensive

are considered a "food supplement" by the Food and Drug Administration; as such, they are not under regulatory control like most pharmaceuticals. Well-established manufacturers in the industry support their products with research; it is essential to use a reputable manufacturer.

A multidisciplinary team specializing in nutrition support should determine the need for EN, type of feeding tube to place, method of delivery, type of formula to use as well as the total volume of formula to provide to meet estimated nutritional needs. This team then monitors the tolerance of the feedings based on symptoms of abdominal pain, nausea, vomiting, and stool output. These symptoms are also indications of other medical problems unrelated to the tube feeding and should be ruled out first prior to adjusting the feeding. Feedings are started slowly and are advanced to the nutritional goal based on tolerance.

PARENTERAL NUTRITION

PN is a complex mixture of up to 40 different nutritional components provided intravenously, which offers a life-sustaining option for patients with intestinal failure when adequate oral intake or EN has failed. ASPEN consensus recommendations for appropriate use identify best practice, guide clinical decisions, and reduce variations in practice to enhance patient safety.[181] PN should be considered in cases of short bowel syndrome, enterocutaneous fistulae where enteral feeding distal to the fistula is not possible, radiation- or chemotherapy-related enteritis resulting in malabsorption, mechanical small bowel obstruction, gut stenosis or stricture, and complex motility disorders of the small bowel leading to impaired nutrient absorption.[181] Inability to achieve and maintain enteral access is another indication. PN is contraindicated when the GI tract is functional and EN is tolerated.

The type of intravenous access determines which type of PN formula to order (Figure 9.15). Peripheral access including midline catheters and other short lines used for PN solutions can only sustain a solution with an UL of 900 mOsmol/L, as the veins are small. These formulations, called peripheral PN (PPN) solutions, come premixed. These solutions may limit the full provision of nutrients with inability to maintain stable blood levels of electrolytes; they may be considered for a shorter length of therapy, 10 to 14 days, and during hospitalization prior to

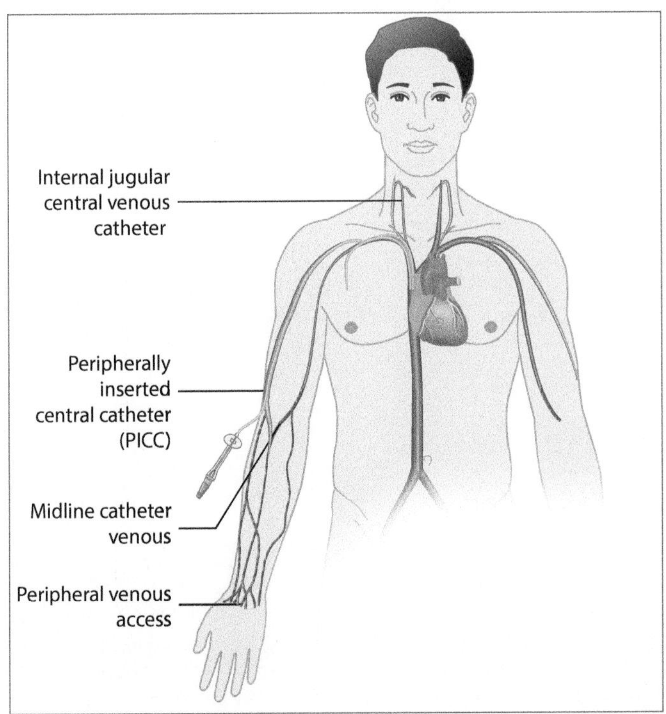

Figure 9.15 **Different locations of venous access for parenteral nutrition. Peripheral catheters, including peripheral intravenous lines and midline catheters, are only appropriate for peripheral parenteral nutrition solution. Peripherally inserted central catheter lines and central venous catheters are the only appropriate access sites for highly concentrated parenteral nutrition solution.**

the placement of an enteral feeding tube. Central venous catheters in which the tip of the catheter is in the superior vena cava, allow for highly concentrated solutions >2,000 mOsmol/L. Obtaining and supporting full nutrition needs is possible with central access. Types of central catheters include peripherally inserted central catheters (PICCs) or surgically placed central lines. After catheter insertion, the placement of the tip of the catheter is confirmed by x-ray prior to use for PN to ensure safe administration of the appropriate solution.

PN formulas are frequently compounded for individual patients, and therefore, individualized adjustments to the PN components, including macronutrients, micronutrients, and medications, can typically be made. Macronutrient sources in PN include crystalline amino acids for protein, dextrose monohydrated solution for carbohydrates, and plant-based lipids, such as soybean oil and medium chain triglyceride oils. Electrolytes, including sodium, potassium, phosphate, magnesium, and calcium, are added to maintain blood serum levels and acid-base balance. A complex of vitamins and minerals are also included. Additional pharmacotherapeutic components may be included in the PN formula on a patient-specific basis, such as regular insulin. Institutional policies may outline the use of insulin when added to the PN formula, as hypoglycemia can occur. PN solution contains sterile water to maintain fluid balance; restricted solution volumes can be ordered if indicated by a patient's volume status. These solutions are made in a pharmacy with a compounding hood and follow strict compounding policies, which outline compatibility of nutrients and sterility in production.[182]

Complications of PN include fatty liver disease, cholestasis, gut mucosal atrophy from lack of use, loss of venous access due to repeated need for catheter insertions, blood clots due to venous access, and bacterial and fungal blood infections from long-term catheter use. An interdisciplinary team of physicians, dietitians, pharmacists, nurses, and advanced practice clinicians should initiate and monitor PN. Healthcare workers can obtain additional certification to utilize PN safely. Monitoring and continuous reassessment of PN are necessary and provide the opportunity to continually reassess the ability to use EN or oral diet. Discontinuation of PN as soon as possible is preferable because of the serious complications than can arise from its use.[183]

COMMON CHIEF COMPLAINTS

APPROACH TO WEIGHT LOSS

Weight loss is a common complaint and can be both intentional and unintentional. Intentional weight loss may be beneficial in patients who are overweight or obese; however, it is critical that intake is nutritionally adequate and in accordance with dietary guidelines. Patients with weight loss should be queried on their current diet to ensure balanced amounts of macronutrients and adequate amounts of micronutrients are obtained; micronutrient serum testing may be of benefit if the patient has disease symptoms or has been consuming a nutritionally inadequate diet for an extended period of time. Patients with unintentional weight loss should be evaluated for an etiology of this weight loss, which may include cancer, autoimmune diseases, eating disorders, and infectious diseases like HIV and tuberculosis. In unintentional weight loss resulting in low body weight and/or malnutrition, care must be taken to restore nutrition carefully.

KNOWLEDGE CHECKS

1. The decision regarding initiation of nutrition support is complex. Compare and contrast indications for enteral and parenteral nutrition.
2. Explain why fat-soluble vitamins are much more likely to be the source of hypervitaminosis than water-soluble vitamins.
3. Patients commonly inquire about what foods are healthy to consume. Discuss the general macronutrient guidelines for healthy adults.

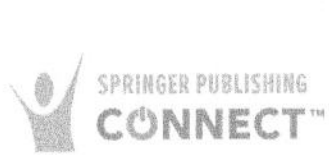

A robust set of instructor resources designed to supplement this text is located at **http://connect.springerpub.com/content/book/978-0-8261-8243-2.** Qualifying instructors may request access by emailing **textbook@springerpub.com.**

REFERENCES

The complete reference list for this chapter appears in the digital version of the chapter, accessible at https://connect.springerpub.com/content/book/978-0-8261-8243-2/chapter/ch09.

Chapter 10

RENAL SYSTEM

JAMES VAN RHEE

LEARNING OBJECTIVES

- Describe the approach to evaluating renal function, including urinalysis.
- Compare hyponatremia and and hypernatremia with regard to pathophysiology, clinical presentation, diagnosis, and management.
- Compare hypokalemia and hyperkalemia with regard to pathophysiology, clinical presentation, diagnosis, and management.
- Describe the pathophysiology, clinical presentation, and management of magnesium disorders.
- Describe the pathophysiology, clinical presentation, and management of calcium disorders.
- Describe the pathophysiology, clinical presentation, and management of phosphate disorders.
- Describe the pathophysiology, clinical presentation, and management of dehydration.
- Describe the pathophysiology, clinical presentation, and management of fluid overload.
- Compare metabolic and respiratory acidosis and alkalosis with regard to pathophysiology, clinical presentation, diagnosis, and management.
- Compare acute and chronic renal failure with regard to epidemiology, pathophysiology, clinical presentation, diagnosis, management, and complications.
- Compare nephrotic and nephritic syndromes with regard to epidemiology, pathophysiology, clinical presentation, diagnosis, and management.
- Discuss the epidemiology, pathophysiology, clinical presentation, and treatment of polycystic kidney disease.

INTRODUCTION

In the United States, millions of people have chronic kidney disease and many others develop acute kidney injury and other kidney diseases each year. Renal disorders are seen by all clinicians regardless of practice area. This is important because with early detection and appropriate management, most forms of kidney disease can be prevented or at least the rate of progression can be slowed.

The role of the kidneys is in filtering blood, and a wide range of diseases of other organ systems and systemic diseases may be manifested in the kidney. Renal disease is a common presentation in patients with a history of diabetes mellitus, hypertension, and autoimmune disorders such as systemic lupus erythematosus.

Patients are typically asymptomatic until relatively advanced kidney failure is present. There are no pain receptors within the substance of the kidney, so pain is not a prominent presenting complaint, except in those renal diseases in which the ureter or renal capsule are involved. In the early stages of kidney disease, patients may only have abnormalities of urine volume or composition of the urine. Later, systemic symptoms and signs of lost renal function are noted.

The kidneys have multiple roles in the body, including blood filtration, metabolism and excretion of endogenous and exogenous compounds, and endocrine functions. Most importantly, the kidneys are the primary regulators of fluid, acid-base, and electrolyte balance in the body.

10.1 ELECTROLYTE DISORDERS

OVERVIEW

Fluid and electrolyte balance is key in maintaining homeostasis. There are numerous regulating mechanisms for the equilibrium of electrolytes. Changes in these mechanisms result in electrolyte imbalances that may be life-threatening.

Electrolyte balance is regulated by the hypothalamus, kidneys, and various hormones, including antidiuretic hormone (ADH), aldosterone, and parathyroid hormone (PTH). These disorders can be effectively evaluated with a stepwise approach.

PATHOPHYSIOLOGY

Sodium is the most important electrolyte in the extracellular fluid (ECF). Sodium plays a vital role in maintaining ECF volume and regulation of a cell's membrane potential.

Sodium regulation occurs in the kidneys. Most of the sodium is reabsorbed in the proximal convoluted tubule (67%), followed by the loop of Henle (25%), and then the distal convoluted tubule and collecting duct (8%). Aldosterone plays a major role in sodium control. As sodium levels decrease, aldosterone is released from the adrenal cortex. Aldosterone then stimulates sodium absorption in the renal tubules.

Hyponatremia is the most common electrolyte disorder. The diagnosis is made when the serum sodium level is <135 mEq/L. Neurologic manifestations are common in hyponatremia, and include headache, confusion, nausea, and delirium. Hypernatremia is diagnosed when the serum sodium level is greater than 145 mEq/L. Symptoms of hypernatremia include lethargy, weakness, seizures, and restlessness. Rapid sodium corrections can lead to serious complications such as cerebral edema and osmotic demyelination syndrome (central pontine myelinolysis).

Potassium is an intracellular ion. The sodium-potassium adenosine triphosphatase pump (Na-K-ATPase pump) is responsible for regulating the homeostasis between sodium and potassium. The Na-K-ATPase pump facilitates the active transport of sodium and potassium ions across the cell membrane against their concentration gradients. Once potassium is absorbed, it circulates to the kidneys, where it is regulated through a process of active secretion and absorption in the distal tubule and collecting ducts. In the kidneys, filtration of potassium occurs at the glomerulus, reabsorption takes place at the proximal convoluted tubule and thick ascending loop of Henle, and secretion takes place at the distal convoluted tubule. Aldosterone plays a role in potassium elimination via the kidneys by increasing the density and activity of Na-K-ATPase pump. The net result is an increase in potassium permeability and driving force, which promotes potassium secretion.

Potassium disorders can lead to cardiac arrhythmias. Hypokalemia occurs when serum potassium level is <3.5 mEq/L. Common symptoms of hypokalemia include weakness, fatigue, and muscle twitching. Hyperkalemia occurs when the serum potassium level is >5.5 mEq/L. Common symptoms of hyperkalemia include muscle cramps and muscle weakness.

Calcium is mostly present in the ECF and involved in skeletal mineralization, muscle contraction, nerve impulse transmission, blood coagulation, and hormone secretion. Diet is the main source of calcium, and absorption occurs in the intestine under the control of vitamin D, 1,25-dihydroxy vitamin D3. PTH regulates calcium secretion in the distal tubule of kidneys. Calcitonin acts on bone cells to increase calcium level in blood.

Magnesium is an intracellular cation and is involved in ATP metabolism, muscle contraction and relaxation, neurologic functioning and neurotransmitter release. Hypomagnesemia is defined as a serum magnesium levels <1.5 mg/dL. Ventricular arrhythmias, such as torsades de pointes, are noted in hypomagnesemia.

Phosphorus is an ECF cation. Eighty-five percent of the body phosphorus is in the bones and teeth and the remaining 15% is in the soft tissues. Phosphate plays a major role in metabolic pathways. Phosphate is regulated with calcium by vitamin D3, PTH, and calcitonin. The kidneys are the main source of phosphorus excretion.

10.1A SODIUM DISORDERS

Disorders of sodium are due to changes in body water, not sodium. Sodium homeostasis and water balance are under the hormonal regulation of the renin-angiotensin system and ADH. Renin, produced by the kidney, is released in response to decreases in circulating intravascular volume.

Renin stimulates the production of angiotensin I, which is converted to angiotensin II in the lung. Angiotensin II stimulates the production of aldosterone, a mineralocorticoid hormone, produced in the zona glomerulosa of the adrenal glands. Aldosterone enhances Na reabsorption and K excretion in the distal nephron.

ADH is synthesized in the hypothalamus and secreted from the posterior pituitary. ADH is released in response to increases in serum osmolality and a decrease in plasma volume. ADH enhances renal water absorption by increasing tubular water permeability.

Hyponatremia is defined as serum sodium <135 mEq/L and can be acute or chronic. Acute is defined as hyponatremia that develops in <48 hours, while chronic refers to hyponatremia that is present for >48 hours. Acute hyponatremia is more common in hospitalized patients and frequently has neurologic manifestations and cerebral edema. Chronic hyponatremia is more common in the outpatient setting and neurologic manifestations are minimal and there is no cerebral edema.

Hypernatremia is defined as a serum sodium >145 mEq/L. Hypernatremia is most commonly due to a deficit in free water in the body. Hypernatremia occurs in patients at the extremes of age and those who are debilitated. The incidence of hypernatremia is 1% with a mortality rate of 45% to 60%.[1]

MEDICAL HISTORY AND CLINICAL PRESENTATION

The earliest findings in hyponatremia include nausea and malaise, which may be followed by headache, lethargy, obtundation, and eventually seizures, coma, and respiratory arrest. Symptoms are due to neurologic dysfunction caused by cerebral edema. Neurologic symptoms are less severe with chronic hyponatremia.

A detailed history should be obtained to help identify the underlying etiology. Possible etiologies should be identified such as vomiting, diarrhea, history of small cell lung cancer, central nervous system (CNS) disease, history of diabetes, mannitol infusion, hyperlipidemia, cirrhosis, heart failure, and renal failure. Many drugs are linked to the development of hyponatremia, including tricyclic antidepressants, selective serotonin reuptake inhibitors (SSRIs), phenothiazines, carbamazepine, chemotherapy agents, and diuretics.

Hypernatremia presents with weakness and lethargy. Severe hypernatremia can present with seizures and coma. The history may be positive for diabetes insipidus, hyperaldosteronism, or Cushing disease. The patient's recent history may be positive for diarrhea, burns, polyuria, or excessive sweating.

PHYSICAL EXAMINATION

Hyponatremia patients present with a wide range of findings, depending on the etiology. If the patient has a hypervolemic hyponatremia they may present with edema, ascites, and an elevated jugular venous distention (JVD). With euvolemic etiologies the presentation will be that of the underlying cause. With hypovolemic etiologies the mucous membranes will be dry, skin turgor decreased, and the patient will be hypotensive and tachycardic.

Patients with hypernatremia appear lethargic, weak, and confused. The physical examination findings are related to the amount of volume deficit in the body and neuronal shrinkage because of hypertonicity. The patient may be orthostatic hypotensive and tachycardic, and have dry skin with decreased turgor. For the physical examination findings to become apparent, acute elevation in the serum sodium concentration to >158 mEq/L is required.

DIFFERENTIAL DIAGNOSIS

Hyponatremia is classified into isotonic hyponatremia, hypertonic hyponatremia, or hypotonic hyponatremia based on the serum osmolality.

Isotonic hyponatremia is hyponatremia with normal osmolality. This is most commonly noted in pseudohyponatremia, which is seen in patients with marked elevations in serum lipids or proteins. The elevations in lipids and proteins results in a reduction in the fraction of serum water and an artificially low serum sodium concentration. It can also occur secondary to absorption of glycine or sorbitol irrigation solutions during transurethral resection of the prostate, hysteroscopy, or laparoscopic surgery.

Hypertonic hyponatremia, with a high serum osmolality, occurs in cases with hyperglycemia, such as diabetic ketoacidosis or hyperosmolar hyperglycemia, and with mannitol administration. Hyperglycemia causes osmotic shifts of water from the intracellular to the extracellular space, causing a relative dilutional hyponatremia. The classic correction factor of 1.6 mEq/L for every 100 mg/dL increase in serum glucose was challenged in a paper by Hillier et al. in 1999, and sometimes the factor of 2.4 mEq/L is used.[2]

Hypotonic hyponatremia, with a low serum osmolality, is the most common scenario, in which there is true excess of free water relative to sodium. Hypotonic hyponatremia is further classified according to the volume status of the patient as hypovolemic hyponatremia, euvolemic hyponatremia, or hypervolemic hyponatremia. See Table 10.1 for the etiologies of hypotonic hyponatremia.

Hypernatremia is classified as hypovolemic, euvolemic, and hypervolemic. See Table 10.2 for summary and comparison of these types.

DIAGNOSTIC STUDIES

Laboratory studies vary depending on the various etiologies. Tests may include serum electrolytes and serum osmolality. Urine studies include urine sodium and urine osmolality. Fractional excretion of sodium (FENa) may need to be calculated.

TABLE 10.1 Etiologies of Hypotonic Hyponatremia

Hypovolemia	Normovolemia	Hypervolemia
Gastrointestinal fluid loss	SIADH	Heart failure
Primary adrenal failure	Hypocortisolism	Cirrhosis
Cerebral salt wasting	Hypothyroidism	Nephrotic syndrome
Burns		Renal failure
Diuretics		

SIADH, syndrome of inappropriate secretion of antidiuretic hormone.

TABLE 10.2 Classification of Hypernatremia

Hypovolemic	Euvolemic	Hypervolemic
Body fluid loss (burns, sweating)	Central and nephrogenic diabetes insipidus	Cushing syndrome
Diuretic use	Fever	Hemodialysis
Gastrointestinal loss (vomiting, diarrhea)	Hypoventilation	Hyperaldosteronism
Heat injury	Hypodipsia	Iatrogenic: Salt tablets, salt water ingestion, saline infusions, enteral feedings
Osmotic diuresis	Medications: Amphotericin, aminoglycosides, lithium, phenytoin	
Postobstruction	Sickle cell disease	

EVALUATION

For details on the process of evaluating the patient with sodium abnormalities, see Approach to Sodium Disorders near the end of this chapter.

TREATMENT

Treatment is based on the presence of symptoms, the degree of volume depletion, and whether the condition is acute or chronic.

Acute Hyponatremia

- Sodium <125 mEq/L should be treated emergently because of risk of cerebral edema and encephalopathy.
- Correct with hypertonic saline (0.3% saline) at a rate of 0.5 to 5.0 mL/kg/hour until symptoms resolve.
- Frequent sodium levels should be obtained to make sure not to raise the sodium by more than 6–12 mEq/L the first 24 hours and 18 mEq/L in the first 48 hours.

Chronic Hyponatremia

- Chronic hyponatremia should be treated with caution, as rapid correction can lead to central pontine myelinolysis.
- The degree to which 1 L of a given solution will increase the serum sodium concentration can be estimated from the following Adrogue formula[3]:

$$\text{Change in serum sodium} = \frac{(\text{infusate sodium} + \text{infusate potassium}) - \text{serum sodium}}{\text{Total body water} + 1}$$

- The first step in the treatment of hypovolemic hyponatremia is fluid resuscitation:
  - In patients with vomiting or diarrhea, treatment consists of isotonic saline with additional electrolytes.
  - In patients on diuretics, stop the diuretics and give isotonic saline.
  - In patients with mineralocorticoid deficiency, treatment consists of volume replacement with isotonic saline.
  - In patients with cerebral salt wasting syndrome, treatment consists of isotonic saline until they are euvolemic.

Syndrome of Inappropriate Antidiuretic Hormone Secretion

- Treatment is fluid restriction.
- If is not successful, then drug therapy with demeclocycline can be used.

Hyponatremia, Other Causes

- In euvolemic hyponatremia in patients with malignancy, treat the underlying malignant lesion; this may reduce or stop the production of ADH.
- If secondary to hypothyroidism, treatment consists of thyroid hormone replacement.
- If due to glucocorticoid deficiency, treatment is with glucocorticoid replacement.
- If secondary to low solute intake, treat with proper nutrition with increased content of solute both as electrolytes and protein.
- In patients with primary polydipsia, treatment consists of fluid restriction by behavior modification and pharmacologic therapy for psychiatric disorders.

Hypervolemic Hyponatremia

- Treatment varies with underlying condition.
- Congestive heart failure treatment consists of sodium restriction, fluid restriction to <1 L/day, diuretic therapy such as loop diuretics and neurohormonal blockade with angiotensin-converting enzyme (ACE) inhibitors and beta-adrenergic blockers.
- In cirrhosis, sodium restriction, fluid restriction, diuretic therapy and large volume paracentesis, and spironolactone are effective.
- In nephrotic syndrome, acute and chronic renal failure treatment consists of fluid restriction to amount less than insensible losses to lead to a negative solute free water balance and correction of hyponatremia.
- Arginine vasopressin receptor antagonists (vaptans) of the AVP V2 receptor—such as conivaptan and tolvaptan—are approved for treatment of euvolemic and hypervolemic hyponatremia.
  - These medications compete with ADH for binding at its site of action in the kidney, thereby blocking the antidiuresis caused by elevated ADH levels. The sodium increases by 4 to 8 mEq within 24 to 48 hours, but these medications are not effective if serum creatinine is >2 mg/dL.

Hypernatremia

- Management of hypernatremia requires replacement of free water and intravascular volume if needed.
- The first step is to correct the underlying cause of the hyperosmolar state. This is followed by replacing the patient's water deficit. This is calculated by the following formula:

$$\text{Water deficit} = \text{Total body water} \times \text{Weight in kg} \times \frac{(\text{Plasma sodium} - 140)}{140}$$

- This is the amount of free water required to return the plasma sodium concentration to 140 mmol/L.
- The rate is determined by the acuteness of the hypernatremia onset.
  - In acute symptomatic hypernatremia, onset <48 hours, treatment should be rapid since cerebral shrinkage can result in seizures, subarachnoid hemorrhage, coma, and death. The plasma sodium should be reduced 1 mEq/L/hour in this situation.
  - With hypernatremia of longer duration, slower correction is necessary to minimize the risk of cerebral edema. The correction rate should be 0.5 mEq/L/hour.

10.1B POTASSIUM DISORDERS

Potassium is the predominant intracellular cation. Normal serum potassium levels are between 3.5 and 5.5 mEq/L with intracellular levels that range between 140 and 150 mEq/L. The distribution of potassium levels across cellular membranes helps maintain the resting membrane potential as well as the timing of membrane depolarization. Systems dependent on membrane depolarization for function, such as nerve cells, cardiac cells, and muscle cells, are affected by changes in serum potassium levels.

The kidneys play a major role in maintaining this homeostasis; 90% of ingested potassium is excreted in the urine while the other 10% is excreted in the gastrointestinal tract.

Potassium excretion is achieved through active secretion in the distal collecting ducts of the kidneys. An increase in serum potassium levels leads to the release of aldosterone from the adrenal glands. Aldosterone increases the number of sodium channels in the distal collecting ducts and leads to direct reabsorption of sodium and indirect secretion of potassium. Through this mechanism, the kidneys can maintain homeostasis by matching intake of potassium with active secretion of potassium.

MEDICAL HISTORY AND CLINICAL PRESENTATION

Both hypokalemia and hyperkalemia can be classified according to changes in intake, changes in excretion, and shifts between the intracellular and extracellular spaces.

Causes of hypokalemia due to decreased intake are rare as the kidneys can limit the excretion of potassium. Other causes of hypokalemia are noted in Table 10.3. Causes of hyperkalemia are noted in Table 10.4.

SIGNS AND SYMPTOMS

Hyperkalemia may have no symptoms and may only be detected when checking blood tests. Patients may present with nausea, malaise, palpitations, muscle weakness, and mild dyspnea.

Hypokalemia presents with fatigue, vomiting, constipation, muscle cramps, and paralysis. Symptoms vary depending on degree of hypokalemia and hyperkalemia.

PHYSICAL EXAMINATION

In hypokalemia, the physical examination is generally not helpful. Severe hypokalemia may be accompanied by muscle weakness, decreased deep tendon reflexes, and ileus. Patients with periodic paralysis syndrome present with proximal motor weakness and hyporeflexia in the presence of a normal level of consciousness.

Patients with vomiting may present with findings of volume depletion, including tachycardia, and orthostatic hypotension. Other examination findings that may be noted are those of the underlying etiology.

TABLE 10.3 Etiologies of Hypokalemia

Etiology	Mechanism
Excess Urinary Losses	
Hyperaldosteronism	Aldosterone increases urinary sodium reabsorption, promoting excretion of potassium in the urine.
Polyuria	High urine output may still lead to excessive potassium losses.
Diuretics	Loop diuretics, thiazides, and carbonic anhydrase inhibitors can cause urinary potassium loss.
Metabolic acidosis	Increased bicarbonate in the distal tubules leads to passive excretion of potassium.
Renal tubular acidosis	There is shifting of potassium from the intracellular to the extracellular space and total body depletion of potassium.
Hypomagnesemia	Hypomagnesemia causes increased potassium loss in the urine.
Bartter syndrome	Autosomal recessive condition; there is impaired sodium chloride absorption in the ascending limb of the loop of Henle.
Gitelman syndrome	Mutations in the thiazide-sensitive sodium chloride cotransporter leads to wasting of sodium, potassium, chloride, and magnesium.
Excessive Nonurinary Losses	
Gastrointestinal	Prolonged or severe diarrhea can lead to clinically significant potassium losses and hypokalemia.
Sweat	Potassium levels are 5–10 mEq/L in sweat and clinically significant losses can occur in hot environments, during exercise, and with cystic fibrosis.
Shifting of Potassium to Intracellular Space	
Alkalosis	With alkalosis intracellular hydrogen ions pass into extracellular fluid and to maintain electroneutrality; potassium ions will enter the intracellular space.
Insulin	Insulin increases the transport of potassium into skeletal muscle and hepatocytes.
Beta-adrenergic activity	Endogenous and exogenous catecholamines increase the transport of potassium into cells.
Hypokalemic periodic paralysis	Sudden and rapid shifts of potassium into cells lead to very low serum potassium levels.

TABLE 10.4 Etiologies of Hyperkalemia

Etiology	Mechanism
Decreased Urinary Excretion	
Renal failure	Impaired potassium regulation and excretion in oliguric states when distal renal tubular flow is compromised.
Hypoaldosteronism	Low aldosterone increases urinary sodium reabsorption and potassium excretion.
Distal renal tubular acidosis (RTA)	Type I RTA leads to impaired reabsorption of sodium and then decreased potassium excretion.
Drugs	Spironolactone and ACE inhibitors decrease the renal excretion of potassium.
Shifting of Potassium to Extracellular Compartment	
Metabolic acidosis	With decrease in pH, extracellular hydrogen ions pass into the intracellular fluid. To maintain electroneutrality, potassium ions will leave the intracellular space to replace the entering hydrogen ions.
Beta-adrenergic blockade	Beta blockers decrease the transport of potassium into cells.
Insulin	Decreased insulin leads to reduced transport of potassium into cells.
Increased tissue breakdown	Cellular breakdown can increase serum potassium levels.

ACE, angiotensin-converting enzyme.

Hyperkalemia may have few physical exam findings. Physical examination findings will typically be those of the underlying etiology. Examination findings include various arrhythmias, decreased deep tendon reflexes, decreased muscle strength, or ascending flaccid paralysis.

DIAGNOSTIC STUDIES

Confirmation of hypokalemia and hyperkalemia is made by checking serum potassium levels. With elevated potassium, pseudohyperkalemia must be ruled out. Pseudohyperkalemia occurs with increased trauma during venipuncture, hemolysis of the sample, use of a tourniquet, and drawing blood over a high resistance catheter or needle.

An EKG should be obtained in all patients with hypokalemia or hyperkalemia (Figure 10.1). Hyperkalemia EKG findings include peaked T waves (when potassium >6.0 mEq/L), widening of QRS duration (when potassium >8.0 mEq/L), and prolongation and loss of P waves. Hypokalemia presents with ST segment depression, decreased T wave amplitude, and prominent U waves.

TREATMENT

Hypokalemia

- Treatment is with potassium replacement.
  - If symptomatic paralysis, EKG changes consistent with hypokalemia, or potassium levels <2.5 mEq/L:

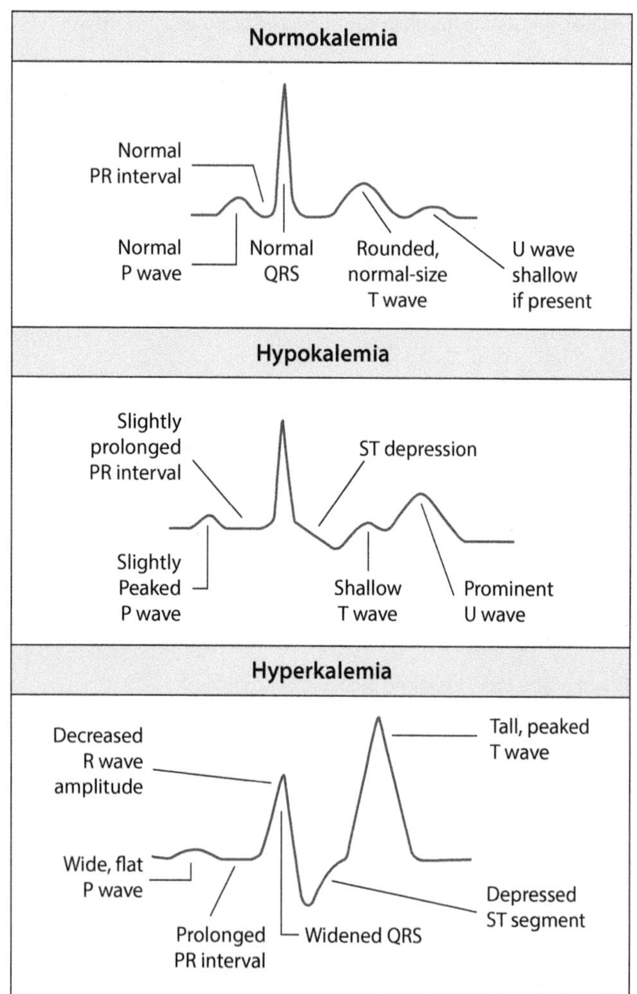

FIGURE 10.1 **EKG changes noted in hyperkalemia and hypokalemia.**

    - Treatment should be started immediately with intravenous (IV) potassium replacement.
      - IV potassium chloride replacement should be started at 0.5 mEq/kg given over 1 to 2 hours, up to 10 to 20 mEq/hour.
      - If higher dose of IV potassium is needed it should be given through a central venous catheter.
      - Monitoring of cardiac function should be done with higher doses of IV potassium replacement.
    - Repeat serum potassium levels should be obtained after each replacement, every 2 to 4 hours.
      - If there is no improvement in potassium level, a magnesium level should be evaluated as hypomagnesemia may be contributing to an intractable hypokalemic state.
  - If no EKG changes, or no clinical manifestations of hypokalemia, or the serum potassium level is 3.0–3.5 mEq/L: Treat with oral replacements or through maintenance IV fluid. Correcting mild hypokalemia can be accomplished by giving 2–3 mEq/kg/day, up to 20 mEq per dose divided into 2 to 4 doses. The risk of developing hyperkalemia with oral replacement is low.

Hyperkalemia

- If serum potassium level is 6.0 to 6.5 mEq/L, a 12-lead EKG should be obtained.
  - If no EKG changes, eliminate all potassium from diet and IV fluid replacement.
- Cardiac monitoring should be obtained, and potassium levels monitored every 12 to 24 hours.
- If serum potassium is >6.5 mEq/L, or there are EKG changes, treatment options include:
  - Calcium gluconate IV peripherally over 3 to 5 minutes or calcium chloride 10 mg/kg IV via a central line over 1 to 5 minutes. If EKG improves, but is not normal, the calcium infusion may be repeated.
  - Sodium bicarbonate IV over 5 to 10 minutes. Sodium bicarbonate is not compatible with calcium gluconate.
  - Insulin combined with dextrose and water can be infused over 30 minutes. This may be repeated 30 to 60 minutes after first dose. Glucose should be monitored.
  - Sodium polystyrene leads to gastrointestinal excretion of potassium by binding potassium in the colon in exchange for sodium; it can be given orally or as a retention enema.
  - Hemodialysis should be considered if hyperkalemia remains severely elevated, >7 mEq/L.

10.1C MAGNESIUM DISORDERS

Magnesium is a very common cation in the body. Half is found in the bone and readily exchanged with magnesium in other parts of the body. The ECF contains 1% of total body magnesium, the rest is intracellular. Normal serum magnesium ranges from 1.5 to 2.5 mEq/L.

Magnesium maintenance is due to dietary intake and effective renal and intestinal conservation. About 70% of serum magnesium is filtered by the kidneys; the rest is bound to protein. Protein binding of magnesium is pH dependent.

Serum magnesium concentration is not closely related to total body magnesium or intracellular magnesium levels.

Magnesium has a major role in enzyme function. Magnesium is required in all enzymatic processes involving ATP and by many of the enzymes involved in nucleic acid metabolism. Magnesium is required to stabilize the structure of DNA and RNA.

Magnesium is also related to calcium and potassium metabolism.

Hypermagnesemia is a serum magnesium concentration >2.5 mEq/dL. The major etiology is renal failure.

Hypomagnesemia is serum magnesium concentration <1.5 mEq/dL. Etiologies include inadequate intake and absorption or increased excretion due to hypercalcemia or drugs such as furosemide.

MEDICAL HISTORY AND CLINICAL PRESENTATION

Symptomatic hypermagnesemia is uncommon. It occurs most commonly in patients with renal failure after ingestion of magnesium-containing drugs. Signs and symptoms include hyporeflexia, hypotension, respiratory depression, and cardiac arrest.

Medications can cause hypomagnesemia. Common medications include prolonged use of proton pump inhibitors and concurrent use of diuretics. Amphotericin B can cause hypomagnesemia, hypokalemia, and acute kidney injury (AKI). Cisplatin can lead to increase renal loss of magnesium; these losses can be severe and persistent. Clinical features are often secondary to the associated hypokalemia and hypocalcemia and include nausea and vomiting, lethargy, tremor, tetany, seizures, and arrhythmias.

PHYSICAL EXAMINATION

The physical examination findings of hypomagnesemia may include the findings noted in hypokalemia and hypocalcemia. Clinical findings include muscle weakness, personality change, tetany with positive Trousseau or Chvostek sign, hyperreflexia, tremor, and muscle fasciculations.

The presence of neurologic signs correlates with the development of concurrent hypocalcemia, hypokalemia, or both. Severe hypomagnesemia may cause generalized tonic-clonic seizures.

DIAGNOSTIC STUDIES

Elevated magnesium levels can lead to EKG abnormalities. At markedly elevated levels the EKG shows prolongation of the PR interval, widening of the QRS complex, and increased T wave amplitude. Deep tendon reflexes disappear as the serum magnesium concentration approaches 10 mEq/L; hypotension, respiratory depression, and stupor develop with increasing hypermagnesemia. Cardiac arrest may occur when blood magnesium concentration is >12 mEq/L.

Severe hypomagnesemia is defined at levels <1.0 mEq/L. Associated hypocalcemia and hypocalciuria are common. Hypokalemia with increased urinary potassium excretion and metabolic alkalosis may be present.

Magnesium deficiency should be suspected even when serum magnesium level is normal in patients with unexplained hypocalcemia or refractory hypokalemia.

TREATMENT

Hypermagnesemia

- Treatment includes cardiac and respiratory support and administration of calcium gluconate 10%. If renal function is normal the patient may be given IV furosemide; furosemide can increase magnesium excretion. Hemodialysis can remove large amounts of magnesium and can be used in severe hypermagnesemia.

Hypomagnesemia

- Treatment includes magnesium salts when patient is symptomatic, or the magnesium concentration is persistently <1.0 mg/dL.
  - Oral magnesium salts, such as magnesium gluconate, are given for 3 to 4 days. Oral treatment is limited by the onset of diarrhea.
  - Parenteral administration is reserved for patients with severe, symptomatic hypomagnesemia who cannot tolerate oral drugs. When magnesium must be replaced parenterally, a 10% magnesium sulfate IV solution is available and a 50% intramuscular (IM) solution is available.
- In severe, symptomatic hypomagnesemia, such as seizures:
  - IV magnesium sulfate is given. If seizures persist, the dose may be repeated up to a total of 10 g over the next 6 hours.
  - When serum magnesium is ≤1.0 mg/dL but symptoms are less severe, IV magnesium sulfate can be given at a slower rate for up to 10 hours.

10.1D CALCIUM DISORDERS

Calcium is involved in several enzymatic and cellular functions. Calcium plays an important role in bone ossification, and about 99% of total body calcium resides in skeletal tissue. Of the fraction found in plasma, 40% is bound to protein, and 10% is complexed with anions. The remaining serum calcium is ionized and unbound. Serum ionized calcium is only a very small fraction of total body calcium but is the most physiologically important. Calcium plays a role in cardiac pacemaker function, muscle contraction, neuronal function, vascular tone, and blood coagulation.

The metabolism of calcium and of phosphate is related. The regulation of both calcium and phosphate is influenced by circulating PTH, vitamin D, and calcitonin.

PTH is secreted by the parathyroid glands and has a major role in calcium balance. The parathyroid gland notes a decrease in serum calcium and responds by releasing PTH into the circulation. PTH increases serum calcium by increasing renal and intestinal absorption of calcium and by bone resorption, mobilizing calcium from bone. Renal calcium excretion parallels sodium excretion and is controlled by the same factors that control sodium transport in the proximal tubule. PTH enhances distal tubular calcium reabsorption independently of sodium. PTH also decreases renal phosphate reabsorption and increases renal phosphate losses.

PTH increases serum calcium by stimulating conversion of vitamin D to calcitriol, the active form of vitamin D. Calcitriol increases the percentage of dietary calcium absorbed by the intestine. Despite this increase in calcium absorption, long-term increases in PTH secretion results in bone resorption by inhibiting osteoblastic function and promoting osteoclastic activity. PTH and vitamin D are both regulators of bone growth and bone remodeling.

Calcitonin is secreted by the thyroid parafollicular cells or C cells. Calcitonin lowers serum calcium concentration by enhancing cellular uptake, renal excretion, and bone formation. The effects of calcitonin are weaker than those of either PTH or vitamin D.

TABLE 10.5 Etiologies of Calcium Disorders

Hypercalcemia	Hypocalcemia
PTH-dependent	**Hypoalbuminemia**
Primary hyperparathyroidism Familial hypocalciuric hypercalcemia Lithium-associated Multiple endocrine neoplasia type 1 and 2A Familial hyperparathyroidism	Hypoparathyroidism—post-surgical/idiopathic Defect in vitamin D metabolism Nutritional Malabsorption Drugs Liver and renal diseases
PTH-independent	**Other**
Acute and chronic renal failure Neoplasms Excess vitamin D Thyrotoxicosis Adrenal insufficiency Drugs: vitamin A overdose, thiazide diuretics, theophylline Immobilization	Metabolic and respiratory alkalosis Sepsis Blood transfusions (massive) Tumor lysis Rhabdomyolysis

PTH, parathyroid hormone.

Etiologies of hypocalcemia and hypercalcemia are noted in Table 10.5.

MEDICAL HISTORY AND CLINICAL PRESENTATION

Most patient with mild hypercalcemia are asymptomatic. Clinical manifestations of hypercalcemia include constipation, anorexia, nausea and vomiting, abdominal pain, and ileus development. Impairment of the renal concentrating mechanism leads to polyuria, nocturia, and polydipsia. Calcium elevation over 12 mg/dL can cause mental status changes including emotional lability, confusion, delirium, psychosis, stupor, and coma. Hypercalcemia can cause neuromuscular symptoms, including muscle weakness. Hypercalciuria with nephrolithiasis is common. Severe hypercalcemia, with values >18 mg/dL may lead to renal failure, shock, and death.

The typical findings in mild to moderate hypocalcemia include fatigue, muscle cramping, weakness, perioral and distal paresthesia, and myoclonic jerks. In severe hypocalcemia findings include tetany, laryngospasm, altered mental status, apnea, and seizures.

PHYSICAL EXAMINATION

Hypocalcemia can present with neurologic manifestations including muscle cramps and encephalopathy. Severe hypocalcemia, serum calcium <7 mg/dL, may cause hyperreflexia, tetany, laryngospasm, or generalized seizures.

Tetany is characterized by sensory symptoms, paresthesia of the lips and distal extremities, carpopedal spasm, muscle aching, and spasm of facial muscles. Tetany typically results from severe hypocalcemia but can result from reduction in ionized serum calcium without marked hypocalcemia, as in severe alkalosis.

Chvostek and Trousseau signs are easily elicited at the bedside to identify tetany.

Chvostek sign is an involuntary twitching of the facial muscles elicited by a light tapping of the facial nerve just anterior to the exterior auditory meatus. It is present in most people with acute hypocalcemia but may be absent in chronic hypocalcemia.

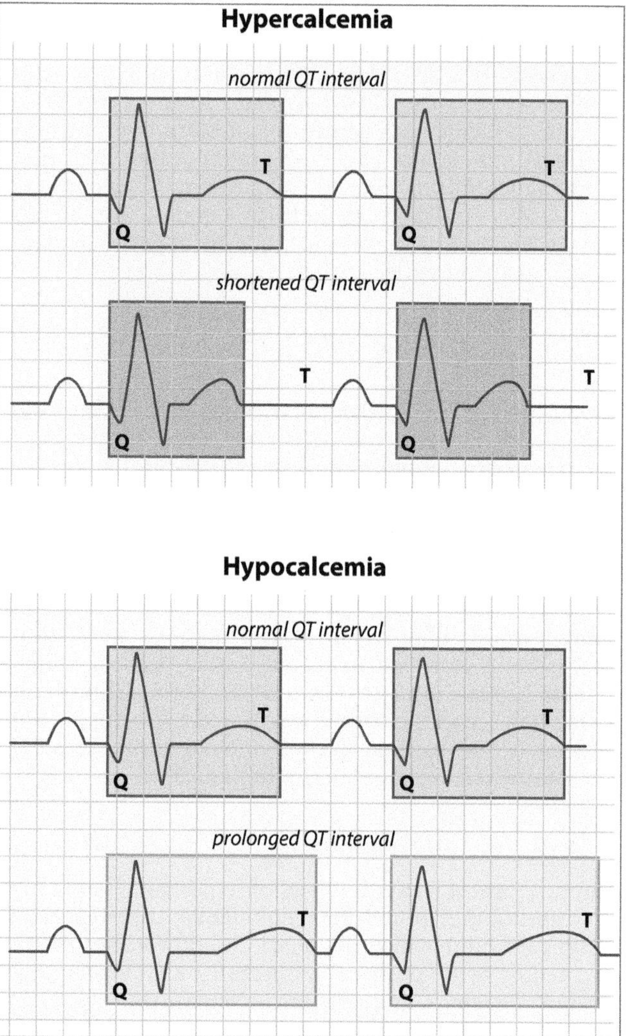

FIGURE 10.2 QT interval abnormalities with hypercalcemia and hypocalcemia.

Trousseau sign is the presence of carpal spasm due to reduction of the blood supply to the hand with a blood pressure (BP) cuff inflated to 20 mm Hg above systolic BP applied to the forearm for 3 minutes. Trousseau sign also occurs in alkalosis, hypomagnesemia, hypokalemia, and hyperkalemia.

Physical examination in patients with hypercalcemia is usually unremarkable. Cardiac abnormalities may be noted such as palpitations.

DIAGNOSTIC STUDIES

Evaluation of hypocalcemia and hypercalcemia should include analysis of total serum calcium and ionized calcium levels. Total serum calcium levels are affected by the levels of serum albumin and should be corrected based on the total albumin level. For every 1 g/dL decrease in albumin, there will likely be a 0.8 mg/dL decrease in total serum calcium.[4]

EKG findings are common in calcium disorders. Hypocalcemia presents with a prolonged QT interval, nonspecific ST and T wave changes, and arrhythmias. In severe hypercalcemia a shortened QT interval is noted along with arrhythmias (Figure 10.2).

TREATMENT

Hypocalcemia

- Symptomatic disease is treated with IV calcium gluconate 100 to 200 mg/kg up to 1 to 3 g maximum over 10 to 20 minutes. If central line access is available, IV calcium chloride can be given 10 to 20 mg/kg up to 1 g over 5 to 10 minutes. The cardiorespiratory system should be monitored when giving IV calcium.
- The asymptomatic patient should be evaluated for hyperphosphatemia and treated.
  - Treatment includes supplementation starting at 50 mg/kg/day of elemental calcium divided into 3 to 4 doses.

Hypercalcemia

- For mild disease (serum calcium <11.5 mg/dL), treat the underlying disorder, restrict calcium from diet, ensuring adequate hydration and voiding.
  - When symptoms are significant, treatment aimed at lowering serum calcium is necessary. Oral phosphate can be used at it binds some calcium, preventing its absorption.
- For total calcium >15 mg/dL immediate treatment should be started.
  - Treatment consists of IV isotonic fluid to restore intravascular volume and ensure adequate urine output. Furosemide 1 mg/kg (10–20 mg max) every 6 hours can be used to improve renal calcium excretion.
  - If there is no improvement, bisphosphonate, denosumab, calcitonin, corticosteroids, or chloroquine should be considered.
    - Bisphosphonates are the drugs of choice for cancer-associated hypercalcemia.
    - Denosumab is a monoclonal antibody inhibitor of osteoclastic activity that can be used for cancer-associated hypercalcemia that does not respond to bisphosphonates.
    - Calcitonin lowers serum calcium by inhibiting osteoclastic activity. Calcium levels can be lowered by 1 to 2 mg/dL within a few hours.
    - Corticosteroids decrease calcitriol production and intestinal calcium absorption in patients with vitamin D toxicity, idiopathic hypercalcemia of infancy, sarcoidosis, and hypercalcemia associated with myeloma, lymphoma, leukemia, or metastatic cancer.
- Chloroquine inhibits 1,25(OH)$_2$D synthesis and reduces serum calcium concentration in patients with sarcoidosis. For severe hypercalcemia (serum calcium >18 mg/dL or with severe symptoms), hemodialysis with low-calcium dialysate may be needed in addition to other treatments.

10.1E PHOSPHATE DISORDERS

Phosphate is one of the major anions found intracellular fluid. Most plasma phosphate is in the ionized form (60%), the rest is bound to plasma proteins, or calcium, sodium, and magnesium. Most phosphorus is found in the bone (85%), followed by soft tissue (14%), and extracellular space (1%).

The typical American diet contains about 1,000 mg of phosphate for females and 1,500 mg for males.[5] Excretion of phosphate in the kidney is equal to gastrointestinal absorption to maintain balance. When the phosphate level decreases the kidneys aid in conserving phosphate. Phosphate in the bone serves as a source of plasma buffer for plasma and intracellular phosphate.

Phosphate plays an important role in aerobic and anaerobic energy metabolism, via adenosine diphosphate (ADP) and adenosine triphosphate (ATP). Via 2,3-diphosphoglycerate (2,3-DPG) in red blood cells phosphate plays an important role in oxygen delivery to tissues.

The normal serum phosphate level in adult patients ranges from 2.5 to 4.5 mg/dL. Because of the role phosphate plays in bone growth the concentration is 50% higher in infants and 30% higher in children.

Hyperphosphatemia, elevated phosphate level, may be due to chronic kidney disease (CKD) secondary to limited phosphate excretion, hypoparathyroidism, metabolic acidosis, or respiratory acidosis.

Hypophosphatemia, decreased phosphate level, is due to decreased dietary intake, hyperparathyroidism, or excess renal loss from renal tubular defects.

MEDICAL HISTORY AND CLINICAL PRESENTATION

Symptoms develop when the serum phosphate level falls below 1.5 mg/dL. Patients may experience muscle weakness, lethargy, paralysis, seizures, and coma. Muscle weakness can lead to respiratory failure. Severe hypophosphatemia can lead to hematologic abnormalities, including hemolytic anemia and impaired leukocyte and platelet function. Drugs such as acetazolamide, cisplatin, and glucocorticoids can lead to hypophosphatemia.

Hypophosphatemia should be suspected in patients who present with seizures, lethargy, muscle weakness, and respiratory depression.

Hyperphosphatemia should be suspected in patients with acute/chronic kidney injury, crush injury, rhabdomyolysis, and tumor lysis syndrome. Elevated phosphate levels typically do not cause any symptoms.

PHYSICAL EXAMINATION

Physical examination findings noted in phosphate abnormalities are typically those of the underlying etiology. Muscle weakness is noted in hyperphosphatemia.

DIAGNOSTIC STUDIES

Hypophosphatemia is diagnosed with a serum phosphate <2 mg/dL and hyperphosphatemia is diagnosed with a serum phosphate >4.7 mg/dL.

TREATMENT

Hypophosphatemia

- Treatment of the underlying cause and oral phosphate replacement make up the first step in treating asymptomatic patients with low phosphate levels. Phosphate-binding antacids and diuretics should be stopped if possible. Correcting hypomagnesemia will aid in correcting low phosphate levels.
- If serum phosphate is <1.5 mg/dL or if patient is symptomatic, IV replacement may be needed. IV potassium phosphate is safe if renal function is normal. If renal function is impaired sodium phosphate should be used.
- Serum calcium and phosphate concentrations should be monitored during therapy, especially when IV phosphate is given, or in patients who have impaired renal function. No more than 7 mg/kg of phosphate should be given over 6 hours.

Hyperphosphatemia

- Treatment is via volume expansion with normal saline, stopping excess phosphate intake and dialysis in patients with kidney injury.
- With advanced CKD treatment consists of avoiding foods high in phosphate and the use of phosphate-binding agents.
    - Calcium carbonate and calcium acetate are used as phosphate binders. But their use should be monitored closely because of possible vascular calcification. Phosphate-binding resins without calcium, including sevelamer and lanthanum carbonate, are used in dialysis patients. While aluminum-containing antacids are effective in binding phosphate they should be avoided in patients with end-stage renal disease (ESRD) because of the risk of aluminum-related dementia and osteomalacia.

KEY POINTS

- Hypernatremia is usually caused by limited access to water or an impaired thirst mechanism.
- Osmotic demyelination syndrome may follow too-rapid correction of hyponatremia.
- Hyperkalemia EKG changes include increased PR interval, shortening of the QT interval, and tall, symmetric, peaked T waves.
- Hypokalemia EKG changes include ST segment sagging, T wave depression, and U wave elevation.
- Hypercalcemia is most commonly due to hyperparathyroidism and cancer.
- Hypocalcemia etiologies include hypoparathyroidism, pseudohypoparathyroidism, vitamin D deficiency, and renal failure.
- The usual cause of hyperphosphatemia is advanced renal insufficiency; hypoparathyroidism and pseudohypoparathyroidism are less common causes.
- Hypomagnesemia may occur in alcoholics, in patients with uncontrolled diabetes, and with hypercalcemia or use of loop diuretics.

10.2 ACID-BASE DISORDERS

OVERVIEW

Regulation of pH and acid-base balance are important for normal physiologic function and cell metabolism. Acid-base disorders are classified into metabolic and/or respiratory processes. Metabolic processes direct change in the level of bicarbonate and respiratory processes direct change in $Paco_2$.

The kidneys have a major role in the metabolic component of acid-base disorders by regulating the bicarbonate concentration. This involves reabsorption of almost all filtered bicarbonate and production of bicarbonate to replace the consumed bicarbonate.

Acid production is a normal part of metabolism. One-third to one-half of acid is excreted by the kidneys in the form of titratable acid. The rest is handled by the excretion of ammonium. The pH becomes alkaline if bicarbonate is reabsorbed and/or acid is secreted into the urine. The pH becomes more acidic when bicarbonate is not reabsorbed, or acid is not excreted into the urine.

The key buffer system in maintaining acid-base balance is the bicarbonate system in the ECF. This system is made up of a weak acid, carbonic acid, and its base, bicarbonate ion. When the hydrogen ion concentration increases, the bicarbonate in this buffer system reacts with the hydrogen ion and any change in acidity is keep to a minimum. This process requires an adequate supply of bicarbonate ions, which is supplied by the kidneys through the generation of bicarbonate buffer and reclaiming filtered bicarbonate in the proximal tubules.

The pulmonary system adjusts pH using expired carbon dioxide. Carbon dioxide forms carbonic acid in the body when combined with water, and the amount of carbon dioxide expired can cause pH to increase or decrease.

The concentration of hydrogen ions increases in two ways, via an increase in $Paco_2$ or a reduction in plasma bicarbonate. The role of ventilation is to remove CO_2 during exhalation. If a patient is breathing rapidly, CO_2 will be lost, while a reduced respiratory drive will retain CO_2. An increased concentration of hydrogen ions, an acidosis, stimulates the respiratory center to increase the rate of breathing, thereby blowing off more carbon dioxide and increasing the pH.

If a primary acid-base disorder is metabolic, the compensatory mechanism is respiratory. The respiratory rate is altered, within minutes, to keep the hydrogen ion concentration normal. If the primary acid-base disorder is respiratory, then the kidneys adapt to counteract the change by altering their handling of hydrogen ions. This process usually takes place over several days.

10.2A METABOLIC ACIDOSIS/ ALKALOSIS

Metabolic acidosis is defined as a low arterial pH and a low serum bicarbonate level. Metabolic acidosis occurs when there is excessive acid in the plasma. The body has a large buffering capacity, with CO_2–HCO_3^- as the major buffer system. The two major routes of acid excretion are CO_2 via the lungs and the nonvolatile acids via the kidneys. Metabolic alkalosis is defined as a high arterial pH and a low Pco_2.

Metabolic acidosis can be caused by one of three mechanisms: increased acid production leading to an elevated anion gap metabolic acidosis, or bicarbonate loss or decreased renal acid excretion leading to a normal anion gap metabolic acidosis. See Table 10.6 for the etiologies of an elevated anion gap metabolic acidosis. See below, under Diagnostic Studies, for anion gap formula.

Normal anion gap metabolic acidosis can be divided into two groups based on serum potassium levels (Table 10.7).

Renal tubular acidosis (RTA) is due to impaired renal hydrogen ion excretion (type 1), impaired bicarbonate resorption (type 2), or abnormal aldosterone production or response (type 4). Type 3 is extremely rare. Patients may be asymptomatic or have the signs and symptoms of electrolyte disorders. Diagnosis is based on laboratory findings, including urine pH and electrolytes. See Table 10.8 for the laboratory findings and etiologies.

Salicylates can also cause an elevated anion gap metabolic acidosis. Salicylates are absorbed in the small intestine and metabolized in the liver. The amount of drug excreted unchanged in the urine is small but can be increased with

TABLE 10.6 Etiologies of Metabolic Acidosis–Elevated Anion Gap

Clinical Process	Substance/ Condition	Acid	Lab Findings
Toxic ingestion	Methanol	Formic acid	Very high osmolar gap, elevated methanol level
	Ethylene glycol	Glycolic acid	Very high osmolar gap, presence of ethylene glycol
	Salicylate	Endogenous acid	Elevated salicylate level
	Paraldehyde	Acetic acid	
	Propylene glycol	Pyruvic acid	
Lactic acidosis	Lactic acid	Lactic acid	Elevated lactate level
Ketoacidosis	Diabetic	Ketoacids	High glucose, positive ketones
	Alcoholic	Ketoacids	High alcohol level, positive ketones
	Starvation	Ketoacids	
Uremia/renal failure	From protein metabolism	Sulfate, phosphate, urate	Elevated blood urea nitrogen and creatinine

TABLE 10.7 Etiologies of Metabolic Acidosis–Normal Anion Gap

Low or Low-Normal Potassium	High or High-Normal Potassium
Diarrhea	RTA type 4
Pancreatic or biliary drainage	Chronic kidney disease
RTA type 1–distal	Hyporeninemic hypoaldosteronism
RTA type 2–proximal	High ileostomy output
Carbonic anhydrase inhibitor	Hydrochloric acid administration
Toluene intoxication	Drugs: NSAIDs, triamterene, amiloride, spironolactone, ACEI/ ARB

ACEI, angiotensin-converting enzyme inhibitor; ARB, angiotensin II receptor blocker; NSAIDs, nonsteroidal anti-inflammatory drugs; RTA, renal tubular acidosis.

alkalization of urine. The mechanism of the metabolic acidosis in salicylate toxicity is thought to be secondary to inhibition of the Krebs cycle and subsequent accumulation of organic acids. Salicylates can also cause a respiratory alkalosis due to respiratory center stimulation.

TABLE 10.8 Etiologies of Renal Tubular Acidosis

	Renal Tubular Acidosis Type 1	Renal Tubular Acidosis Type 2	Renal Tubular Acidosis Type 4
Mechanism	Distal H^+ secretion defect	Proximal HCO_3^- secretion defect	Proximal HCO_3^- reabsorption defect
Serum potassium	Decreased	Decreased	Increased
Urine pH	>5.5	<5.5	<5.5
Urine osmolar gap	<150 mOsm	>150 mOsm	<150 mOsm
Etiologies	Medications Amphotericin NSAIDs Lithium Hyperthyroidism Hyperparathyroidism SLE RA Sjögren syndrome Thyroiditis	Medications Carbonic anhydrase inhibitors Aminoglycosides Antiretrovirals Valproic acid Hyperparathyroidism Vitamin D deficiency Multiple myeloma SLE Sjögren syndrome	Medications Trimethoprim Spironolactone ACEI/ARBs NSAIDs Beta blockers Heparin Sickle cell anemia Adrenal insufficiency Diabetic nephropathy Hypertensive nephropathy

ACEI, angiotensin-converting enzyme inhibitor; ARBs, angiotensin II receptor blockers; NSAIDs, nonsteroidal anti-inflammatory drugs; RA, rheumatoid arthritis; SLE, systemic lupus erythematosus.

Metabolic alkalosis is due either to a gain in bicarbonate, loss of hydrogen ion (H^+) or the loss of fluid that contains Cl^- in higher concentration and bicarbonate in lower concentration than serum. The respiratory compensation, hypoventilation, is due the brainstem sensitivity to interstitial and cellular H^+ changes and the decline in H^+. With simple metabolic alkalosis this respiratory compensation leads to an increase in arterial carbon dioxide content ($Paco_2$). For each 1 mEq/L rise in HCO_3^-, $Paco_2$ rises about 0.7 mm Hg.

Metabolic alkalosis can be divided into two categories: saline-responsive and saline-resistant. See Table 10.9 for the various etiologies of metabolic alkalosis.

MEDICAL HISTORY AND CLINICAL PRESENTATION

A history and physical exam can provide clues to initiating and maintenance factors for metabolic acid-base disorders.

Metabolic acidosis presents with nonspecific symptoms, including headache, chest pain, palpitation, shortness of breath, nausea, vomiting, and muscle weakness. Severe acidosis can lead to seizure, coma, cardiac arrhythmia, and cardiac arrest.

CNS sedation is common in metabolic acidosis from methanol or ethylene glycol. The final metabolite of methanol is formic acid, which is toxic to the retina, and can lead to permanent blindness. The final metabolites of ethylene glycol target the kidney, and lead to acute tubular injury

TABLE 10.9 Etiologies of Metabolic Alkalosis

Saline Responsive	Saline Resistant
Urine chloride <20 mmol/L	Urine chloride >40 mmol/L
Congenital chloride diarrhea	Bartter syndrome
Cystic fibrous	Cushing syndrome
Diuretics–late use	Diuretics–easy use
Gastric fluid loss–vomiting, nasogastric suctioning	Excess bicarbonate administration
Posthypercapnia	Hyperaldosteronism
Villous adenoma	Liddle syndrome

and tubular obstruction from oxalate crystallization and the presence of calcium oxalate crystals in the urine.

Salicylate overdose presents with coma, with or without hyperventilation. Prognosis is related to the salicylate level, patient's age, comorbid illnesses, and degree of clinical decompensation.

Patients with RTA type 1 may present with kidney stones due to high urinary calcium excretion and low urinary citrate excretion.

Most metabolic alkalosis episodes are mild and self-limiting. Systemic alkalosis lowers the risk of arrhythmia by decreasing ionized calcium levels. CNS and peripheral nervous system symptoms may occur due to vasoconstriction of systemic vascular beds.

Hypoventilation may develop due to a decrease in interstitial H^+ in the brainstem respiratory center; the hypoxemia is never clinically severe.

PHYSICAL EXAMINATION

In metabolic acidosis or alkalosis, the physical examination findings are those of the underlying etiology. There may be rapid deep breathing (Kussmaul breathing), anxiety, and change in mental status in patients with metabolic acidosis.

DIAGNOSTIC STUDIES

In metabolic acidosis the arterial pH is low, and the serum bicarbonate is low. In metabolic alkalosis the arterial pH is high, and the serum bicarbonate is high. Serum electrolytes may be needed to calculate the anion gap to separate the elevated anion gap from normal anion gap metabolic acidosis. See below for anion gap formula.

$$\text{Anion gap} = Na^+ - \left(Cl^- + HCO_3^-\right)$$

Osmolar gap may be needed to identify the presence of toxins causing an elevated anion gap metabolic acidosis. See below for osmolar gap formula.

$$\text{MO} = \text{Measured osmolarity (mOsm/L)}$$

$$\text{CO} = \text{Calculated osmolarity (mOsm/L)}$$

$$\text{CO} = 2(Na^+) + \frac{\text{Glucose}}{18} + \frac{\text{BUN}}{2.8} + \frac{\text{Ethanol}}{4.6}$$

(Ethanol level is optional)

$$\text{Osmolar gap} = \text{Measured osmolarity} - \text{Calculated osmolarity}$$

An osmolar gap is defined as a difference of 10 or more between measured and calculated osmolarity.

A normal or small osmolar gap cannot completely exclude a toxic alcohol ingestion. The osmolar gap decreases as the alcohols are metabolized to toxic organic acids, which increases the anion gap due to metabolic acidosis. Markedly elevated osmolar gap (>30) is suggestive of toxic alcohols because other disorders do not cause such marked elevations.

TREATMENT

- Treatment of metabolic acidosis centers on treating the underlying etiology.
- Patients with a pH <7.1 or severe acute acidosis with compromised hemodynamics are considered a medical emergency with a high risk of complications.
- One treatment option is IV bicarbonate. The initial dose will be based on the HCO_3^- deficit. See below.

$$HCO_3^- \text{ deficit} = 0.5 \times \text{body weight (kg)} \times (24 - HCO_3^-)$$

Half of the deficit is given intravenously, over the first 3 to 4 hours. Exogenous bicarbonate should be administered with caution in ketoacidosis and lactic acidosis to prevent overshooting metabolic alkalosis.

Other treatment options include:

- **Lactic acidosis:** Correct the underlying abnormalities, restoring tissue perfusion and treatment of underlying malignancies.
- **Diabetic ketoacidosis:** Treat with regular insulin therapy, aggressive fluid, and electrolyte management.
- **Methanol and ethylene glycol toxicity:** Inhibition of alcohol dehydrogenase by fomepizole and management of airway, breathing, and circulation.
- **Salicylate toxicity:** Treat with alkali therapy to decrease CNS damage.
- **Toluene toxicity:** Treatment is supportive, with hydration, potassium replacement, and bicarbonate therapy in severe cases (pH <7.2). Recovery is usually rapid. Toluene is lipophilic and stored in body fat; therefore, dialysis is not effective.
- **Renal tubular acidosis:** Treat with alkali therapy; large amounts of oral alkali may be needed. Thiazides may reduce the amount of alkali needed. In RTA type 4, dietary potassium restriction and a diuretic for volume control are the mainstay of therapy.

Metabolic Alkalosis

- Treatment of metabolic alkalosis depends on if saline-responsive or saline-unresponsive.
- Saline-responsive is corrected with isotonic saline to replace extracellular volume deficit.
- If fluid resuscitation is not possible, secondary to cardiopulmonary disease, acetazolamide can be used to increase renal bicarbonate excretion.
  - H2-blockers or proton pump inhibitors can be used in patients with alkalosis due to nasogastric suctioning.
- Saline-unresponsive treatment includes surgical removal of any tumors and blockage of aldosterone effect with an ACE inhibitor or spironolactone.

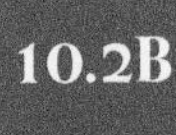

10.2B RESPIRATORY ACIDOSIS/ ALKALOSIS

Respiratory acidosis is due to an increase in Pco_2 caused by hypoventilation with a major complication of hypoxemia. Clinical severity depends on underlying etiology, severity, and rate of change.

The most common causes of increased Pco_2 is a decrease in ventilation, increased CO_2 production without increased ventilation, as noted in sepsis, and those who have increased physiologic dead space (i.e., emphysema).

Respiratory alkalosis is due to a decrease in Pco_2 secondary to hyperventilation. The most common cause of decreased Pco_2 is an absolute increase in ventilation. Decreased CO_2 production without increased ventilation, such as during anesthesia, can also cause respiratory alkalosis.

MEDICAL HISTORY AND CLINICAL PRESENTATION

Respiratory acidosis is due to hypoventilation. Patients may have a history of chronic lung disease, neuromuscular disorders, or sleep disorders. Symptoms include confusion, fatigue, lethargy, shortness of breath, and sleepiness.

Respiratory alkalosis is due to hyperventilation. Patients may have a history of anxiety disorders or neurologic or pulmonary disorders. Symptoms include lightheadedness, syncope, confusion, cyanosis, circumoral paresthesia, and shortness of breath.

PHYSICAL EXAMINATION

Physical examination findings in respiratory acidosis or alkalosis are typically those of the underlying disorder. Physical examination findings in respiratory acidosis include hypoventilation with shallow respirations, hypoxia, muscle weakness, and hyperreflexia. Physical examination findings in respiratory alkalosis include hyperventilation with shallow respirations and perioral or extremity numbness.

DIFFERENTIAL DIAGNOSIS

See Table 10.10 for the etiologies of respiratory acidosis and alkalosis.

DIAGNOSTIC STUDIES

In respiratory acidosis the arterial pH is low, and the arterial Pco_2 is high. In respiratory alkalosis the arterial pH is high, and the arterial Pco_2 is low.

TREATMENT

- Treatment of respiratory acidosis is directed at treating the underlying disorder to improve ventilation.
  - If opioid overdose is possible or there is no obvious cause, a trial of IV naloxone should be considered.
  - If the Pco_2 is >80 mm Hg and the pH <7.10, immediate mechanical ventilation is indicated.
- Treatment of respiratory alkalosis is directed at treating the underlying disorder.
  - If secondary to anxiety, breathing into a paper bag should be avoided as it does not increase Pco_2 and may decrease Po_2.
  - Hyperventilation is usually self-limited because muscle weakness caused by the respiratory alkalosis will decrease ventilation.

TABLE 10.10 Etiologies of Respiratory Acidosis and Respiratory Alkalosis

Respiratory Acidosis	Respiratory Alkalosis
Central nervous system depression Opiates and sedatives Head trauma Cerebrovascular accident	Hypoxia Severe asthma Pneumonia Pulmonary embolus
Airway obstruction Sleep apnea Foreign body Aspiration Bronchospasm	Congestive heart failure/ pulmonary edema/infection Gram-negative sepsis Fever
Respiratory disorders COPD ARDS Pneumonia Pulmonary edema	Increased intracranial pressure Head trauma Stroke Tumor
Neuromuscular disorders Guillain-Barré syndrome Myasthenia gravis Muscular dystrophy Brainstem injury	Anxiety Salicylate toxicity Liver disease Excessive mechanical ventilation

ARDS, acute respiratory distress syndrome; COPD, chronic obstructive pulmonary disease.

KEY POINTS

- Acidosis and alkalosis refer to processes that lead to accumulation or loss of acid and/or alkali; blood pH may or may not be abnormal.
- Acid-base disorders are classified as metabolic if the change in pH is primarily due to an alteration in serum bicarbonate and respiratory if the change is primarily due to a change in Pco_2.
- Initial laboratory evaluation of acid-base disorders includes measurement of arterial blood gases and serum electrolytes and calculation of the anion gap.

10.3 DEHYDRATION

OVERVIEW

Sodium is the major osmotically active ion in the ECF and total body sodium content determines ECF volume. Changes in total body sodium content affect the ECF volume leading to volume depletion or overload. Serum sodium concentration does not necessarily reflect total body sodium.

Total body sodium content is determined by dietary intake and renal excretion. When total sodium content and ECF volume are low, the kidneys increase sodium conservation leading to an increase in volume. When total sodium content and ECF volume are high, the kidneys increase sodium excretion leading to a decrease in volume.

The renin-angiotensin-aldosterone system (RAAS) is the main regulator of renal sodium excretion. In volume-depleted states, glomerular filtration rate (GFR) and sodium delivery to the distal nephrons decrease. This causes the release of renin. Renin cleaves angiotensinogen to form angiotensin I. ACE then cleaves angiotensin I to angiotensin II. Angiotensin II causes:

- Increased sodium retention by decreasing the filtered load of sodium and enhancing proximal tubular sodium reabsorption
- Increased BP
- Increased thirst
- Impaired water excretion
- Stimulated secretion of aldosterone, which increases sodium reabsorption

Aldosterone release is also stimulated by hyperkalemia.

Becoming sodium depleted requires inadequate sodium intake plus abnormal losses from the skin, gastrointestinal tract, or kidneys. Defective renal sodium conservation can be due to primary renal disease, adrenal insufficiency, or diuretic therapy.

Developing sodium overload requires sodium intake greater than excretion; but because normal kidneys can excrete large amounts of sodium, sodium overload also requires a defect in regulation of renal blood flow and sodium excretion; this occurs in heart failure, cirrhosis, or CKD.

Because water crosses plasma membranes in the body via osmosis, loss of sodium quickly results in water loss from the ECF space. Sodium loss always causes water loss. Depending on multiple factors, serum sodium concentration can be high, low, or normal in volume-depleted patients. ECF volume is related to effective circulating volume. A decrease in ECF, or hypovolemia, causes a decrease in effective circulating volume, which in turn causes decreased organ perfusion and leads to clinical sequelae. Causes include vomiting, excessive sweating, diarrhea, burns, diuretic usage, and kidney failure.

SIGNS AND SYMPTOMS

Patients at risk include those with a history of inadequate fluid intake, increased fluid losses, diuretic therapy, and renal or adrenal disorders.

History of fluid intake should be accessed, and losses related to fever, vomiting, polyuria, diarrhea, or nasogastric suctioning. A history of heart failure or renal failure should be noted. Symptoms suggesting dehydration include thirst, syncope, and dizziness.

PHYSICAL EXAMINATION

Clinical features vary depending on the degree of fluid loss of the ECF. When fluid loss is <5% of ECF, this is mild volume depletion, and the major sign is decreased skin turgor. Increased thirst may be noted, and oliguria is common.

When loss is between 5% and 10% of ECF volume—a moderate volume depletion—patients present with orthostatic tachycardia and hypotension. Skin turgor may decrease further.

When loss is >10% of ECF volume—severe volume depletion—signs of shock, such as tachypnea, tachycardia, hypotension, confusion, and poor capillary refill can occur.

If accurate patient weights immediately before and after fluid loss are known, the difference is an accurate estimate of volume loss.

DIAGNOSTIC STUDIES

Diagnosis is made based on clinical findings and laboratory studies including serum electrolytes, blood urea nitrogen (BUN), and creatinine. Volume depletion frequently increases the BUN and serum creatinine concentrations. On occasion plasma osmolality and urine chemistries are needed.

During volume depletion the normal function of the kidney is to conserve sodium. This leads to a urine sodium concentration typically <15 mEq/L; the FENa is typically <1%; and urine osmolality is often >450 mOsm/kg.

If the patient has volume depletion with metabolic alkalosis the urine sodium concentration may be high because large amounts of bicarbonate are spilled in the urine, leading to increased excretion of sodium to maintain ion neutrality. In this case a urine chloride concentration of <10 mEq/L more reliably indicates volume depletion.

Misleadingly high urinary sodium, >20 mEq/L, or low urine osmolality can occur due to renal sodium losses resulting from renal disease, diuretics, or adrenal insufficiency.

10.3A FLUID MANAGEMENT

Fluid management usually involves the IV administration of crystalloid or colloidal solutions and/or blood products. The choice of fluid, the amount to be infused, and rate of infusion are determined by the reason for fluid therapy and the underlying etiology.

Fluid therapy with crystalloid solutions is used to treat hypovolemia, correct free water deficits in dehydrated patients, replace ongoing fluid losses, and meet fluid requirements of patients who cannot take fluids orally.

Colloidal solutions, such as albumin, are used alone or in combination with crystalloid solutions in severe cases of low oncotic pressure. Blood products should be used in cases of severe bleeding.

See Table 10.11 for a summary of the various IV fluid options.

TREATMENT

- Maintenance therapy is indicated in patients who cannot or are not able to take fluids orally.
  - In adults, maintenance dosing is 30 mL/kg of water, 1 g/kg of glucose, 1 to 3 mEq/kg of sodium and chloride, and 0.5 to 1.0 mEq/kg of potassium per day. The fluid rate may need to be adjusted in certain conditions. Increased fluids may be indicated in cases of fever and tachypnea. Decreased rates are indicated in congestive heart failure and low output renal failure.
  - Once the underlying etiology is corrected, fluids are given to replace current volume deficits and any ongoing fluid losses and to provide daily fluid requirements.
- Mild-to-moderate volume deficits can be replaced by increased oral intake of sodium and water when patients are conscious and not vomiting.
- With severe volume deficits or when oral fluid replacement is not possible, IV 0.9% saline or a buffered electrolyte solution (e.g., Ringer lactate) is given. Both are well tolerated and safe.
  - Buffered solutions have lower chloride concentrations and may reduce development of hyperchloremic metabolic acidosis. Both solutions distribute evenly into the

TABLE 10.11 Intravenous Fluids

Solution	Osmolarity (mOsm/L)	pH	Na^+ (mEq/L)	K^+ (mEq/L)	Cl^- (mEq/L)	Ca^{2+} (mEq/L)	Glucose (g/L)	Other
Normal saline	308 (Isotonic)	6.0	154		154			
0.45% Saline	154 (Hypotonic)	6.0	77		77			
3% Saline	1026 (Hypertonic)	5.0	513		513			
Lactated Ringer	273 (Isotonic)	6.5	130	4	109	3		Lactate 28 mEq/L
D_5W	253 (Hypotonic)	4.5					50	
D_5W 0.45% Saline	432 (Hypertonic)	4.0	77		77		50	
D_5W Lactated Ringer	525 (Hypertonic)	5.0	130	4	109	3	50	Lactate 28 mEq/L
Albumin 5%	330 (Isotonic)	7.4	145	<2				Albumin 50 g/L
Albumin 25%	330 (Isotonic)	7.4	145	<2				Albumin 250 g/L

D_5W, 5% dextrose in water.

extracellular space, so three to four times the deficit in intravascular volume needs to be given.

- Circulatory shock and severe intravascular volume depletion requires large-volume IV fluid replacement. In the patient with intravascular volume deficiency compensation is via vasoconstriction, followed by movement of fluid from the extravascular to intravascular compartment. This maintains circulating volume at the expense of total body water. Major volume losses often overwhelm the compensation mechanism.

Fluids

- Crystalloid solutions for replacing intravascular volume are typically isotonic. See Table 10.11.
  - Because water freely moves outside the vasculature, as little as 10% of isotonic fluid remains in the intravascular space.
  - With hypotonic fluid, even less remains in the vasculature. These fluids are not used for resuscitation. In acute brain injury, 0.9% saline is preferred.
- Colloid solutions are effective for volume replacement during major hemorrhage but offer no major advantage over crystalloid solutions.
  - Hydroxyethyl starch has an increased risk of renal injury, and albumin has been associated with poorer outcomes in patients with traumatic brain injury. Both dextran and hydroxyethyl starch may adversely affect coagulation when large volumes are given.
- Blood typically is given as packed red blood cells. Loss of red blood cells diminishes oxygen-carrying capacity.
  - The body will increase cardiac output to maintain oxygen delivery and increases oxygen extraction. Therefore, non–oxygen-carrying crystalloid or colloid fluids may be used to restore intravascular volume in mild to moderate blood loss. In severe hemorrhagic shock, blood products are required.
- Isotonic crystalloid solutions are given for intravascular replacement during shock and hypovolemia. Colloid solutions are not used.
  - Patients with dehydration and adequate circulatory volume typically have a free water deficit, and hypotonic solutions, such as 5% dextrose in water or 0.45% saline, are used. Rapid infusion with a 500–1,000 mL bolus of normal saline or lactated Ringer solution within 15 minutes is indicated. If the patient's response is inadequate the bolus can be repeated.
  - An inadequate response is noted with the following:
    - Low urine output (<0.5 mL/kg/hour)
    - Increased heart rate
    - Low BP

See Table 10.12 for IV fluid guide.

KEY POINTS

- Common causes of dehydration include diarrhea, vomiting, and sweating.
- Physical examination findings include thirst, dry mucus membranes, and decreased urination.

SPECIAL CONSIDERATIONS

- Maintenance therapy is indicated in children who cannot or are not able to take fluids orally. In children, maintenance dosing is based on the Holliday-Segar formula with 4 mL/kg/hour for the first 10 kg plus 2 mL/kg/hour. for the next 10 kg plus 1 mL/kg/hour for the remaining weight.
- In neonates the rate is 150 mL/kg/day.

10.4 VOLUME OVERLOAD

OVERVIEW

Volume overload refers to expansion of the ECF volume. ECF volume expansion occurs in heart failure, kidney failure, nephrotic syndrome, and cirrhosis. Renal sodium retention leads to increased total body sodium content. This increase results in varying degrees of water retention and volume overload. Serum sodium concentration can be high, low, or normal in volume-overloaded patients, despite the increased total body sodium content. Treatment involves removal of excess fluid with diuretics or mechanical fluid removal.

TABLE 10.12 Intravenous Fluid Guide

Type	Uses	Comments
Normal saline (NS) (0.9% NaCl in water)	Increases circulating plasma volume	• Replaces losses without altering concentrations • Used in Na^+ replacement
½ NS (0.45% NaCl in water)	Raises total fluid volume	• Used for daily maintenance • Helpful for establishing renal function • Fluid replacement if extra glucose not needed
Lactated Ringer solution (LR) (Normal saline with electrolytes and buffer)	Replaces fluid and buffers pH	• Often used with surgery
D_5W (Dextrose 5% in water)	Increases total fluid volume	• Provides about 180 kcal/1 L • Physiologically hypotonic as glucose is metabolized
D_5NS (Dextrose 5% in 0.9% saline)	Replaces fluid sodium, chloride, and calories	• Caution: may cause fluid overload
D_5 ½NS (Dextrose 5% in 0.45% saline)	Used in daily maintenance of fluids, nutrition, and for rehydration	• Common postoperative fluid
D_5LR (Dextrose 5% in LR)	Same as LR plus 180 kcal/1,000 mL	• Caution: may cause fluid overload

An increase in total body sodium is the key pathophysiologic event. It increases osmolality, which triggers compensatory mechanisms that cause water retention. When sufficient fluid accumulates in the ECF, usually >2.5 L, edema develops.

MEDICAL HISTORY AND CLINICAL PRESENTATION

Diagnosis is clinical. Clinical features include weight gain and edema. The location and amount of edema are dependent on many factors, including the patient's position. Clinical findings vary depending on the cause. The patient should be assessed for a history of heart failure, kidney failure, nephrotic syndrome, and pregnancy.

PHYSICAL EXAMINATION

Physical examination findings suggestive of volume overload include tachypnea, decreased oxygen saturation, hypertension, increased jugular venous pressure, bilateral crackles, and peripheral edema.

Other findings suggestive of volume overload include increased urine output, ascites, and weight gain.

DIAGNOSTIC STUDIES

Serum sodium concentration can be high, low, or normal in volume-overloaded patients. Urinary sodium will differentiate acute kidney failure from other nonrenal acute causes of volume overload. In renal failure the urinary sodium is >20 mEq/L as compared to <10 mEq/L in heart failure, cirrhosis, and nephrotic syndrome.

TREATMENT

- Treatment should focus on correcting the underlying cause. Treatment includes diuretics and sometimes mechanical fluid removal via methods such as dialysis and paracentesis. Dietary sodium intake should be restricted.
- Response to treatment is monitored by measuring daily weights. The rate of correction of ECF volume overload should be limited to 0.25 to 0.5 kg body weight/day. The rate should be slower in patients with renal insufficiency and hypotension.

10.5 KIDNEY DISORDERS

OVERVIEW

According to the Centers for Disease Control and Prevention (CDC) more than 37 million Americans are estimated to have kidney disease, which is the eighth most common cause of death.[6] Two hundred thousand American children and adolescents have kidney disease. Half a million Americans were on dialysis in the United States in 2014 and another 100,000 declined dialysis and were living with kidney failure.[7]

The kidneys have several important functions, including blood filtration, metabolism and excretion of endogenous and exogenous compounds, and endocrine functions. The kidneys are also the primary regulators of fluid, acid-base, and electrolyte balance in the body.

PATHOPHYSIOLOGY

Several factors contribute the development of kidney disease:

- Because of the high rate of blood flow to the kidneys, renal tissue can be exposed to harmful circulating agents or substances.
- Glomerular filtration is dependent on a high intra- and transglomerular pressure, which makes the glomerular capillaries vulnerable to hemodynamic injury.
- Disruption of the barrier at the glomerular filtration membrane leads to glomerular injury and loss of plasma proteins.
- The nephron microvasculature aids in the spread of glomerular injury to tubulointerstitial compartment in disease.

The main mechanisms of renal injury include immunologic reactions, tissue hypoxia and ischemia, toxic agents, endogenous substances, and genetic defects.

The causes of AKI can be divided into three categories:

- Prerenal: due to decreased renal perfusion, often due to volume depletion
- Renal: caused by a process within the kidneys
- Postrenal: caused by inadequate drainage of urine distal to the kidneys

In patients who already have underlying CKD any of these factors may cause AKI in addition to the chronic impairment of renal function.

10.5A KIDNEY FUNCTION/ EVALUATION

One of the major functions of the kidneys is to handle nitrogenous waste in the form of urea and creatinine byproducts of metabolism. The measuring of serum BUN and serum creatinine reflects this function and recent renal function and can be used to stage renal function.

Several extrarenal factors affect BUN and serum creatinine levels. See Table 10.13 for extrarenal causes of abnormal BUN and serum creatinine.

The BUN: creatinine ratio can be used to narrow down the differential diagnosis to prerenal, intrarenal, or postrenal conditions. See Table 10.14 for the interpretation of the BUN: creatinine ratio.

The gold standard quantitative measure of kidney function is a measured GFR. Measurement of GFR assists in recognition and monitoring of CKD and is a guide for drug dosing. As renal mass declines due to nephron loss or diseases such as hypertension or diabetes, there is a progressive decline in GFR. The rate of GFR decline can be used to predict the risk of complications and time to onset of stage 5 CKD. Measurement of GFR is critical for developing dosage regimens of renally excreted medications to maximize the drug therapeutic efficacy and avoid potential toxicity.

The GFR is expressed as the volume of plasma filtered across the glomerulus per unit time, based on total renal blood flow and capillary hemodynamics. The normal values for GFR are 127 ± 20 mL/min/1.73 m^2 in healthy men and 118 ± 20 mL/min/1.73 m^2 in healthy women. The normal GFR is higher in African Americans.

The measured 24-hour creatinine clearance (CrCl) has been used as an approximation of GFR for years, but it has limited clinical utility. Because of the invasive nature and technical difficulties of directly measuring GFR in clinical settings, many equations for estimating GFR are available.

Most equations utilize factors such as age, gender, weight, and serum creatinine concentration, without the need for urine collection. The most widely used equation is the Cockcroft-Gault equation. This formula uses age and body mass as factors since they contribute to the estimate of CrCl.

$$\text{CrCl (mL / min)} = \frac{(140 - \text{age}) \times \text{Lean body weight (kg)}}{\text{Serum creatinine } \frac{\text{mg}}{\text{dL}} \times 72} (\times 0.85 \text{ if female})$$

Serum creatinine can provide an estimate of GFR.

- Serum creatinine 1 mg/dL is a normal GFR.
- Serum creatinine 2 mg/dL is a 50% reduction in GFR.
- Serum creatinine 4 mg/dL is a 70–85% reduction in GFR.
- Serum creatinine 8 mg/dL is a 90–95% reduction in GFR.

The etiology of kidney disease can be evaluated using several diagnostic tests, including radiography, ultrasonography, MRI, and biopsy. The KUB (kidney, ureters, and bladder) standard radiograph provides a gross estimate of kidney size and identifies the presence of calcifications. The IV pyelogram involves the administration of a contrast agent to visualize the urinary collecting system. It is primarily used in the assessment of structural changes that may be associated with hematuria, pyuria, flank pain, obstruction, or stone formation. Renal angiography utilizes contrast agents to assess for renovascular disease. The captopril (angiotensin-converting enzyme inhibitor [ACEI]) test is used to diagnose renal artery stenosis as captopril reduces the uptake of the contrast agent because the efferent arteriole is dilated, decreasing the perfusion pressure of the affected kidney. In patients with bilateral disease, a decrease in uptake is observed in both kidneys.

CT, spiral or helical, provides a three-dimensional visualization of tissues. CT is utilized in the evaluation of obstructive uropathy, malignancy, and infections of the kidney.

Renal ultrasound can distinguish the renal pyramids, medulla, and cortex, and abnormalities in structure that may occur with obstruction. Renal ultrasound is also used for site localization during percutaneous kidney biopsy.

MRI with contrast agent is useful in the assessment of obstruction, malignancy, and renovascular lesions.

Renal biopsy is used to facilitate the diagnosis when clinical, laboratory, and imaging findings are inconclusive. Functional status of the kidney is not assessed with biopsy, and severity of disease and progression are best measured using quantitative tests. Contraindications include a solitary kidney, severe hypertension, bleeding disorder, severe anemia,

TABLE 10.13 Extrarenal Causes of Abnormal Blood Urea Nitrogen and Serum Creatinine

	Blood Urea Nitrogen	Serum Creatinine
Increased	High-protein diet Gastrointestinal bleed Congestive heart failure Dehydration Shock Fever Rhabdomyolysis	Shock Dehydration Congestive heart failure Rhabdomyolysis Diabetes
Decreased	Liver disease Malnutrition	Decreased muscle mass Low-protein diet

TABLE 10.14 Interpretation of the Blood Urea Nitrogen/Creatinine Ratio

	Prerenal	Renal	Postrenal
Blood urea nitrogen/ creatinine ratio	>20:1	<20:1	10-20:1
Etiologies	Congestive heart failure Dehydration Shock Sepsis	Nephritic Nephrotic Interstitial	Ureter obstruction Nephrolithiasis Bladder tumor Benign prostatic hypertrophy

cystic kidney, and hydronephrosis. Complications include hematuria and perirenal hematoma.

The urinalysis is the most cost-effective and readily available laboratory evaluation. The urinalysis assesses the kidney's work and can identify renal tubular or parenchymal damage but cannot determine the degree of functional loss. See Table 10.15 for an interpretation summary of urinalysis testing.

Urine microscopic examination can identify the presence of cellular components, casts, crystals, and microorganisms. These elements include:

- White blood cells: The presence of bacteria may indicate a urinary tract infection; sterile pyuria may indicate nephritis, nephrolithiasis, or an atypical infection, such as tuberculosis.
- Red blood cells: These may indicate infection, trauma, tumor, or nephrolithiasis.
- Epithelial cells: Presence of transitional or tubular epithelial cells may indicate renal disease. Presence of squamous epithelial cells may indicate contamination.
- Crystals: Presence may indicate an increased risk of or diagnosis of nephrolithiasis.
- Casts: Tamm-Horsfall protein casts can be made up of various cellular elements.
    - Hyaline casts are normal or increased numbers may be noted after exercise.
    - White blood cell casts indicate pyelonephritis.
    - Red blood cells casts are diagnostic of glomerulonephritis or vasculitis.
    - Fatty casts indicate the presence of nephrotic syndrome.
    - Waxy casts are suggestive of urinary stasis and indicate severe chronic renal disease or renal amyloidosis.

TABLE 10.15 Interpretation of Urinalysis Testing

Test	Interpretation
Specific gravity	Related to urine osmolarity and indicator of hydration status, values >1.020 indicate relative dehydration.
pH	Normal urine pH is slightly acidic. Reflects serum pH, except in renal tubular acidosis.
Protein	Measures albumin. Presence of protein in the urine is a hallmark of renal disease.
Glucose	Present when filtered load of glucose exceeds the ability of the tubule to reabsorb it (>180 mg/dL). Noted in diabetes mellitus, Cushing syndrome, liver and pancreatic disease.
Ketones	Products of fat metabolism. Detects only acetoacetic acid. Present in diabetic ketoacidosis and starvation.
Bilirubin	Product of hemoglobin breakdown. Typically, not detected in the urine. Presence may indicate liver dysfunction and biliary obstruction.
Urobilinogen	Small amounts are normal. Elevated in hemolysis and hepatocellular disease.
Blood	Positive result may indicate hematuria, myoglobinuria, or hemoglobinuria.
Nitrite	Positive in the presence of bacteria that can reduce urinary nitrates to nitrites. Noted in many gram-negative and some gram-positive bacteria infections.
Leukocyte esterase	Enzyme present in neutrophils. Positive test indicates pyuria and possible urinary tract infection.

10.5B ACUTE KIDNEY INJURY

AKI, the sudden loss of kidney function, is a common clinical problem. During acute injury the creatinine is not in a steady state, so the calculated GFR will not accurately represent a patient's kidney function.

Several criteria are used to identify AKI. There are the RIFLE criteria (Risk, Injury, Failure, Loss, and End stage kidney disease) and modified RIFLE criteria by the AKI Network (AKIN) that included an absolute increase in creatinine ≥0.3 mg/dL in the diagnostic criteria.[8]

The Kidney Disease: Improving Global Outcomes (KDIGO) group's revised definition of AKI is the preferred definition.[9] They define AKI as:

- Increase in serum creatinine by ≥0.3 mg/dL within 48 hours; or
- Increase in serum creatinine to ≥1.5 times baseline, which is known or presumed to have occurred within the prior 7 days; or
- Urine volume <0.5 mL/kg/hour for 6 hours.

The KDIGO guidelines allow for correction of volume status and obstructive causes of AKI prior to classification. See Table 10.16 for KDIGO staging criteria.

MEDICAL HISTORY AND CLINICAL PRESENTATION

Patient should be evaluated for a history of fluid loss from vomiting, diarrhea, polyuria, and diaphoresis or insufficient

TABLE 10.16 Kidney Disease: Improving Global Outcomes (Criteria for Acute Kidney Injury)

Staging	Criteria
Diagnostic	Increase in serum creatinine of ≥0.3 mg/dL within 48 hours or ≥50% within 7 days Or Urine output of <0.5 mL/kg/hour for >6 hours
Stage 1	Increase in serum creatinine of ≥0.3 mg/dL or 1.5 to 1.9 times baseline Or Urine output of <0.5 mL/kg/hour for 6–12 hours
Stage 2	Increase in serum creatinine to 2.0 to 2.9 times baseline Or Urine output of <0.5 mL/kg/hour for 12–24 hours
Stage 3	Increase in serum creatinine to ≥3.0 times baseline Or Increase in serum creatinine of ≥0.3 mg/dL to ≥4.0 mg/dL Or Urine output of <0.3 mL/kg/hour for ≥24 hours or anuria for ≥12 hours Or Initiation of renal replacement therapy

Source: Kellum JA, Lameire N, Aspelin P, et al. Kidney disease: improving global outcomes. Acute Kidney Injury Work Group. KDIGO clinical practice guideline for acute kidney injury. Kidney Int Suppl. *2012; 2 :1–138. doi:10.1038/kisup.2012.1*

volume intake. Past medical history should be reviewed for cardiac disease, CKD, urologic disorders, or congenital genitourinary abnormalities. History of recent use of renal toxic medications or iodinated contrast material should be obtained.

Review of systems should focus on suprapubic or abdominal pain, hematuria, urinary frequency, foul-smelling urine, and change in urine stream.

PHYSICAL EXAMINATION

Physical examination should be obtained to evaluate the patient's fluid status and identify any underlying etiologies. On examination, determining volume status can be challenging. The presence of a decreased capillary refill time, poor skin turgor, and a dry axilla may indicate volume depletion. Moist mucous membranes and absence of furrows on the tongue help rule out volume depletion.

Signs of heart failure should be evaluated for, including an elevated jugular venous pressure, a displaced apical impulse, an S3 gallop, and a heart rate >100 bpm at rest.

Abdominal examination should be completed including auscultation for an abdominal bruit indicating possible, renovascular hypertension. Flank palpation and costovertebral angle tenderness may indicate pyelonephritis, while pain with palpation of the suprapubic area may indicate cystitis

A prostate examination may demonstrate signs of benign hyperplasia or malignancy that may cause urethral outflow obstruction.

DIFFERENTIAL DIAGNOSIS

AKI can be divided into three major categories (see Table 10.14).

- **Prerenal disease:** Can be due to reduced renal perfusion. Commonly noted in patients with a myocardial infarction, congestive heart failure exacerbation, or hypovolemia. All cause a reduced cardiac output and reduced renal flow leading to prerenal disease.
- **Renal disease:** Intrinsic renal disease including renal vascular disease, glomerular disease, or tubulointerstitial disease can lead to renal cell destruction and AKI.
- **Postrenal disease:** This may be due to obstruction along the urinary tract. Etiologies include nephrolithiasis, trauma, congenital/anatomic abnormalities, and prostate hypertrophy.

DIAGNOSTIC STUDIES

The focus of the laboratory evaluation is to determine renal status and identify underlying etiology.

Urinalysis can be very helpful. The presence of white blood cells in the urine may indicate a urinary tract infection, hematuria can be due to nephrolithiasis, and proteinuria may indicate glomerular disorder. Microscopic examination of the urine may demonstrate muddy brown casts, which are consistent with acute tubular necrosis (ATN). White blood cell casts may indicate pyelonephritis and hyaline casts may indicate chronic renal disease. Dysmorphic red blood cells may be noted if there is a glomerular defect or injury causing the hematuria sometimes found in nephritic syndromes.

The FENa is used to distinguish prerenal issues and ATN. This formula is used in patients not on diuretics. A value <1% suggests prerenal disease, whereas a value >2% suggests ATN.

$$\text{FENa}\,(\%) = \frac{\text{Urine sodium} \times \text{Serum creatinine}}{\text{Serum sodium} \times \text{Urine creatinine}}$$

If the patient is on diuretics a fractional excretion of urea (FEUrea) is calculated. A value <35% suggests prerenal disease and a value >50% suggests ATN.

$$\text{FEUrea}\,(\%) = \frac{\text{Serum creatinine} \times \text{Urine urea}}{\text{Serum urea} \times \text{Urine creatinine}}$$

Radiographic testing may assist in the evaluation of AKI. Renal ultrasound may identify postrenal obstruction with the presence of nephrolithiasis and hydronephrosis. CT scan can be used to identify more detailed morphology characteristics, including signs of inflammation.

A bladder scan, after attempted voiding, should be performed if there is suspicion of urinary retention. Renal artery duplex scan can reveal renal artery stenosis, but this is more commonly noted in CKD.

Renal biopsy is typically not needed in the evaluation of AKI. It may be needed when the diagnosis is unclear.

EVALUATION

After determining if the AKI is prerenal, renal, or postrenal, the next step is determining the cause. If prerenal causes are possible the fluid volume intake should be assessed. Fluid volumes below the minimal amount to maintain appropriate bodily functions may lead to hypoperfusion over time. Certain conditions, such as fever, sweating, or open wounds may lead to increase fluids needs.

The daily maintenance amount, for a healthy adult, can be calculated based on the formula below.

$$\text{Daily maintenance (mL)} = (\text{Lean body weight (kg)} + 40) \times 24$$

While measuring fluid intake is important, so is monitoring urine output. AKI with urine volume of <400 mL in 24 hours or <0.5 mL/kg/hour is considered oliguric renal failure.

If postrenal is possible, a bladder scan and postvoid residuals should be considered. Bladder scans that reveal an increased volume, >800–900 mL, may indicated severe obstruction or neurogenic bladder. Increased postvoid residuals, >250–300 mL, are associated with increased risk of infection and potentially bladder dysfunction.

TREATMENT

- AKI related to prerenal etiologies are best managed with IV fluids.
  - The use of IV fluids is low risk and can be given empirically even when the exact mechanism is unknown.
- Treatment for the renal etiologies of AKI is complex.
  - All nephrotoxic drugs should be stopped and all renally excreted drugs should be adjusted.
  - Sodium and potassium should be monitored, and treatment should be directed at correcting any abnormalities.
  - The underlying etiology should also be treated.
- Postrenal etiologies, including obstruction, are best treated via Foley catheter, percutaneous drainage, and/or cystoscopy.

Hemodialysis or hemofiltration should be initiated in the following situations:

- Severe electrolyte abnormalities not otherwise controlled
- Pulmonary edema not responding to therapy
- Metabolic acidosis not responding to treatment
- Uremic symptoms including vomiting, asterixis, encephalopathy, and seizures
- Overdose of dialyzable toxins such as salicylates, aldehydes, lithium, and theophylline

Dialysis need should not be determined based on BUN and creatinine levels.

PATIENT EDUCATION

- Minimize risk of AKI by maintaining normal fluid balance, avoiding nephrotoxins, and taking precautions such as giving fluids or drugs when contrast or cytolytic therapy is necessary.
- Adjustment of drug dosing should not be based on serum creatinine but on a more specific measurement of GFR.

10.5C ACUTE TUBULAR NECROSIS

ATN, an intrinsic renal cause of AKI, occurs with prolonged ischemic or toxic injury to the kidney resulting in tubular cell injury. The three major causes of ATN include renal ischemia, sepsis, and nephrotoxins. See Box 10.1 for the etiologies of ATN.

Postischemic ATN occurs in the setting of severe renal ischemia from severe prerenal disease, prolonged hypotension, surgery, or sepsis. Postischemic ATN progresses through four phases:

- **Initiation:** Lasts hours to days. The GFR will decrease due to a decrease in renal blood flow.
- **Extension:** The GFR continues to decrease and there is continued ischemic injury to tubule cells and inflammation.
- **Maintenance:** Lasts 1 to 2 weeks. Urine output is at its lowest.
- **Recovery:** Marked by tubular cell repair and regeneration. GFR will slowly improve to premorbid conditions.

Nephrotoxic medications that can induce ATN include aminoglycosides, amphotericin, cyclosporine, sulfa drugs, cisplatin, acyclovir, contrast media, and pentamidine.

Endogenous toxins that can cause ATN include myoglobinuria, hemoglobinuria, crystalline-induced nephropathy, and multiple myeloma.

Using the KDIGO criteria it is estimated that the incidence of hospital-acquired AKI is 21% and that ATN is the most common etiology of AKI, accounting for 38% of cases in hospitalized patients.[10]

Mortality rate associated with ATN is 37% in hospitalized patients and 78% in ICU patients.[11]

BOX 10.1 Etiologies of Acute Tubular Necrosis

Renal hypoperfusion: Hypotension or sepsis
Major surgery
Nephrotoxins: Aminoglycosides, cisplatin, amphotericin B, contrast material, NSAIDs, cyclosporine, vancomycin
Third degree burns: >15% of body surface area
Myoglobin or hemoglobin: Due to rhabdomyolysis or massive hemolysis
Tumor lysis syndrome or multiple myeloma
Ethylene glycol
Pancreatitis

NSAIDs, nonsteroidal anti-inflammatory drugs.

MEDICAL HISTORY AND CLINICAL PRESENTATION

The history is extremely important in determining the cause of ATN as most presenting symptoms are due to the underlying etiology. Evaluation for the signs and symptoms of sepsis should be elicited.

Medication review is important as numerous medications are linked to the development of ATN.

PHYSICAL EXAMINATION

ATN typically presents with no significant physical examination findings. Changes noted on physical exam occur secondary to the underlying etiology.

Uremic findings include pericardial friction rub, asterixis, and skin excoriations. Muscle tenderness may be noted in rhabdomyolysis or orthostatic hypotension noted in dehydration. Urine output should be measured to determine if the patient is oliguric or anuric.

DIFFERENTIAL DIAGNOSIS

ATN needs to be distinguished from another common cause of AKI: prerenal disease.

Prerenal disease is due to a low perfusion state in the kidneys without evidence of tubular damage. Laboratory findings noted in low perfusion state and prerenal disease include low urine sodium, FENa <1.0%, elevated urine osmolality, and elevated BUN/creatinine ratio.

With prolonged hypoperfusion and injury to the tubular cells, ATN develops. Urine sodium and FENa will increase along with a decrease in urine osmolality. The presence of renal tubular epithelial cells, epithelial cell casts, and muddy brown granular casts on microscopic analysis of centrifuged urine will aid in the diagnosis.

The gold standard for distinguishing between prerenal disease and ATN is response to fluid replacement. If sufficient fluid repletion is given to correct volume depletion, and serum creatinine does not return to normal within 1 to 3 days, this represents ATN.

A renal biopsy is usually not needed to make the diagnosis of ATN but may be needed in certain situations. See Table 10.17 for the laboratory findings of ATN and prerenal azotemia.

TABLE 10.17 Laboratory Features of Acute Tubular Necrosis and Prerenal Azotemia

Test	Acute Tubular Necrosis	Prerenal Azotemia
BUN: creatinine ratio	10–15:1	>20:1
Urine osmolarity (mOsm/kg)	<450	>500
Urine specific gravity	≤1.010	>1.020
Urine sodium (mEq/L)	>40	<20
Fractional excretion of sodium (%)	>2	<1
Urine sediment	Muddy brown granular casts, epithelial cell casts, red blood cells	Normal or a few hyaline casts

BUN, blood urea nitrogen.

DIAGNOSTIC STUDIES

The initial evaluation should include:

- **Urine analysis:** Both chemical analysis and microscopic evaluation are needed. The presence of coarsely granular, muddy brown casts or renal tubular epithelial cells on urine microscopy indicates tubular injury and ATN.
- **Urine electrolytes:** Urine sodium and FENa are used to distinguish prerenal disease from ATN. A FENa <1% indicates that the kidney is being underperfused, but that the concentrating ability for the kidney is intact. With tubular injury, the tubules are no longer able to retain sodium and concentrate the urine, leading to an increase in the FENa.

TREATMENT

- The best treatment of ATN is prevention. High-risk patients should be identified and closely monitored. Close monitoring of volume status, management of antihypertensives to avoid large drops in BP, and avoidance of nephrotoxins are vital. Contrast-induced nephropathy should be avoided by utilizing low-volume contrast agent, using IV hydration, and avoiding frequent contrast studies.
- The KDIGO guidelines recommend against using loop diuretics for treatment of AKI except as needed for volume management.
- Discontinuing nephrotoxic medications such as nonsteroidal anti-inflammatory drugs (NSAIDs), aminoglycosides, and contrast dye is necessary.
- If needed, vasopressors should be used to maintain mean arterial pressure. Using "renal-dosed" dopamine has been shown to be ineffective and may cause harm.[12]
  - To prevent recurrent injury maintaining adequate volume status is paramount. Daily weights and strict monitoring of input and output is required.

PATIENT EDUCATION

- Most patients recover from ATN with the renal failure phase lasting 7 to 21 days.
- Prevention is key and includes maintaining euvolemia, avoid nephrotoxic medications, and closely monitoring renal function when renal toxic medications or contrast material is used.

10.5D INTERSTITIAL NEPHRITIS

Two main diseases involve the renal tubules: ATN and tubulointerstitial nephritis (TIN). The term interstitial nephritis is used for TIN that is due to nonbacterial causes of tubular injury such as drugs, viral infections, and autoimmune diseases. The mechanism of injury is due to an inflammatory response and not direct damage.

Acute interstitial nephritis is the third most common cause of AKI.[13] Over two-thirds of acute interstitial nephritis cases are drug-induced and infection-related.[14] The most common medications are antibiotics, such as cephalosporins, quinolones, rifampicin, and sulfa drugs; NSAIDs; gastrointestinal medications H2 antagonists and proton pump inhibitors; acyclovir; phenytoin; allopurinol and bisphosphonates. Less common causes include infections and systemic diseases. Analgesic-induced nephritis is more common in women.[15]

Interstitial nephritis is an immunologic reaction to a variety of medications, infectious agents, or systemic diseases confined to the interstitial compartment of the renal parenchyma. It is mediated by a hypersensitivity reaction to antigens expressed by the tubular cells.

The interstitial infiltrate is predominantly T- and B-lymphocytes, macrophages, and natural killer cells. This infiltrate results in interstitial edema, disruption of tubular basement membrane, and destruction of the interstitial architecture.

MEDICAL HISTORY AND CLINICAL PRESENTATION

Interstitial nephritis develops within days to weeks of drug exposure. Most patients are asymptomatic. If symptoms are present they include edema, hypertension, decreased urine output, and AKI. The classic manifestations of allergic findings including skin rash, arthralgias, fever, eosinophilia, and eosinophiluria are noted in a minority of patients.

PHYSICAL EXAMINATION

There are no physical examination findings specific to interstitial nephritis, and no characteristic findings exist.

DIAGNOSTIC STUDIES

The clinical features of interstitial nephritis are nonspecific; diagnosis is one of exclusion. Blood chemistries may reveal the presence of RTA and hyperkalemia, as well as the degree of renal failure.

Urinalysis may reveal microscopic hematuria, white blood cell casts, and sterile pyuria. The presence of urinary eosinophils is of limited value.[16] Renal biopsy is the only confirmatory test but is rarely needed.

TREATMENT

- Nonspecific therapy includes stopping offending agents, treating the infectious process, and providing disease-specific treatments.
- Corticosteroid use is controversial. There appears to be a more rapid recovery from renal failure with the use of corticosteroids.
- Refractory cases require a renal biopsy to confirm the diagnosis.

PATIENT EDUCATION

- Given the various causes of interstitial nephritis, there is no uniform course.
- The prognosis is poor in disease associated with NSAIDs and acute bacterial infection.

10.5E GLOMERULONEPHRITIS

Glomerulonephritis (GN) is characterized by acute inflammation of glomeruli and due to either infectious or noninfectious etiologies. GN results in AKI and laboratory studies demonstrate proteinuria, hematuria, dysmorphic red blood cells, and red blood cell casts.

The most common cause of GN is IgA nephropathy (Berger disease).[17] GN is a cause of renal impairment accounting for 10% to 15% of cases of end-stage renal failure in the United States, following only diabetes and hypertension.[18]

MEDICAL HISTORY AND CLINICAL PRESENTATION

Symptoms include change in the urine color, hematuria, decreased urine output (typically <400 mL/day), nocturia, hypertension, and fatigue; edema may or may not be present. With secondary etiologies the clinical presentation is consistent with the underlying etiology. Medical history should investigate a history of recent illnesses, symptoms of vasculitis disorders or other organ involvement, and constitutional symptoms.

PHYSICAL EXAMINATION

The physical examination of patients with primary glomerular disease is unremarkable. Findings may include high BP and signs of fluid overload including peripheral or periorbital edema, pulmonary edema, ascites, and jugular venous distention.

DIFFERENTIAL DIAGNOSIS

Nephritic syndrome must be separated from nephrotic syndrome to establish the proper differential diagnosis and appropriate management. Table 10.18 summarizes the differences between nephritic and nephrotic syndrome.

The differential diagnosis of GN can be organized into three categories based on serologic testing.

Anti-glomerular basement membrane GN can either affect the kidneys or renal and pulmonary system.

The immune complex diseases are manifested by antigen-antibody complexes. These can be seen in lupus, endocarditis, membranoproliferative GN, postinfectious GN, IgA nephropathy, and cryoglobulinemia.

Pauci-immune GN is small and medium size-vessel disease and is associated with the antineutrophil cytoplasmic antibody (ANCA) and includes granulomatosis with polyangiitis and microscopic polyangiitis.

DIAGNOSTIC STUDIES

The initial evaluation of acute GN includes a basic metabolic panel, urinalysis with microscopy, and protein/creatinine ratio. Once the diagnosis of acute GN is established, further testing for specific disease entities should be completed.

The first step is to check complement levels. Low complement levels are noted in in a limited number of possible disorders. See Table 10.19 for the major etiologies of acute nephritis based on complement level.

If the complement level is low, further testing can then be used to identify possible etiologies. For example, ANA and double-stranded DNA are positive in systemic lupus erythematous, rheumatoid factor and cryoglobulin are positive in cryoglobulinemia, blood cultures and echocardiogram may be positive in subacute bacterial endocarditis, and antistreptolysin O titers and anti-DNAse B antibodies may be positive in acute poststreptococcal and streptococcal soft tissue infections.

Other laboratory findings in GN include anemia, leukocytosis, and hyperkalemia. Inflammatory markers, erythrocyte sedimentation rate, and C-reactive protein may or may not be elevated. Urinalysis may reveal hematuria, proteinuria, and red blood cell casts (Figure 10.3).

A renal biopsy may be needed to differentiate etiologies of renal disease, monitor disease progression, and determine prognosis.

TABLE 10.18 Differences Between Nephritic Syndrome and Nephrotic Syndrome

Clinical Features	Nephritic Syndrome	Nephrotic Syndrome
Hematuria	Yes	Yes/No
Proteinuria	<3.5 g/24 hours	>3.5 g/24 hours
Red blood cell casts	Yes	No
Hypoalbuminemia	Yes	Yes/No
Hypertension	Yes	Yes/No

EVALUATION

See Table 10.20 for a comparison of the major findings for the various causes of GN.

TREATMENT

- Each etiology has its own specific treatment.
- Immunosuppressive therapy is the center piece of therapy.
- Hypertension is treated with ACEIs, angiotensin receptor blockers (ARBs), or calcium channel blockers.

TABLE 10.19 Major Etiologies of Acute Nephritis

Low Serum Complement	Normal Serum Complement
Systemic lupus erythematosus	Polyarteritis nodosa
Subacute bacterial endocarditis	Hypersensitivity vasculitis
Cryoglobulinemia	Wegener granulomatosis
Acute poststreptococcal	Henoch-Schönlein purpura
Membranoproliferative	Goodpasture syndrome
	IgA nephropathy
	Rapidly progressive
	Anti-glomerular basement membrane disease

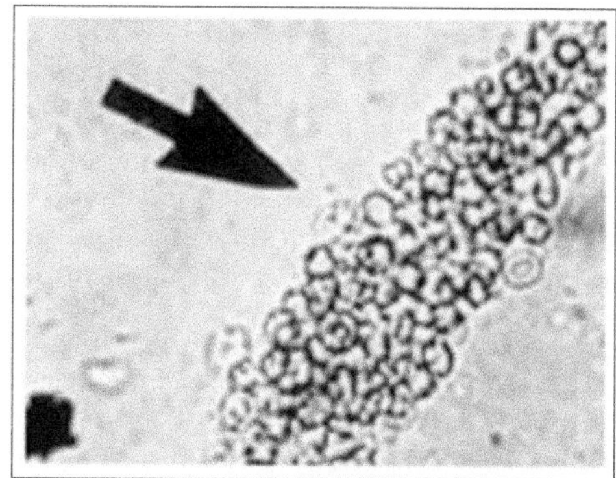

FIGURE 10.3 **Red blood cell cast—present in a number of kidney diseases including glomerulonephritis.**

(Source: Centers for Disease Control and Prevention. Provider-performed microscopy procedures: a focus on quality practices. https://www.cdc.gov/clia/docs/15_258020-A_Stang_PPMP_Booklet_FINAL.pdf)

TABLE 10.20 Summary of Major Causes of Glomerulonephritis

Disease	Clinical Presentation	Associated Diseases	Laboratory Findings	Treatment
Postinfectious		*Streptococcus* infection	ASO positive	Treat underlying cause
IgA nephropathy		Upper respiratory tract infection		ACEI/ARB; steroids; alkylating agent
Goodpasture syndrome	Hematuria; hemoptysis		Anti-GMB positive	Steroids; cyclophosphamide; plasmapheresis
Small vessel vasculitis	Upper respiratory symptoms; hematuria	Sinusitis	ANCA positive	Steroids; cyclophosphamide
Lupus	Rash; oral ulcers; arthritis		ANA positive; dsDNA positive	Steroids
Membranoproliferative	Hypertension	Hepatitis C; SLE; cryoglobulinemia	Low complement	Treat underlying cause
Minimal change disease	Children; facial swelling	Hodgkin lymphoma	Proteinuria; search for underlying cause	Steroids; diuretics
Membranous nephropathy	Hypertension	Renal vein thrombosis; solid organ tumors; hepatitis B	Proteinuria; search for underlying cause; hepatitis panel	Diuretics; statins; ACEI
Focal segmental glomerulosclerosis	Foamy urine; hypertension	HIV	Proteinuria; search for underlying cause	ACEI/ARB; steroids; diuretics

ACEI, angiotensin-converting enzyme inhibitor; ANA, antinuclear antibody; ANCA, antineutrophilic cytoplasmic autoantibody; anti-GBM, anti-glomerular basement membrane; ARB, angiotensin receptor blocker; ASO, antistreptolysin O; IgA, immunoglobulin A; SLE, systemic lupus erythematosus.

TABLE 10.21 Classification of Chronic Renal Failure

Glomerular Filtration Rate		Description	Urinary Albumin-Creatinine Ratio		Description
G1	>90 mL/min per 1.73 m²	Normal	A1	<30 mg/g	Normal or mild increase
G2	60–89 mL/min per 1.73 m²	Mild decrease	A2	30 to 299 mg/g	Moderate increase
G3a	45–59 mL/min per 1.73 m²	Mild to moderate decrease	A3	>300 mg/g	Severe increase
G3b	30–44 mL/min per 1.73 m²	Moderate to severe decrease			
G4	15–29 mL/min per 1.73 m²	Severe decrease			
G5	<15 mL/min per 1.73 m² or treatment by dialysis	Kidney failure			

- Edema is treated with diuretics, such as furosemide.
- Dialysis is rarely needed but must be considered in renal failure.

10.5F CHRONIC KIDNEY DISEASE

CKD is defined as the presence of kidney damage or an estimated GFR (eGFR) <60 mL/min/1.73 m^2, persisting for 3 months or more, irrespective of the etiology. It is progressive loss of renal function resulting in the need for renal replacement therapy. Renal damage consists of pathologic changes noted by imaging studies or biopsy, urinary sediment abnormalities, or increased urinary albumin excretion rates. The 2012 KDIGO CKD classification groups CKD into six categories based on GFR. Staging is also based on levels of albuminuria, with each stage of CKD being subcategorized according to the urinary albumin-creatinine ratio (ACR) in an early morning "spot" urine sample (Table 10.21).

The most common primary diseases causing CKD and ESRD are:

- Diabetes mellitus types 1 and 2
- Hypertension
- Primary GN
- Chronic TIN (CTIN)
- Hereditary or cystic diseases
- Secondary GN or vasculitis
- Plasma cell dyscrasias or neoplasm
- Sickle cell nephropathy

CKD may result from decreased renal perfusion pressure (prerenal); pathology of the vessels, glomeruli, or tubule-interstitium (renal); or obstructive (postrenal).

Decreased renal perfusion occurs in patients with chronic heart failure or cirrhosis; this increases the number of episodes of an intrinsic renal injury, such as ATN, and leads to progressive loss of renal function over time.

The most common renal cause involving vessels is nephrosclerosis. Nephrosclerosis leads to chronic damage to blood vessels, glomeruli, and tubule-interstitium. Another renal vascular disease is renal artery stenosis from atherosclerosis or fibromuscular dysplasia, leading to ischemic nephropathy; it is characterized by glomerulosclerosis and tubulointerstitial fibrosis.

Other causes include nephritic disorders, poststreptococcal GN, infective endocarditis, IgA nephropathy, lupus nephritis, Goodpasture syndrome, vasculitis, and nephrotic issues caused by minimal change disease, focal segmental glomerulosclerosis (FSGS), membranous GN, membranoproliferative GN, diabetic nephropathy, and amyloidosis.

The most common chronic tubulointerstitial disease is polycystic kidney disease (PKD). Other etiologies include nephrocalcinosis, sarcoidosis, Sjögren syndrome, and reflux nephropathy.

Chronic obstruction due to prostate disease, nephrolithiasis, or abdominal/pelvic tumor with mass effect on the ureters are possible etiologies.

MEDICAL HISTORY AND CLINICAL PRESENTATION

Early CKD stages are asymptomatic; symptoms typically manifest in stages 4 and 5. CKD is commonly detected by routine blood or urine testing. CKD can lead to multisystem failure and symptoms across a number of systems. Common signs and symptoms noted in stages 4 and 5 are described in Box 10.2.

PHYSICAL EXAMINATION

Physical examination is typically not helpful, but patients may have skin pigmentation, pericardial friction rub, uremic frost, and funduscopic changes due to underlying etiology.

DIAGNOSTIC STUDIES

When an eGFR of <60 mL/min/1.73 m^2 is noted it needs to be determined if this is due to AKI or CKD. Factors that increase the likelihood of CKD include a history of hypertension, diabetes, prostate disease; presence of skin pigmentation, left ventricular hypertrophy, or fundoscopic changes; abnormal PTH level; or patients with a BUN value >140 mg/dL or serum creatinine >13.5 mg/dL, who appears well and still passing normal volumes of urine.

BOX 10.2 Signs and Symptoms Noted in Chronic Kidney Disease

Nausea and vomiting	Muscle spasms
Loss of appetite	Peripheral edema
Fatigue and weakness	Pruritus
Sleep disturbances	Chest pain/uremic pericarditis
Oliguria	Shortness of breath
Change in mental status	Hypertension

If the distinction between AKI and CKD is unclear, renal function tests should be repeated in 2 weeks of the initial finding of an eGFR <60 mL/min/1.73 m^2. If previous tests confirm that the low eGFR is chronic or the repeat blood test results over 3 months are consistent, CKD is confirmed.

Proteinuria should be assessed by obtaining an early morning urine sample and quantifying ACR.

A renal ultrasound that shows small kidneys with reduced cortical thickness, increased echogenicity, scarring, or multiple cysts suggests chronic disease. Renal ultrasound with Doppler is obtained in suspected renal artery stenosis to evaluate vascular flow.

A low-dose or noncontrast CT is used to diagnose kidney stone disease and evaluate for possible ureteric obstruction.

Voiding cystourethrography is used to evaluate chronic vesicourethral reflux and is used to confirm the diagnosis and estimate the severity of reflux.

A kidney biopsy is used to diagnose the etiology of CKD and provides information regarding the extent of kidney fibrosis.

Urinalysis is of limited value in CKD. In ESRD waxy casts may be noted. Waxy casts are broad casts and develop secondary to urine stasis (Figure 10.4).

TREATMENT

- The best treatment of CKD is prevention.
  - Reversible causes of AKI, such as infection, medications, hypotension, and hypovolemia, should be identified and treated.
- In patients with CKD use of IV contrast studies and nephrotoxic agents such as aminoglycoside antibiotics and NSAIDs should be avoided.
- Factors that cause progression of CKD should be addressed and controlled, such as hypertension, proteinuria, metabolic acidosis, and hyperlipidemia. Hypertension should be managed by establishing BP goals. Other factors that can slow progression include protein restriction, bicarbonate supplements in chronic metabolic acidosis, and intensive blood glucose control.
- Once progression is noted, various options for renal replacement therapy should be considered. Indications for renal replacement therapy include:

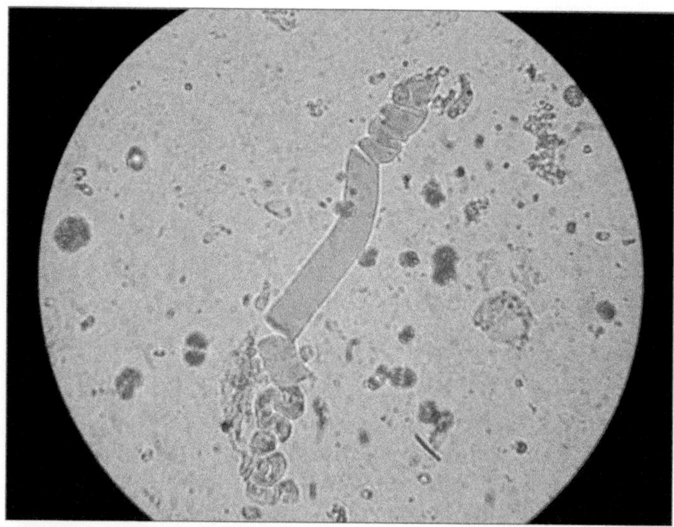

FIGURE 10.4 Waxy cast.
(Source: Jim Van Rhee.)

- Pericarditis or pleuritis (urgently needed)
- Progressive uremic encephalopathy or neuropathy, with confusion, asterixis, myoclonus, and seizures (urgently needed)
- Clinically significant bleeding diathesis attributable to uremia (urgently needed)
- Hypertension poorly responsive to antihypertensive medications
- Fluid overload refractory to diuretics
- Metabolic disorders refractory to medical therapy such as hyperkalemia, hyponatremia, metabolic acidosis, hypercalcemia, hypocalcemia, and hyperphosphatemia
- Persistent nausea and vomiting
- Evidence of malnutrition

- Renal transplantation is the best treatment option of ESRD; long-term survival is better when compared to long-term dialysis therapy. The patients with CKD become eligible for deceased donor renal transplant when the eGFR is <20 mL/min/1.73 m^2.
- Patients with CKD should be referred to a nephrologist when the estimated GFR is <30 mL/min/1.73 m^2.

PATIENT EDUCATION

- The KDOQI guidelines recommend screening high-risk populations including individuals with hypertension, those with diabetes mellitus, and those older than 65 years.
- Screening should include urinalysis, a urine ACR, measurement of serum creatinine, and estimation of GFR.

10.5G RENAL ARTERY STENOSIS

Renal artery stenosis is a decrease in blood flow through one or both renal arteries or their branches. Renal artery occlusion is the complete blockage of blood flow. Stenosis and occlusion are usually due to thromboemboli, atherosclerosis, or fibromuscular dysplasia. Progressive stenosis can cause refractory hypertension and lead to CKD. Renal artery stenosis is considered a disease of the older adult and most commonly affects patients with cardiovascular comorbidities or risks, including diabetes, coronary and peripheral vascular disease, dyslipidemia, hypertension, and smoking.

There are two main pathophysiologic processes in the development of renal artery stenosis. One is atherosclerosis; this progresses just as it does in cardiac or peripheral artery atherosclerosis. The lesions begin as smooth muscle and intimal thickening. Progression occurs with deposition of lipid and macrophages and progression to fibroatheromas. This process is commonly noted in men over 45 years of age. Lesions with >70% stenosis require further investigation and intervention.

Another pathophysiologic process is fibromuscular dysplasia. Fibromuscular dysplasia is due to hyperplasia of any of the vessel wall layers but is most frequently due to medial fibroplasia. This process is seen most often in women younger than 50 years of age.

Atherosclerotic renal artery stenosis affects 0.5% to 7% of the U.S. population over the age of 65 years.[19] It is present in about 5% of patients with CKD.[20] Stenosis may progress in up to half of patients within 2–5 years of diagnosis, but only a small percentage will progress to total occlusion.

MEDICAL HISTORY AND CLINICAL PRESENTATION

Important findings that should raise the suspicion of renal artery disease include:

- Resistant hypertension
- Reduction in eGFR
- Known generalized atherosclerosis

Symptoms of acute occlusion include steady, aching flank pain, abdominal pain, fever, nausea, vomiting, and hematuria.

PHYSICAL EXAMINATION

The patient with clinically significant renal artery stenosis has evidence of secondary hypertension in the setting of renal artery stenosis >70%. Occasionally a renal bruit can be heard.

DIFFERENTIAL DIAGNOSIS

In the patient with refractory or acutely increasing hypertension other causes of secondary hypertension should be considered. This includes pheochromocytoma, obstructive sleep apnea, primary hyperaldosteronism, Cushing syndrome, coarctation of the aorta, hypothyroidism, primary renal disease, and primary hyperparathyroidism.

DIAGNOSTIC STUDIES

The gold standard imaging study for renal artery stenosis is renal arteriography, which is an invasive procedure. Noninvasive imaging has improved; renal artery stenosis is now best diagnosed by noninvasive means.

Digital subtraction angiography is the standard in diagnostic imaging for fibromuscular dysplasia; medial fibroplasia has a typical string and bead appearance.

Magnetic resonance angiography (MRA) is first-line noninvasive screening tool followed by CT angiography in the diagnosis of atherosclerotic renal artery stenosis (Figure 10.5). Both are very specific but less sensitive in diagnosing fibromuscular dysplasia.

Duplex Doppler ultrasonography is another imaging study used to diagnose renal artery stenosis. Ultrasound not only aids in making the diagnosis but is used in calculating a resistive index that can be useful in predicting how a patient will respond to treatment.

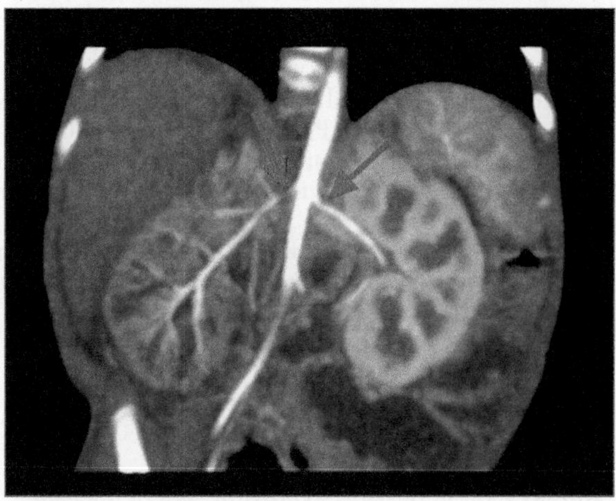

FIGURE 10.5 Renal artery stenosis—Contrast enhanced magnetic resonance angiography showed a high-grade stenosis of the proximal right renal artery.

(Source: Case courtesy of Dr. Roberto Schubert, Radiopaedia.org. https://radiopaedia.org/cases/renal-artery-stenosis-1?lang=us)

TREATMENT

- Medical management is the main treatment option in atherosclerosis renal artery stenosis or cases due to fibromuscular dysplasia.
- First-line medical management is BP control with the use of ACE inhibitors or ARBs.
  - Thiazide diuretics may provide control if the hypertension is due to a hyperactive renin-angiotensin axis and to salt and water retention.
  - Calcium channel blockers and beta blockers should be used for BP control in patients who cannot take or tolerate ACE inhibitors, ARBs, or thiazide diuretics.
- Intervention may be performed if medical management is not effective.
  - A percutaneous transluminal angiography (PTA) with stent placement can help control BP and stabilize or improve renal function.
  - PTA with stent placement should be considered in patients who have a hemodynamically significant lesion, refractory or malignant hypertension uncontrolled with medication, or recurrent episodes of acute pulmonary edema.
  - Patients with fibromuscular dysplasia are often managed with angioplasty without stenting.

PATIENT EDUCATION

- Modification of atherosclerosis risk factors is key to prevention of renal artery stenosis.

10.5H NEPHROTIC SYNDROME

Nephrotic syndrome is caused by a variety of diseases that cause a decrease in the kidney ability to prevent loss of proteins into the filtrate. This leads to protein wasting in the urine and the development of nephrotic syndrome.

Nephrotic syndrome is characterized by the following:

- **Proteinuria:** >3 g in 24 hours or spot urine protein/creatinine ratio >3.5 mg protein/g creatinine
- **Hypoalbuminemia:** Serum albumin <3 g/dL
- **Hyperlipidemia:** Total cholesterol level usually >300 mg/dL

Nephrotic syndrome affects both children and adults.

The pathophysiology of hypoalbuminemia in nephrotic syndrome is multifactorial. Proteinuria plays a role in the pathogenesis of hyperlipidemia. Neurohormonal changes in the RAAS, vasopressin, and sympathetic nervous system are factors in edema formation.

Proteinuria occurs because of changes to capillary endothelial cells and the glomerular basement membrane (GBM), which filter serum protein based on size and charge.

The most common causes are noted in Table 10.22.

TABLE 10.22 Etiologies of Nephrotic Syndrome

Primary	Secondary
Minimal change disease	Diabetic nephropathy
Focal segmental glomerulosclerosis	Amyloidosis
Membranous nephropathy	HIV-associated nephropathy
	Preeclampsia

MEDICAL HISTORY AND CLINICAL PRESENTATION

The hallmark of nephrotic syndrome is edema. The past medical history should be reviewed for a history of renal disease, diabetes mellitus, amyloidosis, HIV, myeloma, lymphoma, and systemic lupus erythematosus (SLE). Medication history should be reviewed for renal toxic drugs, such as NSAIDs, interferons, bisphosphonates, lithium, gold, or penicillamine.

The most common symptoms of nephrotic syndrome include volume overload suggested by presence of edema in the lower extremities, ascites, anasarca, dyspnea, and weight gain; foamy urine due to proteinuria; and fatigue.

PHYSICAL EXAMINATION

Several physical examination findings are diagnostic for nephrotic syndrome. With increasing protein loss in the urine, physical exam findings include diffuse edema including periorbital muscle mass loss and Muehrcke lines on the fingernails.

DIAGNOSTIC STUDIES

The diagnosis of nephrotic syndrome is made by the presence of significant proteinuria, defined as >3.0 g in 24 hours or spot urine protein/creatinine ratio >3.5 mg protein/g creatinine. Urinalysis may reveal oval fat bodies and fatty casts; plain microscopy oval fat bodies can be identified by the appearance of Maltese crosses under polarized light or Sudan orange stain.

Measurement of serum creatinine to assess the degree of renal impairment, serum albumin, and total cholesterol are required.

Other laboratory studies may be indicated based on possible secondary etiologies. This includes ANA and complement levels to help in the diagnosis of SLE; hemoglobin A1c for the diagnosis of diabetes; hepatitis B and C serologies with serum cryoglobulins for the diagnosis of an underlying hepatitis; and serum and urine protein electrophoresis for the diagnosis of multiple myeloma and possibly amyloidosis.

Renal biopsy is indicated in adults to diagnose the etiology of idiopathic nephrotic syndrome. In idiopathic nephrotic syndrome in children it is assumed the etiology is minimal change disease and biopsy is indicated only if the patient fails to improve with a trial of corticosteroids.

TREATMENT

- Treatment should focus on treating the underlying processes and prevention of complications.
- ACE inhibitors or angiotensin II receptor antagonists lower intraglomerular pressures and reduce protein excretion, slowing the progression of disease.
- In minimal change disease, steroids may be beneficial.
- FSGS has a high recurrence rate and progression to ESRD and these patients benefit from steroids and immunosuppression.

PATIENT EDUCATION

- Complications of nephrotic syndrome include infections, thrombotic events, and renal failure.
- Prognosis of nephrotic syndrome is highly dependent on the underlying etiology.

10.5I NEPHROPATHY

Diabetic nephropathy (DN) is characterized by persistent albuminuria, a decline in the GFR, and an increase in arterial BP. Persistent albuminuria (>300 mg/24 hours) in at least two of three consecutive nonketotic urine samples is the hallmark of DN.

DN is the most common cause of nephrotic syndrome in adults and the most common cause of ESRD in the United States.[21] Other risk factors include the duration and degree of hyperglycemia, hypertension, dyslipidemia, smoking, and family history of DN. DN often develops <10 years after the diagnosis of diabetes and renal failure typically develops more than 10 years after the onset of nephropathy.

In the United Kingdom Prospective Diabetes Study (UKPDS), the risk of a patient with type 2 diabetes progressing to microalbuminuria was 2% per year, risk of progressing to macroalbuminuria was 2.8% per year, and the risk of macroalbuminuria to elevated creatinine level was 2.3% per year.[22]

In diabetes mellitus type 1, hypertension is caused by the underlying DN and manifests around the time of the development of microalbuminuria. In diabetes mellitus type 2, hypertension is present at the time of diagnosis in about one third of patients.

The mechanism of hypertension in DN involves excess sodium retention, activation of the sympathetic nervous system, RAAS, endothelial cell dysfunction, and increased oxidative stress. As a result, there is an increase in plasma volume, increase in peripheral vascular resistance, and low renin activity.

Microalbuminuria is usually the first manifestation of DN and progresses gradually over years to overt nephropathy in two-thirds of the patients.

Long-standing hyperglycemia is a significant risk factor for development of DN. Hyperglycemia leads to mesangial expansion, injury, and the development of nephropathy.

MEDICAL HISTORY AND CLINICAL PRESENTATION

Patients with DN can develop the signs and symptoms associated with renal failure, such as edema and weight gain.

Proteinuria in diabetes is occasionally due to a glomerular disease other than DN. Clinical clues suggesting nondiabetic glomerular disease include:

- Significant proteinuria without a long history of diabetes
- No signs of end-organ damage such as retinopathy or neuropathy
- Acute onset of renal disease or nephrotic syndrome
- Presence of active urinary sediment containing red blood cells and cellular casts
- Rapidly rising urinary protein level, or rapidly declining GFR

PHYSICAL EXAMINATION

Most patients are asymptomatic. Peripheral edema may be the first symptom of DN. Fluid retention may be present even with preserved renal function and a slight reduction in serum albumin.

DIFFERENTIAL DIAGNOSIS

The differential diagnosis of nephropathy in a patient with diabetes who has albuminuria and/or renal dysfunction includes:

- Nephrosclerosis
- Renal artery stenosis with/without renovascular hypertension
- Primary or secondary glomerular disease
- Interstitial nephritis
- Amyloidosis
- Chronic urinary obstruction

DIAGNOSTIC STUDIES

Screening and prevention are key in controlling the development of DN. Screening for microalbuminuria should be performed annually in patients with diabetes mellitus type 1 with duration of disease >5 years and in all type 2 diabetics starting at the time of diagnosis.

Urinary albumin can be checked by one of the following:

- Albumin/creatinine ratio on a spot urine sample
- 24-hour urine collection
- Timed urine collections

Normal albumin excretion on a spot collection should be <30 mcg/mg. Microalbuminuria is 30 to 299 mcg/mg, while macroalbuminuria is >300 mcg/mg. With a 24-hour urine collection, normal is <30 mg, microalbuminuria is defined as 30 to 300 mg, and macroalbuminuria is defined as >300 mg.

Transient elevations in urinary albumin excretion can be seen in hyperglycemia, exercise, urinary tract infections, marked hypertension, heart failure, and acute febrile illness.

Diagnosis of DN is based on detection of proteinuria. Patients may also have concurrent hypertension and retinopathy. The diagnosis is established by the following:

- Determination of albuminuria or proteinuria
- BP measurement
- Serum creatinine concentration and measurement or estimation of GFR
- Renal ultrasound
- Ophthalmologic examination

If proteinuria is confirmed it needs to be quantitated. If the patient has typical DN, with type 1 diabetes for >10 years, retinopathy, prior microalbuminuria, no hematuria or red blood cell casts, and normal renal ultrasound; then no further workup is required. If there is no retinopathy, proteinuria without progression through microalbuminuria or has macroscopic hematuria or red blood cell casts, the patient needs to be evaluated further.

A renal ultrasound is obtained to evaluate kidney size. Early in DN the kidney may be enlarged because of hyperfiltration. With progression of diabetic renal disease, the kidney size often decreases because of glomerulosclerosis. It also aids in evaluating the possibility of outlet obstruction as a cause of renal dysfunction.

A renal biopsy may be indicated in the diabetic patient if the following are present:

1. Retinopathy is not present in the type 1 diabetic patient.

2. There is sudden or rapid onset of proteinuria, especially in type 1 diabetic and duration of disease is <5 years or if evolution is atypical.
3. Active urinary sediment or macroscopic hematuria is noted.
4. There is rapid decline of renal function or renal dysfunction without significant proteinuria.

TREATMENT

- Blood glucose and BP control play a significant role in prevention and preventing progression of DN.
- Lifestyle modifications play a central role in managing these patients.
  - Smoking: Increases risk and progression of DN; there is a 1.6-fold increased risk of DN among smokers.
  - Hyperlipidemia: Control of lipids is important because of increased risk of coronary artery disease.
  - Weight reduction: Weight loss can decrease proteinuria; body mass index should be between 18 and 25 kg/m^2.
  - DASH diet plan: Diet should contain increased amount of fruits, vegetables, and low-fat dairy products.
  - Physical activity: At least 30 minutes of aerobic physical activity, most days of the week is recommended.
  - Dietary sodium reduction: Lower sodium intake to <2.4 g sodium.
- The Diabetes Control and Complications Trial has shown that intensive blood glucose control can significantly reduce the risk of developing microalbuminuria and overt macroalbuminuria.[23] Hb A1c of <7% is recommended by ADA guidelines.
- Most sulfonylurea compounds accumulate in renal failure, except glimepiride and gliquidone. Metformin should be discontinued when creatinine is >1.5 mg/dL in males and >1.4 mg/dL in females.
- Recently published guidelines by the American Heart Association and American College of Cardiology recommend a target BP of <130/80 mm Hg in patients with diabetes.[24]
  - The therapy goal is the treatment of hypertension and reduction of proteinuria.
  - After lifestyle modifications, the use of ACEIs or ARBs has become the standard of care in patients with DN.

PATIENT EDUCATION

- If untreated, DN can progress to ESRD.
- The main trigger of DN is hyperglycemia.
- In patients with diabetes mellitus, the main risk factor for coronary artery disease is nephropathy.

10.5J CHRONIC TUBULOINTERSTITIAL DISEASE

CTIN develops when chronic tubular insults cause interstitial infiltration and fibrosis, tubular atrophy and dysfunction, and a gradual deterioration of renal function. Concurrent glomerular involvement (glomerulosclerosis) is more common in CTIN than in acute TIN (ATIN).

The most common causes of CTIN are obstructive uropathy, reflux nephropathy from vesicoureteral reflux, analgesic nephropathy, and heavy metal exposure.

TABLE 10.23 Etiologies of Chronic Tubulointerstitial Nephritis

Etiology	Signs/Symptoms	Laboratory Results
Obstructive uropathy	Polyuria or oliguria; hypertension	Urinalysis—normal or hematuria with pyuria; ultrasound may reveal mass lesions and hydronephrosis
Vesicoureteral reflux	Noted in young children with history of urinary tract infections	Ultrasound may reveal renal scarring and hydronephrosis
Analgesic nephropathy	History of using phenacetin, paracetamol, aspirin, and nonsteroidal anti-inflammatory drugs (NSAIDs); present with hematuria	Urinalysis may reveal blood, protein, and white blood cells
Heavy metals	History of exposure to lead, cadmium, mercury, and bismuth; hypertension; gout due to decreased secretion of uric acid	

MEDICAL HISTORY AND CLINICAL PRESENTATION

Polyuria is common due to tubular damage and inability to concentrate the urine.

Symptoms and signs are generally absent in CTIN unless renal failure develops and vary with underlying etiology. See Table 10.23 for summary of the various etiologies. Edema usually is not present, and BP is normal or only mildly elevated in the early stages.

DIAGNOSTIC STUDIES

Because CTIN is insidious in onset and interstitial fibrosis is common, imaging tests may show small kidneys with evidence of scarring and asymmetry.

Hyperkalemia may be noted, and proteinuria is typically <2 g/day.

Renal biopsy is rarely used for diagnostic purposes but may help characterize the nature and progression of disease. Glomeruli may be normal or destroyed. Tubules may be absent or atrophied. Tubular lumina will vary in diameter and show dilation. Grossly, the kidneys are small and atrophic.

TREATMENT

- Treatment of CTIN requires treating the underlying etiology and supportive measures such as controlling BP and treating anemia associated with kidney disease.
- In patients with CTIN and progressive renal injury, ACE inhibitors or angiotensin II receptor blockers may slow disease progression.

PATIENT EDUCATION

- Prognosis depends on identifying the etiology and stopping the process before irreversible fibrosis occurs.

10.5K POLYCYSTIC KIDNEY

PKD is an autosomal dominant hereditary disorder of cyst formation causing enlargement of the kidneys, with possible progression to renal failure. Autosomal dominant PKD (ADPKD) has an incidence of 1 in 1,000 and accounts for about 5% of patients with ESRD.[25]

Autosomal recessive PKD is very rare; incidence is 1 in 20,000 and frequently causes renal failure during childhood.[26]

In 78% of cases, ADPKD is caused by mutations in the *ADPKD1* gene on chromosome 16; other cases are caused by mutations in the *ADPKD2* gene on chromosome 4.[27] A few familial cases are unrelated to either locus.

MEDICAL HISTORY AND CLINICAL PRESENTATION

ADPKD disease typically causes no symptoms; half of patients remain asymptomatic, never develop renal insufficiency or failure, and are never diagnosed. Most patients who develop symptoms do so by the age of 30.

Symptoms include low-grade flank, abdominal, and lower back pain due to cystic enlargement and symptoms of urinary tract infection or nephrolithiasis. Acute pain is usually due to hemorrhage into cysts or passage of a calculus. Fever is common with acute infection, and rupture of cysts into the retroperitoneal space may cause a fever that can last for weeks.

Signs are nonspecific and include hematuria and hypertension.

PHYSICAL EXAMINATION

An abdominal mass may be noted, and kidneys may be palpable. Up to half of patients have concurrent cysts elsewhere in the body including the liver, pancreas, spleen, and cerebral aneurysms.

DIFFERENTIAL DIAGNOSIS

The differential diagnosis includes simple renal cysts, acquired renal cysts, and medullary sponge kidney. See Table 10.24.

DIAGNOSTIC STUDIES

Diagnosis is made by imaging that reveals extensive and bilateral cystic changes throughout the kidneys. The kidneys are enlarged and have a moth-eaten appearance due to displacement of normal tissue by the cysts.

Ultrasonography is the test of choice. If ultrasonography results are inconclusive, CT or MRI is obtained. MRI is especially useful for measuring cyst and kidney volume.

Urinalysis, BUN, creatinine, and complete blood count (CBC) should be obtained. Urinalysis detects proteinuria and microscopic or macroscopic hematuria. Gross hematuria may be due to the presence of a nephrolithiasis or hemorrhage from a ruptured cyst. Pyuria is common even without bacterial infection; diagnosis of a urinary tract infection should be based on culture results and clinical findings as well as urinalysis. Early in disease the BUN and creatinine are normal or only mildly elevated; they will increase over time, especially in the presence of hypertension. Polycythemia may be noted on CBC.

Patients with cerebral aneurysm require high-resolution CT or MRA. Routine screening for cerebral aneurysm in asymptomatic patients is not recommended. Patients with a family history of hemorrhagic stroke or cerebral aneurysm and ADPKD should be screened for cerebral aneurysm.

Genetic testing for PKD mutations is currently reserved for the following patients:

- Suspected PKD and no known family history
- Inconclusive imaging findings
- Under age 30 with inconclusive imaging results in whom the diagnosis must be made

Genetic counseling is recommended for first-degree relatives of patients with ADPKD.

TREATMENT

- Strict BP control is key.
  - First-line treatment is an ACE inhibitor or ARB. These medications will block angiotensin and aldosterone, growth factors that contribute to renal scarring and loss of renal function.
  - Urinary tract infection should be treated promptly.
  - Aspiration of cysts may relieve severe pain due to hemorrhage or compression but have no long-term effect.
  - Nephrectomy is an option to relieve severe symptoms due to massive kidney enlargement or recurrent urinary tract infections.
- Hemodialysis or kidney transplant is required in patients who develop chronic renal failure.
- Supportive measures include increased fluid intake to suppress vasopressin release.

TABLE 10.24 Differential Diagnosis of Renal Cysts

	Simple Renal Cysts	Acquired Renal Cysts	Autosomal Dominant Polycystic Kidney Disease (ADPKD)	Medullary Sponge Kidney
Prevalence	Common	Noted in dialysis patients	1:1,000	1:5,000
Genetics	None	None	Autosomal dominant	None
Kidney size	Normal	Small	Large	Normal
Cyst location	Cortex and medulla	Cortex and medulla	Cortex and medulla	Collecting ducts
Hematuria	Occasional	Occasional	Common	Rare
Hypertension	No	Varies	Common	No
Renal failure	Never	Always	Frequently	Never

- Tolvaptan, a vasopressin receptor 2 antagonist, slows the increase in kidney volume and decline in renal function. Adverse effects include increase thirst, polydipsia, and polyuria.

PATIENT EDUCATION

- By age 75, over 50% of patients with ADPKD require renal replacement therapy.
- On average, GFR declines by 5 mL/min/year after the fourth decade of life.[28]

10.5L HYDRONEPHROSIS

Hydronephrosis is the enlargement of the kidney and caused by conditions that obstruct urine outflow. The most common causes are nephrolithiasis, vesicoureteral reflux, renal cancer, prostatic hypertrophy and cancer, blood clots, and external compression from pelvic or abdominal masses.

MEDICAL HISTORY AND CLINICAL PRESENTATION

Most patients with hydronephrosis are asymptomatic. The most common symptoms are changes in urine flow, flank pain, hematuria, urge or difficulty urinating, weak urine stream, and hypertension.

The patient's history may be positive for kidney stones, congenital abnormalities, cancer, and prostate enlargement.

PHYSICAL EXAMINATION

Physical examination is typically normal, but the examiner may note pain at the site of the obstruction. Other possible findings include abdominal distention along with a palpable kidney, costovertebral angle tenderness, and a palpable bladder.

DIFFERENTIAL DIAGNOSIS

The differential diagnosis includes pelvic cysts, pyelonephritis, ovarian cysts, and pelvic tumors.

DIAGNOSTIC STUDIES

Patients with hydronephrosis may have an elevated white blood cell count and pyuria if infection is present. The presence of a postrenal azotemia may be noted with an elevated serum creatinine and BUN.

The diagnostic test of choice is the renal ultrasound. Findings on renal ultrasound include:

- Hypoechoic fluid displacing echogenic sinus fat
- Dilation of the proximal renal pelvis due to obstruction
- Dilation of the renal pelvis and calyces due to obstruction
- Thinning of the renal cortex

TREATMENT

- The goal of treatment is to start the flow of urine from the kidney and decrease the swelling and pressure in the kidney and improve renal function.
- Options to improve urine flow include bladder catherization, urethral stenting, pyeloplasty, percutaneous nephrostomy, and percutaneous ureterostomy.
- Treatment of the underlying etiology should be undertaken.

PATIENT EDUCATION

- If left untreated, the kidneys may scar, leading to kidney failure.
- Complications include infections, electrolyte abnormalities, hypertension, and renal insufficiency/failure.
- Prognosis is excellent with a majority of patients recovering.

10.5M RHABDOMYOLYSIS

OVERVIEW

Rhabdomyolysis is a syndrome involving the breakdown of skeletal muscle tissue. Symptoms and signs include muscle weakness, myalgias, and reddish brown urine. Diagnosis is made by history and laboratory findings of an elevated creatine kinase (CK), usually five times greater than the upper limit of normal. Treatment is supportive with IV fluids as well as treatment of the underlying etiology and any complications.

With the breakdown of skeletal muscle, there is release of muscle contents into the circulation. The substances released include CK, myoglobin, the transferases, and electrolytes including potassium. Key causes of rhabdomyolysis include drug-induced, crush injuries, extreme exertion, ischemia, and infections.

When skeletal muscle is broken down there is release of myoglobin. Myoglobin precipitates in the renal tubules leading direct nephrotoxicity and AKI. Renal vasoconstriction can also develop leading to worsening of AKI. AKI is the most serious complications of rhabdomyolysis.

MEDICAL HISTORY AND CLINICAL PRESENTATION

The classic triad of rhabdomyolysis is muscle pain, weakness, and dark-colored urine. Most common is muscle pain. Nonspecific systemic signs and symptoms include malaise, fever, and tachycardia.

Rhabdomyolysis is divided into several categories. These categories should be evaluated in the medical history.

- Drugs and toxins including statins, fibrates, alcohol, and cocaine
- History of traumatic or crush injuries
- Hypoxic from arterial thrombosis, recent procedure with clamping of vessel, or extended immobility
- Exertional from marathon running, intense exercise, or seizure
- Infections with influenza, coxsackievirus, and HIV
- Body temperature extremes such as with heat stroke, malignant hyperthermia, and neuroleptic malignant syndrome
- Metabolic and electrolyte disorders including hypokalemia, hypophosphatemia, and diabetic ketoacidosis
- Others including the inflammatory myopathies, compartment syndrome, and electrical injuries

SIGNS AND SYMPTOMS

Common presenting signs and symptoms are muscle pain, tenderness, and weakness. Nonspecific symptoms include fever and malaise. Patients may note dark-colored urine due to the presence of myoglobin in the urine.

PHYSICAL EXAMINATION

Physical examination findings include muscle pain and weakness. Other findings include fever and tachycardia.

DIFFERENTIAL DIAGNOSIS

The differential diagnosis varies depending on the presentation. The differential diagnosis for the presentation of red-brown urine includes hematuria, hemolysis, renal colic, and various medications. The differential diagnosis for muscle pain includes inflammatory myopathies and immune-mediated necrotizing myopathy. Elevated CK is noted in any condition that causes damage to cardiac or skeletal muscle.

The classic combination of myalgias, elevated CK, and myoglobinuria makes rhabdomyolysis very likely.

DIAGNOSTIC STUDIES

CK is the key laboratory marker used in diagnosing rhabdomyolysis, though it can also be elevated in conditions that cause damage to cardiac muscle. The CK is typically >1,000 U/L.

Other laboratory tests that are elevated in rhabdomyolysis include the alanine aminotransferase (ALT) and aspartate aminotransferase (AST).

Urine tests are useful in diagnosing rhabdomyolysis. A dipstick positive for blood, in the absence of hematuria on urine microscopy, suggests rhabdomyolysis. Pigmented finely granular casts may be seen in rhabdomyolysis.

Imaging is not needed except in cases of possible compartment syndrome.

TREATMENT

- The key to management of rhabdomyolysis is IV hydration. IV hydration works by diluting out the nephrotoxic myoglobin and replacing the fluid deficit. Fluids should be administered at 400–500 mL/hour to maintain a urine output of about 250 mL/hour. Potassium supplements should not be given as patients are already at a risk for hyperkalemia.
    - In patients with markedly elevated CK and a urine pH <7.5, the use of bicarbonate-containing fluids alternating with normal saline should be considered.
- Loop diuretics, such as furosemide, are not indicated unless fluid overload is present. Loop diuretics may lead to hypocalcemia.
- Hemodialysis may be needed to control volume overload, hyperkalemia, acidosis, and uremia.

PATIENT EDUCATION

- AKI is reported in 33% to 50% of rhabdomyolysis complications.[1]

SPECIAL CONSIDERATIONS

- Nephrotic syndrome is common in young children, usually idiopathic, and most often due to minimal change disease. Consider nephrotic syndrome in young children with unexplained edema or ascites.
- Assume minimal change disease if a child with idiopathic nephrotic syndrome improves after treatment with corticosteroids.

KEY POINTS

- Causes of AKI can be kidney hypoperfusion (prerenal), direct effects on the kidney (renal), or urinary tract obstruction (postrenal).
- With AKI, consider ECF volume depletion and nephrotoxins, obtain urinary diagnostic indices, and measure bladder residual volume to identify obstruction.
- ATN can develop after various disorders or triggers decrease renal perfusion or expose the kidneys to toxins.
- Differentiate ATN from prerenal azotemia by the response to volume expansion and by urine and blood chemistry tests and calculations derived from them.
- Confirm nephrotic syndrome by finding spot protein/creatinine ratio ≥3 or urinary protein ≥3 g/24 hours.
- CKD is defined as kidney damage or an eGFR <60 mL/min/1.73 m^2 persisting for 3 months or more irrespective of the cause.
- CKD is usually asymptomatic till stages IV and V.
- Renal artery stenosis or occlusion may be acute, due to thromboembolism, or chronic, due to atherosclerosis or fibromuscular dysplasia.
- Confirm nephrotic syndrome by finding spot protein/creatinine ratio ≥3 or urinary protein ≥3 g/24 hours.
- DN is very common, asymptomatic until late, and should be considered in all patients with diabetes. Periodically screen all patients with diabetes with urinalysis and, if proteinuria is absent, albumin/creatinine ratio calculated from a midmorning urine specimen.
- ADPKD occurs in about 1 in 1,000 people.
- Do not routinely screen asymptomatic patients for ADPKD or asymptomatic patients who have ADPKD for cerebral aneurysms.
- The classic triad of rhabdomyolysis symptoms (myalgias, muscle weakness, and tea-colored urine) is present in <10% of cases.
- A CK level more than five times the upper limit of normal is typically required for rhabdomyolysis diagnosis.
- Rhabdomyolysis treatment is supportive with IV hydration as well as concurrent treatment of the inciting cause and any resulting complications.

COMMON CHIEF COMPLAINTS

APPROACH TO ACID-BASE DISORDERS

Acid-base disorders can be complex and difficult to understand. This section will not include a review of the underlying pathophysiology of acid-base disorders but will focus on the approach. See earlier sections of this chapter on the various etiologies of the acid-base disorders. A patient can have a mixed acid-base disorder and have more than one acid-base disorder at a time.

The first step in the evaluation of arterial blood gases (see Figure 10.6) is to identify the primary acid base disorder.

1. Look at the pH. Whatever side of 7.40 the pH is, the process or processes that caused it to shift in this direction are the primary abnormalities. If the pH is <7.40, then an elevated Pco_2 means a respiratory acidosis; if there is a decreased bicarbonate this means a metabolic acidosis. If the pH is >7.40, then a decreased Pco_2 means a respiratory alkalosis; if there is an elevated bicarbonate this means a metabolic acidosis. Remember that the body does not fully compensate even for a chronic acid-base disorder. Over time the pH will improve but not return to normal. See Table 10.25 for a summary.

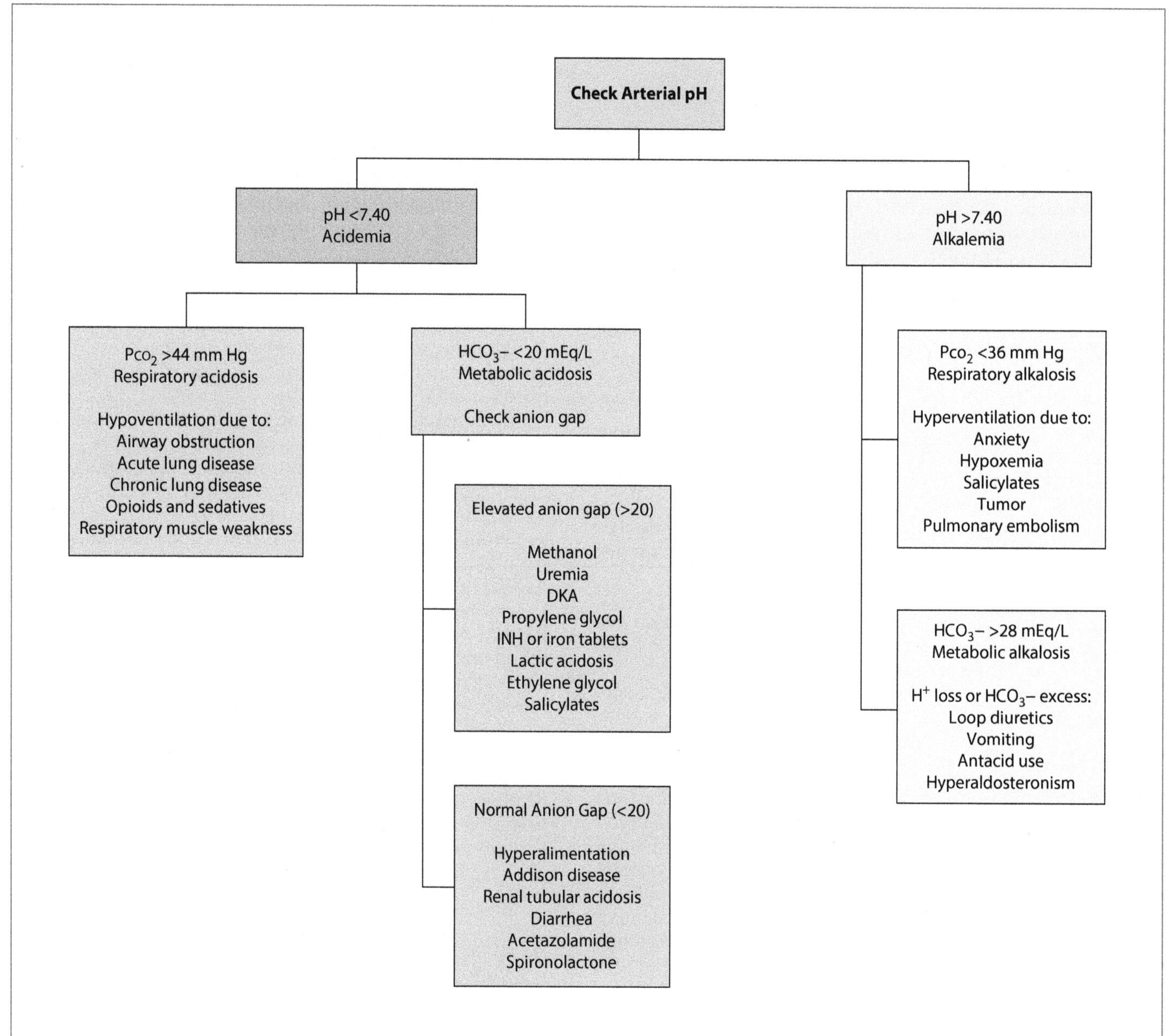

FIGURE 10.6 **Approach to simple acid-base disorders.** DKA, diabetic ketoacidosis; INH, isoniazid.

2. The second step is to calculate the anion gap. See below for anion gap formula.

$$\text{Anion gap} = Na^+ - (Cl^- + HCO_3^-)$$

3. If the anion gap is >20 then an elevated anion gap metabolic acidosis is present regardless of the pH or serum bicarbonate concentration. This increased anion gap is not compensation for an alkalosis. The body does

TABLE 10.25 Primary Acid-Base Disorders

	Primary Disorder	Normal Range (Arterial)	Primary Disorder
pH	Acidemia	7.40	Alkalemia
Pco_2 (mm Hg)	Respiratory alkalosis	35–45	Respiratory acidosis
Bicarbonate (mEq/L)	Metabolic acidosis	22–26	Metabolic alkalosis

not generate a large anion gap to correct a chronic alkalosis.

The third step is to calculate the excess anion gap. See below for formula.

Excess anion gap = (Calculated anion gap − a normal anion gap of 12) + Measured bicarbonate

If the excess anion gap is >30 there is an underlying metabolic alkalosis and if the excess anion gap is <23 there is underlying normal anion gap metabolic acidosis. The basis for this is that for each mmol of acid titrated by the buffer system 1 mmol of bicarbonate is lost. For each mmol decrease in bicarbonate there is a mmol increase in anion gap. In a normal situation, the excess anion gap and the measured bicarbonate should be equal to a normal bicarbonate. If the excess anion gap is greater than a normal bicarbonate (>30) then another disorder, metabolic alkalosis, has added bicarbonate to the extracellular space. If the excess anion gap is less than a normal bicarbonate (<23), then an additional process, a non-anion gap metabolic acidosis, is causing gastrointestinal or renal loss of bicarbonate. See Table 10.26 for a summary.

APPROACH TO SODIUM DISORDERS

Evaluating the patient with hypo- or hypernatremia requires a focused approach. The first step is to assess the level of severity and the sodium level trend over time. This is important in determining possible etiologies and how emergent treatment should be started.

The next step is to determine the patient's clinical status. Is the patient hypovolemic, euvolemic, or hypervolemic? Are there symptoms related to the sodium abnormality?

TABLE 10.26 Acid-Base Interpretation Summary

Step 1	Look at pH. Whatever side of 7.40 the pH is on, this is the cause of the primary disorder.
Step 2	Calculate anion gap. If the anion gap is >20, there is a primary elevated anion gap metabolic acidosis. This is true regardless of pH or bicarbonate level.
Step 3	Calculate the excess anion gap. If the value is >30 there is an underlying metabolic alkalosis and if the value is <23 there is an underlying non-anion gap metabolic acidosis.

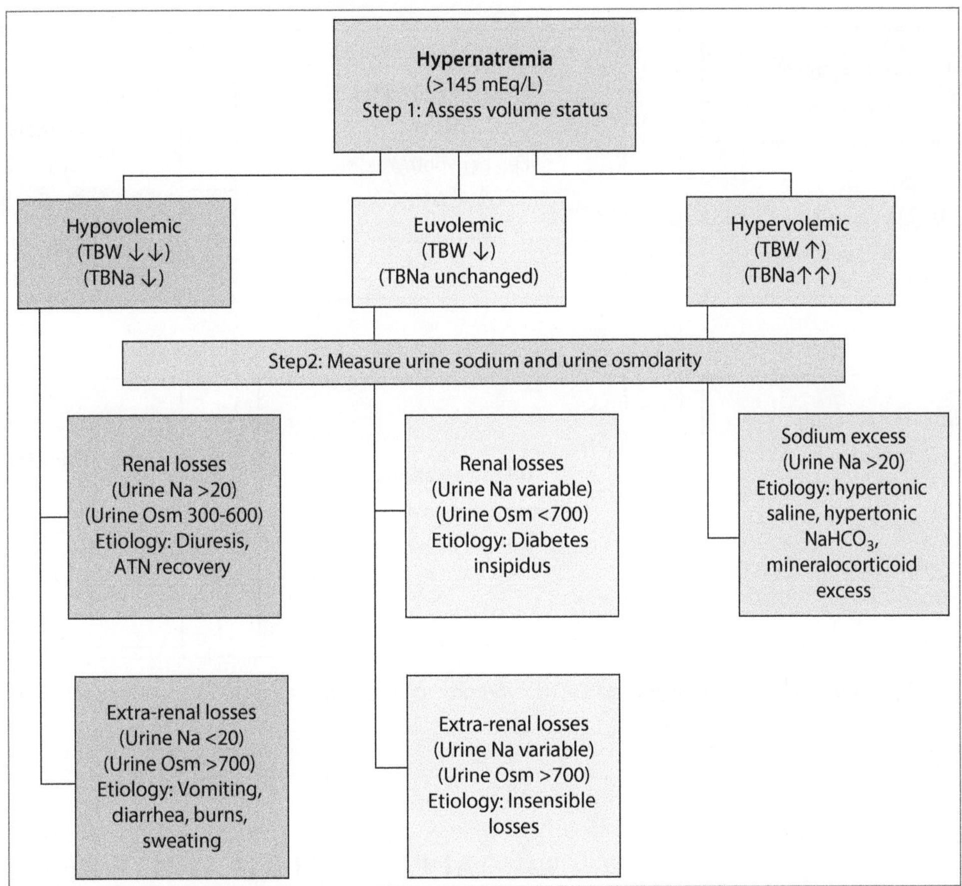

FIGURE 10.7 **Approach to hypernatremia.** ATN, acute tubular necrosis; TBW, total body water; TBNa, total body sodium.

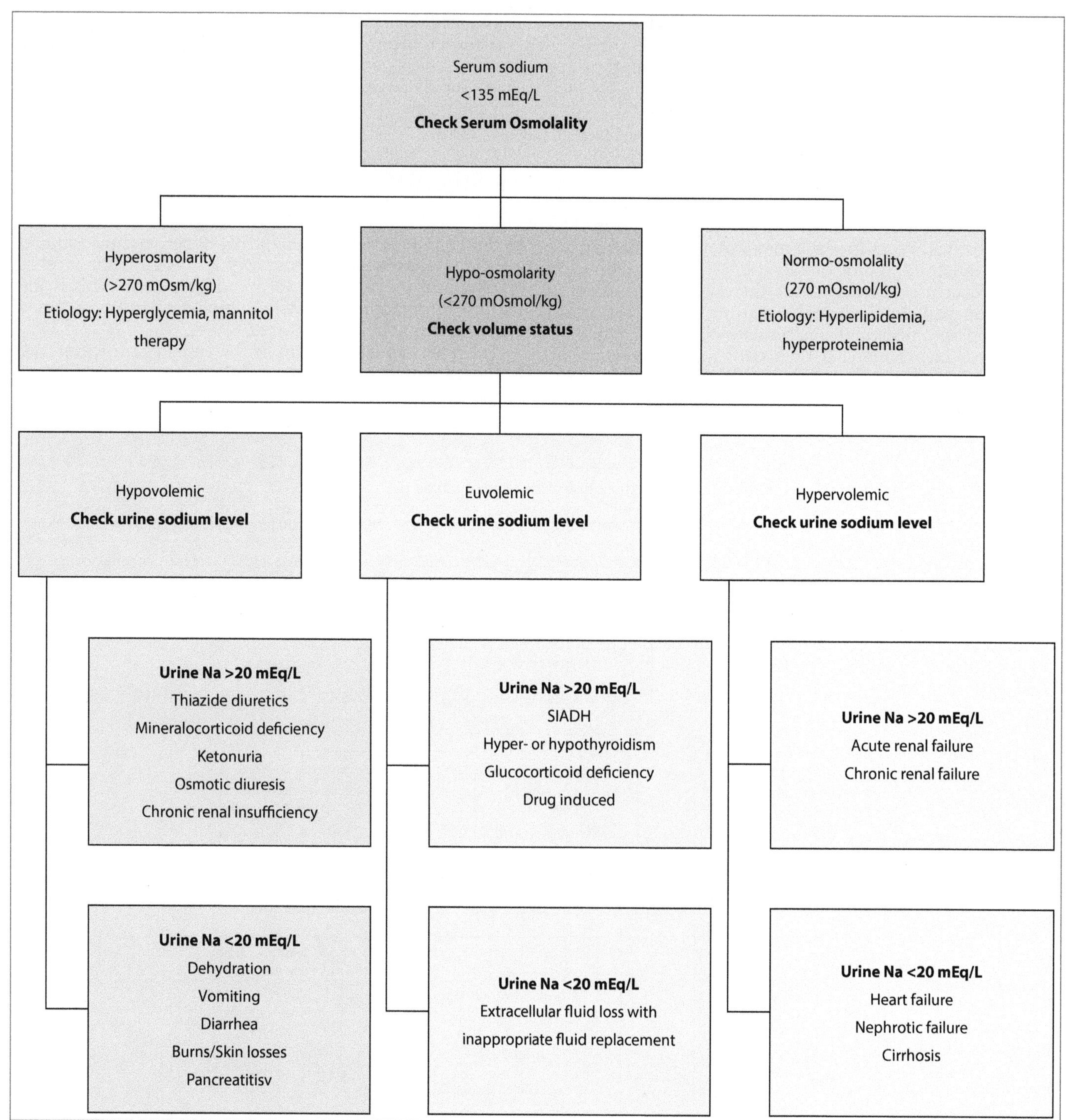

FIGURE 10.8 **Approach to hyponatremia.** SIADH, syndrome of inappropriate secretion of antidiuretic hormone.

This is followed by a detailed medication history. Diuretics and SSRIs can lead to hyponatremia, while loop diuretics and lithium can cause hypernatremia.

After evaluating fluid status and obtaining a history, the laboratory evaluation should include a urine sodium and urine osmolarity. See Figure 10.7 for the evaluation of hypernatremia and Figure 10.8 for the evaluation of hyponatremia.

APPROACH TO ACUTE RENAL INJURY

AKI can be due to multiple etiologies. Determining the etiology is essential to guide management. AKI is typically divided into prerenal, renal, and postrenal to narrow down the differential diagnosis.

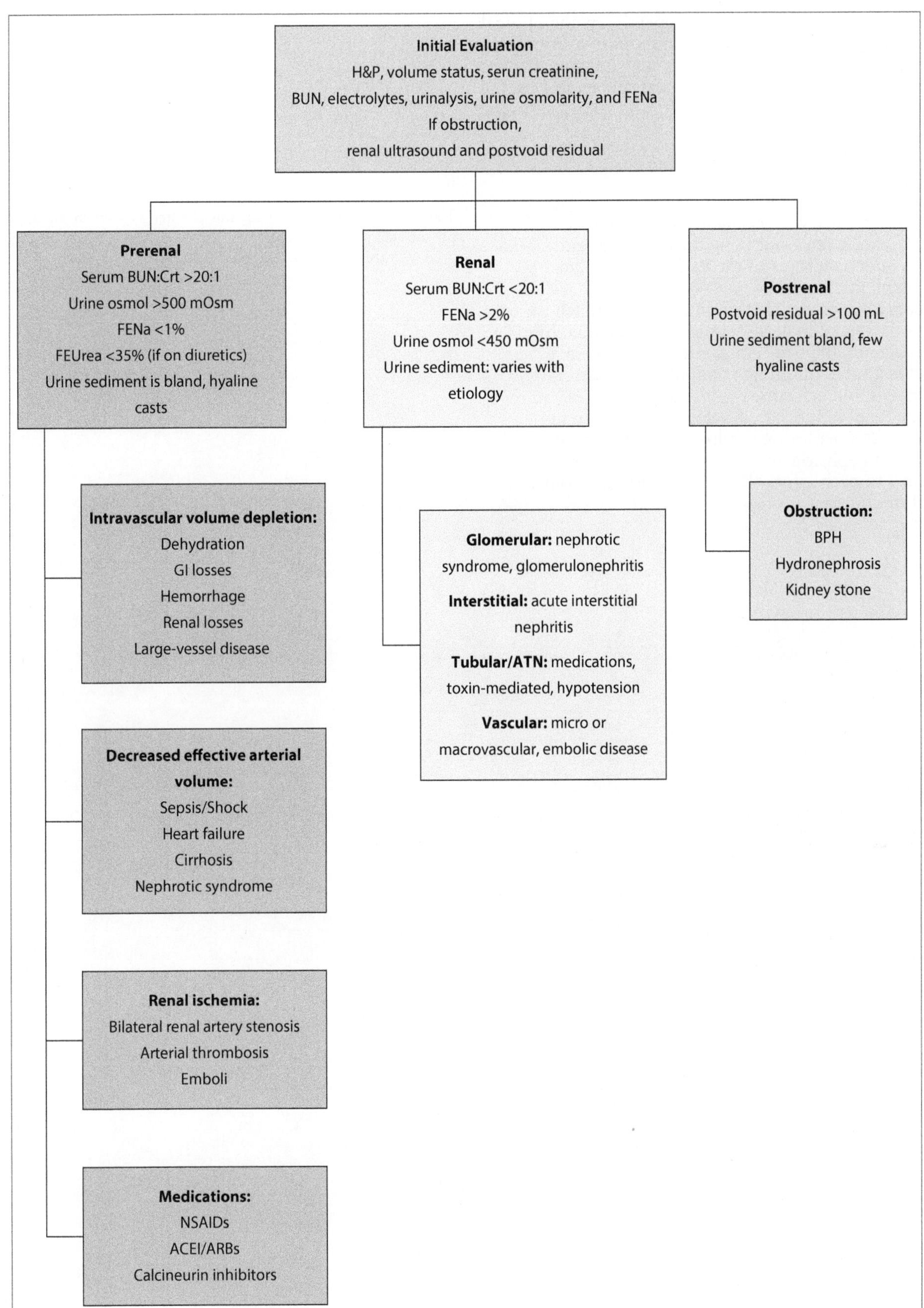

FIGURE 10.9 **Approach to the patient with acute kidney injury.** ACEI, angiotensin-converting enzyme inhibitor; ARBs, angiotensin receptor blockers; ATN, acute tubular necrosis; BPH, benign prostatic hyperplasia; BUN, blood urea nitrogen; Crt, creatinine; FENa, fractional excretion of sodium; FEUrea, fractional excretion of urea; GI, gastrointestinal; H&P, history & physical exam; NSAIDs, nonsteroidal anti-inflammatory drugs; osmol, osmolality.

The diagnostic workup of AKI depends on the clinical context, severity, and duration. At a minimum a urinalysis, examination of the urinary sediment, and imaging studies should be performed, with additional tests depending on the clinical presentation. See Figure 10.9 for the approach to the patient with AKI.

KNOWLEDGE CHECKS

1. Electrolytes are vital in maintaining homeostasis. Create a table outlining the etiologies and signs and symptoms of the various electrolyte abnormalities.
2. Create a flowchart that outlines the approach to hyponatremia, hypernatremia, hypokalemia, hyperkalemia, hypocalcemia, and hypercalcemia.
3. Create a table outlining metabolic and respiratory alkalosis and acidosis.
4. Acute renal failure can develop secondary to nephritic and nephrotic syndromes. Compare and contrast nephritic and nephrotic syndromes in regard to pathophysiology, signs and symptoms, and treatment.

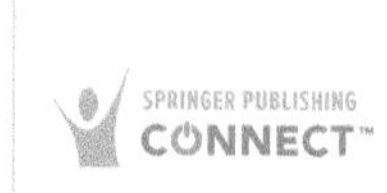

A robust set of instructor resources designed to supplement this text is located at **http://connect.springerpub.com/content/book/978-0-8261-8243-2.** Qualifying instructors may request access by emailing **textbook@springerpub.com.**

REFERENCES

The complete reference list for this chapter appears in the digital version of the chapter, accessible at https://connect.springerpub.com/content/book/978-0-8261-8243-2/chapter/ch10.

CHAPTER 11

GENITOURINARY SYSTEM

JAMES VAN RHEE, LINDA LANG, CHRIS ROMAN, ELIZABETH SCHMIDT, AND MARY RUGGERI

LEARNING OBJECTIVES

- Compare and contrast urethritis, acute and chronic urinary tract infections, and pyelonephritis with regard to the epidemiology, pathophysiology, clinical presentation, diagnosis, and management.
- Compare and contrast prostatitis and epididymitis with regard to the epidemiology, pathophysiology, clinical presentation, diagnosis, and management.
- Discuss the epidemiology, pathophysiology, clinical presentation, diagnosis, and management of nephrolithiasis.
- Compare and contrast the different types incontinence with regard to epidemiology, pathophysiology, clinical presentation, diagnosis, and management.
- Discuss the epidemiology, pathophysiology, clinical presentation, diagnosis, and management of the various testicular disorders.
- Compare and contrast the different penile disorders with regard to epidemiology, pathophysiology, clinical presentation, diagnosis, and management.
- Describe benign prostatic hypertrophy regarding the epidemiology, pathophysiology, clinical presentation, diagnosis, and management.
- Describe the approach to the patient with hematuria, focusing on diagnostic workup and management.

INTRODUCTION

The genitourinary system includes the urinary system and reproductive system. Both systems have a common embryologic origin. They develop from the intermediate mesoderm. Disorders of the genitourinary system range from those that are asymptomatic to those with a full array of signs and symptoms. Causes for these disorders include congenital anomalies, infectious diseases, trauma, and conditions that secondarily involve the urinary structure.

11.1 INFECTIONS

OVERVIEW

Urinary tract infections (UTIs) are common bacterial infections of the bladder and associated urinary tract structures. UTIs are more common in women and are usually caused by *Escherichia coli* and other gastrointestinal (GI) flora. Symptoms commonly include dysuria, hematuria, and urinary frequency/urgency. Fevers and localizing pain can be noted in other areas when the epididymis, kidney, or prostate is involved. Diagnosis generally requires a urinalysis, with a focus on the presence of leukocytes and nitrites, and often culture. Antibiotics are the cornerstone of therapy.

EPIDEMIOLOGY

UTIs occur frequently in females and more seldom in males. There are over 10 million ambulatory care encounters each year in the United States for infections of the bladder (cystitis) and related conditions.[1] Additional risk factors for UTIs include diabetes mellitus, genitourinary anatomic abnormalities, sexual intercourse, and urologic instrumentation. An increasingly important consideration is the rise in antimicrobial resistance among common urinary pathogens.

PATHOPHYSIOLOGY

The bladder is ordinarily a sterile environment. Bacteriuria occurs when bacteria are introduced into the bladder or urinary tract; this can be asymptomatic, and the presence of bacteria alone does not indicate infection. Bacteriuria is generally caused when commensal bacteria from the anogenital region are introduced into the urethra and ascend into the bladder. Friction, as with sexual intercourse, can increase the likelihood of external organisms being introduced into the urethra. Because the urethra is substantially shorter in females compared to males, it is easier for bacteria to get into the bladder in females. This explains the increased prevalence of cystitis in women. In both males and females the infections may ascend or extend into neighboring structures such as the kidney leading to pyelonephritis, and in males extend to the epididymis leading to epididymitis, and the prostate leading to prostatitis.

The normal flora in the anogenital region leads to a relatively small number of pathogens that cause a clear majority of cases of UTI. *Escherichia coli* represents approximately 80% of these infections. When *Staphylococcus saprophyticus* (4.4%), *Klebsiella pneumoniae* (4.3%), and *Proteus mirabilis* (3.7%) are added, these pathogens constitute over 90% of cases.[2] The causative organisms are similar for prostatitis and pyelonephritis; epididymitis is unique in that sexually transmitted pathogens are more common.

11.1A CYSTITIS

MEDICAL HISTORY AND CLINICAL PRESENTATION

Many patients experience recurrent cases of cystitis and will often present quickly after symptom onset. This may follow sexual intercourse, especially with spermicides.[3] Complicated cystitis (see Box 11.1) occurs in individuals who have risk factors for more severe and/or drug-resistant disease. The presence of cystitis in males should prompt evaluation for other contributing factors such as bladder dysfunction, infected stones, anatomic abnormalities, recent urologic manipulation or instrumentation, or prostatitis.

Importantly, older or debilitated/incapacitated individuals may not report urinary symptoms with cystitis or other UTIs. Therefore, a urinalysis is an important part of the initial evaluation of an individual experiencing acute mental status changes.

SIGNS AND SYMPTOMS

Irritative voiding symptoms are nearly always present in cystitis. These include urinary frequency and urgency, as well as dysuria and hematuria. Patients may also report cloudy urine or a change in urine odor, and suprapubic pain may be present. Fever and chills are generally absent in uncomplicated cystitis.

PHYSICAL EXAMINATION

Physical examination for cystitis is often benign, but suprapubic tenderness will be elicited in some patients.

DIFFERENTIAL DIAGNOSIS

See Table 11.1 for differential diagnosis of cystitis.

DIAGNOSTIC STUDIES

Urinalysis is the cornerstone of diagnosis. The urinalysis in a case of cystitis is positive for leukocytes or leukocyte esterase due to bladder inflammation. Many common UTI pathogens, such as the gram-negative rods, convert nitrates to nitrites, which can be detected on a standard urinalysis. Some pathogens, most notably *Proteus mirabilis*, can alkalinize the urine.

Culture is not generally necessary for uncomplicated cystitis but should be considered in patients with recent antibiotic use, frequent/recurrent UTI, or symptoms that are refractory to treatment. New point-of-care tests can identify bacteria in a urine sample. These are becoming widely available but have not yet replaced the urinalysis in conventional practice.

BOX 11.1 Risk Factors for Complicated Cystitis

- Anatomic abnormality of urinary tract
- Catheter or other foreign body
- Diabetes mellitus
- Duration of 7 or more days prior to presentation
- Immunosuppression
- Nosocomial infection
- Pregnancy
- Renal insufficiency
- Renal transplant
- Urinary obstruction

EVALUATION

See Figure 11.1 for the evaluation and treatment of the patient with a possible UTI.

TREATMENT

- Antibiotics are essential in eradicating the offending pathogens. First-line drugs include fosfomycin, nitrofurantoin, and trimethoprim-sulfamethoxazole.
- Fluoroquinolones should be reserved for cases of complicated cystitis or more advanced infections such as pyelonephritis.
- If culture results are available, antimicrobial coverage should be tailored to the drug susceptibilities of the identified pathogen.
- Phenazopyridine can be used to reduce the irritative voiding symptoms associated with cystitis. It is not indicated for use as monotherapy in a UTI.
- Individuals who experience frequent cystitis may be considered for antibiotic prophylaxis. This can be administered postcoitus or regularly if there is not an obvious cause.

PATIENT EDUCATION

- Completing the entire prescribed course of antibiotics is essential to minimize the risks of treatment failure and antimicrobial resistance.
- Use of phenazopyridine should be limited to 2 days so that it does not mask an infection that is failing to respond to antibiotics. Phenazopyridine can darken urine, which is an important point of patient education.
- Nonpharmacologic treatments that can reduce the incidence of cystitis include increasing fluid intake, eliminating the use of spermicides, postcoital voiding to flush the bladder and urethra, and for females wiping from front

TABLE 11.1 Differential Diagnosis for Cystitis

Diagnosis	Description
Interstitial cystitis	Inflammation of the bladder
Pelvic inflammatory disease	Infection of the upper genital tract in women
Prostatitis	Infection and/or inflammation of the prostate gland; can coexist with cystitis
Urethritis	Infection and/or inflammation of the urethra; often due to sexually transmitted pathogens
Vaginitis	Infection and/or inflammation of the vagina

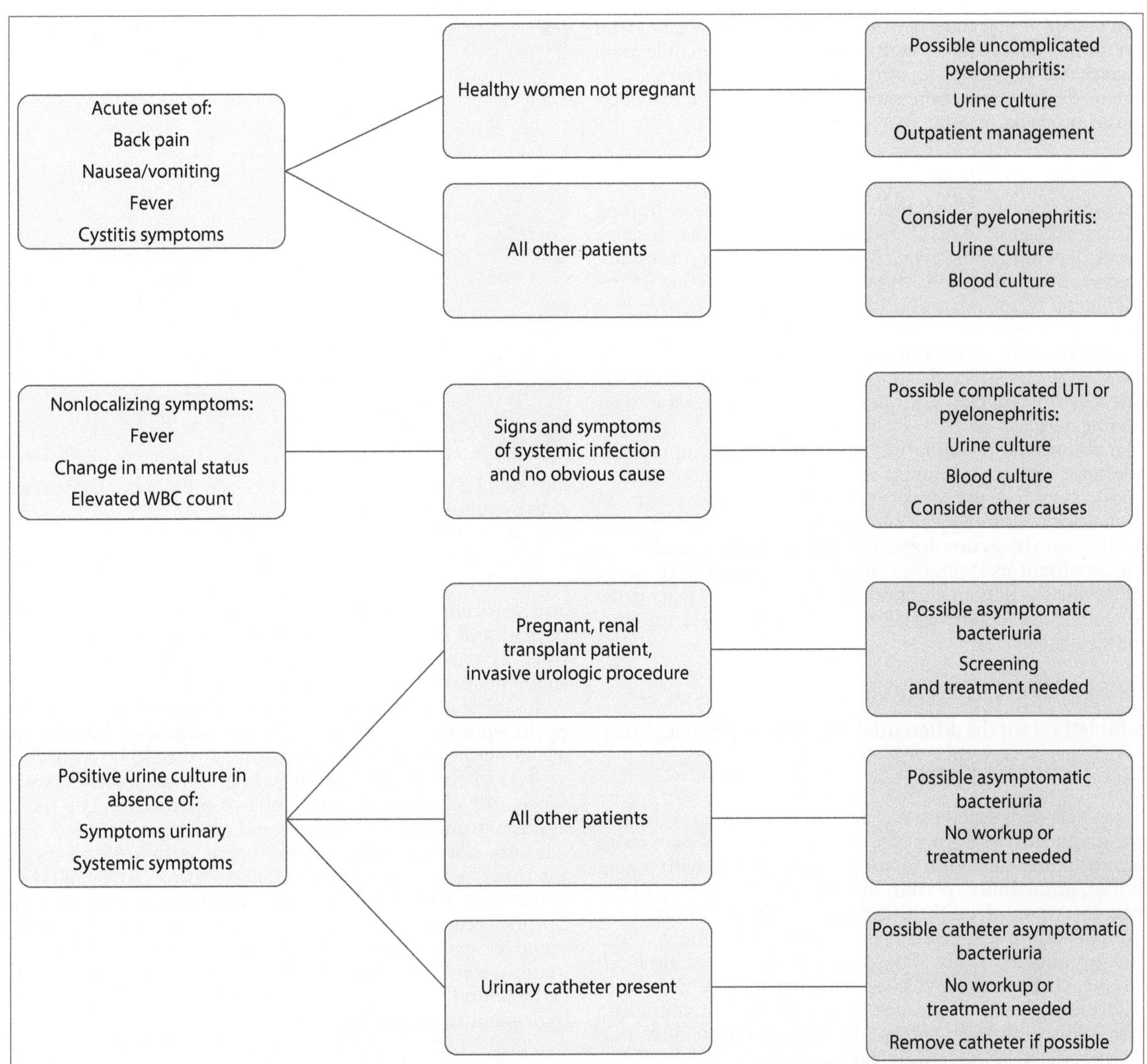

Figure 11.1 Evaluation and treatment of the patient with a possible urinary tract infection. UTI, urinary tract infection; WBC, white blood cell.

to back after emptying the bowel or bladder. In the case of postmenopausal women with recurring cystitis, topical estrogen is often beneficial.

11.1B PYELONEPHRITIS

MEDICAL HISTORY AND CLINICAL PRESENTATION

Acute pyelonephritis is a serious, potentially life- or organ-threatening, inflammatory condition of the renal pelvis and parenchyma resulting from a bacterial infection. Pathogens, most commonly *Escherichia coli* or other gram-negative bacilli, ascend to the kidney from the bladder via the ureter but may also be spread by a hematogenous route. Considered a severe UTI syndrome, pyelonephritis is less common than cystitis, but shares the same risk factors. The classic presentation of acute pyelonephritis includes some combination of fever, flank pain, urinary symptoms, and nausea with or without vomiting. The range of disease severity and patient appearance at the time of the initial examination vary widely, ranging from a general uncomfortable-looking appearance to toxic-appearing. Patients may present to the emergency department due to severity and/or rapid onset of symptoms.

SIGNS AND SYMPTOMS

Patients may or may not experience all the classic symptoms associated with acute pyelonephritis. Flank pain, often unilateral and worst at the costovertebral angle (CVA), varies in intensity from mild to severe. Patients may also report middle and lower back pain as well as suprapubic pain.

While typical symptoms of cystitis may be absent in pyelonephritis, many patients do experience irritative voiding symptoms, which may also include gross hematuria. Anorexia, nausea, and vomiting are also frequently reported, but diarrhea is not.

Several findings that may lead the clinician away from a presumed diagnosis of acute pyelonephritis include pain that radiates to the groin most likely associated with urolithiasis; dyspareunia if present should prompt the consideration of other diagnoses.

PHYSICAL EXAMINATION

Vital signs may be abnormal. Fever is a common finding and may exceed 39.4 °C (103 °F). Tachycardia may also be present depending on fever, hydration status, and presence of sepsis. Marked systolic hypotension in the setting of pyelonephritis is an indication of septic shock or perinephric abscess.

A common finding on physical examination is CVA tenderness over the affected kidney(s). CVA tenderness is easily elicited by the clinician with pressure or fist percussion over the same area.

An abdominal examination is likely to reveal suprapubic tenderness. Other abdominal findings such as rebound tenderness, guarding, or tenderness to palpation at other abdominal locations suggest another diagnosis. Likewise, for women positive gynecologic findings including tenderness on a bimanual examination are not consistent with acute pyelonephritis. In men a digital rectal exam that elicits prostate tenderness is more likely to be indicative of acute bacterial prostatitis.

DIFFERENTIAL DIAGNOSIS

See Table 11.2 for the differential diagnosis of pyelonephritis.

DIAGNOSTIC STUDIES

A urinalysis performed on a clean catch specimen is the primary diagnostic tool for acute pyelonephritis. Where clean catch specimen collection is not possible such as with young children, an inability to void, marked obesity, or very ill patients, intermittent urethral catheterization is indicated for urine collection. Expected urinalysis findings match those of uncomplicated UTIs. The presence of white blood cell (WBC) casts indicates pyelonephritis but may be present in glomerulonephritis. Their presence indicates inflammation of the kidney and are formed by the migration of WBCs across the renal tubular wall (Figure 11.2).

Because of the serious nature of pyelonephritis and the increasing incidence of antibiotic resistance, a urine culture and sensitivity are indicated in all suspected cases, both outpatient and inpatient. A positive urine culture will be identified as growing at least 10,000 colony forming units of a single uropathogen per milliliter of urine.[4]

Imaging is unnecessary in straightforward cases of acute pyelonephritis in patients who are otherwise healthy and are not experiencing complications. It should be considered as part of the initial workup when a patient presents with sepsis, the clinician is suspicious of obstruction, or the diagnosis is unclear. Imaging should also be utilized for those who are not responding to treatment within 48 hours and for those whose condition is deteriorating. Abdominal CT is the study of choice for diagnosing patients with an atypical presentation as well as for isolating the site of infection, identifying abscesses, and determining parenchymal inflammation. Renal ultrasound, while not as sensitive as CT, may be a helpful, less expensive, lower-risk tool for identifying hydronephrosis due to obstruction.[5]

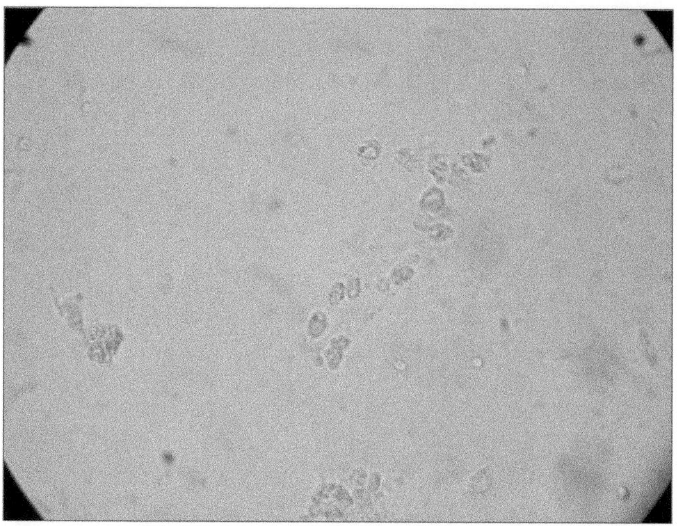

Figure 11.2 White blood cell casts may be present in patients with pyelonephritis.
(Source: James Van Rhee and Janie McDaniel.)

TABLE 11.2 Differential Diagnosis of Pyelonephritis

Diagnosis	Description
Cystitis	See differential diagnosis for cystitis (Table 11.6)
Urolithiasis	Kidney and ureteral stones that may cause urinary tract obstruction.
Rupture or torsion of ovarian cyst	Benign growth on an ovary
Ectopic pregnancy	Implantation of a fetus outside the uterine cavity
Acute abdomen (e.g., appendicitis)	Sudden onset of abdominal pain caused by infection, inflammation, or obstruction of structures within the abdominal cavity

EVALUATION

See Figure 11.1 for the evaluation and treatment of the patient with a UTI.

TREATMENT

- Uncomplicated pyelonephritis in otherwise healthy, nonpregnant patients is typically treated in an outpatient setting.
- All patients who do not meet the above criteria are considered to have complicated pyelonephritis and should be admitted to the hospital for treatment (see Box 11.2).[6]
- Begin empirical treatment with broad-spectrum antibiotic taking into consideration local antibiotic resistance patterns. Fluoroquinolones are considered first-line agents if local resistance is <10%.[4,7] Treatment should align with pathogen and susceptibility once culture results are determined.
- Oral or parenteral administration or a combination of the two routes (initial parenteral followed by oral) are equally effective, and choice can be individualized based on patient presentation.

BOX 11.2 Admission Criteria for Treatment of Acute Pyelonephritis

Severe symptoms
Hemodynamic instability
Unable to tolerate oral pharmacologic therapy
Concern regarding nonadherence
Presence of underlying disease (e.g., diabetes mellitus, urolithiasis)
Pregnancy
Symptoms for more than 7 days

Source: Data from Johnson JR, Russo TA. Acute pyelonephritis in adults. N Engl J Med. *2018;378(1):48–59. doi:10.1056/NEJMcp1702758.*

- Supportive care should also be considered for control of pain, fever, and hydration status. Intravenous fluid resuscitation is appropriate for patients with severe vomiting or signs of sepsis. Nonsteroidal anti-inflammatory drugs and opioids are complementary and recommended for analgesia.
- Complications including hydronephrosis, renal or perinephric abscess, and emphysematous pyelonephritis are more common in patients with urolithiasis, diabetes, chronic kidney disease, sickle cell disease, and immune-compromised states.

PATIENT EDUCATION

- Outpatient treatment of pyelonephritis requires close follow-up; the patient should be seen in 24–48 hours with a low threshold for consideration of hospital admission if symptoms are worsening or not improving.

11.1C PROSTATITIS

MEDICAL HISTORY AND CLINICAL PRESENTATION

Since the pathogenesis of prostatitis depends on typical urinary pathogens being introduced into the prostate, there is often a history of either prostate disease, obstructive urinary symptoms (e.g., urinary hesitancy, weak stream), or intervention/manipulation of the prostate (e.g., cystoscopy, prostate biopsy). Acute infections will manifest with new/evolving symptoms as well as systemic illness.

Bacterial prostatitis may be chronic, which often follows an acute infection.

Nonbacterial prostatitis is common, and generally will present similarly to chronic prostatitis. Testing should include common and uncommon causes of prostatitis, including ruling out infection with *Chlamydia, Mycoplasma*, and *Ureaplasma*, as well as the typical urinary pathogens like *Escherichia coli* that are identified with culture.

SIGNS AND SYMPTOMS

Acute bacterial prostatitis manifests with fever, irritative voiding symptoms, and perineal pain. Any obstructive urinary symptoms that exist due to comorbid disease, such as benign prostatic hypertrophy or prostate cancer, will persist.

Chronic bacterial prostatitis can range from asymptomatic infections to persistent irritative voiding symptoms or pelvic/perineal discomfort. Nonbacterial prostatitis will manifest similarly.

PHYSICAL EXAMINATION

Examination of the anogenital area is key and should include a digital rectal examination to evaluate for prostatic edema and tenderness. The digital rectal examination should be performed gently to minimize pain and the risk of bacteremia due to any pathogens that may be present.

DIFFERENTIAL DIAGNOSIS

The differential diagnosis for prostatitis includes UTI as well as sexually transmitted infections (STIs) and other acute anal and genital pathologic processes (see Table 11.3). These infections can affect multiple parts of the genitourinary system and may coexist.

DIAGNOSTIC STUDIES

Urinalysis with culture and testing for STIs and atypical pathogens, including *Chlamydia, Mycoplasma*, and *Ureaplasma*, should be ordered. A complete blood count (CBC) may reveal leukocytosis with a left shift, and prostate specific antigen levels will often be elevated, though this is not specific for prostatitis.

Prostatic secretions can be expressed by prostate massage, and the cultures of this fluid may be helpful in diagnosing chronic prostatitis. Prostate massage should be avoided in acute prostatitis. Nonbacterial prostatitis is a diagnosis of exclusion.

EVALUATION

See Table 11.4 for differentiation of the various types of prostatitis based on symptoms and physical examination findings.

TABLE 11.3 Differential Diagnosis for Prostatitis

Diagnosis	Description
Benign prostatic hypertrophy (BPH)	Enlargement of the prostate gland
Cystitis	Infection of the bladder
Diverticulitis	Inflammation +/− infection of the colon
Epididymitis	Infection and/or inflammation of the epididymis
Overactive bladder	Detrusor muscle dysfunction leading to urinary incontinence and/or urgency
Prostate cancer	Malignant tumor of the prostate gland
Urethritis	Infection and/or inflammation of the urethra; often due to sexually transmitted pathogens

TABLE 11.4 Summary of the Various Types of Prostatitis

Type	Symptoms	Physical Examination
Acute bacterial (type I)	Urinary urgency, dysuria, hesitancy, obstruction and frequency; systemic fever, malaise, ill appearing, nausea and vomiting	Prostate tender, boggy, enlarged; prostatic massage contraindicated
Chronic bacterial (type II)	Irritative voiding symptoms, low back or perineal pain, recurrent urinary tract infection	Prostate normal, tender, or boggy
Chronic pelvic pain syndrome *Type A: Inflammatory* *Type B: Noninflammatory*	Chronic pelvic pain, possible voiding symptoms	Findings variable
Asymptomatic	No symptoms	None

TREATMENT

- Empiric therapy should be initiated while diagnostic results are pending to reduce the potential for abscess formation, systemic illness, and other complications.
- Antibiotics should be directed at the likely pathogens, and empiric therapy generally consists of a fluoroquinolone or trimethoprim-sulfamethoxazole.
- Prostatitis is unique in that antimicrobial therapy is generally continued for 4–6 weeks.

PATIENT EDUCATION

- Individuals with confirmed or suspected STI should be offered testing for other STIs, including HIV, as well as counseling on STI prevention.
- Symptoms often begin to improve within the first few days of therapy. Patients who do not improve after 3–4 days of therapy should be reevaluated for other causes of their symptoms and/or drug resistance.
- Potential complications include worsening infection, such as abscess formation, and bacteremia.

11.1D EPIDIDYMITIS

MEDICAL HISTORY AND CLINICAL PRESENTATION

The pathogens that cause epididymitis vary based on age and sexual history. Most cases in younger males, <35 years of age, are sexually transmitted, with *Chlamydia trachomatis* and *Neisseria gonorrhoeae* the most common pathogens. In older males, prostate dysfunction, such as benign prostatic hypertrophy, can cause urine retention and reflux into the vas deferens and epididymis. Therefore, cases of epididymitis in the older male population are more likely to be caused by *Escherichia coli* and other common urinary pathogens. Many patients experience recurrent cases of cystitis and will often present quickly after symptom onset. Rarely, epididymitis can be caused by autoimmune or inflammatory disorders, as well as by drugs, such as amiodarone.[8]

SIGNS AND SYMPTOMS

Scrotal erythema and pain are typical, and pain may radiate to the suprapubic area and/or flank. Irritative voiding symptoms may be present, and in cases of STI, urethral discharge may be noted. Pain may worsen with Valsalva maneuver or sexual activity. In severe cases, fever and other signs of systemic toxicity may be present.

PHYSICAL EXAMINATION

Careful examination of the genital area is essential. Urethral discharge suggests an STI, while tenderness of the suprapubic region or bladder can be present in cystitis or prostatitis, respectively. Scrotal erythema on the affected side is common but not universally seen. Palpation of the affected testicle(s) often reveals induration and tenderness around the epididymis on the posterior aspect of the testicle. In some cases, the testicle itself may become involved and will be swollen and tender (this is called *epididymo-orchitis*). The cremasteric reflex is present, which aids in the differentiation from testicular torsion, in which this reflex is absent. Prehn sign, pain relief with elevation of the scrotum, may be positive in patients with epididymitis, which further excludes torsion.

DIFFERENTIAL DIAGNOSIS

The differential diagnosis for epididymitis includes UTIs as well as STIs and other acute genital pathologies (see Table 11.5). Because the pathologies can cause symptoms in several locations, these disorders may coexist. Since some

TABLE 11.5 Differential Diagnosis for Epididymitis

Diagnosis	Description
Fournier gangrene (emergency)	Life-threatening necrotizing infection of the groin/perineum
Orchitis	Infection and/or inflammation of the testicle
Prostatitis	Infection and/or inflammation of the prostate gland; can coexist with cystitis
Testicular torsion (emergency)	The testicle rotates within the scrotum, causing acute severe pain and ischemia
Testicular appendage torsion	The testicular appendage rotates, causing acute severe pain and ischemia; a "blue dot sign," may be visible on the anterior scrotum
Testicular tumor	Can include benign or malignant lesions of the testicle
Urethritis	Infection and/or inflammation of the urethra; often due to sexually transmitted pathogens

acute scrotal disorders can be emergent, a careful evaluation is key to ensure good clinical outcomes.

DIAGNOSTIC STUDIES

Urinalysis with culture and testing for common STIs should be ordered, with treatment dictated by the results. In cases that are severe or when the diagnosis is less clear, scrotal ultrasonography can be invaluable to exclude testicular torsion.

TREATMENT

- In cases that are severe, or when the cause is clear, empiric treatment should be considered. For STIs, empiric therapy would consist of a intramuscular injection of ceftriaxone, followed by azithromycin as a single dose, or 10 days of therapy with doxycycline administered twice daily.
- Treatment should be tailored to the identified or likely pathogens, with a fluoroquinolone or trimethoprim-sulfamethoxazole for empiric coverage of typical urinary pathogens.

PATIENT EDUCATION

- Individuals with confirmed or suspected STI should be offered testing for other STIs, including HIV, as well as counseling on STI prevention.
- Patients who do not improve after 2–3 days of therapy should be reevaluated for other causes of their symptoms.
- Potential complications include infertility or worsening infection, such as abscess formation.

SPECIAL CONSIDERATIONS

- Do not test for or treat asymptomatic bacteriuria except in pregnant women, immunocompromised patients, or before an invasive urologic procedure.

KEY POINTS

- The most common cause of UTIs is *E. coli*.
- Urine culture is indicated in complicated UTI but not in uncomplicated cystitis.
- Chronic bacterial prostatitis and nontoxic acute bacterial prostatitis should be treated with symptomatic measures and fluoroquinolone.
- Patients with acute bacterial prostatitis and possible sepsis should be hospitalized and treated with broad-spectrum antibiotics.
- The most common etiologies of epididymitis are *Neisseria gonorrhoeae* and *Chlamydia trachomatis* in younger men and gram-negative bacilli in older men.
- For most cases of epididymitis, treat pain and infection with antibiotics such as fluoroquinolone, doxycycline, and trimethoprim/sulfamethoxazole.

11.2 INTERSTITIAL CYSTITIS

OVERVIEW

Interstitial cystitis (IC), also known as bladder pain syndrome (BPS), is characterized by chronic bladder pain or discomfort for more than 6 weeks' duration. This condition can be debilitating and greatly impact a patient's quality of life. The pathophysiology is not well known, and the diagnosis of IC is often a diagnosis of exclusion. A variety of symptoms suggest the potential for multiple etiologies, and thus, approaches to treatment will vary from patient to patient.

EPIDEMIOLOGY

IC is more common in women than men; however, the nature of this diagnosis makes establishing prevalence difficult. A survey estimated between 2.7% and 6.5% of women in the United States have symptoms consistent with IC.[9] Only 9.7% of those patients reported having a diagnosis of IC/BPS, which demonstrates the potential for underdiagnosing this condition.[9]

PATHOPHYSIOLOGY

The exact pathophysiology of IC/BPS is unknown; a variety of symptoms suggest the potential for multiple etiologies. Twin studies demonstrate a higher chance of IC with monozygotic over dizygotic twins, suggesting a genetic relationship. Furthermore, first-degree female relatives of patients with IC may have an increased prevalence of IC—17 times that of the general population.[10] Urothelial abnormalities have been observed in patients with IC/BPS and may include:

- Cystoscopy may reveal glomerulations and/or Hunner lesions, disrupting the protective, inner epithelial lining of the bladder.
- Abnormal versions of Tamm-Horsfall proteins may affect the neutralization of toxins in the urine.
- Bladder biopsies in IC patients have shown increased numbers of mast cells, which may play a role in frequency, pain, and fibrosis.
- Epithelial cells in the bladders of some IC patients have been found to produce an antiproliferative factor. This may inhibit the proliferation of normal bladder epithelial cells and contribute to bladder thinning.
- IC patients have an increased incidence of other chronic pain syndromes; nonbladder syndromes causing pelvic pain could sensitize the lower spinal cord resulting in the bladder as the perceived site of pain.

MEDICAL HISTORY AND CLINICAL PRESENTATION

Initially thought to be a disease of young women, more recent data have shown that symptoms of IC/BPS may occur across all ages. IC/BPS should be suspected in patients who have bladder-associated pain for several weeks. Frequent voiding to avoid discomfort with bladder filling and pelvic tenderness increase the clinical suspicion for IC/BPS. With symptoms of hematuria, severe incontinence, or bladder pain not relieved by urination, workup for alternative diagnosis is warranted.

It is important to elicit the characteristics of the pain or pressure as well as any bladder-related medical history (UTIs, pelvic surgery or trauma, neurologic conditions). For patients <30 years of age, frequency, urgency and dysuria are the most common presenting symptoms.[11] For patients 30 to 50 years of age, nocturia, dysuria, and urgency were the most common presenting symptoms.[11] Other common symptoms cited by patients in all age groups include dyspareunia and vulvar pain. As a result of chronic pain and urinary frequency, symptoms can often interfere with home and work life.

IC/BPS appears to be highly associated with other chronic pain syndromes, including fibromyalgia, chronic fatigue, vulvodynia, and irritable bowel syndrome; it is useful to ask about these conditions in the patient's history.

SIGNS AND SYMPTOMS

Patients with IC/BPS have chronic and unpleasant symptoms related to the bladder. Most commonly this includes discomfort with bladder filling and relief upon voiding. Patients may report frequent voiding to avoid discomfort of an increased bladder volume. This is unlike overactive bladder in which frequent voiding occurs to avoid urinary incontinence. Urgency and nocturia are also common symptoms. The discomfort is generally reported as suprapubic or urethral. Onset is often gradual, with symptoms worsening over months; symptoms are typically constant but may vary in severity. Some patients, however, experience an acute onset of severe symptoms. Many patients cannot identify a "triggering" event, some develop symptoms after trauma, surgical procedure, or uncomplicated UTI. Exacerbating factors may include stress, consuming certain foods or drinks, and activities such as sexual activity or exercise.

PHYSICAL EXAMINATION

Common physical exam findings include tenderness of the abdominal wall, pelvic floor, urinary bladder, and urethra. In males, scrotal and penile tenderness may be present. While findings of pain and tenderness may be helpful in the diagnostic process, it is critical to rule out other conditions such as malignancies, masses, hernias, and erosion of surgical mesh. Patients may also experience light touch as being very painful, as is common in other chronic pain conditions; this may make it difficult to perform an adequate pelvic or digital rectal examination.

DIFFERENTIAL DIAGNOSIS

See Table 11.6 for the differential diagnosis of IC.

DIAGNOSTIC STUDIES

As symptoms of IC/BPS may vary, it is important to rule out other possible causes. Urinalysis with microscopy should be performed to exclude an infectious cause and evaluate for hematuria; a urine culture should be ordered for any results suggestive of infection. Sexually transmitted disease (STD) testing may also be performed for patients who are at risk for an STD. A postvoid residual (PVR) urine volume may help to rule out bladder outlet obstruction or neurologic dysfunction. If hematuria is noted in the history or found on urinalysis, cystoscopy should be performed to exclude malignancy. Cystoscopy may be indicated in patients who have failed to respond to various IC/BPS treatment as it may aid in identifying alternative causes of a patient's symptoms.

EVALUATION

The goal of the diagnostic evaluation is to exclude other conditions, including malignancy. IC/BPS should be suspected in patients with pain related to the urinary bladder for several weeks. If evaluations for UTI are negative and the symptoms persist, clinical suspicion is increased. Frequent voiding to avoid discomfort of increased bladder volume as well as pelvic tenderness on examination are consistent with IC/BPS; a clinical diagnosis can be achieved in the setting of an uncomplicated presentation.

TREATMENT

No treatment is effective for all patients; the course of treatment should reflect the characteristics and severity of symptoms as well as clinical judgement and patient preference. Pain management should be assessed for effectiveness because of its impact on one's quality of life. Treatment plans should begin by using conservative options. Generally, surgical treatments should be explored after alternatives have been exhausted.

A stepwise treatment approach is often used[12]:

- **First-line treatments:** patient education, self-care and behavioral modification, stress management, pain management
- **Second-line treatments:** physical therapy, antihistamines, amitriptyline, pentosan polysulfate sodium, intravesical lidocaine or heparin for acute episodes of severe pain, pain management
- **Third-line treatments:** cystoscopy with hydrodistention, treatment of Hunner lesions (if found on cystoscopy), pain management

TABLE 11.6 Differential Diagnosis of Interstitial Cystitis

Diagnosis	Description
Bladder, urethral, or genital cancer	Presence of a mass may cause pelvic pain or pressure as well as urinary symptoms. Malignancies of the organs themselves may cause pain with or without hematuria.
Urinary tract infection	Infection of kidneys, ureters, bladder, or urethra may cause symptoms of pelvic pain, urgency, and frequency.
Sexually transmitted diseases	Infection transmitted by sexual contact may cause pelvic pain and urinary symptoms.
Intravesical pathology	Bladder stones, history of pelvic surgery may result in erosion of surgical mesh or suture into bladder wall.
Benign pelvic masses	Uterine leiomyomas or pelvic organ prolapse may cause bladder pressure or pain.
Neurologic condition	Urinary retention due to neurologic dysfunction; may cause bladder pain.
Chronic pelvic pain syndrome	Noncyclic pelvic pain for 3–6 months or longer. Urinary and gastrointestinal symptoms may be associated with this condition.

- **Fourth-line treatments:** intradetrusor botulinum toxin, neuromodulation, pain management
- **Fifth-line treatments:** cyclosporine, pain management
- **Sixth-line treatments:** diversion with or without cystectomy, substitution cystoplasty, pain management

PATIENT EDUCATION

- IC/BPS is a chronic pain syndrome and the cause is not well understood. The goal of management is to provide symptom relief and improved quality of life.
- No single treatment has been found to work for all patients. Symptom control may require trials of multiple treatment options.
- Self-care and behavioral modifications should be implemented when possible and in conjunction with other treatments. This includes stress management, avoidance of activities or diet that exacerbate symptoms, fluid management, and bladder training.

KEY POINTS

- IC is noninfectious inflammation of the bladder that can cause chronic pelvic pain and urinary frequency.
- IC is diagnosis of exclusion.

11.3 STONE DISEASE

OVERVIEW

Urinary stone disease (USD), commonly known as kidney stones, renal stones, urolithiasis, or nephrolithiasis, is a term that refers to the existence of stones within the urinary tract. Nephrolithiasis are a common problem in general practice, affecting 1 in 11 people in the United States and causing significant morbidity and economic burden.[13,14] Nephrolithiasis incidence rates are rising globally and it is highly prevalent across all demographic groups.[15,16] In their lifetime approximately 12% of men and 7% of women will form at least one kidney stone.[13] Stones can develop due to supersaturation of stone-forming constituents such as calcium oxalate, uric acid, and cystine, as well as decreased urine volume. Environmental and genetic factors have also been identified as risk factors that may contribute to the formation of urinary stones. There are four different stone types: calcium oxalate and calcium phosphate stones (70–85%), uric acid stones (5–10%), struvite (1–5%), and cystine stones <1%.[17] After a first stone, approximately 50% of patients will have stone recurrence within 8 years.[13] Smaller stones <4 mm are usually able to pass spontaneously; stones greater than this size are less likely to do so, and will often require urologic interventions for removal, such as ureteroscopic removal or extracorporeal shock wave lithotripsy (ESWL). Treatment is focused on management of the acute event, followed by long-term strategies to reduce the recurrence rate. This includes educating patients about their diet and fluid intake, and treatment of any underlying metabolic abnormality.

EPIDEMIOLOGY

Kidney and ureteral stones can occur at any age, but the typical time frame for first incidence is 20–49 years. Secondary stone formation is estimated at 50% in 5–10 years, and 75% in 20 years.[18] Nephrolithiasis, affects approximately 12% of the global population[15] with incidence occurring across ethnic groups.[19] Incidence is 1.5 times higher in men than in women, although there is evidence that the incidence ratio is decreasing.[15] Non-Hispanic White men are most affected, followed by Hispanics and Asians. Blacks are typically the least affected; however, incidence rates are rising. The prevalence of stone disease varies significantly by geographic region, with an increased prevalence in areas of elevated temperatures. Southeastern states have the highest prevalence as compared to mid-Atlantic states. In addition to sociodemographic factors, it is possible that inadequate fluid intake contributes to the higher prevalence.

Recent studies indicate that urolithiasis is increasing in prevalence, likely due to changing dietary habits and decreasing physical activity. Decreased fluid intake and resultant decrease in urine volume as well as high protein and salt intake appear to be important factors influencing stone formation. Genetic factors, as well as certain medications, may contribute to stone formation as well. Additionally, research indicates that obesity, diabetes, insulin resistance, and cardiovascular diseases are associated with renal calculi formation.

PATHOPHYSIOLOGY

The main mechanisms that drive kidney stone formation are (1) supersaturated urine, (2) loss of urinary inhibitors in the urine, and (3) acidic pH.

The most common pathway for stone formation of any type is through supersaturation of urine by components such as calcium, oxalate, phosphate, uric acid, and cystine. When the concentration of stone materials exceeds their solubility, crystals form and grow. These crystals then adhere to the urothelium, upon which subsequent stone growth occurs.

Research indicates that the processes within the renal medullary interstitium are a key driver of calcium oxalate stone formation. When calcium phosphate crystals form in the interstitium, they migrate to the renal papillary epithelium, where they form Randall plaques. The plaque then acts as a vector upon which further deposition of calcium oxalate or calcium phosphate occurs. Typically, crystallization is impeded by inhibitors present in urine such as citrate, pyrophosphate, and glycosaminoglycans among others. Stone formers may lack an adequate presence of inhibitors. In cases of stone formation, a critical supersaturation point is reached wherein spontaneous crystallization can occur if the presence of inhibitors is inadequate. There are four different types of renal stones: calcium, uric acid, struvite, and cystine stones.[14] Calcium stones are typically complexed with oxalate or phosphate. Table 11.7 identifies the composition and frequency of different stone types.

TABLE 11.7 Types of Renal Stones

Composition	Frequency
Calcium (oxalate, phosphate, mixed)	70%–85%
Uric acid	5%–10%
Struvite	1%–5%
Cystine	<1%

PREDISPOSING FACTORS

Urinary, dietary, and nondietary risk factors contribute to stone formation in the urinary tract. These risk factors are outlined in Table 11.8.

Urinary risk factors for stone formation are intricately related to urine composition, pH, and volume. High urinary concentrations of stone-forming ions can be spurred by conditions such as hypercalciuria, hyperoxaluria, and hypocitraturia and result in stone formation when the urine becomes supersaturated. The presence of citrate and magnesium can be protective against stone formation. Urinary pH is also a determining factor in stone formation, with persistently low pH contributing to uric acid precipitation and the subsequent formation of uric acid stones. Increased fluid intake is a critical component for reducing the risk of stone formation. Indeed, ≥2 L of fluid intake per day increases urine output and reduces the concentration of urine solute, thereby decreasing the risk of stone formation.

Dietary risk factors for stone formation include animal protein- and sodium-heavy diets. The consumption of significant amounts of animal protein can increase the daily acid load, contributing to oxalate and uric acid stone formation. Increased intake of sodium results in increased calcium excretion, which can promote calcium stone disease. Interestingly, low-calcium diets actually promote calcium oxalate stone formation due to the decreased availability of calcium to bind with oxalate in the intestine. Potassium-rich diets, e.g., those high in fruits and vegetables, can reduce the risk of stone formation through the resultant reduction in urinary calcium and increased urinary citrate excretion, with citrate being a powerful inhibitor of stone formation.

Nondietary risk factors for stone formation include family history and personal medical history. Stone formation increases threefold with a family history of kidney stones.[20] Similarly, stone formation is associated with a personal medical history of hypertension, insulin resistance, primary hyperparathyroidism, gout, chronic metabolic acidosis, and inflammatory bowel disease. Additionally, patients with an anatomic urinary tract abnormality, resulting in urinary stasis, are typically at higher risk of stone formation. Finally, certain medications can also increase the risk of stone formation. Of note, these include the diuretic triamterene, the protease inhibitor drug indinavir, the anticonvulsants topiramate and zonisamide, and high doses of vitamin C (>1,000 mg/day). Risk factors for kidney stone formation are outlined below in Table 11.8

MEDICAL HISTORY AND CLINICAL PRESENTATION

Nephrolithiasis classically presents with unilateral flank pain that may radiate anteriorly and inferiorly to the ipsilateral lower abdomen or groin, depending on the location of the stone as it moves toward the ureterovesical junction. The pain is often of acute onset, typically peaking and plateauing after about 30 minutes and resolving with passage of the stone or stone removal. Gross hematuria, urinary urgency, frequency, nausea, and vomiting may also be present. Nephrolithiasis that presents with fevers, chills, and rigors may signal an obstruction and associated upper UTI. This presentation carries a high risk for the development of severe sepsis.

SIGNS AND SYMPTOMS

Kidney stones cause pain secondary to ureteral spasm as the stone migrates from the renal pelvis, down the ureter, toward the ureterovesical junction. The pain varies in intensity, from a dull pressure or pulling sensation to debilitating pain. Constant pain at the onset signals concern for a more severe obstruction. A stone located in the upper ureter is typically signified by pain that radiates anteriorly to the abdomen. A lower ureteral stone may cause pain to radiate to the ipsilateral testicle or labia in men and women, respectively. Urinary frequency and urgency indicate a stone lodged at the ureterovesical junction.

Stone disease commonly causes hematuria, both macroscopic and microscopic. Hematuria is present in about 90% of patients; however, it is important to note that in 10% of proven kidney stone passage, no hematuria can be detected.[21]

Once the stone passes from the ureter into the bladder, and out in the urine, all symptoms abruptly resolve. The probability of stone passage is related to its size and location in the ureter. Smaller and more distal stones are more likely to pass without intervention. Generally, about 50% of stones >4–6 mm will require urologic intervention. Stones ≥10 mm and stones in the proximal ureter are unlikely to pass spontaneously.[22]

PHYSICAL EXAMINATION

The physical examination can provide useful information for the diagnosis, although further tests are typically required to definitively establish nephrolithiasis as the diagnosis. The patient commonly presents with obvious pain and

TABLE 11.8 Risk Factors for Kidney Stones

Urinary	Dietary	Nondietary
Low urine volume <1 L/day High urine calcium High urine oxalate	Low calcium intake High sodium intake High animal protein intake High oxalate intake Medications: Indinavir Triamterene Vitamin C high dose >1,000/mg/day	Prior history of stone Positive family history for stone Environmental: warm, dry climate Systemic conditions: Recurrent urinary tract infection Hyperparathyroidism Diabetes mellitus Hyperuricemia Renal tubular acidosis Anatomic conditions: Ureteropelvic junction (UPJ) obstruction, solitary kidney, medullary sponge kidney, horseshoe kidney

the inability to position themselves comfortably. Tenderness in the ipsilateral CVA may occur and, in severe cases of obstruction, signs of sepsis may also be present.

DIFFERENTIAL DIAGNOSIS

Table 11.9 outlines the differential diagnosis for nephrolithiasis.

DIAGNOSTIC STUDIES

Diagnosis of nephrolithiasis is made through a combination of patient history, physical examination, and laboratory and imaging studies.

The initial workup should include the following:

Laboratory Findings

- **Urinalysis and urine culture:** Examine the urine to identify evidence of infection (including leukocytes), hematuria, and stone-related crystals. Urinalysis usually reveals gross or microscopic hematuria in majority of patients, ~90%, but its absence does not rule out potential stone diagnosis.[23] The urinary pH should also be noted, as a pH >7 is suggestive of a struvite, or infection stone, which occur in the presence of bacteria that split urease, whereas a urine pH of <5 may indicate potential uric acid calculi. Urine pH between 5.5 and 6.5 suggests a calcium-oxalate-based stone.
- **Routine blood chemistry:** Evaluation of serum creatinine, electrolytes, calcium, uric acid, parathyroid hormone, and phosphorus should be done to assess renal function and evaluate for underlying metabolic derangements. If the patient presents with systemic signs of infection or if an alternate abdominal etiology is suspected, then a CBC with a differential can be considered.
- **Stone analysis:** Analysis for identification of stone type should be conducted, which directs future therapies.

Imaging Studies

- Noncontrast abdominopelvic helical (spiral) CT scan: performed using low-radiation-dose scanning is considered the gold standard for identification of almost all stones, as it is able to diagnose stones as small as 1 mm. It has high sensitivity to small stones, does not require intravenous contrast agent, and can also diagnose other causes of abdominal or flank pain. Ideally, lower dose radiation would be used, as there is an increased risk of malignancy if used repeatedly with repeat stone formers.
- Ultrasound of kidneys and bladder: While less sensitive and specific than CT scans, ultrasounds have good diagnostic ability and can readily detect hydronephrosis and ureteral dilation; however, ultrasounds have limited sensitivity in determining stone size and location. Conducting an initial ultrasound can support patients' preference in avoiding unnecessary radiation exposure via CT scans if the diagnosis can be made by ultrasound alone. Ultrasound is the imaging study of choice in pregnant women.
- Kidney, ureter, bladder (KUB) plain abdominal radiograph: KUB is a plain x-ray of the abdomen and detects opaque calcareous or cystine stones. Less accurate than CT and ultrasound for both stone detection, localization, or identifying hydronephrosis, this method is typically used in combination with ultrasound to follow patients undergoing treatment for nephrolithiasis. KUB's limited sensitivity derives from body habitus, overlying bowel gas, and extragenitourinary calcifications (Figure 11.3).[24]

EVALUATION

Acute renal colic is diagnosed through patient history, physical exam, laboratory, and imaging studies. These methods are aimed at diagnosing and managing the acute event. Following resolution of the acute event, it is recommended that the patient undergo comprehensive evaluation of the underlying causal factors.

TABLE 11.9 Differential Diagnosis of Nephrolithiasis

Diagnosis	Features
Acute abdominal conditions Appendicitis, biliary colic, cholecystitis, and pancreatitis	Stone in distal ureter on right can mimic pain of appendicitis. Stone in the upper ureter can mimic biliary colic. Fever is present in acute abdominal conditions. Fever is absent in renal colic. If peritonitis is suspected patient is motionless as opposed to pacing. Differentiate with urinalysis: hematuria present in 90% of nephrolithiasis, absent in acute abdomen. Liver function tests reveal an obstructive pattern in cholecystitis but are normal in stone disease. CT of abdomen can differentiate nephrolithiasis from appendicitis, cholecystitis, and pancreatitis.
Urinary tract infection Pyelonephritis	Fever, chills, elevated white blood cells, and nitrates usually not present in renal colic; although concurrent stones and infection may coexist. Urine Gram stain and culture needed to determine pathogen in pyelonephritis.
Gynecologic Ectopic pregnancy, ovarian pathology (cyst, torsion)	Gynecologic history is important as well as pregnancy test.
Vascular pathology Abdominal aortic aneurysm	Stone in ureter can mimic an abdominal aortic aneurysm (AAA). AAA present usually in older patient >60 with history of vascular disease. Differentiate with CT, but contrast is necessary for evaluation of AAA as opposed to noncontrast for stone.
Other Musculoskeletal, intestinal obstruction, herpes zoster	

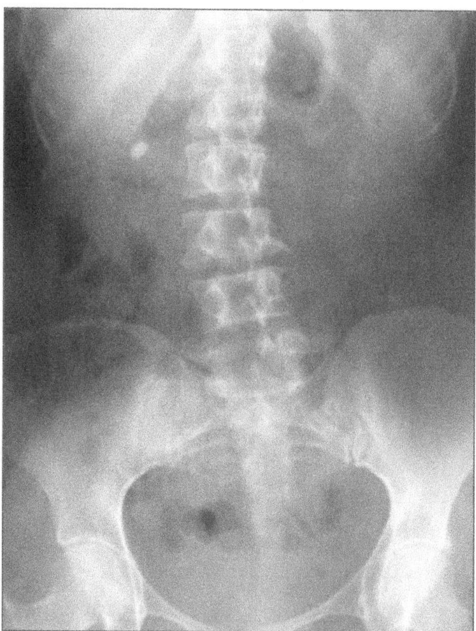

Figure 11.3 **KUB (kidney, ureter, bladder) x-ray of the abdomen showing renal calculus in right lower pole.**

(Source: Saxena V, Kumar R. Bilateral uretic quadruplication with renal calculus. Urology. *2011;77(3):592–593, Fig. 1. doi:10.1016/j.urology.2010.04.004)*

TREATMENT

Acute Management

In the short term, those patients with symptomatic nephrolithiasis can largely be conservatively managed with analgesics and oral or IV hydration until the passage of the stone.

- **Fluids:** This includes oral intake of water or, if the patient cannot intake oral fluids, intravenous normal saline can be used.
- **Pain control:** Nonsteroidal anti-inflammatory drugs (NSAIDs) and opioids are used to control pain in acute renal colic. NSAIDs are typically the preferable option for acute management. Not only do studies indicate that NSAIDs are as effective as opiates, they also decrease ureteral spasm and ureteral smooth muscle tone. Additionally, they typically do not entail side effects such as nausea and/or vomiting as compared to opiates. Similarly, they require less rescue analgesia. Finally, they carry little risk of dependency. However, for those patients with preexisting renal disease or severe volume depletion, NSAIDs should be used with caution as they can further this progression due to their vasoconstrictive properties. Rarely, patients may require narcotic analgesics.
- **Medical expulsive therapy (MET) to facilitate stone passage:** Randomized controlled trials have shown that the use of MET, in conjunction with several medications including alpha blockers and calcium channel blockers, assisted in stone passage for patients being managed conservatively.
- **Urologic intervention:** Stones that are <4 mm in diameter pass spontaneously, stones >4 mm have a progressive decrease in spontaneous passage, while those >10 mm diameter or in the proximal ureter typically require urologic intervention. The choice of modality is dependent on stone size, location, and specific patient characteristics.
    - Ureteroscopy (URS) retrograde is considered first-line treatment for most stones in the mid and distal ureter, stones >10 mm, or in patients with complex renal anatomy, or in patients at increased risk of bleeding.
    - ESWL/URS plays an important role as a second-line therapy for stones in the mid and distal ureter, and stones <10 mm but is contraindicated in pregnancy, those with an increased risk for bleeding, or those with coagulopathy disorders.
    - Percutaneous nephrolithotomy (PCNL) is the cornerstone of management for large, impacted proximal ureteral calculi, staghorn calculi, and large calculi >2 cm.

Chronic Management

- **Stone retrieval and analysis:** Patients should be instructed to strain their urine for several days if following a conservative management course. Any stone material that is passed should then be submitted for analysis. This can guide future dietary and medical interventions for stone prevention.
- **Metabolic evaluation:** Following stone passage, the patient should undergo a comprehensive evaluation for the underlying cause of the stone disease through a combination of 24-hour urine and serum studies, the results of which can then be used to counsel patients on prevention of recurrence. A 24-hour urine collection should be considered in all high-risk first-time stone formers; recurrent stone formers; pediatric patients; patients with solitary kidneys, renal failure, renal transplants, GI bypass, nephrocalcinoisis, chronic kidney disease, or positive family history of stone disease; and immunocompromised patients.
- Response to either dietary therapy or medications is monitored by repeat 24-hour urine collections, which are performed 6 to 8 weeks after treatment commences. If the desired changes are observed, testing is repeated at 6 months and then at yearly intervals.
- Treatments vary depending on the underlying metabolic derangement and stone type. General stone specific therapies are outlined in Table 11.10.

PATIENT EDUCATION

Patients can take several steps to lower the risk of future urinary stone formation, including:

- Increasing fluid intake to increase urine output with a goal of total urine volume in 24 hours >2.5 L/day
- Reduce sodium intake
- Reduce animal protein intake
- Maintain calcium intake
- Reduce oxalate intake
- Avoiding fructose-containing soft drinks as they are associated with an increased urate level

SPECIAL CONSIDERATIONS

- The rise in diabetes, obesity, and hypertension in the pediatric population is resulting in the development of kidney stones in this population.[25] Adolescents are more likely to form stones than younger children. The presentation, underlying causes, and treatment differ in children compared to adults. All children should be referred to a pediatric urologist for further workup and management.

TABLE 11.10 Stone-Specific Therapies

Type of Stone	Therapeutic Options
Calcium oxalate stones	Increase fluid intake Decrease sodium intake Decrease protein intake Maintain normal dietary calcium intake Long-acting thiazide diuretic if hypercalciuric Citrate supplementation Allopurinol or febuxostat if hyperuricosuric Parathyroidectomy if hyperparathyroidism
Calcium phosphate stones	Increase fluid intake Decrease sodium intake Long-acting thiazide diuretics if hyperuricosuric
Uric acid stones	Increased fluid intake Decrease dietary purines by decreasing animal protein intake Increase solubility of uric acid in urine by increasing fluid intake Alkali therapy to raise urine pH to >6.0 Allopurinol
Struvite (staghorn/infection) stones	Removal of infected stone Increase fluid intake Decrease sodium intake Acetohydroxamic acid, effective urease inhibitor, but poorly tolerated
Cystine stones	Rare stone type Increase fluid intake to achieve urinary volume of 3–4 L/day Decrease sodium intake Decrease protein intake Alkali therapy to raise urine pH >7 Thiol-containing drugs (tiopronin or penicillamine)

- Although symptomatic stones during pregnancy are rare, they can occur, particularly during the second or third trimester. Such stones result from the physiologic changes associated with pregnancy. In these cases, renal colic typically radiates to the anterior abdomen or groin. The most common types of stones that occur during pregnancy are calcium phosphate, likely due to a mild increase in urinary calcium excretion, a rise in urine pH, and urinary stasis. The preferred diagnostic tests of choice are renal and pelvic ultrasound to avoid exposing the patient to radiation. Consultation with obstetrics as well as urology is always indicated.
- Elderly individuals are more likely to have atypical presentations, so it is imperative to make the correct diagnosis. The differential diagnosis for the older adult includes abdominal aortic aneurysm and acute myocardial infarction. It is uncommon to have a first-time presentation for renal colic at age 60. If the patient is older than 60 and does not have a prior history of USD, then a high clinical suspicion for an alternate diagnosis is essential.

When to refer:

- Uncontrolled pain, nausea, and vomiting
- Evidence of urinary obstruction and hydronephrosis
- Evidence of sepsis (fever and other signs of infection)
- Anuria
- Anatomic abnormalities, solitary kidney, or chronic kidney disease
- Stones >4 mm in diameter are less likely to pass spontaneously and will require urologic referral and intervention

When to admit:

- Uncontrolled pain, nausea, vomiting
- Obstructing stone with signs of infection

KEY POINTS

- Nephrolithiasis presents with acute onset of severe unilateral flank pain with nausea and vomiting.
- Diagnosis is made by radiologic visualization of stones or by passage or removal of the stone.
- Identifying the underlying causes of stone formation is done through organized evaluation of serum chemistries and urine.

11.4 BLADDER DISORDERS

OVERVIEW

Bladder disorders cause significant health problems with social and economic impact. This section will discuss the following:

- Urinary incontinence—defined as the uncontrolled leakage of urine
- Overactive bladder—presents with frequency, urgency, and urge incontinence
- Vesicoureteral reflux (VUR)—a condition in which urine flows back from the bladder to the ureters and possibly the kidneys

EPIDEMIOLOGY

Incontinence

Urinary incontinence is more common in women. Some degree of incontinence is reported in 25–45% of women and daily incontinence is noted in 9–39% of women over age 60.[26] Risk factors include pregnancy, childbirth, diabetes, and obesity. Prevalence of urinary incontinence in men is approximately half that in women: it is noted in 11–34% of older men, with 2–11% reporting daily symptoms.[26]

Prostate surgery is associated with an increased risk.

Overactive Bladder

The prevalence of overactive bladder increases with age and is more common in women than men. Prevalence is estimated to range from 3% to 43%.[27]

Vesicoureteral Reflux

The prevalence of VUR in normal children has been estimated to be 0.4% to 1.8%.[28]

PATHOPHYSIOLOGY

Incontinence

Incontinence has several different etiologies. Incontinence may be due to bladder dysfunction, sphincter dysfunction, or a combination of both. Sphincter dysfunction leads to stress incontinence and bladder dysfunction leads to urge incontinence. Both sphincter and bladder dysfunction lead to mixed incontinence.

Overactive Bladder

There are two main mechanisms involved in overactive bladder. These mechanisms include an increased sensory (afferent) activity and abnormal management of afferent signals.

Vesioureteral Reflux

VUR is separated into two groups, primary and secondary. Primary VUR is due to a congenital defect that causes inadequate length of the ureter relative to its diameter, which causes inadequacy of the valvular mechanism; secondary VUR is due to the ureters' valvular mechanism being overwhelmed by increased bladder pressures associated with obstruction, which distorts the ureterovesicular junction. The obstructions may be functional or anatomic.

11.4A INCONTINENCE

Urinary incontinence, loss of bladder control, is a common condition and has been reported in up to 45% of women.[26] There are two phases of the bladder function, the filling phase and emptying phase. When these phases are disrupted incontinence can occur.

During the filling phase, the sympathetic nervous system inhibits the parasympathetic activity and assists in bladder filling without a rise in detrusor pressure. The pudendal nerve and sacral efferent nerves control the external urethral sphincter and levator ani muscle during the filling phase. During the emptying phase, inhibition of pudendal and sacral efferent nerves relaxes the external urethral sphincter and levator ani muscle. Loosing of the fascial hammock and descent of the bladder neck occur. The cerebral cortex inhibits sympathetic relaxation of the bladder. The urethra shortens and this lowers resistance to flow, and parasympathetic receptors in the detrusor stimulate bladder contraction.

Stress incontinence is defined as the involuntary immediate loss of urine when the intravesical pressure is higher than urethral pressure. The loss of urine occurs with activities such as coughing, laughing, and exercising. There are typically no associated irritating voiding symptoms. The prevalence of stress urinary incontinence in women ranges from 29% to 75% with a mean of 48%.[29]

Urge incontinence is the loss of urine due to an uninhibited detrusor contraction usually preceded by a strong urge to void. The patient presents with incontinence and has irritating voiding symptoms, such as frequency, urgency, and nocturia. The etiology of urge incontinence is generally thought to be idiopathic. The prevalence of urge incontinence in women is 16.9%.[29]

Mixed urinary incontinence is a combination of stress and urge urinary incontinence. The prevalence of mixed incontinence ranges from 14% to 61%.[29]

Overflow incontinence occurs when urinary retention and overdistention of the bladder leads to a higher intravesical pressure than maximal urethral closure pressure. These patients often have symptoms of spontaneous or continuous leaking. Urinary retention can be due to injury to the sacral portion of the spinal cord or nerves within the cauda equina. Diabetes is a common cause of an overflow incontinence due to peripheral neuropathy and a paralytic bladder.

Risk factors for the various types of urinary incontinence are noted in Table 11.11.

MEDICAL HISTORY AND CLINICAL PRESENTATION

History can aid with the diagnosis of incontinence type. Clinical history of urinary frequency and urgency preceding an incontinence episode has a high sensitivity for diagnosing urge incontinence. A history of only leaking with associated activity, such as coughing and sneezing, is sensitive in 92% diagnosing stress incontinence in women.[30]

A clinical history like stress incontinence but with an inability to empty the bladder without straining is a common symptom noted in overflow incontinence. A clinical history of continuous leaking is commonly associated with a fistula.

PHYSICAL EXAMINATION

Physical examination should focus on signs of medical conditions causing incontinence, such as tumors, stool impaction, and poor reflexes or sensations.

DIFFERENTIAL DIAGNOSIS

The differential diagnosis includes urinary tract fistula, ectopic ureter, and heavy vaginal secretions.

DIAGNOSTIC STUDIES

Diagnostic testing, urodynamics, should be performed in all subjects who fail a trial of conservative therapy or in anyone who may undergo surgical correction. The standard for diagnosing stress urinary incontinence is evidence of leaking of urine with increase in intra-abdominal pressure during urodynamic testing. This includes a simple cough stress test in which the patient's bladder is retrogradely filled through a red rubber catheter to at least 150 mL and visually shows gross urine leak per the urethra during a cough or Valsalva maneuver.

Urge incontinence is diagnosed based on patient's symptoms, after eliminating other conditions. A cystometry demonstrating uninhibited detrusor contractions during the filling phase of the test is confirmatory. Cystometry that documents a bladder capacity that is <250 mL should be referred to a specialist.

TABLE 11.11 Risk Factors for Urinary Incontinence

Stress and Urge	Stress	Urge
Age	Childbirth history	Older age
Obesity	Vaginal delivery	Diabetes mellitus
Family history	Hysterectomy	History of urinary tract infections
Diabetes		High caffeine intake
Hormone replacement therapy		Smoking

Overflow incontinence can be easily diagnosed with obtaining a PVR. A PVR of >300–800 mL would make the diagnosis of overflow incontinence. A PVR of <100 mL is normal.

EVALUATION

The basic evaluation of all patients with incontinence should include a urinalysis, urine culture, renal function tests including a blood urea nitrogen (BUN) and creatinine, and the measurement of PVR.

TREATMENT

Medications can reduce many types of incontinence. Some medications inhibit contractions of an overactive bladder, while others relax muscles leading to more complete bladder emptying during urination. Some drugs tighten muscles at the bladder neck and urethra, preventing leakage, while others cause the muscles involved in urination to function normally. See Table 11.12 for a list of treatment options based on the incontinence type.

Pessaries are medical devices that are inserted into the vagina. The most common is ring-shaped and recommended to correct vaginal prolapse. Pessaries compress the urethra against the symphysis pubis and elevate the bladder neck. This may reduce stress leakage. A possible complication is vaginal infection or UTIs.

Stress incontinence in women may be due to the bladder dropping down toward the vagina. Surgery for stress incontinence involves pulling the bladder up to a more normal position. The procedure of choice in females is a sling procedure. A sling consists of a synthetic mesh material or the patient's own tissue that is placed under the urethra to replace the deficient pelvic floor muscles and provide support under the urethra.

If the incontinence is due to overflow incontinence, a catheter may be used to empty the bladder. Catheters may be used intermittently or on a constant basis. If a long-term catheter is used, UTIs may occur.

Kegel exercises can be used to strengthen or retrain pelvic floor muscles and sphincter muscles to reduce stress leakage. Patients under the age of 60 will benefit the most.

Other treatment options include electrical stimulation, biofeedback, timed voiding, or bladder training.

PATIENT EDUCATION

- Incontinence is not a normal part of aging and should be investigated.
- The basic workup includes renal function tests, urinalysis and culture, and a PVR.
- Management should begin with bladder training and Kegel exercises.

11.4B OVERACTIVE BLADDER

Overactive bladder syndrome is defined as urinary urgency, with or without urgency incontinence, with increased daytime frequency and nocturia. There should be no proven infection or obvious pathology.

Overactive bladder syndrome is a symptomatic diagnosis. This differs from detrusor overactivity, which is characterized by involuntary detrusor contractions during the filling phase.

The prevalence of overactive bladder increases with age and is more common in women than men. Prevalence is estimated to range from 3% to 43%.[27]

MEDICAL HISTORY AND CLINICAL PRESENTATION

A careful history taking, physical exam, and urinalysis are needed in the evaluation of possible overactive bladder. The history should include symptoms such as urgency, urgency incontinence, nocturia, increased frequency, dysuria, hematuria, and lower urinary tract pain.

The major symptom of overactive bladder is urinary urgency. Patients may note leakage due to the urgency; urgency is typically noted at the perineum or the base of penis or vagina/urethra. Urgency urinary incontinence is the involuntary leakage of urine, accompanied or immediately preceded by urgency. Increased daytime frequency is also noted.

PHYSICAL EXAMINATION

The physical examination should include a general assessment with a focus on the abdominal examination for scars, masses such as uterine fibroids, hernias, and distention of the bladder; a neurologic screen for upper motor lesions such as Parkinson disease, and a neurologic screen for lower motor lesions such as sacral nerve root lesions.

A direct rectal examination to determine anal sphincter tone. Fecal impaction distends the distal sigmoid and rectum, resulting in inadequate detrusor activity and compromised bladder emptying.

A vaginal examination may reveal a prolapse of pelvic organs because both cystocele and rectocele may impair bladder emptying and show evidence of urine leakage.

DIAGNOSTIC STUDIES

Laboratory evaluation includes a urinalysis, urine culture, glycosylated hemoglobin (HbA1c), electrolytes, and serum creatinine.

TABLE 11.12 Treatment Options for Incontinence

Vaginal Atrophy	Urge Incontinence	Mixed and Stress Incontinence	Stress Incontinence
Topical/vaginal estrogens	Tolterodine	Imipramine	Pseudoephedrine
	Oxybutynin		Duloxetine
	Propantheline		
	Darifenacin		
	Solifenacin		

PVR urine should be measured using ultrasound or a straight catheter. PVR will be normal on overactive bladder. The residual volume should be <50 mL. Uroflowmetry before and in sequence with the PVR urine test should be obtained; normal is a maximum urinary flow >15 mL/second, with at least 150 mL voided.

Evaluating frequency of voiding and nocturia is carried out by getting the patient to complete a frequency volume chart or bladder diary. In overactive bladder syndrome, the pattern of voided volumes is often erratic.

TREATMENT

The treatment of overactive bladder should start with conservative management and oral pharmacotherapy. Lifestyle interventions include patient education regarding certain aspects, such as volume of fluid intake, smoking cessation, and certain dietary changes. Bladder training and pelvic floor muscle training may reestablish some control over bladder storage.

Drug treatments should be started after conservative methods. Antimuscarinic medications are the main drug class used for treatment. Potential side effects include dry mouth, constipation, cognitive impairment, and visual impairment.

The beta-3-adrenergic agonist, mirabegron, has been shown to help overactive bladder syndrome. Mirabegron works via detrusor relaxation and can be considered for older patients.

Men with overactive bladder syndrome can be given antimuscarinic drugs. If there are concurrent voiding symptoms, they should be given an additional alpha-1-adrenergic blocker as first-line therapy. Side effects include acute urinary retention.

PATIENT EDUCATION

- The causes of overactive bladder are not completely understood, and symptoms may differ among patients.
- A complete cure is rare and the management of an overactive bladder is challenging and should be tailored to the patient's condition.
- Overactive bladder has a major influence on health-related quality of life.

11.4C VESICOURETERAL REFLUX

VUR is defined as the retrograde flow of urine from the bladder into the ureters and kidneys. It is most common in children, occurring in about 0.4–1.8% of children, 2.2% of girls and 0.6% of boys, and 31% of young patients with a UTI.[31]

Primary reflux is noted in a normally functioning lower urinary tract, while secondary reflux is associated with an obstructed or poorly functioning lower urinary tract. This causes abnormally high bladder pressures or an abnormality of the ureterovesical junction.

The most common complication of VUR is the retrograde movement of bacteria from the bladder to the upper urinary tract, which can lead to pyelonephritis and renal scarring.

Primary reflux is a congenital anomaly of the ureterovesical junction; a deficiency of the longitudinal muscle of the intravesical ureter results in an inadequate valvular mechanism. Secondary reflux is caused by bladder outlet obstruction, neuropathic bladder dysfunction, or detrusor sphincter dyssynergia.

MEDICAL HISTORY AND CLINICAL PRESENTATION

VUR is identified in various settings:

- Evaluation of an infant with a history of prenatal hydronephrosis.
- Child who presents with a history of a UTI. In children, symptoms may include complains of lower urinary tract symptoms (LUTS), new onset of urinary incontinence, nausea, abdominal/flank pain, or hematuria. Infants may present with irritability, fussiness, poor oral intake, foul-smelling urine, or fever.
- As part of screening workup of a sibling for VUR.

PHYSICAL EXAMINATION

Physical exam findings may only be significant if the patient has a UTI.

DIFFERENTIAL DIAGNOSIS

The differential diagnosis includes neurogenic bladder, ureteropelvic junction obstruction, UTI, dysfunctional voiding, ureterocele, and ectopic ureter.

DIAGNOSTIC STUDIES

A contrast voiding cystourethrogram (VCUG) is the first step in the evaluation of possible VUR; it allows for the identification of bladder and bladder outlet pathology as well as for the grading of VUR.

Grading is used to determine the likelihood of resolution of VUR (Table 11.13).

EVALUATION

The approach to evaluating VUR begins with a renal ultrasound and VCUG in any child under 5 with a UTI, a child presenting with a febrile UTI, or a boy of any age with a UTI. A VCUG is recommended in a child with prenatally identified hydronephrosis that is confirmed postnatally.

TREATMENT

Because of the high rate of spontaneous resolution, most cases are treated with prophylactic antibiotics and periodic radiologic evaluation. The spontaneous resolution rates for VUR range from 87% for grade I, 77% for grade II, 52% for grade III, 12% for grade IV, and 4% for grade V.[32]

TABLE 11.13 Grading of Vesicoureteral Reflux

Grade	Description
I	Reflux into nondilated ureter
II	Reflux into ureter, renal pelvis, and calyces without dilation
III	Reflux with mild to moderate dilation and minimal blunting of calyces
IV	Reflux with moderate ureteral tortuosity and dilation of pelvis and calyces
V	Reflux with gross dilation of ureter, pelvis, and calyces, loss of papillary impressions and ureteral tortuosity

The most common antibiotic used is amoxicillin, which is used until 8 weeks of age; at 8 weeks children can be switched to trimethoprim-sulfamethoxazole or nitrofurantoin. An alternative option includes cephalexin, used in patients with resistant organisms. Antibiotic prophylaxis may be stopped in older children, over 5–7 years of age, with low-grade VUR and nondocumented renal scarring.

Surgical intervention may be needed in select patients. Indications for surgical intervention include breakthrough UTIs despite prophylactic antibiotics, noncompliance with medical management, severe grades of VUR, and reflux associated with congenital anomalies at the ureterovesical junction.

Surgical treatment consists of open surgical treatment and a minimally invasive approach or cystoscopy and endoscopic injection of dextranomer/hyaluronic acid. Open surgical intervention has the highest success rate but the greatest morbidity. Endoscopic injection therapy is an outpatient procedure with minimal discomfort and has a high success rate depending on the VUR grade.

Short-term complications with intravesical approaches include dysuria, frequency, urgency, and hematuria; these typically resolve in 1 week.

PATIENT EDUCATION

- VUR may spontaneously resolve over time.
- Likelihood of resolution varies with the age of presentation and the grade. The higher the grade and the older the age at presentation, the lower the likelihood of resolution.
- Complications of untreated VUR include pyelonephritis, which can lead to scarring, which can lead to hypertension.

KEY POINTS

- The etiologies of overactive bladder are not completely understood, and symptoms may differ among patients.
- Antimuscarinic agents remain the most effective and simple option to treat the complex symptoms of overactive bladder.
- VUR is often due to congenital abnormalities and diagnosed with a VCUG.

11.5 TESTICULAR DISORDERS

OVERVIEW

As the testis develops a part of the peritoneum constituting the vaginal process projects itself downward into the inguinal canal and emerges at the external inguinal ring. The vaginal process forms a gradually elongating pouch, which reaches the bottom of the scrotum, and behind this pouch the testis is drawn by the growth of the body of the fetus.

By the end of the eighth month the testis has reached the scrotum, preceded by the vaginal process, which communicates with the peritoneal cavity. Just before birth, the upper part of the vaginal process, at the internal inguinal ring, usually becomes closed, and this obliteration extends gradually downward. The process of peritoneum surrounding the testis is now entirely cut off from the general peritoneal cavity and constitutes the tunica vaginalis.

If the internal inguinal ring does not close properly, there is a risk that other contents of the abdominal cavity will protrude through the passageway and cause an indirect inguinal hernia.

Blood supply of the testes and scrotum is separate and distinct. The paired testicular arteries arise directly from the aorta and descend through the inguinal canal; the scrotum and the rest of the external genitalia is supplied by the internal pudendal artery.

Venous drainage is via the paired testicular veins. The veins are formed from the pampiniform plexus in the scrotum. In the retroperitoneal space the left testicular vein drains into the left renal vein, while the right testicular vein drains directly into the inferior vena cava.

11.5A HYDROCELE

Hydrocele is an accumulation of fluid within the process vaginalis/tunica vaginalis. Hydroceles are classified as communicating, noncommunicating, or hydrocele of the cord. Hydroceles are associated with testicular malignancy, so a workup is indicated. Children with a communicating hydrocele are at risk for a hernia.

Most pediatric hydroceles are congenital. The process vaginalis is an outpouching of the peritoneal cavity. It descends with the testes into the scrotum through the inguinal canal and closes shortly after. Peritoneal fluid that surrounds the testis at the time of its descent may become trapped with closure of the process vaginalis. Patent process vaginalis found in term male infants at birth typically close on their own within 18 months of age.

MEDICAL HISTORY AND CLINICAL PRESENTATION

The typical presentation is a painless enlarged scrotum. The patient may report a fullness or heaviness. If pain is noted, this may indicate an accompanying epididymal infection or trauma, or if the pain is severe, testicular torsion.

In children, hydroceles are incidentally identified and present as painless scrotal swelling. The diagnosis of a hydrocele can be confirmed by transillumination of the scrotum.

PHYSICAL EXAMINATION

Physical examination reveals smooth, symmetric enlargement of one side of the scrotum. If the hydrocele is large and tense, it may be difficult to palpate the ipsilateral testis. The size and consistency of hydrocele may vary depending on whether it is communicating or noncommunicating (Figure 11.4).

Communicating hydroceles vary with position; they are smaller in the supine position and increase in size when standing. A Valsalva maneuver can increase the size of a communicating hydrocele. Communicating hydroceles are frequently associated with hernias, which can be elicited or palpated on examination. Unless the cause of the hydrocele is the result of an intrascrotal infectious process, erythema or discoloration is not observed.

Transillumination is usually the first test of choice to evaluate for hydrocele. If a hydrocele is present the light will shine through and light up the scrotum.

DIFFERENTIAL DIAGNOSIS

The differential diagnosis includes testicular tumors, trauma, epididymitis, orchitis, and testicular torsion. A hydrocele is an infrequent complication of varicocele repair.

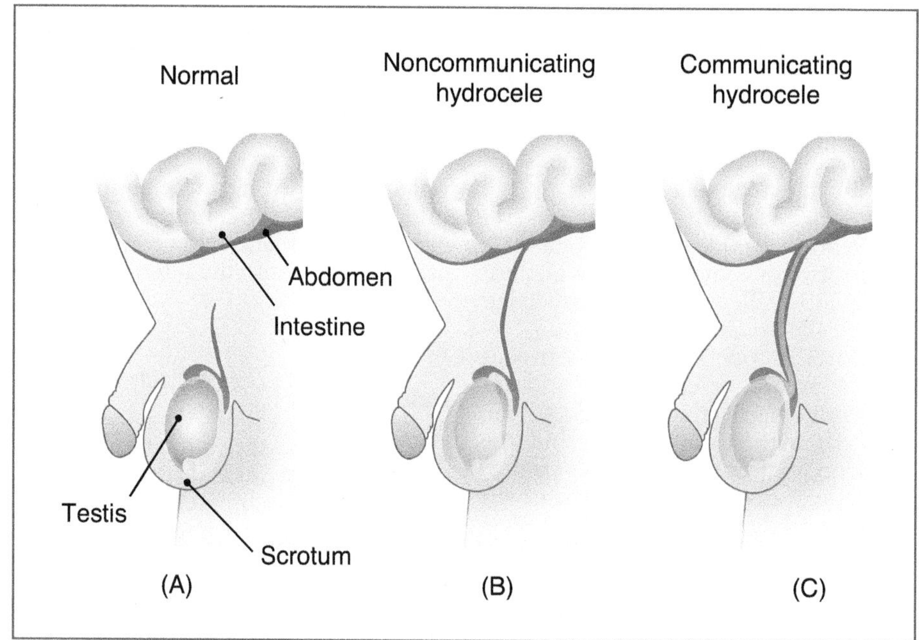

Figure 11.4 Hydrocele. (A) Normal scrotum. (B) Noncommunicating hydrocele. (C) Communicating hydrocele.
(Source: Zeno R, Teall AM. Evidence-based assessment of male genitalia, prostate, rectum, and anus. In: Gawlik KS, Melnyk BM, Teall AM, eds. Evidence-Based Physical Examination. *Springer Publishing Company; 2020:529, Fig. 19.17.)*

DIAGNOSTIC STUDIES

Laboratory tests are not indicated for the evaluation of simple hydroceles. If there is a suspected infectious etiology, epididymitis and/or orchitis, a urinalysis and urine culture should be performed. If testicular tumor is a possible diagnosis, a testicular ultrasound, serum alpha fetoprotein, human chorionic gonadotropin, and lactate dehydrogenase levels should be obtained.

TREATMENT

The first step in the evaluation of the newborn with a hydrocele is to determine if the hydrocele is communicating or noncommunicating. If a noncommunicating hydrocele is demonstrated, observation is indicated because most noncommunicating hydroceles will reabsorb by the first year of life.

If the hydrocele does not reabsorb by the first year of life, inguinal exploration is indicated to ensure that there is no communication and the hydrocele is drained. If the infant has a communicating hydrocele, surgical intervention is indicated because of the risk of an inguinal hernia. If there is an inguinal hernia present, surgical intervention is indicated to prevent incarceration of the hernia.

PATIENT EDUCATION

- Hydroceles can improve with only observation in many patients.
- Surgery has a great success rate; overall, hydroceles have an excellent prognosis

11.5B VARICOCELE

Varicocele is an abnormal enlargement of the scrotum veins that drain the testicles. The testicular vessels start in the abdomen and course down through the inguinal canal as part of the spermatic cord. One-way valves in the veins prevent backward flow of blood and prevent backflow. Defective valves or compression of the vein can cause dilatation of the veins near the testis, leading to the formation of a varicocele.

A varicocele refers to dilatation and tortuosity of the pampiniform plexus. This plexus is a network of veins that drain the testicle. The plexus travels along the posterior portion of the testicle with the epididymis and vas deferens, and then into the spermatic cord. This network then joins the testicular vein. The right testicular vein drains into the inferior vena cava and the left testicular vein drains into the left renal vein.

Varicoceles are present in 15% of the general male population, in 35% of men with primary infertility, and in up to 80% of men with secondary infertility.[33] They are more common in men ages 15–25 years and are most often seen on the left side of the scrotum. Varicoceles are often the cause of infertility in men. The sudden appearance of a left-sided varicocele in an older man may be caused by a kidney tumor, which can block blood flow to a vein. The sudden appearance of a right-sided varicocele could indicate a retroperitoneal mass.

MEDICAL HISTORY AND CLINICAL PRESENTATION

Varicoceles develop slowly. Symptoms of varicocele include an aching pain in the scrotum, feeling of heaviness in the testicle, infertility, atrophy of the testicle, and visible or palpable enlarged vein.

PHYSICAL EXAMINATION

When palpating the scrotum, a nontender, twisted mass along the spermatic cord is felt, the classic "bag of worms." The mass may not be obvious, when lying down, but may be noted with standing. The testicle on the side of the varicocele may or may not be smaller compared to the other side (Figure 11.5).

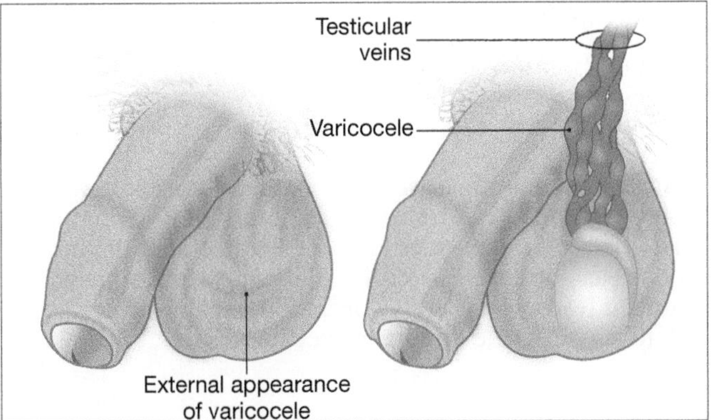

Figure 11.5 Varicocele.
(Source: Zeno R, Teall AM. Evidence-based assessment of male genitalia, prostate, rectum, and anus. In: Gawlik KS, Melnyk BM, Teall AM, eds. Evidence-Based Physical Examination. *Springer Publishing Company; 2020:529, Fig. 19.18.)*

DIAGNOSTIC STUDIES

Varicoceles are diagnosed with ultrasound, which will show dilatation of the vessels of the pampiniform plexus to >2 mm. Patients being evaluated should perform the Valsalva maneuver or stand up during the procedure to increase intra-abdominal venous pressure and increase the dilatation of the veins. Doppler ultrasound will show blood reverse direction in a varicocele with a Valsalva maneuver.

TREATMENT

Varicoceles may be managed with a scrotal support. If pain continues, infertility develops, or there is testicular atrophy, the varicocele may need to be surgically ligated.

Surgical correction with a varicocelectomy can be performed on an outpatient basis. The various approaches include inguinal, retroperitoneal, or subinguinal. Possible procedural complications include hematoma, infection, or injury to the scrotal tissue. An alternative to surgery is embolization, a noninvasive treatment for varicocele. The recovery period is less than with surgery and the risk of complications is minimal. Overall effectiveness is not as high as surgery.

PATIENT EDUCATION

- A varicocele is usually harmless and may require no treatment.
- Varicocele can lead to infertility.

11.5C TORSION

Testicular torsion occurs when the spermatic cord is twisted, cutting off blood supply to the testicle. If not corrected immediately it may result in necrosis of the testicle and surrounding tissues. Testicular torsion can occur at any age, but is seen most frequently in pubertal boys, followed by newborns.

The "bell-clapper" deformity is the lack of fixation of the testis to the scrotal wall because of abnormality of the tunica. The bell-clapper deformity is typically bilateral and noted in 12% of cases.[34]

In adolescents an increase in testes size associated with puberty appears to be a predisposing factor for the development of torsion in the adolescent. Lymphoma involving the testes with the associated testicular enlargement can lead to the development of torsion. In the newborn it maybe due to lack of fixation of the tunica layers to the scrotum.

MEDICAL HISTORY AND CLINICAL PRESENTATION

Acute scrotal pain is a medical emergency. Immediate symptoms are rapid onset of severe local scrotal pain, nausea, and vomiting, followed by scrotal edema and induration. Fever and urinary frequency may be present.

PHYSICAL EXAMINATION

On physical examination the testis is tender and may be elevated and horizontal. The cremasteric reflex is usually absent on the affected side. Scrotum will appear red and swollen and tender to touch. In the newborn it presents as a painless hard intrascrotal mass with some scrotal enlargement.

DIFFERENTIAL DIAGNOSIS

The differential diagnosis includes:

- **Epididymo-orchitis:** inflammation of the epididymis and testes can be secondary to retrograde spread of bacterial infection from the urinary tract. This is the most common cause of scrotal pain in adolescent males.
- **Torsion of the appendix testis:** leads to scrotal pain and acute hydrocele. Typical "blue dot" sign in the scrotum is noted due to the focal nature of the torsion of the testicular appendix.
- **Inguinal hernia:** may present with scrotal pain and swelling. Reduction of the hernia can lead to pain reduction; strangulation of the hernia is a surgical emergency.
- **Varicocele:** present with scrotal swelling; pain is usually chronic if present.
- **Traumatic injury of the testis:** presents with new onset of scrotal enlargement due to an enlarging hematoma.

DIAGNOSTIC STUDIES

Diagnosis of torsion is made with the use of Doppler ultrasound. Ultrasound evaluation can reliably identify any intrascrotal pathology, including trauma, varicocele, epididymitis, hernia, or hydrocele.

No laboratory studies are typically required for diagnosis. A urinalysis and culture may be indicated if epididymitis is in the differential diagnosis.

TREATMENT

If the diagnosis of testicular torsion is a possibility in the adolescent male, immediate surgical exploration is indicated to prevent testis loss. If surgical management is delayed beyond 10 hours, there is little to no chance to save the testicle.

If at the time of surgical exploration, the testis is noted to be nonsalvageable, orchiectomy should be performed. If the testis can be salvaged, orchiopexy is the treatment of choice. The contralateral testis should also be fixed using techniques that will permanently prevent torsion.

PATIENT EDUCATION

- Testicular torsion is a medical emergency and requires immediate surgical management.
- Testicular salvage rates correlate with the duration of the ischemia.
- Despite early surgical management, fertility may be compromised.

11.5D CRYPTORCHIDISM

Cryptorchidism is the absence of at least one testicle from the scrotum. It is the most common birth defect involving the male genitalia. About 3% of full-term and 30% of premature male infants are born with one or both testicles undescended. Approximately 80% of cryptorchid testes descend by the third month of life. This makes the true incidence around 1%.[35]

The undescended testicle can usually be palpated in the inguinal canal. Rarely, the missing testicle may be in the abdomen or be nonexistent.

Undescended testicles are associated with decreased fertility, increased testicular germ cell tumors, testicular torsion, inguinal hernias, and psychological issues.

A normal hypothalamic-pituitary-gonadal axis is required for normal testicular descent. Birth weight and family history are the major risk factors for undescended testes.

In full-term infants, the cause often is not known. Genetics, maternal, and environmental factors may disrupt the hormones and physical changes that influence testicular development and descent.

MEDICAL HISTORY AND CLINICAL PRESENTATION

Signs and symptoms of undescended testicles include the following:

- Reduced fertility, even after orchiopexy.
- Psychological consequences such as disrupted self-esteem.
- Cancer: The risk of testicular cancer if treated before puberty is around two to three times that of the general population and it is five to six times higher when treatment is completed after puberty.[36]

PHYSICAL EXAMINATION

Physical examination will reveal an empty scrotum. The testicle may be noted in the inguinal canal or lower abdomen.

DIFFERENTIAL DIAGNOSIS

The diagnostic challenge is distinguishing a retractile testicle from a testicle that is not spontaneously descending into the scrotum. Retractile testes are more common than undescended testes and do not require surgical correction.

DIAGNOSTIC STUDIES

No laboratory studies are typically required for confirmation of diagnosis.

EVALUATION

Per the American Urological Association (AUA) guidelines: "In the hands of an experienced provider, more than 70% of cryptorchid testes are palpable by physical examination and need no imaging. In the remaining 30% of cases with a nonpalpable testis, the challenge is to confirm absence or presence of the testis and to identify the location of the viable nonpalpable testis."[37]

Currently there is no radiologic test that can conclude with 100% accuracy that a testis is absent.

Hormone levels such as gonadotropins and antimullerian hormone, and a rise of testosterone level with human chorionic gonadotropin stimulation, may confirm hormonally functional testicles worth saving.

TREATMENT

According to AUA Guidelines the use of hormonal therapy to induce testicular descent is not indicated as studies show low response rates and lack of evidence for long-term efficacy.[37]

Surgery is recommended for congenital undescended testes between the ages of 6 and 18 months.[37] For premature babies, corrected age is used to determine surgery timing. Early surgery improves fertility. Patients with bilateral undescended testes who receive orchidopexies as adults are almost always infertile and have azoospermia.

PATIENT EDUCATION

- With proper diagnosis and treatment, prognosis is excellent. Testicular cancer risk and infertility remain increased compared to the general population.
- Orchiopexy is associated with two major complications: atrophy and testicular ascent.

KEY POINTS

- Testicular torsion is a surgical emergency.
- Without surgical correction, an undescended testicle may descend during the first 3 months of life. To reduce risks, undescended testes may be brought into the scrotum with an orchiopexy.

11.6 PENILE DISORDERS

OVERVIEW

Penile disorders can lead to significant morbidity for patients. Prompt recognition and diagnosis of penile disorders can be challenging. Because of the organ's anatomy and physiology, failure or even moderate delays in identifying acute conditions can result in permanent dysfunction and morbidity. Penile disorders fall into two major categories: physiologic and anatomic.

11.6A ERECTILE DYSFUNCTION

Erectile dysfunction (ED) is the inability to attain or sustain an erection satisfactory for sexual intercourse. ED affects 18 million men in the United States. The overall prevalence of ED in men ≥20 years of age is 18.4%.[38]

There are two types of ED: primary, which is defined as the inability to attain or sustain an erection, and secondary, which is defined as dysfunction acquired later in life by a man who previously was able to attain erections.

Primary ED is rare and typically due to psychological factors or clinically obvious anatomic abnormalities. Secondary ED is more common, with a clear majority having an organic etiology. Many with secondary ED develop reactive psychological difficulties that compound the problem.

Psychological factors should be considered in every case of ED. Causes of primary ED include guilt, fear of intimacy, depression, or anxiety. In secondary ED, causes may relate to performance anxiety, stress, or depression.

Organic causes of ED include vascular and neurologic disorders. The most common vascular cause is atherosclerosis of cavernous arteries of the penis. Atherosclerosis and aging decrease the capacity for dilation of blood vessels and smooth muscle relaxation, limiting the amount of blood that can enter the penis.

Neurologic causes include stroke, partial complex seizures, multiple sclerosis, peripheral and autonomic neuropathies, and spinal cord injuries. Diabetic neuropathy and surgical injury are common causes. Prolonged perineal pressure or pelvic or perineal trauma can cause ED.

Testosterone deficiency may decrease libido and cause ED. Numerous drugs can cause ED. See Table 11.14 for the various medications that can cause ED.

MEDICAL HISTORY AND CLINICAL PRESENTATION

A detailed history should include a history of drug and alcohol use, pelvic surgery and trauma, smoking, diabetes, hypertension, and atherosclerosis. Symptoms of vascular, hormonal, neurologic, and psychological disorders should be investigated. A sexual history should assess satisfaction with sexual relationships, including evaluation of partner interaction and partner sexual dysfunction. Each patient should be evaluated for depression, with the Beck Depression Scale or Yesavage Geriatric Depression Scale, as depression may not be apparent.

PHYSICAL EXAMINATION

Physical examination should focus on the genitals and signs of vascular, neurologic and hormonal disorders. Genitals should be examined for signs of hypogonadism and fibrous bands and plaques. Neurologic dysfunction should be considered if poor rectal tone, decreased perineal sensation, or abnormal bulbocavernosus reflexes are noted. Vascular dysfunction is suggested if diminished peripheral pulses are noted.

In young healthy men with abrupt onset of ED, a psychological cause should be suspected. A history of ED with spontaneous improvement suggests psychogenic ED. Men with psychogenic ED usually have normal nocturnal erections and erections upon awakening, whereas men with organic ED often do not.

TABLE 11.14 Common Drugs That Can Cause Erectile Dysfunction

Antihypertensive Agents	Central Nervous System Agents	Others
Beta blockers	Alcohol	Cimetidine
Clonidine	Cocaine	Estrogens
Spironolactone	Anxiolytics	Amphetamines
Thiazide diuretics	Opioids	5-Alpha-reductase inhibitors
	Selective serotonin reuptake inhibitors	Antiandrogens
	Tricyclic antidepressants	Chemotherapeutics

DIAGNOSTIC STUDIES

Laboratory assessment should include measurement of morning testosterone level; if low, prolactin and luteinizing hormone levels should be measured. Evaluation for diabetes, dyslipidemias, hyperprolactinemia, thyroid disease, and Cushing syndrome should be completed based on signs and symptoms.

Duplex ultrasonography after intracavernous injection of a vasoactive drug is used to evaluate penile vasculature. Sleep-entrained erectile events, measured by nocturnal penile tumescence monitors, may help differentiate between organic and psychogenic etiology of ED.

TREATMENT

Treatment of underlying causes, medications discontinued if possible, and reassurance and education should be first steps.

First-line treatment of ED is typically an oral phosphodiesterase inhibitor. Oral phosphodiesterase inhibitors, such as sildenafil, vardenafil, avanafil, and tadalafil selectively inhibit cyclic guanosine monophosphate (cGMP)–specific phosphodiesterase type 5 (PDE5). By preventing cGMP hydrolysis these drugs promote the cGMP-dependent smooth muscle relaxation that is essential for normal erection.

All PDE5 inhibitors cause coronary vasodilation and potentiate the hypotensive effects of other nitrates, as well as recreational amyl nitrate ("poppers"). The concomitant use of nitrates and PDE5 inhibitors should be avoided. Adverse effects of PDE5 inhibitors include flushing, visual abnormalities, hearing loss, dyspepsia, and headache. Patients taking an alpha blocker should wait at least 4 hours before using a PDE5 inhibitor. Rarely, PDE5 inhibitors cause priapism.

Alprostadil (prostaglandin E1) is self-administered via intraurethral insertion or intracavernosal injection and can produce erections with a mean duration of 30 to 60 minutes.

Several mechanical devices are available for treating ED. A constriction ring, around the base of the penis, can be used to help maintain erection. Vacuum erection devices draw blood into the penis via suction, after which an elastic ring is placed at the base of the penis to maintain the erection.

If drugs and vacuum devices fail, surgical implantation of a penile prosthesis can be considered. Prostheses include semirigid silicone rods and saline-filled multicomponent inflatable devices.

PATIENT EDUCATION

- ED can be a normal part of aging.
- Risk factors include chronic health conditions, medications, trauma or surgery, substance abuse, alcohol, and smoking.
- ED can lead to feelings of inadequacy and loss of confidence.

11.6B PARAPHIMOSIS/PHIMOSIS

Paraphimosis, a urologic emergency, occurs in uncircumcised males when the foreskin becomes trapped behind the corona of the glans penis and can lead to strangulation of the glans as well as venous engorgement, edema, and necrosis. Phimosis occurs when the foreskin is unable to be retracted behind the glans of the penis.

In uncircumcised children, paraphimosis is very rare, and less common than phimosis. Paraphimosis is most commonly found in adolescents.

Paraphimosis is an iatrogenic or inadvertently induced condition; coitus as well as penile piercings can lead to paraphimosis. If a constricting band of the foreskin remains retracted behind the glans penis for a prolonged period, this can lead to impairment of distal venous drainage as well as decreased arterial blood flow to the glans. These changes can lead to marked ischemia and potential necrosis of the glans.

Physiological phimosis is secondary to mechanical conditions that prevent retraction of the foreskin. This includes the tip of the foreskin being too narrow to pass over the glans penis and the inner surface of the foreskin is fused with the glans penis. Both are normal findings in children and adolescents. The third condition occurs when the frenulum is too short to allow complete retraction of the foreskin.

Pathologic phimosis is rare, and causes vary.

MEDICAL HISTORY AND CLINICAL PRESENTATION

History is important in the evaluation of the patient with paraphimosis or phimosis. The history should include any recent penile catheterizations, instrumentation, cleaning, or other procedures. History of routine cleaning of the penis and if he or a caregiver routinely retract the foreskin for any reason should be obtained.

Typical paraphimosis symptoms include erythema, pain, and swelling of foreskin and glans due to the constricting ring of the phimotic foreskin.

In physiologic phimosis, ballooning of the foreskin is a common presentation in childhood when the foreskin is still nonretractile. It is self-limiting and resolves once the foreskin becomes more retractile.

PHYSICAL EXAMINATION

The history typically makes the diagnosis, but it will be obvious on direct physical examination. The physical exam should focus on the penis and foreskin. A pink color to the glans is indicative of adequate blood supply; a dark, dusky or black color indicates possible ischemia or necrosis. The physical examination in phimosis will reveal an unretractable foreskin. Paraphimosis presents with acute, distal, penile pain and swelling; pain is not always present (Figure 11.6). The proximal penile shaft is flaccid and unremarkable. A tight band of constrictive tissue is present, often preventing manual reduction of the foreskin over the glans.

By history and physical examination, it should be determined if the patient is circumcised or uncircumcised. It is possible to develop paraphimosis in a patient who has previously been circumcised. This can be due to the patient believing he was circumcised when he was not or excessive remaining foreskin despite the circumcision.

DIAGNOSTIC STUDIES

Laboratory tests and radiography are not typically required in the assessment of paraphimosis or phimosis.

TREATMENT

Mild, uncomplicated paraphimosis can be reduced manually, without sedation or analgesia. Difficult or complicated cases may require local dorsal penile block anesthesia, systemic analgesia, or procedural sedation.

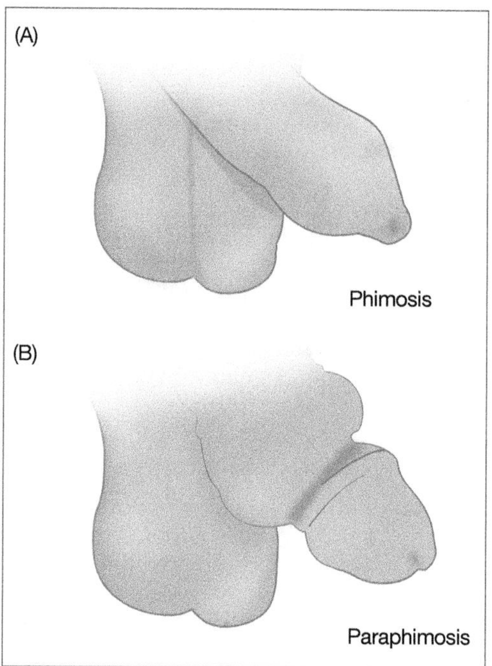

Figure 11.6 (A) Phimosis and (B) paraphimosis.
(Source: Zeno R, Teall AM. Evidence-based assessment of male genitalia, prostate, rectum, and anus. In: Gawlik KS, Melnyk BM, Teall AM, eds. Evidence-Based Physical Examination. *Springer Publishing Company; 2020:529, Fig. 19.15.)*

Manual reduction of paraphimosis can be facilitated by simple compression of the glans and the swollen, edematous foreskin for several minutes before attempting reduction. This will decrease the edematous swelling of the retracted foreskin before attempting repositioning of the foreskin. Surgical treatment of the paraphimosis is required if manual reduction methods are unsuccessful.

Treatment of physiologic phimosis is not indicated, and reassurance of the natural history of the healthy nonretractile foreskin should be provided to concerned parents. Circumcision is the preferred treatment for pathologic phimosis.

PATIENT EDUCATION

- After successful manual reduction, the foreskin should carefully be cleaned. Patients should be instructed to avoid retracting the foreskin for 1 week and avoid any offending activities that contributed to the paraphimosis.
- Physiologic phimosis will resolve spontaneously, resulting in a fully and easily retractable prepuce in almost all boys by the age of 16.

11.6C HYPOSPADIAS/EPISPADIAS

Hypospadias is a congenital anatomic malformation of the male external genitalia. Abnormal development of the urethral fold and the ventral foreskin of the penis causes abnormal positioning of the urethral opening. Epispadias is less common and is a malformation in which the urethral meatus is found on the dorsal side of the penis. Epispadias is most commonly associated with bladder exstrophy.

In hypospadias, the external urethral meatus may present various degrees of malpositioning and may be found with associated penile curvature.

Hypospadias is classified by the location of the abnormal urethral meatus:

- Anterior (subcoronal and glandular)
- Middle (distal penile, proximal penile and midshaft)
- Posterior (scrotal and perineal)

Hypospadias is the second most common congenital disorder in males after cryptorchidism, but is the most common penile congenital malformation. The incidence of hypospadias in the United States has been reported to be 1 out of every 250 males (0.4%).[39] In the United States, the prevalence of classic bladder exstrophy is 3.3 per 100,000 births; male epispadias occurs in 1 in 117,000 births, and female epispadias in 1 in 484,000 births.[40]

MEDICAL HISTORY AND CLINICAL PRESENTATION

A thorough history and physical exam are necessary including a family history of hypospadias and epispadias. The diagnosis of both is made soon after birth.

The key features of hypospadias include a glandular groove and a dorsal hood of the foreskin but in almost all cases the prepuce is incomplete ventrally. The urethral meatus is usually in an abnormal location.

Patients with hypospadias should not be circumcised. The extra tissue of the foreskin may be used to repair the hypospadias. Some patients may have an associated penile curvature, which may be obvious during an erection.

With epispadias the urethra opens on the dorsum of the glans, penile shaft, or at the penopubic junction. In girls, the urethra opens between the clitoris and labia or in the abdomen. Epispadias can be partial or complete; the most severe form occurs with bladder exstrophy. Symptoms and signs of epispadias include incontinence, reflux, and UTIs.

PHYSICAL EXAMINATION

In hypospadias the prepuce is incomplete ventrally and the urethral meatus is noted in an abnormal proximal location. Penile curvature may be apparent or may be discernible only during erection. Proximal hypospadias is associated with a bifid scrotum.

Patients with classic bladder exstrophy or epispadias typically appear as term infants. In classic bladder exstrophy, the bladder is open on the lower abdomen, with mucosa fully exposed through a triangular fascial defect (Figure 11.7). Indirect inguinal hernias are frequent due to wide inguinal rings and the lack of an oblique inguinal canal. In male epispadias, the phallus is short and broad with upward curvature. The glans lies open and flat, and the dorsal component of the foreskin is absent. The urethral meatus is located on the dorsal penile shaft. In female epispadias, the clitoris is often bifid with divergent labia.

DIAGNOSTIC STUDIES

Diagnostic studies are typically not indicated. Imaging studies may be needed to determine extent of structural abnormalities.

TREATMENT

Surgical correction is the mainstay treatment of hypospadias. The main objectives of surgical correction are to straighten the penis with an adequate caliber of the meatus to give an appearance resembling a typical circumcised penis or a penis with a foreskin.

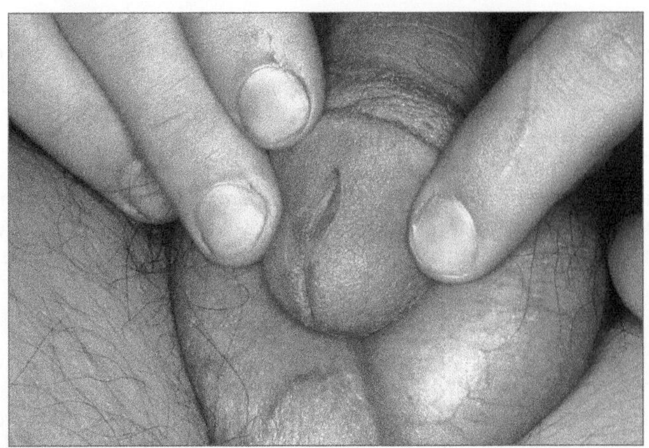

Figure 11.7 Epispadias.
(Source: Centers for Disease Control and Prevention, Gavin Hart, MD.)

In some cases, patients may undergo systemic treatment with testosterone derivatives to increase the penile size and allow better tubularization and avoid or decrease dehiscence before surgical repair.

Surgery is recommended when the patient is between 6 and 18 months of age to limit psychological stress and behavioral problems.

Treatment of epispadias is surgical.

PATIENT EDUCATION

- Exstrophy-epispadias syndrome is a complex anomaly that often requires several surgical procedures and requires lifelong medical follow-up care.

11.6D PEYRONIE DISEASE

Peyronie disease (PD), or congenital penile curvature, is a superficial fibrosing condition of the penis characterized by the presence of fibrotic plaques leading to penile deformity, with or without associated pain. Men with PD most commonly present in their sixth decade of life. PD impacts sexual function and is also associated with psychosocial distress in patients and their partners. PD has a reported prevalence of 0.5–13% in adult men.[41]

The etiology of PD is multifactorial and not completely understood. The most prevalent theory implicates penile trauma, including both acute traumatic events as well as repetitive microtrauma such as that which occurs during intercourse.

MEDICAL HISTORY AND CLINICAL PRESENTATION

PD affects men in the sixth decade of life, with mean age at diagnosis ranging from 52 to 59 years.[41] The hallmark of PD is an acquired penile deformity. PD-related deformity consists of curvature during erection; additional findings include loss of flaccid stretched penile length and an hourglass deformity with erection. The curvature in PD may be in any direction but is most commonly dorsal. Patients with dorsal curvature have more severe curvature than other PD patients.

There are two phases of PD: acute and chronic phase. The acute phase is characterized by progression of penile deformity and may be associated with pain in the erect and/or flaccid states. The length of the acute phase varies from 6 to 18 months. The chronic phase is characterized by stability of penile deformity for at least 6 months, with reduction or resolution of pain.

History should assess the timing of symptom onset, presence of potential inciting incidents, including a history of penile trauma, progression or stability of the deformity, and any interference with intercourse.

PHYSICAL EXAMINATION

Physical examination of the penis should be performed in both the flaccid and erect states. The examination should include a measurement of penile curvature. In the flaccid state, determine stretched penile length and note palpable penile plaque location and size.

DIAGNOSTIC STUDIES

A duplex Doppler penile ultrasound should be obtained to evaluate plaque size, location, and calcification. Ultrasonography after intracavernosal injection is the most accurate assessment tool to determine type and degree of PD deformity.

Laboratory testing is typically not necessary for PD diagnosis. Because of the possible association between PD, diabetes mellitus, and cardiovascular disease, screening for these comorbidities should be considered in at-risk patients.

TREATMENT

Treatment of PD utilizes both medical and surgical approaches.

Surgical intervention should be avoided during the acute phase of PD, as the risk of progression or recurrence of curvature during this phase may interfere with optimal outcomes. Penile deformity and any associated ED should be stable for at least 3–6 months prior to surgical intervention to avoid progressive disease after treatment.

Numerous drugs have been evaluated in the treatment of PD with little proven efficacy. Local injections of verapamil or high-potency corticosteroids into the plaque may be effective; oral corticosteroids are not effective.

PATIENT EDUCATION

- Patients should be made aware that treatment results are unpredictable.

11.6E URETHRAL STRICTURE

Urethral stricture is scarring of the lining of the urethra and surrounding corpus spongiosum that obstructs the anterior urethral lumen. It can be caused by injury, such as straddle or pelvic fracture trauma, or disease such as lichen sclerosis.

Urethral strictures that are caused by trauma such as straddle injury are in the portion of the bulbar urethra proximal to the penis under the scrotum. Trauma can lead to transection of the urethra below the prostate and the attempt at repair leads to the development of scar tissue in the urethra causing narrowing or even closure.

The skin disease lichen sclerosis is an inflammatory disorder that affects the penile skin and can lead to progressive stricture disease. The stricture is just at the tip of the penis. Delay in diagnosis can lead to stricture of the entire anterior urethra.

Other causes of urethral strictures include urethral instrumentation with cystoscopes, hypospadias, complication of surgery to reconstruct the urethra, and infections and STIs. Urethral strictures are rarely congenital.

MEDICAL HISTORY AND CLINICAL PRESENTATION

Symptoms typically do not develop until the urethral lumen diameter has been greatly decreased. Symptoms include a double urine stream; obstructive symptoms including weak urinary stream, hesitancy, or incomplete emptying; or recurrent UTIs. The bladder's capacity may significantly increase due to the inability to completely void.

Urethral strictures may lead to the inability to urinate and may require emergency treatment.

PHYSICAL EXAMINATION

Physical examination is unremarkable. A distended bladder may be noted in the suprapubic region with urinary retention.

DIFFERENTIAL DIAGNOSIS

The differential diagnosis includes urologic conditions that can cause bladder outlet obstruction, such as prostate enlargement.

DIAGNOSTIC STUDIES

Urethral stricture is suspected when urethral catheterization is difficult. Diagnosis of urethral stricture is confirmed by retrograde urethrography, cystoscopy, or urethral ultrasound.

TREATMENT

Treatment is determined by the type of obstruction. One of the most common procedures is dilation or endoscopy, an internal urethrotomy. If the stricture is complicated or persists despite treatment, dilation and endoscopy should be avoided; and daily self-catheterization may be indicated. Open urethroplasty may be indicated if the stricture is localized and causes recurrent problems.

PATIENT EDUCATION

- Overall prognosis is good, repeated treatments may be needed.
- Urinary retention is a medical emergency and should be treated as soon as possible.

KEY POINTS

- ED can be due to vascular, neurologic, psychological, hormonal disorders and using certain drugs can compromise achievement of satisfactory erections.
- Paraphimosis is a urologic emergency, occurring in uncircumcised males, in which the foreskin becomes trapped behind the corona and forms a tight band of constricting tissue.
- Hypospadias is a birth defect in which the opening of the urethra is not located at the tip of the penis but located anywhere from just below the end of the penis to the scrotum.
- PD is commonly caused by minor injury to the penis, often during vigorous sex, sports, or traumatic accidents.

11.7 BENIGN PROSTATIC HYPERPLASIA

OVERVIEW

Benign prostatic hyperplasia (BPH) is nonmalignant adenomatous overgrowth of the prostate gland. Symptoms include weak stream, hesitancy, frequency, urgency, nocturia, incomplete emptying, terminal dribbling, overflow or urge incontinence, and complete urinary retention. Diagnosis is based primarily on digital rectal examination and symptoms. Treatment options include 5-alpha-reductase inhibitors, alpha blockers, tadalafil, and surgery.

EPIDEMIOLOGY

Using the American Urological Symptom score of moderate or high and a prostate volume >30 mL, the prevalence of BPH in men age 55 to 74 without prostate cancer is 19%.[42] Based on autopsy studies, the prevalence of BPH increases from 8% in men age 31 to 40 years to 40–50% in men age 51–60 years and to >80% in men over age 80.[43]

PATHOPHYSIOLOGY

Prostatic enlargement depends on androgen dihydrotestosterone (DHT). In the prostate, 5-alpha-reductase metabolizes circulating testosterone into DHT. DHT binds to androgen receptors in the cell nuclei, potentially resulting in BPH. Other possible factors include the metabolic syndrome, hyperinsulinemia, norepinephrine, angiotensin II, and insulin-like growth factors.

Alpha-1-adrenergic receptors, located in the smooth muscle of the stroma, capsule of the prostate, and the bladder neck, when stimulated cause an increase in smooth muscle tone, which can worsen LUTS.

Multiple fibroadenomatous nodules develop in the periurethral region of the prostate. As the lumen of the prostatic urethra narrows, urine outflow is progressively obstructed. Increased pressure associated with micturition and bladder distention can progress to hypertrophy of the bladder detrusor. Incomplete bladder emptying leads to stasis and predisposes patient to stone formation and infection. Prolonged obstruction can cause hydronephrosis and compromise renal function.

MEDICAL HISTORY AND CLINICAL PRESENTATION

Symptoms of BPH include a group of symptoms that are often progressive, known as LUTS; they include urinary frequency, urgency, nocturia, hesitancy, and intermittency. Pain and dysuria are typically not present. Sensations of incomplete emptying, terminal dribbling, overflow incontinence, or urinary retention may develop. Straining to void can cause rupture of the superficial veins of the prostatic urethra and trigone causing hematuria.

Symptoms can be quantitated by the 7-question AUA Symptom Score.[44] This score also allows monitoring of symptom progression:

- Mild symptoms: Scores 1 to 7
- Moderate symptoms: Scores 8 to 19
- Severe symptoms: Scores 20 to 35

PHYSICAL EXAMINATION

On digital rectal examination, the prostate usually is enlarged and nontender, with a rubbery consistency, and there may be loss of the median furrow. If bladder distention is present the urinary bladder may be palpable during abdominal examination.

DIFFERENTIAL DIAGNOSIS

The differential diagnosis includes prostate cancer, prostatitis, neurogenic bladder, urethral stricture, and overactive bladder.

DIAGNOSTIC STUDIES

To rule out other possible etiologies, laboratory studies such as urinalysis and urine culture and serum prostate-specific antigen (PSA) levels should be obtained.

In patients with moderate or severe symptoms of obstruction a uroflowmetry with measurement of PVR volume by bladder ultrasonography should be obtained. Flow rate <15 mL/second suggests obstruction, and PVR volume >100 mL suggests retention.

The PSA level is moderately elevated in up to half of the patients with BPH, depending on prostate size and degree of obstruction, and is elevated in most patients with prostate cancer, depending on the tumor volume.

In patients without cancer, serum PSA levels >1.5 ng/mL usually indicate a prostate volume ≥30 mL. If the PSA level is >4 ng/mL, other tests or biopsy is recommended.

Transrectal biopsy with ultrasound guidance is indicated if there is suspicion of prostate cancer.

TREATMENT

All anticholinergics, sympathomimetics, and opioids should be stopped, if possible, as these medications can worsen symptoms, and any infection should be treated with antibiotics.

Significant urinary retention requires immediate treatment. Passage of a standard urinary catheter is the treatment of choice followed by a catheter with a coudé tip or flexible cystoscopy. Suprapubic percutaneous decompression of the bladder may be needed if other approaches are not successful.

For patients with mild to moderate obstructive symptoms, alpha-adrenergic blockers, such as terazosin, doxazosin, and tamsulosin, may decrease voiding problems. The 5-alpha-reductase inhibitors, finasteride and dutasteride, may reduce prostate size and decrease voiding problems over months. A combination of both classes of drugs is superior to monotherapy. For men with concurrent ED, tadalafil may relieve both conditions. Many over-the-counter (OTC) complementary and alternative agents, such as saw palmetto, have not been shown to be effective.

Surgery is considered when patients do not respond to drug therapy or develop complications. Transurethral resection of the prostate (TURP) is the standard treatment. Postprocedural complications are rare but include retrograde ejaculation, ED, and incontinence.

Other procedures include microwave thermotherapy, electrosurgery or radiofrequency vaporization, laser techniques, high-intensity focused ultrasonography, transurethral needle ablation, and pressurized heated water injection therapy.

PATIENT EDUCATION

- Treatment options include watchful waiting, medications, and surgery.
- Complications include urinary retention, renal insufficiency, recurrent UTIs, hematuria, and bladder stones.

KEY POINTS

- BPH is extremely common with aging but only occasionally causes symptoms.
- Evaluate patients with a digital rectal examination, urinalysis, urine culture, and PSA test.
- Treatment consists alpha-adrenergic blockers, 5-alpha-reductase inhibitors, tadalafil, or TURP.

COMMON CHIEF COMPLAINTS

APPROACH TO HEMATURIA

Hematuria is defined as blood in the urine. Gross hematuria is noted when looking at the urine, and microscopic hematuria is noted on urinalysis or microscopic examination of the urine.

If gross hematuria is present a microscopic evaluation of the urine should be obtained to confirm presence of red blood cells (RBCs). Other sources should be considered such as urine catheter trauma, menstrual blood contamination, or UTI.

Microscopic hematuria is often due to benign or transient causes but can also be the first sign of a pathologic process such as a glomerulopathy or cancer.

The differential diagnosis for hematuria can be divided into two major categories: glomerular or nonglomerular. See Figure 11.8 for the differential diagnosis of hematuria.

Hematuria can also be categorized by anatomic source:

- **Intrarenal:** Causes include kidney stones, renal cancer, kidney trauma, exercise, glomerulopathies, acute tubular necrosis, acute interstitial nephritis, small vessel disease, renal cyst, polycystic kidney disease, and papillary necrosis.
- **Renal vasculature:** Causes include renal vein thrombosis, renal artery stenosis, and renal arteriovenous fistula.
- **Extrarenal:** Causes include contamination, kidney stones, bladder cancer or infection, prostate cancer/hypertrophy/infection, UTI, Foley catheter trauma, VUR, radiation cystitis, bladder diverticulum, bladder neck contracture, IC, cystocele, urethrocele, and neurogenic bladder.
- **Bleeding disorders:** This is a rare cause and typically there is bleeding at multiple sites.
- **Spurious:** If discolored urine is not due to blood, etiologies include beets, medicine discoloration, and porphyria. If heme-positive urine dipstick is noted but no RBCs on the sediment possible causes include lysed RBCs, myoglobinuria due to muscle breakdown, hemoglobinuria due to hemolysis, or the presence of semen in a postcoital sample.

First step in the evaluation is a urinalysis and microscopic evaluation of the urine sediment to confirm the presence of hematuria. The presence of RBCs and WBCs may indicate infection. The presence of dysmorphic RBCs and RBC casts should also be noted (Figure 11.9).

The presence or absence of proteinuria should be determined. If there is at least 1+ proteinuria on the urinalysis,

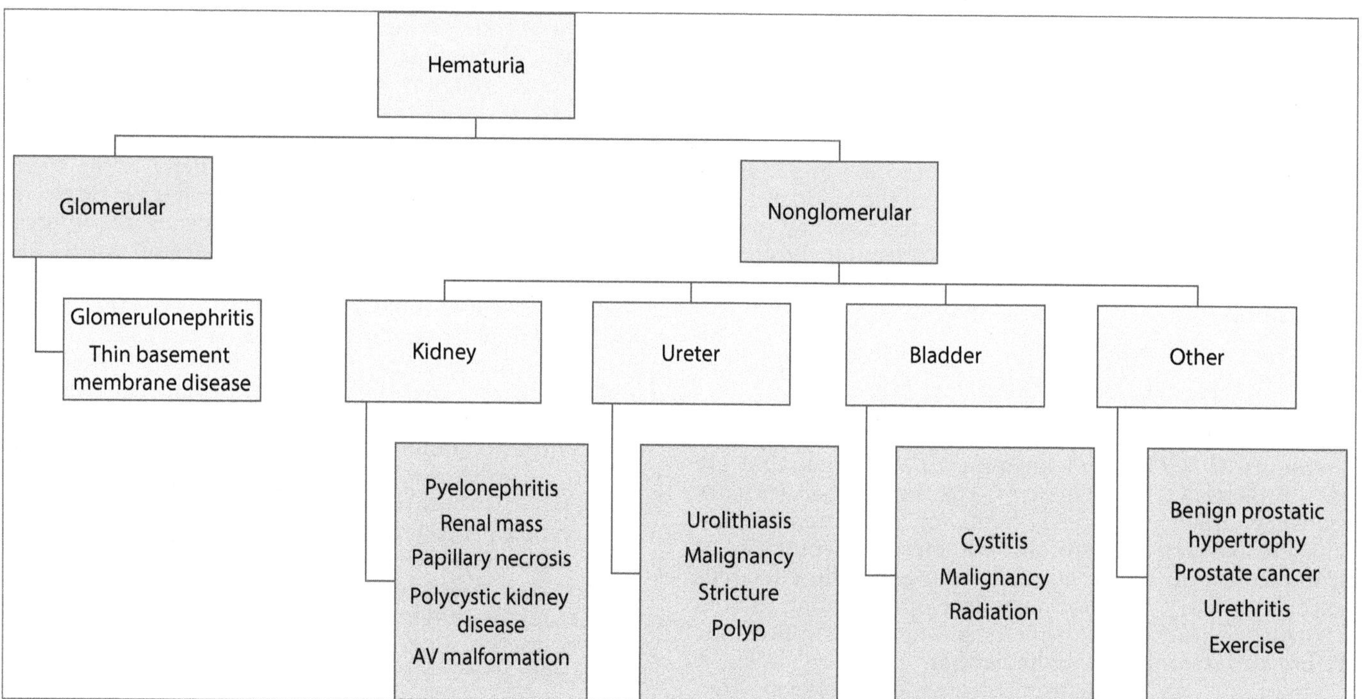

Figure 11.8 Differential diagnosis of hematuria. AV, arteriovenous.

a 24-hour urine protein should be obtained. An abnormal result would be >500 mg/day. A serum creatinine level will help identify any kidney dysfunction.

Depending on the findings, other tests may be needed such as a kidney biopsy, a multiphasic CT urography without and with IV contrast, a cystoscopy, or urine cytology.

The diagnosis of hematuria can also be guided by the age of the patient. See Table 11.15 for the etiologies of hematuria based on age.

For steps in the evaluation of the patient with hematuria see the diagnostic algorithm in Figure 11.10.

Consider the following:

- Characterize the hematuria as gross hematuria versus microscopic hematuria. Gross hematuria should then be characterized as containing clots or not. Clots almost always signify a lower urinary tract issue.
- With nonclotted gross hematuria and microscopic hematuria, the next step is a urinalysis and microscopic evaluation of the urine. Red urine that is both heme-negative on urinalysis and RBC-negative on microscopic analysis is most likely due to a food, a medicine, or porphyria. If heme-positive, but RBC-negative, the most likely etiology is either myoglobinuria or hemoglobinuria, due to rhabdomyolysis or hemolysis; presence of semen causing a false positive heme test; or hematuria in which the RBCs have lysed. If urine is both heme- and RBC-positive, this is true hematuria.
- If true hematuria, the next step is to check for protein in the urinalysis, an increasing creatinine, or evidence of abnormal cells such as dysmorphic RBCs or RBC casts. Proteinuria suggests an intrarenal cause of the hematuria. An increasing serum creatinine helps in confirming that the process is intrarenal. The presence of dysmorphic RBCs or RBC casts is pathognomonic of a glomerulonephritis. Lone persistent glomerular hematuria, without evidence of renal insufficiency or systemic disease, may be IgA nephropathy, Alport syndrome, or thin basement membrane disease.
- Evaluate the urine for presence of WBCs. If >5 WBCs per high-power field (HPF), this indicates pyuria. Pyuria can be divided into culture-positive pyuria or sterile pyuria. Culture-positive pyuria is caused by a UTI. Sterile pyuria may be due to an improperly cultured UTI, contamination of leukocytes from a genital infection, prostatitis, acute interstitial nephritis, glomerulonephritis, analgesic nephropathy, atypical organisms, bladder cancer, or nephrolithiasis.
- Evaluate for risk of cancer. A patient is at greatest risk of cancer as a cause of hematuria if they are over 40–50 years of age, are a smoker, have been exposed to known carcinogens or chemotherapy or radiation, or have a history of chronic analgesic use.
- The next step is imaging of the upper urinary tract with CT and testing of the lower urinary tract with cystoscopy. Gross hematuria is most likely due to bladder cancer and is associated with diagnosing cancer at a more advanced stage.
- If no cause is immediately found, the hematuria should be followed. If the diagnosis continues to be negative, rarer causes of hematuria can be considered such as urinary tract endometriosis, polycystic kidney disease, sickle cell disease, and renal infarcts.

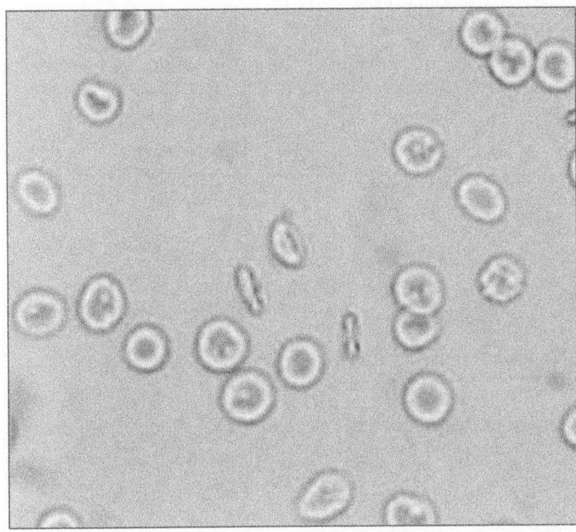

Figure 11.9 Red blood cells on microscopic examination of the urine.
(Source: James Van Rhee.)

TABLE 11.15 Hematuria Etiologies Based on Patient Age

<20 Years of Age	Age 20–60 Years	Over 60 Years, Male	Over 60 Years, Female
Glomerulopathies	UTI	Bladder cancer	Bladder cancer
UTI	Nephrolithiasis	Prostate cancer	Renal cell carcinoma
Congenital malformation	Cancer	Renal cell carcinoma	UTI
Alport syndrome	Endometriosis (if female)	Prostatitis	
Sickle cell disease		UTI	

UTI, urinary tract infection.

KNOWLEDGE CHECKS

1. Differentiate the various infectious diseases of the genitourinary tract in regard to etiology, pathology, diagnosis, and treatment.
2. Separate the various types of incontinence and how each type is diagnosed based on physical examination and testing.
3. Differentiate the various testicular disorders based on etiology, clinical presentation, and long-term complciations.
4. Describe the evaluation and workup of the patient with hematuria.

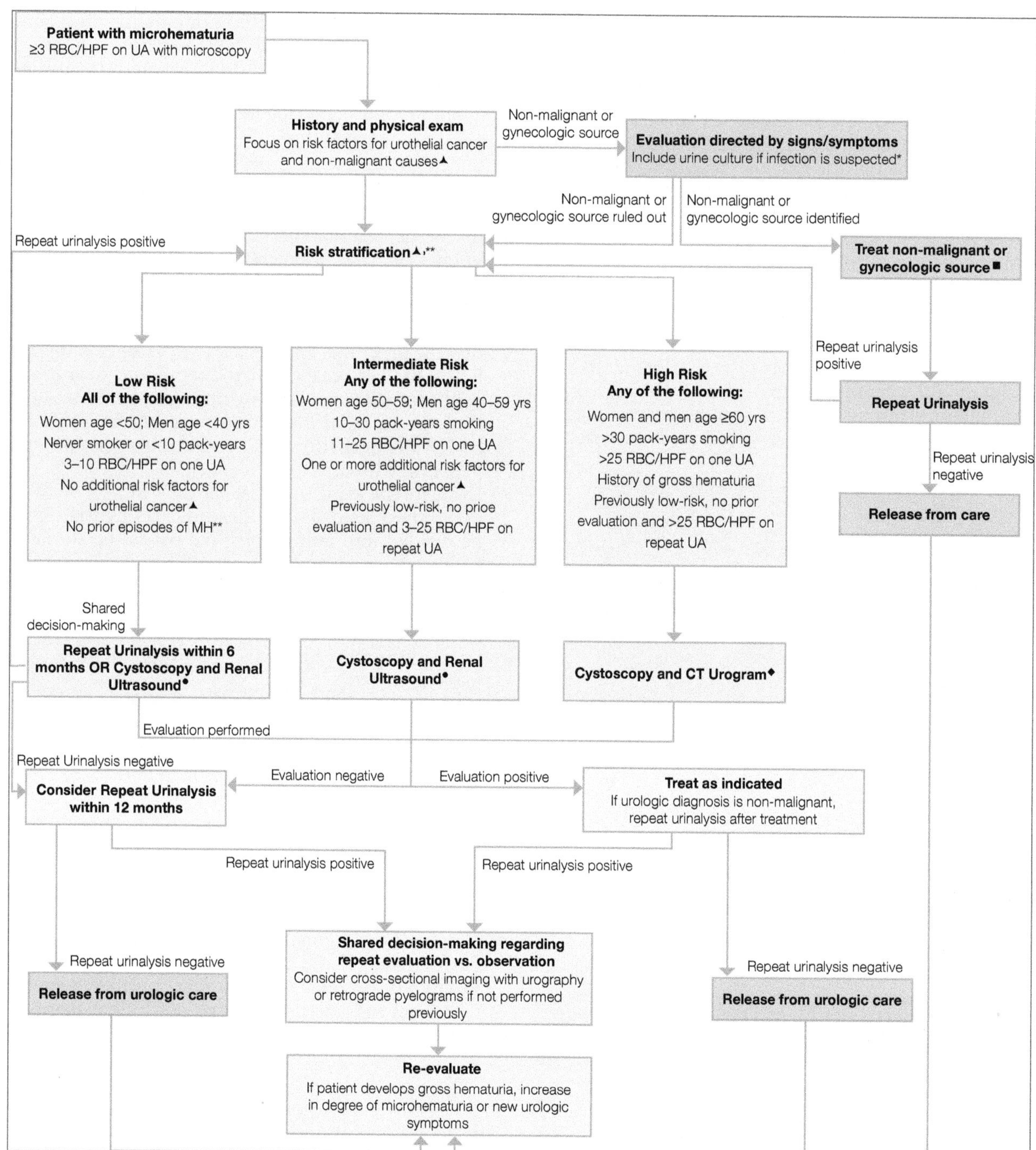

Figure 11.10 Microhematuria evaluation algorithm. CT, computerized tomography; MH, microhematuria; RBC/HPF, red blood cell per high power field; UA, urinalysis

▲ Main risk factors for urothelial cancer are those in the AUA risk stratification system (age, male sex, smoking, degree of microhematuria and history of gross hematuria). Additional risk factors for the urothelial carcinoma include but are not limited to irritative lower urinary tract voiding symptoms, history of cyclophosphamide or ifosfamide chemotherapy, family history of urothelial carcinoma or Lynch syndrome, occupational exposures to benzene chemicals or aromatic amines, history of chronic indwelling foreign body in the urinary tract.

* If medical renal disease is suspected, consider nephrologic evaluation, but pursue concurrent risk-based urological evaluation.

** Patients may be low risk at first presentation with microhematuria but may only be considered intermediate- or high-risk if found to have persistent microhematuria.

■ There are nonmalignant and gynecologic sources of hematuria that do not require treatment and/or may confound the diagnosis of MH. Clinicians can consider catheterized urine specimen in women with vaginal atrophy or pelvic organ prolapse. Clinicians must use careful judgment and patient engagement to decide whether to pursue MH evaluation in the setting of chronic conditions that do not require treatment, such as the aforementioned gynecologic conditions, nonobstructing stone or BPH.

● Clinician may perform cross-sectional imaging with urography or retrograde pyelograms if hematuria persists after negative renal ultrasound.

◆ MR urogram or noncontrast imaging plus retrograde pyelograms if contraindications to CT urogram.

(Source: Reproduced with permission from Barocas DA, Boorjian SA, Alvarez RD, et al. Microhematuria: AUA/SUFU guideline. J Urol. *2020; 204:778.)*

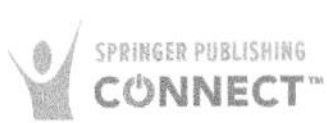

A robust set of instructor resources designed to supplement this text is located at **http://connect.springerpub.com/content/book/978-0-8261-8243-2.** Qualifying instructors may request access by emailing **textbook@springerpub.com.**

REFERENCES

The complete reference list for this chapter appears in the digital version of the chapter, accessible at https://connect.springerpub.com/content/book/978-0-8261-8243-2/chapter/ch11.

CHAPTER 12

REPRODUCTIVE SYSTEM

STEPHANIE NEARY

LEARNING OBJECTIVES

- Differentiate among the most common gynecologic complaints encountered in clinical practice.
- Formulate a differential diagnosis based upon common presenting symptoms.
- Create a list of evidence-based testing options for the conditions discussed.
- Construct an evidence-basned management plan for the conditions discussed.
- Integrate the information presented in the chapter to deliver high-quality care to patients with gynecologic complaints.
- Describe the physiology of conception, implantation, and placental formation.
- Describe the function of the placenta.
- Describe the maternal and fetal physical and anatomic changes that occur during each of the peripartum periods and potential for related adverse effects.
- Discuss fetal development by period of gestation and routine fetal assessment based on risk stratifications.
- Discuss the aims and assessments of the maternal preconception and prenatal and postpartum visits, and describe the timelines, physical exams, screening, education, risk stratification, and counseling for each.
- Understand indications for and methods of genetic screenings.
- Describe the rationale for routine screenings and laboratory tests during peripartum visits.
- Educate and manage common peripartum conditions and complications.
- Identify the equipment and indications necessary for fetal development surveillance.
- Identify and manage labor and delivery from beginning to end based on risk stratification.

INTRODUCTION

STEPHANIE NEARY

Although there are fewer PAs working in obstetrics and gynecology practices than almost any other specialty, it is likely that a gynecologic complaint will be encountered at some point in practice, particularly if one works in primary care, urgent care, or emergency medicine. Gynecologic complaints are a leading reason why women visit their OB/GYN clinicians, with prenatal visits being the primary reason. There is a continued paucity of women's health clinicians across the United States, and PAs are well positioned to help alleviate the shortage by providing this care. As such, PAs should have general knowledge about the most common gynecologic problems encountered in clinical practice.

12.1 BENIGN BREAST DISEASE

ELYSE J. WATKINS

OVERVIEW

While the majority of breast masses are benign, malignancy must always be considered and ruled out. As such, it is important to understand the presentation, diagnosis, and treatment of benign breast conditions. This section describes common benign, or nonmalignant, conditions of the breast: fibroadenoma, fibrocystic breasts, mastitis, and breast abscess.

EPIDEMIOLOGY

At some point in their lifetime, approximately 50% of women will have evidence of fibrocystic changes of the breast accompanied by mastalgia, and about 25% of women will develop a fibroadenoma.[1] Lactational mastitis affects around 30% of women who are breastfeeding and about 25% of these women develop an abscess.[2,3] Breast cysts usually occur in younger patients.

PATHOPHYSIOLOGY

Benign breast masses can be categorized by the following: nonproliferative, proliferative without atypia, and atypical hyperplasia. Atypical hyperplastic lesions are associated with an increased risk of breast malignancy and are not discussed in this section.

Fibroadenomas consist of epithelial connective tissue and stromal cells that have receptors for estrogen and progesterone. Fibrocystic changes are also a result of estrogen and progesterone receptors and develop as a consequence of hormonal variations throughout the menstrual cycle.

Lactational mastitis is a superficial infection of the breast usually due to nipple trauma, inadequate milk drainage, and subsequent engorgement. *Staphylococcus aureus* is the most common organism, but methicillin-resistant *Staphylococcus aureus* (MRSA) infections can occur as well.

Breast abscesses develop when a duct becomes clogged and bacteria colonize the stagnant duct.

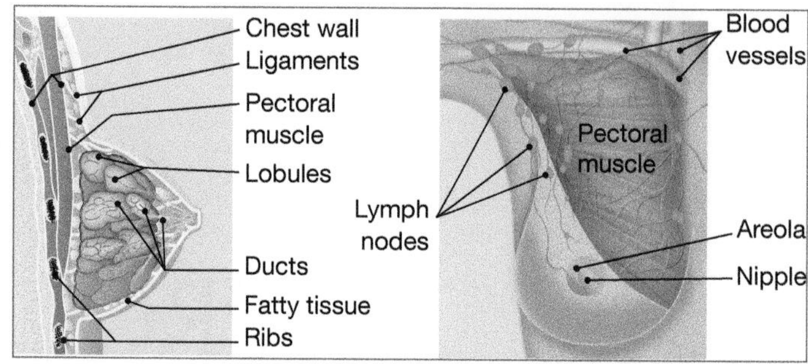

Figure 12.1 Breast anatomy, front (right) and lateral (left) views. The breast is composed of skin, breast tissue, and subcutaneous tissue. The functional or grandular breast tissue, known as the parenchyma, is divided into 15 to 20 lobes that come together at the nipple in a radial configuration.

(Source: Gilmore BM, Hay BB. Evidence-based assessment of the breasts and axillae. In: Gawlik KS, Melnyk BM, Teall AM, eds. Evidence-Based Physical Examination: Best Practices for Health and Well-Being Assessment. *Springer Publishing Company; 2021:484, Fig. 17.1.)*

12.1A FIBROADENOMA

MEDICAL HISTORY AND CLINICAL PRESENTATION

Benign breast conditions usually present during a woman's reproductive years. It is important to determine if the patient is breastfeeding or taking any systemic hormones, and to assess her family history of breast disease. Risk factors for malignant breast disease should always be assessed. A fibroadenoma is a nontender, mobile, solitary, solid lump with rubbery consistency and regular borders.

SIGNS AND SYMPTOMS

Patients with a fibroadenoma may present with a palpable breast mass found incidentally or during a breast self-examination.

PHYSICAL EXAMINATION

All patients with a breast complaint should have a bilateral breast examination (Figure 12.1). Patients are usually supine, but an evaluation of the breasts while the patient is sitting—with arms in various positions to assess for asymmetry—is also helpful. The axillary lymph nodes should always be assessed as well. Nipple discharge may be present. Sanguineous nipple discharge, particularly from a single duct, could indicate malignancy or ductal ectasia and further workup is necessary. Documentation of the physical examination should include position of the lesion as if the breast were a clock face, distance from the nipple/areola, shape, mobility, and consistency.[4] Any skin changes (e.g., dimpling, nipple inversion, erosion, thickening) should be documented as well.

DIFFERENTIAL DIAGNOSIS

Table 12.1 summarizes the differential diagnosis for fibroadenoma.

TABLE 12.1 Differential Diagnosis for Fibroadenoma

Diagnosis	Description
Galactocele	Occurs during breastfeeding Caused by a blocked milk duct Fever, chills, erythema, and induration are not present
Simple breast cyst	Usually occurs during early reproductive years Unilateral mass Usually tender
Fibrocystic breasts	Occurs during reproductive years Bilateral mobile breast masses May be tender prior to menstruation
Breast abscess	Usually occurs in a lactating woman Superficial mass on one breast Erythema Induration Fever
Ductal ectasia	Usually presents in menopausal and postmenopausal patients Nipple discharge Nipple inversion Subareolar mass
Invasive breast cancer	Is usually a solitary mass, may or may not be palpable Can present with nipple discharge, lymphadenopathy, skin changes, nipple inversion

DIAGNOSTIC STUDIES

Ultrasonographic imaging is an invaluable tool to help determine if the mass is solid or fluid-filled, assess a mass's shape, and measure its size. Ultrasound imaging can also provide other information, such as the presence or absence of posterior acoustic shadowing, which could indicate malignancy.

Mammography is another useful tool to help assess a breast mass. Common mammographic findings in breast cancer include speculation, asymmetry, anatomic distortion, and microcalcifications along a duct or lobule. The radiologist will provide a Breast Imaging Reporting and Data System (BI-RADS) category to help guide management.

EVALUATION

The evaluation of a patient with a breast complaint must include a detailed history and physical examination, imaging findings, and need for tissue sampling.

Patients with a solitary breast mass should undergo imaging with a diagnostic mammogram and ultrasound. Most patients will also undergo tissue biopsy. There are three approaches to obtaining tissue: fine needle aspiration, core needle biopsy, and surgical excision. The decision to perform any of these procedures depends upon physical examination, imaging findings, overall risk, and BI-RADS category.

TREATMENT

- No treatment is usually necessary if the fibroadenoma is simple; excision should be considered if histology is complex as there is a slight association with an increased risk of breast cancer. If the lesion grows rapidly or becomes symptomatic, excision is usually undertaken.

PATIENT EDUCATION

- Patients should be given reassurance regarding the benign process.
- Patients should follow clinical practice guidelines regarding breast self-examination and screening mammography.

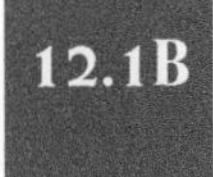

12.1B LACTATIONAL MASTITIS AND ABSCESS

MEDICAL HISTORY AND CLINICAL PRESENTATION

Patients with lactational mastitis will be breastfeeding or recently attempting lactation cessation. Lactational mastitis will reveal erythema of a portion of one breast in a lactating patient. A breast abscess will present unilaterally in a lactating patient with erythema and induration and a tense mass.

SIGNS AND SYMPTOMS

Lactational mastitis will present as a painful, erythematous area of the breast. Patients will usually experience breast swelling, warmth of the breast, and fever. Some patients may experience chills and malaise. A breast abscess is an erythematous, tender, tense, and firm mass that occurs in a breastfeeding patient.

PHYSICAL EXAMINATION

All patients with a breast complaint should have a bilateral breast examination. Patients are usually supine, but an evaluation of the breasts while the patient is sitting can be helpful. The axillary lymph nodes should be assessed as well. Nipple discharge may be present. Sanguineous nipple discharge could indicate malignancy or ductal ectasia and further workup is necessary. Documentation of the physical examination should include position of the lesion as if the breast were a clock face, distance from the nipple/areola, shape, mobility, and consistency.[4] Any skin changes should be documented as well. Sometimes patients will have a secondary fungal infection around the nipple and areola so careful physical examination is required.

DIFFERENTIAL DIAGNOSIS

Table 12.2 summarizes the differential diagnosis for lactational mastitis and abscess.

TABLE 12.2 Differential Diagnosis for Lactational Mastitis and Abscess

Diagnosis	Description
Lactational mastitis	Erythema, induration of an area of the breast Fever +/– Chills Breast engorgement Pain or a burning sensation with breastfeeding
Breast engorgement	Occurs during breastfeeding Erythema, induration, and fever are not present
Galactocele	Occurs during breastfeeding Caused by a blocked milk duct Fever, chills, erythema, and induration are not present
Simple breast cyst	Usually occurs during early reproductive years Unilateral mass Usually tender
Fibrocystic breasts	Occurs during reproductive years Bilateral mobile breast masses May be tender premenstrually
Breast abscess	Usually occurs in a lactating woman Superficial mass on one breast Erythema Induration Fever
Inflammatory breast cancer	Erythema or other skin discoloration Induration Peau d'orange appearance of the skin Edema Nipple inversion (asymmetric or new)
Paget disease of the breast	Usually occurs in women >50 years Eczematous skin changes on the nipple and areola Erythema Pruritus Skin thickening Nipple inversion Sanguineous or yellowish nipple discharge Palpable mass may be present
Invasive breast cancer	A solitary mass Can present with nipple discharge, lymphadenopathy, skin changes, nipple inversion

DIAGNOSTIC STUDIES

Ultrasonographic imaging may help differentiate between mastitis and an abscess, but mastitis and breast abscess are almost always clinical diagnoses based upon physical examination.

EVALUATION

The evaluation of a patient with a breast complaint must include a detailed history and physical examination, imaging findings if present, and need for tissue sampling. The risk for MRSA should be obtained. It is helpful to watch as the patient is breastfeeding to identify and correct any problems that may be present that predispose to tissue injury and predispose the risk of bacterial entry. Sometimes an infant will have a shortened frenulum which can cause difficulty with feeding.

TREATMENT

Lactational mastitis:

- **Antibiotic therapy:** Suggested regimens include dicloxacillin 500 mg orally four times a day for 10 to 14 days, amoxicillin-clavulanic acid 875 mg orally twice a day for 10 to 14 days, cephalexin 500 mg orally four times a day for 10 to 14 days, or if the patient is penicillin-allergic, clarithromycin 500 mg orally twice a day for 10 to 14 days. Clindamycin and trimethoprim-sulfamethoxazole are recommended if MRSA is suspected.
  - Trimethoprim-sulfamethoxazole should only be used if the infant is >1 month old.
- **Analgesia:** Acetaminophen or nonsteroidal anti-inflammatory drugs (NSAIDs) can be used.
- Breastfeeding technique should be assessed to identify and correct common problems.
- Patients who do not respond or worsen on antibiotic therapy should be ruled out for an abscess and inflammatory breast cancer.
- Patients should be considered for intravenous (IV) antibiotics if severe infection is present, the patient is hemodynamically unstable, or the patient is unable to tolerate oral antibiotics.
- Secondary fungal infections can be treated with oral fluconazole or oral nystatin (for the infant as well, if appropriate).

Breast abscess:

- Needle aspiration or incision and drainage is required.
  - Needle aspiration may be undertaken with ultrasound guidance above.
- Antibiotics are advised; see antibiotic therapy for lactational mastitis above.
- Breastfeeding technique should be assessed to identify and correct common problems.

PATIENT EDUCATION

- Lactational mastitis:
  - The patient should continue breastfeeding or pumping.
  - Referral to a lactation consultant may be necessary.
  - Adequate fluid intake is essential.
  - Infections that do not resolve with antibiotics should prompt an evaluation of a possible abscess or malignancy.
- Breast abscess:
  - Prevention of recurrence is critical through identification of underlying breastfeeding problems.
  - Close follow-up to ensure resolution should be encouraged.

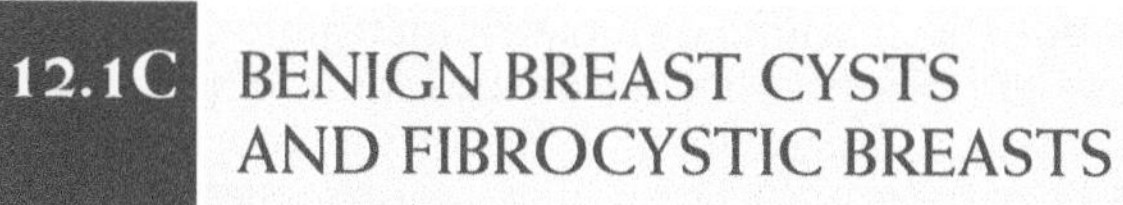

12.1C BENIGN BREAST CYSTS AND FIBROCYSTIC BREASTS

MEDICAL HISTORY AND CLINICAL PRESENTATION

Fibrocystic breasts and a simple breast cyst can be painful when the patient is premenstrual; fibrocystic breasts have palpable mobile breast masses bilaterally. A breast cyst may present as a tender unilateral mass in a patient of reproductive age. Family history may reveal fibrocystic breasts.

SIGNS AND SYMPTOMS

Fibrocystic breasts may present as bilateral, painful breasts with an association to the menstrual cycle. A simple breast cyst will not cause erythema, fever, or chills.

PHYSICAL EXAMINATION

All patients with a breast complaint should have a bilateral breast exam. Patients are usually supine, but an evaluation of the breasts while the patient is sitting can be helpful. The axillary lymph nodes should be assessed as well. Nipple discharge may be present. Sanguineous nipple discharge could indicate malignancy or ductal ectasia and further workup is necessary. Documentation of the physical examination should include position of the lesion as if the breast were a clock face, distance from the nipple/areola, shape, mobility, and consistency.[6] Any skin changes should be documented as well.

DIFFERENTIAL DIAGNOSIS

Table 12.3 summarizes the differential diagnosis for benign breast cysts and fibrocystic breasts.

DIAGNOSTIC STUDIES

Patients with a solitary breast mass should undergo imaging with a diagnostic mammogram and ultrasound. Ultrasonographic imaging is an invaluable tool to help determine if the mass is solid or fluid-filled; assess a mass's shape; and measure its size. Ultrasound imaging can also provide other information, such as the presence or absence of posterior acoustic shadowing, which could indicate malignancy.

Common mammographic findings in breast cancer include speculation, asymmetry, anatomic distortion, and microcalcifications along a duct or lobule. The radiologist will provide a BI-RADS category to help guide management.

EVALUATION

The evaluation of a patient with a breast complaint must include a detailed history and physical examination, imaging findings, and need for tissue sampling. If the clinical findings do not correlate with imaging findings, a decision to perform more invasive testing with tissue sampling is warranted. A simple breast cyst has a very low association with breast cancer, but any atypical findings should be more thoroughly evaluated.

TREATMENT

- Most patients with a breast mass will also undergo tissue biopsy.

TABLE 12.3 Differential Diagnoses for Benign Breast Cysts and Fibrocystic Breasts

Diagnosis	Description
Galactocele	Occurs during breastfeeding Caused by a blocked milk duct Fever, chills, erythema, and induration are not present
Fibroadenoma	Occurs during reproductive years Rubbery Nontender Unilateral breast mass
Simple breast cyst	Usually occurs during early reproductive years Unilateral mass Usually tender
Fibrocystic breasts	Occurs during reproductive years Bilateral mobile breast masses May be tender premenstrually
Breast abscess	Usually occurs in a lactating women Superficial mass on one breast Erythema Induration Fever
Ductal ectasia	Usually presents in menopausal and post-menopausal patients Nipple discharge Nipple inversion Subareolar mass
Invasive breast cancer	Is usually a solitary mass, may or may not be palpable Can present with nipple discharge, lymphadenopathy, skin changes, nipple inversion

- There are three different approaches to obtaining tissue: fine needle aspiration, core needle biopsy, and surgical excision.
  - The decision to perform either of these procedures depends upon physical examination, imaging findings, overall risk, and BI-RADS category.

Fibrocystic breasts:

- No treatment is necessary, but patient education is important (see next section, Patient Education).
- NSAIDs may be used for mastalgia, if present.

Simple breast cyst:

- Aspiration may be considered.
- A follow-up examination in 4 to 6 weeks can be considered to ensure there is no recurrence.
- NSAIDs may be used for mastalgia, if present.

PATIENT EDUCATION

- Fibrocystic breasts:
  - Decreases in caffeine intake may help reduce mastalgia that can accompany fibrocystic breasts, but the evidence is weak.
  - Patients who use systemic estrogens may consider discontinuing such use due to estrogen's effect on breast tissue.
- Simple breast cyst:
  - Patients who use systemic estrogens may consider discontinuing such use due to estrogen's effect on breast tissue; however, combination contraception may help to prevent benign breast cyst development.

SPECIAL CONSIDERATIONS

- Women with known *BRCA* mutations must be referred in a timely manner for evaluation and treatment.
- Women with a family history of breast or ovarian cancer who do not know their *BRCA* status should consider genetic testing. Referral to a breast center may be advised.
- Women who are pregnant and present with a breast mass must be evaluated expeditiously.

KEY POINTS

- All patients who present with a breast mass need to have a thorough history and physical examination.
- Mastitis and breast abscess can be difficult to distinguish; ultrasound can help differentiate between the two.
- Any breast mass palpated by the patient will likely cause significant worry. It is essential to provide appropriate and evidence-based care and patient education.

12.2 GYNECOLOGIC DISORDERS

Mary Ruggeri

Gynecologic disorders are any condition that effects the female reproductive organs. This includes the uterus, fallopian tubes, ovaries, vagina, and vulva. There is a wide range of gynecologic disorders, ranging from surgical emergencies to common, episodic changes in menstruation that may go undiagnosed for years. While pregnancy does affect these reproductive organs, it is not considered a disorder and therefore is discussed separately.

12.2A MENSTRUAL DISORDERS

OVERVIEW

The menstrual cycle is a complex system regulated by hormones secreted by the hypothalamus, pituitary gland, and ovaries. Disruptions to this system can be caused by a wide variety of structural abnormalities, local and systemic diseases, and medications. Menstrual disorders are a common gynecologic complaint and may include abnormal duration, absence or excess of menstruation, and abnormal bleeding or spotting between periods or after menopause. Table 12.4 outlines the most frequent menstrual disorders that will be discussed in subsequent sections.

EPIDEMIOLOGY

There are a variety of menstrual disorders and causes; epidemiology is highly dependent on the specific etiology.

The incidence of primary amenorrhea in the United States is <1%. Chromosomal abnormalities resulting in gonadal

TABLE 12.4 Frequently Encountered Menstrual Disorders

Menstrual Disorder	Description
Primary amenorrhea	Absence of menarche by age 13 when secondary sexual characteristics are absent or absence of menarche by age 15 when secondary sexual characteristics are present
Secondary amenorrhea	Absence of regular menses for ≥3 months or irregular menses for ≥6 months
Abnormal uterine bleeding	Abnormal quantity, duration, or frequency of uterine bleeding
Postmenopausal bleeding	Uterine bleeding postmenopause
Dysmenorrhea	Painful menstruation
Oligomenorrhea	Menstrual bleeding that occurs ≥ every 35 days

dysgenesis or müllerian agenesis are the most common cause of primary amenorrhea. While pregnancy is the most common cause of secondary amenorrhea, estimated frequencies of other causes include hypothalamic disorders (35%), pituitary disorders (17%), ovarian dysfunction (40%), uterine disorders (7%), and other (1%).[5]

A study of premenopausal women in the United States age 18 to 50 years demonstrated an annual prevalence rate of abnormal uterine bleeding (AUB) as 53 per 1,000.[6]

A comprehensive review of dysmenorrhea studies revealed a prevalence range of 16% to 91% in women of reproductive age with severe pain experienced by 2% to 29% of women.[8] The prevalence of primary dysmenorrhea (related to increased prostaglandins) decreases with age, and secondary dysmenorrhea (caused by pelvic pathology) tends to develop later in life.[9]

PATHOPHYSIOLOGY

The menstrual cycle is a complex system regulated by hormones secreted by the hypothalamus, pituitary gland, and ovaries. The hypothalamus releases gonadotropin-releasing hormone (GnRH) in a pulsatile manner stimulating the pituitary gland to produce follicle-stimulating hormone (FSH). The release of FSH stimulates follicle development and the release of luteinizing hormone (LH), which aids in egg maturation, estrogen production, and triggering ovulation. Due to a dominant follicle, increasing levels of circulating estrogen inhibit hypothalamic GnRH release and subsequently pituitary release of LH and FSH, thereby decreasing further follicular maturation. Disruption to this hormonal cascade may result in amenorrhea or abnormal bleeding.

The first 14 days of a normal 28-day menstrual cycle constitutes the follicular phase when the endometrium thickens under the influence of estrogen and a dominant follicle matures in the ovary, leading to ovulation. The second phase, the luteal phase, lasts about 14 days and occurs after ovulation and a high level of estrogen triggers a surge of LH. The ruptured follicle becomes the corpus luteum, secreting progesterone and some estrogen. Progesterone enhances the lining of the uterus to prepare it for implantation. If implantation does not occur, the corpus luteum breaks down, decreasing estrogen and progesterone and leading to menstruation.

Menstrual cycles may vary in length, most falling between 23 and 35 days with a normal distribution centered on 28 days.[9] Typically, a limited amount of blood is expelled during each menstrual period (<5 tablespoons or 80 mL). There is more cycle variability in the first 5 to 7 years after menarche and in the last 10 years before cessation of menses.[12] Excessive bleeding or bleeding between periods is considered AUB and may be caused by a variety of different conditions. All uterine bleeding in postmenopausal women is considered abnormal and requires further evaluation.

12.2B AMENORRHEA

MEDICAL HISTORY AND CLINICAL PRESENTATION

Amenorrhea, or the absence of menses, can be a temporary, intermittent, or permanent condition and can be caused by dysfunction of the hypothalamus, pituitary, ovaries, uterus, vagina, or cervix. It is a normal characteristic in prepubertal, pregnant, and postmenopausal females.

Primary amenorrhea is defined as the failure of menses to occur by age 15 in the presence of normal growth and secondary sexual characteristics or by age 13 if menses has not occurred and signs of puberty (such as breast development) are absent. It is important to assess whether or not the patient has completed other stages of puberty (development of pubic and axillary hair, growth spurt, sweat glands, breast development) as lack of these characteristics could suggest deficient estradiol secretion.

The most common cause of primary amenorrhea is gonadal dysgenesis caused by chromosomal or genetic abnormalities that result in premature depletion of ovarian oocytes and follicles (Table 12.5).[11,12] The most common of these abnormalities is Turner syndrome (chromosome pattern X0).

Secondary amenorrhea is defined as the cessation of menses after menarche for longer than 3 months in those with a history of regular menses or longer than 6 months in those with a history of irregular menses. The leading cause of secondary amenorrhea is pregnancy, so always rule out the possibility with a urine or serum pregnancy test (Table 12.6).

With an initial complaint of the absence of menses, a patient's history and related symptoms may provide clues as to etiology in both primary and secondary amenorrhea workups. In females of reproductive age, pregnancy must be ruled out before further investigation. Depending on whether primary or secondary amenorrhea is suspected, a thorough history may include the questions about the following:

- Development of puberty (pubic and axillary hair, growth spurt, sweat glands, breast development)
- Family history
- Stressors, including illness, eating disorder, change of weight, diet, or exercise
- Symptoms of hyperandrogenism, which include acne, excess body hair growth, and scalp hair loss and may be consistent with diagnosis of polycystic ovary syndrome (PCOS)
- Galactorrhea, which could suggest excess prolactin
- Medication history as some medications may cause amenorrhea, including progestin-secreting intrauterine systems (IUS)

TABLE 12.5 Causes of Primary Amenorrhea

Cause of Primary Amenorrhea[11]	Details
Gonadal dysgenesis (43%)	• Congenital developmental disorder resulting in premature depletion of all ovarian oocytes and follicles. • Turner syndrome (45,X) most common: Oocytes and follicles undergo accelerated apoptosis (often in utero) and ovaries are replaced with fibrous tissue. Without follicles, there is no estrogen secretion from the ovaries. Genitalia, uterus, and fallopian tubes develop normally until puberty when, because of the lack of estrogen, maturation fails. • 46,XY gonadal dysgenesis: cannot secrete antimüllerian hormone resulting in persistent müllerian structures and a female phenotype.
Müllerian agenesis (15%)	• Congenital absence of the vagina with varied uterine development as a result of agenesis or hypoplasia of the müllerian duct system.
Physiologic delay of puberty (14%)	• Chronic systemic disease, acute illness, constitutional delay of puberty. • Can result in decrease of hypothalamic GnRH secretion. Examples: type 1 diabetes, inflammatory bowel disease, and celiac disease.
Polycystic ovary syndrome (7%)	• Often present with oligomenorrhea but can present with amenorrhea. • Typically, but not always, have higher androgen levels, hirsutism, acne, and higher body mass index (BMI).[13]
Gonadotropin-releasing hormone (GnRH) deficiency (5%)	• Complete congenital GnRH deficiency: apulsatile and prepubertal low serum gonadotropin concentrations due to absence of hypothalamic GnRH. • Rare, idiopathic hypogonadotropic hypogonadism or Kallmann syndrome. • Can be inherited as autosomal dominant, autosomal recessive, or X-linked.
Transverse vaginal septum (3%)	• Septae can occur at any level between the cervix and hymenal ring.
Weight loss/anorexia nervosa (2%)	• Contributes to functional hypothalamic amenorrhea (abnormal GnRH secretion).
Hypopituitarism (2%)	• Varied etiologies; results in deficiencies of luteinizing hormone (LH) and follicle-stimulating hormone (FSH).
Less common causes (<1%)	• Hypothyroidism, Cushing disease, imperforate hymen, complete androgen insensitivity, 5-alpha-reductase deficiency, hyperprolactinemia, prolactinoma, other pituitary tumors, congenital adrenal hyperplasia.

TABLE 12.6 Common Causes of Secondary Amenorrhea

Site of Cause of Secondary Amenorrhea	Details
Hypothalamus	• Functional hypothalamic amenorrhea: abnormal hypothalamic GnRH secretion leading to decreased gonadotropin pulsations, low or normal serum LH, absent LH surges, absence of normal follicular development, anovulation, and low serum concentrations of estradiol. FSH often normal.
Pituitary	• Hyperprolactinemia: serum prolactin concentration above normal range in nonpregnant women of reproductive age; can be transiently caused by stress, sleep, exercise, intercourse, medication use, and diet. Can also be caused by certain medications, including metoclopramide, verapamil, and certain antipsychotics such as risperidone. • "Empty sella" syndrome • Cushing syndrome
Ovary	• Polycystic ovary syndrome (PCOS): typically have higher androgen levels, hirsutism, and elevated BMI. • Primary ovarian insufficiency: development of clinical menopause before age of 40 in women with normal karyotype. Typically presents as secondary amenorrhea and can be due to chemotherapy or radiation, autoimmune oophoritis, a genetic mutation or idiopathic.
Uterus	• Intrauterine adhesions (Asherman syndrome) caused by acquired scarring of the endometrial lining. May be secondary to postpartum hemorrhage or infection. Prevents the buildup and shedding of endometrial lining and results in light or absent menses.
Other	• Congenital adrenal hyperplasia, ovarian and adrenal tumors, hypothyroidism, iatrogenic causes, excessive exercise, decreased BMI.

BMI, body mass index; FSH, follicle-stimulating hormone; GnRH, gonadotropin-releasing hormone; LH, luteinizing hormone.

- Changes in libido or ability to reach orgasm
- Gynecologic surgeries

In patients with secondary amenorrhea, ask if this has ever happened before, and if so, the circumstances surrounding the event.

SIGNS AND SYMPTOMS

While the absence of menses is the most common presenting complaint from patients with amenorrhea, there are many other symptoms that may be helpful in the identification a specific etiology. In primary amenorrhea, delayed breast development, growth spurt, and adrenarche are delayed in patients with hypothalamic pituitary failure. With isolated ovarian insufficiency, breast development and pubertal growth spurt are absent or delayed, while adrenarche occurs normally.

Excess hair growth on the face and trunk, hair loss around the temples of the scalp, acanthosis nigricans, and acne may be seen in patients with PCOS. Restrictive eating, excessive exercise, or distorted sense of body image could be indicative of an eating disorder such as anorexia nervosa and may cause functional hypothalamic impairment. Galactorrhea, vision changes, or headaches could be signs of an anterior pituitary adenoma. Vaginal dryness, hot flashes, trouble sleeping, and night sweats may be a sign of premature ovarian failure, also referred to as primary ovarian insufficiency.

PHYSICAL EXAMINATION

A physical examination may help to identify features of the underlying disorders of amenorrhea. An overall assessment of general health (including nutritional status, height and weight, and sexual development) may provide insight into potential etiologies. Hallmarks of Turner syndrome include short stature, webbed neck, pubertal delay, low-set ears or hairline, nail hypoplasia, and cardiac abnormalities. Reduced body mass index (BMI), bradycardia, and hypotension may be observed in patients with anorexia nervosa. In addition, dental erosion, reduced gag reflex, subconjunctival hemorrhage or metacarpophalangeal calluses may indicate frequent vomiting. Patients with PCOS may exhibit hirsutism, acne, and acanthosis nigricans. Thin skin, purple striae, and easy bruising may be signs of Cushing syndrome. Warm, moist skin or tachycardia may be signs of hyperthyroidism.

Assessment of Tanner stage of development is important. Underdeveloped breasts and sparse pubic hair may indicate delayed puberty while underdeveloped breasts with normal pubic hair growth is a sign of gonadal dysgenesis. A pelvic examination can help detect outflow disorders such as imperforate hymen or transverse vaginal septum. It is important to assess emotional maturity and adequately prepare the patient before performing a pelvic examination. It is also advised to have a chaperone present during the examination.

DIFFERENTIAL DIAGNOSIS

Several diagnoses are unique to primary amenorrhea, including chromosomal anomalies (Kallmann syndrome and Turner syndrome), structural anomalies (imperforate hymen, müllerian agenesis, or dysgenesis), and androgen insensitivity syndrome. See Tables 12.5 and 12.6. Always rule out pregnancy.

DIAGNOSTIC STUDIES

A pregnancy test (serum human chorionic gonadotropin, hCG) is the initial step in evaluating a patient with amenorrhea.

The workup for primary amenorrhea should begin with assessing whether breast development is present. Breast development serves as an indicator of estrogen action and thus ovarian function. A pelvic ultrasound may be performed to confirm the presence or absence of ovaries, uterus, and cervix, as well as assess for cervical or vaginal outlet obstruction. If the uterus is absent, a karyotype and serum total testosterone can help differentiate between müllerian agenesis (46,XX), complete androgen insensitivity syndrome (46,XY, female phenotype, serum testosterone in normal male range), or 5-alpha-reductase deficiency (46,XY, serum testosterone in normal male range, virilization at puberty).

For secondary amenorrhea and when the uterus is present in primary amenorrhea, routine endocrine testing of FSH, thyroid-stimulating hormone (TSH), free thyroxine (T4), and prolactin (PRL) can be helpful in the initial workup. In addition, if a patient has signs of hyperandrogenism and PCOS is suspected, sex hormone binding globulin (SHBG), dehydroepiandrosterone sulfate (DHEAS), total and free serum testosterone, and an FSH:LH ratio should be ordered. In patients with suspected primary ovarian insufficiency (premature menopause), antimüllerian hormone and inhibin B can be helpful. Potential lab findings as well as additional testing includes the following:

- FSH: Elevated FSH concentration is indicative of primary ovarian insufficiency. A decreased or normal FSH may suggest a central hypothalamic-pituitary issue, an anatomic outflow abnormality, or endocrine disorder (PCOS, hyperprolactinemia, thyroid disease). In these patients, a repeat FSH along with serum LH should be measured. If both are very low, a GnRH deficiency, constitutional delay of puberty or other etiologies involving the hypothalamic-pituitary axis should be investigated. If LH is low and FSH low/normal, consider causes of functional hypothalamic amenorrhea.
- TSH with reflex to free T4 is a screening tool for thyroid disease. Amenorrhea can be associated with both hypothyroidism and hyperthyroidism.
- PRL can help evaluate for hyperprolactinemia. If elevated, a thorough medication review should be conducted to rule out iatrogenic hyperprolactinemia. If pituitary adenoma is suspected, a pituitary MRI is indicated.
- Serum testosterone and DHEAS should be measured in patients with signs of hyperandrogenism. While PCOS is the most likely cause, androgen-secreting tumors must be ruled out in patients with virilization or severe hyperandrogenemia.
- Serum estradiol (E2) testing with serum FSH may be helpful in evaluating the pituitary-ovarian axis in secondary amenorrhea. Low to normal E2 with an elevated FSH indicates primary ovarian insufficiency. Low to normal E2 with low to normal FSH suggests possible functional hypothalamic hypogonadism or other hypothalamic or pituitary disorder.
- An MRI with contrast of the sella region is indicated in cases of amenorrhea due to hypogonadotropic hypogonadism.
- SHBG will be low in patients with PCOS.
- Antimüllerian hormone will be low or absent in patients with primary ovarian insufficiency.
- Inhibin B will be low or absent in patients with primary ovarian insufficiency.

EVALUATION

The evaluation of an individual with either primary or secondary amenorrhea includes consideration of disorders based upon the level of control of the menstrual cycle: the hypothalamus and pituitary, ovary, uterus, and vagina. For primary amenorrhea, evaluation is indicated with the absence of menses in 15-year-old patients with normal growth and secondary sexual characteristics or in 13-year-old patients with absence of secondary sexual characteristics. For secondary amenorrhea, missing a single menses does not warrant a full workup but ruling out pregnancy is still essential.

TREATMENT

- Management of amenorrhea largely depends upon the underlying etiology, the patient's reproductive goals, and mitigating systemic and psychosocial sequelae.
- Surgery may be required in patients with congenital anatomic abnormalities
- Patients with primary ovarian insufficiency should be counseled on risks and benefits of hormone therapy. For women of reproductive age, hormone replacement can help prevent bone loss and reduce risk of premature coronary heart disease.
- Functional hypothalamic amenorrhea may be reversed by improvement of illness or stressors, weight gain, or reduction of intense exercise.
- For patients with irreversible hypothalamic or pituitary dysfunction, exogenous gonadotropins or pulsatile GnRH can be given.
- The treatment of patients with PCOS requires a multisystem approach to the various metabolic and hormonal derangements. See Section 12.7C on PCOS for a more detailed discussion.
- All patients with primary amenorrhea should be counseled about the specific etiology, treatment options, and reproductive potential. Psychological counseling may be helpful to patients with chromosomal anomalies.
- Patients with secondary amenorrhea who have been ruled out for pregnancy can be given progestin or progesterone for 10 days to induce a menstrual bleed.
- Depending on the etiology, patients who are chronically amenorrheic and still have a uterus must receive progestin or progesterone therapy, daily or sporadically, to protect against endometrial hyperplasia and cancer.

PATIENT EDUCATION

- Menstrual cycle disorders are a common gynecologic complaint. The absence of menstrual periods by the age of 15 or missed periods for 3 consecutive months should be reported to a clinician as they might be a sign of underlying medical conditions.
- Menstrual cycle disorders can be caused by conditions that affect the hypothalamus, pituitary gland, ovaries, uterus, cervix, or vagina.
- Management of amenorrhea includes identifying and treating the underlying cause (when possible), prevention of potential complications, and assisting the patient in achieving her reproductive goals.

12.2C ABNORMAL UTERINE BLEEDING

MEDICAL HISTORY AND CLINICAL PRESENTATION

AUB refers to menstrual bleeding of abnormal quantity, frequency, regularity, or duration. The cause of AUB may be systemic, local, or iatrogenic.

History of a patient with AUB should include a thorough menstrual, sexual, contraceptive, obstetric, and gynecologic surgical history. Information gathered from this line of questioning may provide insight into risk of pregnancy, sexually transmitted infection, scarring, etc. Other pertinent medical history, such as medications, bleeding disorders, endocrine disease, celiac disease, and family history of the same, may provide information to guide further evaluation.

Adolescent patients should be assessed for potential coagulopathies, keeping in mind that irregular menses is common in the first year following menarche. Easy bruising and prolonged bleeding from minor procedures or injuries could indicate von Willebrand disease.

Specific details of volume, timing, and color of bleeding may provide additional insight as to the cause. Heavy bleeding typically comes from the uterus while spotting or light bleeding may be from any site in the genital tract. Postcoital bleeding suggests cervical pathology but may also occur if lesions or friable tissue are present in other areas of the lower tract. Bleeding only during or after urination or defecation may indicate a nongenital source.

Heavy menstrual bleeding (HMB), intermenstrual bleeding, and irregular bleeding are common.

- HMB refers to cyclic (ovulatory) bleeding that is heavy or prolonged. The most common etiologies of HMB include uterine leiomyomas, adenomyosis, cesarean scar defect, or bleeding disorder.
- Intermenstrual bleeding consists of bleeding at irregular intervals, especially between menstrual periods. Common etiologies of intermenstrual bleeding include endometrial polyps, contraceptives, endometrial hyperplasia or carcinoma, endometritis, and pelvic inflammatory disease (PID). Other causes include cervical pathologies such as cervical cancer, polyps, or cervicitis.
- Oligomenorrhea usually signifies anovulatory cycles. Patients may complain of phases of no bleeding and phases with spotting or episodes of heavy bleeding. Irregular bleeding is common among women at the extremes of reproductive age (following menarche or perimenopausal). In addition, PCOS and endocrine disorders are common causes of ovulatory dysfunction.

SIGNS AND SYMPTOMS

Unpredictable, episodic heavy or light bleeding or intermenstrual bleeding may be the primary presenting symptom of AUB. In addition to a thorough patient history, associated symptoms may help narrow possible etiologies. Fever, pelvic pain, or discharge may indicate infection. Urinary or gastrointestinal (GI) symptoms may suggest mass effect or a nongynecologic etiology. Hot flashes, heat or cold intolerance, galactorrhea, hirsutism, or weight loss or gain may suggest an endocrine issue. Illness, stress, extreme changes to diet or exercise, and eating disorders could lead to a hypothalamic dysfunction. Fatigue and shortness of breath could indicate anemia secondary to heavy bleeding or malignant metastasis.

PHYSICAL EXAMINATION

All patients with HMB should have their hemodynamic status assessed. Hemodynamic compromise requires rapid intervention with basic life support interventions. The physical exam should consist of all potential sites of bleeding, including examination of the urethra and anus in addition to the pelvic examination. The pelvic examination should include an inspection of the external genitalia, a speculum examination, and a bimanual examination. The external examination should rule out visible traumatic lesions. The speculum examination should consist of an inspection of the vaginal mucosa as hypopigmentation and decreased rugae indicate a hypoestrogenic state. Examination of the cervix should assess for polyps, friability, mucopurulence, and lesions. A bimanual examination may reveal uterine characteristics suggestive of particular etiologies:

- Reduced uterine mobility may suggest adhesions, a mass, or malignancy.
- A boggy, enlarged, and globular uterus may be due to adenomyosis.
- Uterine tenderness may indicate infection, such as PID or endometritis.
- An enlarged uterus may be present in an intrauterine pregnancy and may also be present with leiomyoma, adenomyosis, or malignancy.

The patient's general appearance may indicate signs of systemic illness. Evidence of hyperandrogenism, enlarged thyroid, or galactorrhea could suggest endocrine etiology. In addition, inspection of the skin may reveal acanthosis nigricans, acne, and hirsutism; palpation of the thyroid may reveal a nodule or thyromegaly; and generalized pallor may indicate anemia.

DIFFERENTIAL DIAGNOSIS

A classification system developed by the International Federation of Gynecology and Obstetrics (FIGO) provides terminology for the various etiologies of AUB: PALM-COEIN (i.e., polyp, adenomyosis, leiomyoma, malignancy and hyperplasia, coagulopathy, ovulatory dysfunction, endometrial, iatrogenic, and not yet classified). Details of these etiologies are outlined in Table 12.7.

It is also important to consider possible trauma, systemic disease, and infection in the differential diagnosis.

DIAGNOSTIC STUDIES

Pregnancy testing (hCG) should be part of the initial workup for patients with AUB as bleeding can be seen in pregnancy in addition to menses. A complete blood count (CBC) and ferritin level should be completed for any patient complaining of heavy or frequent bleeding to assess for anemia.

TABLE 12.7 Differential Diagnosis for Abnormal Uterine Bleeding

Diagnosis	Description
Polyp	Benign endometrial growths. Most commonly presents with intermenstrual bleeding but may present with heavy or prolonged bleeding.
Adenomyosis	Benign invasion of endometrial glands into myometrial wall. Often accompanied by dysmenorrhea or chronic pelvic pain.
Leiomyoma	Benign growths of the myometrial layer of the uterus.
Malignancy	Endometrial carcinoma, uterine sarcoma, ovarian carcinoma, cervical carcinoma.
Coagulopathy	Thrombocytopenia or platelet dysfunction, von Willebrand disease, hematologic malignancy, coagulation factor deficiencies, advanced liver disease.
Ovarian	Bleeding from the ovary often presents as intraperitoneal bleeding while ovarian dysfunction can result in abnormal uterine bleeding.
Endometrial	Endometriosis, endometritis, endometrial hyperplasia, previous endometrial trauma (cesarean scar defect).
Iatrogenic	Medications such as anticoagulants, hormonal contraceptives, intrauterine system.

Low hematocrit and hemoglobin (Hb) can occur with blood loss but may not be apparent in an acute bleeding episode. The CBC may also provide information about platelets and white blood cells (WBCs) if a bleeding disorder or infection, respectively, are suspected. If acute heavy bleeding is present and the patient may require transfusion, a type and cross match should be ordered.

Based on history and physical examination findings, the following tests may be warranted:

- TSH will be elevated with hypothyroidism and decreased in hyperthyroidism.
- Androgen levels will be elevated in PCOS or congenital adrenal hyperplasia.
- PRL level will be elevated in hyperprolactinemia.
- FSH will be elevated and antimüllerian hormone and inhibin B will be low or undetectable in premature ovarian insufficiency. If LH is low and FSH is low/normal, consider causes of functional hypothalamic dysfunction.

If a bleeding disorder is suspected, tests for secondary hemostasis defects (platelet count, prothrombin time [PT], and activated partial thromboplastin time [aPTT]) should be initiated. If these results are normal, testing for von Willebrand factor antigen, fibrinolytic defects, or platelet function abnormalities may be necessary.

If it is difficult to differentiate uterine bleeding from cervical bleeding based on history and exam, patients may need to be screened for cervical cancer and sexually transmitted infections that may cause cervicitis. Urinary analysis and fecal occult blood testing may be warranted if a nongenital source is suspected.

Patients with AUB should have a transvaginal and abdominal ultrasound. Rarely, an MRI may be necessary. Saline-infusion sonography is the preferred method to visualize the endometrium and is often performed with an endometrial biopsy.

Endometrial sampling should be considered in nonpregnant patients with AUB to rule out hyperplasia and malignancy.

EVALUATION

The evaluation of a patient with AUB always starts with a determination of the patient's menopausal status (pre- or postmenopausal). Postmenopausal bleeding (PMB) is always considered abnormal and will be further discussed in Section 12.2D. Premenopausal bleeding requires a thorough history and physical examination and an hCG to rule out pregnancy.

TREATMENT

- Goals of management include control of heavy and/or irregular bleeding and treatment of underlying disorders, treatment of anemia (if present), and maximizing quality of life.
- Management is based on etiology, severity, symptoms, contraceptive or reproductive needs, comorbidities, and patient preference for medical or surgical treatment.
- Infections should be treated with the appropriate antibiotic regimen.
- Structural lesions such as endometrial polyps, submucosal fibroids, and cesarean scar defects may be removed surgically.
- Uterine leiomyomas or adenomyosis can be treated pharmacologically or surgically. Please see Section 12.4 on uterine disorders. Patients with HMB can be treated with

tranexamic acid and NSAIDs if no contraindications exist. Tranexamic acid can be used episodically when heavy bleeding occurs and in episodes of acute heavy bleeding.

- Estrogen and progesterone combinations can be considered if the patient has been ruled out for malignancy and has no contraindications for their use. Otherwise, progesterone only or nonhormonal options should be considered.
- Treatment for patients with bleeding disorders should be individualized based on etiology.
- Endocrine abnormalities may be treated by etiology to restore ovulatory cycles or eliminate bleeding episodes.

PATIENT EDUCATION

- A variety of conditions may cause menstrual bleeding abnormalities. Common causes include uterine fibroids (benign masses in the muscle layer of the uterus), endometrial polyps (smaller growths of tissue that grow on the inside lining of the uterus), and uterine adenomyosis (a condition in which the lining of the uterus grows into the muscle layer of the uterus).
- Abnormal bleeding can also be caused by contraceptives (hormonal birth control), pregnancy, infection, medical illnesses, and bleeding disorders.
- Irregular bleeding is common during the first few months after the first menstrual period as well during perimenopause.
- Bleeding before menarche or after menopause is always considered abnormal.

12.2D POSTMENOPAUSAL BLEEDING

MEDICAL HISTORY AND CLINICAL PRESENTATION

PMB consists of any uterine bleeding in a woman who has been unintentionally amenorrheic for >12 months. Patients presenting with PMB should always be evaluated for endometrial carcinoma.

History questions should aim to elicit bleeding details such as onset, precipitating factors, pattern, duration, quantity, and associated symptoms. In addition, past medical history, medications, and family history may provide additional clues.

SIGNS AND SYMPTOMS

In addition to the complaint of bleeding in the postmenopausal patient, associated symptoms may provide additional information to direct the clinical workup. Unopposed estrogen therapy, tamoxifen therapy, nulliparity, chronic ovulatory dysfunction, obesity, diabetes, or hypertension are risk factors for endometrial cancer.[13] Vaginal dryness and dyspareunia with postcoital bleeding suggest atrophy. Urinary symptoms, vaginal dryness, and dyspareunia are likely due to chronic estrogen deficiency, which is called the genitourinary syndrome of menopause. Urinary symptoms, changes to bowel movements, or bleeding seen only on toilet paper or in the toilet bowl may point to an etiology outside the genital tract.

PHYSICAL EXAMINATION

The physical examination should investigate potential sites of bleeding. Examination of the lower genital tract can serve to identify lesions, foreign bodies, or vaginal atrophy. A bimanual examination can assess the size and contour of the uterus as well as any tenderness. An enlarged uterus may be noted with leiomyomas, adenomyosis, or malignancy, but if a postmenopausal patient presents with new-onset fibroids, she must be ruled out for leiomyosarcoma. The patient's general appearance may also indicate signs of systemic illness.

DIFFERENTIAL DIAGNOSIS

Table 12.8 summarizes the differential diagnosis for PMB.

DIAGNOSTIC STUDIES

Initial evaluation of the endometrium can be performed by either endometrial biopsy or transvaginal ultrasound (TVU). TVU may also be used to evaluate potential uterine pathology such as fibroids or polyps. If the endometrial lining is found to be thicker than 4 mm, or if the patient has persistent bleeding, an endometrial biopsy is indicated.

Cervical cancer screening according to the most recent guidelines is indicated in the evaluation of PMB. All visible cervical lesions should be biopsied.

EVALUATION

The principal goal in the evaluation of PMB is to exclude malignancy.

TREATMENT

- If bleeding is light or self-limited, treatment may be unnecessary after malignancy has been excluded.
- Benign lesions can be treated if bothersome.
- Malignant lesions are evaluated and treated according to associated guidelines.

TABLE 12.8 Differential Diagnosis for Postmenopausal Bleeding

Diagnosis	Description
Polyp	Benign endometrial growths.
Atrophy	Low estrogen levels cause atrophy of vagina and endometrium. Erosions of the epithelial surface can make tissue friable and cause light bleeding or spotting.
Carcinoma	Endometrial cancer is most common, sarcomas of the uterus may also occur. Cancer of the ovary, fallopian tube, cervix, or vagina can also cause bleeding.
Endometrial hyperplasia	Abnormal thickening of the lining of the uterus. Can be a precursor to endometrial carcinoma.
Fibroid/ leiomyoma	Growths of the myometrial layer of the uterus. As these are estrogen dependent, a new presentation of leiomyoma could indicate malignancy.
Adenomyosis	Benign invasion of endometrial glands into myometrial wall. Often accompanied by dysmenorrhea or chronic pelvic pain.
Pathology in other organs	Diseases or inflammation of other organs or organ systems (genitourinary, gastrointestinal) that may cause bleeding.
Medications	Anticoagulants may cause uterine bleeding.

PATIENT EDUCATION

- Bleeding after menopause is always considered abnormal.
- A variety of conditions may cause PMB. Common causes include endometrial polyps (smaller growths of tissue that grow on the inside lining of the uterus), vaginal or endometrial atrophy, endometrial cancer, and hyperplasia.

12.2E DYSMENORRHEA

MEDICAL HISTORY AND CLINICAL PRESENTATION

Dysmenorrhea, or painful menstruation, is a common complaint, can affect normal activities, and impairs quality of life. Primary dysmenorrhea consists of recurrent cramping and lower abdominal pain during menses in the absence of other causes. Primary dysmenorrhea is common among adolescents. Risk factors include family history and high stress, while use of oral contraceptives and increased age and parity were inversely associated.[7] Secondary dysmenorrhea includes similar symptoms; however, they can be explained by an underlying pelvic pathology such as endometriosis, uterine fibroids, or adenomyosis. In general, the prevalence of primary dysmenorrhea decreases with age while incidence of secondary dysmenorrhea increases with age.[8]

A thorough menstrual history and relationship between the pain and the menstrual cycle should be elicited as primary dysmenorrhea typically begins closer to menarche. The timing and characteristics of pain are also pertinent information. Pain that is not cyclical or occurs outside menses is less likely to be dysmenorrhea. It is also important to understand the impact of the pain on daily activities.

SIGNS AND SYMPTOMS

Pain typically starts 1 or 2 days before or with the onset of menstrual bleeding and often recurs with each menstrual cycle. The pain is often located in the lower abdomen and suprapubic area and may be crampy and intermittent or continuous and dull, ranging from mild to severe. Patients may also complain of associated symptoms including nausea, vomiting, diarrhea, headache, and fatigue. Some patients may have pain that radiates into the thighs and low back and often will experience dyspareunia.

PHYSICAL EXAMINATION

For primary dysmenorrhea, there are no related physical examination findings, and a pelvic examination should yield normal findings. In adolescent patients who are not sexually active and whose history and symptoms suggest primary dysmenorrhea, a clinical diagnosis can be made, and a pelvic examination does not need to be performed unless symptoms are resistant to treatment.

In secondary dysmenorrhea, pelvic examination findings may be suggestive of an underlying pathology. A boggy, globular uterus may be indicative of adenomyosis. An enlarged, irregularly shaped, and firm uterus may be caused by fibroids. In patients with endometriosis, lateral cervical displacement due to uterosacral scarring,[14] cervical stenosis, adnexal enlargement, or uterosacral ligament abnormalities may be noted. Cervical motion tenderness, discharge, and fever may be caused by PID.

DIFFERENTIAL DIAGNOSIS

Primary dysmenorrhea is a clinical diagnosis after excluding other potential etiologies, including those that cause secondary dysmenorrhea. The potential etiologies for secondary dysmenorrhea are listed in Table 12.9.

TABLE 12.9 Etiologies of Secondary Dysmenorrhea

Etiologies	Description
Leiomyoma	Benign growths of the myometrium.
Adenomyosis	Areas of endometrial tissue grow into the myometrium of the uterus. May cause hypertrophy and hyperplasia of surrounding myometrium.
Endometriosis	Presence of endometrial tissue outside the uterine cavity. The ectopic tissue responds to cyclical hormonal changes.
Ovarian cysts	Fluid-filled sac that arises in an ovary; most are benign.
Uterine or pelvic adhesions	Bands of scar tissue that attach tissues or organs together irregularly, may occur as a result of surgery, prior inflammation or infection.
Pelvic inflammatory disease (PID)	Infection of upper genital tract including the uterus, fallopian tubes, and/or ovaries.
Endometrial polyps	Small, often benign, growths in the uterus made up of endometrial tissue.
Cervical stenosis	Narrow or closed passageway through endocervical canal.
Intrauterine contraceptive device (IUD)	Common side effects after insertion include abdominal, pelvic, and/or back pain. Risk of IUD also includes device migration, perforation, increased risk of PID, and ectopic pregnancy.
Pelvic congestion syndrome	Chronic pelvic pain due to ovarian vein and pelvic varices.
Uteropelvic junction obstruction	Obstruction at the junction where the ureter meets the renal pelvis.
Chronic pelvic pain	Nonmenstrual pain of 3 months or longer that localizes to the pelvis; pathophysiology not well understood, may be associated with bladder or bowel dysfunction, sexual dysfunction, or other systemic symptoms.

A differential diagnosis for dysmenorrhea should also include:

- **Obstetric causes:** Pregnancy, miscarriage and ectopic pregnancy should be suspected with new onset of pain or menstrual irregularity.
- **Urologic causes:** Urinary tract infection (UTI), interstitial cystitis, or kidney stones may involve crampy pelvic pain. However, this pain generally does not relate to menstruation.
- **Gastrointestinal causes:** Appendicitis, inflammatory bowel disease, irritable bowel syndrome, and diverticulitis may have symptoms of cramping pain. However, these etiologies are often accompanied by GI symptoms such as diarrhea, nausea, and vomiting and are not cyclical with menstruation, and some may be accompanied by fever.

DIAGNOSTIC STUDIES

For primary dysmenorrhea, there are no related imaging findings or diagnostic abnormalities. Sexually transmitted infection testing should be completed in all sexually active patients, and especially when infection is suspected. Urine analysis may be used to rule out UTI. TVU may be used to exclude underlying pathology as it can be helpful in detecting leiomyoma, adenomyosis, adnexal masses. Endometriosis is diagnosed by direct visualization of endometriotic implants with laparoscopy.

EVALUATION

Primary dysmenorrhea is a diagnosis of exclusion. Evaluation should aim to identify any signs and symptoms of pelvic pathology before making this clinical diagnosis.

TREATMENT

- **Primary dysmenorrhea:** Exercise and topical heat may help to alleviate symptoms.[15,16] NSAIDs are first-line therapy as they inhibit prostaglandin-mediated uterine activity and should be used as an initial treatment unless otherwise contraindicated. Patients should be instructed to take NSAIDs for 2 to 3 days before the onset of symptoms for maximum effect. Hormonal contraception, including combined estrogen-progestin and progestin-only options, may also significantly reduce symptoms. For patients who do not experience symptom relief after 3 to 6 months of treatment etiologies of secondary dysmenorrhea should be considered.
- **Pelvic inflammatory disease or tubo-ovarian abscess:** Empiric, broad-spectrum antibiotics are prescribed. Mild to moderate cases may be treated on an outpatient basis, and treatment plans should follow Centers for Disease Control and Prevention (CDC) guidelines.
- **Structural abnormalities of reproductive tract:** These may require surgical intervention to relieve obstruction.
- Secondary dysmenorrhea treatment depends upon the underlying pathology. See Section 12.4 Uterine Disorders for more information.

PATIENT EDUCATION

- Dysmenorrhea, or painful menstruation, is a common problem among females. Often beginning in adolescence, primary dysmenorrhea typically declines with age.
- NSAIDs and hormonal contraception may reduce the pain of dysmenorrhea. It is important to note that women who begin using a hormonal birth control often experience intermittent bleeding or spotting, especially during the first few months of treatment, and this typically decreases with time.
- While many patients experience relief with NSAIDs, more diagnostic testing may be required to identify any underlying conditions.

12.3 VAGINAL AND VULVAR DISORDERS

JENIECE WERT

OVERVIEW

The vagina is a female reproductive organ comprising a fibromuscular tube of smooth muscle of lined with stratified squamous cell epithelium extending from the vestibule to the cervix. The vulva forms the entrance to the vagina and is made up of the labia majora, labia minora, clitoris, vestibule of the vagina, bulb of the vestibule, and the glands of Bartholin. Vaginal symptoms are among the most common complaints among women presenting to their healthcare clinician.[18] Among the common vaginal complaints are vaginal discharge, pruritus, pain, odor, and bleeding. The most common causes of infectious vaginitis are bacterial vaginosis (BV), trichomoniasis, and candidiasis. These infectious causes are typically easily treated but some cases are more complex and even chronic in nature. Vulvar lichen sclerosis (LS; Section 12.3B) is a condition of the surface of the vulva characterized by patches of thin, white skin and, in severe cases, results in complete erosion of vulvar landmarks and scarring. Not only is vulvar LS a concern due to the chronic nature of the disease, it is also a risk factor for vulvar squamous cell carcinoma. Several vaginal and vulvar malignancies will be addressed in Section 12.3C.

EPIDEMIOLOGY

The majority of patients with vaginal complaints are diagnosed with BV, *Candida* vulvovaginitis, or trichomoniasis.[18] BV is the most prevalent of vaginitis cases and is most common in women of childbearing age. *Candida* vulvovaginitis makes up about one-third of vaginitis cases and approximately 75% of women will have at least one episode of *Candida* vulvovaginitis in their lifetime.[19] Trichomoniasis is a sexually transmitted infection caused by the protozoa, *Trichomonas vaginalis*. This can affect both men and women but is more common in women.[20] Vulvar LS typically occurs in perimenopausal or postmenopausal women with a median age of 60 years, with an estimated 14% of women affected by vulvar LS.[21] Though vaginal and vulvar cancers encompass <1% of female reproductive cancers,[22,23] this should be high on the radar for clinicians because of the increased success with early diagnoses.[22] Of the vaginal cancers, squamous cell carcinoma makes up 85%, and 5% to 10% of cases are adenocarcinomas.[22] The rarer histologic types of vaginal cancer are melanoma, sarcoma, and small cell carcinoma. Squamous cell carcinoma makes up 90% of all vulvar cancers with melanoma, adenocarcinoma, and sarcoma accounting for other instances of vulvar cancer.[24]

PATHOPHYSIOLOGY

Normal vaginal microbiology is primarily made up of lactobacilli, most commonly *Lactobacillus acidophilus* and *Lactobacillus fermentum*. Lactobacilli play a role in the inhibition of vaginal bacteria including *Gardnerella vaginalis* and bacterial uropathogens. The vaginal environment is acidic at a pH between 4.0 and 4.5. Sexual activity, tampon use, childbirth, and other events increase the variability and complexity of vaginal flora due to the introduction of enteric flora and can change the vaginal pH. Disturbances in the vaginal microbiology increases the occurrence of vaginal disease processes. For example, decreases in lactobacilli lead to an overgrowth of normal flora such as *Gardnerella vaginalis*, the most common cause of BV. In addition, *Candida albicans* are part of normal vaginal flora in 20% of women and the overgrowth of *C. albicans* and penetration of superficial epithelial cells leads to vulvovaginitis.[20,25] Use of antibiotics, increased estrogen such as in pregnancy, and immunosuppression increase the likelihood of *Candida* vulvovaginitis.[26]

The pathogenesis of vulvar LS is an autoimmune process of which the cause is not known but involves chronic inflammation to the vulva.[27] Vulvar LS, especially those seen in conjunction with vulvar intraepithelial neoplasms (VINs), are a risk factor for vulvar and vaginal malignancy. VIN is a precancerous lesion that occurs when there are dysplastic changes to the skin of the vulva. Typically, VIN occurs when high-risk human papilloma virus (HPV) subtype oncoproteins interfere with the normal cellular function.[28] Differentiated VIN is related to chronic inflammatory changes seen in LS and lichen planus and carries an increased risk of squamous cell carcinoma development.[28] Squamous cell carcinoma is also related to high-risk HPV in 25% of cases, typically HPV16.[29] Since the majority of vaginal and vulvar cancers are squamous cell carcinoma, the changes related to high-risk HPV exposure is significant in the development of these malignancies.

12.3A VAGINITIS

MEDICAL HISTORY AND CLINICAL PRESENTATION

Vaginitis is a term used to describe the collection of disorders that cause infection, inflammation, and/or changes to the normal flora of the vagina. Table 12.10 lists the types of vaginitis and associated features. The focus of this section will be on BV, *Candida* vulvovaginitis, and trichomoniasis as they are the most common causes of vaginitis. The most characteristic feature of vaginitis is vaginal discharge, sometimes associated with pruritus, odor, or discomfort. Typically, this process affects women of childbearing age. In addition, patients with multiple sexual partners are at an increased risk for trichomoniasis as it is sexually transmitted and can live in moist environments for several hours.[30]

TABLE 12.10 Types of Vaginitis and Associated Features

Types of Vaginitis	Associated Features
Bacterial vaginosis	Thin, gray/off-white, malodorous vaginal discharge, "fishy" odor, vaginal odor worsens after intercourse, pruritus
Candida vulvovaginitis	Odorless, pruritic, cottage cheese-like discharge, dysuria, dyspareunia
Trichomoniasis	Frothy, yellow/green, malodorous discharge, pruritus, erythema
Atrophic vaginitis	Vaginal pruritus, pain, and dryness, associated with hormonal changes during menopause
Noninfectious	Erythema, pain and/or itching, due to allergy or irritation such as douching, sprays, spermicides

SIGNS AND SYMPTOMS

Overall, women with vaginitis present with vaginal discharge with each type of vaginitis presenting with different characteristics of discharge. Table 12.10 illustrates the distinguishing features of the vaginitis discharge characteristic of each type. Symptomatic women with BV may complain of "fishy" odor that worsens during menstruation or after sexual intercourse.[31] The dominant feature of *Candida* vulvovaginitis is vulvar pruritus with burning and irritation. It is also common to see dysuria and dyspareunia. In contrast, BV does not typically cause pruritus, dysuria, dyspareunia, or vaginal burning/irritation. A patient with trichomoniasis may present with abdominal pain, dyspareunia, and/or dysuria that typically begins 5 to 28 days after exposure.[32]

PHYSICAL EXAMINATION

In BV, the vulva will appear normal on exam with thin, gray, "fishy-smelling" discharge. In contrast, a patient with *Candida* vulvovaginitis may have vulvar erythema and edema with a normal cervix. Excoriations may be present due to scratching. Erosive vulvovaginitis, characterized by purulent discharge and tenderness with macular erythematous lesions, is suggestive of trichomoniasis, rather than other causes of vaginitis. In addition, strawberry cervix (Figure 12.2) is pathognomonic for trichomoniasis.

DIFFERENTIAL DIAGNOSIS

Table 12.11 summarizes the differential diagnosis for vaginitis.

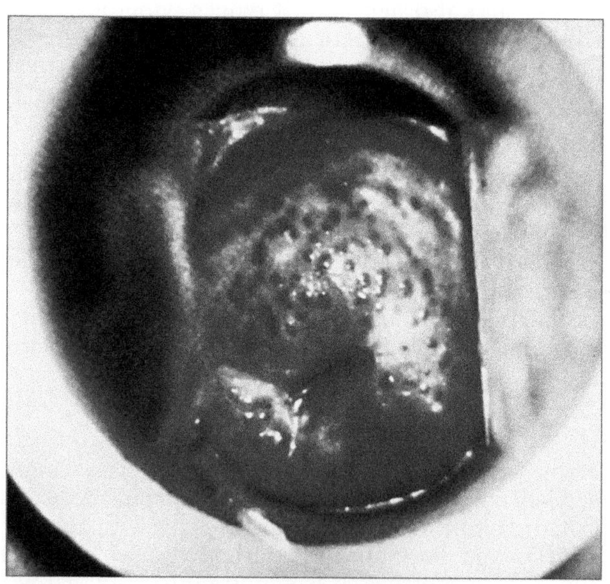

Figure 12.2 "Strawberry" cervix from trichomoniasis. Cervical erythema with petechiae creates the appearance of an overripe strawberry.

(Source: Photo courtesy of the Centers for Disease Control and Prevention.)

TABLE 12.11 Differential Diagnosis for Vaginitis

Diagnosis	Description
Gonorrhea	Mucopurulent vaginal discharge, dysuria, abnormal vaginal bleeding. PCR positive for *Neisseria gonorrhoeae.* Gram stain of vaginal discharge will show gram-negative diplococci.
Atrophic vaginitis	Characterized by vaginal dryness. May have bleeding, burning, itching, discharge, or irritation. Lab test will show a low estrogen. Typically seen in postmenopausal women.
Chlamydia infection	Mucopurulent cervicitis with dysuria and abdominal pain. PCR positive for *C. trachomatis.* Gram stain of vaginal discharge will show gram-negative rods.
Vulvar dermatitis	Vulvar pruritus. Biopsy not routinely performed, but will show spongiosis and dermal infiltrate of lymphocytes with eosinophils.

PCR, polymerase chain reaction.

TABLE 12.12 Diagnostic Findings in Vaginitis

Type of Vaginitis	pH Findings	Wet Prep Findings	Other Studies
Bacterial vaginosis	>4.5	Clue cells, little to no lactobacilli, polymorphonuclear leukocytes	Whiff test will be positive with a fishy odor noted
Candida vulvovaginitis	Normal	Clue cells, budding yeast, hyphae, pseudohyphae Must use 10% KOH	Vaginal swab may be obtained for culture for repeated infections
Trichomoniasis	5.0–6.0	Motile, pea-shaped flagellated protozoa, WBCs	PCR, culture and DNA probe can be performed and will be positive for *Trichomonas vaginalis*

KOH, potassium hydroxide; PCR, polymerase chain reaction; WBCs, white blood cells.

DIAGNOSTIC STUDIES

Vaginal pH and microscopy are the diagnostic tests of choice for vaginitis. Table 12.12 describes the diagnostic findings in vaginitis.

EVALUATION

Complaints of abnormal vaginal discharge, pruritus, and/or vaginal pain should be investigated with evaluation of vaginal discharge and pelvic exam. It is also important to note that pregnant women with BV are at an increased risk for preterm delivery and, therefore, any pregnant patient with abnormal vaginal discharge should be evaluated immediately.[33]

TREATMENT

- BV is treated with a 7-day course of metronidazole either oral or topical gel.
- *Candida* vulvovaginitis is treated with a topical -azole cream, which can be given in a single dose or 1 to 3-day regimens. A single dose of oral fluconazole can also be administered.
- Trichomoniasis is treated with oral metronidazole either a 2 g single dose or a 7-day course of 500 mg.
- The partner(s) of patients diagnosed with trichomoniasis should also be treated at the same time as the patient to prevent reinfection.

PATIENT EDUCATION

- It is important to maintain good vaginal hygiene. Avoid douching, keep vagina dry, avoid tight-fitting clothes, wear cotton underwear, and avoid scented vaginal soaps.
- Trichomoniasis is transmitted sexually, and sexual partners should be notified and treated as well.
- Patients should be advised that condoms should be used during sexual intercourse to prevent the transmission of trichomoniasis.

12.3B VULVAR LICHEN SCLEROSIS

MEDICAL HISTORY AND CLINICAL PRESENTATION

Vulvar LS is characterized by the thinning of the epithelium and inflammation. Instances are higher in women who are immobile and incontinent.[34] The cause of vulvar LS is unknown but about 10% of patients have family members with the same condition.[34]

SIGNS AND SYMPTOMS

The most common presenting symptom of vulvar LS is intense vulvar pruritus that will wake patients from their sleep. Soreness and irritation of the vulva are also common. This also may be associated with anal pain, dyspareunia, and dysuria, due to the thinning of vulvar epithelium and fusion of vulvar landmarks. Though pruritus and irritation are the most common presenting symptoms, some patients are asymptomatic and can be identified only by vulvar architecture and skin changes.

PHYSICAL EXAMINATION

Classic characteristics of early vulvar LS include white, atrophic papules and plaques most frequently affecting the labia minor and/or labia majora (Figure 12.3). Excoriations due to scratching may be noted, as well as secondary lichenification of the affected areas. As the disease progresses, further thinning of the epithelium results in a loss of the distinction between the labia majora and minora, shrinking of the introitus and perineum, as well as clitoral burying under the prepuce (Figure 12.3).

A shiny, "cellophane-like" surface may be seen at this stage and is highly suggestive of LS. The late stage of LS, loss of external vulvar landmarks, results in a pallid, featureless vulva with a classic pinhole orifice (Figure 12.4).

DIFFERENTIAL DIAGNOSIS

Table 12.13 summarizes the differential diagnosis for vulvar LS.

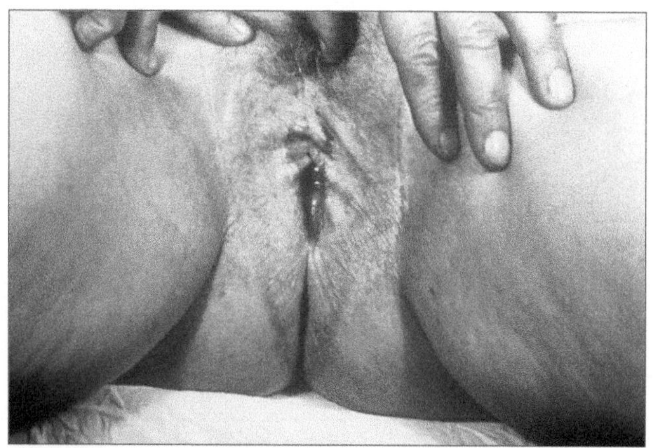

Figure 12.3 **Classic findings of vulvar lichen sclerosis include white, atrophic papules and plaques most frequently affecting the labia minora and/or labia majora.**
(Source: Centers for Disease Control and Prevention/Susan Lindsley.)

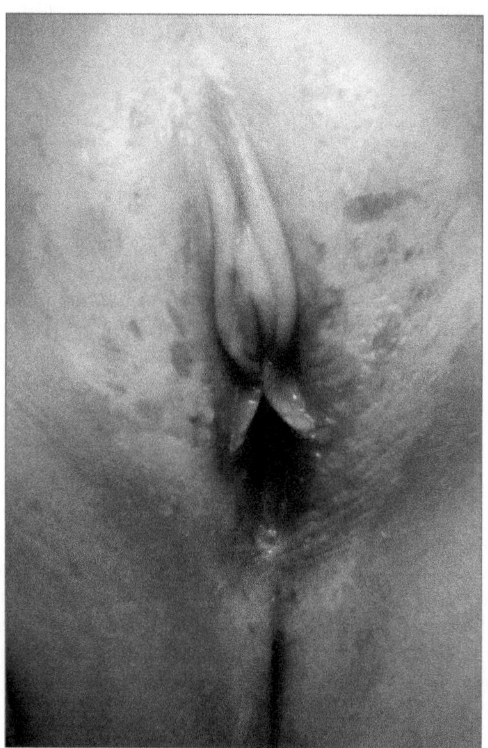

Figure 12.4 **A shiny, "cellophane-like" surface may be seen at the early stage of vulvar lichen sclerosis.**
(Source: Centers for Disease Control and Prevention/Dr. N.J. Fiumara.)

TABLE 12.13 Differential Diagnosis for Vulvar Lichen Sclerosis

Diagnosis	Description
Lichen planus	Similar appearing to LS but typically involves the vagina. Pain is the defining symptom. Biopsy is helpful in distinguishing between the two.
Lichen simplex chronicus	Causes pruritus and irritation where repeated scratching leads to a well-circumscribed area of lichenification.
Vulvar dermatitis	Causes pruritus and irritation resulting in diffuse erythema, scaling, fissures and lichenification. Typically affects the labia majora. Looks similar to early LS.
Candida vulvovaginitis	Results in pruritus and/or burning. Will not have skin changes like LS but may have excoriations due to pruritis.
Vitiligo	Depigmentation of skin similar to the whitening seen in LS but without other symptoms such as itching.

LS, lichen sclerosis.

DIAGNOSTIC STUDIES

Vulvar LS may be diagnosed empirically based on the clinical manifestations; however, the gold standard diagnostic test of choice is a 4-mm punch biopsy of the vulvar lesion. Histology will show areas of hyperkeratosis, epidermal atrophy, and lymphocytic infiltrate of the dermis, and will allow for exclusion of a malignant process.

EVALUATION

All women with pruritus, irritation, and pain should be examined, and lesions should be biopsied. Given the nonspecific early symptoms of vulvar LS, the delay in diagnosis is reported to be around 5 years.[34] However, to prevent severe scaring and erosion of vulvar landmarks, it is important that vulvar LS is diagnosed and treated early. This supports the importance of annual pelvic exams for women. In addition, vulvar LS is associated with an increased risk of vulvar squamous cell carcinoma, especially in the presence of vulvar intraepithelial neoplasia.[21]

TREATMENT

- All patients, including asymptomatic patients, should be treated as early as possible to avoid further progression of this disease.
- Patients should be treated with topical ultrapotent corticosteroid ointment applied nightly to the affected area for 12 weeks initially.[34]
- Patients should be reevaluated after initial therapy.
- Recurrence is common and some patients may need a maintenance regimen.

PATIENT EDUCATION

- Vulvar LS is a chronic condition with frequent recurrences of the signs and symptoms, though the condition is manageable with topical corticosteroids.
- It is important that the patient practice good vulvar hygiene. Hygiene counseling should include avoiding scratching the affected area as this will increase symptoms

and can introduce secondary infections. Patients should also avoid tight-fitting clothing and synthetic materials, scented soaps, douches, sprays, and powders.
- Patients with vulvar LS have an increased risk for vulvar malignancies and should be closely followed for new or worsening symptoms.
- Sexual counseling may be necessary to address associated concerns with sexual function and dyspareunia. Patients should also be counseled that this condition is not contagious and cannot be sexually transmitted.

12.3C VAGINAL AND VULVAR CANCER

MEDICAL HISTORY AND CLINICAL PRESENTATION

The most common clinical presentation of vaginal cancer is vaginal bleeding, though many patients remain asymptomatic. Malignancy-related vaginal bleeding is typically postmenopausal or postcoital. Vaginal discharge that is watery, blood-tinged, and/or malodorous is also a symptom of vaginal malignancy. It is important to note that about one fifth of vaginal cancers are found incidentally during screening for cervical cancer.[35] There are several features (medical history) that contribute to increased risk of vaginal and vulvar malignancies. A major risk factor for vulvar cancer is exposure to high-risk HPV (strains 16, 18, and 31) due to increased occurrence of vulvar intraepithelial neoplasia (VIN) leading to squamous cell carcinoma in the vagina and vulva. Smoking also increases risk due to increased DNA strand breaks and decreased ability to repair mutations.[36] In utero exposure to diethylstilbestrol (DES), a synthetic estrogen used from 1939 to 1971 as a miscarriage and preterm delivery preventive, is a risk factor for vaginal clear cell adenocarcinoma.[37] The average age of those diagnosed with vaginal malignancy is 60 years but could also occur earlier. Vaginal cancer has a 40% 5-year survival rate and a 35% 10-year survival rate.[22] The average age of diagnosis for vulvar cancer is 69 with a 71% 5-year survival rate.[23]

SIGNS AND SYMPTOMS

Vaginal cancers are typically asymptomatic but can cause changes in menstruation, abnormal vaginal bleeding, and vaginal discharge. With the presence of vaginal masses, patients may experience urinary or GI complaints. VIN can be asymptomatic or characterized by itching that will not resolve. Patients with vulvar cancer tend to experience itching, pain, burning, abnormal bleeding, and/or discharge. These malignancies may also be associated with a lump or sore.

PHYSICAL EXAMINATION

A complete pelvic examination should be performed including speculum exam, bimanual exam, and external examination looking for masses and abnormal lesions. Inguinal lymph adenopathy is also common, so palpation of groin lymph nodes is necessary. In vaginal cancer, the most common site for vaginal carcinoma is the posterior wall of the vagina occurring in half of the cases.[38] Because of this, it is important to inspect vaginal walls after the speculum is removed as speculums can obscure view.

DIFFERENTIAL DIAGNOSIS

Table 12.14 summarizes the differential diagnosis of vaginal and vulvar cancer.

DIAGNOSTIC STUDIES

To evaluate a patient for vaginal and vulvar cancers, a biopsy of lesions should be performed, and specimen should be evaluated with histopathologic studies. The vagina and vulva are treated with diluted acetic acid, which causes HPV infected cells to turn white, so these areas are seen more easily. A colposcope may be used to see the surface closely to aid in the ability to biopsy. For small lesions, excisional biopsy is performed for complete removal. Punch biopsy can be used for larger lesions.

EVALUATION

Annual pelvic exams are important to evaluate any skin changes in the vulvar and vaginal area. It is important to note that many early cases of vaginal cancer are asymptomatic and can be diagnosed by the incidental finding of vaginal mass on pelvic exam or during cervical cancer screening histologic studies.[22] Women should also be counseled on the warning signs of vaginal and vulvar malignancies such as abnormal bleeding, vaginal itching, and/or vaginal pain. If any patients experience these symptoms, they should be counseled to present for evaluation.

TREATMENT

- For vaginal tumors, radial hysterectomy, upper vaginectomy, and bilateral pelvic lymphadenectomy are performed. Radiation therapy and chemotherapy may also be required.
- For vulvar cancers, excision of the lesion, vulvectomy, and/or lymphadenectomy may be required. Radiation therapy and chemotherapy may also be required.
- Treatment is determined by staging of tumors and lesions.

PATIENT EDUCATION

- HPV vaccine not only prevents cervical cancer but is also important in preventing HPV-associated vaginal and vulvar squamous cell carcinoma.
- Given that vaginal and vulvar malignancies can be found incidentally on pelvic exam and cervical cancer screening, it is necessary to stress annual pelvic exams and cervical cancer screening every 3 years.

TABLE 12.14 Differential Diagnosis of Vaginal and Vulvar Cancer

Diagnosis	Description
Benign nevi	Border will be well-circumscribed with homogeneous color and <6 mm in diameter.
Syphilitic chancre	Can appear similar to VIN or squamous cell carcinoma. All patients should be screened for sexually transmitted infections.
Vulvar lichen sclerosis	Biopsy will show areas of hyperkeratosis, epidermal atrophy, and lymphocytic infiltrate of the dermis.

VIN, vulvar intraepithelial neoplasia.

- Abnormal bleeding, discharge, vaginal itching, and/or vaginal pain should be evaluated by a clinician.
- Smoking increases risk of vaginal and vulvar cancer and smoking cessation should be encouraged.

SPECIAL CONSIDERATIONS

- Pregnant patients with *Candida* vulvovaginitis should be treated with topical -azole medication rather than oral treatment due to increased risk of miscarriage.[39]

12.4 UTERINE DISORDERS

Elyse J. Watkins

OVERVIEW

Disorders of the uterus can cause a variety of symptoms depending upon the underlying pathology. This section will review two common conditions, leiomyoma (fibroids) and endometriosis.

EPIDEMIOLOGY

Leiomyoma is the most commonly encountered benign mass of the uterus.[48] Risk factors for the development of leiomyoma include age, Black race, family history, and obesity. Less robust data suggest diet, stress, caffeine intake, and tobacco use may increase the risk for leiomyoma. Endometriosis affects about 10% of women during the reproductive years.[49] Risk factors for endometriosis include low waist-to-hip ratios and early age at menarche.

PATHOPHYSIOLOGY

The pathophysiology of endometriosis has largely been attributed to Sampson's theory whereby retrograde menstruation causes ectopic implants. Another theory postulates that during fetal development, coelomic cells that line the abdominal peritoneum and viscera are activated as a result of endogenous or exogenous stimuli. The peritoneum, müllerian ducts, and ovary embryologically derive from coelomic epithelium.[50] Another theory is that stem cells derived from bone marrow and endometrium spread via the lymphatic circulation, vascular circulation, and retrograde menstruation.[50] Endometriotic tissue is highly sensitive to estrogen but resistant to progesterone and can produce its own estradiol. A cascade of events follow including immune cell activation, angiogenesis, and cytokine activation (see Figure 12.5).

The precise pathophysiology of uterine fibroids is unknown, but several theories exist as to why uterine smooth muscle cells transform into abnormal growth resulting in tumor formation through aberrant cell division and extracellular matrix production. The most widely held theory is that a monocyte undergoes neoplastic changes and develops into a benign tumor, but the reason for the transformation is

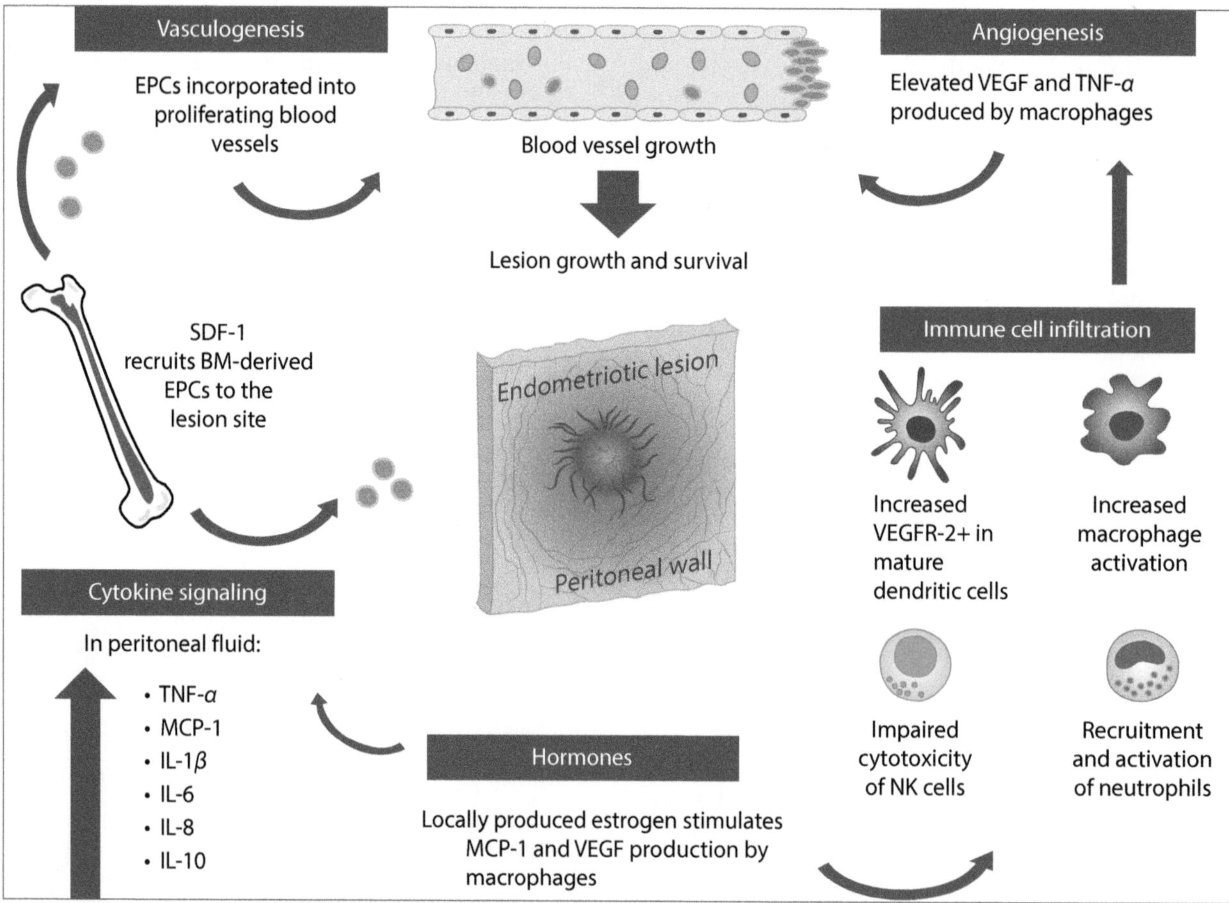

Figure 12.5 Pathophysiology of endometriosis. BM, bone marrow; EPCs, epithelial cells; IL, interleukin; MCP-1, monocyte chemotactic protein-1; NK, natural killer; SDF-1, stromal cell-derived factor 1; TNF, tumor necrosis factor; VEGF, vascular endothelial growth factor; VEGFR, vascular endothelial growth factor receptor.
(Source: Ahn SH, Monsanto SP, Miller C, et al. Pathophysiology and immune dysfunctions in endometriosis. Biomed Res Int. *2015;2015:795976. doi:10.1155/2015/795976)*

contested.[51] It is known that fibroids exhibit a strong affinity for estrogen and progesterone, but newer theories involving genetic mutations, cytokines (particularly tumor necrosis factor-α [TNF-α]), and stem cells are being explored.[52,53]

12.4A LEIOMYOMA

MEDICAL HISTORY AND CLINICAL PRESENTATION

Most women with uterine fibroids will present with pelvic pain or fullness or AUB, but some women will be asymptomatic and the fibroid will be found incidentally. In patients of reproductive age, it is essential to obtain a thorough menstrual and obstetric history, including the date of the last menstrual period (LMP). A family history of fibroids may be present. Some patients may present with anemia due to heavy bleeding or infertility.

SIGNS AND SYMPTOMS

AUB requires a thorough evaluation, but many patients with fibroids will have HMB. Some patients may describe a feeling of pelvic fullness or pressure, depending on the size and location of the fibroid. Constipation and frequent urination may occur, depending again on the location of the mass (Figure 12.6).

PHYSICAL EXAMINATION

A pelvic examination, including bimanual exam, is indicated. A palpable mass may be found but ability to do so often depends upon the patient's body habitus. The classic physical exam finding is an enlarged, firm, irregular, mobile uterus palpated on bimanual exam. However, it can be difficult to differentiate between a fibroid, an adnexal mass, and other abdominal masses, so imaging must occur.

DIFFERENTIAL DIAGNOSIS

Table 12.15 summarizes the differential diagnosis for leiomyoma.

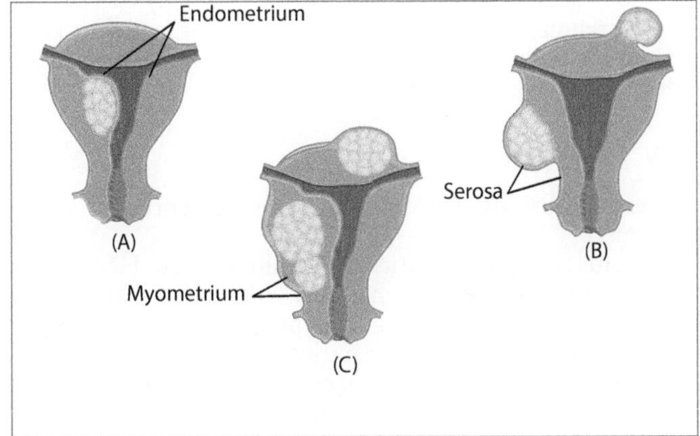

Figure 12.6 Appearance of uterine fibroids: (A) submucous leiomyoma, (B) subserous leiomyoma, and (C) intramural leiomyoma. *(Source: Carcio HA, Secor RM. The physical examination. In: Carcio HA, Mimi Secor R, eds.* Advanced Health Assessment of Women. *4th ed. Springer Publishing Company; 2018:72, Fig. 4.4.)*

TABLE 12.15 Differential Diagnosis for Leiomyoma

Diagnosis	Description
Ectopic pregnancy	Ruled out with a negative β-hCG
Intrauterine pregnancy	Ruled out with a negative β-hCG
Uterine malignancy, sarcomas	Can mimic benign leiomyoma
Uterine malignancy, endometrial carcinoma	Will usually present as abnormal uterine bleeding
Adenomyosis	An enlarged uterus may be seen in adenomyosis
Endometrial polyp	Not palpable on bimanual exam, but could be seen on ultrasound

hCG, human chorionic gonadotropin.

DIAGNOSTIC STUDIES

Ultrasound imaging is the mainstay of diagnosis. Fibroids that extend into the uterine cavity can be detected using saline-infused ultrasonography or hysteroscopy. Leiomyomas that have an atypical appearance should be evaluated with pelvic MRI. A CBC may reveal anemia due to HMB from fibroids.

EVALUATION

The evaluation of a patient includes understanding her desire for future pregnancy, current complaints, desire to maintain the uterus, and desire to avoid surgery.

TREATMENT

- Pharmacologic options include non-steroidal anti-inflammatories, GnRH agonists and antagonists, selective progesterone receptor modulators, combined oral contraceptive pills (COCPs), levonorgestrel-secreting IUS, aromatase inhibitors, and tranexamic acid.
  - **NSAIDs:** Can be used to help decrease pain and bleeding associated with fibroids.
  - **GnRH agonists:** Can cause hypoestrogen side effects including vasomotor symptoms, bone loss; initially causes a flare of symptoms. Use >6 months requires progestin therapy as well.
  - **GnRH antagonists:** Can cause hypoestrogen side effects including vasomotor symptoms, bone loss. No initial flare of symptoms.
  - **Selective progesterone receptor modulators:** Not currently approved for use in the United States.
  - **Combined oral contraceptive pills:** Indicated for HMB.
  - **Levonorgestrel-secreting IUS:** Indicated for HMB; should not be used if fibroids extend into the endometrial cavity.
  - **Aromatase inhibitors:** Not currently Food and Drug Administration (FDA) approved for fibroids.
  - **Tranexamic acid:** Indicated for HMB.
  - The newest option is a combination oral product containing estrogen, progestin, and a selective progesterone receptor modulator.
- Surgical options include myomectomy and hysterectomy.
  - Myomectomy is better for patients who wish to retain fertility, but fibroids tend to recur within 5 years.

- Definitive surgical management is with hysterectomy.
- Other minimally invasive options include uterine artery embolization, magnetic resonance guided focus ultrasound, laparoscopic ultrasound-guided radiofrequency ablation, and endometrial ablation (for HMB).
- Asymptomatic patients can be managed conservatively with routine surveillance.

PATIENT EDUCATION

- Patients should have a clear explanation of their diagnosis and treatment options and potential effect on fertility.
- Patients who desire fertility preservation should opt for more conservative therapies.
- Patients with contraindications for hormone use need to consider other options.

12.4B ENDOMETRIOSIS

MEDICAL HISTORY AND CLINICAL PRESENTATION

Patients with endometriosis are of reproductive age and often present with pelvic pain, dyspareunia, dysmenorrhea, and infertility. Dyschezia can be present if posterior implants are present. However, some patients are asymptomatic and disease is found incidentally. Patients with a history of pelvic pain are at greater risk of having endometriosis. A family history of endometriosis is often elucidated. Irregular menses may present among patients with endometriosis. A thorough menstrual and obstetric history is advised.

SIGNS AND SYMPTOMS

A complete review of systems could elicit dysuria, dyschezia, dysmenorrhea, and dyspareunia. Patients with an acute onset of pain are less likely to have endometriosis, which is a chronic condition.

PHYSICAL EXAMINATION

While endometriosis cannot be diagnosed on a physical examination, it is important to conduct a thorough physical exam to rule out other diagnoses and to document the presence or absence of key findings. Important findings include diffuse tenderness on bimanual examination; nodularity along the uterosacral ligaments, vagina, and posterior cul-de-sac; fixed pelvic structures due to adhesions; and thickening of the pelvic structures. Some patients may experience extreme tenderness even when the speculum is introduced, so careful examination of the cervix and uterus can help eliminate PID or a tubo-ovarian abscess.

DIFFERENTIAL DIAGNOSIS

Table 12.16 summarizes the differential diagnosis for endometriosis.

DIAGNOSTIC STUDIES

Transvaginal and transabdominal ultrasound are useful to rule out other disease processes (see Table 12.16); however, endometriosis cannot be diagnosed by ultrasound imaging. Definitive diagnosis is through direct visualization of endometriotic lesions and histologic sampling of suspicious lesions during laparoscopy.

EVALUATION

The overall evaluation of a patient with possible endometriosis involves careful consideration of the patient's level of pain, impact on daily routine, and desire for preservation of fertility.

TREATMENT

- Treatment options include pharmacologic and nonpharmacologic interventions.
- Nonhormonal pharmacologic options include NSAIDs for pain control.
- Hormonal pharmacologic options include GnRH agonists and antagonists, selective progesterone receptor modulators, aromatase inhibitors, combination hormonal contraceptives, and progestin-only contraceptives.
- Surgical options include laparoscopy with ablation of endometriotic lesions and excision of endometriomas that may be present, and definitive surgical management consists of hysterectomy.
  - Patients who do not desire immediate pregnancy will often be started on a combined contraception or GnRH postoperatively.

PATIENT EDUCATION

- Patients must be educated on their diagnosis of endometriosis and provided with sufficient information that is understandable to the patient in order to share in the decision-making process regarding treatment and prognosis.
- Patients with infertility who are desiring pregnancy should be considered for referral to reproductive endocrinology after treatment is initiated.
- Patients who do not undergo hysterectomy have a high likelihood of recurrence.

SPECIAL CONSIDERATIONS

- Adolescent patients may go undiagnosed. It is important to consider the diagnosis in an adolescent if dysmenorrhea, dyspareunia, and chronic pelvic pain persist in order to mitigate the scarring and potential negative impact on future fertility.

KEY POINTS

- Uterine fibroids are common among reproductive-age women.
- Fibroids can cause significant morbidity due to HMB, pain, and infertility, but some patients will be asymptomatic.
- Treatment of fibroids largely depends upon size and location of the fibroid and the patient's overall expectations.
- There are numerous pharmacologic, minimally invasive, and surgical options for patients with uterine fibroids.
- Endometriosis is a common disease found in reproductive-age females.
- Diagnosis is made through direct visualization of endometriotic lesions and lesion sampling during laparoscopy.

TABLE 12.16 Differential Diagnosis for Endometriosis

Diagnosis	Description
Ectopic pregnancy	Must be ruled out in patients with pelvic pain and a positive β-hCG.
Appendicitis	Can be difficult to differentiate. Patients with endometriosis are generally afebrile unless another process is present. Is usually a more acute process.
Pelvic inflammatory disease	Can be difficult to differentiate. Physical exam should determine if Chandelier sign is present and if mucopurulent cervicitis is present. Is usually a more acute process.
Tubo-ovarian abscess	An adnexal mass will be visualized on ultrasound imaging and may be palpable in bimanual exam. The patient will be febrile.
Ovarian cyst	Can be ruled out with ultrasound.
Pelvic adhesions due to other etiologies	Prior intra-abdominal and pelvic surgeries can cause adhesions, as can inflammatory processes.
Leiomyoma	Can present with pelvic pain and dyspareunia depending on the location and size of the fibroid. Easily distinguished on ultrasound.
Adenomyosis	Usually presents in later reproductive years in parous patients. Ultrasound imaging may assist the diagnosis but is usually found status post hysterectomy.
Interstitial cystitis	Is generally a diagnosis of exclusion. Pelvic pain and chronic dysuria without culture-positive urine specimens strongly suggest the diagnosis.

hCG, human chorionic gonadotropin.

- A multitude of treatment options are aimed at relieving symptoms, reducing the development of adhesions and scarring, and preserving potential fertility.
- Definitive surgical management with hysterectomy will ensure complete resolution and avoid recurrence.

12.5 PELVIC ORGAN PROLAPSE

Jeniece Wert

OVERVIEW

The pelvic diaphragm is made up of a series of muscles that extend across the pelvic cavity in order to support the pelvic organs. Pelvic organ prolapse (POP) describes the herniation and descent of the pelvic organs into or out of the vagina, typically caused by weakening in the supportive pelvic floor organs. POP can be divided into four categories described in Table 12.17 and illustrated in Figure 12.7.

EPIDEMIOLOGY

Approximately one-third of adult women have a degree of POP but many may not be symptomatic or do not seek treatment.[54] The most common type of POP is cystocele, which is twice as likely as a rectocele and three times as likely as a uterine prolapse.[55] Several factors increase likelihood of POP including parity, history of hysterectomy, and obesity. In particular, upwards of 50% of all parous women have some degree of vaginal wall laxity with 20% being symptomatic.[56]

TABLE 12.17 Categories of Pelvic Organ Prolapse

Type of POP	Organ Involvement	Location of Herniation
Uterine or apical prolapse	Uterus, cervix, vaginal vault	Into the vagina
Cystocele	Bladder	Anterior vagina
Rectocele	Rectum	Posterior distal vagina
Enterocele	Small bowel (pouch of Douglas)	Upper vagina

POP, pelvic organ prolapse.

PATHOPHYSIOLOGY

POP occurs when there is weakness in levator ani muscles and enlargement and stretching of the levator hiatus increasing the tension on pelvic fascial support system leading to separations in the pelvic supports. A patient's risk factors increase the likelihood of these separations in the pelvic supports. There is a clear correlation between chronic increased abdominal pressure (due to obesity, chronic constipation, chronic cough, heavy lifting, etc.) and the increased rate of progression of POP.[56] POP is also seen in women who have had multiple pregnancies, especially those who have had multiple vaginal deliveries. The repeated pressure on the pelvic organ support muscles increased the rate of progression of this disease as these supports begin to weaken, resulting in the herniation of pelvic organs. For example, morbid obesity is associated with a 40% increased risk for uterine prolapse, 75% increased risk for rectocele, and 57% increased risk for a cystocele.[54]

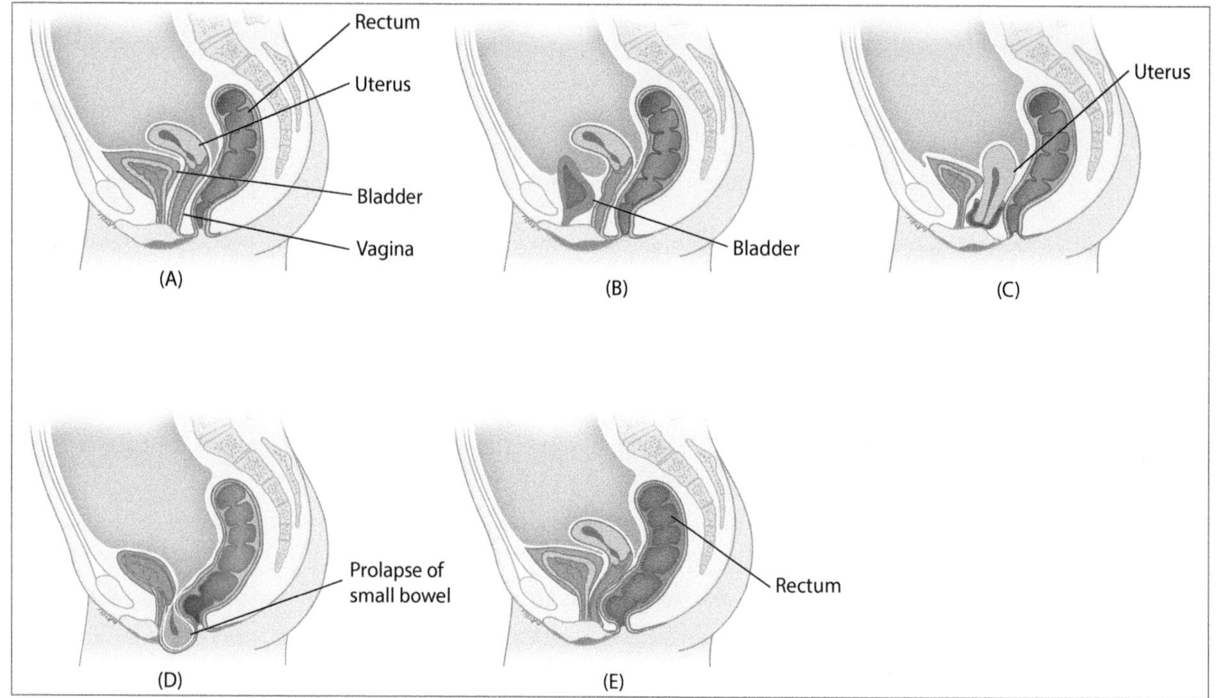

Figure 12.7 Types of pelvic organ prolapse (POP). (A) Normal position of bladder, uterus, vagina, and rectum; (B) cystocele or bladder prolapse; (C) uterine or vaginal prolapse; (D) enterocele or small bowel prolapse; (E) rectocele or rectal prolapse.

MEDICAL HISTORY AND CLINICAL PRESENTATION

Patients describe the feeling as something "falling out" of their vagina or as a heaviness in their vagina. The typical patient is an older woman with a history of hysterectomy, obesity, and/or multiple pregnancies. Patients may also complain of pelvic pressure or lower back pain.

SIGNS AND SYMPTOMS

Patients with POP may experience stress incontinence, especially with cystocele and uterine prolapses due to the prolapsed organ obstructing the urethra resulting in obstructed and incomplete voiding. Defecatory symptoms are common, especially with rectocele. These symptoms consist of fecal urgency, fecal incontinence, and obstructive symptoms. Increased progression of disease is associated with increased sexual dysfunction such as decreased libido, dyspareunia, and inability to reach orgasm. In addition, urinary and/or fecal incontinence during sexual activity is also common.

PHYSICAL EXAMINATION

Physical examination to evaluate POP involves a pelvic visual inspection, speculum exam, bimanual exam, and rectovaginal exam. Each component of this exam should be performed when patient is relaxed and then while the patient performs the Valsalva maneuver. To evaluate for POP with a speculum, the clinician should first insert the speculum and slowly withdraw it to evaluate the descent of the cervix. The clinician can then use a Sims retractor or the posterior blade of the speculum above the cervix (Figure 12.8) to isolate the anterior vaginal wall to evaluate bulges and weaknesses. The same method should be used below the cervix (Figure 12.9) to isolate the posterior vaginal wall for bulges and weaknesses. Retrovaginal examination is used to detect an enterocele and is best performed with the patient standing (Figure 12.10). A positive examination results when the small bowel can be palpated in the cul-de-sac.

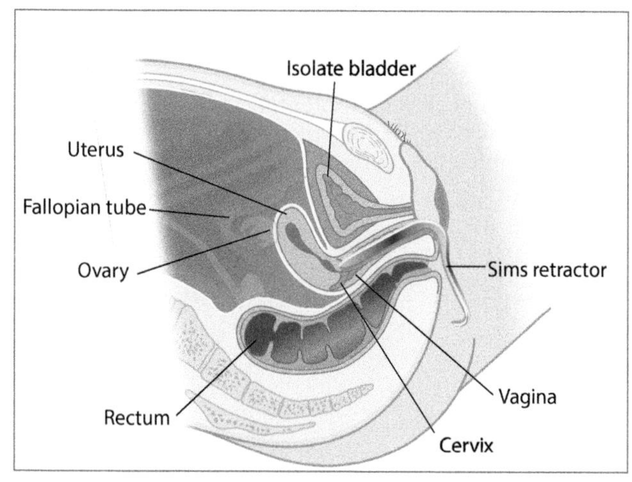

Figure 12.8 Pelvic examination for cystocele. To evaluate for pelvic organ prolapse (POP) with a speculum, the clinician should first insert the speculum and slowly withdraw it to evaluate the descent of the cervix. The clinician can then use a Sims retractor or the posterior blade of the speculum above the cervix to isolate the anterior vaginal wall to evaluate bulges and weaknesses.

DIFFERENTIAL DIAGNOSIS

Table 12.18 summarizes the differential diagnosis for POP.

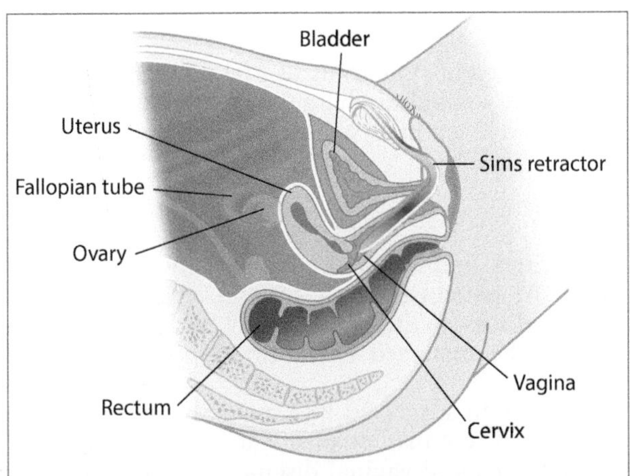

Figure 12.9 Pelvic examination for rectocele. The retractor or the posterior blade of the speculum is used to isolate the posterior vaginal wall to inspect for bulges and weaknesses.

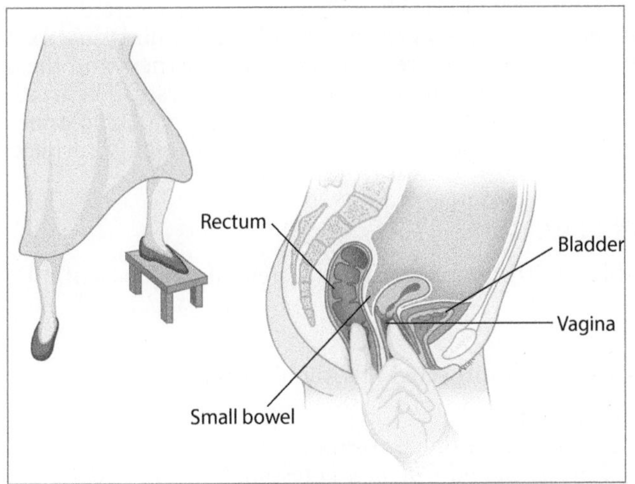

Figure 12.10 Rectovaginal examination for enterocele. Retrovaginal examination is used to detect an enterocele and is best performed with the patient standing; standing can make a minor prolapse more pronounced. A positive examination is when the small bowel can be palpated in the cul-de-sac.

TABLE 12.18 Differential Diagnosis for Pelvic Organ Prolapse

Diagnosis	Description
Bartholin gland cyst or abscess	Will have a mass to the labia majora rather than within the vaginal cavity. Valsalva maneuver will not increase the bulge.
Leiomyoma	On bimanual examination, an enlarged, mobile uterus will be felt. Can also be seen on pelvic ultrasound.
Urethral diverticula	Will manifest as an anterior vaginal wall mass and should be diagnosed with MRI. Frequent urinary tract infections are common with urethral diverticula.
Cervical polyp	May cause dyspareunia and vaginal pressure. Will be seen on speculum examination.

TABLE 12.19 POP-Q Staging Criteria

POP-Q Stage	Criteria
Stage 0	No prolapse
Stage I	More than 1 cm above the level of the hymenal ring
Stage II	Between 1 cm above and 1 cm below the level of the hymenal ring
Stage III	Between 1 cm and 3 cm below the level of the hymenal ring
Stage IV	Complete eversion of organ beyond the level of the hymenal ring

POP-Q, pelvic organ prolapse quantification.

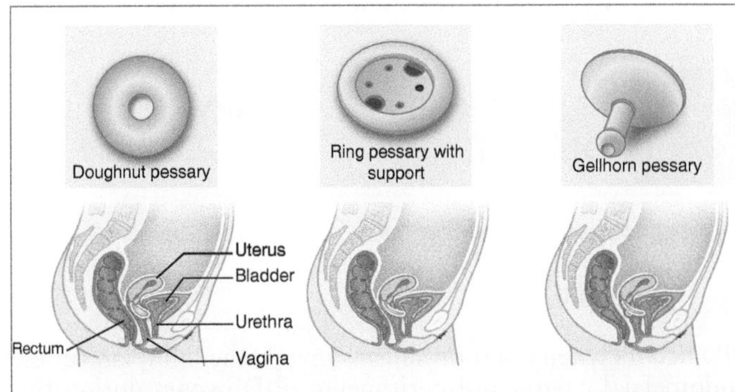

Figure 12.11 Pessary examples: doughnut pessary; ring pessary with support; Gellhorn pessary.

DIAGNOSTIC STUDIES

To stage POP, the POP Quantification (POP-Q) System is used. The measurement is taken when the patient is performing the Valsalva maneuver to determine the maximum point of descent of the pelvic organ. When maximum descent has been achieved, the measurement of the distal portion prolapse organ to the level of the hymen and/or vaginal opening is taken and staged based on the values listed in Table 12.19.

EVALUATION

During annual pelvic examination, women should be asked about the symptoms of POP to determine if further evaluation is needed.

TREATMENT

- Vaginal pessary, pictured in Figure 12.11, is the mainstay of nonsurgical treatment of POP. These are silicone devices inserted into the vagina to provide support to pelvic organs. There are many different shapes and sizes of pessaries and the use of each type will vary based on the patient's needs.
- Physical therapy is recommended for 8 to 12 weeks to strengthen the pelvic muscles.
- Surgical management of POP involves reconstruction of the pelvic area and may include a hysterectomy for uterine prolapse.

PATIENT EDUCATION

- POP is the progressive dropping of the pelvic organs due to loss of vaginal support.
- Weight management and Kegel exercises can be used as preventive measures for POP.

SPECIAL CONSIDERATIONS

- Pregnant patients with POP are always managed conservatively with pelvic floor exercises and/or pessaries.

KEY POINTS

- The key symptom of POP is pelvic pressure or bulges. Commonly, patients describe feeling as though something is falling out of their vagina.
- Risk factors for POP include anything that puts chronic pressure on the pelvic support muscles such as parity, obesity, chronic constipation, and repeated heavy lifting.

12.6 PELVIC INFLAMMATORY DISEASE

Elyse J. Watkins

OVERVIEW

PID occurs when microorganisms invade the fallopian tubes, endometrial cavity, and peritoneum. PID occurs during the reproductive years and should be on the differential diagnosis list for any woman of childbearing age who presents with pelvic pain and fever. It is essential to provide a timely diagnosis and initiate treatment to avoid the sequelae of untreated or inadequately treated PID, such as tubo-ovarian abscess, ectopic pregnancy, chronic pelvic pain, and infertility.

EPIDEMIOLOGY

PID is diagnosed in approximately 2.5 million women between 18 and 44 years of age in the United States.[49]

PATHOPHYSIOLOGY

The most common organisms implicated in PID are *Chlamydia* and *Neisseria gonorrhoeae*; however, other organisms have been found, including *Mycoplasma hominis, Gardnerella vaginalis*, *Streptococcus agalactiae,* and *Haemophilus influenzae.* Untreated or inadequately treated vagino-cervical infections can potentially cause PID as the organisms migrate through the endocervical canal, into the uterus, through the fallopian tubes, and out into the peritoneum. Tubo-ovarian abscess and adhesions can occur. Adhesions can cause chronic pelvic pain and fallopian tube dysfunction leading to infertility. Significant adhesions around the liver can cause perihepatitis, also referred to as Fitz-Hugh-Curtis syndrome.

MEDICAL HISTORY AND CLINICAL PRESENTATION

Patients with PID will present with pelvic or lower abdominal pain. They may present with vaginal discharge as well. Depending on the severity of infection, patients may experience fever, but the absence of fever does not rule out the diagnosis.

SIGNS AND SYMPTOMS

Common signs and symptoms of PID include pelvic or abdominal pain, vaginal discharge, dyspareunia, and fever in a sexually active woman. Women with a history of PID are more likely to develop a subsequent episode of PID.

PHYSICAL EXAMINATION

The physical examination should initially focus on determining if the patient is septic by assessing vital signs and the overall status of the patient. Any patient who appears septic must be managed expeditiously using appropriate interventions.

A patient with suspected PID must always have a pelvic examination. There may be purulent cervical mucus visualized from the os and vaginal discharge present. The cervix itself may be friable, indicating cervicitis. The pathognomonic finding on physical examination is cervical motion tenderness, also called the Chandelier sign. This is evidenced by considerable pain and discomfort when pressure is applied to the cervix. Often, women with PID will experience pain and discomfort when the speculum is inserted past the introitus, but all women should still have a bimanual examination to assess for cervical motion tenderness and the absence or presence of adnexal pain and masses. The triad of cervical motion tenderness, uterine tenderness, and adnexal tenderness in a sexually active woman is highly suspicious for PID.

DIFFERENTIAL DIAGNOSIS

Table 12.20 summarizes the differential diagnosis of PID.

DIAGNOSTIC STUDIES

Patients with suspected PID should have the following:

- Urinalysis
- β-hCG test (urine or serum)
- Gonorrhea and *Chlamydia* testing by PCR or culture
- Saline microscopy of vaginal discharge (patients with PID will have elevated WBCs)

More invasive testing includes the following:

- **Transvaginal ultrasound imaging:** Findings indicative of PID include thickened fallopian tubes, fluid in the fallopian tubes, and fluid in the posterior cul-de-sac. The absence of fluid in the cul-de-sac does not eliminate the possibility of PID. A tubo-ovarian abscess may also be found on ultrasound imaging.
- **Endometrial biopsy:** Findings indicative of PID include endometritis in a patient who is not postpartum.
- **Laparoscopy:** Findings consistent with PID include hyperemia and edema of the fallopian tubes and exudate on adnexal surfaces.
- **C-reactive protein and erythrocyte sedimentation rate:** Both will be elevated in PID but are not sensitive or specific for PID.

EVALUATION

The evaluation of a patient with suspected PID should aim to rule out pathologies that are associated with high mortality rates, such as ectopic pregnancy and ovarian torsion. The entire clinical picture must be assessed, including a thorough sexual history, as there are few tests that are highly sensitive and specific for PID.

TABLE 12.20 Differential Diagnosis for Pelvic Inflammatory Disease

Diagnosis	Description
Ectopic pregnancy	Must be considered in all sexually active women of reproductive age who still have a uterus. A negative β-human chorionic gonadotropin test will eliminate the diagnosis.
Urinary tract infection	Can easily be ruled out with a careful history, physical examination, and urine analysis.
Tubo-ovarian abscess	Adnexal mass present, fever, elevated white blood cell count with a left shift.
Endometriosis	Patients with endometriosis typically do not present with acute pain and are rarely febrile unless there is an underlying infectious process.
Ovarian torsion	Ovarian torsion usually presents as acute pelvic or lower abdominal pain with nausea and vomiting.
Appendicitis	Can be difficult to differentiate between pelvic inflammatory disease and appendicitis, but a careful history and physical exam should provide clues to which is the more likely diagnosis. Patients with appendicitis will often have accompanying anorexia without cervico-vaginal discharge and cervical motion tenderness.
Interstitial cystitis	Typically, pain is insidious and persistent, and the patient is afebrile. Careful history and physical examination will help the PA rule out interstitial cystitis.

TREATMENT

The U.S. Centers for Disease Control and Prevention (CDC) published guidelines on the treatment of PID in the outpatient and inpatient settings.[50]

- The preferred regimen for outpatient settings is:
  - Ceftriaxone 250 mg intramuscularly plus doxycycline 100 mg orally twice daily for 14 days.
  - Metronidazole 500 mg orally twice daily for 14 days if suspicious for an anaerobic organism.
  - An alternative to the above regimen is cefoxitin 2 g intramuscularly plus probenecid 1 g orally for one dose plus doxycycline 100 mg orally twice daily for 14 days.
  - Patients should be followed closely to ensure treatment compliance and improvement of symptoms; failure to see a clinical response within 72 hours necessitates reassessment and admission for IV antibiotics.
- The preferred regimen for inpatient settings is:
  - Cefotetan 2 g intravenously or cefoxitin 2 g intravenously plus doxycycline 100 mg orally or intravenously every 12 hours.
  - An alternative inpatient regimen is clindamycin 900 mg intravenously every 8 hours plus gentamicin 2 mg/kg as a loading dose intravenously, then 1.5 mg/kg every 8 hours.

PATIENT EDUCATION

- Patients should abstain from any sexual activity until treatment is complete and their partners have completed treatment as well.
- Patients who wish to resume sexual activity after treatment is complete should be advised to use condoms.
- Annual screening for *Chlamydia* and gonorrhea is recommended in all sexually active women younger than 25 years and in those who are deemed at higher risk, such as sex workers and women who have multiple partners.[51]
- Patient education should focus on preventing sexually transmitted infections, including discussing vaccination against HPV if the patient has not received her vaccinations.
- Gonorrhea, *Chlamydia*, and *Mycoplasma genitalium* testing is advised 3 to 6 months after treatment is complete.

SPECIAL CONSIDERATIONS

- PID rarely presents in pregnancy after 12 weeks' gestation due to the thickened mucus plug that develops around this time.
- Women who are pregnant and diagnosed with PID should be considered for inpatient management with the elimination of doxycycline in the treatment regimen.
- Women with a true IgE-mediated penicillin allergy may be given an inpatient regimen with clindamycin or gentamicin.
- Patients who are HIV positive are at greater risk of developing a tubo-ovarian abscess. If the patient fails to respond to outpatient treatment within the first few days, she should be admitted for IV antibiotics.

KEY POINTS

- Failure to diagnose and treat PID can cause significant morbidity, including chronic pelvic pain, Fitz-Hugh-Curtis syndrome, and infertility.
- The only confirmatory test for PID is laparoscopy; as such, reproductive-age sexually active women with pelvic or abdominal pain must have a thorough history and physical exam with the entire clinical picture assessed.
- The traditional pathognomonic finding of cervical motion tenderness can help confirm the diagnosis, but women with adhesions and endometriosis can also exhibit tenderness.
- Most patients can be treated as in the outpatient setting but must be watched closely for possible treatment failure.

12.7 OVARIAN DISORDERS

ELYSE J. WATKINS

OVERVIEW

Ovarian pathologies should be considered among children, adolescents, and women who present with lower abdominal and/or pelvic pain. While ovarian cancer is often diagnosed at a later stage, most ovarian processes are not associated with malignancy. This chapter will discuss benign ovarian cysts, PCOS, and ovarian torsion.

EPIDEMIOLOGY

Approximately 70% of ovarian masses will be benign.[52] Incidence of PCOS likely varies due to different diagnostic criteria, but is likely around 7% to 10%.[53,54] Ovarian torsion occurs in about 5.9/100,000 women; however, it is quite common among postmenarchal pediatric patients, and is more likely to present on the right side.[55] Ovarian torsion in postmenopausal women, while uncommon, is associated with ovarian malignancy.[56]

PATHOPHYSIOLOGY

Benign ovarian cysts occur during the reproductive years and are hormonally driven. Follicular ovarian cysts are due to follicular development with failed ovulation. Corpus luteal cysts occur when the corpus luteum does not rupture. Corpus luteal cysts remain during the early weeks of pregnancy and secrete progesterone to help maintain pregnancy. Corpus luteal cysts and follicular cysts can become hemorrhagic. Endometriomas are cysts that are blood-filled or contain endometrial tissue. They can occur in patients with or without endometriosis.

PCOS is a multifaceted endocrinopathy that can result in irregular menses (oligomenorrhea or amenorrhea), androgen excess, insulin resistance, dyslipidemia, hypertension, central adiposity, and infertility. The pathophysiology of PCOS is unknown but may be related to disordered androgen biosynthesis.[57] Studies have found excess responsiveness to 17-hydroxyprogesterone and LH and abnormalities of cytochrome P450c17. Fetal exposure to androgens may play a role in the development of PCOS. In addition, the theca cells of the ovary become hypersensitive to insulin. Insulin resistance results in hyperinsulinemia as a compensatory action, which then causes excess ovarian androgen.[57]

Figure 12.12 depicts the normal menstruation and ovulation process. Figure 12.13 illustrates the steroidogenesis from the ovary and the pathophysiology of insulin resistance and hirsutism in PCOS.

Ovarian torsion occurs when the ovary partially or completely twists on its ligamentous support structures resulting in edema, reduced venous return, hemorrhage, and infarction. Torsion occurs when there is a mass on the adnexa but also can occur in premenarchal females, possibly due to anatomic differences in the infundibulopelvic ligament. Failure to diagnose and surgically correct a torsion will result in ovarian necrosis and could lead to sepsis, peritonitis, and future reproductive compromise.

12.7A OVARIAN CYSTS

MEDICAL HISTORY AND CLINICAL PRESENTATION

Patients with a benign ovarian mass may present with abdominal or pelvic pain or with dyspareunia, or may be asymptomatic. Ovarian cysts are more common among women who are of reproductive age. Patients who take combined oral contraception are less likely to develop benign ovarian cysts. Ovarian cysts can be symptomatic or asymptomatic and are found incidentally on bimanual exam or pelvic imaging. Past medical history may be significant for prior ovarian cysts, PCOS, and infertility.

SIGNS AND SYMPTOMS

Many patients with benign ovarian cysts will be asymptomatic and the cyst is found incidentally. However, some patients will have considerable pain even with smaller cysts.

PHYSICAL EXAMINATION

Patients with benign ovarian cysts may have a palpable adnexal mass on bimanual exam, but this is often limited due to body habitus.

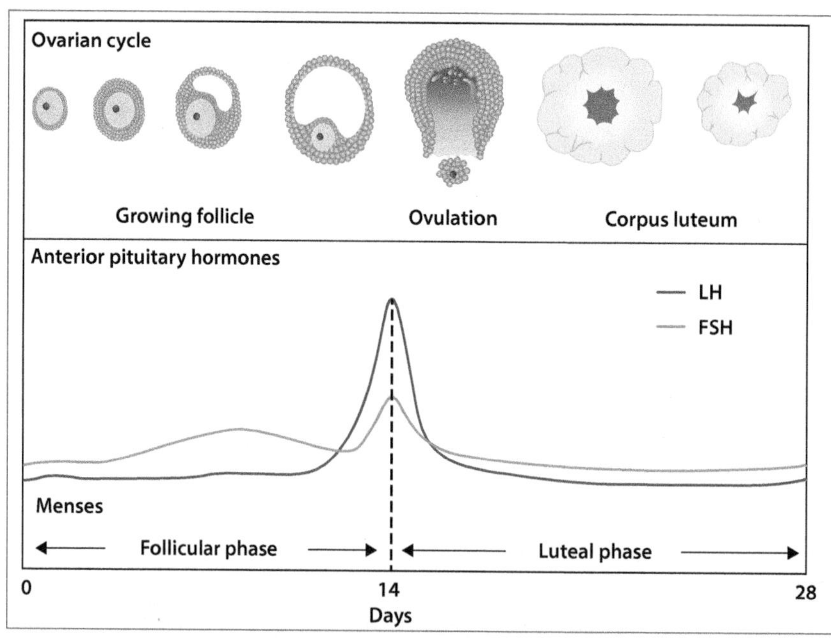

Figure 12.12 Normal menstruation and ovulation. FSH, follicle-stimulating hormone; LH, luteinizing hormone.

(Source: Modified from Koyama A, Hagopian L, Linden J. Emerging options for emergency contraception. Clin Med Insights Reprod Health. *2013;7:23–35. doi:10.4137/CMRH.S8145)*

DIFFERENTIAL DIAGNOSIS

Table 12.21 summarizes the differential diagnosis of an ovarian mass.

DIAGNOSTIC STUDIES

Females of reproductive age should always have a pregnancy test. If the test is positive and pelvic pain is present, ectopic pregnancy must be ruled out. A corpus luteal cyst should be considered as well. Thus, ultrasound imaging is essential in the workup. Common findings of benign adnexal masses include acoustic shadows, smooth unilocular mass, and no blood flow on Doppler.

EVALUATION

An adnexal mass with radiographic findings concerning for malignancy should have a CA-125 and other tumor markers. If negative and the mass is >8–10 cm, the patient should be considered for surgical removal to help prevent ovarian torsion. If the CA-125 is >35 U/mL, prompt referral to a gynecologic oncologist must occur to rule out ovarian cancer. Patients who show signs and symptoms of sepsis and hemodynamic compromise need to be treated expeditiously.

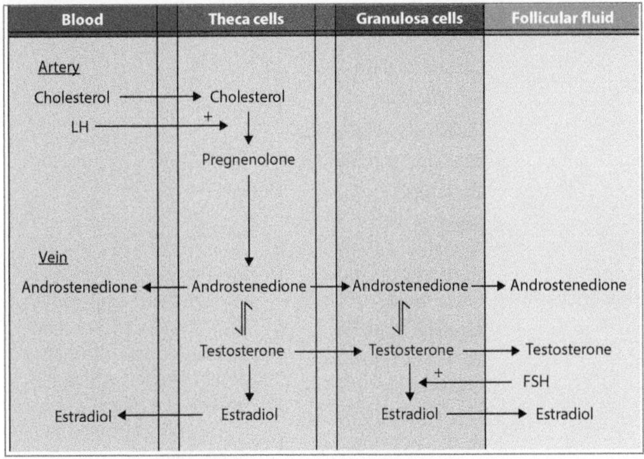

Figure 12.13 Steroidogenesis from the ovary. FSH, follicle-stimulating hormone; LH, luteinizing hormone.

TREATMENT

- The treatment of benign ovarian cysts depends upon the menopausal status of the patient, the amount of pain the patient is experiencing, the size, tumor markers, and radiographic features.
- In postmenopausal women with an ovarian cyst <10 cm and normal CA-125, follow-up ultrasound imaging is recommended.
- In premenopausal women with an ovarian cyst ≥8 cm, surgical intervention should be considered.
- In premenopausal women with an ovarian cyst <8 cm, follow-up imaging after several menstrual cycles can be implemented.
- Opioids should only be used conservatively in select patients for severe pain associated with simple ovarian cysts.
- NSAIDs are appropriate for pain associated with cysts.

PATIENT EDUCATION

- Benign ovarian cysts can recur. Patients should be advised to follow up for any recurring symptoms.

12.7B OVARIAN TORSION

MEDICAL HISTORY AND CLINICAL PRESENTATION

Patients with a history of adnexal masses are at a higher risk of developing a torsion. Often patients will experience acute pain after activity. The pain may radiate to the lower back or legs.

TABLE 12.21 Differential Diagnosis of Ovarian Mass

Diagnosis	Description
Ectopic pregnancy	β-hCG will be positive.
Follicular cyst	Varies in size. Common ultrasound findings: unilocular, smooth thin wall, no solid components or septations.
Corpus luteal cyst	Varies in size. Common ultrasound findings: vascular wall on Doppler ultrasound called a "ring of fire."
Theca lutein cyst	Due to overstimulation of β-hCG. Can be seen in gestational trophoblastic disease and ovarian hyperstimulation syndrome. Tends to be bilateral and multiseptated.
Hemorrhagic cyst	Varies in size. Common ultrasound findings: unilocular, variable wall thickness, low-level echogenicity, no internal vascularity.
Endometrioma	Varies in size. Common ultrasound findings: homogeneous, internal ground-glass echoes, can be multilocular with thin or thick walls.
Mature cystic teratoma (dermoid cyst)	May contain hair, teeth, muscle, and organ tissue. Ultrasound imaging findings depend upon the types of tissue present in the cyst.
Ovarian torsion	Presents with pain, usually accompanied by nausea and vomiting. Ultrasound imaging may reveal adnexal edema, fluid in the cul-de-sac, and reduced blood flow on Doppler.
Ovarian malignancy	See Section 7.6B on malignant disease of the ovary.

hCG, human chorionic gonadotropin.

SIGNS AND SYMPTOMS

The classic signs and symptoms of ovarian torsion include acute onset of pain with nausea and vomiting, but premenarchal females may have a more insidious onset of pain. Pelvic pain may radiate to the thighs or lower back. Less severe intermittent episodes of pelvic pain may be reported occurring days to weeks before the severe acute pain as a result of partial torsion. Fever may be present.

PHYSICAL EXAMINATION

Patients with suspected torsion must be evaluated for hemodynamic compromise. Patients with torsion may have signs of peritoneal irritation on physical examination but usually the physical examination findings are nonspecific.

DIFFERENTIAL DIAGNOSIS

Table 12.22 summarizes the differential diagnosis for ovarian torsion.

DIAGNOSTIC STUDIES

Ovarian torsion can present with decreased Doppler blood flow, but ovarian edema and free fluid in the cul-de-sac are commonly seen.[58] An ovary that is torsed will be enlarged due to the resulting edema. The "whirlpool sign" is common in ovarian torsion whereby the pedicle is vascular and coiled.

EVALUATION

Laboratory evaluation of patients with pelvic pain include a CBC and a pregnancy test if the patient is not postmenopausal. An elevated WBC count can be seen in ovarian torsion. If the patient is hemodynamically compromised, obtaining blood type and crossmatch is recommended.

TREATMENT

- Definitive treatment of ovarian torsion is prompt surgical intervention with detorsion.
- Oophorectomy should be avoided unless the ovary is necrotic.
- Antiemetics and pain medications can be used as needed pending surgical evaluation.

PATIENT EDUCATION

- Patient education for ovarian torsion includes standard postoperative instructions.
- Patients should be advised to report any new pelvic pain as cysts may recur and cause torsion.

TABLE 12.22 Differential Diagnosis for Ovarian Torsion

Diagnosis	Common Physical Exam Findings	Notes
Pelvic inflammatory disease (PID)	Purulent cervicovaginal discharge Fever Chandelier sign	Must be ruled out in patients who are sexually active to help prevent abscess and future fertility impairment.
Tubo-ovarian abscess	See PID above Palpable adnexal mass Peritoneal signs Fever, chills Sepsis	Is usually a consequence of untreated or inadequately treated PID.
Appendicitis	Right lower quadrant pain Periumbilical pain Fever Psoas sign Obturator sign Rosving sign McBurney tenderness Rebound tenderness Guarding Rigidity	Often difficult to differentiate between ovarian torsion and appendicitis. See section on Diagnostic Studies in text.
Ectopic pregnancy	Nonspecific pelvic tenderness Adnexal mass on bimanual may be palpable	Must be considered in all reproductive-age women with first trimester bleeding in a confirmed pregnancy and in women with a history of a missed menses followed by abdominal or pelvic pain. Ruptured ectopic pregnancy could present as hemodynamic compromise.
Pyelonephritis	Abdominal or pelvic pain Nausea Costovertebral tenderness	Fever Chills Pyuria
Nephrolithiasis	Abdominal or pelvic pain Nausea and vomiting Gross hematuria	Nephrolithiasis almost always presents with hematuria.

SPECIAL CONSIDERATIONS

- Corpus luteal cysts are physiologic during early pregnancy as they secrete progesterone to help maintain pregnancy. However, they can persist and cause pain.
- Patients who are pregnant and present with bilateral multiseptated ovarian cysts should be ruled out for gestational trophoblastic disease (GTD).
- Ovarian torsion can occur in pregnancy, although it is rare.
- Adolescents with ovarian torsion should be managed with minimally invasive surgery and an attempt made to preserve as much of the adnexal structure as possible.

KEY POINTS

- Benign ovarian cysts are common among reproductive-age women but may occur in premenarchal and postmenopausal women.
- The menopausal and reproductive status of all women with an adnexal mass must be determined.
- CA-125 serum testing can be useful but must be used appropriately and according to evidence-based guidelines.
- PCOS is a multifaceted endocrinopathy that should be managed holistically.
- Treatment of PCOS aims to protect the endometrial lining, achieve pregnancy when desired, prevent pregnancy

when pregnancy is not desired, and mitigate the long-term effects of insulin resistance and dyslipidemia.
- Ovarian torsion is a must-not-miss diagnosis as delay in diagnosis and treatment can result in loss of reproductive potential and sepsis.

12.7C POLYCYSTIC OVARY SYNDROME

PCOS is one of the most common endocrine disorders in women of reproductive age and the most common cause of anovulatory infertility. It has classically been described as a constellation of excess androgens, irregular anovulatory cycles, insulin resistance, and ovarian cyst development. Symptoms are often acutely distressing for patients, and there is an increased long-term risk of diabetes, cardiovascular disease (CVD), and endometrial cancer for these individuals. Given its ubiquity and potential impact on quality of life in both the short and long term, early identification, diagnosis, and management of PCOS is of paramount importance for the primary care clinician.

MEDICAL HISTORY AND PRESENTATION

Ascertaining a detailed medical history is important if PCOS is suspected, particularly since the diagnosis is one of exclusion. Pregnancy must be ruled out as a cause of secondary amenorrhea in women of reproductive age, and drug-induced hyperandrogenism must also be ruled out. Typically, patients will complain of irregular menses, anovulatory cycles, and infertility. Additionally, a history of hirsutism and cystic acne are common and are often evident upon physical examination. These symptoms can also be a part of normal pubertal development, which may make the diagnosis particularly difficult in adolescent populations. Patients may also report a history of impaired fasting glucose, hyperlipidemia, and hypertension in their past medical encounters.

PHYSICAL EXAMINATION

The vast majority of patients with PCOS are overweight or obese; in the United States, it has been reported that 80% of individuals with PCOS have a BMI ≥30.[59] As previously stated, signs of androgen excess such as hirsutism, cystic acne, and sometimes male-pattern baldness may be present. Physical manifestations of insulin resistance, such as acanthosis nigricans, may be seen, particularly on the nape of the neck and axillary region. If bimanual pelvic examination is performed, ovaries may be enlarged.

DIFFERENTIAL DIAGNOSIS

Table 12.23 summarizes the differential diagnosis of PCOS.

DIAGNOSTIC STUDIES

Currently, the Rotterdam Criteria are regarded as the consensus for diagnosis of PCOS. After other reasons for the clinical symptoms have been excluded, women must fulfill two of the three following criteria:

1. Anovulation or oligo-ovulation
2. Physical or chemical signs of androgen excess
3. Ultrasonographic finds of polycystic ovary morphology (enlarged ovaries with multiple follicles classically described as a "string of pearls")[60,61]

Additionally, a host of lab tests may be helpful in excluding PCOS as a diagnosis as well as for clinical confirmation of the suspected pathology. Table 12.24 delineates some useful studies.

The presence of an elevated ovarian volume >10 mL in the absence of a cyst can be present in PCOS. A combination of diagnostic studies and laboratory exams can be used to support physical exam findings when diagnosing PCOS, but a single definitive diagnosis does not exist.

EVALUATION

After ruling out other causes of symptoms and employing the Rotterdam Criteria for diagnosis, treatment can then ensue based on the individual clinical picture.

TREATMENT

- The treatment of PCOS depends upon the patient's desire for pregnancy.
- Patients with PCOS who are chronically amenorrheic should receive progestin therapy to reduce the risk of endometrial hyperplasia and cancer.
- Because PCOS is associated with risk of cardiovascular complications and type 2 diabetes mellitus (DM), patients with metabolic derangements and elevated blood

TABLE 12.23 Differential Diagnosis of Polystic Ovary Syndrome

Diagnosis	Signs and Symptoms	Diagnostic Tests
PCOS	Anovulation, hirsutism, acne, insulin resistance	Diagnosis of exclusion based on Rotterdam criteria (see Diagnostic Studies)
Hypothyroidism	Weight gain, lethargy, dyslipidemia, anovulation	TSH
Hyperprolactinemia	Galactorrhea, anovulation	Prolactin
Congenital adrenal hyperplasia	Androgen excess, possible ambiguous genitalia, menstrual irregularities	17-Hydroxyprogesterone ACTH stimulation
Cushing syndrome	Abdominal obesity, supraclavicular fat pads, HTN, insulin resistance, striae	24-hour urine cortisol Dexamethasone suppression tests
Androgen-secreting mass	More likely in adolescents with male pattern baldness and clitoromegaly. Mass can be on the ovary or adrenal gland.	Total testosterone ≥200 ng/d

ACTH, adrenocorticotropic hormone; HTN, hypertension; PCOS, polycystic ovary syndrome; TSH, thyroid-stimulating hormone.

TABLE 12.24 Laboratory Studies in Polycystic Ovary Syndrome Workup

Lab	Result	Comment
Androgens (serum testosterone, free testosterone, androstenedione, DHEA-S, SHBG)	Typically elevated with low SHBG	Biochemical evidence of androgen excess may be used as one of the Rotterdam diagnostic criteria for PCOS
Insulin	Elevated	Hyperinsulinemia contributes to multiple facets of PCOS clinical presentation
Fasting glucose, oral glucose tolerance test, HbA1c	Typically abnormal	Impaired fasting glucose, glucose intolerance, and elevated HbA1c fit the picture of insulin resistance, and women with PCOS are 3× more likely to have metabolic syndrome
Total cholesterol, HDL, LDL, TG	Normal or elevated TC/ LDL, low HDL, elevated TG	Elevated TG consistent with insulin resistance, and women with PCOS 3× more likely to have metabolic syndrome
LH:FSH ratio	Elevated (>3:1)	Impaired GnRH secretion results in excess LH and plays a role in chronic anovulation
TSH, FT4	Normal	Rule out hypothyroidism as source of anovulation
17-Hydroxyprogesterone	Normal	Rule out nonclassic congenital adrenal hyperplasia. If results equivocal, progress to ACTH stimulation test
Prolactin	Normal	Rule out hyperprolactinemia as a cause of irregular menses

ACTH, adrenocorticotropic hormone; DHEA-S, dehydroepiandrosterone-sulfate; FSH, follicle-stimulating hormone; FT4, free thyroxine; GnRH, gonadotropin-releasing hormone; HbA1c, hemoglobin A1c; HDL, high-density lipoprotein; LDL, low-density lipoprotein; LH, luteinizing hormone; PCOS, polycystic ovary syndrome; SHBG, sex hormone binding globulin; TC, total cholesterol; TG, triglyceride; TSH, thyroid-stimulating hormone.

pressures should be treated according to the most recent evidence-based practice guidelines.

- Weight loss is advised if the patient is overweight/obese.
- If the patient does not desire pregnancy:
  - Combined hormonal contraception or episodic progestin therapy to help prevent endometrial hyperplasia
  - Metformin for insulin resistance
  - Spironolactone for hirsutism
  - Finasteride for alopecia
  - Management of dyslipidemia
- If the patient desires pregnancy:
  - Folic acid 400 mcg/day
  - Metformin can be used prior to conception and may increase likelihood of pregnancy success in women who are using ovulation inductors.
  - Progestin or micronized progesterone for 10 days to induce a withdrawal bleed if the patient is amenorrheic
  - Ovulation induction with letrozole (an aromatase inhibitor) or clomiphene citrate

PATIENT EDUCATION

Empathetic and compassionate patient education centered on consistently healthy lifestyle choices is of paramount importance in this population. Multiple support groups are also available, such as at pcoschallenge.org, and fostering a positive, collaborative environment among patients can only promote compliance.[61]

SPECIAL CONSIDERATIONS

- Given the diverse range of symptoms, involvement of other clinicians, such as nutritionists, fertility specialists, obstetricians, gynecologists, and endocrinologists, to name a few, may be necessary to optimize outcomes for those with PCOS. Assessment of individual patient risk factors, pertinent family history of diabetes or CVD, and desire for children can direct the clinician regarding potential referral sources.

12.8 INFERTILITY

Joshua Wageman

OVERVIEW

Infertility is a major issue for a large number of couples. Defined as the inability to conceive after 12 months of consistent, unprotected intercourse,[62] the evaluation and management of this problem can become highly nuanced due to the number of factors involved. The clinician must be able to identify both male and female factors that may potentially be implicated and have an understanding of available resources for referral if the problem persists beyond the scope of the primary care setting.

EPIDEMIOLOGY

It is estimated that between 37 and 70 million couples across the world are affected by infertility, including around 9% of married couples in the United States.[63] It is estimated that 12% of U.S. women age 15 to 44 have needed fertility services at some point during their childbearing years.[63] Although there may be more specific physiologic states affecting the fertility of the female partner, it has been reported that 26% to 30% of infertility cases are due to male factors.[62] A 2015 publication from the American Society of Reproductive Medicine reported that the female is solely or contributorily involved 40% of the time, the male is likewise involved 40% of the time, and the remaining 20% of cases are due to unidentifiable causes.[63] Although the data regarding incidence may vary across the literature, infertility is certainly a ubiquitous issue.

PATHOPHYSIOLOGY

The potential pathophysiologic mechanisms are numerous and can be broadly categorized into male and female factors. Male factors can be further categorized as acquired or congenital. Acquired causes of male infertility may be related to infection, exposure to environmental toxins, trauma, or past use of exogenous testosterone or anabolic steroids.[63] Spermatogenesis and sperm quality can be adversely affected by infection, and trauma can result in antisperm antibodies. Exogenous steroid use can disrupt the hypothalamic-pituitary-gonadal axis as well as decrease sperm count (Figure 12.14).[63] Congenital anomalies may include Klinefelter syndrome, Kallmann syndrome, or cystic fibrosis, among others.[62]

The potential factors involved in female reproductive capacity are numerous. Advancing age results in decreased ovarian reserve, and a host of disease states can result in anovulatory cycles.[61] Structural abnormalities in the cervix, fallopian tubes, or uterus may play a role, and disruption of the hypothalamic-pituitary-ovarian (HPO) axis may also inhibit fertility.[62] Indeed, a proper hormonal balance appears essential for optimizing the reproductive environment. Females with too low of a BMI often have amenorrhea, and a lack of insulin is incompatible with reproduction.[64] However, hyperinsulinemia and leptin insensitivity also seem to contribute to the infertility observed in disease states such as obesity and PCOS.[64]

MEDICAL HISTORY AND CLINICAL PRESENTATION

Given the vast array of possible etiologies, ascertaining a detailed history is critical for guiding the workup of infertility. For the male partner, it is important to inquire about a history of past anabolic steroid use, past surgery or trauma to the inguinal or genital region, or history of infection or radiation. Additionally, it is prudent to ascertain a history

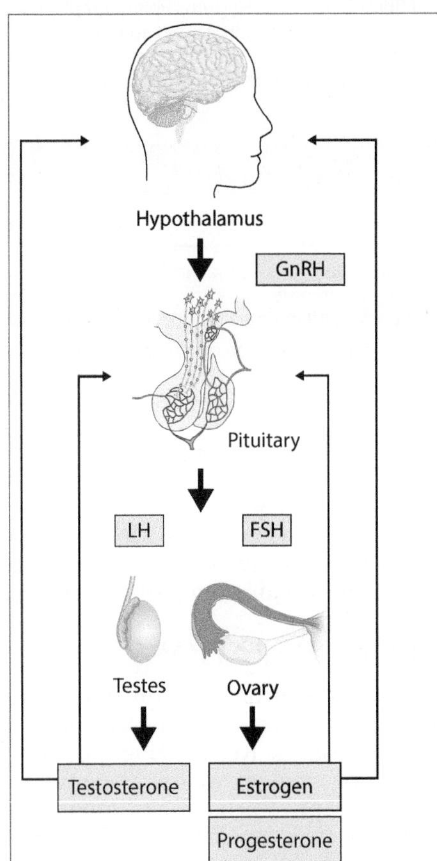

Figure 12.14 Hypothalamic-pituitary-gonadal axis. FSH, follicle-stimulating hormone; GnRH, gonadotropin-releasing hormone; LH, luteinizing hormone.

of sexual development and inquire about any other signs associated with the various differential diagnoses.

Obtaining a detailed history is equally important for the female partner. The clinician must inquire about menstrual history, medication use, substance abuse, sexually transmitted infections, previous pregnancies and outcomes, and any prior surgeries. Additionally, the clinician should conduct a detailed gynecologic and endocrine review of systems.[62]

PHYSICAL EXAMINATION

Clinical presentation will vary widely from couple to couple. Many patients will have a completely normal physical examination, while others may exhibit important signs that may direct the clinician's diagnostic approach. It is important to recognize potentially significant morphologic anomalies in the genitalia of either partner. The body habitus of the female partner may also play a role, as both underweight and overweight patients may have a suboptimal hormonal milieu for conception. The clinician should be aware of any clinical features specific to each differential diagnosis and be capable of identifying these upon examination.

DIFFERENTIAL DIAGNOSIS

Table 12.25 summarizes the differential diagnosis of infertility.

DIAGNOSTIC STUDIES

The diagnostic approach for both partners should be directed by the history and physical examination. In general, however, the initial workup of the male partner should begin with a semen analysis (evaluation and therapy). The male should be instructed to avoid ejaculation for 2 to 3 days prior to the test. If abnormalities such as oligospermia or azoospermia are present, an endocrine issue should be suspected and lab tests such as FSH, LH, total testosterone, and PRL should be obtained.[62]

The diagnostic approach to the female is much more nuanced. Confirming ovulation is an important first step, and this can be done by obtaining a serum progesterone level 7 days prior to onset of menses.[62] If the female is ovulating and has no risk of tubal obstruction, a hysterosalpingography should be ordered as a noninvasive assessment of uterine and fallopian tube structure.[62] If cycles are anovulatory, further labs such as TSH, PRL, midfollicular FSH, and estradiol should be obtained. Once again, the history and physical exam will largely dictate the potential need for more invasive testing or referral to a reproductive specialist.

EVALUATION

After thorough evaluation of both male and female factors, the ensuing treatment regimen will be based on underlying causality, if identified. If initial evaluation yields equivocal or insufficient results, referral to a specialist may be warranted, and the primary care clinician should not hesitate to refer to a trusted clinician with experience in assistive reproductive technology (ART).

TREATMENT

Treatment varies widely and is dictated by the clinical picture of the individuals involved. Rectifying the underlying cause, if identified, usually resolves the inability to conceive. Sometimes, the intervention may be a recommendation to continue attempts at conception, as about 50% of infertile couples with no organic cause are able to succeed given another year of

TABLE 12.25 Differential Diagnosis of Infertility

Diagnosis	Possible Features	Lab and Imaging Results
Male		
CFTR gene carrier (cystic fibrosis)	Vas deferens absent	Semen analysis (will have low volume)
Hypothalamic hypogonadism • Acquired • Kallmann syndrome • Possible testicular atrophy, history of anabolic steroid use • Anosmia, delayed puberty, cryptorchidism		Low FSH, low LH, low testosterone
Klinefelter syndrome	Gynecomastia, developmental delays, small testes, tall stature	Genetic testing (multiple X copies), low testosterone, elevated FSH
Female		
Anovulation • PCOS • Hypothyroidism • Hyperprolactinemia	Irregular or absent menses (all) • Hirsutism, obesity • Fatigue, weight gain, hair loss • Galactorrhea	Mid-luteal progesterone low • Increased LH, increased insulin • Elevated TSH • Elevated prolactin
Endometriosis	Dyspareunia, dyschezia, dysmenorrhea	Imaging typically not helpful. Laparoscopy definitive for diagnosis
Hypothalamic amenorrhea	Low BMI, amenorrhea, possibly female athlete triad, history of disordered eating and/or excessive exercise	Low FSH, low estradiol
Fallopian tube blockage	History of sexually transmitted infections	Hysterosalpingography abnormal
Ovarian failure	History of chemotherapy, early menopause symptoms, amenorrhea	Elevated FSH, low estradiol
Uterine anomalies	Dysmenorrhea, family history of fibroids, palpable tenderness	Hysterosalpingography and/or ultrasound abnormal

BMI, body mass index; FSH, follicle-stimulating hormone; LH, luteinizing hormone; PCOS, polycystic ovary syndrome; TSH, thyroid-stimulating hormone.

TABLE 12.26 Possible Treatment Options for Infertility

Treatment	Indication(s)	Comment
Intrauterine insemination (IUI)	Unexplained infertility	Often used in combination with ovulation induction agents
Clomiphene	Anovulation	Used in combination with IUI or timed intercourse for ovulation induction May result in ovarian hyperstimulation or multiple gestations
In vitro fertilization (IVF)	Failure of IUI/ovulation induction Diagnosis precludes IUI/ovulation	Referral to clinician experienced in assistive reproductive technology (ART) required

unprotected intercourse.[62] Restoration of normal body weight is an important factor in optimizing fertility for both underweight and overweight females.[62] Other specific interventions may also be necessary and are outlined in Table 12.26.

The interventions in Table 12.26 are by no means exhaustive, and if underlying causes have been identified and corrected without resolution of infertility, a referral to a reproductive specialist is in order. Throughout this time, the mental health status of the patient and partner should be considered as infertility can be very emotional and stressful for the couple; referral for counseling should be discussed.

PATIENT EDUCATION

The primary care clinician must educate patients regarding lifestyle modification; correction of suboptimal lifestyle factors can often resolve infertility. Proper nutrition, weight loss or gain as indicated, and avoidance of tobacco and alcohol are critical. A general understanding of timed intercourse, various methods used in ART, and awareness of other options such as gamete donation or surrogate carriers is also helpful when providing empathic care to couples.[63]

SPECIAL CONSIDERATIONS

- Infertility is a major problem with drastic psychosocial implications, and the frustration can lead to significant strain on relationships. Recognizing signs of depression in one or both partners as well as potential red flags indicative of maladaptive behavior is important.[63] The clinician must take into consideration financial burden on the couple as well; ART is often very expensive. Given the complexity of infertility, involvement of other professionals such as counselors, nutritionists, endocrinologists, and reproductive specialists may be necessary to optimally assist patients in their efforts.

12.9 CONTRACEPTION

Elyse J. Watkins

OVERVIEW

Prevention of pregnancy is a common reason for women to visit their primary care clinician. It is important to understand the mechanisms of action, indications and contraindications, and caveats to each method. Every woman should be made aware of her choices and, through shared decision-making, find the option that works best for her.

EPIDEMIOLOGY

Over 72 million women between 15 and 49 years old used contraception from 2015 to 2017.[65] Female sterilization was the most common contraception, followed by the COCP, long-acting reversible contraceptives, and the male condom (Figure 12.15).

MEDICAL HISTORY AND CLINICAL PRESENTATION

The medical history in a patient seeking contraception should be focused on several key elements: gravida and para status, menstrual history, desire to conceive within the next year, risk factors for hormone use, and risk factors for sexually transmitted infections. Other important historical data to elicit includes history of HMB, methods tried previously (with success or failure documented), medical conditions the patient is being treated for, medications currently being taken, and overall risk for thromboembolic events or malignancy if a hormonal contraception is chosen. Social history should include an assessment of the patient's ability to obtain contraception if she needs to go to a pharmacy, ability to pay even if she has a co-pay, and any other issues that could impact compliance.

DIAGNOSTIC STUDIES

It is advisable to rule out pregnancy in a reproductive-age patient who is sexually active even if she is currently using contraception. Women who wish to use an intrauterine system do not need to have sexually transmitted infection testing prior to insertion. Testing can occur at the time of insertion and, if positive, she can be treated accordingly.

EVALUATION

The evaluation of a patient desiring contraception considers her medical history, social history, medications being taken, expectations for future pregnancies, and any other issues that may adversely affect compliance or success in pregnancy prevention.

TREATMENT

There are various options for women to consider (Table 12.27).[66]

PATIENT EDUCATION

- Contraception does not protect against sexually transmitted infections. Use of the condom may help to prevent some sexually transmitted infections.
- It is important to follow all of the instructions for the chosen option.
- The only antibiotic associated with decreased efficacy of contraception is rifampin.

SPECIAL CONSIDERATIONS

- Women with a seizure disorder should not use systemic estrogens as it competes with antiepileptic medications for drug clearance, thus lowering the seizure threshold.
- Women may continue on hormonal contraception until age 50; at that point, a careful risk and benefit discussion should occur.

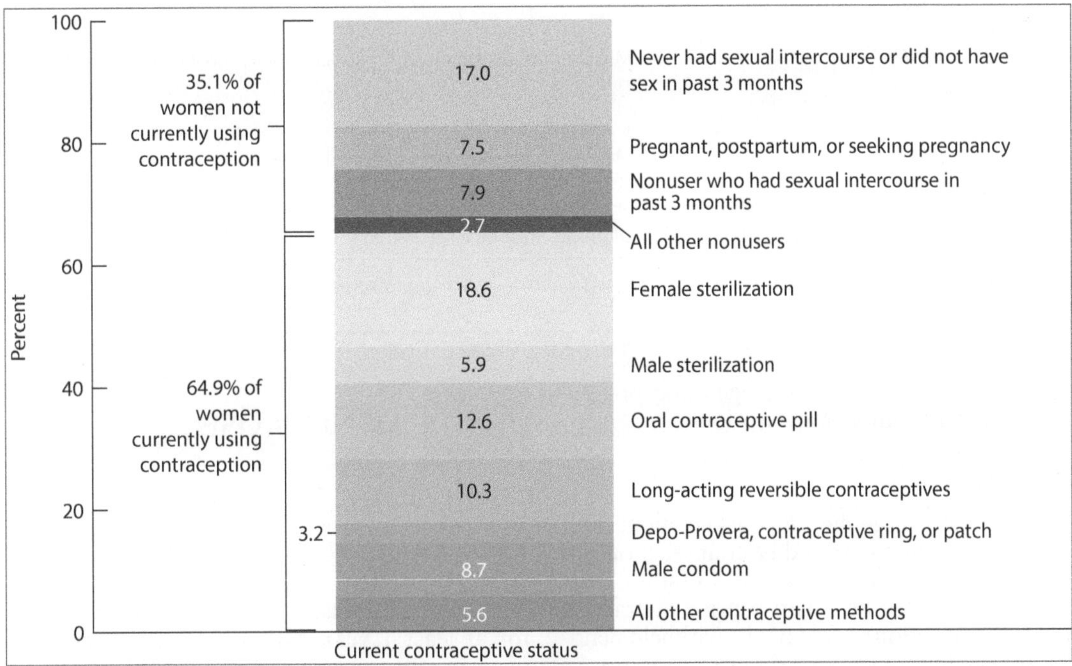

Figure 12.15 Contraceptive use in the United States, 2015–2017.
(Source: Daniels K, Abma JC. Current Contraceptive Status Among Women Aged 15–49: United States, 2015–2017. *NCHS Data Brief No. 327. National Center for Health Statistics; 2018. https://www.cdc.gov/nchs/products/databriefs/db327.htm)*

TABLE 12.27 Contraceptive Options

Method	Effectiveness[66]	Notes
Combined oral contraceptive pill (COCP)	~90% but could be higher with "perfect" use (no missed pills)	Differences in COCPs depend upon the estrogen dose and progestin. In addition, some pills are monophasic, biphasic, or triphasic, meaning the doses could vary throughout the month. Some progestins are androgenic and others are not. Another difference is in the number of placebo days. Must be taken daily. Two missed pills in a month can result in a breakthrough ovulation and subsequent pregnancy. The only antibiotic associated with decreased effectiveness is rifampin.
Progestin-only pill	97% with no missed pills	Also called the "mini-pill." Can be used in breastfeeding women. Must be taken daily.
Combined contraceptive patch	93%–96%; decreased in women with higher body mass index (BMI)	Contains estrogen and progestin. Usually changed each week for 3 weeks. Patients can skip the fourth week in order to have a withdrawal bleed then resume weekly changing of the patch.
Combined contraceptive monthly vaginal ring	93%–96%	Contains estrogen and progestin. The ring is left in the vagina for 3 weeks followed by a week without a ring. Needs to be refrigerated when not in use.
Combined contraceptive annual vaginal ring	96%	Contains estrogen and progestin. Does not need to be refrigerated when not in use.
Intrauterine system (IUS)	99%	Several intrauterine systems are available. Levonorgestrel-containing IUSs contain low amounts of progestin and can help decrease menstrual bleeding. Copper IUSs are indicated for emergency contraception use but may cause heavier menstrual bleeding.
Injectable progestin	93%–96%	Intramuscular injections are given every 12 weeks. May cause weight gain in some women and is associated with decreased bone mineral density when used >3 consecutive years.
Subdermal implant	99%	Implanted in the nondominant upper inner arm. Recommended for 3 years' use.
Sponge	87%	
Diaphragm	87%	
Male condom	87%	Can help prevent sexually transmitted infections.
Spermicide	87%	
Fertility awareness	87%	
Withdrawal	78%	
Breastfeeding (also called lactational amenorrhea method)	~98%	Must breastfeed exclusively, be amenorrheic, and within the first 6 months postpartum.
Sterilization	99%	Male sterilization: Women will need to use a backup method for 3 months.
Emergency contraception pills	87% for levonorgestrel 94%–96% for ulipristal	Levonorgestrel: Must use within 72 hours of unprotected sex. Ulipristal: Must be taken within 120 hours of unprotected sex.
Emergency contraception: intrauterine device	99%	Insert within 5 days of unprotected sex.

- Women with contraindications for estrogen and progestin use should consider nonhormonal options.

KEY POINTS

- All women of reproductive age should be asked about their plans to conceive in the next year and be counseled on options and offered a method that would work best for her.
- Urine pregnancy test should be negative prior to starting contraception. Contraception should not be withheld pending a Pap test or sexually transmitted disease screening.

12.10 MENOPAUSE

Elyse J. Watkins

OVERVIEW

Natural menopause is the unintentional cessation of menses for at least 1 year. Menopause can occur naturally due to ovarian senescence; prematurely due to myriad factors, such as immunologic etiologies; surgically via oophorectomy; iatrogenically with radiation therapy; or induced via GnRH agonists. Premature menopause, also called premature ovarian failure or premature ovarian insufficiency, occurs when menses cease unintentionally before 40 years of age. The average age of natural menopause is 51 years of age. Women who do not experience oophorectomy will undergo a gradual decline in ovarian function resulting in ovarian follicular depletion and subsequent amenorrhea. Prior to the final menses, women may experience perimenopausal symptoms, such as vasomotor flushes, irregular menses, sleep disturbances, and mood changes. Perimenopause usually lasts about 5 years.

EPIDEMIOLOGY

All women who do not undergo oophorectomy will experience natural menopause. Premature ovarian insufficiency or failure occurs in approximately 1% of women before age 40.[67]

PATHOPHYSIOLOGY

Natural menopause is not a pathologic event. Premature ovarian insufficiency or failure can be due to a variety of causes, such as radiation therapy and autoimmune disease. However, in most women there is no known cause; this is called idiopathic premature ovarian failure.

Ovarian senescence is marked by diminishing follicles. FSH will continue being produced from the anterior pituitary, but there are insufficient follicles to respond to the FSH, resulting in a depressed LH surge. Owing to the lack of negative feedback on FSH and LH, serum levels remain elevated well beyond the LMP. In addition, inhibin B decreases due to declining follicles, which removes the negative feedback on FSH. Declines in inhibin B also results in reduced progesterone. Ovulation does not occur, and subsequently estrogen will decline causing a cessation of menses. During the perimenopause, however, estrogen levels may be normal or high as a response to elevated FSH.

MEDICAL HISTORY AND CLINICAL PRESENTATION

The medical history should focus on determining if there is an underlying pathology associated with cessation of menses if women present with premature ovarian failure.

Most women will experience a gradual change in their menses. During the perimenopause, cycles become irregular with missed menses and prolongation between menstrual cycles. In the absence of pathology, bleeding will usually become lighter. Approximately 80% of women will experience vasomotor symptoms.[68]

SIGNS AND SYMPTOMS

The most common signs and symptoms of natural menopause are vasomotor symptoms, irregular menses, mood changes, sleep disturbances, and changes in libido (Table 12.28). Some women will experience dyspareunia, hair thinning, and skin thinning. Women who are postmenopausal may complain of vaginal dryness, decreased lubrication during intercourse, and frequency of urination or stress/urge incontinence. The vaginal and bladder complaints are usually due to loss of estrogen and are termed the genitourinary syndrome of menopause.

PHYSICAL EXAMINATION

There is no specific physical examination for a woman in natural menopause unless she is experiencing the genitourinary syndrome of menopause. If so, a pelvic examination documenting loss of vaginal rugae and the presence or absence of POP will help establish the diagnosis.

DIFFERENTIAL DIAGNOSIS

Table 12.29 summarizes the differential diagnosis for menopause.

DIAGNOSTIC STUDIES

Most patients can be diagnosed by history alone. However, if a patient is suspected of having premature menopause, several laboratory tests can help confirm the diagnosis (see Table 12.30). It is important to keep in mind that during

TABLE 12.28 Findings Along the Menopause Spectrum

Menopausal Status	Duration	Menstrual Cycle	Laboratory Findings
Perimenopause (early)	Varies, can last 5–10 years	Varies; often will lengthen between cycles	FSH: Fluctuations AMH: Low Inhibin B: Low
Perimenopause (late)	1–3 years	Missed menses ≥60 days	FSH: >25 IU/L AMH: Low Inhibin B: Low
Postmenopause (early)	1–6 years	Amenorrhea	FSH: Variable AMH: Low Inhibin B: Low
Postmenopause (late)	Until death	Amenorrhea	FSH: Remains elevated AMH: Very low Inhibin B: Very low

AMH, antimüllerian hormone; FSH, follicle-stimulating hormone.

TABLE 12.29 Differential Diagnosis for Menopause

Diagnosis	Description
Pregnancy	All women of reproductive age who still have a uterus must be ruled out for pregnancy.
Thyroid disease	Poorly managed or undiagnosed thyroid disease can cause menstrual irregularities.
Hyperprolactinemia	Medications that can cause hyperprolactinemia include antipsychotics (particularly older generations), metoclopramide, domperidone, reserpine, monoamine oxidase inhibitors, verapamil, and methadone. Pituitary adenomas can cause hyperprolactinemia.

TABLE 12.30 Common Laboratory Tests for Menopause

Lab Test	Interpretation
Human chorionic gonadotropin (β-hCG)	<5 mIU/mL if patient is not pregnant
Follicle-stimulating hormone (FSH)	Elevated if menopausal
Luteinizing hormone (LH)	Elevated if menopausal
Antimüllerian hormone	Low if menopausal
Inhibin B	Low or undetectable if menopausal

BOX 12.1 Contraindications for Estrogen Use

- Undiagnosed abnormal vaginal bleeding
- Breast cancer
- Endometrial hyperplasia or cancer
- History of a thromboembolic event
- Suspected or known pregnancy
- Hepatic malignancy or dysfunction

the perimenopausal transition, FSH will be variable, so no single FSH test should be used to diagnose menopause. Antimüllerian hormone is the most sensitive test to diagnose the loss of follicles in the aging ovary. Also note that serum estrogen levels are not useful in the diagnosis or management of menopause.

EVALUATION

The evaluation of a perimenopausal or postmenopausal patient involves considering her overall health status. Important areas to focus on include cardiovascular health, sexual health, bone health, breast health, and emotional health.

TREATMENT

- Weight-bearing exercise and aerobic exercise can help prevent bone loss and maintain cardiovascular health.
- Vasomotor symptoms can be treated with systemic estrogens. Systemic estrogens are not recommended to prevent bone loss, CVD, or cognitive decline.
- A clear discussion about the risks, benefits, and alternatives of estrogen use must be discussed with each patient and documented appropriately.
- It is recommended that if no contraindications exist for estrogen use, the prescribed dose should be the lowest to achieve results, continued for no more than 5 years, and not initiated after age 60 (see Box 12.1 for estrogen contraindications).
- Systemic estrogen is not recommended to treat the genitourinary syndrome of menopause in the absence of vasomotor symptoms.
  - Vaginal estrogen preparations are indicated for the treatment of the genitourinary syndrome of menopause.
  - Options also include an FDA-approved selective estrogen receptor modulator, an FDA approved DHEA vaginal insert, ospemiphene, oral estrogen agonist/antagonist, and hyaluronic acid.
- Women who still have their uterus who take systemic estrogen must also be prescribed a progestin or progesterone to help protect the endometrium for hyperplasia and malignancy.
- Transdermal estrogens are preferred over oral preparations.
- Women who take levothyroxine and oral estrogens may need to have their levothyroxine dose adjusted due to estrogen's effect on thyroxine-binding globulin and the subsequent reduction of bioactive thyroxine.
  - Women with hypothyroidism should be considered for transdermal estrogen instead of oral preparations.
- Selective serotonin uptake inhibitors and serotonin norepinephrine reuptake inhibitors are recommended to treat vasomotor symptoms in women who do not wish to use estrogen or who have a contraindication to estrogen use.
- Compounded estrogen is not recommended.
- Yoga and acupuncture may alleviate some of the symptoms of menopause but high-quality evidence is limited.

PATIENT EDUCATION

- Encourage patients to perform weight-bearing and aerobic exercise to help bone strength and cardiovascular health.
- Shared decision-making regarding the treatment plan is recommended.
- Discuss the importance of breast health and current guidelines regarding screening mammography.
- Advise patients to report any unusual vaginal bleeding, pelvic pain, breast masses, or any other new symptom as soon as possible.

SPECIAL CONSIDERATIONS

- Women with premature ovarian failure/insufficiency should be offered estrogen and progesterone therapy to mitigate the long-term effects of hypoestrogenism.

KEY POINTS

- Natural menopause occurs around the age of 51.
- Premenopausal symptoms can begin 5 to 10 years before the final menstrual period.
- FSH, LH, and serum estradiol should not be used to diagnose menopause.
- Antimüllerian hormone and inhibin B are more sensitive and specific indicators of ovarian senescence.
- Women with vasomotor symptoms can be offered treatment with systemic estrogens if no contraindications exist.
- Women with genitourinary symptoms but no vasomotor symptoms should be offered vaginal estrogen, a selective estrogen modulator, an FDA-approved DHEA vaginal insert, or hyaluronic acid.

12.11 PREGNANCY

Stephanie Elko

OVERVIEW

No matter what line of medicine, a clinician has a high chance of treating a pregnant patient. Therefore, every clinician should be prepared to care for patients who are considering pregnancy, are pregnant, or recently have been pregnant.

EPIDEMIOLOGY, BACKGROUND, NOMENCLATURE

Obstetric/perinatal care encompasses care for the mother and the fetus to provide a healthy and safe environment from conception through to labor and delivery as well as the postpartum period. The earlier and more accurately a pregnancy is diagnosed, the higher the chance of a successful outcome. Pregnancy is divided into three trimesters, each of which may present the clinician with unique considerations.

Obstetrics is categorized by timeline to effectively communicate care status and provide optimal care based on the timing. These subcategories begin with differentiating maternal versus fetal medicine, and then understanding that there are two different patients being cared for within one body. This is followed by gestational timelines based on the estimated date of confinement (EDC) or estimated date of delivery (EDD). The timelines are broken down into prepartum, intrapartum, and postpartum. Prepartum, or prenatal period, is further organized into trimesters, based on number of gestational weeks.

Prenatal Subcategories

- Trimesters
  - First trimester is 0 to 12 gestational weeks
  - Second trimester is 13 to 28 gestational weeks
  - Third trimester is 29 to 40+ gestational weeks

Timelines are discussed in terms of weeks and days to provide precise gestational ages (GAs). For example, 29 weeks and 3 of 7 days gestation is often communicated as "29 & 3" and written as GA: 29 & $^{3}/_{7}$.

To effectively communicate a woman's pregnancy history and status, pregnancy nomenclature has been created. The nomenclature improves communication regarding a woman's total number of pregnancies and outcomes. See Table 12.31.

The fetal nomenclature begins with conceptus. The conceptus are the products from the onset of conception to birth. From the beginning of pregnancy, from conception to about 8 weeks' gestation, the fetal conceptus is referred to as an embryo. Following this, and for the remainder of the pregnancy, the fetal conceptus is referred to as a fetus.

TABLE 12.31 Gestational Nomenclature

Term	Definition
Gestational age	Age of fetus in weeks counted from first day of the last menstrual period (LMP) or ultrasound dating
Gravida	Total number of confirmed pregnancies
Para	Number of completed pregnancies
Abortus	Number of abortions; spontaneous, missed, and induced
GTPAL	Total **G**estations, total **T**erm deliveries, total **P**reterm deliveries, total **A**bortions, total **L**iving children

MATERNAL PHYSIOLOGY

During pregnancy, the mother undergoes numerous and profound anatomic and physiologic changes to accommodate the pregnancy state. These changes account for many of the signs and symptoms of pregnancy. Understanding the normal physiology will help to differentiate when an abnormal process may be underway.

Cardiac

During the perinatal state, the cardiovascular system changes to accommodate the increase in demands and protect the mother from risk, such as hemorrhage. By about 8 weeks' gestation, cardiac output (CO) has increased by approximately 20%, and continues to increase to a maximum of 40% to 50% around 28 weeks' gestation.[69,70] It will continue until a short time following delivery, then begin to gradually return to prepregnancy levels. The increased CO is achieved by an increase in stroke volume (SV) in early pregnancy and an increase in heart rate by late pregnancy. The increased SV is thought to be in response to an increase in blood volume from the normal increase in plasma volume and red blood cell mass, and a 35% to 40% reduction in systemic vascular resistance (SVR). By early in the third trimester there is an average increase in left ventricular mass by about 34% above prepregnancy baselines.[70] In the first and second trimesters, it is common to see a slight decrease in blood pressure due to the fall in SVR. However, blood pressure returns back to prepregnancy levels in the third trimester.[69] This is an important distinction when monitoring for hypertensive disease of pregnancy.

Postural hypotensive syndrome is a common, and normal, syndrome that occurs due to uterine enlargement in later pregnancy. The symptoms occur when the mother lies in a supine or right-sided position and the enlarging uterus compresses the inferior vena cava (IVC). This can also happen earlier in pregnancy if the mother has a retroverted uterus. This can create a sharp decrease in cardiac preload leading to maternal hypotension. This hypotension is in response to decreased perfusion and has potential to lead to maternal and fetal compromise. Initial treatment is mantel positioning to decompress the IVC, usually achieved by lying in left lateral decubitus position.[70] If symptoms continue, further intervention is necessary.

Renal

Normal imagery during pregnancy reveals a physiologic increase in kidney size (1–1.5 cm in total) and ureteral dilation without obstruction. There are no histologic changes associated with this increase and often the dilation is asymptomatic. However, occasionally women may have symptoms of hydronephrosis, which may result in the need for invasive interventions, such as drain tube placements.

Lab tests show that the serum creatinine decreases due to a physiologic increase in the glomerular filtration rate, while on urinalysis, mild proteinuria, amino acids, and glycosuria may be noted. These changes are due to the global hemodynamic changes, increased renal perfusion and glomerular filtration rate during pregnancy.[71]

The renin-aldosterone-angiotensin system (RAAS) activates during pregnancy in response to the SVR. Simultaneously, the thirst response and antidiuretic hormone secretions decrease, leading to lower osmolality and serum sodium levels to help mediate the RAAS. Furthermore, the pregnant woman protects against significant rise in SVR and hypokalemia due to various hormonal alterations including a concurrent rise in progesterone levels, which contributes to vasodilation.[72]

Hematology

Blood volume rises during pregnancy to a maximum of about 40% to 50% above prepregnancy levels. However, red blood cells do not rise to these levels, thus leading to physiologic anemia.[73] This anemia can be compounded if iron deficiency anemia or other anemias are present. Increased blood volume can also result in a physiologic murmur.

Respiratory

Oxygen demand increases during pregnancy as a result of increased metabolic rates and requirements as well as increased oxygen consumption.[69] The respiratory tract maintains a state of compensated respiratory alkalosis. This is mainly due to a larger tidal volume with an unchanged respiratory rate. Resting minute ventilation rises almost 50% by gestational term.

Dyspnea during pregnancy is a common complaint. The exact mechanism is unclear, and it is likely multifactorial. The dyspnea usually starts early in pregnancy, thus ruling out increasing abdominal girth and pressure alone; however, later in pregnancy this is often a contributing factor. It should be noted that maternal oxygenation during pregnancy is preserved and warrants further workup if abnormal.[73]

Gastrointestinal

There are physiologic changes throughout the GI tract during pregnancy and several common pregnancy complaints are related to these GI manifestations. Among the most common is nausea, with or without associated vomiting, which is experienced by most women during the first trimester and extends into the second and third trimesters in some women. The exact etiology of nausea/vomiting during pregnancy is unknown and is likely multifactorial. However, there appears to be a link between hCG hormone levels, as well as estrogen levels and the severity of nausea during pregnancy. Because of this, women who are carrying multiples typically experience more nausea and vomiting early in pregnancy than women who are carrying a single fetus. Interestingly, to further this hypothesis, there are lower levels of hCG and estrogen in smokers as well as a lower level incidence of hyperemesis gravidarum (HG); regardless of the effects on nausea, tobacco use is never recommended for a patient. Other hypotheses for nausea and vomiting during pregnancy are evolutionary adaptation and psychological predisposition.[74]

Gut motility is slowed during pregnancy. This phenomenon is thought to be due to hormone changes, physical changes, as well as intra-abdominal pressure changes. These changes result in many pregnancy GI symptoms, including gastroesophageal reflux disease (GERD), bloating, flatus, constipation, incontinence, and hemorrhoids. Slow motility also affects the gallbladder, and hormone changes increase the lithogenicity of bile, leading to an increased risk of cholelithiasis during pregnancy.[75]

Endocrine/Metabolism

As expected, numerous endocrine and metabolic changes occur during pregnancy, and not all are well understood. The thyroxine-binding globulin has increased production by the liver during pregnancy, leading to increased levels of thyroxine (T4) and triiodothyronine (T3). Physiologically important hormones to monitor for euthyroid in the pregnant patient are the serum free T3 and T4.[69]

Cholesterol levels during pregnancy rise to provide for the developing fetus and do not warrant treatment. Hypercholesterolemia during pregnancy is multifactorial, including increased liver synthesis and decreased lipoprotein lipase activity.[69,75] Women who are on statins for hypercholesterolemia prior to pregnancy should cease use several months prior to contraception.

Calcium demands increase during pregnancy, particularly in the third trimester. Most of the calcium demands are from fetal development. Maternal serum ionized calcium levels are maintained, which is a physiologic important component. The increased calcium demands are obtained from dietary absorption, and therefore excreted by urine, leading to an increase risk of kidney stones during pregnancy.[69]

Pregnancy is an insulin-resistant state. Glucose is necessary for the developing fetus, and the mother accommodates this by allowing more for fetal absorption. Both fasting and postprandial glucose levels are elevated. In about 50% of patients, glycosuria will be seen but this should not be used as a marker for gestational diabetes (GDM). However, if the maternal pancreatic function is unable to tolerate this demand, GDM may occur.

Progesterone during pregnancy has many roles; the corpus luteum secretes progesterone to help maintain early pregnancy. If insufficient, spontaneous abortion has high potential to occur. Around 8 weeks' gestation the placenta takes over production of progesterone.

Estrogen concentrations during pregnancy is thought to contribute to uterine contraction and onset of labor, as well as contribute to increasing serum PRL. By full term, the serum PRL levels will increase by 10 times and there is enlargement of the pituitary gland.[69]

LH and FSH are generally not detectable during pregnancy due to a negative feedback loop from estrogen, progesterone, and inhibin.

Oxytocin is not increased during pregnancy, but rather there is an increase of 100- to 200-fold in receptors by term.[76] It contributes to labor and uterine contraction but does not induce labor itself.

Integumentary

Skin changes during pregnancy are common and can be very bothersome to expecting mothers. There can be changes in pigmentation (melasma), vascularization, and connective tissue, such as striae gravidarum (stretch marks). Hair and nail changes also occur. A benign pruritus is a common pregnancy complaint and affects about a quarter of pregnant women. Pregnancy-induced pruritus often affects women in the second half of pregnancy. Symptomatic care is the first line of therapy for this, followed by antihistamines. Patients complaining of full body or generalized pruritus, or a pruritus without evidence of etiology or skin changes, should be evaluated for intrahepatic cholestasis of pregnancy (ICP).[77] ICP can lead to increased risk of fetal morbidity and death if not addressed.[78]

FETAL AND PLACENTAL PHYSIOLOGY

Human embryogenesis begins at the point of fertilization. The fertilized ovum becomes a zygote, typically occurring in the fallopian tubes. Blastomeres are then created by mitotic division of the zygote. These blastomeres increase, and when at approximately 16 blastomeres, they form a solid ball of cells called a morula. The morula continues down the fallopian tube until it reaches the uterus and a fluid-filled cavity is formed, converting the morula into a blastocyte. Blastocytes typically form around days 6 to 7. The blastocyte begins to implant into the uterus, usually in the top two-thirds of the uterus. In some cases, the blastocyte may implant outside the uterus, resulting in an ectopic pregnancy. Once implanted, the blastocyte begins to embed and invade the uterine endometrium. Concurrently the blastocyte has evolved into an outer layer, termed trophoblast, and an inner cell mass. In general, the trophoblast becomes the placenta and the inner cell mass develops into the fetus; however, research has shown there may be some sharing of these developments. During this time, the development of the amniotic sac also begins.[79,80]

Gastrulation occurs when the cells begin to move inward to form the interior of the embryo. During gastrulation, the germ layers differentiate into the ectoderm, mesoderm, and endoderm and eventually become different organ systems.

The placenta rises from the trophoblast and further differentiates into cellular lines that transport nutrients, gases, and waste products between mother and fetus. The placenta also synthesizes steroid hormones and peptides, including hCG, as well as cell lines that proliferate and invade the decidua myometrium allowing for these maternal-fetal communications to occur.[80]

12.11A NORMAL PREGNANCY

The foremost goal of obstetrics is for the patient to carry and birth a healthy infant, while minimizing maternal risk and adverse outcomes. To attain this goal, early and effective prenatal care should be provided. Beyond initiating prenatal care during the preconception period, one of the most effective ways to optimize pregnancy outcomes is with early and accurate diagnosis. The earlier the diagnosis, the more accurate antenatal baseline maternal measurements can be obtained, and the more accurate EDC is established. Furthermore, the earlier any risks can be identified, the sooner intervention can be provided.[81]

DIAGNOSIS

Trophoblast tissue, initially from the early embryo, and eventually from the placenta, produces a chemical called hCG. hCG levels can be detected and measured in several ways. The most sensitive and specific testing is by a maternal plasma serum test. This test quantifies the beta-subunit via immunometric assays. However, the most common, convenient, and affordable way is by hCG urine testing. hCG is excreted in urine, and when hCG concentrations become >20 to 50 mIU/mL, the levels can be detected by most urine pregnancy tests. When there is a concern of pregnancy viability, urine hCG is not sufficient and serial serum hCG testing should be collected. Normally the hCG roughly doubles in concentration approximately every 48 hours through the first 8 weeks of gestation, then falls off around 10 weeks gestation.[82] If the hCG is not rising appropriately, pregnancy viability should be further confirmed early pregnancy ultrasound.[83] Elevated serum hCG during these first 8 weeks can be indicative of multiple gestation.

12.11B PRENATAL CARE

Ideally, prenatal care begins when the mother is in the antenatal or preconception state. This helps assure that the mother will be in optimal health prior to becoming pregnant. Preconception care evaluates a patient's interest in becoming pregnant in the next year and is an opportunity to provide patient education and appropriate screening.

One Key Question—*Would you like to become pregnant in the next year?*—should be asked at all healthcare encounters during a female's reproductive years.[84] If the answer is yes, screening for infectious disease, interpersonal violence, and other health conditions should occur. In addition, it is a good time to review vaccination history, risk of exposure to toxic substances, and any other pertinent psychosocial issues that could affect pregnancy and the first year postpartum. Patients should be advised to take 400 mcg of folic acid daily to help prevent neural tube defects. Review of medications being taken could identify potential teratogens.

INITIAL PRENATAL VISIT

The initial prenatal visit occurs ideally prior to 10 weeks' gestation. The visit should evaluate maternal status and risks based on a history, physical examination, and laboratory results, if available. Typically, the initial prenatal labs are ordered at this visit, and any other testing that needs to be done can be added to the initial obstetric panel. Most clinicians perform a TVU to confirm the presence of a viable pregnancy and the gestational age.

PREGNANCY DATING

The EDD is measured in weeks; 37 0/7 to 38 6/7 is considered early term, 39 0/7 to 40 6/7 is considered full-term pregnancy, and 41 0/7 and beyond is considered late term. Naegele rule calculates the EDD by adding 7 days to the first day of the LMP, then subtracts 3 months. This rule assumes the patient has a regular 28-day cycle. If a patient has irregular menstrual cycles, this rule will likely not be an accurate dating tool, and an ultrasound should be obtained. However, most clinicians will perform an ultrasound at the first visit to document viability and confirm dates. Early obstetric ultrasounds, often transvaginal, have the most accurate dating, and may be used up to 22 weeks' gestation. The most accurate time to date a pregnancy is during the first trimester. After 22+ weeks gestation ultrasound dating is suboptimal.[85]

RISK ASSESSMENT

To identify patients at risk for pregnancy complications a thorough patient history must be obtained (Figure 12.16). Previous obstetric complications may indicate increased risk in the current pregnancy. Some examples of these include large for gestational age fetuses, preterm labor (PTL) and preterm prelabor rupture of membranes, and preeclampsia.

Other risk factors such as socioeconomic risks, safety concerns, and significant stressors should also be discussed. Research has revealed that several pregnancy outcomes may be associated with specific socioeconomic disparities. Non-Hispanic Black females have an approximately 50% increase risk of preterm birth than their non-Hispanic Caucasian peers.[86] Significant stressors that can negatively impact perinatal outcomes must be addressed, such as financial stability, transportation access, caring for a sick person at home, safety at home, and access to food and clean water.

SCREENING

The American College of Obstetrics and Gynecology (ACOG) recommends that all patients should be offered genetic screening and/or diagnostic testing, prior to pregnancy

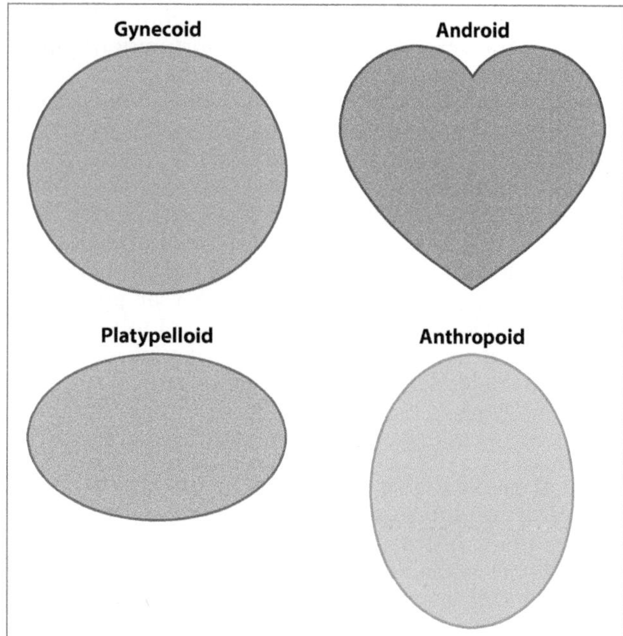

Figure 12.16 **Pelvic types.**

for the carrier testing, during the initial prenatal visit, at specific intervals during the first and second trimester, and all other options.[87] Screening tests include maternal serum testing and ultrasonography. Diagnostic testing includes invasive testing such as chorionic villus sampling and amniocentesis. A more detailed outline of various genetic screenings is outlined in Table 12.32.

TABLE 12.32 Genetic Screening Tests

Screening	Options
Aneuploidy screen offered to all before 20 weeks gestation	**Option 1:** Cell-free DNA from maternal serum sample Trisomy 13, 18, and 21 for fetus Sex aneuploidies Noninvasive Typically completed between 10 weeks' and term gestation If positive, needs further testing **Option 2:** Maternal serum biochemical testing with or without ultrasound marker screening Trisomy 18 and 21 for fetus May detect fetal conditions beyond intended Noninvasive Typically completed between 10 and 13 weeks' gestation If positive, needs further testing **Option 3:** Triple, quad, and penta screening Maternal serum marker testing for certain aneuploidies in second trimester Not as accurate as other screening tests Noninvasive If positive, needs further testing
Diagnostic	
Confirmation testing Only offered to high-risk pregnancy patients	**Chorionic villus sampling** Screening fetal chromosomes for a wide range of aneuploidy dispositions Completed between 10 and 12 weeks' gestation Invasive **Amniocentesis** Screening fetal chromosomes for a wide range of aneuploidy dispositions Usually completed between 15 and 20 weeks' gestation Invasive
Carrier Screening	
Can be completed anytime, including preconception	**Maternal serum genetic screening** Typically screening for maternal markers of many genetic dispositions, including but not limited to cystic fibrosis, spinal muscular atrophy, Tay-Sachs disease, Canavan disease, familial dysautonomia, hemoglobinopathies

Gestational Diabetes Screening

Patients at risk for GDM, as per the American Diabetes Association (ADA) standard criteria for overt diabetes in early pregnancy outlined in Box 12.2 should undergo early pregnancy testing for overt DM type 2.

If early testing is warranted the ADA recommends the following screening test options for diagnosing overt DM in the pregnant patient[88,89]:

- Fasting plasma glucose ≥126 mg/dL, or
- HbA1c of ≥6.5%, or
- Random plasma glucose ≥200 mg/dL with classic symptoms of hyperglycemia

If the early screening test is within normal range, patients should proceed with continued routine GDM screening between 24 and 28 weeks' gestation, as outlined in Box 12.3.

Hypertensive Screening

If a patient is at risk for hypertensive disease in pregnancy, she should have baseline preeclampsia lab tests, including but not limited to a 24-hour urine collection for the creatinine/protein ratio.

Thyroid Disease

A common comorbid disease in the pregnant patient is the presence of thyroid disease. Patients should have a TSH added to the initial prenatal panel as pregnant patients often require modifications of levothyroxine dosing.

Weight/Diet

Weight gain and diet should be outlined for the patient, discussed further below. Nutritional assessment and recommendations are necessary to optimize perinatal outcomes. All patients should be taking a prenatal vitamin, ideally several months prior to conception. Folic acid dose should be 400 mcg, which may need to be adjusted if malabsorption comorbidities exist. Patients should also be advised to increase their dietary intake of calcium, vitamin D, and iron. If deficiencies are suspected, serum testing and supplementation can be considered. Food safety issues should be discussed, including safe handing to avoid infection and limiting certain fish intake, particularly shark and tuna, due to possible mercury contamination.

BOX 12.2 American Diabetes Association Standard Diagnostic Criteria for Overt Diabetes Early Pregnancy Testing

A BMI ≥25 kg/m² (≥23 kg/m² in Asian Americans) plus one or more of the following:
GDM in a previous pregnancy
Hemoglobin A1c ≥5.7%, or impaired fasting glucose previously or random glucose ≥200 mg/dL
First-degree relative with diabetes
History of cardiovascular disease, hypertension, low HDL or significant hypertriglyceridemia
Polycystic ovary syndrome
High-risk ethnicity
Other clinical condition associated with insulin resistance (e.g., acanthosis nigricans)

BMI, body mass index; GDM, gestational diabetes mellitus; HDL, high-density lipoprotein.
Source: Data from American Diabetes Association. Classification and diagnosis of diabetes: standards of medical care in diabetes—2019. Diabetes Care. *2019;42(suppl 1):S13–S28. doi:10.2337/dc19-S002; Durnwald C. Gestational diabetes mellitus: screening, diagnosis, and prevention. In: Post TW, ed.* UpToDate. *UpToDate 2019. https://www.uptodate.com/gestational diabetes mellitus: screening, diagnosis, and prevention.*

BOX 12.3 Gestational Diabetes Screening Options

1. "One-step," a fasting 75 g glucose tolerance test (GTT), or
2. "Two-step," a screening nonfasting 50 g GTT, and if positive followed by a diagnostic fasting 100 g GTT

Source: Data from Durnwald C. Gestational diabetes mellitus: screening, diagnosis, and prevention. In: Post TW, ed. UpToDate. *UpToDate 2019. https://www.uptodate.com/gestational diabetes mellitus: screening, diagnosis, and prevention.*

Substance Use

Avoidance of all illicit drugs, including opiates, should be recommended to all patients. Patients with opioid use disorder should be managed with the appropriate medical assistance per current guidelines to avoid neonatal withdrawal syndrome. Some states require certain protocols and reporting policies with regard to substance use in pregnancy, and PAs should become familiar with these for their area.[90,91]

- Cigarette and E-cigarette smoking can lead to a higher risk of ectopic pregnancy, placenta abruption and placenta previa, small for gestational age, PTL, ogliohydramnios, and preterm prelabor rupture of members (PPROM).
- Alcohol use causes fetal-alcohol syndrome (FAS). FAS is a spectrum disease that has the potential to affect many different systems. The severity is based on the amount consumed during pregnancy; there is no amount of alcohol that is deemed safe in pregnancy.
- Marijuana's effects are controversial. Several studies have provided conflicting outcomes, and more research is needed.
- Cocaine, methamphetamines, and opioids all have risks of significant maternal and fetal complications ranging from placental abruption to cardiovascular to neurodevelopment.

Travel

Maternal travel plans during pregnancy need to be discussed, particularly if the travel is to infectious endemic areas. All travel that requires prolonged sitting puts the patient at the risk of a thromboembolic event. If travel is unavoidable, patients should be counseled to frequently ambulate.

Work

Occupations that may place patients at risk for exposure to chemicals or radiation, heavy lifting, prolonged standing, or infection need to be reviewed. Preventive measures and precautions may need to be implemented. If appropriate, a modified work plan should be advised.

Medication

Medications used during pregnancy must have the risk/benefit ratios considered, including over-the-counter (OTC) drugs and supplements. Owing to rigorous data, OTC supplements should be avoided. Some medications that are contraindicated in pregnancy are shown in Box 12.4.

In 2015 the U.S. Food and Drug Administration (FDA) implemented a radically new pregnancy medication categorizing system for prescription drugs, with no change to OTC medication labeling. The old system was labeled as A (completely safe), B, C, D, and X (teratogenic). The new system is termed the "Pregnancy and Lactation Labeling Rule" or "PLLR" system. The system was introduced to assist the clinician in more informed and up-to-date risk/benefit stratification for patient counseling. The PLLR labeling system separates drugs into three separate categories:

1. Pregnancy and labor and delivery
2. Lactation
3. Reproductive potential for both females and males

BOX 12.4 Various Medications Contraindicated in Pregnancy

Isotretinoin (retinoids)
Tetracyclines
Angiotensin-converting enzyme (ACE) inhibitors
Angiotensin II receptor blockers (ARBs)
Most antineoplastics
Mycophenolate mofetil
Methotrexate (MTX)
Thalidomide
Contraceptives
Androgens
Warfarin
Sulfa
Most antiepileptic drugs (valproic acid, phenytoin, carbamazepine, trimethadione)
Lithium
Methimazole
Cyclosporine
Streptomycin
Diethylstilbestrol (DES)

The pregnancy subsection includes a pregnancy exposure registry for many drugs. This is to collect and compare data and improve safety information and provide real-time data. The lactation subsection also has improved data, providing more clinical information and guidance when working with patients who are breastfeeding. The last subsection provides information about the drug in regard to pregnancy risk, contraception needs, and effect on infertility.[92,93]

PHYSICAL EXAMINATION

A complete physical examination should be completed at the initial prenatal visit. The weight obtained at this office visit will be the reference point for education on pregnancy weight gain recommendations for a singleton pregnancy, which are outlined in Table 12.33. Weight gain recommendations are in place to optimize perinatal outcomes. For example, risks associated with inadequate weight gain are small for gestational age and PTL; with excessive weight gain the risks include maternal hypertensive disorders in pregnancy, GDM, large for gestational age, and macrosomia. In turn, macrosomia may lead to a prolonged stage 2 labor with increase perinatal complications and higher chance for cesarean delivery. If a patient is significantly overweight or obese (BMI 35.0 to >40.0) at the pregnancy outset, approach to weight gain should be individualized. Some studies, albeit with limitations, have revealed that patients in BMI classes II & III may safely have small (<5 kg) weight loss during pregnancy, although further research is needed.[94]

Approximately 90% of pregnant women have a systolic ejection fraction murmur that can be heard on the cardiovascular examination. It may occasionally reveal a bounding and collapsing pulse, as well as a loud first heart sound. Mild peripheral edema may also be noted, though if severe at the pregnancy outset, is likely a more chronic symptom and further investigation may be warranted. The skin exam may reveal increased pigmentation or the appearance of striae on the abdomen in later pregnancy. Upon examination of the reproductive tract in early pregnancy Chadwick sign may be present. This occurs when the cervix turns bluish in color due to increased blood flow or congestion. Cervical assessment should note cervical length (long or short), consistency (firm or soft), dilation (cervical os opening), and effacement (thinning of the cervix). If the cervix has softening, this is termed Hegar sign. Around 6 weeks' gestation the uterus's increased size may be palpated, and by about 12 weeks may be palpated transabdominally. The uterus should be palpated for contour, shape, size, and consistency. There are four basic female pelvic types, demonstrated in Figure 12.16. Although pelvimetry has largely fallen out of favor, certain severe pelvic types with narrow diameters may have more difficultly passing the fetal head through the vaginal canal due to cephalopelvic disproportion. When this occurs, an elective cesarean section should be considered for delivery to reduce perinatal complications.[81]

TABLE 12.33 Pregnancy Weight Chart

Prepregnancy Weight	Prepregnancy BMI Calculated*	Recommended Total Weight Gain, Singleton Pregnancy
Underweight	<18.5	28–40 pounds
Normal weight	18.5–24.9	25–35 pounds
Overweight	25.0–29.9	15–25 pounds
Obese (class 1–3)	≥30.0	11–20 pounds

*BMI (kg/m²) = mass (lb)/height² (in) × 703.
BMI, body mass index.
Source: Adapted from Centers for Disease Control and Prevention. Weight gain during pregnancy 2019. https://www.cdc.gov/reproductivehealth/maternalinfanthealth/pregnancy-weight-gain.htm

COMMON PREGNANCY SIGNS AND SYMPTOMS

Generally, pregnancy symptoms begin in the first trimester, are reduced in the second trimester, and return or worsen in the third trimester.

Nausea/Vomiting

The most common pregnancy complaint is the presence of nausea, with or without vomiting; 50% to 90% of patients will experience nausea in the first trimester but it usually resolves by the second trimester.[95] Supportive measures are the recommended treatment. Less than 3% of patients will develop severe nausea with hyperemesis, or retching. If this occurs and is accompanied by a weight loss of >5% of body weight the patients likely has HG.[74,96] Early intervention will help prevent HG. A differential diagnosis of nausea and vomiting during pregnancy should be considered based on GA of onset and physical findings. Per ACOG, if onset started after 9 weeks' gestation or if there are any other physical findings on examination, alternative etiologies need to be considered. HG patients require further treatment and intervention to avoid adverse perinatal outcomes. These treatments may include antiemetics, IV fluids, and in severe cases hospitalization. There is no known pathogenesis for nausea and vomiting in pregnancy and it is likely multifactorial.

Lightheadedness

Another common complaint is lightheadedness, typically with position changes. This is likely multifactorial and associated with the profound fluid shifts that occur during pregnancy. Adequate hydration is essential to help alleviate this.

Headaches

Headaches commonly occur throughout pregnancy. Etiologies are likely multifactorial, related to hormone changes and dehydration. However, if the headache is unrelenting and not alleviated by acetaminophen, further investigation is warranted.

GERD

Heartburn, or GERD, is most common during the third trimester, though it can occur at any point during pregnancy. First-line treatment should be supportive care, followed by OTC antacids.

Constipation

One of the most bothersome symptoms to patients is constipation. This appears to be a physiologic change that occurs due to decreased GI transit time due to multiple hormonal factors. This slowed transit may possibly be to allow for increased fluid and nutritional absorption during pregnancy. Patients are encouraged to increase their fluids but may also require a fiber supplement. Occasionally stool softeners are needed.

Hemorrhoids

Hemorrhoids are also common during pregnancy and are often associated with constipation. They may also be due to the increased intra-abdominal pressure. Treatment should be supportive.

Leg Cramping

Leg cramps, usually affecting the calves, are common during pregnancy. These frequently occur at night but may occur at any time of day. Treatment recommendations include stretching and strengthening. A Cochrane review revealed no benefit of calcium supplementation in the treatment of leg cramps during pregnancy. However, it did reveal a possible benefit from magnesium supplementation, although more studies need to be completed to confirm this finding.[97] Varicosities are also a common finding.

Round Ligament Pain

During the mid-second trimester a common complaint is pain associated with round ligament stretching. This is often described as a pulling or sharp pain sensation, particularly with rapid maternal movement or position change. This is a normal process and no intervention in necessary.

Falls/Trauma

A less common complaint, but one that can lead to severe consequences, is the change in balance in the pregnant patient. This balance change is due to a variety of factors, including change of center of gravity with the growing uterus and laxity of joints during pregnancy. Patients should take care to avoid falls and trauma.

Back Pain

Back pain may occur during pregnancy, particularly in the last trimester with rapid uterine growth and stretching. Back pain complaints should be investigated, as this may be a warning sign of PTL.

Vaginal Discharge

Pregnant patients frequently report increased vaginal discharge. This is a normal pregnancy phenomenon. Normal discharge is usually described as white and thin, and any deviation from this should be evaluated for infection (change in color, thick, sticky, malodorous, bloody). Vaginal infections, such as sexually transmitted disease and BV have been associated with an increased risk of PTL. If a patient describes a fluid "gush" or clear, nonodorous discharge the differential diagnosis should include premature prelabor rupture of membranes (PPROM). Treatment should be based on findings.

Thromboembolic Events

Though patients may not present complaining of a "venous thromboembolic event," the clinician must be aware of complaints associated with them. These often include complaints such as unilateral calf pain, edema and erythema, or persistent shortness of breath with or without chest pain, and any stoke-like symptoms. During pregnancy patients have a four- to fivefold increased risk of a thromboembolic event over their nonpregnant peers.[98] Preventive measures should be considered in high-risk patients.

Fatigue

Fatigue is a universal complaint among pregnant patients. The etiology is multifactorial, and treatment is supportive. If severe, or associated with other symptoms, further workup may be warranted.

PATIENT EDUCATION

Patient education and counseling take up the bulk of the initial prenatal visit. Often patients have many questions regarding lifestyle, medications, travel, and more. This is an opportunity for the clinician to build rapport and provide disease prevention education. Included in the education should be nutritional guides, weight gain recommendations, exercise and activity guidelines, medication discussion, travel, and infectious disease potentials. Also, a brief discussion on breastfeeding benefits may help the patient consider this more seriously during the postpartum period.

Subsequent Prenatal Visits

Following the initial prenatal visit, routine, healthy patients are generally seen monthly until the third trimester, or 28 weeks' gestation. At this point, the patient is seen biweekly, then weekly starting at 36 weeks' gestation. At any point during the prenatal period if a risk factor or pathologic condition occurs, the patient may need to be seen more frequently. During all visits maternal and fetal well-being should be assessed with vital signs, history, and physical examination of mother, and evaluation of the fetus as necessary. Risk assessment and reductions should be discussed. Furthermore, continued perinatal planning for labor and delivery, postpartum period, and future family planning should all be addressed. Together the patient and clinician should be discussing and anticipating birth plan options, including mode of delivery, risk and complication prevention, and anesthesia. Childbirth classes may also help alleviate fears and answer many questions patients may have about the birthing process. Studies suggest improved perinatal outcomes occur when there is individualized attention during labor, with one-on-one nursing care or a doula.[99] In addition, discussions regarding breastfeeding plans and optimal family planning timing and birth control options should take place prior to delivery.

Maternal Assessments

During second and third trimester prenatal visits patients should have their blood pressure, pulse, weight, and a urinalysis obtained. Assessment should always include an inventory of patient symptoms. All symptoms and complaints should be appropriately evaluated and addressed. Use of laboratory or imaging studies will be based on differential diagnosis.

Between 16 and 22 weeks' gestation fetal movements should begin to be felt by the patient. This is called "quickening." Typically, primigravida patients feel fetal movement later than multigravida patients. Around this same time is when patients most often complain of round ligament pain.

At about 20 weeks' gestation a complete fetal anatomy screen (FAS) with ultrasound is performed. The FAS assesses the fetus for any anomalies, fetal size/weight based on EDD, volume of amniotic fluid, and the maternal anatomy for any anomalies. Gender can often be identified at this time. Occasionally this may be the only ultrasound a patient has during her pregnancy.

Between 24 and 28 weeks' gestation ACOG recommends that Hb and Rh antibody screening laboratory tests are repeated. The Hb is obtained to monitor for anemia that may have developed over the pregnancy. Mild anemia may occur; if Hb levels are much beyond <11 g/dL in the first and third trimesters, and <10.5 g/dL in the second then the CDC defines this as abnormal. If at any point the patient has microcytic anemia, further workup and treatment for possible iron deficiency should take place.

In the Rh D-negative patient, between 26 and 28 weeks' gestation Rho(D) immune globulin (RhoGAM) should be given, after the antibody test has been obtained to avoid false positive tests. Typically, RhoGAM 300 mg intramuscular injection is given once, and protects for 12 weeks. If delivery timing is >12 weeks from the date RhoGAM was given, a repeat dose may be necessary (see Section 12.12F Rh Incompatibility).

Between 24 and 28 weeks' gestation ACOG also recommended GDM screening for all pregnant patients without overt diabetes, including those who may have passed previous DM screening. There are two options for GDM screening during this time in the pregnancy: a glucose tolerance test (GTT) "one-step" option and a "two-step" option (see Box 12.3). Both options have pros and cons, and it is often a regional preference as to which screening tests are used.

In the third trimester patients often begin to feel Braxton-Hicks contractions. These contractions are described as an abdominal tightening without pain, and do not change the cervix. These are thought of as "practice contractions." However, if the patient has any pain associated, or other warning signs, further investigation should be completed.

During the last several weeks of a normal pregnancy, clinicians often begin digital cervical examinations to assess for changes. The assessment should include consistency of cervical tissue (soft, firm), effacement (or shortening and/or thinning of the cervix), dilation (opening of the cervical os), and position within the vaginal vault (anterior vs. posterior). Patients with cervical softness and anterior position are more likely to progress to labor than those with firm or posterior cervical changes.

Cervical effacement is palpated by during the digital cervical examination and is expressed in percentages. Initially the cervix is long, similar to a bottleneck. As the fetal head continues to put pressure on the cervix and effacement progresses the cervix begins to decrease in length and thin out. Cervical dilation occurs when the cervix begins to open wider to allow for the fetus to pass through. Palpation of the external cervical os can be calculated by using digital (finger) measurement in centimeters. A closed os or 0 dilation equates to 0 cm, while fully dilated measures at 10 cm. Fetal position examination should continue to occur during this time, as at this point changes rarely take place; although rare, it has been known that a fetus can turn from breech to vertex at the last minute. Fetal station examination will determine the level of decent the fetus has made into the cervical canal. The measurements are in centimeters from the bony edge of the ischial spines of the pelvis. They range from −5, or 5 cm superior to the ischial spine, to +5, or 5 cm inferior to the ischial spine, or when the fetal head is at the introitus. Engagement occurs when the station is at 0. This is demonstrated in Figure 12.17.

In the last weeks of pregnancy, patients may report a change in vaginal discharge. They occasionally see a thick, "plug-like" collection of vaginal discharge that may or not be tinged with blood. This is called "bloody show" and is the collection of mucus that remains in the cervical os until labor changes occur. Bloody show may present several weeks prior to the onset of labor. No management is necessary for this, other than reassurance to the patient. If there are any other signs or symptoms of labor or infection further workup may be needed.

Common signs of labor include vaginal bleeding, increasing and/or patterned contractions either in abdomen with back pain, or clear fluid "gushes" or continuous leaking. If any of these occur before 38 weeks' gestation, the patient needs to be evaluated appropriately. Heavy vaginal bleeding can indicate placental abruption and needs to be addressed expeditiously.

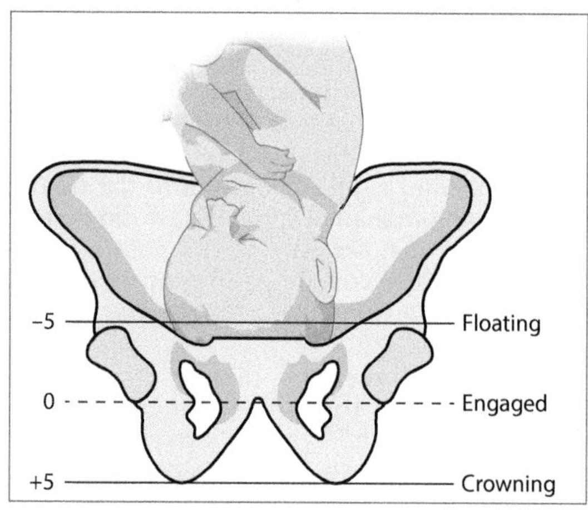

Figure 12.17 **Fetal station.**

Group B streptococcus (GBS) is the leading cause of neonatal infection.[100] The primary vector is maternal colonization and transmission during vaginal delivery. A GBS culture is obtained between 36 $^{0}/_{7}$ and 37 $^{6}/_{7}$ weeks' gestation to assess its presence. It is traditionally obtained via rectovaginal swab. It can also be diagnosed with positive GBS growth on a urine culture at any point during pregnancy, or if the patient has had a previous GBS-infected neonate. ACOG recommends prophylactic IV antibiotics during labor × 4 hours, as oral and intramuscular (IM) have been proved ineffective. The first-line treatment is IV penicillin, with ampicillin an acceptable alternative. Patients with a low-risk allergy to penicillin should have first-generation cephalosporins (e.g., cefazolin). In patients with high-risk penicillin allergies or anaphylaxis, clindamycin IV should be administered.[100]

Fetal Assessments

Fetal well-being and assessment should take place at every prenatal visit. This includes routine maternal abdominal measuring for growth, fetal movement and fetal presentation, depending upon the gestational age.

The fundal height (FH) can be measured abdominally once the uterus can be palpated outside the pelvic cavity, typically around 12 weeks' gestation in a singleton pregnancy. FH is the measured distance (in centimeters) from the pubic symphysis to the top of the uterus, called the fundus. At 20 weeks' gestation the FH should be 20 cm ±2 cm and correspond with the patient's umbilicus. From this point FH will continue to increase approximately 1 cm weekly, corresponding with the number of gestational weeks. For example, at 26 weeks' gestation the FH should measure 26 cm, and 30 weeks' gestation 30 cm with a ±2 cm standard deviation. Any sudden increase or decrease in growth could indicate a fetal issue that requires evaluation. At 36 weeks' gestation, the fetal height may be decreased due to the fetus engaging, or "dropping," into the pelvis to prepare for eventual delivery.

By 26 weeks' gestation, patients should feel consistent fetal movements. The fetus has a sleep-wake cycle, so often there will be brief times when no fetal movement will be palpated. Patients should be instructed to monitor the fetal kick counts daily to help assure fetal well-being. Having the patient choose a time of the day that the fetus is often active and note that activity during this time can be helpful. Fetal movement should be addressed at each prenatal visit after 24 to 28 weeks. If fetal movement is absent or significantly decreased, further investigation is warranted.

Fetal presentation should begin to be assessed in the third trimester. Leopold's maneuvers are a specific palpation technique that allows the PA to determine where the fetus is located within the uterus. The most common and ideal position is cephalic or vertex. This is when the fetus is head down toward the pelvis. Other possible presentations are breech or transverse. Frank breech is when the fetal buttocks are toward the pelvis and head is toward the ribs, whereas footling breech with the head toward the top and buttocks down with the exception of one leg extending down and presenting first during labor. The second leg is curled up toward the head as in frank breech. Transverse is when the fetus is lying with head to either side. See Figure 12.18.

If presentation is difficult to ascertain, a quick transabdominal ultrasound will easily allow visualization of the fetal position.

If malpresentation is present by mid third trimester to 36+ weeks, the fetus may need further evaluation and delivery options should be discussed with the patient. Occasionally the fetus will turn vertex on their own, but if malpresentation is continued into term an external cephalic version or cesarean delivery needs to be considered.

Specialized Assessments

At any point if fetal well-being is in question further investigation must be completed. There are several options to assess the fetus.

- Fetal heart tones (FHTs) with a handheld fetal Doppler is the first option. FHT is the quickest and routinely completed at every subsequent prenatal visit, after 10 to 12 weeks' gestation. FHTs are usually between 110 to 160 bpm. If FHTs are absent or abnormal more extensive evaluation should be completed.[101]

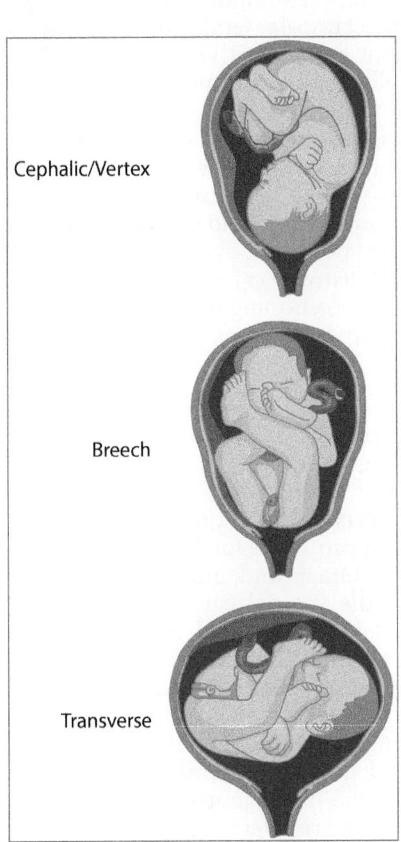

Figure 12.18 **Three common fetal presentations.**

- Nonstress testing (NST) is a noninvasive way of measuring overall health of the fetus. The test involves using a tocodynamometer and placing a dual probe monitor on the gravid abdomen. One monitor is for fetal heart rate, and the other is to measure uterine contractions. The patient presses a button each time she feels movement, and the tocodynamometer automatically records the time the fetal movement was felt so that a correlation between movement and fetal heart rate can be made. Figure 12.19 is an example of a NST tracing. The fetal heart rate should have times of acceleration, or increased heart rate, which may be during movement or stimulation. These accelerations provide feedback of adequate oxygenation and fetal well-being. If these accelerations are not occurring, and unable to be produced, or if decelerations occur, meaning a decrease in heart rate, it may be a sign of fetal hypoxemia and further investigation is warranted. Often the NST will be in combination with biophysical profile (BPP) ultrasound examination for thorough fetal well-being investigation.
- BPPs are transabdominal ultrasound exams that assess for several findings that correlate with fetal well-being. Points are given (either 0 or 2 points) for fetal movement, fetal tone, fetal breathing practices, and amniotic fluid volume. A score of ≥8 assures no signs of hypoxemia at the time of testing. If the score is ≤4 continued investigation must occur for possible fetal compromise.
- Doppler, called cord velocimetry, is useful for evaluating fetal cardiovascular and placental blood flow concerns. This measures blood flow to and from the fetus. It is useful to evaluate for possible intrauterine growth restriction and when Rh incompatibility exists.
- Contraction stress tests (CSTs) are similar to NST, but the patient has induced contractions, either by oxytocin, nipple stimulation, or other. The test monitors fetal well-being during these contractions and if hypoxic injury is present during a contraction.

12.11C EVALUATION OF LABOR

The onset of labor is defined as consistent and regular uterine contractions strong enough to cause cervical dilation and/or effacement. It is thought that once a patient's cervix has dilated to 4 to 6 cm, the patient is entering the active phase of labor (Box 12.5).

At 37 weeks' gestation the pregnancy is considered full term and labor and delivery are considered safe for mom and baby. Usually patients deliver between 37 and 42 weeks. After 42 weeks increased material and fetal complications can occur.

NORMAL LABOR AND DELIVERY

There are three stages of labor. The first stage is the onset of labor to full cervical dilation. The patient is often admitted to the hospital sometime in the middle of this stage. The second stage is the passage of the fetus through the vaginal canal. The third is the delivery of the placenta.

Stage One

The first stage is from the onset of labor to full cervical dilation. This stage is delineated into latent and active phases. The latent stage is the period from onset of cervical changes to the point where regular contractions and rapid cervical changes occur. The change from latent to active phase

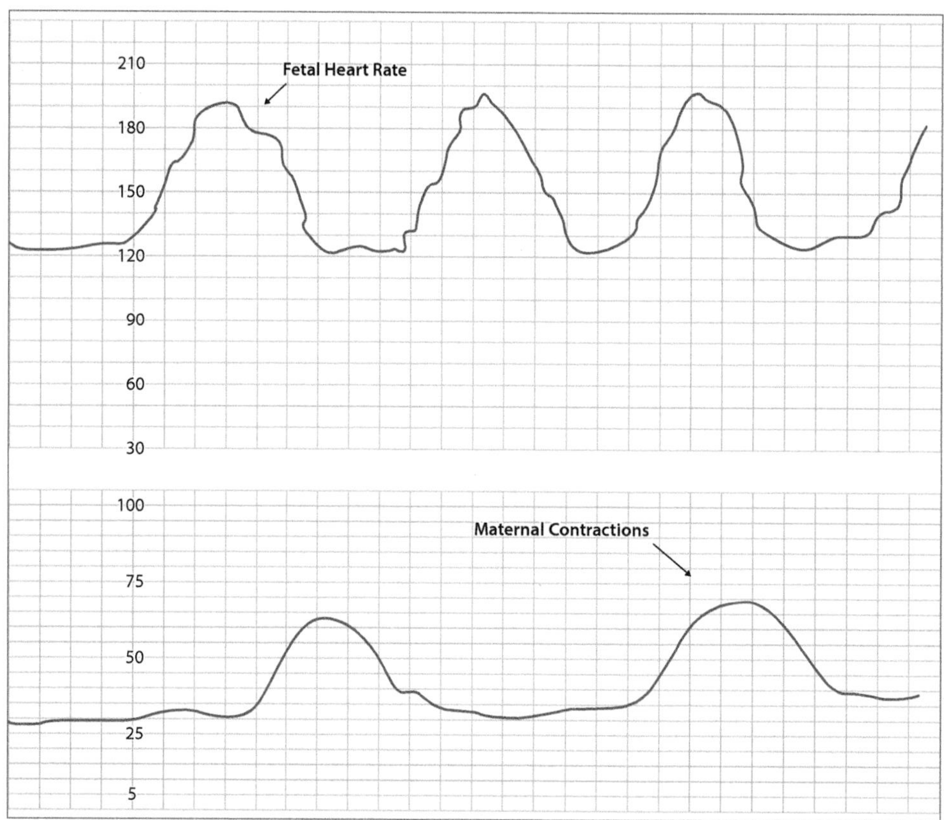

Figure 12.19 **Nonstress test tracing.**

BOX 12.5 Preterm Labor Signs and Symptoms

Contractions, either regular or irregular
Abdominal cramping, often lower abdomen or menstrual-like
Low back pain
Increasing pelvic pressure, usually explained as "feeling like baby will fall out"
Vaginal discharge change
Continuous trickle of clear fluid or a large fluid gush
Vaginal bleeding

generally begins when the patient's cervix reaches between 4 and 6 cm. At this point the patient typically notes regular contractions. Though the patient is actively laboring the phase typically lasts 3 to 6 hours to completion, although it can be longer in nulligravida. Documentation of cervical change and fetal station may be completed by nursing on a partogram (partograph). This is a graph representing the patient's progress of labor.[99]

During the active phase of labor, patients are continuously monitored with the tocodynamometer. In addition, vital signs, cervical change, and fetal station are monitored. The patient should also be assessed for any signs or symptoms of vaginal bleeding that may lead to complications, if fetal membranes are intact or ruptured, fetal station and presentation. Contractions and fetal heart rate may be monitored with cardiotocography or a nonstress test. Per ACOG external fetal monitoring should be reviewed every 30 minutes for patients without complications during the first stage of labor, and every 15 minutes for patients with complications (e.g., preeclampsia, fetal growth restriction).[102]

If the patient has a positive GBS, or if GBS status is unknown at delivery, IV antimicrobials should be initiated 4 hours prior to delivery.[99,100]

Patients without contraindications should have the option to ambulate during this stage to improve maternal circulation, as well as decrease the risk of IVC obstruction from uterine compression and supine hypotensive syndrome. When supine hypotensive syndrome occurs, the fetus may exhibit signs of distress on fetal monitoring due to decreased oxygenation. Repositioning the patient to a left, lateral position should remove the compress on and improve CO.

Stage Two

The second stage of labor is the phase of fetal descent through the vaginal canal. At this point in the process, the clinician should be readily available. The onset of stage two is at full cervical dilation (10 cm) and with fetal station at ≥0, respectively. During this time uterine contractions are involuntary and intense enough to descend the fetus through the vaginal canal for delivery. Patients may help facilitate fetal descent with addition of maternal "pushing" during uterine contractions. At this stage ACOG recommends review of external fetal heart monitoring every 15 minutes in the uncomplicated patients, and every 5 minutes for patients with complications.[103]

During fetal descent, several fetal movements occur to accommodate the passage through the maternal pelvis. These movements are referred to as mechanisms of labor, or cardinal positions, and are demonstrated in Figure 12.20. The movements are as follows: engagement, flexion, descent,

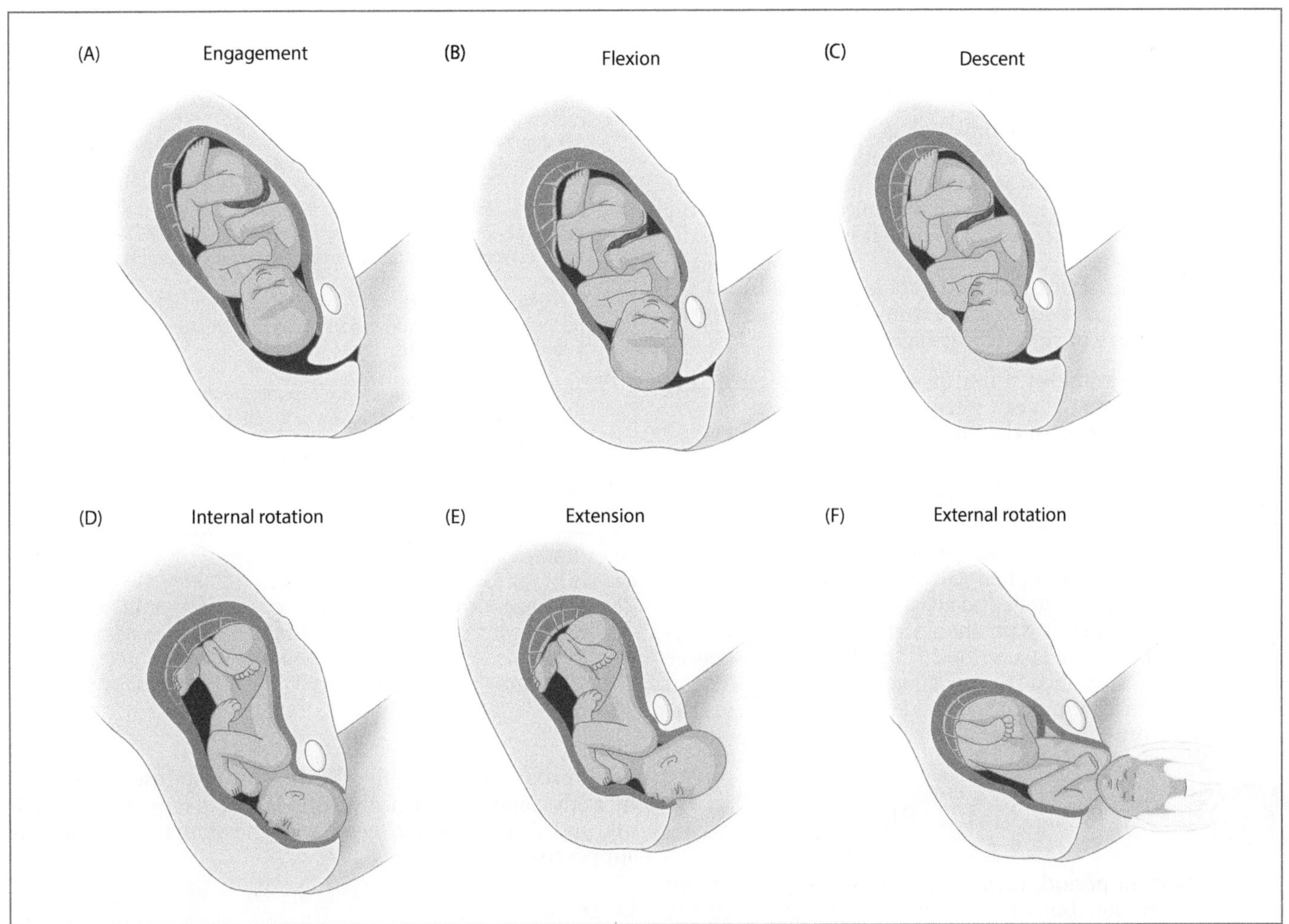

Figure 12.20 Cardinal movements of labor. Engagement (A), flexion (B), descent (C), internal rotation (D), extension (E), and external rotation (F).

internal rotation, extension, external rotation or restitution, and expulsion.[103] During this time, most patients will have complete dilation and fetal head descent, which may be noted by the disappearance of the anterior cervical lip. If this lip persists for >30 minutes, or it becomes edematous, it may be a sign of fetal malposition or labor complication. Perineal massage with lubrication and/or warm compresses to the perineum may help soften the area and reduce risk of trauma. Studies have not revealed any contraindications in otherwise uncomplicated patients for change in maternal position for comfort. Patients who do not use an epidural for anesthesia and who labor in the upright position appear to have a shorter second stage by a few minutes.[104]

There is no specific maximum length of time for the second stage of labor. Though research has shown increased perinatal complications, particularly for the fetus/neonate, occurring in those in stage two for >4 hours with 3 hours of maternal pushing for the nulliparous woman, and >3 hours with 2 hours of active pushing for the multiparous woman.[104]

Second stage labor management goals are to successfully expel the neonate, while reducing maternal perineal trauma. The "hands-on" technique appears to achieve these goals over previous approaches. This technique has the clinician using one had to gentle apply pressure to the neonate's head when crowning, while simultaneously using the other hand to support the patient's perineum. The clinician can then guide the head through delivery with "manual" control and provide perineal support during the entire process. To further this technique the patient may be instructed to take small, expulsive efforts when the head is fully crowning, and delivery is imminent. This helps to prevent rapid expulsion of the neonatal head.[104,105] Once the head is delivered, spontaneous fetal external rotation occurs (Figure 12.20) followed by the anterior shoulder delivery, and then body.[105]

Management of prolongation of the second stage of labor is a clinical judgment based on several factors, including progress to that point and anesthesia type. Generally, if active maternal effort or pushing has been ongoing for 60 to 90 minutes, oxytocin augmentation is reasonable. Ideally, operative interventions are avoided. However, if little progress has occurred with prolonged time frames it may be reasonable to consider operative interventions. Regardless of labor progress, if at any point the fetal heart tracing becomes nonreassuring, prompt operative delivery is indicated.[103,104] An episiotomy is not recommended and should only be performed if absolutely necessary.

If a nuchal cord, or cord around the neonate's neck, is present upon delivery, reduction should take place. Options include slipping the cord off the neonate's head, double clamping and transecting, or by the "somersault maneuver," in which the neonate's head is flexed and held toward the mother's thigh as both shoulders, and then the body, is delivered. In an attempt to reduce the cord, care should be taken to avoid tearing.

Following term deliveries, cord clamping should be completed after 30 to 60 seconds per ACOG.[104]

Stage Three

The third stage of labor is the period from the delivery of the infant to the delivery of the placenta (Figure 12.21). The process of normal placental separation following delivery of the infant is due to myometrial thickening, leading to reduced uterine surface area, and continued uterine contractions resulting in the separation of the placenta. Concurrently these uterine processes result in constriction of the myometrial vessels and reduce blood flow, decreasing the risk of hemorrhage.

Active management of the third stage of labor (AMTSL) has been shown to reduce postpartum hemorrhage (PPH). AMTSL is a series of steps consisting of[105,106]:

- Prophylactic administration of an uterotonic agent before the placenta delivery, plus
- Controlled traction of the umbilical cord, and
- Uterine massage.

If no complications are present, the neonate may be given to the mother for skin-to-skin contact.

Assessment of perineal lacerations and repair following should occur immediately after delivery. The lacerations should be classified based on extent and areas involved, as outlined in Box 12.6. The patient's pain should also be assessed for repair of more extensive lacerations. If third- or fourth-degree lacerations are sustained during delivery, a broad-spectrum antibiotic should be initiated. If fecal content is present, the area needs thorough debridement followed by repair.

BOX 12.6 Perineal Laceration Classification

1st degree: Epithelial injury to perineum and vagina (skin, subcutaneous) without muscle involvement

2nd degree: Injury extends into fascia and muscle of the perineal body, and superficial and deep transverse perineal muscles, sparing the anal sphincter, which remains intact.

3rd degree: Injury extends into the fascia and muscles of the perineal body and involves some or all of the external and internal anal sphincters.

- Further classification is made on whether <50% or >50% of external anal sphincter is torn or if both external and internal sphincters are torn.

4th degree: All perineal structures and rectal mucosa are torn.

Source: Data from Funai EF, Norwitz ER. Management of normal labor and delivery. In: Post TW, ed. UpToDate. *UpToDate; 2019. https://www.uptodate.com/management of normal labor and delivery; Fretheim A, Odgaard-Jensen J, Røttingen J, et al. The impact of an intervention programme employing a hands-on technique to reduce the incidence of anal sphincter tears: interrupted time-series reanalysis.* BMJ Open. *2013;3:e003355. doi:10.1136/bmjopen-2013-003355.*

12.11D POSTPARTUM CARE

The postpartum period, or puerperium, is the period from delivery of the newborn to the return of the body to the nonpregnant state. There is no set time frame for this process, and it has been stated to last anywhere from 6 or 8 weeks to 12 months or longer. Most patients will take between 6 and 12 weeks.

POSTPARTUM PHYSICAL ADAPTATIONS

Shivering

Research has shown that up to 50% of patients in the hour postdelivery will develop vigorous rigors or shivering. The exact etiology is unknown; however, some theories have been proposed including the body's response to a drop in body temperature following labor; postpartum bleeding and coagulation effects; and anesthesia. Treatment is supportive.

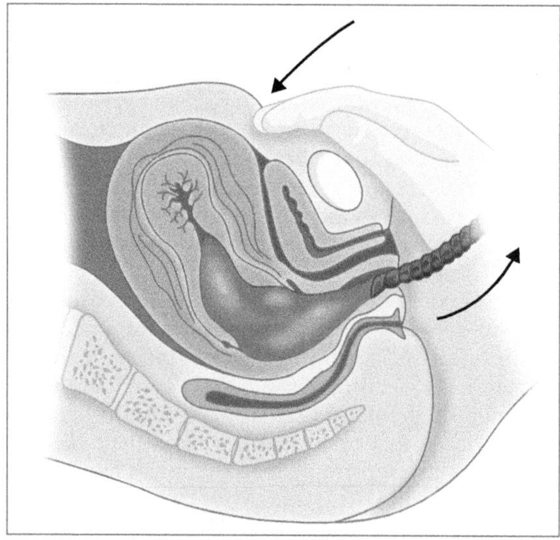

Figure 12.21 **Delivery of the placenta.**

Uterine Involution

Uterine involution begins to occur immediately following delivery. The uterus is typically firm and nontender and palpated between the pubic symphysis and the umbilicus. It then becomes slightly enlarged again, around the umbilicus, approximately 12 hours postdelivery. From here it continues involution at a rate of about 1 cm/day. By the end of postpartum week 2, the uterus is generally not palpable, and it returns to its prepregnancy size by 6 to 8 weeks postpartum.[107]

Lochia

Lochia comprises erythrocytes, leukocytes, decidua, epithelial cells, serous exudate, and bacteria that is shed following delivery. The shedding generally lasts between 3 and 6 weeks postpartum. It begins with lochia rubra, which is darker red to red/brown vaginal discharge or bleeding. This is the shedding of blood and the basal portion of the decidua that remains following separation of the placenta. Several days out from delivery the lochia begins to become much lighter with serous discharge. This is referred to as lochia serosa and is pink to brown. This type of vaginal bleeding or discharge lasts several weeks.

Cervix

Following delivery, the cervix remains slightly dilated and soft. Minor lacerations can often be noted at the external os margins. The cervix dilation will continue to decrease and be <1 cm by the end of the first week postpartum. From a histology perspective the cervix may take up to 3 to 4 months postdelivery to return to baseline.[107] Once completely closed, the cervix will take on a new os shape of transverse instead of the nulliparous cervical os that is round.

Vagina and Pelvic Floor

The pelvic floor undergoes increased pressure during the prenatal period, followed by forcible stretching and compression during the delivery process. Just following delivery, the vagina is extended and smooth. As the edema and vascularity abate, the vagina contracts and rugae return, though will likely never completely return to the nulligravid state. Early postpartum pelvic floor muscle exercises have not proved to decrease the risk of urinary incontinence and may actually be detrimental to patients who have had injury during labor.[107]

Gastrointestinal

Bowel and GI function return to normal following delivery. Frequently the first bowel movement is 2 to 3 days postpartum. Adequate fluids and nutrition will also aid the return of normal GI function.

Human Chorionic Gonadotropin

The hCG beta-subunit will return to negative by 2 to 4 weeks postpartum for the majority of women, although some may take longer.[108] The complication to be on alert for is trophoblastic neoplasms, which are rare, but have high morbidity and mortality if missed. The hallmark that needs further investigation is when the hCG levels do not fall or begin to rise following the typical time frame.

Ovulatory Function

The resumption of ovulation in the majority of patients occurs between 6 and 12 weeks postpartum. This is largely regulated by the postpartum gonadotropins and sex steroids levels, and lactation status. For all women immediately following delivery estrogen levels fall. Estrogen begins to increase again about 2 weeks postpartum in the nonlactating woman. Resumption of ovulation in the lactating patient is regulated by PRL levels, maternal nutrition, and body mass. Lactation increases PRL, which suppresses GnRH. Research has also found that inadequate nutrition during lactation can lead to suppression in GnRH resulting in suppressed ovulation.[107,109]

Breasts/Lactation

The breast changes that occur during pregnancy and the postpartum phase are in preparation for lactation. Lactogenesis has two stages. The first stage is secretory initiation that occurs during the second half of pregnancy. The second stage is secretory activation. This stage is initiated following placental delivery with a drop in progesterone and other hormone levels and increase in PRL, cortisol, and insulin.[110,111] Within 3 to 4 days following delivery the onset of milk production has begun for most patients. Colostrum is the first maternal milk to be produced. Colostrum is present for about 5 days or so, then replaced by maternal milk. Within the first days of lactation, production continues to increase within the breast, causing breast tissue distention. This is termed breast engorgement. Frequently the breasts become full, firm, and tender. If the patient plans to breastfeed, further production is stimulated by expression or continued process of secretion. Continued milk production is stimulated and maintained with regular excretion intervals, either by infant suckling or a breast pump, as well as nipple stimulation. Nipple stimulation initiates the pituitary gland to release PRL and oxytocin, which in turn leads to increased milk production. In turn, if a patient does not plan to breastfeed, decreasing or ceasing expression and nipple stimulation should be avoided. Supportive care, such as cool compresses, may help alleviate the discomfort associated with breast engorgement.

Abdominal Wall

To accommodate the enlarging uterus during pregnancy the rectus abdominis muscles separate. These muscles typically return to normal tone several weeks into the postpartum period. Occasionally, if the rectus abdominis muscles remain separated, diastasis recti occur.

Hematology

During labor and delivery blood loss will occur, thus, a decrease in Hb will also occur. For the normal labor and delivery ACOG does not recommend routine Hb testing postpartum. By approximately 6 to 8 weeks postpartum pregnancy-related hematologic changes return to baseline.

Postpartum patients are at highest risk for venous thromboembolic events (VTEs) than any other time during the perinatal period. In developed countries VTE is the leading cause of maternal death.[107] Patients are at the highest risk during the initial weeks following delivery; the risk gradually reduces and ceases to baseline by 12 weeks postpartum. Clinicians should always be on alert for any symptoms associated with thromboembolic events. All patients should be encouraged to walk around to decrease risk of deep vein thrombosis. If a patient has had severe perineal compromise or has limited mobility, or if patients have a known VTE risk factor, such as previous VTE, coagulopathies, or comorbid conditions known to increase risk, prophylaxis should be initiated per the institution's guidelines.

Cardiovascular

Pregnancy-related cardiovascular modifications begin to amend immediately following delivery. SV and CO increase, heart rate decreases, while blood pressure remains without change. Cardiovascular changes gradually normalize to baselines, including left ventricular size and contractibility.[107]

Integumentary

Some integumentary changes that appear during pregnancy are permanent, specifically striae and laxity of abdominal skin if extensive injury to elastic fibers has occurred. Chloasma resolves with uncertain timing. Hair loss, or telogen effluvium, may last up to a little over 1 year postpartum.[107]

ROUTINE POSTPARTUM CARE

Postpartum care is essential to facilitate healthy maternal and infant outcomes. Some have gone as far as to suggest the postpartum periods should be called the fourth trimester. Research continues to provide guidelines for postpartum care. The Baby-Friendly Hospital Initiative (BFHI) by the World Health Organizations (WHO) and UNICEF is a program that implements research-driven guidelines to promote and support breastfeeding to improve maternal and child health.[107]

Maternal Monitoring

Maternal monitoring while in the hospital should involve routine vital signs, as well as vaginal bleeding assessment, abdominal palpation, and examination of the perineum. Initially, vaginal bleeding may be heavy with mild clotting; however, if the clots are larger than about 2 to 3 cm in diameter, further investigation should be completed. Upon examination the abdomen may be slightly tender, but not overt or acute. The perineum examination should assess for signs of infection or dehiscence. Routine labs are not indicated unless excessive blood loss or signs of infection are present, or for management of chronic illness.

Perineal Care

Perineal care should be discussed with patients. Many patients are apprehensive about having bowel movements following delivery. Reassurance should be provided. Often stool softeners and/or laxatives are helpful, in particular with patients who have had severe perineal injury. Occasionally warm or cool compresses can aid in perineal discomfort. Warm baths without use of soap products may also provide comfort to the patient.

Blood Type

Women who are Rh D-negative and have a child who is Rh D-positive should have anti-D immune globulin administered immediately after delivery and within 72 hours. Women who have had excessive fetomaternal bleeding should be routinely tested for alloimmunization and provided another dose of anti-D immune globulin as necessary.[107]

Pain Management

Postpartum pain can often be sufficiently managed with NSAIDs (e.g., ibuprofen is most commonly used), acetaminophen, and supportive measures. Supportive measures may include warm/cold compresses, warm baths, and witch-hazel pads. Naproxen should be avoided in breastfeeding mothers due to higher risk of accumulation in the infant bloodstream with a long half-life. NSAID use in the patient with hypertension postpartum should be individualized and ideally be avoided. Opioid medications should only be provided on an individual basis after thorough risk evaluation for the mother and infant. Opioids have the potential to decrease infant alertness and suckling response. Prior to any analgesic use, safety use with breastfeeding should be reviewed.

Activity

Activity recommendations is a common question for patients postpartum. Most daily living activities can be resumed as tolerated. If an activity causes increased fatigue or pain, it should be avoided until performed without symptoms. Resumption of sexual intercourse is considered safe once the perineal area lacerations are healed. This is typically around postpartum week 2. Many women will have resumed sexually intercourse by 6 weeks, often when they are seen in clinic for the postpartum follow-up. Therefore, contraception and future pregnancy plans need to be addressed prior to discharge from the hospital.

Contraception

Ovulation has the potential to occur as early as 25 days postdelivery for the nonlactating patient, and usually further out, but less predictable for the lactating patient. Regardless, if contraception is not discussed and started there is potential for unintended pregnancies. Patients choosing a permanent method, such as tubal ligation, can have this completed within 24 hours of delivery, and up to 7 days postpartum. Intrauterine contraception devices (IUDs) may be placed within 10 minutes following placental delivery; however, the frequency of expulsion increases if placed prior to normalization of uterine size.[107,109] The choice of contraceptive method should be a joint decision with the patients, to fit with their life plans, while remaining safe and healthy. The WHO and CDC have different recommendations for the postpartum patient starting a combined systemic hormonal contraception. Overall, data on combined systemic hormonal contraception do not support a significant or ongoing effect on breastfeeding outcomes. Historically, breastfeeding patients were offered progestin-only contraceptives, including the progestin-only pill, depot medroxyprogesterone acetate, subdermal implant, and progestin-secreting IUSs. Evidence has noted that only small amounts of estrogen and progestins are transferred via breast milk to the infant, and no adverse health effects have been suggested by the data; however, high-quality data are lacking and further research is necessary. According to the CDC, if a postpartum patient chooses a combined hormonal contraceptive method, the starting date needs to be delayed at least 3 weeks from delivery due to the VTE elevated risk.[109]

Immunizations

All postpartum patients should have a review of their immunization status and receive updates as necessary. Breastfeeding patients generally follow the same immunization guidelines as the general population. Furthermore, all family living with the newborn infant should have up-to-date immunizations—particularly the tetanus, diphtheria, and pertussis (TDAP) vaccine—to protect the unimmunized infant.

Lactation and Breastfeeding

It has been well documented that maternal milk is the most nutritious for a newborn infant. Therefore, all patients should be educated on the benefits of breastfeeding and recommended to exclusively breastfeed for ideally the first 6 to 12 months. Patients should be taught how to properly place the infant for optimal mouth latch onto the breast. Guidance should be provided on the importance of regular milk expression, either by the suckling infant or by a breast pump extraction, and nipple stimulation for continued milk production. Ideally women will be taught how to breastfeed by a lactation consultant.

Breast engorgement should be treated with excretion of the milk and, if severe, cool compresses and OTC analgesics. If the engorgement continues, the patient may have a galactocele or plugged duct. Treatment is warm nipple compresses and continued expression. If the breast continues with enlargement and tenderness, red "streaks" on breast, and/or fever occurs, the patient may have mastitis. Mastitis is an infection of breast tissue most often due to *Staphylococcus aureus*, and increasingly due to MRSA. Management consists of NSAIDs, cold compresses, continued emptying of the breast, and antibiotic treatment. Breastfeeding can and should safely continue during an episode of mastitis. If symptoms do not improve within 48 to 72 hours further evaluation, usually with ultrasound, for an underlying abscess should be completed.[111]

Postpartum Depression

Postpartum screening needs to be completed with a valid and reliable screening tool at the postpartum follow-up appointment. The Edinburgh Postnatal Depression Scale is frequently used. Ideally postpartum depression screening occurs around days 10 to 14 and again at the 6-week follow-up. If there are signs of depression present, referral to mental health therapy with or without the initiation of antidepressants should be completed.[112]

Weight

Physiologic weight loss is the weight lost from the act of delivery of the infant and placenta, as well as fluid loss. Together this can result in 18–28 pound weight reduction. Typically, by 6 weeks postpartum, gestational weight gain has decreased by 50%, followed by a slower loss thereafter.

Furthermore, chronic disease management and routine health maintenance should be assessed and completed prior to the patient transition out from postpartum follow-up care.[113]

Warning Signs

Early postpartum warning signs and symptoms include severe headaches, elevated blood pressure, seizures, excessive bleeding or hemorrhage, chest pain, dyspnea, severe abdominal pain, and severe perineal edema. If any of these occur, immediate investigation is warranted.

Prior to hospital discharge of the postpartum patient, the obstetric care team should ensure the mother has outside support, a clinician for the infant, and maternal comorbidities have been addressed. It may be beneficial to have a "first call" plan in place for any acute concerns during the postpartum period.

After hospital discharge, routine follow-up care should be continued. There are several models for ideal postpartum follow-up care and evaluation. WHO recommends routine follow-up for mother and baby at 3 days, 1 to 2 weeks, and 6 weeks while ACOG cites that ideally patients will have contact, preferably by office visit, with their clinician within 3 weeks postpartum, and seen in the office by 12 weeks. Anticipatory guidance studies appear to show promise in improvement of maternal well-being, including reduction of depression and increased duration of breastfeeding. During this visit a comprehensive assessment of physical, social, and psychological well-being and a complete physical examination should be performed.[113] These discussions should include evaluation and support for mothers with significant difficulties with sleep and fatigue, coping skills, and resources for help.

Routine Health Maintenance

The postpartum follow-up visit is an opportunity to continue the patient's preventive medicine needs. All comorbid conditions the patient may have should also be addressed. Patients who developed complications during pregnancy should undergo evaluation and repeat screenings as necessary and be educated on any future risk associations. Patients with comorbidities may need to be seen more frequently during the postpartum phase or until improvement or resolution has occurred.

12.12 PREGNANCY COMPLICATIONS

Stephanie Elko and Elyse J. Watkins

12.12A HYPERTENSION IN PREGNANCY

Hypertensive disorders are a leading cause of maternal morbidity and mortality nationally and globally. Hypertensive disorders can be classified into the following categories:

- Preexisting (chronic) hypertension
- Gestational hypertension, previously called pregnancy-induced hypertension
- Acute onset severe hypertension
- Preeclampsia, with or without severe features
- Preeclampsia or eclampsia with superimposed chronic hypertension
- Eclampsia
- HELLP syndrome (hemolysis, elevated liver enzymes, low platelets)

MEDICAL HISTORY AND CLINICAL PRESENTATION

Patients who present prior to 20 weeks' gestation with blood pressures ≥140/90 mm Hg on two separate occasions or ≥160/110 mm Hg on one occasion without a 24-hour urine protein >300 mg or a urine protein/creatinine ratio >0.3 likely have chronic or preexisting hypertension. However, if a patient presents with renal involvement <20 weeks' gestation, preeclampsia should be considered; other diagnoses to be ruled out include molar pregnancy, hemolytic-uremic syndrome, and autoimmune diseases.

Risk factors for gestational hypertension and preeclampsia that should be elicited in the medical history include primiparity, DM, prepregnancy hypertension, advanced maternal age, multiple gestation, obesity, systemic lupus erythematosus, antiphospholipid syndrome, preexisting renal disease, and a history of gestational hypertension, preeclampsia, or thrombocytopenia.

Although less common, patients may present postpartum with a hypertensive disorder of pregnancy. It is important to keep these disorders in the differential diagnosis when evaluating a postpartum patient with headaches, edema, elevated blood pressures, or other signs of cerebral irritation.

SIGNS AND SYMPTOMS

Patients with chronic hypertension, gestational hypertension, and preeclampsia without severe features are often asymptomatic. Patients with severe features will often present with headaches, visual changes (photopsia, scotomata), epigastric or upper abdominal pain, or edema of the feet, legs, and hands. Swelling of the face is almost always a pathologic sign. Patients with HELLP syndrome may or may not have proteinuria or hypertension, but right upper quadrant pain, nausea and vomiting, and malaise are most often present. Patients with eclampsia often experience a prodrome involving manifestations of cerebral irritation. This includes severe headaches, photophobia, blurry vision, and altered mental status.

PHYSICAL EXAMINATION

The physical examination should focus on ruling out other causes of symptoms and documenting the presence or absence of key physical findings that help differentiate between the different categories of hypertensive disorders.

The blood pressure should always be taken with the patient's feet on the floor, arm resting to her side, and using a proper size cuff. The general assessment should specify the patient's level of distress; if cardiorespiratory compromise is evident, emergency action must occur.

Inspect the patient's face and extremities for edema and note if edema is unilateral or bilateral. The presence of pitting edema should also be documented.

Auscultate the lungs for evidence of pulmonary edema and the heart for murmurs or dysrhythmia. Inspect the gravid abdomen and measure FH if gestational age is ≥20 weeks. Auscultate for FHTs. Palpation of the abdomen should seek to identify any tenderness, keeping in mind the normal displacement of organs during advanced stages of pregnancy.

DIFFERENTIAL DIAGNOSIS

Table 12.34 describes each category of hypertensive disorders in pregnancy. The differential diagnosis of each presenting sign and symptom can be extensive. For example, when a patient presents with facial swelling, angioedema should be ruled out, but also consider cellulitis, trauma, cavernous venous thrombosis, myxedema, and periodontal disease.

Patients who present with newly diagnosed hypertension should always be asked about a history of congenital or acquired cardiovascular and rheumatologic disease.

Headaches in pregnancy are common yet an unreliable indicator for the presence or absence of preeclampsia; therefore, it is important to perform a thorough history and physical exam to rule out other pathologies, such as migraine, tension headache, infection, a brain mass, or sequelae of trauma. Severe refractory frontal or occipital headaches with other signs of cerebral irritation could indicate an impending eclamptic seizure.

Pedal edema is also common in pregnancy, particularly during the later stages. It is important to differentiate between dependent pedal edema which is usually bilateral and unilateral lower extremity edema which could indicate a deep vein thrombosis.

Patients who present with abdominal pain in pregnancy should be assessed for nonpregnancy-related etiologies, including cholelithiasis, nephrolithiasis, gastritis/gastroenteritis, peptic ulcer disease, pelvic vein thrombosis, acute fatty liver, ovarian torsion, and pancreatitis. Patients with lower abdominal pain should be evaluated for PTL, UTI, nephrolithiasis, and diverticulitis.

Patients who present with a new-onset seizure should be considered to be eclamptic when other etiologies have been ruled out, such as drug use, infection, and a history of epilepsy.

DIAGNOSTIC STUDIES

Patients who present with elevated blood pressures should be ruled out for preeclampsia. Patients with malaise, nausea and vomiting, and right upper quadrant pain with or without elevated blood pressure should be ruled out for HELLP syndrome (Table 12.35). The presence or absence of proteinuria can be helpful; please see Exhibit 12.1.

EVALUATION

It is essential to consider the entire clinical picture when evaluating a patient for a hypertensive disorder in pregnancy, including risk factors, trimester at presentation, presence or absence of key findings, and overall hemodynamic and neurologic stability of the patient. The health of the mother and the fetus must be considered, so documentation of fetal well-being is essential. Please see the following section on Treatment for more information on assessing fetal well-being.

TABLE 12.34 Categories of Hypertensive Disorders in Pregnancy

Differential Diagnosis	Description
Chronic hypertension	• BP ≥140/90 mm Hg on two separate occasions without renal or hepatic involvement prior to 20 weeks' gestation OR • Previously diagnosed hypertension prior to conception
Gestational hypertension	• BP ≥140/90 mm Hg on two separate occasions or ≥160/110 mm Hg on one occasion without renal or hepatic involvement
Acute onset severe hypertension	• BP ≥160/110 mm Hg for at least 15 minutes
Preeclampsia without severe features	• BP ≥140/90 mm Hg on two separate occasions or ≥160/110 mm Hg on one occasion with proteinuria OR in the absence or proteinuria: • Platelet count <100 × 10^9/L • Serum creatinine concentration >1.1 mg/dL or doubling of serum creatinine concentration in a patient without underlying renal disease • Doubling of upper limit of normal of hepatic transaminases • Pulmonary edema • Headache without other underlying pathology and unresponsive to acetaminophen
Preeclampsia with severe features	• BP ≥140/90 mm Hg on two separate occasions or ≥160/110 mm Hg on one occasion with proteinuria • Platelet count <100 × 10^9/L • Doubling of upper limit of normal of hepatic transaminases or persistent/severe epigastric or right upper quadrant pain not explained by other diagnoses • Serum creatinine concentration >1.1 mg/dL or doubling of the serum creatinine concentration in a patient without underlying renal disease • Pulmonary edema • Headache without other underlying pathology and unresponsive to acetaminophen • Visual disturbances
Eclampsia	• New-onset seizure in a pregnant patient without a known seizure disorder or underlying pathology
HELLP syndrome	• Platelets <100 × 10^9/L • Lactate dehydrogenase ≥600 IU/L • Aspartate aminotransferase and alanine aminotransferase more than twice the upper limit of normal

BP, blood pressure; HELLP, hemolysis, elevated liver enzymes, low platelets

TABLE 12.35 Diagnostic Studies for Hypertension in Pregnancy

Laboratory Test	Results
Complete blood count	Preeclampsia, HELLP: Thrombocytopenia (platelets <100 × 10^9/L)
24-hour urine protein	Preeclampsia: ≥300 mg/dL
Urine protein/creatinine ratio	Preeclampsia: ≥0.30
Serum creatinine concentration	Preeclampsia: >1.1 mg/dL
Aspartate aminotransferase and alanine aminotransferase	Preeclampsia, HELLP: more than twice the upper limit of normal
Lactate dehydrogenase	HELLP: ≥600 IU/L

HELLP, hemolysis, elevated liver enzymes, low platelets

EXHIBIT 12.1 Proteinuria in Pregnancy

Urine protein ≥300 mg/dL in 24 hours

or

Urine protein to creatinine ratio of ≥0.30

or

2+ protein on urine dipstick if quantitative measures are unavailable

TREATMENT

- Low-dose aspirin (81 mg/day) beginning at 12 weeks' gestation should be used to prevent preeclampsia in pregnant patients with chronic hypertension and who are at high risk for developing preeclampsia.
- Patients with blood pressure ≥160/110 mm Hg in the outpatient setting should be referred to inpatient labor and delivery for prompt administration of an antihypertensive and stat laboratory testing.
- Oral nifedipine, IV labetolol, and IV hydralazine are the recommended antihypertensive medications.
  - Most clinicians will begin outpatient oral antihypertensive therapy if the diastolic blood pressure is ≥150 mm Hg.
- Magnesium sulfate is a neuroprotective medication that should be used in patients with acute severe hypertension and preeclampsia with severe features.
  - Patients who are receiving magnesium sulfate should be routinely checked for magnesium toxicity.
  - Hyporeflexia will be the first sign of mild toxicity; more severe toxic levels are manifested by respiratory depression and eventual cardiac arrest.
- The management strategy for patients with gestational hypertension and chronic hypertension involves several different modalities.
  - Weekly or twice-weekly nonstress tests; weekly blood pressure monitoring; weekly urine protein, platelets, and hepatic transaminases; and ultrasound imaging every 2–3 weeks.
- Patients with preeclampsia without severe features are managed depending on the gestational age and with the following recommendations:
  - Weekly or twice-weekly nonstress tests; weekly blood pressure monitoring; weekly urine protein, platelets, and hepatic transaminases; and ultrasound imaging every 2–3 weeks.
  - If blood pressure is <160/110 mm Hg and without severe features, delivery is indicated when the gestational age is 37 weeks 0 days.
  - Delivery is indicated sooner if patients develop HELLP syndrome; have abnormal ultrasound findings (fetal weight <5th percentile or oligohydramnios); have persistently low BPPs (6/10 or less); other maternal or fetal abnormalities; or rupture of membranes.
- Patients with preeclampsia with severe features are managed in labor and delivery with the following recommendations.
  - All patients should be given appropriate antihypertensive therapy and seizure prophylaxis with magnesium sulfate.
  - Patients who are <34 weeks' gestation with severe features should receive continuous fetal monitoring, maternal blood pressure and urine output monitoring, corticosteroid administration, and laboratory evaluation for renal function and the development of HELLP.
  - Patients ≥-34 weeks 0 days should be considered for delivery following a course of antenatal corticosteroids if not yet administered or immediate delivery if there is evidence of fetal distress, ruptured membranes, oliguria, serum creatinine of ≥1.5 mg/dL, pulmonary edema, HELLP syndrome, eclampsia, platelets of fewer than 100 × 10^9/L, coagulopathy, or placental abruption.
- Patients who are eclamptic must receive supportive care, including ensuring adequate oxygenation and minimizing physical harm to the patient.
  - Magnesium sulfate will not arrest the seizure activity but will help prevent further seizures. In refractory cases, or when patients are significantly agitated, the addition of clonazepam, diazepam, or midazolam may be considered.
  - Other important interventions include continuing antihypertensive therapy and evaluating the patient for immediate delivery.
- Patients who develop HELLP syndrome will need to be delivered regardless of gestational age.

PATIENT EDUCATION

- Pregnant patients with a history of a hypertensive disorder in a previous pregnancy may experience it again.
  - Patients at risk should begin taking 81 mg aspirin daily beginning at 12 weeks' gestation.
- Patients who are treated as an outpatient should monitor fetal movements daily and report any new occurrences, such as vision changes, changes in headache intensity and frequency, swelling, abdominal pain, malaise, nausea, vomiting, shortness of breath, and chest pain.
- Preeclampsia and eclampsia can occur during the postpartum period, so close follow-up is essential, including a blood pressure check within 72 hours of hospital discharge.
- Patients with a history of a hypertensive disorder of pregnancy are more likely to develop CVD later in life; risk modification strategies and consistent follow-up is advised.

- Annual blood pressure screenings, lipid evaluations, weight monitoring, and glucose monitoring are often initiated.

12.12B GESTATIONAL DIABETES

DM diagnosed during pregnancy is termed GDM and is a growing epidemic in the United States and globally. This phenomenon is believed to be associated with the growing obesity epidemic. Worldwide, approximately 16.5% pregnancies are affected by GDM.[114]

Normally, pregnancy is considered a diabetogenic state.[69] The purpose of this state is to provide availability of serum glucose to the fetus for development. Exact pathophysiology of GDM is unknown; however, maternal chronic insulin resistance with more acute impairment of the pancreatic beta-cells during pregnancy is thought to be a contributing factor.[114]

All pregnant patients should be routinely screened for GDM. Those at high risk or with risks associated with DM type 2 criteria will require early screening for overt DM type 2. The risk stratification can be based on the same risks for GDM or the ADA criteria for overt DM (see Box 12.2). The most notable risk factors are a personal history of GDM, macrosomia in previous pregnancies, obesity, advanced maternal age, a prepregnancy insulin resistance disposition, hypertension, PCOS, history of CVD, high-risk ethnicity (i.e., African American, Latino, Native American, Asian American, Pacific Islander), and family history of any form of diabetes. Research is active in this area with an association noted between processed meats, high protein diets, and GDM.[88,89,114]

Screening for GDM is crucial in the detection of those at risk; often GDM is asymptomatic or glycosuria may be the only sign or symptom present. If a patient is at high risk for GDM, she should be screened early in pregnancy for overt DM type 2. Overt DM screening should be arranged at the initial OB visit. There are several options for screening:

- Random or fasting serum glucose
- Early glucose tolerance testing as outlined in Box 12.3
- HbA1c level

There are different positive criteria for all options. If any are positive, the patient has overt DM type 2. If the screenings are negative, routine prenatal GDM screenings should be resumed. Routine screening takes place around the late second and early third trimesters with two options outlined in Box 12.3. If the patient does not pass the screening test, a follow-up diagnostic test must be completed. This is typically a 3-hour 100-g glucose loading diagnostic test in which the patient has a fasting serum glucose level tested followed by drinking a 100-g glucose load beverage. Serial serum glucose levels are then drawn every hour × 3. If positive, the patient is diagnosed with GDM. In conjunction to GDM screening, if a patient presents at the initial prenatal visit with signs or symptoms of diabetes, the ADA diagnosis criteria for DM in nonpregnant adults may be used to diagnose overt diabetes in early pregnancy.[88,89]

Women diagnosed with overt diabetes in early pregnancy can be managed similarly to women with pregestational (preexisting) diabetes. If GDM is left untreated there can be significant maternal and fetal consequences. These include increased macrosomia, preeclampsia, polyhydramnios, stillbirth, neonatal morbidity, and long-term maternal CVD risk, diabetes risk, and for child metabolic syndrome and obesity.[88,89,114]

GDM treatment should include consultation with a maternal fetal medicine specialist or an endocrinologist. Good glycemic control is the key to reducing risk of maternal and fetal morbidity and mortality. GDM management is multifactorial and includes glucose monitoring, nutrition therapy, exercise, and, if necessary, insulin. Routine antenatal fetal testing with nonstress test and amniotic fluid index or BPP should be implemented.

In a patient with GDM, delivery timing depends on several factors including overall glycemic control of mother, planned mode of delivery (i.e., cesarean section, vaginal delivery), fetal well-being based on fetal movement and antenatal testing, and gestational size.[88,115]

Following labor and delivery, hyperglycemic effects decrease rapidly and most patients are able to resume a normal diet. To monitor for patients with occult type 2 DM, the Endocrine Society recommends patients continue to check glucose concentrations for 24 to 72 hours postpartum and treat as necessary. Patients with normal fasting postpartum glucose levels should be screened with a 2-hour glucose 75-g oral tolerance test between 4 and 12 weeks' gestation. These patients will carry a lifelong risk of diabetes and, according to the ADA, should be screened every 3 years.[88,115]

12.12C ABORTIONS

Stephanie Elko

There are different types of abortions—spontaneous/missed and induced (or pregnancy termination). Both carry their own risks, workup, and treatment recommendations. WHO has an open-access website to help patients and clinicians locate a safe place to obtain induced abortions.

A spontaneous or missed abortion—also termed a miscarriage by British clinicians in the late twentieth century—is the presence of a nonviable embryo or fetus prior to 20 weeks' gestation.[116] Spontaneous or missed abortions can be further delineated into inevitable, incomplete, and complete. An inevitable abortion is diagnosed when the cervical os is dilated and abdominal pain or vaginal bleeding is present before 20 weeks' gestation. A partial or incomplete abortion is diagnosed when the cervical os is dilated, there is abdominal pain or vaginal bleeding present, and some products of conception have passed through os before 20 weeks' gestation. A complete abortion occurs when the cervical os is closed, there is abdominal pain or vaginal bleeding, and all products of conception have passed before 20 weeks' gestation. Often history alone can decipher if the miscarriage is incomplete or complete, but lab tests and imaging may be used for further determination if necessary. For example, if a woman has a known early pregnancy followed by a period of heavy bleeding and possible tissue passage with cessation of bleeding and is now asymptomatic, the patient is likely experiencing a complete spontaneous abortion. However, if the patient continues to have symptoms and/or bleeding, or if no heavy bleeding or passage of tissue has occurred, the patient may be experiencing a missed or incomplete abortion. These situations require further workup to diagnose. A frequently used tool in these situations is the TVU. TVU can determine an intrauterine pregnancy and, depending upon the gestational age, if a heartbeat is present. Fetal heartbeats can start to be seen between 5 and 6 weeks' gestational age but may not appear until 7 weeks. Another monitoring option is to obtain serial hCG levels, usually weekly, until either progression of a viable pregnancy occurs or a decrease in serum hCG with an eventual return to prepregnancy levels returns. Decreasing serum hCG in early pregnancy is abnormal and signifies a missed abortion. The hCG should be followed back down to the prepregnancy range, or if there is no sign of bleeding or the patient desires faster resolution of missed abortion, a suction dilation and curettage (D&C) can be performed. D&C also allows for the fetal tissue to be sent for pathology. Some clinicians will still have patients follow up for a final hCG to assure complete resolution.

Maternal risk factors for pregnancy loss include the African American race, advanced maternal age, low socioeconomic status, cigarette smoking during pregnancy, maternal comorbid conditions (e.g., DM, hypertension, thyroid disease, inherited thrombophilia, and obesity), multiple gestations of triplets plus, intrauterine device in place, acute and chronic stress, specific medication and substance abuse, and previous pregnancy loss.[117,118] It should be noted that up to 70% of spontaneous abortions occur due to a chromosomal abnormality, and to a much lesser extent due to material anatomic anomalies and significant trauma.[118]

Treatment options are dependent on the abortion type (incomplete or complete) and the preference of the clinician and patient. Complete expulsion of products should be documented by histology. If there is any concern of retained products of conception, intervention by follow-up surgical removal or serial hCG monitoring until negative if the patient declines surgical intervention is recommended. If at any point an hCG level is exponentially high for the gestational age, remains unchanged, or continues to rise despite an identified nonviable pregnancy, GTD must be ruled out.

12.12D ECTOPIC PREGNANCY

Stephanie Elko

An ectopic pregnancy is defined as a pregnancy that implants and develops outside the uterus and is thus a nonviable pregnancy. Ectopic pregnancies occur in about 1 in 50 pregnancies, with the vast majority located in the fallopian tubes. If left untreated, the result could have significant maternal morbidity and even death. The major risk factor for ectopic pregnancy is a history of fallopian tube disruption, including previous ectopic pregnancies, history of sexually transmitted infection or PID, and history of surgery in areas surrounding the fallopian tube.[120]

Typically, patients will present with abdominal pain and cramping, either with known or unknown pregnancy, and may also have associated bleeding. In all patients of reproductive age, a pregnancy test should be performed, even if at low risk for pregnancy with contraception use. An ectopic pregnancy may delay the detection of hCG, leading to false negative urine pregnancy tests. The general consensus is that by an hCG level of approximately 2,000 IU, an intrauterine pregnancy should be identifiable on ultrasound. If an ectopic pregnancy is suspected, an ultrasound should be performed to determine the anatomic location of the pregnancy.[120]

If an ectopic pregnancy is confirmed, the management should be based on gestational age, anatomic location, and maternal symptoms. A ruptured ectopic pregnancy can be life-threatening for the mother. There are three options available to patients with an ectopic pregnancy. The first is a surgical option, in which the products of conception are removed; if located in the fallopian tube, the tube may also be removed while the ovary is often spared. The second option is a medication-induced termination, usually performed with methotrexate (MTX). The third option is expectant management. If the medication termination or the expectant management are chosen, then patients should have their hCG levels monitored until negative to assure expulsion of products of conception to avoid infection and further complications.[121] Each case is managed differently, and all three options may not be viable for every patient.

12.12E GESTATIONAL TROPHOBLASTIC DISEASE

GTD consists of aberrant placenta trophoblast cellular proliferations on a spectrum of premalignant to malignant. The premalignant type is the hydatidiform mole, or molar pregnancy. Molar pregnancies were first described around 400 BCE as "dropsy of the uterus" by Hippocrates.[121] Molar pregnancies can be either partial or complete. Delineation is based on the patients' clinical presentation, chromosomal patterns, and histopathology. Partial molar pregnancies generally have lower hCG levels and have a triploid karyotype while complete molar pregnancies have a marked high level of hCG and the majority consist of absent or inactive maternal chromosomes.[122,123]

The incidence of molar pregnancies has been difficult to ascertain given the low and globally sporadic incidence. However, risk factors are known to include extremes in maternal age (≤15 or ≥35 years old) and a history of previous molar pregnancy. Furthermore, the New England Trophoblastic Disease Center (NETDC) data reveal complete molar pregnancies were greater in Asians than other ethnicities. Patients will often present with typical early pregnancy complaints, such as pelvic pressure, vaginal bleeding, and nausea and/or vomiting. On examination, uterine enlargement may be noted. If a molar pregnancy is suspected, serum hCG level should be obtained along with a TVU. A complete molar pregnancy is easier to confirm, as the corresponding hCG level is typically exponentially higher than with a viable pregnancy. Ultrasound findings of a molar pregnancy are often described as a "snowstorm pattern" or "grape-like cysts" without the visualization of a fetus.

All patients with molar pregnancies should have blood type and crossmatch obtained and be screened for complications, such as anemia, preeclampsia, and hyperthyroidism. Patients who are Rh negative should receive RhoGAM. The treatment is surgical removal of the mass, ideally by suction evacuation and curettage over hysterectomy to preserve the ability to become pregnant again. Furthermore, the hCG level should be monitored weekly to until it returns to prepregnancy levels.

The second type of GTD consists of gestational trophoblastic neoplasms (GTN). These malignant neoplasms comprise abnormal cellular proliferations and include invasive mole, choriocarcinoma, placental site trophoblastic tumor (PSTT), and epithelioid trophoblastic tumor (ETT). The GTN have the ability to act as other invasive neoplasms leading to progression, invasion, and metastases. GNT have a high mortality rate if not identified and treated appropriately.[123,124]

Choriocarcinoma has been known to occur with any pregnancy event but is most common following complete molar pregnancies. Approximately 50% of choriocarcinomas arise from hydatidiform moles, albeit only a small number of molar pregnancies progress into choriocarcinoma. Of the other 50%, approximately 25% follow abortion or ectopic tubal pregnancies and approximately 25% follow preterm or term gestation. Choriocarcinomas are invasive and commonly metastasizes to the lungs, brain, liver, pelvis and vagina, intestines, and spleen.

PSTT is a rare tumor that generally follows nonmolar gestations and is less invasive than choriocarcinoma. The most common metastatic site is lymphatic. The ETT is a rare variant of PSTT and presents some years after a full-term delivery.[123]

GTN risk factors match those of the hydatidiform mole pregnancies. The clinical presentations are similar, but may also include symptoms arising from metastatic disease sites. Diagnosis is clinical with a positive hCG level that corresponds with disease extent. Pathology will confirm the diagnosis.[123]

The American Joint Committee of Cancer, the FIGO, and WHO have all created systems for low- and high-risk GTN stratification. Most often FIGO and WHO systems are used to designate GTN into low or high risk, and treatment is based on these.[124] In general, GTN is highly sensitive to chemotherapy. In accordance with the National Comprehensive Cancer Network (NCCN) and FIGO guidelines, low-risk GTNs should be treated with a single-agent chemotherapy, usually MTX or dactinomycin. Low-risk GTNs are often cured with survival rates reaching 100%, although to reach this rate, additional treatment regimens may be necessary.[125] Treatment of high-risk GTNs, based on FIGO and WHO risk scores, includes combination chemotherapy. However, PSTT and ETT have higher resistance to chemotherapy, leading primary treatment to include a combination of surgery and chemotherapy. Pending response rates, radiation therapy; may be necessary, in addition to chemotherapy, for all GTN patients there should be posttreatment surveillance of hCG levels, at least monthly, until negative and for 12 months thereafter.[125] The patient should be using reliable contraception during this time.

12.12F Rh INCOMPATIBILITY

Rhesus (Rh) D antigen is a protein that may or may not be on erythrocyte surfaces. When the antigen is present, the patient is Rh positive, while when the antigen is absent, the patient is Rh negative. Rh D is inherited, so if both parents are negative, the offspring will be negative, while if both are positive, the offspring will be positive. If the Rh D antigen is different between maternal and paternal, the offspring could be either Rh D-positive or Rh D-negative.

During pregnancy, maternal and fetal circulation remain separate although there can be exposure of maternal blood and fetal blood in certain events, such as hemorrhage or invasive genetic testing. If the maternal blood is Rh D-positive, because the antigen is already present in the blood, no immune response will be elicited. Complications may occur if the maternal blood is Rh D-negative and exposed to fetal blood that is Rh D-positive, due to the maternal creation of Rh D antibodies. When this occurs, the maternal blood begins building antibodies to the new "foreign" Rh D antigen as an immune response. This causes little harm during the current pregnancy; however, subsequent exposures may elicit a maternal immune response to "attack" the foreign Rh D antigen if the fetus is Rh D positive. When maternal antibodies are created it is termed alloimmunization.[126] Other types of alloimmunization exist, but Rh D is the most common.

In the United States since 1970s, the administration of a preventive dose of Rh D immune globulin, or anti-D immune globulin, has significantly reduced the incidence of alloimmunization from about 13% to 16% to 0.5% to 1.8%.[126] In countries where prophylaxis dose is not provided, high fetal morbidity and mortality rates are still seen. In countries using prophylactic Rh D immune globulin, the primary reason for continued alloimmunization is the failure to follow routine antepartum administration guidelines. A sensitizing event is any event in which alloimmunization has potential to occur in an Rh D-negative patient due to cross contamination of fetal and maternal blood. Some common sensitizing events are laid out in Box 12.7. If any of these events occur, Rh D immune globulin should be given within 72 hours. In the United States the standard of care is to administer anti-D immune globulin at 28 weeks' gestation for every Rh D-negative woman with a second dose following delivery after the newborn's Rh D typing is available. The typical anti-D immuneglobulin dose is 300 mcg, given as an IM injection.[126] According to the manufacturers of the anti-D immune globulin drug, the prophylactic period is 12 weeks. Therefore, the patient should have readministration of anti-D immuneglobulin every 12 weeks if a possible sensitizing event has, or will, occur during the remainder of that pregnancy.

If there is uncertainty surrounding a sensitization event, a screening test for fetal-maternal hemorrhage can be performed. If maternal anti-D immuneglobulin antibodies are present in the maternal circulation, subsequent pregnancies may be at risk. These pregnancies will require an obstetrician, and ideally a maternal-fetal medicine specialist, to monitor the fetus throughout the pregnancy. The antibodies can cross the placenta and opsonize the fetal erythrocytes. Results of alloimmunization include hemolytic disease of the fetus and newborn (hydrops fetalis).[127]

ACOG summary of recommendations for the administration of anti-D immuneglobulin are based on scientific evidence that all Rh D-negative patients should be offered anti-D immune globulin at 28 weeks' gestational age and again within 72 hours following the birth of a Rh D-positive infant or possible exposure from a traumatic event such as a fall. Furthermore, anti-D immune globulin should be given to all women with unknown Rh D sensitization.[126]

BOX 12.7 Potential Rh D Sensitizing Events

Abortions (missed, complete, incomplete, induced at any gestational age)
Ectopic pregnancy
Diagnostic fetal genetic testing (amniocentesis, chorionic villus sampling, cordocentesis)
Antepartum hemorrhage for any reason (e.g., placenta abruption)
Intrauterine fetal death
External cephalic version
Delivery

Source: Data from Practice bulletin no. 181: prevention of Rh D alloimmunization. Obstet Gynecol. *2017;130(2):e57–e70. doi:10.1097/AOG.0000000000002232*

12.12G PRETERM LABOR

Preterm birth is the most common obstetric complication leading to antenatal hospitalization and the leading cause of neonatal death.[128] Of preterm births, 40% to 50% are accompanied by PTL, while 20% to 30% have PPROM, and a small percentage are a result of cervical insufficiency. The remaining are due to iatrogenic reasons related to maternal or fetal complications that lead to either spontaneous or clinician-initiated preterm delivery.[129]

Accurately identifying true labor can be challenging at any point during pregnancy. ACOG defines PTL as the initial presentation of a patient with uterine contractions and at least a 2-cm dilation of the cervix, or consistent or regular contractions that produce cervical change, the latter requiring monitoring. Preterm birth is considered birth that takes place between 20 $^0/_7$ weeks of gestation to 36 $^6/_7$ weeks of gestation. Approximately 50% of patients presumed to be in PTL end up delivering at term without any tocolytic intervention. Patients who present with clinical criteria for PTL and deliver within 1 week make up <10% to 13%.[128,130]

No one process is known to trigger PTL, though it may be initiated if any of the following four process are disrupted[129,130]:

- Premature activation of the neuroendocrine stress axis response (either maternal or fetal)
- An inflammatory or infectious process
- Hemorrhage of the decidua
- Pathologic uterine distention

There are numerous risk factors for PTL but many patients have PTL who do not have any known risk factors.[129,131] Box 12.8 outlines a few common PTL risk factors.

CLINICAL PRESENTATION

PTL is often evaluated in a labor and delivery unit in the hospital, or a specific triage center for labor and delivery. Typically, cervical ripening, or cervical changes in preparation for delivery, occurs over days to weeks. True labor cervical change occurs more rapidly and can occur in minutes.

BOX 12.8 Common Preterm Labor Risk Factors

Infection (e.g., UTI, STIs, BV, trichomoniasis)
Vaginal bleeding
Maternal comorbitidies (e.g., high BP, diabetes, coagulopathies, smoking, alcohol, or drug use)
Maternal age and weight extremes, either under or over
Maternal ethnicities (e.g., African American)
Maternal socioeconomic issues (e.g., stress, domestic violence, lack of support, late onset prenatal care)
In vitro fertilization pregnancy
Short interval pregnancies
Certain high-risk pregnancy complications (e.g., placenta previa, increased uterine rupture risk)

BP, blood pressure; BV, bacterial vaginosis; STI, sexually transmitted infection; UTI, urinary tract infection

Source: Data from Robinson JN, Norwitz ER. Preterm birth: risk factors, interventions for risk reduction, and maternal prognosis. In: Post TW, ed. UpToDate. *UpToDate; 2019. https://www.uptodate.com/preterm birth: risk factors, interventions for risk reduction, and maternal prognosis; Eunice Kennedy Shriver National Institute of Child Health and Human Development. What are the risk factors for preterm labor and birth. https://www.nichd.nih.gov/health/topics/preterm/conditioninfo/who_risk*

SIGNS AND SYMPTOMS

- Contractions, either regular or irregular
- Abdominal cramping, often lower abdomen or menstrual-like
- Low back pain
- Increasing pelvic pressure, usually explained as "feeling like the baby will fall out"
- Vaginal discharge change
  - Continuous trickle of clear fluid or a large fluid gush
  - Vaginal bleeding
  - New onset or significant discharge

When a patient presents with the PTL symptoms it is important to review her history for past history of PTL and current comorbid diagnoses that could increase her PTL risk. The gestational age will also help guide risks of possible etiologies and interventions that may need to be taken.

DIAGNOSTIC STUDIES

No one test will diagnose PTL, but several exams and evaluations may help lead to the clinical diagnosis. The patient's history may provide clues to possible etiologies and therefore may guide the tests collected. For instance, if infection is suspected a urinalysis with culture should be obtained along with sexually transmitted disease panel and BV and *Candida* evaluation. If a risk of drug use is suspected, a toxicology screen should be collected.

The speculum examination helps the clinician not only visualize the cervix and surrounding tissue, but also to obtain swabs for possible infection or a fetal fibronectin (fFN) test. The fFN is a protein present at the connection point of the decidua and chorion. If there is disturbance of this interface, fFN will secrete into the vaginal vault and may be detected. If fFN is present, there is an increased risk of PTL in the next 2 weeks. Several factors can lead to false positives, particularly if there has been any act causing disruption to the cervix within the previous 24 hours, including sexual intercourse, digital cervical examination, or TVU.

Following the speculum exam, a digital cervical examination should be performed to assess the cervical length, effacement, consistency, and position. This examination may identify those that fall into the group of PTL with cervical dilation and presence of consistent contractions. PTL patients who are found to have cervical dilation of >3 cm are less likely to respond to PTL cessation interventions.

Ultrasound may also be a supporting tool in the diagnosis of PTL. TVU is a helpful support tool for the diagnosis of PTL. All women with a cervical length that is <3 cm before 34 weeks have an increased risk of preterm birth. Cervical length of ≥3 cm has a negative predictive value of for preterm birth.[130] An obstetric ultrasound examination may also be helpful as it can provide the assessment of the fetal anatomy, position, and weight; maternal and placental abnormalities; and amniotic fluid volume.

Currently, much research is underway surrounding the vaginal microbiome and relation to PTL. It appears the vaginal flora may change during pregnancy to help protect against bacterial associated with PTL.[130]

MANAGEMENT

Before intervention begins the PTL etiology, gestational age, fetal viability, and maternal status and well-being need to be considered. ACOG continually publishes updates on PTL interventions based on new research and expert opinion.

General approaches are based on gestational age and outlined in Table 12.36. If PPROM is present, antibiotic use may be necessary. Bed rest and hydration have also been shown to be ineffective in preventing preterm birth, though the evidence is limited and needs further research.[128]

Cervical Insufficiency

According to ACOG, the definition of cervical insufficiency is the "inability of the uterine cervix to retain a pregnancy in the absence of the signs and symptoms of clinical contractions or labor, or both, in the second trimester."[132] Cervical insufficiency pathophysiology remains obscure, but risk factors are known. The biggest risk factor is a history of cervical trauma, often from previous cervical procedures such as conization, loop electrosurgical excision, rapid mechanical dilating the cervical os, or injury from childbirth. Other less common risk factors include congenital anomalies affecting the cervix, such as mullein anomalies, connective tissue anomalies, or in utero exposure to DES.[133]

Patients with cervical insufficiency are often asymptomatic or have very few, mild symptoms. Symptoms may be of mild pelvic pressure, cramping, low back discomfort, or color change or increase in vaginal discharge during the early second trimester. The diagnosis is clinically based and often challenging without TVU availability. The hallmark of an incompetent cervix patient is a history of two or more consecutive second or extremely early third trimester pregnancy losses without signs or symptoms of labor or other identifiable etiologies for loss.[132,133] If a physical examination is completed, the clinician may note cervical effacement and/or dilation. If not overtly seen, the findings may be elicited from pelvic pressure or Valsalva maneuvers. A TVU can confirm the diagnosis or assist in the finding of an incompetent cervix. A cervix that measures <25 mm before 24 weeks' gestation via TVU may be associated with cervical insufficiency but is not diagnostic without a history of preterm birth or loss.[132]

Management of patients with cervical insufficiency should be based on the patient's history, physical exam finding, as well as mode of diagnosis. The options for management for singleton pregnancies are:

- Monitoring with serial TVU, followed by more invasive treatments as necessary
- Vaginal or IM progesterone supplementation
- Cervical cerclage placement, with or without the above

Despite the patient history, a cervical cerclage placement should be considered if TVU notes cervical funneling or a very short cervix of <10 mm. Cervical cerclage should not be placed if the finding was incidental on TVU and the patient has no risk factors or history of preterm birth, or if the pregnancy has multiple gestation. These patients may be treated with vaginal progesterone alone. Furthermore, a cerclage should not be placed if there are any risks for infection or labor signs/symptoms have begun.[132,133]

12.12H PRETERM PRELABOR RUPTURE OF MEMBRANES

CLINICAL MANIFESTATIONS, DIAGNOSIS, AND MANAGEMENT

There are many reasons membranes rupture during pregnancy, including the normal progression of pregnancy and onset of labor. Preterm rupture of membranes (PROM) refers to an episode of membranes rupture that occurs prior to the onset of labor, whereas preterm prelabor rupture of membranes (PPROM) refers to episodes of membrane rupture before 37 weeks' gestation and prior to onset of labor.[134] Approximately one-third of preterm births is associated with PPROM.[135]

PPROM often occurs without any noted patient risks. However, associated risks have included intra-amniotic infection, short cervical length, second and/or third trimester bleeding, maternal low BMI, cigarette smoking, illicit drug use, and low socioeconomic status. Irrespective of clinical presentation and risks, at least 50% of PPROM patients deliver within 1 week of membrane rupture. Furthermore, the latency period (the time from membrane rupture to labor) is inversely related to the gestational age at time of rupture.[134]

DIFFERENTIAL DIAGNOSIS

Differential diagnosis includes urinary incontinence, increased vaginal secretions associated with pregnancy, increase

TABLE 12.36 General Approaches to Preterm Labor Based on Gestational Age

Gestational Age	Intervention	Reasoning	Timing
23 weeks	Corticosteroids, single dose	Decreased risk of respiratory distress syndrome and necrotizing enterocolitis	If at risk of delivery within 7 days
24–34 weeks	Corticosteroids, single dose	Decreased risk of respiratory distress syndrome and necrotizing enterocolitis	If at risk of delivery within 7 days. OK to repeat dose if previous dose was 14 days earlier. Rescue dose may be given if last was 7 days prior in certain clinical situations.
24–34 weeks	First-line tocolytics (beta-adrenergic agonist therapy, calcium channel blockers, or NSAIDs)	For short-term pregnancy prolongation (up to 48 hours) to allow antenatal steroids	
<32 weeks	Magnesium sulfate	Neuroprotection, reduces risk of cerebral palsy	

NSAIDs, nonsteroidal anti-inflammatory drugs.

Source: Data from American College of Obstetricians and Gynecologists Committee on Practice Bulletins—Obstetrics. Practice bulletin no. 171: management of preterm labor. Obstet Gynecol. *2016;128(4):e155–e164. doi:10.1097/AOG.0000000000001711; Robinson JN, Norwitz ER. Preterm birth: risk factors, interventions for risk reduction, and maternal prognosis. In: Post TW, ed.* UpTo-Date. *UpToDate; 2019. https://www.uptodate.com/preterm birth: risk factors, interventions for risk reduction, and maternal prognosis; Lockwood CJ. Preterm labor: clinical findings, diagnostic evaluation, and initial treatment. In: Post TW, ed.* UpToDate. *UpToDate; 2019. https://www.uptodate.com/preterm labor: clinical findings, diagnostic evaluation, and initial treatment*

discharge production in the presence of vaginal infection, and exogenous fluids (semen or from douching).

DIAGNOSTIC STUDIES

PPROM can be diagnosed by patient history and physical examination. Patients will often report fluid "gushes" or continuous leaking. If suspected, sterile speculum exam is recommended, as digital examination may increase risk of infection. On exam a direct visualization of cervical os fluid leaking or vaginal vault pooling at the posterior fornix may be seen. Analysis includes nitrazine testing, which uses pH to distinguish between amniotic fluid and other fluids (specifically urine and vaginal secretions). This is performed by placing a nitrazine test strip on the speculum used for the examination. Based on the vaginal fluids present the nitrazine test will remain yellow or change to blue if the pH is >6.0. Amniotic fluid pH is approximately 7.0, urine around 6.0, and vaginal secretions around 3 to 4.0; therefore, a blue test strip indicated the presence of amniotic fluid.

The fern test is another test for amniotic fluid presence and is more reliable than the nitrazine test. For this examination, a small amount of the speculum fluid can be placed on a slide and allowed to dry at room air. Once dry, the sodium chloride in the amniotic fluid takes on a fern-like pattern, with multiple fine branches, whereas cervical mucus has a thick appearance and does not produce this fern pattern.

Ultrasonography may also help guide the diagnosis. Specifically, ultrasound can look for oligohydramnios. As with all diagnostic tests, none are specific for PPROM, and therefore, none are 100% accurate. However, with the help of multiple tests and a patient history and/or physical exam consistent for PPROM, the diagnosis can be made.[100]

MANAGEMENT

Management of PPROM is dependent on gestational age.

- PPROM before 22 to 24 weeks' gestation is often associated with higher risk of perinatal death, as well as pulmonary hypoplasia and fetal deformations. This is often a result of prolonged oligohydramnios. Maternal complications within this time frame include intra-amniotic infection, endometritis, placental abruption, and retained placenta. A discussion with the patient regarding expectant delivery versus induction should occur. Antibiotics may be considered. Before viability GBS, corticosteroids, magnesium sulfate, and tocolysis are not recommended.[134,135]
- PPROM that occurs between 24 and 33 6/7 weeks of gestation (preterm) should include expectant management, antibiotics if latency is prolonged and if no contradictions, single course steroids, and GBS prophylaxis as indicated.[134,135]
- PPROM between 34 and 36 6/7 weeks of gestation (late preterm) follows the same guidelines as PROM.
- PROM 37+ weeks' gestation should proceed to delivery and follow GBS routine guidelines.[134,135]

The most common maternal complication is infection, which can occur in up to one-quarter of PPROM patients. The earlier the gestational age at time of PPROM, the higher the risk of infection. The primary fetal risk is prematurity, specifically respiratory immaturity, and to lesser extent risks of sepsis, intraventricular hemorrhage, and necrotizing enterocolitis.[134,135]

12.12I ABRUPTIO PLACENTAE

Placental abruption, or abruptio placentae, although an infrequent complication, is one of the leading causes of maternal morbidity and perinatal mortality.[136] The *American Journal of Obstetrics and Gynecology* defines placental abruption as the "premature separation of the implanted placenta before the delivery of the fetus."[136,137] The uterine muscle is relatively pliable; however, the placenta is not. Separation occurs when the placenta begins to come apart from the uterine wall. The separation that occurs can be discussed by extent, partial or complete, and delineated by location within the uterus. It can also be a closed or open system of bleeding, depending if the bleeding is concealed and contained within the uterus or if there is an opening allowing blood to drain out, thereby causing vaginal bleeding. Placental abruption most often occurs before 37 weeks' gestation. The etiology remains unknown, but strong risk factors have been identified, as outlined below[136,138]:

- Maternal history
  - Smoking
  - Cocaine use during pregnancy
  - Advanced maternal age
  - Hypertension, chronic
  - History of previous pregnancy with placental ischemic event/disease
    - Previous placental abruption (high risk factor for recurrence)
    - Fetal growth restriction
    - Preeclampsia
- Current pregnancy event
  - Multiple gestations
  - Polyhydramnios
  - Pregnancy-induced hypertension, preeclampsia, eclampsia
  - Latent premature rupture of membranes
  - Chorioamnionitis
- Acute events
  - Abdominal trauma
    - Motor vehicle accidents
    - Lap seatbelt injury
    - Falls
    - Domestic violence

When the placenta separates or detaches from the uterus it leads to vascular disruption of the structures that deliver oxygen and nutrients to the fetus, thereby leading to fetal/neonatal compromise, asphyxia, and possibly death. Maternal complications include significant uterine hemorrhage, bleeding disorders such as disseminated intravascular coagulopathy, postpartum pituitary gland necrosis, and death.[136]

Diagnosis of placental abruption is made clinically. Clinical signs and symptoms may vary depending on extent and location of placental separation, as described above. Often placental abruption has a rapid onset. Painful vaginal bleeding in the third trimester is the most common complaint and may be mild to severe; uterine contraction may be present. The uterus becomes tender despite contraction presence. Fetal compromise is seen as heart rate abnormalities, or the absence of FHTs with fetal demise. It should be noted that if there are FHT abnormalities and a tender uterus and discomfort, despite the presence of vaginal bleeding, placental abruption should be considered due to the possibility of a concealed bleed. Diagnostic studies may help support the diagnosis, specifically the presence of a hematoma on ultrasound.[138]

DIFFERENTIAL DIAGNOSIS

The differential diagnosis includes placenta previa, PTL, and uterine rupture.

MANAGEMENT/TREATMENT

Management of placental abruption will depend on the extent and location. All patients need a blood type and screen at diagnosis, given the high probability of blood transfusion. Maternal vital signs should be monitored closely, and fluids administered. Expectant management may be appropriate for mild to moderate bleeding and preterm gestation, but delivery is recommended for severe abruption and/or hemorrhage. Rarely a condition called uteroplacental apoplexy, or Couvelaire uterus, is seen upon cesarean section with severe placental abruptions. This condition occurs when the peritoneal cavity serosa turns blue or purple in color due to the penetration of blood through the uterine wall from the placental abruption.[138]

12.12J PLACENTA PREVIA

Placenta previa is defined as placental location over the internal os of the cervix, whereas a low-lying placenta occurs when the placenta is not covering the os, but the placental edge is within 2 cm of the internal cervical os. Often patients are asymptomatic and it is found incidentally on routine prenatal ultrasound. Some patients may experience painless vaginal bleeding.

DIAGNOSTIC STUDIES

Diagnosis is made by ultrasound with direct visualization of the placenta over the internal os. If found early in pregnancy, it is reasonable to monitor for placenta movement up the uterine wall as the pregnancy progresses. Conversely, if diagnosed later in pregnancy, the chances of placenta movement decrease.

Placenta previa is associated with placenta previa-accreta, fetal malpresentation, vasa previa, and velamentous umbilical cord. Placenta previa-accreta occurs when the patient has placenta previa and the placenta tissue invades into the uterine myometrium. This should be considered upon diagnosis of placenta previa, especially in women with previous cesarean sections.[139]

Management of placenta previa begins with the assessment of the patient and her symptoms. If a patient is asymptomatic, monitoring for placental position movement with ultrasound and reducing risk of bleeding are main goals. Anecdotal expertise, which research has neither supported nor refuted, has led to patients being advised to begin "pelvic rest" to reduce the risk of hemorrhage. Pelvic rest is just a term to recommend that patient avoid behaviors that could disrupt the cervix and potentially induce bleeding. These include digital cervical exams, penetrative sexual activity, particularly with orgasm, moderate to strenuous exercise, lifting >20 pounds, and prolonged periods of standing. If placenta previa remains as the pregnancy progresses, comorbid conditions (e.g., placenta accreta) should be identified, and cesarean delivery should become the management strategy.[140]

If the patient is having acute bleeding associated with placenta previa, the main goal should be to stabilize the mother, monitor the fetus, and transfuse as necessary. Indications for cesarean delivery include:

- Active labor
- Nonreassuring fetal tracing despite resuscitative interventions
- Severe and persistent vaginal bleeding, when maternal stability cannot be attended despite intervention, or severe vaginal bleeding after 34 weeks' gestation[140]

In preparation of delivery, magnesium sulfate for neuroprotection and, depending upon the gestational age at the time of labor or presence of vaginal bleeding, corticosteroids for fetal lung maternity may be advised. Tocolytic agents have not shown a benefit for the management of placenta previa and may cause harm if uterine contractions are ceased with promotion of placental separation and bleeding. Therefore, the use should be weighed on an individual basis.[139]

12.12K POSTPARTUM HEMORRHAGE

Worldwide, PPH remains the leading cause of material mortality. ACOG reVITALize programs refers to PPH as the occurrence of ≥1,000 mL cumulative blood loss, or symptomatic hypovolemia accompanied by blood loss, that occurs within 24 hours following the birth process.[141] In 2017 ACOG updated this definition, while continuing to state that a vaginal delivery blood loss >500 mL cumulatively within 24 hours following a vaginal delivery is considered abnormal and needs further investigation for etiologies.[142] Furthermore, if a patient's hematocrit is <22% or Hb is <7 g/dL the patient requires intervention.[98]

In the postpartum period, upon placental separation, hemostasis is regulated by a combination myometrium contractions and local clotting factors. When either of these mechanisms are disrupted, PPH has potential to occur. The most frequent etiology is uterine atony, either focal or diffuse, followed by trauma ensued during the birthing process and coagulopathies or other bleeding disorders.

Table 12.37 outlines PPH etiologies in relation to risk factors followed by evaluation and interventions based on the etiologies.[101,141–143]

PPH is an emergency and should be conducted as such. Upon recognition, management should proceed with alerting personnel, stabilization of the patient and rapid assessment and etiology identification, and targeted interventions in order to reduce risk of morbidity and mortality. Though PPH often occurs in high-risk populations, it may occur in patients without any known risk factors.

12.12L CORD PROLAPSE

An umbilical cord prolapse (UPC) is an emergent obstetric event that can become fatal if not properly identified and addressed. UPC occurs when the umbilical cord is present between the cervix and presenting fetal parts and can be either overt or occult. If overt, the cord is past the presenting fetal part, while if occult it is alongside the presenting fetal part.[144] UPC causes compression of the umbilical cord thereby decreasing fetal oxygenation. This can lead to significant fetal morbidity and mortality if not managed emergently.

TABLE 12.37 Postpartum Hemorrhage Outline

Mechanism of Action (MOA)	Etiology	Risk Factors	Immediate Interventions*	Continued Interventions†
Disrupted myometrium contractions	Uterine atony	Induction of labor, augmentation of labor using oxytocin, failure to progress during the second stage of labor increasing chorioamnionitis, oxytocin augmentation, LGA (macrosomia), polyhydramnios, multigestations, uterine anomalies (fibroids) or inversion, general anesthesia (uterine atony)	Perform bimanual massage, administer uterotonics.	Review records for risk factors. Document in detail.
Coagulopathy disruption	Trauma ensued during the birthing process	Operative/instrumental delivery or precipitous delivery leading to episiotomy, genital tract lacerations, uterine rupture	Repair any lacerations and hematomas. No blindly placed sutures. Pack area and monitor for hematoma stability. Assess for clotting and treat as needed.	Assess for clotting with coagulation profile as needed (may need to be done STAT), review records, treat appropriate factor replacement, monitor for emboli. Document in detail.
Coagulopathy disruption	Coagulopathies	Maternal coagulopathies or other bleeding disorders, hypertensive disease of pregnancy	Repair any lacerations and hematomas. No blindly placed sutures. Pack area and monitor for hematoma stability. Assess for clotting and treat as needed.	Assess for clotting with coagulation profile as needed (may need to be done STAT), review records, treat appropriate factor replacement, monitor for emboli. Document in detail.
Both MOA	Placental abnormalities: retained, placenta accreta, infection	Per etiology	Retained placenta: manual removal, u/s assessment and guidance for complete removal, suction curettage. Placenta accreta: maternal stabilization with surgical intervention, alert anesthesia and team for surgery. Infection: begin antibiotic treatment.	Review records for risk factors. Treat infection as necessary. Document in detail.

**General management. Assess hemodynamic status, begin maternal stabilization, perform bimanual exam (atony), palpate for retained products/rupture, perform speculum exam (lacerations).*

†Review records for risk factors. Document in detail. Blood transfusions may be necessary if significant blood loss or symptomatic. Surgical intervention may be warranted.

LGA, large for gestational age.

Source: Data from Beckmann C, Casanova R, Ling F, et al. Obstetrics and Gynecology. *7th ed. Lippincott Williams & Wilkins; 2014; Committee on Practice Bulletins-Obstetrics. Practice bulletin no. 183: postpartum hemorrhage.* Obstet Gynecol. *2017;130(4):e168–e186. doi:10.1097/AOG.0000000000002351; Belfort MA. Overview of postpartum hemorrhage. In: Post TW, ed.* UpToDate. *UpToDate; 2019. https://www.uptodate.com/overview of postpartum hemorrhage; Sheiner E, Sarid L, Levy A, Seidman DS, Hallak M. Obstetric risk factors and outcome of pregnancies complicated with early postpartum hemorrhage: a population-based study.* J Matern Fetal Neonatal Med. *2005;18(3):149–154. doi:10.1080/14767050500170088*

Upwards of 50% of UPC cases occur due to iatrogenic reasons, such as amnioinfusion, fetal blood sampling, external cephalic version, internal scalp electrode placements, and with induction of labor, such as with insertion of cervical ripening balloon or use of instrumentation during delivery. Other maternal risk factors include fetal malpresentation, low lying placenta, maternal pelvic or uterine anomalies, external fetal tumors, multiparity, prematurity, twin gestation, polyhydramnios, and prolonged labor.[145]

Overt UPC can be diagnosed either by visualizing the prolapsed cord or by palpation of it. However, when UPC is occult, the diagnosis can become more difficult. UPC should be suspected with any of the above risk factors, and clinical presentation usually includes signs of fetal distress as evidenced by rapid onset of significant, prolonged fetal bradycardia or moderate to severe decelerations in a previously normal tracing. Ultrasound with color flow Doppler may help ascertain the UPC location.[144]

The Royal College of Obstetrics and Gynecology reports to optimize perinatal outcomes the decision-to-delivery interval should be <30 minutes, the delivery should be by cesarean section and vaginal/instrumentation delivery only if faster than cesarean delivery, and the location of the prolapsed cord should be considered to initiate manual compression alleviation as able.[144]

Upon diagnosis of UPC, the following steps should be initiated:

1. Call for assistance
2. Delivery method decision. If in first stage of labor, a cesarean section is the fastest way to delivery, so clinicians should be alerted and preparations made. If in second stage and delivery is imminent, the decision to use instrumentation should be considered.
3. Continuous fetal monitoring started/continued
4. Maternal supplemental O_2 by mask
5. Begin maneuvers to decrease cord compression, such as manual elevation of fetal presenting parts via two fingers or hand through the vagina, patient repositioning to steep Trendelenburg, exaggerated Sims position, bladder filling with 500mL or more of saline.

6. Avoid excessive cord manipulation, which can lead to umbilical artery vasospasm and further decrease fetal oxygenation.[144]

Given UCP may never be completely unavoidable, having knowledge of risk factors and prevention strategies should be acknowledged. Simulation training has also been shown to be useful in managing UCP emergent events.[144]

12.12M SHOULDER DYSTOCIA

Shoulder dystocia is an unpredictable and unpreventable obstetric emergency.[146] Therefore, all delivering clinicians need to be prepared for the possibility of shoulder dystocia as well as its management and consequences.

Several studies have tried to look at incidence and risk factors for shoulder dystocia; however, only a few consistencies have been identified. The factor with the highest incidence associated with shoulder dystocia is fetal macrosomia, or birth weight of >4,000 to 5,000 g at the time of delivery. The macrosomia may be due to a variety of etiologies, such as maternal diabetes (GDM or chronic), excessive maternal weight gain, or postterm pregnancy. Other potential risk factors include prolonged second stage labor and precipitous delivery. Women with a history of shoulder dystocia in a previous pregnancy are also at higher risk for recurrence. However, it should be noted that the majority of shoulder dystocia cases occur during delivery with mothers without diabetes and in infants without macrosomia.[146,147]

Once risk factors are identified, management and delivery planning options should be shared and discussed with the patient. If a woman has a history of diabetes and fetal macrosomia of >4,500 g, or without maternal diabetes but with fetal macrosomia of >5,000 g, an elective cesarean section should be considered.

Shoulder dystocia is encountered during the intrapartum period and the clinician needs to be aware of signs associated with it. One sign is resistance following the delivery of the head. Another is termed the "turtle sign," which is seen when, following the delivery of the head, there is tension and retraction onto the maternal perineum.[101]

If shoulder dystocia occurs during delivery, there are several options to intervene. The most common is the McRoberts maneuver (Figure 12.22), which is performed when the mother hyperflexes her legs close to the abdomen. Another option is externally applying downward pressure on the fetal anterior shoulder with maternal suprapubic pressure laterally toward the fetal sternum.[123] If both maneuvers are unsuccessful, the recommended next maneuver is to attempt to deliver the posterior arm, although attempts at rotational maneuvers may also be attempted, as well as an episiotomy. More aggressive approaches may be warranted if severe shoulder dystocia continues despite the above attempts.[146]

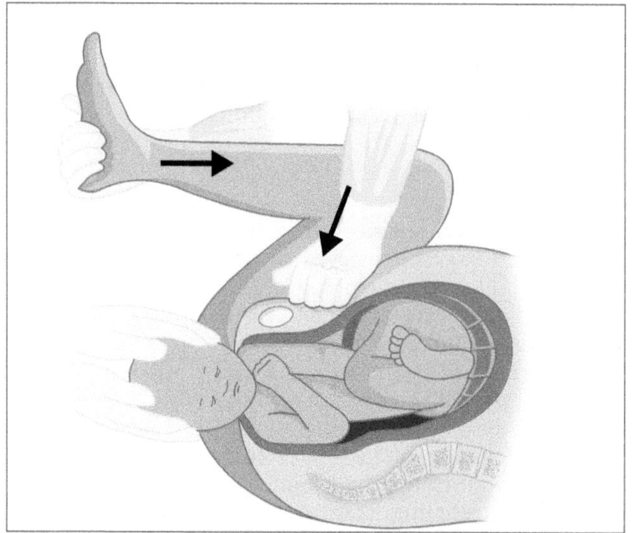

Figure 12.22 **McRoberts maneuver.**

Often there is no fetal injury following shoulder dystocia if it is corrected. If there are consequences, however, they can be severe for the mother and infant. Maternal complications include increased risk for PPH, perineal lacerations, and obstetric anal sphincter injuries. When more aggressive maneuvers have been tried, there have been increased risks of significant maternal morbidity, and therefore these approaches should only be attempted by the experienced obstetric clinician. The most common fetal/infant injury due to shoulder dystocia are brachial plexus injuries and clavicle and/or humerus fractures. Rarely do other sequelae arise, such as neonatal encephalopathy or demise.[146,147]

COMMON CHIEF COMPLAINTS

Elyse J. Watkins

APPROACH TO MISSED MENSES

Missed menses is a common complaint among reproductive-age women (Figure 12.23). While pregnancy must always be ruled out, there are other etiologies to consider in the differential diagnosis. Diagnosis begins by differentiating primary from secondary amenorrhea, which can be done based on timeline and patient age (Table 12.38).

Primary amenorrhea is usually due to an underlying pathology or chromosomal abnormality. The most common cause of secondary amenorrhea is pregnancy, but other nonpathologic conditions can cause secondary amenorrhea, such as menopause or breastfeeding. HPO axis abnormalities can also result in primary or secondary amenorrhea (see Table 12.39).

Causes of primary amenorrhea can result from either anatomic, enzyme, or receptor abnormalities. See Table 12.40.

The differential diagnoses for primary amenorrhea can be classified as pregnancy-related, congenital/genetic disorders, or acquired (see Table 12.41).

A urine pregnancy test is the first step in diagnosing primary amenorrhea. If negative, a bimanual pelvic examination should be performed, followed by transabdominal ultrasound to identify any anatomic disorders. If an adrenal or pituitary mass is suspected, MRI of the sella turcica or adrenals would be indicated. Laboratory evaluation is essential in differentiating the multiple possible hormonal causes of primary amenorrhea (see Table 12.42).

SECONDARY AMENORRHEA

Patients who present with secondary amenorrhea should be asked about their sexual practices and risk of pregnancy (Figure 12.24). A missed menses in a reproductive-age female is most frequently caused by pregnancy. Absence of menses for

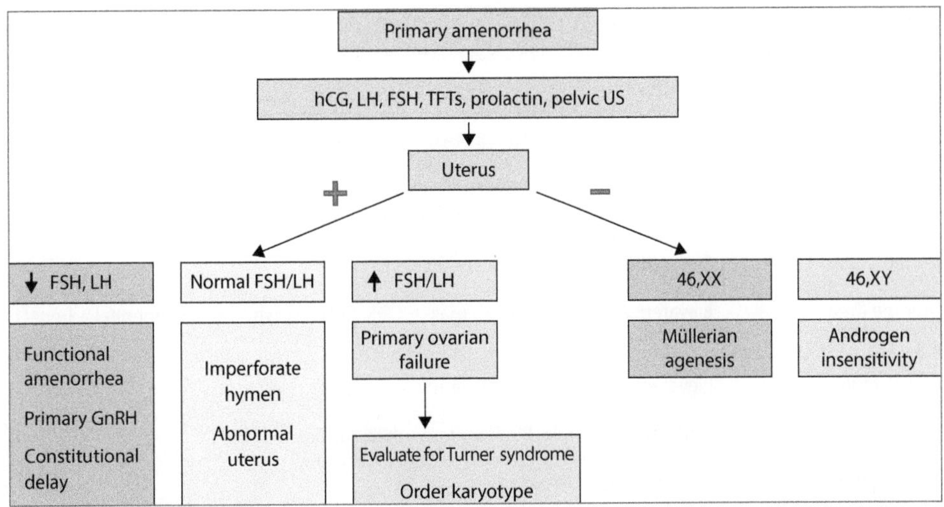

Figure 12.23 Approach to primary amenorrhea. FSH, follicle-stimulating hormone; GnRH, gonadotropin-releasing hormone; hCG, human chorionic gonadotropin; LH, luteinizing hormone; TFTs, thyroid function tests; US, ultrasound.

TABLE 12.38 Definitions of Primary and Secondary Amenorrhea

Primary Amenorrhea	Secondary Amenorrhea
Absence of menses by 14 years of age and no breast development	The absence of menses for ≥3 months when menses were previously monthly
Absence of menses by 16 years of age with breast development	The absence of menses for >6 months when menses were previously irregular

TABLE 12.39 Common Causes of Amenorrhea in the Hypothalamic-Pituitary-Ovarian Axis

Hypothalamic	Pituitary	Ovary
Anorexia nervosa	Hyperprolactinemia	Gonadal dysgenesis
Chronic severe stress	Pituitary adenoma	Turner syndrome (45,X)
Hypo/hyperthyroidism	Cushing disease	Primary ovarian insufficiency
Galactosemia	Craniopharyngioma	Swyer syndrome (45,XY with gene mutations)
Kallmann syndrome	Empty sella syndrome	Polycystic ovary syndrome
	Pituitary infarct	Menopause
	Chronic kidney disease	

TABLE 12.40 Anatomic, Enzyme, and Receptor Abnormalities in Primary Amenorrhea

Anatomic	Enzyme	Receptor
Müllerian dysgenesis	17-Alpha-hydroxylase deficiency	Androgen insensitivity syndrome
Imperforate hymen	5-Alpha-reductase deficiency	
Transverse vaginal septum		

3 consecutive months in a female with a history of monthly menses requires investigation, starting with a urine pregnancy test. Important questions to ask in the medical history include gravida and para status, a complete menstrual history, past medical history of any chronic diseases, medications being taken, and any history of severe stress or surgery.

TABLE 12.41 Differential Diagnosis of Primary Amenorrhea

Diagnosis	Description
Pregnancy	Easily ruled out with a pregnancy test.
Congenital/genetic disorders	Anatomic disorders: imperforate hymen, transverse vaginal septum Turner syndrome Müllerian dysgenesis Kallmann syndrome Enzyme deficiencies Receptor deficiencies
Acquired	Hypo/hyperthyroidism Severe anorexia nervosa Chronic illness (e.g., autoimmune disease, Cushing syndrome, adrenal insufficiency, chronic kidney disease) Radiation therapy Hyperprolactinemia (pituitary adenoma, medications)

Pregnancy test should be followed by a complete physical examination, including a pelvic exam. Visual field defects could indicate a pituitary mass. Thyroid masses or enlargement could indicate thyroid disease. Bradycardia can be found in anorexia nervosa. Striae and a buffalo hump are indicative of Cushing syndrome. Acanthosis nigricans, central adiposity, and hirsutism can indicate PCOS. Virilization, such as clitoromegaly, could indicated an androgen-secreting tumor or late onset congenital adrenal hyperplasia. Once pregnancy and anatomic abnormalities have been ruled out, laboratory evaluation is needed. (Table 12.43).

Consider the following:

1. Is this primary or secondary amenorrhea?
2. Is the patient pregnant?
3. If not, are there physical exam findings that support an anatomic cause?
4. If not, are there physical exam findings that support an underlying endocrine disorder?
5. Perform ultrasound and screening lab tests.
6. Consider MRI to rule out pituitary mass if indicated by lab results.

TABLE 12.42 Laboratory Evaluation in Primary Amenorrhea

Test	Results
17-Hydroxyprogesterone	Elevated: Congenital adrenal hyperplasia, late onset
Follicle-stimulating hormone (FSH)	Elevated: Turner syndrome, primary ovarian insufficiency Low: Functional hypothalamic dysfunction
Luteinizing hormone (LH)	Elevated FSH:LH ratio indicates PCOS
Serum testosterone (free and total)	Elevated: Adrenal or ovarian mass, PCOS, Cushing syndrome, congenital adrenal hyperplasia
Testosterone: DHT ratio	Elevated: 5α-Reductase deficiency
Prolactin	Hyperprolactinemia: Pituitary mass, medications
Thyroid-stimulating hormone	Elevated: Hypothyroidism Low: Hyperthyroidism
5α-Reductase type 2 gene (*SRD5A2*)	Mutation: 5α-Reductase deficiency
Karyotype	Turner, Kallmann, androgen insensitivity syndrome, other rare genetic disorders

DHT, dihydrotestosterone; PCOS, polycystic ovary syndrome.

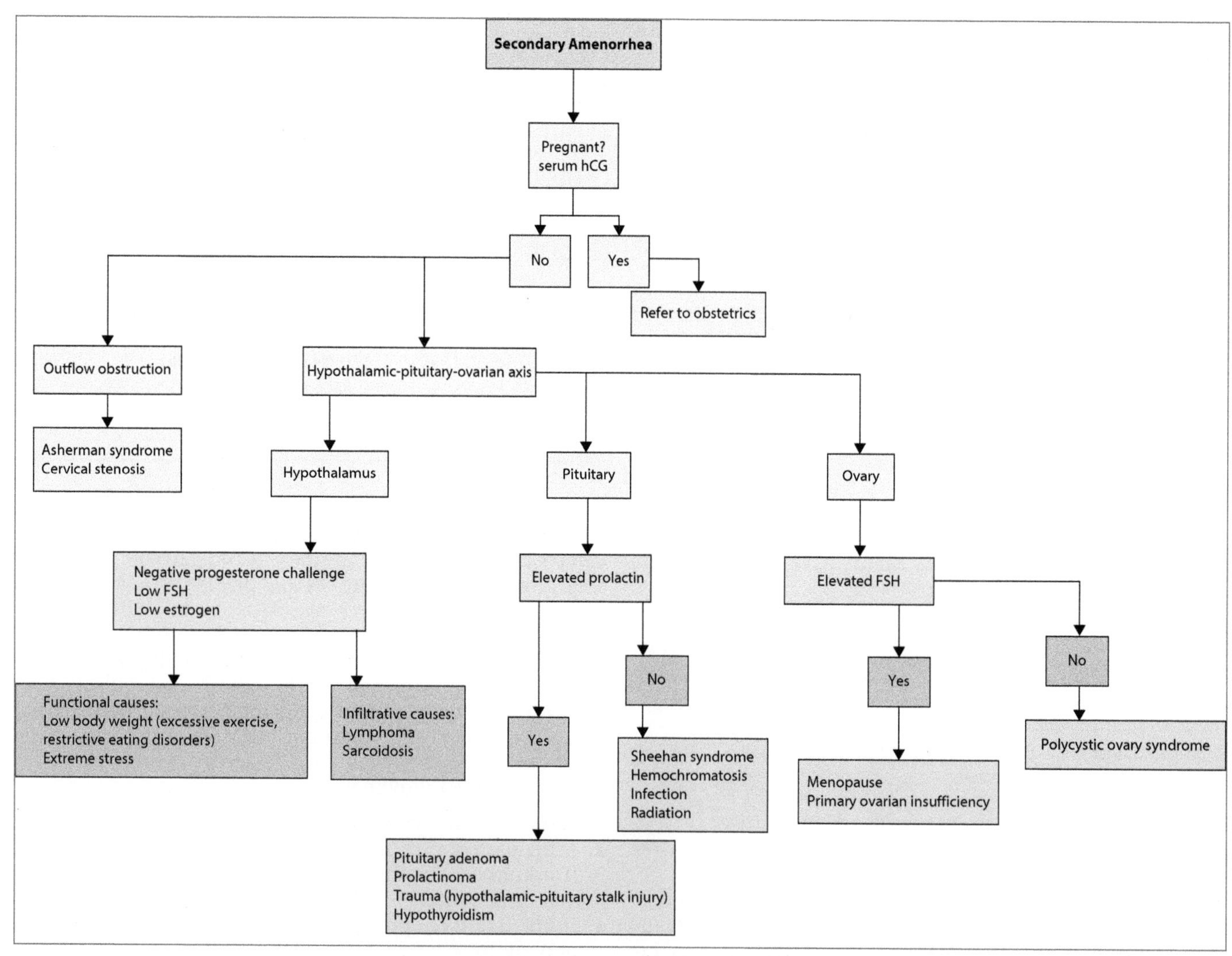

Figure 12.24 **Approach to secondary amenorrhea.** FSH, follicle-stimulating hormone; hCG, human chorionic gonadotropin.

TABLE 12.43 Laboratory Evaluation for Secondary Amenorrhea

Test	Notes
β-hCG (serum or urine)	<5 mIU/mL is negative.
Antimüllerian hormone	Low or undetectable in ovarian insufficiency and menopause.
Follicle-stimulating hormone (FSH)	Variable during perimenopause. Elevated late postmenopause. Low or normal in functional hypothalamic amenorrhea.
Luteinizing hormone (LH)	Variable during perimenopause. Elevated FSH:LH ratio indicates PCOS. Low or normal in functional hypothalamic amenorrhea.
Dehydroepiandrosterone-sulfate (DHEA-S)	Elevated in congenital adrenal hyperplasia. Can be elevated in PCOS.
Sex hormone binding globulin (SHBG)	Low in PCOS.
Prolactin	Elevated is hyperprolactinemia by definition.
Thyroid-stimulating hormone	Elevated: Hypothyroidism Low: Hyperthyroidism
Serum 17-hydroxyprogesterone	Elevated: Should have adrenocorticotropic hormone stimulation testing for 21-hydroxylase deficiency.
Testosterone (free and total)	Elevated: Could be PCOS, adrenal mass, rarely androgen-secreting tumor.

β-hCG, beta-human chorionic gonadotropin; PCOS, polycystic ovary syndrome.

KNOWLEDGE CHECKS

1. Pelvic pain is a common chief complaint. When considering the differential diagnosis, what are key historical facts that can help guide the evaluation?
2. If a patient presents with an adnexal mass, what critical physical examination and imaging findings help guide the evaluation?
3. When a patient presents with a breast mass, what key historical, physical examination, and imaging findings help guide the evaluation and diagnosis?

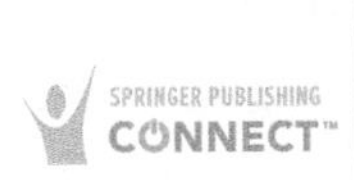

A robust set of instructor resources designed to supplement this text is located at **http://connect.springerpub.com/content/book/978-0-8261-8243-2.** Qualifying instructors may request access by emailing **textbook@springerpub.com.**

REFERENCES

The complete reference list for this chapter appears in the digital version of the chapter, accessible at https://connect.springerpub.com/content/book/978-0-8261-8243-2/chapter/ch12.

CHAPTER 13

MUSCULOSKELETAL SYSTEM

CHRISTINE BRUCE

LEARNING OBJECTIVES

- Identify red flag signs and symptoms and evaluation strategies for the patient presenting with neck or back pain.
- Describe the physical examination findings of a patient with various low back and neck pain syndromes.
- Develop an evaluation and treatment regimen for patients presenting with shoulder, hip, wrist, knee, elbow, or ankle pain.
- Determine appropriate referral for orthopedic surgical conditions.
- Differentiate between the anatomic site of hip fracture and the treatment along with determination of risk factors for poor outcomes and complications that occur with hip fractures and dislocations.
- Discuss the mechanism of injury, presenting signs and symptoms, and treatment for knee injuries including ligament, meniscus, and cartilage damage.
- Describe the clinical presentation, diagnostic evaluation, treatment, and prognosis for wrist and ankle complaints.
- Describe the clinical presentation, diagnosis, and treatment of various fractures and dislocations of the upper and lower extremities.
- Discuss the epidemiology, clinical presentation, diagnosis, treatment, and complications of glenohumeral instability, glenohumeral dislocations and acromioclavicular joint separation, rotator cuff tears, and subacromial impingement syndrome.
- Outline the epidemiology, pathophysiology, clinical presentation, diagnostic evaluation, and treatment of Osgood-Schlatter disease, slipped capital femoral epiphysis (SCFE), and developmental dysplasia.
- Compare and contrast lumbosacral strain/sprain, disc herniation, and spinal stenosis regarding pathophysiology, clinical presentation, diagnostic evaluation, and treatment.
- Describe the pathophysiology, clinical presentation, and treatment of cauda equina syndrome.

INTRODUCTION

The musculoskeletal system involves joints, bones, muscles, and extra-articular soft tissues. Arthritis is the primary joint manifestation involved with musculoskeletal disease and this can be secondary to trauma, infection, autoimmune disorders, or crystal-induced inflammation. Bone involvement includes fractures, Paget disease, and tumors. Extra-articular tissue involvement includes fibromyalgia, and periarticular soft tissue involvement can involve bursitis, sprains, and tendinitis.

13.1 PAIN DISORDERS

CHRISTINE BRUCE

OVERVIEW

The cervical spine consists of seven vertebrae (C1–C7) that support the weight of the head, which is approximately 14 pounds. The first two vertebrae are called the axis and atlas and do not have a disc between them but are closely bound together by a complex of ligaments. The C1 (atlas) ring rotates around the odontoid process, or dens, of the axis, allowing for almost 50% of the total cervical rotation. The spinal canal is housed within the cervical vertebrae and is widest between C1 and C3, where it narrows as it progresses caudally.[1]

Most neck and back pain is caused by disorders of the spine, most of which are mechanical. Nonmechanical causes of pain include infection, inflammation, cancer, and osteoporosis-related fragility fractures. Most mechanical spine disorders that cause neck or back pain are due to nonspecific mechanical derangements such as muscle strain, spasm, poor posture, decreased strength of stabilizing muscles, or decreased flexibility. Structural lesions leading to pain include disc herniation, compression fractures, lumbar spinal stenosis, osteoarthritis, and spondylolisthesis. Neck and back pain can be attributed to a generalized myofascial pain syndrome such as fibromyalgia, which is noted as having multiple areas of trigger point pain.

Cervical radicular pain occurs along a dermatomal pattern that is caused by the irritation of a nerve root. It is mediated by phospholipase A2, interleukins 1 and 6, tumor necrosis factor alpha, and nitric oxide. Cervical radicular pain is a separate entity from cervical radiculopathy and is often associated with nerve root compression and involves a sensory or motor deficit from a dysfunctional nerve pathway. Diagnostic nerve blocks, electromyography (EMG), and imaging studies can help to determine the exact nerve root level that is causing the pain. Treatment options include conservative medical treatment, physical therapy (PT), cervical epidural steroid injections, and spinal cord stimulation.[2] Cervical radicular pain is most commonly seen at C6 and C7.

EPIDEMIOLOGY

The estimated lifetime prevalence of a significant episode of neck pain is 40% to 70% and the prevalence of neck pain is 4.9%.[3] While most people will recover from an episode of neck pain within 1 year, relapses are common and up to 20% of acute neck pain will become chronic.[4] Predictors for chronic neck pain are high body mass index (BMI), frequent neck extension during a workday, high initial pain intensity, and high psychological job demands.[4] Injury is a strong predictor of chronic neck pain.[5] Other independent baseline risk factors for subsequent neck pain include the number of children, poor self-assessed health, poor psychological status, and a history of low back pain. History of neck injury is an independent and distinct risk factor.[5]

The lifetime incidence of low back pain is 58% to 84% while 11% of men and 16% of women have chronic low back pain. Back pain accounts for 7% of primary care visits and more than 30% of people still have clinically significant symptoms a year following sciatica.[6]

PATHOPHYSIOLOGY

There is an association between mechanical neck pain (MNP) and dysfunction of the muscles of the cervical spine. There are changes in the physical structure which include fatty infiltration and alterations in the muscle fibers as well as changes in the behavior—including the timing and the activation levels—of the cervical muscles. This leads to an impaired capacity of the cervical muscles to generate, sustain, and maintain precision of the required levels of torque needed for optimal function. This leads to the deleterious consequences for the cervical region, which relies heavily on muscles for mechanical stability.[7]

Back pain has multiple underlying etiologies with different pathophysiologic processes contributing to this pain. These are discussed in detail in Section 13.1B Acute Back Pain.

13.1A NECK PAIN

MEDICAL HISTORY AND CLINICAL PRESENTATION

Neck pain can be classified into four categories[8]:

- **Grade 1:** No signs of major pathology and little interference with daily activities.
- **Grade 2:** No signs of major pathology but pain may impact daily activities.
- **Grade 3:** Neck pain with neurologic signs or symptoms (radiculopathy).
- **Grade 4:** Neck pain with major pathology such as fracture, myelopathy, neoplasm, or spinal infection.

SIGNS AND SYMPTOMS

Myofascial pain is a common etiology for acute cervical pain. Myofascial pain can be referred through trigger points and can be seen in other locations as well. These trigger points are believed to result from foci of muscular strain. The mainstay of treatment for myofascial pain focuses on conservative care with PT, heat, and nonsteroidal anti-inflammatory drugs (NSAIDs). Injections of trigger points can also be utilized.[9]

Occupational history is important as patients with jobs requiring physical labor have a higher risk of chronic neck syndromes. Patients with increased mental stress, those with previous injury to the neck, and those with poor self-image have an increased risk for the development of neck pain. Additionally, psychological factors may predict those who will go on to develop chronic neck pain.

PHYSICAL EXAMINATION

The clinician should inspect the neck and back for any visible deformity, areas of redness, or vesicular rash (possible herpes zoster). Palpate the spine itself and the vertebral muscles for tenderness, spasm, and features of myofascial pain, which may include tight bands, trigger points, and pressure sensitivity. Test gross range of motion (ROM) and examine the shoulders to determine possible referred pain from the shoulders into the neck. In the setting of low back pain, primarily evaluate the hip ROM along with pain in various anatomic areas.

The neurologic examination assesses the function of the entire spinal cord, including motor strength, sensation of both light touch and deep pain, and deep tendon reflexes. Patients with active neurologic symptoms will need to be assessed for sensation and sacral nerve function by evaluation of rectal tone during rectal examination, the anal wink reflex, and the bulbocavernosus reflex. Reflexes are compared contralaterally. Corticospinal tract abnormalities are indicated by extensive plantar response and Hoffman sign. To assess for Hoffman sign, the clinician taps the nails or flexes the volar surface of the third finger observing for thumb flexion, which connotes a positive test in the setting of corticospinal tract dysfunction.

Examination of the neck includes observation for abnormal posturing, palpation for tenderness, and ROM. The upper extremities are also assessed for sensation, motor function, and reflexes. Muscle tone and spasticity are also noted.

Differentiating the cause of pain and dysfunction due to cervical spine versus shoulder pathology is challenging as the patient may report an anatomic region of pain that can mislead the clinician. This is an important differentiation to make because successfully treating these patients requires a careful and complete history and physical examination with appropriate provocative maneuvers in order to make the appropriate diagnosis. If advanced imaging does not reveal a definitive source of pathology, there is a role for EMG and selective injections, which can be revealing when the patient responds to those injections.[10]

Provocative tests of the neck, during which the neck and arm are positioned to either aggravate or relieve arm symptoms, are commonly used in clinical practice to assess patients with suspected cervical radiculopathy. The tests with the highest sensitivities include Spurling test, traction/neck distraction, and Valsalva maneuver.[11]

Little evidence exists to support the use of clinical tests in evaluating the anatomic integrity of the cervical spine in adults with neck pain and its associated disorders. However, the use of extension/rotation tests is reliable with adequate validity in ruling out pain that arises from facet joints. Other physical examination maneuvers that are reliable in ascertaining pain originating from the cervical spine include the neurologic exam, Spurling maneuver, and upper limb neurodynamic tests utilizing Doppler studies to evaluate cervical arteries.[12]

Spurling maneuver was first described in 1944 as a method of identifying cervical radiculopathy. Several modifications of this maneuver have been noted. The maneuver consists of extension, lateral bending, and axial compression and has the best evidence for identifying cervical radiculopathy. Although most revealing, these maneuvers were also the least tolerable. Whenever cervical radiculopathy is suspected, it is recommended that staged provocative maneuvers be performed, first to include extension and lateral bending, followed by the additional axial compression if previous maneuvers are inconclusive.[13]

DIFFERENTIAL DIAGNOSIS

The differential diagnosis for neck pain is summarized in Table 13.1.[14]

DIAGNOSTIC STUDIES

There is a limited role for laboratory assessment in the evaluation of neck pain unless infection, malignancy, or inflammatory arthritis is suspected. In these cases, an erythrocyte sedimentation rate and C-reactive protein can be performed. Complete blood count (CBC) should also be done in the setting of suspected infection. Lumbar puncture should be done if meningitis is suspected and the patient does not have increased intracranial pressure.

Cervical CT is universally accepted as the initial diagnostic study, making flexion and extension neck x-rays of little value in the evaluation of a patient with persistent neck pain. It is recommended that flexion-extension films can be excluded from cervical spine clearance protocol in neurologically intact, awake patients who have undergone CT.[15]

In the patient without red flag symptoms, a cervical spine x-ray film series includes anteroposterior (AP), lateral, and open-mouth views. Cervical spine images can be performed in patients older than 50 with a new onset of neck pain or those who have symptoms or signs consistent with an infection. Patients with discitis will have endplate destruction where the infection occurs.[16]

Cervical spine symptoms are frequent complaints in visits to general, spinal orthopedic surgeons, and primary care clinicians. CT scan is accurate but there is a great deal of associated radiation exposure, so these should be pursued with caution. MRI is a highly effective imaging tool but is very expensive. The Spurling maneuver can help to identify patients who require advanced imaging as the sensitivity of the Spurling maneuver has been shown to identify nerve root pathology 95% of the time with a specificity of 94%.[17]

CT myelography is used similarly to MRI to visualize neurologic encroachment. CT is indicated only if an MRI cannot be done. Cervic MRI is the definitive test used in the evaluation of patients for cervical radiculopathy or cervical myelopathy. This is indicated in the setting with neurologic symptoms or signs of cord compression, progressive neurologic dysfunction, and the lack of response to therapy.[18]

CT angiography and MR angiography can identify cervical artery dissection as can digital subtraction angiography.[19]

EVALUATION

Neck pain can occur spontaneously or following significant trauma. It is vital that significant underlying etiologies be evaluated as failure to identify red flag symptoms can result in neurologic compromise for patients. Patients presenting after trauma should be evaluated for cervical spine injury. High-risk conditions include patients over the age of 65, paresthesias in the extremities, altered mental status, diving accident, significant head or facial injury, or when multiple other fractures are identified that indicate the level of trauma.

The cervical spine should be immobilized in any patient with a suspected cervical spine injury until the patient is cleared through examination or imaging. Screening imaging is performed before neck movement is done. CT is the study of choice for suspected spine injury in the setting of multiple trauma with a high-risk mechanism of injury. MRI of the cervical spine will identify ligamentous injury. Cervical spine x-rays (flexion and extension) can be performed in the patient with low risk for significant injury. Patients may be screened via chest x-ray if they have no tenderness at the posterior midline on palpation, no focal neurologic deficits, and no distracting injuries with pain that occupies the patient's attention; demonstrate normal mentation; and are not under the influence of medications or substances.

TREATMENT

Conservative treatment with analgesics with or without muscle relaxants are traditionally given for patients with cervical radiculopathy since spontaneous resolution of all or at least most symptoms typically occurs within 2 to 8 weeks in most patients. Anti-inflammatory medications and referral to PT can be helpful. Narcotic medication is avoided as patients can respond to other treatments without the concern of addiction that narcotics can cause. Cervical spine manipulation is generally avoided as quadriparesis, herniation of intervertebral disc, stroke, or vertebral fracture can occur. If nonsurgical treatment is ineffective or if patients develop muscle atrophy, motor weakness, or signs of myelopathy, surgical evaluation is warranted.

Cervical spondylosis is treated with conservative care and reassurance with the caveat that the symptoms may last several months or become chronic. NSAIDs are first-line therapy. There is a role for PT in helping these patients. Surgical decompression with or without fusion may be necessary for patients with intractable pain, progressive neurologic findings, or symptoms of spinal cord compression. Patients with intractable neck pain that does not respond to conservative treatment, or patients with progressive neurologic symptoms, should be referred to a specialist.

Patients with cervical spine pain secondary to muscular strain such as that with a whiplash injury should be given reassurance regarding the natural progression of this condition. For the first 1 to 2 weeks following the incident, NSAIDs are indicated with consideration for muscle relaxants if the patient experiences spasms. Narcotic medication should be restricted for this condition. PT can help with the patient's limited mobility or tight muscles through stretching

TABLE 13.1 Differential Diagnosis for Neck Pain

Diagnosis	Description
Myofascial pain	Myofascial pain can result in the formation of trigger points that can contain a band of muscle, which may also have a nodular component as well. Pain localized to the neck is most likely to be myofascial pain. Myofascial pain is commonly described as deep, aching, or sharp.
Nociceptive pain	Cervical strain is categorized as an axial neck pain, which is a type of nociceptive pain. This pain can result from direct stimulation of nerve endings.
Referred pain	Referred pain is pain perceived in the location in the body other than the one in which the stimulus causing the pain originates. Poorly localized pain is likely to be referred pain from the neck.
Radicular pain	Radicular pain is described as electric, lancinating, or shooting. Radicular pain radiates in a narrow, characteristic distribution. Pain radiates down from the neck to the ipsilateral upper extremity with numbness with or without associated weakness. Radiation of pain and numbness occurs in a dermatomal pattern. Spurling test is positive on the side where the head is rotated.
Fracture	Bone pain can occur from fracture of the cervical vertebral body that can occur with trauma or significant osteoporosis with compression fracture, which is more common in the thoracic rather than the cervical spine. Fracture may occur from a fall from a height, diving injuries, motor vehicle collision occurring at a high speed, or collision involving motorized recreational vehicle or bicycle.
Infection	Bacterial meningitis can cause neck pain along with headache, neck stiffness, and mental status changes. Epidural abscess can present with fever and spinal pain with urgent need for neurosurgical decompressive surgery. May have a history of illicit drug use or recent spinal surgery. MRI will show discitis with abscess or intraspinal abscess.
Osteoarthritis	Repetitive work or injury can lead to degeneration in the neck with formation of osteophytes. Decreased range of motion and neck soreness in symptomatic patients. Spondylosis may be seen on neck x-ray.
Acute whiplash	Flexion-extension injury to the neck that typically occurs in motor vehicle collision.
Atlantoaxial subluxation	Most likely to occur in patients with rheumatoid arthritis in which there is osteochondral destruction of C1 and C2 leading to instability. Caution with trauma to the neck or during endotracheal intubation.
Carotid artery dissection	Ipsilateral neck pain, facial pain, weakness and sensory loss, and possible amaurosis fugax. May progress to Horner syndrome with ipsilateral myosis, ptosis, and anhidrosis. Atherosclerosis and acute elevation of blood pressure can lead to a tearing sensation in the neck. Patients present with neck pain and urgent diagnosis is needed to identify this condition.
Vertebral artery dissection	Ipsilateral neck pain and facial pain, vertigo, ataxia, dysarthria, diplopia, and motor and sensory deficits. Ipsilateral cranial nerve palsy and contralateral motor or sensory limb dysfunction, constituting a similar presentation to posterior circulation stroke.[14]
Cervical facet syndrome	Pain referred to the head, neck, shoulders, and back without a dermatomal pattern. May occur in patients whose neck x-ray is typically normal.
Spastic torticollis	Unilateral contraction of neck muscles resulting in head tilt toward the side of the contracture without any neurologic focal findings. Can be congenital or inherited.
Neoplastic	Can be the site of bone metastatic disease from prostate, thyroid, breast, lung, or kidney most commonly. Localized point tenderness found. Bone scan will show abnormal increased uptake in cervical spine. MRI may identify metastatic lesion with bony destruction. Can also occur as a primary bone cancer.
Cervical myelopathy	Slowly progressive symptoms with clumsiness of hands and feet, ambulatory problems, paresthesias of upper and lower extremities followed by symptoms of poor coordination, progressive gait difficulty, or alteration in bowel or bladder habits. Increased muscle tone with hyperreflexia of the lower extremities, clonus, and positive Babinski sign. MRI reveals encroachment of spinal cord from spondylosis with central herniation.

Source: Data from Merwick Á, Werring D. Posterior circulation ischaemic stroke. BMJ. *2014;348:g3175. doi:10.1136/bmj.g3175*

and strengthening exercises and the establishment of a home exercise program.

Fractures of the cervical spine are treated with immobilization acutely. Intravenous (IV) steroids are given if there is an associated spinal cord injury. Specialty referral typically inherits the care of these patients.

PATIENT EDUCATION

Various factors will impact participation in physical activity for adults who have chronic cervical spine pain. Key factors affecting physical activity in patients with chronic neck pain include those who are actively in pain, those who fear movement, those who smoke, those with lower socioeconomic status, and those with fewer leisure or work time activities.[20]

Patients who have cervical spine pain due to cervical spine metastasis may be helped by percutaneous vertebroplasty. This procedure not only relieves spinal pain but also can stabilize the vertebral body.[21]

There is a relationship between temporomandibular disorders and cervical spine disorders. Patients with cervical spine pain have shown improvement as a result of viscosupplementation with hyaluronic acid when they have had both cervical spine pain and temporomandibular joint (TMJ) osteoarthritis. By giving this viscosupplementation, pain improved not only in the TMJ area, but also in cervical spine ROM and cervical pain relief.[22]

SPECIAL CONSIDERATIONS

- Patients who are immunocompromised may not develop fever in the setting of epidural abscess or discitis.
- Clinicians should exercise a high index of suspicion for infection of the central nervous system; missing this diagnosis and delaying treatment can have devastating consequences.

KEY POINTS

- The majority of neck and back pain is caused by mechanical spinal disorders, which are usually nonspecific and self-limited.
- Patients who have focal neurologic deficits implicating spinal cord compression should have MRI or CT urgently.
- Patients who have acute nonradicular back pain can begin conservative therapy without extensive evaluation to search for specific underlying cause.

13.1B ACUTE BACK PAIN

MEDICAL HISTORY AND CLINICAL PRESENTATION

Acute back pain is a common complaint seen in the ED. Chronic pain lasting more than several months can be indicative of an underlying back condition such as nucleus pulposus herniation, spinal stenosis, or cervical spondylosis in the case of neck pain.

PHYSICAL EXAMINATION

The clinician should assess whether the patient has symptoms of spinal cord or root compromise, which would include limb weakness, radicular pain and numbness (including saddle anesthesia), or bowel, bladder, or erectile dysfunction. These patients should be evaluated for spinal and paraspinal tenderness, and straight leg raise test should be performed.

DIAGNOSTIC STUDIES

Straight leg raise test is used to confirm sciatica. The patient lies supine with both knees extended and the ankles dorsiflexed. Passive straight leg raising is performed with symptoms occurring between 10 and 60 degrees of elevation in the setting of sciatica. For the cross straight leg test, the clinician raises the opposite leg and pain that occurs on the affected, opposite leg indicates a positive finding. These tests are then repeated with the patient performing these actions rather than clinician. The seated straight leg raise test is done while the patient is seated with a hip flexed at 90 degrees and the lower leg slowly raised until the knee is fully extended. If sciatica is present, the pain in the spine occurs as the leg is extended.

Lab tests can include a CBC and inflammatory markers such as erythrocyte sedimentation rate and C-reactive protein, which help in detecting an underlying infectious or inflammatory etiology. Imaging can include plain x-rays, CT, and MRI scans.

Plain films do not identify abnormalities in the soft tissue or nerve tissues, which are the most common and most serious causes of low back pain. Because x-ray findings do not identify common or serious causes of low back pain, they do not impact patient management and are therefore not routinely recommended. Testing is guided by physical examination findings and is based upon the differential diagnosis for the most common etiology.

Patients with neurologic deficits, especially those for whom spinal cord compression is suspected, should have CT or MRI urgently. Patient for whom infection is suspected should have white blood cell count, erythrocyte sedimentation rate, or C-reactive protein as a screen. CT, MRI, or bone scan can assess for possible metastatic or primary cancer to the spine. If aneurysm is suspected, CT angiography or ultrasound can be performed. If aortic dissection is suspected, angiography, CT, or MRI is performed.

TREATMENT

Specific treatments depend upon the underlying cause and range from conservative measures with medications for analgesia and muscle relaxation along with PT progressing to more interventional options such as local or regional anesthetic blocks and spinal epidural steroid injections. If there is significant, active neural compromise, surgery may be indicated.[23] Treatment should be targeted at the underlying cause. Analgesics, heat and cold application, and reassurance along with judicious use of NSAIDs can constitute treatment. Extensive evaluation should be avoided in patients without red flag symptoms as most patients with low back pain will respond to the tincture of time. PT can be utilized for lumbar stabilization and strengthening the abdominal and low back muscles and helping with posture. Corticosteroids are unproven for acute back pain as the results of steroids are not sustained.[24]

Acetaminophen is ineffective for acute low back pain and NSAIDs are helpful for acute back pain but have fewer benefits for chronic low back pain. Duloxetine, an antidepressant, is effective for chronic low back pain but benzodiazepines are ineffective for radiculopathy. Skeletal muscle relaxants are effective for short-term pain relief and acute low back pain but at the expense of causing sedation. The evidence is insufficient to determine the effects of antiseizure medications. Opioids used for chronic low back pain may have modest benefit, but clinical trials have not assessed the serious harms that occur with the long-term use of these agents in the setting of chronic low back pain.[25]

A brief initial period of 1 to 2 days of decreased activity may be helpful for patient comfort acutely. Prolonged bed rest, spinal traction, and lumbar braces have not been found to be beneficial. Patients should be given reassurance regarding the favorable prognosis of low back pain with the advice on returning to normal activities along with the use of NSAIDs and weak opioids only for short period of time. Patients with chronic low back pain can continue with NSAIDs with supplementation of antidepressants, exercise therapy, and psychosocial interventions. Referral to a specialist is recommended for patients who have no improvement after 4 weeks or those with concerning symptoms.[26]

Spinal manipulation can help relieve pain due to muscle spasm or following an acute neck or back injury. There is some inherent risk with this technique and overaggressive manipulation should be avoided.[27] One theory as to why this form of treatment is successful is that it provides individualized care, psychological support, and reassurance for improvement.

Reassurance is an essential part of treatment for low back pain and should be incorporated as part of the overall treatment of this condition. Reassurance can provide patients who are at psychological risk such as those having depression, anxiety, catastrophizing, or fear avoidance with providing counseling that this is a short-term, limited, and curable condition. Reassurance has been shown to positively affect satisfaction, disability, pain, and mood on a long-term basis.[28]

13.1C LUMBAR SPINAL STENOSIS

MEDICAL HISTORY AND CLINICAL PRESENTATION

Lumbar spinal stenosis is a narrowing of the lumbar spinal canal, which results in pressure on the cord or sciatic nerve roots prior to their exit from the foramina. This condition can be congenital or acquired. It is most commonly seen in middle-aged and older patients. Underlying causes are osteoarthritis, degenerative disc disease, spondylosis, and spondylolisthesis. There is an increased risk for lumbar spinal stenosis development in patients who have ankylosing spondylitis.

Degenerative lumbar spinal stenosis is usually associated with the three joint complex degeneration (superior and inferior vertebral end plates and disc herniating into vertebral body). Schmorl nodes are vertical herniations of the disc into the vertebral body through a weakened part of the endplate that leads to disc degeneration. These nodes can adversely affect spine unit stability and are found more commonly in patients with degenerative lumbar spinal stenosis.[29]

SIGNS AND SYMPTOMS

Positional back pain, symptoms of nerve root compression with radiculopathy, and lower extremity pain during walking or weight bearing are classic findings.

PHYSICAL EXAMINATION

Patients with lumbar spinal stenosis have pain that occurs in the buttocks, thighs, or calves during ambulation, climbing stairs, and even standing erect. Flexing the back relieves the discomfort and leaning on a grocery cart for support tends to decrease the pain. Physical examination may show weakness and diminished reflexes ipsilaterally and symptoms can include pain, paresthesias, and weakness.

DIFFERENTIAL DIAGNOSIS

Calf claudication can be confused with peripheral arterial disease-related claudication. This can be differentiated as patients with spinal stenosis experience relief with rest and flexion position change. Additionally, they do not display skin atrophy, abnormalities in pulses, capillary refill, or abnormal ankle-brachial index, all of which are seen in vascular claudication. Calf claudication caused by spinal stenosis is also termed pseudoclaudication or neurogenic claudication as there is no vascular component contributing to this condition. In its worst form, cauda equina syndrome can occur.

DIAGNOSTIC STUDIES

Diagnosis can be based on clinical assessment. Diagnosis can be confirmed with MRI or EMG studies. Electrodiagnostic studies include nerve conduction studies and EMG. Patients with moderate-to-severe lumbar central spinal stenosis have lower distal amplitudes of motor action potential in both the peroneal and tibial nerves. Positive sharp waves and fibrillation potentials are seen on EMG in patients with severe spinal stenosis. The studies may be helpful to diagnose radiculopathy caused by lumbar central spinal stenosis and helping to differentiate this from other causes of radiculopathy.[30]

AP and lateral lumbar spine views may demonstrate spondylolisthesis or a significant narrowing of the intervertebral disc.

DIFFERENTIAL DIAGNOSIS

The differential diagnosis for spinal stenosis is summarized in Table 13.2.

TREATMENT

Treatment of spinal stenosis includes encouraging activity as tolerated, use of analgesics, and medications to relieve neuropathic pain. There is a role for PT with stretching and strengthening of abdominal and back muscles to relieve pressure on the lumbar spine. There has not been a significant improvement in physical functioning when patients with lumbar spinal stenosis are given surgery versus PT.[31]

Epidural corticosteroid injections have a role in mitigating pain. Patients who failed to respond to these conservative methods may be treated with spinal surgery. Surgery involves decompression of nerve root entrapment by the vertebral canal and foraminal encroachments. Laminectomy or laminotomy is the typical procedure with or without spinal fusion. Spinal fusion is performed in the setting of an unstable spine or in those with severe, well-localized arthritic changes in one or more vertebral interspaces. The use of surgical decompression alone to treat lumbar spinal stenosis declined in the United States where there is an increase in the use of a combined procedure of decompression and fusion by a factor of 15 in this time frame. Evidence demonstrating the benefit of adding fusion to decompression surgery is lacking, even in patients who have demonstrated degenerative spondylolisthesis.[32]

TABLE 13.2 Differential Diagnosis for Spinal Stenosis

Diagnosis	Description
Abdominal aortic aneurysm	Pulsatile abdominal mass, may have associated bruit. Most commonly occurring in men over age 65, especially if there is a smoking history.
Vascular or arterial insufficiency	Intermittent claudication with activity, with relief of pain after rest, decreased pulses and thin, atrophic skin. Dependent rubor can occur with the leg in a dependent position. Patients typically will have pain occurring at predictable distances due to vascular claudication and inability to perfuse the extremity.
Cellulitis	Unilateral leg involvement with redness, indistinct skin border surrounding the redness, edema, and low-grade fever.

13.1D DISC HERNIATION

MEDICAL HISTORY AND CLINICAL PRESENTATION

The intravertebral disc is composed of the nucleus pulposus, which is a gel-like material that acts as cushion during axial compression, the annulus fibrosis, a specialized ligamentous structure surrounding nucleus pulposus helping to stabilize the spine, and the superior and inferior cartilaginous endplates. Lifting and twisting increase pressure on the nucleus pulposus. Lumbar disc herniation usually develops over time as the weaker posterolateral portion of the annulus fibrosis develops fissures that permit egress of the disc components, which herniate into the lumbar canal adjacent to the exiting lumbar nerve root. Pain occurs from direct mechanical compression of the nerve root and from chemical irritation of the nerve root from the extracted substances within the nucleus pulposus.

SIGNS AND SYMPTOMS

The pain associated with disc herniation is aggravated by sitting, walking, standing, coughing, and sneezing. Patients have difficulty finding a position of comfort and they lie on their back with a pillow under the knees or lie on the side in the fetal position.

Disc herniation of the lumbar spine is a common cause of sciatica. Sciatica is a symptom rather than a specific diagnosis. Inflammation and compression are needed for the nerve root to become symptomatic.

Compression of nerve roots in the lower back results in sciatica, which is pain along the sciatic nerve. In addition to intervertebral disc herniation, other causes of sciatica include osteophytes and spinal stenosis. Symptoms include pain radiating from the buttocks down the ipsilateral lower extremity.

PHYSICAL EXAMINATION

Sciatica is mainly diagnosed through history taking and physical exam. Patients report pain that radiates along the course of the sciatic nerve, most commonly down the buttocks and the posterior aspect of the ipsilateral lower extremity to below the knee. The pain is described as burning, lancinating, or stabbing and it may occur with or without low back pain. The pain can be exacerbated with the Valsalva maneuver when it is due to disc herniation. Patients may also have complaints of numbness and weakness on the ipsilateral leg. The most commonly affected locations are L5–S1 and L4–L5 (Table 13.3).

TABLE 13.3 Locations of Disc Herniation and Associated Physical Examination Findings

Site of Injury	Physical Exam Findings
L3–L4 disc (L4 nerve root)	Weakness in the anterior tibialis, numbness in the shin, pain in the thigh, and an asymmetric knee reflex.
L4–L5 disc (L5 nerve root)	Weakness in the great toe extensor, numbness on the dorsum of the foot and first webspace, and pain in the posterolateral thigh and calf. There is no corresponding reflex.
L5–S1 disc (S1 nerve root)	Weakness in the great toe flexor as well as in the gastrocnemius-soleus complex. Patients will have an inability to sustain tiptoe walking, numbness in the lateral foot, pain and ache in the posterior calf, and an asymmetric ankle reflex.

Straight leg raising is positive when the lower extremity is raised above 60 degrees producing pain radiating down the leg. This pain can be replicated when the contralateral leg is lifted, a test known as the crossed straight leg raise test. This test is more specific for sciatica.

The evaluation of sciatica begins with assessing the strength, reflexes, and sensation of each dermatome. If neurologic focal deficits are noted or if symptoms last longer than 6 weeks, there may be a role for imaging and electrodiagnostic studies. Structural abnormalities such as spinal stenosis can be diagnosed by MRI or CT.

DIFFERENTIAL DIAGNOSIS

The differential diagnosis for patients with lumbar radiculopathy is summarized in Table 13.4.

TABLE 13.4 Differential Diagnosis for Lumbar Radiculopathy

Diagnosis	Description
Cauda equina syndrome	Perianal numbness, urinary/fecal overflow incontinence or retention, reduced anal sphincter tone, bilateral leg weakness. Considered neurosurgical emergency.
Hip or knee arthritis	Decreased internal rotation of the hip with groin pain; effusion of knee with decreased range of motion. Pain following rest and with continued ambulation.
Lateral femoral cutaneous nerve entrapment	Etiology from tight belt around the waist. Affects sensory only with numbness or pain of the lateral thigh.
Spinal stenosis	Neurogenic claudication with intermittent calf pain with activity. Pain relieved by flexing the back and leaning forward. Seen mostly in the older population and stooped gait may be seen.
Trochanteric bursitis	Pain in the lateral hip that can radiate down the lateral thigh and leg, exquisite tenderness over the greater trochanter. May have increased pain at night.
Vascular claudication, peripheral arterial disease	Decreased dorsalis pedis or posterior tibialis pulses, decreased ankle to brachial index, smooth shiny atrophic skin, claudication with activity typically at a predictable distance. There may be decreased capillary refill in the toenails.

DIAGNOSTIC STUDIES

Diagnosis can be clinical based on presenting signs and symptoms with the diagnosis being confirmed with MRI or CT. Electrodiagnostic studies can identify the affected level.

Nerve root compression can cause sensory, motor, or reflex deficits. L5–S1 disc herniation may affect the ankle jerk reflex and L3–L4 herniation affects the patellar reflex.

TREATMENT

For the first 6 to 8 weeks following an acute event, treatment is conservative. Treatment modalities include PT, NSAIDs, epidural corticosteroid injections, and transforaminal periradicular injections of steroids, along with advice for the patient to maintain physical activity. Discectomy has benefits in the short term but in the long run, it is not more effective than prolonged conservative care.[33]

Further treatment includes keeping the patient as active as tolerated, using analgesics for pain control and PT for mobilization and stretching. Acute pain relief can occur within 24 to 48 hours after the patient has brief bed rest in a semi-Fowler position (30-degree elevation). Adjunctive medications can include antidepressants such as duloxetine, antiepileptics such as gabapentin, or tricyclic antidepressants such as amitriptyline. Muscle spasm can be relieved with heat or cold along with PT. Epidural corticosteroid injections can accelerate pain relief but are not first-line treatment.

Surgery is indicated for cauda equina syndrome (see Section 13.1E) or for persistent disc herniation symptoms not responsive to conservative care such as muscular weakness, progressive neurologic deficits, or intractable pain. Microdiscectomy or laminotomy can be performed to relieve the pressure on the disc. There is no longer a role for chemonucleolysis.[34]

13.1E CAUDA EQUINA SYNDROME

MEDICAL HISTORY AND CLINICAL PRESENTATION

Cauda equina syndrome involves damage to nerve roots at the caudal end of the spinal cord. This condition mimics conus medullaris syndrome in that they both cause distal leg paresis and sensory loss in and around the perineum and anus along with numbness causing saddle anesthesia. The distal end of the spinal cord, the conus medullaris, terminates at the L1–L2 level. Below this level, the spinal canal is filled with the L2–S4 nerve roots known as the cauda equina. Compression of the roots distal to the conus medullaris causes paralysis without spasticity.

The cauda equina syndrome typically occurs from a sudden reduction in the volume of the lumbar spinal canal the causes compression of multiple nerve roots leading to muscle paralysis if untreated. The sacral nerve roots, S2–S4, control the bladder and anal function and these nerve roots are particularly vulnerable to injury. Etiologies for cauda equina syndrome include central disc herniation, epidural abscess, epidural hematoma, and trauma to the spine with retropulsion of a portion of the vertebral burst fracture.

SIGNS AND SYMPTOMS

Symptoms include bladder or bowel dysfunction with bowel frequency or incontinence, erectile dysfunction, loss of rectal tone, and abnormal bulbocavernosus and anal wink reflexes.

Radicular pain and numbness typically involve both legs even if one leg is more severely involved. Perineal numbness in the saddle distribution is also typically found. Lower extremity pain may diminish as the paralysis progresses. Leg weakness may cause the patient to have a stumbling gait, difficulty arising from a chair, or foot drop. There may be difficulty voiding or incontinence of urine and feces. The symptoms can occur after lifting or following recent spine surgery with the patient complaining of increased back and leg pain.

TABLE 13.5 Differential Diagnosis for Cauda Equina Syndrome

Diagnosis	Description
Guillain-Barré syndrome	Sensation is intact with ascending weakness and normal MRI finding. Can be a complication of infection such as *Campylobacter jejuni*.
Herniated lumbar disc	Unilateral radiculopathy with motor weakness, normal rectal tone, and normal perineal sensation.
Primary or metastatic cancer	Pathologic fracture can be seen, lytic lesions on imaging, abnormal increased activity on bone scan.
Multiple sclerosis	Gait abnormalities, uveitis, urinary retention/incontinence in a patient whose MRI enhanced with gadolinium shows various lesions in time and space.
Spinal cord tumor	Positive Babinski reflex, spasticity, and paresthesias.

PHYSICAL EXAMINATION

Physical examination reveals the patient to have decreased muscle tone and deep tendon reflexes. The patient may have an inability to rise from a chair due to quadriceps and/or hip extensor weakness and will be unable to walk on the heels or toes, which suggest multiple nerve root dysfunctions. Patients may have poor anal tone on rectal exam and loss of an anal wink.

DIFFERENTIAL DIAGNOSIS

The differential diagnosis for cauda equina syndrome is summarized in Table 13.5.

DIAGNOSTIC STUDIES

MRI or CT can confirm the diagnosis of this condition. AP and lateral films can identify structural problems such as a fracture or spondylolisthesis.

TREATMENT

The onset of cauda equina can be immediate as seen with a fracture or can occur over a few hours or days with other conditions. Urgent surgery is performed to relieve the nerve root compression and to stop the progression of neurologic deficits. Even with appropriate treatment, recovery of neurologic function is often incomplete with failure to improve bowel and bladder dysfunction.

13.1F COMPLEX REGIONAL PAIN SYNDROME

MEDICAL HISTORY AND CLINICAL PRESENTATION

Complex regional pain syndrome (CRPS) was formerly known as reflex sympathetic dystrophy, Sudeck atrophy, and causalgia. This condition is a clinical diagnosis consisting of pain, autonomic dysfunction, trophic changes, and functional impairment. CRPS is identified as type I if there are no identified etiologies or type II if there is an identified nerve lesion. CRPS has pain that is out of proportion to what would have been expected from the original injury. This pain persists despite ongoing cellular damage or death. CRPS is an abnormal prolongation of normal postinjury physiologic responses that also involves receptor dysfunction. This process is initiated in the extremity but becomes affected by spinal cord and cortical events.

CRPS is probably a disease of the central nervous system (CNS) that manifests as peripheral inflammatory processes.[35] CRPS occurs in about 7% of patients who have limb fractures, limb surgery, or other injuries. Initially, there are inflammatory characteristics causing a "warm complex regional pain syndrome" which progresses to "cold complex regional pain syndrome" in which autonomic features dominate. This syndrome is diagnosed purely on the basis of clinical signs and symptoms.[36]

CRPS can be seen in the upper or lower extremity. Injuries precipitating CRPS include fracture of the distal radius and injuries of the infrapatellar branch of the saphenous nerve. This can occur after a contusion injury or arthroscopy. Some patients develop CRPS without apparent injury. If trauma precipitates CRPS, the trauma may only be minor. IV fluid infiltration has also been identified as a cause of this condition.

SIGNS AND SYMPTOMS

Pain is the cardinal symptom of CRPS. Patients who develop CRPS typically become symptomatic between 3 and 10 days after the initiating event. Initial symptoms include painful hot swelling, painful cold extremity, or stiff atrophic changes in the affected extremity. Patients will continue to have pain, swelling, cold sensitivity, hypersensitivity, allodynia, and sleep difficulty. Hallmark complaints include burning, tearing, searing, and throbbing pain. Allodynia is pain that is caused by a normally nonpainful stimulus. This severe pain may not respond to narcotic therapy. Extremities can be hot and swollen or cold and stiff. Over time, pain can become dull, boring, and aching.

PHYSICAL EXAMINATION

Physical examination signs include swelling, hypersensitivity, abnormal sweating, stiffness, contracture formation, and atrophy of the hair, skin, and soft tissues.

DIAGNOSTIC STUDIES

Diagnostic tests include plain x-rays showing spotty areas of osteopenia or demineralization in the bones of the affected extremity. Bone scans can show increased uptake in the extremity.

TREATMENT

Treatment includes early recognition and prompt treatment which includes PT, use of biofeedback, parenteral medication, and surgery. Analgesics include NSAIDs and narcotics for short-term use. Antidepressants, anticonvulsants, and calcium channel blockers may be used. PT includes passive ROM leading to encouragement of active ROM. Contrast baths and transcutaneous electrical nerve stimulation (TENS) may be used. Psychological counseling can be used adjunctively for the patient to learn coping techniques and biofeedback to control the autonomic function of the body to regulate sweating, skin temperature, and blood flow.

Early treatment of CRPS includes physical and occupational therapy to decrease pain and increase limb function and mobility. Secondary treatment goals include reduction of edema, decreasing muscle guarding, and functional improvement with daily activities. Functional therapy concentrates on improving the ROM and functional dexterity to improve the activities of daily living. Medications that can be used include prednisone, bisphosphonates,[37] tricyclic antidepressants, anticonvulsants, and topical local anesthetics. Additional therapy for chronic CRPS includes all the above along with TENS.[38]

Stellate blocks utilizing parenteral medications such as bupivacaine and sympathetic blockade can also be used.[39] Botulism toxin injection can also be used for prolonged sympathetic blockade.[40] Intrathecal injection of clonidine has also been shown to reduce pain in this condition.[41] The use of IV magnesium in treating pain associated with this condition has not been shown to have benefit.[42]

13.2 SHOULDER DISORDERS

Paul Kuhlman

13.2A SHOULDER IMPINGEMENT

OVERVIEW

Shoulder pain is often caused by subacromial impingement. The acromion and surrounding structures like the coracoacromial ligament, acromioclavicular (AC) joint, and coracoid process can all cause impingement on underlying bursa and tendons, specifically, the biceps tendon and rotator cuff tendons. This syndrome is synonymous with rotator cuff tendinitis, biceps tendinitis, and subacromial bursitis.

MEDICAL HISTORY AND CLINICAL PRESENTATION

Shoulder impingement generally has a gradual onset as it is typically an overuse injury. Often, the patient will present with a history of anterior and/or lateral shoulder pain that has been persistent for several months. Pain can often be elicited with certain movements, including a throwing motion or internal rotation of the shoulder. Most patients will complain of pain at night and have difficulty sleeping on the affected side. They may also complain of some "catching" or other mechanical symptoms within the shoulder. Depending on duration of symptoms, they may also complain of some muscle loss on the affected shoulder.

Shoulder impingement is often caused by overuse injuries resulting in an inflammatory process within the subacromial space. Some people are more susceptible to impingement depending on their profession, anatomy, and what activities they participate in recreationally. For example, someone who does a lot of overhead activity for their occupation is more likely to have impingement. Also, a person with a type III (hooked) acromion is more likely to impinge with overhead activity than someone with a type I (flat) acromion. Recreational activities involving an overhand throwing motion will also cause impingement. The history will play an important role when making the diagnosis of shoulder impingement.

SIGNS AND SYMPTOMS

- Anterolateral shoulder pain with overhead pain and internal rotation
- Night pain when sleeping on affected shoulder
- "Catching" in shoulder with ROM
- Anterior and lateral shoulder point tenderness to palpation

PHYSICAL EXAMINATION

On inspection, the patient may have atrophy to the supraspinatus/infraspinatus fossa. The patient may have shoulder dyskinesis or scapular winging on inspection. They will likely have tenderness to palpation over the anterolateral aspect of the shoulder. They may have tenderness over the greater tuberosity or within the bicipital groove. The patient should have full ROM with impingement syndrome; however, they will likely have pain with internal rotation of the shoulder. The Neer and Hawkins tests are specific for shoulder impingement. The rotator cuff strength should always be tested bilaterally for comparison. This will help differentiate a rotator cuff tear versus impingement.

DIFFERENTIAL DIAGNOSIS

The differential diagnosis for shoulder impingement is summarized in Table 13.6.

DIAGNOSTIC STUDIES

Diagnostic studies relevant to shoulder impingement are summarized in Table 13.7.

TREATMENT

Rest and NSAIDs are the mainstay treatment for impingement and involve mostly conservative treatment. The patient should avoid any offending activities. It is important to stretch and run the shoulder through a full ROM multiple times daily. If rest and NSAIDs are ineffective, a subacromial corticosteroid injection can be performed. A corticosteroid injection with rest can be effective and give long-lasting pain relief. This injection should not be repeated multiple times as it can increase risk of rotator cuff rupture. If no improvement is seen with the above measures, referral for PT is advised.

TABLE 13.6 Differential Diagnosis for Shoulder Impingement

Diagnosis	Description
Acromioclavicular osteoarthritis	Patient will have point tenderness over the AC joint. This will be evident on plain radiographs.
Glenohumeral osteoarthritis	Pain with most ROM and generally decreased ROM. This will be evident on plain radiographs.
Rotator cuff tear	Patient will have weakness on affected shoulder. The supraspinatus muscle is most commonly involved.
Adhesive capsulitis	Decreased ROM.
Suprascapular nerve entrapment	Patient will have atrophy of the supraspinatus and infraspinatus muscles.
Herniated cervical disc	Deltoid weakness, absence of biceps reflex (reflexes are unaffected with impingement), neck stiffness, possible sensory loss.

AC, acromioclavicular; ROM, range of motion.

TABLE 13.7 Diagnostic Studies for Shoulder Impingement

Diagnostic Test	Features and Findings
X-ray—Four radiographic views	• Anteroposterior scapula view—rule out glenohumeral osteoarthritis. • Anteroposterior acromioclavicular view—shows acromioclavicular joint osteoarthritis and shows inferior bone spurs. • Scapula Y view—Evaluates the acromion shape (type I, II, or III). • Axillary lateral view—rule out glenohumeral osteoarthritis and evaluate for os acromiale.
MRI	• Will show full and partial thickness tears of the rotator cuff and tendinosis of the rotator cuff or biceps tendon.
Ultrasound	• Less sensitive than MRI. • Will show rotator cuff thickening or tendinosis. • Less expensive than MRI.

PATIENT EDUCATION

Patients should be instructed to avoid offending activities for their shoulder symptoms. They should continue with stretching to prevent shoulder stiffness. Patient should follow up if there is no improvement with conservative treatment.

13.2B ROTATOR CUFF INJURIES

OVERVIEW

The rotator cuff is a major stabilizer of the shoulder joint. It consists of four muscles: supraspinatus, infraspinatus, teres minor, and subscapularis (SITS), as seen in Figure 13.1. Rotator cuff tears can also be a cause of shoulder impingement. People can continue activities with a partial thickness tear with minimal symptoms, although a full thickness rotator cuff tear can be very debilitating. It is rare to see rotator cuff tears in younger patients. The occurrence of cuff tears generally starts in patients in their 40s and then increases exponentially with each decade of life.

MEDICAL HISTORY AND CLINICAL PRESENTATION

Occasionally, a patient will present immediately after an acute injury. More often, the patient will present with a history of shoulder pain for several months. A cuff tear differs from impingement in that patients can generally refer to a specific incident predicating onset of symptoms. Patients also complain of night pain and are unable to sleep on the affected side. Similar to impingement, the patient will have complaints of both pain and mechanical symptoms. However, pain is generally elicited by overhead motion rather than internal rotation. Weakness is a chief complaint with rotator cuff tears as well.

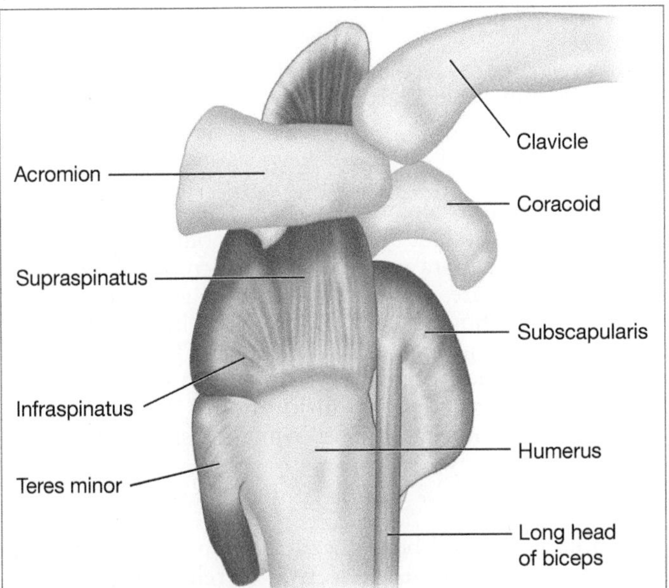

Figure 13.1 The rotator cuff.
(Source: Myrick KM. Advanced health assessment of the musculoskeletal system. In: Myrick KM, Karosas LM, eds. Advanced Health Assessment and Differential Diagnosis: Essentials for Clinical Practice. *Springer Publishing Company; 2021:395, Fig.12.6.)*

Acute rotator cuff tears occur generally from a fall landing on an outstretched arm. They can also occur with a sudden direct pulling on the shoulder. General wear on the rotator cuff can occur with chronic repetitive motions overhead or lifting things. This is more likely to start as a partial thickness tear and progress over time. A full thickness tear is typically more symptomatic and often requires surgical intervention. Untreated, it can progress to rotator cuff arthropathy.

SIGNS AND SYMPTOMS

- Weakness with resisted strength test
- Difficulty lifting arm over head
- Limited ROM and pain with overhead activity
- "Catching," or other mechanical symptoms
- Night pain or pain from lying on affected shoulder

PHYSICAL EXAMINATION

On inspection, the patient may have atrophy of the supraspinatus and infraspinatus muscles. This will be more obvious with chronic rotator cuff tears. Often, there is tenderness to palpation over the greater tuberosity. The most significant finding will be weakness with a resisted strength test. Patient may have difficulty lifting their arm overhead.

DIFFERENTIAL DIAGNOSIS

The differential diagnosis for rotator cuff injuries is summarized in Table 13.8.

EVALUATION

Patients may do well with conservative treatment for partial thickness tears, but full thickness tears will often need surgical intervention. Recovery and return to activity is dependent on the extent of the tear.

TABLE 13.8 Differential Diagnosis for Rotator Cuff Injuries

Diagnosis	Description
Subacromial bursitis	Pain with impingement exam
Adhesive capsulitis	Decreased ROM with both active and passive ROM
AC joint osteoarthritis	Point tenderness over AC joint, will be evident on x-ray
Glenohumeral osteoarthritis	Pain and decreased ROM, will be evident on x-ray
Thoracic outlet syndrome	Paresthesias, especially in ulnar nerve distribution

AC, acromioclavicular; ROM, range of motion.

TREATMENT

Conservative treatment includes rest and NSAIDs. PT is often required for strengthening and stretching. Avoiding the offending activity or overhead activities is beneficial. Subacromial corticosteroid injections are also helpful, but generally not definitive. Repeat injections are contraindicated as they can weaken the rotator cuff tendons and lead to progression of the tear. Surgical intervention for arthroscopic rotator cuff repair is often needed if symptoms are severe enough and the patient wants to undergo surgery. Patients often do better with surgical repair the sooner they have the surgery. Over time the muscle will atrophy and the cuff tissue is more difficult to repair, so early referral to orthopedics is important.

PATIENT EDUCATION

Patient should be instructed to avoid offending activities. It is important to continue stretching to prevent a frozen shoulder (adhesive capsulitis). Developing a frozen shoulder can worsen outcomes or delay treatment if surgical intervention is required.

13.2C SHOULDER DISLOCATION

OVERVIEW

The shoulder is a ball and socket joint. Unlike the hip, the glenohumeral joint is not nearly as stable — it is like a golf ball sitting on a golf tee. The shoulder joint relies heavily on the rotator cuff for stability because it is such a shallow joint. The humeral head (ball) is supposed to be centered on the glenoid (socket). Patients who have glenohumeral instability are unable to keep this centered. Labral injuries are often associated with shoulder instability injuries. An incomplete dislocation is often referred to as subluxation and a complete dislocation involves the humeral head slipping completely off the glenoid.

MEDICAL HISTORY AND CLINICAL PRESENTATION

Patients often report that the shoulder is "slipping" out of the socket. It is important to distinguish subluxation versus dislocation. A traumatic dislocation will often result after a fall on an outstretched arm or other traumatic injury. Atraumatic dislocations often occur in people who do repetitive motions that cause microtrauma to the shoulder. Over time, the persistent microtrauma results in laxity of the shoulder joint. This generally presents in athletes who do overhead or throwing activities in sports such as baseball, volleyball, swimming, and gymnastics. This is often an anterior dislocation and happens with the arm in a throwing position—arm abducted and externally rotated.

It is important to obtain a detailed medical history as well. Certain genetic disorders can cause joint hyperlaxity like Marfan syndrome or Ehlers-Danlos syndrome. It is important to know if it is the first dislocation or if the patient previously had a diagnosed shoulder dislocation. The majority (95%) of shoulder dislocation and instability occur in the anterior dislocation.[43] Posterior dislocations are much less common and are generally a result of a high-energy injury, electrocution, or convulsions.

SIGNS AND SYMPTOMS

- Pain and apprehension when the arm is in throwing position, abducted and externally rotated
- Obvious deformity of the shoulder joint compared to contralateral shoulder
- Patient that presents when holding the shoulder while the arm is externally rotated
- Pain relieved with reduction
- "Sliding" sensation

PHYSICAL EXAMINATION

A shoulder dislocation is often obvious on inspection as there is gross deformity. This is then confirmed with x-ray. Shoulder instability is examined with specific tests.

- **Apprehension test:** This exam tests anterior shoulder instability. The clinician puts the patient's arm in throwing position with the arm in abduction and externally rotated and applies stress to it. Patient will have the sensation that the arm is "slipping" or is going to dislocation. This is a positive result.
- **Sulcus sign:** This exam tests inferior shoulder instability. The clinician pulls the arm downward while stabilizing the scapula. A positive result will demonstrate indentation between the acromion and humeral head.
- **Laxity exam:** This exam is used to test capsular laxity. It will be positive in the "double-jointed" patient.

DIFFERENTIAL DIAGNOSIS

The differential diagnosis for shoulder dislocation is summarized in Table 13.9.

TABLE 13.9 Differential Diagnosis for Shoulder Dislocation

Diagnosis	Description
Rotator cuff tear	Rule out with arthrogram or MRI
Shoulder impingement syndrome	Positive impingement on exam
Glenohumeral osteoarthritis	Rule out with plain radiographs

DIAGNOSTIC STUDIES

Studies relevant to the diagnosis of shoulder dislocation are summarized in Table 13.10.

EVALUATION

It is important to evaluate the patient's neurovascular function when they present. The shoulder should be reduced as soon as possible. X-rays should be performed following relocation as fractures can occur with these activities. Patient should rest the shoulder for 2 to 4 weeks following an initial dislocation. Patients age <21 years have a 70% to 90% risk of repeated dislocation; patients over the age of 40 have a 20% to 30% risk of repeated dislocation.[43] Return to activity will depend on instability following a dislocation.

TREATMENT

The shoulder should be reduced as soon as possible. The Stimson procedure is very effective for relocation of an anterior dislocation (Figure 13.2). The patient can lie prone on a table with the arm hanging off the edge. They should lie in this position for 20 to 30 minutes with gentle traction on the arm. The shoulder can then be manually reduced with slight axial traction on the arm and countertraction to the trunk. Shoulder reductions are often done in the ED with light sedation. Patients should rest the arm for 2 to 4 weeks performing only pendulum exercises to maintain motion. To maintain strength and ROM, early PT is recommended, especially in the older population who tend to lose motion more quickly. Younger patients can wait a couple weeks to start PT. If there is persistent instability or subsequent dislocations or if there is an associated fracture or soft tissue injury, referral is necessary for surgical intervention.

PATIENT EDUCATION

Patients should be instructed to avoid offending activities of shoulder instability. Rehabilitation with PT is important to strengthen the shoulder to prevent instability. Patients can be instructed on how to reduce the shoulder if they have recurrent dislocations and are avoiding surgery.

TABLE 13.10 Diagnostic Studies for Shoulder Dislocation

Diagnostic Test	Features and Findings
X-ray	• Anteroposterior and axillary scapular views—rule out fracture and observe the location of the humeral head in relation to the glenoid. • Orthogonal view—assesses for a posterior dislocation. • X-ray is helpful to identify bony injuries and assess for a Hill-Sachs lesion.
MRI	Useful to assess soft tissue injuries. Often used after a traumatic dislocation or subsequent dislocation to assess for labral tear or associated rotator cuff tears.
MRI arthrogram	Best imaging to assess labral tears associated with a dislocation.
3D CT scan	Can be useful to assess bone loss.

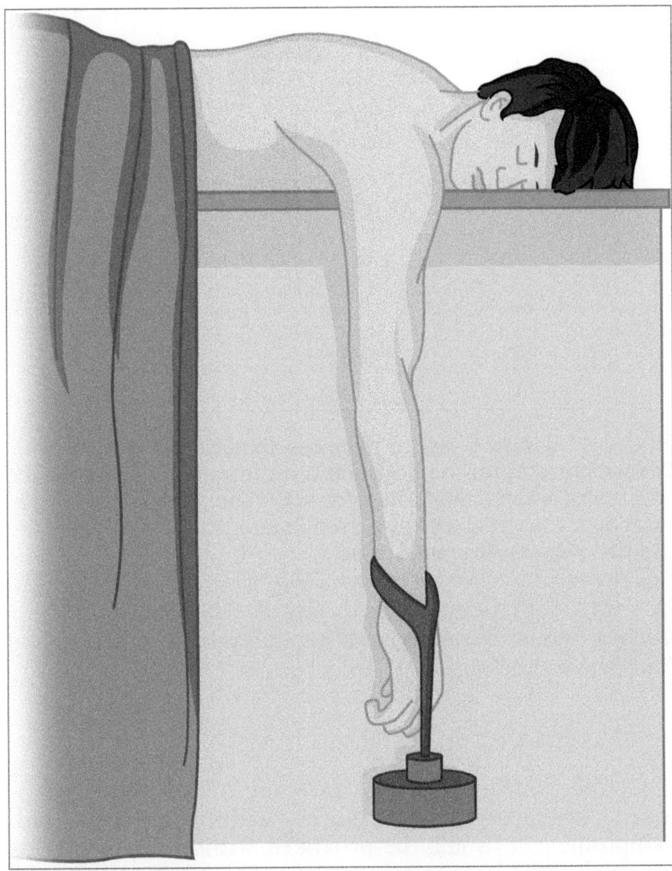

Figure 13.2 **Stimson procedure.**

13.2D ADHESIVE CAPSULITIS

OVERVIEW

Adhesive capsulitis is synonymous with frozen shoulder or a stiff shoulder. The cause is generally unknown but often some inflammatory process within the shoulder is the culprit. Generally, if the patient is experiencing pain, they do not move the arm, and thus, the shoulder gets stiff. Lean women between the ages of 40 and 65 years are at higher risk for a frozen shoulder. Other medical conditions associated with a frozen shoulder include clinical depression, type 1 diabetes mellitus, hypothyroidism, Parkinson disease, recent myocardial infarction, and recent neurosurgical procedure. Adhesive capsulitis can be debilitating with a prolonged recovery period.

MEDICAL HISTORY AND CLINICAL PRESENTATION

Patients present with shoulder stiffness without a specific cause being identified. Often they will be perimenopausal women and they may have endocrine disorders as mentioned above. They often will feel that the shoulder is weak, although strength is generally limited secondary to pain. The nondominant arm is affected more often. There are three different phases with adhesive capsulitis: the "inflammatory" phase, "freezing" phase, and "thawing" phase. The "inflammatory" phase is typically 4 to 6 months. As the name states, there is underlying inflammation within the shoulder. Generally, there is no specific cause for the inflammation, meaning there is no trauma, fracture, cuff tear, or other injury. The "freezing" phase is the stiffening phase. This also lasts about 4 to 6 months. The "thawing" phase is the recovery portion. This can take 1 to 2 years to regain ROM with conservative treatment.

SIGNS AND SYMPTOMS

- Painful shoulder with minimal or no specific trauma to the shoulder
- Significant stiffness during the "freezing" phase that recovers during the "thawing" phase
- Limited external rotation with the arm at the side
- Lean women of perimenopausal age

PHYSICAL EXAMINATION

Patient will have significant decreased active and passive ROM to the affected side compared to contralateral arm. A rotator cuff tear will only have decreased active ROM because of rotator cuff weakness. They will still have full passive ROM. Patients will often have stiffness in their fingers from lack of use as well. The patient will not likely be able to push their palms together in a "praying" position. They may have decreased strength, but this is often secondary to pain.

DIFFERENTIAL DIAGNOSIS

The differential diagnosis for adhesive capsulitis is summarized in Table 13.11.

DIAGNOSTIC STUDIES

X-ray is the most relevant diagnostic test for adhesive capsulitis. AP, axillary, and lateral glenohumeral radiographs are beneficial to rule out osteoarthritis as this can be a cause of decreased active and passive ROM.

EVALUATION

Adhesive capsulitis can be debilitating and take up to 3 years to resolve. Therefore, many follow-ups are required to assess resolution. A physical therapist will be evaluating the patient most frequently and should report results

TABLE 13.11 Differential Diagnosis for Adhesive Capsulitis

Diagnosis	Description
Impingement syndrome	Patient will still have decent ROM despite pain.
Glenohumeral osteoarthritis	Decreased ROM but OA will be evident on radiographs.
Proximal humerus fracture	Traumatic incident and will be evident on radiographs.
Rotator cuff tear	Patient will have decreased AROM but normal PROM on exam.
Shoulder instability	Normal PROM.
Tumor	Rare but this will be apparent on the plain radiographs or MRI.

AROM, active range of motion; OA, osteoarthritis; PROM, passive range of motion; ROM, range of motion.

of progress. If no progress is made with PT, manipulation under anesthesia may be necessary to speed up the recovery.

TREATMENT

During the "inflammatory" phase, conservative treatment consists of NSAIDs, PT, and possible corticosteroid injections. Oral prednisone can also be used. If conservative treatment fails, then manipulation under anesthesia is beneficial. One major risk with manipulation is fracture. Arthroscopic release of the capsule or adhesions can also be beneficial if conservative treatment fails. It is important to start PT immediately after manipulation or arthroscopic release to maintain motion.

PATIENT EDUCATION

Patient should be instructed to stretch every day to prevent loss of shoulder motion gained with PT. They should continue oral anti-inflammatories to help with pain. Patients can use ice for inflammation and sometimes heat is effective before stretching.

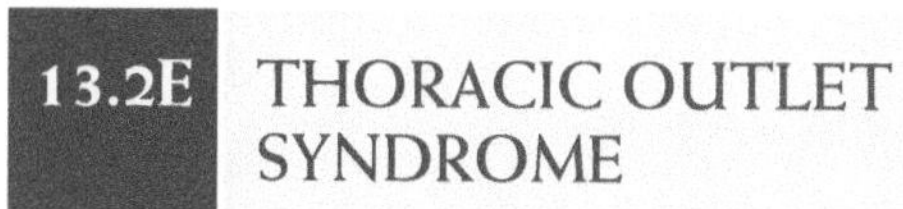

13.2E THORACIC OUTLET SYNDROME

OVERVIEW

Thoracic outlet syndrome (TOS) is caused by compression of neurovascular structures of the upper arm as they exit between the shoulder girdle, including the anterior and middle scalene muscles and first rib, which can be a normal first thoracic rib or a cervical rib. The neurovascular structures include the brachial plexus and the subclavian artery or vein. These structures can be compressed individually or as a group. The compression often occurs with overhead activity. The brachial plexus is often the culprit in >90% of cases.

MEDICAL HISTORY AND CLINICAL PRESENTATION

The patient will generally present with pain, swelling, weakness, and paresthesias in the upper extremity. This is dependent upon which structures are being compressed. The symptoms can present anywhere from the neck to the fingers. As the brachial plexus is most often involved, patients may complain of numbness in the fourth and fifth digits (ulnar nerve distribution). When the artery is involved, the patient will often complain of pallor in digits when the arm is elevated overhead or sensitivity to cold in the fingers. In severe (and rare) cases, the patient can experience gangrene of the fingers. When the vein is affected, the patient will complain of edema, engorgement, or cyanosis in fingers.

SIGNS AND SYMPTOMS

- **Brachial plexus:** Paresthesias in fourth and fifth digits, weakness, and muscle atrophy
- **Subclavian artery:** Pallor of fingers with arm elevation, sensitivity to cold, and gangrene of digits
- **Subclavian vein:** Edema, cyanosis, and engorgement of fingers
- Pain in upper arm, shoulder, and neck area

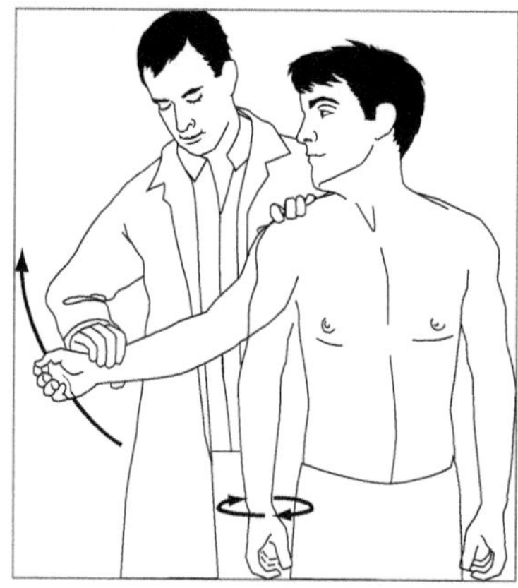

Figure 13.3 Adson test to diagnose thoracic outlet syndrome. The patient extends the neck and turns toward the symptomatic arm, which is abducted 30 degrees at the shoulder and maximally extended. The patient takes a deep breath and holds it while the clinician palpates the radial pulse.

(Source: Freeman TL, Johnson EW, Freeman ED, et al. Electrodiagnostic medicine and clinical neuromuscular physiology. In: Cuccurullo SJ, ed. Physical Medicine and Rehabilitation Board Review. *4th ed. Springer Publishing Company; 2019:386, Fig. 5.79.)*

PHYSICAL EXAMINATION

On inspection, patient may have any of the above symptoms. These symptoms often occur with the arm overhead. Symptoms can usually be provoked within 60 seconds by instructing the patient to elevate arms in a "stick-em-up" position (i.e., abducted 90 degrees in external rotation) (Papadakis, 2014, p. 832). Generally, the upper extremity reflexes are still present in TOS. Occasionally, the radial pulse will be absent with certain maneuvers of the arm, but this does not occur in most cases of TOS. Palpation over the brachial plexus can reproduce paresthesias in the hand. Common tests used include the Adson test, costoclavicular maneuver, and elevated arm stress test (Figure 13.3).

DIFFERENTIAL DIAGNOSIS

The differential diagnosis for TOS is summarized in Table 13.12.

TABLE 13.12 Differential Diagnosis for Thoracic Outlet Syndrome

Diagnosis	Description
Brachial plexus neuritis	Sudden onset with severe pain.
Carpal tunnel syndrome	Paresthesias on the radial aspect of the wrist in median nerve distribution. Patient will have a positive Phalen and Tinel test with CTS.
Impingement syndrome	Shoulder pain with positive impingement test.
Ulnar nerve entrapment	Positive Tinel sign at the elbow. This is confirmed with a nerve conduction study.
Herniated cervical disc	Symptoms on radial aspect of hand (similar to CTS).
Pancoast tumor	Venous congestion. Rule out with chest radiography.

CTS, carpal tunnel syndrome.

TABLE 13.13 Diagnostic Studies for Thoracic Outlet Syndrome

Diagnostic Test	Features and Findings
X-ray	• AP and lateral radiographs of cervical spine. • Chest radiography will show a cervical rib as the cause. Also beneficial to rule out tumor or infection.
MRI	MRI with arms in different positions can show impaired blood flow. This can also rule out a cervical disc rupture or cervical spondylosis.
Angiography	Confirms intra-arterial and venous obstruction of blood flow with vascular involvement.
Nerve conduction studies	Does not confirm TOS but can rule out other causes for paresthesias in the upper extremity.

AP, anteroposterior; TOS, thoracic outlet syndrome.

DIAGNOSTIC STUDIES

Studies relevant to the diagnosis of TOS are summarized in Table 13.13.

EVALUATION

It is important to identify structures being compressed during examination. Patient will need therapy and to avoid offending activities and often this alone can manage TOS.

TREATMENT

PT is most important, emphasizing muscle strength. Core strengthening is important as well as teaching proper posture. PT should be maintained for a minimum of 3 months and the patient should continue with a home exercise program. Offending activities should be avoided. This often includes overhead activities, strenuous activities, carrying heavy objects, or sleeping on affected side. Placing straps over the affected side should also be avoided. This can include a bra strap, purse, or seatbelt. NSAIDs and muscle relaxants can decrease symptoms. TENS units can also be beneficial to decrease symptoms. PT and conservative treatment may not be helpful in the presence of a congenital anomaly like a cervical rib. These patients will likely need surgical intervention. However, surgical outcomes are variable with high complication rate so conservative treatment should be tried initially.

PATIENT EDUCATION

Patients should be instructed on activity modification to prevent TOS symptoms along with PT for strengthening, which is important in relieving symptoms. It is vital that the patient continue with a home exercise program after completion of formal PT.

13.3 ELBOW DISORDERS

Morgan Wilson

OVERVIEW

Elbow disorders may arise from any of the structures in and around the joint. While some disorders are acute, such as most fractures and ligament injuries, other disorders are due to chronic conditions. Inflammation of the tendons is a common cause of chronic elbow pain. Nerves branch from the brachial plexus and travel though the elbow prior to continuing to the hand and may become entrapped distally, which may also elicit pain at the elbow. A full examination is needed to determine the underlying cause of pain in every patient.[44]

EPIDEMIOLOGY

Elbow pain is a common complaint in adult patients and is often related to occupation activity. While the traumatic injuries occur more often in the younger population, they still occur in the adult population. Chronic and overuse injuries are seen much more frequently in adults, 1% to 3% of whom are diagnosed with lateral epicondylitis per year.[45] However, the elbow is the second most commonly dislocated large joint caused by trauma or injury. Posterior dislocations account for 90% of elbow dislocations. Over half of elbow dislocations per year occur in children between the ages of 10 and 20 years. In children, supracondylar humerus fractures make up over 55% of elbow fractures.[46]

PATHOPHYSIOLOGY

Any injury or pathology around the elbow may disrupt the structures of the joint causing pain, decreased motion, numbness, and loss of function.[47,48] The elbow is a complex joint that comprises the humerus, radius, and ulna bones (Figure 13.4). The bones are stabilized by the ulnar collateral ligament, lateral collateral ligament (LCL), and the joint capsule. There are 23 muscles that make up the dynamic motion of the elbow joint and allow for flexion, extension, supination, and pronation. The flexor muscles originate from the medial epicondyle of the humerus and the extensor muscles originate from the lateral epicondyle. The ulnar nerve, radial nerve, and medial nerve run along the elbow and continue into the hand.

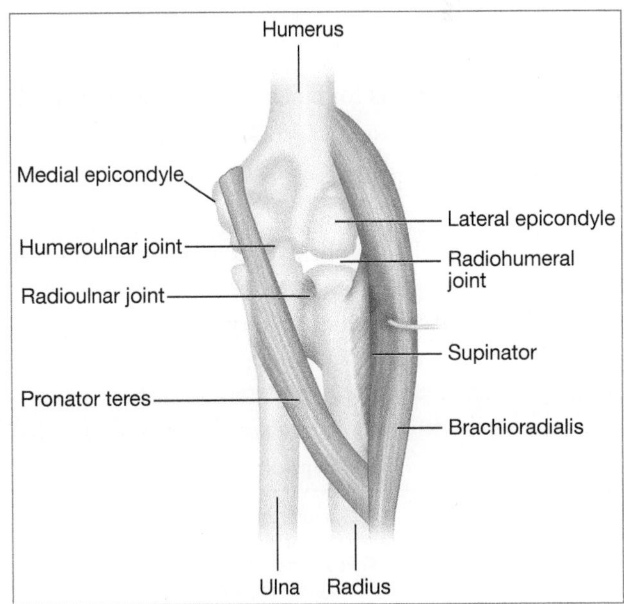

Figure 13.4 Muscles and joints of the elbow.
(Source: Myrick KM. Advanced health assessment of the musculoskeletal system. In: Myrick KM, Karosas LM, eds. Advanced Health Assessment and Differential Diagnosis: Essentials for Clinical Practice. *Springer Publishing Company; 2021, Fig. 12.12.)*

13.3A EPICONDYLITIS

MEDICAL HISTORY AND CLINICAL PRESENTATION

Epicondylitis is a common source of pain in middle-aged patients. Epicondylitis is caused by inflammation at the medial or lateral epicondyle of the elbow, which is the origin for the wrist flexors and extensors. "Tennis elbow" and "golfer elbow" are common terms for lateral and medial epicondylitis, respectively. The condition has a 12- to 18-month self-limiting course. However, some cases persist. This is often a chronic condition caused by overuse.[49]

SIGNS AND SYMPTOMS

Epicondylitis often presents as a gradual increase in pain. Patients will likely describe pain with flexion/extension of the wrist that may radiate down from the forearm into the wrist. The pain is often aggravated by activity. With lateral epicondylitis, the posterior interosseous nerve (PIN) may become irritated causing a burning sensation. Underlying arthritis or bony abnormalities may cause increased inflammation and lead to secondary epicondylitis.

PHYSICAL EXAMINATION

Epicondylitis is often diagnosed clinically and does not require further imaging or tests. The patient will have tenderness to palpation along the epicondyle. For medial epicondylitis, patients will exhibit pain with resisted wrist flexion and passive wrist extension. The opposite findings can be seen in patients with lateral epicondylitis.

Special tests to consider include the following:

- **Maudley test:** Pain with resisted wrist extension
- Decreased grip strength
- **Thomson maneuver:** Pain at elbow with passive flexion of wrist

DIFFERENTIAL DIAGNOSIS

The differential diagnosis for epicondylitis is summarized in Table 13.14.

DIAGNOSTIC STUDIES

Epicondylitis is typically a clinical diagnosis. The following studies may be useful as confirmation and to rule out other diagnoses:

- X-ray to rule out bony abnormality
- Ultrasound/MRI

TABLE 13.14 Differential Diagnosis for Epicondylitis

Diagnosis	Description
Bony abnormality	• Fracture, arthritis, OCD lesion, etc.
Elbow Instability	• Posterolateral instability, collateral ligament instability, etc.
Bursitis	• Inflammation in the bursa.
Nerve impingement	• Cervical radiculopathy, PIN entrapment, cubital tunnel.

OCD, osteochondritis dissecans; PIN, posterior interosseous nerve.

- Diagnostic injection
- EMG to rule out nerve impingement

EVALUATION

Clinical evaluation of epicondylitis is often adequate for diagnosis. The condition is often self-limiting and improves with rest and other conservative treatments.

TREATMENT

- PT
- Steroid injection
- Wrist brace; avoid counterforce brace, which can cause secondary PIN impingement, leading to further pain and burning
- Over-the-counter oral and topical analgesics
- Surgery[50]

PATIENT EDUCATION

- This condition is most often self-limiting and resolves with activity modification and conservative treatment.

13.3B ELBOW FRACTURES

MEDICAL HISTORY AND CLINICAL PRESENTATION

Elbow fractures, much like other fractures, occur following a trauma. The most common mechanisms of injury associated with elbow fractures are a direct blow, valgus stress, or falling onto an outstretched arm. The patient usually presents with immediate pain at the elbow joint and/or increased pain with attempted motion. Increased edema, ecchymosis, or obvious deformity may also be present.

SIGNS AND SYMPTOMS

Patients with elbow fractures exhibit signs of pain, edema, ecchymosis, tenderness to palpation, and decreased motion. The patient may present with guarding of the elbow by holding it close to the body in a position of comfort.

PHYSICAL EXAMINATION

A complete physical examination is needed when a patient presents after an injury or with increasing pain around the elbow joint. A complete physical examination should include assessment of neurovascular status, evaluation of skin, strength testing, and ROM. The elbow joint is one of the most complex joints in the body, with multiple nerves that encompass the elbow as they pass distally to the hand. It is important to note that a fracture around the elbow could significantly damage nerves, causing both temporary or permanent paralysis to the hand. For this reason, it is important to note the neurovascular examination before and after any necessary manipulation.

DIFFERENTIAL DIAGNOSIS

The differential diagnosis for elbow fractures is summarized in Table 13.15.

TABLE 13.15 Differential Diagnosis for Elbow Fractures

Condition	Differentiating Features
Supracondylar fracture	• Account for 60% of pediatric fractures • X-rays and long arm immobilization • Monitor for neurologic changes
Medial epicondyle avulsion fracture	• Referred to as "Little League elbow" • Occurs in skeletal immature patients • X-rays and long arm immobilization
Radial head/neck fracture	• Make up 30% of elbow fractures • Nondisplaced fractures are often treated nonoperatively • X-rays and long arm immobilization • Displaced fracture often requires surgery
Olecranon fracture	• Secondary to trauma • Nonoperative with immobilization • Surgical fixation

DIAGNOSTIC STUDIES

Diagnostic studies to consider include the following:

- **X-ray:** The first-line diagnostic study of choice
- **CT scan/MRI:** May be done to further evaluate fracture pattern or occult fracture if the fracture is intra-articular
- **DEXA (dual energy x-ray absorptiometry) scan/laboratory workup:** A fracture after a low energy fall should lead to bone density workup

EVALUATION

Evaluation of an elbow fracture begins with a thorough physical examination. Evaluation of the shoulder and wrist is necessary to determine if other injuries have occurred. The patient is often in significant pain and is unable to perform motion, strength testing, or even correct positioning for imaging.

TREATMENT

- Immobilization
- Surgery if indicated
- Oral analgesics, ice, elevation
- Occupational therapy

PATIENT EDUCATION

- Because of the complex nature of the elbow joint, patients can lose full motion of the joint and should therefore be educated about the need to initiate PT immediately to minimize loss of function.
- Monitor for neurologic changes.
- Therapy is most often needed.

SPECIAL CONSIDERATIONS

Occult fractures occur more frequently in the pediatric population. The clinician should pay close attention to displacement of the fat pad on the lateral radiographs of the elbow. This is referred to as "sail sign" and is suspicious for occult fracture. This is to be treated as a fracture until otherwise ruled out. Further imaging may be required.[51]

13.3C ELBOW DISLOCATIONS

MEDICAL HISTORY AND CLINICAL PRESENTATION

Elbow dislocations are rare; however, when they do occur, they are usually caused by falling or trauma. Traumatic force may cause a dislocation, fracture, or both. The elbow is a complex joint allowing for fluid motion along many planes. Although there are various types of elbow dislocations, the most common is the posterior dislocation. Immediate medical attention is needed as surrounding blood supply and nerves can be damaged. Patients with a connective tissue disorder, such as Ehlers-Danlos syndrome, have an increased risk of dislocation with low-energy injuries due to their ligamentous laxity.

SIGNS AND SYMPTOMS

Similar to elbow fractures, a patient will present usually with a history of trauma and have immediate pain, edema, and decreased motion. Guarding will occur and the elbow is placed in the position that is the most comfortable. The patient may be unable to extend or rotate the forearm due to the displacement of the bones. They patient may also complain of numbness or tingling due to a stretch, compression, or damage to the nerve.[52]

PHYSICAL EXAMINATION

A full physical examination is warranted any time there is a traumatic accident. Elbow dislocations often occur with higher velocity traumas. After inspecting the skin for puncture wounds and abrasions, visualize the elbow. There may be edema, ecchymosis, gross deformity, decreased motion, or open skin. Evaluation of neurovascular status is important to determine if there is damage to the nerve and vessels.[52]

DIFFERENTIAL DIAGNOSIS

The differential diagnosis for elbow dislocation is summarized in Table 13.16.

TABLE 13.16 Differential Diagnosis for Elbow Dislocation

Differential Diagnosis	Description
Posterior elbow dislocation	• Account for 80% of elbow dislocations • Often after axial load on arm • Ulna displaces posteriorly • Reduction and splinting • Evaluate for fracture
Anterior elbow dislocation	• Rare injury • Often with associated fracture • Reduction, surgery if indicated, splint
Terrible triad	• Posterior dislocation with associated radial head and coronoid fractures • Surgery for reduction and stabilization • High-energy trauma commonly with associated injuries
Monteggia fracture dislocation	• Proximal third ulna fracture with associated radial head dislocation • Reduction, surgery, splinting

DIAGNOSTIC STUDIES

- **X-ray:** Evaluate disruption of bony anatomy. If reduction is attempted a postreduction x-ray in splint is indicated.
- **CT scan/MRI:** Imaging may be needed for further evaluation of bony and associated ligamentous injuries as indicated.

TREATMENT

- Reduction
- Surgery if indicated
- Splinting
- Therapy

PATIENT EDUCATION

- Surgery may be required.
- Stiffness is a complication that may occur with both operative and nonoperative treatment.
- Early PT and early motion are often indicated.
- Damage to nerves and arteries may lead to severe functional loss that affects daily function.
- Volkmann contractures are known complications of supracondylar fractures of the humerus.
- Brachial artery and median nerve injuries are most likely to occur in the setting of elbow injuries.[53]

KEY POINTS

Epicondylitis:

- Most courses of epicondylitis resolve after 12 to 18 months.
- Activity modifications and therapy often improve epicondylitis.
- Avoid counterforce braces because of potential for secondary PIN irritation in epicondylitis.

Elbow fracture:

- Pain after direct blow or trauma in suspicious for an elbow fracture.
- Significant guarding and decreased ROM may be present in elbow fractures.
- Neurovascular changes need to be considered and well documented pre- and postmanipulation for elbow fractures.
- Elbow stiffness is very common after elbow injury and can be debilitating.

Elbow dislocation:

- Loss of terminal extension is common with elbow dislocations. Early active ROM is important to maintain full motion.
- Residual instability may be present with elbow dislocations.
- Monitor for neurovascular compromise in setting of elbow dislocations.[54]

13.4 WRIST AND HAND DISORDERS

OVERVIEW

Hand and wrist injuries range from sprains, strains, nerve compressions, tendon injuries, fractures, dislocations, and lacerations.[55] Hand injuries will be seen in a large realm of practices from ED, urgent care, primary care, and occupational health clinics. Hand and wrist conditions affect all ages and populations. Sports-related injuries commonly occur in children and adolescences. The geriatric population is at a higher risk for the development of more chronic conditions.

EPIDEMIOLOGY

Hand and wrist injuries account for 20% to 30% of ED visits annually. Wrist and hand injuries occur in all ages and populations.[56] These injuries account for around $740 million per year in healthcare costs and are the most costly injury types over all other orthopedic injuries.[57]

PATHOPHYSIOLOGY

The hand and wrist consist of a complex system of bones, nerves, muscles, ligaments, soft tissues, and vascular structures (Figure 13.5). The wrist is made up of the radius and ulna, which articulate with the carpal bones. There are eight carpal bones arranged in proximal and distal rows. The distal row articulates with the metacarpals. The metacarpals provide the base for the fingers, which are composed of phalanx bones. The bones are held together by various ligaments. The ligaments provide the stability for these structures.

The extrinsic muscles originate in the forearm and terminate in the hand and allow movement of the hand and wrist. A pulley system of soft tissue allows leverage for the tendons to function. The intrinsic muscles of the hand provide fine motor function.

The muscles and skin are innervated by the median, radial, and ulnar nerves. These branch from the brachial plexus. Blood supply arises from the radial and ulnar arteries, which join to form the arches of the hands.[58]

Trauma or overuse to the hand and wrist can cause disruption or inflammation in the structures of the wrist and hand. This leads to pain and decreased function.

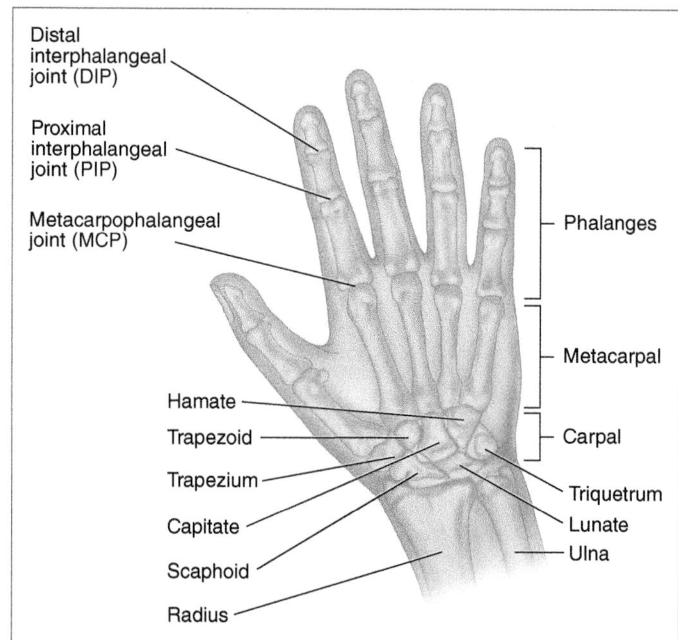

Figure 13.5 Bones of the hand and wrist.
(Source: Myrick KM. Advanced health assessment of the musculoskeletal system. In: Myrick KM, Karosas LM, eds. Advanced Health Assessment and Differential Diagnosis: Essentials for Clinical Practice. *Springer Publishing Company; 2021, Fig. 12.14.)*

13.4A CARPAL TUNNEL SYNDROME

MEDICAL HISTORY AND CLINICAL PRESENTATION

The carpal tunnel is formed from the carpal bones (acting as the floor and sides) and the transverse carpal ligament as the roof (Figure 13.6). Nine tendons and the median nerve all pass through the carpal tunnel. Carpal tunnel syndrome occurs as the median nerve is compressed as it passes through the carpal tunnel. This usually is progressive and a chronic condition; however, acute carpal tunnel can occur with trauma and other etiologies.[59] Risk factors include female sex, pregnancy, genetic predisposition, and underlying medical conditions that cause inflammation such as diabetes mellitus, chronic alcohol use, and smoking.[60]

SIGNS AND SYMPTOMS

Carpal tunnel syndrome affects the median nerve which supplies sensation to the thumb, index, long, and radial half of the ring finger as seen in Figure 13.6. The motor branch of the median nerve supplies motor function to the thenar eminence. Typical signs and symptoms include numbness affecting the median nerve distribution, atrophy, pain, and decreased strength, which can lead to complaints of dropping objects. Early symptoms are often noticed at night and cause difficulty sleeping and improvement of symptoms with hand movement such as shaking the hand vigorously.

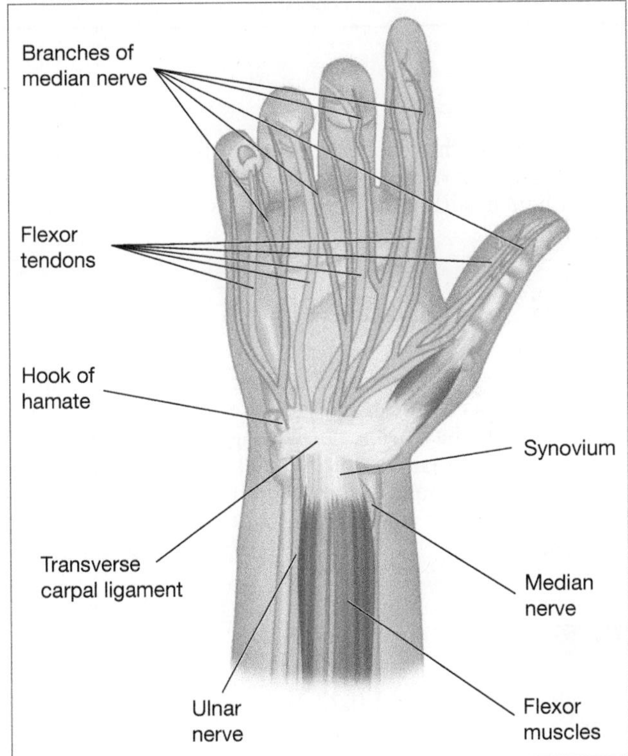

Figure 13.6 The carpal tunnel with median nerve.

(Source: Myrick KM. Advanced health assessment of the musculoskeletal system. In: Myrick KM, Karosas LM, eds. Advanced Health Assessment and Differential Diagnosis: Essentials for Clinical Practice. Springer Publishing Company; 2021,Fig. 12.18.)

Women who are pregnant may have symptoms that improve after pregnancy.[61]

PHYSICAL EXAMINATION

A thorough physical examination relies upon a neurologic exam. Decreased sensation along the median nerve distribution, loss of one- versus two-point discrimination, thenar atrophy, and decreased thumb opposition strength are all signs consistent with carpal tunnel syndrome. Further special tests to consider include the following[60]:

- **Tinel test:** Pain or re-creation of symptoms while tapping along the carpal tunnel
- **Phalen test:** Passive wrist flexion to 90 degrees re-creates symptoms

DIFFERENTIAL DIAGNOSIS

The differential diagnosis for carpal tunnel syndrome is summarized in Table 13.17.

DIAGNOSTIC STUDIES

- **EMG:** A nerve conduction study may be needed to evaluate for carpal tunnel syndrome. An EMG will test severity of compression as well as confirm the area of compression.
- **X-ray:** This imaging is used to evaluate any underlying cause such as arthritis or previous injury that would cause compression to carpal tunnel.
- **Laboratory:** Basic laboratory work may be used to rule out other causes.[62]

EVALUATION

There are many causes for hand numbness and the origin is often not due to compression at the hand. A full upper extremity neurologic examination is warranted. Similarly, underlying chronic diseases can also cause neurologic symptoms and should be ruled out prior to referral. Referral to a subspecialist should be made if needed. Conservative treatment is often the first step.

TREATMENT

- Nighttime wrist extension braces
- Steroid injection
- Occupational therapy
- Surgical release[59]

TABLE 13.17 Differential Diagnosis for Carpal Tunnel Syndrome

Diagnosis	Description
Thoracic outlet syndrome	Compression of the brachial plexus and vascular structures as it passes under the clavicle; usually vascular symptoms are present
Cervical nerve root compression	Compression of the nerve root as it exits the spinal column
Peripheral neuropathy	Decreased sensation due to underlying medical conditions such as diabetes and vitamin deficiency

PATIENT EDUCATION

- Carpal tunnel syndrome can be cured with conservative treatment.
- Night splinting is the first line of treatment in mild cases.
- The syndrome may progress requiring further diagnostics and possibly surgery.

13.4B WRIST AND HAND FRACTURES

MEDICAL HISTORY AND CLINICAL PRESENTATION

Wrist and hand fractures often occur after falling on an outstretched arm or a direct blow. Fractures may be displaced or nondisplaced. The patient's age, activity level, fracture pattern, and other factors may determine treatment options.

SIGNS AND SYMPTOMS

Fractures to the hand or wrist most often occur after trauma. The patient usually is able to describe an incident or trauma followed by immediate pain. They often endorse increased pain with motion of the hand, wrist, or elbow with improvement with immobilization. Edema, ecchymosis, and obvious deformity are accompanying signs.[63]

PHYSICAL EXAMINATION

Physical examination of fractures will elicit tenderness to palpation along the fracture site. Guarding, loss of function, edema, ecchymosis, and obvious deformity may be seen. Decreased sensation may occur due to a stretching or compression of the nerve. This is most times a transient neuropraxia.

DIFFERENTIAL DIAGNOSIS

The differential diagnosis for wrist and hand fractures is summarized in Table 13.18.

DIAGNOSTIC STUDIES

- **X-ray:** This is the first-line diagnostic study of choice.
- **CT scan:** This may be done to further evaluate fracture pattern or occult fracture, especially if the fracture is intra-articular.
- **DEXA scan/laboratory workup:** A fracture after a low-energy fall should lead to bone density workup.

EVALUATION

Evaluation of the patient as well as imaging will determine treatment options. Many factors play a role in the treatment including age, dominant versus nondominant hand, activity level, amount of displacement, and underlying medical conditions.

TREATMENT

- Immobilization
- Surgery if indicated
- Oral analgesics, ice, elevation
- Occupational therapy

TABLE 13.18 Differential Diagnosis for Wrist and Hand Fractures

Diagnosis	Description
Scaphoid fracture	• Most commonly fractured carpal bone. • Tenderness in the anatomic snuff box • May not show on imaging until 10–14 days after fracture • Risk of avascular necrosis due to blood supply • Splint: Thumb spica
Distal radius fracture (Colles/Smith)	• Most commonly after falling on an outstretched arm • Often present with deformity • Splint: Sugar tong
Galeazzi fracture	• Displaced distal radius fracture with ulna dislocation • Needs reduction and surgical fixation • Splint: Sugar tong
Torus fracture (buckle fracture)	• Pediatric injury only • Stable fracture • Splint: Sugar tong vs. wrist brace
Metacarpal fracture	• Often after direct blow or striking an object with a closed fist • "Boxer's fracture" is a fifth metacarpal neck fracture • Splint: Ulnar gutter or radial gutter
Phalanx fracture	• Mechanism of injury: Finger caught in an object or direct blow • Ulnar/radial gutter, volar splint, buddy finger splint

PATIENT EDUCATION

- Depending on the fracture pattern, full return to preinjury ROM may not occur.
- Compliance with splinting and activity modifications is important.

SPECIAL CONSIDERATIONS

If a patient present with tenderness to palpation in the anatomic snuff box, yet there is no fracture on x-ray, this should still be treated as a fracture. Place the patient into a thumb spica splint and have repeat imaging in 10 to 14 days to identify callus formation or the fracture line. Undiagnosed scaphoid fractures have a higher chance for nonunion, malunion, or avascular necrosis of the proximal pole if left untreated.[64]

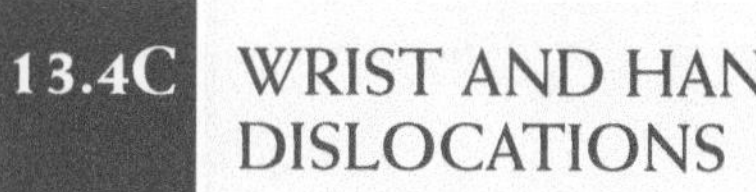

13.4C WRIST AND HAND DISLOCATIONS

MEDICAL HISTORY AND CLINICAL PRESENTATION

Much like fractures of the hand and wrist, dislocations often occur after trauma or a direct blow. Fractures and dislocations often coincide and are not isolated. When a dislocation occurs, there is often collateral damage to the bony structures when displaced out of normal alignment. If the normal anatomy of the wrist is disrupted, there may also be a disruption to neurovascular supply. Nerves and arteries may be placed on a stretch which compromises blood flow and sensation. Reduction of the wrist is indicated to decrease irreversible effects.[65]

SIGNS AND SYMPTOMS

Again, the signs and symptoms of a dislocation are often associated with the signs and symptoms of a fracture. Increased pain, edema, obvious deformity, guarding, and decreased function may occur. Patients often have complaints of paresthesias in the hand. This is due to a compression or stretch of a nerve.

PHYSICAL EXAMINATION

The patient's physical examination may be limited in an acute injury. Patients generally present with significant guarding. Examination may reveal edema, ecchymosis, or obvious deformity. Patients who have sustained a carpal dislocation exhibit "fullness" in the wrist due to the displacement of the bones. A neurovascular examination is indicated to document adequate blood flow and sensation.

DIFFERENTIAL DIAGNOSIS

The differential diagnosis for wrist and hand dislocations is summarized in Table 13.19.

DIAGNOSTIC STUDIES

- **X-ray:** Evaluate disruption of bony anatomy; if reduction is attempted a postreduction x-ray in splint is indicated.
- **CT scan:** Used for surgical planning or to obtain additional information not available with just plain film.
- **MRI:** Used in evaluating soft tissue injury.

EVALUATION

Dislocations are frequently missed on x-ray. Proper diagnosis and quick reduction of the injury will lead to better outcomes. Referral to hand surgeon is indicated.

TABLE 13.19 Differential Diagnosis for Wrist and Hand Dislocations

Diagnosis	Description
Perilunate dislocations	• Capitate dislocated dorsally • Treatment: Reduction, splinting, surgery
Lunate dislocation	• Lunate dislocated volar • "Spilled tea-cup" sign on lateral x-ray • "Piece of pie" sign of posteroanterior x-ray • Treatment: Reduction, splinting, surgery
Scapholunate dissociation	• Widening space between the scaphoid and lunate • Treatment: Splinting and surgery if indicated
Galeazzi fracture	• Displaced distal radius fracture with ulna dislocation • Treatment: Reduction and surgical fixation • Splint: Sugar tong

TREATMENT

- Reduction
- Surgery
- Splinting
- Therapy

PATIENT EDUCATION

- Wrist and hand dislocations have associated ligament damage. Although the ligaments can be repaired surgically, there is a risk for long-standing instability and need for subsequent surgeries. This may include ligament reconstruction, fusion, and excision of carpal bones.
- Early osteoarthritis may occur.
- Monitor for compartment syndrome.
- Monitor for acute carpal tunnel symptoms.
- If patient is taken to the operating room for surgical intervention, carpal tunnel release is performed to prevent median nerve entrapment.[65]

KEY POINTS

Carpal tunnel syndrome:

- Carpal tunnel syndrome affects the thumb, index, long, and half of the ring finger.
- Pain, paresthesia, achy hand, dropping objects, and nocturnal pain are common symptoms.
- Neurologic examination and positive compression maneuvers are useful in evaluation.
- Further workup includes x-rays, EMG, and laboratory work.
- Treatment options include night splinting, occupational therapy, steroid injection, and surgical release.

Wrist and hand fractures:

- Pain after trauma and decreased motion is highly suspicious of a fracture.
- Obtain x-rays and immobilize properly for best treatment outcomes.
- Refer to an orthopedic surgeon.
- Tenderness to palpation in the anatomic snuff box is treated as a scaphoid fracture until repeat x-rays after 10 to 14 days are obtained for further evaluation.

Wrist and hand dislocations:

- Reduction, splinting, and referral to hand surgery in a timely manner are important.
- Even with proper treatment, there may be long-term effects such as instability, osteoarthritis, pain, stiffness, and need for subsequent surgeries.

13.5 HIP DISORDERS

Christine Bruce and Carey A. Wheelhouse

OVERVIEW

Hip fractures can occur at a variety of different locations including the head, neck, and intertrochanteric portion of the femur. Those in the geriatric population are the most likely to sustain a hip fracture, with this risk increasing even more in the setting of osteoporosis. It is not just contact with the ground that causes a hip fracture but rather an osteoporotic bone may not be able to support the weight of the body with resultant fracture of the hip causing the fall. A patient with a fractured hip may have shortening of the lower extremity with external rotation. Diagnosis can be made with AP and lateral x-rays. Occult fracture of the hip that is not readily apparent on a hip film can be diagnosed with an MRI.

Hip fracture affects an estimated 1.6 million persons annually and the consequences of hip fracture are significant with more than half of those sustaining a fracture either dying or not returning to functional abilities in order to function independently.[66] Alzheimer disease and other cognitive impairment processes pose major risks for hip fracture to occur.[67] Hypoalbuminemia is another known risk factor for increased mortality and longer length of hospitalization for patients who sustain hip fracture.[68] Patients with a positive attitude regarding this injury have better functional recovery after hip fracture than those who are clinically depressed.[69]

Diagnosis of a hip fracture is made with demonstration of the fracture on x-ray with the patient history usually being specific for either a fall or trauma. Hip fractures often lead to increased risks for morbidity and mortality that may not be directly related to the fracture itself. Many patients do not fully recover ambulation capabilities following a hip fracture. An older patient who sustained a hip fracture may not be able to get up from the fall with resultant complications such as rhabdomyolysis, blood loss leading to hypotension and shock, and kidney injury as a result of poor perfusion and increased cellular elements arriving in the kidney.

EPIDEMIOLOGY

The primary risk factors for hip fracture are aging and osteoporosis. Significant trauma to the hip from external forces can also result in both hip fracture and/or dislocation. Falling to the ground can traumatize the hip or an osteoporotic hip may not be able to support the body weight and fracture, leading to a fall. Hip fractures can occur in the femoral head, femoral neck (often called subcapital), intertrochanteric, and subtrochanteric areas.

PATHOPHYSIOLOGY

Bones that have less density or abnormal chemical components have an increased risk for fracturing. Trauma stronger than bone force resistance can also lead to fracture. Metastatic cancer to the bone replaces the strong cellular elements leading to abnormal architecture with tendency to pathologically fracture. Pathologic fracture is any fracture that occurs through abnormal bone architecture, which would include osteoporosis, metastatic disease of the bone, or primary bone tumor.

13.5A HIP FRACTURES

MEDICAL HISTORY AND CLINICAL PRESENTATION

These fractures are most likely to occur in the older population with 80% of these fractures occurring in females who also have a higher rate of osteoporosis with the average age of 80 years.[70] Patients with hip fracture will complain of pain located in the groin and typically will not be able to ambulate. Hip fracture pain can also radiate into the knee, which is why joints are checked proximal and distal to the site of the pain. Depending on the amount of displacement, the patient may not be able to ambulate. Transportation to the healthcare center can be done via wheelchair or litter as most patients will not be ambulatory. The typical patient will have sustained a fall or will have received trauma directly to the hip leading to the hip injury.

SIGNS AND SYMPTOMS

Groin pain from hip fracture can be significant and will occur immediately after the fall. Patients with displaced fractures will not be able to walk, but patients with impacted fractures may be able to continue to ambulate with only mild to moderate pain. Patients keep the affected lower extremity motionless as any movement will cause significant pain with displaced fractures.

PHYSICAL EXAMINATION

Patients with displaced fractures of the hip present with external rotation and abduction of the hip with the leg appearing to be shortened.[70] Patients with an impacted femur fracture will not be able to perform a straight leg raise against resistance. Palpation of the hip will elucidate pain with increased pain with any attempt at logrolling the lower extremity, which is essentially performing internal and external rotation of the hip.

DIFFERENTIAL DIAGNOSIS

The differential diagnosis for hip fractures is summarized in Table 13.20.

TABLE 13.20 Differential Diagnosis for Hip Fractures

Diagnosis	Description
Hip dislocation	Can occur anteriorly (most likely post total hip arthroplasty with flexion and abduction) or posteriorly (significant force applied to a flexed hip mostly seen with significant trauma).
Trochanteric bursitis	Lateral hip pain; minimal pain with internal and external rotation of the hip. Stretching of hip capsule relieves pain.
Osteoarthritis of hip	Groin pain with impaired internal and external rotation of the hip. Joint space narrowing with osteophyte production on imaging.
Aseptic necrosis of hip	Increased risk in the setting of sickle cell disease, prolonged steroid use, or atherosclerosis.
Ischial bursitis	Buttocks pain that is worsened with sitting on hard surfaces
Acetabular fracture	Diagnosed most commonly with x-ray. Can occur in setting of posterior hip dislocation.
Femoral shaft fracture	Increased swelling in the thigh from bleeding at the fracture site. X-rays demonstrate this fracture.
Septic hip	Signs of sepsis can be found. Hip is red, tender, and warm. Aspiration of joint demonstrates pus with increased WBC count.
Pubic ramus fracture	Patients have pain in the groin similar to the pain felt with hip fracture. X-rays differentiate between these two conditions.

WBC, white blood cell.

DIAGNOSTIC STUDIES

Plain film is typically sufficient to make the diagnosis. An AP pelvic x-ray along with AP and lateral views of the affected hip are indicated. An x-ray of the femur can be ordered if either femoral fracture or distal extension of the fracture in the hip is suspected. If this x-ray is normal and there is still an index of suspicion for a hip fracture, CT or MRI can identify the fracture site.

MRI of the pelvis is ordered if hip fracture is still under consideration with positive MRI findings for fracture showing marrow edema and a fracture line on this very sensitive test. CT can be used if MRI is unavailable. CT can confirm a suspicious finding on a plain x-ray or can confirm a fracture when fracture of the hip is suspected but routine x-rays are negative.

EVALUATION

Since the diagnosis is primarily made by x-ray, additional laboratory studies are not needed except for helping to determine the patient's preoperative risks prior to undergoing surgery. Keeping the patient comfortable after sustaining a hip fracture is of prime importance. Stabilizing the fracture site until more definitive therapy can be done is necessary. Urgent surgical intervention occurs following medical stabilization since the patient's medical condition tends to deteriorate with the patient being in a bedbound state.

Following confirmation of the hip fracture, the patient is taken to the operating room for appropriate surgical intervention after optimal medical stabilization is performed.

TREATMENT

Operative treatment for hip fractures is more likely to result in fracture healing without leg shortening, requires a shorter hospital stay, is associated with an increase in the return of patient back to the original residence, and often results in a patient being able to begin ambulating—in some cases bearing full weight—immediately after surgery, when compared to patients treated conservatively with bed rest and traction.[71] Multidisciplinary team management including orthopedic surgeons, medical support clinicians, physical therapists, and social workers can provide improvement in perioperative medical care, expedited preoperative evaluation, and cost savings for patients in facilities that have sufficient volume of patients needing these services.[72]

Preoperative traction is not recommended due to lack of benefit for pain relief, ability to obtain reduction, or the quality of reduction at the time of surgery.[73]

The treatment of hip fractures is dependent upon the specific type of hip fracture. Intracapsular or undisplaced femoral neck fractures are treated with open reduction and internal fixation (ORIF) using a dynamic hip screw or multiple cannulated screws. Patients who are given operative treatment rather than conservative care have reduced length of stay in the hospital and improved rehabilitation potential.[74]

Patients who are younger than 60 years of age with a femoral neck fracture undergo urgent ORIF in order to lessen the risk of avascular necrosis to the femoral head, although urgent surgical timing has not been definitively proved. Internal fixation can be done with multiple screws or dynamic hip screws or can be done with hip implant to the affected area if blood supply is compromised. Patients with a history of alcohol abuse, renal disease, or respiratory disease should have hemiarthroplasty considered as an alternative treatment as these patients are most likely to have nonunion and avascular necrosis when they are under 60 years of age and sustain a displaced fracture of the femoral neck.[75]

Patients with femoral neck fracture who are between the ages of 60 and 80 have less need for revision surgery at 1 year with no change in mortality if they undergo arthroplasty rather than ORIF but they have an increased risk of infection and blood loss.[76,77]

Intertrochanteric fractures of the hip or extracapsular fractures that are undisplaced are treated with internal fixation with dynamic hip screws and nailing or percutaneous (minimally invasive) fixation. Displaced intertrochanteric fractures can be treated in the same manner in order to restore the anatomy of the proximal femur in order to allow for early rehabilitation.

In patients undergoing surgery for closed fracture fixation, single dose antibiotic prophylaxis significantly reduces deep surgical site infection, superficial surgical site infections, urinary infections, and respiratory infections. Single dose prophylaxis with ceftriaxone has been found to be a cost effective intervention.[78] Following surgery, patients are typically given PT and rehabilitation. Weight bearing and ROM activities are encouraged in order to allow the patient to recover, return home, and resume normal activities. The best predictors for rehabilitation success are the instrumental activities of daily living and cognition of the patient undergoing rehabilitation.[79] Scheduled analgesic regimens can improve functional outcome in geriatric patients undergoing rehabilitation.[80]

In addition to prophylactic antibiotics, patients with hip fractures are also given deep vein thrombus prophylaxis, preferably low-molecular-weight heparin.[70]

PATIENT EDUCATION

Prevention of hip fractures resides in the prevention of osteoporosis as low bone mineral density is a primary risk factor for the development of this condition. In addition to preventing bone loss that naturally occurs with aging, prevention of falls is also essential in mitigating the risk of hip fracture. In hospital falls can be mitigated, even in patients who have cognitive impairment.[81] Avoidance of benzodiazepines is a useful strategy in preventing falls in the hospitalized patient. It is estimated that 84% of all adverse events in the hospitalized patient are related to falls.[82]

Other preventive strategies against hip fracture include the management of osteoporosis, adequate nutrition including sufficient calcium and vitamin D intake, reduction of alcohol intake, and smoking cessation. Home assessments to prevent falls include removing tripping hazards and installing grab bars in the shower and toileting area. Medication assessment includes eliminating medications that cause impairment in cognition, those with high anticholinergic activity, and those that are known to cause orthostatic hypotension. Patients who wear hip protectors have marginal benefit with their use.[83]

Complications of hip fractures include avascular necrosis, which is caused by damage to the blood supply of the femoral head. Risk of avascular necrosis increases if the femoral neck fracture is displaced or if the fracture has significant valgus angulation.[84] Nonunion of the fracture site and fixation failure are the two most common reasons for reoperation and this situation is more likely to occur with femoral neck fractures in older adults who are treated with internal fixation rather than arthroplasty and this is more likely to be seen in women and in the older age population.[85]

Osteoarthritis is another long-term complication for patients who have had significant hip injuries and in those with congenital development dysplasia of the hip.

13.5B HIP DISLOCATIONS

Hip dislocation in the adult population is most commonly posterior and is most likely to occur in trauma situations such as having a flexed hip contact a dashboard during a motor vehicle collision. These posterior hip dislocations can result in stretching of the sciatic nerve over the posteriorly dislocated femoral head. Fragments of bone from a posterior wall acetabulum fracture can also cause injury to the sciatic nerve.[86]

Anterior hip dislocation can also result in injury to the femoral artery, vein, or nerve.

Significant trauma leads to hip dislocation so concomitant injuries often occur to the ipsilateral knee, patella, and femur. There also may be associated pelvic fractures and spinal injuries.[87]

Reduction of a dislocated hip is performed as a closed reduction as soon as possible as muscles go into spasm interfering with relocation of the joint and also delayed closed reduction increases the risk of avascular necrosis.

Two techniques are used to relocate the hip, which is done under sedation with or without muscle relaxation: The Allis technique involves flexing the hip to 90 degrees and applying vertical traction to the femur. This technique worked best when the patient is lying on a rigid backboard or put onto the floor. The Captain Morgan technique entails holding a bedbound patient's hips down by a sheet or belt and then flexing the dislocated hip. Clinicians place their knee under the patient's knee and lift up while applying vertical traction to the femur. Following either of these techniques, a CT is performed to identify fracture or intra-articular debris.

Following total hip replacement, the prosthetic hip dislocates in up to 2% of patients. Posterior dislocations are most common. Closed reduction is used to relocate the prosthetic hip after the first episode but recurrent dislocations of prosthetic hips often require revision surgery to prevent future occurrences.

KEY POINTS

- Hip dislocations can result in pain, swelling, decreased ROM or inability to move the joint, and shortening with internal rotation of the hip, with the hip being held in flexion and abduction.
- Anterior hip dislocation patients have the hip held in external rotation with mild flexion and abduction.
- AP and lateral x-rays can be used to confirm the dislocation.
- Since these injuries occurred as a result of high-velocity traumatic events, searches for injury to other structures such as the pelvis and femur should be performed.

13.5C OSGOOD-SCHLATTER DISEASE

OVERVIEW

Osgood-Schlatter disease (OSD) is an overuse condition, resulting from repetitive strain on the quadriceps muscles and subsequent injury to the tibial tuberosity. Patients typically present with anterior knee pain in adolescence, often following period of rapid growth.[88,89] OSD is self-limiting and symptoms typically resolve with conservative management.[88–90]

EPIDEMIOLOGY

OSD affects approximately 20% to 25% of the adolescent population, most commonly adolescents participating in athletics especially in sports that require jumping such as gymnastics and basketball or baseball catchers who perform repetitive squatting.[88] Onset of OSD is earlier in females than males, typically presenting in 8- to 13-year-old females and 10- to 15-year-old males.[88–90] Prevalence of OSD was previously thought to be more common in males; however, as the number of female athletes has increased, more recent data suggest a similar prevalence in both males and females.[88]

PATHOPHYSIOLOGY

OSD results from stress on the tibial tubercle. Repetitive extension of the knee coupled with forceful contraction of the quadriceps femoris muscle, as often seen in sports involving running and jumping, results in extensor mechanism overuse.[88,90] Extensor mechanism overuse subsequently leads to the patellar tendon placing traction on the tibial tubercle apophysis, resulting in microavulsion or avulsion fractures.[88] OSD often occurs around adolescent growth spurts, suggesting periods of rapid growth contribute to patellar tendon strain on the tibial tubercle apophysis. Recent research has suggested tightness or shortening of the rectus femoris muscle contributes to the development of OSD.[88,91]

MEDICAL HISTORY AND CLINICAL PRESENTATION

Patients with OSD present with gradual onset of anterior knee pain localized inferior to the patella, over the patellar tendon and tibial tuberosity.[89,90] Onset typically begins in adolescence following a period of rapid growth.[88–90] Anterior knee pain usually presents unilaterally, though OSD may present bilaterally in approximately 20% to 30% of patients.[88] Knee pain in OSD is aggravated by running, jumping, and kneeling, and is alleviated with rest.[88–90]

SIGNS AND SYMPTOMS

Localized knee pain inferior to the patella is the most common presenting symptom of OSD. Anterior knee pain may begin as an intermittent, mild ache and over time progress to severe, continuous pain that limits activities.[90] Patients presenting with OSD may also report anterior knee swelling, difficulty with ambulation, or a limp.[88,90]

PHYSICAL EXAMINATION

Inspection may reveal a prominent tibial tuberosity on the affected knee.[88,89] There is localized tenderness to palpation of the tibial tuberosity and, in some cases, the distal patellar tendon.[90] In chronic cases of OSD, a firm mass may be palpated over the tibial tuberosity.[88] Swelling and tenderness of the patellar tendon may also be noted upon palpation, though pain is more pronounced over the tibial tuberosity. Active ROM often elicits anterior knee pain.[89] In acute cases, active ROM may be limited, but passive ROM remains intact.[88] Pain is reproduced with resisted extension of the affected knee.[89] Patients with severe OSD may also have gait abnormalities.[88] Ligamentous stability of the affected knee remains intact.[88]

DIFFERENTIAL DIAGNOSIS

OSD should be distinguished from other sources of anterior knee pain. Patellar tendinitis may present with similar features and is distinguished from OSD by tenderness to palpation of patellar tendon as opposed to the tibial tuberosity. Acute avulsion fractures of the tibial tuberosity present with sudden onset of pain, whereas OSD pain has a gradual onset.[92] Ligamentous instability, effusion, or mechanical symptoms should lead the clinician to consider patellar dislocation or injuries to the meniscus, cruciate ligaments, or collateral ligaments.[88] Knee pain in osteochondritis dissecans is reproduced with palpation medial to the inferior pole of the patellar tendon, performed with the knee in a flexed position, differentiating it from the pain of OSD.[93] Nighttime pain or presence of systemic symptoms, such as fever, malaise, or weight loss, may be related to bony tumors or infection.[88,89] Children presenting with knee pain should also undergo examination of the hip; knee pain with associated loss of hip ROM may indicate hip pathology as the source of pain.

DIAGNOSTIC STUDIES

The diagnosis of OSD is often made by history and physical examination. However, plain radiographs may help rule out other diagnoses in patients who present with additional symptoms. Radiographic findings consistent with a diagnosis of OSD are best seen in lateral views of the knee. Radiographic findings of OSD include elevation or fragmentation of the tibial tuberosity, a superficial ossicle in the patellar tendon, soft tissue swelling anterior to the tibial tuberosity, and thickening of the patellar tendon.[88] Ultrasound has been used to aid in the diagnosis and management of OSD, though most cases are successfully diagnosed and managed without sonography. Ultrasound may provide greater visualization of soft tissue than plain radiographs, demonstrating distal patellar tendon thickening, pretibial soft tissue swelling, and fragmentation of the tibial tuberosity ossification center.[88,91] While not necessary for the diagnosis and management of OSD, MRI has been useful in atypical or refractory presentations of OSD.[88,94]

TREATMENT

In the majority of cases, treatment of OSD includes activity modification and NSAIDs.[88,90] In rare cases, surgical management is required.[88,89]

- Activity modification
  - Reduction in frequency, duration, and intensity of exercise for a limited time
  - Avoid high-impact activities, such as running and jumping.
  - Avoid kneeling or provide padding to the tibial tuberosity.
  - Low-impact activities, such as swimming or cycling, may be performed as long as the patient is able to do so without pain.
  - When symptoms resolve, the patient may begin a gradual return to play.
    - If symptoms return, modify the frequency, duration, and intensity until symptoms resolve.
- NSAIDs
  - These may be used for pain relief and swelling reduction as needed for short periods of time.
- Referral to specialists
  - Patients with severe or intolerable symptoms, refractory symptoms, or symptoms that persist into adulthood should be referred to a specialist for consideration of surgical management.

PATIENT EDUCATION

Patients should be educated on the pathophysiology as well as the self-limited nature of OSD. Provide patients with the reassurance that, while OSD may recur for 12 to 18 months, the condition will likely fully resolve within a few years, after completion of their growth spurt.[88–90] However, failure to treat OSD may result in chronic pain and nonunion of the tibial tuberosity.[88]

Patients should be provided information on appropriate physical activities, including strengthening and stretching exercises to promote muscle balance, maintenance of physical activities that do not produce pain, and gradual return to higher intensity activities as symptoms tolerate.[88,89] Rarely, conservative management may not fully resolve symptoms, and approximately 10% of patients continue to experience symptoms into adulthood.[89,90] If patients have persistent symptoms that do not resolve with conservative treatment or continue to persist into adulthood, they should be referred to a specialist for further evaluation and treatment recommendations.[88,89]

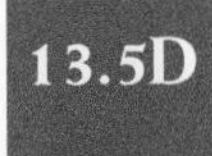

13.5D SLIPPED CAPITAL FEMORAL EPIPHYSIS

OVERVIEW

SCFE is a disorder characterized by capital femoral epiphysis displacement from the metaphysis through the physis. It is most common in overweight adolescents, particularly males. Common symptoms of SCFE include a limp and pain in the hip, groin, thigh, or knee. Patients with SCFE often have limited hip ROM, and radiographic findings demonstrate the epiphyseal displacement. Surgical treatment of SCFE is intended to reduce further progression of the slip and prevent the development of complications.

EPIDEMIOLOGY

SCFE is a hip disorder occurring most commonly in adolescence. The incidence of SCFE is approximately 10 per 100,000 U.S. adolescents.[95,96] SCFE occurs more frequently in overweight adolescents, with roughly half of patients diagnosed with SCFE having a BMI in the 95th percentile or higher.[95] The incidence of SCFE is higher among male adolescents than female, occurring at a rate of 13.35 per 100,000 males and 8.07 per 100,000 females.[96]

Over the past few decades, the age of onset has been gradually decreasing in both males and females, likely in relationship to earlier maturation of both genders.[96] Current research suggests the average age of onset is 12.7 for males and 11.2 for girls, approximately 1 year earlier than previous studies.[95,96] Earlier age of onset is often correlated with obesity.[95,96] SCFE is more common in Pacific Islanders, Blacks, Native Americans, and Hispanics than Caucasians.[95,96]

PATHOPHYSIOLOGY

SCFE occurs when the capital femoral epiphysis is displaced from the metaphysis through the physis. In this displacement, the metaphysis moves anterosuperior to the acetabulum, displacing it from the epiphysis, which is held in the acetabulum by the ligamentum teres.[95,97] The pathophysiology of SCFE is likely multifactorial, including both biochemical and biomechanical factors. Because SCFE is often associated with obesity, pathophysiology is thought to be associated with biomechanical changes related to obesity. Obesity is associated with approximately a 10- to 11-degree decrease in femoral anteversion relative to nonobese adolescents, termed relative retroversion.[95,97] Relative retroversion subsequently increases the shear stress across the physis. Additional research suggests children with SCFE have a deeper acetabulum than children without SCFE, again creating greater shear stress across the physis.[97]

Other considerations of SCFE pathophysiology include hormonal changes related to puberty. Accelerated growth often occurs around the age of onset for SCFE, and researchers have suggested growth hormone may widen and subsequently weaken the epiphysis.[95,97] SCFE occurs more frequently in males and occurs rarely in females after menarche, suggesting that testosterone may also weaken physeal strength.[97] Additionally, incidence of SCFE has been noted to be higher in children with hypothyroidism, those with hypogonadism, and those undergoing growth hormone supplementation, suggesting a possible association with endocrine dysfunction.[95,97]

MEDICAL HISTORY AND CLINICAL PRESENTATION

The typical presentation of SCFE includes hip pain and abnormal gait. Pain may present as pain of the hip, groin, thigh, or knee.[95,97] Gait abnormalities often include a limp on the affected side.[95,97] The presentation of these symptoms differs based on the classification of SCFE, which may be classified by presentation pattern, stability, or severity.[95,97]

SIGNS AND SYMPTOMS

SCFEs categorized by presentation include pre-slip, acute, chronic, or acute on chronic. Chronic SCFE is the most common presentation, occurring in about 85% of SCFE cases. Acute SCFE occurs in approximately 10–15% of cases.[95,97]

Patients in the pre-slip phase commonly present with leg weakness and groin or knee pain upon exertion. Prolonged standing will exacerbate symptoms of SCFE in the pre-slip stage. Patients with acute slip present with severe pain that limits weight bearing, external rotation deformity, and decreased ROM. To classify as acute, symptoms are present for 3 weeks or less. Patients with chronic SCFE often have intermittent bouts of hip, groin, thigh, or knee pain that presents over months to years. Intermittent limping and leg-length discrepancy may also be noted in chronic SCFE. Acute on chronic SCFE initially presents with symptoms similar to chronic SCFE, but patients subsequently develop a sudden increase in symptoms due to an acute slip.[95,97]

Alternatively, SCFEs can also be classified by stability and radiographic severity. SCFE classifications include stable versus unstable. A stable SCFE is one in which the child or adolescent is able to maintain weight bearing and ambulation without assistive devices, such as crutches. Contrarily, an unstable SCFE is one in which the child or adolescent is unable to bear weight or ambulate, or otherwise requires assistive devices to do so. Classification of SCFE by stability is predictive of prognosis, with roughly 50% of unstable SCFE cases developing osteonecrosis.[95,97]

Radiographic classifications of SCFE are based on the severity of the slippage, and may be mild, moderate, or severe (Box 13.1). Further discussion of radiographic classification is found below under Diagnostic Studies.

BOX 13.1 Categories of Clinical Presentation and Stability Classifications of Slipped Capital Femoral Epiphysis

Clinical Presentation Classification
Pre-slip
Acute
Chronic
Acute on chronic
Stability Classification
Stable
Unstable

PHYSICAL EXAMINATION

Physical examination should include general inspection of body habitus. Observation of gait may reveal antalgic gait including external rotation of the affected limb, shortened steps to decrease pain, waddling gait, or inability to bear weight. Leg-length discrepancies may show the affected limb to be shorter than the unaffected hip. Hip ROM may be decreased, ranging from mild limitations in movement to severe pain and loss of internal rotation, abduction, and flexion on the affected side. It is important to assess both lower extremities, as bilateral symptoms may occur in up to 60% of cases.[95,97]

DIFFERENTIAL DIAGNOSIS

SCFE should be differentiated from other causes of antalgic gait or limp in child and adolescent patients. Late diagnosis of developmental hip dysplasia may also lead to leg-length discrepancies, hip pain, and antalgic gait; however, radiographic features show dysplasia of the femoral head, acetabulum, or both. Legg-Calve-Perthes disease, or idiopathic avascular necrosis of the hip, may also present with hip pain in children or adolescents. However, diagnosis of Legg-Calve-Perthes disease usually occurs at an earlier age than SCFE, with a peak incidence in 5- to 7-year-olds.[98] Bone scan or MRI of Legg-Calve-Perthes disease will show decreased perfusion of the femoral head.[99] Other considerations of acute hip pain and loss of motion may include septic arthritis or osteomyelitis, in which patients will likely present with systemic symptoms such as fever, and diagnosis is made upon aspiration of hip fluid.

DIAGNOSTIC STUDIES

Initial evaluation of SCFE includes plain hip radiographs, consisting of AP and lateral views of both hips. Patients with stable SCFE may undergo frog-leg lateral views, which may be best at detecting early symptoms.[95] However, patients with acute and unstable SCFE symptoms are at risk of

TABLE 13.21 Classification of Slipped Capital Femoral Epiphysis Severity Based on Radiographic Findings

Severity	AP View	Lateral View
Mild	Displacement of epiphysis is <33% of the diameter of the femoral neck	Degree of slip is <30%
Moderate	Displacement of epiphysis is 33%–50% of the diameter of the femoral neck	Degree of slip is 30%–50%
Severe	Displacement of epiphysis is >50% of the diameter of the femoral neck	Degree of slip is >50%

AP, anteroposterior.

further displacement with frog-leg lateral views and should undergo true lateral hip radiographs instead.[100]

AP radiographs of bilateral hips may demonstrate a widening of the physis as well as signs of remodeling in the metaphysis and retroversion deformity of the femoral neck. Additional findings on AP radiographs may include the metaphyseal blanch sign of Steel and Klein's line. The metaphyseal blanch line of Steel is seen as a double density, in which the posteriorly displaced epiphysis is superimposed on the medial metaphysis. Klein's line is drawn along the anterosuperior aspect of the femoral neck on the AP view of the hip. In a normal hip, Kline's line will intersect with the epiphysis. However, in SCFE, the epiphysis is often just flush with or below Klein's line.[95,97] Lateral views often better demonstrate the posterior displacement of the epiphysis on the femoral neck.

Radiographic severity measurement includes mild, moderate, or severe. Severity on the AP view is determined by the size of displacement of the epiphysis (Table 13.21). On the lateral view, the severity is determined by the angle of the slip. The degree of the slip angle is calculated by subtracting the epiphyseal-shaft angle on the unaffected side from the epiphyseal shaft angle on the affected side.[95,97] Additional studies may include MRI or bone scan if the child is at risk of osteonecrosis. CT scanning provides three-dimensional visualization of SCFE but is not necessary to make the diagnosis.[97]

TREATMENT

Treatment of SCFE serves two major purposes: (1) prevent progression of the slip and (2) avoid complications including osteonecrosis, chondrolysis, and degenerative joint disease.[95,97,101] Treatment of SCFE is often surgical. Once diagnosed with SCFE, patients should be non-weight-bearing status, using crutches or a wheelchair, and referred for orthopedic evaluation. Patients with unstable or bilateral SCFEs require urgent orthopedic referral and hospital admission due to their higher risk of complications. Multiple surgical interventions exist, though the most widely accepted is the single-screw fixation.[95,97] Patients with single-screw fixation may have a 6- to 8-week non-weight-bearing period following surgery.

PATIENT EDUCATION

- Surgical treatment is recommended to reduce further progression of the slip and avoid complications.
- Complications of SCFE include osteonecrosis, chondrolysis, and degenerative joint disease.
- Single-screw fixation is the most widely accepted surgical intervention, with lower rates of complications than other surgical methods.
- After surgical fixation, patients should expect to be non-weight-bearing for 6 to 8 weeks.
- Prophylactic pinning of the contralateral hip is controversial, and patients should have discussion with their orthopedic surgeon for further recommendations.

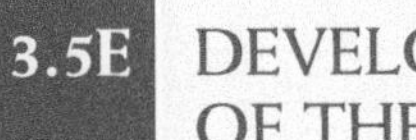

13.5E DEVELOPMENTAL DYSPLASIA OF THE HIP

OVERVIEW

Developmental dysplasia of the hip (DDH) refers to a spectrum of abnormalities of the femoral head, acetabulum, or both present at the time of birth. Untreated DDH leads to early onset of hip osteoarthritis and has been documented as the underlying cause in up to 29% of all hip replacements in patients under the age of 60.[102,103] Early identification and treatment of DDH are associated with improved prognosis and decreased risk of long-term complications. The American Academy of Pediatrics (AAP) recommends universal screening for DDH with physical examination in the newborn to 12-month-old child.[103] Children with risk factors for or symptoms of DDH should be referred to an orthopedic specialist for further evaluation and treatment. Early treatment options include flexion-abduction splinting and are associated with a decreased likelihood of developing osteoarthritis of the hip.[102–104]

EPIDEMIOLOGY

Approximately 1 in 1,000 infants are born with a dislocated hip, whereas up to 28.5 infants per 1,000 may have dysplasia or instability of the hip.[102–105] The left hip is most commonly affected, occurring in 60% of DDH cases.[103,104] DDH occurs more commonly in firstborn children, females, and infants with breech presentation.[103–105] Additionally, 12%–33% of patients with DDH have a family history positive for DDH.[104] Risk of DDH increases with the number of affected family members. Patients with a sibling who has DDH are at a 6% greater risk of developing DDH. Patients with a parent who has DDH are at a 12% greater risk of developing DDH.[104] The risk further increases to 36% in patients who have both a parent and sibling with DDH.[104]

PATHOPHYSIOLOGY

Pathophysiology of DDH is thought to be both biologic and environmental. Risk factors for DDH include intrauterine position, sex, race, family history, and the postnatal environment. In utero position is thought to contribute to DDH through forces on the position of the hip and knee during gestation. In utero, the left hip is commonly adducted against the mother's spine, which likely contributes to higher rates of left hip DDH. In firstborn children, the mother's uterus has not yet been stretched, and is suspected to influence the positioning of the child's limb in utero and subsequent hip instability. Breech positioning is associated with in utero knee extension, which may lead to hip instability through a continuous strain on the hamstrings.[103,104]

Researchers speculate estrogen may increase ligamentous laxity, explaining the higher incidence of DDH in females.[104,105] Other risk factors for DDH, including oligohydramnios, large for gestational age birth weight, metatarsus adductus, and torticollis, are less understood.[103,104] DDH is more common in cultures that swaddle their infants. Swaddling places the hip into an adducted and extended position, placing the child at risk for abnormal developmental of the femoral head or acetabulum.[103]

MEDICAL HISTORY AND CLINICAL PRESENTATION

All children should undergo a thorough history to identify risk factors for DDH. Because DDH consists of a spectrum of hip abnormalities ranging from mild dysplasia to complete dislocation, the initial presentation of symptoms may vary in both age of symptom presentation and symptom severity. Early identification of DDH often results in improved treatment results and decreased risk for long-term complications.[103,104]

SIGNS AND SYMPTOMS

In children younger than 2 months, symptoms of DDH are most often elicited on screening during the physical examination. Screening includes Ortolani and Barlow maneuvers, manipulations of the hip joint that result in a palpable clunk in infants with DDH.[102,103] As children reach 2 to 3 months of age, presenting symptoms may include decreased abduction in one or both hips. Mild cases of DDH may not be caught on early examination, and children may present with a range of symptoms including leg-length discrepancies, a unilateral flat appearing buttocks, asymmetrical skin folds on the thigh, difficulty crawling, late onset walking or tip-toe walking, difficulty straddling a bicycle, and limp.[102,103]

PHYSICAL EXAMINATION

While the American Academy of Family Physicians (AAFP) and the U.S. Preventive Services Task Force (USPSTF) have found insufficient evidence to recommend screening for DDH, the American Academy of Pediatrics (AAP) recommends universal physical examination screening for neonatal DDH as well as a focused examination of the hips at all well visits from birth to 12 months.[103] Assessment of infants ages 0 to 3 months should include Ortolani and Barlow maneuvers (Box 13.2). Positive Ortolani and Barlow maneuvers on examination warrant further evaluation.[103,104]

Ortolani and Barlow maneuvers are less reliable with increasing age, and physical examination of infants age 2 to 12 months should include assessment of hip abduction. Limitations in hip abduction may be indicative of DDH. Hip abduction is considered abnormal when, with the hip flexed to 90 degrees, abduction is <60 degrees.[104] Galeazzi sign is another physical examination finding associated with DDH. To assess for Galeazzi sign, the examiner places that patient supine while flexing both hips and knees. The examiner then stands at the patient's feet and inspects the height of the knees simultaneously. Galeazzi sign is present when the height of one knee is shorter than the other.[104,105]

BOX 13.2 Ortolani and Barlow Maneuvers

Ortolani and Barlow maneuvers are used to assess developmental dysplasia of the hip (DDH) in children age newborn to 2 months.

Ortolani maneuver is a physical examination used to assess for DDH by attempting to reduce a posteriorly dislocated hip. To perform the Ortolani maneuver, the infant's hip should first be placed into 90 degrees of flexion. Once in flexion, the thumb is placed on the medial surface of the thigh, and the index and long fingers are placed on the lateral surface of the thigh, with the finger pads over the greater trochanter. The hip is then abducted, using the index and long fingers to place pressure on the greater trochanter, pressing the proximal femur anteriorly. The Ortolani maneuver is positive when an audible or palpable clunk occurs upon pressing the proximal femur anteriorly.

Barlow maneuver is another physical examination used to assess for DDH by attempting to identify an unstable hip through posterior displacement. In this maneuver, the hip should be flexed to 90 degrees, with the thumb placed along the medial thigh and the index and long finger placed along the lateral proximal femur. Using light to moderate pressure, the examiner then attempts to push the proximal femur posteriorly, assessing for posterior instability. The Barlow maneuver is positive when an audible and palpable clunk occur upon releasing posterior pressure.

If the diagnosis is made later in development, additional physical examination findings may include leg-length discrepancies or asymmetrical skin folds on the thigh. Asymmetrical skin folds are not specific to DDH and should not be used to make the diagnosis alone.[103–105] Children who have delayed ambulation, present with a limp, or demonstrate tip-toe walking may also have a missed diagnosis of DDH, and should undergo further evaluation.[104,105]

DIFFERENTIAL DIAGNOSIS

DDH should be differentiated from other causes of leg-length discrepancy in infants. Radiographic findings often differentiate the diagnoses (Table 13.22).

DIAGNOSTIC STUDIES

Currently, there is insufficient evidence to recommend universal screening of DDH with imaging. The AAP recommends use of imaging to evaluate high-risk infants, including infants with evidence of instability on examination and infants with two or more risk factors for DDH regardless of the presence or absence of instability.[103,104] Ultrasonography

TABLE 13.22 Differential Diagnosis for Developmental Dysplasia of the Hip

Diagnosis	Description
Proximal femoral focal deficiency	Absence or hypoplasia of the femoral head
Coxa vara	Angle between femoral neck and shaft is <120 degrees
Limb deformity	May occur as part of a genetic syndrome or sacral agenesis

is the preferred imaging study in infants under 4.5 to 6 months of age.[103–105] After 4.5 to 6 months of age, plain radiographs of the AP pelvis may aid in the diagnosis of dislocation, subluxation, or dysplasia.[103–105] Additionally, CT and MRI may be useful in monitoring treatment and follow-up.

EVALUATION

Initial assessment of DDH includes assessment of risk factors as well as Ortolani and Barlow maneuvers within 24 hours of birth (Box 13.2). Patients with breech position, two or more other risk factors, or findings of instability on examination should be referred to an orthopedic specialist and undergo ultrasonography. Neonates with mild instability may be monitored until 6 weeks of age. If the instability continues to persist at 6 weeks of age, the child should be referred to an orthopedic specialist and undergo ultrasonography.[103]

Children without risk factors and instability upon initial examination should be assessed for hip instability at all routine visits until 12 months of age. If signs and symptoms of DDH are present, children under 6 months should be referred to an orthopedic specialist and undergo ultrasonography since the hip may not be fully ossified and will not appear on plain x-rays. Children over 6 months of age with signs and symptoms of DDH on examination should be referred to an orthopedic specialist for further evaluation.[103]

TREATMENT

Treatment for DDH is dependent on the age of diagnosis. Earlier identification and treatment are associated with better long-term outcomes.[103,104]

- Infants <6 months of age with dislocatable hips or persistent instability beyond 6 weeks of age are placed in a flexion-abduction splint.
  - Initial flexion-abduction splinting includes a Pavlik harness for up to 6 to 12 weeks.
  - Persistent hip instability despite splinting may require closed reduction and placement of a hip-spica cast for 6 weeks.
  - DDH that is refractory to hip-spica casting may require open surgical fixation.
- Children >6 months of age with DDH should undergo closed reduction and hip-spica casting for up to 12 weeks.
  - DDH that is refractory to hip-spica casting may require open surgical fixation.

PATIENT EDUCATION

- Early identification and treatment of DDH reduce long-term complications, such as osteoarthritis.[103,104]
- Risk of treatment includes development of avascular necrosis, occurring in 0% to 14% of patients treated with splinting and 5% to 60% of patients requiring surgical intervention. The risk of avascular necrosis is <2% when treatment begins in early infancy.
- After treatment, patients with DDH should undergo follow-up evaluation with radiographic imaging until skeletal maturity.

13.6 KNEE DISORDERS: LIGAMENT INJURIES

Tad Schrader

OVERVIEW

The ligaments of the knee are the primary source of intrinsic stabilization of the joint. Each ligament is designed specifically to give stability and support via proprioception of the knee joint while moving through an array of motions and activities. This stability is what helps preserve the meniscus and articular cartilage of the knee. Without a stable intra-articular ligament complex it places much more stress on the dynamic stabilizers (extra-articular muscles), and therefore earlier wear of the articular surfaces leading to osteoarthritis.

EPIDEMIOLOGY

Ligament injuries are among the most common reasons for knee pain and instability, especially in younger patients (<40 years of age). The incidence rate for ligament injuries is approximately 1,193 per 100,000. These injuries result in both surgical and nonsurgical treatment options. The most common of these injured is the anterior cruciate ligament (ACL), followed by the medial collateral ligament (MCL), LCL, and finally the posterior cruciate ligament (PCL). These injuries are more commonly seen in men than women and are most prevalent from ages 16 to 40 years.

PATHOPHYSIOLOGY

Ligament injuries occur when there is a stretching, partial rupture, or full rupture of the ligament at either of its inversions or through the body of the ligament.

The ACL inserts proximally on the fossa of the medial surface of the lateral femoral condyle. Distally it inserts on the anterior medial aspect of tibial spine.

The PCL inserts proximally to the fossa of the lateral aspect of the medial femoral condyle. Distally it inserts to the posterior central and lateral aspect of the tibial spine and posterior cortex of the tibial plateau.

The MCL inserts proximally on the medial aspect of the medial femoral condyle. Distally it inserts medial to the tibial tuberosity distal to the anterior medial aspect of the tibial crest.

The LCL inserts proximally on the lateral aspect of the lateral femoral condyle. Distally it inserts on the fibular head in common conjunction with the insertion of biceps femoris.

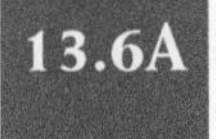

13.6A ANTERIOR CRUCIATE LIGAMENT RUPTURE

MEDICAL HISTORY AND CLINICAL PRESENTATION

Most commonly, ACL injuries are caused from a noncontact sudden change in direction of the knee joint (e.g., cutting, pivoting, hyperextension, valgus stress); see Figure 13.7. Occasionally these injuries can occur from traumatic contact injuries. ACL injuries can frequently occur with MCL

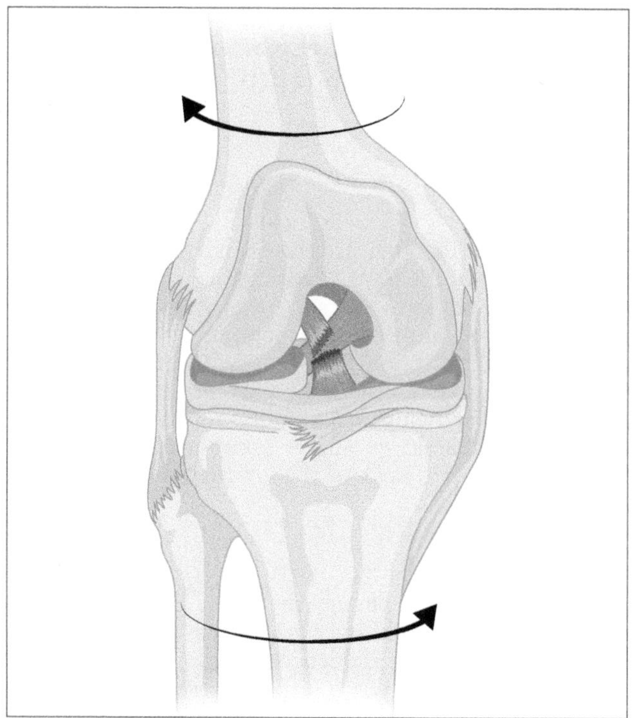

Figure 13.7 **Anterior cruciate ligament rupture. Mechanism of injury involves sudden change in direction of the knee joint (e.g., cutting, pivoting, hyperextension, valgus stress).**

injuries as well as lateral meniscus tears (terrible triad). Patients often present with complaints of pain, feeling of instability, clicking, popping, intermittent swelling, and weakness.

SIGNS AND SYMPTOMS

Symptoms include feeling of instability, intermittent effusions, weakness, popping, and clicking. Patients often say their knee "gives out" without notice. Signs are often effusion (+/– how acute the injury is), quad weakness, and quad atrophy.

PHYSICAL EXAMINATION

Physical examinations will often be limited by patient pain and swelling. If the patient is cooperative with allowing a full exam without guarding (relaxing extrinsic stabilizers to allow for exam) exam can be incredibly useful in accurate diagnosis without imaging.

Nonspecific exam findings would be effusion, jointline tenderness to palpation, and decreased ROM. Special tests for the ACL are anterior drawer test and Lachman test. Both the anterior drawer and Lachman exam would show increased anterior tibial translation when compared to the contralateral side. Patients with ACL tears will not have a clear end point when performing these maneuvers. It is always important to check the translation of the contralateral side as each patient will have a different baseline.

DIFFERENTIAL DIAGNOSIS

The differential diagnosis for ACL rupture is summarized in Table 13.23.

TABLE 13.23 Differential Diagnosis for Anterior Cruciate Ligament Rupture

Diagnosis	Description
Medial meniscus tear	Refer to meniscus injury section (13.7A). Twisting injury, pivoting as mechanism of injury.
Hairline fracture or contusion of tibia or femoral condyle	Likely seen on MRI in form of bony edema without evidence of ligament tear. Occurs with direct trauma to affected bone.
Patellofemoral osteochondral defect	See patellofemoral pain section (13.8)

DIAGNOSTIC STUDIES

Initial knee x-rays will likely be normal showing no defect. On occasion there will be some evidence of joint effusion. Only ACL avulsion fractures can be visualized on x-ray.

Gold standard study of choice is an MRI without contrast. This will give further insight to ACL rupture type (avulsion versus midsubstance) as well as other potential intra-articular injuries.

EVALUATION

For most nonsurgical ligament injuries, the primary evaluation focuses on pain, swelling, strength, and perceived stability. Return to normal activity is dependent on how the patient feels. Their return to activity should be slow and should only progress if feeling well during activity.

If surgery is needed, rehabilitation will be based on a very strict return to activity protocol.

TREATMENT

Treatment of ACL injuries is very dependent on the extent of the ACL injury. For ACL sprains therapy includes conservative management for pain and swelling control. This would also be followed by extensive PT to ensure further extrinsic stabilization and ACL protection. These injuries would also benefit from a functional ACL brace as patients who are braced are more likely to return to full activity faster than a surgical candidate. For partial ACL tears roughly 50% are able to improve and get rid of symptoms of instability and pain with the aforementioned conservative approach. The other 50% of these will progress to needing surgical intervention. Complete acute ACL ruptures are nearly all surgical. Surgical treatment of ACL injuries includes ACL reconstruction or repair. ACL repair is becoming much more popular with certain types of ACL avulsion ruptures. These interventions are followed by extensive PT and limited activity while the patient returns to full strength and healing of their surgical reconstruction or repair.

PATIENT EDUCATION

- Appropriate management of ACL injuries is vitally important to continue to conserve native joint cartilage.
- Most ACL tears will likely require surgery for full return of activity, and all should undergo formal PT.
- Long-term bracing after ACL injuries can be helpful to the patient but is not always required.

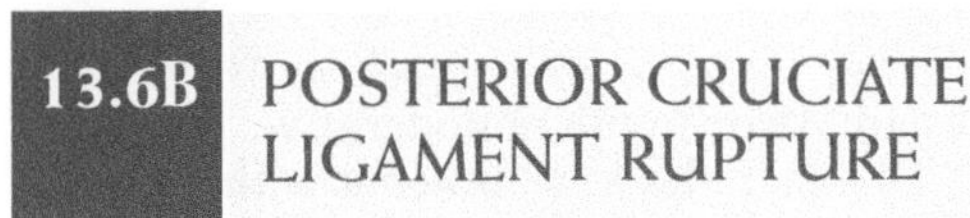

13.6B POSTERIOR CRUCIATE LIGAMENT RUPTURE

MEDICAL HISTORY AND CLINICAL PRESENTATION

Unlike ACL injuries, PCL injuries are caused most commonly by direct trauma to the knee causing the tibia to translate posterior to the femur (Figure 13.8). Some of the most common causes of PCL injuries are dashboard injuries (where the knee slams into a car dashboard forcing the tibia to translate posteriorly) and posterior knee dislocations. Landing on another person's foot after jumping that causes posterior tibial translation is another mechanism for PCL injury. In most instances when a force is strong enough to cause a significant PCL injury, other knee injuries typically occur including but not limited to ACL injuries, meniscus injuries, potential tendon rupture, potential neurovascular injuries, fracture, and osteochondral injuries.

SIGNS AND SYMPTOMS

Like ACL injuries, most patients with PCL injuries will have a significant sensation of knee instability, clicking or locking sensation, pain, a constant or intermittent effusion, and weakness. Decreased ROM is also common secondary to weakness and effusion.

PHYSICAL EXAMINATION

Examination of the PCL is very similar to the ACL. Common nonspecific findings are effusion, weakness, guarding, and nonspecific tenderness to palpation.

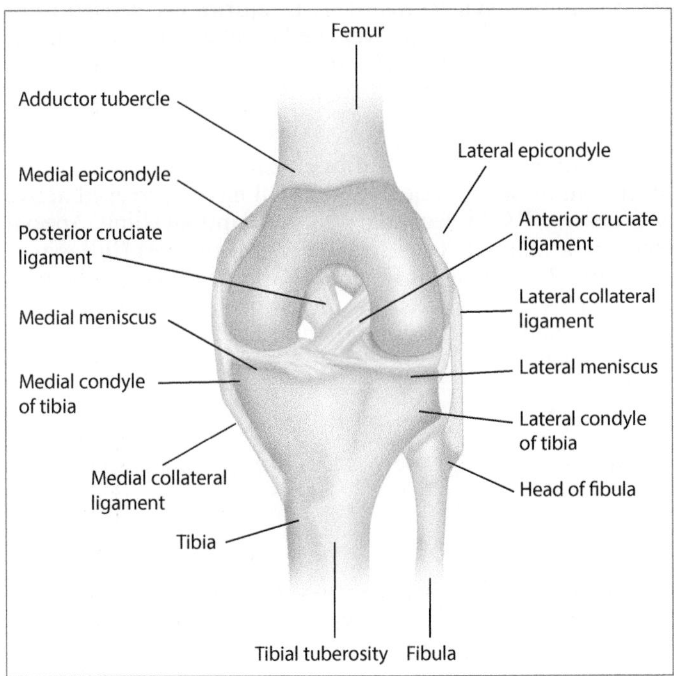

Figure 13.8 **Anterior view of the bones and ligaments in the knee.** *(Source: Myrick KM. Advanced health assessment of the musculoskeletal system. In: Myrick KM, Karosas LM, eds.* Advanced Health Assessment and Differential Diagnosis: Essentials for Clinical Practice. *Springer Publishing Company; 2021, Fig. 12.28.)*

Special tests aimed at isolating PCL injuries include the posterior drawer test and posterior sag (or step off) sign. With these exams, it is important to evaluate the contralateral uninjured knee in the same fashion to establish a baseline.

DIFFERENTIAL DIAGNOSIS

The differential diagnosis for PCL rupture is summarized in Table 13.24.

DIAGNOSTIC STUDIES

X-rays are always the first-line study to help rule out fracture and knee dislocation. However, as with ACL injuries, MRI without contrast of the knee is the gold standard imaging for diagnosing PCL tears, and is useful to help diagnose other injuries that have likely occurred as well.

EVALUATION

For most nonsurgical ligament injuries the primary evaluation focuses on pain, swelling, strength, and perceived stability. Return to normal activity is dependent on how the patient feels. Their return to activity should be slow and should only progress if feeling well during activity.

If surgery is needed, rehabilitation will be based on a very strict return to activity protocol.

TREATMENT

PCL tears almost always require surgical intervention due to the nature of the mechanism of injury. The PCL reconstruction is followed by intense PT and careful protection of the reconstructed ligament, slow return to play protocol, and bracing for an extended period of time.

PATIENT EDUCATION

- PCL injuries are most commonly caused by significant trauma.
- They will also likely require a long postsurgical recovery prior to being able to return to play or full recreation activity.

TABLE 13.24 Differential Diagnosis for Posterior Cruciate Ligament Rupture

Diagnosis	Description
Meniscus tear	Refer to meniscus injury section (13.7B). Twisting injury, pivoting as mechanism of injury.
Fracture or contusion of tibia or femoral condyle	Likely seen on MRI in form of bony edema without evidence of ligament tear. Direct trauma to bone.
Tendon rupture	Rupture of extrinsic knee stabilizers such as sartorius, popliteus, or gastrocnemius muscles.
Bakers cyst	Fluid collection in the popliteal fossa can often be mistaken for structural problems. Tends to parallel inflammation occurring in knee.

13.6C MEDIAL COLLATERAL LIGAMENT INJURY

MEDICAL HISTORY AND CLINICAL PRESENTATION

MCL injuries are very similar to ACL injuries in that they can be caused by both contact and noncontact injuries. Generally isolated MCL injuries are traumatic injuries with a valgus force applied to a planted and firm knee joint. When caused by noncontact injuries, these injuries are often found in conjunction with ACL injuries. Similarly to other ligament injuries patients will complain of knee pain with instability, and a sense of the knee "giving out."

SIGNS AND SYMPTOMS

Most common symptoms of MCL injuries are sensation of knee instability, bruising over the medial aspect of the knee, edema of medial knee, knee effusion, popping, and clicking.

PHYSICAL EXAMINATION

As with other ligament injuries, effusion, edema, and ecchymosis can be found. Patients often will have decreased active and passive ROM secondary to pain and swelling. Special tests are a manual valgus stress test at 0 degrees (full extension) and 30 degrees of flexion. Both knees need to be tested. A valgus stress test is considered positive with increased laxity compared to the contralateral side. Pain is not considered a positive test.

DIFFERENTIAL DIAGNOSIS

The differential diagnosis for MCL injuries is summarized in Table 13.25.

DIAGNOSTIC STUDIES

Similar to other ligament injuries, baseline diagnostic studies should include knee x-rays to rule out fracture. MRI is the gold standard for full evaluation of the MCL injury.

EVALUATION

For most nonsurgical ligament injuries, the primary evaluation focuses on pain, swelling, strength, and perceived stability. Return to normal activity is dependent on how the patient feels. Their return to activity should be slow and should only progress if feeling well during activity.

If surgery is needed rehabilitation will be based on a very strict return to activity protocol.

TABLE 13.25 Differential Diagnosis for Medial Collateral Ligament Injuries

Diagnosis	Description
Meniscus tear	Refer to meniscus injury section (13.7A). Twisting or pivoting injury.
Fracture or contusion of tibia or femoral condyle	Likely seen on MRI in form of bony edema without evidence of ligament tear
ACL tear	See ACL injury section (13.6A). Noncontact planting and twisting injury with valgus stress.

ACL, anterior cruciate ligament.

TREATMENT

Most MCL injuries are treated with nonoperative, conservative management. This includes knee bracing with a hinged knee brace, NSAIDs, ice, compression, and PT. PT should include conservative slow-moving strength and motion modalities. Any type of valgus activities should be avoided for at least 3 to 4 weeks after injury. The best way to ensure this is to educate patients that "figure 4" knee motion should be the only motion used.

PATIENT EDUCATION

- These patients are treated very successfully without surgical treatment, but most will need PT.
- Most times treatment is short in duration (4–6 weeks to full recovery).

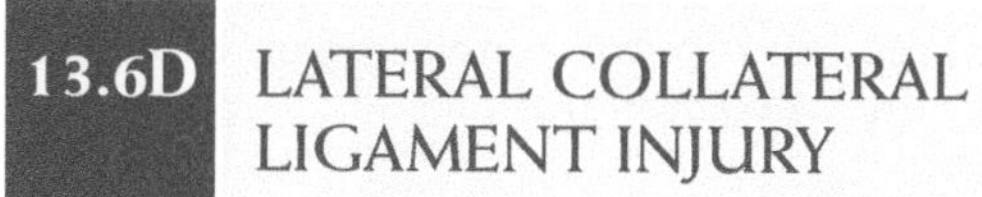

13.6D LATERAL COLLATERAL LIGAMENT INJURY

MEDICAL HISTORY AND CLINICAL PRESENTATION

LCL injuries are primarily caused by traumatic force applied to the inside of the knee while the knee remains planted in the ground. This would be a varus force applied to the knee. Patients will have immediate and consistent pain. They will feel as if their knee remains unstable especially with activities such as climbing stairs, running, and even walking.

SIGNS AND SYMPTOMS

Most common symptoms of LCL injuries are sensation of knee instability, bruising over the lateral aspect of the knee, edema of medial knee, knee effusion, popping, and clicking.

PHYSICAL EXAMINATION

As with other ligament injuries effusion, edema, and ecchymosis can be seen. Patients often will have decreased active and passive ROM secondary to pain and swelling. Special tests are a manual varus stress test at 0 degrees (full extension) and 30 degrees of flexion. Both knees need to be tested. A varus stress test is considered positive with increased laxity compared to the contralateral side. Pain is not considered a positive test.

DIFFERENTIAL DIAGNOSIS

The differential diagnosis for LCL injuries is summarized in Table 13.26.

DIAGNOSTIC STUDIES

Similar to other ligament injuries, baseline diagnostic studies should include knee x-rays to rule out fracture. MRI is the gold standard for full evaluation of the LCL injury.

EVALUATION

For most nonsurgical ligament injuries the primary evaluation focuses on pain, swelling, strength, and perceived stability. Return to normal activity is dependent on how the patient feels. Their return to activity should be slow and should only progress if feeling well during activity.

TABLE 13.26 Differential Diagnosis for Lateral Collateral Ligament Injuries

Diagnosis	Description
Lateral meniscus tear	Refer to meniscus injury section (13.7B). Twisting knee injury with pain on lateral knee.
Fracture or contusion of tibia or lateral femoral condyle	Likely seen on MRI in form of bony edema without evidence of ligament tear
ACL tear	See ACL injury section (13.6A). Noncontact planting and twisting injury with valgus stress.
Popliteus tendon injury	One of the main extrinsic stabilizers of the knee. This muscle shares a lateral insertion with the proximal lateral cruciate ligament

ACL, anterior cruciate ligament.

TREATMENT

LCL injuries are primarily nonsurgical. Most patients do very well with bracing and PT. Patients typically will need a minimum of 4 weeks of limited strenuous activity. As with most musculoskeletal conservative management, these patients will benefit from the RICE protocol (Rest, Ice, Compression, Elevation). Patients with grade 3 tears (complete retraction after injury) occasionally will need surgery to provide an anchoring area for the ligament to heal.

PATIENT EDUCATION

- LCL tears are often a result of direct varus trauma to the knee and heal well with conservative management.
- Rarely is surgery needed for LCL repair; however, most important is to limit activity for a minimum of 1 month after injury.

KEY POINTS

- Ligament injuries can occur with both contact and noncontact injuries.
- Often nonsurgical management with RICE, bracing, and limited activity is effective for mild ligament injuries.
- MRI is the gold standard evaluation for all ligament injuries.

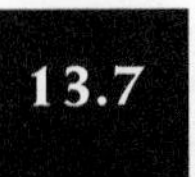

13.7 KNEE DISORDERS: MENISCUS TEARS

TAD SCHRADER

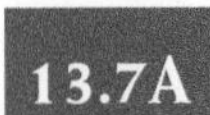

13.7A MEDIAL MENISCUS TEARS

MEDICAL HISTORY AND CLINICAL PRESENTATION

Meniscus injuries are most consistently caused by noncontact hyperextension, twisting, or locking mechanisms. Medial meniscus tears occur more commonly than lateral meniscus tears. Patients typically complain of knee instability, swelling, and intermittent pain.

SIGNS AND SYMPTOMS

The most common symptoms of meniscus tear are popping, clicking, locking (knee getting caught in flexion or extension), swelling, and sensation of knee "giving out." Occasionally, they will also have weakness and decreased ROM. Ecchymosis and atrophy can occur but are not as frequently seen.

PHYSICAL EXAMINATION

Physical examination can show effusion, decreased passive motion, and weakness. However, most commonly, there will be tenderness to palpation over the medial joint line and medial aspect of the knee. The special test for the meniscus is the McMurray maneuver (Figure 13.9). Patients with medial meniscus tear will have pain and locking or catching sensation when stressing the medial compartment with the McMurray test.

DIFFERENTIAL DIAGNOSIS

The differential diagnosis for medial meniscus tears is summarized in Table 13.27.

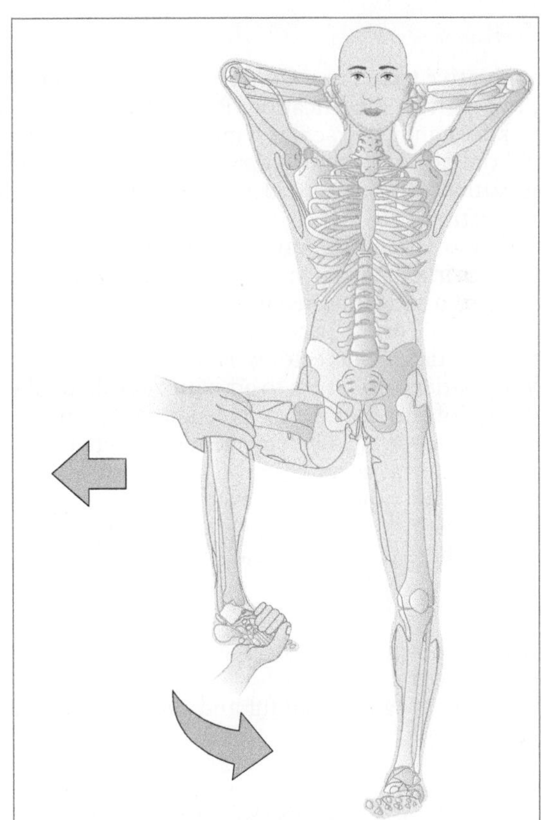

Figure 13.9 McMurray test for meniscal injuries. Patients with medial meniscus tear will have pain and locking or catching sensation when stressing the medial compartment as shown here.
(*Source: Stutzman Z, Gawlik K. Evidence-based assessment of the musculoskeletal system. In: Gawlik KS, Melnyk BM, Teall AM, eds.* Evidence-Based Physical Examination: Best Practices for Health and Well-Being Assessment. *Springer Publishing Company; 2021, Fig. 15.41.*)

TABLE 13.27 Differential Diagnosis for Medial Meniscus Tears

Diagnosis	Description
ACL tear or injury	Refer to ACL injury section (13.6A)
Fracture or contusion of tibia or femoral condyle	Likely seen on MRI in form of bony edema without evidence of ligament tear occurring after direct trauma to bone
Osteoarthritis	See osteoarthritis section of Chapter 14, Rheumatology

ACL, anterior cruciate ligament.

DIAGNOSTIC STUDIES

Plain film x-rays of the knee can be helpful to rule out fracture and potentially visualize joint effusion. However, soft tissue of the meniscus cannot be visualized with plain x-rays.

MRI without contrast is the gold standard for evaluation of meniscus tears. Three main types of meniscus tears are radial (or bucket handle), horizontal, and root tears.

EVALUATION

Repeat evaluation of meniscus tears is symptom-based. If the patient's symptoms are improved, treatment is considered successful. However, the meniscus does not heal itself and it is always possible for symptoms to return.

TREATMENT

- **Nonoperative treatment:** Conservative management with rest, ice, activity modification, PT, and steroid injections of the knee can help to calm symptoms. Steroid injections should only be performed every 3 to 4 months, and only if the patient gets at least 3 to 4 months of relief from their injection.
- **Operative treatment:** Surgical intervention includes meniscus repair or partial meniscectomy. Meniscus repair takes up to a year-long recovery with activity protection and about an 8-week period of non-weight-bearing after surgery. Partial meniscectomy is a much faster recovery allowing patients to return to activities as tolerated within a few days of surgery. Meniscus repair versus meniscectomy operation is typically dependent on where the tear has occurred. Central tears have very poor blood flow and have a difficult time healing even when repaired. Blood supply to each meniscus is posteromedial so this is the best area where repair will heal.

PATIENT EDUCATION

- Meniscus tears are successful with both operative and nonoperative treatment.
- Meniscus tears can be painful and can significantly limit activities.

13.7B LATERAL MENISCUS TEARS

MEDICAL HISTORY AND CLINICAL PRESENTATION

Meniscus injuries are most consistently caused by noncontact hyperextension, twisting, or locking mechanisms. Lateral meniscus tears are relatively uncommon but are a part of the terrible triad of injuries that can occur (ACL tear, MCL injury, lateral meniscus tear). Patients typically complaint of knee instability, swelling, and intermittent pain.

SIGNS AND SYMPTOMS

The most common symptoms of meniscus tear are popping, clicking, locking (knee getting caught in flexion or extension), swelling, and sensation of knee "giving out." Occasionally patients will also have weakness and decreased ROM. Ecchymosis and atrophy can occur but are infrequent.

PHYSICAL EXAMINATION

Physical examination can show effusion, decreased passive ROM, and weakness. However, most commonly there will be tenderness to palpation over the lateral joint line and lateral aspect of the knee. The special test for the meniscus is the McMurray maneuver (see Figure 13.9). Patients with lateral meniscus tear will have pain and locking or a catching sensation when stressing the lateral compartment with the McMurray test.

DIFFERENTIAL DIAGNOSIS

The differential diagnosis for lateral meniscus tears is summarized in Table 13.28.

TABLE 13.28 Differential Diagnosis for Lateral Meniscus Tears

Diagnosis	Description
ACL tear or injury	Refer to ACL injury section (13.6A)
Fracture or contusion of tibia or femoral condyle	Likely seen on MRI in form of bony edema without evidence of ligament tear
Osteoarthritis	See osteoarthritis section in Chapter 14, Rheumatology

ACL, anterior cruciate ligament.

DIAGNOSTIC STUDIES

Plain film x-rays of the knee can be helpful to rule out fracture and potentially visualize joint effusion. However, the soft tissues of the meniscus cannot be visualized with plain x-rays.

MRI without contrast is the gold standard for evaluation of meniscus tears. There are three main types of meniscus tears: radial (or bucket handle), horizontal, and root tears.

EVALUATION

Repeat evaluation of meniscus tears is symptom-based. If the patient's symptoms are improved, treatment is considered successful. However, the meniscus does not heal itself and it is always possible for symptoms to come back.

TREATMENT

- **Nonoperative treatment:** Conservative management with rest, ice, activity modification, PT, and steroid injections of the knee can help calm symptoms. Steroid injections should only be performed every 3 to 4 months, and only if the patient gets at least 3 to 4 months of relief from of their injection.
- **Operative treatment:** Surgical intervention includes meniscus repair or partial meniscectomy. Meniscus repair can involve up to a year-long recovery with activity protection

and about an 8-week period of non-weight-bearing after surgery. Partial meniscectomy allows a much faster recovery permitting patients to return to activities as tolerated within a few days of surgery. Meniscus repair versus meniscectomy operation is typically dependent on where the tear has occurred. Central tears have very poor blood flow and have a difficult time healing even when repaired.

PATIENT EDUCATION

- Meniscus tears are successful with both operative and nonoperative treatment.
- Meniscus tears can be very painful and can significantly limit activities.

SPECIAL CONSIDERATIONS

Meniscal tears treated nonoperatively provide some short-term relief of pain and instability; however, this treatment generally does not last longer than a few months as the tears are easily reaggravated.

KEY POINTS

- Meniscus tears can either be isolated or in conjunction with other knee injuries. Their most successful long-term treatment plan often consists of surgical treatment.

13.8 KNEE DISORDERS: PATELLOFEMORAL PAIN

Tad Schrader

MEDICAL HISTORY AND CLINICAL PRESENTATION

Pain of the patellofemoral joint (or kneecap) can occur for a variety of reasons. For young patients, this can be caused by a patellar dislocation (of the kneecap outside the trochlear groove to the lateral aspect of the knee), anatomic variant of the knee joint, and weakness of the quadriceps muscles. All of these can lead to slow developing or chronic arthritis (chondromalacia) as well as a single acute osteochondral defect (osteochondral fracture). Females and overweight patients are the most common demographic to have patellofemoral issues. Kneecap dislocation can be caused by a traumatic injury and can also be a predisposed issue due to anatomic variant or quadriceps weakness. The anatomic variant that can cause this is due to either a flattened lateral femoral condyle, which does not allow for a deep enough trochlear groove, which makes it easier for the patella to sublux out of the patellofemoral joint, or a patellar alignment variation, which can predispose to dislocation. The vastus medialis is the primary muscle responsible for keeping the patella in the patellofemoral joint. When the vastus lateralis muscle is significantly stronger than the vastus medialis it can lead to a disproportionate traction of the patella leading to lateral patellar subluxation.

SIGNS AND SYMPTOMS

Most commonly patients will have continued weakness and the sensation that their kneecap is going to dislocate at any moment. In patients with chronic dislocations, the cartilage on the underside of the kneecap will become worn with each dislocation. This will lead to chronic chondromalacia (or patellofemoral arthritis). If it is a patient's first dislocation, there is a high likelihood they have an acute injury to their patellar cartilage. If these acute injuries are caught and treated quickly, the patient can avoid long-term arthritis as much as possible.

Aside from the sensation and fear of repeat dislocations patients complain of anterior knee pain, which is described as constant, deep, achy pain that is worse with movement or exercise.

PHYSICAL EXAMINATION

Physical examination can demonstrate knee effusion and tenderness to palpation over the anterior knee and patella. Testing patellar stability can be done by having the patient's knee flat on the table and applying medial and lateral pressure to the kneecap. If there is not a good end point, or it seems the kneecap can be easily dislocated, the patient likely suffers from patellar instability. Signs consistent with this diagnosis include a patellar osteochondral defect, a chondromalacia palpable crepitus of the kneecap with passive flexion and extension of the knee and manual patellar testing. This crepitus is most often painful and re-creates the pain the patient has with active weight-bearing motion.

DIFFERENTIAL DIAGNOSIS

The differential diagnosis for patellofemoral pain is summarized in Table 13.29.

DIAGNOSTIC STUDIES

Standard knee films will help rule out patellar fracture. These x-rays can also be helpful in determining the joint space of the patellofemoral joint for chronic chondromalacia of the kneecap.

For an acute injury of the cartilage of the knee an MRI would be the gold standard study. MRIs will be able to diagnose acute osteochondral defects of the patella as well as potential anatomic variants.

Strength testing with PT can help diagnose vastus medialis weakness in comparison to vastus lateralis strength.

EVALUATION

Repeat x-rays can be helpful to continue to evaluate joint space and chronic wear of the joint. PT can perform reevaluation of strength testing and repeat testing for patellar stability.

TREATMENT

- **Patellar instability:** The most important treatment of patellar instability is PT. This will help give isolated exercise to the vastus medialis and help provide for medial stability to the patella. For patients with chronic dislocation rupture of the medial patellofemoral ligament (MPFL) surgical reconstruction may give more static stability to the kneecap.

TABLE 13.29 Differential Diagnosis for Patellofemoral Pain

Diagnosis	Description
ACL tear or injury	Refer to ACL injury section (13.6A)
Fracture of patella	Can be seen on lateral and possibly sunrise views of knee x-rays
Partial quadriceps tendon tear	Diagnosed on MRI if a partial tear

ACL, anterior cruciate ligament.

- **Osteochondral defect (fracture):** When these are diagnosed early, the best treatment is surgery. In this situation, surgical approach can consist of ORIF of the displaced chondral piece. When diagnosed late, an osteochondral allograft transfer (cartilage transfer known as OAT) can be performed to replace the damaged cartilage defect.
- **Chronic chondromalacia:** This can be treated both operatively and nonoperatively. Nonoperative management includes intra-articular steroid injections, NSAIDs, ice, compression, PT, and activity modification. Operative management could be either a partial knee replacement if the cartilage wear occurs on both the patella and trochlea, and an OAT can be reserved for patients who fail conservative therapy.

PATIENT EDUCATION

- Kneecap pain and injuries are common injuries that occur at all ages. Risk reduction is by good exercise programs that include closed-chain exercises (e.g., squats, lunges, leg press) while maintaining good form.
- Early treatment of patellofemoral issues is usually best, especially when considering long-term outcomes.
- Both surgical and nonsurgical options can produce good outcomes of patellofemoral pain; however, for some problems, surgery has much better long-term results.

13.9 ANKLE AND FOOT DISORDERS

Paul Kuhlman

13.9A ANKLE SPRAINS

OVERVIEW

Ankle sprains are one of the most common sports-related injuries. It is important to rule out fracture initially, but once ruled out, ankle sprains can often be treated conservatively. Ankle pain, swelling, bruising, and ecchymosis are very common after an acute ankle injury. Inversion injuries are most common and affect the anterior talofibular ligament (ATFL) and calcaneofibular ligament (CFL). Eversion injuries are less common. These are considered "high" ankle sprains. Ankle sprain often includes the ATFL and syndesmotic injury. Tenderness over the deltoid ligament medially can indicate syndesmotic injury in the setting of distal fibular fracture as well (Figure 13.10).

MEDICAL HISTORY AND CLINICAL PRESENTATION

Patients will present with pain over the ankle after an acute injury. They will often describe the injury as having "rolled" their ankle. The patient will have swelling and bruising within the ankle and often experience decreased function on the affected side. The patient may complain of a "pop" at the time of the injury, which can be either a severe sprain or possible fracture. They may complain of some instability after the injury, but they generally have pain with weight bearing.

SIGNS AND SYMPTOMS

- Ankle pain with point tenderness over the affected ligament
- Swelling and associated decreased ROM
- Bruising/ecchymosis
- Pain with weight bearing, especially worse with eversion ankle sprains

PHYSICAL EXAMINATION

The patient will either present limping or unable to bear weight on the affected ankle. On inspection, there will be swelling, bruising, and ecchymosis. Ankle ROM should be tested both passively and actively. This is often limited secondary to pain and swelling. The patient will have tenderness to palpation over the affected ligament. This will also help rule out other injuries to the foot and ankle. The clinician should first inspect the skin for open wounds and

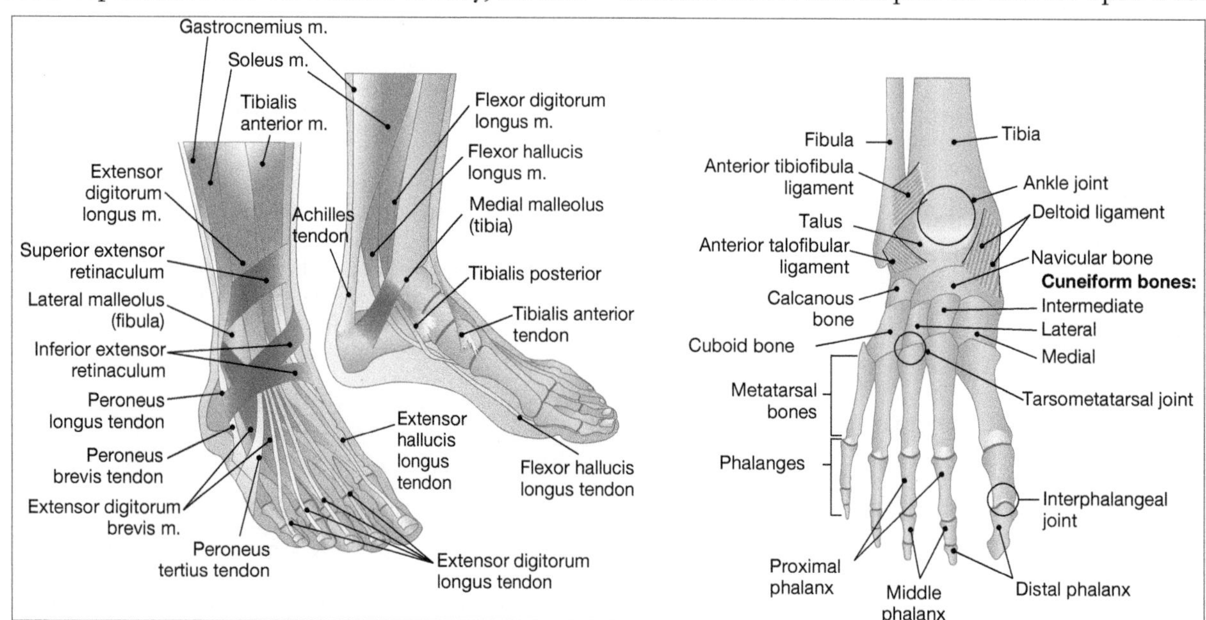

Figure 13.10 Ankle anatomy.

(*Source: Stutzman Z, Gawlik K. Evidence-based assessment of the musculoskeletal system. In: Gawlik KS, Melnyk BM, Teall AM, eds.* Evidence-Based Physical Examination: Best Practices for Health and Well-Being Assessment. *Springer Publishing Company; 2021, Fig. 15.12.*)

perform a neurovascular examination prior to proceeding with physical examination.

Palpate over the ATFL, posterior talofibular ligament, CFL, anterior tibiofibular ligament, and deltoid ligament. Also palpate over the tendons of the ankle including the Achilles, peroneals, posterior tibialis, and flexor hallucis longus. Neurovascular status should be assessed before proceeding with any specialized stress tests.

Ankle strength should then be tested. The patient may have some weakness on exam secondary to pain. Resisted ankle dorsiflexion, plantar flexion, inversion, and eversion should each be tested independently.

Other tests can be used to test stability of the ankle. The anterior drawer test is positive if there is increased translation anteriorly. Therefore, there is a loss of end point of the anterior tibiofibular ligament with a positive test. The contralateral ankle is used for comparison of increased laxity. The subtalar tilt test is used to check increased laxity for the CFL. The clinician inverts the calcaneus while stabilizing the tibia with the other hand. A normal exam is approximately 30 degrees of talar tilt. If the subtalar joint has inversion >10 degrees compared to the unaffected side, it is a positive test. Lastly, an external rotation stress test is used to test for syndesmotic injury. In similar fashion, the tibia is stabilized with one hand. With the other hand, the clinician will dorsiflex and externally rotate the ankle. This will reproduce pain, indicating syndesmotic injury.

DIFFERENTIAL DIAGNOSIS

The differential diagnosis for ankle sprains is summarized in Table 13.30.

DIAGNOSTIC STUDIES

Diagnostic tests include AP, lateral, and oblique (mortise) x-rays to rule out fracture. If there is concern for syndesmotic injury, a stressed mortise view may be necessary. MRI is not typically used initially but is the best modality to visualize ligamentous injuries. This is beneficial for patients who fail conservative treatment.

TABLE 13.30 Differential Diagnosis for Ankle Sprains

Diagnosis	Description
Avulsion fracture of foot/ankle (calcaneus, talus, lateral malleolus, medial malleolus, base of fifth metatarsal)	These will be ruled out with plain radiographs.
Proximal fibular fracture (Maisonneuve fracture)	Rule out with plain radiographs. It is always important to get imaging of the entire tibia/fibula.
Neuropraxia of the superficial or deep peroneal nerve	Patient will have numbness or tingling over the top of the foot or a foot drop.
Osteochondral fracture of the talar dome	Often seen on plain radiographs, but CT scan or MRI may be necessary.
Peroneal tendon tear or subluxation	Rule out with MRI.
Subtalar joint sprain	Increased pain and laxity on subtalar tilt test.
Syndesmotic injury	Patient will have positive external rotation stress test. Will see widening between the distal tibia and fibula on a stressed mortise view.

EVALUATION

Ankle sprains can generally be diagnosed in the clinical setting with a good examination. Imaging is important to rule out fractures. Patients will often do well with conservative treatment and will need to modify their activities temporarily. Most people can return to normal activities rather quickly but more severe sprains can take a few months to resolve.

TREATMENT

Immediate treatment includes modifying activities, rest, ice, elevation, and support. For more severe sprains, protected weight bearing with crutches can be beneficial but not necessary. Patients can take NSAIDs for pain and inflammation. Early motion is important to prevent any ankle stiffness. PT is beneficial for strengthening, proprioception, and balance exercises. This is helpful to restore function. This will also help prevent future sprains. An ankle support brace can be beneficial with activities if susceptible to subsequent ankle sprains. If patient fails conservative treatment after a few months, they may need an MRI of the ankle to assess for tear that may need to be repaired surgically.

PATIENT EDUCATION

Patient should be instructed to rest the ankle after the initial sprain. Ice, elevation, and compression can help with swelling in the ankle. They should be instructed on early mobilization to prevent stiffness. This will be easier as the swelling decreases. Patient should be advised that they may have increased ankle swelling for several months with activity that should decrease overnight. A support brace is important for active patients to prevent subsequent ankle sprains.

13.9B ANKLE FRACTURES

OVERVIEW

Ankle fractures involve the medial, lateral, and posterior malleoli; the collateral ligamentous structures; and the talar dome. Ankle fractures can be stable, involve only one malleolus, and have no ligament structures. Unstable ankle fractures involve two malleoli or the distal fibula with ligamentous disruption. The patient is at risk for displacement, instability, and posttraumatic arthritis with unstable fractures, and immediate reduction is vital.

MEDICAL HISTORY AND CLINICAL PRESENTATION

Patients with ankle fracture may present similarly to those with ankle sprains. They will likely present unable to bear weight on the affected side or limping on the fractured ankle. There will be swelling and bruising within the ankle. Dislocation of the ankle is possible for unstable fractures. The patient will generally report a specific trauma to the ankle with some specific rotation or twisting of the ankle.

SIGNS AND SYMPTOMS

- Ankle swelling, pain, bruising, and petechiae
- Extreme point tenderness at the fracture site and associated ligamentous structures
- Unable to bear weight on the affected side or antalgic gait

PHYSICAL EXAMINATION

Patient will present with ankle swelling, bruising, and petechiae on inspection. They often are unable to bear weight on the affected ankle. There is extreme tenderness to palpation at the fracture site. With a lateral malleolus fracture and tenderness over the deltoid, a stress view should be taken to assess syndesmotic injury and check if the deltoid ligament is torn. The proximal fibula should be palpated to assess for Maisonneuve fracture. Neurovascular exam includes checking the posterior tibial pulse and dorsalis pedis pulse. Plantar sensation should be assessed for possible posterior tibial nerve injury. It is important to get plain radiographs if fracture is suspected in order to confirm the diagnosis.

DIFFERENTIAL DIAGNOSIS

The differential diagnosis for ankle fractures is summarized in Table 13.31.

DIAGNOSTIC STUDIES

Diagnostic tests include AP, lateral, and oblique (mortise) x-ray views. It is important to incorporate the proximal fibula on AP and lateral views if tenderness is present in this area. A stressed mortise view should be obtained if deltoid and syndesmotic injury is suspected. CT can be beneficial for more complex fractures involving the articular surface or lateral portion of the distal tibia, and for surgical planning with complex fractures.

EVALUATION

After initial assessment, it is important to get imaging quickly to confirm presence of ankle fracture. Distal fibula fractures are most common with ankle fractures. Distal fibular fractures are often described as type A, B, or C Weber fractures. This will play a part in how to treat these fractures as well. The treatment and length of recovery are then dependent on severity/complexity of the ankle fracture. Return to activities will be sooner for stable fractures versus unstable fractures.

TREATMENT

Stable fractures involving one malleolus and no ligamentous involvement are often treated with a weight-bearing cast or boot for 6 weeks. Generally, the patient will be non-weight-bearing with crutches for the first couple weeks and then progress as tolerated. Prolonged immobilization should be considered with patients who have peripheral neuropathy. Unstable fractures should be referred to orthopedic specialty for further management. These will often need surgical fixation for best outcomes.

TABLE 13.31 Differential Diagnosis for Ankle Fractures

Diagnosis	Description
Ankle sprain	Fracture will be confirmed with x-ray.
Forefoot, midfoot, and hindfoot fractures	Rule out with x-ray.
Osteochondral fracture of the talar dome, lateral process of the talus, and anterior process of the calcaneus	Rule out with x-ray of the foot and ankle.

PATIENT EDUCATION

Patient should be advised to rest the ankle and elevate for pain/swelling. They will likely need to be non-weight-bearing for a short period with stable fractures until they are more comfortable. They can then progress their weight-bearing status as tolerated in the boot or walking cast. They may need PT for strengthening and ROM around 6 weeks when they are able to discontinue the boot/cast. It is important to educate the patient about the possibility of nonunion, malunion, and posttraumatic osteoarthritis. Any unstable fractures should be referred to orthopedic specialty for further workup and treatment.

13.9C FOOT FRACTURES

OVERVIEW

The foot is divided into three different sections: the hindfoot, midfoot, and forefoot. Fractures in each area are often treated differently. The hindfoot contains the talus and calcaneus. They are very strong bones and typically only fractured with severe trauma. The patients generally present after a car accident or fall from height landing on the foot. The midfoot contains the tarsal bones: cuneiforms, navicular bone, and cuboid bone. Injuries of the midfoot are often traumatic and result in disruption of the tarsometatarsal joints. This can involve a fracture or dislocation. Midfoot fractures are often associated with a Lisfranc fracture-dislocation. The forefoot contains the metatarsals and phalanges. These often present as a singular fracture or multiple fractures. Fracture of the proximal fifth metatarsal is considered a Jones fracture and is treated differently than other metatarsal fractures. Phalangeal fractures are often less debilitating and heal uneventfully.

MEDICAL HISTORY AND CLINICAL PRESENTATION

- **Hindfoot fracture:** Patient will present unable to bear weight on the affected foot. They generally have a history of a significant trauma including a car accident or fall from a height. The patient will have swelling and ecchymosis around the heel and complain of extreme pain.
- **Midfoot fracture:** Patients often complain of pain over the dorsum of their foot. They will typically complain of an ankle sprain or "rolling" the ankle. Often, there is a history of trauma, fall, or "rolling" injury, especially in athletic activities. They will also present with pain, swelling, and bruising on the foot.
- **Forefoot fracture:** Patient will complain of pain with weight bearing as well as swelling and bruising. These injuries often appear less traumatic at presentation. Fractures of metatarsals generally occur with twisting injury or direct impact of dropping something on the foot. Stress fractures of the metatarsals often occur after starting a new training program or excessive running and walking. With phalangeal fractures, the patient will often complain of direct impact or stubbing the toe.

SIGNS AND SYMPTOMS

- Pain with weight bearing
- Swelling, bruising, and petechiae within the foot

PHYSICAL EXAMINATION

On inspection, the patient will often have bruising and swelling within the foot. They often will present either unable to bear weight on the affected side or with a significant limp. For hindfoot, midfoot, and forefoot fractures, the patient will have tenderness to palpation over the affected area. Midfoot injuries can be misdiagnosed as an ankle sprain. Therefore, it is important to pay attention to the area of maximum tenderness. These patients will be more tender along the tarsometatarsal joint rather than ankle ligaments. Also, patient will have severe pain over the midfoot with a Lisfranc injury with rotating and abducting the foot while stabilizing the heel. When symptoms are present, fracture should be confirmed with plain radiographic imaging.

DIFFERENTIAL DIAGNOSIS

The differential diagnosis for foot fractures is summarized in Table 13.32.

DIAGNOSTIC STUDIES

Diagnostic tests include AP, lateral, and oblique x-rays. MRI and CT are generally not necessary for the diagnosis of foot fractures but can be beneficial for stress fractures not observed on plain radiographs. CT can be helpful on hindfoot fractures to assess intra-articular fractures. CT/MRI can both be beneficial with midfoot fractures if plain radiographs are normal but physical examination findings are positive.

EVALUATION

Hindfoot and midfoot injuries are often traumatic, therefore, these patients will often have some residual pain into the foot for a longer duration. Most forefoot injuries are less traumatic and the patient can return to normal activities much sooner. Patients will generally present similarly for all foot injuries with pain, swelling, and bruising. Therefore, plain radiographs of the entire foot should be taken to differentiate where the fracture is. Return to activities is dependent on the site of each fracture.

TREATMENT

Immediate treatment often consists of a well-padded splint, non-weight-bearing, and elevation. Hindfoot injuries often require surgical fixation, so early referral is important. Midfoot fractures can also be placed in a well-padded splint initially and then cast or boot. Patient will be non-weight bearing to the affected limb for 6 to 8 weeks with nondisplaced fractures. They may need a rigid arch support to the affected foot for another 3 months following initial immobilization. Fracture-dislocation, or Lisfranc, injuries often need surgical fixation and referral should be made to orthopedic specialty. Most single metatarsal fractures can be treated with a walking boot or postoperative shoe. These patients will often be non-weight-bearing initially and then progress as tolerated. The only exception is with Jones fractures, which are at higher risk for nonunion and require a longer period of non-weight-bearing. If multiple metatarsals are involved with displacement, these often need surgical repair and patient should be referred to podiatry or orthopedic specialty. Phalangeal fractures should be reduced if needed. The affected toe can be buddy-taped to the adjacent toe if more comfortable. Patient can continue full weight bearing as tolerated.

TABLE 13.32 Differential Diagnosis for Foot Fractures

Diagnosis	Description
Hindfoot Fractures	
Associated lumbar spine fracture	Patient will have referred pain to the foot and these often result from high-energy traumatic injuries.
Malleolar fracture	Swelling into foot and ankle. Rule out with plain radiographs.
Medial/lateral ankle injuries	Ankle swelling and instability. Rule out with plain radiographs.
Midfoot Fractures	
Ankle fracture	Rule out with plain radiographs.
Ankle sprain	Rule out with plain radiographs. Patient will have focal pain over the involved ankle ligament.
Metatarsal fractures	Rule out with plain radiographs.
Metatarsal Fractures (Forefoot)	
Lisfranc dislocation/sprain/fracture	Rule out with imaging checking the tarsometatarsal joint. May need to image contralateral foot for comparison.
Metatarsalgia	Pain over the plantar aspect of the metatarsal head with no fracture on plain imaging.
Morton neuroma	Plantar pain, often "burning" in the forefoot without fracture on x-ray.
Phalangeal Fractures (Forefoot)	
Freiberg infraction	Imaging will show osteonecrosis of the metatarsal head. Occurs only in pediatric population.
Ingrown toenail/paronychia	Clinical diagnosis and there will be no fracture on plain radiographs.
Metatarsalgia	Pain over the plantar aspect of the metatarsal head with no fracture on plain imaging.
Metatarsophalangeal synovitis	Metatarsophalangeal joint tenderness with no fracture on imaging.

PATIENT EDUCATION

Patient should be educated about which type of fracture they have. Elevation is important for foot/ankle injuries as there is often significant swelling. This will help alleviate pain as well. Depending on injury, they should be instructed on weight-bearing status. This is important for injuries for which the patient is at higher risk for nonunion. Hindfoot injuries can have more adverse outcomes, so patient should be educated about this early on.

13.9D FOOT/ANKLE DISLOCATIONS

OVERVIEW

Foot and ankle dislocations are often associated with intra-articular fractures and tears in the surrounding ligaments. A dislocation is displacement of bone from the joint. For the foot, this often occurs with Lisfranc injuries. In the ankle, the "plafond" is considered the distal tibial articular surface over the talus. The plafond is often involved with ankle dislocations. The deltoid ligament is the main stabilizer against lateral displacement of the talus and the fibular collateral ligaments provide lateral support to the ankle. The fibular collateral ligaments are not as strong as the medial complex that makes up the deltoid ligament. "The normal ROM of the ankle in dorsiflexion is 30 degrees, and in plantar flexion it is 45 degrees; motion analysis strides reveal that a minimum of 10 degrees of dorsiflexion and 20 degrees of plantar flexion are required for normal gait".[106]

MEDICAL HISTORY AND CLINICAL PRESENTATION

Patients typically present after some trauma for an ankle dislocation. They will likely be non-weight-bearing on the affected extremity. Assessment for open fracture is important as this is a medical emergency for surgery and immediate orthopedic consultation is needed. There is generally gross deformity to the affected ankle and the ankle should be reduced immediately. These patients will often present to an ED setting. Neurovascular exam should be done immediately. The ankle should be reduced immediately in order to preserve neurovascular integrity. This will also prevent tenting of the skin that can lead to an open fracture. Ankle can often be reduced after either local anesthetic or light sedation.

SIGNS AND SYMPTOMS

- Ankle deformity
- Skin tenting or open fracture
- Swelling, petechiae, and bruising
- Possibly compromised neurovascular exam
- History of traumatic injury

PHYSICAL EXAMINATION

Ankle dislocation is often noted immediately on inspection. Neurovascular status should be checked immediately. Reduction of the ankle should also be performed immediately. Neurovascular status should be checked again after reduction. Reduction should be performed before any imaging to prevent skin tenting, fracture blisters, and to maintain neurovascular integrity. Patient will have diffuse tenderness to palpation.

DIFFERENTIAL DIAGNOSIS

The differential diagnosis for foot and ankle dislocations include open ankle fractures and osteochondral fractures of the talar dome, lateral process of talus, or anterior process of calcaneus, all of which are confirmed with plain radiographs. Open ankle fractures will have broken skin or puncture wounds and are often associated with a dislocation.

DIAGNOSTIC STUDIES

Diagnostic tests include AP, lateral, and mortise radiographs following ankle reduction. Occasionally, images of contralateral ankle are necessary for surgical planning. Coronal and sagittal CT views are important to assess articular surface and are also beneficial for surgical planning.

EVALUATION

Patients will present non-weight-bearing, often after a traumatic injury. Concomitant injuries are common because these injuries typically occur from high-energy injuries and other injuries should be ruled out during early evaluation. Ankle fracture-dislocations often have adverse outcomes. There is much higher risk for infection if the fracture is open. Patient is likely to have some posttraumatic osteoarthritis as the articular surface is involved. Patient should also be evaluated for compartment syndrome as these are often high-energy injuries as well. Return to activities can take many months and sometimes up to a year.

TREATMENT

Initial treatment includes immediate reduction to maintain neurovascular integrity and prevent any soft tissue injuries. Early reduction can help prevent fracture blisters and necrosis of the skin. It can also help restore blood flow to the ankle if compromised. Most ankle fracture-dislocations will need surgical intervention so early referral is necessary. However, surgery is generally postponed 1 to 2 weeks to allow soft tissue swelling to decrease. The ankle soft tissue envelop is very thin so making a surgical incision before soft tissue is ready can increase the patient's risk exponentially for infection and wound issues. Patient should ice/elevate to help with swelling. Analgesics and occasionally narcotics are necessary for pain control.

PATIENT EDUCATION

Patient should be educated on the severity of their injury. They should be instructed to continue non-weight-bearing as the ankle joint is unstable. Strict ankle elevation is important to decrease swelling for surgical fixation. Follow-up with orthopedic surgeon is very important for improved outcomes.

13.10 COMPARTMENT SYNDROME

Paul Kuhlman

OVERVIEW

The muscles and neurovascular structures are divided into compartments. The pressures within the compartments can build and eventually reach dangerous levels that can affect the muscles and neurovascular structures. Compartment syndrome can be either acute, which is more dangerous, or chronic. Acute compartment syndrome is what is more commonly described and more often presents in lower extremities. It usually presents after a severe trauma and is a medical emergency. If not treated immediately, it can cause permanent muscle damage. Chronic compartment syndrome is not a medical emergency. It is synonymous with exertional compartment syndrome, and as the name points out, it often occurs with athletic exertion.

The muscles, nerves, and blood vessels of extremities are grouped into compartments by fascia. The fascia does not expand easily, so when there is substantial increased swelling, the compartments get very tight and compartment syndrome is the result. If undiagnosed, compartment syndrome can lead to muscle necrosis and loss of function. The leg is the most common location to get a compartment syndrome and is divided into four compartments: anterior compartment, lateral compartment, deep posterior compartment, and superficial posterior compartment (Figure 13.11).

With increased swelling and bleeding into the compartments after a severe injury, the compartments get tight and disrupt the blood flow to the muscles and nerves within the compartment. Since the muscles and nerves are not getting oxygen and nutrients from blood supply, this results in nerve and muscle cell damage. Pressure needs to be released immediately to prevent further damage of cells and, eventually, tissue death and permanent disability, if blood supply is not restored by releasing pressures.

These same events do not happen with chronic compartment syndrome. Generally, the compartment has some swelling, causing symptoms. Other compartments in the arms, hands, buttocks, and feet can be affected, although the lower leg is most often affected.

MEDICAL HISTORY AND CLINICAL PRESENTATION

A patient with acute compartment syndrome often presents to the ED after a trauma. Generally, they have a fracture, severely bruised muscle, or history of a crush injury. The patient may have a history of taking anabolic steroids, which can be a risk for compartment syndrome. Constricting bandages can cause compartment syndrome as well. This is why patients will often go into a splint rather than a cast after a fracture to allow for swelling. Once the swelling has decreased, the patient can now be converted to a cast for nonoperative fracture treatment.

A patient with chronic compartment syndrome will often present complaining of pain and cramping into the affected compartments. This is generally reported with exercise or some exertion and then subsides when the activity is discontinued. It most commonly occurs in the lower leg as well. Patient may complain of some numbness or difficulty lifting the foot. The patient might describe foot drop after walking or running.

SIGNS AND SYMPTOMS

- Acute compartment syndrome (5 Ps)
  - Pain—patient will have extreme pain with passive ROM.
  - Paresthesias—patient will often complain of tingling sensation.

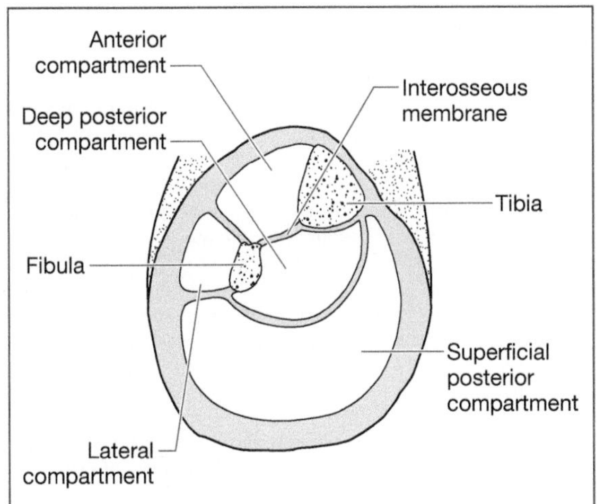

Figure 13.11 Lower leg in cross section. (Note fascial compartments.) *(Source: Brown DP, Freeman ED, Cuccurullo SJ, et al. Musculoskeletal medicine. In: Cuccurullo SJ, ed.* Physical Medicine and Rehabilitation Board Review. *4th ed. Springer Publishing Company; 2019: 386, Fig. 4.114.)*

  - Pallor—patient will have discoloration (pale skin tone) of affected limb.
  - Pulsenessness—pulse mat be either absent or very faint.
  - Paralysis—weakness with movement of affected limb. This is a late finding in compartment syndrome and often indicates that there is permanent tissue damage.
- Chronic (exertional) compartment syndrome
  - Cramping during exercise
  - Numbness and tingling
  - Visible muscle bulging
  - Difficulty moving the foot or visual foot drop
  - Most symptoms resolve with cessation of activity.

PHYSICAL EXAMINATION

Initial exam is often done in the ED. Neurovascular exam and assessment of tissue swelling is most important. Patient will have extreme pain out of proportion with passive ROM to the affected limb. Compartment syndrome is generally a clinical diagnosis based on the above signs and symptoms; however, compartment pressures can be tested using handheld manometer. A normal pressure is 0 mm Hg to 8 mm Hg within the compartment. Pressures within 30 mm Hg of the patient's diastolic blood pressure indicate a compartment syndrome. At this pressure, the extremity is not being adequately perfused and fasciotomy is needed. The compartment pressures should be measured before and after exercise when testing for exertional compartment syndrome, although this is generally a clinical diagnosis as well.

DIFFERENTIAL DIAGNOSIS

The differential diagnosis for compartment syndrome is summarized in Table 13.33.

DIAGNOSTIC STUDIES

Compartment syndrome is primarily a clinical diagnosis. Imaging may show fracture as it is often associated with a compartment syndrome due to some trauma. Handheld manometry can be used to measure compartmental pressures.

EVALUATION

Patient is often initially evaluated in the ED. However, compartment pressures can increase over time and may be delayed following the initial trauma. This is a medical emergency and surgery is needed immediately so early consultation from orthopedics is needed.

TREATMENT

Fasciotomy is the treatment for an acute compartment syndrome. This is a medical emergency, and the patient needs to have release of the compartment urgently to allow perfusion to the nerves and muscles. After fasciotomy is performed, the skin can sometimes not be closed and a Jacob's ladder or vacuum-assisted wound closure may be needed for a short period until primary wound closure can be performed. Otherwise, the skin is closed after the fascia is released, if allowed.

Chronic compartment syndrome can include PT and NSAIDs to help alleviate symptoms. Otherwise, activity modification or avoiding specific activities causing the symptoms completely is effective. Occasionally, cross-training or changing the exercise surface (concrete versus grass) can relieve some symptoms. Surgical intervention is an option after failed conservative treatment. The fascia is released similarly to an acute compartment syndrome.

TABLE 13.33 Differential Diagnosis for Compartment Syndrome

Diagnosis	Description
Cellulitis	Swelling with erythematous skin. Patient will generally not have pain with passive ROM.
Deep vein thrombosis (DVT)	Patient generally does not have paresthesias. Rule out with duplex ultrasound.
Necrotizing fasciitis	Wound or eschar is present. Patient will have other signs of infection like fever, chills, hypotension. This is also a medical emergency.
Gas gangrene	Will see gas on plain x-ray.
Peripheral vascular injury	Can be associated with a compartment syndrome.
Fracture	Can be associated with a compartment syndrome. Fracture on x-ray and patient will have pain. However, should not have other symptoms of compartment syndrome.
Rhabdomyolysis	Compartment syndrome can be a complication of rhabdomyolysis. Rule out with labs, physical examination findings.

ROM, range of motion.

PATIENT EDUCATION

Patient should be instructed to rest, ice, and elevate following an acute compartment syndrome to allow swelling to decrease. Depending on the severity of the compartment syndrome, they may have some permanent damage to nerves and muscles and can have long-lasting symptoms. For patients with chronic compartment syndrome, the patient should be instructed on activity modification and cross-training. Changing the surface they exercise on can be beneficial. Referral to orthopedics should be made for patients who fail conservative treatment.

COMMON CHIEF COMPLAINTS

JAMES VAN RHEE

APPROACH TO LOW BACK PAIN

Low back pain is very common, about 85% of people suffering from it at some point in their lives.[107] It is a leading cause of lost time at work and disability. In the United States, total cost related to low back pain is over $100 billion with two-thirds related to lost wages and decreased productivity.[108]

Back pain is divided into three categories based on symptom duration.

- Acute back pain is defined as pain that has been present for 6 weeks or less.
- Subacute back pain has 6- to 12-week duration.
- Chronic back pain lasts longer than 12 weeks.

Backache is usually self-limited, resolving in 4 to 8 weeks in over half of patients, but recurrence rate is high. The differential diagnosis of acute low back pain can be divided into three groups: intrinsic, systemic, and referred. See Table 13.34 for the differential diagnosis of low back pain.

The history and physical examination are first and foremost in the evaluation of acute low back pain. There are several red flags associated with low back pain that may indicate more severe etiologies. See Table 13.35 for the historical elements and red flags of low back pain.

Laboratory evaluation is not required in most patients with acute low back pain. If infection or malignancy is suspected, an erythrocyte sedimentation rate or C-reactive protein may be indicated.

Imaging is not indicated in patients with nonspecific low back pain. The presence of any of the red flags of low back pain may be an indication for imaging.

Treatment of acute low back pain includes patient education regarding prognosis and activity level and NSAIDs or acetaminophen. Other options to consider include a muscle relaxant, short course of opioid therapy if pain is severe, and referral to PT.

An approach to the assessment of the patient with low back pain is provided in Figure 13.12.

TABLE 13.34 Differential Diagnosis for Acute Low Back Pain

Diagnosis	Description
Intrinsic	
Compression fracture	Trauma history, point tenderness, pain worsens with flexion
Herniated disc	Leg pain greater than back pain and worsens with sitting, radiation of pain related to specific nerve root
Sprain/strain	Diffuse back pain, worsens with movement and improves with rest
Spinal stenosis	Leg pain greater than back pain and worsens with standing, improves with rest and flexion
Spondylolisthesis	Leg pain greater than back pain and worsens with standing, improves with rest and flexion
Spondylolysis	Back pain in adolescents, pain worsens with spine extension and activity
Systemic	
Inflammatory	Pain at night is intermittent, morning pain and stiffness
Malignancy	Pain worse in prone position, spinous process tenderness, weight loss, fatigue
Discitis/osteomyelitis	Pain constant, spinous process tender, normal CBC, maybe no fever, elevated sedimentation rate
Referred	
Abdominal aortic aneurysm	Abdominal discomfort, pulsatile mass
Gastrointestinal conditions	Abdominal discomfort, nausea/vomiting
Herpes zoster	Unilateral dermatome pain, vesicular rash; pain occurs prior to onset of rash
Pelvic conditions	Lower abdominal, pelvis, or hip discomfort
Retroperitoneal conditions	CVA tenderness, possible fever

CBC, complete blood count; CVA, costovertebral angle.

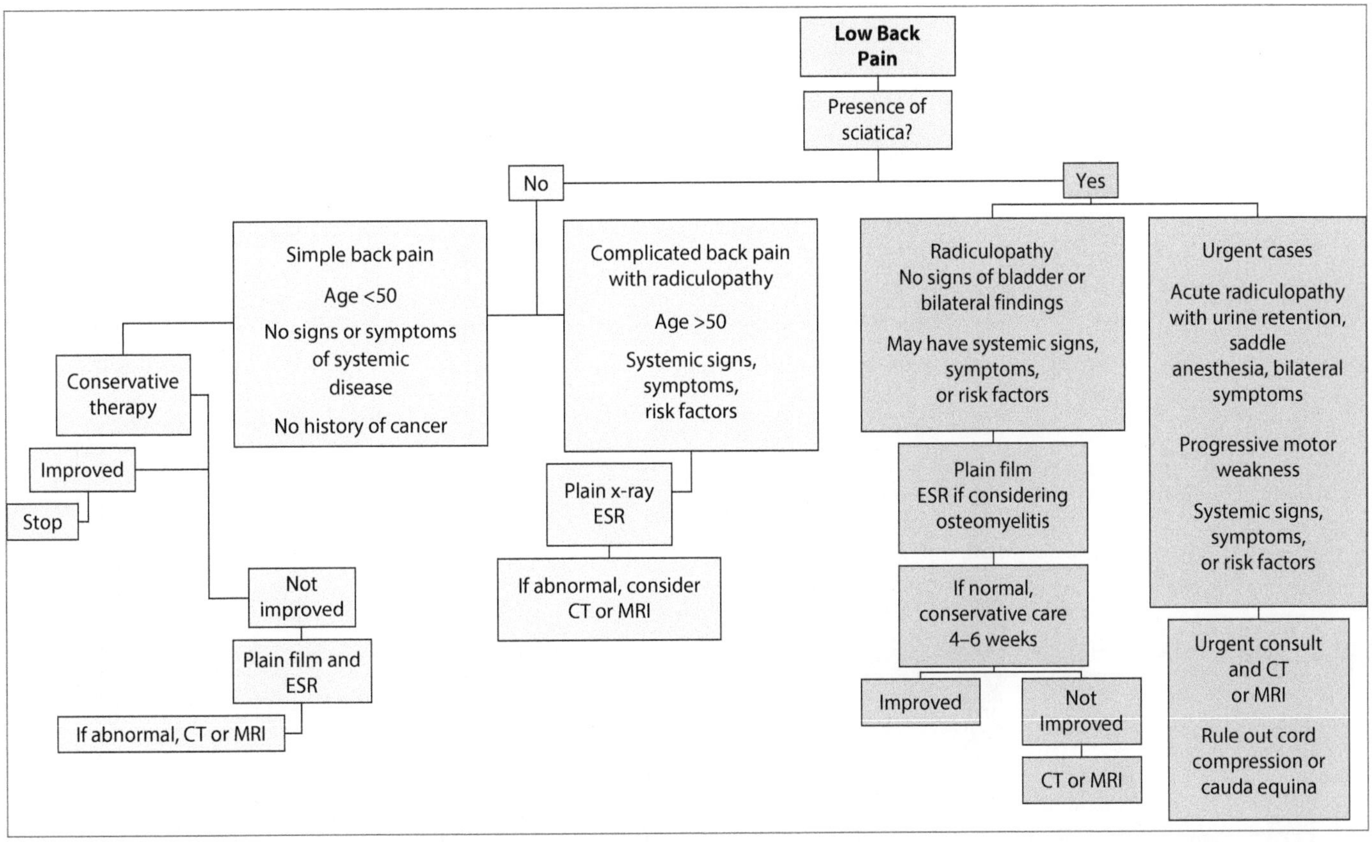

Figure 13.12 **Algorithm for the approach to low back pain.** ESR, erythrocyte sedimentation rate.

TABLE 13.35 History and Red Flags of Low Back Pain

Pertinent History	Red Flags
Onset and duration of pain	Age over 50
Location and radiation of pain	History of cancer
Character of pain	Weight loss
Aggravating and alleviating factors	Pain lasting >1 month
Associated symptoms: numbness, weakness, bowel/bladder dysfunction	Pain unrelieved by rest
History of injury	Acute trauma
	History of intravenous drug use
	Fever
	Corticosteroid use
	Bowel or bladder incontinence
	Neurologic findings

KNOWLEDGE CHECKS

1. Explain why patients younger than 70 years of age with a femoral neck fracture may be treated with internal fixation versus older patients with femoral neck fracture who are treated with joint arthroplasty.
2. Explain why patients with hip fracture are urgently given surgical intervention.
3. Describe the mechanism of action for posterior hip dislocation.
4. Detail the most common presentation for anterior hip dislocation.
5. Describe a clinical scenario for a patient who is developing cauda equina syndrome.
6. Explain why a patient feels better leaning forward or bending over when they are suffering from spinal stenosis.
7. Identify the cancers that are most likely to cause metastatic disease to the vertebral bodies.

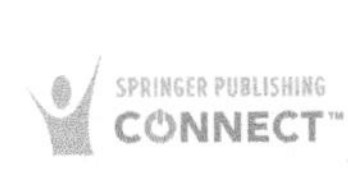

A robust set of instructor resources designed to supplement this text is located at **http://connect.springerpub.com/content/book/978-0-8261-8243-2.** Qualifying instructors may request access by emailing **textbook@springerpub.com.**

REFERENCES

The complete reference list for this chapter appears in the digital version of the chapter, accessible at https://connect.springerpub.com/content/book/978-0-8261-8243-2/chapter/ch13.

CHAPTER 14

RHEUMATOLOGY

CHRISTINE BRUCE, CARRIE BEEBOUT, SYLVIE M. FADRHONC, AND BENJAMIN J. SMITH

LEARNING OBJECTIVES

- Compare the various types of rheumatologic disease and discriminate between inflammatory and noninflammatory joint involvement.
- Describe the underlying pathophysiologic problems and physical examination findings of patients with rheumatologic disease.
- Develop an evaluation strategy for patients suspected of having rheumatologic disease that includes laboratory, radiographic, and ultrasound findings.
- Formulate a treatment plan for the various types of rheumatologic diseases that includes disease-modifying antirheumatologic medications, biologics, and the role for nonsteroidal anti-inflammatory medications and steroids.
- Develop an evaluation strategy for patients who present with a painful joint.
- Explain the physiologic process of monosodium urate crystals deposited in a joint including the precipitants and risk factors for the development of gout.
- Differentiate calcium pyrophosphate deposition disease acute arthritis from gout, rheumatoid arthritis, and osteoarthritis.
- Describe the pathophysiology and systemic effects of rheumatoid arthritis.
- Explain the relationship between giant cell arteritis and polymyalgia rheumatica.
- Describe the pathophysiology, presentation, and pertinent findings associated with polyarteritis nodosum, granulomatosis with polyangiitis, cryoglobulinemia, and vasculitis.

INTRODUCTION

Patients with rheumatologic disease can present in a variety of ways with musculoskeletal complaints typically being the most common presenting symptom. Patients may complain of pain from inflammation in their joints or from systemic involvement from their rheumatologic condition.

Inflammatory rheumatologic disorders need to have systemic evaluation in addition to performance of a careful musculoskeletal exam as these conditions have underlying systemic causes and symptoms. Symptoms of joint inflammation include pain, redness of the affected joints, warmth, and swelling.

Any concern about a septic joint should lead to aspiration of the joint and examination of the aspirated fluid. Septic joints will have increased neutrophils and positive Gram stain/culture that identifies the bacterial pathogen. Joint involvement in rheumatologic disease should have assessment for whether a single joint or multiple joints are involved. Any monoarticular arthritis should be assessed for possible septic joint since the time frame for identifying a septic joint is quite limited before joint destruction occurs. If the patient has more than one joint involvement, it should be noted whether the joint involvement is symmetric, which is classically associated with rheumatoid arthritis (RA).

Patients who have a history of trauma to the joint are more likely to develop postinjury traumatic arthritis with degenerative joint disease (osteoarthritis [OA]) developing. Patients with Lyme disease can progress to develop monoarticular arthritis with the knee being the most commonly affected joint. Gout typically has an initial predilection for the first metatarsophalangeal (MTP) joint and is classically monoarticular in presentation. Pseudogout, deposition of calcium pyrophosphate crystals into a joint, also causes a monoarticular arthritis with the knee also being the most commonly affected joint.

Degenerative joint disease with OA typically will involve destruction of the articular cartilage with the erosion of the cartilage exposing the bone to ongoing trauma. Weight-bearing joints are most commonly affected. Patients with OA develop osteophytes as a kind of bone bridge to protect exposed bone from further damage. RA, on the other hand, typically involves synovitis along with periarticular osteopenia. Patients with RA classically will have symmetric involvement of the small joints bilaterally including the proximal interphalangeal (PIP) joint, the metacarpophalangeal joints, and the wrist. RA patients have elevation of inflammatory markers since this is a systemic disease that has a predilection for joint involvement.

Systemic lupus erythematosus (SLE) is a systemic disease that not only affects the joints but can cause a malar rash, kidney involvement, and increased susceptibility to infection. Patient suspected of having SLE should be screened with an antinuclear antibody, which is highly sensitive but not specific for this condition. Patients with SLE need to have additional blood work, which consists of finding double-stranded DNA antibodies along with anti-Smith antibody.

Acute polyarthritis typically involves at least five joints concurrently with a predilection for the small joints of the hands and/or feet. Various viral infections can lead to polyarthritis, including parvovirus B19, HIV, rubella, and hepatitis B infection.

Autoimmune disease seen in the setting of RA has a much higher incidence in the female population with the exception of ankylosing spondylitis. Because rheumatologic diseases often have a systemic component, extra-articular manifestations occur. Patients can have a low-grade fever along with stiffness after rest lasting at least an hour, which is known as gelling. Fatigue occurs frequently with these patients and sleep is often nonrestorative. Eye involvement with rheumatologic diseases include episcleritis, scleritis, and dryness, which is especially prominent in Sjögren syndrome. Retinal ischemia can occur in the setting of giant cell arteritis, which often coexists with polymyalgia rheumatica, which is seen almost exclusively in patients over 50 years of age. Conjunctivitis can be seen in the setting of reactive arthritis along with urethritis and arthritis in patients having an underlying human leukocyte antigen (HLA)-B27 allele.

There are several associations between rheumatologic disease and heart involvement. Pericarditis is frequently seen with RA, and pediatric Kawasaki disease can lead to the development of coronary artery aneurysms and vasculitis. Valvular heart disease can also be associated with various rheumatologic diseases.

Lung involvement in the setting of RA includes serositis and rheumatoid nodules. Interstitial lung disease can occur in the setting of cutaneous systemic sclerosis. Patients with lupus who carry antiphospholipid antibodies have an increased risk for the development of blood clots as a result of this hypercoagulable state. Sarcoidosis, often classified as a rheumatologic disease, classically has hilar adenopathy in the mediastinum.

With regard to the kidney, SLE has a recognized association with the kidney that includes glomerulonephritis and renal infarcts as a result of the antiphospholipid antibodies.

Several laboratory tests measure inflammation in the body, specifically erythrocyte sedimentation rate (ESR) (Sed rate) and C-reactive protein (CRP). These tests are sensitive in identifying the markers of inflammation but they are not specific in that they do not identify where the inflammation is occurring. The level of elevation of these tests also parallels the clinical course of the disease. Owing to their poor specificity, elevation of these tests can also occur in the setting of malignancy and chronic infection. Older women may have an unexplained elevation in the ESR without underlying pathology causing this inflammation. Sed rates typically allow a higher normal value for women compared to men.

Autoantibodies can directly damage tissue and can also lead to the formation of immune complexes, that lead to complement activation, and tissue inflammation and destruction. Complement measurements are acute phase reactants that increase in the setting of many inflammatory conditions. However, whenever immune complexes are formed, such as that seen with lupus nephritis, complement levels decrease, reflecting immune complex formation with complement consumption. Low complement levels are associated with active kidney disease as complement is consumed.

RA can be diagnosed based on clinical grounds, although laboratory studies can support this diagnosis when autoantibodies are found. RA autoantibodies consist of rheumatoid factor (RF) and anti-cyclic citrullinated peptide (anti-CCP) antibodies, which are more specific but less sensitive for RA. RF is an immunoglubulin M (IgM) antibody that is directed against the Fc portion of immunoglobulin G (IgG). Patients who are RF positive tend to have a more aggressive disease than those without this factor being present. The level of RF elevation, however, does not necessarily parallel disease activity so it is not useful in following the course of the disease.

Antinuclear antibodies (ANA) are the sensitive test used in the identification of lupus. Higher titers of ANA by dilution increase the likelihood of SLE being present along with the appearance of these antibodies when microscopically examined. The ANA test should be used as a screen for lupus in the appropriate clinical setting, and if normal, lupus is effectively ruled out. ANA should not be ordered unless the patient has clinical evidence of SLE since this can be positive in patients without SLE. Follow-up studies with a greater likelihood of detecting SLE include the anti-double-stranded DNA antibody and the anti-Smith antibody. Anti-Ro/SSA and anti-La/SSB are seen with Sjögren syndrome while anti-La/SSB can be seen in the setting of systemic sclerosis. Anti-Jo antibodies are seen in the setting of polymyositis. Anti-histone antibodies are seen in the setting of drug-induced lupus. Cryoglobulins are seen in the setting of vasculitis, hepatitis C, SLE, and RA.

Classic radiographic findings include bony erosions and periarticular osteopenia with RA and asymmetric joint space narrowing with osteophyte formation and subchondral sclerosis being seen with OA. Patients with ankylosing spondylitis have sacroiliitis with squaring of the vertebral bodies. Progression of ankylosing spondylitis can lead to a bamboo appearance of the vertebral bodies. Psoriatic arthritis affecting the hands causes a pencil in cup deformity of the distal interphalangeal (DIP) joints with destructive arthritis being seen with erosions and osteophytes.

There is a growing role for ultrasound to be used in the assessment of joint involvement as this is readily available, inexpensive, and without radiation exposure with the limitation being that ultrasound is dependent upon the skills of the operator. In addition to identifying joint and soft tissue abnormalities, ultrasound can be used to help to guide aspiration and joint injections.

14.1 OSTEOARTHRITIS

Christine Bruce

OVERVIEW

OA is a major source of pain, disability, morbidity, and socioeconomic cost worldwide.[1] OA is the most common joint disorder.[2] OA increases with aging and the joints with the greatest disease burden secondary to OA are the knees and hips (Figure 14.1).[3]

OA is the result of both biologic and mechanical events primarily affecting the articular cartilage. Joints become less stable and biomechanics are affected as a result of the interruption in the articular cartilage. In addition to the articular cartilage, OA affects the entire joint including subchondral bone, pericapsular muscles, capsule, and synovium. OA progresses to cause loss of cartilage, sclerosis of the subchondral bone, formation of osteophytes, and subchondral cysts. All these factors result in joint pain, stiffness, and functional limitation.[4]

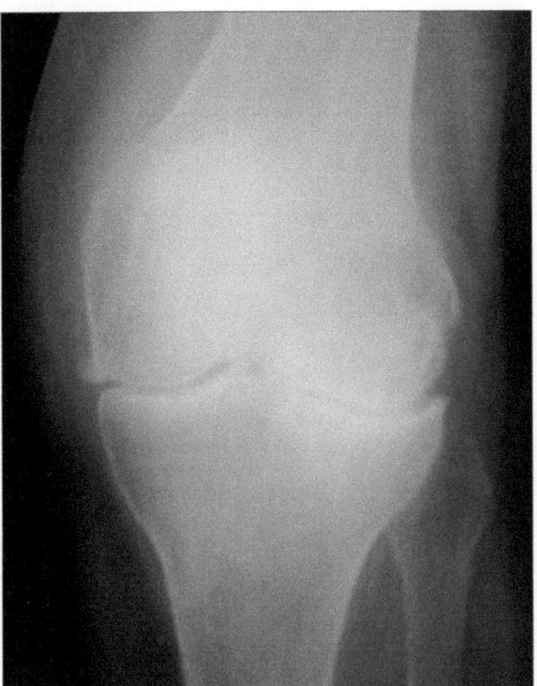

Figure 14.1 Osteoarthritis of the left knee. Note the osteophytes, narrowing of the joint space, and increased subchondral bone density.
(Source: Courtesy of James Heilman, MD.)

EPIDEMIOLOGY

The epidemiology of the disorder is complex with genetic, biologic, and biomechanical components.[1] Obesity is the primary risk factor for the development and progression of OA affecting the knee joints.[5] The incidence of OA is on the rise; the aging population and the obesity epidemic contribute to this surge of cases.[6] Symptomatic knee OA occurs in 10% of men and 13% of women age 60 years or older.[7] Systemic and local factors play a role in causing OA. Risk factors for OA include old age, female sex, overweight and obesity, previous injury to the affected joint, repetitive use of joints, increased bone density, muscle weakness, and joint laxity.[7]

PATHOPHYSIOLOGY

Pathologically, OA relates to degeneration of articular cartilage, limited intra-articular inflammation with synovitis, and changes in periarticular and subchondral bone. Mechanical influences play a role in the development of OA, as do the effects of aging on the cartilage matrix composition and structure. Genetic influences also impact this condition. Initial stages of OA involve increased cell proliferation and synthesis of matrix proteins, proteinases, growth factors, cytokines, and other inflammatory mediators by chondrocytes. Synovium and subchondral bone also contribute to the pathogenesis of OA. The chondrocyte maintains cartilage with a low turnover of matrix states but it has little capacity to regenerate the original cartilage matrix architecture.[8]

OA pathogenesis has been expanded to assess the role that synovitis, inflammatory mediators such as cytokines and prostaglandins, and subchondral bone plays in the development and progression of OA. Current research examines the role that inflammation plays, which differs substantially from the long accepted "wear and tear" component of OA. Subchondral bone has a substantial role in the OA process, serving as a source of inflammatory mediators and pain as it degrades the deep layer of cartilage. OA is theorized to be a much more complex disease with inflammatory mediators released by cartilage, bone, and synovium.[9]

MEDICAL HISTORY AND CLINICAL PRESENTATION

OA causes joint pain, stiffness, and limitation of joint function. The knee is the most commonly affected joint.[10] Obesity, especially in the female population, is a major risk factor for the development of knee OA and may even exacerbate the effects of trauma on the articular cartilage.[11] Along with environmental and clinical factors, genetics also play a significant role in the development of OA.[12]

SIGNS AND SYMPTOMS

Patients with OA are typically older than 50 years of age; the major risk factor for this condition is aging. Patients with previous traumatic joint injury can develop secondary OA at a younger age due to altered joint biomechanics as a result of the injury. Aging has also been shown to increase the incidence of hand OA.[13]

PHYSICAL EXAMINATION

The physical examination of the joints affected by OA can show enlargement of the affected joint as compared to the joint without OA (Figure 14.2). Heberden nodes are bony deformities and swelling of the DIP joints while Bouchard nodes are swelling of the proximal interphalangeal (PIP) joints. The ***base of the thumb*** is the most commonly affected joint in the hand and there may be increased pain at the base of the thumb or pain on palpation when the patient performs range of motion of the thumb (Figure 14.3). In addition to the increased bone formation at the affected joints, there may also be effusion in the joint that can be identified on physical examination, ultrasound, or x-ray.

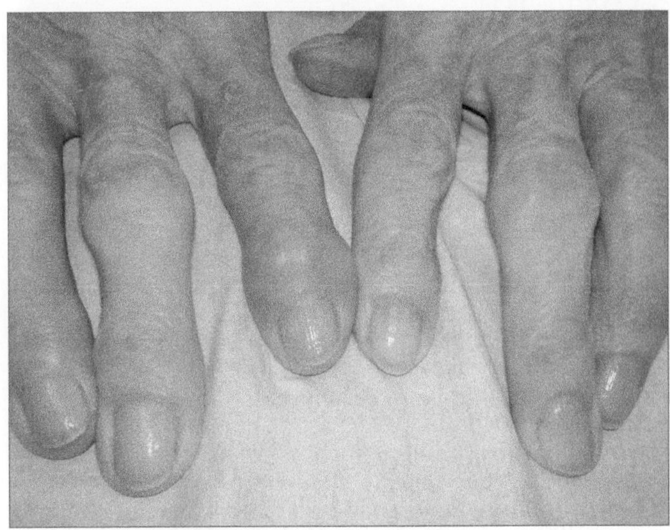

Figure 14.2 Osteoarthritis of hands with distal interphalangeal and proximal interphalangeal joint involvement.
(Source: Courtesy of Drahreg01)

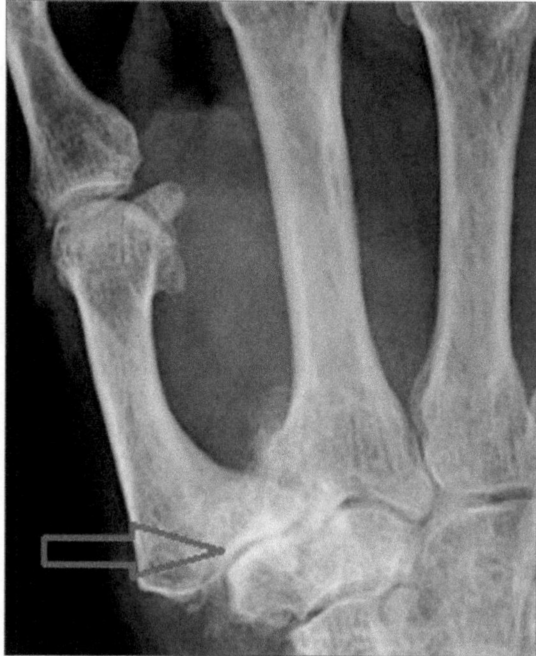

Figure 14.3 **Osteoarthritis of the carpometacarpal joint of the thumb**.
(Source: Courtesy of Maartenv)

Active and passive range of motion may also be significantly limited as a result of OA. Patients may have flexion and/or extension contractures in the setting of advanced OA. Patients with hip OA will have pain in the groin and internal rotation rather than pain in the lateral hip, which may be found in a patient with trochanteric bursitis. Examination of the patient in sitting and standing positions permits the clinician to identify misalignment that occurs as a result of this condition.

OA joints may be tender on palpation especially over the joint line, and crepitation may be felt over the joint when range of motion is performed.

DIFFERENTIAL DIAGNOSIS

The differential diagnosis for OA is summarized in Table 14.1.

DIAGNOSTIC STUDIES

The diagnosis of OA is clinical. There is widespread overuse of imaging methods as there is not a strong correlation between the amount of pain that the patient experiences and the actual x-ray findings.[14] X-rays of the involved joint with OA shows the narrowing of joint space, which is caused by progressive cartilage degeneration along with alterations in subchondral bone in the synovial membrane. Articular disturbances lead to pain, disability, and loss of joint architectural integrity.[15]

Inflammatory markers such as ESR or CRP are not necessary to order unless inflammatory arthritis is suspected. No laboratory study is definitive for OA. RF and anti-citrullinated peptide antibody could be ordered to assess for possible RA so that appropriate treatment can be pursued.

TABLE 14.1 Differential Diagnosis for Osteoarthritis

Condition	Description
Rheumatoid arthritis (RA)	Joint involvement in RA is typically symmetric with primary involvement in the small joints of the hands and feet. Hand involvement is primarily of the MCP and PIP joints rather than the DIP and PIP joints, which are seen with OA. Since RA is a systemic disease, RA patients are more likely to have generalized symptoms of fatigue and feeling generally unwell. RA patients have joint pain and stiffness lasting >1 hour (phenomenon known as the gel sign) while OA patients have joint pain and stiffness lasting <30 minutes.
Gout	Gout typically has acute onset of monoarticular arthritis that is most likely to affect the first metatarsophalangeal joint. The joint is red, warm, and acutely swollen. Joints affected by gout are acutely tender versus the typical slowly progressive discomfort in an OA joint. Tophi, the collection of monosodium urate crystals in bursae and joints, occur in the setting of hyperuricemia, something that does not occur with OA.
Pseudogout	Joint involvement in pseudogout typically has pain evolving over several hours which can also be seen in the setting of exacerbation of acute OA. Pseudogout is also typically monoarticular and aspiration of the joint will show crystal formation made of calcium pyrophosphate. If pseudogout occurs secondary to hemochromatosis, MCP joints of the hand are typically involved.
Bursitis	Trochanteric bursitis of the hip produces pain in the lateral hip while hip OA patients complain of groin pain. Past anserine bursitis in the knee causes pain and swelling over the medial aspect of the knee. There is more stiffness and feeling of the joint instability for patients with knee OA.
Psoriatic arthritis	Psoriatic arthritis affecting the hands primarily affects the DIP joints just like OA. There may be nail involvement with pitting in patients with psoriatic arthritis. X-rays will be helpful to differentiate between these conditions as psoriatic arthritis will show erosive changes along with the classic pencil-in-cup deformity on hand x-ray.

DIP, distal interphalangeal; MCP, metacarpophalangeal; PIP, proximal interphalangeal; OA, osteoarthritis.

EVALUATION

OA is a clinical diagnosis. When patients have a history of ongoing joint pain and stiffness in weight-bearing joints or in their hands or feet, OA should be suspected. The initial tests typically include x-rays of the affected joints but they should be ordered cautiously in the setting of a patient not considering joint replacement. These x-rays can also identify other pathologic processes affecting the joint.

If inflammatory arthritis such as RA or psoriatic arthritis is suspected, CRP or ESR can be ordered.

MRI of the affected joint is more sensitive in the detection of joint damage in OA. MRI should only be done after plain film imaging. MRI is also indicated in the setting of suspected spinal OA especially if neurologic deficits are present. Nerve root impingement and status of intervertebral discs are well delineated on MRI.

TREATMENT

The goal of treatment in managing OA is to control joint pain and stiffness, maintain function, and prevent disability. Management of OA includes pharmacologic, nonpharmacologic, and surgical therapy. Nonpharmacologic modalities include patient education, exercise, weight loss if overweight, use of ambulatory assist devices and braces, and application of ice to the affected joint. Quadriceps strengthening exercises and walking programs may help to limit the pain in knee OA.[16] Treadmill walking without elevation of the walking surface has been shown to mitigate pain, improve joint function, and maintain thigh muscle strength for obese patients with knee OA.[17]

Weight loss has also been found to improve pain scores in patients with knee OA and should be encouraged as part of the treatment for OA.[18] Knee orthotic braces that off-load the joint may also have a role in treatment. These braces are especially useful in medial compartment arthritis and have been shown to reduce joint pain and even delay the need for knee replacement.[19] Contralateral use of a cane for knee or hip arthritis also unloads the joint and can help alleviate pain.

Pharmacologic modalities include the use of acetaminophen, tramadol, duloxetine, and nonsteroidal anti-inflammatory drugs (NSAIDs), which can be given topically or orally. Although once considered to be the initial medication of choice for OA, acetaminophen is inferior for pain resolution in OA.[20] Duloxetine, a selective serotonin-norepinephrine receptor blocker, is also effective in the management of OA.[21] Tramadol—a schedule IV medication—is a central opioid agonist that binds to mu receptors and weakly inhibits serotonin and norepinephrine uptake; it has been proved to be effective to treat joint pain related to knee and spine OA.[22]

The use of hyaluronic acid injections for knee OA has fallen out of favor due to studies demonstrating that patients receiving these injections have more OA-related treatment than patients who do not receive them.[23] There are conflicting guidelines for the use of hyaluronic acid injections and their role in mitigating pain associated with OA.[24] Research on the use of combination glucosamine and chondroitin demonstrates that these therapies have no advantage in the management of knee OA.[25] Initial trials promoting the benefits of these agents were of lower quality and tended to exaggerate the benefits.

Platelet-rich plasma injections have been used in the treatment of knee OA but positive effects wane 6 to 9 months after treatment.[26] Most insurance companies will not provide coverage, viewing this treatment as experimental and unproven, so patients opting for this treatment typically must pay out of pocket.

Intra-articular corticosteroids are recommended for both hip and knee OA. Patients who have joint effusions are most likely to respond to intra-articular joint injections. Joint replacement is recommended for treatment failures and patient preference based on potential for disability.[27]

The use of intra-articular steroid injection for OA of the knee has been shown to be effective at pain mediation without causing deterioration of the joint or having deleterious anatomic effects even with repeated injections.[28]

Surgical correction with joint replacement is effective treatment for symptomatic end-stage disease. Joint preserving interventions, including lifestyle modification, are utilized before definitive surgical replacement. Currently, there are no proven methods to arrest or delay disease progression.[1]

PATIENT EDUCATION

Alteration in diet leading to weight loss, with or without exercise, decreases the mechanical load on the knee joint while walking and this influences joint biomechanics more than exercise alone. Mechanical alignment influences whether damage to the meniscus will occur, which is seen in patients who sustain degenerative meniscal tears without significant trauma.[29]

KEY POINTS

- OA is the most common cause of joint pain with its incidence increasing with age and obesity.
- No effective treatments are proven to prevent or stop the progression of OA, yet recommendations for increased exercise and weight loss for overweight patients can help to mitigate pain.
- NSAIDs, intra-articular joint injections, tramadol, and duloxetine are the current medications recommended for pain relief for OA.
- Total joint replacement "cures" OA, but recovery is challenging and costly to the healthcare system.

14.2 CRYSTAL-INDUCED ARTHRITIS

14.2A GOUT

Christine Bruce

OVERVIEW

Gout is the most common inflammatory arthritis in adults in the Western world. Gout occurs as a result of hyperuricemia, which causes both acute and chronic inflammation in joints and bursa. In addition to acute monoarticular arthritis, gout can also lead to a chronic type of arthritis. Environment and genetics play significant roles in the causation of gout.[30]

Gout is heralded by an acute onset of severe joint pain that typically occurs in just one joint. Affected joints are red, warm, swollen, and acutely tender. If arthrocentesis is performed, monosodium urate crystal deposition is identified in the joints. Gout can also affect the kidney and bursa leading to tophi development.[30] Acute management involves NSAIDs, colchicine, and corticosteroids. In addition to acute treatment, preventive therapy will stop the formation of uric acid, interfere with the chemical metabolism related to uric acid, or cause increased excretion of uric acid. Gouty arthritis can progress to cause joint destruction, kidney disease, and nephrolithiasis.

EPIDEMIOLOGY

Gout is more common in the male population until women reach menopause, at which point the incidence of gout in women increases dramatically. Dietary intake plays a role in the development of an increased uric acid level. Gout is more common in aging populations, which may be reflective of less uric acid clearance by the kidney as the kidney ages. Diuretics, especially thiazide diuretics, interfere with the release of uric acid into the urine increasing serum uric acid levels leading to the development of gout.

Gout affects 1% to 2% of adults in developed countries making it the most common inflammatory arthritis in men. Diet and the inability of kidneys to excrete urate are the main factors causing primary gout.[31]

PATHOPHYSIOLOGY

New insights in the development of gout include the role of NALP3 inflammasome-induced inflammation.[30] There is also release of interleukin 1 (IL-1) beta in acute gout flares.[32] Monosodium urate crystals also activate other pain mediators including tumor necrosis factor (TNF), IL-6 and IL-8, and leukotrienes.[33] Gout and hyperuricemia are associated with hypertension, diabetes, metabolic syndrome, and kidney and cardiovascular disease.[31]

MEDICAL HISTORY AND CLINICAL PRESENTATION

The first phase of gout is characterized by acute attacks that spontaneously resolve over a period of 7 to 10 days followed by asymptomatic periods between attacks. If hyperuricemia is not adequately treated, the second phase of gout occurs and is manifested as chronic tophaceous gout involving polyarticular attacks, symptoms between attacks, and deposition of crystals in soft tissues or joints in the form of tophi. Recurrent attacks are common.[33]

The risk of gout increases in persons with an increased intake of dietary purines (particularly meat and seafood), ethanol (especially beer and spirits), and soft drinks containing fructose.[34] The risk of gout is decreased with intake of coffee, dairy products, and vitamin C, which lowers urate levels.[35] The vitamin C lowering of uric acid is the reason that intake of cherries is commonly recommended to patients with hyperuricemia.

Gout can be precipitated by various events and medications. The use of diuretics is a well-known precipitant[36] as well as increased alcohol intake.[37] Abrupt changes in the level of uric acid in the body and joints is another trigger for an acute gout attack, so some clinicians advocate giving colchicine as a preventive strategy when initiating urate-lowering therapy.[38]

The initial presentation of acute gout is joint pain that escalates within 24 hours in a peripheral joint where there is a lower temperature causing crystal formation in the setting of increased saturation of monosodium urate. This is exemplified in the first MTP joint, termed podagra.

Gout should be suspected in patients who have a rapid onset of severe monoarticular joint pain. Patients can tell the clinician exactly when the pain began and they may also note that this is the worst pain that they have ever experienced. While the first MTP joint is most commonly affected, gout flares may involve other foot joints or even the ankle.

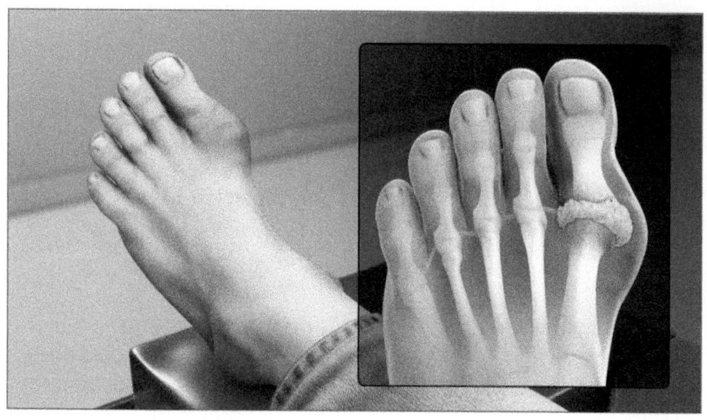

Figure 14.4 Foot affected by gout.
(Source: Scientific animations. http://www.scientificanimations.com/wiki-images)

SIGNS AND SYMPTOMS

Gout affects the peripheral joints much more frequently than the axial joints in the body.[39] The primary complaint for these patients is acute and dramatic joint pain that overshadows any other complaint that the patient may have.

PHYSICAL EXAMINATION

The joint affected by gout will be red, warm to hot, tender, and swollen (Figure 14.4). The range of motion of the affected joint will be limited by pain. Tophi may be present over the extensor surface joints, especially the elbows, knees, and Achilles tendon, and the helix of the ears. When palpated, tophi are hard, subcutaneous nodules. Most commonly, a single joint is involved but patients may also have an oligoarthritis with four or fewer joints involved.

DIFFERENTIAL DIAGNOSIS

The differential diagnosis for gout is summarized in Table 14.2.

DIAGNOSTIC STUDIES

The gold standard in gout diagnosis is joint aspiration revealing monosodium urate crystals. These crystals are needle-shaped and negatively birefringent under polarizing light. Because it is difficult to convince patients with a highly inflamed joint to have needle aspiration performed, diagnosis is often made on the basis of the history and physical examination rather than joint aspiration.[40] Serum uric acid level is not necessarily reliable in determining whether gout is present in the joint because there may not be a consistency between the serum uric acid level and the amount of monosodium urate crystals in the joint.

EVALUATION

Patients who are clinically suspicious for acute gout should have a careful history and physical examination of all joints performed. Although joint aspiration is the gold standard, it is typically not performed unless there is confusion as to whether the joint pain, redness, and swelling are caused by gout or by a septic joint. Elevated serum uric acid levels can suggest that gout is present but a normal uric acid level does not rule out gout in a joint.

There is little role for x-rays in this condition but they may be helpful in identifying other conditions causing

TABLE 14.2 Differential Diagnosis of Gout

Condition	Description
Pseudogout	Another crystal-induced arthritis made of calcium pyrophosphate crystals that are positively birefringent under polarized light. The knee rather than the first toe is the most commonly affected joint. The crystals of gout are negatively birefringent under polarized light and are needle-shaped while pseudogout crystals are positively birefringent and rhomboid shape.
Septic joint	Presents as acute monoarticular arthritis with a red, warm, tender, swollen joint. Any joint can be affected. Aspiration, Gram stain, and culture will identify the bacterial pathogen. Patient may have a toxic appearance and show other signs of systemic infection. Erythrocyte sedimentation rates and C-reactive protein levels can be elevated in both conditions although the degree of elevation is typically higher in a septic joint. Septic joints need to be treated emergently in order to prevent joint destruction, which can occur in as few as 24 hours following infection.
Reactive arthritis (formerly Reiter syndrome)	Typically causes oligoarthritis rather than a single joint. May have preceding urogenital or gastrointestinal infection. Increased risk for patients who have HLA-B 27 allele. Can have coexisting conjunctivitis/iritis, rash, and urethritis.
Psoriatic arthritis	Can occur in patients with history or psoriasis but can also occur without any skin manifestations. Joint involvement is asymmetric and predilection for DIP joints also noted. Arthritis is erosive and there may be a pencil-in-cup deformity in the DIP joints on hand x-rays.
Acute trauma to joint	Patient history of previous injury to affected joint. Appearance of joint is swelling but lacking redness or warmth.

DIP, distal interphalangeal.

acute joint pain and swelling.[41] Classic joint x-ray findings demonstrate joint swelling and erosions along with tophi that develop calcifications over time. Ultrasound tends to be a better diagnostic acumen in identifying joint erosions and linear urate deposits over hyaline cartilage.[42]

TREATMENT

Overall, the target serum urate level is <6 mg/day for urate-lowering therapies.[30] Many patients need medications in order to reach this goal. A full understanding of the mechanism of action for different gout medications is needed for maximum therapeutic benefit to be achieved. Lowering of serum uric acid leads to crystal dissolution and suppression of future flares.[32]

Treatment of acute gout flares involves the use of anti-inflammatory medications such as NSAIDs, corticosteroids that can be given orally or intra-articularly, and colchicine.[43] Colchicine can be effective if given soon after the appearance of symptoms. Cold compress helps with the acute inflammation.[44] Colchicine is given in 0.6 mg tablets with two tablets given at the onset of pain followed by one tablet in 1 hour, then twice daily dosing.[45] The daily prophylactic colchicine dose is 0.6 mg/day. Acute treatment duration is typically 7 to 10 days with gradual reduction of the anti-inflammatory medications.[46]

Oral steroids have been shown to have equivalent effects in pain reduction when compared to naproxen, an NSAID.[47] If providing intra-articular steroid injections, ultrasound imaging can be used as an aid to guide this steroid injection.[48]

For patients experiencing a first gout attack or those for whom gout infrequently occurs, acutely initiating urate-lowering therapy is not recommended.[43] Urate-lowering therapy can be initiated 2 to 3 weeks following the resolution of the acute gout flare. Allopurinol reduces the production of uric acid and this medication is typically started at 100 mg daily with an increase of 100 mg per week until the serum uric acid level is at 6 mg/dL or below. Chronic urate-lowering therapy with allopurinol, a xanthine oxidase inhibitor, should have a dosage reduction in the setting of chronic kidney disease.[49] Consideration should be given to administering colchicine or NSAIDs during the initiation of the urate-lowering therapy in order to prevent a gout flare during the first 6 months of urate-lowering treatment since alteration in serum uric acid levels is a known precipitant for gout.

Allopurinol can be associated with allopurinol hypersensitivity syndrome, which is characterized by Stevens-Johnson syndrome, toxic epidermal necrolysis, eosinophilia, leukocytosis, fever, hepatitis, and renal failure.[50]

As an alternative to allopurinol, febuxostat, a nonpurine selective xanthine oxidase inhibitor can be given as a second-line agent if allopurinol cannot be given or for treatment failure or intolerance to allopurinol. There is a concern with the use of this agent due to increased cardiovascular risk for death and overall higher mortality when compared to allopurinol.[51]

Intravenous pegloticase, a pegylated recombinant mammalian uricase agent, is reserved for those patients who have refractory tophaceous gout that has not responded to other treatments. Gout flares are less common when this agent is given every 2 weeks rather than monthly.[52]

If patients cannot tolerate traditional urate-lowering therapy, a uricosuric medication such as probenecid can be given. This agent increases the renal excretion of uric acid resulting in a lowering of serum uric acid. This agent should not be given to those with renal failure or to patients who previously had a uric acid kidney stone. It should also not be started in patients with an acute gout attack.

PATIENT EDUCATION

Gout attacks are painful and debilitating but are typically self-limiting. Many patients with one gout attack will go on to have a second attack if the underlying cause is not treated. Many patients will never have additional gout attacks even if no therapy is given. Once a patient has a third attack of gout, the recommendation is to provide urate-lowering treatment at that time. Complications of gout include permanent arthritis and tophi deposits. Serum uric acid levels should be decreased to 6 mg/dL but urate-lowering therapy should not be instituted until several weeks after the acute attack. Consideration should be made for giving prophylactic agents such as NSAIDs or colchicine when urate-lowering therapy is undertaken. Although most underlying causes of gout are due to underexcretion of uric acid, urate-lowering therapy is typically done to prevent the formation of uric acid.

KEY POINTS

- Gout is the most common joint disease in the male population.
- Although the gold standard for diagnosing gout is joint aspiration, this is typically not done due to patient reluctance to have this procedure.
- Risk factors for gout include use of diuretics; alcohol, meat, or seafood intake; cyclosporine use; or following chemotherapy as a result of successful cancer therapy producing a high cell turnover.

14.2B PSEUDOGOUT

OVERVIEW

Pseudogout is also known as calcium pyrophosphate deposition disease (CPPD), which can affect joints. It is caused by deposition of calcium pyrophosphate crystals in the affected joints. When CPPD occurs before the seventh decade, the cause for this crystal deposition may be secondary to other metabolic problems such as parathyroid disease or hemochromatosis. This condition can lead to both acute and chronic arthritis. Chondrocalcinosis is the term used when x-rays or ultrasound demonstrates CPPD in the joints.[50]

Calcium pyrophosphate deposition can lead to acute monoarticular arthritis due to deposition of these crystals within the joint. Knees, wrists, shoulders, ankles, elbows, and hands are most commonly affected. The chronic form of CPPD arthritis is clinically similar to both OA and RA. Patients with this condition have a variable degree of inflammation.

EPIDEMIOLOGY

CPPD is typically found in patients over the age of 60; the incidence increases with aging. About 8% of older adults in both European and U.S. populations show x-ray signs consistent with chondrocalcinosis.[53] This number increases to 44% of patients showing chondrocalcinosis over the age of 84.[54]

Although CPPD is most likely to occur with aging, the risk is also increased due to multiple metabolic conditions, including hyperparathyroidism, hemochromatosis, hypomagnesemia, hypophosphatemia, and OA.[55] Hypoparathyroidism has been identified as a risk factor for the development of CPPD in the setting of hungry bone disease, which occurs following parathyroid manipulation either with or without osteoporosis being present.[56]

PATHOPHYSIOLOGY

The deposition of calcium pyrophosphate crystals occurs in the articular hyaline and fibrocartilage. This condition starts with the overproduction of inorganic pyrophosphate and ions by chondrocytes. The interaction of the cation calcium, and the negative anion inorganic pyrophosphate leads to CPPD crystal formation within the joint.[57,58]

These crystals result in inflammatory-mediated damage caused by activation of the immune system. The degenerative changes to chondrocytes and cartilage predisposes to pathologic crystal deposition. Hyperparathyroidism, hypophosphatemia, hypomagnesemia, and hemochromatosis are predisposing factors to crystal deposition due to increased inorganic pyrophosphate levels in the synovium.[59] Once crystals are formed, the inflammatory cycle is activated starting with the secretion of cytokine IL-1 beta. Neutrophils are also activated and a prolonged neutrophilic inflammatory response occurs with pseudogout-associated inflammatory calcium pyrophosphate dihydrate microcrystals -induced formation of neutrophil extracellular traps.[60] CPPD deposits within the synovium cause chronic changes in the joint similar to that seen in OA.

MEDICAL HISTORY AND CLINICAL PRESENTATION

Risk factors for the development of pseudogout include hyperparathyroidism, use of loop diuretics, RA, thiazide diuretic use, and chronic renal failure.[61] The most commonly affected joints are the knees, wrists, shoulders, ankles, elbows, and hands (especially the second and third metacarpophalangeal [MCP] joints when this condition is caused by hemochromatosis). The development of CPPD acutely has also been linked with the use of bisphosphonates, especially in the female population.[62]

The most common presentation of acute CPPD arthritis is monoarthritis, particularly the large joints and especially the knee or wrist. Elbow involvement is less frequently the presenting symptom.[50]

SIGNS AND SYMPTOMS

Patients can have severe and sudden inflammation with painful swelling. Attacks can last from 10 days up to several weeks. Oligoarthritis, polyarthritis, and migratory arthritis can also occur but are a less common presentation. Another alternative presentation is the involvement of multiple small joints with the initial outbreak, especially the MCP joints, while also affecting the large joints.[50] Fever may also occur and this could raise suspicion for septic arthritis if monoarthritis is present. Presentation may be very similar to a patient with RA with regard to abruptness of presenting symptoms.

The axial skeleton can be involved including the atlantoaxial junction, facet and intervertebral joints, and discs. Patients may present with severe neck pain, neck rigidity, and fever.

PHYSICAL EXAMINATION

The physical examination of the patient with acute CPPD classically will show monoarticular joint redness, tenderness, warmth, and decreased range of motion of the involved joint. The knee is the most commonly affected joint so it is likely that the patient will present with knee pain. Other features that would make one suspect CPPD are involvement of the second and third MCP joints of the hands. Joint involvement is typically not symmetric and does not typically involve the joints of the foot. The hips are not as commonly involved in CPPD even though the hips are weight-bearing joints.

There may be some crossover between joints with OA and CPPD as patients with degeneration in their joints are more likely to be susceptible to CPPD as a result of the damage to the articular cartilage that occurs with aging. Occasionally, signs of systemic disease such as fever, chills, tachycardia, or tachypnea may be present and if present, the first consideration to rule out is a septic joint rather than CPPD.

DIFFERENTIAL DIAGNOSIS

The primary differential diagnosis with CPPD is gout, OA, and RA.

Presentation of CPPD is nearly identical to that of acute gout. Gout is most likely to affect the small joints of the lower extremity especially the first MTP joint, which is not commonly affected with CPPD.

Owing to the abruptness of the acute joint inflammation and pain, RA should be considered. The types of joints involved with RA, however, are different in the sense that RA is most likely to be symmetric in presentation and there is prolonged stiffness (gel sign) lasting >1 hour occurring only with RA. Additionally, RA is a systemic disease and there are more systemic signs of inflammation with RA than with CCPD.

CPPD can result in a chronic OA-like syndrome that is more likely to be confused with OA. In order to differentiate between these conditions, the sites of joint involvement with CPPD include the shoulder at the glenohumeral joint, metacarpal joints, wrists, and elbows, which are not joints typically seen with OA.[63] Hand involvement with OA is typically at the base of the thumb along with the DIP joints and PIP joints but not the MCP joints that are seen in the setting of CPPD. OA x-rays will show joint space narrowing and osteophyte formation while chondrocalcinosis with CPPD exhibits calcification of the cartilage, something that is not seen with OA.

Septic arthritis should be considered for all patients with monoarticular arthritis. Aspiration of the joint will identify the pathogen responsible and immediate treatment is necessary in order to prevent destruction of a joint by a pathogen.

DIAGNOSTIC STUDIES

The gold standard for making the diagnosis of CPPD is finding positively birefringent, rhomboid-shaped crystals under polarized light in the synovial fluid of affected joints. Analysis of the synovial fluid also reveals highly inflammatory cells with elevated white blood cell (WBC) counts during an acute attack.[64]

X-rays will show findings consistent with chondrocalcinosis, which illustrates the radiographic appearance of CPPD crystals. This appearance will show heavily rounded calcifications within the fibrocartilage. Ultrasound may help to differentiate chondrocalcinosis with calcium pyrophosphate crystal deposition from monosodium urate deposition that occurs with gout. On ultrasound, CPPD shows hyperechoic rounded deposits within the substance of the cartilage, whereas monosodium urate crystals will provide a more linear deposit on the surface of the cartilage.[65]

EVALUATION

CPPD may be diagnosed from joint aspiration identifying calcium pyrophosphate crystal within the joint. Since its appearance is almost identical to gout, joint aspiration can discriminate between these two conditions. Acute gout joint aspiration reveals monosodium urate crystal formation. The location of the monoarticular arthritis, can also be a primary differentiating feature as knee involvement is more common with CPPD and MTP joint involvement most commonly occurs with gout.

Patients with risk factors for CPPD can lead the clinician to suspect this condition when joint inflammation occurs. Patients with hemochromatosis, hyperparathyroidism, osteoporosis, hypophosphatemia, or hypomagnesemia have a higher risk for the development of CPPD as the underlying cause for the joint involvement.

X-rays of the affected joint will show cartilage calcification especially in the small joints, which is known as chondrocalcinosis. There is no specific laboratory study that can identify CPPD but the likelihood of CPPD is increased when patients have low serum calcium, magnesium, or phosphate levels. ESR or CRP may be elevated because of the underlying inflammation that occurs with CPPD but these are nonspecific findings for this condition.

TREATMENT

Treatment of CPPD arthritis has been based mainly on clinical experience rather than controlled trials and range from observation alone all the way through to the use of IL-1 inhibitors.[66] Monoarticular arthritis pain caused by CPPD in the joint may respond to cold compress, rest of the involved joint, and intra-articular steroid injections.[67] Asymptomatic patients do not require therapy.[67]

Acute arthritis from CPPD is painful because of inflammation and activation of the immune system. There is crossover with gout because of a similar underlying inflammatory process, and treatment for CPPD arthritis is similar to the treatment of acute gouty arthritis. There may be a role for intra-articular steroid injection with CPPD.[67] Patients with polyarticular presentations may need treatment with systemic corticosteroids as joint injections may be too numerous to perform.[68] Inflammation may also be relieved by NSAIDs and colchicine.[69]

Chronic CPPD arthritis poses many more difficulties for treatment given that there is typically degenerative joint disease coexisting in these older patients. Treatments that have been tried include colchicine,[70] IL-1 inhibition,[67] and hydroxychloroquine.[71]

There are no established standards for the treatment of pseudogout.[50]

PATIENT EDUCATION

Following a diagnosis of acute CPPD arthritis, patients can be told that their symptoms will gradually diminish over days to weeks. Some patients may have recurrent disease with acute exacerbation of joint pain. Since the affected joints may also have some underlying OA, some patients may not return to their baseline prior to the acute attack. Depending on the treatment selected for this condition, the clinician should educate the patient regarding the side effects of colchicine, NSAIDs, and steroids. Patients are encouraged to maintain function so that the joint does not further deteriorate.

KEY POINTS

- CPPD is caused by calcium pyrophosphate crystals being deposited in the articular cartilage.
- The presentation and treatment of CPPD is similar to that for gout.
- The knee is the most commonly affected joint.

14.3 FIBROMYALGIA

OVERVIEW

Fibromyalgia is a syndrome consisting of persistent and widespread pain, fatigue, stiffness, cognitive difficulties, psychiatric symptoms, and sleep disturbance.[72] The etiology underlying the syndrome is unknown, as is the specific pathophysiology. It typically affects young or middle-aged women, though it can affect male and female patients of any age. Fibromyalgia is the most common cause of chronic widespread musculoskeletal pain.[73]

EPIDEMIOLOGY

Fibromyalgia has been diagnosed in countries around the world and does not exhibit a predilection for a certain ethnic group or culture. A study conducted in the United States estimated the prevalence to be 6.4% of the population, with women making up 7.7% and men 4.9%. Similarly, data from France, Italy, Germany, Portugal, and Spain estimated the prevalence in Europe to be at 4.7%.

In the adult population, women are more likely to develop fibromyalgia than men. However, in the pediatric population, the difference in incidence between genders is minimal. Males with the syndrome tend to have more physical limitations and lower health perception than do females. Females with fibromyalgia, however, have greater pain sensitivity, which may impact their activities of daily living more profoundly.[74] Though usually thought of as a disease of middle age, fibromyalgia can develop at any age. In the pediatric population, it most often affects adolescents.[75] In adults, the peak prevalence is not seen until the sixth decade in women.[76]

PATHOPHYSIOLOGY

The pathophysiology of fibromyalgia is not completely understood but is believed to be a result of disordered central pain processing, or aberrant sensitivity. Evidence of altered chemistry and functional connectivity in the brain's pain-processing system has been linked to the disorder.[77] Researchers suggest that patients with fibromyalgia may have a lower threshold for pain as well as for other stimuli, such as noise, heat, and strong odors. It has also been suggested that hypersensitivity may develop as a result of neurobiologic changes affecting the perception of pain.

MEDICAL HISTORY AND CLINICAL PRESENTATION

The primary symptoms of fibromyalgia are generalized pain, sleep disturbances, and fatigue that have been present consistently for at least 3 months and for which there is not another explanation. The chronic widespread pain of fibromyalgia is most commonly the primary complaint upon initial presentation. The pain is present on both sides of the body, above and below the waist, and typically affects at least six tenderpoint sites, such as the head, arms, chest, abdomen, upper back, lower back, and legs. Figure 14.5 shows the most commonly affected sites. Patients often state that they hurt all over or feel like they always have the flu. Though the pain is most often described as affecting the muscles, in some cases patients will describe joint pain and may even experience joint swelling.

Patients with fibromyalgia describe fatigue and sleep disturbances as moderate to severe. Pain and fatigue are often aggravated by seemingly minor activities, although prolonged sedentary behaviors also worsen symptoms. Even after having slept for 8 to 10 hours, patients will awake feeling unrefreshed and stiff.

The majority of patients with fibromyalgia also describe cognitive disturbances often dubbed "fibro fog." Problems with attention and difficulty completing tasks that require rapid changes in thought are especially common. In addition, depression and/or anxiety are present in up to half of all patients at the time of diagnosis with the disorder. Approximately 50% of patients diagnosed with fibromyalgia have a personal lifetime history of major depression.[78] In addition, anxiety disorders, posttraumatic stress disorder, and bipolar disorder are more common in patients with fibromyalgia, as well as traits such as alexithymia and catastrophizing.[79,80]

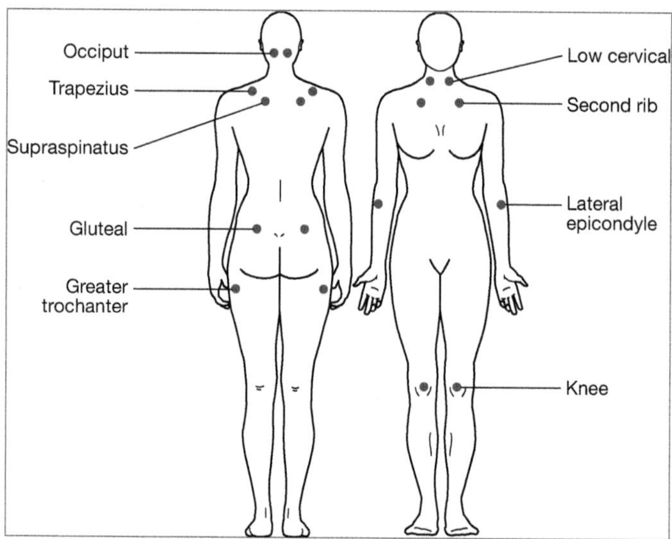

Figure 14.5 Sites commonly affected in fibromyalgia.
(Source: Nucatola TR, Freeman ED, Bagay L, et al. Rheumatology. In: Cuccurullo SJ, ed. Physical Medicine and Rehabilitation Board Review. *4th ed. Springer Publishing Company; 2019:141, Fig. 3.5.)*

Various other symptoms are common in those who suffer from fibromyalgia. Headaches, including migraine and tension types, are present in over half of all patients.[81] Paresthesias, especially of the arms and legs, are also common, as are irritable bowel syndrome, gastroesophageal reflux disease, and dry eye syndrome.[82]

Approximately one third of patients with fibromyalgia identify a specific event, such as an illness, injury, or extreme stress, that precipitated the development of the disease. However, the majority of patients develop symptoms spontaneously, without an identifiable stressor.

SIGNS AND SYMPTOMS

Widespread pain, fatigue, and sleep disturbance are the core symptoms of fibromyalgia. The pain is present above and below the waist on both sides of the body, and typically affects at least six sites, such as the head, arms, chest, abdomen, upper back, lower back, and legs. Cognitive disturbances, psychiatric symptoms, headaches, irritable bowel symptoms, gastroesophageal reflux disease, and dry eye syndrome are also common.

PHYSICAL EXAMINATION

Physical examination in patients with fibromyalgia is typically benign, with the exception of tenderness with palpation of soft tissue sites. These sites, known as tender point locations, are found at the upper mid-trapezius muscle, the greater trochanter, the lateral epicondyle, and at a number of other locations. Tenderness overlying the joints is not found in fibromyalgia patients, and swelling or erythema of the joints or soft tissue is uncommon. Muscle strength is also preserved.

DIFFERENTIAL DIAGNOSIS

A number of disease processes can present with symptoms similar to fibromyalgia. However, a thorough history and physical examination, in addition to limited laboratory studies, can help to support the diagnosis of fibromyalgia, and rule out other diagnoses. In particular, systemic autoimmune disorders, spondyloarthritis, systemic inflammatory arthropathies, polymyalgia rheumatica, hypothyroidism, and inflammatory myopathies should be considered.

DIAGNOSTIC STUDIES

There is no specific laboratory or imaging study that confirms the diagnosis of fibromyalgia. Testing is primarily done to rule out another illness that may present similarly to fibromyalgia or to identify a comorbid condition. Fibromyalgia does not cause any abnormal findings in routine imaging or in laboratory testing.

EVALUATION

Fibromyalgia is a diagnosis of exclusion. Careful history and thorough physical examination in patients who present with the widespread muscle pain, sleep disturbance, and fatigue lasting longer than 3 months can help to support the diagnosis as well as ruling out other causes. Other diseases may present similarly, such as RA and SLE, which have objective physical exam findings as well as abnormalities on laboratory or imaging studies.

In patients in whom fibromyalgia is suspected, limited laboratory studies are indicated. The role of these studies is to eliminate other potential causes for the patient's symptoms. Complete blood count (CBC), and either CRP or ESR are all that are typically ordered. A normal finding on CRP or ESR is reassuring that an occult inflammatory disorder is not likely. In patients with history and physical exam findings consistent with thyroid dysfunction, thyroid function testing is indicated.

TREATMENT

There is no cure for fibromyalgia. Education, lifestyle modifications, and appropriate medications can improve symptoms significantly. Initial management of fibromyalgia should focus on nonpharmacologic therapies and be tailored to each patient's specific needs. For example, psychological therapies may be helpful in treating depression and anxiety, while pharmacotherapy may be indicated for sleep disturbances. Aerobic exercise, a balanced diet, and stress management have all been found to be beneficial in those diagnosed with the disease.

Three medications have been approved by the Food and Drug Administration for the treatment of fibromyalgia: duloxetine (Cymbalta), pregabalin (Lyrica), and milnacipran (Savella). Though these drugs are specifically indicated to treat the symptoms of fibromyalgia, many patients still find them to be minimally beneficial. NSAIDs and acetaminophen are also minimally effective at reducing pain. Opioid analgesics and corticosteroids have no significant effect on fibromyalgia pain, and so should be avoided.

PATIENT EDUCATION

There is no known cure for fibromyalgia; however, there are measures that can be taken to improve symptoms. Maintaining a balanced diet, exercising daily, limiting stress, and practicing good sleep hygiene may lead to significant improvement in overall symptoms. Though the disease is chronic in nature, it is not progressive. Once patients are educated on the disease, they are more likely to be compliant with treatment and to take an active role in disease management.

14.4 AUTOIMMUNE DISEASE

Autoimmune disease occurs when the body fails to recognize self versus nonself and forms an antibody against antigens that are naturally present in the body. This section will concentrate on autoimmune disease from a rheumatologic standpoint.

Autoimmune disease has a female prevalence and can occur in the juvenile to geriatric population. Autoimmune disease in humans involves an immunologic response, which is protective when foreign antigens are introduced by allowing the body to fight infection; however, autoimmune disease is maladaptive in the sense that it works too well and starts to produce antibodies against the body's own natural antigens and immunoglobulins. Autoimmune disease involves both T-cell and B-cell responses but instead of being directed against foreign antigens that threaten the host, these substances are now directed against the host itself.

Autoimmune disease can be recognized by demonstrating autoantibodies that the body produces. Autoantibodies are produced by immunocompetent individuals during the course of infection, inflammation, or cancer. The recognition of autoantibodies against self helps to confirm the diagnosis of various autoantibody diseases. Autoantibodies typically predate the development of symptoms in patients.

When autoantibodies are formed, there is evidence of destructive inflammatory and reactive features that occur as a result of cell-mediated and antibody-driven reactions of the patient against the host's own tissues. Autoimmune disease involves both cell-mediated and antibody system activation and this seems to exist in the context of HLA alleles.[83]

Once an autoimmune disease is present, management strategies are shifting toward downregulation of the autoimmune response in order to limit the self-directed inflammatory process by limiting harmful messenger molecules that participate in tissue injury.[83]

Autoantibody disease has a higher prevalence among family members, so history is an important component in determining an increased risk for autoantibody rheumatologic diseases. Sections covered under this chapter include RA, SLE, antiphospholipid syndrome, Raynaud phenomenon, systemic sclerosis, myopathies including polymyositis and dermatomyositis, Sjögren syndrome, and rhabdomyolysis. Environmental triggers are assessed as potential risk factors as these have been clearly identified in SLE, Sjögren syndrome, and dermatomyositis.[84]

This section will discuss the classic presentation, evaluation strategies, risk factors, and management of these various entities.

14.4A RHEUMATOID ARTHRITIS

RA is a systemic, inflammatory, autoimmune disorder. It is now better understood how environmental factors interact with susceptibility genes in the immune system and how this may contribute to RA.[85] RA results in persistent synovitis, systemic inflammation, and formation of autoantibodies, especially to RF and CCPs.[86]

RA occurs when there is a combined genetic susceptibility (such as HLA-DR1 or HLA-DR4) along with an environmental trigger resulting in joint inflammation. Joint inflammation occurs in joints in a symmetric fashion. Hands, wrists, and feet are commonly affected with hand involvement occurring primarily in the MCP and PIP joints. As in other autoimmune diseases, the body fails to recognize self and forms autoantibodies that adversely affect the joints and other body systems such as the eyes, heart, and lungs.

OVERVIEW

RA typically affects 0.5% to 1% of the general population with an increased incidence in women and elderly.[86] Genetic factors have a role in increasing the risk for RA specifically in the HLA groups, especially HLA-D alleles with genetics contributing to about 50% of those affected.[86] Many of these genes alter the immune response causing the inability of the body to recognize self with the resultant formation of autoantibodies.

EPIDEMIOLOGY

Genetic predisposition plays a significant role but there may be other factors at play, including environmental triggers. Smoking is the primary environmental risk for RA development.[86] Smoking is thought to precipitate RA by increasing formation of citrullinated proteins, leading to autoimmunity to these proteins and subsequently the development of clinically apparent RA in genetically susceptible individuals.[87]

Chronic stimulation of the immune system by bacterial antigens within periodontal tissue is associated with several autoimmune conditions, including RA.[88] The prevalence of periodontal disease has increased twofold in patients with RA compared to the general public.[89] *Porphyromonas gingivalis* produces the enzyme peptidylarginine deiminase that induces citrullination of various autoantigens, and levels of anti-CCP antibodies are higher in RA patients who have periodontal disease, suggesting that periodontitis may contribute to the pathogenesis of RA.[89]

PATHOPHYSIOLOGY

RA patients with seropositivity, as measured by autoantibodies against RF and citrullinated proteins, tend to have more aggressive disease than those without those antibodies, with more severe symptoms, joint destruction, and increased mortality.[90] Autoantibodies against citrullinated peptides (ACPs) form immune complexes that subsequently bind to RF which can lead to abundant complement activation.[91]

There is a triggering of antigen presenting cells activating CD4 helper cells, which stimulate B cells, which are made into plasma cells, which make autoantibodies. T-cells secrete cytokines, which are responsible for joint destruction and erosions. Primary cytokines in this condition include various types of IL along with TNF. It is these cytokines in which disease-modifying drugs in RA (DMARDs) are directed against. RA has marked synovial tissue involvement with synovitis and pannus formation, which is made up of various inflammatory cells, which damage articular cartilage and soft tissues of the joint.

MEDICAL HISTORY AND CLINICAL PRESENTATION

The history and physical examination are of utmost importance in the evaluation and management of a patient with RA.[92]

The most common sites of symmetric joint involvement include PIP, MCP, wrists, elbows, knees, ankles, and MTP joints. Joint destruction is primarily related to pannus formation, joint erosions, and osteopenia of the bones surrounding the joint. Rheumatoid joints typically have soft tissue swelling and there may be joint effusions noted as well. Joints may be warm but they are not hot. With longstanding rheumatoid disease, there may be tender nodules noted primarily on the extensor surfaces.

SIGNS AND SYMPTOMS

Signs and symptoms of RA include symmetric joint stiffness and swelling lasting >1 hour, which is known is the gel sign. Although patients with OA can have stiffness after rest, these symptoms resolve within 30 minutes. As the joint warms up with activity, patient movement becomes easier.

The symmetric involvement of joints includes the small joints of the hand including the MCP joints, the PIP joints, and the MTP joints of the feet. Other joint involvement includes the wrists, elbows, shoulders, hips, knees, and even ankles. Although both sides of the body have joint involvement, patients may not have the same amount of pain on both sides.

Patients who have extra-artricular manifestations of RA have a more aggressive and severe course.[93] Table 14.3 summarizes sites of extra-articular involvement and their manifestations.[94-97]

Syndromes associated with RA including Felty syndrome, which consists of splenomegaly, RA, and neutropenia making these patients susceptible to bacterial infection. Caplan syndrome consists of RA with occupational exposure to coal dust and silica with the development of pneumoconiosis and rapid development of basilar nodules and obstructive airway disease.[98]

PHYSICAL EXAMINATION

Palpation of the involved joints reveals bogginess and some warmth but not truly hot joints. Rheumatoid nodules may be palpated. Physical examination signs can involve the above-mentioned organs.

DIFFERENTIAL DIAGNOSIS

The differential diagnosis for RA is summarized in Table 14.4.[99-104]

DIAGNOSTIC STUDIES

Laboratory testing includes presence of RF and positive anti-CCP antibodies, which tend to be more specific for RA than RF. Autoantibodies directed against citrulline-containing proteins have a specificity of nearly 100% in patients with RA and have been suggested to be involved in the disease pathogenesis.[105] RA can be diagnosed without these lab abnormalities as RA can be diagnosed on clinical grounds. Patients with positive RF and anti-CCP antibodies tend to have more aggressive disease. Patients with a positive RF do not necessarily have RA since this is not a specific test and RF can be present in other autoimmune diseases. Because inflammation occurs with this condition, there will be an elevated ESR or CRP level.

X-rays of the hands and feet should be performed early when RA is suspected. X-ray findings consistent with RA

TABLE 14.3 Manifestations of Extra-Articular Involvement of Rheumatoid Arthritis

Site of Extra-Articular Involvement	Manifestation
Cervical spine	C1–C2, or atlantoaxial joint, which is a very important consideration when patients are being intubated as hyperextension of the neck can result in subluxation and paralysis.
Lungs	Interstitial lung disease as a result of pulmonary fibrosis and small air trapping; interstitial lung disease is more common with increased age of patient, smoking, and positive anti-CCP antibodies.
Vasculitis	Skin ulcers and peripheral arterial disease.
Skin	Rheumatoid nodules present in up to 30% of patients with seropositive RA and increased risk for nodule development in RA patients who smoke. Nodules are typically located on the extensor surfaces or bony prominences.
Eyes	Dry eyes are the most common eye manifestation (known as secondary Sjögren syndrome) being present in about one-third of patients with resultant decreased corneal sensitivity, but scleritis, uveitis, and episcleritis can also occur.
Heart	Cardiovascular disease remains a common cause of death for patients with RA.
Hematology	Anemia of inflammation commonly found since RA is a common cause of ongoing, chronic inflammation. Anemia is typically normochromic, normocytic.

anti-CCP, anti-cyclic citrullinated peptide; RA, rheumatoid arthritis.
Source: Data from Krauss WE, Bledsoe JM, Clarke MJ, Nottmeier EW, Pichelmann MA. Rheumatoid arthritis of the craniovertebral junction. Neurosurgery. *2010;66:A83–A95. doi:10.1227/01.NEU.0000365854.13997.B0; Salaffi F, Carotti M, Di Carlo M, Tardella M, Giovagnoni A. High-resolution computed tomography of the lung in patients with rheumatoid arthritis prevalence of interstitial lung disease involvement and determinants of abnormalities.* Medicine. *2019;98:e17088. doi:10.1097/MD.0000000000017088; Nyhäll-Wåhlin B, Jacobsson LTH, Petersson IF, Turesson C, BARFOT study group. Smoking is a strong risk factor for rheumatoid nodules in early rheumatoid arthritis.* Ann Rheum Dis. *2006;65:601–606. doi:10.1136/ard.2005.039172; Kim IG, Lee JH, Kim SS. Reduced corneal sensitivity in patients with rheumatoid arthritis.* Cornea. *2012;31:1381–1385. doi:10.1097/ICO.0b013e31824d0e22*

TABLE 14.4 Differential Diagnosis for Rheumatoid Arthritis

Condition	Description
Osteoarthritis (OA)	Can be difficult to differentiate between OA and RA when hand involvement is present. Prolonged gel times are seen with RA. RA is also more likely to respond to acute prednisone therapy. More periarticular osteopenia and synovitis with osteophyte bridging associated with OA. RA in hands involve MCP and PIP joints with OA predominately involving the DIP joints.
Gout	Single joint involvement is typical with gout although a small subset of patients may have polyarticular involvement. Tophi from monosodium urate collection is seen only in gout. Joint erosions are not typical for gout patients. Aspiration of joint will show monosodium urate crystals and serum uric acid level is also typically above 7 mg/dL. More joint cartilage damage, bone edema, and synovitis with gout versus RA.
Systemic lupus erythematosus (SLE)	Both RA and SLE can present with involvement of multiple joints in the hands and feet. SLE arthritis is not deforming. SLE has high antinuclear antibody titers while RA may have RF and anti-CCP antibodies.
Psoriatic arthritis (PsA)	Psoriatic arthritis involves the small joints of the hands and feet but it is less symmetric than RA. Oligoarthritis is the rule with PsA and involvement may include the DIP joints, which are typically not involved with RA. PsA is typically seronegative. There is less bone loss (osteoporosis) with RA than PsA.
Reactive arthritis (ReA; formerly Reiter syndrome)	ReA can cause symmetric hand and feet arthritis along with conjunctivitis, rash, and urethritis. These patients can be predisposed by carrying the HLA-B27, but it is not necessary for making the diagnosis. Initial infection with reactive arthritis is from the gastrointestinal or genitourinary system with joint involvement occurring several weeks later. ReA most commonly occurs as a result of infection with *Chlamydia trachomatis*. ReA is classified as seronegative arthritis with inflammatory back pain, migratory oligoarthritis, and extra-articular symptoms.
Septic arthritis	Fever, systemic signs of infection, and monoarthritis are seen with septic arthritis while RA has symmetric joint involvement, especially of the small joints.

CCP, cyclic citrullinated peptide; DIP, distal interphalangeal; MCP, metacarpophalangeal; PIP, proximal interphalangeal; RA, rheumatoid arthritis; RF, rheumatoid factor.
Source: Data from Kiltz U, von Zabern C, Baraliakos X, et al. Diagnostic value of a 3-day course of prednisolone in patients with possible rheumatoid arthritis—the TryCort study. Arthritis Res Ther. *2017;19:73–79. doi:10.1186/s13075-017-1279-z; Popovich I, Lee AC, Doyle A, et al. A comparative MRI study of cartilage damage in gout versus rheumatoid arthritis.* J Med Imaging Radiat Oncol. *2015;59:431–435. doi:10.1111/1754-9485.12306; Paolino S, Botticella G, Casabella A, et al. THU0421 Rheumatoid versus psoriatic arthritis: similar or different bone loss?* Ann Rheum Dis. *2014;72:A307; Hannu T. Reactive arthritis.* Best Pract Res Clin Rheumatol. *2011;25:347–357. doi:10.1016/j.berh.2011.01.018; Carter JD, Inman RD. Chlamydia-induced reactive arthritis: hidden in plain sight?* Best Pract Res Clin Rheumatol. *2011;25:359–374. doi:10.1016/j.berh.2011.05.001; Selmi C, Gershwin ME. Diagnosis and classification of reactive arthritis.* Autoimmun Rev. *2014;13:546–549. doi:10.1016/j.autrev.2014.01.005*

include joint erosions, symmetric joint space narrowing, and periarticular osteopenia. When comparisons are made between sides, there is typical symmetric joint involvement. Synovitis can be picked up via ultrasound.

Ultrasound of the joints, a noninvasive study, has been shown to be more accurate in identifying joint disease than physical examination of the joints even early in the course of the disease.[106] Ultrasound can detect joint fluid, early erosions, synovial thickening, and increased vascularity. MRI can be used to identify early synovitis and tenosynovitis in the PIP joints and can be useful to identify patients with early disease, even before RA becomes symmetric.[107] MRI can also measure bone marrow edema, synovitis, and joint erosions.

EVALUATION

An updated classification system for RA has been developed in order to define criteria for diagnosing RA based upon number of joints, laboratory studies, and duration of synovitis.[108] Points are awarded that put the patient at low, moderate, and high risk for RA and higher levels of these findings are associated with increased severity of disease and mortality.[109]

TREATMENT

New therapeutic strategies now promote the early use of disease-modifying drugs with tight disease control in order to halt joint destruction. With better understanding of the pathophysiology of RA, treatments are now individualized in the early phases of the illness with the potential goal of even being able to prevent RA.[85] As treatments are individualized, response to the biologic agents may be impacted if patients continue to smoke.[110]

Although NSAIDs may help with pain relief and inflammation, they do not affect the natural course of the disease. Intra-articular glucocorticoid injection may provide symptomatic relief but do not change the course of the disease. The approach to treatment is with early use of DMARDs. Methotrexate, the first DMARD that is typically used is given as a once weekly dosing and can be used as monotherapy or in combination with other medications. Patients taking methotrexate should be given additional folic acid as methotrexate is a folate inhibitor.

Patients taking methotrexate should have a pregnancy test prior to starting as pregnancy is strictly prohibited due to its teratogenicity. Pregnancy avoidance is essential and women who wish to conceive while being treated should consider other treatments. Other tests that should be done as a baseline include a CBC with differential, renal function and liver function studies, and chest x-ray. Methotrexate is continued indefinitely since stopping of this medication will lead to a rebound effect and flare of joint pain and disease progression.

Hydroxychloroquine, leflunomide, and sulfasalazine are other DMARDs that might be used. Patients taking hydroxychloroquine should have serial physical examinations looking for retinopathy along with monitoring QT interval on the EKG since it may be prolonged with the use of this agent. Patients taking sulfasalazine should have CBCs performed as this medication can cause leukopenia and neutropenia. Patients taking leflunomide are monitored for liver enzyme elevation and for blood pressure measurements as hypertension can occur with the use of this medication.

Biologic therapy is associated with successful control of RA symptoms with TNF-alpha inhibitors being added as biologic DMARD therapy if control of the condition is not successful with the use of DMARDs such as methotrexate. Biologics and methotrexate are successful drug combinations that improve symptoms and slow the progression of RA. Patient should be checked for tuberculosis prior to starting these immunomodulating agents since these agents could reactivate latent tuberculosis. Prior to DMARD therapy, patients should also be checked for hepatitis B and hepatitis C along with baseline measurements for liver function and CBCs.

Corticosteroids may be used while waiting for DMARDs to result in symptomatic improvement. They can also be used on a short-term basis in order to help control flares of RA pain.

The TNF-alpha inhibitors may be associated with pancytopenia, drug-induced lupus-like syndrome, and demyelinating disease. TNF-alpha inhibitors can also cause heart failure type of symptoms. T-cell modulators are also approved for moderate to severe RA. Other biologic therapies include B-cell modulators, IL-6 inhibitors, and oral Janus kinase (JAK) inhibitors.

Another immunosuppressant that can be utilized in order to modify the progression of RA joint destruction is cyclophosphamide. This medication can cause hemorrhagic cystitis, so patients should be made aware of this unusual complication.

PATIENT EDUCATION

Modern treatment for patients with RA includes aggressive DMARD medications early in the course in order to reduce symptoms and joint destruction and stop its progression. The goal is to prevent disability and to control the inflammation, which may also help with lowering cardiovascular disease risk, which is the most common cause of death for patients with RA. Flares can occur even in patients with overall good control. These flares may be well controlled with the use of corticosteroids on a short-term basis.

Ongoing monitoring for response to therapy and to assess for adverse drug reactions is serially performed. Treatment is individualized and will be guided by patient response symptomatically and for joint response to the intended treatment.

Patients should be counseled to not stop therapy as disease flare is likely to occur if therapy is stopped. Control of this condition is likely given the advances in treatment, but cure is not expected. All patients should be told about the relationship of smoking and exacerbation of disease and patients who smoke should be counseled to stop smoking.

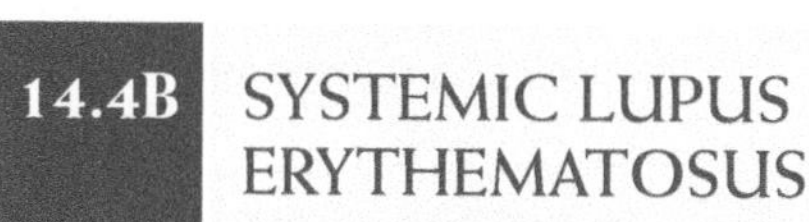

14.4B SYSTEMIC LUPUS ERYTHEMATOSUS

OVERVIEW

SLE is a chronic autoimmune disease affecting multiple organ systems. Though virtually any organ system in the body can be affected by the disease, most commonly involved sites are the skin, joints, blood cells, kidneys, and nervous system. Clinical manifestations and severity can vary widely, with some patients having only mild joint and skin involvement while others develop fulminant disease. Abnormalities of the immune system include the presence of various ANAs, which are a common finding in those with SLE.

EPIDEMIOLOGY

The incidence of SLE has drastically increased over recent years due to improved detection of mild disease, with an estimated incidence rate of 1 to 25 per 100,000 currently in North America, South America, Asia, and Europe.[111,112] Over 90% of cases of SLE occur in women, with the onset most typically occurring after puberty in the 20s and 30s.[113] The prevalence of SLE varies by race, but also by location. Black women have a higher rate of the disease than women of any other race, with Asian women also having a higher incidence than White women. Black women in the United States are two to four times more likely to develop the disease than are White women.[114] However, Black women in Africa have relatively low reported rates of SLE. The disease also appears to be more common in those who live in urban areas as compared to people from rural areas.[115]

PATHOPHYSIOLOGY

The etiology of SLE is unknown, but there are clearly multiple factors involved. Genetic, immunologic, ethnic, hormonal, and environmental factors each appear to play a role in the development of the disease. The formation of antibodies and creation of immune complexes are directly or indirectly responsible for the clinical manifestations of SLE. These antibodies may precede the onset of symptoms by many years.[116] In active SLE, immune complexes form within the microvasculature, leading to activation of complement and subsequent inflammation. Some autoantibodies have been found to be related to the development of specific clinical manifestations. For example, those SLE patients with antiribosomal P antibodies were found to be at increased risk of developing lupus psychosis.[117]

MEDICAL HISTORY AND CLINICAL PRESENTATION

SLE may affect virtually any organ system in the body, and symptoms can range from mild and intermittent to life-threatening. Therefore, it is critical to gather a thorough history from those patients in whom SLE is suspected. Joint pain, which occurs in over 90% of patients with SLE, is typically one of the earliest manifestations, often leading the patient to seek medical care.[118] The arthralgias and arthritis are moderately painful, and tend to be symmetric, polyarticular, and migratory. The arthritis does not usually cause erosions and is rarely deforming. Most commonly involved are the knees and wrists, as well as the joints of the hands. A swan-neck deformity of the fingers may occur but is usually reversible. A history of Raynaud phenomenon (RP) precedes the diagnosis of SLE in up to 50% of patients.[119]

At some point in the course of the disease, constitutional symptoms, such as fatigue, weight loss, and fever, are experienced by most patients. Of these complaints, fatigue is the most prevalent and for some patients, the most disabling. Weight loss may be attributed to decreased appetite, gastrointestinal (GI) disease resulting from the SLE, or may be a side effect of a medication. Weight gain may also be seen in those with the disease, often resulting from corticosteroid use or salt and water retention. Over half of patients with SLE will develop fever, though it can be difficult to determine if this is due to secondary infection or a result of disease flare.[119]

Lesions on the skin and mucous membranes develop at some point during the course of the disease for most patients with SLE. The characteristic "butterfly" rash (Figure 14.6), with erythema appearing in a malar distribution over the cheeks and nose, occurs in fewer than half of patients. This malar rash, which spares the nasolabial folds, develops after sun exposure. Discoid lupus (Figure 14.7), a chronic rash that may develop in those with SLE, also occurs in sun-exposed areas. These lesions are plaque-like and may lead to scarring.

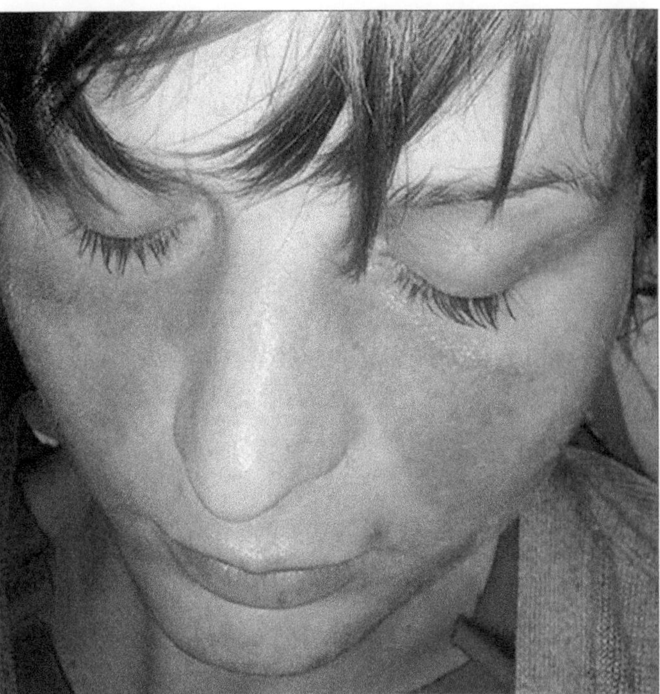

Figure 14.6 **The malar rash of systemic lupus erythematosus.**
(Source: Courtesy Doktorinternet)

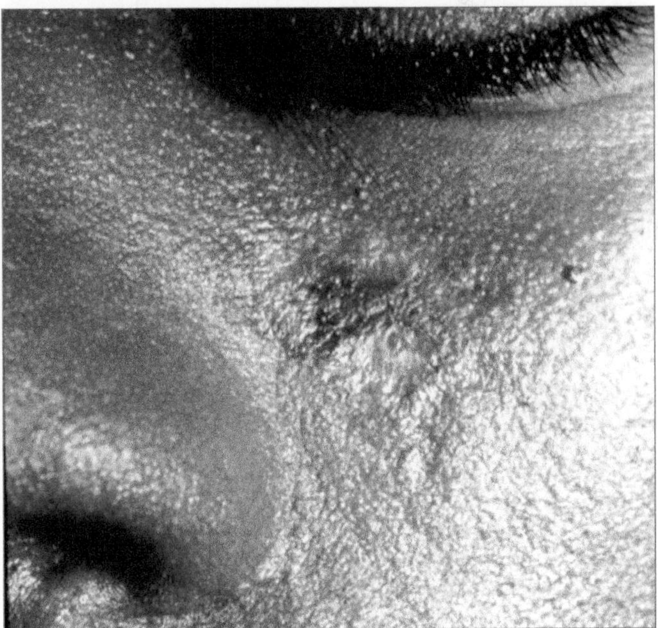

Figure 14.7 **Discoid lupus.**
(Source: Leonard C. Sperling, MD, COL, MC, USA, Department of Dermatology, Uniformed Services University.)

Panniculitis, livedo reticularis, alopecia, and mucosal lesions may also develop, but are not specific to the disease.

Cardiac manifestations in those with SLE are common, with roughly 25% of patients experiencing pericarditis at some point during the course of their disease.[120] The myocardium, valves, coronary arteries, and conduction system may also be affected. Vasculitis is also more prevalent than in the general population, with the small vessels being more commonly affected.

Pulmonary involvement may include pneumonitis, pleuritis, pulmonary hypertension, and interstitial lung disease. Alveolar hemorrhage is a rare complication, but is life threatening when it does develop. Respiratory infections are also more common for those on immunosuppressive therapy.

A significant cause of death and morbidity, renal involvement is found in approximately 50% of patients with SLE, most commonly in the form of glomerulonephritis.[121] SLE-related GI manifestations include those related to esophagitis, acute pancreatitis, protein-losing enteropathy, intestinal pseudo-obstruction, lupus hepatitis, and mesenteric ischemia or vasculitis. Hematologic manifestations result from effects of the disease on all three blood cell lines, with leukopenia and anemia of chronic disease being common.[122] Eye involvement is also quite common, with keratoconjunctivitis sicca and retinal vasculopathy being the most common and second most common ophthalmologic diagnoses, respectively.[123]

A wide range of neuropsychiatric manifestations are related to SLE. Seizures, which can be generalized or partial, may occur. Demyelinating syndrome, cerebrovascular disease, autonomic disorders, and mononeuropathy all may develop. In addition, mood disorders and anxiety disorders may occur, as well as frank psychosis manifesting with hallucinations or paranoia.[124]

SIGNS AND SYMPTOMS

SLE can affect nearly every organ system, leading to a wide range of signs and symptoms. RP is often the first clinical manifestation of the disease, frequently appearing years prior to other symptoms. Fatigue, weight loss, and fever occur at some point in the disease in most patients. Arthralgias and arthritis are common in those with the disease, and tend to be symmetric, polyarticular, and migratory. Skin manifestations are also frequently noted, with malar rash, discoid lupus, alopecia, and mucosal lesions developing in many patients at some point in the course of the disease.

Additional signs and symptoms may be present either acutely during disease flares or chronically. A thorough history and physical exam should investigate the existence of manifestations in all body systems. Routine follow-up and thorough examination of all body systems is encouraged, as clinical manifestations can change significantly over the course of the disease.

PHYSICAL EXAMINATION

In patients with SLE, a thorough physical exam is warranted, as the disease may affect any organ system. The presence of constitutional symptoms should be evaluated by monitoring weight, temperature, and level of fatigue. The skin and mucosa must be inspected for the presence of lesions, and the joints for indications of arthritis. Auscultation of the lungs may reveal abnormalities if pleural effusion or interstitial lung disease is present. Careful examination of the cardiovascular, ophthalmologic, and GI systems should also be included. The presence of hypertension or hematuria may indicate renal involvement, therefore screening for both should be done routinely. Neuropsychiatric evaluation should be comprehensive.

DIFFERENTIAL DIAGNOSIS

The diagnosis of SLE can be difficult to arrive at due to the wide range of signs and symptoms, which can cause the clinical presentation to vary drastically from patient to patient. Other possible diagnoses to be considered in a patient with suspected SLE should be based on that particular patient's clinical presentation. Other rheumatologic disorders, such as RA, fibromyalgia, polymyositis, and scleroderma should be considered. Additionally, infectious processes include Lyme disease, infectious mononucleosis, hepatitis C, and infective endocarditis.

It has been found that some medications can cause a transient form of SLE known as "drug-induced lupus." The most common culprits are hydralazine, procainamide, and isoniazid, though there are many others that may cause this. Therefore, it is critical to gather information about current and recent medications from those presenting with suspected SLE. In those patients who experience drug-induced lupus, discontinuation of the offending medication typically leads to complete resolution of symptoms.

DIAGNOSTIC STUDIES

Though diagnostic criteria do exist for SLE, they are chiefly used to categorize patients in research studies. There is no single diagnostic test that confirms the diagnosis of SLE, but there are studies that are highly specific, and so can be used to support the diagnosis. The ANA test is positive in almost all patients with SLE at some point in the course of their disease. Specific autoantibodies, if positive, may support the diagnosis, or provide insights into severity (Table 14.5).[125,126]

Additional laboratory testing should be done to evaluate disease progression. A CBC and differential may reveal anemia, leukopenia, or thrombocytopenia. A serum creatinine level and urinalysis will help to identify renal involvement, while a serum protein electrophoresis may reveal hypergammaglobulinemia suggestive of systemic inflammation. Additional testing should be done based on the clinical presentation.

Diagnostic studies may also be warranted to rule out other possible causes. RF and anti-CCP antibodies may help to exclude the diagnosis of RA in patients with arthritis or arthralgias. Creatine kinase (CK), when elevated, is indicative of myositis rather than SLE. Additionally, testing for hepatitis C virus, human parvovirus B19, Lyme disease, and Epstein-Barr virus infection may also be indicated, depending on the clinical presentation.

TABLE 14.5 Specific Antibodies in Relation to Systemic Lupus Erythematosus Diagnosis

Autoantibody	Sensitive/Specific	% Positive
Anti-dsDNA antibodies	Highly specific	70%
Anti-Sm antibodies	Highly specific	30%
Anti-Ro/SSA and anti-LA/SSB antibodies	Highly specific	30%
Antiribosomal P protein antibodies	Highly specific; when +, increased risk for central nervous system involvement[117]	Variable
Anti-U1 RNP antibodies	Lacks specificity (seen with mixed connective tissue disease)[126]	25%

RNP, ribonucleoprotein.

Source: Data from Riemakasten G, Hiepe F. Autoantibodies. In: Wallace DJ, Hahn BH, eds. Dubois' Lupus Erythematosus and Related Syndromes. *8th ed. Elsevier; 2013:282.*

EVALUATION

In a patient who presents with signs and symptoms suggestive of SLE, demographics, including gender, age, race, and ethnicity, should be considered. A complete and through history and physical exam are an absolute requirement due to the heterogeneity of clinical presentations seen with SLE. Special attention should be paid to the patient's list of current and recent medications, as drug-induced lupus may be responsible for their current symptoms.

Though there is no one test that confirms the diagnosis of SLE, laboratory studies can help to support the diagnosis. The ANA test is the preferred initial study to perform. Though some patients with SLE will have a negative result, they are still in the minority. The high specificity of the anti-double-stranded DNA and anti-Smith tests make them ideal for further supporting the diagnosis. Diagnostic studies targeted at ruling out other possible diagnoses should be based on clinical presentation. Additional evaluative methods should focus on determining the impact and severity of the disease.

TREATMENT

Treatment of SLE should be tailored to match each patient's clinical presentation and disease severity. However, all patients with SLE should avoid sun exposure to decrease the likelihood of developing or exacerbating cutaneous symptoms due to photosensitivity. Many patients with SLE have been found to have decreased levels of vitamin D, leading to the recommendation that those with the disease take a daily vitamin D supplement.

Hydroxychloroquine, an antimalarial, has been shown to not only prevent disease flares, but also to decrease risk of mortality.[127] Corticosteroids are indicated for more serious manifestations including glomerulonephritis, pericarditis, hemolytic anemia, alveolar hemorrhage, and central nervous system (CNS) involvement. In cases resistant to corticosteroids, immunosuppressive agents such as azathioprine and cyclophosphamide are used.

PATIENT EDUCATION

For most patients with SLE, the disease follows a relapsing and remitting pattern. However, in some patients the disease pursues a much more virulent course. In these patients, serious impairment of vital structures, including heart, brain, lungs, and kidneys, may occur. Fortunately, the use of corticosteroids and immunosuppressive medications has considerably decreased the morbidity and mortality rates of SLE over the past decade.

Patients with SLE should generally have their care managed by a rheumatologist who specializes in the disease. Family planning is an important consideration due to the potential for disease flares during pregnancy and the teratogenic risks of some medications used to treat SLE. Vitamin D supplementation is advised, as there is a high prevalence of vitamin D deficiency in patients with the disease. Chronic inflammation in those with SLE accelerates the development of atherosclerosis in many patients, putting these individuals at a much higher risk of myocardial infarction than the general population. Therefore, patients with SLE should avoid cigarette smoke and follow other recommendations for a healthy lifestyle. As patients with SLE are also at a higher risk for developing malignancy, routine cancer screenings should be completed per the recommended schedule. Avoidance of sun exposure is also strongly recommended to decrease cutaneous symptoms.

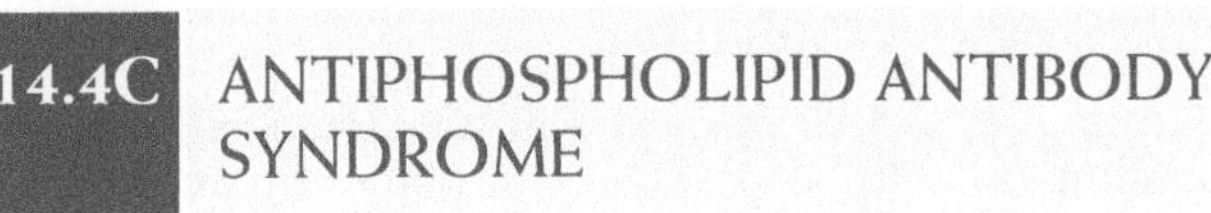

14.4C ANTIPHOSPHOLIPID ANTIBODY SYNDROME

OVERVIEW

Antiphospholipid antibody syndrome (APLA) is a condition that puts a patient at risk for unprovoked thrombosis and recurrent fetal loss. It is caused by the presence of autoantibodies that are most commonly seen with SLE, but these autoantibodies can also occur in the setting of other autoimmune diseases, cancer, or the use of certain medications.

APLA should be suspected in all of the following circumstances: unprovoked venous thromboembolism; unexplained or unprovoked arterial thromboembolism in patients <50 years of age; when thrombosis occurs at unusual sites; late pregnancy loss; or any thrombosis during pregnancy.[128]

Other clinical scenarios that could be associated with the presence of the lupus anticoagulant or APLA includes an incidentally found prolonged activated partial thromboplastin time (aPTT) in asymptomatic patients, patients with recurrent spontaneous early pregnancy loss, and provoked venothrombotic disease in young patients.[128]

The term "lupus anticoagulant" is actually a misnomer. While patients with "lupus anticoagulant" have prolongation of the aPTT, this does not protect the patient against thrombosis and it actually makes monitoring treatment with anticoagulants much more difficult to perform.[129]

EPIDEMIOLOGY

APLA is an important underlying cause of acquired thrombophilia. It can be associated with autoimmune diseases, medication use (especially estrogen), malignancy, or as a primary disease. APLA consists of different autoantibodies: antiphospholipid antibodies which are directed against beta-2 glycoprotein-1 and anticardiolipin antibodies and patients can also have the lupus anticoagulant.[128] Lupus anticoagulant is seen more frequently with fetal loss during pregnancy.

PATHOPHYSIOLOGY

Anticardiolipin antibodies react with proteins associated with cardiolipin. Anticardiolipin antibodies can be measured directly in the lab by looking at both IgM and IgG. Antiphospholipid syndrome is suspected with unprovoked thrombosis and recurrent pregnancy loss.[128]

The presence of the lupus anticoagulant or either of the two primary antiphospholipid antibodies (anticardiolipin and anti-beta-2 glycoprotein-1) are the best known autoantibodies seen with APLA. At least 30 other different antibodies have been identified as playing a role in antiphospholipid syndrome. These autoantibodies may be directed to platelets, glycoproteins, various coagulation factors, and cell surface markers.[130]

The term *lupus anticoagulant* designates that antiphospholipid antibodies inhibit coagulation, impairing prothrombinase activation of prothrombin. Lupus anticoagulant is typically seen in the plasma of patients with SLE. This inhibitor is thought to be directed against phospholipids. The lupus anticoagulant associated prothrombotic condition can also arise in the absence of lupus or other connective tissue disorders.[128]

DIAGNOSTIC STUDIES

Autoantibodies can be measured in the serum as lupus anticoagulant or antiphospholipid antibodies against beta-2 glycoprotein-1, or against anticardiolipin antibody.[131] Lupus anticoagulants are antiphospholipid antibodies that prolong the aPTT. In the clinical laboratory, this aPTT is not corrected when adding other elements to the blood sample. The presence of a lupus anticoagulant is confirmed by measuring a Russell viper venom time or a kaolin clotting time.[132]

Since acute insults to the body such as trauma or infection can alter these autoantibodies, these tests need to be repeated after the patient recovers from the acute situation with 12 weeks after the event being the suggested time frame.

More than 90% of patients with the lupus anticoagulant have elevated anticardiolipin antibody levels. Lupus anticoagulant is considered the most important acquired risk factor for both thrombosis and fetal loss. Lupus anticoagulant consists of autoantibodies that inhibit phospholipid-dependent coagulation reactions in the absence of specific coagulation factor inhibition.[128]

Individuals with lupus anticoagulant have circulating autoantibodies that inhibit blood coagulation. These autoantibodies are of IgG or IgM isotype and are directed against phospholipid-binding plasma proteins. Lupus anticoagulant is a well-recognized risk factor for venous and arterial thromboembolism and pregnancy loss.

SIGNS AND SYMPTOMS

Thromboembolic complications, venous thromboembolism including deep vein thrombosis with or without pulmonary embolism, and cerebral ischemia causing transient ischemic attack or stroke are the most common manifestations of APLA.[128]

Antiphospholipid antibodies lead to a hypercoagulable state causing both venous and arterial thrombosis. Arterial thrombosis is more common in males causing acute coronary syndrome, stokes, and limb ischemia. *Libman-Sachs endocarditis* is a nonbacterial cause of endocarditis that causes vegetations to form on the mitral valve.[133] These patients can present with dyspnea on exertion as a result of this mitral valve pathology. Deep vein thrombosis is more common in females with antiphospholipid antibodies; they have the increased risk for pulmonary embolism and stroke to develop.

Antiphospholipid syndrome is caused by swelling of the venules from the clots obstructing them, which leads to the appearance of purplish discoloration of the skin. Women affected by antiphospholipid syndrome tend to have pregnancy- related complications of miscarriage but this is not completely understood. APLA is thought to cause neurologic symptoms such as headaches and seizures and, in rare cases, antiphospholipid syndrome leads to rapid organ failure due to generalized thrombosis catastrophic antiphospholipid syndrome.[129] Diagnosing antiphospholipid syndrome requires meeting at least one clinical and one laboratory diagnostic criteria or two criteria of history of thrombosis and pregnancy complications.

Patients with APLA are at increased risk for recurrent vascular occlusive disease including strokes, migraines, and deep venous thrombosis (DVT) along with myocardial infarction, mitral valve endocarditis, and pulmonary embolism. They are at high risk for vaso-occlusive disease when anticoagulants are discontinued prior to surgery.[129] APLA is an independent risk factor for the development of cerebrovascular events.[134] Patients without cirrhosis who develop portal vein thrombosis should be tested for APLA.[135]

Complications and progression of APLA can include *catastrophic antiphospholipid antibody syndrome (CAPS)*. This condition may only be recognized at autopsy, since it is associated with a high mortality rate. CAPS can occur when anticoagulation is stopped by the patient with APLA. Management of these patients after thrombosis can be challenging because many of them have coexisting thrombocytopenia. It should be emphasized that patients with APLA should not discontinue anticoagulation and these patients may have special challenges when undergoing surgery with the anticipated need for heparin bridging therapy.[136]

TREATMENT

Patients who are lower risk for clotting due to antiphospholipid syndrome can prevent thrombosis with aspirin in order to inhibit platelet activation along with avoiding risk factors like smoking and using oral contraceptives. Patients with recurrent venous clots or first event arterial clot are treated with a combination of aspirin and high-intensity anticoagulants.[137] Pregnant patients may benefit from the use of hydroxychloroquine, which has been shown to lower morbidity of the fetus and have fewer complications associated with pregnancy when this medication is used throughout pregnancy.[138] Anticoagulation during pregnancy is by low-molecular-weight heparin since warfarin is considered to be teratogenic. There may be a role for the direct oral anticoagulants in managing patients with APLA.[138]

There may be improvement in lessening APLA titers with the use of modulators of B-cell function such as belimumab and abatacept.[139]

PATIENT EDUCATION

Patients with APLA syndrome need lifelong anticoagulation/antiplatelet therapy. Patients should avoid dehydration, long travel, smoking, oral contraceptives or estrogen replacement, and immobilization as these factors are also clot-producing. Patients with APLA who undergo surgery will need additional treatment and monitoring as discontinuing anticoagulation prior to surgery increases the risk for venous and arterial thrombosis. The risks of bleeding versus clotting should be considered and expert consultation should be sought in order to allow the patient to have the best outcomes possible. Patients with APLA will need lifetime anticoagulation/antiplatelet therapy and are at high risk for clotting if therapy is missed.

14.4D RAYNAUD PHENOMENON

OVERVIEW

Raynaud Phenomena (RP) refers to episodic color changes of distal extremities, often related to cold or emotional stress. It was first described by French medical student Maurice Raynaud in his 1862 thesis as a transient vasospasm induced by cold exposure not caused by underlying vascular disease that in severe cases could cause gangrene.[140] RP was felt to indicate exaggerated response of normal physiologic vasomotor reaction to cold and stress. RP can be primary (not caused by underlying rheumatologic disease) or secondary to an underlying rheumatologic disorder such as mixed connective tissue disease (MCTD) or scleroderma.

EPIDEMIOLOGY

RP affects 5% to 20% of women and 4% to 14% of men and generally occurs more in younger females and individuals with a family history of RP.[141–144] It is less common in African American individuals (3.8%).[145] RP is seen more commonly in patients living in colder climates. It may be a symptom of another rheumatologic disease (secondary) though the majority of patients with RP do not have any underlying rheumatologic process (primary) (Table 14.6).

PATHOPHYSIOLOGY

RP is felt to be caused by overactivation of a normal physiologic response to cold exposure and emotional stress. Blood flow is reduced to peripheral tissues to preserve adequate core body temperature. Mechanisms causing RP can be divided into vascular, neural, and intravascular abnormalities.[146] Vascular abnormalities include activation of endothelial cells, which are responsible for regulating vascular tone. Endothelial cells can secrete vasodilating agents such as such as prostacyclin and nitric oxide and vasoconstricting agents such as endothelin and angiotensin. Patients with systemic sclerosis are known to have overactivation of endothelin-1, which leads to increased risk for vasoconstriction and risk for intravascular thrombus. Neural transmitters can also affect vascular tone as blood vessels can be innervated from sympathetic vasoconstrictor neurons, sympathetic or parasympathetic vasodilator neurons, and sensory neurons that regulate dilation of blood vessels. Release of norepinephrine, somatostatin, and neuropeptide Y lead to vasoconstriction while release of substance P, vasoactive intestinal peptide, calcitonin gene-related peptide, and neurokinin A lead to vasodilation.[146] Intravascular abnormalities that cause RP include activation of platelets, reduced fibrinolysis, activation of WBCs, reduced red blood cell deformability, and oxidative stress.[146] Smoking in adults can also increase risk of RP as can chemical/drug exposures (use of amphetamines, cocaine, LSD, ecstasy, antihistamines, CNS stimulants and attention-deficit hyperactivity disorder [ADHD] therapeutics, and ergotamine).

TABLE 14.6 Characteristics of Primary Versus Secondary Raynaud Phenomenon

Primary Raynaud Phenomenon	Secondary Raynaud Phenomenon
Female	Male
Onset between 15–30 years	Age >40 years
Symmetric symptoms	Asymmetric symptoms
Normal nailfold capillaries	Abnormal capillary nailfold changes
Lack of digital ulcerations	Digital ulcerations
Shorter duration of painful attacks	Ischemic changes proximal to fingers or toes
Family history of primary Raynaud phenomenon	Color changes involving thumbs, nose, ears
	History of thrombosis
	Abnormal labs suggesting secondary rheumatologic disease (MCTD, SLE, APL syndrome)

APL, acute promyelocytic leukemia; MCTD, mixed connective tissue disease; SLE, systemic lupus erythematosus.

MEDICAL HISTORY AND CLINICAL PRESENTATION

Patients with RP typically present with a history of recurrent discoloration of the hands and feet with exposure to cold or emotional upset. Pallor and cyanosis of the extremities are described, often involving a single finger or toe with sharp demarcation (Figure 14.8). Patients often report numbness, tingling, or aching sensation of the affected digit (index, middle and ring fingers most commonly). While fingers and toes are most commonly affected, patients may also report cutaneous vasospasm of the auricles of the ears, tip of the toes, tip of the tongue, and rarely the nipples. Skin discoloration begins as pallor caused by decreased blood flow from transient vasospasm. As oxygen is depleted from tissue, skin may appear cyanotic. Episodes of discoloration usually last minutes and are reversible with rewarming of the affected tissue. Patients often report pain during the rewarming phase as blood flow is exaggerated causing increased redness, flushing, and sometimes swelling or itching of the affected skin. In some cases of RP, patients may develop tender, painful subcutaneous nodules known as pernio. In severe cases of RP, digital ulcerations may occur from chronic recurrent local tissue ischemia. Prolonged tissue ischemia can lead in rare cases to autoamputation of digits.

SIGNS AND SYMPTOMS

Painful discoloration of the fingers and toes with exposure to cold or stress are the most common signs/symptoms of RP. Index, middle, and ring fingers are most commonly affected. RP is characterized by triphasic white, blue, and red color changes (in that order) in which the red phase is

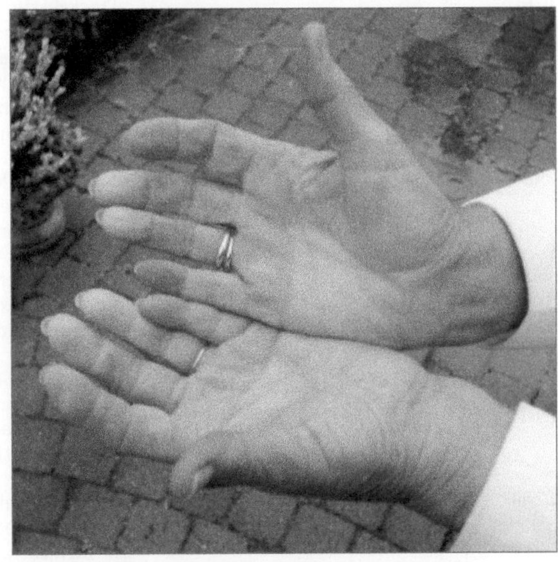

Figure 14.8 Adult female with characteristic findings of Raynaud phenomenon. Note white, red, and blue color changes and distribution more on second, third and fourth fingers.
(Source: Courtesy of Jamclaassen)

associated with a rapid blushing or pink coloring of the skin during rewarming. Patients often report numbness during the white phase of discoloration and pain with rewarming (red phase) of affected tissues.

PHYSICAL EXAMINATION

Examination of a patient with RP often shows poor circulation in the hands and feet with delayed capillary refill. Patients may have red, purple, or splotchy fingers and toes at baseline during clinical evaluation that become white with cold exposure. Digital ulcerations on the fingers or toes would provoke concern for tissue ischemia from prolonged lack of blood flow. Nailfold capillary microscopy (handheld magnifier with a low-power microscope used at bedside) may show tortuous distorted capillary loops suggestive of RP. Abnormal nailfold capillaries are more common in secondary RP than primary RP. Patients may have discoloration episodes but may not be actively symptomatic during clinical evaluation.

DIFFERENTIAL DIAGNOSIS

RP should be differentiated from a thrombotic event through careful history to differentiate prolonged discoloration from transient ischemia as well as to identify the history of potential occlusive vascular disease. Differential diagnosis for RP includes acrocyanosis, excessive cold sensitivity, peripheral neuropathy, reflex sympathetic dystrophy syndrome or complex regional pain syndrome (RSD/CRPS), pernio/chilblains, and erythromelalgia (EM).

Table 14.7 summarizes the differential diagnosis for RP.

DIAGNOSTIC STUDIES

Primary RP is diagnosed by history and physical exam along with the exclusion of systemic symptoms. Lab tests are not indicated for patients with primary RP and can be misleading. If there is a high clinical suspicion for secondary RP (male gender, onset of symptoms in patients >40 years or prepubertal, evidence of digital ulcerations, asymmetric attacks, abnormal nailfold capillaries, comorbid vascular disease, comorbid arthritis, and rashes suggestive of connective tissue disease), laboratory testing should be ordered and should include screening for associated rheumatologic illness such as APLA, MCTD, SLE, and scleroderma. Tests include CBC with differential, ESR, CRP, comprehensive metabolic panel (CMP), ANA with reflex to extractable nuclear antigens (paying particular notice of ribonucleoprotein antibodies, Scl 70 antibodies, and anticentromere antibodies), C3, C4, anticardiolipin antibodies, beta-2 glycoprotein, and lupus anticoagulant panel.

TREATMENT

Treatment for RP depends on the severity of manifestations and whether it is primary or secondary. Primary RP can often be managed conservatively without medication by avoiding sudden cold exposure, reducing emotional stress, dressing appropriately for cold weather (i.e., layering on the core, wearing mittens instead of gloves, using wool and moisture-wicking fabrics), and using gentle rewarming techniques if color changes have started to occur (e.g., running hands under warm water, swinging arms, placing hands in axillae for warmth). Cigarette smoking and use of CNS stimulants (decongestants, ADHD medications) should be avoided. Treatment for secondary RP is aimed at treating the underlying condition but will often include pharmacologic treatment to improve distal circulation. More severe cases of primary RP may also require pharmacologic treatment. The most common medications used to treat RP are calcium channel blockers (CCB) such as amlodipine and nifedipine. Patients who start a CCB should take medication at night with sufficient water and should monitor their blood pressure within 3 days

TABLE 14.7 Differential Diagnosis of Raynaud Phenomenon

Condition	Description
Acrocyanosis	Symmetric painless, persistent blue-to-black discoloration of the hands and feet. More commonly affects the entire hand or foot and not isolated digits. Extends proximally without sharply demarcated boundaries of color change. Precipitated by exposure to cold and stress like Raynaud phenomenon (RP), but does not improve with vasodilator treatment.
Cold sensitivity	Lacks the hallmark color changes seen in RP. Common for individuals, especially women and older patients, to report sensitivity to cold but in the absence of painful demarcated white, blue, and red color changes.
Peripheral neuropathy	Similar intolerance to cold with numbness, tingling, and color changes of fingers and toes. Differs from RP on exam as patients show decreased sensation to sharp, dull, and temperature, as well as decreased proprioception of the hands and feet.
Reflex sympathetic dystrophy (RSD)/Complex regional pain syndrome (CRPS)	Typically presents with paresthesias, unilateral color changes, and temperature changes of an affected extremity in the setting of significant allodynia/hyperalgesia and potential refusal to move the affected limb. Pain is persistent in patients with RSD/CRPS and not transient as is seen in patients with RP.
Pernio/chillblains	Patients develop painful, tender blisters or nodular lesions most commonly on the fingers and toes with exposure to cold. These lesions do not blanch, whereas color changes in patients with RP do blanch.
Erythromelalgia (EM)	Patients develop erythema, warmth, and occasional swelling of their hands and feet with exposure to warm temperatures. Affected patients report relief of symptoms with cold exposure or application of ice/cold water. EM is sometimes considered the opposite of RP.

of starting medication to assess for hypotension. Patients who do not respond to CCBs or who cannot tolerate CCBs may try treatment with direct vasodilators such as nitroglycerin (oral or topical), hydralazine, or minoxidil. Indirect vasodilators such as sildenafil, prazosin, fluoxetine, captopril, losartan, and bosentan have also been shown to be effective.

PATIENT EDUCATION

Patients with RP should be educated on primary versus secondary RP and signs and symptoms to be aware of that would be concerning for underlying rheumatologic disease. All individuals with RP should be educated on potential triggers and how to mitigate this (avoiding sudden cold exposure, dressing appropriately, reducing stress, avoiding smoking and medications known to exacerbate RP).

14.4E SYSTEMIC SCLEROSIS

OVERVIEW

Systemic sclerosis is a chronic disease affecting multiple organ systems. It is characterized by progressive fibrosis of the skin and internal organs as well as widespread vascular dysfunction. The term "scleroderma" refers to the presence of thickened and hardened skin, which is the hallmark feature of systemic sclerosis. There are two generally recognized forms of the disease, with limited systemic sclerosis affecting primarily the face and hands, while the diffuse form affects those areas as well as the trunk and proximal extremities. In those patients diagnosed with systemic sclerosis, approximately 80% have the limited version, while the remaining 20% have diffuse disease. The prognosis for those with the limited form of the disease is more favorable, since the kidneys and lungs are not impacted as severely as they are in those who have diffuse disease.

EPIDEMIOLOGY

Systemic sclerosis is a rare disease that occurs in women two to three times more often than in men. However, diffuse systemic sclerosis occurs at equal rates in both genders. Though cases have been diagnosed in childhood, symptoms usually do not appear until the third to fifth decades of life.

PATHOPHYSIOLOGY

Systemic sclerosis is an autoimmune disease, though the pathophysiology is not fully understood. In addition to an autoimmune component, genetic, environmental, and vascular factors are all believed to play a role in the pathogenesis of the disease. Hardening and tightening of the skin results from an overproduction of collagen. Collagen deposition in the skin and organs as well as disturbances in its degradation lead to the characteristic signs and symptoms.

MEDICAL HISTORY AND CLINICAL PRESENTATION

Patients with systemic sclerosis often experience fatigue and pain in addition to major organ involvement.[147] Pain most commonly presents as arthralgias or results from RP and skin-related discomfort to include ischemic digital ulcers. The fatigue experienced is considered significant and can be compared to that of a patient with SLE or RA.[148]

Major organ involvement in systemic sclerosis can include nearly every organ system. Cutaneous manifestations are almost always present and include thickening and hardening of the skin, which can vary in severity and extent. The areas affected first are typically the fingers, hands, and face, with erythema and edema preceding induration. Patients may also experience pruritus, dryness, changes in pigmentation, and loss of appendicular hair in the affected areas. In later disease, skin ulcerations may be present over the finger joints, and ulcers may form at the digital tips. RP, which is almost always present in those with systemic sclerosis, may occur in prolonged episodes, which can last 30 minutes or longer. This can lead to progressive permanently impaired blood flow due to structural changes in the small blood vessels over time. The result is often ischemic pain, trophic changes, digital ulcerations, and even ischemia and infarction.

Musculoskeletal manifestations are common in those with systemic sclerosis and develop as a result of fibrosis around tendons and other structures in both large and small joints. Joint pain, immobility, and contractures may initially affect the small joints of the hands, but the wrists, elbows, and ankles may also be involved. Contractures of the fingers may develop.

Evidence of GI involvement is present in almost 90% of patients with systemic sclerosis, regardless of the subtype.[149] However, roughly half of those affected are asymptomatic. The most frequently affected section of the GI tract is the esophagus, though any part may be involved. In those patients who do experience GI symptoms, dysphagia, heartburn, choking, hoarseness, early satiety, and alternating diarrhea and constipation are common.

The vast majority of those with systemic sclerosis develop some degree of pulmonary involvement. Interstitial lung disease and pulmonary vascular disease are the most common clinical manifestations. Dyspnea on exertion and a nonproductive cough are the most common symptoms, though symptoms may be absent or go unnoticed in early disease. Pulmonary arterial hypertension may develop in those systemic sclerosis patients with pulmonary vascular disease as a late complication and can lead to cor pulmonale as well as right-sided heart failure. Another common complication, thrombosis of the pulmonary vessels, is a frequent cause of death in those in the late stages of the disease.

While cardiac involvement is common in those with systemic sclerosis, men are likely to experience more severe manifestations, leading to a poorer prognosis.[150] Pericardial disease, myocardial fibrosis, myocardial ischemia, and conduction system disturbances and arrhythmias are also common.

Scleroderma renal crisis (SRC) is seen more commonly in patients with diffuse systemic sclerosis and is more likely to occur early in the disease process. Abrupt onset of severe hypertension and development of acute oliguric renal failure characterize SRC. Even in those who do not develop SRC, kidney involvement is common, with microalbuminuria, hypertension, and mild elevation of the plasma creatinine concentration demonstrating the effects of the disease on the renal system.

SIGNS AND SYMPTOMS

The signs and symptoms of systemic sclerosis are summarized in Table 14.8.

TABLE 14.8 Signs and Symptoms of Systemic Sclerosis

Sign/Symptom	Significance
Raynaud phenomenon	Appears years prior to systemic sclerosis
Malaise, weight loss, and polyarthralgia	Seen with diffuse systemic sclerosis
Skin thickening, pruritus, loss of normal skin folds, changes in pigmentation, and telangiectasias	Seen with diffuse and local systemic sclerosis
Progressive dysphagia for solids	GI involvement commonly seen along with abdominal pain
Shortness of breath	Seen with pulmonary involvement

GI, gastrointestinal.

TABLE 14.9 Diagnostic Studies for Systemic Sclerosis

Laboratory Study	Significance
The antinuclear antibody (ANA)	Positive in 95%
Anticentromere antibody (ACA)	Positive with limited systemic sclerosis
Antitopoisomerase I (anti-SCL-70) and anti-RNA polymerase III antibody[151]	Seen with diffuse systemic sclerosis; highly specific but only moderately sensitive
Complete blood count (CBC)	Anemia resulting from iron deficiency, malabsorption, or blood loss through the GI tract
Serum creatinine, urinalysis	Abnormal with renal involvement
Creatine kinase (CK) level	Identifies myositis, myopathy
Hand x-rays	Calcinosis cutis; soft tissue calcifications of the distal phalanges

GI, gastrointestinal.

PHYSICAL EXAMINATION

In patients with systemic sclerosis, physical examination of the face and neck reveal thickening of the skin, changes in pigmentation, loss of normal skin folds, and telangiectasias. Tightening of the skin surrounding the mouth may lead to a decreased oral aperture. Inspection of the fingers may reveal sclerodactyly, ulcerations, and atrophy. Depending on the severity of disease, lung findings may be consistent with restrictive lung disease due to diffuse pulmonary fibrosis and pulmonary vascular disease.

DIFFERENTIAL DIAGNOSIS

The diagnosis of systemic sclerosis often takes considerable time and a high incidence of suspicion early in the disease process. RP, which often precedes other symptoms of the disease by years, is a common disorder, which can occur alone or in conjunction with other rheumatologic conditions. Some medications, such as those used to treat metastatic breast cancer, may cause a similar presentation of symptoms. Additionally, other rare diseases, such as eosinophilic fasciitis, scleromyxedema, and lichen sclerosis should be considered.

DIAGNOSTIC STUDIES

Diagnostic studies relevant to systemic sclerosis are summarized in Table 14.9.[151]

EVALUATION

The ANA test is the preferred initial study to perform, as a negative result is a reliable indicator that the patient's symptoms are due to another cause. The high specificity of the anticentromere antibody (ACA), anti-SCL-70, and anti-RNA polymerase III tests make these ideal for further supporting the diagnosis, as well as helping to differentiate between the limited and diffuse forms.

TREATMENT

There is no known medication or therapy that is effective in decreasing the overproduction and deposition of collagen found in systemic sclerosis. Therefore, treatment is targeted at the involved organ systems and is supportive in nature. Moderate to severe RP should be treated with calcium channel blockers, vasodilatory medications, or intravenous prostaglandins. Esophageal dysfunction may improve with the use of proton pump inhibitors and H2 blockers. Antibiotics may be indicated if bacterial overgrowth of the digestive tract leads to malabsorption. Angiotensin-converting enzyme inhibitors administered intravenously in an inpatient setting are the preferred treatment of hypertensive crises caused by SRC. Owing to an increased risk of organ failure and other complications, patients with diffuse skin and severe inflammatory organ involvement (including myocarditis and interstitial lung disease) are treated more aggressively with systemic immunosuppressive therapy.

PATIENT EDUCATION

Patients with diffuse systemic sclerosis have a poorer prognosis than those with limited disease.[152] Because the severity and organ systems affected can vary greatly from patient to patient, management of the disease should be tailored to the individual. Symptoms from RP may be avoided or ameliorated by dressing in loose layered clothing including gloves and socks, and by avoiding exposure to the cold. Smoking should be discouraged due to worsening of symptoms and negatively impacting the overall prognosis. For those patients who experience GI symptoms, eating smaller meals, remaining upright for at least 2 hours after eating, and crushing medications or taking them in liquid form may be beneficial. Patients suffering from a rapidly progressing or severe form of the disease should be treated in centers specializing in systemic sclerosis management.

14.4F MYOPATHIES

OVERVIEW

A myopathy is a muscle disease that is not related to a disorder of the neuromuscular junction or innervation. Etiologies vary widely and include idiopathic, inherited, infectious, inflammatory, endocrine, drug-induced or toxic, and metabolic. Muscle weakness, the most common symptom, leads to difficulty in accomplishing daily activities for many patients. Though there are a number of inflammatory myopathies, ***polymyositis*** and ***dermatomyositis*** are among the most common.

EPIDEMIOLOGY

The inflammatory myopathies are rare, with polymyositis and dermatomyositis having a combined incidence estimated at 2 per 100,000 people annually.[153] Both diseases occur in women twice as often as men. The peak incidence is between age 40 and 50, though dermatomyositis may also occur in children. In the pediatric population, the peak incidence is between ages 5 and 10.[154]

PATHOPHYSIOLOGY

The pathophysiology of polymyositis is not entirely understood. Evidence suggests that defective cellular immunity leads to an immune-mediated reaction in which T cells are directed against muscle antigens. Similarly, the pathophysiology of dermatomyositis is poorly understood. However, injury to both capillaries and myofibers is a well-established finding, although the mechanism remains unknown. In both polymyositis and dermatomyositis research suggests that there may be a number of factors responsible for development of each disorder including environmental, genetic, infectious, and immunologic factors.

MEDICAL HISTORY AND CLINICAL PRESENTATION

Though the predominant feature of both dermatomyositis and polymyositis is proximal skeletal muscle weakness, a wide variety of clinical manifestations affecting multiple organ systems occurs.[155] Patients with dermatomyositis also develop characteristic dermatologic manifestations. Heart, lung, and esophageal diseases may develop as a result of either disorder. Adults with dermatomyositis appear to be at a higher risk of developing malignancy.[156]

Muscle weakness is the primary feature of both dermatomyositis and polymyositis and is often why individuals seek medical care. Patients typically provide a history of gradually worsening muscle weakness developing over several months with activities such as climbing stairs, rising from a chair, picking up a child, or carrying heavy items being reported. The muscle weakness is typically symmetric in a proximal distribution, with the hip flexors and deltoids most profoundly affected. The flexor muscles of the neck may also be weakened. Some patients will experience distal muscle weakness, but this is typically mild without negatively impacting daily activities. Skin manifestations may precede or accompany weakness in those with dermatomyositis. Some patients may experience mild myalgias as well as muscle tenderness. Muscle atrophy is a late finding of the diseases.

Dermatologic manifestations include several distinct skin eruptions in those with dermatomyositis. In some patients dermatologic findings may be subtle and more challenging to see, while in others they may be quite conspicuous. Though skin changes may occur in patients with polymyositis, they are not specific for the disease. Gottron papules and the heliotrope rash, both of which are described below, are pathognomonic features of dermatomyositis.

Pulmonary disease develops in roughly 10% of those with polymyositis and dermatomyositis, typically in the form of interstitial lung disease. This may rapidly progress to respiratory failure, and even death. Diaphragmatic and chest wall muscle weakness may also contribute to respiratory insufficiency, especially with exertion.

Dysphagia is present in about one third of patients with polymyositis and dermatomyositis and results from weakness of the striated muscle that forms the superior portion of the esophagus.[157] In addition, weakness of the oropharyngeal muscles leads to nasal regurgitation. Aspiration increases the risk of bacterial pneumonia, especially in older patients, who are more likely to have esophageal involvement.[158]

Subclinical cardiac involvement including rhythm disturbances and conduction abnormalities can occur as sequela in those with polymyositis and dermatomyositis.[159] These patients are also at increased risk for experiencing myocardial infarction.[160] Heart failure and other symptomatic cardiac manifestations are less common.[161]

SIGNS AND SYMPTOMS

Proximal muscle weakness is typically the earliest and most pronounced clinical manifestation of polymyositis and dermatomyositis. The weakness is progressive and involves the muscle groups of the proximal upper and lower extremities as well as the neck. Difficulty rising from a chair and climbing stairs are typically noted earlier than upper extremity symptoms. Characteristic skin findings, as described below, may precede or accompany the muscle weakness in dermatomyositis. Difficulty swallowing, dyspnea with exertion, and aspiration pneumonia can develop depending on the severity of disease.

PHYSICAL EXAMINATION

In patients with dermatomyositis or polymyositis, physical examination will reveal symmetric proximal muscle weakness of the upper and lower extremities. Though some patients may experience mild tenderness with palpation of the affected muscles, most will not. Sensory deficits are not present, and deep tendon reflexes remain normal. Additionally, facial, and ocular muscles are unaffected. Weakness of the neck muscles may make holding the head up difficult. In late disease muscle atrophy and decreased deep tendon reflexes may be observed. Systemic symptoms such as fever, malaise, and fatigue are not typical and so should lead to a search for other causes.

Patients with dermatomyositis may present with a wide array of dermatologic findings. Gottron papules and heliotrope rash are the hallmark features of the disease, though other skin eruptions are also common. Gottron papules (Figure 14.9) develop symmetrically over the dorsal aspects of the MCP, DIP, and PIP joints. The papules have a flattened top and range in color from erythematous to violaceous in those with lighter skin tones. In patients with darker skin tones, the papules may appear hyperpigmented. Scaling may be present, giving the lesions a psoriasis-like appearance. Heliotrope rash (Figure 14.10) can range from erythematous to violaceous and is most prominent on the upper eyelids. In some patients the eruptions will be accompanied by edema of the eyelids. While the heliotrope eruption may be prominent in some patients, it can be considerably less vivid and difficult to observe in others.

Not to be confused with Gottron papules, Gottron sign (Figure 14.11) is the presence of macules, patches, or papules on the extensor surfaces of joints other than on the hands. These lesions, which range from erythematous to violaceous, most commonly occur on the knees, elbows, and

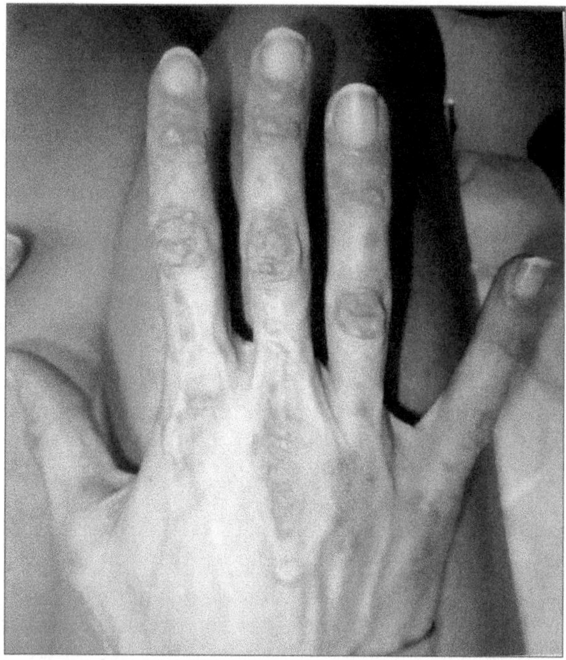

Figure 14.9 **Gottron papules.**
(Source: Courtesy of Mohammad2018)

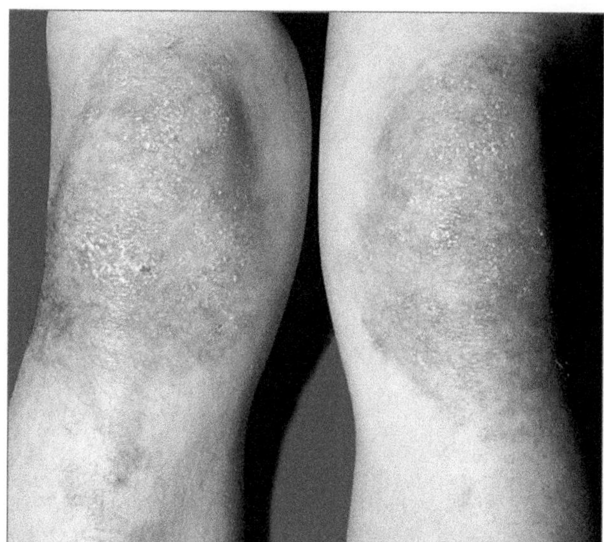

Figure 14.11 **Gottron sign overlying the knees in a pediatric patient with dermatomyositis.**
(Source: Dugan EM, Huber AM, Miller FW, Rider LG, the International Myositis Assessment and Clinical Studies (IMACS) Group. Photoessay of the cutaneous manifestations of the idiopathic inflammatory myopathies. Dermatol Online J. *2009;15(2). https://escholarship.org/uc/item/1f04d17z)*

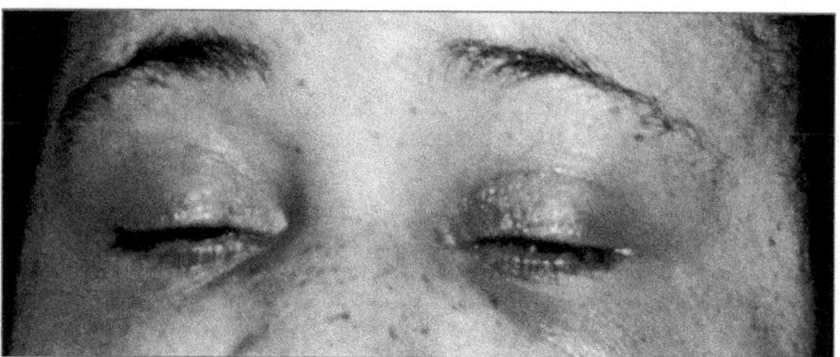

Figure 14.10 **Heliotrope rash.**
(Source: Dugan EM, Huber AM, Miller FW, Rider LG, the International Myositis Assessment and Clinical Studies (IMACS) Group. Photoessay of the cutaneous manifestations of the idiopathic inflammatory myopathies. Dermatol Online J. *2009;15(2). https://escholarship.org/uc/item/1f04d17z)*

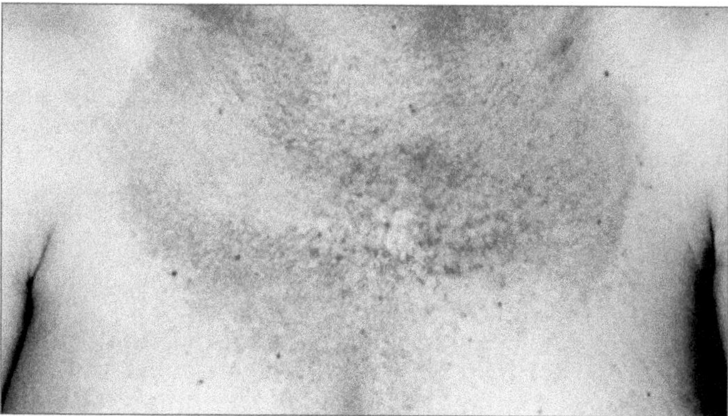

Figure 14.12 **Poikiloderma of the upper chest and neck.**
(Source: Dugan EM, Huber AM, Miller FW, Rider LG, the International Myositis Assessment and Clinical Studies (IMACS) Group. Photoessay of the cutaneous manifestations of the idiopathic inflammatory myopathies. Dermatol Online J. *2009;15(2). https://escholarship.org/uc/item/1f04d17z)*

ankles. In some patients the lesions will thicken, causing them to have a psoriatic appearance.

Some less common skin findings may develop in those with dermatomyositis but are not considered to be hallmarks of the disease. Midfacial erythema, similar to the malar rash seen in SLE, may develop. Additionally, poikiloderma may develop on photo-exposed sites. Skin demonstrating poikiloderma will be both hypopigmented and hyperpigmented, with visible telangiectasias and epidermal atrophy. In those with dermatomyositis, there may be a violaceous hue. The classic areas where poikiloderma is likely to be observed is on the upper back, which is known as the "shawl sign," and the V of the upper chest and neck (Figure 14.12). These eruptions may be significantly pruritic, which helps to distinguish them from those found in SLE. Many patients with dermatomyositis develop diffuse scalp involvement that may resemble seborrheic dermatitis or psoriasis. Periungual erythema and dilation of nailfold capillaries are often accompanied by an overgrowth of nail cuticles, referred to as "ragged cuticles."

DIFFERENTIAL DIAGNOSIS

A number of disease processes can present with symptoms similar to polymyositis. Amyotrophic lateral sclerosis (ALS), polymyalgia rheumatica, fibromyalgia, hyper- or hypothyroidism, Cushing syndrome, sarcoidosis, and SLE are part of the differential diagnosis. Other forms of myositis, such as inclusion body myositis and focal myositis, should be considered, as well as myasthenia gravis, muscular dystrophy, and various myopathies. For patients with suspected dermatomyositis, causes of similar cutaneous manifestations should be considered. This includes psoriasis, rosacea, discoid lupus erythematosus, and lichen planus. Some medications such as azole antifungals, statins, colchicine, and some antimalarials can lead to myopathy in certain patients; therefore, it is important to inquire about current and recent medication use.

DIAGNOSTIC STUDIES

Though laboratory studies and electromyography may help to support the diagnosis, the only specific test for polymyositis and dermatomyositis is biopsy of involved muscles. Histopathology can distinguish between the two diseases as well as excluding other forms of myopathy. Lymphoid inflammatory infiltrates are found in both polymyositis and dermatomyositis; however, in dermatomyositis they are perivascular and interfascicular, while in polymyositis they are primarily intrafascicular with necrosis of scattered individual muscle fibers.

Serum levels of muscle enzymes are elevated in most patients with polymyositis or dermatomyositis. Serum CK levels may be elevated up to 100 times the upper limit of the reference range. Aldolase, aspartate aminotransferase (AST), alanine aminotransferase (ALT), and lactic dehydrogenase (LDH) levels may also be elevated. Though the severity of the muscle weakness may correlate with the height of elevation in muscle enzymes, the degree of muscle dysfunction may be significant in patients with only moderate elevations in enzyme levels.[155]

A positive ANA result is common in both polymyositis and dermatomyositis but is not required for diagnosis. A number of autoantibodies are seen exclusively in patients with myositis, and so are termed myositis-specific antibodies (MSAs). They are found in approximately 30% of those with polymyositis or dermatomyositis. Anti-Jo-1 antibodies are more commonly found in patients with polymyositis and are associated with pulmonary involvement, which includes interstitial lung disease. Anti-Mi-2 antibodies are highly specific for dermatomyositis, though sensitivity is low. Anti-SRP antibodies are found in a small subset of patients with polymyositis and are associated with acute onset of severe weakness and increased incidence of cardiac involvement leading to higher mortality rates.

Electromyography in patients with polymyositis or dermatomyositis will frequently show changes indicating a myopathic rather than neurogenic cause of weakness; however, these findings are not specific for either disease. MRI is often preferred over electromyography as it can show areas of edema, inflammation, and scarring. This may also help to identify the most appropriate site for muscle biopsy.

Once the diagnosis of polymyositis or dermatomyositis is strongly suspected or confirmed, testing should be done to determine the impact of the disease. Electrocardiography, pulmonary function studies, and esophageal manometry may be indicated to evaluate heart, lung, and GI involvement. Further testing to rule out occult malignancy may include imaging, laboratory testing, and cancer screenings such as colonoscopy and Pap smear.

EVALUATION

In patients who present with the complaint of muscle weakness, history and physical exam should be targeted at determining which muscle groups are involved, if the involvement is symmetric, and if there is pain. Polymyositis and dermatomyositis should be suspected in any patient with proximal muscle weakness of the upper and lower extremities, who is experiencing minimal or no pain. Characteristic dermatologic findings may support the diagnosis of dermatomyositis, but the workup is the same for both diseases. Initial diagnostic studies should be done to rule out metabolic and endocrine causes. Muscle enzymes, particularly CK, are likely to be elevated, and MSAs may not only support the diagnosis, but also provide insight as to prognosis. Definitive diagnosis is through muscle biopsy, which differentiates between polymyositis and dermatomyositis if the clinical picture is unclear.

TREATMENT

Corticosteroids are the first-line treatment for both polymyositis and dermatomyositis. High-dose prednisone, 40 to 60 mg or more per day continued over a 4- to 8-week period, is typically effective at decreasing muscle enzyme levels back to within reference range. Muscle strength and endurance improve gradually as CK levels decrease. The prednisone dose is then tapered by 5 to 10 mg monthly while muscle strength and enzyme levels are monitored.

Immunosuppressive or cytotoxic agents are often added as adjunctive therapy early in the course of treatment in an attempt to minimize the harmful side effects of high-dose prednisone. Methotrexate and azathioprine are two commonly used agents that have been found to be effective in controlling the diseases long-term. Though these medications do have some side effects, they can be used safely in most patients. Other alternative or adjunctive therapies include intravenous immune globulin, rituximab, or mycophenolate.

For patients with skin involvement, minimizing sun exposure is critical. Patients should be encouraged to wear photoprotective clothing, avoid direct sunlight, and use sunscreens. Additionally, topical corticosteroids and oral hydroxychloroquine may provide relief.

PATIENT EDUCATION

There is no known cure for polymyositis or dermatomyositis; however, medication can help to control the symptoms. Patients should be cared for by a clinician familiar with the treatment and monitoring of these diseases. Routine monitoring is important to detect disease reactivation and adjust medications appropriately. In addition, monitoring for involvement of other body systems, including the heart and lungs, is beneficial for long-term management of the disease.

Physical and occupational therapy should begin soon after the diagnosis of polymyositis or dermatomyositis is made. Regular exercise can help to preserve and regain muscle strength and flexibility. In addition, the prevention of the development of contractures is critical.

The prognosis for patients with polymyositis and dermatomyositis is variable, with some patients experiencing only mild weakness that responds well to treatment while others have a rapid progression of symptoms that do not respond to even the most advanced therapies. Patients who are quickly diagnosed and treated tend to have a better outcome. Patients who experience difficulty swallowing, who have involvement of the heart or lungs, or who are found to have an occult malignancy have a poorer prognosis.

14.4G SJÖGREN SYNDROME

OVERVIEW

Sjögren syndrome is a chronic systemic autoimmune disease characterized by lymphocytic infiltration of exocrine glands, especially of the eyes and mouth.[162] Patients with Sjögren syndrome present with mouth and eye dryness, fatigue, and pain.[163] Primary Sjögren syndrome presents in isolation without other rheumatic diseases being present while secondary disease occurs as part of other rheumatologic diseases, especially RA and SLE. Autoantibodies attack glands producing lubrication in the mouth and eyes and patients with Sjögren syndrome have increased levels of cytokines in the tears that they do produce.[164]

Middle-aged women are most commonly affected with this condition, with women outnumbering men at a 9:1 ratio.[165]

SPECIAL CONSIDERATIONS

- There are multiple antibodies seen in Sjögren syndrome including anti-SSA/Ro and anti-SSB/La antibodies, RF, cryoglobulins, and ANA.[162]
- Anti-Ro/SSA and anti-La/SSB are considered hallmarks of the disease and are associated with systemic disease, but are also present in patients with SLE. These antibodies can precede the manifestations of the disease by decades.[166] Antimuscarinic-3 receptor antibodies can be found in up to 80% of patients with Sjögren syndrome.
- Women with Sjögren syndrome are twice as likely to develop hypertension and hypertriglyceridemia elevating their risk for subsequent cardiovascular disease.[167] Due to the high variability of the presentation for Sjögren syndrome, labial salivary gland biopsy can be used to confirm the diagnosis.[168] Biopsy will show lymphocytic infiltration of the glandular acini.[169]
- Patients with Sjögren syndrome who also have low vitamin D levels are more likely to develop lymphoma secondary to chronic lymphocytic activation.[170]

14.5 VASCULITIS SYNDROMES

14.5A POLYMYALGIA RHEUMATICA

OVERVIEW

Polymyalgia rheumatica is a chronic inflammatory rheumatic condition characterized by pain and stiffness in the shoulders, hips, and neck. It occurs in patients >50 years of age. There is a relationship between polymyalgia rheumatica and giant cell arteritis, but the exact nature has yet to be clearly established.

EPIDEMIOLOGY

Polymyalgia rheumatica occurs exclusively in those over the age of 50. The prevalence of the disease progressively increases with advancing age, with the median age at the time of diagnosis is 72 years.[171] Women are two to three times more likely to be affected than men. The disease is more common in those of Northern European descent than those of Asian, African American, or Latino descent.[172]

PATHOPHYSIOLOGY

The etiology of polymyalgia rheumatica is unknown. Increased prevalence in those of Northern European descent and occurrence in siblings suggest that genetics play a role in the pathophysiology. Specific alleles of HLA-DR4 have been associated with both polymyalgia rheumatica and giant cell arteritis. There is also a similar distribution of circulating $CD4^+$ T-cell subsets found in both diseases, and elevated levels of proinflammatory cytokine IL-6 are found in both as well. It is the presence of this proinflammatory cytokine that is believed to be responsible for the constitutional manifestations of both diseases.

Though the word "polymyalgia" implies that there is a myopathic process involved in the disease, the muscle in those affected remains histopathologically normal. Rather, it is the articular and periarticular structures, primarily the tendons and bursae, that are affected. This has been demonstrated repeatedly via various forms of radiographic imaging.[173]

MEDICAL HISTORY AND CLINICAL PRESENTATION

The primary symptoms of polymyalgia rheumatica are pain and stiffness of the shoulders, hips, and neck. Most patients describe an acute onset of symptoms, often beginning in the upper arms and shoulders prior to affecting other areas. Hip pain is typically reported as affecting the lateral aspects of the hips and the groin, with radiation to the posterior thighs. At onset, the symptoms may be unilateral but become symmetric within a few weeks. At presentation patients will often report having difficulty with such things as pulling on a shirt, putting on socks or shoes, reaching overhead, and rising from a sitting position. Stiffness of the affected joints—also known as "gelling"—is a key feature, and typically lasts for >1 hour upon rising in the morning or after having long periods of inactivity. Patients may also complain of pain during the night impacting their sleep. Distal symptoms, which are generally mild, and most commonly affect the wrists and MCP joints, may also be reported. The knees are occasionally affected, but the feet and ankles are not.

Such nonspecific systemic manifestations as fatigue, malaise, anorexia, weight loss, low-grade fever, and depression may also be present. High spiking fever is rare in polymyalgia rheumatica, which should prompt evaluation to rule out giant cell arteritis as well as potential infectious causes. Approximately 15% of patients will develop giant cell arteritis either before, along with, or after polymyalgia rheumatica.[174] History should include questions about symptoms suggestive of giant cell arteritis, to include jaw claudication, scalp tenderness, and visual changes, due to the potential morbidity involved with this disease process.

SIGNS AND SYMPTOMS

Acute or recent onset of shoulder, hip, and neck pain and stiffness are the most common symptoms of polymyalgia rheumatica. Patients will typically identify activities of daily living that have been negatively impacted by their symptoms, such as putting on clothing, reaching overhead, putting on shoes or socks, and rising from a seated position. Reports of muscle weakness or long-standing symptoms should encourage the clinician to search for other causes.

PHYSICAL EXAMINATION

Physical examination in patients with polymyalgia rheumatica will produce characteristic findings. Range of motion of the shoulders, hips, and cervical spine are typically limited. A finding that is considered classic for the disease is the inability to abduct the shoulders past 90 degrees. Muscle strength is not affected, though this can be difficult to gauge due to pain. Approximately 50% of patients have distal findings, including mild synovitis of the wrists and MCP joints.[175] Minor knee effusions may be found, but the ankles and feet are never affected. Neurologic examination will not reveal any focal abnormalities.

DIFFERENTIAL DIAGNOSIS

Other causes of similar manifestations should be considered as part of the differential diagnosis. RA can have a late onset; however, it typically affects the small joints of the hands and feet, and this is not present in polymyalgia rheumatica. Laboratory testing can help to rule out the diagnosis. Other causes of localized joint pain including infectious arthritis, bursitis, tendinitis, and OA should be considered. In addition, other rheumatologic disorders, such as polymyositis, dermatomyositis, crystalline disease, and ankylosing spondylitis should be considered. Fibromyalgia and malignancy should be ruled out.

DIAGNOSTIC STUDIES

In virtually all patients with polymyalgia rheumatica, acute phase reactants are elevated. In >92% of patients, the ESR is >30 mm/hour, while the CRP is elevated in 99% of patients.[176] Serologic testing, to include RF, ANA, and CCP antibodies, are typically negative, and CK is always normal. CBC may reveal a normocytic anemia, but this is a nonspecific finding.

While characteristic findings on imaging are not required to make the diagnosis of polymyalgia rheumatica, they can help to support it. MRI results of the shoulders consistent with this condition includes subacromial or subdeltoid bursitis and biceps tenosynovitis. These findings, when they appear bilaterally, are considered the radiographic hallmark of the disease.

EVALUATION

There is no single test that is specific for the diagnosis of polymyalgia rheumatica. A careful history and thorough physical examination in patients who present with stiffness and pain of the shoulders and hips is warranted. Complaints of sleep disruption, morning stiffness, and systemic symptoms, to include fever and weight loss, should all be explored. In addition, the presence of signs and symptoms of giant cell arteritis, such as headache, scalp tenderness, jaw claudication, and visual changes, must be identified. Characteristic physical examination findings of symmetry of joint involvement, and decreased range of motion of the hips and shoulders, along with normal strength and neurologic findings, supports the diagnosis of polymyalgia rheumatica.

Elevation of the CRP or ESR supports the diagnosis, while a normal finding virtually excludes the disease. For any patient in which the diagnosis is in question, MRI of the shoulders is indicated. Subacromial/subdeltoid bursitis and biceps tenosynovitis that appears bilaterally is strongly supportive of the diagnosis.

TREATMENT

The therapeutic goals for patients with polymyalgia rheumatica are control of pain, improvement of joint stiffness, and resolution of constitutional symptoms. Most patients would add the goal of improvement of ability to perform daily activities, but this is realized as the three stated goals are accomplished. Corticosteroids are the mainstay of treatment as they have been found to lead to near-complete resolution of symptoms and reduction of ESR and CRP back to normal.

Prednisone is the most common corticosteroid used in the treatment of polymyalgia rheumatica. A starting dose of 12.5 to 25 mg of prednisone per day, or other equivalent corticosteroid and dose, is recommended by the American College of Rheumatology.[177] In most patients, relief of symptoms occurs within the first 24 to 72 hours of beginning pharmacotherapy. If symptoms are not well controlled within 1 week of starting treatment, the corticosteroid dose should be increased. Resistance to treatment is an indication that comorbid giant cell arteritis should be investigated. Once symptoms have been effectively treated, a gradual taper of the prednisone is recommended. Decreasing by <1 mg per month has been found to result in fewer relapses. Upon reaching 10 mg/day, the taper should be slowed to 1 mg every 2 months.[178]

PATIENT EDUCATION

The prognosis for patients with polymyalgia rheumatica is excellent since it typically responds well to treatment with corticosteroids. Patients should be advised to begin calcium and vitamin D supplementation to counter the effects of corticosteroid therapy. Activity restriction is generally not indicated. For those patients who are having difficulty in regaining mobility, physical therapy may be helpful.

14.5B GIANT CELL ARTERITIS

OVERVIEW

Giant cell arteritis is a chronic vasculitis affecting large and medium-sized arteries most commonly in the temporal and external carotid arteries and its branches. Patients with giant cell arteritis have an increased risk of developing aortic aneurysms and aortic dissection, which may be fatal.[179]

Giant cell arteritis and polymyalgia rheumatica are closely related disorders affecting people >50 years of age. Because of their frequent appearance together, a search for the other condition should be done when either one of these conditions is identified. Genetic and environmental factors may play a role in the development of these conditions.[180]

Giant cell arteritis can be complicated by visual loss, headache, scalp tenderness, jaw claudication, stroke, aortic arch syndrome, thoracic aortic aneurysm, and aortic dissection.[180]

Glucocorticoids are the cornerstone of treatment for both polymyalgia rheumatica and giant cell arteritis. Glucocorticoids may need to be given for several years. Steroid sparing regimens have not been proved to be highly efficacious.[180]

EPIDEMIOLOGY

Giant cell arteritis is also called temporal arteritis because giant cell arteritis commonly affects the superficial temporal arteries along with the ophthalmic, posterior ciliary, and vertebral arteries. In these affected vessels, arteritis causes intimal hyperplasia leading to stenosis or occlusion resulting in a variety of cranial ischemic manifestations. The aorta and its proximal branches can also be affected by this type of inflammation. Upper extremity vasculitis of giant cell type has been known to affect the subclavian, axillary, and proximal brachial arteries.[179]

Giant cell arteritis is rare before age 50 with a peak age of 70 for those affected with this condition.[179]

PATHOPHYSIOLOGY

There are genetic predispositions for this condition with an environmental trigger, which probably contributes to this condition in patients who are >50 years of age.

There has been some evidence of microorganisms being present in temporal artery biopsies for patients who have giant cell arteritis. *Propionibacterium acnes* and *Escherichia coli* are the most abundant microorganisms found in patients who have positive biopsies.[181] This condition typically has a chronic, relapsing course with relapse most commonly occurring within the 2 years of diagnosis.[182]

SIGNS AND SYMPTOMS

Polymyalgia rheumatica symptoms are related to synovitis of the proximal joints, and giant cell arteritis primarily affects the aorta and its extracranial branches.[180]

Patients may present with jaw claudication, diplopia, and tenderness over the temporal artery. Patients may also have headache located over the temporal artery or on the scalp.

PHYSICAL EXAMINATION

Patients may have tenderness on palpation of an inflamed, slightly indurated, thickened temporal artery. Scalp tenderness may be present. Bruits may be heard over involved arteries. Patients may have achiness and stiffness in the neck, shoulder, hips, and proximal extremities since there is a crossover between polymyalgia and giant cell arteritis.[183]

DIAGNOSTIC STUDIES

Initial tests include ESR or CRP. Elevation of these levels will prompt further investigation, either temporal artery biopsy or temporal artery ultrasound. Positive biopsy results show granulomatous inflammation in a focal and segmental pattern.

In the past, therapy was held until surgical biopsy was performed to reveal giant cell arteritis. Currently, several strategies have been employed in order to identify patients with giant cell arteritis as early as possible without surgical biopsy being carried out. Fast track evaluations include clinical examination, laboratory results, and ultrasound findings. Presence of hypoechoic ring around the vessel wall along with noncompressible halo sign is considered a positive ultrasound finding for the existence of giant cell arteritis.[184]

This fast-track approach allows patients to be evaluated within 24 hours followed by immediate initiation of treatment for patients having positive fast track evaluations. Under this protocol, ultrasound studies have been able to replace surgical biopsy with surgical biopsy being reserved for patients who have negative or inconclusive findings on ultrasound. As a result of fast track evaluation, fewer patients have permanent sight loss compared to patients who followed the traditional pathway that included surgical biopsy, which typically has delayed findings for about 1 week.[184]

If large vessel involvement is suspected, aortic arch angiography can be done to identify this large vessel involvement.[185]

TREATMENT

Corticosteroids are the cornerstone of treatment but these agents have significant adverse effects with long-term use. Prednisone is given up to 80 mg/day with a gradual taper over a 6- to 12-month period. The average duration of treatment is about 3 years after initial diagnosis is made. For patients with vision-threatening onset, intravenous (IV) methylprednisolone can be administered daily for 3 days. Several different medication classes have been used in order to assess whether remission is maintained after the initial 12 weeks of therapy, with prednisone. Abatacept, a T-cell costimulator modulator and DMARD, has been shown to maintain remission and did not have a higher rate of toxicity compared to continued prednisone therapy, so there are ongoing studies for the use of this agent in giant cell arteritis.[186] Toclizomab, an IL-6 antagonist and DMARD, can be utilized as steroid sparer in patients who cannot take glucocorticoids or who fail to respond. Methotrexate can be considered for those who do not respond to glucocorticoids.

Patients who have a relapsing course need additional glucocorticoid administration, which increases the patient's risk for osteoporosis.[182] It is recommended that patients be given treatment to prevent osteoporosis with the long-term use of corticosteroids.

Aspirin can be considered to prevent ischemic complications of giant cell arteritis. Aspirin may also lower the risk of vision loss and cardiovascular accidents.[187]

PATIENT EDUCATION

While it is well known that giant cell arteritis affects large vessels, there are also increased risks for myocardial infarction, stroke, and peripheral vascular disease.[188] The most common serious complication of giant cell arteritis is permanent blindness. If vision loss has occurred prior to treatment, it is typically irreversible. Vision loss anterior optic ischemic neuropathy occurs more frequently in patients older than 75 and who also have jaw claudication.[189]

14.5C POLYARTERITIS NODOSUM

OVERVIEW

Polyarteritis nodosum (PAN) is a vasculitis of small and medium size arteries in the dermis and subcutaneous tissue without systemic involvement. There is a cutaneous PAN that involves painful, recurrent ulcerations and polyneuritis. Multiorgan system disease can also occur with PAN.[190]

EPIDEMIOLOGY

Hepatitis B infection is the underlying cause of PAN in about one third of the patients. PAN has become less common due to the decrease in incidence of hepatitis B virus as a result of immunization programs and improved screening for this condition with subsequent treatment. If PAN is not related to infection, the etiology is typically unknown. There is a suggested immune underlying cause as immunosuppressive therapy is an effective treatment.

PAN most commonly occurs between the ages of 40 and 60.

PATHOPHYSIOLOGY

Small to medium-sized vessels are involved with PAN. Pathology reveals focal and segmental transmural necrotizing inflammation with fibrinoid necrosis within the vessels.

MEDICAL HISTORY AND CLINICAL PRESENTATION

Clinical manifestations of PAN include fever, skin involvement, kidney involvement but without glomerulonephritis, neurologic involvement, GI involvement, cardiac involvement, and pulmonary involvement.[191] Patients may have unintentional weight loss, myalgias and arthralgias, paresthesias, muscle tenderness, and abdominal pain. Skin manifestations may include livedo reticularis, skin ulcers, vesicular eruptions, and purpura. These skin findings are not specific to PAN. Coronary artery involvement may lead to chest pain or heart failure as a result of impaired coronary artery function.[191]

Neurologic involvement consists of both peripheral neuropathy and mononeuritis multiplex. Neurologic involvement can be demonstrated by wrist and foot drop. Kidney involvement occurs as a result of renal artery microaneurysms with tissue infarcts or hematomas. Kidney manifestations include hypertension, hematuria, and proteinuria but not glomerulonephritis. GI involvement is in the form of mesenteric ischemia, which could lead to intestinal perforation, pancreatitis, cholecystitis, appendicitis, and GI bleeding. Patients with GI involvement can present with acute abdomen. Testicular involvement results in the orchitis that is usually unilateral.[192]

SIGNS AND SYMPTOMS

PAN has a wide range of clinical presentations. The spectrum of this condition ranges from involving a single organ to multiple organ failure. The main organ that is spared is the lungs.[192] Symptoms are typically not specific for PAN but rather include symptoms similar to any of the vasculitis or other rheumatologic diseases. High index of suspicion should put PAN as part of a differential diagnosis in any patient suspected of having vasculitis.

PHYSICAL EXAMINATION

No specific physical examination findings identify PAN. Neurologic involvement with mononeuritis multiplex can be demonstrated by the patient having wrist or foot drop. Testicular involvement with tenderness secondary to orchitis can also be a symptom that may be encountered.

DIFFERENTIAL DIAGNOSIS

The differential diagnosis for PAN is summarized in Table 14.10.

DIAGNOSTIC STUDIES

Patients suspected of having PAN should be evaluated in an expedited manner because delay in treatment may increase morbidity and mortality. There are no specific diagnostic tests used to diagnose PAN but there are test results that are consistent with this condition.

Because PAN is a systemic vasculitis, there will be elevation in CRP or ESR. Fibrinogen, an acute phase reactant, will be elevated with active disease. Renal involvement will cause an elevated serum creatinine level but urinalysis will show a bland urine without cellular elements. Glomerular disease is not typically a feature of PAN so there should not be red blood cell casts or significant proteinuria. Abnormal liver function studies can suggest hepatitis but this is less frequent today with immunization and screening. The CBC can show anemia from either chronic inflammation or ongoing GI blood loss.

TABLE 14.10 Differential Diagnosis of Polyarteritis Nodosum

Condition	Description
Granulomatosis with polyangiitis	Associated with antineutrophil cytoplasmic antibody (ANCA) associated small vessel vasculitis versus PAN, which affects medium-sized and small vessels. This condition will have glomerulonephritis if the kidney is involved, something that PAN does not have.
Churg-Strauss syndrome	Patients typically will have a history of asthma, allergic rhinitis, or sinusitis, which is not typically seen with PAN. Both conditions share mononeuritis multiplex with foot drop and wrist drop as manifestations. This condition will have glomerulonephritis, something that PAN does not have.
Giant cell arteritis	Affects large and medium-sized vessels, especially the temporal artery. This condition lacks skin involvement and involvement of the kidneys, something that PAN does involve.
Rheumatoid arthritis	Joint involvement of small, symmetric joints in hands and feet. Vasculitis can occur with both conditions.
Systemic lupus erythematosus	Antinuclear antibody is present in nearly all cases. Physical exam signs consistent of a malar rash, alopecia, and renal involvement.
Thromboangiitis obliterans (Buerger disease)	Male dominant disease primarily seen in smokers. Symptoms include claudication, Raynaud phenomenon, and gangrene of the extremities. Small and medium-sized vessels of the hand and feet are primarily involved. No involvement in the GI tract or kidneys.

GI, gastrointestinal; PAN, polyarteritis nodosum.

As part of the evaluation, patient should be evaluated for hepatitis B and hepatitis C. Since this is a type of vasculitis, antinuclear cytoplasmic antigen or antineutrophil cytoplasmic antibodies (ANCA) should be used to assess for other types of vasculitis. RF and antibodies to cyclic CCP can be drawn if the patient has features consistent with RA. ANA can be used to screen for lupus. HIV testing is recommended since this infection is associated with PAN.

CT or MR angiography is performed if patients are suspected of having PAN.[193] Findings consistent with this disorder are small, multiple aneurysms, vessel ectasia, and occlusive lesions in medium-sized vessels, especially the renal and mesenteric arteries. Doppler studies can identify renal and hepatic aneurysms that occur in the setting of PAN.

Surgical biopsy can be performed if the disease is still in question. Biopsy results consistent with PAN are focal and segmental transmural necrotizing inflammation.

EVALUATION

Diagnosis of PAN requires utilization of clinical, angiographic, and biopsy findings.[192]

TREATMENT

Treatment of PAN involves a combination of glucocorticoids and cyclophosphamide. There may also be a role for plasmapheresis. If PAN is the result of hepatitis B infection, the primary treatment approach will be for eradication of this pathogen. PAN limited to the skin can be treated with NSAIDs over a short period of time.[192]

PATIENT EDUCATION

Patients with PAN should continue their medications as instructed. Since triggers for relapse have not yet been identified, education for preventing relapse is in the form of general lifestyle modification recommendations. Patient should avoid smoking to prevent further endothelial vessel damage. Patient should avoid high-risk encounter for infection as the use of corticosteroids and immunomodulating agents place the patient at risk for infection.

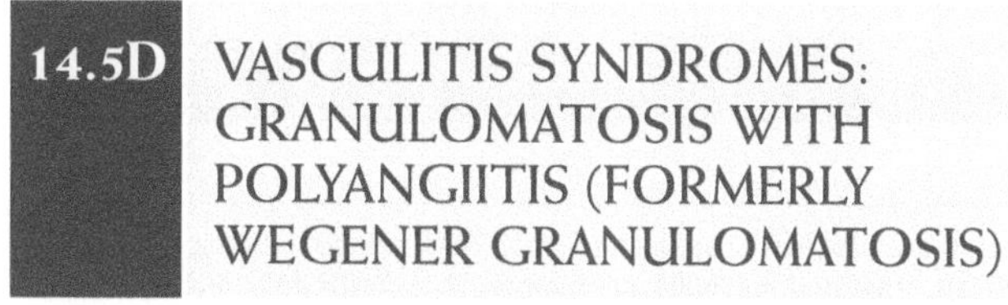

14.5D VASCULITIS SYNDROMES: GRANULOMATOSIS WITH POLYANGIITIS (FORMERLY WEGENER GRANULOMATOSIS)

OVERVIEW

Graulomatosis with polyangiitis (GPA), formerly known as Wegener granulomatosis, is a rare autoimmune disease primarily affecting the small vessels (rarely affects medium-sized vessels) affecting the upper respiratory tract, lungs, and kidneys.[194] The majority of patients (63%) present with isolated ear, nose, and throat abnormalities, which typically causes a delay in making this diagnosis since these kinds of complaints are commonly encountered in clinical practice.[195] When this condition occurs, it typically has a relapsing, chronic course.

GPA typically involves the upper and lower respiratory tract and can cause glomerulonephritis. Organ involvement can include the skin, eyes, muscles, and nerves. Ear, nose, and throat involvement is most common.

EPIDEMIOLOGY

GPA can occur at any age with the vast majority of patients being between 40 and 60 years of age. Disease is most commonly seen in the Caucasian population with higher incidence seen in Sweden and countries north of the equator.[196]

PATHOPHYSIOLOGY

ANCA play a major role in the development of GPA. In addition to ANCA, the cellular immune system contributes to the pathogenesis of the disease. ANCA-mediated degranulation of neutrophils causes vasculitic damage, T cells produce granulomas, and overall vasculitis damage is promoted through several different pathways. All these processes further enhance autoantibody production by the B cells. Complement plays a role in this overall process.[197]

MEDICAL HISTORY AND CLINICAL PRESENTATION

The most common presentation for GPA involves the upper respiratory tract. Patients may have recurrent sinusitis, nasal crusting, cough, and recurrent upper respiratory tract infections. Because these symptoms overlap with many other common conditions, there typically is a delay in diagnosis.

SIGNS AND SYMPTOMS

The signs and symptoms of PGA include fatigue, unexplained weight loss, recurrent fever, dyspnea, numbness in extremities, bruising, persistent cough, painful joints and muscles, coryza, recurrent sinusitis, trace amounts of blood in nasal mucus, sputum, or urine, and recurrent ear infections.[198]

PHYSICAL EXAMINATION

Heart involvement can cause pericarditis, myocarditis, or conduction disorders. Ear, nose, and throat involvement reveals crusting, rhinorrhea, sinusitis, otitis media, chondritis of ears and nose with saddle nose deformity, and nasal septal perforation. GI involvement reveals ulceration when it occurs. Kidney involvement reveals glomerulonephritis with red blood cell casts and protein in the urine. Lung involvement shows alveolar hemorrhages, nodules, and tracheal or subglottic stenosis. Ocular involvement involves scleritis, episcleritis, and retinal involvement. Skin involvement can be demonstrated by palpable purpura, nodules, pyoderma gangrenosum, and mucosal ulcerations. Neurologic involvement can demonstrate mononeuritis multiplex and peripheral neuropathy with wrist and foot drop

DIFFERENTIAL DIAGNOSIS

As a rare autoimmune disease, GPA should be differentiated from the other causes of autoimmune disease, especially those that are associated with vasculitis. c-ANCA is most helpful in differentiating GPA from PAN, which typically will have a positive p-ANCA. Additionally, GPA will involve the kidneys causing glomerulonephritis while PAN can have kidney involvement but not a glomerulonephritis type of involvement.

DIAGNOSTIC STUDIES

GPA has a positive cytoplasmic/ANCA (antiproteinase-3 antibodies) in almost all affected patients. The histology on biopsy shows pauci-immune necrotizing granulomatous vasculitis.[199]

GPA is a systemic disease associated with the autoantibody c-ANCA (cytoplasmic, directed against the neutrophil proteinase). This is a pattern of immunofluorescent staining. Enzyme-linked immunosorbent assays are used to confirm antibody positivity.[200]

ANCA may play a direct role in vessel damage by hyperactivating already primed neutrophils leading to vessel endothelial inflammation and damage. The presence of granulomatous inflammation in some forms of ANCA-associated vasculitis suggests a role for cell-mediated immunity.

The pattern of ANCA can predict long-term outcomes. Cytoplasmic antibody associated vasculitis or c-ANCA is associated with this granulomatous polyangiitis.[200] A biopsy remains the gold standard for making this diagnosis.[201]

The diagnosis of GPA ultimately relies on the constellation of radiographic findings, laboratory findings, and patient clinical history and physical examination.[202]

EVALUATION

For patients suspected of having GPA, the first test to order is the ANCA. This test is helpful in being consistent with the diagnosis but it is not helpful in monitoring response to treatment. Biopsy will provide definitive diagnosis.

TREATMENT

Recommendations for treating GPA includes starting immunosuppressive therapy in combination with glucocorticoids in order to induce remission. Maintenance medications are then issued to retain remission after it is obtained. Patients with life-threatening or organ-threatening conditions are treated with plasma exchange especially in the setting of rapidly progressive renal failure or severe diffuse pulmonary hemorrhage.[203]

Cyclophosphamide and rituximab are the mainstay of remission induction, but some patients can also be treated with methotrexate and mycophenolate. Rituximab works by depleting the B cells, which interferes with the inflammatory response. Remission can be maintained with either azathioprine or rituximab. Remission maintenance therapy should be continued for minimum of 2 years after which time tapering could be considered.[201]

PATIENT EDUCATION

As a result of the improvements in both the direction and treatment of GPA, mortality risk has dramatically improved. Patients should be counseled about the importance of continuing treatment in order to attain and maintain clinical remission in this chronic and relapsing condition. When death occurs as a result of GPA, it is typically due to renal failure, infection, and vasculitis.[204]

14.5E CRYOGLOBULINEMIA

OVERVIEW

Cryoglobulinemia refers to the presence in the serum immunoglobulins that precipitate only in cold temperatures. Type I cryoglobulins are single monoclonal immunoglobulins that occur in various hematologic disorders. Type II and III are mixed cryoglobulins composed of monoclonal or polyclonal IgM, respectively. These particular immunoglobulins have RF activities that bind to polyclonal immunoglobulins. Mixed cryoglobulinemia (MC) syndrome is a consequence of immune complex mediated vasculitis and is characterized by purpura, weakness, and arthralgias. Multiple organs may be involved, especially the kidney and the peripheral nervous system.[205]

Hepatitis C is by far the most common precipitant of cryoglobulinemia. The most common autoimmune conditions associated with cryoglobulinemia are Sjögren syndrome, SLE, systemic sclerosis, undifferentiated connective tissue disease, and vasculitis.[206]

EPIDEMIOLOGY

Cryoglobulinemia can cause vasculitis that primarily involves the skin, joints, peripheral nervous system, and the kidneys. MC is involved in type II and III cryoglobulinemia and is primarily caused by hepatitis C viral infection with MC accounting for almost 90% of all of the subtypes with hepatitis C being responsible as a precipitant in 90% of these cases.[207]

PATHOPHYSIOLOGY

The pathophysiology of MC consists of deposition of immune complexes on the walls of small vessels followed by the subsequent activation of the complement cascade.[208]

MEDICAL HISTORY AND CLINICAL PRESENTATION

MC can be asymptomatic or lead to the clinical manifestations of purpura, arthralgia, and weakness. Some patients with this condition develop a more serious vasculitis with both neurologic and renal involvement.[208] Clinical presentation of MC is varied but typically will include arthralgia, purpura, skin ulcers, glomerulonephritis, and peripheral neuropathy.[209]

SIGNS AND SYMPTOMS

Patients may complain of arthralgias, weakness, and skin changes. Weakness is actually considered to be one of the hallmark symptoms of MC. Skin symptoms include complaints consistent with Raynaud phenomenon, ulcers, skin necrosis, and livedo reticularis in addition to the palpable purpura, which occurs mostly in the lower extremities.[210] Although the skin findings are the dominant findings, other findings will include peripheral neuropathy, arthritis, and glomerulonephritis.

PHYSICAL EXAMINATION

Physical examination of a patient with MC can reveal palpable purpura on the skin. The patient may have increased discomfort with range of motion of the affected joints. Some affected patients may have skin ulcerations. When purpura are felt, they are most likely to be in the lower extremities. Skin discoloration may also occur.[210]

DIFFERENTIAL DIAGNOSIS

Cryoglobulinemia is a small vessel vasculitis so it should be differentiated from all of the other small and medium-sized vessel vasculitic conditions. It is important to identify vasculitis early on as this condition can be life-threatening, especially if multiorgan failure is present.

DIAGNOSTIC STUDIES

Cryoglobulinemia consists of cryoglobulins, which are immunoglobulins that precipitate out in temperatures lower than 37 °C.[211] Other studies that should be considered as part of the evaluation are the ESR and CRP, which can be elevated in the setting of vasculitis. Urinalysis can demonstrate active urinary sediment, hematuria, or proteinuria when the kidney is involved with this condition.[210] RF may be positive since the IgM immunoglobulin has RF activity. Patient should also be checked for hepatitis C and hepatitis B as both of these conditions can precipitate cryoglobulinemia.[210]

Because of complement activation, a low C4 complement may be found, if tested.[207]

When the skin is involved, skin biopsy can be performed and will show leukocytoclastic vasculitis in the setting of MC.

EVALUATION

Because of vasculitis symptoms may not occur for several years after hepatitis C infection, any patient who tests positive for hepatitis C should have a consideration for MC. Since universal hepatitis C testing is now recommended for all adults above age 18, there may be an ability to recognize MC even prior to the onset of vasculitis.

Since cryoglobulins only precipitate at temperatures <37 °C, it is imperative that the blood sample be handled under appropriate conditions in order to prevent false negative test results.

TREATMENT

Treatments for MC are directed at the underlying cause such as treating hepatitis C infection or controlling the underlying systemic autoimmune disease. Patients who do not have a clear etiology for their cryoglobulinemia, also known as idiopathic cryoglobulinemia, are treated with corticosteroids and immunosuppression. There is also a role for B-cell depleting anti-CD20 biologic agents such as rituximab.[212] Asymptomatic patients are monitored for progression of their disease but are not actively treated.

Mild cryoglobulinemia patients are treated with 10 to 20 mg of prednisone on a daily basis. Rituximab, a monoclonal antibody against CD20, is given by specialists when patients have severe disease or in those who do not respond to corticosteroid treatment.[212]

PATIENT EDUCATION

Patients who are diagnosed with MC need to have close monitoring for the development of organ involvement and vasculitis. Special attention is focused on the skin as this typically is the most common physical manifestation. Patients should keep their body warm, especially the extremities, since this condition is sensitive to a cold environment.

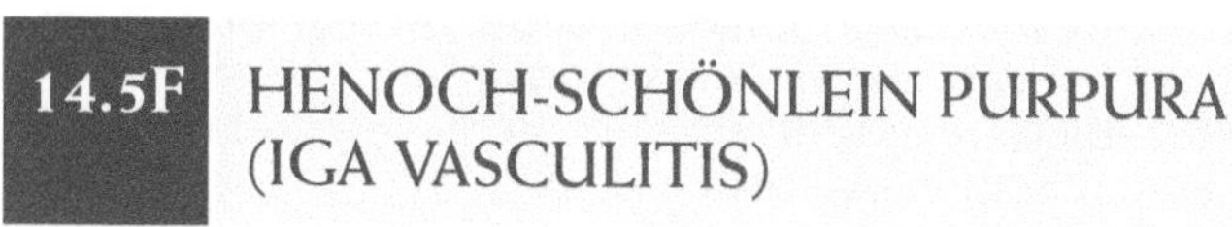

14.5F HENOCH-SCHÖNLEIN PURPURA (IGA VASCULITIS)

OVERVIEW

Henoch-Schönlein purpura (HSP) is a vasculitis caused by IgA. This condition is seen overwhelmingly in children in whom it has a benign course. When HSP occurs in the adult population, the course of the disease can be associated with morbidity.[213] Approximately one-half of the patients with HSP have renal involvement, which is chronic but does not tend to progress to end-stage kidney failure.[213]

HSP is thought to be a specific immune-mediated entity induced by environmental factors, especially infection.[214]

EPIDEMIOLOGY

HSP is the most common type of systemic vasculitis in childhood.[215] Glomerulonephritis occurs in up to half of these patients, in whom it tends to be mild although there are a few patients who progress to chronic kidney disease and nephrotic syndrome.[216] The exact etiology for this condition remains unknown. There is a true seasonal variation with fall and winter seasons predominating.[214]

PATHOPHYSIOLOGY

HSP nephritis is caused by the glomerular deposition of immunoglobulin A (IgA) containing immune complexes in the mesangium, the subepithelial, and the subendothelial spaces.[216] Mesangial proliferation and renal damage are triggered by these immune complexes, which are deposited in the kidneys. This process involves the activation of the complement system.[216]

MEDICAL HISTORY AND CLINICAL PRESENTATION

HSP vasculitis can affect the joints, GI tract, lungs, scrotum, and rarely the CNS.[213]

SIGNS AND SYMPTOMS

Children with HSP present with abdominal pain, arthritis, renal impairment, and nonthrombocytopenic purpura.[213] Clinical features of HSP includes the presence of purpura or petechiae especially in the lower limb, abdominal pain, arthritis or arthralgia, and renal involvement.[217]

PHYSICAL EXAMINATION

The presence of purpura is an essential feature in making the diagnosis of HSP. This purpura is distributed symmetrically over the extensor surfaces of the lower limbs, buttocks, and forearm with occasional involvement of the trunk and face.[218]

DIFFERENTIAL DIAGNOSIS

Differential diagnosis for HSP includes drug reactions, idiopathic or immune thrombocytopenia purpura, Rocky Mountain spotted fever, disseminated gonococcal disease, and urticarial vasculitis.[213] Other considerations include cryoglobulinemia, HIV infection, and rheumatic diseases such as lupus that can present with cutaneous vasculitis. Because patients can present with acute abdominal pain, other conditions that cause abdominal pain should be included in this differential.[214]

DIAGNOSTIC STUDIES

There are no disease-specific laboratory abnormalities specific for HSP. If and when biopsy is performed, histopathologic changes are fairly specific for this condition but these changes can also occur with IgA vasculitis.[214]

Biopsy of the vessel shows deposition of IgA and C3 in small vessel walls along with polymorphonuclear neutrophilic infiltration around and in the vessel walls. Other lab findings reveal increased serum levels of IgA along with protein inflammatory cytokines during the acute stage.[219]

EVALUATION

The platelet count is either normal or increased in the setting of HSP. During acute inflammation, a mild leukocytosis with a shift to the left can be noted. Inflammatory cytokines are elevated in the acute state but this is nonspecific IgA may also be elevated.[219]

TREATMENT

Corticosteroid therapy reduces the duration and severity of abdominal and joint pain but this does not prevent the development of nephritis or alter the natural history of HSP. There is still no clear best treatment identified for severe nephritis.[220]

Treatment is conservative because the disease course is typically benign and self-limited.[219]

PATIENT EDUCATION

While children with HSP tend to have a more benign course, relapse is more common in patients who have the diagnosis of HSP made while they are complaining of GI complaints and joint pain.[221] Treatment should be based upon the degree of inflammation and those with mild disease may only need to be monitored and have their renal function serially followed.

14.5G BEHÇET SYNDROME

OVERVIEW

Behçet syndrome is a multisystem, immunologically mediated autoimmune disease causing inflammatory infiltration of multiple organs. Small vessel vasculitis also occurs in this condition. The principal clinical features are oral and genital aphthous ulcers, uveitis, and retinal vasculitis along with skin lesions, which include erythema nodosum and acneiform pustules or folliculitis. Other features of Behçet syndrome include inflammatory arthritis, arterial and venous occlusion and arterial aneurysms, and GI and neurologic lesions.[222]

EPIDEMIOLOGY

Behçet syndrome is most commonly seen in Asia and less commonly seen in North America. The disease is more prevalent in men, who also have a more severe disease course. HLA-B51 is associated with this disease.[223] This condition is seen most frequently in the second and third decades, being rare prior to puberty or after age 50.[224]

PATHOPHYSIOLOGY

Pathophysiologic mechanisms for Behçet syndrome are incompletely understood. There is an interaction between patients with specific genetic tendencies along with an environmental or infectious factor that contributes to the immune dysregulation that characterizes this disease.[225]

MEDICAL HISTORY AND CLINICAL PRESENTATION

Patients typically present with oral ulcers that are most commonly located on the inside of the mouth. These ulcers do not usually occur on the outer surface of the lips, which distinguishes these painful ulcers from the ulcer seen with herpes simplex. Painful genital ulcers can also occur and can heal with deformity. Skin complaints are with lesions similar to acne along with folliculitis. Erythema nodosum is associated with this condition. Eye involvement can lead to the development of a hypopyon, which is seen as a white layering of inflammatory cells in the anterior chamber of the eye and is a marker for severe inflammation.

SIGNS AND SYMPTOMS

Recurrent oral ulcerations are present in 98% of patients diagnosed with Behçet syndrome. Recurrent genital ulcerations are seen in 80% of affected patients. Of the skin lesions, folliculitis occurs in 71% of patients and erythema nodosum in 47% of the patients. Arthritis or arthralgia is seen in about half of these patients.[226]

Oral ulcerations are painful and may be accompanied by a tender, submucosal nodule. Large ulcers can lead to mucosal scarring. Mouth ulceration may be the earliest manifestation of Behçet syndrome and may be the presenting feature in clinical practice.[227]

Eye manifestations can include iritis with hypopyon and retinal vasculitis.[228] Joint involvement typically includes the knees as the most commonly affected joint followed by ankles, wrists, elbows, small joints of the hands and wrists, shoulders, feet, and hips.[229]

Vasculitis in Behçet syndrome can be in the form of superficial thrombophlebitis, deep vein thrombosis, arterial occlusion or aneurysm formation, and vena cava occlusion.[230]

Pulmonary involvement includes pleural effusion, hilar enlargement, cavitating lesions, apical fibrosis, and calcified lesions along with emphysema.[231]

Neurologic manifestations include spinal cord lesions, focal brain lesions, headaches, and thrombosis, all of which are caused by underlying vasculitis.[232]

Ulcerative lesions of the GI system can affect the entire length of the GI tract.[233]

PHYSICAL EXAMINATION

Physical exam characteristic features of Behçet syndrome include recurrent painful oral and genital mucosal ulcerations along with inflammatory eye disease. Patients may have other clinical manifestations including venous thrombosis affecting the large veins. CNS involvement can be demonstrated by patients complaining of headache and diplopia. GI involvement includes symptoms consistent with inflammatory bowel disease.[222]

DIFFERENTIAL DIAGNOSIS

Behçet oral ulcers are located on the inner mucosal surface versus the external lips, as seen with herpes simplex stomatitis. While aphthous ulcers can be painful, these patients do not have any other symptoms nor do they have genital ulcers. Abdominal pain can occur with the ulcer formation so Crohn disease is a consideration but patients with Crohn disease do not have genital ulcer involvement. Skin lesions with Behçet syndrome are identical to acne vulgaris but patients with acne will not have the other manifestations typically seen with Behçet syndrome. Erythema nodosum can be seen with Crohn disease, infection, and sarcoidosis. Joint involvement can mimic RA but ulcer formation typically does not occur.

DIAGNOSTIC STUDIES

Pathergy test is important in making the diagnosis of Behçet syndrome. In this test a sterile needle pricks the skin and a positive result is the appearance of pustules forming within 48 hours of the sterile needle prick. Positive tests are consistent with vasculitis in the dermis. Positive tests can be a clue predicting disease severity and course of the disease.[234]

Since there is a genetic link with this condition, patients may have a positive HLA-B51 genetic marker. In order to rule out other conditions, laboratory testing in Behçet syndrome should be negative for RF, ANA, and ANCA. If hemoptysis is part of the patient presentation, high-resolution CT scan can be performed to evaluate for a pulmonary aneurysm.

EVALUATION

Evaluation should be undertaken when patients have recurrent oral ulcers along with the presence of genital ulcers or skin or eye lesions. Pathergy test can be helpful when positive. Laboratory tests other than HLA-B51 are not very helpful. Patient presentation should guide further evaluation; those suspected of having Behçet syndrome need aggressive evaluation and treatment for signs of organ involvement.

TREATMENT

Oral and genital ulcers may be treated with topical glucocorticoids. Colchicine is the drug of choice for preventing recurrent mucocutaneous lesions and acute arthritis.[235] Recurrent disease may be treated with immunosuppressants such as azathioprine, interferon alfa, or tumor necrosis alpha inhibitors. Glucocorticoids are also used in the setting of acute exacerbations.

Goal of treatment for Behçet syndrome is to promptly suppress inflammatory exacerbations and recurrences in order to prevent irreversible organ damage. Optimal care is provided by multiple disciplinary team approach. Treatment needs to be individualized and based upon age, gender, type and severity of organ involvement, and patient preferences.[236] Skin, mucosa, and joint involvement cause the most impairment in the quality of life but permanent damage does not typically occur when these structures are affected. On the other hand, untreated eye, vascular, nervous system, and GI system involvement cause significant morbidity and even death.[236] Treatment should be based upon how Behçet syndrome affects the patient's quality of life compared to the risks associated with medical treatment.[236] Organ involvement needs to have rapid suppression of the inflammation with the hope of preventing relapses and the loss of function. Organ involvement will typically need immunosuppressant treatment. When this condition wanes, therapy can be tapered and even ultimately stopped.[224]

Ocular involvement is one of the most disabling complications of this condition leading to a loss of vision and progressing to blindness if untreated. Treatment involves rapid suppression of inflammation during the attacks and prevention of recurrent attacks. Treatment includes immunosuppressives, corticosteroids, and biologic agents. Surgery may be required if the patient does not respond to treatment.[237]

PATIENT EDUCATION

Patients should be told that many patients with Behçet syndrome will go into remission and the disease will improve with time. Patients need to continue immunosuppressants when the disease is active in order to control the disease and to enable remission to occur. Patients failing to respond to immunosuppression can have surgery as a last resort. Ongoing monitoring will be needed to follow progression of disease and to look for side effects associated with the use of these medications. Patients should have annual ophthalmologic exams performed.

14.6 SPONDYLOARTHROPATHIES

OVERVIEW

Spondyloarthropathies are a group of disorders that share certain clinical manifestations and genetic similarities. Ankylosing spondylitis, psoriatic arthritis, and reactive arthritis are among the most common spondyloarthropathies. These diseases occur more frequently in males than females, and usually appear prior to age 40. Common symptoms include inflammatory arthritis of the sacroiliac joints and spine, asymmetric oligoarthritis, especially of the large joints of the lower extremities, dactylitis, and uveitis. Enthesopathy, inflammation at the point where ligaments, tendons, and joint capsules insert into bone, is a hallmark finding for the spondyloarthropathies. RF is typically negative in these diseases, causing them to be known as "seronegative spondyloarthropathies." The HLA-B27 gene is believed to be the single largest genetic contributor to these diseases; however, the presence of HLA-B27 is not an absolute requirement for any of the spondyloarthropathies. HLA-B27 is a major histocompatibility complex (MHC) class I molecule involved in the presentation of T-cell antigen.

14.6A ANKYLOSING SPONDYLITIS

EPIDEMIOLOGY

Ankylosing spondylitis is the most common spondyloarthropathy, occurring in 0.1% to 1% of the general population.[238] It is more common in Whites and has a higher prevalence in those from northern Europe than in equatorial regions. The age of symptom onset in ankylosing spondylitis is typically prior to age 16, though diagnosis may be delayed by years if the symptoms are mild or the patient is asymptomatic.[239] Males are affected more than females, at a ratio of 3:1.

PATHOPHYSIOLOGY

The etiology of the ankylosing spondylitis is unknown, but a combination of environmental and genetic factors works together to produce clinical disease.[240] The primary pathology is enthesitis with chronic inflammation, which includes both $CD4^+$ and $CD8^+$ T lymphocytes and macrophages. In addition, cytokines, such as tumor necrosis factor-α (TNF-α) and transforming growth factor-β (TGF-β), contribute to the inflammatory process, leading to fibrosis and eventual ossification at the sites of enthesitis.[241] Two seemingly paradoxic processes occur as inflammation destroys bone through an osteoclastic process, while new bone formation via an osteoblastic process leads to syndesmophytes. In some patients this new bone formation converts the entire vertebral column into a rigid spine that appear similar to bamboo in radiologic imaging.

MEDICAL HISTORY AND CLINICAL PRESENTATION

Patients with axial spondyloarthritis present with chronic back pain usually prior to the age of 45 that can be associated with synovitis, enthesitis, and dactylitis. Other features include uveitis, psoriasis, inflammatory bowel disease, and an HLA-B27 positive status. The subtypes of axial spondyloarthritis include both ankylosing spondylitis and nonradiographic axial spondyloarthritis with the difference being patients having ankylosing spondylitis having x-ray abnormalities consistent with sacroiliitis, which is lacking in the other subtype.

Chronic pain and stiffness are the most common presenting symptoms in patients with ankylosing spondylitis. Inflammatory back pain is the first manifestation and the most common symptom in 75% of patients.[242] The pain is poorly localized to the sacroiliac and gluteal areas and is described as dull. The back pain typically has an insidious onset and has been present intermittently over months or years. Patients commonly describe morning stiffness, which lasts for at least 30 minutes, and improves with moderate physical activity. Radiation of pain into both buttocks is also frequently described. Stiffness and pain that awakens the patient in the early morning are fairly common in ankylosing spondylitis and should help to differentiate it from other musculoskeletal disorders.

Joint involvement tends to occur in the first 10 years of the disease, and affects the hips and shoulders, as well as the acromioclavicular and sternoclavicular joints. Joint damage of the hips and shoulders may be evidenced in radiographic imaging. Decreased range of motion of the chest wall due to costovertebral and costotransverse joint involvement can lead to complaints of chest tightness or difficulty breathing. Over half of all patients with ankylosing spondylitis complain of fatigue that is moderately severe.

SIGNS AND SYMPTOMS

Low back pain and stiffness are typically the earliest and most pronounced clinical manifestations of ankylosing spondylitis. Involvement of the sacroiliac joints is also present, with stiffness and pain in the buttocks being the primary symptom. Hip involvement is common and may present as groin or knee pain. The shoulders may also be affected, as well as the joints of the chest wall. In addition, patients may experience arthritis in the peripheral joints other than the hips and shoulders. Enthesitis may also be noted.

Extra-articular manifestations are common in ankylosing spondylitis, and can affect the eyes, heart, lungs, kidneys, nervous system, and GI tract. The most common extra-articular manifestation is uveitis, which affects 20% to 30% of patients with ankylosing spondylitis.[243] The presentation is typically acute with unilateral pain, photophobia, blurred vision, and increased lacrimation, which resolve after 2 to 3 months of treatment. Patients with long-standing disease may develop shortness of breath as a result of limited chest expansion. Atlantoaxial subluxation, fractures of fused spine, and cauda equina syndrome may lead to neurologic complications in patients with severe long-standing disease.

PHYSICAL EXAMINATION

In patients with ankylosing spondylitis, spinal mobility may be limited due to structural abnormalities of the vertebrae. Chest expansion may also be limited in more severe or long-standing cases. In addition, abnormal posture may be noted on physical exam, with hyperkyphosis resulting from wedging of the thoracic vertebrae.[244] Both active and passive range of motion of the axial and peripheral joints may be decreased and tenderness with palpation of the sacroiliac joints is common. Enthesitis may be identified by swelling and tenderness at the areas of tendon and ligament insertion, such as the insertion of the Achilles tendon or the plantar fascia on the calcaneus.

Unilateral anterior uveitis may be noted on physical examination, with decreased visual acuity, conjunctival injection, photophobia, and increased lacrimation all being present. Though not as common, aortitis of the ascending aorta may develop, leading to distortion of the aortic ring and eventually aortic valve insufficiency. Restrictive lung disease may be found in patients with long-standing disease due to limited chest expansion. Patients should undergo a thorough neurologic exam to assess for signs of cervical myelopathy, spinal fractures, and cauda equina syndrome.

DIFFERENTIAL DIAGNOSIS

Any disorder or disease process that can cause back pain should be considered in the differential diagnosis of ankylosing spondylitis. In addition, other potential diagnoses should be added based on the patient's presenting symptoms. Degenerative disc disease, herniated nucleus pulposus, congenital spinal deformity, spinal fractures and dislocations, OA, spinal stenosis, spondylosis, spondylolisthesis, and spondylolysis should all be considered. Additionally, psoriatic arthritis and reactive arthritis have similar presentations, and so should be prominent on the differential diagnosis list.

DIAGNOSTIC STUDIES

Imaging and laboratory studies are both helpful in supporting the diagnosis of ankylosing spondylitis. While there are no laboratory studies specific for the disease, there are a number of findings that are commonly discovered. Over half of patients with ankylosing spondylitis have an elevation in their acute phase reactants, specifically CRP and ESR.[245] In severe disease, mild elevation of serum alkaline phosphatase levels may be seen and are associated with greater structural damage in the spine, and sacroiliac joints.[246] HLA-B27 is present in the majority of patients with ankylosing spondylitis, though it is not an absolute requirement for the diagnosis. Synovial fluid findings are consistent with inflammatory arthritis, with a WBC count that is elevated and contains an overabundance of polymorphonuclear leukocytes.

Various imaging modalities may be used to evaluate the spine and sacroiliac joints, to include conventional radiographs, CT, and MRI. Radiographic findings consistent with ankylosing spondylitis can range from subtle joint space narrowing of the sacroiliac joints, to sclerosis, erosive changes, and even fusion (ankylosis).[247] Imaging of the spine may show squared off vertebral bodies early in the disease process. Later disease findings include ankylosis of the facet joints, and syndesmophytes, and eventually bamboo spine as seen in Figure 14.13.

EVALUATION

A thorough history and physical exam can help to narrow down potential causes of back pain. When the sacroiliac joints are involved, and morning stiffness is a major factor, ankylosing spondylitis should be further investigated. Imaging studies are more likely to reveal spinal and sacroiliac findings consistent with the disease. Laboratory studies including the HLA-B27 are not specific for ankylosing spondylitis, but may help to support the diagnosis.

TREATMENT

Early diagnosis is critical, and patient education can help the patient to understand the course and treatment of the disease. A combination of pharmacologic and

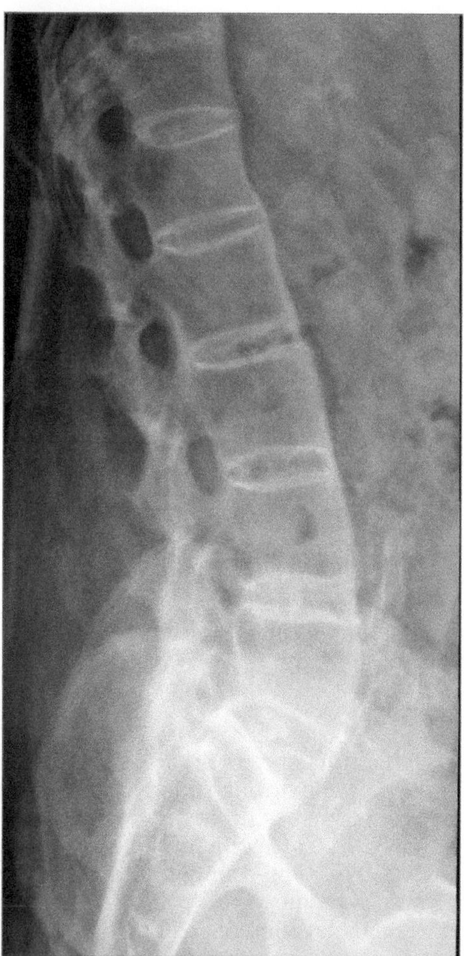

Figure 14.13 **MRI showing increased bone formation and fusion of ankylosing spondylitis.**

nonpharmacologic therapies provide the best approach. Manifestations such as uveitis should be treated according to current recommendations.

Pharmacologic therapy can help to reduce functional limitations that may result from disease activity. NSAIDs, other analgesics, DMARDs, and biologics may be indicated. Oral glucocorticoids have not been found to be beneficial in the treatment of ankylosing spondylitis, and so should not be used.

Nonpharmacologic therapy should center on reducing symptoms and maintaining function. Physical therapy and routine exercise can help to preserve both strength and flexibility. Posture training is critical to slow or prevent the development of hyperkyphosis.

PATIENT EDUCATION

There is no known cure for ankylosing spondylitis. The primary goals of treatment include relief of symptoms, maintenance of function, and prevention of complications. It is important that disease activity is regularly monitored and the therapeutic plan adjusted accordingly. Physical therapy and an exercise program should begin soon after the diagnosis of ankylosing spondylitis is made. Regular exercise can help to preserve and regain muscle strength and flexibility. In addition, posture training should be initiated shortly after diagnosis.

14.6B PSORIATIC ARTHRITIS

OVERVIEW

Psoriatic arthritis is a form of seronegative spondyloarthritis that develops in patients with psoriasis. It is a chronic inflammatory arthritis affecting the joints and entheses of both the peripheral and axial skeleton. As with the other spondyloarthropathies, extra-articular manifestations, such as uveitis, are common.

EPIDEMIOLOGY

Psoriatic arthritis is relatively rare, with a prevalence in the general population of approximately 1 to 2 per 1,000.[248] Approximately 20% of patients with psoriasis have or develop psoriatic arthritis.[249] Women and men are affected equally, and Whites appear to be affected more commonly than those from other racial groups. While psoriatic arthritis can develop at any age, adult onset is most common between the ages of 35 and 55, while pediatric onset is between ages 9 and 11 years.

PATHOPHYSIOLOGY

Although the pathogenesis of psoriatic arthritis is not fully understood, research strongly suggests that there are genetic and environmental factors, along with the complex actions of immune-mediated inflammation. Susceptibility to the development of psoriasis and psoriatic arthritis shows a strong genetic tendency, with approximately 40% of patients with either disorder having a positive family history in at least one first-degree relative.[250] There are a number of HLAs that have been found to occur with increased frequency in patients with psoriatic arthritis.[251] While patients with psoriatic arthritis show an increased frequency of HLA-B27 as compared to those with uncomplicated psoriasis, it is not as frequently found as in ankylosing spondylitis or reactive arthritis. To further complicate matters, some patients with psoriasis and spondyloarthropathy are actually HLA-B27 negative, while many patients with psoriatic arthritis who are positive for HLA-B27 do not have any spinal symptoms. Environmental factors are believed to play a role in the etiology of psoriatic arthritis through a process where superantigens react with autoantigens. Both bacterial and viral pathogens, as well as trauma, have been implicated in the pathogenesis of psoriasis and psoriatic arthritis. The inflammatory process involved in psoriatic arthritis leads to similar synovial fluid findings as are found in RA, suggesting some similarities. However, specific variations in the proinflammatory cytokines involved in each condition suggest different underlying mechanisms.[252]

MEDICAL HISTORY AND CLINICAL PRESENTATION

Psoriasis precedes the onset of psoriatic arthritis in the majority of patients by an average of 7 to 8 years, though in some cases it has been by as long as 40 years.[253] In approximately 14% of patients, arthritis begins prior to skin disease, and in an additional 15%, the two present simultaneously.[254] However, researchers point out that in the latter two instances, it is possible the skin disease has been relatively mild or hidden and was therefore undiagnosed.

Pain and stiffness in the affected joints are the most common presenting symptoms in most patients with psoriatic arthritis. In most cases there is an insidious onset, though as many as one-third of patients report the onset as acute. Accompanying fatigue occurs in 22% of patients.[255] A thorough medical history should focus on history of skin disease, description of the joints involved, symptoms of enthesitis, involvement of the fingers and/or eyes, and any history of inflammatory back pain. In addition, a family history should be obtained, especially as related to psoriasis, psoriatic arthritis, or other rheumatologic disorders.

SIGNS AND SYMPTOMS

Psoriatic arthritis may affect axial joints, peripheral joints, or both. The most common presentation is as a polyarthritis. Tenosynovitis, enthesitis, and dactylitis are also common. There are five commonly recognized clinical patterns of psoriatic arthritis:

- Symmetric polyarthritis resembling RA, but usually with fewer joints involved
- Distal arthritis, most commonly affecting the DIP joints, often with nail pitting and onycholysis
- Asymmetric oligoarthritis, typically affecting fewer than five joints
- Arthritis mutilans with severely deforming arthritis and marked osteolysis
- Spondyloarthritis with spinal involvement and sacroiliitis

Patients may present with one of the above clinical patterns but change to a different pattern during the course of the disease.[256] Additional musculoskeletal manifestations include enthesitis, tenosynovitis, and dactylitis or "sausage digit." This uniform swelling of the soft tissues of the fingers occurs in almost 50% of patients with psoriatic arthritis and is a predictor of progressive joint damage.[257]

The fingernails are affected in 80% to 90% of patients with psoriatic arthritis as compared with <50% in those with uncomplicated psoriasis.[251] Pitting, onycholysis, splinter hemorrhages, and hyperkeratosis are common. These findings are identical to the nail findings typical of uncomplicated psoriasis. Pitting edema of the hands or feet is sometimes present.

Ocular inflammation occurs in some patients and includes conjunctivitis and uveitis. Conjunctivitis occurs more frequently, affecting approximately 20% of patients.[258] Uveitis may present acutely with painful injection, or insidiously with impaired visual acuity. In contrast to the uveitis seen in other forms of spondyloarthropathies, the uveitis of psoriatic arthritis is more frequently bilateral and posterior to the lens.

PHYSICAL EXAMINATION

Affected joints are tender with effusions, often in asymmetric distribution.[259] Marked joint deformity may be present without a significant degree of pain. Dactylitis may be present, as well as enthesitis, especially involving the Achilles tendon. Tenderness of the spine and sacroiliac joints may be elicited with palpation or manipulation.

Inspection of the skin and nails may reveal findings consistent with psoriasis. Some patients will present without history or overt signs of psoriatic skin disease. Careful examination of skin surfaces, to include the gluteal cleft, umbilicus, and scalp, may reveal a single hidden psoriatic patch.

A thorough ophthalmologic examination should be done to assess for uveitis, conjunctivitis, and other ocular manifestations.

DIFFERENTIAL DIAGNOSIS

The differential diagnosis of psoriatic arthritis must take into account the pattern of symptoms and objective findings. When psoriatic arthritis presents with polyarthritis, it can be difficult to distinguish from RA. However, asymmetrical distribution of joint involvement, spondyloarthritis, dactylitis, dermatologic findings, and nail manifestations all suggest psoriatic arthritis.[260] History of a preceding genitourinary or GI infection helps to differentiate psoriatic arthritis from reactive arthritis since there is crossover of symptoms with these two condition. Similarly, ankylosing spondylitis may be difficult to distinguish from psoriatic arthritis, but the presence of psoriasis and some characteristic radiologic findings may help to differentiate between the two disorders. In addition, cervical spine involvement is more common in psoriatic arthritis while lumbar spine involvement occurs less frequently. Other causes of joint pain, such as gout and OA, should also be considered.

DIAGNOSTIC STUDIES

The diagnosis of psoriatic arthritis is a clinical diagnosis, based on history and physical exam, and supported by the results of diagnostic studies. Distinguishing psoriatic arthritis from other forms of inflammatory arthritis can present challenges. There is no single diagnostic study that confirms the diagnosis.

Laboratory findings in psoriatic arthritis are nonspecific. Autoantibodies such as ANA, RF, and anti-CCP antibody are typically not present. Acute phase reactants, such as ESR and CRP, are elevated in fewer than half of patients. Uric acid levels may be high due to the active turnover of affected skin. Testing for HLA-B27 may be helpful when this is found as it indicates increased risk of spondylitis, which may be asymptomatic early in its course.

In those patients who present with joint effusion, arthrocentesis and examination of the synovial fluid should be done to rule out other diagnoses such as septic arthritis and crystalline disease. Cell count and differential, Gram stain and culture, and examination for the presence of crystals should all be included in this evaluation. In those with psoriatic arthritis, findings are characteristic of inflammatory arthritis and nonspecific for the disease.

Imaging in patients with suspected psoriatic arthritis can reveal characteristic changes typically not seen in other forms of inflammatory arthritis. The coexistence of new bone formation and erosive changes, either in the same joint, or in different joints in the same digit, is common. Lysis of the terminal phalanges, mutilation of isolated joints, fluffy periostitis, and a "pencil-in-cup" appearance are common radiographic findings. Axial radiographs may show changes identical to those seen in patients with ankylosing spondylitis. MRI may be more sensitive at detecting subtle axial changes in those who are early in the disease process.

EVALUATION

The diagnosis of psoriatic arthritis can typically be made in a patient who has psoriasis and inflammatory arthritis in a pattern consistent with this disease. Patients with psoriasis can develop other forms of arthritis, to include OA, RA, and reactive arthritis; therefore, it is important to establish the pattern of joint involvement, and to perform appropriate laboratory testing and imaging. Extra-articular findings typical of the disease, especially affecting the eyes, skin, and nails, may help to support the diagnosis.

TREATMENT

Treatment of psoriatic arthritis is directed toward controlling the inflammatory process. NSAIDs are usually sufficient in mild cases. For those patients who do not get adequate relief for their peripheral arthritis with the use of NSAIDs, DMARDs are indicated, with methotrexate being the most commonly used. In those with severe disease, including joint erosion and functional limitation, TNF inhibitors are considered first-line therapy. In patients with axial disease, NSAIDs are indicated for mild symptoms. For axial symptoms that fail to respond to NSAID therapy or for those patients with more severe pain and prolonged morning stiffness, a TNF inhibitor is recommended. Patients who are experiencing eye pain or visual disturbance or who have abnormal eye findings on physical exam should be referred to an ophthalmologist for evaluation and treatment.

PATIENT EDUCATION

Patients should be evaluated for comorbidities which are prevalent in psoriatic arthritis such as diabetes,, coronary artery disease, metabolic syndrome, depression, and fatty liver.

The course of psoriatic arthritis may vary considerably from patient to patient. Though there is no cure for the disease, a minority of patients will experience remission. In others, pharmacologic therapy can lead to a significant decrease in symptoms. Despite a wide array of medications used in treatment, a subgroup of patients will progress to significant joint damage.

14.6C REACTIVE ARTHRITIS

OVERVIEW

Reactive arthritis is a form of spondyloarthritis that develops either soon after or during an infection elsewhere in the body. The causative pathogens can be separated into two varieties: GI and urogenital. GI causative agents include *Salmonella*, *Shigella*, *Yersinia*, *Campylobacter*, *Escherichia coli* and *Clostridioides difficile*.[261] *Chlamydia trachomatis* and *Chlamydia pneumoniae* are the known urogenital pathogens that cause this condition.[262] When reactive arthritis results from a sexually transmitted infection, it is referred to as sexually acquired reactive arthritis (SARA).[263] It is important to note that the causative microorganism cannot be recovered from the affected joint, which can make it difficult to identify the specific pathogen.[264]

EPIDEMIOLOGY

Reactive arthritis is relatively rare and occurs most frequently in younger adults. Incidence of reactive arthritis in patients recently infected by *Salmonella*, *Shigella*, or *Campylobacter* ranges between 9 and 12 patients per 1,000.[265] When *Chlamydia* is the causative pathogen, 3% to 8% of patients will go on to develop reactive arthritis.[266]

PATHOPHYSIOLOGY

Though the pathophysiology of reactive arthritis is not fully understood, research strongly suggests that there is a genetic link. The gene for HLA-B27 is the single largest genetic contributor to reactive arthritis, though it is not an absolute requirement, as other HLA and non-HLA genes are also involved. Approximately 75% of patients with reactive arthritis are positive for HLA-B27.[267]

The specific process by which the causative organism interacts with the host, leading to the development of reactive arthritis, is unknown. It is suspected that a cross-reaction between microbial antigens and self-proteins stimulates an autoimmune response mediated by type 2 T helper (Th2) cells. Additionally, a Th2 cytokine profile leading to decreased clearance of bacteria has been associated with joint damage and chronic disease.[102] The synovitis present in reactive arthritis is mediated by proinflammatory cytokines. Though cultures of the synovial fluid are negative for enteric organisms or *Chlamydia*, IL-17 can be found in elevated levels in patients with reactive arthritis.[268]

MEDICAL HISTORY AND CLINICAL PRESENTATION

Reactive arthritis typically presents acutely as an asymmetric mono- or oligoarthritis affecting one to four joints. This usually occurs 1 to 4 weeks after the inciting GI or urogenital infection.[261] The causative pathogen and severity of the preceding infection do not predict the severity of the condition.[269] In some cases, the preceding GI or urogenital infection is clinically silent. This is especially true when *Chlamydia* is the causative organism.[102] For at least 50% of patients, the symptoms will resolve in under 6 months.[269]

A classic triad of symptoms related to reactive arthritis includes arthritis, noninfectious urethritis, and conjunctivitis. All three manifestations are found in only one-third of patients. When present, the triad has a sensitivity of 50.6% and a specificity of 98.9%.[270]

SIGNS AND SYMPTOMS

Signs and symptoms of the infection preceding reactive arthritis are characteristic of the causative pathogen, with enteric organisms causing diarrhea and genitourinary organisms causing urethritis. At the onset of the disease, many patients complain of fatigue, malaise, and fever. Myalgias may also be noted early in the course. The remaining signs and symptoms of reactive arthritis can be divided into two categories; musculoskeletal and extra-articular.

Musculoskeletal manifestations of reactive arthritis include arthritis, enthesitis, back pain, and dactylitis.[271] Acute-onset oligoarthritis is asymmetric and affects the lower extremities most typically, though about half of patients will have upper extremity complaints. Some patients may also experience polyarthritis in the small joints.[271] The knee is commonly affected. Enthesitis occurs when the site of insertion of tendons, ligaments, joint capsule, or fascia to bone becomes inflamed. Heel swelling, pain, and localized tenderness at the insertion of the Achilles tendon and the plantar fascia on the calcaneus are characteristic of enthesitis. As many as 90% of patients with reactive arthritis experience enthesitis.[271] Inflammatory back pain, especially of the lower back, is also commonly reported. Dactylitis, or "sausage digits," may also develop. For those patients in whom *Chlamydia* was the causative organism, the incidence of dactylitis is as high as 40%.[272]

Extra-articular manifestations of reactive arthritis can be categorized as ocular, genitourinary, GI, skin and mucosal, and cardiac. Ocular manifestations may include conjunctivitis, anterior uveitis, keratitis, and episcleritis, with conjunctivitis occurring most frequently. Genitourinary tract symptoms, which can occur even when the causative organism was enteric, include dysuria, urethritis, pelvic pain, cervicitis, cystitis, prostatitis, or salpingo-oopheritis.[273] Diarrhea is the most common GI symptom. Skin and mucosal manifestations can include keratoderma blennorrhagicum (Figure 14.14), which affects the palms and soles, and painless shallow ulcers on the glans penis and urethral meatus known as circinate balanitis (Figure 14.15). Similar circinate lesions may be present on the tongue. Cardiac manifestations are not common, but may include valvular disease, particularly of the aortic valve, leading to aortic insufficiency.[274]

PHYSICAL EXAMINATION

Affected joints are tender, warm, and swollen, and may also be erythematous. Distribution is typically asymmetric, with the weight-bearing joints of the lower extremities, including the hip, knee, and ankle being the most common sites affected. The shoulder, elbow, and wrist may also be involved. Dactylitis may be present, as well as enthesitis, especially involving the Achilles tendon. Tenderness of the spine and sacroiliac joints may be elicited with palpation or manipulation.

Inspection of the skin and mucosal surfaces may reveal cutaneous eruptions and other changes. Hyperkeratotic skin on the palms and soles may contain vesicles, macules, papules, and nodules characteristic of keratoderma blennorrhagicum and shallow circular lesions on mucosal surfaces may be present. The nails may become ridged and thickened and may crumble or shed.

Conjunctivitis is a common finding in patients with reactive arthritis, especially early in the disease. Conjunctival injection is often intense in color, and commonly bilateral. Edema and purulent discharge may or may not be present. Symptoms range from completely painless or minimal discomfort to severe photophobia and blepharospasms. A thorough ophthalmologic exam should be done to rule out anterior uveitis, scleritis, episcleritis, and keratitis.

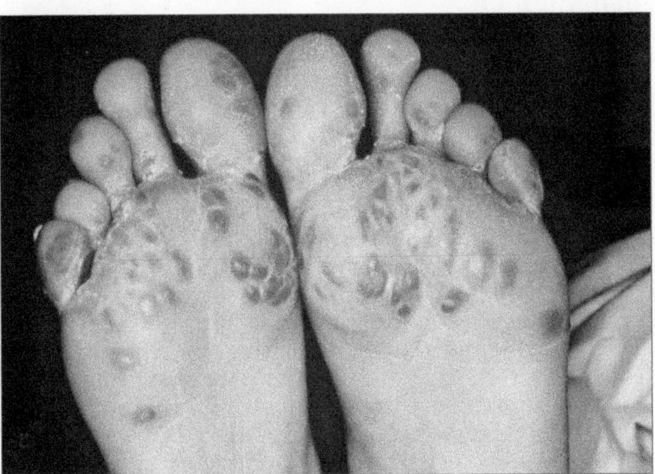

Figure 14.14 Keratoderma blennorrhagicum in a patient with reactive arthritis.
(Source: Centers for Disease Control and Prevention/Dr. M. F. Rein. https://phil.cdc.gov/details.aspx?pid=6950)

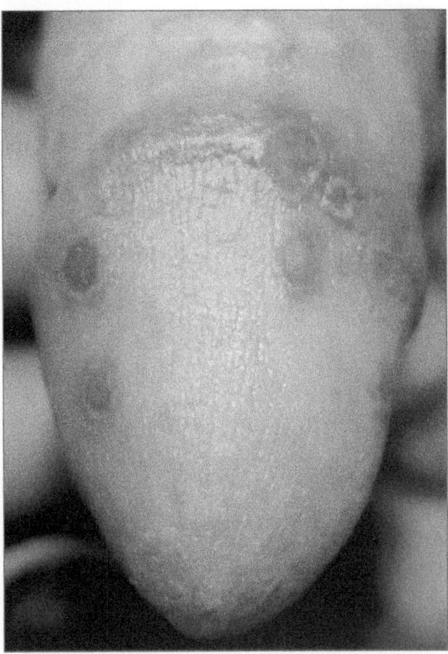

Figure 14.15 Circinate balanitis in a patient with reactive arthritis.
(Source: Courtesy of Freakedenough)

Examination of the genitourinary tract should include inspection of the urinary meatus for edema, erythema, and discharge. Prostatitis should be ruled out in males. Vulvovaginitis, cervicitis, and salpingo-oophoritis should be ruled out in female patients.

DIFFERENTIAL DIAGNOSIS

The differential diagnosis of reactive arthritis must take into account the pattern of symptoms and findings. Common causes of joint pain, including trauma, OA, crystalline arthropathies, Lyme arthritis, and septic arthritis, should be considered. Additional diagnoses should be determined based on the presenting symptoms.

DIAGNOSTIC STUDIES

The diagnosis of reactive arthritis is a clinical diagnosis, based on the history and physical exam as well as the exclusion of other diseases. There is no single diagnostic study that confirms the diagnosis. Though validated diagnostic criteria have not been established, the diagnosis should be suspected in patients who exhibit characteristic musculoskeletal findings, evidence of preceding infection, and lack of evidence of another cause.

Laboratory studies that may help to support the diagnosis include acute phase reactants, such as ESR and CRP, which may be elevated. A normal finding does not rule out the disease. Test results for RF and ANA are negative. HLA-B27 is not found in all patients who have reactive arthritis, but a positive finding makes the diagnosis more likely. A negative finding does not exclude the diagnosis.

Cultures are indicated depending on the clinical presentation. In patients who present with active diarrhea, stool cultures should be tested for the presence of *Salmonella*, *Shigella*, *Yersinia*, and *Campylobacter*. Patients who present with genitourinary symptoms should be tested for chlamydial infection either via a urine sample or swab. In those patients who do not present with history of GI or genitourinary symptoms, *Chlamydia* should be ruled out.

In those patients who present with a joint effusion, arthrocentesis and examination of the synovial fluid should be done to rule out other diagnoses such as septic arthritis and crystalline disease. In those with reactive arthritis, findings are characteristic of inflammatory arthritis and nonspecific for the disease. Leukocyte counts are typically elevated and show a predominance of neutrophils. WBC counts have a wide range between 2,000 and 64,000 WBCs/mm^3.[275]

Imaging in patients with suspected reactive arthritis is aimed at ruling out other causes of joint pain. Plain radiographs may reveal stress fractures or other forms of arthritis. In those reactive arthritis patients who are early in the disease process, radiographic findings are often absent. In more severe or long-standing disease, radiographic changes are nonspecific.

EVALUATION

Reactive arthritis is diagnosed clinically, based on history and physical exam findings. The disease should be suspected in those patients who experience characteristic musculoskeletal findings after a preceding GI or genitourinary infection. Extra-articular findings typical of the disease, especially affecting the eyes and skin, help to support the diagnosis. Exclusion of other possible causes through diagnostic testing ultimately leads to the diagnosis of reactive arthritis.

TREATMENT

Treatment of reactive arthritis is directed at the preceding infection if still present, along with musculoskeletal symptoms, and any extra-articular symptoms. Antibiotic therapy is indicated in patients with ongoing genitourinary infection and should follow the current guidelines for the treatment of chlamydial infection. Antibiotics are not indicated for the treatment of uncomplicated enteric infections. However, in patients who are immunocompromised, older, or with severe infection, antibiotic therapy may be indicated. In those with chronic reactive arthritis, antibiotic therapy has not been found to be beneficial.[271]

NSAIDs are the mainstay of treatment for acute reactive arthritis, unless contraindicated. Anti-inflammatory doses of naproxen, diclofenac, or indomethacin can significantly improve the symptoms, though there is no evidence that they shorten the course of the disease. Because of the self-limited nature of reactive arthritis, and the infrequency with which joint damage occurs, NSAIDs are often the only treatment needed.

In patients with persistent symptoms and inadequate relief from NSAID therapy, intra-articular glucocorticoid injections may be effective in reducing joint inflammation and improving symptoms. An oral glucocorticoid may be used in patients who do not experience improvement after a trial of NSAIDs and intra-articular glucocorticoid injection, or for those who have a large number of joints involved. Treatment with DMARDs is reserved for those patients whose symptoms are not adequately improved with NSAIDs and glucocorticoid therapy. DMARDs are also indicated in patients with chronic reactive arthritis, typically defined as those having disease for longer than 6 months who do not respond to NSAID and glucocorticoid therapies. In these patients, a nonbiologic DMARD, such as sulfasalazine or methotrexate, is most commonly used.

Patients who are experiencing eye pain or visual disturbance or who have abnormal eye findings on physical exam should be referred to an ophthalmologist to determine if uveitis or other ocular manifestations are present. Lesions of the skin and mucous membranes may be mild and require no treatment. In those with symptomatic keratoderma blenorrhagicum, topical steroids may be beneficial. Topical vitamin D and retinoids may also be used.

PATIENT EDUCATION

The course of reactive arthritis may vary considerably from patient to patient. The causative organism and the genetic background of the patient are both thought to influence the severity and course of the disease.[275] The disease is typically self-limited, lasting 3 to 5 months in most patients. Those who are HLA-B27 positive and those who present with the triad of arthritis, conjunctivitis, and urethritis may be more likely to develop chronic disease and therefore have a poorer prognosis.

14.7 INFECTIONS

14.7A SEPTIC ARTHRITIS

OVERVIEW

Septic arthritis, a medical emergency, is an infection of a joint caused by a bacterial or fungal organism. Septic arthritis has also been termed infectious, pyogenic, suppurative, or purulent arthritis. The need to recognize and treat septic arthritis emergently is due to the potential of this condition to cause destructive joint changes and substantial morbidity and mortality. While viral infections can lead to arthritic symptoms, virally caused arthritis will not be discussed in this section.

EPIDEMIOLOGY

The incidence of septic arthritis is reported as 2 to 6 per 100,000 people per year.[276,277] Certain patient populations are noted to be at increased risk for septic arthritis (Box 14.1).[278]

PATHOPHYSIOLOGY

The primary method by which offending microbial agents enter the joint is by hematogenous spread. The joint synovium is highly vascular and lacks a protective basement membrane. Inflammatory conditions such as RA increase vascular flow to a joint suggesting one possible reason why these conditions are a risk factor for septic arthritis. Previous joint damage and the use of immunosuppressive medications to treat these inflammatory conditions may also lend to increase septic arthritis risk. Direct means of joint inoculation such as trauma, surgery, or arthrocentesis are known causes of septic joints. Septic arthritis may also occur as a result of an adjacent osteomyelitis or overlying cellulitis. Human or animal bites are also causes of septic arthritis.

BOX 14.1 Increased Risk Factors for Developing Septic Arthritis

Age >80 years
Diabetes mellitus
Rheumatoid arthritis
Presence of a prosthetic joint
Recent joint surgery
Intravenous drug use
Skin infections
Prior intra-articular corticosteroid injections
HIV-1 infection

The invading microbe causes an inflammatory response that can affect articular structures and bone and lead to secondary degenerative joint changes. The potential destructive inflammatory process is driven by cytokines and proteases.[279]

MEDICAL HISTORY AND CLINICAL PRESENTATION

Persons with septic arthritis will often present with a monoarthritis. The patient may describe an acutely painful, swollen, and warm joint with difficulty with range of motion. Fever is not a universal finding. The presence of fever is likely due to a person's individual immune response as medical research to date has not associated causative pathogens with increased incidence of fever.[280] ***Knees*** are the most commonly affected joint followed by the shoulders, wrists, hips, and ankles in adults. ***Hips*** are the most commonly affected joint in children.[281,282] Other joints such as sacroiliac joints and symphysis pubis may be involved and should be considered in the appropriate clinical patient presentation. Sacroiliac joint and symphysis pubis infectious arthritis may present with pain in these areas occurring with ambulation and fever.

SIGNS AND SYMPTOMS

When clinical suspicion of septic arthritis is present, the examiner must evaluate the patient's symptoms. The finding of a monoarticular flare with swelling, warmth, and erythema should lead a clinician to consider septic arthritis When septic arthritis occurs in a weight-bearing joint, patients may have difficulty with ambulation or be unable to ambulate. Oligoarticular presentations of septic arthritis should also be considered, particularly in patients with multiple risks factors.

PHYSICAL EXAMINATION

Because of patient discomfort and the emergent situation, the examiner must urgently examine persons with suspected septic arthritis. Evaluating the affected joint for swelling, warmth, and erythema is needed. A more comprehensive joint examination and periarticular exam are also needed when considering other potential causes for the patient's presenting symptoms. At minimum, examining joints above and below the affected joint and the same joint on the contralateral side should be done.

DIFFERENTIAL DIAGNOSIS

The differential diagnosis for septic arthritis includes other conditions that may cause monoathritis and conditions that may cause a monoarticular flare of polyarticular disease. Box 14.2 contains a list of conditions to consider in the differential diagnosis based on the patient's presenting signs and symptoms.

DIAGNOSTIC STUDIES

The diagnostic approach to septic arthritis includes both laboratory and radiographic studies. Arthrocentesis that leads to synovial fluid analysis is essential. The evaluation of the aspirated synovial fluid should include a WBC count, Gram stain, culture, and crystal examination by polarized light microscopy. Results of these studies can influence initial treatment. Synovial fluid cultures may take 2 days to several weeks for results dependent upon the causative organism. A WBC count of >50, 000 should raise suspicion of a septic arthritis diagnosis (Table 14.11).

Synovial fluid culture results provide a more targeted approach to antibiotic treatment. Synovial fluid for culture should be obtained prior to beginning the antibiotic treatment regimen. The most common bacterial cause of septic arthritis is *Staphylococcus aureus* followed by groups A and

BOX 14.2 Differential Diagnosis for Septic Arthritis

Systemic inflammatory arthritis (rheumatoid arthritis, seronegative spondyloarthropathy)
Crystal arthritis (gout, pseudogout, other crystal), can coexist with septic arthritis
Systemic lupus erythematosus
Reactive arthritis
Lyme disease
Sickle cell disease
Transient synovitis of the hip
Foreign body synovitis
Pigmented villonodular synovitis
Hemarthrosis
Neuropathic arthropathy
Osteoarthritis
Intra-articular injury (fracture, internal derangement of meniscus or cartilage)

TABLE 14.11 Synovial Fluid Analysis

Condition	Color	Clarity	WBC Count*	Crystals	Culture and Sensitivity
Osteoarthritis	Amber	Clear	200–2,000	(–)	(–)
Trauma	Pink-red	Clear-opaque	<2,000	(–)	(–)
Inflammatory	Yellow	Cloudy	2,000–100,000	(–/+)	(–)
Infection	Purulent	Opaque	>50,000 (>90% PMNs)	(+)	

**WBC count in cells/mm^3.*
PMNs, polymorphonuclear leukocytes; WBC, white blood cell.

B streptococci.[283–285] The two most common gram-negative bacterial causes of septic arthritis include *Neisseria gonorrhoeae* and *Neisseria meningitidis*.[283] Gonorrheal septic joint infections may also be associated with disseminated gonococcal infection with additional manifestations including painless macules, papules and pustules, tenosynovitis, and, less commonly, gonococcal genitourinary symptoms. Other gram-negative septic arthritis infections are seen more frequently in immunocompromised patients and IV drug abusers. Less common causes of septic arthritis include associations with tuberculosis (may require synovial biopsy), brucellosis, and Lyme disease.

Other laboratory studies such as acute phase reactants (ESR and CRP) may be elevated in septic arthritis patients. A total WBC elevation in serum samples may also be noted. In the synovial fluid sample, glucose may be low while protein and lactic acid levels may be elevated. It must be noted that these laboratory results are nonspecific and should be considered in the appropriate clinical context.

A growing number of bacterial species may be detected by polymerase chain reaction (PCR) including *N. gonorrhoeae* and *Borrelia burgdorferi*.[286]

Plain film radiography of the affected joint is the initial imaging study that should be obtained. X-ray findings suggestive of septic arthritis may include joint space widening, periarticular fat pad displacement, loss of the white cortical line over extended and continuous segments, and erosive changes.[287] Periarticular osteopenia may be an early finding of septic arthritis. Other imaging studies such as ultrasonography, CT, scintigraphy, and MRI may be considered depending on the clinical presentation and the results of the initial plain x-rays.

EVALUATION

Arthrocentesis is essential for persons presenting with monoarthritis. Consultation with the orthopedics service is appropriate.

TREATMENT

- There are two primary treatment approaches to septic arthritis treatment: antimicrobials and synovial fluid drainage.
- Initial antibiotic choice may be determined by patient demographics, comorbidities, and Gram stain results.
- Vancomycin is generally the initial antibiotic treatment choice. A third-generation cephalosporin may be added to the initial treatment regimen for IV drug abusers or immunocompromised patients.
- IV ceftriaxone is considered for suspected gonococcal infections.
- The antibiotic treatment regimen is adjusted according to culture and sensitivity results when available.
- IV antibiotics are generally administered for 14 days followed by oral antibiotics for a similar duration. The duration of treatment is determined by patient response to treatment.
- As septic arthritis is a closed infection, synovial fluid drainage is needed. Synovial fluid drainage may be achieved by aspiration, arthroscopic drainage, or open surgical drainage. The method of drainage is determined by extent of infection, duration of infection, location of affected joint, procedural availability, and clinician preference.[280]

PATIENT EDUCATION

- Patients and their support care team should be educated concerning the emergent nature of septic arthritis.
- Patients with inflammatory arthritis should be educated to report any intense or unusual monoarticular flares of their joint disease.
- Patients should be educated on the importance of completing their prescribed treatment regimen for septic arthritis.

14.7B OSTEOMYELITIS

OVERVIEW

Osteomyelitis, by definition, is an infection of bone that can be described as acute or chronic. Acute and chronic osteomyelitis may be distinguished by the presence or absence of osteonecrosis. Location and underlying etiology assist in determining optimal treatment approach. High clinical suspicion is needed to diagnose osteomyelitis.

EPIDEMIOLOGY

The overall incidence of osteomyelitis is fairly low, in part, due to bone being resistant to infection by virtue of its structure. Factors increasing the risk of osteomyelitis include the following: diabetes mellitus, decubitus ulcers, surgery, trauma, intravenous drug abuse, and open fractures.[288]

PATHOPHYSIOLOGY

Osteomyelitis may occur by three primary routes. In children, hematogenous osteomyelitis mostly affects long bones commonly affecting the metaphysis.[289] Hematogenous osteomyelitis in adults may present as vertebral osteomyelitis or discitis. In young adults, osteomyelitis secondary to trauma or surgery is most common. In older adults, contiguous osteomyelitis is most commonly related to joint arthroplasty, diabetes mellitus, vascular disease, or decubitus ulceration. Contiguous osteomyelitis may commonly be polymicrobial.

Staphylococcus aureus is the most common bacterial cause of osteomyelitis. Coagulase-negative *Staphylococcus* species, beta-hemolytic streptococci, viridans streptococci, enterococci, and aerobic gram-negative bacilli are also common causes of osteomyelitis.[290]

MEDICAL HISTORY AND CLINICAL PRESENTATION

Although patients with osteomyelitis may present with vague symptoms, it is vital that clinicians obtain a through history when considering this diagnosis. Location of symptoms, duration of symptoms, and history of trauma should be included in the initial details. Comorbidities such as diabetes and diabetic complications should be documented.

A patient may describe pain, erythema, swelling, or drainage from a symptomatic site. Often patients note that symptoms may cyclically improve if pus passes through a fistula.[288]

Acute, subacute, or chronic onset of symptoms may occur.

SIGNS AND SYMPTOMS

The underlying etiology and affected location of a patient's osteomyelitis influences the clinical presentation. When a hematogenous cause is present, patients may have subacute or chronic pain at the involved site. When trauma or surgery is the underlying cause, patients may present with soft tissue erythema, swelling, with sinus tract drainage or with a slow to heal wound. A patient presenting vertebral osteomyelitis may present with pain or neurologic dysfunction with signs of cord compression or compromise dependent upon the degree of the effects of the infection. Vascular insufficiency associated causes of osteomyelitis may demonstrate ulceration, erythema, swelling, or drainage. Each of these potential osteomyelitis causes may or may not present with constitutional symptoms such as fever and chills.[290]

PHYSICAL EXAMINATION

The physical examination will support a clinician's suspicion of osteomyelitis. A finding of exposed bone, visible surgical hardware, or a draining fistula raises the suspicion for osteomyelitis.[288]

A common physical examination technique used in diabetic foot ulcers to detect osteomyelitis is the probe to bone technique. When a foot ulcer is present, an examiner places a sterile, blunt probe into the ulcerated lesion. A patient is not commonly expected to feel this probing in the setting of diabetic neuropathic changes. A rock-hard structure felt with the probe would be indicative of bone and should lead the examiner to consider osteomyelitis.[291]

DIFFERENTIAL DIAGNOSIS

The differential diagnosis for osteomyelitis is summarized in Box 14.3.

BOX 14.3 Differential Diagnosis for Osteomyelitis

- Soft tissue injury/disease (sprain, strain, infection)
- Charcot arthropathy
- Osteonecrosis of a noninfectious cause
- Crystal arthritis
- Fracture
- Bone malignancy (primary or secondary)
- Sickle cell vaso-occlusive pain crisis
- Complex regional pain syndrome
- Osteoarthritis
- SAPHO (synovitis, acne, pustulosis, hyperostosis, and osteitis)

DIAGNOSTIC STUDIES

A bone biopsy is the gold standard for osteomyelitis diagnosis, which includes culture and pathology examination of the bone. Other ancillary tests may support the osteomyelitis workup when a biopsy is not performed.

Superficial cultures may be obtained; however, the clinician must realize that the culture organism may not be the organism causing the osteomyelitis.

Laboratory tests, while nonspecific, may be supportive of a diagnosis of osteomyelitis. A serum WBC count may be elevated, particularly in hematogenous or acute osteomyelitis. ESR and CRP may also be elevated, but are neither sensitive nor specific. Blood cultures may be positive in hematogenous osteomyelitis, but negative in chronic osteomyelitis.

Radiographic studies initially include plain radiography, which may not be sensitive to early osteomyelitic changes. Plain film radiography is helpful to rule out other causes of the patient's symptoms. CT may be helpful to identify bony changes such as sequestra (necrotic bone separated from living bone by granulation tissue). MRI is more sensitive for detecting early osteomyelitis changes. Scintigraphy can also be helpful.

EVALUATION

A clinician utilizes the history and physical examination when determining laboratory, radiographic, and procedural approaches in the setting of suspected osteomyelitis.

Consideration should be provided for special patient populations presenting with osteomyelitis symptoms: diabetics, patients who have experienced trauma, patients with sickle cell disease (consider *Salmonella* as causative agent), patients who abuse intravenous drugs, and patients being treated with hemodialysis.[290]

TREATMENT

- Osteomyelitis treatment often includes both surgical and medical approaches.
- Surgical treatment provides an opportunity for obtaining culture and tissue samples, debridement, and orthopedic

hardware and dead tissue removal if indicated, along with localized antibiotic placement.
- Antibiotic treatment is guided by the underlying bacterial causative agent. Vancomycin and a third-generation cephalosporin or beta-lactam/beta-lactamase inhibitor are often given for empiric treatment. Adjustments to the antibiotic treatment regimen are made based on culture and sensitivity results. Four to 6 weeks of IV antibiotics are generally recommended for acute osteomyelitis. Chronic osteomyelitis usually requires a longer duration of antibiotic treatment depending on causative organism and a patient's comorbidities. This period treatment may be reduced if clean margins are found when bone is debrided.[290]
- The use of hyperbaric oxygen therapy in the treatment of osteomyelitis may be used in specific situations such as anaerobic pathogens causing osteomyelitis.

PATIENT EDUCATION

- Bone infections can occur and are more prevalent in certain patient populations.
- Confirming a bone infection may require several diagnostic tools.
- Completion of a prescribed antibiotic regimen is necessary for optimal outcomes in the treatment of osteomyelitis.

COMMON CHIEF COMPLAINTS

APPROACH TO JOINT PAIN

Patients with the various types of rheumatologic disease typically complain of joint pain and stiffness especially after prolonged rest. Since these conditions are systemic, fatigue and an overall sense of poor health typically accompany the various rheumatologic disorders. Many organs may be involved with autoimmune disease and several of these rheumatologic diseases have specific predilection for certain organs. Dryness of the mouth and eyes are key features of Sjögren syndrome. Jaw claudication and pain over the temporal artery are seen with giant cell arteritis. Chronic aching and a subjective achiness and feeling of weakness in the shoulder and hip girdle areas that occurs in patients over age 50 are seen in the setting of polymyalgia rheumatica.

Malar rash and kidney involvement are classically associated with SLE. Actual muscle weakness and pain with elevation of CPK is seen with polymyositis. Active muscle inflammation with the rash is seen with dermatomyositis and these patients are considered to have a higher risk for underlying malignancy.

Patients with underlying HLA-B27 allele are more likely to develop ankylosing spondylitis, which is a male-dominated disease, causing sacroiliitis and progressing to fusion of the vertebral bodies and resultant restrictive lung disease due to the inability of the ribs to expand with deep inhalation. Patients with HLA-B27 allele are at increased risk for the development of reactive arthritis when exposed to pathogens such as enteric organisms or *Chlamydia*, leading to conjunctivitis, urethritis, and a rash development.

Patients with fibromyalgia have multiple trigger point areas of tenderness along with nonrestorative sleep. There has not been laboratory abnormalities identified in these patients and there is a crossover with these patients having irritable bowel syndrome or chronic fatigue. At this time, active inflammation cannot be measured and there is controversy about whether fibromyalgia should be listed among the rheumatologic diseases.

The number of joints that are painful for patients along with which joints are involved are key historical elements that should be ascertained when evaluating patients with joint complaints. Monoarticular joint involvement should have a consideration for septic joint since this condition is considered an emergency. If there is any question as to whether joint involvement has an infectious etiology, joint aspiration and examination of this fluid is essential so that a septic joint is never missed.

Involvement of the first MTP joint of the foot is classically associated with gout as monosodium urate crystals can precipitate in a joint when they are at increased concentration and if the joint is cool as coolness tends to precipitate monosodium urate into crystals.

Patients with previously traumatized joints have an increased risk for the development of degenerative joint disease making this history relevant. Weight-bearing joints and joints with previous overuse are more likely to develop OA, which is considered degenerative but not inflammatory. Weight-bearing joints are also more susceptible to degeneration in patients with high body mass index. RA typically has symmetric involvement and prolonged stiffness lasting at least 1 hour. The DIP joint is most commonly involved with OA as these bony abnormalities are known as Heberden nodes. Bouchard nodes are seen in the PIP joints in the setting of OA. MCP joint and wrist involvement are seen with RA. The second and third metacarpal bones and other joints may be manifestations of hemochromatosis.

Knees are commonly involved with OA, Lyme disease, and pseudogout.

Patients with joint involvement should also be questioned with regard to systemic involvement. With autoimmune disease, there can be organ involvement involving the eyes, heart, lungs, skin, and kidneys in addition to joint involvement.

The goal of treatment of patients with autoimmune disease is a return to the patient's baseline and achievement of remission. Patients with RA have an increased risk for the development of cardiovascular disease so prevention strategies are appropriate. Cardiovascular disease is the most common cause of death for patients with autoimmune disease and these patients also have an increased risk for infection, especially if biologic treatment is given as part of the treatment regimen.

Current management of patients with rheumatologic disease involves early institution of DMARDs. These medications may arrest the progressive joint destruction that invariably occurs with autoimmune joint involvement. NSAIDs are utilized for controlling pain until the DMARD becomes fully effective. NSAIDs carry a black box warning for cardiovascular disease. Celecoxib induces this same cardiovascular risk but has a lower incidence of GI-related complications.

APPROACH TO INTERSTITIAL LUNG DISEASE

About 10% of patients with RA develop interstitial lung disease and these patients tend to have a more severe disease course and higher mortality.[292] Patients may develop cough as part of the pulmonary manifestations in the development of interstitial lung disease.[293] Patients can also develop bronchial hyperresponsiveness, bronchiectasis, brochiolitis, and recurrent respiratory infections.[293] Renal involvement includes tubulointerstititial disease and immune complex damage to the glomerulus.[294]

Peripheral neuropathy seen in Sjögren syndrome can be manifested by bilateral leg weakness as a pure motor syndrome.[295]

Symptoms of dryness are treated with artificial tears in the eyes and gels in the mouth to mimic saliva. Cyclosporine is approved for helping with the dry eye sensation. Meticulous dental care is needed. Sugar-free candies can stimulate saliva flow. Vaginal symptoms of dryness can be treated with topical lubricants or estrogen. There is a role for immunosuppression in combating dryness but response to treatment has been disappointing.[296]

KNOWLEDGE CHECKS

1. Differentiate between joint pain and stiffness in the setting of osteoarthritis versus rheumatoid arthritis.
2. Explain why the base of the thumb is a common site for the development of osteoarthritis.
3. Determine why acetaminophen may not provide as much benefit as NSAIDs in treating pain due to osteoarthritis.
4. Explain why patients with elevated serum uric acid may have acute gout precipitated when urate-lowering therapy is initiated.
5. Provide an explanation as to why the first metatarsophalangeal joint of the toe is the most commonly affected joint for acute gout to occur.
6. Although joint aspiration of an inflamed joint to obtain fluid for analysis is considered the gold standard, why is this technique infrequently used in order to differentiate between gout and pseudogout affecting a joint?
7. Determine what laboratory studies are needed to perform in the setting of fibromyalgia.
8. Explain the role, if any, for the use of antidepressants in the setting of fibromyalgia.
9. In addition to SLE, which rheumatic condition has a positive anti-Ro antinuclear antibody diagnostic study?
10. What is the earliest pathologic change that occurs in the setting of rheumatoid arthritis?
11. Describe the monitoring that should be done when hydroxychoroquine is used in the management of SLE.
12. Talk about the role for corticosteroids in the setting of rheumatoid arthritis.

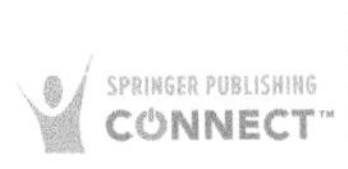

A robust set of instructor resources designed to supplement this text is located at **https://connect.springerpub.com/content/book/978-0-8261-8243-2.** Qualifying instructors may request access by emailing **textbook@springerpub.com.**

REFERENCES

The complete reference list for this chapter appears in the digital version of the chapter, accessible at https://connect.springerpub.com/content/book/978-0-8261-8243-2/chapter/ch14.

CHAPTER 15

NEUROLOGIC SYSTEM

MELINDA MOORE GOTTSCHALK

LEARNING OBJECTIVES

- Accurately diagnose and treat head and facial pain disorders recognizing the warning signs indicating emergent care.
- Evaluate and manage seizure disorders ordering the necessary tests and medications.
- Describe cognitive disorders. Able to develop and implement a treatment plan to address both patient and family needs as the disorder progresses.
- Recognize cerebrovascular accidents and importance of initial treatment, the appropriate treatment plan, and rehabilitation protocols.
- Understand the signs and symptoms of movement disorders and neurodegenerative disorders. Know the appropriate testing and treatment protocols.
- Recognize the symptoms of infectious disorders of the nervous system. Understand the immediate treatments and diagnostic tests.
- Evaluate and treat acute injuries to the nervious system. Understand treatment and rehabilitation protocols for acute injuries.

INTRODUCTION

The neurologic system affects every system in the body and comprises the central nervous system (brain and spinal cord) and the peripheral nervous system. This chapter will discuss vascular, structural, functional, degenerative, and infectious disorders of the nervous system.

15.1 HEADACHES

MELINDA MOORE GOTTSCHALK

OVERVIEW

"Headache" is the broad term that encompasses all head and facial pain. *The International Classification of Headache Disorders,* 3rd edition[1] describes headaches as primary headaches, secondary headaches, and painful cranial neuropathies, other facial pain, other headaches. This section explores four common headaches: migraine, tension-type, cluster, and post-traumatic headaches.

EPIDEMIOLOGY

When considering the epidemiology of headaches, the 5 Ws of epidemiology (who, what, when, where and why), can be as varied as the headaches themselves. The epidemiology depends on whether the headache is a primary headache, secondary headache, or a painful cranial neuropathy, facial pain, or other headache (Table 15.1). The epidemiology of migraine, tension-type, cluster, and post-traumatic headache is discussed in their respective sections.

The history of the headache can provide the most helpful criteria in diagnosis. The clinician should always assess the "red flags" for a secondary headache at each visit, regardless of underlying headache disorder, by using the SNNOOP acronym: Systemic symptoms, Neoplasms, Neurologic deficits, Onset sudden or following Valsalva maneuver, Older age, Prior history.

15.1A MIGRAINES

Migraines are a primary headache. Migraines are classified with or without aura. Migraines without aura are the more common. According to the National Center for Health Statistics,[2] migraines affected 15.5% of adults over the age of 18 between 2015 and 2018. Migraine can affect any age or gender but is most common in women between 20 and 60 years of age.[3] There are many comorbidities with migraines, including vascular, neurologic, psychiatric, and nonmigraine pain conditions.

PATHOPHYSIOLOGY

The mechanism for migraine remains largely unknown, but it is thought to be caused by abnormal brain activity affecting the nerves and blood vessels in the brain. Cortical spreading depression from occipital, sensory, and motor cortex is the most common explanation for a migraine, although there remains much to learn about the exact mechanism causing activation of the trigeminal pathway. Cortical spreading also causes changes in the vasculature causing constriction of the cortical surface arteries. 5-Hydroxytryptamine 1B/D

TABLE 15.1 Classifications of Headaches

Primary Headache	Secondary Headaches
Migraine	Outside factors Trauma
Tension-type	Medication withdrawal or overuse
Trigeminal autonomic cephalalgias	Vascular disorder or intracranial disorder
Other primary headaches	Infection or homoeostasis
	Psychiatric disorder
	Facial pain: face, mouth, eyes, ears, nose, sinus, teeth, or cervical structure

TABLE 15.2 Clinical Presentation of Migraines

Patient	Migraine History	Symptom
Female > Male	Increasing over the years	Usually unilateral pain; throbbing
12–70 years old	Worse before, during, or after menstrual cycle Onset after menarche	Facial (forehead/cheeks) pain, ear pain, temporal pain, occipital pain, scalp pain
	Positive family history	Nausea and/or vomiting
	History of head trauma	Sensitivity to lights, smells, and sounds Moderate to severe intensity and made worse with physical activity

receptors mediate multiple mechanisms that are thought to contribute to the development of migraines. Additionally, data suggest the hypothalamus plays a role in the prodrome stage of a migraine by communication with the trigeminal pathway or in areas related to pain transmission or autonomic function.[4]

MEDICAL HISTORY AND CLINICAL PRESENTATION

Taking a detailed history will help develop the diagnosis and reveal the risk factors the patient might have to develop a migraine. Past medical history, family history, medications, and social history are especially helpful for diagnosing migraine.

- **Past medical history:** Endocrine disorders, menstrual irregularities, psychological diagnosis, vitamin deficiencies, gastrointestinal (GI) problems, cardiac problems
- **Family history:** Migraine history in family, psychological history, endocrine, early menopause
- **Medications:** Some antidepressants, proton pump inhibitors (PPIs), testosterone, Accutane, some antihypertensives
- **Social history:** History of physical or emotional abuse or trauma, smoking history, alcohol history, daily caffeine intake, sleep habits, military history—specifically exposure to blast or shock waves, toxins
- **Environment:** Workplace (smells, odors, lights, noise), stress, excessive temperature changes

Some risk factors will be decreased and even eliminated if the patient adheres to a comprehensive treatment plan. Risk factors are classified as modifiable or nonmodifiable. Caffeine, snoring, and medication overuse can all trigger migraines. Educating the patient about the risk factors they can control is an important part of the migraine treatment plan.

Clinical presentation of migraine summarized in Table 15.2.

SIGNS AND SYMPTOMS

To meet the criteria of a migraine, the patient must have a unilateral headache, nausea with or without vomiting, photophobia, and phonophobia. The headache pain is typically described as stabbing, severe pressure, pulsating, or throbbing.[1]

Migraines are described as having phases (Figure 15.1).[4] The first phase of the migraine cycle is the "prodrome." The classic symptoms during this phase are photophobia, phonophobia, and nausea; however, a prodrome can consist of any symptom the patient has consistently days to hours before the headache begins, including sweating, yawning, fatigue, loss of concentration, hunger, and/or a stiff neck.

While migraine without aura is more common, in some patients, the second phase of the migraine is the "aura." The aura has more neurologic symptoms than the prodrome. The aura can present as visual disturbances ranging from blurred vision, spots, or squiggly lines to total blindness.

The third phase of the migraine is the actual headache. The migraine lasts 4–72 hours and is dependent on medication to abort the migraine and the underlying trigger. The fourth phase of the migraine is the postdrome, a newly recognize phase of a migraine. The postdrome was once known as the "migraine hangover" and consists of lethargy, irritability, nausea, difficulty with concentration, any of the symptoms the patient had during the prodrome. If the headache or symptoms do remain despite treatment, the postdrome can cycle into the prodrome and the cycle starts again.

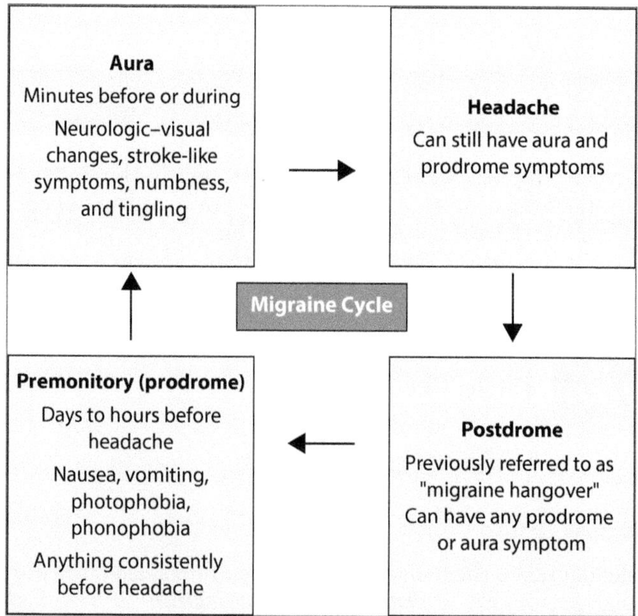

Figure 15.1 **Migraine with aura cycle.**

PHYSICAL EXAMINATION

The neurologic examination[5] begins with observation of the patient and how they present themselves. Are they wearing sunglasses or in a darkened room? Are they well groomed, confident, normal weight? Are they alone, and if not, is the patient giving the history? These are clues of possible underlying factors that are contributing to the migraine.

A migraine physical examination is head to toe, including a full neurologic and musculoskeletal examination.

1. Palpation of the scalp, beginning in the frontal region and palpating to the occipital region, cervical spine, and upper trapezius muscles noting areas of tenderness or tension.
2. Cranial nerves II-XII: Although CNII is important, a migraine is often triggered by fundoscopic examination. If the patient is currently suffering from a migraine, this part of the examination can be deferred; however, the patient should make appointment with ophthalmology for a complete examination with dilation within in the next few days. It is important for the optic nerve to be visualized for a comprehensive migraine workup. Test the other cranial nerves and document.
3. Sensation, including light touch and temperature in all four extremities as well and both sides of face. Vibratory testing at wrist and ankles. Romberg sign.
4. Strength testing and range of motion of arms, hands, fingers, legs, feet, and toes. Patients should show they can lift on their toes and back on their heels. Deep tendon reflexes are tested and include Hoffman sign and test for clonus.
5. Range of motion of neck and back in extension, flexion, rotation, side to side, noting deficiencies and limitations secondary to pain.
6. Tandem and casual gait noting arm swing and if the patient can get out of the chair unassisted. Note if they have a cane or walker or are aided by another person in standing or walking.
7. Perform a mini-mental status examination. As you talk to the patient you will be able to determine if you need to do a more extensive mental status examination.
8. Pulmonary and cardiac examinations, including carotid arteries, are important.

DIFFERENTIAL DIAGNOSIS

When developing the differential diagnosis, consider all the demographic and historical information as well as family history. Migraines have a strong family determinant. Post-traumatic headaches often convert to migraine headaches if not resolved in 6 months. Emotional problems, alcohol or physical abuse history, smoking, or overuse of headache rescue medications complicate the migraine diagnosis but should be addressed to successfully treat the migraine. Sinus infections and cluster headaches are important considerations. Tension headache can trigger migraine and migraine can trigger tension headaches.

DIAGNOSTIC STUDIES

Unless it is an emergency, the preferred study for migraine in a patient with red flag symptoms is a brain MRI with or without contrast. However, in the ED, order a CT scan without contrast due to its sensitivity for detecting a subarachnoid hemorrhage. Lab tests are ordered in conjunction with the MRI to determine the renal status, blood urea nitrogen (BUN), and creatinine. Testing should match the diagnoses being treated or being referred for treatment.

Other testing is determined by the history but could include:[1,3,6–10]

- **Blood tests:** Thyroid-stimulating hormone (TSH), complete blood count (CBC), comprehensive metabolic panel (CMP), vitamin B12, vitamin D, C-reactive protein (CRP), erythrocyte sedimentation rate (ESR) to rule out secondary cause of headaches.
- **Electroencephalogram (EEG):** Ordered if seizures are part of the headache history.
- **Sleep study:** Ordered if history of headache in the morning or waking with headache at night. Snoring can contribute to the morning headaches, and if treated, can reduce early morning headaches.
- **Venogram (MRV) and angiogram (MRA):** If concern for vascular components
- **Cervical studies:** Include flexion and extension if pain with those motions and or bilateral obliques if arm pain is present.

EVALUATION

Assuming all testing is normal, a patient with unilateral head pain, nausea with photophobia, and phonophobia is diagnosed with a classic migraine.[1] Contributing factors could be untreated sleep apnea, depression, poorly controlled diabetes, vitamin deficiencies, or other health issues. Correcting the underlying problems is essential to control the migraine.

TREATMENT

Prevention

Migraine specialists recommend preventive medications if the patient has at least three or more headache days a month.[1,6–9] The treatment can start with supplements, but effectiveness of the supplements can take 3 months. Prescription medication most often recommended are in three classes: antidepressants, antiepileptics, and beta blockers. Patients who fail these medications qualify for onabotulinumtoxinA therapy or calcitonin gene-related peptide (CGRP) inhibitors. Strict criteria for onabotulinumtoxinA and CGRP inhibitors necessitate documentation of failure of at least two of the three classes of medications for prevention.

- **Supplements:** Magnesium glycinate 400–550 mg daily, CoQ10 400 mg daily, vitamin B2 400 mg daily
- **Antidepressants:** Tricyclics are frontline treatment option for prevention of migraine.
- **Antiepileptics:** Topiramate is the frontline treatment option for prevention of migraine. Caution in patients with history of kidney stones. Precautions for women of childbearing age, extra contraceptive measures to avoid pregnancy secondary to topiramate's teratogenicity properties.
- **Beta blockers:** Propranolol and metoprolol are frontline treatment for prevention of migraine. Contraindicated with patients on immunotherapy for allergies, or if heart ailments check with cardiologist before starting beta blockers.

Other treatments include physical therapy with migraine specific modalities, psychological counseling for patients with depression, anxiety, or psychological trauma, sleep study for patients with sleep apnea.

Acute Treatment

An occasional migraine can convert to a "chronic" migraine (occurring 15 or more days per month) if the acute headache is not treated thoroughly and early in the headache cycle. The American Headache Society (AHS) recommends nonsteroidal anti-inflammatory drugs (NSAIDs) for mild migraines. If the NSAIDS do not work, or the adult patient with an established migraine diagnosis has a migraine with sudden onset, present in the morning or with nausea, the treatment that is considered Level A is a triptan. If the patient fails that treatment, the clinician can prescribe one of the new emerging therapies (fast-acting CGRPs or gepants). Studies have shown that gastroparesis may be the cause of the nausea, the most common complaint with the migraine syndrome. The AHS recommends treating the acute migraine with nonoral triptan, intranasal or injectable, if the patient has nausea and or vomiting.

PATIENT EDUCATION

The patient should receive education on the phases of a migraine and triggers for their migraines.[7,8,10,11] The importance of keeping a headache diary is stressed. The recommendation is to provide information on sleep hygiene and sleep apnea as well as tips to include the importance of avoiding dehydration, caffeine, alcohol given in writing to the patient. At the end of the visit a written "game plan" with the medications (vitamin, minerals, prescriptions) and information on medication overuse headache is important to include in a comprehensive headache plan.

15.1B CLUSTER HEADACHE

MEDICAL HISTORY AND CLINICAL PRESENTATION

A cluster headache is a trigeminal autonomic cephalalgia.[1] Cluster headaches can happen in relation to other types of headaches; determining the cluster headache's relationship to the other headache will help determine whether the cluster is a primary or secondary headache disorder, or both. The medical history would include history of previous headaches or cluster headaches, either episodic or chronic. Episodic cluster headache will occur for 7 days to a year and then cease for at least 3 months. Chronic cluster headaches occur for 1 year or more and cease <3 months between episodes. All secondary causes of headaches are ruled out using SNNOOP.[6]

The typical patient with a cluster headache is a male 20 to 40 years of age at first attack. The attacks are severe, often debilitating, and unilateral. The pain centers around one eye, supraorbital, in the temporal region, or in all three regions. The attacks range from 15 minutes to hours and can occur once a day or many times a day. Allodynia, hyperalgesia, anxiety, and depression are often present in the patient with cluster headaches.[12]

SIGNS AND SYMPTOMS

The patient with cluster headache experiences autonomic symptoms and often has psychological comorbidities.[12] Aside from unilateral head pain, the patient may present with either nasal congestion or rhinorrhea, lacrimation, conjunctival injection, eyelid edema, sweating, miosis or ptosis, restlessness, agitation, anxiety, or depression.[1,12]

PHYSICAL EXAMINATION

The patient must undergo a thorough physical examination with special attention to the neurologic and musculoskeletal examination. A mini-mental status examination expanding into a more comprehensive examination may be necessary if psychological factors are present.[5]

DIFFERENTIAL DIAGNOSIS

Cluster headaches may coexist with migraine or tension headaches or trigeminal neuralgia. An ophthalmologist[13] should examine the patient with only eye pain to rule out optic neuritis, uveitis, and other eye disorders.

DIAGNOSTIC STUDIES

Studies are determined by the history of the headache. If this is a new cluster headache order a brain MRI with and without contrast. Consideration of an MRA and MRV is dependent upon the history. Order a toxicology screen in patients with erratic behaviors, most often seen in the ED setting. If the headache is not new and the patient states the headache frequency and intensity have not increased, there is no need to order a diagnostic study. Care to document the history as stated by the patient is important for future headache attacks.[1,8]

EVALUATION

Criteria for a cluster headache according to *The International Classification of Headache Disorders,* 3rd edition[1]:

1. Five attacks with severe unilateral eye, supraorbital, or temporal pain
2. Agitation and/or restlessness or at least one of the following ipsilateral to the headache: conjunctival injection and/or lacrimation, nasal congestion or rhinorrhea, eyelid edema, forehead and facial sweating, miosis, and/or ptosis
3. Frequency of an attack every other day or eight per day
4. Not better accounted for with another headache type

TREATMENT

First-line treatment for prevention of cluster headache is verapamil.[14] Lithium is a frontline medication, but the side effect profile makes it intolerable for most patients. Second-line treatments with dihydroergotamine, topiramate, divalproex acid, and gabapentin have all shown efficacy in treating cluster headaches. Steroids are used in acute attacks, but exercise caution. Frequent use of steroids causes complications affecting the overall health of the patient. First-line therapy for acute attacks is 100% oxygen or subcutaneous sumatriptan 6 mg. For resistant cases, use intranasal lidocaine, oral ergotamine, and IV dihydroergotamine.

PATIENT EDUCATION

Provide a clear treatment plan for the patient at each visit outlining medications and other instructions. Educating patients includes caution that an attack can be triggered after alcohol intake or napping, as well as use of medications like nitroglycerin and some vasodilating antihypertensives. Patients should contact the clinician if the headaches have a severe increase in frequency and intensity. Close follow-up is needed until achieving headache control.

15.1C TENSION-TYPE HEADACHE

MEDICAL HISTORY AND CLINICAL PRESENTATION

Like the cluster headaches, tension-type headaches (TTHs) can be primary, secondary, or both and are episodic and chronic. TTHs are common and occur equally in males and females. The ages range from early childhood to geriatric patients. Evaluate the patient using SNNOOP[6] to rule out secondary causes of headache. TTHs last 30 minutes to 7 days. Description of this headache is mild-moderate pain that is not worse or aggravated by physical activity.[15]

SIGNS AND SYMPTOMS

The patient with only a TTH will complain of a bilateral frontal pain, described as pressure or a tight band around their head. The patient will not have any other complaints except scalp and upper trapezius tenderness. If there are other complaints, then evaluate for additional headache type, treating as indicated by the diagnosis.

PHYSICAL EXAMINATION

The patient must undergo a thorough physical examination with special attention to the neurologic and musculoskeletal examination. A mini-mental status examination expanding into a more comprehensive examination may be necessary if psychological factors are present.[5] Pay special attention to palpation of the scalp and upper trapezius muscles, and if tender this will aid in the diagnosis.

DIFFERENTIAL DIAGNOSIS

Migraine without aura and TTHs often coexist. Other types of headache would depend on the presenting symptoms.[15]

DIAGNOSTIC STUDIES

The medical history will determine the need for testing. If this is a new headache or if the headache is worsening, the clinician should order a brain MRI with and without contrast. If the headache is a known issue, no studies are needed unless there has been a change in intensity and frequency. The yield and correlation to laboratory tests are debatable but order laboratory tests if needed to rule out secondary causes of headaches.[15] See Section 15.1A Migraines for a list of laboratory tests.

EVALUATION

If testing does not reveal a secondary cause of headache, the diagnosis for the patient with only bilateral head pain—described as pressure or a "tight band" around the head—is a TTH. The patient may not have any other symptoms. If other symptoms are present, the clinician will begin an investigation for a secondary cause of headache.[1,15]

TREATMENT

Treat TTHs with over-the-counter (OTC) analgesics or prescription NSAIDs. Medication with butalbital have some positive evidence but have negative reports of increasing headaches. Triptans are not effective unless the patient also has migraines. Tricyclics for prevention and muscle relaxers for prevention and acute attacks are helpful in TTHs.[15]

Lifestyle changes and behavior modification are helpful in TTHs. Biofeedback, acupuncture, and relaxation techniques are helpful behavior modifications. Lifestyle changes including exercise, sleep hygiene, eating regular meals, and avoidance of triggers are helpful in controlling TTHs.[15]

PATIENT EDUCATION

Education includes avoidance of triggers and the need to incorporate lifestyle changes and behavior modifications into their daily routine to control the TTH. Patients should contact the clinician if the headaches have a severe increase in frequency and intensity.

15.1D POST-TRAUMATIC HEADACHE

MEDICAL HISTORY AND CLINICAL PRESENTATION

Post-traumatic headaches come from a trauma to the head or neck from various insults. The majority of post-traumatic headaches spontaneously resolve within a few days or weeks after the trauma.[1] Post-traumatic headaches resemble TTH and migraine headache in character, quality, and associated symptoms. Whiplash, injuries in motor vehicle accidents, and traumatic brain injuries have been shown to cause post-traumatic headaches.[16] The diagnosis is dependent on the history. *The International Classification of Headache Disorders,* 3rd edition[1] states the headache must be reported as starting "within 7 days of the trauma, within 7 days of regaining consciousness, and within 7 days of being able to sense and report pain." The patient may complain of other symptoms related to the post-traumatic headache and will tell you they had loss of consciousness, nausea, vomiting, dizziness, confusion, gait disturbance, and/or memory loss at the time of injury.[17] Occurrence is equal in males and females and the patient can be any age that is able to report a headache.[17]

SIGNS AND SYMPTOMS

The patient presents with a headache they connect with a traumatic event. They may say their head hurts at the point of trauma or all over. The patient's headache may now have symptoms like migraine or tension-type headaches. The patient may also have a component of medication overuse headache from trying to treat the headache with OTC medications prior to seeking medical help for the headache.[1,17]

PHYSICAL EXAMINATION

The patient must undergo a thorough physical examination with special attention to the neurologic and musculoskeletal examination. A mini-mental status examination expanding into a more comprehensive examination if cognitive or memory symptoms are present.[5]

DIFFERENTIAL DIAGNOSIS

The differential diagnosis for the post-traumatic headache is determined by the history. Migraine and TTH are often present.[1,17] A careful analysis using SNNOOP[6] is used to rule out secondary headaches.

DIAGNOSTIC STUDIES

The history and availability of the records will determine diagnostic studies. A new diagnostic study is not needed if a recent diagnostic study is available and the patient does not report an increase in intensity and frequency since the most recent study. The trauma history and the medical history of underlying conditions will determine laboratory studies.[1,17] The American College of Radiology (ACR) Appropriateness Critera can be used to determine the best imaging study.

EVALUATION

Evaluate the patient for migraine, tension-type, post-traumatic, and any other headache or disorders indicated by the history, physical examination, and/or results from labs or diagnostic studies.[17]

TREATMENT

The U.S. Food and Drug Administration (FDA) has not approved any medications specifically for post-traumatic headaches. However, studies have shown that many of the medications used for migraine and TTH have some efficacy in post-traumatic headaches that have converted to a migraine or TTH syndrome. OTC acetaminophen and ibuprofen can be beneficial if not taken in excess. Tricyclics and gabapentin seem to be the most efficacious of the migraine preventive agents in treating post-traumatic headaches. Behavior modifications and lifestyle changes have, as in other headache disorders, been beneficial to patients with post-traumatic headaches.[17]

PATIENT EDUCATION

See Section 15.1C Tension-Type Headache.

SPECIAL CONSIDERATIONS

Pregnancy

- Consult with the patient's obstetrician before continuing or starting new medications. In the pregnant patient, the clinician must weigh the risk verses benefit before starting or continuing medication for the pregnant patient. Investigate secondary headaches using SNNOOP.[6]

Nursing patients

- As in the pregnant patient, consult with the patient's obstetrician or the child's pediatrician before starting medications. Investigate secondary headaches using SNNOOP.[6] Many of the same considerations for pregnant patients continue in the nursing mother. Some medications require the patient to "pump and dump" for a set time after taking the medication.

Children

- Investigate secondary headaches using SNNOOP.[6] Most common headaches for children are migraine and TTH. Other types of headaches such as cluster, idiopathic intracranial hypertension (IIH), and, although exceedingly rare, increased pressure intracranially with space-taking lesion. Perform a thorough workup with a careful history, physical examination, and testing as in the adult patient.[18,19]

Geriatric patients

- Investigate secondary headaches using SNNOOP.[6] If a geriatric patient presents with no history of headache, start an immediate workup with the appropriate diagnostic test according to the symptoms.

KEY POINTS

- All headaches begin with a thorough workup to determine if the headache is a primary headache, a secondary headache, or other facial pain.
- Using SNNOOP[6] will help determine secondary headaches and need for studies.
- Lifestyle changes and behavior modifications are essential in all headache types.
- Providing patients with a preventive plan decreases headaches by enabling the acute medications to be more effective, by desensitizing the nervous system, and avoiding medication overuse headaches.
- If the geriatric patient presents with first headache after age 50 to 65, this is a red flag and demands immediate workup.
- Symptoms that indicate giant cell arteritis (GCA) or temporal arteritis necessitate immediate lab work with ESR and CRP, a brain MRI, and starting the patient on a high-dose steroid. Delay in treatment could lead to blindness or death.[10]

15.2 TRIGEMINAL NEURALGIA

Joshua Wageman

OVERVIEW

Trigeminal neuralgia (TN) is an enigmatic and exquisitely painful condition affecting the sensory branches of the trigeminal distribution. The pain is classically described as a unilateral "stabbing," like an "ice pick," and "electric shock-like." While brief in nature, TN can drastically impact quality of life for patients.[20]

These paroxysms, usually lasting a few seconds or less, may recur throughout the day in response to mundane stimuli such as chewing, speaking, or light touch to the face. Given the capricious and debilitating nature of these symptoms, it is important that clinicians recognize, diagnose, and manage this condition.

EPIDEMIOLOGY

There is significant variability in epidemiologic data surrounding TN; however, there appears to be a greater prevalence in women compared to men and incidence increases with advancing age. The average age at diagnosis for primary TN is 53 years, while secondary TN due to other conditions such as multiple sclerosis or tumor, is 10 years younger.[20]

The right side of the face is slightly more affected than the left side, and the V2 and V3 branches are affected significantly more often than the first branch of the trigeminal distribution. This is a rare condition, as lifetime prevalence is estimated at 0.16% to 0.3%.[20]

PATHOPHYSIOLOGY

The current consensus is that classical TN is caused by neurovascular compression, usually by an artery, or other morphologic changes to the nerve itself.[20] There is some evidence that localized demyelination of afferent fibers may also lead to neuronal hyperexcitability, thus leading to aberrant and repetitive depolarization. For secondary TN, the cause may be due to demyelination at the nerve root from multiple sclerosis or compression from a space-occupying lesion such as a meningioma, aneurysm, or arteriovenous malformation.[20]

MEDICAL HISTORY AND PRESENTATION

As in the case of any facial pain, a detailed history must be ascertained; the vast majority of maxillofacial pain is due to a dental or oral mucosal issue.[21]

Patients with TN will describe sudden onset of unilateral, lancinating, short-lived pain, typically in the maxillary (V2) and mandibular (V3) divisions of the trigeminal nerve. They may first present to the dentist citing tooth pain as the cause of their symptoms. Triggers can be mechanical in nature, such as with toothbrushing or chewing, and symptoms are often provoked by light touch. Autonomic symptoms are absent, and other etiologies should be suspected in younger patients, those with bilateral symptoms, or if any focal neurologic deficits are present. Additionally, any history of facial trauma or complaint of unrelenting pain should raise suspicion for other conditions. Around 2% of patients with multiple sclerosis will develop secondary TN, and this may be characterized by bilateral involvement.[21]

PHYSICAL EXAMINATION

Physical examination may be unremarkable, but if in acute paroxysm, patients typically will wince in pain for the duration of the episode. This manifestation was the basis for TN originally being referred to as "tic douloureux."[20]

Additionally, sensory testing of the trigeminal nerve may elicit symptoms or reveal regions of hypoesthesia to light touch.[22]

In any case, a neurologic assessment is mandatory if TN is suspected. Any abnormalities in motor function, dysautonomia, or an examination revealing focal neurologic signs should warrant further workup for other pathologic states.

DIFFERENTIAL DIAGNOSIS

The differential diagnosis of TN is summarized in Table 15.3.

DIAGNOSTIC STUDIES

There is no definitive laboratory or imaging test for the diagnosis of TN; the diagnosis is clinical and based on the International Classification of Headache Disorders (ICHD-3 beta) criteria. This includes the following:[20]

1. At least three attacks of unilateral facial pain in one or more divisions of the trigeminal nerve with three out of the four following characteristics:
    a. Severe intensity
    b. Recurrent episodes lasting a split second to 2 minutes
    c. Provoked by innocuous stimuli
    d. Having a quality described as "shooting, electric shock-like, stabbing, or sharp"
2. No neurologic deficits on physical examination
3. No other diagnosis that would better explain the symptoms

Although the diagnosis is clinical, MRI of the brain is helpful in determining any areas of neurovascular compression and the degree to which nerve morphology has been affected. Any secondary causes of TN can also be elucidated with MRI, and this imaging is essential should the patient be considered as a surgical candidate. Neurophysiologic studies such as trigeminal evoked potentials may also be conducted to identify any lesions.[21]

TABLE 15.3 Differential Diagnosis of Trigeminal Neuralgia

Condition	Location	Symptoms	Demographic	Treatment
Trigeminal neuralgia	Unilateral, typically V2 and V3 distribution	Severe, stabbing, electric-shock-like pain lasting a second to 2 minutes Recurrent	Women > men Risk increases with age	Sodium channel blockers
Cluster headache	Unilateral, periorbital, temporal, or frontal	Episodes lasting 15 minutes to 3 hours, ptosis, lacrimation, miosis	Young men 18–40	100% oxygen Verapamil prophylaxis
Herpes zoster	Typically V1 distribution if trigeminal nerve affected	Constant, burning pain followed by eruption of vesicles in dermatomal pattern	Males and females age 60–70	Antivirals
Glossopharyngeal neuralgia	Tongue, tonsils, ear, larynx	Paroxysms similar in quality to trigeminal neuralgia	Women > men	Sodium channel blockers

Source: Maarbjerg S, Di Stefano G, Bendsten L, Cruccu G. *Trigeminal neuralgia—diagnosis and treatment.* Cephalalgia. *2017;37(7):648–657. doi:10.1177/0333102416687280*

EVALUATION

After secondary causes of symptoms have been ruled out and diagnosis of TN has been made, treatment can commence with medical therapy.

TREATMENT

First-line therapy of TN is pharmacologic intervention with sodium channel blockers. Carbamazepine has historically shown the greatest efficacy, but often high doses are needed for therapeutic effect and side effects may lead to intolerability. Serious side effects include aplastic anemia, hyponatremia, transaminitis, and a risk for Stevens-Johnson syndrome if positive for the HLA-B*15-02 allele.[21]

Consequently, regular monitoring with a CBC, metabolic panel, and liver function tests are important for all patients taking carbamazepine, and Asian patients should be screened for the aforementioned allele prior to commencing therapy. Oxcarbazepine is also considered first-line and has fewer medication interactions and better tolerability. Other antiepileptic drugs (AEDs), such as lamotrigine, may be added or used as monotherapy if carbamazepine or oxcarbazepine are ineffective or poorly tolerated.[21]

If pharmacologic intervention fails, various surgical options can be explored. Microvascular decompression has shown the greatest efficacy in symptom reduction but is highly invasive.[22]

Less invasive, but potentially less efficacious interventions involve percutaneous destruction of the Gasserian ganglion or gamma knife surgery to the trigeminal root.[22]

The pros and cons of each procedure must be discussed with the surgeon prior to any elective surgery.

PATIENT EDUCATION

Much of the patient education in TN revolves around the potential side effects of the pharmacologic agents employed and the necessity for frequent monitoring.

SPECIAL CONSIDERATIONS

Often, the debilitating and unpredictable nature of symptoms can lead to depression in patients with TN. In one report, 34% of patients with TN were even deleteriously impacted in their vocations, and many patients have reported fear and anxiety related to basic activities of daily living.[22]

Understanding the degree to which normal functioning can be impaired by this condition is of critical importance for the primary care clinician.

15.3 SEIZURE DISORDERS

Julie DesMarteau

OVERVIEW

Seizures are isolated episodes of neuronal dysrhythmia. A seizure disorder is an enduring predisposition to have recurrent seizures. The terms "seizure disorder" and "epilepsy" are generally used interchangeably.

The International League Against Epilepsy (ILAE) defines epilepsy as having had two unprovoked seizures, a single unprovoked seizure and an additional risk factor that indicates the person has at least a 60% chance of additional seizure activity unless treated, or the diagnosis of a specific epilepsy disorder.[23] Epilepsy is defined as a propensity for unprovoked seizures but it includes the interface between seizures and numerous neurobiologic, cognitive, emotional, and psychosocial comorbidities.

Epileptic seizures are divided into two categories: generalized and focal. Generalized seizures involve substantial parts of both cerebral hemispheres at the onset of the seizure and are believed to arise from broad dysfunction within the thalamocortical network. Focal seizures begin in one localized area of the brain that may or may not spread to involve more of the cortex. An individual can have more than one source of focal seizures, referred to as "multifocal epilepsy." Occasionally, an individual patient will have both types of seizures.

A new classification scheme was introduced by the ILAE in 2017, detailing the various types of seizures, epilepsies, and epilepsy syndromes (Table 15.4).[24,25] The new scheme makes it clear that focal and generalized seizures can present with identical symptoms.

Once the type of seizure is determined, the clinician can determine which type of epilepsy an individual may have, and in some cases, which epilepsy syndrome is present. The ILAE defines epilepsy syndromes as "a cluster of features incorporating seizure types, EEG, and imaging features that tend to occur together." Syndromes may have particular ages of onset and/or remission, seizure triggers, diurnal variation, and prognosis. They may also have characteristic comorbidities such as developmental or intellectual disabilities.[25]

Whether seizures are focal or generalized, they are considered "intractable," or "medically refractory" if the seizures remain uncontrolled despite therapeutic trials of two appropriate seizure medications used at therapeutic doses, concurrently or sequentially. Approximately one-third of cases of epilepsy are considered refractory to medication.

TABLE 15.4 International League Against Epilepsy 2017 Classification of Seizure Types

Focal Onset		Generalized Onset	Unknown Onset
Aware	Impaired Awareness	Motor Onset • Tonic-clonic • Clonic • Tonic • Myoclonic • Myoclonic-tonic-clonic • Myoclonic-atonic • Atonic • Epileptic spasms Nonmotor Onset • Typical • Atypical • Myoclonic • Eyelid myoclonia	Motor • Tonic-clonic • Epileptic spasms Nonmotor • Behavior arrest
Motor Onset • Automatisms • Atonic • Clonic • Epileptic spasms • Hyperkinetic • Myoclonic • Tonic Nonmotor Onset • Autonomic • Behavior arrest • Cognitive • Emotional • Sensory			Unclassified
Focal to bilateral tonic-clonic			

Source: Adapted with permission from Fisher RS, Cross JH, French JA, et al. Operational classification of seizure types by the International League Against Epilepsy: position paper of the ILAE Commission for Classification and Terminology. Epilepsia. *2017;58(4):522–530. doi:10.1111/epi.13670*

Treatment options for both intractable and nonintractable epilepsies are discussed below.

EPIDEMIOLOGY

According to the World Health Organization (WHO), 50 million people worldwide suffer from epilepsy.[26] A meta-analysis of international studies published in 2016 reported the point prevalence of active epilepsy was 6.38 per 1,000 persons, and the lifetime prevalence was 1.60 per 1,000. The annual incidence was 67.77 per 100,000 persons. The prevalence and incidence of epilepsy are higher in low and middle income countries.[27]

The Centers for Disease Control and Prevention (CDC) reported that 1.2% of the population in the United States reported having active epilepsy in 2015. This equates to roughly 3 million adults and 470,000 children with self-reported doctor-diagnosed epilepsy who were under treatment or reported a seizure within 12 months of the interview.[28] Similarly, results from the 2010–2013 National Health Interview Survey estimates approximately 1% of the U.S. population has active epilepsy.[29]

Incidence of epilepsy is highest in children and the elderly. Prevalence, however, is relatively low in childhood but increases through adolescence, adulthood, and old age. While some childhood-onset epilepsies persist throughout the lifetime, a number of epilepsy syndromes of childhood will resolve before adulthood. Incidence starts increasing again in older age due to risk factors such as stroke, or fall-related head injuries.[27,29–31]

PATHOPHYSIOLOGY

The pathophysiology of epilepsy is complex and varies from one case to the next. In general, seizures are the result of an imbalance between excitatory and inhibitory forces acting on neurons. The underlying cause of this imbalance is also variable. Any congenital or acquired condition may be epileptogenic if it increases brain tissue's propensity for abnormal excitation and synchronicity. Acquired conditions such as traumatic brain injuries (TBIs), strokes, anoxia, neoplasia, and infections can permanently alter brain tissue's propensity for abnormal excitation. Congenital causes are genetic disorders or developmental lesions (e.g., cortical dysplasia, heterotopia).

15.3A SEIZURE TYPES AND EPILEPSY

MEDICAL HISTORY AND CLINICAL PRESENTATION

Determining the age of onset can be helpful in determining if a particular epilepsy syndrome may be present. For example, childhood absence epilepsy typically presents between the ages of 4 and 8 years of age, while juvenile absence epilepsy has peak onset between the ages of 10 and 16.[32]

Risk factors for epilepsy include history of prematurity, febrile seizures, perinatal or traumatic brain injury, stroke, infection of the central nervous system (CNS), and a family history of seizures. However, in many cases the patient has no risk factors at all.

One concept that is confusing for patients is that of seizure provocation. By definition, epileptic seizures are "unprovoked," meaning that there is no major, acute force that is the direct, primary cause of neuronal misfiring. Nevertheless, the preexisting propensity for epileptic seizures can be exacerbated by particular stimuli such as illness, alcohol consumption, extreme stress, or sleep deprivation. Patients with "reflex" epilepsy will have seizures triggered by certain movements, noises, or other stimuli. While these seizures are elicited by circumstances, they would not occur without the underlying propensity of seizure activity to occur in the first place. This is what separates epileptic seizures elicited by provocative factors from purely "provoked seizures," seen in the context of acute head injury, CNS infection, withdrawal syndromes, medication nonadherance or other acute phenomena.

Timing, both in terms of the time of day and duration of the episode can also provide the clinician with clues as to the type of epilepsy an individual may have and whether their episodes are epileptic seizures at all. The majority of epileptic seizures will spontaneously end in <5 minutes. Additionally, certain seizure types and epilepsy syndromes have a diurnal variation. Primary generalized epilepsies with tonic-clonic and myoclonic seizures often manifest in the early morning hours. Seizures that occur shortly after falling asleep at night are often associated with frontal lobe epilepsy. Certain epilepsies, such as autosomal dominant nocturnal frontal lobe epilepsy (ADNFLE), manifest with seizures almost exclusively in sleep.

In addition to a detailed semiology, every visit note should reference the reported frequency of seizure activity. Patients should be encouraged to keep a seizure diary to facilitate accurate reporting. There are many "apps" available to track seizures. Keeping the information in a smart phone also decreases the chance that the patient will forget to bring it to the visit.

Finally, for patients with known epilepsy, inquiring about medication tolerance and compliance is of the utmost importance. Missed doses of AEDs is a common cause of status epilepticus and a risk factor for sudden unexpected death in epilepsy (SUDEP).[33,34] Failing to address medication side effects or barriers to compliance jeopardizes the patient's safety and quality of life.

SIGNS AND SYMPTOMS

The seizure semiology, which is a description of preictal, ictal, and postictal signs and symptoms of a seizure, is one of the most valuable pieces of information available to the clinician. There has been considerable data collection in this area, allowing clinicians to make educated determinations about the likely epileptogenic zone of the cortex. It is often necessary to interview both the patient and witnesses of the ictal event to obtain a comprehensive, detailed semiology. Whenever it is safe to do so, video recording of seizure events by friends and family members can be helpful.

Obtaining a detailed semiology can help the clinician determine if an individual has focal or generalized epilepsy (Tables 15.5 and 15.6). If focal, the semiology can also hold clues about the lateralization (left versus right) and localization of the lobe or specific structure from which the seizure may be originating.[35,36]

It is critical to document any injuries the patient has sustained as a result of their episodes, including tongue lacerations, joint dislocations, and damage from seizure-induced falls. Incidence of urinary and bowel incontinence should also be noted in the record. Make note of any urgent/emergent care visits between regular follow-ups. This history is

TABLE 15.5 Semiology of Focal Seizures and Corresponding Localization and Lateralization

Aura/Focal Seizure Without Loss of Awareness		Localizing	Lateralizing
Somatosensory (e.g., numbness or tingling)	Unilateral/small area	Primary sensory cortex	Contralateral
	Bilateral/larger area	Supplementary sensorimotor area (SSMA) or second somatosensory area (sylvian fissure/ posterior insula)	Not applicable (N/A)
Visual	Flashing lights in one particular visual field	Occipital lobe (primary and secondary visual cortex)	Contralateral
Auditory	Simple noises like a buzz	Temporal lobe (Heschl gyrus)	N/A
Olfactory	Smell	Mesial temporal lobe (especially amygdala)	N/A
Gustatory	Taste	Insula	N/A
Autonomic	Sweating, palpitations, piloerection	Insula	N/A
Abdominal	Many types of sensations in the abdomen; usually begins in the midline/epigastric area then rises up	Temporal lobe epilepsy; less frequently with frontal lobe or insula	N/A
Psychic	Complex hallucinations or sensations involving different senses (e.g., "out of body," deja vu, jamais vu, fear, ecstasy, unreality)	Most associated with temporal lobe epilepsy	N/A

considered when medical records are reviewed as part of disability determinations and can prompt the clinician to recommend specific safety measures, such as wearing a helmet.

In addition to giving a description of the episode(s) of presumed seizure activity that led the individual to seek medical attention, the patient may also report symptoms of depression, anxiety, and problems with concentration or memory. Insomnia and hypersomnolence are also common complaints, as are headaches. Especially once the diagnosis is clear, the chief complaint often shifts from the seizures to these other issues that tend to be more problematic on a day-to-day basis.

PHYSICAL EXAMINATION

Many patients with epilepsy present with a nonfocal neurologic examination. A complete examination must be conducted, however, as subtle findings, such as a unilaterally decreased nasolabial fold, can suggest an occult lesion, substantiating the need for imaging. If the epilepsy is due to a traumatic or perinatal brain injury, stroke, or similar cause, then deficits can exist concordant with those injuries. These sorts of deficits are often obvious to the clinician and known to the patient.

The examination should not be limited to the neurologic system. Certain genetic conditions associated with seizures can also cause abnormal findings in other systems, such as the pathognomonic skin lesions seen on patients with tuberous sclerosis and Sturge-Weber syndrome. The clinician must also complete at least a basic cardiovascular examination to assess for risk factors that could contribute to the formation of a seizure focus (e.g., arrhythmia or bruit suggesting higher stroke risk).

When patients present with a sudden exacerbation of a known seizure disorder, the clinician should check for signs and symptoms of ear, nose, throat, or bladder infections. Even minor infections can be a trigger for worsening seizure activity.

Certain AEDs may be responsible for abnormal exam findings, particularly when the levels are high. Nystagmus and ataxia can indicate AED toxicity. Patients on phenytoin should also be checked for gingival hyperplasia. Weight is important to monitor with valproate, which frequently contributes to weight gain, and topiramate/zonisamide which are more likely to contribute to weight loss. Tremor and mild peripheral edema are also side effects of several common AEDs.

DIFFERENTIAL DIAGNOSIS

When a patient presents with new-onset seizure-like activity, the first priority is to identify any provocative factors that require emergency treatment. Examples include fever in children, acute injury, alcohol/drug withdrawal, eclampsia, uremia, metabolic derangement, CNS infection, very low or very high blood glucose, or hypoxemia. Once a "provoked seizure" has been ruled out in the acute care setting, the clinician can turn the focus to other common conditions that are easily mistaken for epileptic seizures.

Nonepileptic attack disorder (NEAD) is also referred to as nonepileptic events (NEE), pseudoseizures, and psychogenic nonepileptic seizures (PNES). Psychiatric comorbidities, history of abuse or trauma, fibromyalgia, family dysfunction, and vague somatic complaints are common in patients with NEAD.

In addition to patient characteristics, qualities of the episodes themselves can offer clues as to whether an episode is a seizure or nonepileptic attack (Box 15.1). While helpful, these qualities are not diagnostic.

Differentiating NEAD from epilepsy is complicated by the fact that around 10% of people with NEAD will also have documented epilepsy (reports vary from 5% to 50%).[37] This particular patient population presents a major challenge to the clinician. Even when their epileptic seizures are well controlled, these "mixed type" patients have very poor quality of life outcomes when their NEAD is not treated.

NEAD may be the most common mimicker of epilepsy (especially among adolescents and adults), but there are multiple physiologic conditions that may also be difficult to differentiate from epilepsy. Breath-holding spells and benign shudder attacks are mostly limited to the pediatric population, while transient ischemic attacks (TIAs) and transient

TABLE 15.6 Semiology of Generalized Seizures and Corresponding Localization and Lateralization

Seizure Type	Description	Localizing	Lateralizing
Myoclonic	Short (<200 ms) muscle contractions Usually seen in generalized epilepsies, but can be associated with focal epilepsy	N/A	Not applicable (N/A)
Tonic	Sustained muscle contractions creating a sustained, rigid posture	Frontal lobe > parietal; occipital > temporal	Contralateral (if seizure contractions are unilateral); contralateral to the arm raised in "fencing posture" and the arm extended in "sign of four" posture
Clonic	Rapidly recurring, rhythmic myoclonic contractions	If clonus begins before the impairment of awareness it is more likely that the seizure focus is within the primary motor strip. The face, eyes, and hands tend to be impacted before the lower extremities when clonic activity occurs with temporal lobe seizures.	Focal seizures with clonus may begin on the side contralateral to the seizure focus and, conversely, end with greater clonic activity on the ipsilateral side.
Tonic-clonic	A seizure with a tonic phase that progresses to clonic contractions	"Pure" tonic clonic seizures are associated with generalized epilepsies. Focal seizures can have tonic and clonic components, but it is usually preceded by other types of seizure activity and is often asymmetric.	N/A
Atonic	A sudden loss in postural tone causing a fall or head drop	Usually generalized but has been seen in focal epilepsy, especially frontal and temporal; usually the fall is not as fast/hard with focal atonic seizures as it is when generalized	N/A
Akinetic	Inability to perform movements in an otherwise conscious and cooperative patient	Negative motor areas in the mesial frontal and inferior frontal gyri	N/A
Epileptic spasm	Relatively symmetric tonic or myoclonic contractions favoring the proximal axial muscles	Usually generalized but has been seen in focal epilepsy, especially with parieto-occipital onset	N/A
Hyperkinetic	Involve a lot of large, complicated movement such as thrashing or thrusting movements, bicycling of legs, running, etc.	Most associated with orbital and mesial frontal regions, but can occur with temporal and insular epilepsies	N/A
Automotor/ automatisms	Much more subtle than hyperkinetic movement, these involve distal regions such as hands, feet, and tongue (fumbling motions in hands, lip smacking, etc.)	Temporal and frontal lobe epilepsies. Temporal lobe automotor seizures tend to be longer than those from the frontal lobe.	If movements are unilateral, they are usually ipsilateral to the seizure focus. In the rare case of an automotor seizure with preserved consciousness, the non-dominant mesial temporal lobe is usually the focus.

BOX 15.1 Characteristics of Nonepileptic Attacks

- Prolonged events
- Single patient reports many different semiologies
- Biting tip of tongue instead of the side
- Crying during the event
- Closing the eyes during the event
- Head shaking side to side
- Asynchronous alternating right-left movements
- Not responding to antiseizure medication
- Pelvic thrusting
- Prolonged major bilateral motor manifestation without loss of awareness

global amnesia (TGA) are more common in older adults. Panic attacks, migraines, parasomnias, movement disorders (e.g., tics, dystonia), syncope, and cardiac arrhythmia may all present with signs and symptoms that could suggest an epileptic disorder.

Additionally, it is critical to consult cardiology if there is any concern for arrhythmia.

DIAGNOSTIC STUDIES

Neurophysiology

ELECTROENCEPHALOGRAM

EEG is arguably the most important study in the evaluation of epilepsy. Electrodes glued to the scalp are used to record the electrical waves generated by neuronal activity. Trained neurophysiologists can detect particular discharges or patterns from the EEG that may indicate what sort of seizure disorder a person has. There is also usually a single EKG lead to monitor heart rhythm. This diminishes the chance of missing a seizure that is induced by an arrhythmia and detects peri-ictal bradycardia or other abnormalities that could signal a higher risk of SUDEP.

The main weakness of EEG is that it has a low detection rate of seizures without loss of awareness. This makes it very difficult to distinguish between "focal aware" seizures and mimickers of epilepsy. Another limitation is that an EEG without abnormalities does not exclude the possibility of an epileptic disorder. Many patients with epilepsy do not have consistent epileptiform abnormalities between seizures. A single routine interictal recording has only a 50% to 55% sensitivity.[38]

While EEG tracings provide objective data, they are reviewed and summarized by a physician. There is a considerable degree of subjectivity in that review process. It is common for readers to have different opinions about the significance of the EEG, even at expert levels.

VIDEO EEG

Video EEG (VEEG) is the gold standard test for the diagnosis of epilepsy. This test is usually completed over a longer time period (several hours or days) and creates a visual and auditory recording of the patient along with the EEG.

HIGH DENSITY EEG

Standard EEG recordings utilize 21 electrodes placed at prespecified locations on the scalp. High-density EEGs (HD EEGs) are systems of over 250 electrodes that can be efficiently secured to the scalp and face for optimal source localization of epileptiform discharges. Because the volume of data generated is so large, additional staff training and time is needed. This extra data can be helpful in the pre-surgical evaluation process to assist in confirming the likely focus of seizure onset.

INTRACRANIAL EEG

It is not always possible to determine the seizure focus using EEG electrodes glued to the scalp. If initial studies have generated a strong hypothesis about the location of a seizure focus, surgical electrodes can be placed directly on the brain. This greatly reduces the chance of a seizure falsely localizing or lateralizing on scalp EEG due to a complicated neural pathway. Grids or strips of electrodes can be used to monitor and map areas of cortex. In addition to localizing seizure onset, stimulating the different electrodes helps the epileptologist determine which areas are safe to resect, and which might involve critical motor areas or eloquent cortex. Thin depth electrodes can be used to assess deeper structures with a technique referred to as stereo EEG (SEEG).

Imaging

BRAIN CT

CT is of limited use in the comprehensive evaluation of seizures. However, CT scans are useful in urgent care settings when patients present with a focal neurologic deficit following an acute onset of seizure activity. A CT scan may also be necessary if a patient is known or suspected to have suffered a head injury as the result of a seizure. Many patients will present in postictal stupor, unable to participate in a neurologic examination. Rapid imaging of the head is appropriate in this circumstance to rule out a serious injury or hemorrhage.

BRAIN MRI

MRI is the most frequently used imaging technology in the evaluation of epilepsy. Many of the lesions that cause focal epilepsy are subtle and require high-resolution scans for detection. Imaging is worth repeating in refractory patients if previous "normal" scans are outdated or lower resolution. Even when generalized epilepsy is strongly suspected, an MRI is usually performed to rule out a deep focus that could lead to generalized findings on an EEG.

POSITRON EMISSION TOMOGRAPHY

Studies have demonstrated [^{18}F]fluoro-2-deoxyglucose (^{18}F-FDG) PET imaging of brain glucose metabolism has reasonable sensitivity in the lateralization and localization of epileptogenic zones in refractory focal epilepsy.

SINGLE PHOTON EMISSION COMPUTED TOMOGRAPHY

Single photon emission computed tomography (SPECT) imaging for focal epilepsy measures blood flow to brain by injecting radionucleotides at the onset of a seizure. The nucleotide uptake by brain cells is directly related to the amount of blood flow at the time of injection. Any areas of hyperperfusion may suggest a seizure focus. This image is referred to as the ictal SPECT scan. The same study is usually repeated on a different day when the patient has not had any recent seizures to determine perfusion differences. This second study is referred to as the interictal SPECT scan.

MAGNETOENCEPHALOGRAPHY

Magnetoencephalography (MEG) is reserved for focal epilepsy. MEG uses hundreds of magnetic sensors to directly measure neuronal function. MEG can assess spontaneous activity (e.g., epileptiform discharges) or be used to map brain function (e.g., motor, language, and visual mapping). MEG technology is not widely available but is utilized at some epilepsy centers.

WADA TEST

A Wada test (WAH-dah, named for Japanese physician, Dr. Juan Wada) is sometimes referred to as an intracarotid sodium amobarbital test, although sodium amobarbital is not always the anesthetic used.

FUNCTIONAL MRI

Functional MRI (fMRI) is being used more frequently as part of the presurgical evaluation for patients with focal epilepsies. Lateralization of language dominance to the left or right hemisphere is readily accomplished with fMRI, but memory assessment can be difficult with this modality. Some epilepsy centers have developed protocols to assess memory using semantic language tasks as a proxy. Research on these protocols is ongoing.

Other

GENETICS

Genetic testing was once limited to academic interests, or to bring the peace of knowledge to patients and families struggling to come to terms with a diagnosis. More recently, genetic testing has started to guide patient care plans, and is becoming more helpful in giving an accurate prognosis. A clinician specializing in epilepsy must stay informed of updates concerning phenotypes related to various genetic epilepsies.

NEUROPSYCHOLOGY

The purpose of the neuropsychological evaluation is to learn about the patient's cognitive abilities using a variety of validated assessment tools. Areas of focus are usually memory, executive functioning, and language skills. The patient's psychological status is also assessed, as depression and anxiety are prevalent in patients with epilepsy. A number of "effort measures" are embedded in the evaluation to screen for indications of non-neurologic explanations for poor performance, including malingering.

EVALUATION

The evaluation of a patient with epilepsy is a highly individualized process. Patients who respond to medications with no bothersome side effects may require only a very brief assessment to ensure the underlying cause of the seizures is not life threatening (e.g., imaging to rule out a tumor). Patients with a clinical history and EEG suggesting generalized epilepsy do not require imaging in most cases although patient expectations often compel the clinician to obtain a routine MRI. When epilepsy proves to be refractory, a multidisciplinary evaluation is essential to provide comprehensive care and efficacious, evidence-based treatment. This type of evaluation is completed at a Comprehensive Epilepsy Center accredited by the National Association of Epilepsy Centers. Patients who continue to have seizures after 1 year under the care of a general neurologist should be referred to an epileptologist.

TREATMENT

While there are many considerations to keep in mind when selecting treatments for seizures, it is essential to center discussion of all possible therapies around the patient's concerns and priorities. When appropriate, involvement of family and caregivers can offer further guidance to ensure the care plan reflects not only evidence-based practice, but the patient's values and autonomy as well.

Many of the treatments below can be used for focal and generalized epilepsies. Medications used for focal, generalized, or both types of epilepsy are discussed below. Surgery to remove a seizure focus and responsive neurostimulation are only appropriate for patients with focal epilepsy. In the United States, vagus nerve and deep brain stimulators currently have FDA indications for focal epilepsy, but both modalities have clinical utility for generalized epilepsy as well. Vagus nerve stimulation in particular is frequently used for both focal and generalized epilepsy.

Lifestyle Modifications (Focal and Generalized Seizures)

Behavioral choices can impact seizure control in many ways. Patients are encouraged to avoid common triggers such as excessive alcohol consumption and sleep deprivation. Behaviors such as maintaining personal hygiene and getting timely vaccinations can minimize the risk of seizure-inducing infections. Research shows improved seizure control in patients who practice relaxation techniques (e.g., deep breathing, visual imagery) on a regular basis as well as when they experience signs of oncoming seizure activity. Multiple studies have linked a high sense of self-efficacy with improved self-management of seizure disorders. There are several validated programs that focus on enhancing individual self-efficacy and self-management abilities.[39,40]

Medications (Focal and Generalized Seizures)

While the importance of lifestyle modification is too often underestimated, it is usually not sufficient to prevent further seizure activity in someone with epilepsy. Medications are typically the first line of defense against seizure recurrence. Table 15.7 features a summary of medications for focal and generalized seizures. The arsenal of anticonvulsant medications contains a variety of options for both focal and generalized types of seizure disorders. Despite the increasing number of medications available, the overall percentage of patients not responding to any single or combination of medications has remained static at 30% to 35%. Newer generation AEDs tend to be superior in terms of tolerability but are not necessarily more effective than their predecessors.

When determining what medication to prescribe, the clinician considers many factors, such as the type of epilepsy needing treatment (focal, generalized, or undetermined), concerns about tolerability, comorbidities, teratogenicity, likelihood of compliance, compatibility with other medications, and cost. Most seizure medications can be used for focal onset seizures. In contrast, there are several medications that are best avoided in cases of generalized epilepsy, especially when the patient has myoclonic seizures. It is best to stick with broad-spectrum agents when the classification of epilepsy is uncertain.

The most desirable end point in the treatment of seizure disorders is "no seizures, no side effects." This may not always be attainable, but independent of seizure control, preventing or minimizing adverse effects of medications is a priority when developing a care plan. Any mediation can cause any side effect, in anyone, at any time, and at any dose. Reducing the dose and following a slower titration, taking the medication with food, and using a longer acting version of the medication if available are all common strategies to enhance tolerability.

Lack of adherence to prescribed anticonvulsant medications is a frequent cause of seizures in people with otherwise controlled epilepsy. Patients can be educated on medication management strategies for optimal medication compliance (e.g., pill organizers, reminder alarms) and family and friends should double check (Box 15.2).

In the United States, all AEDs have a black box warning about suicidality due to a correlation found between AED use and suicide attempts. At this time, patients should be advised to contact their clinician right away if they experience thoughts of self-harm. When necessary the patient should be contracted for safety and advised of emergency resources in case of suicidality.

Resective Surgery (Focal Seizures Only)

It is sometimes possible to identify the source of focal seizures. When an individual has a single seizure focus, it may be possible to surgically resect or ablate that portion of brain tissue. Extensive testing is required to ensure the seizure focus is accurately identified and determine that the individual is unlikely to suffer significant cognitive deficits from the resection. The latter is a point of some conjecture, as chronically uncontrolled epilepsy is known to contribute to cognitive deficits as well. In some cases, the cognitive risks posed by surgery may be favorable to the cognitive decline anticipated with ongoing uncontrolled seizure activity. The risk to benefit analysis requires consideration of each patient's presurgical abilities and postsurgical goals. Surgical procedures for epilepsy have historically required a craniotomy. At this time, some laser technologies are available that can offer a less invasive approach. While healing time is reduced, less is known about the long-term efficacy of this approach.

TABLE 15.7 Common Drugs and Side Effects for Focal and Generalized Seizures

Drug	Primary Use	Side Effects	Pharmacology
Brivaracetam Tablet Liquid IV	Focal but may have potential for broader use	*Common*: GI distress, headache, fatigue, dizziness, nystagmus, poor coordination *Serious*: angioedema, leukopenia, neutropenia, psychosis	MOA: high and specific affinity for synaptic vesicle protein 2A (SV2A) in the brain which modulates neurotransmitter release Half-life: 9 hr
Carbamazepine Liquid Tablet Chewable Capsule	Focal May worsen myoclonus	*Common*: anemia, anorexia, diarrhea, elevated LFTs (especially with concomitant valproate use), fatigue, dizziness, poor coordination, sleep disruption *Serious*: angioedema	MOA: neuronal inhibition via synaptic and extrasynaptic GABA channels, modulation of intracellular calcium, and possible anti-inflammatory effects related to interaction with adenosine Half-life: 56–61 hr
Cannabidiol Oil	Severe epilepsy (mainly LGS and Dravet syndrome)	*Common*: GI distress, hyponatremia, rash, fatigue, dizziness, headache, diplopia or blurred vision, fluid retention *Serious*: agranulocytosis, bone marrow suppression, SIADH, SJS/TEN, liver failure, pancreatitis, iatrogenic lupus, hypogammaglobulinemia	MOA: promote fast inactivation of Na channels Half-life: initial: 25–65 hr immediate release, 3–40 extended release; later: 3–20 hr in children, 12–17 hr adults
Clonazepam Tablet ODT	Myoclonic, atonic	*Common*: drowsiness, ataxia, behavior problems, dizziness, cognitive impairment, slurred speech, paradoxical reaction (agitation, hostility), withdrawal syndrome *Serious*: leukopenia, thrombocytopenia, respiratory depression	MOA: binds at the benzodiazepine site of the GABAA receptor to potentiate GABAergic neurotransmission Half-life: 20–40 hr
Clobazam Tablet Liquid Oral film	Broad spectrum mostly for intractable epilepsy	*Common*: drowsiness, drooling, aggression, respiratory infection, fever, poor coordination, slurred speech, withdrawal syndrome *Serious*: angioedema, eosinophilia, hallucination, hypothermia, increased liver enzymes, leukopenia, SSJ/ TEN, thrombocytopenia, urinary retention, respiratory depression	MOA: binds at the benzodiazepine site of the GABAA receptor to potentiate GABAergic neurotransmission Half-life: 16 hr pediatric, 36–42 hr adult; Active metabolite: 36–42 hr
Eslicarbazepine Tablet	Focal May worsen myoclonus	*Common*: GI distress, hyponatremia (usually mild), rash, dizziness, drowsiness, headache, poor coordination, vision change, tremor *Serious*: SJS, DRESS, prolonged PR interval, angioedema, AV block	MOA: inhibition of Na channels Half-life: 10–16 hr pediatric, 13–20 hr adult
Ethosuximide Capsule Liquid	Absence (generalized)	*Common*: GI distress, sleep disturbance, drowsiness, headache *Serious*: agranulocytosis, SJS/TEN, aplastic anemia, liver failure	MOA: inhibition of voltage-sensitive sodium and calcium channels, reduction of glutamergic transmission through modulation of NMDA receptors, and potentiation of GABA transmission Half-life: 30–60 hr
Felbamate Tablet Liquid	Broad spectrum (usually for specialist use only)	Common: anorexia, weight loss, GI distress, insomnia, somnolence, headache Serious: rare aplastic anemia, irreversible liver failure	MOA: blocks glycine from NMDA receptors Half-life: 14–23 hr
Gabapentin Tablet Liquid Capsule	Focal	*Common*: weight gain, somnolence, dizziness, ataxia, GI distress, peripheral edema, hyponatremia Serious: multiorgan hypersensitivity, angioedema, DRESS, erythema multiforme, SJS, rhabdomyolysis	MOA: modulates release of excitatory neurotransmitters from presynaptic calcium channels with alpha-1 delta-2 subunit Half-life: 5–9 hr
Lacosamide Tablet Liquid IV	Focal	*Common*: GI distress, ataxia, dizziness (especially when used concomitantly with other Na channel blockers), headache, diplopia, fatigue *Serious*: Atrial fibrillation/flutter, PR prolongation (1st degree block), multi-organ hypersensitivity (rash, eosinophilia, stupor, hepatitis, fever), neutropenia	MOA: selective Na channel slow inactivation, binding to CRMP-2 Half-life: 13 hr
Lamotrigine Tablet Chewable ODT	Broad spectrum May worsen myoclonus	*Common*: fatigue, drowsiness, tremor, headache, nausea, diplopia, nystagmus *Serious*: SJS (high risk if rapidly titrated)/TEN, multiorgan hypersensitivity, aseptic meningitis, hypogammaglobulinemia	MOA: blocks Na channels and blocks release of glutamate Half-life: 12–50 (up to 70 hr when co-administered with valproate)
Levetiracetam Tablet Liquid IV ODT	Broad spectrum	*Common*: irritability, anxiety, depression, somnolence, dizziness *Serious*: SJS/TEN, angioedema, psychosis, pancytopenia, hypogammaglobulinemia	MOA: inhibits calcium channels; facilitation of GABA; reduction of delayed potassium current; and/or binding to synaptic proteins which modulate neurotransmitter release Half-life: 7 hr

TABLE 15.7 Common Drugs and Side Effects for Focal and Generalized Seizures *(continued)*

Drug	Primary Use	Side Effects	Pharmacology
Oxcarbazepine Tablet Liquid	Focal May worsen myoclonus	*Common*: headache, drowsiness, GI distress, dizziness, hyponatremia, psychomotor slowing, ataxia, visual changes *Serious*: SJS/TEN, multiorgan hypersensitivity, agranulocytosis, pancytopenia, leukopenia	MOA: modulate Na channels Half-life: 1–2.5 hr, metabolite 12 hr
Perampanel Tablet	Focal and generalized tonic-clonic	*Common*: dizziness, headache, fatigue, hyponatremia, UTI, muscle/joint pain, hypertriglyceridemia, GI distress, weight gain, gait problems/falls *Serious*: hostility & aggression, psychosis, DRESS	MOA: noncompetitive antagonist of the (AMPA) glutamate receptor on postsynaptic neurons Half-life: 105 hr
Phenobarbital Tablet Liquid IV	Broad spectrum	*Common*: mood changes, ataxia, confusion, dizziness, drowsiness, hallucination, headache, impaired cognition, insomnia, urinary retention *Serious*: SJS, bradycardia, agranulocytosis, thrombocytopenia, megaloblastic anemia, laryngospasm, respiratory depression, decreased bone density with long-term use	MOA: enhances GABA-mediated chloride channel opening Half-life: 40–140 hr
Phenytoin Capsule Chewable Liquid IV	Broad spectrum May worsen myoclonus	*Common*: gingival hyperplasia, hirsuitism, coarsening features, acne, folate deficiency, rash, nystagmus, ataxia, lethargy *Serious*: SJS/TEN, agranulocytosis, aplastic anemia, liver failure, DRESS, hypersensitivity reaction, adenopathy, neuropathy, iatrogenic lupus, pseudolymphoma	MOA: modulate Na channels Half-life: 5–34 hr
Pregabalin Capsule	Focal	*Common*: peripheral edema, increased appetite, weight gain, constipation, xerostomia, ataxia, dizziness, somnolence, visual changes *Serious*: myopathy, angioedema, rhabdomyolysis, hypersensitivity reaction	MOA: binds to the alpha(2)-delta site; reduces the Ca-dependent release of several neurotransmitters Half-life: 6–7 hr
Primidone Tablet	Broad spectrum	*Common*: dizziness, headache, fatigue, hyponatremia, UTI, muscle/joint pain, hypertriglyceridemia, GI distress, weight gain, gait problems/falls *Serious*: hostility & aggression, psychosis, DRESS	MOA: primidone has two active metabolites, phenobarbital and phenylethylmalonamide (PEMA); PEMA may enhance the activity of phenobarbital Half-life: 3–7 hr (metabolites: PEMA 30–36; phenobarbital 40–140 hours)
Rufinamide Tablet Liquid	Broad spectrum (most often used with LGS)	*Common*: headache, somnolence, ataxia, dizziness, gait changes, nausea, diplopia *Serious*: SJS/TEN, multiorgan hypersensitivity reaction, QT shortening (usually not significant unless patient has preexisting short QT syndrome)	MOA: prolongs inactivation of Na channels Half-life: 6–10 hr
Topiramate Tablet Capsules	Broad spectrum	*Common*: cognitive slowing, impaired word finding, somnolence, anorexia, weight loss, diarrhea, hyperthermia, acute myopia, closed angle glaucoma, paresthesia (especially in fingers), anxiety/mood problems *Serious*: urolithiasis, SJS/TEN, acute myopia and closed angle glaucoma, oligohidrosis and hyperthermia	MOA: blocks Na channels, enhances GABA, antagonizes AMPA/kainite glutamate receptors Half-life: 21 hr
Valproic Acid Tablet Capsules Liquid IV	Broad spectrum	*Common*: weight gain, GI distress, alopecia, bruising, tremor *Serious*: agranulocytosis, SJS/TEN, aplastic anemia, hypersensitivity reaction, thrombocytopenia, liver failure (high risk in <2 yr old), pancreatitis, bruising, PCOS, hypogammaglobulinemia	MOA: promotes GABA in several ways (including inhibiting GABA-T which breaks down GABA and activating GAD for GABA synthesis), blocks sodium channels and to a lesser degree blocks T-type calcium channels Half-life: 7–13 hours children 2 m–2 y, 9 hr ages 2–14, 9–19 hr adults
Vigabatrin Tablet Powder sachets	Infantile spasms & intractable focal seizures (specialist use only)	*Common*: weight gain, drowsiness, headache, dizziness, ataxia, behavior problems, weight gain, infection, insomnia, sedation, rash, GI distress, tremor, fever, nystagmus *Serious*: permanent loss of peripheral visual fields, MRI abnormalities of unknown clinical significance, mood problems, psychosis, SJS/TEN, multiorgan failure, malignant hyperthermia	MOA: reduces breakdown of GABA by inhibiting GABA-T Half-life: 5–6 hours in infants, 5–10 hr children; 10.5 hr adults
Zonisamide Capsules	Broad spectrum	*Common*: anorexia, weight loss, GI distress, somnolence, agitation, mood problems, dizziness, paresthesia, vision changes *Serious*: aplastic anemia, oligohidrosis with hyperthermia (especially in children), psychosis, urolithiasis, leukopenia, metabolic acidosis	MOA: modulates Na and T-type Ca channels Half-life: 50–68 hr

AMPA, a-amino-3-hydroxy-5-methyl-4-isoxazolepropionic acid; AV, atrioventricular; CRMP-2, collapsin response mediator protein-2; DRESS, drug reaction with eosinophilia and systemic symptoms; GABA, gamma-aminobutyric acid; GABA-T, GABA transaminase; GAD, glutamic acid decarboxylase; GI, gastrointestinal; IV, intravenous; LFTs, liver function tests; LGS, Lennox-Gastaut syndrome; MOA, mechanism of action; NMDA, N-methyl-D-aspartate; ODT, orally dissolving tablet; PCOS, polycystic ovary syndrome; SIADH, syndrome of inappropriate antidiuretic hormone secretion; SJS, Stevens-Johnson syndrome; TEN, toxic epidermal necrolysis; UTI, urinary tract infection.

BOX 15.2 Education About Antiepileptic Drugs

Include the following recommendations:
Avoid activities requiring alertness/coordination until drug effects are realized.
Avoid sudden discontinuation of drug in non-emergent situations.
If drug is stopped for more than a day or two, do not restart without first consulting a healthcare professional.
Do not take within 2 hours of antacids.
Medications are generally better tolerated when taken with food.
Take medication as consistently as possible.
If you miss a dose take it as soon as you realized it was missed unless it is only 2 hours until the next dose, in which case you should take the next dose early.
Note red flag signs of any serious side effects, and follow instructions on next steps if they occur.

Stimulators

There are several approved methods for treating medically refractory epilepsy with neurostimuation. The focus of these devices is to improve seizure frequency and intensity. They are all valuable weapons in the arsenal for fighting epilepsy, but they have low likelihood of resulting in seizure freedom. It is recommended that they be used adjunctively with medication, not as stand-alone therapies. Responsive neurostimulation is only appropriate for patients with focal epilepsy. In the United States, vagus nerve and deep brain stimulators currently have FDA indications for focal epilepsy, but both modalities have clinical utility for generalized epilepsy as well.

Vagus Nerve Stimulators

In the United States this use is approved for the treatment of refractory partial onset seizures in patients age 12 and older. In clinical practice, however, the vagus nerve stimulators (VNS) is often used successfully in much younger patients and for generalized epilepsy as well.[41,42]

Responsive Neurostimulators

Use of responsive neurostimulators (RNS) is approved for treatment of refractory focal onset epilepsy in patients age 18 and up but has been used in children as well. Unlike other stimulators, RNS cannot be used in the treatment of generalized epilepsy.

Diet (Focal and Generalized Epilepsy)

Ketogenic diets for epilepsy were created as a means of "tricking" the brain into the same pattern of energy utilization that it relies on during times of starvation. This has the desirable impact on neuronal function but prevents malnutrition by providing adequate calories and a reasonable amount of protein. The registered dietitian ensures that the calorie and protein goals are met through the diet, and micronutrients are supplied through a variety of nutritional supplements. Long-term compliance is poor in older patients, but the diet can be effective in any age group.[43]

PATIENT EDUCATION

When initiating patient education, seizure safety precautions and first aid must be prioritized. Adults and adolescents with uncontrolled seizures must be counseled on the driving restrictions in their state, province, or country. Potential consequences of failing to comply with these regulations should be explicitly reviewed. Restrictions related to heavy machinery should typically apply to driving. Other advisable restrictions are to avoid being at heights unless appropriately restrained, avoid hot surfaces and open flames, and avoid water in which one could drown (including baths) unless appropriately supervised by someone capable of performing a water rescue. Many clinicians will explicitly caution against using firearms or working in tight spaces where suffocation could occur or rescue would be impeded.

People with seizures should be counseled to avoid activities in which a sudden loss of awareness or motor control would result in serious injury occurring to themselves or others. This constant risk/benefit analysis contributes to anxiety. "Seizure worry" often causes distress and may negatively impact quality of life of both the patient and their loved ones.[44] Helping the patient to find a balance between reasonable safety precautions and excessive worry is one of the most difficult but vital tasks for the compassionate clinician.

Education of women of childbearing potential with epilepsy is a topic that has gained much-needed attention. Proper education and prophylactic measures for this population is covered by the Quality Measurement Set supported by the American Academy of Neurology. The AAN advises that women with epilepsy be counseled on the impact of epilepsy on contraception and/or pregnancy at least annually, and that this population be supplemented with folic acid. Rates of unintended pregnancy among women with epilepsy are 55% to 65%, significantly higher than in the general population. The reasons are multifactorial, but the impact of many AEDs on oral contraceptive efficacy is a major factor. It is the clinician's responsibility to advise patients about the relationship between contraceptives and AEDs. Progesterone-based contraceptives tend to have fewer worrisome drug–drug interactions.

The AAN guidelines also emphasize the importance of counseling women about the potential for AEDs to cause congenital malformations as well as cognitive delays and behavioral issues.[45]

One of the most difficult conversations a clinician must initiate relates to sudden unexpected death in epilepsy (SUDEP). This topic was overlooked for many years out of concern that it would cause unnecessary distress to the patients and their families. However, SUDEP is now well documented and, if properly educated, patients can take steps to minimize their risk.

SUDEP describes the following scenarios[46]:

- A person with epilepsy dies suddenly or unexpectedly.
- Death may be witnessed or unwitnessed.
- Death is not due to trauma, drowning, and/or status epilepticus.
- Postmortem examination does not reveal a cause of death.

- Death is usually (but not always) preceded by a seizure, and frequently occurs during sleep.

In the absence of a postmortem examination, the death may be termed "probable SUDEP." If there is an alternative explanation for the death in addition to SUDEP, it may be termed "possible SUDEP."

Most cases of SUDEP occur during or immediately after a seizure. Thorough a complicated multidirectional pathophysiologic pathway, breathing patterns are disrupted, resulting in bradycardia and then asystole.[46]

Nonmodifiable risk factors include age (20–40), gender (M>F), genetic predisposition, epilepsy onset before age 16, epilepsy duration >15 years, and intellectual disability. Other risk factors include treatment-resistant seizures, nocturnal seizures, sleeping alone and unmonitored, sleeping in prone position, history of three or more convulsions within 12 months, poor compliance with treatment and/or subtherapeutic AED levels, sudden and frequent changes in AEDs, excessive alcohol use, and other psychiatric comorbidities.[33]

Steps patients and families can take to reduce risk of SUDEP include:

- Minimizing seizures by avoiding triggers and adhering to treatment regimen
- Avoidance of alcohol
- Getting enough sleep, not sleeping on stomach
- Consider a seizure monitor or other device to alert others if you have a seizure
- Training those who interact with patients with epilepsy in seizure first aid and cardiopulmonary resuscitation (CPR)

15.3B STATUS EPILEPTICUS

MEDICAL HISTORY AND CLINICAL PRESENTATION

Status epilepticus (SE) is seizure activity that extends beyond the time frame when seizures typically resolve spontaneously. The failure of usual seizure-ending mechanisms may lead to one prolonged seizure, or multiple seizures without return to baseline in between ictal events. The ILAE recognizes two distinct time points when describing SE: T1 and T2. T1 is the point in time when the typical mechanisms that lead to seizure cessation are deemed to have failed and external intervention is warranted. T2 is the point in time when the prolonged seizure is anticipated to cause neuronal injury, death, or other long-term alteration in function.[47] The commonly used practical definition of SE is the occurrence of more than 5 minutes of continuous seizure activity, or multiple seizures without a complete recovery between seizures.

EPIDEMIOLOGY

SE and epilepsy have much in common, but they are not synonymous. Fewer than half of people with SE have epilepsy, and only about 15% of people with epilepsy will ever experience SE. Studies from a number of developed countries have reported 10 to 20 cases per 100,000 persons per year, but some studies report 40 or more cases per 100,000 persons per year.[34,48]

The frequency of etiologies of SE will vary by age. Febrile seizures account for over half of the cases of SE in children, while acute stroke, hypoxia, and metabolic derangements are the most common causes among older adults. The most common cause of SE among people with epilepsy is subtherapeutic levels of their anticonvulsant medication (usually attributed to noncompliance). Occasionally, an episode of SE may be the presenting seizure in a case of new onset epilepsy.[34,48,49]

When handling SE, treating any identifiable underlying causes is of utmost importance. Sometimes, however, the etiology of SE is unknown. This is the case with new-onset refractory status epilepticus (NORSE). With this life-threatening condition, a person without previous history of seizures will begin seizing for the first time and develop refractory SE within several days. If the individual has a history of fever of any duration within the 24 hours to 2 week period prior to developing NORSE, it is referred to as FIRES (febrile infection-related epilepsy syndrome). Both conditions have a poor prognosis and require an extensive multidisciplinary evaluation, aggressive treatment, and intense supportive care.[49,50]

Estimates of mortality from SE range from 10% to 50%. Generalized convulsive status epilepticus (GCSE) and nonconvulsive status epilepticus (NCSE) with coma are the most serious forms of SE, demanding immediate and aggressive intervention. Cases that are unresponsive to first- and second-line interventions have a poor prognosis (i.e., refractory SE). An additional category of superrefractory SE is used to describe SE that does not respond to third-line agents. Not surprisingly, patients in this category have the worst prognosis.[49,51]

SIGNS AND SYMPTOMS

Just as there are different types of seizures, there are different types of SE. GCSE has garnered the most attention in research and has the highest mortality and morbidity rates. For these reasons, GCSE is the primary focus of the following sections, unless NCSE is specifically mentioned. As the name suggests, the patient presents with enduring generalized convulsions and loss of awareness. Focal motor SE also involves ongoing convulsions, but they are limited to one focal area, such as a single limb, or at least to one side of the body. Awareness may or may not be impaired when the convulsions are unilateral. Myoclonic SE and tonic SE are other, less common forms of convulsive SE.

For GCSE, the ILAE proposal specifies that T1 and T2 are 5 and 30 minutes, respectively. For other types of status epilepticus, the most appropriate time intervals for T1 and T2 have not been well defined and are far more speculative, particularly for NCSE. The ILAE suggests using a T1 and T2 of 10 and >60 minutes for focal status epilepticus with impaired consciousness, respectively. For absence SE, the T1 is 10 to 15 minutes; data are insufficient to designate any particular T2.[47]

In most cases of SE, the patient will not be able to provide extensive history. Whenever possible, a history should be obtained from any witnesses who may have insight about the duration of SE prior to presentation for medical care. Family and friends may also be able to provide information about recent drug ingestion or patterns of alcohol use that could contribute to prolonged seizure activity, or if the patient has a known history of epilepsy.

PHYSICAL EXAMINATION

Physical examination for SE focuses on assessing alertness and the patient's respiratory and circulatory status. The patient should be assessed for fever, rash or other signs of sepsis, uremia, and meningitis. The patient should be evaluated for signs of head injury as well.

DIFFERENTIAL DIAGNOSIS

Convulsive types of SE tend to be easily distinguished from other conditions, although they can appear similar to some movement disorders. Focal motor SE, for example, might resemble dystonia.

Uncontrolled myoclonic jerking may result from pathways that are pathophysiologically distinct from the neuronal misfiring associated with seizure activity. This "action myoclonus" is often an outcome of anoxic or metabolic injury and is not associated with the spike or sharp waves on EEG that are seen in myoclonic SE.

Psychogenic status "nonepilepticus" is not very common, but it does occur. A psychogenic etiology must be considered for individuals who present with enduring bilateral motor movements without loss of awareness.

Unlike convulsive status, NCSE may be symptomatically indistinguishable from other causes of altered mental status. It has been reported that about 5% of cases presenting with altered mental status are attributable to NCSE.[52] In patients with a known history of isolated focal seizures, the presentation of seizure activity during SE may be different from the stereotypical event they usually have. This is especially true the longer NCSE lasts, as it tends to be increasingly subtle in semiology as time goes by.

DIAGNOSTIC STUDIES

Diagnostics may need to be performed after an initial round of empirical treatment is administered. It would not be feasible or safe to perform most of the following tests on a patient actively convulsing or too confused to cooperate.

Laboratory evaluation (often serum studies and urinalysis) is conducted to assess for underlying triggers of seizure activity, or for other causes of altered mental status in the case of NCSE. This usually includes a fingerstick glucose, CMP, magnesium, phosphorus, toxicology, and levels of any previously prescribed AEDs. Creatine kinase, troponin, lactate, and an arterial blood gas also help screen for and assess the degree of systemic illness. A lumbar puncture is critical if there is any concern for an infectious or autoimmune etiology. Blood, urine, and cerebrospinal fluid cultures are prudent when infection is suspected.

EEG/VEEG is the best modality to distinguish seizure activity from its mimickers, but readings may be obscured by EMG artifact during convulsive SE. Given the high morbidity and mortality rate of GCSE, it is also not practical to insist on confirming the diagnosis of GCSE before treating empirically. In cases of altered mental status of unknown etiology, or when it persists despite the correction of presumed causes, an EEG should be performed to assess for NCSE.

Brain imaging such as CT or MRI are warranted to rule out hemorrhage, ischemia, or mass, especially when the patient has no known history of seizure activity.

TREATMENT

In 2016, the American Epilepsy Society (AES) published an algorithm for the treatment of convulsive SE in adults and children. The schematic specifically addresses GCSE, which is the primary focus of this section. The AES breaks the treatment of prolonged seizure activity into four separate phases.[53]

The initial stage, referred to as the Stabilization Phase, accounts for the first 5 minutes of the seizure and addresses prevention of SE. Of course, in many cases, the seizure will not start in the presence of a clinician, which is why the patients' families and caregivers need to be briefed on a community-based approach to seizure first aid (see "Patient Education" below). When a seizure does occur in the health-care setting, the clinicians' immediate focus is typically circulation, airway, breathing, and any supportive care needed. Timing the seizure, checking a fingerstick blood glucose, and monitoring vital signs should begin as soon as possible. Oxygen can be administered via nasal cannula or mask, and an EKG may be initiated. IV access should also be obtained as soon as possible to permit initial labs (see "Diagnostic Studies" above) and treatment of hypoglycemia or electrolyte disturbance. Adults are generally treated empirically with IV thiamine (100 mg) in case the seizure is related to chronic alcohol abuse. Antipyretics are called for if the patient is febrile.

The AES Initial Therapy Phase accounts for minutes 5 to 20 of the seizure and is the first stage when the seizure is considered SE using the ILAE T1 cutoff for GCSE. A high level of evidence supports use of an intravenous (IV) or intramuscular (IM) benzodiazepine at this point. IV phenobarbital can also be administered but is generally reserved for situations when benzodiazepines are not available. Many patients may have emergency supplies of rectal or intranasal benzodiazepines, and these are frequently used in community settings (see "Patient Education").

The Second Therapy Phase includes minutes 20 to 40, when the episode is considered refractory SE. The AES algorithm acknowledges there is less evidence to support the next step in phamacotherapeutic intervention, but recommends IV fosphenytoin, valproate, or levetiracetam. Some authors have reported success with other agents such as lacosamide or topiramate, but these are usually reserved for research protocols or when the patient has not responded to fosphenytoin, valproate, or levetiracetam.

The Third Therapy Phase refers to cases of super refractory SE. At this point, a different agent from the Second Therapy Phase could be attempted, followed by anesthetic doses of barbiturates (thiopental, pentobarbital), midazolam, or propofol. Ketamine is another agent that has garnered much research attention for its utility at this point in the treatment plan. Other agents being scrutinized in SE research include perampanel, brivaracetam, cannabidiol, and fenfluramine.

SE triggered by an autoimmune disorder is a rare but increasingly recognized phenomenon. Autoimmune seizures and SE may or may not be a symptom of a paraneoplastic process. Routine use of immunosuppression is not currently supported by research, but may be prudent when this is suspected as a possible cause of SE. When suspicion for this is high or confirmed, plasmapheresis, intravenous immune globulin (IVIG), and agents such as rituximab may be included in treatment.[54]

PATIENT EDUCATION

For patients with a history of seizures, education should begin before the first incident of SE. Poor compliance with AEDs is a major risk factor for SE in people with epilepsy. Fortunately, SE due to AED noncompliance tends to have better outcomes than SE due to other etiologies. Nevertheless, a single episode of SE in a person with epilepsy can lead to a costly emergency and even long-term care and risks long term cognitive consequences.

In addition to focusing on medication compliance, clinicians often prescribe "rescue" medication that a patient or family member can administer in case of any seizure activity lasting more than 5 minutes. These medications are usually various formulations of benzodiazepines. In cases of SE without loss of awareness, the individual may be able to safely swallow tablets. However, "at home" treatments for GCSE usually involve rectal, buccal, or intranasal benzodiazepines.

The patient and family should keep these medications close at hand and be educated on the best methods for administration. Specific documentation with exact protocols for administration should be provided to anyone who may have occasion to provide the emergency intervention.

Parents of children with febrile seizures should be educated to begin antipyresis as soon as there is reason to suspect the child may be at risk for developing a fever. They are also often provided with a prescription for rectal diastat to be administered in the case of a prolonged febrile seizure in the future.

15.4 CEREBROVASCULAR DISORDERS

Rayne Loder

OVERVIEW

Stroke, or cerebrovascular accident, refers to acute neurologic dysfunction from injury to cerebral tissue. Stroke encompasses both ischemic and hemorrhagic etiologies, and treatment differs for the two subtypes. Transient ischemic attack (TIA) refers to an episode of neurologic deficit which is caused by cerebral ischemia and which completely resolves within 24 hours without resultant infarction on brain imaging. Subarachnoid hemorrhage is a type of intracranial hemorrhage that usually results from a ruptured brain aneurysm and causes bleeding into the subarachnoid space. An aneurysm is a protrusion of an intracerebral arterial wall and can be related to vascular risk factors or can be familial. An arteriovenous malformation is usually a congenital cerebrovascular abnormality that can cause hemorrhage, seizure, headaches, focal neurologic deficits, or can be diagnosed incidentally on brain imaging.

EPIDEMIOLOGY

Stroke is the most prevalent manifestation of cerebrovascular disease. According to the CDC, 7.8 million American adults have had a stroke, which accounts for 3.1% of the adult population; 146,383 adults die of stroke in the United States every year.[55]

PATHOPHYSIOLOGY

Blood is supplied to the brain via the carotid arteries and vertebrobasilar arteries. The internal carotid arteries provide oxygenated blood to the anterior cerebrum, while the vertebrobasilar arteries provide oxygenated blood to the posterior cerebrum, part of the cerebellum, and brain-stem.

The carotid and vertebrobasilar arteries form a circle at the base of the brain known as the circle of Willis, from which the anterior cerebral artery, middle cerebral artery, and posterior cerebral artery arise.

The disorders discussed in this section arise from dysfunction of the cerebrovascular system and disruption of blood supply, which can lead to a variety of neurologic syndromes.

15.4A TRANSIENT ISCHEMIC ATTACK

TIA refers to an episode of focal neurologic deficit that resolves completely within 24 hours without evidence of infarction on subsequent brain imaging. TIAs are sometimes referred to as "mini strokes," which reflects that the initial presentation is very similar to stroke. Although TIAs, by definition, result in complete resolution of neurologic symptoms, as many as 20% of ischemic strokes are preceded by TIAs, so urgent evaluation is important to identify and treat causative conditions with the aim of preventing a future cerebrovascular accident.[56]

MEDICAL HISTORY AND CLINICAL PRESENTATION

While ischemic strokes can be caused by either thrombosis or embolization, TIAs are more commonly associated with embolization. Cardiogenic emboli can develop due to atrial fibrillation, valvular disease, and complication of heart failure and cardiac ischemia. The presence of passageways between the right and left sides of the heart (e.g., atrial-septal defect or patent foramen ovale) can allow venous thromboemboli to travel into cerebral circulation. Asking questions about history of abnormal heart rhythms, heart murmurs, heart disease, and IV drug use can help to determine a possible cardiac cause of TIA. Areas of atherosclerotic disease in the vessels of the neck and head, particularly at the carotid bifurcations, can act as embolic origins and so asking about risk factors for vascular disease is helpful as well.

While embolism is the more common cause of TIA, causes of TIA can also include inflammatory vascular disorders (e.g., giant cell arteritis), hypercoagulability disorders, and subclavian steal syndrome.

SIGNS AND SYMPTOMS

The signs and symptoms of TIA vary depending on etiology and vascular territory involved. Symptoms typically start suddenly and resolve suddenly but by definition must resolve within 24 hours of onset.

PHYSICAL EXAMINATION

A full neurologic examination to assess for any unresolved neurologic deficit is indicated in patients who present with suspected TIA, as well as a careful cardiovascular examination to assess for possible etiology. The NIH Stroke Scale should be used to evaluate the patient (www.stroke.nih.gov/documents/NIH_Stroke_Scale_508C.pdf).

DIFFERENTIAL DIAGNOSIS

The differential diagnosis for TIA is summarized in Table 15.8.

TABLE 15.8 Differential Diagnosis for Transient Ischemic Attacks

Diagnosis	Description
Stroke (cerebrovascular accident)	Episode of neurologic dysfunction caused by cerebral infarction
Seizure	Episode of abnormal electrical activity in the brain that can result in temporary focal neurologic findings
Migraine	Headache subtype that can manifest with visual changes and focal neurologic abnormalities
Hypo/hyperglycemia	Abnormally low or elevated blood sugar can cause altered mental status due to metabolic abnormalities

DIAGNOSTIC STUDIES

Noncontrast head CT or head MRI within 24 hours of symptoms is important to exclude intracranial hemorrhage, which is important when determining treatment as intracranial hemorrhage is a contraindication to thrombolytic administration. Noncontrast head CT is highly sensitive for hemorrhage. MRI is more sensitive for infarction than CT in the initial 6 to 12 hours after onset of neurologic symptoms, which makes it helpful in establishing the diagnosis of TIA versus stroke.

CT or MR angiography of the head can assess for intracranial vasculopathy, and assessment of the vessels of the neck can be performed using either ultrasound or CT/MR angiography. The North American Symptomatic Carotid Endarterectomy Trial (NASCET) criteria should be used to determine severity of internal carotid artery stenosis. Using NASCET criteria, stenosis is categorized as either mild (0%–49%), moderate (50%–69%), or severe (70%–99%).

EKG is indicated to assess for abnormal rhythms, particularly atrial fibrillation. Echocardiogram is performed to assess for cardiogenic embolic source.

Laboratory studies including CBC, blood glucose determination, lipid studies, coagulation studies, and toxicology screening should be considered. Blood cultures should be obtained if infective endocarditis is suspected.

EVALUATION

In addition to the diagnostic tests listed above, noninvasive blood pressure monitoring, continuous cardiac monitoring, and regular surveillance for change in neurologic status are often included in stroke evaluation. Continuous cardiac monitoring is especially germane in TIA to evaluate for paroxysmal atrial fibrillation (PAF). Ambulatory cardiac monitoring can be considered in patients in whom PAF continues to be suspected despite normal cardiac monitoring during a hospital course.

TREATMENT

The goal of TIA treatment is to prevent further attacks and to prevent stroke. Cardiovascular risk factors should be identified and addressed. For instance, smoking cessation and weight reduction should be encouraged and hypertension and diabetes mellitus managed.

The decision to hospitalize a TIA patient is dependent upon multiple factors. In general, hospitalization should be considered for patients at high risk for a subsequent stroke; those who are unlikely to have a thorough diagnostic evaluation within 24 to 48 hours of the episode; or those who have other comorbid conditions that would benefit from hospitalization.

For patients who are found to have had a TIA related to the presence of atrial fibrillation, initiation of anticoagulation is indicated. Patients who do not have an indication for anticoagulation should be considered for antiplatelet therapy.

Patients for whom carotid artery stenosis is believed to be the cause of TIA (refer to NASCET criteria) should be referred to a vascular surgeon to discuss carotid endarterectomy.

In general, treatable etiologic conditions (e.g., infective endocarditis, hypercoagulable disorders) should be treated.

PATIENT EDUCATION

Education is paramount for any patient with TIA who is treated as an outpatient. These patients need to be carefully counseled that they are at risk for stroke. They should be educated regarding the signs and symptoms of stroke and instructed to call 911 immediately if they develop any further neurologic symptoms. If they are started on antiplatelets or any other medications, they should be counseled to take their medication as directed. They should be counseled for compliance with recommended lifestyle changes to reduce risk of further neurologic events.

15.4B STROKE

Cerebrovascular accident, commonly known as stroke, is the fifth leading cause of death in the United States.[55] The lifetime risk of stroke in adults worldwide is estimated to be 25%.[57] Stroke results from acute damage to cerebral tissue with resultant acute neurologic dysfunction and is an umbrella term under which two pathologic processes are encompassed: ischemia and hemorrhage. Early identification of etiology is crucial in stroke, as treatment of ischemic stroke and hemorrhagic stroke are significantly different.

The majority of strokes (estimated 80%) are caused by an ischemic process. There are two primary mechanisms by which cerebral ischemia can occur: thrombosis or embolism. Thrombosis refers to the development of an in situ blood clot in an artery of the brain and is most frequently a result of atherosclerotic disease. Embolism refers to a piece of clot or other material that was formed in and traveled from a distal site in the body before causing obstruction in an artery of the brain. Emboli that cause stroke commonly originate in the heart (valves or chambers).

Hemorrhagic stroke can be divided into two subtypes: intracerebral hemorrhage and subarachnoid hemorrhage. Intracerebral hemorrhage usually consists of bleeding from smaller arteries or arterioles and is most commonly associated with hypertension, amyloidosis, or coagulopathies. Subarachnoid hemorrhage will be discussed in detail in a subsequent section.

MEDICAL HISTORY AND CLINICAL PRESENTATION

The most important historical question to ask a stroke patient is "When did the symptoms start?" This information can also be obtained from bystanders by asking, "When was

TABLE 15.9 Signs and Symptoms for Ischemic Stroke by Vascular Territory

Vascular Territory	Signs and Symptoms
Anterior cerebral artery	Motor weakness and sensory deficits in the contralateral leg and, sometimes, arm; grasp reflex; abulia; and paratonic rigidity
Middle cerebral artery	Contralateral hemiplegia, sensory loss, and visual field deficit (homonymous hemianopia); aphasia (if dominant hemisphere involved)
Posterior cerebral artery	Contralateral sensory disturbance, homonymous hemianopia
Vertebrobasilar	Cranial nerve palsies; vertigo; nystagmus; ataxia; dysphagia; coma

the patient's last known normal?" or "At what time was the patient last observed to be at their baseline neurologic function?" The answer to this question determines treatment in patients with ischemic stroke, which is the most common stroke type.

Assessment for stroke risk factors is also important when taking a medical history in a patient who presents with an acute neurologic deficit suspicious for stroke. Risk factors for stroke include hypertension, hyperlipidemia, diabetes mellitus, history of tobacco use, atrial fibrillation, atherosclerosis.

SIGNS AND SYMPTOMS

Signs and symptoms of stroke will depend on etiology but, in general, stroke presents as acute neurologic dysfunction. Signs and symptoms of ischemic stroke will reflect vascular territory involved and are summarized in Table 15.9.

Intracerebral hemorrhage generally presents with focal neurologic findings that occur over minutes to hours as the blood forms a hematoma over brain tissue and can be accompanied by headache and/or nausea and vomiting as intracranial pressure increases.

PHYSICAL EXAMINATION

Neurologic examination findings in stroke will vary depending on etiology. The National Institutes of Health Stroke Scale, a tool that standardizes the neurologic examination of stroke patients, is used by many clinicians and healthcare systems that care for acute stroke patients.

In addition to a thorough neurologic examination, the physical examination of a stroke patient should include auscultation for carotid bruits and cardiac auscultation to assess for murmurs or abnormal rhythms.

DIFFERENTIAL DIAGNOSIS

The differential diagnosis of stroke includes transient ischemic attack (TIA), seizure, migraine, hypo/hyperglycemia, and drug toxicity (Table 15.10).

TABLE 15.10 Differential Diagnosis for Stroke

Diagnosis	Description
Transient ischemic attack	Transient episode of neurologic dysfunction characterized by complete resolution of symptoms and lack of infarct on imaging
Seizure	Episode of abnormal electrical activity in the brain that can result in temporary focal neurologic findings
Migraine	Headache subtype that can manifest with visual changes and focal neurologic abnormalities
Hypo/hyperglycemia	Abnormally low or elevated blood sugar can cause altered mental status due to metabolic abnormalities
Drug toxicity	Drug toxicity can cause altered mental status

DIAGNOSTIC STUDIES

A CT scan of the head without contrast should be obtained as soon as possible in patients who present with acute neurologic dysfunction thought to be secondary to stroke. CT scanning is highly sensitive for hemorrhage and allows clinicians to differentiate whether stroke is of the ischemic or hemorrhagic type and can therefore guide acute treatment.

CT scanning is *not* sensitive for acute ischemia in the initial 6 to 12 hours after onset of symptoms. MRI of the brain with diffusion-weighted sequences can help to identify infarcted area and extent of infarction in the acute period.[58]

CT angiography of both the head and neck allows for assessment of source of ischemic stroke and, if large vessel obstruction is present, can identify patients who are candidates for endovascular therapy.

In addition to brain imaging, laboratory studies including CBC, blood glucose, lipid studies, coagulation studies, and toxicology screening should be considered. An EKG must be considered to evaluate for cardiac rhythm abnormalities. Echocardiography allows for evaluation of structural cardiac abnormalities, such as patent foramen ovale (PFO), which can increase risk of stroke.

EVALUATION

In addition to brain imaging, laboratory studies, and cardiac studies as described in the previous section, noninvasive blood pressure monitoring, continuous cardiac monitoring, and regular surveillance for change in neurologic status are often included in stroke evaluation.

TREATMENT

Treatment of stroke depends on whether stroke is ischemic or hemorrhagic. If stroke is ischemic:

- IV thrombolytic therapy with alteplase (tissue plasminogen activator, or tPA) is indicated if patient does not have contraindication to thrombolytic treatment (see Box 15.3) and last known normal time is <3 to 4.5 hours. The primary risk of tPA administration is hemorrhage, which is reflected in the list of contraindications. tPA is effective at decreasing likelihood of neurologic disability up to 4.5 hours after last known normal time. Use of tPA between 3 and 4.5 hours after symptoms onset is considered off-label, but is common. Beyond 4.5 hours, the risk of thrombolytic-related hemorrhage is thought to outweigh benefit.

BOX 15.3 Contraindications to Thrombolytics

Head trauma or stroke within past 3 months
Symptoms of subarachnoid hemorrhage
Recent arterial puncture at noncompressible site
History of intracranial hemorrhage
Intracranial mass or arteriovenous malformation
Recent brain or spine surgery
Active internal bleeding or coagulopathy
Glucose <50 mg/dL
Large area of infarction on CT
Blood pressure >185/110 mm Hg (can be lowered with intravenous antihypertensives)
Relative contraindications: Symptoms minor, concurrent seizure, pregnancy, major surgery within 2 weeks, internal bleeding within 3 weeks, myocardial infarction within 3 months

- Patients with large vessel occlusion can be considered for mechanical embolectomy/thrombectomy up to 24 hours after time of symptom onset.[59] Endovascular mechanical embolectomy/thrombectomy can be considered even in patients who have been administered thrombolytic therapy.
- Aspirin is given immediately unless patient has received thrombolytic. Aspirin therapy can be initiated 24 hours after thrombolysis after follow-up CT rules out thrombolytic-related hemorrhage.
- Anticoagulants can be initiated if indicated based on suspected etiology (e.g., atrial fibrillation).
- Hypertension is common and generally allowed in the acute period following stroke to ensure adequate cerebral circulation, unless lowering blood pressure would allow patient to become a candidate for thrombolytic treatment.

If stroke is hemorrhagic:

- Blood pressure should be treated with IV antihypertensives with a target systolic pressure of <140 mm Hg.
- Thrombocytopenia and coagulopathies should be addressed.
- Increased intracranial pressure should be addressed with head of bed elevation and IV osmotics.
- Neurosurgical consultation to discuss hematoma evacuation or decompression may be indicated.

PATIENT EDUCATION

Patients who survive stroke can benefit from physical therapy, occupational therapy, and speech therapy. Patients and family should be counseled that depression is common following stroke and that mental healthcare is an important part of recovery. Patients can also develop urinary incontinence after stroke and can be counseled that this is also common and, many times, temporary. Discussion should also include risk of secondary stroke and prevention measures.

15.4C SUBARACHNOID HEMORRHAGE

Subarachnoid hemorrhage (SAH), along with intracranial hemorrhage, is one of the two primary types of hemorrhagic stroke. Subarachnoid hemorrhage refers to bleeding within the subarachnoid space, which is filled with cerebrospinal fluid (CSF). Subarachnoid hemorrhage occurs most commonly due to trauma but can also occur spontaneously due to rupture of an aneurysm or from an arteriovenous (AV) malformation.

MEDICAL HISTORY AND CLINICAL PRESENTATION

SAH, along with intracranial hemorrhage, is one of the two primary types of hemorrhagic stroke. SA refers to bleeding within the subarachnoid space, which is normally filled with CSF. SA occurs most commonly due to trauma but can also occur spontaneously due to rupture of an aneurysm or from an arteriovenous (AV) malformation. Aneurysmal SA impacts 10–15/100,000 people in the United States,[60] which represents approximately 5% of all strokes,[61] and is most common in patients between ages 50 and 60.[62] SA can lead to death or to significant morbidity for those who survive.

SIGNS AND SYMPTOMS

In addition to complaining of a thunderclap headache, patients with SA may develop symptoms of intracranial pressure, including nausea, vomiting, and altered mental status.

PHYSICAL EXAMINATION

Because the subarachnoid space contains CSF, patients may have nuchal rigidity as a result of meningeal irritation. Patients commonly experience deterioration of mental status with eventual loss of consciousness. Focal neurologic abnormalities are not common.

DIFFERENTIAL DIAGNOSIS

SA should be a high diagnostic consideration in any patient presenting with a thunderclap headache (Table 15.11).

TABLE 15.11 Differential Diagnosis for Subarachnoid Hemorrhage

Diagnosis	Description
Encephalitis/meningitis	Infection of brain or meninges, can cause headache and nuchal rigidity, usually also presents with fever
Intracerebral hemorrhage	Type of hemorrhagic stroke, usually related to hypertension, if headache is present usually of an insidious onset
Acute hypertensive crisis	Headache can be a result of end-organ damage/encephalopathy, present with markedly elevated blood pressure, symptoms improve as blood pressure is lowered, is diagnosis of exclusion
Cervical artery dissection	Usually presents with headache and neck pain, often a history of trauma or inciting event
Cerebral venous thrombosis	Presentation can be similar to subarachnoid hemorrhage, but more typically includes papilledema and seizures

DIAGNOSTIC STUDIES

CT scan of the brain without contrast is the initial imaging examination of choice to assess for presence of hemorrhage. If noncontrast CT scan is negative for hemorrhage but clinical suspicion for SA remains high, CSF analysis should be performed to assess for xanthochromia and increased red blood cell count.

EVALUATION

CT or MR angiography is used to evaluate for source of bleeding. When catheter-based angiography is performed under the guidance of an interventional radiologist, it is possible for the procedure to be diagnostic as well as therapeutic if the radiologist is able to treat an aneurysm or AV malformation endovascularly.

TREATMENT

Patients with SA should be hospitalized, usually requiring admission to an ICU. Measures to reduce intracranial pressure should be implemented (e.g., keeping systolic blood pressure <140 mm Hg, raising head of bed, preventing straining with bowel movements, treating anxiety). Treatment of the underlying cause, including surgical clipping or endovascular embolization of aneurysm if present, decreases likelihood of recurrent hemorrhage.

PATIENT EDUCATION

Patients who survive a SA may make a full recovery, though many do not survive and many who do survive may suffer from permanent disability. Of those who suffer an aneurysmal SA, 11% die in minutes and 40% die within a month. Up to 50% of survivors may never return to their baseline level of cognitive function.[63] Patients and family members should be counseled that the patient may have long-term memory deficits, cognitive impairment, mood changes, or difficulty with speech or mobility and should be referred to appropriate resources to address any permanent impairments.

KEY POINTS

Stroke

- Acute focal neurologic deficit secondary to cerebral ischemia and infarct
- Caused by either ischemic or hemorrhagic process
- Asking about last known normal time is most important historical question
- Fast CT head without contrast is vital to differentiate ischemic from hemorrhagic stroke.
- Ischemic stroke can be treated with thrombolytic or mechanical embolectomy.
- Hemorrhagic stroke is treated with intracranial pressure reduction, reversing coagulopathies, neurosurgical intervention.

TIA

- Episode of acute focal neurologic deficit that completely resolves in 24 hours and does not result in infarct
- Frequently embolic in etiology
- Patient with TIA are at high risk to have subsequent stroke; evaluation for and treatment of cause should be done quickly, and TIA often requires hospital admission.

SA

- Hemorrhage into subarachnoid space due to trauma or spontaneous rupture of aneurysm or arteriovenous malformation
- Presents with "thunderclap" headache, "worst headache of my life"
- If initial brain imaging is negative, CSF evaluation should be done to assess for xanthochromia.
- Treatment includes ICP reduction and surgical or endovascular repair of aneurysm or arteriovenous malformation.

Intracerebral Aneurysm

- Abnormalities of cerebral arterial walls related to vascular risk factors or genetic conditions
- Usually asymptomatic, diagnosed incidentally or on screening studies
- Rupture leads to subarachnoid hemorrhage.
- Treatment goal is to prevent rupture; treatment can be addressed surgically or endovascularly.

Arteriovenous Malformations

- Cerebrovascular malformation in the brain
- Usually congenital and nonfamilial, though there is a known link with hereditary hemorrhagic telangiectasia (HHT)
- Can present with hemorrhage, seizure, headache, focal neurologic deficits, or can be found incidentally on imaging
- Diagnosed with imaging and angiography
- Patients should be referred to neurosurgery to discuss treatment options.

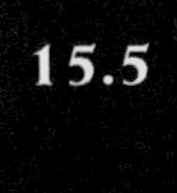

15.5 IDIOPATHIC INTRACRANIAL HYPERTENSION (PSEUDOTUMOR CEREBRI)

Jonathan Kilstrom

OVERVIEW

Idiopathic intracranial hypertension is also commonly referred to as pseudotumor cerebri. It is a nonmalignant condition that results in increased intracranial pressure which produces signs and symptoms of headache, vision loss, and papilledema. The symptoms of idiopathic intracranial hypertension can wax and wane anywhere from weeks to years.

EPIDEMIOLOGY

Idiopathic intracranial hypertension affects 1 to 2 people per 100,000. Obese women ages 15 to 44 are at highest risk of developing idiopathic intracranial hypertension.[64–66] In one study, 92% of patients were women and 94% were obese.[67]

Idiopathic intracranial hypertension can less commonly present in the elderly, children as young as 4 months, males, and healthy weight individuals; however, secondary causes of intracranial hypertension should be carefully ruled out prior to making the diagnosis of idiopathic intracranial hypertension.[68]

Up to 25% of patients with idiopathic intracranial hypertension may be at risk for severe, permanent loss of vision.[69]

PATHOPHYSIOLOGY

The exact cause of idiopathic intracranial hypertension is unknown, but when considering all potential causes the high incidence in obese females of childbearing years is significant. Weight gain, endocrine changes, hypercoagulable states, obstructive sleep apnea, and some medications have been associated with the development of idiopathic intracranial hypertension.[70]

MEDICAL HISTORY AND CLINICAL PRESENTATION

The classical presentation of idiopathic intracranial hypertension is an obese female of childbearing years presenting with a chief complaint of headache and visual changes.

SIGNS AND SYMPTOMS

The most common presenting symptom of idiopathic intracranial hypertension is headache. The headache is often described as severe, intermittent or persistent, unilateral and throbbing in character.

Patients may also report visual changes including transient loss of vision, sustained vision loss, and diplopia. Other symptoms include nausea and vomiting, pulsatile tinnitus, photopsia, back pain, and retrobulbar pain.[65,66]

If left untreated, idiopathic intracranial hypertension can result in optic atrophy and permanent vision loss.

PHYSICAL EXAMINATION

The hallmark feature of idiopathic intracranial hypertension is papilledema on fundoscopic examination. Patients may also present with visual field loss and a sixth cranial nerve palsy (abducens paralysis) resulting in diplopia when looking at objects side by side and a deficit of abduction on examination. This may be unilateral or bilateral.[65,71]

DIFFERENTIAL DIAGNOSIS

The differential diagnosis for idiopathic intracranial hypertension is summarized in Table 15.12. The majority of secondary intracranial hypertension causes can be ruled out by MRI or MR venography.

TABLE 15.12 Differential Diagnosis for Idiopathic Intracranial Hypertension

Diagnosis	Description
Secondary intracranial hypertension	Occurs as the result of a specific condition that may increase intracranial pressure and lead to papilledema. These can include intracranial mass lesions, venous outflow obstruction, hydrocephalus, malignant hypertension, decreased cerebrospinal fluid (CSF) absorption, and increased CSF production.
Migraine	Typically results in headache to one particular area that varies in intensity. Often accompanied by nausea, vomiting, photosensitivity, and phonosensitivity. Does not typically cause papilledema.
Stroke	Acute condition that can result in severe headache. Also, can cause difficulty with ambulation and speaking. Often results in unilateral weakness or numbness. Does not result in papilledema.
Lyme disease	Typically causes flu-like symptoms, including headache, due to *Borrelia burgdorferi* bacteria. Bulls-eye rash is a common finding. Does not result in papilledema.

DIAGNOSTIC STUDIES

The modified Dandy criteria is used to diagnose idiopathic intracranial hypertension. Each of the following must apply:[72,73]

- Signs and symptoms of increased intracranial pressure (headache, vision changes, papilledema)
- No additional neurologic deficits on examination
- An awake and alert patient
- Elevated intracranial pressure with normal CSF composition on lumbar puncture in the lateral decubitus position
- Normal neuroimaging study that shows no other etiology for symptoms
- No other cause of increased intracranial pressure identified

An abnormal CSF opening pressure is >20 cm H_2O in nonobese and >25 cm H_2O in obese patients.

EVALUATION

Any patient presenting with headache and papilledema should be examined for increased intracranial pressure. MRI with MR venography (MRV) is the preferred test to exclude secondary causes of increased intracranial pressure.[74] Those with contraindications to MRI should have a CT scan with contrast performed.

Lumbar puncture will show an elevated opening pressure with a normal CSF composition. To record an accurate opening pressure, the procedure should be performed with the patient in the lateral decubitus position with legs extended. https://www.medscape.com/answers/80773-32948/how-is-measurement-of-the-opening-pressure-taken-during-a-lumbar-puncture-lp

A complete ocular examination should be performed on all patients with suspected idiopathic intracranial hypertension to include visual field examination, dilated fundus examination, and optic nerve evaluation. Referral to an ophthalmologist should be considered.[75]

Potential medical conditions or medications that may worsen idiopathic intracranial hypertension should be addressed or discontinued.

TREATMENT

- Treatment is aimed at alleviating symptoms and preserving vision.
- Serial lumbar punctures may be useful at temporarily reducing symptoms but should be avoided if possible due to potential complications of the procedure.[76]
- Weight loss by means of a low-sodium diet should be encouraged for all obese patients with idiopathic intracranial hypertension.[66]
- Carbonic anhydrase inhibitors such as acetazolamide may reduce the rate of CSF production.[77] Topiramate can also be used to lower intracranial pressure.
- Loop diuretics may be useful in conjunction with carbonic anhydrase inhibitors at reducing CSF production, CSF pressure, and papilledema.[78]
- Corticosteroids have been recommended, but are typically avoided due to significant side effects.[79]
- Optic nerve sheath fenestration can be performed on patients who continue to have visual deficits despite medication treatment. This can stabilize or improve visual field loss secondary to papilledema.[79]
- A CSF shunt, either ventriculoperitoneal or lumboperitoneal, can be surgically placed in patients who fail

medication therapy. This procedure can help relieve headache, visual disturbances, and papilledema.[79]

PATIENT EDUCATION

- The exact cause of idiopathic intracranial hypertension is unknown, but obese females of childbearing age are at highest risk.
- Treatment is aimed is alleviating symptoms and preserving vision.
- Frequent follow-up visits with serial visual examinations are required until the condition is stabilized.
- Obese patients should be encouraged to lose weight.
- Idiopathic intracranial hypertension can be treated with prescription medications to help decrease the production of CSF.
- If pharmacologic therapy is not successful, CSF shunt placement and/or optic nerve fenestration can be performed to alleviate symptoms and preserve vision.

15.6 MOVEMENT DISORDERS

Jacqueline Cristini, Kathy Pedersen, Traci Hornbeck, Christa Cooper, Lori Fauquher, Daniel Sturm, and Stephanie Neary

The term "movement disorders" has been coined for diseases characterized by abnormal or excessive movements occurring in conscious patients. The term "extrapyramidal disorder" is an older classification of central motor disturbance not involving the corticospinal pathway.[80,81] Clinicians are able to readily identify *abnormal* movements in patients because they are accustomed to observing *normal* movements. Observing and describing a patient's gait as they walk from the waiting room into the examination room and speech and language used while taking a history provide significant clinical information. Most movement disorders are associated with pathologic alterations in the basal ganglia or their connections.[81] Not all movements are classified as "hyperkinetic," which is technically abnormal *excessive* movements. Other abnormal movements are classified as "hypokinetic," characterized by a partial or complete loss of muscle movement due to a disruption in the basal ganglia.[81,82] Examples of *hyperkinetic* movement disorders include chorea (Huntington disease), dystonia, restless legs syndrome, tics (Tourette syndrome), and tremor. *Hypokinetic* movement disorders would typically include Parkinson disease (parkinsonism), apraxia, hesitant or freezing gaits, rigidity, and muscle stiffness.

Lewy bodies (LB), discovered in 1912 by Frederic Lewy, remain the pathologic hallmark of Parkinson disease (PD). Neuronal cell loss in PD appears first in the dopaminergic cells of the substantia nigra pars compacta (SNc).[83] It is estimated that approximately 50% to 70% of dopaminergic neurons are lost at the time of a diagnosis of PD. The average age of onset is 65 and males are affected more than females by a ratio of 1.5:1. PD remains a clinical diagnosis; the three cardinal symptoms are tremor, bradykinesia, and rigidity. A DaTscan, an FDA approved nuclear medicine test can support a diagnosis of PD.

Essential tremor differs from the tremor typically seen in a patient with a diagnosis of PD, which is typically classified as a tremor at rest or *resting tremor* with unilateral onset. Essential tremor is the most common form of tremor and the most commonly diagnosed movement disorder. Tremor is a *hyperkinetic* movement disorder characterized by rhythmic oscillations of one or more body parts and most frequently affects the hands and arms. Essential tremor is an *action* tremor, mainly postural and kinetic, with a bilateral and symmetric onset. Phenomenologic classification of tremor would include rest tremor, action tremor such as postural tremor, kinetic tremor, and intention tremor. A *tremor at rest* generally starts in an asymmetric pattern and if accompanied by bradykinesia and/or muscle rigidity, a diagnosis of idiopathic PD should be included in the differential.

Dystonia is a neurologic disorder with an extremely broad range of clinical manifestations that may emerge at any age.[84] Dystonia is a *hyperkinetic* movement disorder. *Dystonia is a syndrome of sustained muscle contractions, frequently causing twisting and repetitive movement or abnormal postures.*[85] Torsion dystonia can be classified by age of onset, anatomic distribution, and etiology. Example of focal dystonia might be writer's cramp or tardive dyskinesia. Segmental dystonia involves two contiguous body regions, such as oromandibular dystonia and blepharospasm; a multifocal dystonia is more diffuse and generalized dystonia involves more extensive anatomic areas. Focal dystonia is the most common form of dystonia with cervical dystonia being the most common focal dystonia. The physical examination focuses on the body parts affected and whether there are associated findings that might point to a specific syndrome or identifiable cause.[84]

Huntington disease (HD) is an autosomal dominant inherited neurodegenerative disease characterized by progressive motor, behavioral, and cognitive decline, resulting in death within 15 to 20 years after diagnosis.[83] The typical clinical triad in HD is a progressive motor disorder, progressive cognitive disturbance culminating in dementia, and psychiatric disturbances including depression. *Chorea,* or the dance-like movements, is the clinical hallmark of this neurodegenerative disorder. Although chorea is only a small part of motor dysfunction in HD, it remains its most recognizable feature.[83] In less dramatic forms, chorea may pass for fidgetiness.[81,83] It is important to obtain an accurate family history; however, the lack of a positive family history does not exclude a diagnosis of HD as patients may present with symptoms more typical of parkinsonism.

Tourette syndrome is characterized by multiple motor tics plus one or more phonic tics that wax and wane over time.[84] Tics are quite common and often benign in the general population.[86] A clinical diagnosis is usually straightforward and other than the presentation of a motor or phonic tic, the remainder of physical exam is usually normal. Symptoms typically begin in childhood and are associated with behavioral comorbidities such as attention-deficit/hyperactivity disorder (ADHD) and obsessive-compulsive disorder (OCD). The treatment approach to patients with a diagnosis of Tourette syndrome should be multidisciplinary include cognitive behavioral therapy, psychotherapy, and counseling.

Gait disorders are common and may be the presenting feature in some neurologic disorders. Gait is an important motor function that is unconscious, automatic, and a fundamental skill that is basic to the quality of life. Walking requires considerable motor coordination. The classification and diagnosis of gait disorders is essentially based on observational analysis that can be challenging. Like many movement disorders, it is generally a clinical diagnosis based on a careful history and physical/neurologic examination. Gait ataxia can be classified as either cerebellar ataxia or sensory ataxia. The word origin of ataxia is *without order*. There are some distinctive physical clues that may aid the examiner in narrowing down the diagnosis, such as a positive Romberg sign or a positive retropulsion pull test.

Restless legs syndrome (RLS) is a common sensorimotor neurologic disorder. Obtaining an accurate medical and family history will aid in forming a diagnosis. In attempting to describe the symptoms of RLS, patients use countless terms such as the sensation of *bugs crawling on their legs*, a strong urge to move their legs, a throbbing sensation. Symptoms are present when they are asleep or falling asleep and are frequently absent during the day. The syndrome is more common in the geriatric population and is not uncommon in patients with PD. Patients may have a family history of RLS. RLS can be disabling, is sometimes resistant to treatment, and has a significant negative impact on patients' quality of life. Serious sleep disturbances are frequently associated with RLS.

15.6A PARKINSON DISEASE

OVERVIEW

Parkinson disease (PD) is one of the most common age-related neurodegenerative disorders, second in frequency only to Alzheimer disease. *Idiopathic* PD is the most common cause of degenerative parkinsonism. In the United States at least 500,000 people are diagnosed as having PD, and the frequency is predicted to triple over the next 50 years as the average age of the population increases.

Diagnosis of PD is usually attained by conducting a thorough history and physical examination; essentially, it remains a clinical diagnosis. The most commonly observed cardinal motor symptoms are a resting tremor, rigidity, bradykinesia, and postural instability (postural instability is usually a late-stage manifestation in idiopathic PD). Regrettably, by the time these features are obvious, extensive loss of dopamine has already occurred. It has been postulated that approximately 70% of the neurotransmitter dopamine is lost before motor symptoms manifest. The etiology of idiopathic PD remains unknown.

EPIDEMIOLOGY

PD is a heterogeneous neurodegenerative disorder that affects an estimated 10 million sufferers worldwide.[87]

PD is more common in men than women. Generally, White people in Europe and North America have a higher prevalence, around 100 to 350 per 100,000 population.[88] Individuals diagnosed with PD under the age of 40 are considered to be early-onset or young-onset PD and constitute approximately 10% to 15% of the PD population.

PATHOPHYSIOLOGY

Parkinsonism is considered to result primarily from abnormalities of basal ganglia function. The motor signs of PD are thought to result in large part from reduction of dopamine in the basal ganglia. The key role of basal ganglia in the initiation and integration of movement is shown by the effects of the pathologic changes that occur in illnesses such as PD. The selective loss of dopaminergic cells in the substantia nigra pars compacta in PD and the subsequent fall in caudate-putamen dopamine content led to a better understanding of the functional integration of basal ganglia circuitry. In PD, the degeneration of dopaminergic neurons and their projections to the striatum is a slowly evolving process that may take decades to develop.[89]

Anatomically, the term basal ganglia refers to the deep gray masses within the telencephalon. The key role of dopamine deficiency in PD led to the description of multiple dopamine receptor subtypes within basal ganglia. A key component of the classic model of basal ganglia organization is that D1 dopamine receptors are selectively localized to the cell bodies of the direct output pathway, while D2 receptors are selectively found on the cell bodies of the indirect pathway.

Parkinsonism

- **Idiopathic Parkinson disease (IPD):** Most common form of parkinsonism (85%)
    - Nearly all studies of PD show that there is a 3:2 ratio of males to females. While there is no obvious explanation for this observed male preponderance, exposure to toxins, head trauma, neuroprotection by estrogen, mitochondrial dysfunction, or X-linked genetic factors have been suggested.[90] This classification also includes young-onset PD (diagnosed under the age of 40) and juvenile parkinsonism, which is arbitrarily defined as parkinsonian symptoms and signs presenting prior to 21 years of age. Levodopa-responsive juvenile parkinsonism that is consistent with diagnostic criteria for PD is most often caused by mutations in the PARK-Parkin, PARK-PINK1, or PARK-DJ1 genes.
    - Research suggests that the pathophysiologic changes associated with PD may start before the onset of motor features and may include several *nonmotor* presentations, such as sleep disorders, depression, and cognitive changes. Evidence for this preclinical phase has driven the enthusiasm for research that focuses on protective or preventive therapies.[91]
    - IPD is a progressive neurodegenerative disease with a rather insidious onset in many cases. Significant dopamine depletion from the substantia nigra occurs prior to onset of motor symptoms. The three cardinal motor symptoms are tremor at rest, bradykinesia, and rigidity. Onset of symptoms is typically asymmetric with gradual progression to bilateral symptoms. Although a resting tremor (e.g., pill rolling) is the symptom that most clinicians associate with a diagnosis of PD, many patients do not present with a tremor but may only manifest symptoms of bradykinesia and rigidity in an asymmetric pattern. PD without tremor is commonly mistaken for a musculoskeletal condition, particularly in the older population.
- **Progressive supranuclear palsy (PSP):** Also referred to as Parkinson-plus disorders
    - The most common form of atypical parkinsonism. As with any form of parkinsonism, the onset is insidious. Clinical features include postural instability (unheralded falls), vertical gaze palsy, rigidity and retrocollis (abnormal posturing of neck), and dementia. Two retrospective studies found gait disturbance, often unheralded falls, to be a presenting feature in 90% and 62%, respectively.[81]

- **Multiple-system atrophy (MSA):** A syndrome characterized clinically by features of parkinsonism with dysautonomia
  - Prominent features include orthostatic syncope, impotence in males, and urinary incontinence in females. Usually symptomatic orthostatic hypotension develops rather early on as well as urinary dysfunction. Several primary distinguishing factors that may help in differentiating IPD from MSA are early postural instability, rapid progression, and typically, a poor response to dopaminergic therapy.
- **Vascular parkinsonism (multi-infarct/VP):** Symptoms are usually symmetric, patients are elderly with a history of hypertension and/or stroke(s).
  - VP is classically described as an entity characterized by predominant lower-body parkinsonism, postural instability, shuffling or freezing gait, absence of rest tremor, absent or poor response to dopamine, and presence of corticospinal tract signs.[92] Patients are typically older and more likely to present with a wide-based ataxic gait and poor balance. A history of falling with upper body motor function preserved is not uncommon.
- **Drug-induced parkinsonism (DIP):** Antipsychotic or neuroleptics are well-recognized causes
  - A number of drugs can induce parkinsonism. The most commonly prescribed offending agents include antipsychotics, neuroleptics, and antiemetics. DIP is likely the most common drug-induced movement disorder and one of the most common *nondegenerative* causes of parkinsonism. Any medication that interferes with dopamine transmission may cause parkinsonism. If the patient is under the care of a psychiatrist, the clinician should advise the patient to bring any involuntary motor movements they are experiencing to their clinician's attention. The psychiatrist or clinician may choose a less offensive antipsychotic or lower dose, but in many instances the patient's current psychiatric medications are effective in controlling their psychiatric symptoms, making this a judgement call. The prototypical drugs are dopamine receptor blocking agents, specifically those that block D2 (Table 15.13).[93]

TABLE 15.13 Common Offending Drugs of Dopamine Blocking Agents

Atypical antipsychotics (second generation)	Risperidone (Risperdal)
	Clozapine (Clozaril)
	Olanzapine (Zyprexa)
	Quetiapine (Seroquel)
	Ziprasidone (Geodon)
	Aripiprazole (Abilify)
	Paliperidone (Invega)
	Lurasidone (Latuda)
Antiemetics	Metoclopramide (Reglan)
	Promethazine (Phenergan)
	Prochlorperazine (Compazine)

A thorough neurologic examination and medical history will usually provide a diagnosis. One of the reasons that IPD is misdiagnosed or is a missed diagnosis is due to the rather insidious onset and somewhat vague symptoms. It is not uncommon for patients to be referred for shoulder surgery due to their complaint of worsening stiffness and pain in one shoulder without realizing that it is actually a neurologic condition. Likewise, patients are referred to osteopathic specialists for a complaint of back stiffness that is affecting their gait. Ironically, tremor-dominant PD bodes a much better prognosis and the tremor does not usually affect a person's ability to function due to the nature of the tremor.

MEDICAL HISTORY AND CLINICAL PRESENTATION

An accurate medical history is extremely helpful in diagnosing any form of parkinsonism. In addition to the commonly recognized cardinal motor symptoms of PD such as tremor at rest, bradykinesia, and rigidity there are a multitude of clinical clues that may be able to guide one to a more accurate diagnosis (Figure 15.2). There are numerous nonmotor symptoms that may provide further diagnostic clues that are frequently unrecognized by clinicians and remain untreated. Some of the more common nonmotor symptoms may occur early on, and in some instances many years prior to the manifestation of a motor symptom. These include a history of hyposmia, vivid dreams or other sleep disturbance, depression/anxiety, constipation, gastroparesis, erectile dysfunction, cognitive changes, pain, and fatigue. Patients do not typically consult a neurologist until an obvious motor symptom is present though they may have been experiencing nonmotor symptoms of PD for many years. Typically, PD patients experience orthostatic hypotension, particularly those with a diagnosis of multiple-system

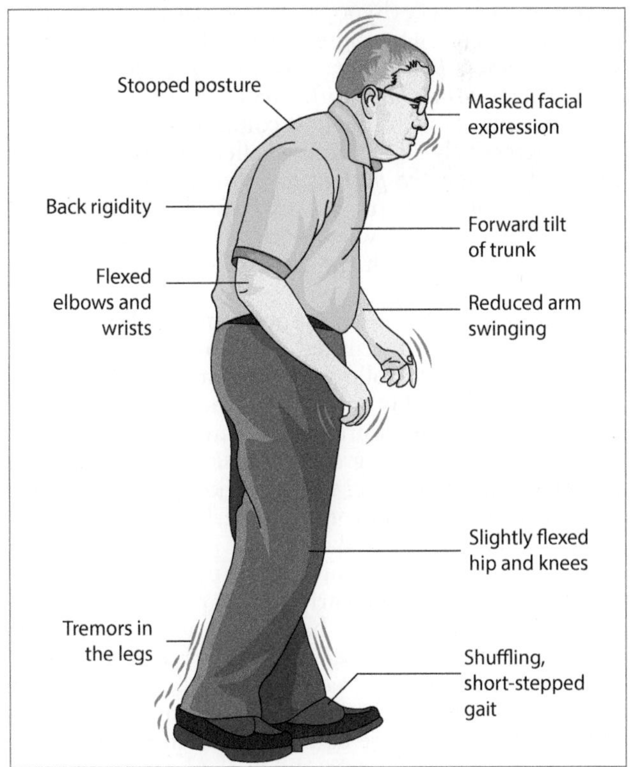

Figure 15.2 **Typical appearance of Parkinson disease.**

atrophy. Orthostatic blood pressure measurements can provide useful information in any parkinsonian disorder. MSA patients will commonly provide a history of fatigue, lightheadedness, and perhaps syncopal episodes, as well as urinary incontinence or erectile dysfunction. The clinician may not elicit cardinal motor signs such as tremor or rigidity, but more likely bradykinesia, postural instability, and slowed gait will be present.

PHYSICAL EXAMINATION

A comprehensive physical examination is paramount. Not every patient will present with a resting hand tremor or stooped posture. There are numerous clinical pearls to be aware of that will aid in a timely diagnosis and are generally elicited through careful observation.

Listed below are practical questions a clinician might ask as well as some very distinctive physical clues that may further help narrow down the differential diagnosis. A thorough history of the use of neuroleptics or antipsychotics is of particular importance to rule out DIP. The motor symptoms may be difficult to sort through. Observe for any involuntary motor movements that might indicate the onset of tardive dyskinesia, secondary to the use of any dopamine-blocking medications.

- **Sense of smell:** Has the patient been aware of a diminished sense of smell? This may be present for many years. *Can they smell coffee brewing, fire burning, or the scent of strong perfumes and colognes?* Hyposmia is one of the most common and best-characterized conditions that is also one of the first nonmotor features of PD.[94]
- **Facial expression:** This may be difficult as most patients cannot state whether or not their facial expression is diminished (hypomimia or masked facies). If it is not clearly observable by the examiner, *ask the patient to look at photographs from the past as to whether they notice a less animated facial appearance.*
- **Voice:** Is the voice hypophonic? Is there a history of the voice becoming progressively soft? *Ask the patient whether others have asked them to repeat things several times because they have difficulty being heard.*
- **Handwriting:** One of the most common symptoms of PD is a progressively slower and smaller handwriting or micrographia. *Ask the patient to write a sentence such as "what time of the day do you wake in the morning"* three times. Observe as to whether they experience difficulty by the time they reach the third repetition. Is it slower, smaller?
- **Eye movements:** Cardinal eye movements should be full in all directions. Diminished eye movements or slowed saccades (ability to follow movement from left to right smoothly and quickly) may be an indication of atypical parkinsonism such as progressive supranuclear palsy. *Is the patient experiencing blurred vision, diplopia, or dry eyes?* Commonly, decreased eye blinking is present which may cause dry eye syndrome and perhaps blurred vision. Note any *diminished upward gaze.*
- **Gait:** In the most common form of parkinsonism (IPD), gait is usually preserved early on and patient may exhibit only mild symptoms that have gone unrecognized. *Ask the patient if they ever feel as though their feet are glued or nailed to the floor (freezing of gait).* As you test the patient's gait, be particularly aware of their arm swing. Arm swing changes are common even in the early stages of PD. An asymmetric, diminished arm swing may be slight and easy to miss but in fact be the presenting initial motor symptom. The patient should be able to stand without using their arms to push off and initiate gait without hesitation. Observe posture for erectness and whether one foot scrapes the floor when ambulating. Be aware of the stride length, particularly whether there are small, shuffling steps and perhaps hesitation when turning. A festinating gait (gradual increase in speed) is a classic PD gait. *Is the patient able to turn fluently or do they require stepping in place (turning en bloc) as if standing on a block of wood?* This may be the only opportunity to observe an asymmetric resting hand tremor as it may occur only during ambulation. A normal gait is familiar, so differences or deviations are usually obvious to the observer. MSA patients may have a bradykinetic gait with postural instability but posture is usually reasonably erect. Vascular parkinsonism (VP) gait is typically slow, wide-based, and hesitant with difficulty picking up the feet; a shuffling gait is not uncommon (upper extremities are within normal range and asymptomatic).
- **Posture:** Typically, the posture of a patient with IPD is stooped or flexed slightly forward. If the posture is erect with slight extension of the neck (retrocollis), it is more typical of a Parkinson-plus syndrome such as progressive supranuclear palsy.
- **Tremor:** Tremor at rest is the classic tremor of PD and other parkinsonian syndromes. It disappears with action. The most common anatomic site for a rest tremor is the distal parts of the upper extremities. The tremor may not initially be obvious. In order to elicit a tremor at rest, ask the patient to perform a mental task that may cause a minor stress such as *reciting the months of the year starting with December and going backward. Ask the patient to draw an Archimedes spiral which will be distinctly different from a patient with essential tremor (increased with activity).* Both of these tasks will help to provoke a resting tremor and are otherwise referred to as distracting techniques. Deep brain stimulation (DBS) surgery is very effective in controlling tremor, whereas medications provide only limited benefit. Various studies have shown that tremor-dominant PD implies a better prognosis overall.[95]
- **Bradykinesia:** Though this may seem a challenge, it is one of the easiest motor symptoms to elicit on examination. *Ask the patient to open and close each hand separately as fast as they can.* Notice any asymmetry in the speed in which they open and close each hand and whether the movements became slower and smaller over a 15 second time interval. The patient should then tap each heel on the floor individually. Again, observe the speed and whether they were able to pick up each heel at least 3 inches off the floor. *Are the movements smooth and symmetric bilaterally?*
- **Rigidity:** Test for any increased tone in all four limbs as well as asymmetry. Check for cogwheel rigidity—where movement of limbs occurs with ratchet-like start and stop movements—particularly at the wrist and elbow joints where cogwheeling is more prominent. If present, note any asymmetry.

DIFFERENTIAL DIAGNOSIS

The differential diagnosis of parkinsonism is summarized in Table 15.14.

TABLE 15.14 Differential Diagnosis of Parkinsonism

Diagnosis	Signs and Symptoms	Response to Levodopa Therapy	History of Abrupt, Unexplained Falls	Unilateral Onset
Idiopathic Parkinson disease	Tremor Bradykinesia Rigidity (2 out of 3 motor symptoms is a clinical diagnosis)	**Robust**	No	**Yes**
Progressive supranuclear palsy (PSP)	Motor symptoms (bradykinesia, rigidity, tremor can vary) Ophthalmoparesis (slow saccades, vertical gaze palsy) Rigidity Retrocollis	Minimal, absent	**Yes**	Variable
Multiple system atrophy (MSA)	Motor symptoms (bradykinesia, rigidity, tremor can vary) Orthostatic hypotension (syncope) Bladder dysfunction (females) Impotence (males)	Minimal, absent	No	Variable
Vascular parkinsonism (multi-infarct)	Predominantly lower body parkinsonism Shuffling, freezing, wide-based gait Vascular risk factors (myotonic dystrophy, hypertension) Imaging: lacunar infarcts in basal ganglia	Variable	No	**No**

DIAGNOSTIC STUDIES

The diagnosis of PD remains a challenge in patients who have abnormal symptoms or show a lack of response to medication. The true definitive diagnosis of the parkinsonian syndrome (PS) disorders can only be made from a postmortem examination of the brain.[96] Although parkinsonism is essentially a clinical diagnosis, several diagnostic tests can help narrow down the differential diagnosis.

- **DaTscan:** Approved by the FDA in 2013, the DaTscan can help diagnose PD. It can be helpful when differentiating essential tremor from PD or when patients present with atypical symptoms. The results are either positive for parkinsonism (IPD, MSA, PSP) or negative. On imaging, "commas" are negative, "periods" are positive. This scan is usually negative if the diagnosis is DIP.
- **MRI of the brain:** This is not diagnostic for parkinsonism and used generally to rule out other neurologic or structural abnormalities. Typically, it is normal unless the patient has a history of cardiovascular disease, in which case, the imaging may reveal ischemic changes in multiple vascular areas, periventricular white matter changes, and cortical atrophy.
- **MSA:** The "hot cross bun" sign (HCBS) is a radiologic finding describing a cruciform T2 hyperintense signal on axial MRI of the pons.[97]
- **PSP:** "Hummingbird sign and mickey mouse" sign. Midbrain atrophy on MRI is highly suggestive of PSP and is described as hummingbird sign. This sign is very helpful in differentiating PSP from PD.[98]

Autonomic function testing is useful, particularly when considering a diagnosis of MSA. Routine serum laboratory tests should include vitamin B12, thyroid function tests, and ceruloplasmin.

EVALUATION

The Unified Parkinson's Disease Rating Scale (UPDRS) is the most commonly used scale to evaluate the course of PD in patients over a longitudinal period. It rates both motor and nonmotor symptoms. The lowest number is 0 (normal); the highest is 199 (severe).

TREATMENT

- **Pharmacology:** The mainstay and gold standard of treatment for parkinsonism continues to be *carbidopa/levodopa*. Levodopa is the precurser of dopamine, the neurotransmitter depleted in the substantia nigra in PD. Due to the preponderance of gastroparesis in PD, the bioavailability of levodopa fluctuates immensely. The half-life of most of the formulations is short, at approximately 90 minutes and requires multiple dosing throughout the day. The typical starting dose of carbidopa/levodopa is 25/100 mg three times daily. The most common side effects that may lead to intolerability are nausea and *dyskinesia* (involuntary movements). It is important to start low and go slow. If the patient has IPD, the response should be robust but depending on the severity of symptoms, a higher dose may still be required. There are various formulations of carbidopa/levodopa, including extended release capsules and inhaled levodopa, which bypasses the gastric tract thereby allowing levodopa to cross the blood-brain barrier more efficiently. Another form of levodopa is an enteral suspension formulation and is delivered through a percutaneous endoscopic gastrostomy with jejunal extension (PEG-J). There are numerous dopaminergic medications to treat symptoms of PD. The selection of the appropriate drug depends on several factors including classification of parkinsonism, age of patient, predominant symptoms, cognitive impairment and the presence of dementia and/or hallucinations.

- **Surgical intervention:** Deep brain stimulation surgery (DBS) involves placing a thin electrode (about the diameter of a piece of spaghetti) into one of several possible brain targets on one or both sides of the brain. The electrode is connected to a battery, which is implanted under the skin in the chest below the collarbone. All parts of the stimulator system are internal; there are no wires coming out through the skin.[99] Unfortunately, many patients with IPD are not aware of this extremely effective management option. The clinician uses a programming computer during routine office visits to adjust the settings for optimal symptom control. DBS was approved in 2002 for the management of PD. Patients are provided with a patient programmer, enabling them to make minor changes to their DBS settings as necessary. Pyschiatric screening should be performed prior to DBS as there may be possible psychiatric complications.[100]

PATIENT EDUCATION

Numerous resources are available for information regarding PD. The American Parkinson's Disease Association (APDA), Parkinson's Disease Foundation (PDF), The Michael J. Fox Foundation, and the National Parkinson's Foundation are just a few of the most widely used resources. These organizations support education and research for patients and caregivers. They are easily accessible through the internet. Educating not only patients and caregivers but also clinicians regarding the various resources available is vitally important in helping patients to understand the disease state and achieve an improved quality of life. The clinician should strongly urge patients to seek out local PD support groups as these are invaluable supportive resources.

SPECIAL CONSIDERATIONS

All patients with a diagnosis of parkinsonism should be referred for physical, occupational, and speech therapy. There are specific therapeutic programs designed to focus on the distinctive and disabling symptoms of PD. The "BIG" physical therapy program addresses gait, balance, and generalized movement, with an emphasis on exaggerated movements, such as big steps. Local programs can be found through the website (https://www.lsvtglobal.com/LSVTBig).

The Lee Silverman Voice Treatment (LSVT) program is particularly helpful for patients with PD since the voice tends to get softer as the disease progresses. Patients become very frustrated and less social due to the inability to express themselves verbally. The benefits from a regular exercise program cannot be overemphasized. LSVT BIG is derived from the Lee Silverman Voice Treatment and focuses on intensive exercising of high-amplitude movements.

15.6B TREMOR

OVERVIEW

Tremor is a rhythmic and oscillatory movement produced by alternating contractions of antagonistic muscles. It is the most common form of involuntary movement.[101] Tremor can be intermittent or constant. The amplitude of tremor can vary from mild to severe and the frequency can vary depending on the classification of the tremor. Tremor can be idiopathic, or it can occur secondary to another medical disorder. There are many causes of tremor and finding the cause involves an investigation of multiple factors, starting with identifying the tremor's characteristics and determining the most accurate classification.

Tremor can be phenomenologically classified into two major categories: rest and action tremor. Rest tremor occurs when the muscles are at rest, fully supported against gravity. This type of tremor can sometimes be referred to as a "pill-rolling" tremor because it appears as though the patient is rolling a pill between the thumb and index finger. It can occur while hands are resting in the patient's lap, on a table, when legs are at rest in a seated position, or when distal arm muscles are at rest while walking. This type of tremor will diminish upon activating the muscles of the affected body part such as lifting the affected hand off a lap or table in order to use it. Action tremor is the second major category and it involves tremor of the affected body part that occurs during voluntary contraction of those muscles. Action tremor can be further subdivided into postural and kinetic tremor. Postural tremor occurs during voluntarily maintenance of a position of the affected limb against gravity, such as tremor seen in an outstretched arm. Kinetic tremor occurs due to muscle activation during voluntary movement of the affected limb as seen in asking a patient to move their finger during the "finger to nose" test, when reaching for an object, or when performing specific tasks such as writing. Intention tremor is a type of kinetic tremor that is characterized by an increase in the amplitude of the tremor when the affected body part approaches its target.[102]

EPIDEMIOLOGY

Essential tremor (ET), which has also been referred to as "benign essential tremor" or "familial tremor," is the most common movement disorder. The estimated prevalence worldwide is 1%, and of adults over the age of 60 years, it is approximately 5%. The prevalence of ET is similar in males and females, although some studies report a slight male predominance.[103,104] ET can be inherited or sporadic. Family history of tremor is present in 30% to 70% of individuals with ET and can be as high as 80% in those with onset before the age of 40 years.[105,106] Studies suggest an autosomal dominant inheritance with reduced penetrance.[107–111]

PATHOPHYSIOLOGY

Pathophysiologic mechanisms of ET are thought to be due to neural firing abnormalities within the olivocerebellar pathways, relayed via the thalamus and motor cortex to the spinal cord.[112] A general and simplified overview of the local anatomy and physiology is that the motor cortex sends information to the cerebellum and the basal ganglia, a network of nuclei deep in the white matter of the cerebral cortex, and both structures send information back to cortex via the thalamus. The output of the cerebellum is excitatory, while the basal ganglia are inhibitory. The balance between these two systems allows for smooth, coordinated movement, and a disturbance in either system will manifest as a movement disorder such as ET.[113]

MEDICAL HISTORY AND CLINICAL PRESENTATION

ET is a disorder manifesting primarily as an action tremor that occurs in the hands. It can also have associated tremor in other locations of the body, almost always in conjunction with the hands tremor. In order from most to least frequent, these areas can include head, voice, leg, jaw, face, and trunk.[114–116] The tremor in the extremities is often bilateral and asymmetric, with one side being more severe than the other.[117] Individuals with ET experience tremor to varying degrees. Postural tremor is present and occurs during activation of the affected muscles while maintaining the limb in a posture against gravity. There can also be a kinetic tremor present as well while activating the affected muscles during movement, which usually is a chief complaint of the patient when the tremor occurs during common activities of daily living such as holding utensils for eating, drinking from a cup, and writing. To a much lesser degree, intention and rest tremor can also be present in more advanced stages.[118–120]

Tremor develops at any age but most often in the midlife. One study revealed that the age of onset for ET showed a bimodal distribution with peaks in the second and sixth decades.[114] The tremor's onset is mild, and it tends to be slowly progressive over many years. Because of this, many of these individuals do not seek medical attention for the tremor until many years after its onset.

In ET, as compared to other disorders that include tremor, the frequency is moderate to high (4 to 12 Hz).[121] Over an individual's lifetime, as the tremor progresses, it can become higher in amplitude and lower in frequency.[117] The amplitude of the tremor can vary significantly between affected individuals, ranging from being a minor annoyance in some patients to being severely disabling in others, rendering the affected individual unable to perform independent activities of daily living such as eating and hygiene-related tasks. Tremor can be exacerbated by emotional and physiologic stressors, medications, and caffeine and can increase in severity while performing specific tasks.

DIFFERENTIAL DIAGNOSIS

The differential diagnosis for tremor is broad. Classification of the tremor as well as considering its characteristics and location(s) and identifying associated symptoms are essential. An estimated 30% to 50% of ET diagnoses are incorrect, and the true diagnosis in those patients is often PD or other tremor disorders.[122]

Enhanced physiologic tremor, the most common tremor in patients presenting to primary care clinicians, can be sometimes mistaken for mild ET.[123,124] Physiologic tremor is present in all humans due to the interaction between local mechanical-reflex mechanisms and central oscillators. It is a high-frequency (10 to 12 Hz), low-amplitude tremor.[123,125]

Tremor associated with PD versus ET can be a common diagnostic diagnostic challenge for clinicians and tends often to be a concern of patients. A cardinal feature of PD is rest tremor.

Primary orthostatic tremor is a postural tremor that has similar features to ET; however, it is a slightly higher frequency (14 to 18 Hz), and it occurs only in the legs and trunk and only while standing. This type of tremor can be associated with cramping of the calf muscles and unsteadiness.

Task-specific or site-specific tremor may look similar to ET but often represents a form of dystonia tremor. This includes primary writing tremor, which is an action tremor that occurs while writing only. It has a lower frequency (5 to 6 Hz) and larger amplitude than the typical ET action tremor.

Cerebellar outflow tremor can manifest as increasing oscillations during the middle of the kinetic phase and decrease as the affected limb reaches its target. It can include postural, kinetic, and intention tremor. The frequency of this tremor is low (3 to 8 Hz) and the clinician should also look for other signs associated with cerebellar disorders such as ataxia, wide-based gait, and dysmetria.[119,126,127]

Neuropathic tremor is typically a postural or kinetic tremor due to a large fiber peripheral neuropathy. It is typically a low-frequency (3 to 6 Hz) tremor in the upper extremities.

Functional tremor, also known as psychogenic or somatoform tremor, is tremor due to a conversion disorder and accounts for about 4.1% of patients who present with tremor.[128]

MEDICAL HISTORY AND CLINICAL PRESENTATION

Evaluating the patient with tremor involves a thorough history and physical exam. The diagnosis of ET is clinical, meaning no one particular diagnostic study will elucidate the diagnosis; rather, it is the identification of the pattern seen within the history and physical exam that reveals characteristic features of ET and recognition of atypical features that usually indicate an alternative cause for the tremor. Also, it is a diagnosis of exclusion, meaning all other reasons for tremor are worked up appropriately and ruled out definitively. It is important to accurately identify the cause of the tremor, in order to assure that the patient is receiving the most beneficial therapy.

The following attributes of tremor are typically found in a diagnosis of ET (inclusions):

- Bilateral postural tremor with or without kinetic tremor of upper extremity
- Tremor duration >5 years, slowly but progressively worsening over time
- Asymmetry, both extremities may be involved but typically one side is worse
- Possible involvement of other body parts
- Amplitude may fluctuate
- Tremor +/– disability
- Tremor may involve other body parts in addition to the upper extremities

The following attributes or associations with the tremor are found in diagnosis other than ET (exclusions):

- Presence of any cardinal features of PD
- Factors present that may cause enhanced physiologic tremor
- Exposure to tremor-inducing drugs
- Central or peripheral nervous system lesion or injury
- Concern for psychogenic origin
- Sudden onset or nonlinear deterioration

The medical history for workup of ET should identify patterns that fit into the aforementioned categories. The information about the tremor's onset can be vitally important to understand the trajectory of the disease course. This includes age of onset, severity at onset, involved body parts, degree of progression over time, associated symptoms, whether there is a family history of tremor, relieving factors, exacerbating factors, associated symptoms, and degree of disability. Tremor in ET is often improved after drinking alcohol, and while this is not considered an appropriate treatment, inquiring about this alcohol responsiveness can be helpful to distinguish ET versus other forms of tremor.

PHYSICAL EXAMINATION

Clinical examination of the tremor should include identification of the frequency, amplitude, pattern, and distribution of the tremor.[129] The frequency and amplitude of the tremor are most often assessed clinically. Electromyography (EMG) or other motion-analyzing equipment is available and can be used if the clinical assessment is unclear. However, this is not typically necessary. Associated neurologic findings may help distinguish patients with the two diseases. Laboratory testing may provide information that further aids in differentiating the two diseases. A comprehensive neurologic examination in ET should be otherwise normal, although signs of mild cerebellar dysfunction can be seen.[130]

Evaluating cognition or inquiring about changes in cognition can be helpful to evaluate for any neurogenerative disorders. In neurology clinics, patients are usually asked to hold the arms out in front of them for several seconds to evaluate for postural tremor. In order to assess kinetic tremor, the patients are asked to draw a spiral, provide a handwriting sample, or pour a full cup of water into another cup in order to evaluate the tremor's severity and to look for characteristic consistent frequency of the tremor as it is revealed in the handwriting samples.

Evaluating the patient's hands at rest during the interview can reveal rest tremor. It is also important to look for any signs of parkinsonism such as cogwheel rigidity, bradykinesia, or shuffling gait, which can manifest with reduced stride length and step amplitude. It is important to make sure ataxia is not present, which could indicate a number of alternative causes of tremor. Evaluating reflexes and looking for any focal motor or sensory deficits can elucidate other causes such as lesions or peripheral neuropathy.

DIAGNOSTIC STUDIES

Laboratory testing can be evaluated for excluding enhanced physiologic tremor such as electrolytes such calcium and thyroid function testing. Brain imaging is not necessary if ET is strongly suspected. Although not necessary for the diagnosis of ET, striatal dopamine transporter imaging using ioflupane I-123 single-photon emission computed tomography (SPECT; DaTscan) can be helpful in distinguishing between ET and PD in patients who have typical features of ET and also subtle parkinsonism when the diagnosis remains unclear despite a trial of levodopa administration to evaluate for PD.

TREATMENT

Treatment of ET is not required and is only necessary if the patient desires tremor reduction, which is most often due to impairment in function or social concerns causing psychological distress. Primary care clinicians can manage ET as long as it remains responsive to the most commonly prescribed medications.

For patients who want situational tremor control (i.e., when trigger is exacerbated by public speaking) and do not feel the need to take continuous therapy, propranolol is the preferred choice because it is quick acting. It can cause bradycardia or other side effects such as fatigue in large doses. The recommended starting dose for taking it in this intermittent manner is 10 to 20 mg.[131]

A low-dose benzodiazepine is used by some clinicians, but caution must be taken as it carries the risk of cognitive impairment and dependence.[132]

For patients who want continuous therapy, it is recommended to start with one medication, which can be propranolol initiated at 20 to 40 mg once or twice per day (the mean dose is 185.2 mg/day with a dose range of 60 to 320 mg/day) or primidone initiated at a dose of 25 or 50 mg once per day for 1 to 2 weeks, then increased by 25 to 50 mg each week with a mean dose of 481.7 mg/day and a dose range of 50 to 1,000 mg daily, each of which reduces tremor amplitude by about 50%. Propranolol achieved this after 1 week. Primidone has a slower onset of action, taking about 2 weeks. These medications are not effective for all ET patients.

Second-line medications may be tried, including gabapentin and topiramate; however, they are not as effective. These medications can be used in conjunction with first-line agents, but the patient should be monitored for common side effects such as fatigue, sedation, memory difficulty, dizziness, ataxia, parasthesias, and weight changes.[133] The dosage should be titrated slowly and should not exceed any significant side effect thresholds. Additional second-line agents can include benzodiazepines and other beta blockers.

Nonmedication management can be considered for medically refractory tremor. This includes botulinum toxin injections into the involved muscles, including neck muscles for head tremor and forearm muscles for hand tremor.

Chronic DBS involves stereotactic implantation of a lead, via intracranial burr holes, into the ventral intermediate nucleus of the thalamus. This operation has been considered the gold standard for surgical treatment of disabling, medically refractory ET for many years. In the hands of an experienced movement disorders neurosurgery program, patients have good outcomes and the operation tends to be tolerated well with the small risks associated with intracranial surgical procedures, including but not limited to a 1% risk of hemorrhage and 3% to 5% risk of infection and a low risk of cognitive changes, parasthesias, dysarthria, or ataxia.

PATIENT EDUCATION

The treatment of ET depends mostly on the severity and the level of disability the patient experiences from the tremor. Often, in tremor that is not severe and not bothersome to the patient, simple reassurance is adequate.

15.6C HUNTINGTON DISEASE

OVERVIEW

HD is a rare, progressive, neurodegenerative disease that can impact a person's motor abilities, cognition, and mood. It was described by George Huntington in 1872 after observing a family affected by the same illness over multiple generations. In his essay "On Chorea" he described an inherited, relentlessly progressive disease that caused abnormal movements and inappropriate behaviors.[134] HD is an autosomal dominant disease with children of an affected parent having a 50% risk of inheriting the faulty gene. The gene encodes for a protein called *huntingtin,* which accumulates in cells and causes dysfunction and cell death.

Diagnosis of HD can be made by a thorough neurologic exam and family history. Symptoms usually develop between the ages of 30 and 50 and progress over the course of 10 to 25 years. Genetic testing confirms the diagnosis but is not necessary to make a diagnosis of HD in a symptomatic individual. Genetic testing can also be done in asymptomatic individuals who have a family history of HD and are interested in learning their genetic status. All clinicians should follow the Huntington's Disease Society of American (HDSA) published guidelines for presymptomatic testing. These guidelines are discussed in depth later in this section.

EPIDEMIOLOGY

Currently there are >40,000 people living with HD in the United States and there are another 200,000 people at risk for inheriting the disease. The prevalence of HD has seemingly increased over the past two to three decades most likely because of the availability of genetic testing. In some areas of the world the prevalence is much higher and this is due to a "founder effect." A founder effect occurs when a small group of individuals becomes isolated from the larger population causing less genetic variation among the group. A good example of this effect occurred in Lake Maracaibo, Venezuela where there is a much larger population of people affected with HD (700/100,000). Compare this to North America, which has approximately a 7.33 per 100,000 population risk of HD.[135]

Genetics

A diagnosis of HD impacts the entire family. When a person is first diagnosed, they may be experiencing many different emotions including sadness, guilt, fear, or anxiety. *The decision to perform genetic testing should not be made hastily and should involve the expertise of a genetic counselor.* There is a lot of misinformation and misunderstandings about the HD gene and how to interpret the results. The gene was discovered in 1993 and is located on the short arm of chromosome 4. The mutation causes an abnormally long repetition of DNA base pairs, CAG. This is referred to as a trinucleotide repeat. The HD gene encodes for the production of huntingtin protein, whose normal function is not entirely known but is necessary for life. Overproduction of huntingtin protein, which is the issue in HD, leads to accumulation in neurons and eventual cell dysfunction and death.

Every person has two HD alleles and only one faulty gene needs to be present to be affected by the disease. This autosomal dominant inheritance pattern means males and females are at equal risk. A child born to one parent with HD has a 50% risk of inheriting the disease themselves.

The HDSA has published guidelines on testing at-risk individuals who are currently not displaying any symptoms of HD. This is commonly referred to as "predictive testing" as it can predict if the person will develop symptoms of HD in the future. Currently only about 10% of at-risk individuals decide to get predictive testing. Common reasons cited for undergoing predictive testing are family planning or to guide decisions about their future. Box 15.4 lists the current HDSA guidelines for predictive testing, which includes a telephone call prior to the first in-person visit, meeting with a genetic counselor, mental health assessment, neurologic exam, and only giving the results in person.

BOX 15.4 HDSA Recommendations for Huntington Disease Predictive Testing

1. Telephone contact
2. Visit one:
   a. Genetic counseling
   b. Sign informed consent document
   c. Mental health assessment
   d. Neurologic examination
   e. Draw blood
3. Visit two:
   f. Disclosure of results in person
   g. Arrange postresult follow-up
4. Follow-up:
   a. Prearranged phone call or in-person visit

HDSA, Huntington's Disease Society of America.
Source: Huntington's Disease Society of America. Genetic Testing Protocol for Huntington's Disease. *Huntington's Disease Society of America; 2016. http://hdsa.org/wp-content/uploads/2015/02/HDSA-Gen-Testing-Protocol-for-HD.pdf*

MEDICAL HISTORY AND CLINICAL PRESENTATION

HD is known to cause a clinical triad of symptoms impacting motor, psychiatric, and cognitive abilities. Patients can vary in their presentations and even first-degree relatives do not always have the same course or presentation of disease.

- **Motor symptoms:** Not all patients will experience the same motor symptoms. Occulomotor slowing is often the first, very subtle, motor abnormality present in HD but goes unnoticed by patients. Chorea is more commonly seen as the first motor abnormality in adult-onset HD and is the most characteristic motor symptom of HD. Juvenile-onset HD does not typically present with chorea but rather has a more parkinsonian presentation with bradykinesia, rigidity, and dystonia.
  - **Chorea:** Rapid irregular muscle jerks that occur involuntarily and unpredictably in different parts of the body. Can affect all areas of the body including limbs, trunk, upper face, and lower face. Mild chorea can be present in the fingers and toes and can be misinterpreted as fidgeting, nervousness, or the inability to sit still. Chorea often worsens temporarily during times of heightened emotions (e.g., anger, anxiety, joy).
  - **Dystonia:** Sustained inappropriate contraction of a muscle resulting in an abnormal posture. Dystonia can be present in the neck (cervical dystonia), trunk, or limbs. It can be accompanied by pain in some circumstances.
  - **Myoclonus:** Sudden, rapid, twitch-like muscle contraction. These movements are very quick and jerky, unlike chorea, which is more fluid, slower, and dance-like.
  - **Occulomotor abnormalities:** Can be a subtle first sign of motor symptoms. This may manifest as restricted range of motion (ROM) of extraocular movements or slowed/jerky saccades. As the disease progresses patients may not to be able to initiate saccades at all or have severely restricted ROM of their eyes.
  - **Rigidity:** Stiff or inflexible muscles. Muscles are unable to relax and this can lead to decreased ROM as the disease progresses. This is often present earlier in the course of juvenile HD and in later stages of adult-onset HD.
  - **Bradykinesia:** Can be present in both juvenile and adult-onset HD; however, it is more commonly seen earlier in the course of juvenile HD.
  - **Motor impersistence:** Inability to sustain a voluntary muscular effort. It is tested in HD by asking patients to open their mouth and stick their tongue out. A test is considered normal if the patient can sustain this posture for at least 10 seconds. If the patient's tongue

returns to their mouth before 10 seconds, they are considered to have motor impersistence. Patients may complain of dropping items frequently such as their phone or dishware. This occurs because their hand involuntarily opens from the gripped position.
    - **Speech and swallowing:** Commonly impacted in HD. Dysarthria is common and can occur in earlier stages of disease whereas dysphagia usually presents in mid to late stage of HD.
- **Psychiatric symptoms:** May be more impactful to daily life than motor symptoms in some patients. An estimated 40% of HD patients suffer from major depression or anxiety. Psychiatric symptoms tend to worsen as the disease progresses with apathy being a common symptom throughout all stages of disease. The suicide rate is 5% to 10% higher in the HD community compared to the general population. There are typically two times when suicide rates peak in HD; after genetic testing and in mid-stage disease. This is very important to remember when considering testing a patient for HD. Before genetic testing is completed it is imperative that the patient meet with a mental health professional to rule out suicidal ideation.
    - Other psychiatric symptoms seen in HD include hallucinations, delusions, obsessions, and compulsions. Hallucinations are most commonly visual and can cause behavioral issues and distress for the patient. HD patients who develop hallucinations or delusions should be evaluated for causes such as metabolic or neurologic derangements, intoxication or drug withdrawal, or delirium. If these possibilities have been ruled out, then neuroleptics are used for treatment.
- **Cognitive symptoms:** HD can impact many areas of cognition including memory, language, and executive functions. Mild cognitive impairment can be seen very early in the course of the disease and almost inevitably progresses to dementia over time. One common symptom that makes HD particularly difficult to treat in the early and mid-stages is anosognosia. Anosognosia is described as a "lack of insight" and impairs a person's ability to perceive and understand their own symptoms. Unfortunately, this can be a barrier to care as patients do not perceive themselves as having any difficulties due to HD symptoms. This "lack of insight" can also cause arguments between patients and their loved ones. Changes in personality including irritability, temper outbursts, impulsive behaviors, and obsessions are also common with cognitive decline. Clinicians should be sensitive to family members caring for a loved one with HD and offer support and resources to ease the burden of care. Social workers are a key part of the healthcare team and can help support and find resources for families impacted by HD.

PHYSICAL EXAMINATION

Patients may present to the clinic before symptoms occur if they have a known family history of HD. There are different classifications for patients who are at risk, prodromal, or with manifest HD (Table 15.15). For patients with confirmed HD the Unified Huntington's Disease Rating Scale (UHDRS) is typically performed at every appointment. This helps track progression of symptoms over the course of the disease. It can also help pick up subtle signs suggesting a previously presymptomatic patient has now become a prodromal or motor-manifest HD patient. The UHDRS includes assessments of eye movements, tongue protrusion, speech, dystonia, chorea, rigidity, bradykinesia, gait, tandem gait, and postural instability.

TABLE 15.15 Different Classifications of Huntington Disease Based on Symptoms and Genetic Testing

HD Genetically Confirmed	Signs and Symptoms	HD NOT Genetically Confirmed
Presymptomatic HD (genetically confirmed HD but no symptoms)	• No clinical motor signs or symptoms • No cognitive signs or symptoms • May or may not have changes in imaging, quantitative motor assessments, or other biomarkers • No symptomatic treatment indicated	Clinically at-risk (not genetically tested, no symptoms, parent affected with HD)
Prodromal HD (HD genetically confirmed, prodromal/subtle symptoms)	• Subtle motor signs and/or subtle cognitive signs or symptoms • Apathy or depression or other behavioral changes related to HD may be present • Usually changes in imaging and quantitative motor assessments • May or may not need symptomatic treatment (e.g., for depression)	Clinically prodromal HD (HD not genetically confirmed, prodromal symptoms)
Manifest HD (HD genetically confirmed and obvious symptoms present)	• Presence of clinical motor and/or cognitive signs and symptoms that have an impact on life • Decreased in functional capacity • Symptomatic treatment appropriate	Clinically manifest HD (HD not genetically confirmed but obvious symptoms present)

HD, Huntington disease.

DIFFERENTIAL DIAGNOSIS

Lack of family history does not automatically rule out an HD diagnosis in a symptomatic patient. Death at an early age, misdiagnosis, adoption, or false paternity may result in a "new" diagnosis of HD in the family. Table 15.16 is an overview of some conditions that should be on the differential diagnosis list. Clinicians working in an urgent care or ED setting should be aware patients with HD are sometimes mistaken for being intoxicated. There have been unfortunate incidents between police and HD patients because abnormal movements, wobbly gait, and slurred speech were interpreted as alcohol intoxication rather than recognized as symptoms of HD.

TREATMENT

- **Pharmacology:** Currently there are no disease-modifying treatments available to slow the progression of HD. Treatment is therefore focused on improving symptoms and quality of life. When starting treatment for chorea

TABLE 15.16 Differential Diagnosis for Huntington Disease

Differential Diagnosis by Category	Specific Disease Examples
Autosomal dominant	Huntington disease-like types 1 and 2; spinocerebellar ataxia types 1, 2, 3, and 17; idiopathic basal ganglia calcification (Fahr disease)
Autosomal recessive	Ataxia with oculomotor apraxia types 1 and 2; Friedreich ataxia; phenylketonuria
X-linked	McLeod syndrome; Lesch-Nyhan disease
Maternal inheritance	Mitochondrial disorders
Autoimmune or inflammatory	Antiphospholipid antibody syndrome; sarcoidosis; Sydenham chorea
Cerebrovascular	Arteriovenous malformation; moyamoya disease
Infection	Creutzfeldt-Jakob disease; progressive multifocal leukoencephalopathy
Metabolic or endocrine	Hypoparathyroidism; hyperthyroidism; renal failure
Neoplasia	Paraneoplastic syndrome, basal ganglion involvement
Toxic	Alcohol intoxication or withdrawal; carbon monoxide

clinicians should consider other symptoms the patient is experiencing and start a medication that will have dual purposes. Neuroleptics, for example, can be used to treat psychosis and chorea. Some neuroleptics can also help increase appetite or improve sleep. There are currently only two FDA-approved medications for the treatment of chorea in HD, tetrabenazine and deutetrabenazine. Both medications are classified as VMAT2 inhibitors (vesicular monoamine transporter-2 inhibitors). Their mechanism of action is to reduce the release of dopamine which in turn reduces stimulation of dopamine receptors in the brain. Clinicians should use VMAT2 inhibitors with caution in patients with uncontrolled depression or history of suicide as worsening mood and increased suicidal thoughts can be unintended side effects. Table 15.17 lists symptoms that may be present along with chorea and medications that should be considered. For treatment of mood symptoms (e.g., depression, anxiety), antidepressants such as fluoxetine, paroxetine, or sertraline are good options. These can also help with irritability or at higher doses selective serotonin reuptake inhibitors (SSRIs) can help with obsessions. Consultation with a psychiatrist is often necessary as the disease progresses and psychiatric symptoms become more problematic. Many HD centers have a psychiatrist as part of the team that is familiar with the unique features of HD. There is little convincing evidence that any medications improve cognition in HD, but many clinicians will try donepezil, rivastigmine, or memantine in appropriate patients.

- **Therapies:** Allied health professionals are an integral part of HD patient care. Physical and occupational therapists are extremely helpful for motor symptoms and activities of daily living. Speech therapists help with communication and can evaluate swallowing function. As swallowing function declines a video swallow study will be necessary to make recommendations about diet and thickening liquids. Dietitians can help by making nutritional assessments and providing counseling. Social workers aid with the disability process, management of social crises, advance directives, nursing home placement, accessing community resources, and mental health counseling (if licensed).

TABLE 15.17 Medication Considerations in Huntington Disease With Troublesome Chorea

Accompanying Symptoms	Drugs to Consider
No other symptoms	Tetrabenazine, amantadine, deutetrabenazine
Weight loss	Olanzapine, cannaanoids
Psychosis, aggression, or impulsivity	Aripiprazole, haloperidol, olanzapine, risperidone, or other neuroleptic
Anxiety	Benzodiazepines
Depression	Aripiprazole and avoid tetrabenazine/deutetrabenazine
Apathy	Amantadine or stimulating medications and avoid neuroleptics
Prominent dystonia	Amantadine, benzodiazepines, focal neurotoxin injection, and avoid neuroleptics

- **Research:** Trials are ongoing to find a disease-modifying agent that can slow down the progression of HD. Antisense oligonucleotides are "huntingtin lowering" therapies aimed to slow progression of HD by reducing production of huntingtin protein. They have shown promise in animal studies and in phase 1a/2b human trials but have not yet been proved to slow down HD progression. Another option being researched for HD is gene therapy. One type of gene therapy involves delivery of a viral vector directly into the brain. The viral vector contains a modified piece of RNA that reduces the production of huntingtin protein. This has proved successful in animal models and is in the early stages of human trials. No vitamins, supplements, or alternative treatments have been proved to slow the progression of HD. Many patients are looking for hope and clinicians must be able to provide gentle guidance on the potential harm from unproven "treatments."

SPECIAL CONSIDERATIONS

- It is extremely important that every patient meet with a genetic counselor prior to genetic testing to be educated on all potential ramifications. The Genetic Information Nondiscrimination Act (GINA) protects against discrimination based on genetic information.[136] However, this act only covers discrimination in the workplace and for

health insurance and there is no guarantee that it will not be changed or overruled in the future. Even with GINA, HD patients can still legally be discriminated against with regard to life insurance and long-term care insurance.
- Testing minors is a complex issue that should not be done without input from an HD specialist. A presymptomatic minor who receives a positive test result will live the rest of their life knowing they will eventually develop HD. Testing for symptomatic minors is recommended only after following with a neurologist (preferably an HD specialist) for at least 6 months. The neurologist will need to perform a physical examination at the initial visit and again at least 6 months later before testing is recommended.
- For other complex scenarios (e.g., testing pregnant women, one twin wants to be tested and the other does not, testing unborn fetuses, testing adult children before their parent) it is best to refer the patient to an HDSA Center of Excellence. If there are none in your geographic area it may be worthwhile to reach out to the nearest Center of Excellence for guidance and support. You can find contact information for
  - **HDSA Centers of Excellence:** https://hdsa.org/find-help/clinical-care-services/hdsa-centers-of-excellence/.
  - **HDSA Chapters:** 53 chapters across the United States provide support for community social workers who can be of service to any potential HD patient and their healthcare team (https://hdsa.org/about-hdsa/chapters-affiliates/)

15.6D TOURETTE SYNDROME

OVERVIEW

Tourette syndrome is a childhood-onset neurologic movement disorder characterized by the presence of both motor and phonic (vocal) tics. The disorder generally presents before adulthood, most often between 2 and 15 years of age.

EPIDEMIOLOGY

The exact prevalence of Tourette syndrome is not known, but estimations average approximately 0.77%. Boys are more likely than girls to be affected, with the average male-to-female ratio being 4:1.[137]

PATHOPHYSIOLOGY

Tourette syndrome is thought to result from a complex interaction between social, environmental, and genetic abnormalities. Accumulating evidence suggests that abnormalities in the basal ganglia and corticostriatal thalamacocortical circuits contribute to the pathogenesis of the disorder.[137]

MEDICAL HISTORY AND CLINICAL PRESENTATION

The physical examination is generally normal except for the presence of tics and is most important for ruling out other diagnoses. Comorbidity with other neurobehavioral disorders, such as ADHD, conduct or oppositional defiant disorders, and OCD, is common.

Tics are the clinical hallmark of the disorder and may not be easily observed during the initial examination. Tics are sudden, repetitive movements (motor tics) or sounds (phonic tics) that typically mimic some aspect of normal behavior. They are often brief and occur in bouts. Tics are considered involuntary but can be voluntarily suppressed temporarily. They are often exacerbated by stress, anxiety, emotional upset, or fatigue. Many patients describe premonitory feelings or sensations, which are relieved by the execution of the tic. The severity of tics usually peaks between ages 10 and 12, and by age 18, 50% of patients are essentially free of tic symptoms.

Simple motor tics involve a single muscle or group of muscles. Complex motor tics involve multiple muscle groups and are usually of longer duration (Table 15.18).

Simple phonic tics are vocalizations of sounds, where as complex phonic tics are vocalizations of words and/or complex phrases (Table 15.19).

DIFFERENTIAL DIAGNOSIS

Tourette syndrome and related tic disorders generally must be distinguished from other movement disorders due to medical conditions, such as HD, stroke, Wilson disease, and multiple sclerosis. Transient tics of childhood occur in about 25% of normal children and usually last about 1 year.[138] The ability to temporarily suppress tics and premonitory sensations often help to differentiate it from other hyperkinetic movement disorders, such as dystonia, chorea, and myoclonus.

EVALUATION AND DIAGNOSIS

Diagnosis of Tourette syndrome is made based on the history and clinical presentation. A careful review of the medical, social, and family history for tics or tic-related disorders is essential. The diagnosis is made based on history and clinical features of the disease, particularly the presence of multiple motor tics and phonic tics, with onset prior to age 18 to 21 (depending on the guidelines used). Tic severity and progression can be measured using a validated scale, such as the Yale Global Tic Severity Table.[138] There are no diagnostic laboratory tests or imaging studies to confirm the diagnosis of Tourette syndrome.

TABLE 15.18 Simple Versus Complex Motor Tics

Simple Motor Tics	Complex Motor Tics
Eye blinking	Jumping or shaking
Nose sniffing	Touching oneself or others
Neck/arm twitching	Performing obscene gestures (copropraxia)
Shoulder shrugging	Mimicking of gestures (echopraxia)

TABLE 15.19 Simple Versus Complex Phonic Tics

Simple Phonic Tics	Complex Phonic Tics
Throat clearing	Repeating one's own words or phrases
Grunting or snorting	Repeating the last-heard word (echolalia)
Coughing or barking	Rarely: uttering socially unacceptable words or phrases (coprolalia)

TREATMENT

The goals of treatment are to improve social functioning, self-esteem, and quality of life. A multimodal treatment approach is most effective, including both nonpharmacologic interventions and pharmacotherapy when appropriate. There is no cure for tics, and treatment is purely symptomatic. Patients are more likely to be impaired by the manifestations of comorbidities than the tics themselves, and choice of initial treatment depends largely on the most disabling symptoms for each patient. Neurologic and psychiatric evaluation and treatment may be useful for other primary disorders and comorbid conditions (ADHD, OCD, depression). Environmental modifications, identifications of triggers, and cognitive-behavioral therapy (CBT) may be helpful nonpharmacologic measures for management of tics.

When initiating pharmacotherapy in patients, monotherapy is preferred. Goals should be aimed at reducing the severity of tics while minimizing side effects of the medications, as most patient will not experience complete resolution of tic symptoms. Frontline treatment options include dopamine D2 receptor antagonists, typical or atypical antipsychotics, and alpha-2 adrenergic receptor agonists.

15.5E GAIT DISORDERS

OVERVIEW

Gait is an important motor function that is unconscious and automatic. Gait is a fundamental skill and is basic to the qualify of life. Walking requires considerable motor coordination. Disorders of gait are common and may be the presenting feature in some neurologic disorders. Gait disorders are particularly important in the elderly because they compromise independence and contribute to the risk of falls and injury.

It is important to distinguish between balance and stance. Stance is the posture of standing, which normally is in the upright position, whereas balance is the ability to maintain stance. The causes of gait disorders include neurologic conditions (e.g., sensory or motor impairments), orthopedic problems (e.g., osteoarthritis and skeletal deformities), and medical conditions (e.g., heart failure, respiratory insufficiency, peripheral arterial occlusive disease, and obesity).[139]

PATHOPHYSIOLOGY

There is a great deal of interest in the pedunculopontine nucleus (PPN) of the brain as a locomotor center; it sits at the convergence of several motor pathways. The PPN projects to the brainstem and spinal cord. The dorsal midbrain (home of the PPN) is among the areas activated by walking as shown in SPECT imaging. The PPN is an important integrator of activity from the basal ganglia, cerebellum, and motor cortex. Many gait disorders result from pathology in the forebrain, which includes the basal ganglia, motor cortex, and frontal subcortical circuits. Several neurologic systems are involved in ambulating, including the frontal lobes, basal ganglia, diencephalon and midbrain, spinal cord, peripheral nervous system, vestibular system, and cerebellum.

MEDICAL HISTORY AND CLINICAL PRESENTATION

The classification and diagnosis of gait disorders are essentially based on observational analysis that can be challenging. Following is a list of abnormal gait patterns that may provide the observant clinician with a working diagnosis. Attention should be paid to specific aspects of gait, such as the stride length and cadence, deviations from the direction of progression, stride width, stiffness, and the ability to turn smoothly. In addition to normal ambulation, patients should be asked to walk a straight line, heel to toe. The "pull test" is generally helpful in identifying a problem with balance and is an important diagnostic clue when considering PD.

If an elderly patient presents with the *triad* of a parkinsonian gait, acute cognitive impairment, and urinary incontinence, MRI of brain is typically ordered to rule out normal pressure hydrocephalus (NPH). If NPH is present, the MRI will reveal cerebral atrophy and enlarged ventricles. A useful diagnostic tool for NPH is performing a lumbar puncture and drawing off approximately 50 mL of CSF. If gait improves following lumbar puncture the diagnosis is positive for NPH; if there is no improvement in gait, it is not typically due to NPH.

Weakness is commonly due to neuropathy or myopathy. Ataxia looks mostly clumsy, while chorea often has a dancing quality. Veering gait defined as a deviation from a direct line of progression is due to either vestibular or cerebellar disorders.[83]

PHYSICAL EXAMINATION

- **Romberg sign:** Ask the patient to stand with feet close together and closed eyes. A slight sway is not abnormal but marked swaying or falling is indicative of a *proprioceptive* deficit (positive Romberg sign). These patients may have trouble navigating familiar places (bedroom to bathroom) in the dark or maintaining balance while in the shower (due to reduced visual input). A person with *cerebellar* dysfunction will sway with their eyes open.
- **Retropulsion pull test:** This test traditionally is used to assess balance. Instruct the patient as to what is about to happen. The clinician stands behind the patient and pulls their shoulders backwards. Patients are instructed to stand erect, eyes open and feet comfortably apart. They should not shift their weight forward in anticipation of the pull. The clinician stands behind the patient with enough room to allow the patient to take several steps if needed to recover their balance but close enough to support the patient if needed. The pull test is part of the UPDRS and is performed during the motor examination. In a normal test the patient maintains balance without taking any steps backward. One or two steps are also considered to be in the normal range; three to five steps would indicate slight disease progression. The rating score is 0–4. The higher the number, the more advanced the disease. This enables clinicians to follow the patient's balance longitudinally.

Common Patterns of Gait Disorders

- **Cautious gait:** The pattern of reduced stride, wider base, shorter swing phase with preservation of rhythmic stepping is, in essence, an adaptation to perceived imbalance. This is a common disorder, particularly in the elderly who may have already experienced a fall(s). It may resemble how a normal person would "walk on ice." It is usually wide-based, slow with short steps. The patient tries to reach out for something to hold on to for support. Fear of falling is a primary contributor to a cautious gait and worsens following a fall, particularly if it resulted in an injury. A cautious gait usually responds very well to physical therapy.

- **Stiff-legged gait/spastic gait:** This is a disorder observed among patients with cerebral palsy, demyelinating diseases such as multiple sclerosis, and spinal disorders. Legs may scissor and shoes often reflect uneven wear due to toes turning in and scraping floor.
- **Parkinsonian gait:** Parkinsonian patients usually have a stooped posture with marked flexion at the trunk. Balance is poor, gait is distinctive for short, shuffling steps and can be associated with *festination*, which is a hastening of gait and turning en bloc (as if turning around on a block of wood). One of the easiest and usually first observed changes in gait is diminished arm swing, typically asymmetric. Freezing of gait (FOG) is a distinctive phenomenon of PD. FOG is a major cause of falls in PD due to the forward momentum of the upper body and the inability to pick up the feet to follow this movement. The patient may appear to walk somewhat reasonably well but hesitate when turning or when coming to the threshold of a doorway. The frequency of FOG increases as disease progresses. The patient will describe their *feet feeling like they have been "glued or nailed" to the floor*. Once patients initiate the first step, they overcome the motor block. Motor blocks can be overcome with the aid of sensory or visual cues. A visual cue may be simply asking the patient to visualize a log in front of their feet and in order to walk, they need to step over it. Patients are able to navigate walking up a staircase without difficulty due to the horizontal lines of the steps. If a patient has FOG at doorways when home, a clinician might recommend that they lay down several horizontal strips of adhesive tape on either side of the doorway threshold; this is usually helpful in overcoming motor blocks and reducing falls. There are canes and walkers available specifically designed to aim a *laser light beam* across the floor in front of the patient's feet. By focusing on the beam, they are usually able to overcome the motor block.
- **Dystonic gait:** This gait may be focal or generalized. Usually the examiner will notice inversion of the foot while walking. Whatever the cause, dystonia can produce rather unusual disorders of gait with so much abnormal movement, it may resemble the dancing choreic gait of HD chorea. The gait may completely disappear if the patient is asked to walk backward.
- **Ataxic gait:** The word origin of "ataxia" is "without order."
  - ***Cerebellar* ataxia:** Characterized by irregularity of stepping, in direction, distance, and timing. The patient may lurch in different directions. Balance, which is the ability to maintain stance, is poor and it is broad-based. Gait ataxia is probably the most common manifestation of cerebellar damage; it is often the first clinical sign of damage to the cerebellum and is also one of the most troublesome symptoms for patients.
  - ***Sensory* ataxia:** This may be observed in patients with a history of peripheral neuropathy that may be due to a number of disorders including cobalamin (vitamin B12) deficiency, paraproteinemia (multiple myeloma), diabetes, multiple sclerosis, spinal cord compression, and autoimmune or paraneoplastic disorders. Sensory ataxia differs slightly from cerebellar ataxia in that the patient will usually look down; gait is slow and high-stepping; Romberg testing is usually positive and a history of frequent falls is typical. Patient may appear to be "walking on pillows" and have absent proprioception of limbs on clinical examination.
- **Apraxia:** The word origin of "apraxia" is inability to perform particular purposive actions.
  - *Apraxic gait*: Apraxia is traditionally defined as a disorder of voluntary movement that cannot be explained by weakness, spasticity, rigidity, akinesia, sensory loss, or cognitive impairment.[83] These patients typically have normal leg function when seated or in the supine position. They can imitate riding a bicycle while in the supine position and make circles in the air with their feet. When standing, lower limb movement is impaired and appears unsure. Patients maintain normal upper limb movement. Gait is commonly broad-based with short shuffling and hesitating steps. The patient's steps may resemble a parkinsonian gait with the exception that it is a symmetric movement. Patients are unable to mimic steps and do not respond to visual cues. Other clues may be brisk reflexes, urinary incontinence, and no response to administration of levodopa. The differential diagnosis should include frontal lobe disease and normal pressure hydrocephalus.

DIFFERENTIAL DIAGNOSIS

Some very distinctive physical clues may further help narrow down the differential diagnosis. The clinician can perform physical exam and observe for clinical features (Table 15.20)

TABLE 15.20 Clinical Features of Gait Disorders

Clinical Features	Diagnostic Considerations
Positive Romberg sign	Cerebellar ataxia
Positive retropulsion pull test, stooped posture, shuffling steps, diminished arm swing, freezing of gait	Parkinsonism
Decreased stride, wider base, resembles "walking on ice"	Cautious gait, elderly, history of falls
Stiff-legged, spastic	Cerebral palsy, multiple sclerosis, spinal disorder
Foot inversion, normal gait walking backward	Dystonia (focal or generalized)
Ataxia (cerebellar)	Stroke, cerebral palsy, multiple sclerosis
Ataxia (sensory)	Neuropathy, vitamin B12 deficiency, diabetes mellitus, multiple sclerosis
Apraxic gait (normal upper limb function)	Frontal lobe disease, normal pressure hydrocephalus
Dancing/choreic	Huntington chorea

DIAGNOSTIC STUDIES

- Serum vitamin B12, CBC, thyroid function testing: diagnostic for common causes of peripheral neuropathy such as vitamin B12 deficiency, diabetes mellitus, and hypothyroidism
- Neuromuscular testing such as EMG and nerve conduction study (NCS): for abnormalities such as peripheral neuropathies and radiculopathies
- Imaging studies: MRI and/or CT to exclude intracranial disorders that include lesions, normal pressure hydrocephalus, and stroke

TREATMENT

Management of gait disorders will be highly varied and dependent on the underlying pathophysiology.

15.6F RESTLESS LEGS SYNDROME

MEDICAL HISTORY AND CLINICAL PRESENTATION

RLS, also called Willis-Ekborn disease, is a common neurologic sensory disorder that affects sleep. It is estimated to affect 5% to 15% of the general population.[140] Despite RLS's prevalence, it is thought to be underdiagnosed by clinicians due to a lack of understanding about the disorder and an absence of uniform diagnostic criteria. The pathophysiology of RLS is poorly understood, but dopamine dysfunction and a low concentration of iron in the basal ganglia may play a role.

RLS may be referred to as either primary or secondary. Primary RLS is idiopathic but has a genetic component as several gene loci have been implicated. Additionally, primary RLS often has an onset before the age of 40. Regardless of age or cause, RLS worsens over time. Secondary RLS occurs in the presence of certain medical conditions. Pregnancy, renal failure, anemia, low ferritin levels, neuropathy, PD, sleep apnea, and multiple sclerosis are common comorbid conditions. Environmental factors including diet, anxiety, stress, and the use of certain medications may contribute to the severity of symptoms. These medications have been shown to exacerbate symptoms:

- Alcohol, caffeine, nicotine
- Antihistamines (diphenhydramine)
- Antinausea medications
- Antipsychotic medications
- Antidepressants (tricyclics, SSRIs)

SIGNS AND SYMPTOMS

Patients with RLS experience uncomfortable sensations in the legs coupled with a strong compulsion to move the legs. These sensations vary by individual, but common descriptors include itchy, tingly, throbbing, "creepy-crawly," or a generalized feeling of discomfort. These sensations are relieved by moving the limbs. Symptoms occur or significantly worsen during periods of inactivity, particularly in the evening or throughout the night. During the daytime, symptoms disappear or improve significantly. Symptoms may wax and wane and may disappear for weeks, months, or years before returning.

Many patients with RLS experience involuntary jerking movements of the legs during sleep. This is called periodic leg movements of sleep (PLMS). PLMS symptoms in the absence of RLS is called periodic limb movement disorder (PLMD).

Patients with RLS may suffer from significant sleep disturbances, which may include insomnia, poor sleep quality, and daytime somnolence. It is unclear if the symptoms from RLS or the motor activity from the PLMS cause the sleep disturbances. Impaired work performance and cognitive function adversely affects the quality of life for those with RLS.

PHYSICAL EXAMINATION

Physical exam findings are normal in RLS. However, a neuromuscular exam should be completed to rule out parkinsonism, radiculopathy, neuropathy, or claudication.

DIFFERENTIAL DIAGNOSIS

The differential diagnosis for RLS is summarized in Table 15.21.

EVALUATION

RLS is a clinical diagnosis that requires a careful history and physical examination. Patient questionnaires for RLS are available to assess the impact on the quality of life for those affected. The iron status of all patients with RLS should be evaluated and corrected if deficient. This should include a CBC, serum ferritin level, transferrin saturation, and a total iron binding capacity. Those with low levels of ferritin (<50 µg/L) respond to oral iron supplementation. Consider checking renal function if clinically indicated; uremia may worsen symptoms of RLS. Additional laboratory testing to consider may include magnesium, folate, vitamin B12, and glucose levels.

A polysomnography (sleep study) should be considered to identify the presence of sleep apnea and/or to quantify the severity of PLMS since both may contribute to poor sleep quality.

TREATMENT

Iron supplementation should be given to all patients who are anemic or have low serum ferritin levels (<50 µg/L). Ferrous sulfate 325 mg once or twice a day is sufficient.

TABLE 15.21 Differential Diagnosis for Restless Legs Syndrome

Diagnosis	Description
Leg cramps	Usually unilateral; associated with physical changes in the muscle like hardness/firmness
Claudication	Associated with decreased temperature of the skin and reduced pulses
Neuropathy/radiculopathy	Associated with atrophy, decreased strength, impaired deep tendon reflexes, impaired primary sensation (light touch, pain discrimination)
Akathisia	A feeling of restlessness or urge to move without any sensory symptoms; a common adverse reaction from long-term use of first-generation antipsychotic medications

Coadministration with 200 mg of vitamin C will improve absorption. Owing to the potential side effects and risks of parenteral iron, parenteral iron administration should be reserved for patients with complete intolerances to oral iron, those with malabsorption issues, or in cases of severe symptoms from large ferritin deficiencies. Iron therapy is ineffective in patients without laboratory evidence of iron deficiency (low ferritin and/or transferrin saturation) and should be avoided.

First-line pharmacologic therapy for RLS has traditionally included dopamine agonists (pramipexole, ropinirole, rotigotine). The lowest effective dose should be used, because long-term continuous use of these drugs may worsen symptoms, a phenomenon known as augmentation. Augmentation will resolve when the medication is withdrawn. To prevent augmentation, pulse therapy (taking the medication only a couple of days per week and/or during flare-ups) may be helpful. Side effects of dopamine agonists include daytime sleepiness or unexpected sleeping attacks. This is more common with higher doses. Prior to initiation of therapy with a dopamine agonist, clinicians should inquire if the patient has had a previous history of impulse control disorders (e.g., gambling, shopping, and eating) since these medications may affect these disorders. An alpha-2-delta ligand, gabapentin enacarbil has recently been approved as first-line therapy for RLS.[141] Augmentation does not appear to be a problem with gabapentin enacarbil and appears to improve sleep quality. Side effects include drowsiness, dizziness, weight gain, and suicidal ideations. Other alpha-2-delta ligands (gabapentin and pregabalin) have some data to support their use in treating RLS but are not approved by the FDA at the time of this writing.

Benzodiazepines and opioids may be helpful in the short-term management of RLS but should be avoided long-term due to the risks of tolerance and abuse.

Nonpharmacologic therapy for RLS may be considered first-line in patients with mild and/or intermittent symptoms given the complicated side effect panels of the pharmacologic therapies. These may include:

- Moderate exercise
- Leg massages
- Warm baths, heating pad
- Cold packs
- Reducing alcohol, caffeine, and nicotine intake
- Discontinuing medications that are known to exacerbate symptoms

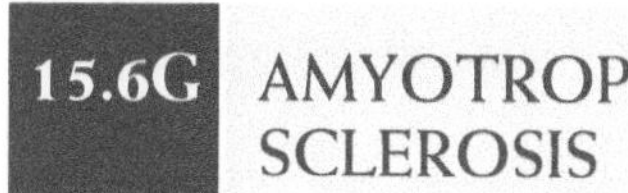

15.6G AMYOTROPHIC LATERAL SCLEROSIS

OVERVIEW

Amyotrophic lateral sclerosis (ALS), also known as Lou Gehrig disease, is a neurodegenerative disease characterized by muscle weakness and progressive disability. ALS progresses rapidly, causing significant morbidity throughout the course of disease and often leads to death within 3 to 5 years. However, about 10% of people with ALS do live beyond 10 years after diagnosis.[142]

EPIDEMIOLOGY

ALS is divided into two main categories: sporadic and familial. Sporadic ALS makes up >90% of all cases, while familial accounts for the remaining <10%. Non-Hispanic White Americans are more frequently diagnosed with ALS than other racial and ethnic groups.[143] Males have slightly higher incidence rates than females and risk increases with each decade of life, with peak onset occurring after the age of 40; however, cases have been reported in patients in their 20s.[142] The only known risk factors are age and family history.

PATHOPHYSIOLOGY

The pathophysiology of ALS is complex; however, overlap with frontotemporal dementia (FTD) has been clearly defined. ALS can be distinguishable from other motor neuron diseases based on the degree of anterior horn cell and corticomotor neuron involvement. In ALS, motor neurons degenerate leading to gliosis, the dense proliferation of glial cells in response to central nervous system injury. Characteristic findings include cortical motor cell degeneration, white matter changes, atrophic spinal cord, and loss of myelination of motor nerves. When present with FTD, degeneration of frontal and/or temporal cortical neurons is also appreciated.[144]

Identifying involved genetic mutations is an area of ongoing research; a defect in the *C9ORF72* gene has been linked to about 40% of cases of familial ALS.[142]

MEDICAL HISTORY AND CLINICAL PRESENTATION

A slow and often subtle onset of symptoms is characteristic of most patients with ALS. Patients may not notice their symptoms at first or present only after symptoms begin to progress or interfere with activities of daily living (ADLs). Upon reflection, patients frequently comment on noticing fasciculations, muscle cramping, weakened grip strength, and difficulty with chewing and swallowing. Patients often present when symptoms have progressed to the point where they have difficulty buttoning shirts or turning a key to unlock a door. The rate and order of progression of symptoms remain highly varied among patients. Unlike symptoms seen in multiple sclerosis, symptoms are constant and progressive rather than relapsing and remitting.

SIGNS AND SYMPTOMS

Unlike many neurologic conditions, ALS presents with a combination of upper and lower motor neuron symptoms (Table 15.22). Upper motor neuron lesions are characterized by stiffness and spasticity while lower motor neuron

TABLE 15.22 Clinical Presentation of Amyotrophic Lateral Sclerosis by Motor Neuron Level

Upper Motor Neuron Findings	Lower Motor Neuron Findings
Weakness	Weakness
Hyperreflexia	Hyporeflexia
Spasticity	Fasciculations
Rigidity	Atrophy
Abnormal reflexes present (Babinski)	Foot drop
Pseudobulbar affect	

lesions are characterized by atrophy and fasciculations. In rare cases, patients may present with only upper motor neuron symptoms (primary lateral sclerosis) or only lower motor neuron symptoms (progressive muscular atrophy), but both conditions may progress to true ALS.[145]

Despite large deficits in motor functioning, patients maintain cognitive functioning. Because of this, many patients develop severe depression and anxiety as they are fully aware of their declining physical abilities. Progressive weakness eventually begins to affect respiration, resulting in respiratory depression so severe that patients become dependent on a ventilator for breathing. This also leaves patients at an increased risk of pneumonia.[142]

PHYSICAL EXAMINATION

A complete neurologic exam is the foundation of diagnosing ALS and, depending on the stage of progression, will reveal weakness, atrophy, and spasticity. Patients may have hyper- or hyporeflexia and abnormal reflexes, such as Babinski, are often present. Gait testing often reveals unsteadiness. Mini-mental status exam (MMSE) will show maintained cognitive functioning and the sensory portion of a physical examination is also typically normal. Additionally, extraocular muscle (EOM) function is maintained. Pseudobulbar affect, characterized by inappropriate emotions of laughing or crying, may be observed.

DIFFERENTIAL DIAGNOSIS

The differential diagnosis for ALS includes multiple sclerosis, post-polio syndrome, spinal cord tumor, Lyme disease, and myasthenia gravis.

DIAGNOSTIC STUDIES

There is no one, definitive test for diagnosing ALS. The revised El Escorial World Federation of Neurology criteria (El Escorial criteria) have been widely accepted to aid in proper and efficient diagnosis of ALS.[146] The El Escorial criteria include the presence of upper and lower motor neuron signs and symptoms in one limb/body segment, EMG evidence of lower motor neuron disease in two body segments, and continued progression of disease in the absence of pathologic evidence of another condition.[146] While the simultaneous presence of both upper and lower motor neuron disease is highly suggestive of ALS, a thorough physical examination and diagnostic testing to rule out related diseases must be performed. EMG can help to differentiate peripheral neuropathies from ALS. MRI, which is usually normal in patients with ALS, can reveal other possible causes of symptoms, such as spinal cord tumors or multiple sclerosis. As ALS can cause extreme muscle wasting and malnutrition, conditions like HIV infection, leukemia, and polio must also be considered. Additionally, as early symptoms are typically mild, myasthenia gravis (MG) should be considered. MG can be ruled out through EMG and lab testing for acetylcholine receptor antibodies.

EVALUATION

Continued evaluation through neurologic testing, imaging studies, genetic testing, and routine laboratory analysis is often needed. Patients should be closely monitored for progression of disease, and intervention is focused on maintaining independence as long as possible.

TREATMENT

- No cure for ALS has been identified. Currently treatments are aimed at maintaining independence, reducing complications, and improving the ability to perform ADLs.
- Riluzole and edaravone are both FDA approved for use in ALS.
- Additional treatment can be used to manage symptoms associated with depression, muscle cramping, sleep disturbances, and spasticity.
- Physical therapy and speech therapy should be started very early in disease progression.
- Nutritional support and respiratory support are often required.

PATIENT EDUCATION

- ALS is a chronic and progressive disease with no cure, but research is being done on ways to improve quality of life.
- Mental health help for both the patient and caregivers/family should be encouraged early in the disease progression.
- An interdisciplinary and collaborative effort between the patient, family, and medical team is needed for optimal care.

15.7 INFECTIOUS DISORDERS

Rayne Loder

OVERVIEW

Meningitis and encephalitis are both infectious disorders of the CNS. Meningitis is inflammation of the meninges and is most frequently bacterial or viral in etiology. While viral meningitis generally has a benign and self-limited disease course, bacterial meningitis is a major cause of morbidity and death if not promptly diagnosed and empiric antibiotic therapy quickly initiated. Encephalitis is inflammation of the brain itself and has both infectious and noninfectious causes, though infectious encephalitis is the focus of this section. Encephalitis is most commonly viral in etiology, although there are myriad potential causative organisms. CSF analysis, including viral PCR and serology, is diagnostically important. Empiric antiviral treatment should not be delayed.

EPIDEMIOLOGY

Epidemiologic information germane to meningitis and encephalitis are discussed in the respective subsections.

PATHOPHYSIOLOGY

Pathophysiology of meningitis and encephalitis, including common infectious organisms, are discussed in the respective subsections.

15.7A MENINGITIS

OVERVIEW

Meningitis refers to acute inflammation of the meninges, the membranes that line the central nervous system. Infectious meningitis can be caused by a variety of organisms and is generally categorized into septic meningitis (bacterial) and aseptic meningitis. Bacterial meningitis requires rapid diagnosis and initiation of treatment. Morbidity and death are considerable with this condition and likelihood of poor outcome increases as treatment is delayed.

MEDICAL HISTORY AND CLINICAL PRESENTATION

Bacterial meningitis can occur in patients of any age, though the incidence of meningitis in children has decreased due to the introduction of childhood vaccines against three causative organisms: *Haemophilus influenzae* type b, *Streptococcus pneumoniae*, and *Neisseria meningitidis*. In neonates, the most common causative organism is *Streptococcus agalactiae* (group B streptococcus [GBS]), which is usually transmitted from mother to child during a vaginal birth. Querying mothers about prenatal GBS testing and, if GBS positive, whether or not correct maternal antibiotic treatment was initiated during labor is an important part of obtaining a medical history in an infant in whom meningitis is suspected.

Streptococcus pneumoniae is the most common cause of bacterial meningitis in children and adults, followed by *Neisseria meningitidis*. *Listeria monocytogenes* is linked to cases of meningitis in neonates, the elderly, and the immunocompromised. Infection can occur due to hematogenous spread, local infection spread (including from otitis media or sinusitis), or as a postsurgical or post-traumatic complication.

Aseptic meningitis refers to meningeal inflammation that is not caused by a bacterial infection and is most frequently caused by enteroviral infection. Less common causes of aseptic meningitis include other viral infections (including herpes simplex virus), fungal infections, medication effects, and malignancy. Aseptic meningitis is more prevalent in summer and early fall when enterovirus is most prevalent.

SIGNS AND SYMPTOMS

Patients with meningitis classically present with fever, headache, neck pain and stiffness (nuchal rigidity), and/or altered mental status. They may also complain of photophobia, nausea with or without vomiting, cranial nerve palsies, or seizure.

PHYSICAL EXAMINATION

Patients with meningitis will be frequently febrile. Mental status can be assessed using the Glasgow Coma Scale. Nuchal rigidity, which manifests as an inability for patient to either passively or actively flex the neck and touch chin to the chest, is an indicator of meningeal inflammation (meningismus). Other physical examination signs that may indicate meningismus include the Brudzinski sign (spontaneous flexion of the hips during attempted passive flexion of the neck) and Kernig sign (inability or reluctance to allow full extension of the knee when the hip is flexed 90 degrees); while commonly discussed, sensitivity and specificity remain low for both exams. A headache that becomes more severe with rapid horizontal rotation is referred to as jolt accentuation and is a classic examination finding in meningitis. A petechial rash is sometimes present and indicates *Neisseria meningitidis* (meningococcal) infection. Papilledema may be present on fundoscopic examination.

Infants may be found to have a bulging anterior fontanelle and may present with poor feeding, irritability, vomiting, and/or lethargy.

DIFFERENTIAL DIAGNOSIS

At its highest level, the diagnosis of meningitis involves differentiating whether the etiology is bacterial or otherwise, which will be discussed in the diagnostic studies and evaluations subsections.

Other diagnostic considerations in patients presenting with fever, headache, nuchal rigidity, and altered mental status include whether the patient is suffering from concurrent encephalitis, or inflammation of the brain. Encephalitis is discussed in Section 15.7B.

DIAGNOSTIC STUDIES

All patients suspected of having meningitis should have routine bloodwork performed including CBC, chemistries, and blood cultures. Lumbar puncture to obtain CSF sample should be performed and CSF samples sent for cell count, protein, glucose, culture, Gram stain, and selected viral PCR studies.

Lumbar puncture should be obtained as quickly as possible unless there is concern for elevated intracranial pressure. Performing lumbar puncture on patients with elevated intracranial pressure could lead to brain herniation. Patients who have altered level of consciousness, focal neurologic abnormalities, papilledema, seizure, or who are immunocompromised should have CT of the head performed prior to lumbar puncture to rule out space-occupying lesion.

EVALUATION

Patients with meningitis will frequently have leukocytosis. Blood cultures may be positive for the causative organism. Typical CSF findings for bacterial versus viral meningitis are detailed in Table 15.23.

TREATMENT

Empiric antibiotic treatment of suspected bacterial meningitis should be initiated within 1 hour of presentation to reduce morbidity and chance of death. Obtaining blood cultures and performing lumbar puncture prior to initiation of antibiotic therapy should be the aim. However, in patients requiring CT scanning prior to lumbar puncture, administering antibiotic before lumbar puncture may be necessary. CSF culture and Gram stain can remain positive for 4 hours after administration of antibiotic, and so lumbar puncture should be performed as soon as possible after antibiotic administration so that CSF results are minimally affected.

There is also evidence[147] to suggest that the administration of dexamethasone can reduce the incidence of long-term neurologic sequelae in patients with bacterial meningitis, specifically streptococcal infection. If streptococcus is

TABLE 15.23 Cerebrospinal Fluid Findings in Bacterial Versus Viral Meningitis

	Glucose	Protein	WBC Count
Bacterial	<40 mg/dL	>200 mg/dL	>1,000/μL
Viral	>40 mg/dL	<200 mg/dL	5–1,000/μL

WBC, white blood cell.

suspected as the causative organism, dexamethasone should be administered just prior to the first antibiotic dose.

Patients with bacterial meningitis should be admitted to the hospital.

Viral meningitis generally has a milder course than bacterial meningitis and is self-limited. Viral meningitis due to the herpes simplex virus can be more severe and can benefit from treatment with antiviral agents. Most patients with viral meningitis can be treated as outpatients but should be given careful instructions to return to the hospital with any changing or worsening symptoms.

PATIENT EDUCATION

Patients should be educated that vaccination can help prevent several types of bacterial meningitis. Household contacts of patients infected with bacterial meningitis should be referred to their clinicians to discuss prophylactic treatment in order to prevent disease transmission.

15.7B ENCEPHALITIS

Encephalitis refers to inflammation of the brain. Infectious encephalitis is usually virally mediated. Encephalitis must be differentiated from encephalopathy, which is a general term for altered mental status without focal neurologic deficit that can result from a number of etiologic processes. Like meningitis, prompt diagnosis and treatment of encephalitis are necessary to reduce risk of death and long-term sequelae.

MEDICAL HISTORY AND CLINICAL PRESENTATION

Over 100 viruses have been determined to cause encephalitis, but the most prevalent infectious organisms in North America are herpes simplex virus-1(HSV-1) and West Nile virus. HSV-1 encephalitis tends to affect patients <20 and >50 years of age and does not have a seasonal prevalence.[148] Encephalitis caused by West Nile virus, a type of arbovirus, should be considered in endemic areas and during times of year in which mosquitos are active as mosquitos are the primary vectors of transmission to humans. Asking about recent travel, exposure to ticks or mosquitos, recent animal bites, HIV status, and immunocompromised status can help shorten the list of potential causative organisms.

SIGNS AND SYMPTOMS

Patients with encephalitis typically present with fever, headache, and altered mental status. Altered mental status can manifest as confusion, personality changes, or obtundation. There may be history of seizure and new focal neurologic deficit. The main differentiator between encephalitis and meningitis is the absence of meningismus in encephalitis, though meningoencephalitis can occur.

PHYSICAL EXAMINATION

Altered mental status is the hallmark of encephalitis, the severity of which can be rated with the Glasgow Coma Scale. Patients with encephalitis will be frequently febrile and seizures are common. Papilledema may be present on fundoscopic exam. Focal neurologic deficits may be present and could include hemiparesis, cranial nerve palsies, and abnormal reflexes.

DIFFERENTIAL DIAGNOSIS

A number of noninfectious etiologies can present similarly to infectious encephalitis and must be considered in the patient suspected of having a central nervous system infection (Table 15.24).

DIAGNOSTIC STUDIES

All patients suspected of having encephalitis should have routine bloodwork performed including CBC, chemistries, and blood cultures. Lumbar puncture to obtain CSF sample should be performed and CSF sent for cell count, protein, glucose, culture, Gram stain, and selected viral polymerase chain reaction (PCR) studies.

Lumbar puncture should be obtained as quickly as possible unless there is concern for elevated intracranial pressure, in which case a CT scan of the head should be performed prior to lumbar puncture to prevent brain herniation. Discussion of criteria for CT prior to lumbar puncture was included in the meningitis subsection.

Chest x-ray, electroencephalography (EEG), and MRI of the head are also frequently utilized diagnostic studies in the evaluation of patients suspected to have encephalitis.

EVALUATION

Characteristic CSF findings in encephalitis resemble the characteristic findings of viral meningitis (discussed in the previous section). HSV and enterovirus PCR studies should be included in the CSF evaluation of all patients suspected of having encephalitis. Serologic testing for West Nile IgM antibodies is also a prudent consideration. HIV testing should be considered in any patient presenting with a central nervous system infection.

TREATMENT

Empiric coverage of HSV-mediated encephalitis with intravenous antiviral (acyclovir) therapy is standard of care and should be initiated as soon as possible after initial presentation.

Treatment otherwise focuses on supportive care. Patients with encephalitis are admitted to the hospital for monitoring of intracranial pressure, seizure activity, fluid requirements, electrolyte levels, and cardiac and respiratory function.

PATIENT EDUCATION

Patients can reduce risk of West Nile virus transmission by being advised to eliminate areas of stagnant water in

TABLE 15.24 Differential Diagnosis of Encephalitis

Diagnosis	Description
Malignancy	Presence of neoplastic masses on imaging
Medication effects	Absence of alternative explanation and known exposure to offending agent
Autoimmune process	Most commonly anti-NMDA receptor encephalitis
Paraneoplastic process	Cancer-related

NMDA, N-methyl-D-aspartate.

which mosquitos can breed and by taking measures to minimize mosquito bites, such as covering their body with clothing, using mosquito repellents, and staying indoors after dark.

SPECIAL CONSIDERATIONS

Immunocompromised patients are at increased risk of cryptococcal meningitis and toxoplasmic encephalitis and these organisms should be considered on the differential when central nervous system infection is suspected in this population of patients.

KEY POINTS

Meningitis

- Inflammation of the meninges leading to fever, headache, neck stiffness, and altered mental status
- Can be caused by bacteria (*S. pneumoniae* or *N. meningitidis*) or viruses (enterovirus most common)
- Bacterial (septic) meningitis is most severe form and can be life threatening if not promptly treated.
- Prompt lumbar puncture and CSF collection aids in diagnosis of bacterial meningitis but should not delay antibiotic administration.
- Viral (aseptic) meningitis can often be managed on an outpatient basis.

Encephalitis

- Inflammation of the brain leading to fever, headache, and altered mental status
- Usually viral in etiology (HSV-1 and West Nile virus most common), though noninfectious types of encephalitis are differential considerations.
- CSF should be obtained and sent for viral PCR and serologies.
- Empiric treatment with IV acyclovir is standard of care.

15.8 DEMENTIA

Anna Swanson

OVERVIEW

Dementia is an umbrella term used to describe neurodegenerative processes that are primarily characterized by a progressive decline in memory, problem-solving, behaviors, language, and the ability to take care of oneself. These deficits fall outside the normal aging process and begin to interfere with the patient's job performance, social functions, and ADLs. There are several different kinds of dementia including but not limited to Alzheimer disease, vascular dementia, frontotemporal dementia, Lewy body dementia, and PD dementia. These are distinguished from one another based on presenting symptoms, rate of progression, cognitive testing, and neuroimaging. Alzheimer disease accounts for approximately 60% to 80% of dementia cases, with vascular dementia being the second most common form.[149] Patients may be diagnosed with mild cognitive impairment rather than dementia after a formal evaluation and cognitive testing. This occurs when the patient does, in fact, exhibit cognitive disturbances on testing, but he or she is still able to independently function in day-to-day activities with minimal or no assistance.

EPIDEMIOLOGY

According to WHO, there are currently around 55 million people worldwide who have dementia, with an estimated 10 million new cases every year.[150] The incidence of dementia in the population increases exponentially after the age of 65. There is approximately a 7% global prevalence of dementia in patients older than 65 years of age. The prevalence of dementia is slightly higher in developed countries at 8% to 10% due to longer lifespans.[151]

PATHOPHYSIOLOGY

The pathophysiology varies for each type of dementia. Most forms of dementia are the result of abnormal protein accumulation and deposition within the brain, leading to neuron cell death and neurodegeneration. This presents clinically as the cognitive deficits detailed below. There are different types of proteins implicated in each disease and some forms of dementia have overlap of the proteins involved. For the sake of this review, the proposed pathophysiology of Alzheimer disease and vascular dementia will be covered.

Alzheimer disease is theorized to be caused by the extracellular aggregation of β-amyloid peptides and intracellular presence of hyperphosphorylated tau neurofibrillary tangles throughout the brain, specifically in the medial temporal lobe and neocortical structures. β-Amyloid peptides are pro-aggregatory molecules that clump together to form oligomers (Figure 15.3). Some of these oligomers are naturally cleared from the brain, but when they are not, they continue to clump together forming larger structures called fibrils. These fibrils attract other proteins and cellular products, resulting in the development of insoluble plaques. These plaques trigger neurotoxic cascades that ultimately lead to cell death. Hyperphosphorylation of microtubule tau proteins leads to cytoskeletal modifications and eventual synapse and neuronal cell death.

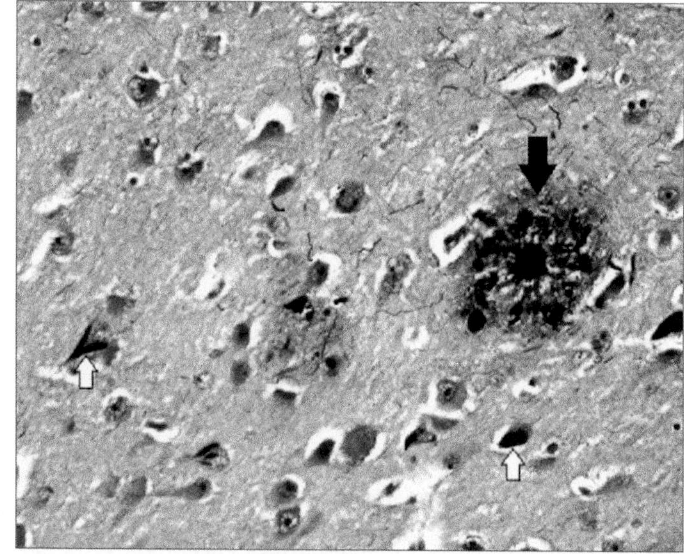

Figure 15.3 Amyloid plaques and neurofibrillary tangles seen in Alzheimer disease. A section of hippocampus with visible neurofibrillary tangles of tau protein aggregates (white arrow) and neuritic plaque of beta-amyloid protein (black arrow).

(Source: Gale SA, Acar D, Daffner KR. Dementia. Am J Med. *2018;1164; Courtesy of Gad A. Marshall, MD, Brigham and Women's Hospital, Boston, MA.)*

Vascular dementia does not occur due to abnormal protein accumulation but instead is the result of vessel changes within the brain. This can occur suddenly after a stroke or slowly over time as atherosclerotic disease accumulates and causes microvascular changes. Uncontrolled diabetes and hypertension can also contribute to these changes. Multiple small strokes in the subcortical region can cause damage, which may lead to progressive cognitive dysfunction.

15.8A ALZHEIMER DISEASE

MEDICAL HISTORY AND CLINICAL PRESENTATION

Alzheimer disease is the most common form of dementia in the world. Typical onset is at the age of 65 or older; however, it can present before the age of 65 and would then be classified as early-onset Alzheimer disease. Typical patient presentation for Alzheimer disease begins with episodic memory loss that slowly progresses over time to involve other cognitive domains. This results in executive dysfunction, changes in language, and visuospatial deficits. Early in the disease, patients may be aware of their deficits, while others may be unaware or attribute symptoms to "getting older." Family members and patients typically present for evaluation when a modest decline in memory or function occurs. It is important to ask questions about the patient's ability to independently perform basic ADLs (e.g., bathing, grooming, dressing, toileting) and functional activities of daily living (e.g., shopping, paying bills, cleaning the house, cooking). Coupled with a thorough history, medication review, and physical examination, cognitive testing will help guide the clinician in making a diagnosis.

SIGNS AND SYMPTOMS

Memory loss is usually the primary chief complaint for individuals later diagnosed with Alzheimer disease. Episodic memory, the ability to recall specific events that occurred at a specific time or place, is affected early in the disease course. Examples include recalling what you ate for breakfast or where you were on 9/11. This type of memory relies significantly on the hippocampus, which is affected in Alzheimer disease. The patient may also have difficulty recalling recent events. Executive dysfunction, judgment deficits, or problem-solving difficulties may present with initial memory impairment or shortly after. Patients may have a lack of insight into their deficits, anosognosia, while others may be aware of their shortcomings early in the disease. Patients with knowledge of their deficits are more likely to develop depression. It is important to always have a family member, or someone who knows the patient well, at these visits so the clinician can compare the patient's interview to the informant's report.

Later in the disease process, patients will begin to exhibit language deficits and behavioral changes including word finding difficulty, agitation, apathy, irritability, wandering, and psychosis. Their memory deficits will also worsen and begin to include learned information, or semantic memory, and immediate recall (Box 15.5). Examples of semantic memory include knowing that the sky is blue or that football is a sport.

BOX 15.5 General Stages of Alzheimer Disease

Early stages: Cognitive problems interfere with day-to-day activities. Patients may have significant difficulty working a job. Changes in the environment can destabilize a patient.

Middle stages: Patients are unable to work and have increased difficulty performing basic activities of daily living (e.g., walking, dressing, grooming) because of apraxia (i.e., inability to perform once learned motor skills). Visuospatial deficits—the inability to distinguish where objects are in space—interfere with their ability to complete these activities as well. They likely require daily assistance and supervision due to wandering behaviors and getting lost in familiar environments. Language also becomes impaired.

Late stages: Patients begin to develop delusions and disinhibition becomes evident. There is a loss of judgment and reasoning. Sleep-wake cycle disturbances lead to nighttime wandering. Patients may develop muscle rigidity and are ultimately bedridden.

PHYSICAL EXAMINATION

A thorough neurologic examination and cognitive testing should be completed in all patients presenting with cognitive complaints. Several standardized forms may be used for cognitive testing—the two most often used are mental state exams (e.g., Mini-Mental State Examination [MMSE]) and the Montreal Cognitive Assessment (MoCA). The MoCA is slightly more sensitive for executive function and language. A score ≥25 out of 30 is considered normal for the MMSE. Scoring ≥26 out of 30 on the MoCA is considered normal; an extra point is given if the patient has 12 or fewer years of education. The MoCA is freely accessible at www.mocatest.org with several different versions and languages.

The physical examination may be normal in patients in the early stages of the disease. As Alzheimer disease progresses, the clinician can expect to see signs of apraxia and visuospatial deficits, difficulty following complex commands, and disorientation. Muscle rigidity, myoclonus, and seizures may present later in the disease as well.

DIFFERENTIAL DIAGNOSIS

There are some patients, usually early-onset cases, who do not present with typical progressive amnestic memory loss. Instead, they may present initially with word finding difficulties or visual impairment. Posterior cortical atrophy (PCA) is a progressive form of cortical visual impairment. Patients with this diagnosis may develop visual hallucinations and have signs of homonymous hemianopia, dysgraphia, acalculia, and simultanagnosia. Antegrade memory is typically spared in these patients. Logopenic primary progressive aphasia (PPA) is a neurodegenerative disorder with progressive language deficits most commonly defined as word-finding speech hesitations without comprehension deficits or grammar difficulties. It is important to note PPA is usually classified as a form of frontotemporal lobar degeneration; however, the logopenic variant is most commonly associated with Alzheimer disease pathology (Table 15.25).

TABLE 15.25 Distinguishing Vascular Dementia from Alzheimer Disease

Diagnosis	Description
Vascular dementia	This is the second most common form of dementia and can sometimes occur with Alzheimer disease. Vascular changes seen in brain imaging include hemorrhagic stroke, ischemic stroke, or chronic small vessel ischemic changes. Neurologic examination may reveal signs of stroke. Patients with chronic small vessel ischemic changes may not have neurologic signs on physical exam.

DIAGNOSTIC STUDIES

Table 15.26 summarizes diagnostic studies for Alzheimer disease.

EVALUATION

The patient's medication list should be evaluated because medications with anticholinergic properties are likely to cause cognitive impairment in patients 65 years or older. If any are identified, the clinician should discontinue these if possible. The patient should improve over time if medication side effects are the sole cause of cognitive impairment. Examples of common anticholinergic medications include amitriptyline, nortriptyline, cyclobenzaprine, dicyclomine, hycosamine, diphenhydramine, doxylamine, meclizine, oxybutynin, solifenacin, and tolterodine.

Memory labs should also be drawn. These include vitamin B12, vitamin B1, TSH, free T4, HIV, syphilis antibody, CBC, and CMP. Any abnormalities should be addressed and corrected.

Neuropsychological testing is a great tool for clinicians. These long visits perform more thorough testing that otherwise could not be performed at a regular appointment. This testing is especially useful for patients with multiple contributing factors (e.g., depression and obstructive sleep apnea), atypical presentations, or whose history and routine cognitive testing do not provide a clear diagnosis. A clinician can always refer the patient to a neurologist or memory care center at any point for further workup and management.

A definitive diagnosis for Alzheimer disease is usually obtained at autopsy as it is confirmed through histopathologic examination. The National Institute on Aging and the Alzheimer's Association created criteria for the diagnosis of probable Alzheimer disease seen in Exhibit 15.1.

TABLE 15.26 Diagnostic Studies for Evaluating a Patient with Memory Impairment and the Expected Findings for Alzheimer Disease

Studies	Findings
MoCA	Average score for patients with AD is between 11–21. Most prominent cognitive domains affected early in the disease are usually delayed recall and executive function. Later most, if not all, of the cognitive domains are involved as the disease progresses.
MRI brain	Atrophy will be seen in the hippocampi or medial temporal lobes early in the disease with eventual involvement of the lateral temporal lobes, parietal lobes, and frontal lobe. *Differential diagnosis:* PCA—parietal involvement is predominant Logopenic PPA—left posterior sylvian atrophy or left parietal atrophy
PET scan FDG-PET	Positive for amyloid deposits in AD. This is not typically covered by insurance and can produce false positives in older generations. *Differential diagnosis:* PCA—hypometabolism in the parietal, parieto-occipital, and temporo-occipital regions Logopenic PPA—hypometabolism in the left temporal and parietal lobes
CSF studies	Low cerebrospinal Aβ42 or (Aβ42: Aβ40 ratio) Elevated total tau and phosphorylated tau

AD, Alzheimer disease; CSF, cerebrospinal fluid; FDG-PET, fluorodeoxyglucose-positron emission tomography; MoCA, Montreal Cognitive Assessment; PCA, posterior cortical atrophy; PPA, primary progressive aphasia.

EXHIBIT 15.1 Probable Alzheimer Disease Dementia: Core Clinical Criteria

Probable Alzheimer disease (AD) dementia is diagnosed when the patient meets criteria for dementia and has the following characteristics:

A. Insidious onset. Gradual onset of symptoms occurs over months to years, not sudden over hours or days.
B. There is a clear-cut history of worsening of cognition by report or observation.
C. The initial and most prominent cognitive deficits are evident on history and examination in one of the following categories.
   a. **Amnestic presentation:** Impairment in learning and recall of recently learned information. There should also be evidence of cognitive dysfunction in at least one other cognitive domain.
   b. Nonamnestic presentations:
      i. **Language presentation:** Most prominent deficits are in word-finding. Deficits in other cognitive domains should be present.
      ii. **Visuospatial presentation:** Most prominent deficits are in spatial cognition, including object agnosia, impaired face recognition, simultanagnosia, and alexia. Deficits in other cognitive domains should be present.
      iii. **Executive dysfunction:** Most prominent deficits are impaired reasoning judgment, and problem-solving. Deficits in other cognitive domains should be present.
D. The diagnosis of probable AD dementia should not be applied when there is evidence of core or prominent feature of other neurodegenerative disorders of substantial concomitant cerebrovascular disease.

Source: McKhann GM, Knopman DS, Chertkow H, et al. The diagnosis of dementia due to Alzheimer's disease: recommendations from the National Institute on Aging-Alzheimer's Association workgroups on diagnostic guidelines for Alzheimer's disease. *Alzheimer's Dement.* 2011;7(3):263–269. doi:10.1016/j.jalz.2011.03.005

TREATMENT

Unfortunately, there is currently no cure for Alzheimer disease. Medication therapies are aimed at reducing symptoms and improving quality of life for the patients and caregivers.

- Cholinesterase inhibitors (e.g., donepezil, rivastigmine, galantamine)
  - Mechanism of action: These agents inhibit the enzyme cholinesterase thereby increasing cholinergic transmission.
  - Utilized as first-line agents. Rivastigmine is available as a transdermal patch if the patient is unable to tolerate oral medications.
  - The clinician should monitor for bradycardia, QT prolongation, and torsades de pointes in at-risk patients, especially with donepezil.
- N-methyl-D-aspartate (NMDA) receptor antagonists (e.g., memantine)
  - Mechanism of action: NMDA receptor is activated by excitatory neurotransmitters. Overstimulation of these receptors can cause neuronal damage/death. These drugs block the NMDA receptor and reduces the number of excitatory neurotransmitters that can bind.
  - They are utilized as add-on therapy in moderate to severe dementia.
- SSRIs can be utilized for depression.
- Trazodone can be considered for sleep difficulties as well, but always try melatonin first.

PATIENT EDUCATION

- Mild cognitive impairment places the patient at a significant risk for dementia but does not always progress to dementia. In some cases, a patient's mild cognitive impairment may stay the same or the patient may revert to their cognitive baseline.
- Patients with a diagnosis of amnestic mild cognitive impairment (MCI) have a higher risk of converting to Alzheimer disease than the general population.
- Patients should be informed they can no longer drive. If they protest, they should be referred for a formal driving safety evaluation.
- Delirium can cause acute behavioral changes. Patients should always be screened for an underlying urinary tract infection or other infection by their primary care clinician to rule out delirium as an underlying cause of these changes.
- Genetic testing is not typically recommended in evaluating patients with Alzheimer disease.
- To help maximize their thinking abilities, it is generally recommended that patients should stay mentally and physically active, eat a well-rounded diet, write down tasks and focus on one task at a time, and manage stress.

15.8B FRONTOTEMPORAL DEMENTIA

MEDICAL HISTORY AND CLINICAL PRESENTATION

Frontotemporal lobar degeneration (FTLD) consists of a clinical group of neurodegenerative disorders marked by frontal and temporal lobe degeneration. Behavioral variant frontotemporal dementia (bvFTD), nonfluent and semantic primary progressive aphasia, frontotemporal dementia with motor neuron disease (FTD-MND), corticobasal syndrome (CBS), and progressive supranuclear palsy syndrome (PSP) are all considered to fall within the FTLD spectrum. The disorders are characterized by progressive changes in the patient's personality, behavior, and/or speech. Motor symptoms are seen in CBS and PSP. Occasionally, there are signs and symptoms of a motor neuron disease in patients with bvFTD. These disorders generally develop when patients are in their 40s to 60s with bvFTD being the most common FTD syndrome. For this reason, the remainder of this section discusses the presentation of bvFTD.

SIGNS AND SYMPTOMS

Patients with bvFTD present with symptoms of personality changes, socially inappropriate behavior, apathy, compulsive behaviors, a lack of insight to the changes in their behavior, poor judgment or decision-making, and changes in diet. They may have frequent and sudden mood changes.

PHYSICAL EXAMINATION

The physical examination in patients with early stages of bvFTD may be relatively normal, outside of inappropriate comments or behaviors. In later stages, their language may become impaired, parkinsonism features may appear, and compulsive or inappropriate behaviors are replaced by apathy. Memory and visuospatial function are relatively spared early in the disease. Assessing for fasciculations, strength, speech, and respiratory function is important because some patients with bvFTD end up developing motor neuron disease. Pseudobulbar affect, inappropriate laughing or crying not consistent with the patient's actual mood, can also be seen in this disorder.

DIFFERENTIAL DIAGNOSIS

The differential for bvFTD includes delirium, alcohol or drug dependence, Alzheimer disease, vascular dementia, chronic traumatic encephalopathy, and structural brain disorders. Psychiatric conditions should also be considered including bipolar disorder, depression, personality disorder, and late-onset schizophrenia.

DIAGNOSTIC STUDIES

Neuroimaging is of utmost importance in supporting a diagnosis of bvFTD. Early in the disease, the imaging may appear normal. Brain MRI may reveal focal frontal or temporal atrophy while fluorodeoxyglucose-positron emission tomography (FDG-PET) may reveal bilateral frontal and/or temporal lobe hypometabolism.

EVALUATION

It is important to remember individuals may be misdiagnosed with a psychiatric disorder due to the prominent behavioral changes. The diagnosis of bvFTD is usually clinically based with neuroimaging findings acting as supportive evidence. A definitive diagnosis is usually not obtained until autopsy when histopathology can be performed.

TREATMENT

- There is no cure for FTD or method to slow down the disease process. For this reason, treatment is based on symptom management.

- SSRIs are useful for depression, irritability, excessive eating, agitation, aggression, and compulsions.
- Cholinesterase inhibitors used in Alzheimer disease may worsen behavioral symptoms in FTD, and therefore, are not recommended for use in bvFTD.
- Atypical antipsychotics can be utilized after a patient has failed behavioral modifications and SSRIs. This medication class carries a black box warning by the FDA for an increased risk of death when used in patients with dementia. For this reason, it is recommended that the patient be referred to a geriatric psychiatrist for management of medications if possible.

PATIENT EDUCATION

- Life expectancy after diagnosis is approximately 8 to 10 years. Patients with concomitant motor neuron disease have a shorter life expectancy.
- Over half of patients with FTD have a sporadic form, meaning there is no family history of a neurodegenerative disorder.
- The patient should be informed that they should no longer drive.
- As the disease progresses and functional abilities become more limited, the clinician should discuss placement options for the patient or employing home care to help alleviate caregiver burden.

15.8C DEMENTIA WITH LEWY BODIES

MEDICAL HISTORY AND CLINICAL PRESENTATION

Dementia with Lewy bodies (DLB) is one of the most common neurodegenerative disorders. It is classified pathologically by the presence of Lewy bodies deep in the cortical layers of the brain. Several distinct features of a patient's history help with the clinical diagnosis of DLB in addition to the presence of dementia. These features include visual hallucinations, rapid eye movement (REM) sleep behavior disorder, parkinsonism, dysautonomia, and sensitivity to antipsychotics.

SIGNS AND SYMPTOMS

Dementia must be present for a patient to be diagnosed with DLB. Caregivers may report the patient becomes lost in familiar areas or is unable to perform his or her job well. Cognitive domains affected early in the disease include visuospatial, executive, and attention. In later stages, the patient develops memory difficulties. This is unlike Alzheimer disease, in which memory impairment occurs early in disease presentation. A patient may have fluctuations in their level of alertness or cognition, reporting symptoms of "blanking out," acting in strange ways, or briefly losing motor or speech function. The spouse may report the patient acts out his or her dreams, with the spouse likely being hit in some way, and they no longer sleep in the same room. Families may report there are falls without a mechanical reason or the patient has lost their sense of smell. Visual hallucinations are also a common occurrence in DLB patients. Hallucinations may range from distorted shapes to insects to people.

PHYSICAL EXAMINATION

Examination will likely reveal parkinsonism features including bradykinesia, cogwheel rigidity, and a shuffling gait. Tremors are less common in LBD than PD. Cognitive testing reveals deficits in the visuospatial domain, executive domain, and attention domain. Autonomic dysfunction may be manifested by orthostatic hypotension when reviewing vitals.

DIFFERENTIAL DIAGNOSIS

The differential diagnosis for DLB is summarized in Table 15.27.

DIAGNOSTIC STUDIES

Diagnostic biomarkers for DLB are not yet clinically available. However, the following findings on imaging may be helpful:

- Brain MRI: generalized atrophy with lesser involvement of the hippocampi when compared to Alzheimer disease
- SPECT: generalized hypoperfusion, most noticeable in the occipital lobes
- PET scan: generalized hypometabolism most noticeable in the occipital lobes
- EEG: helpful if needing to rule out seizures as cause of myoclonus or "blanking out" episodes

EVALUATION

For full evaluation, perform cognitive testing, order lab studies discussed in Section 15.8A Alzheimer Disease, and perform neuroimaging. Treatable conditions should be excluded before diagnosing a patient with any form of dementia. Like other neurodegenerative disorders, definitive diagnosis is usually obtained at autopsy. Diagnosis is usually made by a history and examination, which reveal the core clinical features discussed above.

TREATMENT

Treatment is aimed at symptom management. There are no disease-modifying treatments available right now.

- Cholinesterase inhibitors can be helpful in treating cognitive disturbances in DLB patients.

TABLE 15.27 Differential Diagnosis for Lewy Body Dementia

Diagnosis	Description
Parkinson disease dementia	This diagnosis is similar to dementia with Lewy bodies; however, patients are typically diagnosed with Parkinson disease first and then develop dementia 1 year or later after initial diagnosis.
Normal pressure hydrocephalus	Patients present with cognitive decline, gait changes (magnetic gait), and urinary incontinence; however, NPH does not exhibit REM sleep behavior disorder, psychiatric disturbances, or symptoms of autonomic dysfunction like dementia with Lewy bodies.

NPH, normal pressure hydrocephalus; REM, rapid eye movement.

- Carbidopa-levodopa is sometimes utilized to treat parkinsonism symptoms. This medication can worsen hallucinations and confusion experienced by patients with DLB, so proceed with caution and close monitoring.
- Physical therapy should be considered to help with gait dysfunction and reduce fall risks.
- SSRIs can be utilized to treat depression.
- Melatonin may be used to treat REM sleep behavior disorder.

PATIENT EDUCATION

- DLB is a neurodegenerative process, meaning the patient will continue to worsen and their life span will be shortened as a result.
- The patient needs be informed that they should no longer be driving due to the cognitive impairments.
- Families should consider implementing a regular routine and employing another caregiver to help alleviate caregiver stress and burnout if possible.

15.8D DELIRIUM

OVERVIEW

Delirium is defined as an acute and fluctuating impairment in cognition and the patient's level of alertness. Individuals with delirium typically have a reduced ability to focus, maintain, or shift attention. Delirium develops over a short period of time and will last from hours to days. It is important to ensure the cognitive changes are not the result of a worsening dementia process. Precipitating factors include infection, dehydration, polypharmacy, malnutrition, and immobility. The underlying etiology is usually a medical illness, medications, or substance use. Alcohol or substance withdrawal are the most common causes of delirium in the hospital setting. If the underlying cause is treated, delirium is typically reversible. Patients who have been diagnosed with delirium are at an increased risk of hospital readmission and skilled nursing facility placement.

EPIDEMIOLOGY

Delirium is relatively uncommon in the outpatient setting and is typically seen wherever there are sick patients, most often in ICUs, EDs, and hospice units. Elderly patients are at a greater risk for developing delirium with severe medical illnesses and cognitive decline noted as contributing risk factors. Delirium affects up to 50% of hospitalized seniors, and one review shows the occurrence rate of delirium in general medicine and geriatric wards to be between 29% and 64%.[152]

PATHOPHYSIOLOGY

Delirium is considered acute brain dysfunction and the pathophysiology behind it is not fully understood at this time. Metabolic dysfunction (e.g., too much or too little sodium or potassium, glucose levels outside normal limits, uremia), dehydration, and hepatic dysfunction can all cause or contribute to an individual developing delirium. Infection is also a big risk factor due to the development of inflammatory cascades that trigger cytokine activation, blood flow reduction, and neuronal death. See Box 15.6 for more examples of common factors in the development of delirium.

BOX 15.6 Common Factors in the Development of Delirium

Risk Factors
Advanced age
Cognitive impairment or dementia
Functional impairment or debility
Sensory impairment or hearing/visual loss
TIA or stroke
Alcohol abuse or dependence
Major depression
Comorbidity level or complex multimorbidity
Precipitating Factors
Polypharmacy (five or more medications)
Psychoactive or sedative medications
Infection
Surgery or trauma
Indwelling urinary catheter
Use of physical restraints
Coma
Metabolic or physiologic derangements

TIA, transient ischemic attack.
Source: Adapted from Setters B, Solberg LM. Delirium. Prim Care. *2017; 44(3):541–559. doi:10.1016/j.pop.2017.04.010*

15.9 MULTIPLE SCLEROSIS

Brittany R. Lueking

OVERVIEW

Multiple sclerosis (MS) is an immune-mediated inflammatory demyelinating disease of the central nervous system characterized by demyelinating lesions disseminated in space and time. The cause of MS is unknown; however, several genetic and environmental factors may contribute. Clinical manifestations of MS can vary greatly. As a result, delayed diagnosis is very common, which may lead to progressive accumulation of disability. Misdiagnosis on the other hand may lead to unnecessary exposure to the risks of treatment. Therefore, it is important to possess an adequate understanding of the disease process and develop an appropriate approach to diagnosis and management.

Diagnosis is made using the 2017 McDonald Criteria, integrating patient history, physical examination, neuroimaging, and sometimes CSF analysis to demonstrate dissemination of demyelinating lesions in space and time. MS may be categorized as clinically isolated syndrome, relapsing remitting MS, secondary progressive MS (active or inactive), or primary progressive MS. The former three categories can be considered a spectrum of relapsing disease, while primary progressive MS has a unique clinical course, prognosis, and management. Management of a patient with multiple sclerosis generally includes monitoring for clinical and radiographic disease progression, disease-modifying therapy, symptomatic therapy, and management of acute exacerbations.

EPIDEMIOLOGY

MS classically is a disease of the young, with onset between ages 15 and 45. It can, however, develop earlier or later in life. A small percentage of cases begin during adolescence, and very rarely before the age of 10. MS is more common in women than in men; however, primary progressive MS generally presents at a later age than does relapsing remitting MS and affects men and women more equally.

Although the cause of MS is unknown, it is widely considered at least in part autoimmune in nature; thus, the incidence is higher in individuals with a family history of autoimmune disorders. Individuals with other autoimmune diseases are more likely to develop MS, just as individuals with MS more likely to develop other autoimmune diseases.

The role of genetics in developing MS is still being explored. The strongest observed associations occur with certain major histocompatibility complex (MHC) alleles. The frequency of familial MS varies greatly among studies, but those with a first-degree family member are at increased risk of developing MS compared to the general population. The lifetime risk for monozygotic twins is much greater, further supporting the role of genetic susceptibility in developing MS.

Geographic patterns have been observed as well, specifically a latitude effect. MS is most commonly encountered in the northern areas of Europe and North America. In contrast, MS is markedly less prevalent in the tropics. The explanation for this latitude effect is not definitively known, but vitamin D deficiency is known to be associated with an increased risk of developing MS. Vitamin D may interact with select MHC alleles to increase the risk of developing MS. It is theorized that the ultraviolet-B radiation from the sun in the tropics, which is critical to the biosynthesis of vitamin D, is protective against developing MS.

Other environmental factors appear to play a role in developing MS as well, although these factors are less well developed. Certain viruses such as Epstein-Barr virus (EBV) and varicella-zoster virus (VZV) have been associated with an increased risk of developing MS. On the contrary, infection with cytomegalovirus (CMV) appears to be protective against developing MS. Other proposed factors that may contribute to the risk of developing MS include tobacco smoking, childhood obesity, and birth month.

PATHOPHYSIOLOGY

MS is characterized by plaques of demyelination and gliosis throughout the CNS, sparing the peripheral nervous system. These plaques are multifocal in nature, and can occur in the optic nerves, supratentorial and infratentorial brain, and the spinal cord. MS has historically been considered a disease of white matter, but it is now understood to involve gray matter as well. Although the cause of MS remains unknown, the main mechanisms that lead to the clinical manifestations of the disease include inflammation, demyelination, and axonal degeneration.

In the acute phase, there is inflammation and disruption of the blood-brain barrier. The inflammatory component is thought to be more predominant in relapsing than in progressive forms of MS. This disruption of the blood-brain barrier allows for migration of T cells, B cells, and macrophages into the central nervous system. This inflammatory phase of a demyelinating event can be seen radiographically as gadolinium enhancement of lesions on MRI and is a characteristic finding of an MS exacerbation.

The myelin sheath of oligodendrocytes in the central nervous system are attacked, forming a lesion, also called a plaque. In myelinated axons, nerve conduction occurs in a saltatory manner, allowing for significantly faster nerve conduction compared to unmyelinated axons. When the myelin sheath is disrupted, the signal may be delayed or completely disrupted, leading to clinical symptoms. There is partial preservation of axons in such a demyelinating event; however, even early in the disease course of MS, axonal damage does occur.

With time, ongoing axonal damage and atrophy lead to progressive accumulation of disability. Later in the disease course, disease progression is characterized less by inflammatory and immune-mediated mechanisms, and more by microglial activation and neurodegeneration. Although axons may be able to adapt to demyelinating events initially, this axonal damage and cerebral atrophy are irreversible, and in time are often associated with cognitive decline.

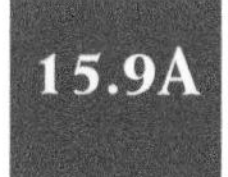

15.9A RELAPSING REMITTING MULTIPLE SCLEROSIS

MEDICAL HISTORY AND CLINICAL PRESENTATION

Relapsing remitting multiple sclerosis (RRMS) is the most common type of MS. RRMS is characterized by acute relapses (also known as exacerbations or attacks) and periods of remission. In an acute relapse, new symptoms develop over days to weeks. Patients with RRMS often experience complete resolution of these symptoms with time, or at least partial recovery. Between attacks, RRMS is characterized by periods of clinical stability, without progression or accumulation of disability. However, many patients with RRMS do eventually reach a secondary progressive phase of disease.

SIGNS AND SYMPTOMS

An MS attack, or exacerbation, is an episode with patient-reported symptoms and objective clinical evidence representing a CNS demyelinating event. Symptoms may develop over hours to days and last a minimum of 24 hours. The neurologic deficit may persist for weeks, but is usually followed by a partial or complete recovery in the setting of RRMS. A true MS exacerbation occurs in the absence of fever/infection; however, worsening of MS-related symptoms in the context of illness, fever, stress, or environmental overheating is referred to as a pseudoexacerbation. A pseudoexacerbation does not represent disease progression.

The quality and severity of symptoms of an MS exacerbation vary greatly depending on the location of a lesion and the degree of damage. Sensory disturbance is the most common initial symptoms of MS and is experienced to a degree by most patients with MS at some point in their lives. Such sensory disturbance may be described as numbness, tingling, or burning. Symptoms also may be described as feeling swollen, wet, tight, or itching. Sensory examination is somewhat unreliable; however, decreased light touch, temperature, vibratory, or pain sensation may be noted on neurologic examination. Decreased facial sensation, and trigeminal neuralgia, can also be seen in MS. Lhermitte syndrome is a transient electric shock-like pain that occurs with neck flexion due to lesions in the cervical cord.

Motor symptoms are also common in MS and can be debilitating. One may experience paraparesis or paraplegia. Motor weakness may be described as loss of strength, muscle fatigue, or slowed movements. Focal motor weakness may be noted on clinical examination. One may also experience spasticity, which can be painful and make transfers and other ADLs quite difficult. Motor symptoms may correlate with increased muscle tone, hyperactive deep tendon reflexes, clonus, and Babinski sign on exam.

Visual symptoms are another common initial presentation of MS. Optic neuritis can present as decreased visual acuity, color desaturation, and dimness. Central vision is most affected, and symptoms are usually unilateral. Bilateral optic neuritis is possible but rare in the context of MS, and should raise concern for an alternative diagnosis. These visual disturbances may be accompanied by pain with eye movements. Fundoscopic examination may initially reveal optic disc edema, and later optic disc pallor. A relative afferent pupillary defect is commonly seen in the affected eye.

MS can cause eye movement disorders through a variety of mechanisms, which may be experienced by the patient as diplopia, difficulty focusing, or blurred vision. Nystagmus and limitations in extraocular movements may be observed on physical examination. Internuclear ophthalmoplegia, observed as impaired adduction of one eye accompanied by horizontal nystagmus of the contralateral abducting eye, is due to a lesion of the medial longitudinal fasciculus on the side of the eye with impaired adduction. Palsies of the sixth or less commonly third or fourth cranial nerves may also occur.

Cerebellar lesions may lead to symptoms of ataxia. Patients may experience gait disturbance, imbalance, incoordination, cerebellar tremors, or difficulty speaking. Dysmetria, intention tremor, saccadic eye movements, and scanning speech may be noted on clinical examination. Vertigo can occur with lesions in vestibular pathways of the brainstem. In advanced disease, other brainstem symptoms such as dysphagia, dysarthria, or difficulty clearing secretions can occur.

Bladder and bowel dysfunction can also occur. Urinary urgency is most common, but urinary incontinence and retention can also occur. Neurogenic bladder may involve detrusor overactivity, reduced detrusor contractility, sphincter dyssynergia, and abnormal bladder sensation. Constipation and bowel incontinence can also occur. Sexual dysfunction may occur due to decreased genital sensation, impotence, or decreased libido.

Other common symptoms include fatigue, depression, cognitive dysfunction, and heat sensitivity. Although MS can cause symptoms involving a number of body systems, most individuals affected by MS do not have evidence of another associated systemic process.

DIFFERENTIAL DIAGNOSIS

MS is commonly misdiagnosed.[153] Symptoms of other conditions such as complicated migraine, hemiplegic migraine, or fibromyalgia are commonly mistaken for symptoms of MS. Other disorders of neuroimmunology including neuromyelitis optica spectrum disorders, myelin oligodendrocyte glycoprotein (MOG) antibody-associated disease, neurosarcoidosis, or lupus can also be considered. The differential diagnosis may also include vascular disease, central nervous system lymphoma, or conversion disorder. Atypical features such as onset during childhood or after age 50, acute or transient neurologic deficits, and signs of systemic illness should prompt one to consider alternative diagnoses. Radiographic characteristics such as longitudinally extensive transverse myelitis, optic neuritis spanning more than half of the optic nerve, bilateral optic neuritis, and only nonspecific lesions or lack of lesions on brain MRI are also atypical of MS.

DIAGNOSTIC STUDIES

There is no single test to confirm the diagnosis of MS. The diagnosis is clinical based on the 2017 Revised McDonald Criteria. A diagnosis of MS requires objective evidence of one or more clinical attacks, dissemination in space, dissemination in time, and no other explanation for the clinical findings. Objective clinical evidence may include an abnormality on physical examination, neuroimaging, or neurophysiologic testing. Dissemination in space may be observed as a separate clinical site implicating a different site in the CNS, or one or more T2-hyperintense lesions on MRI in two or more typical regions (periventricular, juxtacortical, infratentorial, and spinal cord). Dissemination in time can be observed as development of a separate clinical attack, new lesion consistent with an MS plaque on follow-up MRI, or simultaneous presence of gadolinium-enhancing and nonenhancing lesions on MRI. For patients who meet radiographic criteria for dissemination in space, the presence of oligoclonal bands in the CSF can substitute for radiographic or clinical evidence of dissemination in time in order to meet diagnostic criteria and confirm the diagnosis.

MRI of the brain and spinal cord is the initial test of choice for evaluation of a patient with suspected MS. Lesions are multifocal and may appear in the supratentorial or infratentorial white matter, optic nerves, or spinal cord. MS lesions are classically ovoid in appearance, and oriented perpendicular to the corpus callosum. These classic MS plaques are referred to as "Dawson's fingers" when seen on sagittal imaging. Spinal cord lesions typically span no more than two vertebral segments and are associated with little to no cord swelling. MS plaques are hyperintense on T2-weighted imaging. Some plaques may be seen as hypointense on T1-weighted imaging, suggestive of axonal loss. This is more commonly seen in chronic, long-standing MS. Postcontrast imaging is useful to identify active demyelination in the setting of an acute exacerbation. Acute lesions are often larger and more poorly circumscribed due to associated edema. Disruption of the blood-brain barrier during this inflammatory phase allows gadolinium contrast to accumulate in plaques. Therefore, lesions demonstrating postcontrast enhancement, which may persist for a few weeks, are consistent with active disease.

Many patients will meet diagnostic criteria for MS based on clinical presentation and radiographic features alone, and do not need any additional workup. However, analysis of CSF can be useful for patients who meet McDonald Criteria for dissemination in space but not time. While oligoclonal bands in the CSF is highly sensitive for MS, it should be noted that it is possible to meet diagnostic criteria for MS without the presence of oligoclonal bands in the CSF, and oligoclonal bands are not specific for MS. They may be seen in other mimicking disorders such as lupus, CNS infections, and various neuropathies. The CSF profile is often remarkable for an elevated IgG index, but otherwise is grossly normal. Other diagnostic studies that may be used to support the diagnosis include visual evoked potentials and optical coherence tomography.

TREATMENT

The first-line treatment for an acute MS exacerbation is high-dose corticosteroids, typically methylprednisolone 1,000 mg administered intravenously for 3 to 5 consecutive days. Alternatively, high doses of oral prednisone can be used. Administration of corticosteroids during an acute exacerbation is thought to reduce inflammation and restore the integrity of the blood-brain barrier. Treatment with methylprednisolone often hastens partial or complete recovery from an exacerbation; however, it does not significantly affect long- term disability. Thus, preventing relapses with disease-modifying therapy (DMT) is of utmost importance to prevent progressive accumulation of disability.

The goal of treatment with DMT is to reduce relapse rate, decrease the development of MRI lesions, and prevent accumulation of disability. DMT does not cure MS, nor does it prevent relapses and disease progression altogether, but it does slow down the rate at which these developments occur. Early intervention with DMT is recommended, even if clinical and radiographic disease burden is mild, to maintain functional status and to prevent or delay conversion to secondary progressive MS. It should be clearly communicated to patients that DMTs are not intended to cure the disease or improve the symptoms of MS. When selecting a DMT for a patient, one must take into account safety, efficacy, and tolerability of the treatment. This should be a joint decision between the patient and the clinician to ensure appropriate compliance with treatment. There are injectable, oral, and infusion therapy options available, each with differing mechanisms of action.

The injectable DMTs include interferon beta-1a, interferon beta-1b, pegylated interferon beta-1a, and glatiramer acetate. These are some of the first medications FDA approved for the treatment of MS, and therefore, they have the most long-term safety data. The interferons are administered as a subcutaneous or intramuscular injection. Different variations may be administered as frequently as once every other day, or as infrequently as once every other week. Common side effects include flu-like reactions, injection site reactions, depression, and transaminitis. Interferons in general are considered a foundational class of MS medications; however, the side effects can be difficult to tolerate and efficacy is modest at best. Glatiramer acetate is a subcutaneous injection that can be administered in different doses either daily or three times weekly. Side effects of glatiramer acetate include postinjection reactions (transient chest pain, flushing, anxiety, palpitations, and shortness of breath), injection site reactions, and lipoatrophy around the injection site. Serious adverse effects of glatiramer acetate are not common. Glatiramer acetate can be continued throughout pregnancy and breastfeeding.

Ofatumumab

There are multiple oral DMT options that offer a convenient approach to preventing relapses and disease progression which many patients prefer. However, the oral medications do have the potential for serious adverse effects including infections and rare cases of progressive multifocal leukoencephalopathy. Fingolimod, siponimod, and ozanimod are sphingosine-1 phosphate receptor modulators that sequester lymphocytes to the lymph nodes. Both medications are administered once daily. In addition to infection, safety concerns also include bradyarrhythmias, macular edema, lymphopenia, transaminitis, and severe relapse and disease progression upon discontinuation. Both medications are contraindicated in patients with acute coronary syndrome, stroke, or transient ischemic attack within the last 6 months, as well as individuals with heart failure, second or third AV block, sick sinus syndrome, or prolonged QT interval. Fingolimod requires a 6-hour first dose observation during which vital signs are monitored and an EKG is obtained before and after. Siponimod requires screening for certain CYP genotypes, which affect how the drug is metabolized. Depending on the genotype, siponimod may be contraindicated or require dose adjustment to prevent dangerously high plasma levels of siponimod. Dimethyl fumarate and diroximel fumarate are also oral DMTs that are dosed twice daily. Lymphopenia, liver injury, and serious infections can also occur during treatment. Common side effects include GI upset, flushing, and itching; however, these side effects often improve with time and by taking the medication after a large meal. Teriflunomide is a pyrimidine synthesis inhibitor that is administered once daily. Hepatotoxicity and teratogenicity are serious safety concerns related to treatment with teriflunomide. Common side effects include hair thinning, GI upset, and transaminitis. Cladribine tablets are typically reserved for individuals who have failed other DMTs. Cladribine is administered for 4 or 5 consecutive days for four treatment cycles. The first two treatment cycles are separated by 4 weeks, and the last two treatment cycles occur 1 year later. Adverse effects related to treatment with cladribine include serious infections, malignancy, and lymphopenia.

Several intravenously administered DMTs are highly effective and also ideal in the event that adequate compliance has been difficult to achieve with injectable or oral medications. Natalizumab is a monoclonal antibody administered once every 4 weeks. Common side effects include infusion reactions. In addition to increased risk of infection in general, the main safety concern with natalizumab is the potential development of progressive multifocal leukoencephalopathy (PML), which can result in death or significant disability. Although there have been cases of PML with many DMTs, natalizumab has rendered many more cases than alternative treatments. PML is caused by the migration of the John Cunningham virus (JCV) from its benign presence in the kidneys to its potentially fatal presence in the central nervous system as a result of immunosuppression. Risk factors that contribute to the development of PML include prior immunosuppressive therapy, length of time on natalizumab, and measurement of JCV index. JCV index should be monitored periodically to better stratify the risk of development of PML, and a high titer may require discontinuation of the medication. Nonetheless, natalizumab remains a very effective treatment in quieting aggressive disease. Ocrelizumab is another monoclonal antibody and is administered once every 6 months. Infusion reactions are also common with treatment with ocrelizumab, and rarely can be life threatening. Treatment with ocrelizumab may increase risk of infection and malignancy, and there have been rare cases of PML during treatment with ocrelizumab as well. Alemtuzumab is also a monoclonal antibody administered for 5 consecutive days, followed by a second treatment course of 3 consecutive days 1 year later. Like cladribine, alemtuzumab is typically reserved for patients who have failed alternative medications with a more benign safety profile. Alemtuzumab increases the risk of serious infections, development of other autoimmune diseases, and malignancies. Specifically, autoimmune thyroiditis, idiopathic thrombocytopenic purpura, thyroid cancer, bladder cancer, and thrombocytopenic are of concern. Alemtuzumab requires monthly laboratory monitoring for 4 years following the last dose of the medication, and annual skin examinations to screen for skin cancers.

Because DMT does not improve established symptoms of MS, symptomatic therapy is equally as important to address to maximize quality of life. Fatigue is often one of the most debilitating symptoms of MS. Lifestyle modifications including diet and exercise are first line, but medications are sometimes required. Amantadine, modafinil, armodafinil, and other stimulants can be used. Paresthesias and neuropathic pain can be managed with gabapentin and pregabalin. Tricyclic antidepressants and other antiepileptics can be considered for refractory cases. Spasticity can be managed with muscle relaxants including baclofen, tizanidine, cyclobenzaprine, metaxalone, or diazepam. Baclofen pumps and botulinum toxin injections can also be considered in patients who do not adequately respond or are unable to tolerate oral muscle relaxants, and for patients with severe contractures. Gait instability is principally managed with physical therapy and orthotic devices. Dalfampridine is a potassium channel blocker that can be beneficial for gait instability secondary to weakness. Dalfampridine can, however, lower seizure threshold and cause potentially irreversible increased spasticity, and kidney function should be monitored. Bladder dysfunction can often be well managed with lifestyle modification including scheduled bathroom breaks, but medications such as oxybutynin, tolterodine, and mirabegron can be helpful. Botulinum toxins or self-catheterization may also be needed. A urology referral is often indicated for the management of neurogenic bladder. Constipation should be initially managed by increasing fiber and fluid intake as well as increased exercise; however, stool softeners and laxatives may be required. Bulking agents that slow transit time, anticholinergics, and antispasmodics are sometimes used for management of bowel incontinence.

PATIENT EDUCATION

Individuals living with MS often feel that their disease course is unpredictable and have difficulty discerning what is and is not related to their disease or considered an acute exacerbation. Patients should be educated on the natural history of MS, including the possibility of relapses, potential for recovery, and possible transition to a progressive stage of disease. Much care should be taken to explain the purpose of and manage expectations for DMT to increase the likelihood of compliance. Likewise, the role of steroids including the risks and benefits in an acute exacerbation should be explained. Steroids should not be used for symptomatic management in the absence of an acute exacerbation. Patients should also be taught how to recognize a possible relapse, and when to call the office or go to the ED.

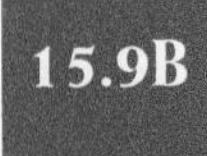

15.9B SECONDARY PROGRESSIVE MULTIPLE SCLEROSIS

MEDICAL HISTORY AND CLINICAL PRESENTATION

Secondary progressive multiple sclerosis (SPMS) can be considered a disease state on the same spectrum as clinically isolated syndrome and RRMS. Some patients do continue a relapsing remitting course of disease throughout their lives without ever converting to a secondary progressive course. Many, however, begin to experience fewer relapses, and more gradual progression of disease, 10 to 20 years following the onset of disease. SPMS is characterized by this gradual progression rather than clinical stability following a previously relapsing remitting course. SPMS may be classified as active SPMS, that is, still having acute exacerbations with a gradually progressive baseline, or inactive SPMS, meaning one gradually progresses without clear relapses.

SIGNS AND SYMPTOMS

Individuals with SPMS can present with any of the clinical symptoms or physical examination findings seen in RRMS. In general, individuals with SPMS have more prominent gait disturbance, which gradually worsens with time. Cognitive complaints such as memory loss, brain fog, and difficulty computing or maintaining attention are also more common in the secondary progressive phase of disease. SPMS is characterized by slow, gradual progression of symptoms, although acute exacerbations as seen in RRMS can still occur in active sSPMS.

DIAGNOSTIC STUDIES

There is no specific test to confirm one has transitioned to SPMS. The diagnosis is often made retrospectively, after the patient and clinician have observed this change over the course of a few years. Over time, one may see more brain parenchymal volume loss on MRI, and fewer new lesions. Radiographic disease activity does not correlate as clearly with disease progression in SPMS as it does in RRMS.

TREATMENT

The treatment for active SPMS is similar to the treatment for RRMS. Most DMTs are FDA approved for the treatment of relapsing forms of MS, to include clinically isolated syndrome, RRMS, and active SPMS. These DMTs include glatiramer acetate, interferon beta-1a, pegylated interferon beta-1a, interferon beta-1b, fingolimod, siponimod, dimethyl fumarate, diroximel fumarate, teriflunomide, cladribine, natalizumab, ocrelizumab, and alemtuzumab. There is no FDA-approved treatment for the management of inactive SPMS. Thus, one must consider the risks and benefits of continued treatment in these individuals. Symptomatic therapy is also important to address and does not greatly differ from symptom management in RRMS for these patients.

15.9C PRIMARY PROGRESSIVE MULTIPLE SCLEROSIS

MEDICAL HISTORY AND CLINICAL PRESENTATION

Primary progressive multiple sclerosis (PPMS) is less common than RRMS, but is usually associated with a more aggressive disease course. There is progressive accumulation of disability from the onset of disease. Although individuals may still experience relapses with minor improvements and occasional periods of clinical stability, the disease course of PPMS is characterized primarily by ongoing progression of disability without significant improvement.

SIGNS AND SYMPTOMS

PPMS can present with any of the same complaints or physical examination findings as RRMS; however, most commonly present with spinal cord signs and symptoms that worsen over time. These individuals tend to have a higher level of disability, and one may see a significant decline in the ability to ambulate over the years, such that many patients with PPMS eventually become nonambulatory.

EVALUATION

The 2017 Revised McDonald Criteria can also be applied to individuals who present with gradual progression consistent with PPMS. Diagnosis requires disease progression over a 1-year period, plus two of the three diagnostic criteria. These criteria include one or more characteristic MS plaques in the supratentorial or infratentorial brain, two or more MS plaques in the spinal cord, and presence of oligoclonal bands in the CSF.

TREATMENT

While there are many options for the treatment of relapsing forms of MS, treatment options for PPMS are more limited. Ocrelizumab is the only medication that has demonstrated a statistically significant reduction in the risk of disease progression and accumulation of disability compared to placebo. Ocrelizumab is the only FDA-approved treatment for PPMS and as such is generally considered the first-line therapy. Ocrelizumab is contraindicated in patients with active hepatitis B infection, and safety concerns include serious infusion reactions, infections, and development of malignancies. Prior to the FDA approval of ocrelizumab, other immunosuppressants were used, and are still sometimes used, although evidence of the efficacy of these treatments is lacking. Such treatments include methotrexate, azathioprine, mycophenolate mofetil, and rituximab. Pulse methylprednisolone and IVIG have also been used, again with very limited evidence for efficacy.

SPECIAL CONSIDERATIONS

Clinically isolated syndrome (CIS) is essentially the first clinical episode consistent with MS, without evidence of prior demyelination and without meeting criteria for dissemination in space and time. CSF analysis can be useful in determining risk of progression to MS. The majority of patients, but not all, with CIS and MRI lesions do progress to develop MS. Individuals with CIS and without MRI lesions are less likely to develop MS. Acute symptoms can be managed as an MS exacerbation with high-dose glucocorticoids. Long-term management of CIS is based on clinical judgment and risk factors for progression to MS. Options include monitoring for development of new MRI lesions or clinical signs or symptoms consistent with MS, or early initiation of DMT for those at higher risk for developing MS. Many of the DMTs discussed for the management of RRMS are also FDA approved for clinically isolated syndrome.

Cases in which MRI findings are highly suggestive of MS, but the patient is asymptomatic and without any clinical findings suggestive of CNS demyelination, are referred to as radiologically isolated syndrome (RIS). In these cases, an MRI is typically ordered for an unrelated reason, such as trauma or headaches, and the findings are incidental. There is limited data regarding the conversion of RIS to CIS or MS. RIS is generally managed with close follow-up to monitor for the development of signs or symptoms consistent with demyelinating disease.

Pregnancy is generally protective against MS exacerbations, as the immune system is naturally suppressed to protect the fetus. Most individuals have fewer relapses during pregnancy than otherwise if off DMT. However, the risk of relapse and disease progression is higher following delivery. Glatiramer acetate is sometimes initiated during or continued throughout pregnancy and breastfeeding in conjunction with the guidance of the obstetrician and pediatrician to prevent postpartum relapse.

15.10 MENTAL STATUS CHANGES/COMA

John Ramos

OVERVIEW

Consciousness is conceptually defined by Plum and Posner, as "the state of full awareness of the self and one's relationship to the environment."[154] Content and arousal are the major components of consciousness. Content refers to cerebral mediated cognitive behaviors and affective responses (e.g., thinking, awareness, expression, language, and emotions). Arousal refers to wakefulness and alertness and is assessed by response to internal and external stimulation. The conceptual definition of consciousness assumes a patient has no underlying psychiatric disease and has intact sensory and motor functions (e.g., a patient with lower extremity neuropathy with decreased response to sharp touch because of insensate feet). Common variations include acute changes in arousal and content (delirium), dysfunctional arousal and content (coma), and chronic changes in arousal (depression) and content (dementia).[155]

Coma is a state of deep unconsciousness in which a patient is alive but lacks the ability to respond to internal and external stimulation. In order of descending frequency, coma is commonly caused metabolic disorders, exogenous toxins, or head injuries. Coma rarely lasts more than 2 to 4 weeks. Patients who survive coma may regain functional consciousness, but more commonly progress to a vegetative state (VS) or sometimes a minimally conscious state (MCS). VS is characterized by cycling states of arousal and eye opening with or without external stimuli; however, there is no spontaneous speaking or response to commands.[156] VS is considered persistent after a period of 30 days, and no clear criteria exist to diagnose permanent VS.[157,158] MCS is a condition of severely lowered consciousness with minimal but definite evidence of responses to external or internal stimuli. After stabilizing comorbid emergent conditions (e.g., dialyzing an offending toxin or evacuating a subdural hematoma), management of patients in coma, VS, or MCS consists of supportive care (e.g., nutrition, oral hygiene) and prevention of infection (pneumonia is the leading cause of death), venous thromboembolism, pressure sores, and musculoskeletal deformities. Patients in MCS may have better long-term functional outcomes with focused therapy.

EPIDEMIOLOGY

The incidence of acute changes in mental status is not well studied given its variable presentation and the association with a variety of conditions. In the pediatric population acute changes in mental status are most commonly caused by infection, trauma, metabolic disorders, and poisoning. In the young adult population poisoning and trauma are more common etiologies than infection. Mental status changes in the elderly are most commonly caused by stroke, infection, poisoning, medication interactions, or alterations in living environment. Delirium is common among hospitalized elderly patients, estimated to be present in 10% to 25% of hospitalized patients at time of admission.[155] Prognosis, morbidity, and mortality related to acute mental status changes are best defined by the underlying etiology. For example, one study on patients in Massachusetts with nonfatal opioid overdose found mortality rates of 1.1% and 5.5% within 1 month and 1 year from date of ED discharge, respectively.[159]

Epidemiologic literature on coma, VS, and MCS is limited, but distinctions are made based on the etiology of coma. The most common causes of nontraumatic coma are stroke, anoxic brain jury, poisoning, and metabolic disorders.[160] The most common causes of traumatic coma are traumatic brain injuries. Coma most commonly progresses to brain death, and the most common primary causes of brain death are traumatic brain injury, ruptured cerebral aneurysm, intracerebral hemorrhage, ischemic stroke, hypoxic-ischemic encephalopathy, and hepatic encephalopathy.[154] Coma rarely lasts longer than 2 to 4 weeks; those who survive progress to VS and sometimes MCS. Some evidence suggests that VS is considered permanent after 3 months with nontraumatic injuries and 1 year with traumatic injuries.[161] The most common cause of death in a patient who is in coma or VS is infection.

There is a generally better prognosis for comatose patients with traumatic brain injuries. With regard to mortality one study found ranges of 40% to 50% for patients with traumatic injuries compared to 54% to 88% in comatose patients secondary to cardiopulmonary arrest.[162] Traumatic coma also has better prognosis for recovery with one study finding recovery of independent function at 6 months in 39% of patients compared to only 16% of patients in nontraumatic coma.[163,164] In one longitudinal study of pediatric patients in MCS after a traumatic brain injury most recovered functional independence.[165]

A more favorable prognosis exists for patients who progress from coma to VS or MCS. In one study of patients in VS 1 month after traumatic coma, 52% of adults and 62% of children recovered consciousness within 1 year. Patients in VS 1 month after a nontraumatic coma were less likely to recover consciousness (15% of adults and 13% of children studied). There are differences observed in time to recovery of consciousness from VS, with recovery from traumatic coma occurring most commonly within 6 months. It is very unlikely for patients to recover from VS following traumatic coma after 6 months or from atraumatic coma after 3 months.[161,162] Lastly, a few studies have shown improved life expectancy and improved Disability Rating Scale measurements for patients in MCS compared to patients in VS at 1 year after both traumatic and nontraumatic injury. There is no correlation between duration of time in MCS and emergence from MCS or functional recovery.[166]

PATHOPHYSIOLOGY

Reticular activating system (RAS) is a collection of ascending polysynaptic neurons that are essential for arousal and maintenance of wakefulness. RAS neurons are located within the brainstem reticular formation, which extends from the lower medulla through the paramedian pons to the central midbrain. Prominent extensions of RAS project to functionally related thalamic nuclei and the inferomedial frontal lobes (although RAS projections extend to nearly all parts of the cerebral cortex). There are unique differences in the anatomic concentration of RAS. Within the infratentorial brainstem RAS is concentrated in small areas, in contrast to the sparse RAS fibers that project to the supratentorial cerebral hemispheres and thalamic nuclei. Thus, dramatic changes in alertness and arousal can result from infratentorial lesions that are relatively small compared to larger supratentorial lesions. Localizing physical examination findings may identify lesion location, as supratentorial lesions may be accompanied by focal motor/sensory deficits and infratentorial lesions tend to be accompanied by cranial nerve palsies and motor deficits.

Space-occupying lesions, or mass lesions, cause intracranial tissue displacement (mass effect), which may manifest changes in mental status. The cranial cavity is externally restricted by the skull bones and internally divided into compartments by infoldings of dura mater. The two cerebral hemispheres are separated by the falx. The tentorium separates the anterior and posterior fossae. Herniation occurs when a space-occupying lesion displaces brain tissue into a contiguous compartment that the tissue does not normally occupy.

Transtentorial herniation is the most common form of herniation, in which tissue is displaced from supratentorial to infraterorial through the tentorial opening. Supratentorial compression on the diencephalon (thalamus, hypothalamus) manifests as decorticate (extensor) posturing and mitotic pupils (interruption of descending sympathetic autonomic fibers). Uncal transtentorial herniation occurs when the anterior medial temporal gyrus is displaced through the tentorial opening, compressing the parahippocampal gyrus, midbrain, RAS fibers, and cranial nerve III. Autonomic fibers are spatially arranged on the periphery of cranial nerves with autonomic functions, compared to the motor and sensory fibers, which are arranged centrally. Compressive forces on cranial nerve III first affect the more superficial autonomic fibers, and so an ipsilateral enlarged pupil is an early sign of herniation. The compressed midbrain may displace laterally against the opposite cerebral peduncle, manifesting in a Babinski sign and Kernohan-Woltman sign (hemiparesis contralateral to the hemiparesis that resulted from the mass). Herniated tissue may compress the anterior and posterior cerebral arteries resulting in brain infarction.

Central transtentorial herniation refers to inferior displacement of the thalamus through the tentorial opening with subsequent upper midbrain compression. Compression of the midbrain (the location of the cranial nerve III nucleus, in addition to RAS fibers) manifests as miotic pupils and drowsiness.

Central and uncal herniation cause progressive rostral to caudal compression of the brainstem. Compression of the midbrain manifests as unreactive pupils and decerebrate (extensor) posturing. Compression of the pons manifests as gasps and prolonged pauses with inspiration (apneustic breathing). Compression of the pons and medulla manifests as no motor movement and ultimately respiratory failure.

Transfalcial herniation occurs as the cingulate gyrus is compressed under the falx and across the midline. Foraminal herniation occurs when the cerebellar tonsils are displaced caudally into the foramen magnum.

Cerebral neurons depend on cerebral blood flow for the delivery of oxygen and glucose. Brain glucose reserves can provide energy for about 2 minutes after blood flow is interrupted, and simultaneous hypoxia and ischemia more quickly exhaust glucose supply. Tissue hypoxia-ischemia and cellular apoptosis occur with inadequate cerebral perfusion pressure, which is dependent on intracranial pressure and mean arterial pressure. In space-occupying lesions, intracranial pressure is increased, and cerebral perfusion pressure is inadequate unless blood pressure is increased. Cardiovascular insults such as arrythmias or hypotension decrease mean arterial pressure and thus cerebral perfusion.

Metabolic (nonstructural) conditions are more commonly responsible for changes in mental status and coma, especially for patients presenting without a history of trauma. Substrate deficiencies may impair neuronal function (e.g., hypoglycemia, hypoxemia, hypercapnia, hyperosmolarity). Although not completely understood the mechanism of cellular insult from substrate deficiencies is likely related to changes in ion flux across neuronal and glial cell membranes and/or decreased adenosine triphosphate or neurotransmitter production. In contrast to tissue hypoxia, metabolic disorders produce minor neuropathologic changes and full recovery is often achieved with correction of the underlying derangement. Of course, anoxic brain injury can occur with impaired cardiorespiration resulting from metabolic or toxicologic conditions.

Exogenous toxins are also commonly responsible for changes in mental status among patients with or without a history of trauma.

MEDICAL HISTORY AND CLINICAL PRESENTATION

Recent changes in mental status require a careful historical account of symptom onset and duration, exacerbating or relieving factors, medical history, and especially history of medications (prescribed, OTC, and herbal supplements) and illicit substance use. Patients with mental status changes can be challenging historians. Whenever safe and feasible, information should be obtained from collateral sources (e.g., caregivers, parents, children, friends, bystanders). Obtaining a complete list of medications is essential and may require consultation with local pharmacies or controlled substance databases.

Antecedent events or symptoms and timing and duration of mental status changes provide great insight into the ultimate diagnosis. Antecedent events or symptoms such as traumatic injuries, drug administration, syncope, near syncope, vertigo, headache, chest pain, or vomiting do aid in investigation, but can be difficult to ascertain from the primary historian. Acute changes (minutes to hours) in mental status suggest vascular etiologies (e.g., cerebral, cardiac, or peripheral vascular occlusion or dissection, or aneurysm rupture), traumatic brain injury, epileptic activity, or drug overdose. Subacute changes may suggest systemic illness, infection, intracranial mass (traumatic or neoplastic), or degenerative disorders. Establishing a chronologic timeline is important for patients with baseline disordered arousal, alertness, cognition, and memory. Historical fluctuations in mental status, including onset, duration, frequency, and interventions may also offer insight into the underlying disorder. It is important to consider changes in environment (e.g., caregivers, seasons, exposure to lightness and darkness) or medication history (e.g., new medications, changes in dose or frequency, medication interactions).

The historical evaluation of an acutely comatose patient is similar to the approach to changes in mental status. In the setting of trauma:[167]

- Allergies
- Medications currently used
- Past illnesses/pregnancy
- Last meal
- Events/environment related to the injury

The acute stabilization of initial injuries and coma occurs in the hospital setting, and the persistent VS or MCS are likely the most common presentation in the primary care setting. Evaluating a patient with a history of coma in the primary care setting should initially focus on the hospital course and disease-specific risk factors. Patients in coma can have complex hospital management and essential information to ascertain include:

- Etiology of coma (structural, trauma, metabolic, poisoning)
- Length of time in a state of coma
- Time to recovery or progression to VS or MCS
- Length of time in ICU
- Respiratory support (necessity of mechanical ventilation, and length of time on ventilator)
- Neurosurgical interventions
- Nutrition (enteral or indications for parenteral)
- Infectious (before or acquired during admission)
- Prophylaxis for and/or incidence of infection, GI ulcers, venous thromboembolism, pressure sores

SIGNS AND SYMPTOMS

An awake and alert person is fully responsive to stimuli and aware of their self and environment. Patients presenting with altered mental status or altered levels of consciousness may have varied changes in mood, behavior, or cognitive function.

PHYSICAL EXAMINATION

A general approach to the patient with mental status changes or coma is to assess level of consciousness, breathing patterns, pupillary size and reactivity, eye movements and oculovestibular responses, and skeletal motor responses. Numerous conditions present with altered mental status, and more detailed and specific physical examination findings can be found with associated diagnoses in other chapters of this book.

Impaired consciousness is categorized by awareness of and responsiveness to external and internal stimuli. Table 15.28 defines some common descriptions and diagnoses associated with altered consciousness or mental status. Although terms such as obtunded, lethargic, and drowsy exist, there is more clinical utility describing consciousness by specifying level of arousal and responses evoked by stimuli. For example, patients with severe depression or catatonia may appear "stuporous" but can be aroused with stimulation and once aroused have relatively little cognitive impairment. The sleeping patient may appear "obtunded" with eyes closed, reduced alertness, and slow responses to stimulation, but sleep is a recurrent physiologic process that is easily reversed and does not persist with external stimulation.

Altered mental status is a common presentation for patients with toxic ingestions or medication interactions.[168] Toxidromes are a constellation of signs and symptoms associated with specific classes of toxins. Recognizing the most common toxidromes greatly aids diagnosis and management when toxic ingestions are suspected, particularly with patients who are unreliable historians (Table 15.29). Co-ingestions are common and, as with any syndrome, a patient may not present with all the classic signs of any particular toxidrome.

The original Glasgow Coma Scale (GCS) was published in 1974 as a diagnostic and prognostic tool for patients with traumatic head injuries.[169] Since 1974 it has been validated as an effective tool for diagnosing altered levels of consciousness in patients with traumatic and atraumatic brain injuries. Serial examinations are necessary, as outcome and severity of brain injury are based on trends rather than an isolated score. Other valuable assessment tools include the Mini-Mental State Exam (MMSE), Quick Confusion Scale, and Confusion Assessment Method (CAM).[155,170,171]

TABLE 15.28 Descriptions of States of Altered Consciousness

State	Description
Drowsiness or lethargy	Reduced spontaneous physical and mental activity. Alertness/wakefulness sustained only with external stimulation. Mildly impaired concentration and attention.
Clouding of consciousness	Minimally reduced wakefulness or awareness. May be associated with hyperexcitability, alternating drowsiness in daytime, and irritability at nighttime.
Obtundation Latin: "to beat against or blunt"	Mild to moderate reduction in alertness and reduced interest in external environment. Slow responses to stimulation.
Stupor Latin: "to be stunned"	Profoundly reduced wakefulness and behavioral unresponsiveness. Arousal only achieved and sustained with repeated vigorous external stimulation. Persistent inactivity with stimulus withdrawal. Significantly impaired concentration and attention.
Comatose	Unresponsiveness without arousal to external or internal stimuli. Early findings may include moaning with noxious external stimulation. Loss of sleep-wake cycles. No volitional movements. Loss of autonomic reflexes like swallowing, coughing, pupillary and corneal reflexes.
Vegetative state (unresponsive wakefulness syndrome)	Variable spontaneous arousal, no clinical evidence of self-or environmental awareness, cycling of arousal states, periods of eye opening, and no purposeful movement.
Locked-in syndrome	Fully awake without volitional limb movement or speech production. Normal mental activity, self-awareness and sleep-wake cycles. Eye movements preserved.
Akinetic mutism	Decreased consciousness without spontaneous motor activity or evidence of awareness.
Delirium Latin: "to go out of furrow"	Misperception of sensory stimuli, reduced ability to focus, sustain or shift attention. May have associated memory deficits and altered speech. Environmental disorientation to time is most commonly observed, followed by place then person.
Dementia	Chronic condition with no effect on level of wakefulness, alertness, or awareness, except in severe cases. Progressive impairment of memory and cognitive domains (planning motor tasks, recognition, language, executive function).

DIFFERENTIAL DIAGNOSIS

Table 15.30 summarizes the differential diagnosis for altered mental status.

DIAGNOSTIC STUDIES

The diagnostic approach to changes in mental status is to investigate common reversible causes. The underlying disorder or offending agent leading to altered mental status may be achieved with a thorough medical history and physical exam. In certain circumstances diagnostic studies may not be necessary to confirm a diagnosis. With regard to exogenous toxins, diagnostic tests may not be readily available or clinically useful, and response to treatment may confirm the cause of mental status changes. Selection of appropriate studies should always be informed by the patient's medical history, their examination, and associated risk factors. Of course, patients with altered mental status may not be reliable historians, and clinicians should maintain a high index of suspicion for serious pathology when evaluating the acutely intoxicated patient. In other words, the primary care setting is likely not appropriate for a patient with altered mental status who may likely require serial laboratory studies, EKG, radiographic imaging, or hospitalization.

Diagnostic studies may not elucidate the underlying cause of mental status changes but are certainly useful in identifying sequelae from the underlying etiology or associated injury. A CBC with differential, a CMP (including glucose), and an EKG are often useful initial tests. Other circumstantially useful tests include TSH, free T3 and T4, ammonia, serum osmolality, among others. Serum substance concentrations (alcohol, acetaminophen, salicylate) may be valuable when they are appropriately ordered, readily available, and have a high likelihood of changing management. Of note, serum alcohol concentrations do not correlate with clinical intoxication and cannot diagnose sobriety. In the setting of altered mental status and suspected medication reaction or poisoning, serum concentrations (lithium, phenytoin, carbamazepine, digoxin) can evaluate subtherapeutic, therapeutic, and toxic levels. Of note, hyperammonemia may occur with supratherapeutic or therapeutic doses of valproic acid and is not dose dependent. Urinalysis may aid in the diagnosis of infection and is sometimes helpful with exogenous toxins.

Caution should be exercised with the interpretation of urine toxicology screens. Assay sensitivity may limit substance detectability (synthetic opiates, designer drugs). Urine tests often rely on substance metabolites, and the concentration of metabolites may be affected by time of ingestion and physiologic differences in metabolism. False positives are common.

The decision to obtain radiographic imaging should be informed by history, physical exam, and risk factors. Noncontrast studies of the head are useful for identifying some space-occupying structural lesions. Vascular abnormalities are better identified with contrast enhanced CT. MRI is the study of choice for many vascular conditions including posterior circulation strokes, vertebrobasilar insufficiency, and dural sinus thrombosis.

There have been several small studies on the use of diagnostic tests in patients in VS and MCS. Structural injuries within the corpus callosum and dorsolateral brainstem identified on MRI significantly predicted nonrecovery from VS.[172] Global decreases in cerebral metabolism have been identified in patients in VS using quantitative FDG-PET, but early identification offers relatively little insight on patient outcomes.[173] A low *N*-acetyl aspartate-to-creatine ratio in the thalamus has been identified with magnetic resonance spectroscopy in patients in VS who do not recover; however, the small sample of patients studied limits its application in clinical practice.[174] EEG evidence of long-latency auditory cortical potentials and mismatch negativity event-related potentials has been suggested as a predictor of recovery from VS.[175] Neuroimaging for MCS is limited to academic research, although there is some evidence that patients in MCS had appropriately associated cortical activity when prompted to visualize an object, and command following is a hallmark of MCS.[176] Ultimately there is no consensus recommendation for neuroimaging or EEG in the diagnosis of VS or MCS.

TABLE 15.29 Toxidromes, Associated Toxic Agents, and Signs and Symptoms

Toxidrome and Examples of Toxic Agents	Signs and Symptoms
Anticholinergic • First-generation antihistamines Atypical antipsychotics Tricyclic antidepressants Atropine Scopolamine Benztropine • Trihexyphenidyl • Cyproheptadine • Tramadol Jimson weed Datura Belladonna	Dilated pupils (mydriasis), decreased sweating, elevated temperature (<38.8° C), decreased micturition and bowel movement, mental status changes, illusions, or hallucinations. Blind as a bat (mydriasis), hot as a hare (elevated temperature), dry as a bone (decreased sweating, salivation, lacrimation), fast as a fox (tachycardia), full as a flask (decreased bowel sounds and urinary bladder enlarged), mad as a hatter (illusions or hallucinations, mental status changes).
Cholinergic • Carbamates • Choline Nicotine • Organophosphate compounds (pesticides) • Pilocarpine	Overactivation of target organs, followed by fatigue. Miosis, seizures, wheezing, twitching, bradycardia, excessive secretory output (bronchial secretions, sweat, saliva, tears, vomiting, bladder/bowel incontinence).
Opioid • Natural opiates Semisynthetic opioids • Fully synthetic opioids	CNS depression, pinpoint pupils (miosis), and central nervous system and respiratory depression.
Sedative-hypnotic • Atropine Anticonvulsant medications • Anxiolytics • Benzodiazepines • Ethanol • GHB • Ketamine • Rohypnol	CNS depression leading to a decreased level of consciousness progressing to comas, depressed respirations, and ataxia.
Sympathomimetic • Amphetamines • Ephedrine • Cathinone derivatives • Cocaine • Caffeine, theophylline • Bupropion	Characterized by catecholamine excess and CNS excitation. Confusion, panic, mydriasis, diaphoresis, and increased pulse, respiration, and blood pressure.
GABA-ergic withdrawal • Alcohol • Barbiturates • Benzodiazepines	Elevated temperature, heart rate, respirations, blood pressure. Lethargy, confusion, delirium. Diaphoresis, mydriasis, increased bowel sounds.
Knockdown toxidrome • Inert gases (helium, argon, neon, radon, etc.) • Methemoglobin inducers (local anesthetics [lidocaine, benzocaine, prilocaine], antimicrobials [sulfonamides, trimethoprim, dapsone, chloroquine], among others) • Carbon monoxide • Cyanide	Tissue perfusion decreased secondary to oxygen displacement (inert gases), impaired oxygen transport (carbon monoxide, methemoglobinemia), and/or mitochondrial inhibition (cyanide). Altered consciousness, fatigue, lightheadedness, dyspnea, seizures, coma, arrhythmias, cardiac arrest.
Salicylate • Aspirin • Bismuth subsalicylate • Methyl salicylates	Elevated temperature, heart rate, blood pressure, and respirations. Shallow breathing, diaphoresis. Agitation, confusion, coma. Normal pupils and bowel sounds.
Serotonin syndrome • Monoamine oxidase inhibitors • Selective serotonin reuptake inhibitors • Lithium • Meperidine • Dextromethorphan • Linezolid	Sudden onset of signs/symptoms (<24 hours). Elevated temperature, heart rate, blood pressure, bowel sounds, and respirations. Mydriatic pupils. Delirium, agitation, coma. Tremors, myoclonus, clonus, hyperreflexia.
Neuroleptic malignant syndrome • Dopamine antagonists • Dopamine withdrawal	Slower onset of signs/symptoms (days to weeks). Elevated temperature (>41.1° C), heart rate, blood pressure, bowel sounds, and respirations. Normal or mydriatic pupils. Delirium, agitation, neuromuscular hypoactivity (bradykinesia, lead-pipe rigidity), hypoactive bowel sounds.

CNS, central nervous system; GABA, gamma-aminobutyric acid; GHB, gamma-hydroxybutyrate.

TABLE 15.30 Differential Diagnosis for Altered Mental Status

	Primary Intracranial	Systemic Disease Effect on CNS	Exogenous Effects	Withdrawal States
Neuro/CNS	Intracranial hemorrhage (SAH, pontine, cerebellar) Ischemic stroke Status epilepticus Primary or metastatic brain tumor Venous sinus thrombosis Concussion Cerebral contusion			
Infectious	Bacterial or viral meningitis/ encephalitis Brain abscess	Sepsis Septic shock		
Metabolic		Hypoglycemia Hyperglycemia Thiamine deficiency Hyponatremia Hypernatremia Hypocalcemia Hyperammonemia Myxedema coma Thyrotoxicosis Uremia		
Toxic			Acetaminophen Alcohol Amphetamines Anticonvulsants Aspirin Benzodiazepines Beta blockers Calcium channel blockers Cardiac glycosides Cocaine GHB Heroin/opiates Isoniazid Lithium LSD Marijuana Psychedelic mushrooms PCP SSRIs TCAs NSAIDs	Alcohol Benzodiazepines SSRIs
Environmental		High altitude cerebral edema Heat stroke Hypothermia Malignant hyperthermia Dysbarism	Carbon monoxide Cyanide Organophosphates Neuroleptic malignant syndrome	

CNS, central nervous system; GHB, gamma-hydroxybutyric; NSAIDs, nonsteroidal anti-inflammatory drugs; LSD, lysergic acid diethylamide; PCP, phencyclidine; SAH, subarachnoid hemorrhage; SSRIs, selective serotonin reuptake inhibitors; TCAs, tricyclic antidepressants.

Source: Patti L, Gupta M. Change in mental status. In: StatPearls. StatPearls Publishing; 2019. https://www.ncbi.nlm.nih.gov/books/NBK441973

EVALUATION

The evaluation of the acutely comatose patient is generally outside the scope of primary care practice, and there is no role for screening patients for altered mental status or coma.

TREATMENT

- Treatment should address the underlying conditions contributing to altered mental status or coma.
- Treatment plans should address the goals of the patient.
- Treatment of the persistent VS is largely supportive and prophylactic
- Clinicians should have a high index of suspicion for polypharmacy.

PATIENT EDUCATION

- Surrogates should be informed that coma may be permanent, although some patients may progress to a VS.
- Surrogates should be informed that progression to the VS does not indicate additional improvement or recovery.
- Surrogates should be informed that during the VS, sleep-wake cycles, blinking, eye movements are not purposeful.

SPECIAL CONSIDERATIONS

MCS is a transitional state of severely impaired consciousness with minimal objective evidence of behavioral evidence of self and environmental awareness. Patients may transition to MCS during recovery from coma or deteriorate to MCS from worsening neurologic disease. The concept of MCS is relatively recent and the Aspen Workgroup developed recommendations for diagnosis and neurocognitive evaluation. Patients may remain in MCS permanently, but there is evidence that emergence from MCS (at the least the ability to consistently engage others) is more likely than for patients in VS. Criteria for diagnosis are listed in Exhibit 15.2 and recommendations for assessment in Exhibit 15.3.

KEY POINTS

- Consciousness is the state of full self and environmental awareness.
- Coma is a state of deep unconsciousness in which a patient is alive, but lacks the ability to respond to internal and external stimulation.
- Coma is commonly caused metabolic disorders, exogenous toxins, or head injuries.
- Coma rarely lasts more than 2 to 4 weeks.
- A more favorable prognosis exists for patients who progress from coma to VS or MCS.
- Traumatic, metabolic, vascular, and toxic causes are the most common causes of altered mental status.

EXHIBIT 15.2 Criteria for the Clinical Diagnosis of the Minimally Conscious State

To make the diagnosis of minimally conscious state, limited but clearly discernible evidence of self- or environmental awareness must be demonstrated on a reproducible or sustained basis by one or more of the following behaviors:

1. Following simple commands
2. Gestural or verbal yes/no responses (regardless of accuracy)
3. Intelligible verbalization

Purposeful behavior, including movements or affective behaviors that occur in contingent relation to relevant environmental stimuli and are not due to reflexive activity. Some examples of qualifying purposeful behavior include appropriate smiling or crying in response to the linguistic or visual content of emotional but not to neutral topics or stimuli; vocalizations or gestures that occur in direct response to the linguistic content of questions; reaching for objects that demonstrates a clear relationship between object location and direction of reach; touching or holding objects in a manner that accommodates the size and shape of the object; pursuit eye movement or sustained fixation that occurs in direct response to moving or salient stimuli.

Source: Giacino JT, Ashwal S, Childs N, et al. The minimally conscious state. *Neurology*. 2002;58(3):349–353. doi:10.1212/WNL.58.3.349. Used with permission.

EXHIBIT 15.3 Recommendations for Behavioral Assessment of Neurocognitive Responsiveness

Differential diagnosis among states of impaired consciousness is often difficult. The following steps should be taken to detect conscious awareness and to establish an accurate diagnosis:

1. Adequate stimulation should be administered to ensure that arousal level is maximized.
2. Factors adversely affecting arousal should be addressed (e.g., sedating medications and occurrence of seizures).
3. Attempts to elicit behavioral responses through verbal instruction should not involve behaviors that frequently occur on a reflexive basis.
4. Command-following trials should incorporate motor behaviors that are within the patient's capability.
5. A variety of different behavioral responses should be investigated using a broad range of eliciting stimuli.
6. Examination procedures should be conducted in a distraction-free environment.

Source: Giacino JT, Ashwal S, Childs N, et al. The minimally conscious state. *Neurology*. 2002;58(3):349–353. doi:10.1212/WNL.58.3.349. Used with permission.

15.11 HEAD INJURIES

Brooke Jackson Gerlach

OVERVIEW

Head injuries are vaguely described in the literature so there is not a clear definition, which can make diagnosis difficult. The workup and treatment should include an interdisciplinary team when at all available. Depending on the degree of the injury, they may involve a temporary or permanent neurologic or physical deficit, which may present itself as a functional or psychological change. Head injuries occur when there is direct trauma to the head or if there is an acceleration/deceleration force to the head or neck.

Mild traumatic brain injuries (TBIs) are called concussions. Currently, the concussion diagnosis is based on clinical presentation. Concussions can be determined by physical examination findings and a thorough history of present illness. Glasgow Coma Scale (GCS) can also be used 30 minutes after the injury to determine the level of injury. Using the GCS, a score of 13–15 would indicate a mild injury, 9–12 is moderate, and <9 is severe. There are also several verified tools that can be used to assess concussion symptoms and improvement. With mild TBIs, a full recovery to baseline is usually expected. With moderate to severe TBIs, understanding which parts of the brain were damaged is important to be able to offer the patient and their family the best care possible. This can often be determined by head imaging and the use of GCS. Initial head imaging should always be done without contrast. If a head trauma is suspected to be more than mild based on your examination, or if there are any concerning symptoms, patients should be evaluated in the ED.

EPIDEMIOLOGY

The number of concussions and head injuries are currently increasing in the United States, and the CDC has taken it upon themselves to try to help address this national problem. According to a study by the CDC in 2014, 2.87 million ED visits, hospitalizations, and deaths occurred from head injuries; 837,000 of these events were with children. This is up 53% from 2006. An estimated 2.5 million people (including 812,000 children) visit the ED with a TBI annually. Most of those seen in the ED presented with a fall, motor vehicle crash, or unintentionally being struck by an object. These visits were proportionally larger for patients over 75 years, 0 to 4 years, and 15 to 24 years; 288,000 of these ED visits led to hospitalization. Most patients hospitalized were admitted after a fall or multivehicle crash (MVC). Unfortunately, the CDC states that more than 50,000 people die from head injuries each year.[177]

PATHOPHYSIOLOGY

Head injuries are typically caused by falls, car crashes, physical assaults, sports injuries, or by being hit by an object. Damage can occur by a brain bleed or a direct crushing of the brain. Damage to the brain or any head injury can also result in brain edema or a change in blood flow such as a dissection or compression, which can cause further damage after the initial insult. The pathophysiology for head injuries is divided into primary injury and secondary injury.

Primary Injury

This injury occurs at the immediate point of the trauma such as a contusion or hematoma. Contusions are typically found in the temporal or frontal area of the brain, based on point of contact. Hematomas or hemorrhages typically occur in the subdural or subarachnoid space and occur with moderate to severe head injuries. Hemorrhages are the tearing of vessels; these vessels are most likely veins that communicate in these spaces. It can also include the shearing of white matter tracts. This is also called diffuse axonal injury (DAI). DAI can occasionally be seen on MRI if it is done close to the date of the head trauma. As a result of any of these injuries, the brain can also experience swelling or edema.

Secondary Injury

A secondary injury is a cascade of events that lead to neuronal injury due to the head trauma. The mechanism of the cascade is still somewhat unknown, but it likely involves free radical injury to cell membranes, inflammation, and cell death. This cascade can in turn lead to edema or increased intracranial pressure. The cascade of events can worsen with second injury during the healing process. For this reason, it is very important for patients to be educated to avoid further head injuries and athletes should not return to play until cleared to do so.

MEDICAL HISTORY AND CLINICAL PRESENTATION

A patient's medical history should include some mechanism of injury. A patient may present to a primary care center and often not know they have sustained a concussion. They also may present after being evaluated in the ED or significant time after the injury due to continued symptoms. A clear history of present illness should include mechanism of injury (coup and contrecoup), any amnesia that occurred before or after injury, and any symptoms that a patient has been experiencing since the head injury. As a general rule, especially with mild head injuries, symptoms should diminish over time. A patient should also detail if they have had any prior head injuries as it will likely alter their recovery time.

If the incident was a car crash, it should be determined if there was a "seat belt sign" or any contusions. This can help determine the severity of the injury and should alert a clinician to assess for a more serious head injury. However, this should not be the only factor that is taken into account. It should be known if there was any loss of consciousness and for how long. It should also be documented if there was any amnesia before or after the head injury; getting an account of the event and the patient's symptoms from an eyewitness or trusted source can be helpful in getting an accurate history. After these things are determined, it is important to find out if the patient sought medical attention. If they did, document what was done, including scans and testing. If a patient has risk factors for a more serious injury and they were not evaluated in an ED or urgent care setting, a low threshold for imaging should be kept.

SIGNS AND SYMPTOMS

As part of the medical history, it is important to assess signs and symptoms. Head injuries can cause many symptoms, and these will result as postconcussion syndrome. Symptoms can include headaches, dizziness, nausea, photophobia, phonophobia, confusion, numbness, and tingling, and feeling "off." Signs will include slow reaction to commands, flat affect, and moving clumsily.

If any other signs are present, such as loss of vision, change in visual fields, weakness, trouble swallowing, dysarthria, confusion that worsens, repetitive vomiting, change in pupil size, seizures, lethargy, a more serious brain injury may have occurred and imaging and immediate emergent evaluation should be obtained.

PHYSICAL EXAMINATION

Physical examination is one of the most important features of assessing a TBI along with a thorough history.

- It is important to assess overall appearance. If the patient is being seen right after the insult, they should be assessed for any visible bleeding. Bleeding on the head, in the ear, or behind the ear is an indication of an urgent injury. The patient should be sent for evaluation in the ED for a brain bleed or skull fracture.
- If there are no signs of bleeding, a detailed neurologic examination should be performed. It is important to establish if there is any cranial nerve deficit or any changes in strength, especially unilateral.
  - Visual fields should be assessed, and the optic nerve should be visualized. If there is a change in the visual fields, it should be noted as to where the defect is localized. If there is any swelling or visual change noted, the patient should be evaluated in the ED if they have not already been seen.
  - An ophthalmologic exam can also be helpful, especially if optical coherence tomography (OCT) and visual field testing is used. Pupils should be equal and reactive to light; they may be sluggish with new head injuries or moderate to severe.
  - If there are pupil discrepancies, further evaluation is needed. Extraocular movements should be assessed, including convergence. Often, patients with postconcussion syndrome will have delayed convergence. If this is indicated, vision therapy may be helpful. Strength testing should be done of all extremities.
  - Any clonus should also be noted. Besides strength, sensation should also be assessed. Any abnormalities should be noted and localized to a dermatome if possible.
  - Gait and balance should be evaluated. This can be done with Romberg sign and tandem walk. Changes in balance can direct what kind of therapy may be needed such as vestibular therapy.
- It is important to keep in mind that brain injury should be differentiated from other physical injury. Strength may be affected by pain from another injury that was sustained in the insult. If the brain injury was mild, there should not be any substantial unilateral weakness unless there is also a spinal cord injury.
- If a spinal cord injury or vertebra fractur is suspected, proper imaging and referrals need to be obtained.
- Cervical fractures should be immediately evaluated in the ED. Pain to cervical midline palpation and/or signs of myelopathy raises the suspicion of this. Signs of myelopathy can include increased reflexes and pathologic reflexes. These include Babinski and Hoffmann reflexes.

DIFFERENTIAL DIAGNOSIS

The differential diagnosis for head injuries is summarized in Table 15.31.

TABLE 15.31 Differential Diagnosis for Head Injuries

Diagnosis	Description
Stroke	Hemorrhagic stroke and brain bleed may appear similar in both imaging and clinical imaging. People with hemorrhagic strokes usually have risk factors that make them susceptible to a brain bleed.
Subdural hematoma	This can usually be seen on head imaging. A subdural hematoma is bleeding located between the dura mater and the arachnoid mater in the meninges. If this is seen, the injury is automatically categorized as moderate to severe traumatic brain injury (TBI). This can be a deadly manifestation of a head injury.
Cerebral aneurysm	This is a focal dilation of an artery in the brain. It is a weak area and is at high risk of rupture. If it ruptures, it can cause a brain bleed.
Epilepsy	Seizures are usually followed by a postictal period. If the seizure is accompanied by a fall and a head injury occurs, there may be an overlap of concussion symptoms like confusion and postictal state. Postictal state will typically conclude with a return to baseline within 24 hours while a concussion may have lingering symptoms.
Functional neurologic disorder	This is a difficult diagnosis to distinguish. Usually this diagnosis is determined after normal testing. Typically, with functional disorders, there are inconsistencies with physical exam. This can be noted as weakness that corrects with encouragement or variable results on repeat testing of abnormal findings with different results.
Hydrocephalus	Hydrocephalus may occur for various reasons and is usually seen on imaging. It occurs when the cerebrospinal fluid in the ventricles build up and put pressure on the brain. This can be confused with brain edema that results after a brain injury.

DIAGNOSTIC STUDIES

Initial diagnostic studies are often done in the ED setting. With head injuries that result in physical examination symptoms or with a low GCS score, a head CT without contrast should be ordered. Sodium should be assessed as low levels could indicate cerebral salt wasting or SIADH (syndrome of inappropriate antidiuretic hormone secretion). Elevated levels may indicate dehydration or diabetes insipidus. Magnesium should also be evaluated acutely as it can be an antioxidant and may help improve outcomes. There are also several blood markers that are currently being evaluated to be able to better assess if a mild-to-severe head injury has been sustained. Glial fibrillary acid protein (GFAP) is one of these markers. A certain ubiquitin derivative can be used in combination with GFAP. Many of these blood tests are still being validated. These tests are very promising and will be of great help when trying to distinguish a concussion from malingering or somatization.

If postconcussion symptoms linger >6 to 12 months, a brain MRI can be used to rule out any other causes of prolonged symptoms. This should be a brain MRI with contrast, if possible, especially if dizziness is the main complaint.

EVALUATION

Head injury evaluation should include a thorough history of present illness and physical examination. These two steps will determine if further imaging is needed. Most patients that present to a primary care setting after a head injury and are looking for explanation and treatment of their symptoms. It is important that a thorough neurologic exam is done so a patient can be reassured or evaluated further. Most symptoms from a concussion should be resolved within a few months but can subside within days. Symptoms do not typically last longer than 6 months unless one or more prior head injuries have been sustained. Reminding a patient that with time and rest, symptoms will resolve can be very therapeutic.

TREATMENT

- **Nausea:** Treat with antinausea medication.
- **Dizziness:** If there is a delay in convergence, vision therapy would be beneficial. Unfortunately, not all insurance will cover this; if balance is an issue, vestibular therapy would benefit.
  - Nausea medication may also help with some dizziness symptoms.
- **Headache:** Consider a tricyclic antidepressant (especially if sleep is a problem), a beta blocker, or gabapentin.
  - Topiramate may also be considered if there is a migraine component and the patient has no contraindications.
  - Opioids should never be the primary option.
  - If headaches present from the neck area, cervicalgia should be considered. Physical therapy would be beneficial.
    - Imaging should be considered if there is a positive Lhermitte sign.
  - OTC pain medications as well as prescription pain medications should be limited to no more than twice a week to avoid rebound headache.
  - If a brain bleed occurred or is suspected, NSAIDs should be avoided.
- **Fatigue:** Sleep should be encouraged to be between 7.5 and 9 hours.
- **Limit screen time:** Helpful to set phone, computer, and TV time limits to 10 minutes or less per day if patient is symptomatic. This can be increased as tolerated and reduced as symptoms return.
- **Exercise:** Encourage walking around 10 to 20 minutes a day as tolerated.
- **Photophobia:** Blue light filtering glasses or FL-41 may be beneficial.
- Overstimulation should be reduced at it may aggravate symptoms.
- Patient should be brought down to a level of activity at which they are generally symptom-free before increasing activity and stimulation. This can be very difficult when translating this to a working environment. A clinician must use their best judgment on how to implement this in the workplace.
- **Confusion or memory problems:** Speech language cognitive therapy may be beneficial if available. Neuropsychology may also be utilized.
- **Depression or anxiety:** CBT should be used if available. Behavioral medicine services can help reduce any of these symptoms that may prolong reversible head injury symptoms.
  - SSRIs should be considered.

PATIENT EDUCATION

- Mild traumatic brain injuries should return to baseline over time. Symptoms may be prolonged if there are any other underlying conditions.
  - These may include prior head injuries, neck injury, depression, mental health, stress in various forms.
- The patient should be reminded that things will get better with therapy, medication, and time.
- Patients should be educated about warning signs of when things may be more severe and when to go to the ED. This is especially important within the first few days of the injury.
  - Warning signs:
    - Loss of vision, change in visual fields, weakness, trouble swallowing, dysarthria, confusion that worsens, repetitive vomiting, change in pupil size, seizures, and lethargy
- Moderate to severe head injuries should be monitored. It is important that a caregiver is well informed of what areas of the brain were affected and what symptoms are expected due to the brain injury.
- Great care should be taken to avoid future head injuries. Further head injuries can take more time to recover from upon each incident.
- Many patients with multiple head injuries will be concerned about chronic traumatic encephalopathy (CTE). There is no evidence as to how many head injuries lead to this. So far, it seems CTE appears in people who participate in contact sports, such as football and boxing. This is likely due to the numerous head injuries sustained. CTE can present as dementia and behavior changes. Definite diagnosis can only be made at autopsy.

15.12 PERIPHERAL NEUROPATHIES

Erin Salcido

OVERVIEW

Peripheral neuropathies involve damage to the peripheral nervous system. Peripheral neuropathy (PN) can affect one nerve (mononeuropathy), two or more nerves in different areas (multiple mononeuropathy), or many nerves (polyneuropathy). PNs are classified based on which structure is affected. Examples include axonal degeneration or paranodal or segmental demyelination. The distinction is usually discovered by neurophysiologic studies; nerve conduction velocity (NCV) and EMG. In axonal neuropathies, conduction velocity is normal or mildly reduced whereas EMG provides evidence of denervation. In demyelinating neuropathies, conduction is slowed or completely blocked in some cases, and EMG is normal.

There are many different causes of PN, including diabetes, chemo-induced, metabolic/vitamin and nutritional deficiencies, hereditary disorders, inflammatory infections, autoimmune diseases, exposure to toxic chemicals, and certain medications.

Symptoms of PN may develop suddenly or progress over time, depending on the etiology. Symptoms range from mild to disabling. In some instances, the symptoms improve on their own. In addition, symptoms vary depending on the type of nerves that are damaged: motor, sensory, or autonomic. Most PNs affect all three types of nerve fibers. Common symptoms are numbness, tingling sensation, sharp burning pain, muscle weakness, or paralysis.

The diagnosis of PN depends greatly on the history and physical examination, including a complete neurologic examination. Occasionally, blood tests can aid in the diagnosis or help to exclude other causes. Additionally, neurophysiologic studies help to determine the nature and extent of the neuropathy.

- NCV test measures signal strength and speed along specific large motor and sensory nerves. It can detect whether symptoms are caused by degeneration of the myelin sheath or the axon. During the exam, a probe electrically stimulates a nerve fiber, generating an electrical impulse. An electrode placed further along the nerve's pathway measures the speed of signal transmission along the axon. Slow transmission rates indicate damage to the myelin sheath, while a reduction in the strength of impulses at normal speeds is a sign of axonal degeneration.
- EMG involves inserting very fine needles into specific muscles to record their electrical activity at rest and during contraction. EMG tests irritability and responsiveness, detects abnormal muscular electrical activity in motor neuropathy, and can help differentiate between muscle and nerve disorders.

Treatment of PN greatly depends on the type of nerve damage, symptoms, and locations. Correcting the underlying causes, in some instances, can result in the neuropathy completely resolving. Other cases involve anti-inflammatory or immunosuppressive medications, surgery, occupational or physical therapy.

TABLE 15.32 Pathophysiology of Peripheral Neuropathy

Reaction	Pathology	Type	Etiology
Wallerian degeneration	The axon degenerates distal to a focal lesion the interrupts the continuity of the axon	Focal mononeuropathies	Trauma, nerve infarction
Axonal degeneration	Occurs at the most distal extent of the axon, symmetric, degeneration occurs distal-to-proximal	Generalized polyneuropathies	Metabolic
Segmental demyelination	Focal degeneration of myelin sheath, sparing of the axon	Focal mononeuropathies, generalized sensorimotor or predominately motor neuropathies	Immune-mediated or inflammatory

EPIDEMIOLOGY

PN occurs as a component of several common and many rare diseases. It is heterogeneous in etiology, diverse in pathology, and varied in severity.[178] As a group, PNs are common and affect 1% of the population, but the prevalence increases to 7% with advancing age.[179] PNs are more common in people older than age 55. The most common condition associated with polyneuropathy is diabetes, seen in 66% of type 1 diabetics and 59% of type 2 diabetic patients.[180] By reviewing each cause of PN separately, increased knowledge of epidemiologic features may lead to better understanding of the disease itself. In addition, with the diabetes and obesity pandemic, the prevalence of PN is increasing.[181]

PATHOPHYSIOLOGY

Peripheral nerves exhibit three distinct pathologic reactions to an insult or disease: wallerian degeneration, axonal degeneration, and segmental demyelination. The specific mechanisms by which these occur are unknown (Table 15.32).

15.12A CARPAL TUNNEL SYNDROME

MEDICAL HISTORY AND CLINICAL PRESENTATION

Carpal tunnel syndrome (CTS) is a disorder characterized by pain, paresthesias, and weakness of the hand resulting from compression of the median nerve. It is the most common compressive PN seen in clinical practice. The carpal tunnel is formed by the transverse carpal ligament, or flexor retinaculum, superiorly and the carpal bones inferiorly. The median nerve travels through this anatomic tunnel and compression of this nerve can lead to nerve ischemia. Several factors can lead to median nerve compression such as synovitis of the tendon sheaths, recent fracture, tumors, and edema. CTS is common in pregnancy due to fluid retention and in those who use their hands in repetitive motion. CTS is also noted in many systemic diseases such as rheumatoid arthritis. CTS is more frequent in women with the female-male ratio of approximately 3:1.

SIGNS AND SYMPTOMS

Initially, patients may complain of pain, burning, and tingling in the distribution of the median nerve. Occasionally, patients complain of radiation of pain to the forearm, shoulder, and less commonly, the neck. Pain is exacerbated by activity and worsens at night. Some patients complain they are awakened at night by the symptoms. Symptoms are often worsened by extreme wrist flexion that would compress the median nerve further. They are also provoked by wrist extension or by activities that raise the arms, such as driving, reading, typing, and holding a phone. Bilateral CTS can also occur. Motor symptoms usually occur later in the disease and patients will complain of weakness or clumsiness when holding objects, turning keys, buttoning shirts, or opening jar lids.

PHYSICAL EXAMINATION

On physical examination, the patient may elicit sensory disturbances in the distribution of the median nerve. However, their absence does not rule out the diagnosis of CTS. Muscle weakness is limited to the muscles of the thenar eminence and is manifested as weakness of thumb abduction and thumb opposition. Atrophy of the thenar eminence may be noted.

Special maneuvers for CTS include the Phalen and Tinel sign. The most common way to test for Phalen sign is to have the patient flex the wrists to 90 degrees while the backs of their hands are against each other. A positive Phalen sign is defined as pain and/or paresthesia in the distribution of the median nerve within 1 minute of wrist flexion (68% sensitivity and 73% specificity).[182]

Tinel sign is achieved by percussion over the median nerve that produces pain and/or paresthesia of the median-innervated fingers (50% sensitivity and 77% specificity).[182]

The carpal compression test induces direct pressure over the carpal tunnel. It is positive if paresthesia occurs within 30 seconds of applying pressure (63% sensitivity and 84% specificity.[182]

DIFFERENTIAL DIAGNOSIS

There are several neurologic, musculoskeletal, and vascular conditions that can present with pain, paresthesia, sensory loss, or weakness of the upper extremity (Table 15.33).

DIAGNOSTIC STUDIES

Imaging studies such as ultrasound are useful in the evaluation of CTS if a structural abnormality, such as a tumor, deformity, or other bone or joint disease, is considered. MRI can be used to detect abnormalities of the median nerve, flexor tendons, vascular structures, and transverse carpal ligament but is reserved for unusual cases.

Electrodiagnostic testing, such as NCS and EMG, are standard in the evaluation of CTS. They are useful for gauging the severity of median nerve injury and for excluding other conditions.[183] In mild CTS, the nerve conduction may not be impaired. As the condition progresses and the median nerve is more compressed, focal demyelination can occur resulting in a conduction delay. With severe compression, axonal damage occurs resulting in a reduction of motor or sensory amplitude. EMG is most often used to exclude other conditions and evaluate the severity of CTS if surgical decompression is considered.[184] In the case that patients have classic presentation of CTS and confirmatory findings on NCS, and surgery is not an option, EMG is not completed.

TABLE 15.33 Differential Diagnosis of Carpal Tunnel Syndrome

Condition	Description
Cervical radiculopathy	Presence of neck pain, exacerbation of symptoms with neck movement, radiation of pain from the neck into the shoulder or arm, reduced reflexes, weakness of proximal arm muscles
Cervical spondylotic myelopathy	Bilateral sensory loss and motor dysfunction in the hands
Brachial plexopathy	Symptoms outside the median nerve distribution
Median neuropathy	Forearm pain and sensory loss involving the entire lateral palm, sensory loss over the thenar eminence, which is spared in CTS, and weakness of thumb flexion, wrist flexion, and arm pronation, which are median-innervated muscles proximal to the carpal tunnel
Motor neuron disease	The absence of pain argues against CTS. More importantly, ALS essentially never presents with weakness of a single muscle

ALS, amyotrophic lateral sclerosis; CTS, carpal tunnel syndrome.

EVALUATION

The diagnosis of CTS is clinical and is suspected when the characteristic signs and symptoms are present. The most important of these are nocturnal pain or paresthesias along the distribution of the median nerve.[185]

The likelihood of diagnosis is thought to correlate with the number of standard symptoms and provocative factors (Table 15.34).[185]

The combination of electrodiagnostic study findings and symptom characteristics provides the most accurate information for classification of CTS.[186]

TREATMENT

Treatment is directed at relieving pressure on the median nerve. Conservative management includes splinting, NSAIDs, steroid injections, therapeutic ultrasound, and ergonomic positioning. Nonsurgical options are reasonable in patients who have mild clinical symptoms.

Nightly wrist splinting has shown some evidence for efficacy.[187] The splints should be worn for a minimum of 4 weeks and the wrist should be in neutral or slight extension. This approach is low cost and carries a low risk for adverse effects. NSAIDs may benefit some populations of patients; however, the American Academy of Orthopaedic Surgeons state that oral agents are not more beneficial than placebo. Steroid injections, on the other hand, seem to improve both the neurophysiologic and symptomology in patients with CTS.[188]

Those who fail initial nonsurgical treatment or have evidence of significant nerve damage on NCV studies should undergo decompressive surgery, by release of the transverse carpal ligament. Surgical treatment relieves symptoms significantly better than splinting.[189] The procedure provides high success rates with low rates of complications.

PATIENT EDUCATION

Patients who are treated conservatively should have a follow-up visit within 4 to 6 weeks to determine efficacy.

TABLE 15.34 Characteristic Signs and Symptoms of Carpel Tunnel Syndrome

Standard symptoms	Dull, aching discomfort in the hand, forearm, or upper arm
	Paresthesia in the hand
	Weakness or clumsiness of the hand
	Occurrence of any of these symptoms in the median distribution
Provocative factors	Sleep
	Sustained hand or arm positions
	Repetitive actions of the hand or wrist
Mitigating factors	Changes in hand posture
	Shaking the hand

Those who have not experienced symptomatic relief should be referred for surgical intervention.

CTS is a progressive disorder and can lead to permanent median nerve damage if left untreated. Approximately 90% of patients with mild to moderate CTS respond to conservative management.

It is prudent to avoid factors that cause or aggravate the symptoms of CTS, such as repetition, posture, or vibration through the wrist.

15.12B MONONEUROPATHIES

MEDICAL HISTORY AND CLINICAL PRESENTATION

Mononeuropathies are a type of PN that affects an individual peripheral nerve. They are diagnosed clinically based on signs and symptoms that correlate with an individual nerve distribution. They are characterized by focal sensory disturbances and/or motor deficits. Mononeuropathies occur due to direct trauma, compression, angulation, or stretching injury. Patients generally present with pain and sensory disturbances distal to the site of the lesion. Percussion of the nerve at the site of the lesion may cause parasthesias in the distal distribution. Depending on the site and extent of injury, symptoms may resolve rapidly and spontaneously in some cases, while becoming progressive and disabling in others.

Radial nerve palsies have several etiologies. Humeral nailing during a surgical procedure to stabilize an acute humeral fracture has been known to cause direct injury to the nerve.[190] Palsies can occur from compression of the nerve in the axilla, such as in the case of crutches or direct pressure at the spiral groove when the arm hangs over the back of a chair, termed "Saturday night palsy." Patients with radial nerve palsy most commonly present with weakness of wrist dorsiflexion (i.e., wrist drop) and finger extension. Sensory disturbances are present but depend on the site of injury.

Entrapment of the ulnar nerve is the second most common entrapment neuropathy in the upper extremity, after entrapment of the median nerve.[191] The most common site is at or near the elbow region, in the cubital tunnel or in the epicondylar groove. Ulnar nerve entrapment can also occur at or near the wrist, in a structure called the canal of Guyon. Patients will present with pain, paresthesias, and weakness in the hand and digits.[192]

In the lower extremity, the most common mononeuropathy is of the peroneal nerve. Injury to this nerve occurs as a result of direct compression as the nerve winds around the neck of the fibula and has a superficial course. It is also susceptible to a stretch injury as the nerve dives distally into the peroneus longus muscle. Patients typically present with a foot drop, pain at the site of compression, and sensory disturbances distal to the lesion.

SIGNS AND SYMPTOMS

- **Radial nerve lesions:** The most common reported symptom is wrist drop. If the lesion is above the elbow, the patient may complain of numbness in the forearm and hand. If the lesion is at the wrist, patients report paresthesias over the back of the hand without motor weakness.
- **Ulnar nerve lesions:** Patients report sensory changes: numbness, tingling or burning, in the fifth and medial half of the fourth digits and along the medial border of the hand. Occasionally, patients will complain of pain in the elbow and it may radiate into the hand or up to the shoulder. Weakness may also be a presenting complaint and the patient may describe difficulty opening jars or turning doorknobs.
- **Peroneal nerve lesions:** Patients will present with frequent tripping due to a foot drop. They may experience night cramps in the anterior lower leg and pain at the site of compression. Numbness and tingling may occur in the lateral lower leg and foot.

PHYSICAL EXAMINATION

- Radial nerve lesions
  - Patients with radial neuropathy will have weakness of wrist dorsiflexion and finger extension.
  - Injury to the radial nerve in the axilla leads to weakness or paralysis of all the muscles supplied by the nerve, including the triceps. On examination, the triceps and brachioradialis reflexes are decreased. In addition, sensation is decreased over the triceps muscle, the posterior part of the forearm, and dorsum of the hand.
  - Compression at the spiral groove leads to weakness of all radial-innervated muscles except the triceps. The brachioradialis reflex is decreased and patients experience sensory loss over the radial dorsal part of the hand and the posterior part of the forearm.
  - If the lesion is at the wrist, the patient does not experience motor weakness. However, they will have numbness of the dorsal hand but sparing of the fifth digit.
- Ulnar nerve lesions
  - Patients with ulnar neuropathy usually have a positive Tinel sign at the elbow, which is specific for ulnar entrapment. To perform Tinel sign, the examiner taps a reflex hammer over the ulnar nerve in the ulnar groove and cubital tunnel. The patient will experience paresthesias in the ulnar portion of the hand. Another diagnostic exam is the elbow flexion test, which is considered the best diagnostic test for cubital tunnel syndrome.[193] During this exam, the patient flexes the elbow past 90 degrees, supinates the forearm, and extends the wrist. Results are positive if pain or paresthesia occurs within 60 seconds.
  - It is also important to test for muscle weakness and sensation along the forearm, hand, and fingers. The examination may illicit intrinsic muscle weakness of the hand and decreased sensation and 2-point discrimination along the ulnar nerve distribution.
- Peroneal nerve lesions
  - If the lesion is severe, a complete foot drop will be noted. The foot drop spares plantar flexion and foot inversion. The patient will have a high-stepping gait with "foot slapping." The patient may complain of pain and tingling with tapping of the nerve at the fibular head. Distribution of sensory changes and type of lower extremity weakness aid in localizing the lesion.

DIFFERENTIAL DIAGNOSIS

The diagnosis of mononeuropathies include a thorough physical examination, eliciting the sensory and/or motor disturbances along the peripheral nerve distribution (see Table 15.35).

TABLE 15.35 Differential Diagnosis for Radial, Ulnar, and Peroneal Mononeuropathies

Diagnosis	Description
Radial Nerve	
Ulnar neuropathy	Motor and sensory changes along ulnar nerve distribution.
Median neuropathy	Motor and sensory changes along median nerve distribution.
Ulnar Nerve	
Alcohol-related neuropathy	Generally begins in the feet and legs with paresthesias and burning pain. Progresses slowly. Symmetric, bilateral.
Amyotrophic lateral sclerosis	Neurologic disease in which the patient loses the ability to control voluntary muscle movement. For many patients, the first sign of ALS is upper extremity weakness.
Cervical spondylosis	Common degenerative disease of the cervical spine. Patients experience neck and shoulder pain, radicular pain to the upper extremities, and paresthesias or weakness to upper limbs.
Peroneal Nerve	
L4-L5 lumbar disc herniation, spinal stenosis, or degenerative disease	Presents with back pain radiating to the lower extremity. Strength reduced in dorsiflexion, toe extension, foot inversion and eversion. Sensory loss to lateral shin and dorsum of foot.
Diabetic neuropathy	Nerve damage relating to high glucose. Symptoms usually begin in the legs and feet. Numbness, tingling, and pain are common symptoms.
Nutritional neuropathy	Peripheral neuropathies due to nutritional deficiencies, such as in the case of alcohol neuropathy, thiamine deficiency, niacin, and more. Sensory disturbances are bilateral, symmetric glove-and-stocking distribution.
Uremic neuropathy	Sensorimotor polyneuropathy caused by uremic toxins. Compressive mononeuropathy may be present in the median, ulnar, or peroneal nerve distribution.
Vasculitic neuropathy	Peripheral neuropathy as a result of ischemic infarction caused by inflammatory occlusion of the blood vessels which leads to wallerian degeneration of nerves. Presents with asymmetric or multifocal sensorimotor neuropathy. Exam findings vary depending on the location of the nerve(s) involved.

ALS, amyotrophic lateral sclerosis.

DIAGNOSTIC STUDIES

Routine lab studies for mononeuropathies are aimed at excluding other diagnoses. For example, a CBC; urinalysis; fasting blood glucose; vitamins B12, B1, and B6 and folate levels; and renal function tests may help to exclude acquired neuropathies from diabetes, uremic, or nutritional etiologies.

Radiographs of the cervical spine and lumbar spine are useful if cervical or lumbar pathology is suspected. Radiographs of the elbow and wrist are necessary in the evaluation of ulnar nerve entrapment and radial compression. X-rays may show masses or bony lesions, such as fractures, dislocations, callus formation or osteophytes, that could be compressing the nerve.

Ultrasound evaluation of peripheral nerves is able to identify structural lesions and inflammatory changes in the nerve. It can determine the change in diameter of a nerve at the site of compression. Just proximal to the site of compression, swelling of the nerve can be seen.[194]

MRI is valuable in the diagnosis of PN. In most cases, history, physical exam, and electrophysiologic testing are sufficient to make the diagnosis of mononeuropathy. However, MRI is helpful for evaluation of the soft tissue surrounding the nerve and more direct imaging of the nerve.[195] MRI can detect abnormalities or variations in the soft tissue that can lead to nerve compression. In one study, the authors found that MRI was "more sensitive" than electrophysiologic tests.[196]

Electrodiagnostic testing is a standard part of the evaluation for PNs. They are used to confirm diagnosis, establish baseline results, and determine severity and location of the lesion.[197]

EVALUATION

The clinical diagnosis of a peripheral mononeuropathy can be made with a careful history, thorough physical examination, and knowledge of the anatomy underlying the peripheral motor and sensory symptoms. In most cases, the diagnosis can be confirmed by electrodiagnostic testing.

TREATMENT

- Radial neuropathy
  - Treatment of radial neuropathy is dependent on the site and cause of injury. For example, if injury is due to external compression at the spiral groove, treatment is removing the source of compression. If the lesion is due to a humeral fracture, the fracture must be carefully reduced and set to avoid further injury. Surgical exploration is indicated for chronic compressive lesion or transection.
- Ulnar neuropathy
  - It is generally recommended that patients with ulnar neuropathy at the elbow should avoid leaning on the elbow and prolonged elbow flexion. In addition, nonsurgical treatments, such as medications, splinting, and physical therapy, can provide significant help.[195] NSAIDs, tricycylic antidepressants, anticonvulsants and vitamin B6 supplements have shown limited benefits for pain and sensory symptoms.
  - Occupational therapy aimed at promoting smoother movement of the nerve within the cubital tunnel and reducing adhesions has shown benefits in patients.
  - An elbow pad or night splinting for 3-month trial is recommended. If symptoms do not improve, daytime immobilization for 3 weeks should be considered. Subsequently, if a patient fails conservative management, surgical release is generally warranted. Surgery consists of nerve transposition if the lesion is in the condylar groove, or a release procedure if it is in the cubital tunnel.

- Peroneal neuropathy
  - Most peroneal nerve lesions respond to conservative management with rest and elimination of triggering factors. Physical therapy and the use of an ankle foot orthosis (AFO) is helpful in recovery of function for foot drop. Surgical management is indicated only if there is a mass compressing the nerve, the nerve is tethered and needs release, or the nerve was severely or completely transected.

PATIENT EDUCATION

Patients may be referred to physical therapy to help with functional movement of a limb after nerve injury or repair. Recovery of a nerve injury is related to the degree and type of injury. In most cases of mild injury, recovery after several months is expected. Factors for unfavorable outcome include age older than 50 years, comorbidities, especially diabetes, and surgical repair.

15.12C GUILLAIN-BARRÉ SYNDROME

MEDICAL HISTORY AND CLINICAL PRESENTATION

Guillain-Barré syndrome (GBS) is described as a polyradiculoneuropathy that often follows an infection. It is considered to be immune-mediated in that antibodies produced in response to an infectious agent attack the myelin in the peripheral nervous system. Two-thirds of patients report a history of a recent bacterial or viral illness prior to the onset of neurologic symptoms.[198] Most often, patients experience benign upper respiratory infections or GI illness. Infection with *Campylobacter jejuni*, which can cause respiratory and GI infections, has been attributed to the development of GBS. CMV infections are the second most commonly reported infections preceding GBS.[199] The onset of GBS has also been associated with certain vaccinations, other infections such as Zika or *Haemophilus influenzae*, surgical procedures, and trauma.

Typically, patients present 2 to 4 weeks following illness with proximal muscle weakness of the lower extremities. The weakness is symmetric and ascends superiorly. It may progress over hours to days to involve the upper extremities, truncal and respiratory muscles, and cranial nerves. The patient often experiences sensory changes such as paresthesias or numbness, which may precede the weakness.

SIGNS AND SYMPTOMS

- **Weakness:** The weakness experienced by patients with GBS is ascending and symmetric. The lower limbs are generally affected before the upper extremities. The patient may have pronounced ataxia or may not be able to stand.
- **Sensory changes:** Most patients complain of paresthesias or numbness, which usually precedes the weakness. Patients experience loss of vibration, proprioception, and touch. Patients may also report pain described as achy or throbbing in nature.
- **Autonomic changes:** Dysfunction of the autonomic and parasympathetic nervous systems is also identified in patients with GBS. These include the following:
  - Tachycardia or bradycardia
  - Facial flushing
  - Paroxysmal hypertension
  - Orthostatic hypotension
  - Cardiac arrhythmias
  - Anhidrosis and/or diaphoresis
  - Urinary retention
  - Constipation
- **Cranial nerves:** Cranial nerves III-VII and IX-XII may be affected. These symptoms may manifest after the trunk and limbs are affected. Common complaints are the following:
  - Facial droop
  - Diplopia
  - Dysarthria
  - Dysphagia
  - Ophthalmoplegia
  - Pupillary disturbances
- **Respiratory involvement:** Upon presentation, almost half of patients have respiratory or oropharyngeal weakness. They typically complain of the following:
  - Dyspnea on exertion
  - Shortness of breath
  - Difficulty swallowing
  - Slurred speech

PHYSICAL EXAMINATION

As a result of the autonomic dysfunction, vital signs may be abnormal, severe, and life-threatening. This includes tachycardia or bradycardia. Blood pressure may be altered as well, and the patient could have hypertension or hypotension. The patient's temperature may be elevated or low. Respiratory rate may be elevated and could be a sign of progressive respiratory failure.

On neurologic examination, symmetric lower extremity weakness is appreciated. The patient has adequate strength but may be unable to stand or walk. There is minimal muscle atrophy. Facial weakness is the most frequently observed deficit of the cranial nerves. Other cranial nerve deficits include facial droop, dysphagia, dysarthria, and oculomotor dysfunction, such as decreased extraocular movements (CN VI) and ptosis (CN III).

Hyporeflexia or areflexia of involved areas are common findings early in the disease course.

DIFFERENTIAL DIAGNOSIS[200,201]

GBS can be differentiated from many disorders with a thorough history and physical examination. Some serologic studies will help to exclude etiologies such as toxic and infectious neuropathies. See Table 15.36 for a complete description of the differential diagnosis.

DIAGNOSTIC STUDIES

The diagnosis of GBS in the emergent setting is generally made clinically. Basic laboratory studies, such as a CBC, basic metabolic panel, liver function studies, and ESR, are usually normal and are of limited values. In patients with GBS, the CSF will reveal an elevated protein (>400 mg/L) with a normal white blood cell count.

Electrodiagnostic studies, such as EMG and NCS, can aid in the diagnosis of GBS and provide information regarding the prognosis. They can be normal in acute disease. Occasionally, these studies may show evidence of demyelination.

TABLE 15.36 Differential Diagnosis of Guillain-Barré Syndrome

Condition	Description
Botulism	Neuroparalysis due to neurotoxin *Clostridium botulinum*; symmetric descending weakness and paralysis
Cauda equina	Lower extremity neuromuscular disturbances
Chronic inflammatory demyelinating polyradiculoneuropathy	Insidious onset, slow progression, proximal and distal limb weakness, and sensory disturbances
Myasthenia gravis	Autoimmune disorder; causes reduced muscle strength; bulbar muscles commonly affected
Heavy metal toxicity	Uncommon diagnosis; lead or iron toxicity, history of exposure, gastrointestinal symptoms common
Lyme disease	Vector-borne illness caused by *Borrelia burgdorferi*, commonly presents as flu-like illness, tender local adenopathy, and a rash
Metabolic myopathies	Group of rare disorders characterized by abnormalities of muscle energy metabolism that result in skeletal muscle dysfunction
Multiple sclerosis	Central nervous system disease that classically affects different anatomic locations at various times
Nutritional neuropathy	Peripheral neuropathies caused by alcohol exposure or vitamin deficiencies
Vasculitic neuropathy	Asymmetric or multifocal painful sensorimotor neuropathy

Imaging with gadolinium-enhanced MRI of the spine may show thickening of the intrathecal spinal nerve roots and cauda equina.[202]

EVALUATION

Diagnostic criteria for GBS is widely used in clinical practice and was developed by the National Institute of Neurological Disorders and Stroke (NINDS). Features needed for the diagnosis of GBS are progressive weakness in legs and arms (sometimes initially only in legs) and areflexia in weak limbs.[203,204] Additional features that strongly support the diagnosis are as follows:

- Progressive phase lasts from days to 4 weeks (usually <2 weeks)
- Relative symmetry of symptoms and signs
- Relatively mild sensory symptoms and signs
- Cranial nerve involvement, especially bilateral facial palsy
- Autonomic dysfunction
- Muscular or radicular back or limb pain
- Increased protein level in CSF; normal protein levels do not rule out the diagnosis
- Electrodiagnostic features of motor or sensorimotor neuropathy

TREATMENT

All patients suspected of having GBS or who are diagnosed with GBS require hospital admission. Approximately one-third of patients require admission to an ICU at presentation, due to respiratory involvement, including respiratory failure and the need for mechanical ventilation.[205] Initially all patients require supportive care due to the risk of respiratory failure and autonomic dysfunction. Frequent monitoring of blood pressure, heart rate, and vital capacity is essential. Intubation is considered if the forced vital capacity reaches 15 mL/kg. Supportive treatment continues until it is determined that the disease has reached a plateau or symptoms have started to reverse.

Both plasma exchange and IVIG have been effective in the treatment of GBS and have been found to decrease recovery time.[206] Corticosteroids are ineffective, do not hasten recovery or affect the outcome. Patients may need analgesia with NSAIDs or narcotics. Patients will need to undergo chest physical therapy to prevent atelectasis. Low-dose heparin is recommended to prevent venous thromboembolism.

Physical and occupational therapy should be included in the patient's treatment plan and begun early in the course of the disease. The goals of therapy are to reduce functional deficits and prevent long-term disability. Speech therapy may be initiated for patients who had significant oropharyngeal weakness, dysphagia, and dysarthria to promote speech and safe swallowing skills.

PATIENT EDUCATION

Most patients eventually make good recovery and some studies have reported continued improvements in strength beyond 2 years.[207] The proportion of patients with GBS who walk independently at 6 months and 12 months after diagnosis is approximately 80% and 84%, respectively.[208] Some patients may complain of fatigue-related problems after achieving physical recovery. Relapses with increased weakness occur in up to 10% of patients with GBS.

KEY POINTS

- There are many different causes for PNs and the specific cause needs to be evaluated to determine best course of treatment.
- NCV and EMG testing are helpful in the diagnosis of most PNs.
- Surgical release of the transverse carpal ligament provides relief of symptoms in CTS.
- GBS can be life-threatening and the patient must be adequately monitored in the hospital.

15.13 BELL'S PALSY

Erin Salcido

OVERVIEW

Bell's palsy, often referred to as idiopathic facial paralysis (IFP), is the most common neurologic disorder affecting the cranial nerves. It is a palsy the lower motor neuron of the facial nerve (cranial nerve VII). Most cases of Bell's palsy gradually resolve on their own. The cause remains unknown, although many believe it to be a polyneuritis with possible viral, inflammatory or immune etiologies.

EPIDEMIOLOGY

In the United States, Bell's palsy affects 34/100,000 persons annually. It tends to occur more frequently on the right side and has a recurrence rate of 4% to 14%.[209] It can affect bilateral facial nerves about 23% of the time.[210] Bell's palsy is more common in diabetic, immunocompromised, and pregnant patients. Women in their third trimester and first week postpartum are at greatest risk. It affects men and women equally. The greatest incidence is in people age 60 or older.

PATHOPHYSIOLOGY

The facial nerve courses through the facial canal at the temporal bone. The first segment of the canal, the labyrinth, is the narrowest at 68 mm in diameter. If there is any inflammation or edema of the facial nerve, it is in this segment that compression and nerve ischemia is thought to occur, as evidenced by enhancement on MRI.[211]

The most widely accepted viral cause of Bell's palsy is reactivation of herpes simplex virus or varicella-zoster virus. It is believed that the virus spreads to the axons and multiplies leading to inflammation, demyelination, and palsy.

The increased risk of Bell's palsy in the third trimester of pregnant women may be due to fluid retention of pregnancy that causes increased edema and compression in the canal.

MEDICAL HISTORY AND CLINICAL PRESENTATION

The diagnosis of Bell's palsy can be made clinically after a very thorough history and physical examination. It is a diagnosis of exclusion and occasionally diagnostic studies may be needed to rule out more serious causes.

Patients will typically present with complaints of sudden onset (0 to 72 hours) of unilateral facial paralysis or paresis. In addition, they will not have any signs or symptoms of CNS, ear, or cerebellar disease.

SIGNS AND SYMPTOMS

Most commonly patients with Bell's palsy complain of unilateral facial paralysis that came on suddenly. They will state difficulty closing the eye on the affected side and diminished tearing. They commonly also complain of a droopy smile on the same side.

Patients may also report increased salivation, taste disturbance, hyperacusis, and numbness to the face on the same side as the paralysis. Some patients complain of posterior auricular pain for 1 to 2 days prior to the onset of the paralysis.

PHYSICAL EXAMINATION

Paralysis of the facial nerve affects both the upper and lower part of the same side of the face. A careful physical examination will exclude other more serious conditions. Common physical examination findings include eyebrow sagging, inability to raise the eyebrow, inability to completely close the eye, disappearance of the nasolabial fold, and drooping at the affected corner of the mouth (Figure 15.4).

A complete neurologic examination is necessary. This includes a complete cranial nerve exam, peripheral motor and sensory examination, and cerebellar testing. Any neurologic abnormalities warrant additional testing such as CT or MRI of the brain.

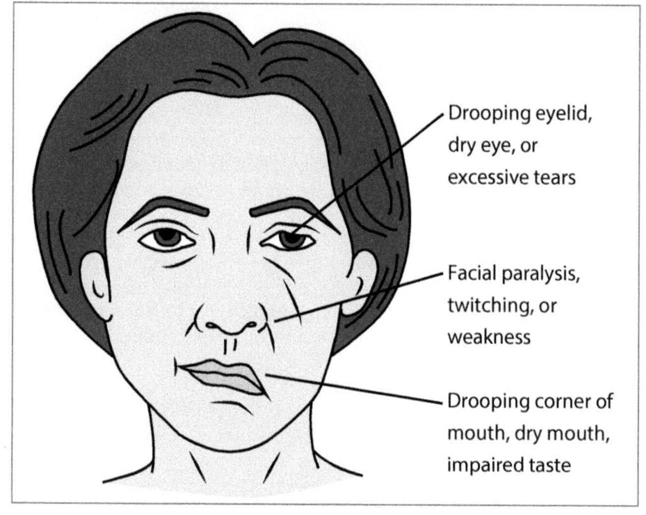

Figure 15.4 Facial features of Bell's palsy.

DIFFERENTIAL DIAGNOSIS

In most cases, the diagnosis of Bell's palsy is straightforward. Careful attention must be given to the history and performance of a complete physical examination.

Bell's palsy can be differentiated from a cerebrovascular accident (CVA) by the presence of lower motor neuron findings. In addition, a stroke or other CNS lesion will not cause hyperacusis or taste disturbance. They generally spare the forehead and present with other focal neurologic deficits, such as involvement of the extremities.

Tumors involving the seventh cranial nerve, temporal bone, internal acoustic canal and others can present with ipsilateral facial weakness. However, the course is usually prolonged, slowly progressive, relapsing, or persistent without recovery.

Bell's palsy can be differentiated from GBS by the bilateral and symmetric nature of the disease. Unilateral facial palsy is a very rare occurrence in GBS.

Facial nerve palsy is a common presentation in Lyme disease. Involvement of the facial nerve can be unilateral or bilateral. Often, patients will present with painless, nontender swelling and erythema of the face, which precedes the facial palsy. Patients will also have a history of travel or live in an endemic area for Lyme disease.

Facial paralysis can also occur as a complication of herpes zoster. However, in such a condition, vesicles are noted on physical exam.

DIAGNOSTIC STUDIES

Recommendations from the American Academy of Otolaryngology-Head and Neck Surgery Foundation state that clinicians should not obtain routine laboratory testing, perform diagnostic imaging, or perform electrodiagnostic testing in patients with new-onset Bell's palsy.

Imaging studies such as CT or MRI of the brain are indicated in patients whom paralysis does not improve or worsens or in patients with history or physical exam findings suspicious of another etiology.

Nerve conduction testing and EMG are useful to evaluate a patient with persistent or severe/complete paralysis. The tests demonstrate the location and extend of nerve injury and can aid in prognosis. They are usually performed 1 to 2 weeks after the onset of paralysis.

Laboratory testing is indicated in order to rule out other potential conditions or to identify potential viral etiologies.

In such cases, serologic studies for HSV or Lyme titers should be performed.

EVALUATION

Diagnosis can be made clinically in patients with a typical presentation and absence of CNS disease. The minimum criteria for diagnosis are sudden onset of unilateral facial paralysis/paresis, involvement of the upper and lower facial muscles, and absence of other neurologic deficits. A thorough history and physical examination should exclude other causes (see Differential Diagnosis).

TREATMENT

It is important to note that many patients with Bell's palsy will completely recover within 3 to 4 months without intervention. Pharmacologic treatment is often initiated to increase the likelihood of complete recovery and if started within 72 hours of symptom onset, may have better outcomes. The goals of treatment are to improve facial nerve function and protect the eye. The American Academy of Otolaryngology-Head and Neck Surgery Foundation strongly recommends treatment with glucocorticoids within 72 hours of symptom onset. They recommend against oral antiviral monotherapy but suggest combination therapy of antivirals (valacyclovir or acyclovir) and steroids, within 72 hours of symptom onset, may be beneficial. The recommended dose of prednisone is 1 mg/kg or 60 mg/day for 6 days, followed by a taper for a total of 10 days. If a viral etiology is suspected, combination treatment with prednisone and acyclovir (400 mg, five times a day for 10 days) or valacyclovir (500 mg twice daily for 5 days) is recommended. If varicella-zoster virus is suspected, higher doses of antivirals may be necessary.

One of the important nonpharmacologic treatments is appropriate eye care. Because Bell's palsy causes poor eyelid closure and reduced tearing, the cornea easily becomes dry and can result in a corneal abrasion. Eye protection includes artificial tears, protective glasses or goggles or an eye patch.

The American Academy of Otolaryngology-Head and Neck Surgery Foundation does not have a recommendation for surgical decompression of the facial nerve or physical therapy. Surgery may be considered for patients with severe paralysis as identified by nerve testing. Physical therapy may help to restore facial muscle function.

Specialist referral is recommended for any of the following: new or worsening neurologic findings at any point, development of ocular symptoms, or incomplete facial recovery 3 months after initial onset.

PATIENT EDUCATION

Although there is no cure for Bell's palsy, the medications prescribed will help to reduce swelling and improve chances for complete recovery.

In a vast majority of patients, facial paralysis will completely resolve. Most people start to notice a difference within the first 3 weeks of symptoms. It can take up to 6 months to get completely back to normal. Some people do not fully recover and will experience some residual paralysis or paresis.

Recurrence is rare but possible and is likely to happen in the first 10 years after initial disease.

Patients should be educated on appropriate eye care to decrease the chance of corneal abrasion.

KEY POINTS

- Bell's palsy is a palsy of the lower motor neuron of the facial nerve (CN VII) causing unilateral facial paralysis.
- The most likely etiology is viral.
- Bell's palsy must be differentiated from more serious central nervous system lesions.
- Treatment with glucocorticosteroids within 72 hours of symptom onset generally produces a favorable outcome.
- Most patients achieve complete recovery.

15.14 PLEXUS LESIONS

John Ramos

OVERVIEW

A plexus is a functional network of sensory, motor, and autonomic nerve fibers that is anatomically defined by the convergence of spinal nerve roots that branch into peripheral nerves. The C5-T1 nerve roots contribute to the brachial plexus, and the L1-S4 nerve roots contribute to the lumbosacral plexus. Traumatic and nontraumatic injuries of a plexus most commonly present asymmetric signs and symptoms of motor, sensory, or reflex abnormalities in multiple contiguous nerve root distributions. Acute brachial plexus injuries are most commonly traumatic and present with pain, and subacute to chronic injuries are typically less painful with an insidious onset of progressive motor and sensory deficits.[212,213] Lumbosacral plexus injuries are more commonly traumatic, and present motor, sensory, or autonomic and/or skeletal muscle reflex abnormalities.[214,215] Motor weakness without pain or sensory involvement strongly suggests motor neuron disease. Urinary bladder or bowel incontinence and saddle anesthesia are highly suspicious for cauda equina syndrome. Imaging and electrodiagnostic studies are commonly used to distinguish plexopathies from competing primary neurologic diagnoses like neuropathies and radiculopathies. Imaging may also aid in diagnosing secondary causes of neurologic deficits, as plexopathies may be the initial presentation of neoplasm, arterial aneurysm, retroperitoneal hemorrhage, psoas major lesions, or compressive arteriovenous malformations. Treatment of plexopathies is determined by underlying cause and is usually supportive, although medical or surgical specialists may be necessary.

EPIDEMIOLOGY

The epidemiology of plexopathies is specific to underlying pathology and is not well researched. Neuralgic amyotrophy (immune-mediated brachial plexus neuropathy, Parsonage-Turner syndrome, acute brachial plexitis) is relatively uncommon with an estimated annual incidence of 2–3 per 100,000 and affects males 2:1.[212,216,217] Hereditary conditions are rare.[213,218] Radiation-induced brachial plexopathy affects 2% to 4% of cancer patients treated with radiation.[219] True neurogenic thoracic outlet syndrome is rare with estimated incidence of 1 per 100,000 with female-male ratio of 9:1.[220]

Lumbosacral plexus lesions are most commonly nontraumatic, with diabetes mellitus being the most common cause.[215,221] In the largest population study to date the annual incidence of lumbosacral radiculoplexus neuropathy (LRPN) in Olmsted County, MN was 4.16 per 100,000 in general, and 2.79 and 1.27 per 100,000 among patients with diabetes and without diabetes, respectively. In this study, the median age at diagnosis was 70 years but ranged 24 to 88 years.[215]

PATHOPHYSIOLOGY

The brachial plexus is formed by the anterior rami of nerve roots C5-T1 and exits between the anterior and middle scalene muscles along the subclavian artery. The dorsal scapular nerve and long thoracic nerve exit before the remaining fibers form the superior, middle, and inferior trunks. The trunks form three anterior and three posterior divisions. The anterior divisions innervate the anterior (flexor) compartments of the arm and forearm while the posterior divisions innervate the posterior (extensor) compartments of the arm and forearm. The divisions give rise to three cords anatomically named by their relative position to the axillary artery (lateral, medial, and posterior). The brachial plexus terminates in the musculocutaneous, median, ulnar, radial, and axillary nerves. The brachial plexus also contains postganglionic sympathetic nerve fibers from vertebral ganglia.

The lumbosacral plexus contains the lumbar and sacral plexuses. The lumbar plexus contains fibers from the anterior rami of the L1 through L4 nerve roots. The rami pass inferiolaterally along the psoas major muscle and within the muscle divide into the anterior and posterior branches. The anterior branches become the obturator nerve and the posterior branches (which contain fibers from L2–L4) become the femoral nerve. The lumbar plexus also contributes to the lateral femoral cutaneous, iliohypogastric, ilioinguinal, and genitofemoral nerves. Some L4 nerve root anterior rami and all L5 anterior rami converge in the lumbosacral trunk. The lumbosacral trunk courses over the sacral ala and joins the sacral plexus, which contains anterior rami of S1–4 nerve roots. The sacral plexus divides into anterior and posterior branches which form the lateral and medial divisions of the sciatic nerve, respectively. The sacral plexus also contributes to the pudendal, posterior cutaneous thigh, and inferior and superior gluteal nerves.

There are several common mechanisms of injury in plexopathies. Nerve fibers may become transected with high force blunt trauma, which may also cause nerve root avulsion. In the brachial plexus, C8 and T1 are the two lowest nerve roots and more susceptible to root avulsion, which is usually unamenable to surgical repair. Nerve fibers may also be compressed by trauma or local masses. Neoplasm may compress nerve fibers, but more commonly plexopathies arise from metastatic invasion from local bone or soft tissue cancers.[222] Axonal damage can also be caused by ischemia due to large and small blood vessel pathology.[223] Small intraneural vessels called vaso vasorum are more commonly affected in nonstructural causes of brachial plexopathies. Damage to the intraneural blood vessels is poorly understood pathologically but may be the mechanism underlying metabolic and inflammatory causes of plexopathies. Aneurysms, dissections, and hematomas of large blood vessels are relatively rare causes of plexopathies but are more commonly seen in lumbosacral plexopathies (LSP).

15.14A BRACHIAL PLEXUS LESIONS

MEDICAL HISTORY AND CLINICAL PRESENTATION

Brachial plexus lesions are most commonly caused by traumatic injuries in children and adults.[213] Motor vehicle and motorcycle crashes, industrial accidents, falls, and sports-related injuries are common blunt traumatic brachial plexus injuries, while gunshot wounds, lacerations, and animal bites account for the majority of penetrating traumatic injuries. Iatrogenic causes are implicated in 7% to 10% of all brachial plexopathies.[213,224] Nontraumatic brachial plexus injuries are less common, but etiologies include inflammation, infection, radiation, and neoplasm. Radiation-induced brachial plexopathy typically presents within 6 years (mean) of last radiation dose, is more likely with doses >6,000 cGy, and is more likely with cancers of the breast, followed by lung and lymphoma.[219,222,223] Brachial plexopathy secondary to neoplasm is more frequently associated with cancers of the breast and lung.

Hereditary brachial plexopathy is an autosomal dominant condition resulting from a mutation in the septin nine gene (SEPT9) on chromosome 17q25. The condition commonly presents in childhood and has a relapsing/remitting course characterized by triggered or unprovoked attacks that resolve spontaneously with residual weakness. Hereditary neuropathy with predisposition to pressure palsies (HNPP, tomaculous neuropathy) is an autosomal dominant condition associated with PMP22 deletions. HNPP is an episodic demyelinating neuropathy and symptoms most often appear in the second decade of life.[218]

SIGNS AND SYMPTOMS

Traumatic injuries to the brachial plexus may present with various neurologic complaints, and pain is frequently reported. Root avulsions and plexopathies are common with high-energy traction injuries and may present with permanent motor and sensory deficits.[213] Blunt trauma to the neck, commonly seen in athletic contact sport injuries, produces a burner or stinger syndrome of transient burning and stinging sensations in the upper extremity. Backpack palsy is a syndrome of extremity weakness associated with prolonged upper trunk compression from backpacks or child-carrying harnesses. Usual symptoms are unilateral painless upper extremity weakness in the distribution of the affected plexus, and there may be associated sensory loss in the same distribution.

With nontraumatic brachial plexus injuries, timing and progression of symptoms may help distinguish the underlying cause. The acute onset of symptoms without a history of trauma favors a metabolic or inflammatory disease process.

Neuralgic amyotrophy classically presents with rapid or subacute onset unilateral shoulder girdle and lateral arm pain. Often symptoms wake patients from sleep at night. Bilateral symptoms are reported in 29% of patients. Sensory symptoms may also be present, often hypesthesia and/or paresthesia. Pain is followed by weakness within 24 hours of symptom onset in one-third of patients, and more than 2 weeks in one-fourth of patients.[217]

Brachial plexopathies associated with breast and lung cancers typically present with shoulder and axilla pain, and the lower plexuses (inferior trunk and medial cord) are most commonly invaded. Radiation-induced brachial plexopathy shares a similar presentation.

Postoperative brachial plexopathies have unique presentations.[213,224] Traction or pressure during surgery may compress the upper brachial plexus and present with painless weakness. Postmedian sternotomy plexopathy presents with weakness and paresthesia involving the fourth and fifth fingers.

PHYSICAL EXAMINATION

Physical examination findings of plexopathies include sensory loss, weakness, and atrophy. Neurologic deficits may be present in the distribution of one or more nerves, and physical examination alone is generally insufficient to distinguish plexopathies from mono- or polyneuropathies, or radiculopathies. Weakness may be difficult to appreciate when effort is reduced secondary to pain, but tendon reflexes may be reduced in truly weak muscles. Muscle atrophy may not appear for several weeks, limiting its utility in the acute setting. Isolated motor weakness without sensory deficits should prompt suspicion for motor neuron disease.

There are several eponymous syndromes associated with plexopathies.[225] Erb palsy classically presents with the affected upper extremity hanging at the side and internally rotated ("bellhop's tip" position) without hand muscle weakness. Erb palsy results from high plexus injuries (C5 and C6 root damage from glenohumeral dislocation or peripartum shoulder dystocia). Klumpke palsy presents with a "claw hand" deformity, resulting from injuries to C8 and T1 roots. Apical lung tumors typically compress the lower brachial plexus and thus sympathetic nerve fibers which innervate the iris dilator muscle, Müller muscle (a smooth muscle of the eyelid assisting in upper lid elevation and lower lid retraction), and sweat glands of the face. Unilateral tumor compression may cause sympathetic paresis called Horner syndrome (miosis, ptosis, anhidrosis).

DIFFERENTIAL DIAGNOSIS

The differential diagnosis for brachial plexopathy is summarized in Table 15.37.

TABLE 15.37 Differential Diagnosis for Brachial Plexopathy

Diagnosis	Description
Trauma	Most common cause of brachial plexopathies
Idiopathic	Neuralgic amyotrophy
Hereditary	Autosomal dominant Septin 9 gene mutation, provoked or unprovoked, relapsing/remitting course with residual weakness
HNPP	Autosomal dominant, episodic demyelinating neuropathy
Neoplasm	Breast and lung cancer most common
Radiation induced	Difficult to distinguish from neoplasm, typical onset is within 6 years of last radiation, more likely with doses >6,000 cGy, and with cancers of the breast and lung, and lymphoma
Motor neuron disease	Isolated motor weakness with no sensory deficits, and often painless
Infection	Multiple organisms
Iatrogenic	Postoperative, postmedian sternotomy
Diabetes	Rarer cause of brachial plexopathy Laboratory evidence of insulin resistance Usually presents with nerve root involvement and/or other upper or lower extremity mono/poly neuropathy Symptoms may be unilateral or bilateral
True neurogenic TOS	Motor and sensory abnormalities in the distributions of C8 and T1 nerve roots

cGy, centigray; HNPP, hereditary neuropathy with predisposition to pressure palsies; TOS, thoracic outlet syndrome.

DIAGNOSTIC STUDIES

Laboratory studies are primarily indicated to exclude alternative diagnoses including diabetes, malignancy, Lyme disease, syphilis, and HIV infection. CSF analysis is indicated when there is clinical suspicion for alternative diagnoses including neoplasm, GBS, and neurosyphilis, among others. MRI is typically indicated for all patients with signs and symptoms of brachial plexopathy to identify or exclude a mass lesion. Nerve conduction studies are indicated for all patients and may exclude more common mononeuropathies. Needle EMG is useful for identifying denervation pattern. Neurogenic thoracic outlet syndrome is characterized by motor and sensory conduction abnormalities affecting C8 and T1 nerve fibers.[213,214,226]

EVALUATION

Any patient with clinical symptoms of a brachial plexopathy should be evaluated. Neurology and/or neurosurgery referrals are often necessary for neuroimaging and electrodiagnostic study interpretation. There is currently no indication for screening asymptomatic patients.

TREATMENT

- Improvement from traumatic brachial plexopathies without surgery may occur within 6 months. Surgical intervention may be indicated when there is no documented improvement after 3 to 4 months.[227]
- Patients with early presentations of neuralgic amyotrophy may benefit from high-dose glucocorticoids.[214]
- For neuralgic amyotrophy, physical therapy may improve range of motion.[214]

PATIENT EDUCATION

- Traumatic brachial plexus injuries can cause a variety of symptoms (numbness, tingling, weakness, pain) that typically resolve within 6 months.
- Nontraumatic brachial plexus injuries can cause a variety of symptoms; pain is usually the most common presenting symptom. Pain may progress to weakness. Pain and weakness may improve or resolve in months to years, but at least half of patients with hereditary or idiopathic brachial plexopathies have permanent, sometimes decreased, pain and weakness.

15.14B LUMBAR PLEXUS LESIONS

MEDICAL HISTORY AND CLINICAL PRESENTATION

Diabetic lumbosacral radiculoplexus neuropathy (DLRPN, Bruns-Garland syndrome, diabetic amyotrophy) is the most common lumbosacral plexus disease and affects 1% of patients with diabetes.[228] Small studies have revealed some relevant clinical findings.[221,229] The median age at diagnosis was 65 years old and median duration of diabetes was 4 years. In 21% of patients DLRPN was the presenting feature of diabetes. The most frequently reported symptoms at onset are pain and weakness. Compared to patients with diabetic sensorimotor polyneuropathy, patients with DLRPN are less likely to initially present with other microvascular complications like diabetic retinopathy or nephropathy.[229]

In one small study of 42 patients with idiopathic LRPN, only two (5%) developed diabetes after being diagnosed with LRPN.[230] In another study 48% of patients with diabetic LRPN required wheelchair assistance at some point during illness and only 6% reported full recovery.[221]

Neoplasm and trauma are the other common causes of LSP. Among patients with LSP, one-third of patients developed symptoms within 1 year of primary tumor diagnosis and the other two-thirds within 3 years.[231] Only 15% of patients developed LSP symptoms prior to primary tumor diagnosis. Radiation-induced LSP is relatively uncommon, may occur within 3 to 30 years after exposure, and can be difficult to distinguish from a recurrent tumor.[232] The incidence of LSP in the setting of trauma is not well studied, although one study reported electrodiagnostic confirmation of LSP in 0.7% of pelvic and acetabular fractures and 2% of sacral fractures.[233] In a postmortem study of 42 victims with fatal pelvis fractures, plexus damage was identified in 20 (48%).[234]

While relatively uncommon causes of LSP, vascular etiologies frequently require emergent and/or surgical intervention.[235] Retroperitoneal hemorrhage typically has an acute onset and should be considered in the setting of trauma or patients with bleeding disorders or therapeutic anticoagulation. Hemorrhage into the retroperitoneal space more often compresses the femoral nerve or lumbar plexus, and less frequently the entire lumbosacral plexus. In addition, aneurysm, pseudoaneurysm, and dissection of the abdominal aorta, iliac arteries (common, external, internal), gluteal arteries (inferior and superior), and hypogastric arteries have been reported to cause LSP, especially in postoperative patients. Aortic dissection may present with acute pain and neurologic deficits secondary to ischemia of the lumbosacral plexus.

SIGNS AND SYMPTOMS

LSP classically present unilateral pain, weakness, and sensory deficits in the distribution of multiple contiguous nerve roots.[221,229] Most commonly symptoms are confined to the proximal lower extremity. Lesions of the lumbar plexus tend to cause weakness with hip adduction and knee extension, while weakness with hip abduction and knee flexion are more common with lumbosacral trunk and upper sacral plexus lesions. Sensory symptoms include numbness, dysesthesia and/or paresthesia. Sensory disturbances in the anterior/medial thigh and medial leg are usually signs of lumbar plexus involvement, while those involving the posterior thigh, perineum, leg, and dorsal foot are more characteristic of a lumbosacral trunk and/or plexus lesion. The acute onset of bilateral symptoms is rare, but progression to bilateral symptoms is common in patients with and without diabetes, and commonly occurs within 1 to 3 months after symptom onset.

Weight loss (>10 pounds) and autonomic symptoms (e.g., orthostatic hypotension, tachycardia, urinary incontinence, constipation, diarrhea, and sexual dysfunction) are common. Notably, urinary bladder and/or bowel incontinence and perineal numbness are highly suspicious for sacral metastases and/or cauda equina syndrome.

Neoplasm can cause LSP, and most commonly from direct invasion from primary or metastatic disease in organs in close proximity (e.g., colorectal, reproductive organs, renal, vertebrae). LSP may also develop from metastatic cancers of the breast, lung, stomach, and thyroid. Among patients with LSP secondary to neoplastic invasion, pain is the most commonly reported initial symptom and may be worsened at night, lying supine, or straining with bowel movements. Sensory and motor disturbances are common while autonomic symptoms are rare, although up to 40% of patients have epidural tumor extension. Radiation-induced LSP is painless in 50% of patients and primarily sensory disturbances are most frequently reported.[232]

PHYSICAL EXAMINATION

A general and neurologic examination is useful, with careful attention to functional sensation, strength, and reflexes of the bilateral lower extremities. Neurologic deficits may be present in the distribution of one or more nerves, but physical examination alone is generally insufficient to distinguish plexopathies from mono- or polyneuropathies or radiculopathies.

Lumbar plexus lesions frequently present weakness with hip adduction and flexion and knee extension, decreased sensation at the top and inner proximal leg, and decreased patellar tendon reflexes. Sacral plexus lesions result in complete inability to abduct the proximal leg at the hip, weakness with hip extension and knee flexion and decreased sensation at the posterior proximal leg and lower leg (below the knee). The sacral plexuses are in relatively close anatomic proximity compared the lumbar plexuses, and sacral lesions are therefore more likely to present with bilateral findings. Decreased rectal tone and pudendal sensory loss should prompt suspicion for sacral metastases and/or cauda equina syndrome. Metastatic compression at the level of the conus medullaris may cause bowel and bladder incontinence without sensory deficits.

DIFFERENTIAL DIAGNOSIS

The differential diagnosis for lumbosacral plexopathy is summarized in Table 15.38.

DIAGNOSTIC STUDIES

In a patient with clinical evidence of LSP, laboratory and electrodiagnostic studies are the best initial tests.[236] Routine laboratory studies include a CBC, coagulation profile, fasting blood glucose, hemoglobin A1c, and ESR. Nerve conduction studies and needle EMG are particularly useful in identifying the level of plexus involvement or identifying or excluding radiculopathy or polyneuropathy. MRI is the imaging study of choice and gadolinium contrast enhancement is particularly useful when infectious, neoplastic, inflammatory, or postoperative conditions are suspected or should be excluded (e.g., a patient with symptoms of LSP with elevated sedimentation rate). CT angiography is indicated when there is suspicion for vascular etiologies. Undifferentiated LSP requires additional blood testing for infectious, postinfectious, and autoimmune disorders. If additional blood testing is not helpful, lumbar puncture may be helpful to identify an occult infectious or neoplastic disease. Abdominal and pelvic organ tissue biopsy is the gold standard for diagnosis of neoplastic or infiltrative diseases.

TABLE 15.38 Differential Diagnosis for Lumbosacral Plexopathy

Diagnosis	Description
Diabetes	Most common cause of LSP, but usually presents with nerve root involvement and/or other upper or lower extremity mono/polyneuropathy. Type II most common. Classic presentation is acute and asymmetric pain followed by weakness of the proximal leg. Autonomic symptoms and weight loss also commonly associated. Bilateral or distal leg symptoms may occur.
Idiopathic	Clinical and electrodiagnostic evidence of LSP without clinical or diagnostic evidence of insulin resistance, or infectious, postinfectious, or autoimmune disease.
Neoplasm	Most commonly direct invasion from tumors in close proximity. With metastatic cancer the most common primary tumors are colorectal, cervical, and breast. Presents severe pain with or without radicular symptoms. Symptoms may be worsened with position (classically, lying supine). Neoplastic epidural spinal cord compression commonly presents as severe pain and then radicular symptoms, may progress to paraplegia.
Conus medullaris syndrome	Back pain and urinary bladder and bowel symptoms with no motor or sensory deficits, secondary to tumor compression.
Cauda equina syndrome	Urinary bladder and bowel incontinence, and pain, paresthesia, sensory, and motor deficits in the distribution of one or more nerve roots, secondary to compression (tumor and/or trauma).
Trauma	Isolated LSP from trauma infrequently reported. Retroperitoneal hemorrhage presents with acute pain in the setting of trauma.
Motor neuron disease	Isolated motor weakness with no sensory deficits, and often painless.
Vascular	Patients with surgical arterial instrumentation or those with risk factors for aneurysm (age, hypertension).
Common peroneal neuropathy	Most commonly secondary to trauma or other compressive injury. Presents with anterior tibialis weakness ("foot drop"). May be distinguished from L5 radiculopathy in which foot eversion is spared with intact S1 innervation.
Herniated disc	Common presentation of low back pain. May have worsened pain with straight leg raise test; on the symptomatic side, examiner extends the thigh at the hip with the foot dorsiflexed. Usually no evidence of microvascular complications (retinopathy, nephropathy) at presentation.
Infectious	Rare cause of LSP, but may be secondary to infection with CMV, HIV, EBV, VZV, Lyme disease, syphilis.
Autoimmune, postinfection	Rheumatic conditions, Guillain–Barré syndrome.

CMV, cytomegalovirus; EBV, Epstein–Barr virus; LSP, lumbosacral plexopathy; VZV, varicella-zoster virus.

EVALUATION

Any patient with clinical symptoms of a lumbosacral plexopathy should be evaluated. Neurology and/or neurosurgery referrals are often necessary for neuroimaging and electrodiagnostic study interpretation. There is currently no indication for screening asymptomatic patients.

TREATMENT

- There is no proven or effective treatment for LSP with diabetic or idiopathic etiologies, although there is some limited evidence of glucocorticoids and immunomodulator therapies.[219]
- Analgesics are recommended for pain in the initial phase of the disease.[219]

PATIENT EDUCATION

- Symptoms of LSP may include pain and may progress to weakness.
- Symptoms of LSP may improve over months to years, or they could be permanent.
- Most patients will need ambulatory aids at some point in their illness.

SPECIAL CONSIDERATIONS

Neonatal brachial plexus injury is an uncommon injury resulting from shoulder dystocia during delivery. Injuries to C5 and C6 manifest as adduction and internal rotation of the arm and forearm extension, with preserved hand and wrist movement. Injury to C7 presents with abnormal flexion of the wrists and fingers (Erb palsy). Complete arm paralysis is caused by total brachial plexus injury and may be accompanied by Horner syndrome.

KEY POINTS

- Trauma is the most common cause of brachial plexopathy, and the majority of patients improve without surgery by 6 months.
- Idiopathic and hereditary brachial plexopathies are rare.
- Brachial plexopathy secondary to malignancy is most commonly associated with breast and lung cancers.
- Apical lung tumor compression may cause a symptomatic paresis (Horner syndrome).
- LSP is most commonly caused by diabetes but only affects 1% of diabetic patients.
- Patients with diabetes may have mono/polyneuropathies and radiculopathies presenting with uni- or bilateral upper or lower extremity symptoms.

- LSP secondary to neoplasm occurs by direct invasion from primary or metastatic origins, and most commonly from organs in close anatomic proximity.
- Idiopathic and hereditary brachial plexopathy, and patients with diabetic or nondiabetic LSP generally have some degree of residual pain and weakness that is permanent.
- Motor weakness without sensory deficits or pain is highly suspicious for motor neuron disease.
- Urinary bladder or bowel incontinence is concerning for conus medullaris syndrome, or cauda equina syndrome when motor/sensory deficits are present.

15.15 NEUROMUSCULAR DISORDERS

Julia Karnoski and Ashley Bell

15.15A MYASTHENIA GRAVIS

OVERVIEW

Myasthenia gravis (MG) is an acquired autoimmune disorder of the neuromuscular junction characterized by fatigable motor weakness that affects the muscles of the eyes, oropharynx, respiratory system, and proximal limbs. Manifestation of the disease is variable and can range from self-limiting to rapidly progressive. Symptoms are treatable with medication and, in some cases, remission can be achieved with surgical intervention.

EPIDEMIOLOGY

MG is a relatively rare condition, with approximately 40,000 to 60,000 cases in the United States. The global prevalence is estimated between 14 and 20 people per 100,000 and the disease is slightly more prevalent in females, with a 3:2 female-to-male ratio.[237] Age at symptom onset varies widely but typically occurs earlier in women than in men, with females presenting in the second and third decades of life and most males presenting after 60 years of age. The incidence does not seem to predominate in any specific racial or ethnic groups. Mortality rate was once estimated to be as high as 40% but has decreased to 3% to 4% in the past 50 years due advances in diagnosis and treatment.[238]

PATHOPHYSIOLOGY

To initiate muscle contraction, motor neurons release acetylcholine into the neuromuscular junction, which binds nicotinic acetylcholine receptors (nAChR) on the postsynaptic membrane. This causes a cation channel to open, allowing for the influx of sodium ions and the efflux of potassium ions. If this increases the membrane potential to its threshold, it will trigger an action potential down the muscle fiber and result in muscle fiber contraction.

In MG, the body produces autoantibodies against acetylcholine receptors, which manifests in the patient as impaired skeletal muscle contraction. The etiology of immune dysregulation is not fully understood, but a clear link between thymus abnormalities and MG has been established. Immature T cells are housed in the thymus, and it is thought that they become sensitized to acetylcholine receptors on thymic myoid cells (the only nonmuscle cells with ACh receptors). This autoimmunization results in the production of anti-AChR antibodies, and once released into circulation, they attack the acetylcholine receptors of the neuromuscular junction. When an anti-AChR antibody binds a nicotinic receptor, that receptor is no longer able to bind acetylcholine and no longer able to participate in the cascade of events that results in muscle contraction. In addition, this process activates the complement pathway, which damages the muscle cell and reduces the number of nicotinic receptors on the cell surface. The net result is a decrease in both the number and function of nicotinic acetylcholine receptors; once the receptors are reduced to about 30% of normal function, the decrease in stamina of skeletal muscles becomes clinically apparent. With initial activation, acetylcholine binds the available nicotinic receptors resulting in normal muscle contraction, but with repetitive or sustained activation, there are insufficient receptors to maintain an adequate response and strength deteriorates. This explains the fatiguability of MG: while the neuromuscular apparatus is capable of producing normal muscle contraction, the decrease in functional acetylcholine receptors prevents the muscle fiber from maintaining sustained or repetitive action.

Notably, a small number of MG patients are seronegative for the anti-AChR antibody, and they instead have antibodies against muscle-specific tyrosine kinase (MuSK), an enzyme responsible for clustering acetylcholine receptors at the end plate of the muscle cell membrane. As these anti-MuSK antibodies effectively reduce the amount of acetylcholine receptors available, the symptomology is indistinguishable from those with anti-AChR antibodies.

MEDICAL HISTORY AND CLINICAL PRESENTATION

Many patients have a personal and/or family history of autoimmune disorders, including systemic lupus erythematosus, rheumatoid arthritis, and Graves disease. This correlation hints at a genetic predisposition, most likely having to do with certain HLA subtypes. The disease has been linked with small cell lung cancer, Hodgkin lymphoma, and hyperthyroidism. In addition, many pharmacotherapeutics have been implicated in the development or exacerbation of myasthenic symptoms, including penicillamine, antibiotics, antiarrhythmics, anticholinergics, lithium, chloroquine, prednisone, and neuromuscular blocking agents. In these patients, thymectomy often results in significant improvement of symptoms or even complete remission.

Because both the severity of illness and manifestation of symptoms are widely variable, MG can be further classified into several subtypes (class I through V). An important distinction is whether symptoms are predominantly ocular or more generalized, defined as affecting muscles of the axial skeleton, proximal limbs, oropharynx, and the respiratory system. But even in *generalized* myasthenia, patients do not complain of *generalized* fatigue or muscle weakness. They instead report distinct episodes of weakness in identifiable muscle groups. The symptoms are often transient at first, fluctuating between periods of remission and exacerbation. Sometimes weeks will go by with no symptoms at all. During early exacerbations, patients typically wake up symptom-free and develop weakness throughout the day, with noticeable muscle fatigue after sustained or repetitive use. Symptoms are also exacerbated by physiologic stress, such as viral infections, pregnancy, thyroid dysfunction, extreme heat, surgery, and tapering of immunosuppression.

Within the first few years, approximately one-third of patients will have spontaneous remission, but the remainder will progress to more persistent or more widespread disease.

SIGNS AND SYMPTOMS

Not unlike other neuromuscular disorders, MG presents with skeletal muscle weakness, but the hallmark of the disease is pronounced fatiguability. Myasthenic weakness is significantly exacerbated by activity, especially repetitive movements, and is relieved with rest. The symptoms also fluctuate drastically over time, and the disease is characterized by periods of exacerbation and remission. A majority of patients present with predominant ocular symptoms (class I), most commonly complaining of asymmetric ptosis that worsens throughout the day. Many complain of binocular diplopia, meaning either vertical or horizontal double vision while both eyes are open due to extraocular muscle weakness and misalignment; monocular vision is unaffected. Patients may simply report blurry vision if they are unable to appreciate true diplopia, and they may also report halos and photophobia. Of these patients who present with isolated ocular symptoms, just over half will progress to more widespread disease, usually within the first 3 years of symptom onset. More generalized disease can present with fatigable weakness of the axial and proximal extremity muscles. MG also frequently affects the bulbar muscles (including the tongue, pharynx, larynx, and neck muscles), causing difficulty with speech, chewing, and swallowing. Patients may report a nasal quality to their voice, with frequent throat clearing and nasal regurgitation of food. They may also complain of slurred speech after talking for extended periods of time, jaw fatigue, frequent choking, and possibly even aspiration. The most dangerous feature of MG is "myasthenic crisis," which is defined as respiratory and/or bulbar weakness severe enough to necessitate intubation. It affects 10% to 20% of patients with MG and carries a mortality rate of 5%.[239] Myasthenic weakness is typically heralded by a worsening of existing weakness, and as the respiratory muscles become affected, patients experience orthopnea, dyspnea, and respiratory insufficiency, which can rapidly progress to life-threatening respiratory failure. Patients typically require mechanical ventilation for a mean duration of 2 weeks, and myasthenic crisis can precipitate complications such as infection, venous thromboembolism, myocardial infarction, and cardiac arrest.

PHYSICAL EXAMINATION

Given the variability of symptoms in MG and the nature of fatigability, physical findings may be absent on examination. On general inspection, patients have been described as looking tired or sad with a sagging or expressionless face. Attempts to smile can result in a horizontal smile, termed the "myasthenic snarl," and patients will often not be able to puff out their cheeks against force. Unilateral ptosis is common, and compensatory hypercontraction of the frontalis muscle may be noted. Manual elevation of the eyelid with ptosis may cause a dropping of the contralateral lid, known as enhanced ptosis. Also, in 80% of patients, ptosis will improve transiently after application of ice to the affected eye—the "ice pack test." EOM weakness will be asymmetric and will not be limited to muscles innervated by a single cranial nerve, which would be more indicative of a central etiology. While testing EOMs, have the patient hold the upward gaze for 60 to 180 seconds and observe for fatigability. Then have the patient hold a downward gaze and then return to looking straight ahead – the upper eyelid may overshoot the gaze revealing sclera between the limbus and upper lid before settling into the neutral position; this is called "Cogan's lid twitch." Sustained lateral gaze of 60 seconds may elicit diplopia. When the patient attempts to forcefully shut their eyes, the orbicularis oculi will fatigue with time, and a sliver of sclera will be visible, this is called the "peek sign." Orbicularis oculi weakness can also be tested by trying to pry the eyes open while the patient is forcefully shutting them. Pupillary response will be normal. The clinician might note a hypophonic voice with a somewhat nasal quality, and having the patient hold a high-pitched "eee" sound might reveal hoarseness. A unique feature of MG is weakness with jaw closure, but not with jaw opening. Neck muscle weakness is common, and the clinician may note a head drop or weakness of neck flexion and extension on exam. When testing extremity muscles, have the patient perform repeated or sustained contractions to provoke weakness. The most common muscles involved are the deltoids, wrist and finger extensors, hip flexors, quadriceps, and hamstrings. Reflexes are not classically involved, and although they will be normal at first, the strength of response may wane with repeated testing. Difficulty counting to 20 in a single breath may represent impaired vital capacity, and spirometry is helpful in evaluation. Any evidence of weakness in the respiratory muscles is an emergency as it may indicate impending myasthenic crisis; do not be comforted by a normal oxygen saturation. MG does not affect sensation, coordination, or cognition. In suspected or known MG, evaluate the patient for any signs of concurrent autoimmune disease.

DIFFERENTIAL DIAGNOSIS

MG must first be distinguished from conditions that cause generalized weakness or fatigue, as myasthenic weakness affects specific skeletal muscle groups. Of the several conditions that can present with motor weakness of the ocular, bulbar, or proximal muscles (Table 15.39), MG is the only one among them that causes *fatigable weakness*. Next, it is important to note that MG does not cause pain and will not affect sensation, coordination, or cognition, so presence of these findings suggests an alternate diagnosis. Although the patient's history and physical examination will aid in narrowing the differential, laboratory tests, nerve conduction studies, and advanced imaging of the brain must be done to exclude some diagnoses.

DIAGNOSTIC STUDIES AND EVALUATION

There is no one single diagnostic test for MG, but rather, the diagnosis is made following a thorough physical examination and a series of specialized tests, including electrodiagnostics, pharmacologic testing, antibody testing, and imaging to search for thymus disease.

Nerve conduction studies can be very helpful in the evaluation of a patient with possible MG. Neuron integrity will prove normal, but repetitive nerve stimulation will reveal a decrease in action potential amplitude in over 50% of patients. Single-fiber electromyography (SFEMG) is the most accurate test for MG, with a sensitivity of 100% and the potential to reach a specificity of 99% if more than one muscle is tested. Therefore, if the SFEMG test is normal, MG is effectively ruled out.[240]

TABLE 15.39 Differential Diagnosis for Myasthenia Gravis

Diagnosis	Description
Chronic progressive external ophthalmoplegia (CPEO)	An inherited disease of the mitochondria that causes progressive ophthalmoplegia and ptosis. It may also cause generalized skeletal muscle weakness. Diagnosed via muscle biopsy.
Oculopharyngeal muscular dystrophy (OPMD)	An inherited disorder that causes progressive muscle wasting of the eyelids and throat. Presents with ptosis and dysphagia. Diagnosed by testing for the correlating genetic mutation.
Lambert-Eaton myasthenic syndrome (LEMS)	An autoimmune disorder of the neuromuscular junction, often associated with small cell lung cancer, that presents very similarly to myasthenia gravis (MG). The most prominent feature of LEMS is proximal limb weakness, as opposed to ocular weakness in MG. Autonomic dysfunction is also common, causing orthostasis and dry mouth.
Amyotrophic lateral sclerosis (ALS)	A neuromuscular disease that causes rapidly progressive motor weakness and paralysis. Diagnosis is difficult, and it often requires the exclusion of other neuromuscular disorders.
Multiple sclerosis (MS)	An autoimmune disorder affecting myelin of the brain and spinal cord. The distinguishing characteristic of MS vs. MG is that it affects both sensory and motor neurons, as well as the autonomic nervous system.
Chronic fatigue syndrome	An idiopathic disorder characterized by profound fatigue, malaise, and pain that is exacerbated by activity, but not improved by rest. Symptoms are generalized and unpredictable, as opposed to the specific reproducible weakness in the affected muscle groups.

Pharmacologic testing with a short-acting acetylcholinesterase inhibitor can also help to identify abnormal neuromuscular transmission as the source of weakness. Commonly referred to as the "Tensilon test," administration of intravenous edrophonium (Tensilon) will cause objective improvement in most patients with MG, but the test is not very sensitive nor specific.

The anti-acetylcholine receptor antibody test has high specificity, but false positive results have been reported in Lambert-Eaton syndrome, small cell lung cancer, thymoma, and in a small percentage of unaffected individuals over 70 years old. Sensitivity is at about 85% for patients with generalized MG, and about 50% for those with isolated ocular involvement.[241] Other antibodies that might be found in patients with MG are the anti-MuSK antibody, anti-lipoprotein-related protein 4 (LRP4) antibody, anti-agrin antibody, anti-striational antibody, and the anti-cortactin antibody.

Once the diagnosis of MG has been made, the next step is to determine if a thymoma is present. A plain chest radiograph is a reasonable place to start, as a thymoma may be appreciable as an anterior mediastinal mass. But eventually, a CT scan of the chest is warranted in all cases of MG in order to definitively rule in or rule out the presence of a thymoma or thymus enlargement.

TREATMENT

- Thymectomy is standard of care in all patients with thymoma as well as in those with generalized MG. In patients with isolated ocular symptoms, delay thymectomy for about 2 years, as many patients will spontaneously recover.
- Acetylcholinesterase inhibitors (pyridostigmine) are considered the mainstay of symptomatic treatment, as they increase the availability of acetylcholine in the synaptic cleft.
- If acetylcholinesterase inhibitors fail to meet treatment goals, the next step in symptomatic management is immunosuppression with corticosteroids (methylprednisolone) or nonsteroidal immunosuppressants (azathioprine).
- In life-threatening situations, such as myasthenic crisis, IVIG and plasmapheresis are used as short-term therapy.
- Myasthenic crisis also necessitates intubation and mechanical ventilation.
- Patients with dysphagia and recurrent aspiration may benefit from a feeding tube.

PATIENT EDUCATION

- Explain the potential for myasthenic crisis and instruct patients to seek immediate medical attention if they develop any respiratory difficulty or significant worsening of symptoms.
- The symptoms of MG fluctuate in severity and are exacerbated by activity, so patients need to rest frequently when they engage in exercise. Encourage patients to start an aerobic exercise regimen and adhere to a healthy diet.
- Emotional or physiologic stress, as well as extreme heat, may also exacerbate symptoms.
- Chewing may become difficult, so patients may need to avoid tough meats and hardy vegetables.
- For patients with dysphagia, nasal regurgitation and aspiration are more likely with thin liquids, therefore recommend that patients drink thickened beverages.
- In patients of child-bearing potential, explain that pregnancy could possibly exacerbate their symptoms and their newborn may have transient myasthenic weakness while the maternal acetylcholine receptor antibodies remain in circulation.

15.15B LAMBERT-EATON MYASTHENIC SYNDROME

OVERVIEW

Lambert-Eaton myasthenic syndrome (LEMS) is a rare autoantibody-mediated disorder of the neuromuscular junction that results in profound muscle weakness. A diagnosis of LEMS often indicates an underlying malignancy or autoimmune disease and should therefore prompt a thorough clinical investigation.

EPIDEMIOLOGY

LEMS is a very rare condition; the incidence is estimated at 0.5 case per 1 million people, and the prevalence is roughly 2.5 per 1 million.[242] This demonstrates the high rate of mortality in patients with LEMS, largely due to an underlying malignancy. In 50% of LEMS cases, it is found to be a paraneoplastic disorder caused by a small cell lung carcinoma (SCLC). And roughly 3% of patients with SCLC have LEMS.[243]

PATHOPHYSIOLOGY

LEMS is characterized by autoimmune-mediated dysfunction of neuromuscular transmission. As the action potential propagates along the cholinergic neuron, it depolarizes the presynaptic terminal membrane and causes voltage-gated calcium channels (VGCC) to open. The influx of calcium triggers acetylcholine-containing vesicles to fuse with the presynaptic membrane, releasing acetylcholine into the synaptic cleft. The acetylcholine then binds receptors on the muscle cell, resulting in depolarization and muscle contraction. In LEMS, autoantibodies promote removal of the presynaptic VGCC, reducing the amount of acetylcholine released into the synaptic cleft. This results in insufficient activation of the acetylcholine receptors, and an attenuated response in the muscle fiber. With repeated activation, each action potential will release more and more acetylcholine into the synaptic cleft, eventually allowing the postsynaptic membrane to reach its threshold. Therefore, the weakness described in LEMS improves with repetitive stimulation, which is in stark contrast to the fatigable weakness of MG.

MEDICAL HISTORY AND CLINICAL PRESENTATION

Over half of patients with LEMS are found to have an underlying malignancy, most with SCLC, but it has also been linked with prostate cancer and lymphoproliferative malignancies. In this population the mean age of symptom onset is 60 years with a greater incidence in males than females, likely reflective of the male affinity for smoking. Those with non-SCLC LEMS typically present earlier than their counterparts and have equal distribution among the sexes. Many have HLA haplotypes that carry a predisposition for autoimmunity.[244] The prognosis is variable, and morbidity and mortality are usually related to the underlying autoimmune disease or malignancy. The weakness of LEMS does, however, affect the quality of life of patients and can significantly impair functionality.

SIGNS AND SYMPTOMS

LEMS is characterized by a triad of proximal muscle weakness, loss of deep tendon reflexes, and autonomic dysfunction. The most common presenting complaint is symmetric weakness of the proximal extremity muscles, with the lower extremities affected more often than the upper extremities. Symptoms are slowly progressive, and patients often report difficulty rising from a chair or climbing stairs. Many also complain of myalgias, muscle cramping, and stiffness. Very rarely do patients initially present with ocular or bulbar weakness, although one-quarter of patients will eventually develop diplopia, ptosis, dysphagia, or dysarthria.[245] LEMS also causes dysfunction of the autonomic neurons, which can manifest as dry mouth, postural hypotension, or impotence. Symptoms are exacerbated by certain medications and increased temperatures, including environmental exposure, fever, and hot baths. Paradoxically, patients may note that their strength improves after exercise, whereas the weakness of MG worsens with activity. Unlike MG, the respiratory system is not typically affected.

PHYSICAL EXAMINATION

Patients with LEMS typically have a nonspecific presentation and physical exam findings are often unimpressive. The mild weakness noted on physical exam is often incongruent with the patient's reported extent of weakness and dysfunction. This discrepancy can lead to a delay in diagnosis, misdiagnosis, or even a dismantling of the patient's perceived reliability.

On examination, the patient will have mild weakness in the proximal muscles of the extremities, which may produce a waddling gait and limited mobility of the shoulders. Distal muscle strength is typically preserved, and sensation is not affected. Strength often improves with repeated testing, which can confound the clinical picture. Similarly, deep tendon reflexes will be decreased or absent on initial exam but will reappear after isometric muscle contraction for 15 seconds. This phenomenon is called *postactivation facilitation* and is considered a defining feature of LEMS. This phenomenon is also evidenced in the examination of patients with ptosis and can help to differentiate LEMS from MG. Upon sustained upward gaze, patients with LEMS will have paradoxical eyelid elevation, as compared to the fatiguing of muscles and exacerbation of ptosis seen in patients with MG.

DIFFERENTIAL DIAGNOSIS

In patients presenting with symmetric proximal muscle weakness, the initial workup should exclude common causes of generalized weakness and fatigue such as anemia, electrolyte imbalance, hypothyroidism, and psychiatric illness. If a true neuromuscular process is suspected, more sophisticated diagnostic tests are required to narrow down the list of differentials (Table 15.40).

DIAGNOSTIC STUDIES AND EVALUATION

A diagnosis of LEMS is not often one that is found incidentally, and the clinician must be intentional in their diagnostic workup. Repetitive nerve stimulation studies will initially show a low-amplitude compound muscle action potential, but when tested after voluntary contraction of the muscle in question, the amplitude will often double in size, a facilitation unique to LEMS. Antibody assays are also an important component of the workup, and most patients with LEMS will have antibodies to VGCC. Although antibodies to acetylcholine receptors are usually indicative of MG, some patients with LEMS will have these antibodies as well. Convention states that if a patient has anti-acetylcholine receptor antibodies and a known malignancy, the diagnosis is most likely LEMS and not MG.

TREATMENT

- In cases of LEMS associated with SCLC, first treat the underlying malignancy. Effective cancer therapy often results in a profound improvement of symptoms, and further treatment may not be necessary.

TABLE 15.40 Differential Diagnosis for Lambert-Eaton Myasthenic Syndrome

Diagnosis	Description
Amyotrophic lateral sclerosis (ALS)	A neuromuscular disease that causes rapidly progressive motor weakness and paralysis. Diagnosis is difficult, and it often requires the exclusion of other neuromuscular disorders.
Guillain-Barré syndrome (GBS)	An acute inflammatory demyelinating polyradiculoneuropathy characterized by sensory changes, areflexia, and ascending motor weakness. Usually follows a benign upper respiratory or gastrointestinal infection.
Myasthenia gravis	An autoimmune destruction of acetylcholine receptors at the neuromuscular junction, resulting in fatigable motor weakness.
Polymyalgia rheumatica (PMR)	A chronic inflammatory condition that causes pain and stiffness of the hip and shoulder girdles, but is not associated with true muscle weakness. PMR is closely linked with giant cell arteritis.
Spinal muscular atrophy	A collection of genetic diseases characterized by progressive lower motor neuron weakness and muscle wasting.

- Initial symptomatic treatment includes a medication that increases the release of acetylcholine into the synapse (3,4-DAP or amifampridine), along with an acetylcholinesterase inhibitor (pyridostigmine) as adjunctive therapy.
- More severe cases may warrant plasmapheresis or IVIG for acute management, with a transition to immunosuppressants for maintenance therapy.

PATIENT EDUCATION

- Engage in physical therapy and exercise in order to maintain muscle tone and strength.
- Avoid hot showers and baths as increased body temperatures can exacerbate symptoms.
- Avoid medications that can exacerbate symptoms. Neuromuscular blocking agents, such as those used in general anesthesia, can cause prolonged weakness or apnea. Many antibiotics, some antiarrhythmics, and iodinated IV contrast agent can also exacerbate weakness.

15.15C CEREBRAL PALSY

MEDICAL HISTORY AND CLINICAL PRESENTATION

Cerebral palsy (CP) represents a group of congenital, permanent, nonprogressive motor disabilities. It is the most common cause of childhood disability, occurring in about 1 of 500 live births.[246] While nonprogressive, the clinical presentation may change over time with the maturation of the central nervous system. In addition to motor challenges, those with CP may develop seizure disorders, and could have deficits in sensory systems, communication, intellectual ability, and behavioral milestones.

CP is typically first diagnosed between ages 12 and 24 months. Patients with a history of prematurity, multiple gestation, low birth weight, abnormal pre- or perinatal history or other complications at birth are most at risk. CP can be caused during fetal development, during birth, or during infancy. It usually involves a hypoxic, hemorrhagic or infectious insult to the CNS, a congenital or chromosomal abnormality, or kernicterus.[247–249]

Obtaining a thorough medical and family history is paramount to making a diagnosis of CP. Many disorders, some progressive, present similarly to and may be misdiagnosed as CP. Any report of loss of previously attained developmental, neurologic, or sensory skills, dysmorphic features, symptoms worsening during illness or fasting, oculomotor abnormalities, or the absence of any risk factors for CP should prompt a search for possible alternative diagnoses.[250]

Multiple subtypes of CP exist and are commonly classified by the location of injury and the type of motor abnormalities; however, this classification may be interpreted subjectively (Table 15.41).

SIGNS AND SYMPTOMS

Initial suspicion relies heavily on reports from the child's caregivers. Excessive irritability, decreased interaction, weakness, difficulty feeding, rigid body positions, or hypotonia are common concerns that when paired with supporting history should prompt a consideration of CP.[246,251]

Dyskinetic CP patients may have one or more forms of involuntary movement; some children with spastic CP may have forms of dyskinesia as well. Caregivers may report unusual, stiff, or jerky movements. Patients with dystonic CP may have symptoms that cease during some activities or with sleep.[252]

The signs and symptoms of ataxic CP are highly variable, including feeding problems, hypotonia, delayed speech and motor skills, and can be difficult to discern from simple incoordination common in young children. Signs and symptoms overlap with other subtypes of CP.[253]

TABLE 15.41 Spastic, Dyskinetic, and Ataxic Cerebral Palsy Subtypes

Cerebral Palsy Type	Presentation
Spastic Cerebral Palsy	
Spastic diplegia	Spasticity, motor difficulties; legs affected more than arms, bilateral
Spastic hemiplegia	Spasticity, motor difficulties, arms affected more than legs, unilateral
Spastic quadriplegia	Spasticity, motor difficulties, all extremities, often upper affected more than lower extremities
Dyskinetic Cerebral Palsy	
Dystonic	Hypokinesia, hypertonia, twisting, stiff/repetitive movements
Choreoathetotic	Hyperkinesia, hypotonia; uncoordinated writhing, jerky movements
Ataxic Cerebral Palsy	Hypotonia, loss of coordination, unsteadiness, language difficulty

Sources: Graham HK, Rosenbaum P, Paneth N, et al. Cerebral palsy. Nat Rev Dis Primers. *2016;2:15082. doi:10.1038/nrdp.2015.82; Wimalasundera N, Stevenson VL. Cerebral palsy.* Pract Neurol. *2016;16(3):184–194. doi:10.1136/practneurol-2015-001184*

PHYSICAL EXAMINATION

Cerebral palsy can mimic other neurologic and musculoskeletal disorders; as such, a thorough exam of each system should be conducted. Mental status, head circumference, posture, reflexes, muscle tone, strength, and gait should be tested.[255]

Physical examination findings depend on the subtype of CP and the degree to which the patient is affected, which can be minimal or severe. Spastic CP presents with both "positive" and "negative" physical exam findings of an upper motor neuron syndrome.

"Positive" findings involve *increased* muscle activity or movement. In response to passive limb movement, muscle resistance increases; in severe forms, this spasticity occurs in both flexion and extension. Extrapyramidal features, such as ataxia, cause the patient to have difficulty making precise and controlled movements. Other positive signs include clonus, hyperreflexia, and a positive Babinski reflex outside age-appropriate windows.

"Negative" findings involve *decreased* muscle activity or control. In spastic CP, these may include fatigue, weakness, slow movements, and lack of dexterity and fine-motor skills.

Patients with dystonia may present with sustained, involuntary muscle contractions that cause tilted or twisted body positions. Choreoathetotic CP causes an antagonistic action of opposing muscle groups, such as flexion/extension or pronation/supination, caused by any number of stimuli—emotion, change in posture, movement, or others.[252]

Ataxic CP typically affects motor milestones and language skills most severely. This is the most difficult type of CP to diagnose due to its rarity and variability in signs, symptoms, and examination findings. Ataxic CP often presents similarly to progressive neurodegenerative disorders; however, ataxic CP verbal skills can sometimes improve over time, while progressive diseases do not.[253]

DIFFERENTIAL DIAGNOSIS

The differential diagnosis for CP is summarized in Table 15.42.

TABLE 15.42 Differential Diagnosis for Cerebral Palsy

Diagnosis	Description
Hereditary spastic paraplegia	Inherited disorder, characterized by progressive weakness and spasticity of the legs.
Tethered cord	Often associated with spina bifida, this may cause pain, weakness, deformities, bowel/bladder problems, gait problems.
Rett syndrome	Primarily in females; characterized by repetitive hand movements, slowed development, intellectual disability, gait difficulties, seizures.
Pyruvate dehydrogenase deficiency	Genetic condition causing buildup of pyruvate, converting to lactic acid, leading to neurologic issues including intellectual disability, seizure, hypotonia, gait difficulties.
Lesch-Nyhan syndrome	Primarily in males; genetic deficiency in ability to recycle purines, leading to overproduction of uric acid; gouty arthritis, dystonia, chorea, ballismus, self-injury.
Niemann-Pick type C	Genetic progressive disorder that causes inability to transport lipids, causing accumulation in various tissues; decreased muscle tone, learning disabilities, difficulty swallowing, slurred speech, developmental regression, psychiatric symptoms, jaundice, seizures, gait problems.
GLUT1 deficiency syndrome	Genetic disorder affecting glucose transport, causing seizures, microcephaly, involuntary eye movements, intellectual disability, spasticity, ataxia, dysarthria; worse when fasting.
Zellweger syndrome	Group of genetic disorders that prevent peroxisomes from forming, which are responsible for the breakdown of fatty acids and the production of lipids used in digestion and the nervous system. This leads to hypotonia, feeding problems, hearing/vision loss, seizures, multiorgan issues, and skeletal issues.
Pontocerebellar hypoplasias	Group of genetic mutations causing maldevelopment of the pons and the cerebellum, microcephaly and usually causing death in childhood. Hypotonia, contractures, vision impairment, breathing issues, feeding problems, lack of motor skills, seizures, dysphagia, speech issues, clonus, chorea, dystonia, and/or spasticity may be present.
Angelman syndrome	Inherited disorder causing delayed development, intellectual disability, speech impairment, ataxia, seizures, microcephaly, and an overly excitable presentation; patients often appear very happy, with frequent laughter, hand-flapping, hyperactivity, short attention spans, difficulty sleeping, and a fascination with water.
Leigh syndrome	Mitochondrial DNA mutation causing impaired energy production and cell death, leading to progressive loss of cognitive and motor abilities; hypotonia, vomiting, diarrhea, dysphagia, ataxia develop; results in death within 2–3 years, usually from respiratory failure.
Joubert syndrome	Multiple genetic mutations produce proteins that interfere with cilia, interrupting chemical signaling during development. Structures near the cerebellum and brainstem are commonly affected. Hypotonia, ataxia, breathing problems, abnormal eye movements, intellectual disability, and delayed development are common. Distinctive facial features include widely spaced eyes, ptosis, arched eyebrows, a broad forehead, low-set ears, and a triangle-shaped mouth.
Muscular dystrophies	Over 30 different progressive disorders with varying degrees of severity, disability, age of onset, life expectancy, and clinical features; however, most involve some degree of muscle wasting/weakness or inability to relax muscle groups.
Metachromatic leukodystrophy	Genetic mutation causes accumulation of sulfatides in cells, which are toxic to nervous system; destroys myelin-producing cells, causing progressive destruction of central and peripheral nervous system.

GLUT1, glucose transporter 1.

DIAGNOSTIC STUDIES

CP is largely a historical and clinical diagnosis. However, some diagnostic studies are useful to rule out alternative diagnoses and pinpoint locations of injury.

MRI is preferred for discovering abnormal neuroanatomy that may lead to the determination of the cause of CP.[249] In neonates, cranial ultrasound may be useful to identify intraventricular hemorrhage and periventricular leukomalacia. While not diagnostic of CP at this stage of life, these findings on ultrasound may signal a risk for later diagnosis of CP.[254]

If the patient is suspected of having seizures, an EEG should be ordered. Any patient suspected of having a stroke or ischemic event should have a thrombophilia screening done, although it has not been determined if there is a clear link between hereditary thrombophilia and CP.[255]

Patients who have progression in symptoms should undergo testing to search for alternative diagnoses, as CP is not a progressive disorder. These diagnostics may include metabolic panels, lumbar punctures, further neuroimaging, or additional genetic testing.[250]

EVALUATION

While there are limited laboratory and radiologic studies that can assist in making a diagnosis of CP, some assessment tools are useful when attempting to make an early diagnosis. The Hammersmith Infant Neurological Examination (HINE), a scorable neurologic examination tool for infants between 2 and 24 months of age, has a 90% sensitivity for the detection of CP.[256] The Prechtl Qualitative Assessment of General Movements (GMs) has a 98% predictive validity prior to 5 months' corrected age. When used in combination with a thorough clinical and family history, as well as MRI, these tools improve accuracy of predictions and diagnoses.[257]

Once the diagnosis of CP has been established, the gross motor function classification system (GMFCS) for children can be applied to describe the patient's level of disability. This scale can also serve as a predictive tool for the level of function the child is likely to have later in development. After age 5, motor ability plateaus, so if the child is at a more severe GMFCS level at around age 5, they are unlikely to improve much past that level.[258]

TREATMENT

- Requires multiple specialists, including primary care, orthopedics, neurology, physical therapy, occupational therapy, speech therapy, behavioral health, social workers, and others[251]
- Botulinum toxin and benzodiazepines for pain and spasticity[252]
- Anticholinergics, speech therapy or surgery for sialorrhea[259]
- Surgical management options:
  - Baclofen pump, tendon releases, selective dorsal rhizotomy—for severe spasticity
  - Spinal fusion
  - Deep brain stimulation[252]
- Stem cell trials are in progress.
- Postnatal head cooling following known hypoxic injury can improve disability outcomes.[258]

PATIENT EDUCATION

- Life expectancy correlates to the severity of disability; in mild to moderate impairment, life expectancy is only marginally reduced, while in severe and/or multiple disabilities, life expectancy is shortened.[258]

15.16 MUSCULAR DYSTROPHIES

Ashley Bell

OVERVIEW

Muscular dystrophy is a group of approximately 30 genetic disorders that cause muscle weakness and breakdown. These disorders are progressive and have varying ages of onset, life expectancy, degree of disability, and clinical features.

The muscular dystrophies are typically organized into eight subtypes: Duchenne/Becker (DMD/BMD), myotonic (DM), limb-girdle (LGMD), facioscapulohumeral (FSHD), congenital (CMD), distal (DD), oculopharyngeal (OPMD), and Emery-Dreifuss (EDMD).

EPIDEMIOLOGY

DMD is the most common childhood inherited muscle disease and is found in about 8.3 per 100,000 boys. BMD is found in about 7.3 per 100,000 boys. FSHD affects about 3 per 100,000 people.[260,261] Myotonic dystrophy is the most common form of muscular dystrophy in adults and affects about 10.6 per 100,000 people. LGMD affects about 1 in 20,000.[262] OPMD prevalence is highest in Quebec, Canada, at 1:1,000 and among Bukhara Jews living in Israel at 1:600. Most OPMD patients in the United States are of French-Canadian background but large numbers have also been noted in California and Texas, and in those with Jewish Ashkenazi backgrounds.[263] The prevalence of EDMD is 1.3–2 in 100,000 individuals.[264] For CMD, there are at least 30 different subtypes, which makes providing prevalence difficult; however, a gross estimate has been stated at 1 in 100,000 births.[265] DD also makes up a group of multiple subtypes, with some occurring more frequently in European families, some in Japanese families, and some in Middle Eastern families.[266]

PATHOPHYSIOLOGY

Muscular dystrophies may be X-linked, autosomal, or sporadic mutations (Table 15.43).

MEDICAL HISTORY AND CLINICAL PRESENTATION OF MUSCULAR DYSTROPHIES

The age of onset and location of muscle weakness are dependent on the specific classification of the patient's muscular dystrophy (Figure 15.5).

DMD and BMD present with pelvic followed by shoulder girdle weakness. As DMD progresses, weakness moves to the limb and respiratory muscles. In LGMD, patients typically have pelvic or shoulder girdle weakness, and as the disease progresses, weakness in one moves to also include the other. FSHD first involves the face and shoulder girdle, then moves to the pelvic area and legs. DM affects the face, neck, and distal limbs. The distribution of EDMD is humeroperoneal or scapuloperoneal. OPMD presents with ptosis, external ophthalmoplegia, and dysphagia. DD has onset in the distal extremities and moves proximally later in the disease.[261,262,266,267]

TABLE 15.43 Inheritance, Pathophysiology, and Progression of Selected Muscular Dystrophies

Muscular Dystrophy Subtype	Inheritance	Pathophysiology	Progression
Duchenne	X-linked recessive	Dystrophin deficiency, causing muscle wasting	Rapid
Becker	X-linked recessive	Dystrophin deficiency (less severe than Duchenne)	Slow
Myotonic	Autosomal dominant	Weakness of voluntary muscles and inability to relax muscles at will	Slow
Limb-girdle	Autosomal recessive, dominant, or sporadic mutation	Pelvic and/or shoulder muscle wasting caused by deficient or nonfunctioning proteins	Variable
Facioscapulohumeral	Autosomal dominant	Inappropriate expression of *DUX4* gene on chromosome 4 causes excessive protein and toxicity in muscle cells	Slow
Congenital	Autosomal recessive	Weakness present at birth; multiple causes, most involving mutations in glycoproteins which interfere with normal muscle function and cause injury from normal muscle contraction	Variable
Distal	Autosomal dominant or recessive	Multiple; some involving a deficiency in dysferlin, a protein involved with skeletal muscle repair	Slow
Oculopharyngeal	Mostly autosomal dominant but can be autosomal recessive	Defect in *PABPN1* gene causes protein to collect in muscle cell nuclei, impairs function of muscle cells and causes cell death	Slow

SIGNS AND SYMPTOMS

DMD patients are boys typically in early childhood who have weakness, difficulty climbing stairs, and/or toe walking. Many have cognitive disabilities. As the disease progresses, patients will become nonambulatory and will have diminished respiratory function, progressing to difficulty coughing, sleep apnea, and daytime hypoventilation.[261] Females may carry the abnormal dystrophin gene and few develop symptoms of muscle weakness, but generally the cases are not as severe as males and more closely resemble that of BMD.[268]

Compared with DMD, Becker (BMD) patients are usually older children and have milder, though similar, symptoms. They are usually ambulatory until late adolescence or into adulthood.[269]

DM usually presents during adolescence or adulthood, but in some forms can present in infancy or childhood. It affects multiple systems, causing facial, arm, and leg muscle weakness and loss. The heart is commonly affected, leading to heart block. Cataracts, difficulty swallowing, and intellectual disabilities are also sometimes found. Delayed muscle relaxation after contraction (myotonia) is a frequent finding in DM patients. DM patients often suffer from respiratory and cardiac issues as their disease progresses.[260,267]

Most patients with LGMD begin showing muscle weakness as young adults, although some phenotypes may show symptoms in the first decade of life. Interestingly, patients with some variants of LGMD actually show athletic giftedness as young children and teens. Once clinical symptoms begin, proximal weakness is present, and some patients may have calf weakness or hypertrophy as well. They may lose the ability to ambulate as the disease progresses. Muscle cramps, contractures, and cardiac arrhythmias occur in some patients.[262]

FSHD patients display facial, shoulder, scapular, and arm weakness; classically, weakness appears in early adulthood, but a childhood form many cause challenges with intellectual disabilities, seizures, ambulation, and hearing loss. Both forms lead to the inability to close the eyes to sleep, to smile, or to show facial expression; vision and hearing are often affected as the disease progresses. While the progression is slow and the lifespan is usually normal, the patient often becomes significantly disabled due to weakness in the shoulders and hips and may have weakness of the wrists and ankles as well.[270]

CMD often presents at birth with "floppy baby" hypotonia; joint contractures may be present, as well as eye and brain abnormalities. Other signs and symptoms depend on the phenotype and may include seizures, respiratory difficulties, skin abnormalities, and cardiac arrhythmias.[265]

DD may present at any age, depending on the phenotype, but commonly presents in mid-life. Distal weakness sometimes spreads proximally and in some phenotypes there may be cardiac involvement. Finger weakness, foot drop, calf weakness, and wrist extension problems are common findings.[267]

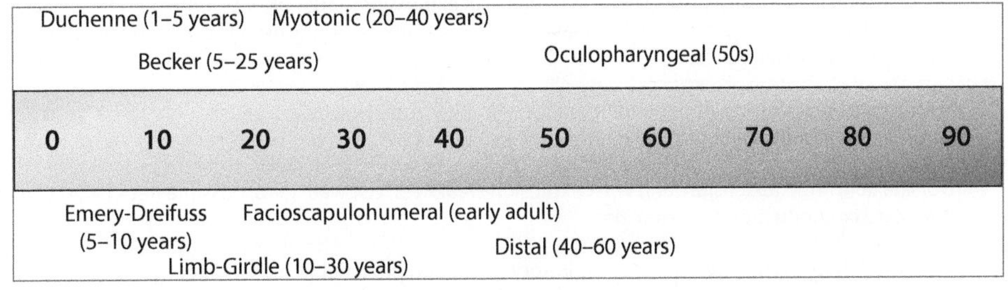

Figure 15.5 **Common ages of onset for muscular dystrophy subtypes.**

OPMD typically presents in adults in their 50s with ptosis, dysphagia, and eventually proximal muscle weakness. As the disease progresses, respiratory issues due to dysphagia may develop.[267]

EDMD presents in childhood or adolescence with contractures of the Achilles tendons, the elbows, and the posterior cervical muscles, followed by muscle weakness and wasting, usually starting in the arms. Occasionally, facial weakness can be seen. The heart is commonly affected, causing cardiac arrhythmias.[267]

PHYSICAL EXAMINATION

Table 15.44 summarizes the physical examination findings of muscular dystrophies.

DIFFERENTIAL DIAGNOSIS

Table 15.45 summarizes the differential diagnosis for muscular dystrophies.

DIAGNOSTIC STUDIES

While initial suspicion is based on clinical presentation, most patients will be definitively diagnosed by genetic testing after telltale clinical features are noted. For cases in which these features are unclear, EMG and muscle biopsy may be done prior or in addition to genetic testing.[267] Elevated creatine kinase (CK) levels are seen in some muscular dystrophies, but elevated CK, carnitine, lactate, and pyruvate levels can also be seen in some metabolic myopathies, so these should be considerations in the diagnostic process as well. For some CMD patients, MRI of the brain and lower extremities may be useful in determining a specific subtype diagnosis.[260,271]

In DMD, CK concentrations are elevated prior to the appearance of any signs or symptoms, even in some affected newborns. CK is typically 10 to 20 times normal and peaks by age 2 years in these patients. Transaminases are also elevated.[269]

Muscular dystrophy patients should have baseline cardiac and respiratory evaluations at diagnosis and at regular intervals depending on their specific diagnosis.[260,271]

TABLE 15.45 Differential Diagnosis for Muscular Dystrophies

Diagnosis	Description
Toxic myopathies	Drug-induced myopathies, reversible at early stages
Endocrine myopathies	Result from abnormal endocrine activity; treatable
Autoimmune myopathies	Dermatomyositis, immune-mediated necrotizing myopathy, antisynthetase syndrome, polymyositis; symmetric proximal muscle weakness; responsive to immunosuppressive therapy
Metabolic myopathies	Disorders in processing various nutrients/chemicals, causing buildup and damage in muscles
Myasthenia gravis	Autoimmune disorder of neuromuscular transmission; fluctuating weakness
Spinal muscular atrophy	Loss/degeneration of motor neurons in the spinal cord, leading to weakness and atrophy in muscles
Progressive bulbar palsy	Lower motor neuron disorder affecting swallowing, jaw/facial muscles, speech, tongue muscle atrophy, weak limbs; may progress to amyotrophic lateral sclerosis

EVALUATION

As muscular dystrophy is a progressive disease, evaluation is guided by response to supportive treatment. Muscular dystrophy requires a multidisciplinary management team including educational specialists, occupational therapists, psychologists, behavioral therapists, orthopedic specialists, neurologists, cardiologists, primary care providers, and more. Early in the disease, modifications may be minor and

TABLE 15.44 Physical Examination Findings of Muscular Dystrophies

Muscular Dystrophy	Physical Examination
Duchenne (DMD)	Proximal weakness, hypertrophied calves, toe walking, difficulty walking up stairs, delayed motor milestones; Gower sign: using hands and arms to walk up one's own body from a squatting position.
Becker (BMD)	Similar to DMD, but usually milder and later age of onset.
Myotonic (DM)	Muscle loss in face, arms, legs; heart block; cataracts; may have joint problems or difficulty swallowing; excessive daytime sleepiness; myotonia.
Limb-girdle (LGMD)	Proximal weakness; some patients may have calf hypertrophy/weakness and contractures. Scapular winging in some phenotypes. Cardiac arrhythmias/cardiomyopathy in some patients.
Facioscapulohumeral (FSHD)	Facial weakness, difficulty closing eyes, making facial expressions; possible vision/hearing loss, weakness in shoulders, upper arms, and hips; later stages may show weakness of wrists/ankles; adults usually can ambulate until later stages but children may lose ability to ambulate.
Congenital (CMD)	Hypotonia; otherwise varies depending on the phenotype; may include scoliosis, rigid spine, contractures, respiratory issues, cardiac arrhythmias, keloids, hyperkeratosis pilaris.
Distal (DD)	Dorsiflexion, finger extension, and wrist extension weakness; calf weakness, possible neck flexion and facial weakness; may have cardiac conduction abnormalities.
Oculopharyngeal (OPMD)	Ptosis and dysphagia in early stages; respiratory issues and proximal weakness later.
Emery-Dreifuss (EDMD)	Contractures, most prominent in spine, elbows, and ankles; muscle wasting that usually starts in arms, followed by legs.

gradual; however, as interventions become more involved, it is important that all those involved in the patient's care fully recognize the scope of the patient's situation. Patients, parents, and caregivers should understand the typical course of their disease and have the opportunity to make decisions regarding treatments, location of care, palliative support, end-of-life care, and resuscitation options.

TREATMENT

- Glucocorticoids are the primary treatment for DMD and BMD, as they increase strength, muscle function, and lung function, as well as delaying the progression of scoliosis.[272]
- Multiple therapies are in development, including gene modification therapies, dystrophin restoration therapies, drugs targeting myostatin, medications to improve mitochondrial function, and others for DMD.[272]
- For most other forms of muscular dystrophy, no disease modifying therapy is available.
- Pacemakers are implanted in patients with cardiac involvement.
- Stretching exercises are recommended to prevent contractures.
- Feeding tube placement may be necessary if swallowing ability is affected.
- For many complications, treatment is aimed at managing symptoms.

PATIENT EDUCATION

- Muscular dystrophy has varying degrees of severity, and many patients can lead active lives.
- Many organizations, such as the Muscular Dystrophy Association, have resources and contacts for networking and support available.
- Muscular dystrophy affects not only one's ability to move the arms and legs, but also can affect the ability to swallow, breathe, and can cause heart problems.
- Muscular dystrophy is a progressive disease.

SPECIAL CONSIDERATIONS

- Parents may need guidance regarding discussions about the disease with their children, especially as it relates to progression and the terminal nature.
- Genetic counseling should be recommended for anyone with a family history of muscular dystrophy or those who are known carriers.
- Pregnancy in patients with muscular dystrophy is high-risk. Compared to those unaffected by muscular dystrophy, pregnant patients with muscular dystrophy are more likely to have preeclampsia, preterm labor, require a cesarean section, suffer a venous thromboembolism, require a transfusion, and suffer a cardiac dysrhythmia during delivery. Neonates are more at risk of being born premature, having a congenital malformation (including having a muscular dystrophy), and having an intrauterine growth restriction.[273]

KEY POINTS

- Muscular dystrophies are inherited and progressive.
- Life expectancy, age of onset, rate of progression, and severity of disability vary depending on the specific subtype of disease.
- Diagnosis is mostly clinical and is made through genetic testing.
- With few exceptions, treatment is aimed at managing symptoms and preventing complications.

COMMON CHIEF COMPLAINTS

APPROACH TO HEADACHE

MELINDA MOORE GOTTSCHALK

Headaches come in five distinct classifications: primary headaches, secondary headaches, painful cranial neuropathies, other facial pain, and other headaches.[1] When a patient presents with a headache, taking a detailed history will determine the next step.

The interview begins with headache and general health questions to discover if other medical problems or medications are the reason for the headaches. A detailed history would include:

- **When** did the headache start?
- **Where** is the pain located on the head?
- **What** makes the headaches better or worse?
- Are there **associated symptoms?**
- Is there a **family history** of headache?
- **Medications** and past **medical/surgical** history

If the patient's symptoms seem to indicate they have a primary headache, such as a migraine, tension, or a cluster headache, the next steps will depend on the length of time the headache has been present and if the headache has changed recently in intensity and frequency. Any time a headache changes, it may necessitate a diagnostic study. The "red flags" in headaches will help determine the need for a diagnostic study (Figure 15.6).

SNNOOP is the acronym for the red flags in headaches (see Table 15.2). SNNOOP helps diagnosis secondary causes of headaches. After a secondary cause of headache is discovered, the underlying condition must be addressed.

Example of a "red flag": A patient presents saying, "This is the worse headache of my life!" This patient should immediately go to the ED for a head CT to rule out a subarachnoid hemorrhage, aneurysm, stroke, or other intracranial disorder. Delaying treatment in this situation is life-threatening.

Keeping an accurate headache diary enables the patient to report the frequency and severity of their headaches to their clinician. Capturing the migraine phases in the headache diary—prodrome, aura, headache, and postdrome—helps determine changes to the treatment plan. Starting migraine abortive medications at the earliest recognized phase of the migraine allows the patient the have more success in stopping the headache, while using fewer medications. However, tension and cluster headaches do not have a prodrome, aura, and postdrome.

If there are no underlying disorders, start preventive migraine treatment: recommended supplements and one of the three medication classes specifically indicated for migraine. A tension headache and a migraine headache are often present at the same time or one may be the cause of the other headache. Because the two headaches are often together, the medications used for migraine prevention and acute treatment are used for tension headache prevention and acute treatment. A muscle relaxer is added to treat a tension headache while an antiemetic is added for a migraine. Cluster and postconcussion headaches are treated with the same medication classes as migraine/tension, but with a few variations.

To judge efficacy of the headache medications, the medication should be taken for 3 months unless there are side effects. Keeping a careful record of medications that have been tried

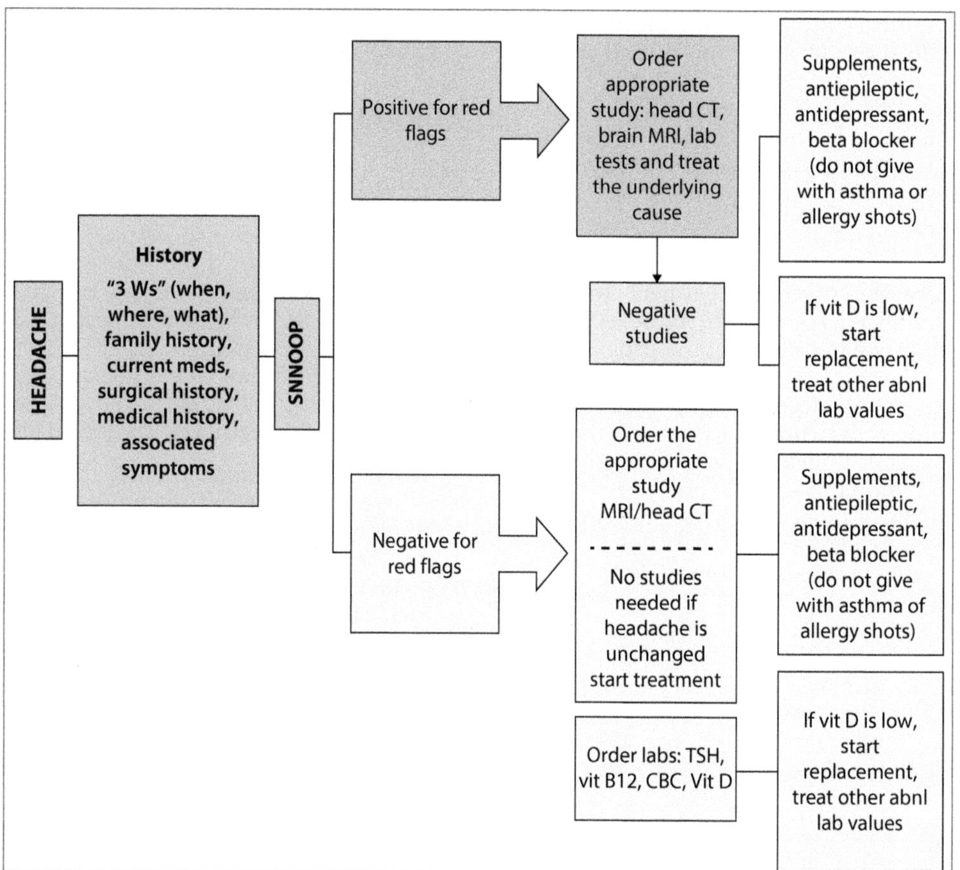

Figure 15.6 **Algorithm for approach to headache diagnosis.** abnl, abnormal; CBC, complete blood count; SNNOOP, Systemic symptoms, Neoplasms, Neurological deficits, Onset (sudden or following Valsalva maneuver), Older age, Prior history; TSH, thyroid-stimulating hormone; vit, vitamin.

and failed will enable the clinician to move onto more expensive headache medications with fewer insurance barriers.

APPROACH TO DIZZINESS

Rayne Loder

Dizziness is a common chief complaint encountered in clinical practice. Dizziness is also a highly subjective descriptor that may mean very different things to different patients. It is the job of the clinician to ask careful historical questions to clarify the nature of the patient's reported dizziness.

Dizziness can generally be thought of in four categories: vertigo, disequilibrium, presyncope, and lightheadedness. Each category has its own differential considerations list that will guide the physical exam and general diagnostic approach (Figure 15.7).

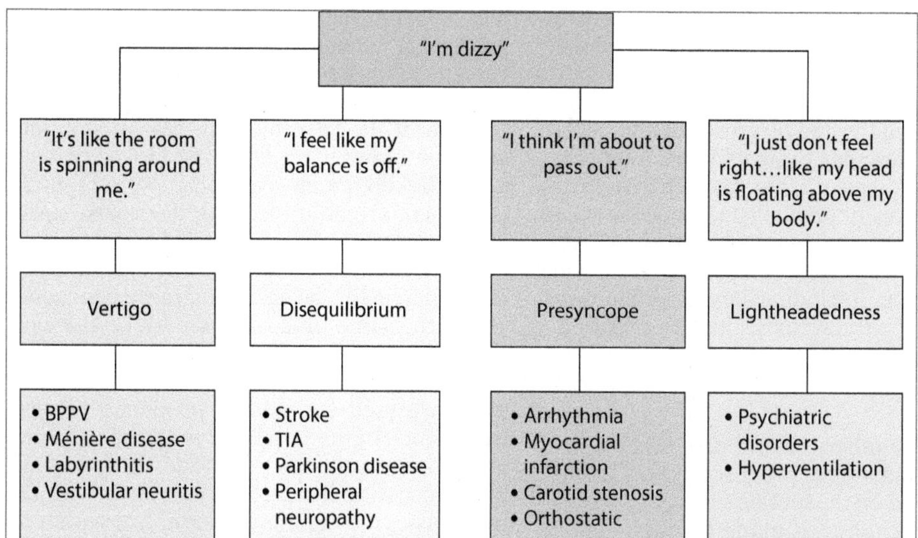

Figure 15.7 **Algorithm for approach to dizziness as a chief complaint.** BPPV, benign paroxysmal positional vertigo; TIA, transient ischemic attack.

Vertigo is the most common cause of dizziness and refers to a sensation often described as "room-spinning." Vertigo is related to disorders of the ear or vestibular system, including benign paroxysmal positional vertigo (BPPV), Ménière disease, labyrinthitis, and vestibular neuritis. BPPV and Ménière disease generally cause episodic vertigo, while labyrinthitis and vestibular neuritis cause sustained vertigo. Ménière disease and labyrinthitis are associated with hearing loss, while BPPV and vestibular neuritis are not. Nystagmus, swaying to one side during Romberg testing, and an abnormal head impulse test can all be indicative of a vertiginous cause of dizziness. The Dix-Hallpike maneuver can be used in the office to diagnose BPPV.

Disequilibrium refers to a sense of imbalance. This can be due to a central nervous system cause such as stroke or transient ischemic attack. Disequilibrium can also be related to peripheral neuropathies and movement disorders. A careful neurologic examination, including gait observation, is helpful to differentiate this chief complaint.

Presyncope refers to the sensation that one is on the verge of passing out or losing consciousness. When dizziness is presyncopal in nature, cardiovascular causes must be entertained and include arrhythmias, cardiac ischemia, carotid stenosis, and orthostatic hypotension. Checking orthostatic vital signs on exam and performing a careful cardiovascular examination is helpful in the differentiation of this complaint.

Lightheadedness is the most nebulous of the four categories of dizziness and refers to a vague sense of being disconnected from one's surroundings. Lightheadedness is frequently psychiatric in etiology, and hyperventilation syndrome is another common diagnosis. Asking about psychiatric history and current symptoms is important in the differentiation of this chief complaint.

APPROACH TO DEMENTIA/DELIRIUM

Anna Swanson

When evaluating a patient with cognitive disturbances, whether acute or chronic, a clinician should always try to

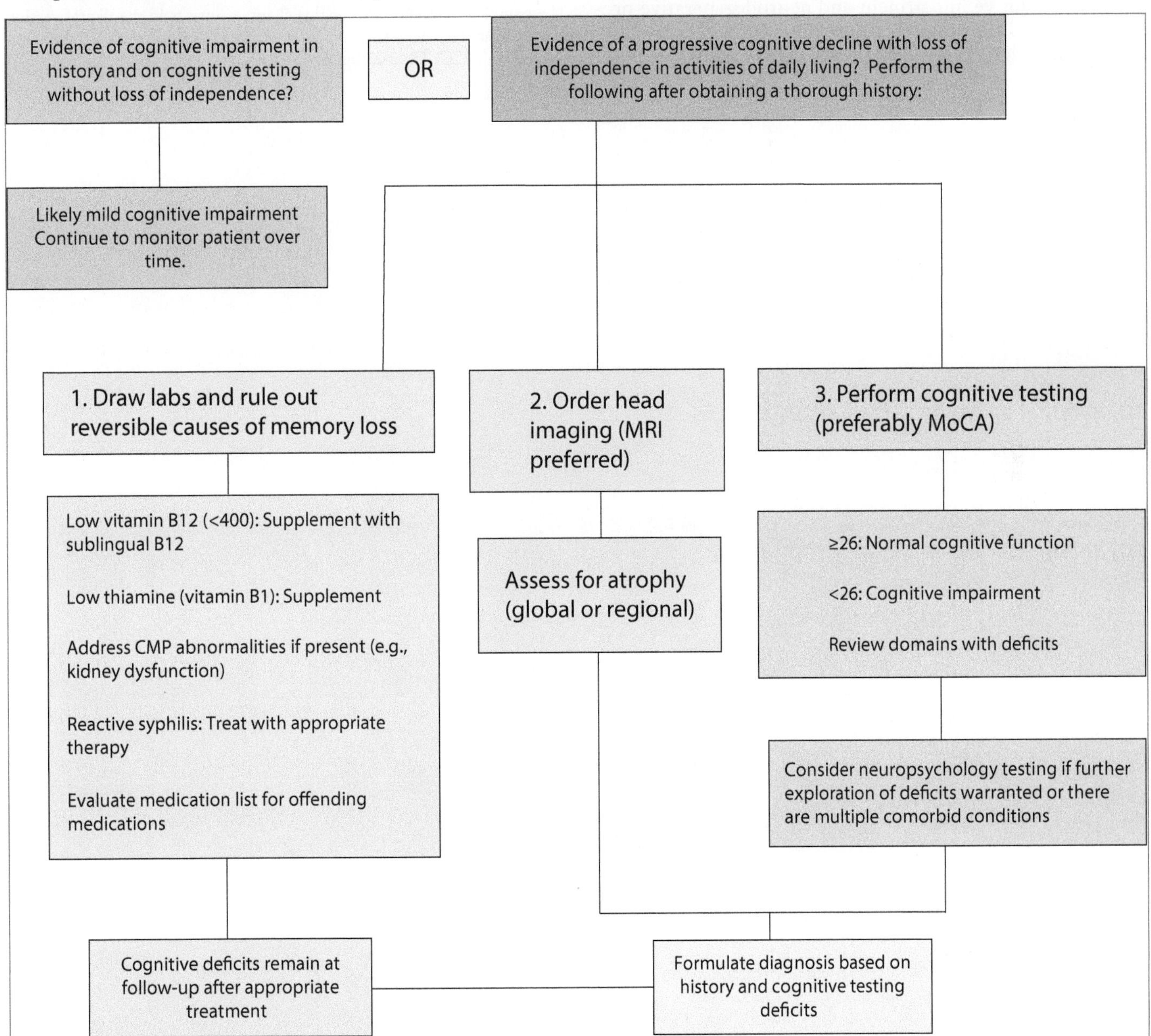

Figure 15.8 Algorithm for approach to dementia after obtaining history. CMP, comprehensive metabolic panel; MoCA, Montreal Cognitive Assessment.

obtain a history from a caregiver or family member who knows the patient's baseline cognitive status. Ask about activities of daily living, both basic and instrumental (e.g., managing finances, shopping for groceries, preparing a meal). Is the patient fully independent or do they rely on someone to complete the majority of instrumental or basic activities of daily living? What are some of the biggest changes the patient or family has noticed? Are there any new behavioral symptoms? Go over the patient's medication list with the family and look for medications that have strong anticholinergic properties. After obtaining a history, perform cognitive testing. There are several ways to evaluate cognitive decline. If the decline is acute, then screening for infection and metabolic abnormalities should be done first. Electrolyte abnormalities, liver dysfunction, and kidney dysfunction can be identified by a complete metabolic panel. A urinary tract infection or upper respiratory infection can cause a demented patient to develop an acute confusional state. If cognitive changes are more of a slow progressive decline, then the patient should be evaluated for reversible causes of cognitive impairment and neurodegenerative processes. Figure 15.8 provides a flowchart for a general clinician's approach to evaluating progressive cognitive decline.

KNOWLEDGE CHECKS

1. What unique characteristic differentiates dystonia from spasticity or rigidity or other movement disorders?
2. What are the most important tools in diagnosing dystonia?
3. When should surgery be considered as a treatment for dystonia?

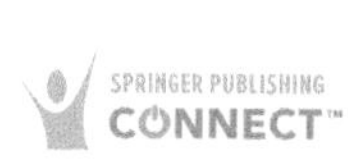

A robust set of instructor resources designed to supplement this text is located at **https://connect.springerpub.com/content/book/978-0-8261-8243-2.** Qualifying instructors may request access by emailing **textbook@springerpub.com.**

REFERENCES

The complete reference list for this chapter appears in the digital version of the chapter, accessible at https://connect.springerpub.com/content/book/978-0-8261-8243-2/chapter/ch15.

CHAPTER 16

ENDOCRINE SYSTEM

STEPHANIE NEARY AND GINA HOGG

LEARNING OBJECTIVES

1. Describe normal positive and negative hormone feedback loop pathophysiology with regard to hypothalamus, pituitary gland and target organ function.
2. Compare and contrast the various causes of hormone deficiency disorders with regard to epidemiology, pathophysiology, clinical presentation, diagnosis, and disease management.
3. Compare and contrast the various causes of hormone excess disorders with regard to epidemiology, pathophysiology, clinical presentation, diagnosis, and disease management.

INTRODUCTION

The endocrine system is made up of a complex, interrelated network of glands and hormones that communicate with organ systems throughout the body and serve to regulate reproductive function, bone metabolism, human growth, and metabolism. For clinicians, understanding the role of positive and negative feedback loops is paramount when diagnosing and managing endocrine disorders. Simply measuring serum hormone concentrations is often enough to determine the site of dysfunction and the initial treatment approach. Most hormone testing is rather straightforward; typically, if a deficiency is expected, a stimulation test is helpful, whereas if excess is expected, a depression test is helpful. Once the disorder is diagnosed, management is achieved through hormone replacement therapy for deficiency disorders and either surgical removal of the tumor or gland or pharmacologic hormone reduction for excess disorders.

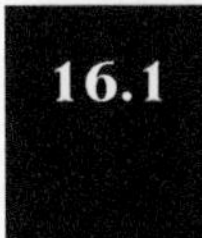

16.1 DISEASES OF THE HYPOTHALAMUS AND PITUITARY GLAND

OVERVIEW

Hormones work as messengers throughout the body and carry information to receptors located on target organs. The system of glands and hormones that make up the endocrine system cannot be defined by basic anatomic constraints like many other body systems; rather, the endocrine system can be viewed as the communication pathway that links organ systems. Achieving and maintaining homeostasis requires an intricate series of feedback loops involving the hypothalamus, pituitary gland, and multiple target organs throughout the body. There are countless causes for hormonal dysregulation ranging from intrinsic abnormalities such as adenomas and vascular infarcts to external factors such as increased stress and medication use.

EPIDEMIOLOGY

Pituitary dysfunction is relatively rare, with specific rates of incidence varying widely by condition. Pituitary adenomas account for approximately 10% to 15% of all intracranial lesions, with incidentalomas occurring in approximately 10% of autopsies.

PATHOPHYSIOLOGY

The pituitary gland, divided into anterior and posterior pituitary lobes, is at the core of the endocrine system. The anterior pituitary produces six major hormones: prolactin (PRL), growth hormone (GH), adrenocorticotropic hormone (ACTH), luteinizing hormone (LH), follicle-stimulating hormone (FSH), and thyroid-stimulating hormone (TSH; Table 16.1). The pulsatile release of anterior pituitary hormones is regulated by hormones secreted from the hypothalamus via the hypothalamo-hypophyseal portal vessels, a network of blood vessels that create a direct pathway from the hypothalamus to the pituitary gland through the infundibulum. There are six releasing hormones of the hypothalamus: anti-diuretic hormone (ADH; vasopressin), gonadotropin-releasing hormone (GnRH), thyrotropin-releasing hormone (TRH), prolactin-releasing hormone (PRH), GH-releasing hormone (GHRH), and corticotropin-releasing hormone (CRH).

The posterior pituitary—also referred to as the neurohypophysis—stores two hormones that are produced in the hypothalamus: oxytocin (OT) and ADH (also referred to as vasopressin; Table 16.2).

To discuss hypothalamus and pituitary disorders, the physiology of both negative and positive feedback loops must first be understood. The defined hormone regulation pathway between the hypothalamus, pituitary gland, and target organ is called an axis (Table 16.3).

Examples of negative feedback control include the following (Figure 16.1):

Table 16.1 Anterior Pituitary Hormones, Function and Target Organ(s)

Hormone	Target Organ(s)	Key Function
Prolactin (PRL)	Mammary glands, ovaries	Milk production, estrogen/progesterone secretion
Growth hormone (GH)	Liver, adipose tissue	Growth promotion
Adrenocorticotropic hormone (ACTH)	Adrenal gland	Secretion of glucocorticoids, mineralocorticoids, and sex corticoids
Luteinizing hormone (LH)	Gonads	Sex-hormone production
Follicle-stimulating hormone (FSH)	Gonads	Reproductive system growth (ovarian follicles growth, spermatogenesis)
Thyroid-stimulating hormone (TSH)	Thyroid gland	Secretion of thyroid hormones

Table 16.2 Posterior Pituitary Hormones, Function and Target Organ(s)

Hormone	Production Location	Target Organ(s)	Key Function
Antidiuretic hormone (ADH; vasopressin)	Hypothalamic paraventricular nucleus	Kidneys (collecting ducts)	Stimulates water reabsorption
Oxytocin	Hypothalamic supraoptic nucleus	Uterus, mammary glands	Females: Promotes contractions during labor, milk ejection

Table 16.3 Overview of Hormone Axes and Effects

Hypothalamus Releasing Hormone	Pituitary Hormone	Target	Effects
		Anterior Pituitary	
GnRH	LH	Gonads	Stimulation of sex-hormone production
GnRH	FSH	Gonads	Stimulation of follicle growth (female) and spermatogenesis (male)
TRH	TSH	Thyroid gland	Metabolism regulation through stimulation of thyroid hormone release
PRH	PRL	Mammary glands	Promotion of milk production
GHRH	GH	Liver, bone, muscle	Stimulation of growth and metabolism through production of insulin-like growth factors (IGF) at targets
CRH	ACTH	Adrenal glands	Regulation of metabolism and stress through production of glucocorticoids
		Posterior Pituitary	
Hypothalamus Releasing Hormone	**Pituitary Hormone**	**Target**	**Effects**
ADH	ADH storage	Renal collecting ducts	Water reabsorption
—*	OT	Uterus, mammary glands	Promotes uterine contractions during labor, milk ejection

**Oxytocin does not have a hypothalamic releasing hormone; it is produced in the hypothalamus and stored in the posterior pituitary.*
ACTH, adrenocorticotropic hormone; ADH, antidiuretic hormone, vasopressin; CRH, corticotropin-releasing hormone; FSH, follicle-stimulating hormone; GH, growth hormone; GHRH, GH-releasing hormone; GnRH, gonadotropin-releasing hormone; LH, luteinizing hormone; OT, oxytocin; PRH, prolactin-releasing hormone; PRL, prolactin; TRH, thyrotropin-releasing hormone; TSH, thyroid-stimulating hormone.

- Thyroid hormone regulation of the TRH-TSH axis
- Cortisol regulation of CRH-ACTH axis
- Gonadal steroid regulation of the GnRH-LH/FSH axis
- Insulin-like growth factor-1 (IGF-1) regulation of the GHRH-GH axis

All of these pathways, or axes, include both positive and negative components. For example, Figure 16.2 displays the impact of cortisol on the CRH-ACTH axis. Small increases in circulating cortisol levels cause decreased production of CRH by the hypothalamus and decreased release of ACTH

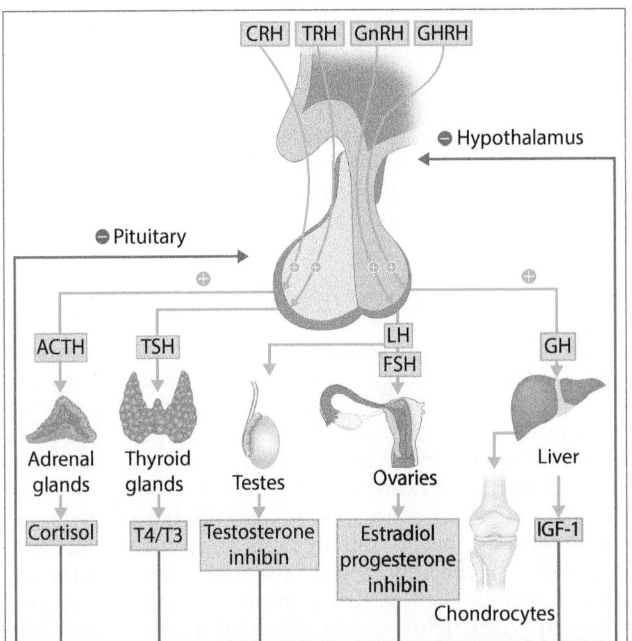

Figure 16.1 Examples of negative feedback loop. ACTH, adrenocorticotropic hormone; CRH, corticotropin-releasing hormone; FSH, follicle-stimulating hormone; GH, growth hormone; GHRH, GH-releasing hormone; GnRH, gonadotropin-releasing hormone; IGF-1, insulin-like growth factor 1; LH, luteinizing hormone; T3, triiodothyronine; T4, thyroxine; TRH, thyrotropin-releasing hormone; TSH, thyroid-stimulating hormone.

by the anterior pituitary. These decreased hormone levels signal the adrenal glands to decrease cortisol production (negative feedback). Likewise, a decrease in circulating cortisol level results in an upregulation of the axis causing increased levels of CRH and ACTH and resulting in increased adrenal production of cortisol to restore homeostasis. Disruption of feedback loops can occur for many reasons. Exposure to exogenous steroid, such as dexamethasone, will downregulate the CRH-ACTH axis in the same way increased circulating cortisol will. Because of this, low-dose (1 mg) dexamethasone suppression testing is a common screening test when hypercortisolism is suspected as the administration of 1 mg exogenous dexamethasone should result in decreased cortisol production. If cortisol levels remain elevated despite the administration of dexamethasone, endogenous overproduction of cortisol can be confirmed. Additionally, endogenous excess cortisol production from an adrenal adenoma can result in the same downregulation of the CRH-ACTH system while maintaining elevated cortisol levels. Likewise, a pituitary adenoma can cause increased ACTH production, resulting in increased cortisol production despite an otherwise normal functioning adrenal gland. Because of these feedback loops, dysfunction at the hypothalamic or pituitary level causes disruption of target organ function as well, and levels of circulating hormones from the hypothalamus, pituitary gland, and target organ can together be used to determine the level of disruption of the axis. The specifics of these scenarios will be further discussed in the following sections of this chapter.

Positive feedback control is far less common, with the hallmark example being the role of OT in labor. As the fetus pushes against the mother's cervix, nerve impulses are sent to the hypothalamus triggering the release of OT from the mother's posterior pituitary gland, where it is stored after being produced in the hypothalamus. Estrogen that is released during labor from the ovaries induces OT receptors on the uterus and stimulates uterine contraction and the production of prostaglandins from the placenta. Prostaglandins

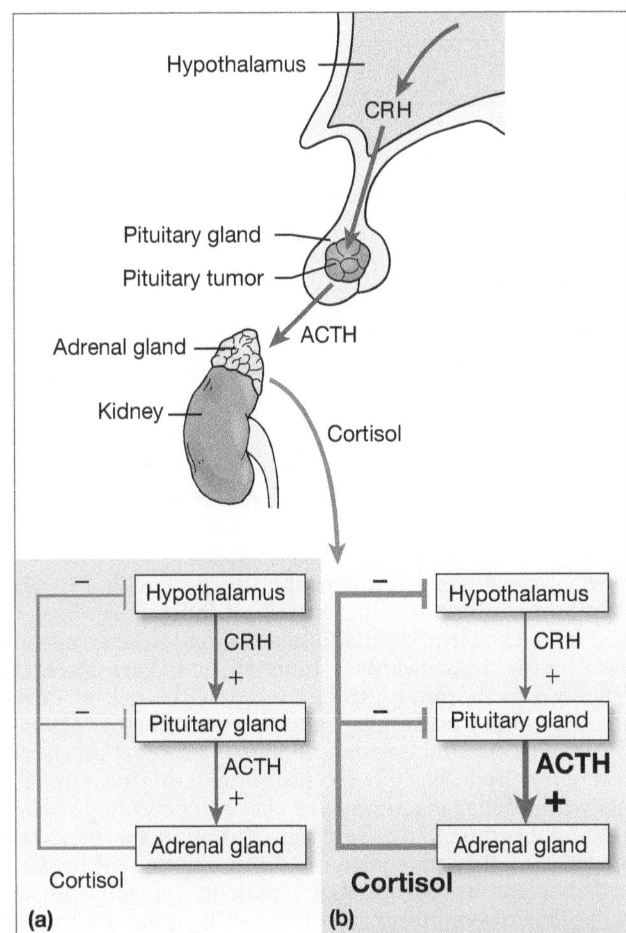

Figure 16.2 ACTH-stimulated cortisol production. The HPA axis and negative feedback. (a) In the normal HPA axis, hypothalamic CRH stimulates pituitary release of ACTH, resulting in stimulation of cortisol synthesis and secretion, and growth promotion of all of the adrenal gland layers. Cortisol also provides negative feedback to the pituitary and hypothalamus, inhibiting excessive ACTH and CRH secretion. (b) In Cushing disease, an ACTH-secreting pituitary adenoma continuously secretes supranormal amounts of ACTH, driving adrenal gland hyperplasia and excessive cortisol secretion. Negative feedback via increased cortisol inhibits hypothalamic CRH secretion, but is ineffective at reducing ACTH secretion from the autonomously activated tumor cells. ACTH, adrenocorticotropic hormone; CRH, corticotropin-releasing hormone; HPA, hypothalamic-pituitary-adrenal.
(Source: Yedinak C, Hurtado CR, Leung AM, et al. Endocrine system. In: Tkacs NC, Hermann LL, Johnson RL, eds. Advanced Physiology and Pathophysiology. *Springer Publishing Company; 2020:677.)*

stimulate additional uterine contractions as well as the release of more OT from the posterior pituitary gland (positive feedback). Additionally, the release of OT stimulates myoepithelial cell contraction in the breast and milk ejection. Once the infant is born, suckling reinforces this positive feedback loop, resulting in continued OT release (Figure 16.3).

16.1A ADENOMA

MEDICAL HISTORY AND CLINICAL PRESENTATION

Approximately 90% of sellar masses in adults over the age of 30 are pituitary adenomas, which make up about 10% of all intracranial neoplasms. Pituitary adenomas are benign

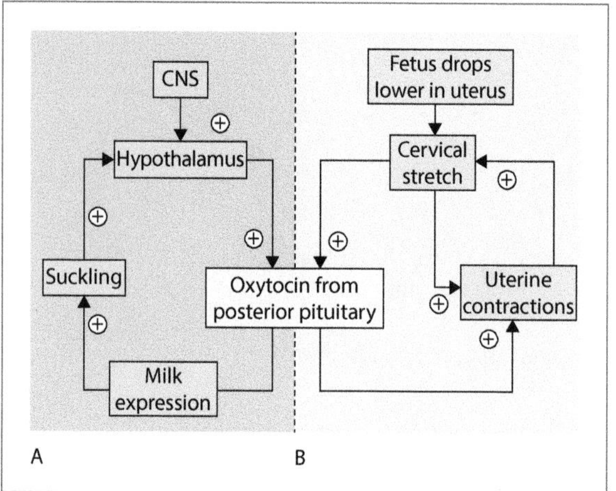

Figure 16.3 Positive feedback loop for oxytocin. CNS, central nervous system.

tumors of the anterior pituitary and present with a myriad of symptoms given the impact on multiple hormones released from the pituitary gland in addition to the symptoms caused by the mass itself (see Table 16.1). In rare cases, the following genetic mutations can increase the risk of developing a pituitary adenoma: multiple endocrine neoplasia-1 (MEN1), guanine nucleotide stimulatory protein (Gs-alpha), and andaryl hydrocarbon receptor-interacting protein. Patients with a sellar mass may present with neurologic symptoms and hormonal dysregulation (usually due to excess disorders), or they may remain asymptomatic and be diagnosed incidentally. Symptomatic patients typically present complaining of symptoms associated with pituitary hormone hypersecretion or visual defects due to mechanical pressure from the tumor on the optic chiasm (Table 16.4). In rare cases, macroadenomas can cause mechanical compression of the posterior pituitary resulting in decreased ADH (vasopressin) release. If sustained, this can result in the development of diabetes insipidus (DI), a condition characterized by polydipsia and high volumes of very dilute urine (see Section 16.1C). Over 80% of individuals with nonfunctioning adenomas (typically gonadotroph adenomas) present with a complaint of impaired vision in the temporal fields due to suprasellar extension of the mass, which results in compression of the optic chiasm. This specific pattern of visual loss, called bitemporal heminopia, may result in varying degrees of deficiency in each eye. Any unexplained pattern of visual deficiency should be further evaluated for a sellar mass. Because of the slow growth rate of most tumors, and therefore the slow onset of symptoms, patients may delay seeking treatment for months to years.

SIGNS AND SYMPTOMS

Because of the multiple target organs of pituitary hormones, the presence of pituitary adenomas can cause a variety of presenting symptoms. Table 16.4 reveals the key presenting symptoms associated with each classification of pituitary adenoma. Gonadotroph adenomas are typically considered nonfunctioning adenomas and rarely present with symptoms associated with hormone (LH, FSH) hypersecretion; because of this, visual impairment caused by mechanical compression of the adenoma on the optic chiasm is the leading chief complaint. Bitemporal heminopia (decreased vision in the temporal fields) is the most common visual disturbance resulting from this mechanical compression. Rarely, patients with pituitary adenomas, specifically gonadotroph adenomas, present with gonadotropin deficiency, which presents as hypogonadism. In males, hypogonadism is characterized by erectile dysfunction and in women by changes in menstruation (typically secondary amenorrhea). In both men and women, hypogonadism can cause decreased libido, fatigue, hot flashes, muscle weakness, and irritability. In addition to the findings in Table 16.4, neurologic symptoms more general to sellar masses are frequently found. The onset of headaches, diplopia, pituitary apoplexy, cerebrospinal fluid (CSF) rhinorrhea, and Parinaud syndrome should all be further investigated for the possible presence of a sellar mass, specifically a pituitary adenoma.

PHYSICAL EXAMINATION

Similar to the presenting signs and symptoms, physical examination findings will vary with adenoma type. See Table 16.4 for associated clinical findings.

Table 16.4 Adenoma Type, Excess Anterior Pituitary Hormone, Clinical Findings and Associated Conditions

Adenoma Classification	Hormone in Excess	Clinical Findings	Associated Condition
Prolactinomas or lactotroph	Prolactin (PRL)	Women: amenorrhea, galactorrhea, decreased libido, infertility, osteoporosis; Men: gynecomastia, erectile dysfunction, decreased libido, infertility, osteoporosis	–
Somatotroph	Growth hormone (GH)	Children: rapid growth, joint pain, increased sweating; Adults: skull, hand, and feet growth, voice deepening, joint pain, increased sweating	Children: acromegaly Adults: gigantism
Corticotroph	Adrenocorticotropic hormone (ACTH)	Central adiposity, abdominal striae, hirsutism, acne, buffalo hump	Cushing disease
Gonadotroph	Luteinizing hormone (LH)/ Follicle-stimulating hormone (FSH)	Women: irregular menstruation; Men: low testosterone, decreased libido*	–
Thyrotroph	Thyroid-stimulating hormone (TSH)	Palpitations, menstrual irregularities (females), heat intolerance, tachycardia, insomnia	Secondary hyperthyroidism

**Many patients remain asymptomatic, and these adenomas are considered nonfunctional.*

DIFFERENTIAL DIAGNOSIS

The differential diagnosis includes craniopharyngioma, lactotroph hyperplasia (during pregnancy), meningiomas, and malignant tumors (primary or metastatic).

DIAGNOSTIC STUDIES

Diagnostic studies are useful in further classifying neoplasms into microadenomas (<1 cm) or macroadenomas (>1 cm). Furthermore, as adenomas can arise from any cell type found in the anterior pituitary, six subclassifications exist (see Table 16.4 for associated clinical findings):

- Gonadotroph adenomas
- Thyrotroph adenomas
- Corticotroph adenomas
- Lactotroph adenomas
- Somatotroph adenomas
- Lactotroph/somatotroph adenomas

MRI is necessary for diagnosing a pituitary adenoma. If performed correctly, no additional confirmatory imaging is required. MRI typically reveals a large mass that extends outside the sella. MRI will differentiate an adenoma from other types of pituitary lesions as pituitary adenomas have a similar signal to that of other central nervous system (CNS) tissue. Craniopharyngiomas typically have low-intensity signals due to their cystic nature. Conversely, meningiomas produce a more homogeneous and brighter signaling that adenomas. Gadolinium-enhanced imaging is not indicated as pituitary adenomas, craniopharyngiomas, and meningiomas have similar degrees of uptake, making these masses indistinguishable. Lactotroph hyperplasia should only be considered during pregnancy.

In addition to imaging studies, hypothalamic-pituitary hormone function should also be evaluated, and laboratory tests vary based on the suspected adenoma type (Table 16.5).

EVALUATION

When a patient presents with clinical findings suggesting hormonal hypersecretion, associated screening lab tests should be ordered (see Table 16.6). It is important to differentiate between a pituitary versus a target organ cause of excess hormone secretion, and screening lab tests are straightforward in assisting with this differentiation. In a global perspective, if the hormones secreted from the target organ are elevated, stimulating hormones from the pituitary gland should be ordered. If there is a primary disease (stemming from the target organ), the target organ hormone will be elevated but the stimulating hormone from the pituitary will be appropriately downregulated and appear low. If there is secondary disease (stemming from the pituitary), both the target organ hormone and the pituitary stimulating hormone will remain elevated as the expected downregulation of the axis caused by excess circulating hormone is dysfunctional. Hypothalamic releasing hormones can be used to distinguish tertiary disease from secondary disease; if the problem occurs at the hypothalamic level, releasing hormones will also be elevated, but if it occurs in the pituitary, releasing hormones will be appropriately downregulated. For example, primary hypercortisolism due to adrenal hyperplasia can be responsible for excess cortisol secretion that will result in an elevated 24-hour urine cortisol level. Follow-up testing of ACTH levels will be decreased in a (failing) attempt to downregulate the adrenal gland function. Conversely, if both 24-hour urine cortisol and ACTH levels are elevated, dysfunction is coming from the pituitary, hypothalamus, or an ectopic ACTH-secreting tumor rather than the adrenal

Table 16.5 Hormonal Hypersecretion Screening Lab Tests by Adenoma Type

Adenoma Classification	Screening Lab Tests
Prolactinomas or lactotroph	Elevated serum prolactin
Somatotroph	Elevated insulin-like growth factor-1 (IGF-1)
Corticotroph	Elevated 24-hour urine cortisol with elevated adrenocorticotropic hormone (ACTH) concentration
Gonadotroph	Considered nonfunctioning and rarely raise serum gonadotropin (luteinizing hormone [LH], follicle-stimulating hormone [FSH]) concentrations
Thyrotroph	Elevated serum free thyroxine (T4) and triiodothyronine (T3) with inappropriately elevated thyroid-stimulating hormone (TSH)

Table 16.6 Percentage of Patients With Signs and Symptoms of Acromegaly

Clinical Sign or Symptom	Percentage of Patients With Acromegaly Affected
Facial changes, soft tissue swelling	100
Excessive sweating	83
Carpal tunnel syndrome	68
Tiredness, lethargy	53
Headaches	53
Oligo- or amenorrhea or infertility (in women)	55
Erectile dysfunction or decreased libido (in men)	42
Arthropathy	37
Impaired glucose tolerance or overt diabetes	37
Goiter	35
Ear, nose, throat, and dental problems	32
Congestive heart failure or arrhythmias	25
Hypertension	23
Visual field defects (primarily bitemporal heminopia)	17

Source: With permission from Carroll PV, Jenkins PJ. Acromegaly. In: Feingold KR, Anawalt B, Boyce A, et al, eds. Endotext. *MDText.com; 2017).*

gland. Elevated CRH levels will show the problem is stemming from the hypothalamus, whereas normal or decreased CRH levels will show the problem is stemming from the pituitary gland or an ectopic tumor. In this situation, an MRI or inferior petrosal sinus sampling is typically indicated to diagnose the cause of hypercortisolism. This same lab pattern holds true in reverse for hyposecretion (discussed in Section 16.5).

Given the frequency of the adenoma's extension beyond the sella, evaluation of the mass in relation to the optic chiasm and cavernous sinuses should also be performed. It is recommended that all adenomas >1 cm be evaluated with MRI, visual field testing, and hormone hypersecretion and hyposecretion biochemical evaluation.

TREATMENT

- Asymptomatic incidentalomas do not typically require treatment, but monitoring should be continued.
- Most pituitary adenomas require transsphenoidal resection, resulting in hormonal insufficiency in approximately 7% to 20% of patients.
  - Intraoperative and perioperative glucocorticoids may be needed until adrenal function returns to normal.
  - Close monitoring of fluid intake and output, serum sodium, and urine osmolality should be performed in the days following surgery as patients are at an increased risk of experiencing syndrome of inappropriate antidiuretic hormone secretion (SIADH) and/or DI (see Section 16.1C).
  - Postoperative rhinorrhea should be tested for beta transferrin to rule out a CSF leak.
- Lactotroph adenomas may initially be treated with dopamine agonists in attempts to lower prolactin levels. Transsphenoidal resection should be performed when dopamine agonists produce intolerable side effects, symptoms persist despite treatment, or in female patients who desire to become pregnant.
- With persistent or recurrent disease, repeat resection is often indicated.

PATIENT EDUCATION

- The patient and family should be educated that the prognosis for pituitary adenomas is very good and that transsphenoidal resection is relatively low risk and often successful in treating the condition.
- Postoperative follow-up will be important, and the patient should be made aware of common signs and symptoms of hormone hypersecretion and hyposecretion and advised to return to clinic if signs and symptoms present.

16.1B ACROMEGALY

MEDICAL HISTORY AND CLINICAL PRESENTATION

Acromegaly is defined by the hypersecretion of GH from the anterior pituitary gland, typically as a result of a benign pituitary adenoma. Other, very infrequent causes of acromegaly include excessive ectopic GHRH from a peripheral neuroendocrine tumor or from excessive hypothalamic GHRH secretion. The normal negative feedback pathway that regulates GH secretion includes hypothalamic secretion of GHRH leading to pituitary release of GH and hepatic release of IGF-1. GH also has direct effects on bone, muscle, and adipose tissues (Figure 16.4). Ghrelin is a GH secretagogue found in highest concentrations in the stomach. Ghrelin levels decrease after eating and increase with fasting, leading endocrinologists to believe that the increased GH levels measured during fasting and overnight can be partially attributed to ghrelin regulation. GH secretion is also closely linked to other hormone systems by mechanisms that are still not fully understood (Table 16.7).

When excess GH is secreted in childhood, before growth plates have closed, gigantism results. When this occurs in adulthood, after the closing of growth plates, the result is acromegaly. If multiple family members are affected, genetic testing may be indicated as genetic causes of acromegaly make up about 5% of all cases and include MEN1 syndrome, McCune-Albright syndrome, familial acromegaly,

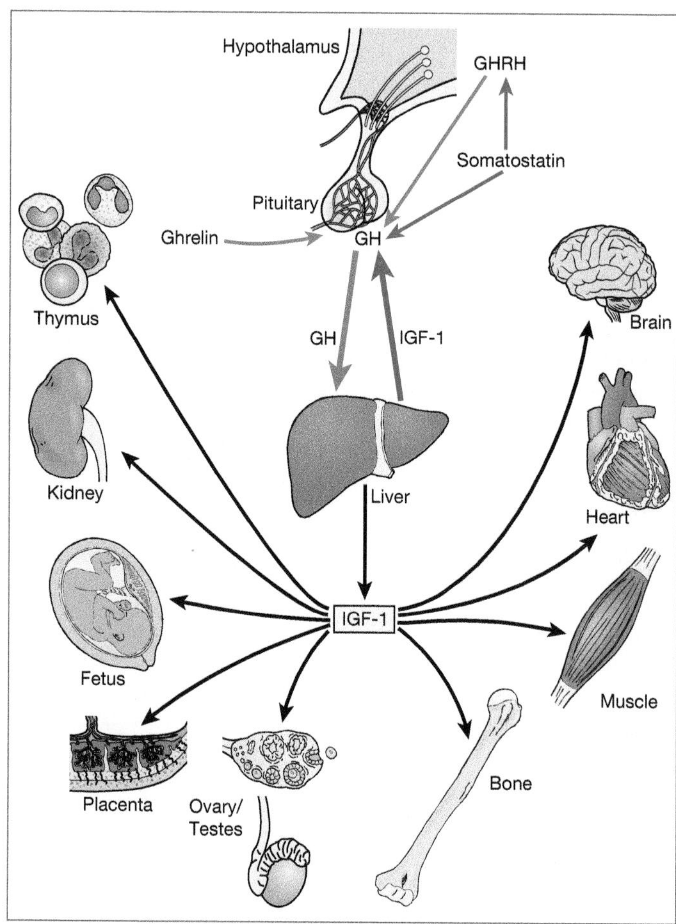

Figure 16.4 **Effects of growth hormone. GH has wide-ranging effects beginning with prenatal growth and development of the placenta, fetal growth and development, and maintenance of thymus, kidney, gonads, heart, and brain. The most pronounced effects of GH on development and maintenance are on bone and muscle. Linear growth in childhood is dependent on GH stimulation, and GH deficiency is associated with short stature, whereas GH excess in children is associated with attainment of extreme height. Many GH effects are mediated by IGF-1, produced by the liver in response to GH stimulation.** IGF-1, insulin-like growth factor 1; GH, growth hormone; GHRH, GH-releasing hormone.

(Source: Yedinak C, Hurtado CR, Leung AM, et al. Endocrine system. In: Tkacs NC, Hermann LL, Johnson RL, eds. Advanced Physiology and Pathophysiology. *Springer Publishing Company; 2020:681.)*

Table 16.7 Peripheral Hormone Regulation of Growth Hormone Secretion

Associated Condition	Impact on Growth Hormone (GH) Secretion
Hypothyroidism	Reduced GH and insulin-like growth factor 1 (IGF-1)
Cushing syndrome (or exogenous corticosteroid use)	Reduced GH secretion
Hyperglycemia	Reduced GH secretion
Hypoglycemia	Increased GH secretion
Puberty	Increased GH secretion

Carney syndrome, and familial isolated pituitary adenoma (FIPA). The incidence and prevalence of acromegaly worldwide are 3 to 4 cases per 1 million population per year and 60 per 1 million, respectively; in 2017, this translated to approximately 1,500 cases across the United States. Men and women are equally affected, with typical age of onset between 20 and 40 years. The condition was first formally identified and named in 1886 by Pierre Marie, using the Greek words of akron (extremities) and megas (large).[1]

Acromegaly typically presents slowly, with growth occurring over a period of years. Patients typically present complaining of a change in facial features; increased hand, head or feet size; or fatigue.

SIGNS AND SYMPTOMS

As the majority of GH-secreting benign pituitary adenomas are >1 cm in diameter, they are classified as macroadenomas. Given their size, macroadenomas often present with symptoms of mass effect that are unrelated to the presence of increased GH levels and include headache, hydrocephalus, bitemporal heminopia, and ophthalmoplegia. About 25% of patients with acromegaly will have galactorrhea due to coexistent excess prolactin secretion. A delay in diagnosis of several years is common as symptoms typically present very slowly. Changes in facial features over time is a common presenting clinical symptom, primarily consisting of broadening of the nose, thickening of the lips, and increased spacing between front teeth. Frequently, hands, head, and feet are enlarged, and patients may report hats, gloves, rings, or shoes no longer fitting. Joint pain presents due to accelerated joint degeneration along with frequent median nerve neuropathy resulting in carpal tunnel syndrome. Muscular hypertrophy with simultaneous weakening has also been noted. Cardiac enlargement (cardiomegaly) and colon enlargement have been well documented, but analysis of additional organ enlargement has shown mixed results. Patients may complain of excessive fatigue as a result of sleep apnea, a common comorbid condition in patients with acromegaly. Table 16.6 highlights the frequency of various clinical signs and symptoms in patients with acromegaly.

PHYSICAL EXAMINATION

Physical examination of a patient with acromegaly will most notably reveal "soft, dough-like" skin over the face, palms, and soles of the feet. Characteristic, prominent facial findings also exist, including lower lip and nose enlargement, wide-spacing teeth, enlarged pores and increased acne, thickening of the eyelids, prominent tongue, and cutis verticis gyrata (thick folds on the scalp resembling gyri). Additionally, examination may reveal skin tags, excessive hair growth, hypertension, and galactorrhea. The airway should be evaluated for possible obstruction.

DIFFERENTIAL DIAGNOSIS

See Table 16.8 for summary of the differential diagnosis for acromegaly.

DIAGNOSTIC STUDIES

Because of the pulsatile nature of the release of GH, single sampling of circulating hormone levels is ineffective in measuring GH. Additionally, measuring urine levels of GH is also ineffective as there are multiple situations and comorbid conditions that can increase normal circulating levels of GH including sleep, malnutrition, periods of fasting, stress, exercise, hypoglycemia, uncontrolled type 1 diabetes mellitus, and cirrhosis of the liver.[1] Serum IGF-1 levels are accepted as a marker of serum GH concentration and are preferred for screening patients who have a prior diagnosis of acromegaly. Additional consideration should be given to patients who are pregnant as IGF-1 levels will naturally be two to three times above normal. Additionally, increased age, poorly controlled diabetes, liver disease, and kidney disease can all cause a decline in IGF-1 levels.[2] GH is used to confirm the diagnosis of acromegaly with failure of a GH suppression test: 75 g oral glucose load is given and within 1–2

Table 16.8 Differential Diagnosis for Acromegaly

Differential Diagnosis	Description
Familial tall structure	Patients are proportionately tall and have grown along a consistent growth curve throughout developmental years.
Beckwith-Wiedemann syndrome	Present with macroglossia, enlarged adrenal glands, macrosomia, and abdominal wall defects.
Marfan syndrome	Autosomal dominant. Clinical features include tall, thin body habitus, disproportionately long extremities and fingers, visual defects.
Pseudoacromegaly	Seen in patients with severe insulin resistance. Patients present with the clinical features of acromegaly but lack elevated growth hormone (GH) or insulin-like growth factor 1 (IGF-1).
Pachydermoperiostosis syndrome	Clinical features include finger clubbing, enlargement of the extremities, hypertrophic skin changes, periosteal bone formation.

Note: Acromegaly should also be considered as one component of a larger diagnosis such as seen with Carney complex or McCune-Albright syndrome.

hours, GH fails to measure <0.04 mcg/L, indicating that the suppression attempt was not successful. Administering a glucose load should, through negative feedback, inhibit the release of GH. In the case of acromegaly, GH remains elevated despite the administration of an oral glucose load.

EVALUATION

Upon diagnosing acromegaly through a GH suppression test, MRI of the pituitary should be performed to determine the size and location of the pituitary adenoma. CT scan can be used if MRI is contraindicated but will not provide as sensitive results and may miss small adenomas. In the event that a pituitary adenoma is not detected, the much less common (<1%) presence of an ectopic source should be determined. Potential tumor sites should be evaluated with CT for diagnosis.

The patient should also be evaluated for common comorbid conditions by the associated screening test(s):

- **Hyperprolactinemia:** Prolactin levels
- **Insulin resistance/diabetes mellitus:** Hemoglobin A1c or oral glucose tolerance testing
- **Hyperthyroidism/hypothyroidism:** TSH and thyroxine (free T4)
- **Colon polyps/colon cancer:** Colonoscopy
- **Sexual dysfunction:** LH and FSH

If unmanaged, acromegaly can decrease life expectancy by 10 years when age-matched to a control population.

TREATMENT

The overarching goal of treatment of acromegaly is to reduce excess hormone production and associated symptoms.

- Transsphenoidal resection of the pituitary adenoma (if present) is considered first-line therapy. If successful, patients can begin to experience some symptom relief within days.
- If surgery is unsuccessful, medical management can be used.[2]
  - Somatostatin analogs (SSAs) reduce GH production, resulting in GH and IGF-1 level reduction up to 70%, and may reduce pituitary adenoma size by 50%. They are sometimes used prior to surgical resection in patients with particularly large adenomas.
  - GH receptor antagonists (GHRAs) interfere with GH action and result in normal IGF-1 levels in up to 90% of patients. GHRAs have no impact on lowering GH levels.
  - Dopamine agonists are considered third-line medication therapy as they are effective in only a minority of patients.
- After resection and medication management, patients who remain symptomatic may undergo radiation therapy.

PATIENT EDUCATION

- Acromegaly has little impact on life expectancy when well managed.
- Many comorbid conditions could be a result of acromegaly, increasing the motivation to properly diagnose and treat the condition.
- First-line therapy is typically surgical removal of the tumor (pituitary adenoma).

16.1C DIABETES INSIPIDUS

MEDICAL HISTORY AND CLINICAL PRESENTATION

DI, although closely related by name to diabetes mellitus (discussed in Section 16.7), is a completely independent condition. DI is further classified as central DI (CDI) or nephrogenic DI based on the pathophysiology of the disease. Despite physiologic differences, both conditions are a result of decreased levels of ADH, also called arginine vasopressin (AVP), leading to polyuria and increased thirst. ADH helps to concentrate urine, so in the absence of adequate ADH, due to either decreased secretion or increased resistance, the result is large volumes of very dilute urine.

There are two known receptor sites for ADH: V1 and V2. V1 is responsible for vasoconstriction and increased prostaglandin release while V2 manages antidiuretic response, peripheral vasodilation and endothelial cells release of factor VIIIc and von Willebrand factor.[3] In broad terms, CDI results from a dysfunction in the brain and nephrogenic DI results from a dysfunction in the kidney. In CDI, there are many possible locations of dysfunction responsible for contributing to decreased ADH secretion: hypothalamic osmoreceptors, supraoptic or paraventricular nuclei, superior portion of the supraopticohypophyseal tract.[4]

In about half of patients with CDI there is no known cause; however, current research suggests an autoimmune process may be involved in the destruction of ADH-secreting cells located in the hypothalamic nuclei.[5] When the cause can be found, primary or secondary tumors, infiltrative diseases such as Langerhans cell histiocytosis, transsphenoidal resection of a sellar mass, or trauma are typically to blame.[6] There are a few familial and congenital disorders that can lead to the development of CDI: familial CDI, Wolfram syndrome, congenital hypopituitarism, and septo-optic dysplasia. During pregnancy, the placenta releases increased amounts of vasopressinase, an enzyme that catabolizes ADH, which can lead to the initial diagnosis of disease or exacerbate existing symptoms of known disease.

Nephrogenic DI, like CDI, typically presents with polyuria but in these patients, hypothalamic production of ADH is maintained, and dysfunction occurs in the renal response to circulating ADH, most frequently a result of increased resistance to ADH in the collecting tubules.[4] There are multiple possible causes of nephrogenic DI:

- Decreased renal function seen with increased age, illness or chronic kidney disease (CKD)
- Hereditary (X-linked) nephrogenic DI resulting in vasopressin V2 receptor gene mutations
- Lithium toxicity
- Hypercalcemia
- Hypokalemia
- Pregnancy (gestational diabetes insipidus)

Any patient presenting with polyuria should be further evaluated for DI.

SIGNS AND SYMPTOMS

Polyuria is the hallmark symptom of DI, with output in some patients reaching up to 15 quarts per day (average adult output is usually 1 to 2 quarts per day). Patients present complaining of polyuria, including nocturia, and as a result, increased thirst. As patients are typically mildly hypernatremic due to excessive urine losses, the thirst response remains present in attempt to compensate. In advanced disease, patients may also present with decreased bone mineral density (BMD), but the relation of ADH to bone loss is still largely unclear. Pediatric patients may not be able to voice their symptoms as well, so parents should be aware of an increase in very heavy or wet diapers, nocturnal enuresis, or increased thirst.

PHYSICAL EXAMINATION

Physical examination should include evaluation for dehydration including decreased weight, decreased skin turgor, increased capillary refill time, dry oral mucosa, orthostatic hypotension, and tachycardia. Mental status is usually unaffected. Physical exam can aid in ruling out other possible causes of polyuria or polydipsia. Patients with new-onset diabetes mellitus may also present with polydipsia; patients with type 2 diabetes mellitus (T2DM) may be overweight or obese and have thick, dark patches of skin (acanthosis nigricans) and patients with new-onset type 1 diabetes may appear cachectic. Benign prostatic hypertrophy as a cause for polyuria can be evaluated with digital rectal exam revealing a smooth, diffusely enlarged prostate. Primary polydipsia is a diagnosis of exclusion that can be made after ruling out other possible causes of increased fluid intake.

DIFFERENTIAL DIAGNOSIS

See Table 16.9 for summary of differential diagnosis of DI.

Additional secondary causes of polydipsia and polyuria should also be ruled out including CKD, drug use, primary or secondary tumors, and Langerhans cell histiocytosis.

DIAGNOSTIC STUDIES

The presence of polyuria should be confirmed in all patients who present complaining of increased urinary output and thirst (Figure 16.5). Polyuria is confirmed when output exceeds 50 mL/kg/24 hours or >3–4 L/day. Once confirmed, urine osmolality should be measured; a diagnosis of hypotonic polyuria is defined as <800 mOsm/kg. Normal or high serum sodium (≥146 mmol/L) along with plasma osmolality of ≥300 mOsm/kg are highly indicative of either CDI or nephrogenic DI, and sometimes a diagnosis can be made at this stage of testing. If the diagnosis remains unclear, water deprivation testing, baseline plasma copeptin levels, and hypertonic saline infusion testing can be used to diagnose and differentiate DI.[7] Patients with DI are typically euvolemic with mild hypernatremia; however, patients who are unable to freely access water to match their increased thirst may have severe hypernatremia. This can be seen in both children and elderly patients with concurrent dementia.

Although most cases of CDI are idiopathic, MRI can be helpful in determining a cause if present. With autoimmune destruction, which remains the likely cause of many idiopathic cases of CDI, MRI typically reveals thickening of the pituitary stalk and posterior pituitary. Although this is a suggestive finding, it is nonspecific and should not be used for diagnosis.

Table 16.9 Differential Diagnosis of Diabetes Insipidus

Differential Diagnosis	Description
Diabetes mellitus	Must be ruled out as a cause of polydipsia and polyuria, which result from osmotic diuresis
Benign prostatic hypertrophy (in men)	Must be ruled out as a cause of urinary frequency, although total daily volume output is typically normal
Primary polydipsia	Patients intake excessive amounts of water with no known physiologic stimulus to increased intake.

EVALUATION

Once a patient's sodium level becomes normal and the patient is no longer symptomatic while taking desmopressin, monitoring of serum sodium should occur every 6 to 12 months. If at any point while taking desmopressin symptoms begin to return, a 24-hour urine test is necessary to capture total volume output.

TREATMENT

Treatment is aimed at reducing symptoms of polyuria, polydipsia, and nocturia.

Central Diabetes Insipidus

- Desmopressin, typically taken before bed, is the preferred first-line treatment.
  - If excessive fluid intake continues, hyponatremia may result due to nonsuppressible ADH activity.
  - Serum sodium should be measured at 2 days after initiation and again at 4 days if normal.[8]
- In very mild cases or when a patient is resistant to taking desmopressin, thiazide diuretics may be used.
- Low-solute diets (low-sodium, low-protein) are rarely used. If warranted, they are typically used in combination with a thiazide diuretic.
- In infants and small children, subcutaneous desmopressin or diluted intranasal desmopressin administered buccally may be necessary.
- Individuals who either do not have an intact thirst mechanism or who do not have free access to water for adequate replacement may require intravenous (IV) dextrose and water. Administering fluids without dextrose may result in central pontine hemolysis.

Nephrogenic Diabetes Insipidus

- The decision to treat is managed on an individual level depending heavily on the patient's symptoms, as thirst typically increases intake enough to maintain plasma sodium levels in a near-normal range.
- Treatment typically consists of a low-sodium, low-protein diet in combination with nonsteroidal anti-inflammatory drugs (NSAIDs) and/or a thiazide diuretic.
- If cause can be attributed to medication use, a medication change should be considered.
- In infants, water should be made accessible throughout the day.
- If ADH resistance is a primary cause, intranasal desmopressin may help relieve symptoms.

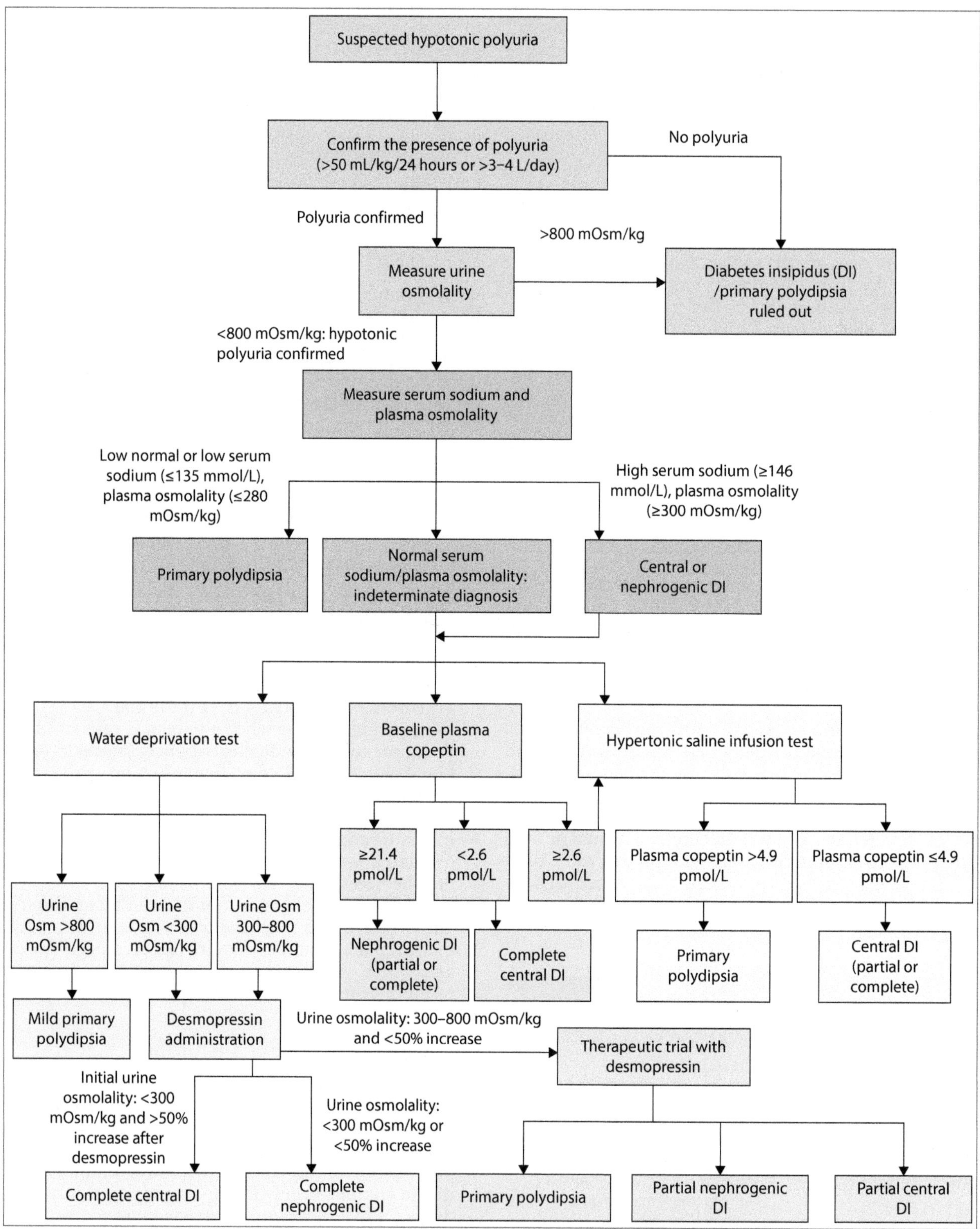

Figure 16.5 **Approach to suspected hypotonic polyuria.**

PATIENT EDUCATION

- Patients treated with desmopressin should be well-informed of the early signs and symptoms of hyponatremia (nausea, vomiting, headache).
- Medication (desmopressin) will need to be continued as long as the patient remains symptomatic.
- Fluid restriction to reduce urinary output should be avoided in all patients.

16.1D ACHONDROPLASIA

MEDICAL HISTORY AND CLINICAL PRESENTATION

Dwarfism, sometimes referred to as "short stature" or "little people," is characterized by an adult height of <4 feet 10 inches and further categorized into disproportionate dwarfism and proportionate dwarfism. GH deficiency is a common cause of proportionate dwarfism. Achondroplasia, the most common form of disproportionate dwarfism, is a chondrodysplasia resulting from a mutation in fibroblast growth factor receptor 3 (*FGFR3*) gene (100% penetrance) from either a sporadic mutation (80% of cases) or autosomal dominant inheritance (20% of cases). The condition affects 1:26,000–1:28,000 live births.[9] The name achondroplasia, meaning "without cartilage formation," is a misnomer for the actual pathophysiologic process occurring with the condition.[9] The problem occurs with ossification, the conversion of cartilage to bone, not with the presence or absence of cartilage itself. This dysfunction in ossification occurs most notably in the long bones of the arms and legs, leading to the hallmark disproportionate short stature. Individuals with achondroplasia present with short stature, attributed primarily to short extremities as trunk size remains average. The condition is typically diagnosed in infancy. Infants may present with hypotonia accompanied by atypical and delayed reaching of motor milestones. Adult females reach an average height of 4 feet 1 inch and adult males reach an average height of 4 feet 4 inches. Despite the many characteristic physical findings, individuals typically maintain normal intelligence.

SIGNS AND SYMPTOMS

Achondroplasia should be considered in any individual of short stature with disproportionately short arms and legs, especially those who have a family history of the condition (Box 16.1). In infancy, patients typically present with hypotonia, disproportionately short arms and legs, macrocephaly, and short fingers.

PHYSICAL EXAMINATION

Key findings for physical examination for a patient with achondroplasia include an average-size trunk, disproportionately short arms and legs, macrocephaly with forehead prominence, and trident appearance of the hands characterized by divergence of digits three and four. As there are many possible health complications that can result from the physical abnormalities found in patients, special attention must be given during exams (Box 16.2). Given the increased frequency of ear infections in adult patients due to midface hypoplasia, otoscope exam should always be performed when a patient presents with sinus congestion or cold-like symptoms. A complete and thorough musculoskeletal exam should also be performed given the high incidence of orthopedic malformations.

BOX 16.1 Common Signs and Symptoms of Achondroplasia Presenting at Any Age

Short extremities
Average-size trunk
Macrocephaly
Elbow extension limitation
Brachydactyly
Trident hand formation

Source: Data from Legare JM. Achondroplasia. In: Adam MP, Ardinger HH, Pagon RA, et al, eds. GeneReviews. *University of Washington; 1993–2019. https://www.ncbi.nlm.nih.gov/books/NBK1152*

BOX 16.2 Medical Conditions Frequently Associated With Achondroplasia

Apnea
Obesity
Acute otitis media
Lordosis
Genu varum
Kyphosis
Lumbago
Spinal stenosis

Source: Data from Genetics Home Reference, National Institutes of Health. Achondroplasia. https://ghr.nlm.nih.gov/condition/achondroplasia

DIFFERENTIAL DIAGNOSIS

Table 16.10 summarizes the differential diagnosis for achondroplasia.[10,11]

DIAGNOSTIC STUDIES

Physical examination findings of characteristic features is the first step in diagnosing a patient with achondroplasia (Box 16.2; Table 16.10). Once suspected, x-ray images may reveal[9]: short and robust tubular bones, narrowing of the interpedicular distance of the caudal spine, square ilia and horizontal acetabula, narrow sacrosciatic notch, proximal femoral radiolucency, and mild and generalized metaphyseal changes. Individuals who have both the characteristic physical examination findings as well as the suggestive radiographic findings require no further testing for diagnosis. If diagnosis is still unclear, genetic testing to identify the presence of a mutation in the *FGFR3* gene can be performed.

EVALUATION

After the diagnosis of achondroplasia is made, the extent of disease must be established as clinical manifestations vary

Table 16.10 Differential Diagnosis of Achondroplasia

Differential Diagnosis	Description
Thanatophoric dysplasia	Characterized by short limbs, redundant skin on extremities, narrow chest, lung underdevelopment, macrocephaly, wide-spaced eyes[10]
Hypochondroplasia	Possible overlap with radiographic and clinical phenotypes, also caused by variants of the fibroblast growth factor receptor 3 (*FGFR3*) gene
SADDAN syndrome	Characterized by *s*evere *a*chondroplasia, *d*evelopmental *d*elays, and *a*canthosis *n*igricans[11]

greatly among individuals. All patients should be referred to a genetic counselor, a neurologist, and a pediatric specialist well versed in managing chondrodysplasias. Patients should be regularly monitored for height, weight, and head circumference using achondroplasia-specific growth standards rather than the typical Centers for Disease Control and Prevention (CDC) growth standards, in addition to achondroplasia-specific developmental milestone timelines. Soon after birth, CT should be performed to visualize and evaluate the craniocervical junction to determine the likelihood of requiring decompression surgery as well as establish baseline ventricular size for future comparison if needed. Likewise, polysomnography should be performed to evaluate for apnea. Audiologic evaluation should be completed as a newborn, as with all newborns, and repeated again 1 year after birth. Any delays in development warrant a prompt referral to an audiologist for further evaluation and management.

TREATMENT

With achondroplasia, care is focused on the management of symptoms and associated conditions rather than treatment as the underlying cause is due to a genetic mutation that cannot be treated.[9]

- **Hydrocephalus:** Ventriculostomy shunting may be necessary.
- **Craniocervical junction constriction:** Suboccipital decompression may be necessary.
- **Obstruction sleep apnea:** Therapy includes adenotonsillectomy, positive airway pressure, weight reduction.
- **Middle ear dysfunction:** Maintain a high index of suspicion for ear infections; therapeutic options include tympanostomy tubes, referrals to audiology.
- **Short stature:** Exogenous use of GH and extended limb lengthening may be used, but remain highly controversial.
- **Obesity:** Routine dietary and exercise counseling; patients should be monitored using achondroplasia-specific growth charts.
- **Spinal and orthopedic deformities:** Adaptive braces can be used for posture, gait, and joint laxity.
- **Adaptive needs:** Once in school, all students should have an individualized education program (IEP). Examples include size-appropriate school desks, step stools, and weighted pens.
- **Immunizations:** All routine immunizations should be given along with increased emphasis on respiratory-related immunizations.
- **Socialization:** Support groups can be very helpful for both children and families.

PATIENT EDUCATION

- Children should remain in rear-facing car seats as long as height and weight restrictions allow because of the increased risk of neck injuries.
- Children should avoid activities that increase the risk of spinal cord injury at the craniocervical junction, as macrocephaly and weak ligaments pose an increased risk of injury. Examples include contact sports, jumping on trampolines, and hanging upside down from monkey bars.
- Pregnancy is possible and will always require cesarean delivery due to pelvic size of the mother. Genetic counseling should be highly recommended in the early stages of family planning.[9]

16.1E HYPOPITUITARISM

MEDICAL HISTORY AND CLINICAL PRESENTATION

Hypopituitarism is a broad term referring to decreased secretion of pituitary hormones. There are many possible causes of hypopituitarism and a universal decrease in function is called panhypopituitarism. One well-known cause of panhypopituitarism is Sheehan syndrome, which results from pituitary infarct after hemorrhage following childbirth. The most common causes of hypopituitarism are a pituitary adenoma or the result of surgical resection of a pituitary adenoma. In the case of a pituitary adenoma that causes excessive growth of one portion of the pituitary gland, mechanical compression of other regions of the gland can occur. This process can damage the pituitary gland and result in decreased hormone production from other regions of the pituitary gland. Other possible causes of pituitary dysfunction include trauma, neurosurgery, lack of oxygen due to cerebrovascular accident (CVA), and infections like meningitis or neurosyphilis. Developmental hypopituitarism can be seen in Kallmann syndrome, Bardet-Biedl syndrome, leptin receptor mutations, and Prader-Willi syndrome. Additionally, decreased hormone secretion from the pituitary gland can result from pituitary dysfunction or from improper secretion of hypothalamic-releasing hormones that typically signal pituitary hormone secretion. Hypothalamic-releasing hormones and corresponding pituitary hormones can be found in Table 16.3.

As opposed to pituitary adenomas that typically result in a variety of hypersecretion symptoms depending on which hormones are secreted in excess, the clinical presentation of hypopituitarism is highly dependent on the hormones that have decreased secretion. Given the relationship between the pituitary hormones and the function of the target organ discussed in the opening of this chapter (Figure 16.3), the clinical presentation of hypopituitarism typically mimics the clinical presentation of a decrease in the target organ function, making it difficult to differentiate primary versus secondary disease based on clinical presentation alone. In secondary hypothyroidism, for example, TSH levels are decreased, resulting in decreased stimulation of the thyroid gland. This leads to subsequent decrease in secretion of thyroid hormone, and the patient will present with symptoms of hypothyroidism. In primary hypothyroidism, TSH levels are elevated in attempts to stimulate the thyroid gland but the thyroid gland is not responding and unable to secrete the necessary amount of thyroid hormone, also resulting in

TABLE 16.11 Hormone-Specific Clinical Findings Associated With Pituitary Hormone Hyposecretion

		Anterior Pituitary
Hypothalamus Releasing Hormone	**Pituitary Hormone**	**Effects of Hyposecretion**
GnRH	LH	**Women**: irregular menstruation or amenorrhea, decreased libido, infertility **Men**: erectile dysfunction, decreased facial hair, weakness, decreased libido
GnRH	FSH	
TRH	TSH	Fatigue, weight gain, irregular menstruation (women), dry skin, increased cold sensitivity
PRH	PRL	Weakness, weight gain, anxiety or depression, decreased milk production (women)
GHRH	GH	**Child**: short stature, delayed puberty, lack of hair growth, immature facial features **Adult**: fatigue, central adiposity, insulin resistance, hair loss, decreased libido, decreased muscle mass
CRH	ACTH	Fatigue, weight loss, hypotension, hypoglycemia, salt cravings, GI discomfort
		Posterior Pituitary
Hypothalamus Releasing Hormone	**Pituitary Hormone**	**Effects of Hyposecretion**
ADH	ADH storage	Polyuria, polydipsia
-	OT	Changes in mood, decreased lactation (women)

ACTH, adrenocorticotropic hormone; ADH, antidiuretic hormone, vasopressin; CRH, corticotropin-releasing hormone; FSH, follicle-stimulating hormone; GH, growth hormone; GHRH, growth hormone-releasing hormone; GI, gastrointestinal; GnRH, gonadotropin-releasing hormone; LH, luteinizing hormone; OT, oxytocin; PRH, prolactin-releasing hormone; PRL, prolactin; TRH, thyrotropin-releasing hormone; TSH, thyroid-stimulating hormone.

symptoms of hypothyroidism. The clinical picture of these two patients would appear the same, both presenting with signs and symptoms of hypothyroidism, but the physiologic process leading to these symptoms differs. The rate at which pituitary cells are affected, the severity of hormonal deficiency, and the number of cells affected all impact the clinical presentation of disease.

SIGNS AND SYMPTOMS

Additional details regarding specific conditions associated with hyposecretion can be found throughout the chapter, but Table 16.11 summarizes these findings.

PHYSICAL EXAMINATION

Physical examination findings will vary depending on the pituitary hormones that are insufficient and the degree of insufficiency. The often insidious onset of the disease can result in vague physical examination findings. Individual chapter sections for disorders resulting from hormone deficiency should be referenced for specific physical examination findings.

DIAGNOSTIC STUDIES

Immunoassay testing of anterior pituitary hormones and their target hormones is a reasonable first step in diagnosing hypopituitarism. Basal (morning fasting) hormone levels can be used to differentiate primary target organ disease from pituitary hypofunction for prolactin, LH, FSH, and TSH but are unreliable for GH and ACTH. The expected relationship between target organ, pituitary, and hypothalamic hormones at basal levels and with stimulation testing can be found in Table 16.12. Additionally, brain MRI can be used to further determine pituitary versus hypothalamic causes of dysfunction in the event of a pituitary adenoma.

IGF-1 can be used to diagnose GH deficiency as measuring GH levels is not sufficient. An IGF-1 value of <77.2 mcg/L is considered specific for GH deficiency, although normal values by age range should be reviewed.[12] Some sources will state that an insulin tolerance test (ITT) is the gold standard for diagnosing, but it is not recommended because it can induce dangerous hypoglycemia and is very unpleasant for the patient. In an ITT, 0.1 unit of insulin per kilogram of body weight is administered to the patient intravenously and serum glucose and GH are measured before administration and again at 15, 30, 60, 90, and 120 minutes after administration. ITT attempts to stimulate GH production; in the event that GH fails to rise to normal levels, GH deficiency can be diagnosed (<5.1 ng/mL).[13] Provocative tests such as ITT should be performed under close supervision of a trained endocrinologist and be reserved for cases in which IGF-1 results are equivocal.

Diagnosis of adrenal insufficiency has three main features that are outlined below and further discussed in Section 16.5 (Figure 16.6):

1. Establishing the presence of low cortisol levels
2. Determining whether low cortisol levels are dependent or independent of ACTH deficiency
3. Determining the primary cause of the deficiency

EVALUATION, DIFFERENTIAL DIAGNOSIS, TREATMENT, AND PATIENT EDUCATION

These sections will be highly varied and specific to the individual hormones that are found to be insufficient. Conditions associated with hormone insufficiency are discussed throughout the chapter and should be referred to for evaluation, differential diagnosis, treatment approach, and patient education.

TABLE 16.12 Diagnostic Evaluation of Hypopituitarism

	Basal		Stimulatory		
	Pituitary Hormone	Target Gland Hormone	Pituitary Hormone	Hypothalamic Hormone	
			Target Gland Hormone	Pituitary Hormone	Target Gland Hormone
Normal	N	N	N	N	N
Target gland disease	↑	↓↓	↓↓	↑↑	↓↓
Pituitary disease	↓↓	↓	N-↑	↓↓	↓↓
Hypothalamic disease	N-↓	↓	N-↑	N-↑	N-↑

N, normal concentration; ↑, increase; ↑↑, further increase; ↓, decrease; ↓↓, further decrease.
Source: With permission from Kim SY. Diagnosis and treatment of hypopituitarism. Endocrinol Metab (Seoul). *2015;30(4):443–455. doi:10.3803/EnM.2015.30.4.443*

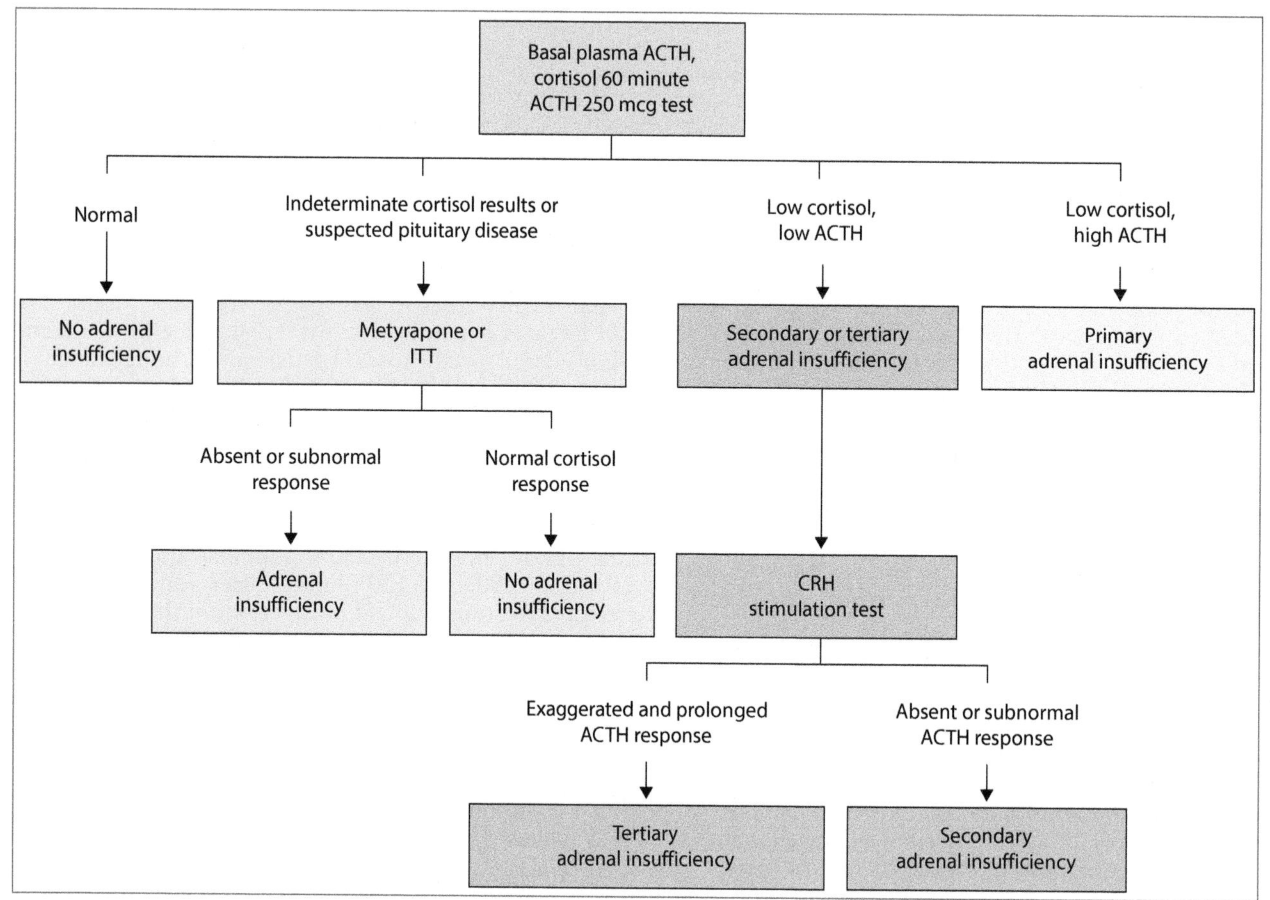

Figure 16.6 Diagnostic approach to adrenal insufficiency. ACTH, corticotropin; CRH, corticotropin-releasing hormone; ITT, insulin tolerance test.

KEY POINTS

- Pituitary adenomas are typically benign and can result in a variety of symptoms depending on which hormones are being hypersecreted.
- Over 99% of acromegaly cases are caused by a GH- secreting pituitary adenoma and are managed by transsphenoidal resection.
- Sporadic mutation in *FGFR3* gene accounts for 80% of cases of achondroplasia, with the remaining 20% resulting from autosomal dominant inheritance of the *FGFR3* mutation.
- DI is often idiopathic in nature and treatment is determined at the individual level, with an emphasis on symptom management.

16.2 THYROID DISEASE

OVERVIEW

The thyroid gland is located in the anterior neck, resting anterior to the trachea and inferior to the larynx. This butterfly-shaped gland weighs 10–20 g and is responsible for metabolism regulation throughout the body. In infants, thyroid hormone also aids in CNS development. Given this important role, large amounts of circulating thyroid hormone are kept in reserve and the gland is very sensitive to even minor changes in concentrations, allowing levels to be kept within very tight limits for optimal function. Thyroid dysfunction is very common to encounter in clinical practice and Table 16.13 outlines the most frequently seen conditions.

Laboratory testing is an essential step in diagnosing thyroid disease and very typical result patterns appear for both hyper- and hypothyroidism (Table 16.14). These lab results can be used to differentiate primary disease from secondary disease as well as subclinical disease from overt disease. Both hypothyroidism and hyperthyroidism are discussed further in sections 16.2A and 16.2B, respectively.

EPIDEMIOLOGY

Given the large scope of possible causes of thyroid dysfunction, epidemiology is highly dependent on the specific condition being considered. Hypothyroidism affects approximately 1 in 300 U.S. adults, with increased prevalence with age and female sex and there are an estimated 13 million cases that remain undiagnosed.[14] Conversely, the prevalence of hyperthyroidism is only about 1.3% in the United States, broken into 0.5% overt hyperthyroidism and 0.8% subclinical or undiagnosed hyperthyroidism.[15,16]

TABLE 16.13 Most Frequently Encountered Types Thyroid Dysfunction

Thyroid Dysfunction	Description
Hypothyroidism	Thyroid hormone deficiency
Hyperthyroidism	Thyroid hormone excess
Goiter	Diffuse thyroid gland enlargement
Thyroid nodule	Focal enlargement of the thyroid gland
Abnormal thyroid function tests	Testing is abnormal, clinically the patient remains euthyroid

PATHOPHYSIOLOGY

As discussed in Section 16.1, the thyroid gland functions as part of an axis comprising the hypothalamus, pituitary gland, and thyroid gland. Circulating levels of thyroid hormone are controlled through a negative feedback loop (Figure 16.7). In a normally functioning axis, when circulating thyroid levels decline, TRH is released from the hypothalamus and signals the pituitary gland to release TSH, which signals the thyroid gland to release thyroid hormone from thyroid follicular cells. As circulating thyroid hormone levels return to normal, the axis is downregulating and TRH production declines, thereby reducing TSH and thyroid hormone levels. Because of this axis, thyroid dysfunction can occur due to dysfunction within the thyroid gland itself (primary disease) or as a result of pituitary gland or hypothalamic dysfunction (secondary disease). Combination of free thyroxine (T4) and TSH testing, as well as multiple thyroid hormone antibodies, can help differentiate the origin of disease and guide follow-up imaging and biopsy.

Thyroxine (T4) and 3,5,3′-triiodothyronine (T3) are the two forms of thyroid hormones and both can be found in circulation as well incorporated into thyroglobulin within the thyroid gland. T3 is more potent than T4 but only about 20% of T3 is produced by the thyroid gland itself. The remainder of T3 is created peripherally when T4 is deiodinated.[17] Thyroglobulin is a protein that is responsible for both the synthesis and storage of T3 and T4; this method of keeping the hormones in reserve allows for more immediate release in response to very small variations in circulating levels. T3 is produced by many tissues throughout the body and T4 is only produced by the thyroid gland. Despite large amounts of circulating T3 and T4, the vast majority (>99%) of these hormones are circulating bound to proteins: thyroxine-binding globulin (TBG), transthyretin (TTR), albumin, and lipoproteins. Because of this, small changes in these proteins can result in large changes in T3 and T4. Fortunately, free T4 and T3 concentrations can also be measured, more accurately depicting the amount of bioavailable thyroid hormone. Along with T3 and T4 that is incorporated into thyroglobulin, these binding proteins also allow immediate availability of thyroid hormone when needed, allowing for tight control.

Much about thyroid disease is still unknown, but there is thought to be a large autoimmune component to the most common diseases encountered. Three primary antigens have been identified, allowing autoantibody testing to help confirm disease (Table 16.15).

TABLE 16.14 Screening Lab Results for Hyperthyroidism and Hypothyroidism

Condition	Thyroid-Stimulating Hormone (TSH) Level	Free Thyroxine (T4) Level
Overt hypothyroidism	Elevated	Decreased
Subclinical hypothyroidism	Elevated	Normal/near normal
Overt hyperthyroidism	Decreased	Elevated
Subclinical hyperthyroidism	Decreased	Normal/near normal
Secondary hypothyroidism	Decreased	Decreased
Secondary hyperthyroidism	Elevated	Elevated

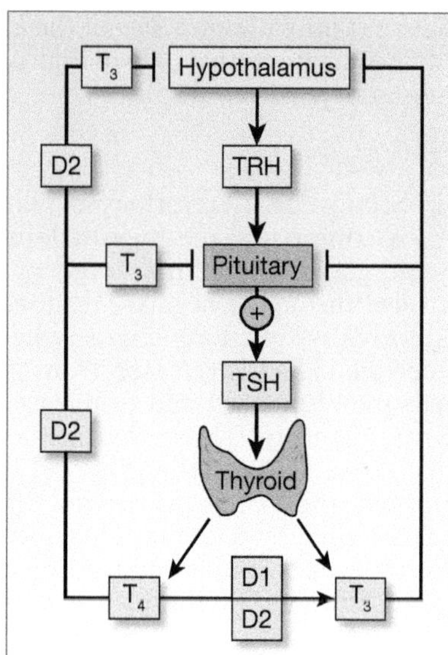

Figure 16.7 **Negative feedback control of thyroid hormone through the hypothalamic-pituitary-thyroid axis. The hypothalamus secretes TRH, which stimulates the pituitary to secrete TSH. TSH stimulates the thyroid gland to produce T4 and, to a lesser extent, T3. T4 is then converted to T3 in target tissues by the type I (D1) and type II (D2) deiodinases. T3 exerts genomic and nongenomic actions of thyroid hormone in target tissues and exerts negative feedback on TRH and TSH secretion.** T_3, triiodothyronine; T_4, thyroxine; TRH, thyrotropin-releasing hormone; TSH, thyroid-stimulating hormone. *(Source: Yedinak C, Hurtado CR, Leung AM, et al. Endocrine system. In: Tkacs NC, Hermann LL, Johnson RL, eds.* Advanced Physiology and Pathophysiology. *Springer Publishing Company; 2020:701.)*

TABLE 16.15 Thyroid Antigens and Related Thyroid Autoantibodies

Thyroid Antigen	Thyroid Autoantibody Testing
Thyroglobulin (Tg)	Tg antibodies
Thyroidal peroxidase (TPO)	Anti-TPO antibodies
Thyroid-stimulating hormone (TSH) receptor	Thyrotropin receptor antibodies (TRAbs): thyroid-stimulating immunoglobulins (TSI) or TSH receptor-binding inhibitor immunoglobulin (TBI)

16.2A HYPOTHYROIDISM

MEDICAL HISTORY AND CLINICAL PRESENTATION

Hypothyroidism is the result of insufficient thyroid hormone production from the thyroid gland. The majority of the time, hypothyroidism is caused by disease of the thyroid gland (primary hypothyroidism) but it can also be caused by a dysfunction of the pituitary gland or hypothalamus (secondary hypothyroidism; Table 16.16). Autoimmune thyroid disease (e.g., Hashimoto thyroiditis) is the most common cause of hypothyroidism. Primary hypothyroidism can be further subclassified as overt or subclinical. In overt disease, lab values reflect hypothyroidism (elevated TSH and reduced free T4) whereas in subclinical disease, TSH is elevated but T4 remains normal and the patient does not experience symptoms associated with hypothyroidism. In subclinical disease, the thyroid gland is able to still maintain normal T4 levels but requires additional stimulation from the pituitary to do so. Individuals with subclinical hypothyroidism are at risk for developing overt hypothyroidism in the future.

If untreated, hypothyroidism can lead to a variety of unpleasant symptoms but also to long-term effects including hypertension, dyslipidemia, and infertility.[14] The severity of presenting clinical symptoms typically corresponds to the severity of disease, and once treatment has begun, the return of symptoms can be used to prompt retesting. Clinical symptoms associated with both primary and secondary hypothyroidism are similar as both are characterized by decreased thyroid hormone, but patients with secondary disease typically also present with symptoms of pituitary dysfunction. Hallmark symptoms of hypothyroidism include fatigue and cold intolerance. As hypothyroidism is more common in women and prevalence increases with age, many women attribute initial symptoms to decreased metabolism that comes with aging and may therefore delay seeking medical attention.

SIGNS AND SYMPTOMS

While fatigue and cold intolerance are the most common presenting complaints from individuals with hypothyroidism, many other symptoms can occur. Figure 16.8 shows the common clinical symptoms for adult patients with hypothyroidism. Cognitive decline may be the only, or most pronounced, clinical symptom in elderly patients, whereas infants and children may present with failure to thrive.

PHYSICAL EXAMINATION

Physical examination findings will support many of the presenting signs and symptoms depicted in Figure 16.8. Common findings include obesity, dry skin, peripheral edema, thinning of the lateral half of the eyebrows, delayed deep tendon reflexes (DTRs), brittle and thin hair, and goiter.[14] It is important to differentiate severe hypothyroidism from septic shock as both may present with pericardial effusion, pleural effusion, megacolon, hemodynamic instability, and possible coma.[14] The thyroid gland is typically diffusely enlarged with a pebbly texture in hypothyroidism.[18] Any rapidly growing thyroid gland should be further evaluated with fine needle aspiration for primary thyroid lymphoma given the increased incidence in individuals with a history of Hashimoto thyroiditis.

DIFFERENTIAL DIAGNOSIS

See Table 16.17 for a summary of the differential diagnosis of hypothyroidism.

DIAGNOSTIC STUDIES

Laboratory testing is key for diagnosing hypothyroidism due to the highly varied clinical picture. The hallmark of hypothyroidism is decreased thyroid hormone. In primary disease, TSH is elevated and free T4 is decreased, and in secondary disease, TSH and free T4 are both decreased (see

TABLE 16.16 Causes of Primary and Secondary Hypothyroidism

Cause of Hypothyroidism	Further Classification of Cause
Primary hypothyroidism	
Chronic autoimmune thyroiditis (Hashimoto thyroiditis)	
Iatrogenic	Thyroidectomy, radioiodine therapy, external irradiation
Irregular iodine levels	Iodine excess, iodine deficiency
Drug-induced	Thionamids, lithium, amiodarone, interferon-alpha, interleukin 2, tyrosine kinase inhibitors, checkpoint inhibitor immunotherapy
Infiltrative disease	Fibrous thyroiditis, hemochromatosis, sarcoidosis
Transient hypothyroidism	Painless thyroiditis, subacute granulomatous thyroiditis, postpartum thyroiditis, subtotal thyroidectomy, post-radioiodine therapy for Graves hyperthyroidism
Congenital disease	Thyroid agenesis, thyroid dysgenesis, hormone synthesis defects
Secondary hypothyroidism	
Thyroid-stimulating hormone (TSH) deficiency	See Section 16.1
Thyrotropin-releasing hormone (TRH) deficiency	

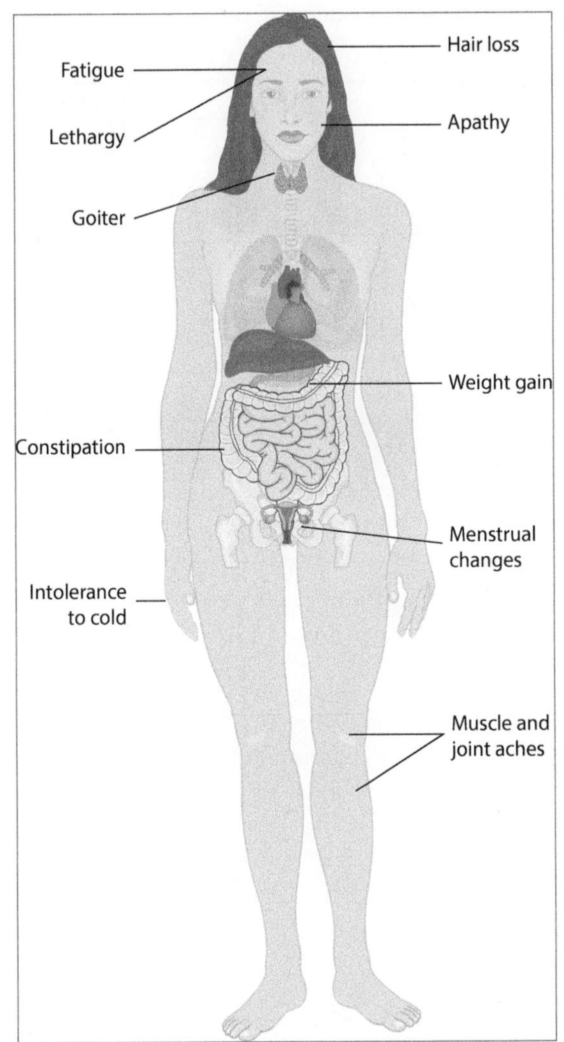

Figure 16.8 **Clinical symptoms of adults with hypothyroidism.**

TABLE 16.17 Differential Diagnosis of Hypothyroidism

Differential Diagnosis	Description
Depression	Refer to the *Diagnostic and Statistical Manual of Mental Disorders (DSM-5)* for diagnostic criteria; TSH and free T4 remain normal.
Pituitary adenoma	Primary cause of secondary hypothyroidism. TSH and free T4 will both be decreased.
Anemia	Normocytic anemia is common in hypothyroidism. When TSH is normal and anemia is present, consider alternative causes.
Alzheimer disease	TSH and free T4 remain normal. Head CT shows brain atrophy.

T4, thyroxine; TSH, thyroid-stimulating hormone.

Table 16.16) as dysfunction originates in the pituitary gland or hypothalamus. Thyroid peroxidase (TPO) antibodies are typically positive in Hashimoto thyroiditis.

Additionally, lab tests may reveal[14]:

- Elevated C-reactive protein
- Hyperprolactinemia
- Hyponatremia
- Increased creatine kinase
- Increased low-density lipoprotein (LDL) cholesterol
- Increased triglycerides (TGs)
- Normocytic anemia
- Proteinuria

EKG may reveal bradycardia, flattened T waves, and low voltage.[14] When severe hypothyroidism leads to decreased function in multiple organs, myxedema coma results. Myxedema coma is very rare but carries a high mortality rate, so it should always be considered.

EVALUATION

Any patient who presents with clinical symptoms of hypothyroidism should be evaluated. The United States Preventive Services Task Force (USPSTF) and the American Academy of Pediatrics (AAP) do not recommend screening asymptomatic adults for hypothyroidism. Screening may be considered for asymptomatic adults on a case-by-case basis for individuals who are particularly high risk, especially those with a history of autoimmune disease, subclinical hypothyroidism, neck radiation, radioactive iodine therapy, presence of goiter, family history of hypothyroidism, or use of drugs that have a known impact on thyroid function.[14]

TREATMENT

- Levothyroxine is considered the first line therapy for primary hypothyroidism, and treatment is typically required lifelong.
- Once treatment is started, repeat TSH and free T4 testing within 8 weeks and titrate accordingly.
- Typical starting dose of levothyroxine for nonpregnant adults is 1.6 mcg/kg per day, whereas elderly patients require a typical starting dose of 25–50 mcg.
- Individuals with subclinical hypothyroidism do not typically need treatment.

PATIENT EDUCATION

- Hypothyroidism can have an insidious onset which may delay diagnosis.
- Treatment for hypothyroidism is typically lifelong.
- If symptoms return, patients should notify their clinician and repeat lab testing before adjusting medication dosing.

16.2B HYPERTHYROIDISM

MEDICAL HISTORY AND CLINICAL PRESENTATION

Hyperthyroidism is defined by an excess of thyroid hormone produced by the thyroid gland. Graves disease, toxic multinodular goiter, and toxic adenoma are the most common causes of excessive thyroid hormone production leading to hyperthyroidism. Graves disease, an autoimmune disorder and the most common cause of hyperthyroidism, results from the activation of TSH receptors by thyroid-stimulating antibodies. This activation triggers the synthesis of thyroid hormone. Women and individuals with a positive family or personal family history of autoimmune disease carry the highest risk for developing Graves disease.[15] Toxic multinodular goiter is also relatively common, but most frequently occurs in individuals who are iodine deficient. Over time, either a single nodule, called toxic adenoma, or multiple nodules can arise. Additionally, hyperthyroidism can result from the autoimmune destruction of thyroid follicles; this process is referred to as transient thyroiditis. Transient thyroiditis can occur after childbirth, as seen with postpartum thyroiditis, or results from drug use, including lithium and amiodarone.[15] There are multiple other less common causes of hyperthyroidism that should also be considered including metastatic thyroid cancer, struma ovarii, and human chorionic gonadotropin (hCG)-producing trophoblastic tumors. Rarely, patients will intentionally induce a hyperthyroid state through exogenous thyroid hormone intake, primarily to achieve weight loss.[19]

Hyperthyroidism can present with a broad clinical picture, directly correlated to the severity of hormone excess. Elevated thyroid hormone most commonly presents with an elevated metabolism manifesting with cardiac palpitations, diaphoresis, and tremor. As symptoms progress, weight loss, increased appetite, and lid lag can present. In extreme excess, thyroid storm can result. Thyroid storm typically follows a stressful event such as trauma, surgery, emotional distress, or CVA and presents with tachycardia, hypertension, and hyperthermia; prompt diagnosis and early intervention are critical as thyroid storm carries a high mortality rate.

SIGNS AND SYMPTOMS

Palpitations, diaphoresis, and tremor are the primary presenting symptoms of hyperthyroidism, but multiple body systems can be affected, as shown in Figure 16.9. Adrenergic symptoms include palpitations, tachycardia, anxiety, tremors, diaphoresis, heat intolerance, lid lag, and hyperdefecation.[15] These symptoms represent a hypermetabolic state, in contrast to the hypometabolic state seen with hypothyroidism. Additional hypermetabolic signs include weight loss and, during thyroid storm, fever. Orbitopathy (exophthalmos or periorbital edema), pretibial myxedema, and thyroid acropachy are considered pathognomonic signs for Graves disease.[15] Older patients with hyperthyroidism

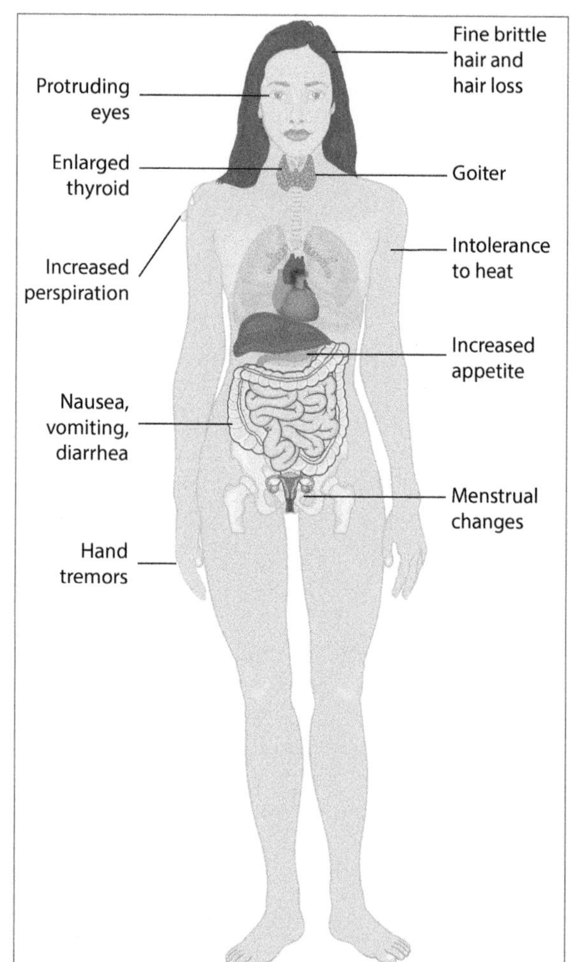

Figure 16.9 **Signs and symptoms of hyperthyroidism.**

tend to present with more weight loss and cardiopulmonary symptoms including tachycardia, dyspnea on exertion, and edema compared to younger adults.[20]

PHYSICAL EXAMINATION

Physical examination findings will support the presenting signs and symptoms of hyperthyroidism as previously outlined. Physical examination may reveal generalized hyperactivity and weight loss in addition to the following, organ system-specific symptoms (Table 16.18):

- **Skin:** Warm, moist, thinning and fine hair
- **Ear, nose, throat:** Lid lag, exophthalmos,* periorbital and conjunctival edema,* thyroid goiter
- **Cardiac:** Tachycardia, irregularly irregular pulse if concurrent atrial fibrillation, systolic hypertension
- **Musculoskeletal:** Tremor, proximal muscle weakness, hyperreflexia

*These symptoms are seen only in patients with Graves disease.

DIFFERENTIAL DIAGNOSIS

See Table 16.19 for a summary of the differential diagnosis for hyperthyroidism.

DIAGNOSTIC STUDIES

Thyroid hormone labtests are essential in diagnosing hyperthyroidism. In primary disease, TSH will be decreased and free T4 will be elevated. In secondary disease, both TSH and free T4 will be elevated. If free T4 is elevated, thyroid radioactive iodine uptake and scan are also indicated to further determine the cause of disease. When hyperthyroidism is in the differential diagnosis, TSH should first be ordered with reflex to free T4 for further diagnosis if TSH results are abnormal. Subclinical hyperthyroidism occurs when TSH levels are decreased and free T4 levels remain normal and clinically, the patient remains euthyroid. Thyroid ultrasound exam should be reserved for patients with a palpable thyroid gland, regardless of thyroid function test results.[15]

Establishing the presence of hyperthyroidism is the first step in diagnosis, but the cause must also be identified. If the diagnosis of Graves disease cannot be readily determined based on presentation and physical exam, it is necessary to pursue further testing to determine a cause. Thyrotropin receptor antibodies, color-flow Doppler ultrasonography to measure thyroidal blood flow, and radioactive iodine uptake can all be used. Positive thyrotropin receptor antibodies can be used to confirm the diagnosis of Graves disease. In the presence of hyperthyroidism, low iodine uptake typically points to thyroiditis, excess exogenous thyroid hormone, or struma ovarii whereas diffusely high uptake typically points to Graves disease, toxic multinodular adenoma, a pituitary adenoma, or trophoblastic disease. High uptake indicates excess hormone production, whereas low uptake indicates inflammation or destruction of thyroid tissue. It should be noted that radioactive iodine uptake is contraindicated during pregnancy and breastfeeding.

TABLE 16.18 Thyroid Gland Physical Exam Finding by Condition

Condition	Thyroid Gland Findings
Graves disease	Diffuse enlargement ranging from minimal to massive
Toxic multinodular goiter	Palpable, multinodular goiter
Thyroid adenoma	Single, palpable nodule

TABLE 16.19 Differential Diagnosis for Hyperthyroidism

Differential Diagnosis	Description
Euthyroid hyperthyroxinemia	Abnormalities in serum thyroid-binding proteins cause an elevation in total serum T4 concentrations and typically normal T3 and TSH levels.
Glucocorticoid therapy	High-dose glucocorticoid therapy can lead to decreases in TSH, but free T4 and free T3 are also low or normal.
Biotin therapy	Ingestion of biotin can cause falsely low TSH with falsely elevated T4, T3, and TSH receptor-binding inhibitor immunoglobulin (TBII).

T3, triiodothyronine: T4, thyroxine; TSH, thyroid-stimulating hormone.

EVALUATION

As serum TSH levels may remain low for weeks after treatment has begun, frequent early monitoring of free T4 is most reliable for establishing a euthyroid state. Subclinical hyperthyroidism should continue to be monitored, but typically treatment is not indicated. Patients taking thioamides should have free T4 levels monitored every 4 to 6 weeks until maintenance dosing has been achieved. After radioiodine ablation, free T4, total T3, and TSH should be measured at 4 to 6 weeks, then free T4 and TSH every 4 to 6 weeks. This screening should be continued until the patient has been diagnosed as hypothyroid and reached therapeutic levels of levothyroxine; if this has not occurred within 6 months of ablation, screening can be discontinued and only restarted if symptoms of hyperthyroidism or hypothyroidism present. Following a thyroidectomy, free T4 should be measured prior to discharge and TSH should be measured 6 to 8 weeks after surgery; levothyroxine dosing should be adjusted accordingly.

TREATMENT

- Methimazole is considered the first-line therapy for hyperthyroidism, with propylthiouracil (PTU) considered first-line during pregnancy.
- Beta blockers should also be administered to reduce symptoms, but do not treat the underlying condition.
- Radioiodine and surgical ablation are also viable options, especially after a trial of antithyroid medication use or in patients with a high risk of hyperthyroid complications. Patients should first obtain a euthyroid state prior to seeking ablative therapy.

PATIENT EDUCATION

- Hyperthyroidism is a manageable disease but requires lifelong monitoring of hormone levels to remain asymptomatic.

16.2C THYROIDITIS

MEDICAL HISTORY AND CLINICAL PRESENTATION

Thyroiditis is an umbrella term encompassing many disorders that all cause inflammation of the thyroid gland. Thyroiditis can be further categorized into painful thyroiditis and painless thyroiditis (Table 16.20). Conditions that cause painful thyroiditis include subacute thyroiditis, acute (suppurative) thyroiditis, and radiation-induced thyroiditis. Conditions that cause painless thyroiditis include Hashimoto thyroiditis, postpartum thyroiditis, subacute lymphocytic thyroiditis, and drug-induced thyroiditis. The most common cause of thyroiditis is Hashimoto thyroiditis, an autoimmune disease resulting in hypothyroidism. Conversely, thyroiditis can also cause hyperthyroidism as seen with postpartum hyperthyroidism.

Subacute thyroiditis is also called giant cell thyroiditis or de Quervain thyroiditis. Like most thyroid conditions, it occurs more in women than in men with peak incidence between the ages of 40 and 50 years. Acute (suppurative) thyroiditis is very rare and typically bacterial in nature. The most common pathogens are *Streptococcus pyogenes, Staphylococcus aureus,* and *Streptococcus pneumoniae*. Only about half of patients with thyroiditis have a history of thyroid disease and incidence increases with age and immunosuppression.[18] Radiation-induced thyroiditis occurs within about a week following radiation therapy and can become fibrotic in <18 weeks. Patients will have a known history of radiation exposure.

TABLE 16.20 Type of Thyroiditis, Clinical Presentation, and Course of Disease

Type of Thyroiditis	Clinical Presentation	Course of Disease
Hashimoto thyroiditis	Hypothyroidism	Typically permanent in nature
Postpartum thyroiditis	Hyperthyroidism followed by hypothyroidism*	Must occur after delivery of baby; Typical, resolution within 12–18 months
Painless thyroiditis	Hyperthyroidism followed by hypothyroidism*	Must not occur after delivery of baby; Typically, resolution within 12–18 months
Drug-induced thyroiditis	Can manifest as hyperthyroidism or hypothyroidism	Typically resolves shortly after cessation of medication use
Infectious thyroiditis (subacute thyroiditis, acute thyroiditis)	Painful thyroid gland, prodrome of myalgias, fever, and fatigue	Subacute: transient hyperthyroidism lasting 3–6 weeks, subacute hypothyroidism lasting up to 6 months, with euthyroid levels achieved by 6–12 months

**Only about one-third of patients experience each hyperthyroid symptom and hypothyroid symptom.*

Hashimoto thyroiditis is the most common cause of hypothyroidism and the most common type of painless thyroiditis. It is discussed further in Section 16.2A, but its characteristic presentation includes fatigue, weight gain, and cold intolerance. Patients with postpartum thyroiditis have a positive history of delivery within the past 2 to 6 months and present with a small, nontender but firm goiter. Patients are more likely to also have a history of hypothyroidism or comorbid autoimmune disease, supporting the suggestion to screen these at-risk mothers.[18] Individuals with a history of iodine deficiency are at a particular risk of developing subacute lymphocytic thyroiditis, a likely autoimmune condition presenting with a goiter that is only differentiated from postpartum thyroiditis by the lack of preceding delivery; it can be further differentiated from Graves disease by physical exam findings, including the lack of a thyroid bruit. A specific drug history should be obtained from all patients in whom thyroiditis is suspected, looking for a positive history of medications that are known to cause thyroid destruction (e.g., amiodarone, interferon, and lithium).

SIGNS AND SYMPTOMS

Individuals with subacute or acute thyroiditis typically report a prodrome of cold-like symptoms including myalgias, fever, and fatigue. A diffusely tender "woody" thyroid may also be reported in subacute thyroiditis. Those with acute (suppurative) thyroiditis present with a very tender, erythematous thyroid gland. Fever, dysphagia, and dysphonia are also common. Patients with Hashimoto thyroiditis present with fatigue, cold intolerance, and weight gain, whereas those with postpartum thyroiditis will present with either symptoms of hypothyroidism or hyperthyroidism, depending on the manifestation of disease.

PHYSICAL EXAMINATION

As physical examination findings for hyperthyroidism and hypothyroidism have been previously discussed, this section will focus on differentiating different causes of thyroiditis. Physical examination findings can be used to further differentiate subacute thyroiditis and Graves disease. Findings of exophthalmos and pretibial myxedema, both pathognomonic for Graves disease, are not found in subacute thyroiditis. Likewise, an enlarged thyroid can be found in both conditions, but the thyroid is typically only tender to palpation with subacute thyroiditis. Additionally, a thyroid bruit may be found in Graves disease, but is not typically found in subacute thyroiditis.[18] In postpartum thyroiditis, physical exam will reveal a nontender, firm goiter.

DIFFERENTIAL DIAGNOSIS

Table 16.21 summarizes the differential diagnosis for thyroiditis.

As thyroiditis is a broad term referring to inflammation of the thyroid gland, further differentiation must be made once thyroiditis is suspected.

DIAGNOSTIC STUDIES

Individuals with subacute thyroiditis may also present with elevated erythrocyte sedimentation rate (ESR), anemia, and leukocytosis. As subacute thyroiditis is not autoimmune in nature, antithyroid antibodies are not elevated. Thyroid hormone labtests typically remain normal for acute thyroiditis, but ESR is elevated and marked leukocytosis with

TABLE 16.21 Differential Diagnosis for Thyroiditis

Differential Diagnosis	Description
Thyroid lymphoma	B-cell non-Hodgkin lymphoma, can be a complication of Hashimoto disease
Graves disease	Autoimmune, present with hyperthyroidism

a left shift is also present. Diagnosis should be confirmed with Gram stain and culture, which is also useful in guiding treatment approach. Labtests for Hashimoto thyroiditis will reveal a typical hypothyroidism pattern of decreased free T4 and elevated TSH. Antithyroid peroxidase antibodies are present in >90% of patients, whereas antithyroglobulin antibodies and TSH-receptor-blocking antibodies are not as helpful in diagnosing because of their decreased sensitivity.[18] As postpartum and subacute lymphocytic thyroiditis can present with either hyperthyroidism, hypothyroidism, or hyperthyroidism followed by hypothyroidism, serum TSH and free T4 are essential to diagnosis. ESR and white blood cell count tend to remain normal, while antithyroid peroxidase antibodies are typically elevated. Physical exam findings should be used to further differential postpartum thyroiditis from Graves disease.

EVALUATION

As there are many types of thyroiditis, evaluation will be determined by the severity of symptoms. Evaluation of hyperthyroidism and hypothyroidism (Sections 16.2A and 16.2B) should be used to help guide monitoring.

TREATMENT

- **Subacute thyroiditis:** NSAIDs for pain control; expect pain resolution within 5 weeks. Consider prednisone if no improvement within 1 week of starting NSAIDs.
- **Acute (suppurative) thyroiditis:** Empiric antibiotics, using Gram stain and culture to guide further treatments. Surgical drainage may be necessary depending on severity and response to therapy.
- **Radiation-induced thyroiditis:** NSAIDs for pain control; rarely, prednisone taper is needed. A beta blocker can be started if patient is experiencing hyperthyroid symptoms.
- **Hashimoto thyroiditis:** Levothyroxine is the treatment of choice.
- **Postpartum and subacute lymphocytic thyroiditis:** If hyperthyroid, beta blockers should be used for symptom relief but must be used with caution in breastfeeding mothers. If hypothyroid, levothyroxine therapy should be initiated.
- **Drug-induced thyroiditis:** Symptoms should begin to resolve with discontinuation of medication. Beta blockers or levothyroxine may be necessary in persistent dysfunction.

PATIENT EDUCATION

- About 50% of patients with postpartum thyroiditis will develop permanent hypothyroidism within 9 years of diagnosis.[21]
- Individuals taking a medication that is known to cause drug-induced thyroiditis should be counseled preemptively on the symptoms of hyperthyroidism and hypothyroidism and see their medical clinician if symptoms present.
- It is important to continue seeking follow-up care as directed in order to prevent further progression of disease.

KEY POINTS

- TSH and free T4 are essential for diagnosing hyperthyroidism and hypothyroidism; once established, imaging and thyroid antibodies can be used for further classification.
- Close monitoring of thyroid levels should be followed until euthyroid state has been achieved for all disorders of thyroid dysfunction.
- Patients diagnosed with an autoimmune disease should be educated on the early presenting signs and symptoms of hyperthyroidism and hypothyroidism, as most cases are autoimmune in nature.

16.3 PARATHYROID DISEASE

OVERVIEW

The parathyroid glands are a series of four 3- to 4-mm glands located in the neck anteriorly to the trachea and posteriorly to the thyroid gland, with two glands behind each lobe of the thyroid. Approximately 10% of people have ectopic parathyroid glands, located in various locations ranging from near the esophagus to the chest; this results from incorrect movement of the glands during fetal development. The primary function of the parathyroid glands is to control the body's calcium levels, which is achieved through tight regulation of parathyroid hormone (PTH). PTH works to maintain calcium homeostasis through three key processes: bone resorption, intestinal absorption, and renal filtration. When blood calcium levels drop, bone resorption of calcium and intestinal absorption of calcium increase while renal filtration of calcium decreases, leading to an overall increase in blood calcium levels. When blood calcium levels rise, bone resorption and intestinal absorption decrease and the kidneys take up less calcium, all resulting in decreased blood calcium levels. Disease can be primary (at the level of the parathyroid gland) or secondary (typically caused by renal failure). Primary hyperparathyroidism (PHPT) is the most common parathyroid disease, with 80% of individuals having only a single adenoma alongside three normally functioning glands.

EPIDEMIOLOGY

Hyperparathyroidism is twice as common in women than in men, affecting approximately 28/100,000 U.S. adults. It is more common in older adults, with an average age at diagnosis of 65 years. Additionally, only 5% of cases can be attributed to an inherited syndrome, most commonly associated with multiple endocrine neoplasia type 1 and type 2, leaving 95% of cases to be deemed sporadic. Hypoparathyroidism affects approximately 37/100,000 U.S. adults and most commonly is a result of a thyroidectomy or parathyroidectomy.[22] Primary parathyroid cancer is very rare, affecting only 1 in 2 million people.

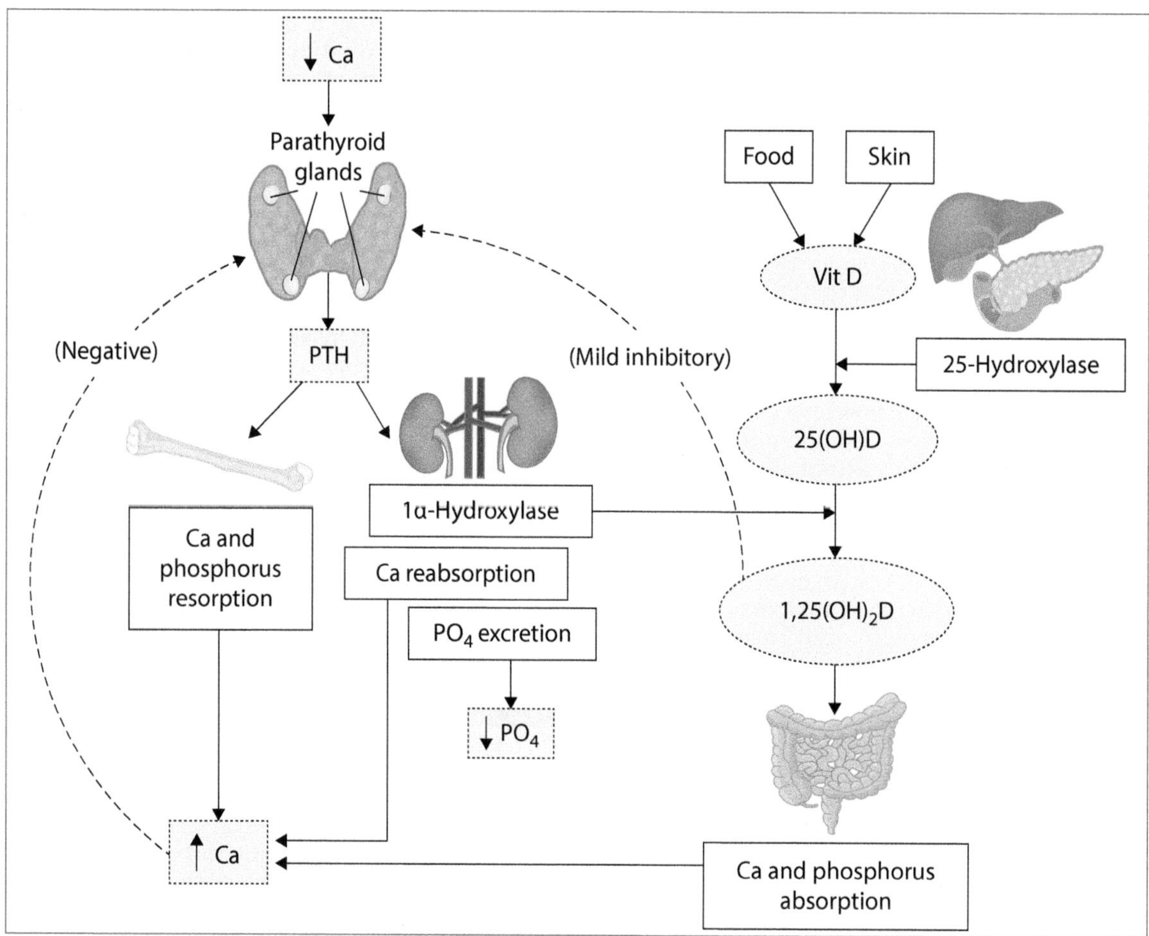

Figure 16.10 Parathyroid hormone function in response to hypocalcemia. Ca, calcium; 25(OH)D, 25-hydroxyvitamin D; $1,25(OH)_2D$, 1,25-dihydroxyvitamin D; PO_4, phosphate; PTH, parathyroid hormone.
(Source: With permission from Song L. Calcium and bone metabolism indices. Adv Clin Chem. *2017;82:1–46, Fig. 1.)*

PATHOPHYSIOLOGY

PTH works to maintain homeostasis of both serum calcium and phosphate. Calcium is primarily controlled by a balance of resorption and excretion in the kidneys, absorption in the intestines, and bone resorption, all regulated primarily by PTH and 1,25-dihydroxyvitamin D ($1,25(OH)_2D$). Phosphate homeostasis is maintained by both PTH and $1,25(OH)_2D$, but also by fibroblast growth factor 23 (FGF 23; see Figure 16.10). Because of this integrated control, both hypercalcemia and hypophosphatemia can result from PHPT, whereas hypocalcemia and hyperphosphatemia result from primary hypoparathyroidism. Secondary hyperparathyroidism typically results from CKD and causes both hypercalcemia and hyperphosphatemia. The most common cause of secondary hypercalcemia is CKD; when the kidneys begin to fail, they are unable to filter enough phosphorus or create enough vitamin D, which both lead to the development of hypocalcemia. When serum calcium is low, the parathyroid glands are activated to assist in raising serum calcium levels through the secretion of PTH. This chronic hyperstimulation of the parathyroid glands can lead to the development of a parathyroid adenoma, resulting in secondary hyperparathyroidism. Secondary hypoparathyroidism typically results from a secondary process that causes elevated calcium (such as malignancy) that downregulates the function of the parathyroid gland through negative feedback, resulting in decreased PTH secretion (Table 16.22).

16.3A HYPERPARATHYROIDISM

MEDICAL HISTORY AND CLINICAL PRESENTATION

The most common cause of PHPT is a benign parathyroid adenoma. Most frequently, patients with PHPT only present

TABLE 16.22 Lab Findings for Primary Versus Secondary Hyperparathyroidism and Hypoparathyroidism

Condition	Parathyroid Hormone	Serum Calcium	Serum Phosphate
Primary hyperparathyroidism	Elevated	Elevated	Decreased
Secondary hyperparathyroidism	Elevated	Elevated	Elevated
Primary hypoparathyroidism	Decreased	Decreased	Elevated
Secondary hypoparathyroidism	Decreased	Elevated	Elevated

with asymptomatic hypercalcemia on routine screening. If undetected long enough and calcium levels begin to rise, patients may present with classic symptoms of hypercalcemia, including weakness, fatigue, muscle pain, nausea, vomiting, confusion, headaches, nephrolithiasis, and depression (commonly remembered as "bones, stones, abdominal moans, psychic groans and fatigue overtones"). The severity of symptoms also seems to be somewhat related to the speed at which hypercalcemia develops, rather than solely linked to the serum calcium level. Additionally, individuals who have vitamin D deficiency and hyperparathyroidism tend to have more pronounced clinical symptoms.[23] In patients with asymptomatic hyperparathyroidism, serum calcium levels typically remain around or below 1.0 mg/dL. In some very rare situations, patients may be screened for elevated PTH after finding low bone density, when serum calcium is normal. This is a relatively newly recognized phenomenon and causes of secondary hyperparathyroidism must be ruled out, including CKD, calcium malabsorption, and medication use (e.g., loop diuretics, bisphosphonates).

Approximately 1% to 2% of patients with PHPT will develop a parathyroid crisis, characterized by serum calcium levels that can rise above 15 mg/dL and symptoms of hypercalcemia, with changes in mental status being very common.[24]

The increased bone resorption seen with PHPT manifests classically as osteitis fibrosa cystica, a condition with multiple, specific findings on imaging, but incidence has decreased in recent years as it is historically seen with more severe cases of PHPT. Radiographic findings consistent with osteitis fibrosa cystica include brown tumors of the long bones, a "salt and pepper" appearance of the skull, subperiosteal bone resorption of the radial aspect of the middle phalanges, and tapering distal clavicles. Renal osteodystrophy remains a significant problem for individuals with secondary hyperparathyroidism due to CKD.[25]

SIGNS AND SYMPTOMS

Symptomatic patients typically present with classic findings of hypercalcemia, with symptoms becoming more pronounced as serum calcium levels rise. Common symptoms include weakness, fatigue, muscle pain, nausea, vomiting, confusion, headaches, nephrolithiasis, and depression ("bones, stones, abdominal moans, psychic groans and fatigue overtones"). Additionally, patients may present with polyuria and polydipsia. In any patient presenting with hypercalcemia, both malignancy and hyperparathyroidism should be thoroughly worked up.

PHYSICAL EXAMINATION

Asymptomatic PHPT does not typically have any associated characteristic physical exam findings, as parathyroid adenomas are rarely palpable on exam. Patients with hypercalcemia may exhibit decreased DTRs and decreased Mini-Mental State Examination (MMSE) scores due to confusion.

DIFFERENTIAL DIAGNOSIS

Table 16.23 summarizes the differential diagnosis for hyperparathyroidism.

TABLE 16.23 Differential Diagnosis for Hyperparathyroidism

Differential Diagnosis	Description
Malignancy	Common cause of hypercalcemia
Sarcoidosis	Common cause of hypercalcemia
Chronic kidney disease	Cause of secondary hyperparathyroidism

DIAGNOSTIC STUDIES

Hyperparathyroidism is diagnosed by elevated PTH on laboratory studies in a patient with hypercalcemia. As screening is usually only done after incidental findings of hypercalcemia, confirming hypercalcemia through repeat testing concurrently with testing PTH is necessary. In addition to elevated PTH, serum calcium is also typically elevated or on the high end of normal. Normocalcemic PHPT is a variant of PHPT that was discovered in 2009, and little is known about this condition.[26] Hypercalcemia with normal or high-normal PTH may be the result of exogenous (IV) calcium causing suppression of PTH or from non-PTH mediated hypercalcemia. When PTH is the low end of normal in the presence of confirmed hypercalcemia, non-PTH mediated disease should be considered.

Serum phosphate levels will also be low or on the low end of normal in PHPT due to limited phosphate reabsorption in the proximal tubules that progresses as the disease become more overt. Additional lab findings may include elevated serum calcitriol, elevated magnesium, metabolic acidosis, and normochromic, normocytic anemia.

EVALUATION

Once diagnosed with hyperparathyroidism, additional screening must take place. The 24-hour urine calcium excretion can be measured to assess for renal function in asymptomatic patients as well as to evaluate for risk of nephrolithiasis through a stone risk profile. BMD should also be measured, as this is an essential part of disease management. Decreased BMD is common in the forearms, hips, and spine and an independent diagnosis of osteoporosis may be found. Lastly, the high prevalence of vitamin D insufficiency in patients with PHPT should prompt routine screening of 25(OH)D levels, with repletion indicated typically for levels that are below 20 ng/mL.[27]

TREATMENT

- Surgical resection of the parathyroid adenoma is recommended when:
  - Serum calcium remains >1 mg/dL above the upper limit of normal.
  - BMD testing reveals a T-score of –2.5 or less.
  - A vertebral fracture is present.
  - Creatinine clearance is below 60 mL/min.
  - A kidney stone is detected.[27]
- For patients for whom surgery is not indicted, DXA scans should be completed every 1 to 2 years, with calcium and PTH levels measured each year. Additionally, patients should be on replacement vitamin D to reach a sustained serum level of 25(OH)D >20 ng/dL.
- Pharmacologic management is controversial and not well supported. In some cases, bisphosphonates, specifically alendronate, may be used to improve BMD with minimal impact on serum calcium or PTH concentrations. Cinacalcet can be used to reduce serum calcium levels.[28]

PATIENT EDUCATION

- Hyperparathyroidism requires close monitoring.
- Often, no intervention is needed aside from monitoring.
- Patients should be educated on early symptoms of hypercalcemia and instructed to return to clinic if symptoms present.

16.3B HYPOPARATHYROIDISM

MEDICAL HISTORY AND CLINICAL PRESENTATION

Insufficient PTH secretion is the hallmark of hypoparathyroidism. Just as hyperparathyroidism results in hypercalcemia, hypoparathyroidism results in hypocalcemia. Most frequently, hypoparathyroidism is secondary to a parathyroidectomy, which accounts for about 75% of cases, but only 7%–8% of relevant neck surgeries result in hypoparathyroidism, and about 75% of these cases are transient, lasting <6 months.[22] Prevalence of hypoparathyroidism in the United States is about 37 per 100,000 person-years, with a mean age of 58 years and females accounting for 71% of patients.[22] Hypoparathyroidism can be linked to underlying genetic disease, in the case of DiGeorge syndrome, or autoimmune destruction of the parathyroid gland. In rare cases, the problem may lie in resistance to PTH, resulting in pseudohypoparathyroidism. Patients typically remain asymptomatic until hypocalcemia develops.

SIGNS AND SYMPTOMS

Symptoms of hypoparathyroidism are directly linked to calcium levels, with increasing severity as calcium levels decrease. Primary symptoms include numbness and tingling in the hands and feet, circumoral numbness, muscle cramping and spasm, facial twitching, tetany, and seizures. Additionally, hypocalcemia may result in laryngospasm, cognitive impairment, and prolonged QT intervals.

PHYSICAL EXAMINATION

The presence and severity of physical exam findings are directly correlated to the severity of hypocalcemia present. Neck scarring consistent with prior surgery may be found and a neck examination is expected to be otherwise normal. Chvostek and Trousseau signs are consistent with hypocalcemia and are therefore associated with hypoparathyroidism but are not unique to the disease. Chvostek sign, twitching of the upper lip, is elicited by tapping over the facial nerve, while Trousseau sign, carpopedal spasm, is elicited by placing a blood pressure cuff over the patient's brachial artery and inflating it above their normal systolic pressure for 3 minutes. In cases of severe hypocalcemia, spastic paraplegia, dysphagia, or tetany may be present.

DIFFERENTIAL DIAGNOSIS

Table 16.24 summarizes the differential diagnosis for hypoparathyroidism.

If hypocalcemia is discovered, it should first be confirmed by a second test. If serum calcium is confirmed low upon this second test, follow-up lab tests include PTH, phosphate, magnesium, serum creatinine, estimated glomerular filtration rate (eGFR), 25(OH)D, amylase, and creatinine kinase.[22] In the presence of confirmed hypocalcemia, the following lab results can be used to help guide the differential diagnosis[22]:

TABLE 16.24 Differential Diagnosis for Hypoparathyroidism

Differential Diagnosis	Description
Pseudohypoparathyroidism	Characterized by hypocalcemia as a result of parathyroid hormone receptor resistance
Chronic kidney disease	Increases serum phosphorus and decreased 1,25-dihydroxy vitamin D production can lead to hypocalcemia
Hypomagnesemia	Decreases production and release of parathyroid hormone

- **Elevated PTH, decreased phosphate:** vitamin D deficiency, acute pancreatitis, bisphosphonate use
- **Elevated PTH, elevated phosphate:** CKD, pseudohypoparathyroidism, tumor lysis
- **Decreased PTH, elevated phosphate:** hypoparathyroidism (reversible or irreversible)
  - **Reversible causes:** hypomagnesemia, cinacalcet use, neonatal hypocalcemia
  - **Irreversible causes:** parathyroid loss due to agenesis, surgical resection, or autoimmune destruction

DIAGNOSTIC STUDIES

Diagnosis of hypoparathyroidism relies on laboratory testing and is characterized by hypocalcemia (serum adjusted calcium <2.2 mmol/L), hyperphosphatemia, and hypoparathyroidism. Additionally, $1,25(OH)_2D$ concentrations and alkaline phosphatase activity, a marker of bone turnover, are typically decreased. Critically ill patients may benefit from measuring ionized calcium rather than corrected serum calcium, as changes in serum pH can alter calcium-albumin binding.

EVALUATION

Patients with hypothyroidism should be asked about any family history of the disease or prior head or neck surgery. Complications of hypoparathyroidism are typically the result of hypocalcemia, hyperphosphatemia and/or calcium and vitamin D levels.[22] EKG is indicated to identify potential cardiac changes, with intermittent prolonged QT interval being the most common finding. As calcium supplementation is the primary method of management, the patient should be monitored for the development of hypercalcemia and its related complications, including nephrolithiasis.

TREATMENT

- Acute management of hypocalcemia[29]:
  - When serum calcium is measured <1.9 mmol/L or ionized calcium is measured <1 mmol/L, IV calcium gluconate is indicated.
  - Oral calcium supplements may also be necessary.

  - Correct any underlying magnesium deficiency or alkalosis.
  - Cardiac monitoring is necessary during calcium supplementation as arrhythmias may result.
- Chronic management of hypocalcemia[29]:
  - Goals of management include maintaining serum calcium and serum phosphorus within normal limits while avoiding hypercalcemia with supplementation and mitigating patient symptoms of hypocalcemia.
  - Oral calcium (typically calcium carbonate or calcium citrate) and vitamin D supplementation are recommended.
  - Correct underlying hypomagnesemia.
  - Treat underlying cause of vitamin D deficiency, if present.
  - Thiazide diuretics can be helpful in decreasing urinary calcium excretion and are most effective when combined with a low-salt and low-phosphorus diet.
  - PTH supplementation may be necessary in rare cases but is not currently a mainstay of treatment, making hypoparathyroidism treatment unique from other endocrine disorders of hormone deficiency for which direct replacement is typically the favored treatment approach.

PATIENT EDUCATION

- It is important to follow up as directed with primary care for close monitoring of laboratory tests.
- Monitor for signs and symptoms of hypercalcemia.

KEY POINTS

- Hyperparathyroidism and hypoparathyroidism are typically asymptomatic and discovered through either elevated or decreased serum calcium levels, respectively, and confirmed with repeat testing and analysis of PTH levels.
- Symptoms of hyperparathyroidism and hypoparathyroidism are directly linked to calcium levels.
- Management of hyperparathyroidism and hypoparathyroidism requires close monitoring of calcium, phosphate, and vitamin D levels.

16.4 OSTEOPOROSIS

OVERVIEW

It is now known that osteoporosis is a primary disorder of the skeleton and is related to metabolic disruption throughout the body. Osteoporosis is defined as decreased bone mass per unit volume of anatomic bone and is characterized by decreased bone strength caused by a disruption in bone remodeling and an increased risk of fracture. The process of bone remodeling occurs at targeted sites where repair is needed; bone resorption is achieved by osteoclasts, whereas new bone is made by osteoblasts. When this system is out of balance, osteoporosis can occur. Bone mass reaches its peak in the third decade of life and then decreases throughout the remainder of life. This decrease in bone density that occurs with age is most likely caused by functional impairment of stem cell differentiation into the osteoblast lineage. This results in increased marrow adipogenesis and increased bone resorption.[30] Despite the close relationship with BMD, decreased BMD and osteoporosis should not be used interchangeably as osteoporosis is a disease of bone fragility, and decreased BMD is only one risk factor. Along with decreased BMD, increased femoral neck size, increased cortical porosity, and decreased osteocyte viability are contributing factors to decreased bone strength. Additional risk factors for osteoporosis include tobacco use, family history of osteoporosis or fracture, age >65 years, and low body mass index (BMI). Multiple secondary causes of osteoporosis should be considered including long-term glucocorticoid use, type 1 and type 2 diabetes, rheumatoid arthritis, liver disease, multiple myeloma, and gluten enteropathy. Despite the multifactorial etiology of osteoporosis, primary osteoporosis is typically attributed to either postmenopausal estrogen loss or age-related microarchitecture deterioration.[30] Individuals with osteoporosis are at an increased risk for fractures in age-compared analysis. Along with increased age, the most notable risk factors for fractures include sex hormone deficiency, lipid oxidation, decreased weight-bearing exercise, long-term glucocorticoid use, and increased fall risk. Additionally, the inverse relationship between fracture risk and BMD has no threshold limit.[30]

EPIDEMIOLOGY

Age-adjusted estimates of osteoporosis in the United States at either the spine or femur neck among those over age 65 are about 25% in women and about 6% in men.[31] Risk factors for osteoporosis include history of fracture as an adult, history of fragility fracture in a first-degree relative, low BMI, current tobacco use, and chronic use of oral corticosteroid therapy. Independent risk factors that have been shown to increase the risk of fractures in postmenopausal women include age, history of maternal hip fracture, decreased body weight, poor overall health, history of hyperthyroidism, tachycardia, and benzodiazepine use.[32]

PATHOPHYSIOLOGY

The pathophysiology of osteoporosis is complex, with many contributing factors still unclear. Coupling—the process of bone resorption followed by bone formation—is a continuously occurring process throughout the body. Typically, this occurs due to microtrauma and the result is improved bone strength despite frequent, small insults. There are two types of bone strength: tensile and compressive. Tensile strength is determined by collagenous proteins, whereas compressive strength is determined by mineralized osteoid. Increased calcium concentration is directly linked to improved compressive strength, hence the need for calcium supplementation as one form of osteoporosis prevention. This coupling process relies on proper functioning of osteoclasts for bone resorption and osteoblasts for bone formation, but these processes also seem to work together in an intricate fashion with osteoblasts controlling osteoclasts' function. The process of bone resorption is regulated by the nuclear factor-kappa B ligand (RANKL)/receptor activator of nuclear factor-kappa B (RANK)/osteoprotegerin (OPG) system. Fusion, differentiation, activation, and survival of osteoclasts are all results of RANKL binding to RANK. RANKL cytokine is produced by osteoblasts and activated T-cells in the bone marrow. OPG serves as a "decoy," sequestering RANKL and inhibiting RANK-RANKL limit bone resorption. When coupling is disturbed, as seen in osteoporosis, the slow process of bone formation (months) is unable to keep pace with bone resorption (weeks). In other words, osteoclast function begins to far outpace osteoblast function, resulting in a perpetual cycle of bone loss.[33] As newly remodeled areas of bone are temporarily less densely mineralized and therefore weaker, the risk of fracture during these times is high.

Coupling disturbance accounts for only a fraction of cases of decreased BMD and osteoporosis, with genetics accounting for up to 80% of peak bone mass variance.[34] The pathophysiology of osteoporosis is multifactorial:

- Estrogen deficiency reaches its peak in postmenopausal women and accelerates bone resorption and decreases bone formation as osteoblasts, osteocytes, and osteoclasts all have estrogen receptors. Additionally, increased sensitivity to bone effects of PTH are seen with estrogen deficiency.
- Osteoblast supply declines as a part of normal aging beginning in about the third decade of life.
- Secondary hyperparathyroidism caused by decreased calcium absorption from the gut or by vitamin D deficiency can trigger calcium resorption from bone.
- Long-term glucocorticoid use can inhibit osteoblast function while increasing apoptosis, leading to decreased bone formation.
- Epigenetics is offering new insight into the importance of prenatal and postnatal factors in the development of peak bone mass later in life, with increased birth weight and rate of growth before age 1 both associated with increased bone mass in the six and seventh decades of life.[35,36]

MEDICAL HISTORY AND CLINICAL PRESENTATION

A thorough medical history should be obtained to rule out potential causes of secondary osteoporosis or risk of malignancy, as bone metastasis is a common cause of fractures. Patient history and clinical presentation may reveal no abnormalities because osteoporosis is asymptomatic; it is the associated fractures that cause symptoms and typically lead to diagnosis when screening has not been performed. The "signs and symptoms" section outlines the clinical presentation for individuals with osteoporotic fractures.

SIGNS AND SYMPTOMS

Osteoporosis typically remains clinically silent until a fracture occurs and even then, many vertebral fractures do not cause pain. Table 16.25 outlines common presenting fractures for patient with osteoporosis.

PHYSICAL EXAMINATION

Physical exam findings for osteoporosis are specific to presenting fractures as the condition itself does not have any specific physical exam findings. Point tenderness over the affected vertebra may be present with a vertebral fracture as well as thoracic kyphosis and diminished lumbar lordosis. Compression fractures may also result in an overall loss of height. Flexion in abduction and external rotation (FABER) testing may reveal limited range of motion with hip fractures, as well as antalgic gait upon ambulation. Colles fracture may reveal point tenderness over the ulnar aspect of the wrist and pain with wrist flexion and extension.

TABLE 16.25 Signs and Symptoms of Common Osteoporotic Fractures

Fracture Type	Common Signs and Symptoms
Vertebral fracture	• Fall followed by localized, specific pain • Increased pain with movement • Paravertebral spasms
Hip fracture	• Groin, thigh, or medial knee pain when attempting to bear weight • Reduced hip range of motion • Hip rests in external rotation
Collesfracture	• Pain with wrist flexion and extension • Point tenderness over ulnar aspect of wrist

DIFFERENTIAL DIAGNOSIS

Table 16.26 summarizes the differential diagnosis for osteoporosis.

DIAGNOSTIC STUDIES

Timely screening is necessary for individuals at risk for osteoporosis because until a fracture occurs, most patients remain asymptomatic. Dual-energy x-ray absorptiometry (DXA) or quantitative CT (QCT) are used to measure bone mass and are a necessary part of diagnosis. For every 1 standard deviation (SD) an individual's bone density falls below the normal mean BMD at any skeletal site, there is a two-fold greater risk of a hip fracture.[30] The World Health Organization uses a T-score of −2.5 (<2SD below the mean) to diagnose osteoporosis. A T-score of −1 to −2.5 SD diagnoses osteopenia, whereas a T-score of <−2.5 SD or the presence of a fragility fracture is diagnostic for severe osteoporosis. BMD screening should be performed on all women 65 years and older, as well as postmenopausal women who are younger than 65 years who also have risk factors for fracture as discussed above. Men over 50 who have identified risk factors and both men and women over 50 who have adult-age fractures should also be screened.[37] DXA screening can also provide Z-scores, which compare age-, sex-, and race-adjusted values with a cutoff point of −2.0 SD to indicate below the expected range for age. Although Z-scores can be helpful clinically, they cannot be used alone for making a diagnosis of osteoporosis. Recent studies encourage clinicians to use this quantitative analysis but also factor in qualitative findings such as bone turnover, mineralization,

TABLE 16.26 Differential Diagnosis for Osteoporosis

Differential Diagnosis	Description
Osteomalacia	Decreased bone mineralization leading to fragility
Metastatic bone disease	Can cause compression fractures
Osteonecrosis	Decreased blood flow to bone leading to expedited bone break down

and trabecular connectivity, as osteoporosis is not only a problem of decreased BMD. As fractures are the most common presenting sign of osteoporosis, individuals should also undergo x-ray imaging studies appropriate for the suspected fracture.

EVALUATION

As decreased BMD only accounts for approximately 50% of the risk of fractures associated with osteoporosis, an independent analysis of fracture risk must be performed. The Fracture Risk Assessment Tool (FRAX) score should be used to estimate the 10-year probability of hip and major osteoporotic fracture in both men and women who are 40 years or older. Major osteoporotic fractures are defined as spine, forearm, hip, and humerus. The FRAX takes into account both measured and self-reported data to calculate a total score, with elevated probabilities predetermined to be 3% or greater for hip fracture and 20% or greater for the other, major osteoporotic fractures listed above.[38] While the original algorithm required a T-score input, updated versions no longer require this value.

Baseline laboratory tests should also be performed so that abnormalities that may increase the risk for osteoporosis can be identified. Thyroid dysfunction, vitamin D insufficiency, and hypercalciuria have been linked to osteoporosis as well as multiple myeloma. In males, hypogonadism has also been associated with osteoporosis. Because of this, TSH, 25-hydroxyvitamin D, serum protein electrophoresis, 24-hour urine calcium, testosterone (total and/or free), LH, and FSH should all be ordered.

Per National Osteoporosis Foundation recommendations, vertebral imaging should be performed for all women age 70 and over and all men 80 and over who have a T-score in any location of −1.0 SD or below and for all women age 65 to 69 years and all men age 70 to 79 years who have a T-score in any location of −1.5 SD or below.[37] As falls are the leading cause of hip fractures, fall risk assessment should be performed on all patients who are found to have osteoporosis or decreased BMD.

TREATMENT

- Lifestyle modifications are a key part of fracture prevention with osteoporosis. Clinicians should work with patients to develop plans that are safe and reduce the risk of injury.
  - Routine weight-bearing exercise
  - Routine strength training
  - Optimize calcium and vitamin D intake
- Pharmacologic therapy can be used, but recommendations are reserved for postmenopausal women and women 50 years or older who also have a personal history of[37]:
  - DXA T-score of −2.5 SD or below (indicating osteoporosis)
    - Secondary causes of decreased BMD must first be ruled out.
  - DXA T-score of −1.0 to −2.5 SD and a FRAX result of 3% or greater for a hip fracture or 20% or greater for a major osteoporosis-related fracture
  - Hip or vertebral fracture
- When pharmacologic treatment is indicated, bisphosphonates are the first-line therapy[39]

PATIENT EDUCATION

- Osteoporosis is usually asymptomatic until a fracture occurs, so screening according to established guidelines is important in identifying risk and forming a diagnosis.
- Patients should be counseled on the importance of fracture prevention through fall risk assessment and prevention as well as lifestyle modifications including increased weight-bearing exercise.

KEY POINTS

- All patients with osteoporosis must be evaluated for both BMD and fracture risk (FRAX) and secondary causes of osteoporosis must be ruled out.
- Fracture prevention is the mainstay of management.

16.5 ADRENAL GLAND DISORDERS

OVERVIEW

The adrenal glands are two small, triangle-shaped glands that sit on the superior aspect of the kidneys. They are an essential part of the endocrine system and help to regulate metabolism, blood pressure, stress response, and immune response through the production of cortisol and sex steroids. Each adrenal gland has two distinct parts, the medulla and the cortex, and the cortex is further divided into three zones: zona glomerulosa, zona fasciculata, and zona reticularis. The medulla is responsible for the secretion of epinephrine and norepinephrine, essential regulators of the flight-or-fight response. The zona glomerulosa secretes aldosterone, which is controlled by renin and assists in maintaining sodium balance. The zona fasciculata secretes cortisol, which is controlled by ACTH and has many different functions, including regulating the sleep/wake cycle and the suppression of inflammation. The zona reticularis secretes dehydroepiandrosterone (DHEA), which is controlled by androgen-stimulating hormone and helps produce androgen and estrogen.

Excess cortisol (hypercortisolism) due to a pituitary adenoma is called Cushing disease, which falls under the umbrella diagnosis of Cushing syndrome (see Section 16.5B). Primary corticoadrenal insufficiency, which results in hypocortisolism, is referred to as Addison's disease (see Section 16.5A) and excess aldosterone production from the adrenal glands (hyperaldosteronism) is referred to as Conn's syndrome. Pheochromocytoma is a rare condition that is caused by a chromaffin cell tumor of the adrenal glands that results in excessive catecholamine secretion (epinephrine and norepinephrine). Pheochromocytoma is a secondary cause of hypertension, and symptoms of headache, sweating, and palpitations are often misdiagnosed as a panic attack.

As adrenal disorders are conditions of hormone excess or insufficiency, screening and diagnosis rely heavily on hormone testing. As a general rule, if the concern is hormone excess then a suppression test should be ordered, and if the concern is hormone insufficiency then a hormone stimulation test should be ordered.

EPIDEMIOLOGY

Worldwide estimates of Addison's disease prevalence are about 144 million, and estimates of congenital adrenal hyperplasia are about 1 in 14,000 live births. There is no one distinct predisposing factor for the development of adrenal insufficiency and no one group of individuals is at a higher risk of developing the associated disorders.[40] Reports of incidence of Cushing syndrome are highly varied depending on source. Women and men are equally likely to develop Cushing disease as well as Cushing syndrome caused by an ectopic ACTH-secreting tumor, considered a paraneoplastic syndrome largely associated with lung cancer. Cushing disease typically presents in the third to fifth decades of life.

PATHOPHYSIOLOGY

The pathophysiology of adrenal disorders is highly dependent on the specific condition. The adrenal glands are part of the hypothalamic-pituitary-adrenal (HPA) axis and are regulated through an extensive network of feedback loops; disruption at any level of this cycle can result in oversecretion or undersecretion of adrenal hormones (see Section 16.1). Primary adrenal insufficiency is most commonly caused by autoimmune destruction of the adrenal cortex. Secondary adrenal insufficiency is caused by a problem at the level of the pituitary gland and most frequently results from traumatic brain injury or panhypopituitarism but can also be caused by a pituitary adenoma (discussed in Section 16.1E). Pituitary dysfunction causes decreased secretion of ACTH, resulting in decreased stimulation of the adrenal glands and ultimately insufficient cortisol production. Tertiary adrenal insufficiency, typically caused by exogenous glucocorticoid use, causes hypothalamic production of CRH, which leads to decreased anterior pituitary release of ACTH and decreased stimulation of the adrenal glands. Hemorrhagic adrenal gland infarction and infectious agents can also cause decreased hormone production. Additionally, congenital adrenal hyperplasia can cause adrenal insufficiency (decreased cortisol and/or aldosterone in the presence of androgen excess) that leads to precocious puberty in males and the development of male characteristics in females.

Adrenal crisis is a life-threatening complication for all patients with adrenal insufficiency as both mineralocorticoid and glucocorticoid deficiencies can precipitate the event. Mineralocorticoids are necessary to maintain proper sodium retention and promote vasoconstriction, and glucocorticoids are necessary to maintain proper vascular response to angiotensin II and norepinephrine as well as synthesis of renin substrate. Because of this, both mineralocorticoid and glucocorticoid levels must be maintained, or an adrenal crisis may occur.[41]

Cushing syndrome is the most common cause of hypercortisolism and can either be ACTH dependent (~80% of cases) or ACTH independent (~20% of cases), with Cushing disease making up close to 70% of all Cushing syndrome diagnoses.[42] Cushing disease is defined as hypercortisolism as the result of a pituitary adenoma causing hypersecretion of ACTH that results in excess cortisol secretion from the adrenal glands (zona fasciculata). Iatrogenic Cushing syndrome occurs as a result of long-term exogenous glucocorticoid administration and is commonly seen in treatment for autoimmune disorders. ACTH-dependent Cushing syndrome results in bilateral adrenocortical hyperplasia due to chronic overstimulation of the adrenal glands. Causes include pituitary hypersecretion of ACTH (Cushing disease), nonpituitary tumor causing ectopic ACTH secretion, nonhypothalamic tumor causing ectopic secretion of CRH hypersecretion, or administration of exogenous ACTH. All causes of ACTH-dependent Cushing syndrome are the result of a problem above the level of the adrenal glands where increased ACTH causes cortisol hypersecretion from the adrenal glands. In a healthy patient, cortisol hypersecretion would downregulate the release of CRH from the hypothalamus and ACTH from the anterior pituitary through negative feedback. In the case of ACTH-dependent Cushing syndrome, this feedback system is dysfunctional and despite attempted downregulation, the adrenal glands continue to be hyperstimulated either through ectopic ACTH secretion or hypersecretion from the pituitary gland itself (Cushing disease).

ACTH-independent Cushing syndrome is most frequently the result of exogenous synthetic glucocorticoid use, which mimics the effects of cortisol, with high-dose chronic prednisone being the biggest culprit. This exogenous glucocorticoid use downregulates the HPA axis, suppressing adrenal gland stimulation by ACTH and decreasing endogenous cortisol levels. Long-term use may cause adrenal gland atrophy as ACTH stimulation is required to maintain homeostasis; when this exogenous glucocorticoid administration is discontinued, adrenal insufficiency may result. ACTH-independent Cushing syndrome may also be caused by primary adrenocortical disease, primary disease indicating there is a problem in the adrenal glands. Adrenal adenomas are very effective at producing cortisol and result in hypercortisolism; increased levels of cortisol downregulate the HPA axis, resulting in decreased CRH and ACTH levels but this does not regulate the secretion of cortisol caused by the adenoma.

16.5A ADRENAL INSUFFICIENCY

MEDICAL HISTORY AND CLINICAL PRESENTATION

Adrenal insufficiency is an umbrella term covering many different independent diagnoses. The most common disorder is primary adrenal insufficiency, also known as Addison's disease. In the case of chronic primary adrenal insufficiency, patients have a history of glucocorticoid, mineralocorticoid, and androgen (women only) deficiencies, whereas patients with secondary or tertiary adrenal insufficiency will only present with symptoms of mineralocorticoid deficiency. The clinical picture is often confounded by the frequently insidious onset of nonspecific symptoms. The majority of patients present with chronic fatigue and weight loss, often precipitated by decreased intake and dehydration.[43] Patients should also be questioned regarding use of chronic glucocorticoids, as prolonged use often causes ACTH depression resulting in secondary adrenal insufficiency.

SIGNS AND SYMPTOMS

Despite the cause, most patients with adrenal insufficiency report similar symptoms that include weight loss, decreased appetite, frequent nausea and/or vomiting, and excessive fatigue.[43] If left untreated, patients may develop psychiatric symptoms including depression and memory impairment.[44]

Women may also complain of decreased libido due to decreased androgen production. The characteristic bronze skin, postural hypotension, and salt cravings associated with Addison's disease are not present in other forms of adrenal insufficiency.[43] As secondary adrenal insufficiency can be caused by a pituitary tumor, headache and bitemporal heminopia may be present. All patients with adrenal insufficiency are at a high risk of adrenal crisis, a life-threatening disorder characterized by seizures, shock, and coma.

PHYSICAL EXAMINATION

Patients with chronic primary adrenal insufficiency (Addison's disease) who are not in an adrenal crisis may present with skin hyperpigmentation due to an increased production of proopiomelanocortin (POMC) that becomes multiple biologically active hormones including both ACTH and melanocyte-stimulating hormone (MSH). Additionally, decreased skin turgor and postural hypotension may be appreciated. In women, decreased axillary and pubic hair is common due to decreased androgen production; this is not a common finding in men as most androgens are made in the testes.

There is no increase in POMC production in secondary or tertiary adrenal insufficiency; therefore, there is no additional production of MSH and skin bronzing does not occur. Additionally, dehydration, hypotension, and gastrointestinal (GI) upset are far less common in secondary and tertiary disease, but hypoglycemia is more common due to the frequently accompanying loss of GH secretion.

Patients in adrenal crisis typically present in shock, but may have additional symptoms including nausea, vomiting, weakness, lethargy, and confusion. Because there is typically an acute stressor that causes an adrenal crisis, a thorough evaluation should be done to identify the precipitating event. Common precipitating events include trauma, sepsis, infection, myocardial infarction, and severe emotional stress.[45]

DIFFERENTIAL DIAGNOSIS

Table 16.27 summarizes the differential diagnosis for adrenal insufficiency.

TABLE 16.27 Differential Diagnosis for Adrenal Insufficiency

Differential Diagnosis	Description
Sepsis	Adrenal crisis typically manifests as shock, which can be confused with septic shock
Shock	Adrenal crisis typically manifests as shock
Dehydration	Patients frequently present with symptoms of severe dehydration
Gastrointestinal (GI) malignancy	Patients often complain of fatigue, weight loss, and GI upset

DIAGNOSTIC STUDIES

Laboratory studies most frequently reveal hyponatremia, hyperkalemia, and normocytic anemia, with hyponatremia being present in ~75% of patients.[43] Hypoglycemia may be present after long periods of fasting but is more commonly found in patients who have both type 1 diabetes mellitus and Addison's disease. Laboratory testing is needed to confirm adrenal insufficiency. The three pillars of diagnosing adrenal insufficiency are identifying low cortisol secretion, determining ACTH dependency, and identifying a cause. Establishing decreased serum cortisol is the first step in diagnosing adrenal insufficiency. Once a cortisol deficiency has been established, these diagnostic steps should be followed (Figure 16.11):

1. Standard high-dose ACTH stimulation test:
   a. Perform 250 mcg IV corticotropin stimulation test.
      i. Adrenal insufficiency is confirmed when cortisol levels are below 500 nmol/L at 30 or 60 minutes after bolus.
   b. If standard corticotropin stimulation test is not available, decreased morning cortisol with elevated ACTH is suggestive of primary adrenal insufficiency and decreased morning cortisol with decreased ACTH is suggestive of secondary or tertiary adrenal insufficiency. Corticotropin stimulation testing should still be used to confirm diagnosis when available.
2. Plasma ACTH level:
   a. This can be done at the same time as the ACTH stimulation test.
      i. Primary adrenal insufficiency is confirmed when plasma ACTH is more than twice the upper limit in the established reference range.
      ii. If ACTH is not elevated, consider secondary or tertiary adrenal insufficiency.
         1. CRH testing: if elevated, confirms secondary adrenal insufficiency (problem of the pituitary) and if decreased, confirms tertiary adrenal insufficiency (problem of the hypothalamus)
3. If primary adrenal insufficiency is established, order plasma renin and aldosterone to rule out subsequent mineralocorticoid deficiency.
4. Cause should be determined.

In patients in whom the cause of adrenal insufficiency remains unclear, HIV testing should be performed.

EVALUATION

Upon diagnosis, patients should be referred to an endocrinologist for management, typically requiring annual appointments for adults and quarterly appointments for pediatric patients. In patients who have an autoimmune cause of adrenal insufficiency, periodic monitoring for the development of additional autoimmune disease should also be performed. Because of the nonspecific nature of presenting symptoms of adrenal crisis, a high index of suspicion must be maintained at all times.

TREATMENT

- Glucocorticoid replacement is the mainstay of treatment, with hydrocortisone the treatment of choice for long-term management.
- Mineralocorticoid replacement may be required if the patient has an aldosterone deficiency.
- If undergoing surgery, stress-dose glucocorticoids are needed before and after the procedure.
- Management of adrenal crisis requires a multidisciplinary team approach and a high index of suspicion. IV or intramuscular (IM) hydrocortisone and IV fluids are required, with the addition of IV dextrose often needed.

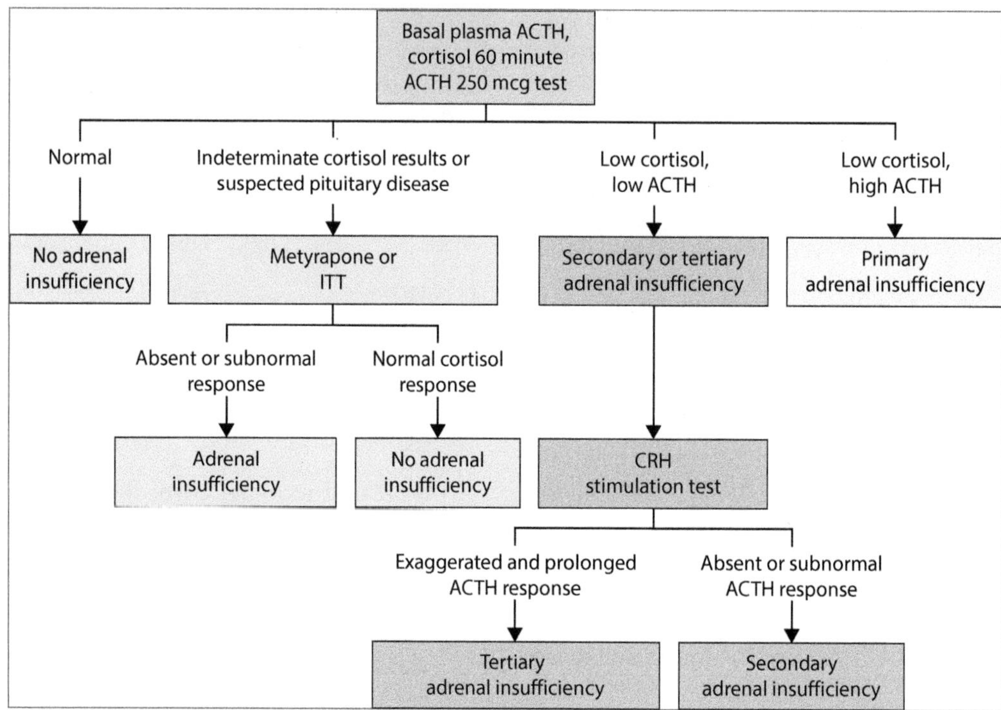

Figure 16.11 Diagnostic approach for suspected adrenal insufficiency. ACTH, adrenocorticotropic hormone; CRH, corticotropin-releasing hormone; ITT, insulin tolerance test.

- Any patient on long-term glucocorticoid therapy that is causing ACTH deficiency should be slowly tapered off medication if stopping as abrupt withdrawal can result in severe symptom exacerbation.[46]

PATIENT EDUCATION

- Patients should be made aware of the signs and symptoms associated with glucocorticoid under- and over-replacement and advised to follow up with a clinician as soon as they present.
- Risk of adrenal crisis in patients with adrenal insufficiency is high and patients should understand the risks involved with lapses in medication management.
- Patients should be counseled on the need for increased dosage of glucocorticoid therapy during illness, fever, or stress (dosing determined by endocrinologist).[46]

16.5B CUSHING SYNDROME

MEDICAL HISTORY AND CLINICAL PRESENTATION

Cushing syndrome is the result of excess cortisol presentation varies significantly with the cause, degree, and duration of hypercortisolism. In the event of iatrogenic Cushing syndrome, patients will have a history of chronic exogenous glucocorticoid use. If the cause is a pituitary adenoma (Cushing disease), patients may present with headache, bitemporal heminopia, or signs and symptoms of hypersecretion of other pituitary hormones. Patients most frequently present with proximal muscle weakness with extremity wasting, central adiposity, and facial plethora. Independently, the presenting signs and symptoms of Cushing syndrome appear vague and possibly unrelated, so grouping symptoms that have their onset in a similar time frame is important for early recognition.

SIGNS AND SYMPTOMS

Whether exogenous or endogenous in nature, increased exposure to glucocorticoids causes the signs and symptoms associated with Cushing syndrome. Characteristic signs and symptoms of hypercortisolism include proximal muscle weakness with extremity wasting, central adiposity, facial plethora (moon face), abdominal striae, and supraclavicular fat pads.[47] Although these are the most common group of presenting complaints, hypercortisolism causes systemic effects that may also be appreciated:

- Menstrual irregularities in females due to GnRH suppression[48]
- Increased ecchymosis due to loss of subcutaneous tissue loss
- Skin atrophy and striae as a result of stratum corneum thinning and skin that is stretched rapidly to accommodate central adiposity
- Tinea versicolor, primarily on the trunk
- Hyperpigmentation of the skin due to increased ACTH production, primarily the presence of an ectopic ACTH-secreting tumor
- Glucose intolerance, hyperglycemia, and/or diabetes mellitus as a result of cortisol's stimulation of gluconeogenesis as well increased peripheral resistance to insulin due to obesity
- Osteoporosis due to decreased intestinal and renal calcium absorption and decreased bone formation
- Obesity, primarily in the trunk, face, and abdomen, resulting in the characteristic "buffalo hump," "moon face," and central adiposity
- Depression

Patients who gain weight with Cushing syndrome are at risk for obesity-related conditions including hypertension, cardiovascular disease (CVD), and sleep apnea.

Adrenal adenomas (ACTH-independent Cushing syndrome) typically only secrete glucocorticoids, whereas causes of ACTH-dependent Cushing syndrome result in androgen excess in women due to ACTH-stimulated hyperandrogenism. Adrenal carcinoma most commonly results in hyperandrogenism and patients present with hirsutism, acne, and decreased libido. These same symptoms do not present in men, as the testes are responsible for the majority of androgen production in males versus the adrenal glands in females. When hypercortisolism is caused by adrenal carcinoma, weight loss, rather than the characteristic weight gain, may be present.

PHYSICAL EXAMINATION

Physical exam findings will support the signs and symptoms outlined above.

DIFFERENTIAL DIAGNOSIS

Table 16.28 summarizes the differential diagnosis of Cushing syndrome.

DIAGNOSTIC STUDIES

In addition to those presenting with the typical signs and symptoms of Cushing syndrome, young adults with hypertension or osteoporosis and patients with adrenal incidentalomas should be screened for Cushing syndrome. Before any screening, use of exogenous glucocorticoids must also be excluded, as well as common causes of physiologic hypercortisolism that include pregnancy, severe obesity, and major depressive disorder. Additionally, factitious Cushing syndrome, the purposeful self-administration of excessive exogenous glucocorticoids, must be excluded. Because of variability in screening laboratory results, a diagnosis is not confirmed until at least two positive, first-line tests are unequivocally abnormal. After a diagnosis is confirmed through two tests, the cause must then be established (see Table 16.29).

Cortisol levels are typically lower at night than during the day. Late-night salivary cortisol testing is used to evaluate hypercortisolism because in a healthy patient, cortisol levels should be decreased during this time. In patients with Cushing syndrome, this physiologic decrease does not occur, and levels remain elevated. The 24-hour urinary free cortisol (UFC) excretion requires urine collection over 24 hours and measures aggregate cortisol levels for the entire day. Overnight 1 mg dexamethasone suppression test (DST) requires patients to take 1 mg of dexamethasone at 11:00 pm followed by laboratory testing for serum cortisol levels at 8:00 am the following morning. In a healthy individual, the administration of exogenous glucocorticoids (in the form of dexamethasone for this test) will suppress endogenous secretion of cortisol from the adrenal glands through negative feedback at both the hypothalamus (CRH suppression) and anterior pituitary gland (ACTH suppression). In patients with Cushing syndrome, serum cortisol levels remain elevated (>1.8 mcg/dL) despite the administration of exogenous glucocorticoids.

Once hypercortisolism is established, ACTH levels can be measured to help determine the source of the problem. If ACTH levels are decreased, an adrenal tumor is likely the cause as negative feedback at the hypothalamus and pituitary glands are properly attempting to downregulate the system. If ACTH levels are high or normal, the problem is likely a pituitary tumor or an ectopic ACTH-secreting tumor. CRH stimulation testing can be used to attempt to further elevate ACTH and cortisol levels; if ACTH and cortisol rise with CRH administration, a pituitary tumor, versus an ectopic tumor, is likely. Additionally, high-dose DST can be used to differentiate a pituitary tumor from an ectopic tumor. If cortisol levels decline after high-dose dexamethasone administration, a pituitary tumor is likely the cause, whereas continuously elevated cortisol levels point toward an ectopic tumor. Regardless of tumor location, it must be visualized and both CT and MRI scanning can be beneficial. In the event that a pituitary tumor is suspected and does not appear on imaging, petrosal sinus sampling can be used.[49]

TABLE 16.28 Differential Diagnosis for Cushing Syndrome

Differential Diagnosis	Description
Obesity	Frequent presenting sign of Cushing syndrome
Depression	Can present with weight gain, decreased mood
Polycystic ovary syndrome (PCOS)	Patients present with obesity, hirsutism, and irregular menstruation

TABLE 16.29 Diagnostic Approach for Cushing Syndrome

Level of Suspicion	Diagnostic Tests	Diagnostic Considerations
Low index of suspicion	Select **one** of the following: 1. Late-night salivary cortisol 2. 24-hour urinary free cortisol (UFC) excretion 3. Overnight 1mg dexamethasone suppression test (DST) *If first is positive, select another to confirm*	• UFC: results should be 3x upper limit of normal • DST: upper limit of normal for serum cortisol concentration should be <1.8 mcg/dL • If low suspicion and negative, no further testing needed • If low suspicion and only one test is positive, refer to endocrinology • If high suspicion and negative (for one or both tests), refer to endocrinology
High index of suspicion	Select **two** of the following: 1. Late-night salivary cortisol 2. 24-hour UFC excretion 3. Overnight 1 mg DST	

EVALUATION

Patients who are diagnosed with Cushing syndrome should be further evaluated for obesity-related conditions including diabetes mellitus, hypertension, and hypercholesterolemia. Additionally, as surgery is typically required for disease treatment and patients are at an increased risk for thrombotic events, risk must be evaluated, and prevention measures put in place prior to undergoing any procedures.

TREATMENT

- Effective management of Cushing syndrome first requires determining the cause of increased cortisol production.
- Exogenous Cushing syndrome requires a slow taper off of glucocorticoids to mitigate symptoms of hypothalamic-pituitary-adrenal insufficiency that may follow the discontinuation of therapy.
- Cushing disease requires removal of the pituitary adenoma, typically performed by transsphenoidal resection.
- Ectopic ACTH-producing tumors should be removed surgically, with possible need for chemotherapy or radiation treatment.
- Primary adrenal tumors typically require an adrenalectomy.
- Patients should receive dietary and exercise counseling due to the increased risk of obesity-related conditions.
- Management of any related conditions such as diabetes, depression, and hypertension is also necessary.

PATIENT EDUCATION

- Healthy diet and routine exercise are an important part of Cushing syndrome management due to the increased risk of obesity-related disease.
- After effective treatment, physical signs and symptoms of Cushing syndrome typically resolve within 1 year.
- Metabolic syndrome-related conditions may not fully resolve with surgical treatment alone.

SPECIAL CONSIDERATIONS

Patients with primary adrenal insufficiency who are pregnant should be instructed to report any symptoms associated with glucocorticoid over- or under-replacement as soon as they arise. Formal in-office review should occur at least once per trimester in conjunction with a routine prenatal appointment. Increased hydrocortisone therapy may be needed in the third trimester, with stress doses during labor. Children with primary adrenal insufficiency often require divided doses of hydrocortisone and close monitoring of growth velocity, blood pressure, and energy levels.[46]

In children, Cushing syndrome may result in growth retardation and should be considered in any child who has an unexpected drop in height percentile and increase in weight percentile. For pregnant patients in whom Cushing syndrome is suspected, DST should not be used as a diagnostic test.

KEY POINTS

- High index of suspicion for adrenal crisis is needed for all patients with a history of adrenal insufficiency or who present with shock.
- Stress dose glucocorticoid therapy is required in many situations for patients with adrenal insufficiency and patients should be managed by an endocrinologist.
- Patients with a sudden increase in central adiposity paired with facial edema and striae should be tested for Cushing syndrome.
- Cushing syndrome must be differentiated into ACTH-dependent and ACTH-independent Cushing syndrome.

16.6 MULTIPLE ENDOCRINE NEOPLASIA

OVERVIEW

Multiple endocrine neoplasia (MEN) syndromes are the result of heritable gene mutations that cause excessive growth of various endocrine glands, predisposing patients to benign and malignant tumors. MEN syndromes consist of three independent, but sometimes overlapping, patterns: 1, 2A, and 2B. Although other endocrine glands can be affected, MEN1 most commonly affects the parathyroid gland, resulting in PHPT (see Section 16.3A), the anterior pituitary gland, and pancreatic islet cells. MEN2 most commonly causes medullary thyroid cancer (MTC), pheochromocytoma, and primary parathyroid hyperplasia, affecting all organs where the *RET* proto-oncogene is expressed. Mutations are inherited in an autosomal dominant pattern and despite the high degree of penetrance, symptoms vary greatly by patient as a single mutant gene can result in multiple different effects. The affected endocrine gland determines the presenting signs and symptoms, and patients typically have effects in more than one gland.

- MEN1 expressions (in order of most to least common):
  - PHPT
  - Entero-pancreatic tumors (e.g., gastromas, insulinomas)
  - Anterior pituitary adenomas
  - Adrenal cortical tumors, foregut carcinoid tumors.
    - *The foregut carcinoid and adrenal cortical tumors are typically nonfunctioning. The presence of these tumor types aid in the clinical diagnosis of MEN1.*
- MEN2A subclassifications:
  - MEN2A classical: MTC, pheochromocytoma, PHPT
  - MEN2A with cutaneous lichen amyloidosis (CLA)
  - MEN2A with Hirschsprung disease (HD)
  - Familial MTC (FMTC)
- MEN2B expressions:
  - MTC
  - Pheochromocytoma
  - Less commonly: mucosal neuromas, intestinal ganglioneuromas, marfanoid habitus

EPIDEMIOLOGY

MEN1 has an estimated prevalence of only 2 cases per 100,000. MEN2 (2A and 2B) has an estimated prevalence of 1 in 30,000.

PATHOPHYSIOLOGY

MEN syndromes follow an autosomal dominant inheritance pattern but cannot always be traced back to a single gene mutation. The *MEN1* gene was named in 1988 after discovering the genetic linkage between a specific region on the long arm of chromosome 11 (11q13) and the heritable syndrome. Much information regarding how menin, the protein product of the *MEN1* gene, directly impacts tumorigenesis is still largely unknown. It is thought that, as individuals typically only inherit one affected copy of the *MEN1* gene, there is a frequently occurring suppressive function of the remaining, unaffected gene (see Figure 16.12).

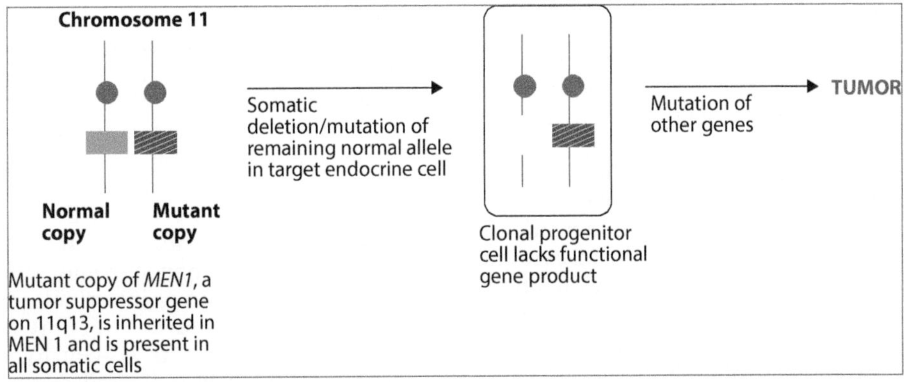

Figure 16.12 **The formation of tumors in patients with MEN1 (multiple endocrine neoplasia type 1).**

However, some individuals who present with the typical clinical picture do not test positive for this known defect, leaving researchers to believe other genetic mutations may rarely be responsible for the same phenotypic presentation as seen with MEN1. Emerging research has shown a MEN1-like condition caused by cyclin-dependent kinase (CDK) inhibitor gene mutation (CDKN1B mutation) that has been named MEN4. It is thought that 1–2% of patients previously thought to have MEN1 but in whom genetic mutations of the *MEN1* gene cannot be identified, may actually have MEN4.

About 95% of individuals with MEN2B have a single amino acid substitution in the RET protein on chromosome 10, but about 50% of these substitutions are de novo mutations, so patients will not have a family history of disease. In both MEN2A and MEN2B, the amino acid substitution causes *RET* proto-oncogene-mediated cellular process activation; development of related tumors depends on the specific *RET* mutation, with MTC having close to 90% penetrance.

MEDICAL HISTORY AND CLINICAL PRESENTATION

The 3Ps mnemonic can be used to remember the primary effects of MEN1: parathyroid, pancreatic islet, and anterior pituitary tumors. Additionally, carcinoid tumors and lipomas are more common than the general population. By age 50, almost all individuals affected by MEN1 have parathyroid gland tumors, manifesting as PHPT. Hyperparathyroidism caused by familial MEN1 does differ in some regard from sporadic PHPT: men and women are affected equally in MEN1 (versus female predominance), presentation in the second to fourth decades (versus fourth to sixth decades), and high rates of recurrent disease despite initially successful subtotal parathyroidectomy. An incidental finding of hypercalcemia on routine labtests, followed by findings of elevated serum PTH levels, is the most common presentation for familial MEN1 PHPT. If the disease progresses and patients become symptomatic, patients may have decreased BMD, nephrolithiasis, polyuria, polydipsia, and constipation (see Section 16.3A).

Pituitary adenomas, most commonly lactotroph, also occur as a result of MEN1. Lactotroph adenomas result in hyperprolactinemia and patients may present with galactorrhea. In patients with MEN1, macroadenomas and hormone levels that are resistant to therapy are more common than sporadic adenomas.

Pancreatic islet cell tumors and GI endocrine cell tumors are also more prevalent in patients with MEN1. Zollinger-Ellison syndrome (ZES) is the leading cause of severe peptic ulcer disease and diarrhea as a result of elevated serum gastrin levels. Additionally, radiographic screening has proved an increased risk of nonfunctioning pancreatic neuroendocrine tumors that have malignant potential and frequent liver metastases. In addition to ZES, insulinomas may occur causing patients to present with uncontrollable bouts of hypoglycemia.

The clinical presentation of MEN2A depends highly on the affected organs but with nearly 100% penetrance of MTC, it can be expected that this finding will be present in the vast majority of patients. Patients with FMTC are at an increased risk for MTC but do not have the same predisposition to pheochromocytoma or parathyroid hyperplasia as seen in classical MEN2A. Most frequently, FMTC presents in the third decade of life with a solitary thyroid nodule and with or without cervical lymphadenopathy. Pheochromocytomas typically present late in the third decade of life and are usually identified during early screening in patients with known MEN2. Pheochromocytomas are rarely the first presenting sign of MEN2.

SIGNS AND SYMPTOMS

As multiple different endocrine glands can be affected in MEN types 1, 2A, and 2B, the signs and symptoms of disease will vary greatly by individual. Understanding the signs and symptoms of endocrine gland hyperfunction as outlined throughout this chapter can be helpful in determining affected glands.

Possible signs and symptoms of MEN1 tumors:

- **Parathyroid tumors:** Polyuria, polydipsia, constipation, abdominal pain, decreased BMD
- **Pituitary (lactotroph) adenomas:** Galactorrhea
- **Pancreatic islet cell and gastrointestinal endocrine cell tumors:** Peptic ulcers, dyspepsia, diarrhea, hypoglycemia

Possible signs and symptoms of MEN2 tumors:

- **Medullary thyroid cancer:** Cervical lymphadenopathy, thyroid nodule
- **Pheochromocytomas:** Paroxysmal attacks of anxiety, headache, sweating, palpitations, and tachycardia
- **Parathyroid tumors:** Polyuria, polydipsia, constipation, abdominal pain, decreased BMD

PHYSICAL EXAMINATION

Physical examination should be guided by the presenting signs and symptoms and findings will vary greatly based on the affected endocrine glands. In patients with MEN1 or MEN2 in whom PHPT is suspected, asymmetric parathyroid gland enlargement may be appreciated, but normal neck findings should not rule out suspicion or prevent further diagnostic evaluation (see Section 16.3A). Pituitary adenomas may be asymptomatic, but physical exam may reveal bitemporal heminopia due to physical compression of the optic chiasm by the mass. Additional physical exam findings will be consistent with the specific hormone that is being hypersecreted. For example, a lactotroph adenoma may cause galactorrhea.

MTC is the most common presenting tumor associated with MEN2. Patients most frequently present with a palpable solitary thyroid nodule with or without cervical lymphadenopathy. In patients with pheochromocytomas, physical exam may reveal weight loss, fever, tremor, or tachycardia, although symptoms are typically paroxysmal with many only appreciated during acute attacks.

DIFFERENTIAL DIAGNOSIS

Box 16.3 summarizes the differential diagnosis for MENs.

DIAGNOSTIC STUDIES

The clinical diagnosis of MEN1 requires the presence of two or more primary MEN1 tumor types in an individual without a positive family history of MEN1, or one primary MEN1 tumor type in a patient with a positive family history of MEN1. Genetic testing can be used to aid in diagnosis of patients with a mixed clinical picture or who do not have a known family history of disease. Additionally, it can aid in identifying individuals who are genetically predisposed to developing clinical manifestations of MEN1. Individuals and families should work closely with a genetic counselor before undergoing screening studies, as there is no established benefit to screening patients who are at risk for MEN1 prior to the presentation of symptoms. Workup for symptoms of specific gland dysfunction is the same as in sporadic disease.

- **Primary hyperparathyroidism:** Elevated serum calcium, elevated PTH (for more details, see Section 16.3A)
- **Pituitary adenoma:** Serum hormone levels associated with suspected disease (lactotroph adenomas: elevated serum prolactin), positive MRI (for more details, see Section 16.1A)
- **ZES:** Elevated fasting serum gastrin levels, low gastric pH

BOX 16.3 Differential Diagnosis for Multiple Endocrine Neoplasias

Sporadic hyperparathyroidism
Peptic ulcer disease
Hypoglycemia
Panic attack

Whereas genetic testing is of controversial value in diagnosing MEN1, it is considered necessary in diagnosing MEN2. The diagnosis of MEN2 requires one or two classical clinical findings and either the presence of an identified *RET* mutation or identification of classical symptoms in a first-degree family member. Without an identified *RET* mutation or a clear autosomal dominant inheritance pattern, a clinical diagnosis of MEN2B can be made when at least two classical features are present. Classical features include MTC, pheochromocytoma, mucosal neuromas, marfanoid habitus, intestinal ganglioneuromas, and myelinated corneal nerves. MTC is frequently diagnosed in the preneoplastic state (C-cell hyperplasia) in patients in whom screening is indicated due to known family history of MTC. Additionally, basal serum calcitonin levels are typically elevated in patients with a palpable thyroid tumor. It can be very difficult to differentiate the FMTC variant of MEN2A from classical MTC variant of MEN2A; vigilant screening for the presence of pheochromocytomas and a thorough family history are imperative, making differentiation more difficult in smaller families. Pheochromocytomas are diagnosed through catecholamine testing followed by abdominal CT or MRI; bilateral pheochromocytomas are much more common in patients with MEN2 than sporadic disease. Much like in MEN1, PHPT in MEN2A is typically multiglandular and patients are diagnosed through findings of elevated serum PTH and elevated hypercalcemia.

EVALUATION

Enteropancreatic neuroendocrine tumors, such as pancreatic islet cell tumors, now pose the biggest threat to life for patients with MEN1 as effective management or treatment for hyperparathyroidism and pituitary adenomas tends to be more readily available. Patients should be counseled on the early presenting signs and symptoms of disease, although many patients have pancreatic and carcinoid tumors present at diagnosis of MEN1. Once a diagnosis of MEN2 is established, specific *RET* mutation analysis should be performed, along with meetings with a genetic counselor to initiate familial screening recommendations. For patients with known MEN2, increased awareness of early symptoms of pheochromocytoma and annual screening of plasma fractionated metanephrines is indicated. Additionally, serum calcium levels should be monitored annually in patients with MEN2A for early detection of hyperparathyroidism; patients with MEN2B do not require serum calcium screening as hyperparathyroidism is not present in this condition.

TREATMENT

MEN1

- **Parathyroid tumors:**
    - Surgical recommendations for patients with PHPT due to MEN1 are similar to those with sporadic PHPT. Patients who are experiencing symptoms of hypercalcemia, such as nephrolithiasis or decreased bone density, are strong candidates for parathyroidectomy. Patients who are asymptomatic may delay surgery until symptoms present.

- **Gastrinomas:**
  - Management of hypercalcemia associated with hyperparathyroidism by parathyroidectomy can secondarily also reduce gastrin levels and improve symptoms associated with ZES.
  - Proton-pump inhibitors may be used to suppress symptoms related to peptic ulcers.
  - Partial pancreatectomy or duodenectomy may be indicated in resistant disease.
- **Insulinomas:**
  - Differing from sporadic insulinomas as multiple tumors are typically found throughout the pancreas, MEN1 insulinomas may require local excision of tumors in the head of the pancreas in addition to a subtotal distal pancreatectomy to increase the chances of removing all affected cells.
- **Pituitary adenomas:**
  - Treatment guidelines are very similar to sporadic adenomas, with hormonal control first being treated pharmacologically through suppression mechanisms if possible, with the majority of patients requiring transphenoidal resection of the adenoma.

MEN2

- Prophylactic thyroidectomy is indicated in all patients with a positive *RET* mutation.
- Pheochromocytomas, if present at the time of diagnosis, should be surgically removed prior to thyroidectomy.
- Parathyroidectomy is indicated in patients diagnosed with PHPT.

PATIENT EDUCATION

- Patients with a family history of MEN1 should see a genetic counselor before undergoing genetic screening as it is not indicated in all patients.
- Almost all patients with MEN2 will require a thyroidectomy as MTC has nearly 100% penetrance.
- Patients with a personal diagnosis or known family history of MEN2 should meet with a genetic counselor before becoming pregnant to discuss screening options and early detection.
- Patients with MEN2 require routine screening for MEN2-related tumors; close monitoring and early detection are imperative.

KEY POINTS

- Genetic screening is not always indicated for family members of patients diagnosed with MEN1 but is required with MEN2.
- Early detection of MTC leads to an excellent prognosis.

16.7 DIABETES MELLITUS

OVERVIEW

Type 1 diabetes (T1DM), formerly known as juvenile diabetes or insulin dependent diabetes, is typically diagnosed before the patient reaches adulthood, although some cases are diagnosed later in life. According to the American Diabetes Association (ADA), 1.25 million Americans currently have T1DM and nearly 40,000 more will be diagnosed with it this year. With T1DM, the patient's pancreas does not properly produce insulin and the patient must rely on exogenous insulin. This leads to the need for frequent monitoring of blood glucose and adjustment of insulin to maintain euglycemia. While T1DM is far less common than T2DM, the complications that result from the disease are very similar.

T2DM is a major health epidemic worldwide and has become the seventh leading cause of death in the United States. Additionally, having T2DM is a major risk factor for having comorbid CVD. T2DM is far more common in the U.S. population than T1DM, with 90% to 95% of people with diabetes having type 2 according to the CDC.[50] T2DM is the leading contributor to renal failure, adult blindness, and nontraumatic lower limb amputations in the United States. Diabetes is a costly disease for the patient and for taxpayers. For the patient, the growing cost of insulin and testing supplies is a burden many patients cannot bear. For taxpayers, the cost associated with prolonged hyperglycemia is staggering.

EPIDEMIOLOGY

Type 1 Diabetes Mellitus

As of 2015, 1.25 million people in the United States were living with T1DM. Nearly 85% of those diagnosed, are diagnosed before 20 years of age with rates of incidence starting at birth and increasing around puberty (ages 10 to 14 years of age). This decreases after age 14 and stabilizes between the ages of 15 and 29.[51] Worldwide, there does not appear to be any gender disparity as males and females are diagnosed in equal numbers. The SEARCH for Diabetes in Youth study was founded to determine if race was a factor in incidence of T1DM; it was unable to show that T1DM was predominant in any particular race.[51]

Type 2 Diabetes Mellitus

As of 2015, there were 30.3 million Americans with T2DM in the United States and another 84.1 million with prediabetes.

- Prevalence varies with level of education; 12.6% of people with less than a high school diploma have diabetes. Those with a high school diploma make up 9.5% of patients with diabetes.[50]
- More men (36.3%) than women (29.3%) have prediabetes.
- More than 25% of seniors over 65 years of age have T2DM.
- More than 193,000 youth under the age of 20 now have T2DM.
- Prevalence is varied according to ethnicity:
  7.4% of non-Hispanic whites
  8.0% of Asian Americans
  12.1% of Hispanics
  12.7% of non-Hispanic blacks
  15.1% of American Indians/Alaskan Natives[52]

Diabetes has become the seventh leading cause of death in the United States with diabetes listed as a contributing cause of death on more than 252,000 death certificates in 2015. It was listed as the cause of death for 79,535 people. The cost of diabetes in the United States alone is staggering. In 2017, T2DM accounted for $237 billion in direct medical costs and another $90 billion in reduced productivity.[52]

PATHOPHYSIOLOGY

Type 1 Diabetes Mellitus

T1DM is a chronic autoimmune disorder occurring in genetically susceptible individuals, although environmental factors may play a part in the patient developing diabetes. The immune system is triggered to mount an autoimmune defense against altered beta cell antigens that resemble a viral protein; 85% of patients have circulating islet cell antibodies that are detectable in the blood. The majority of these patients also have circulating anti-insulin antibodies. Most islet cell antibodies are directed against glutamic acid decarboxylase (GAD) within pancreatic beta cells.With the immune attack against the pancreatic beta cells, the number of beta cells declines, and so does the ability to produce insulin for circulation in the body. Once 80% to 90% of the beta cells have been destroyed, the pancreas no longer possesses the ability to produce enough insulin and hyperglycemia occurs.

Type 2 Diabetes Mellitus

T2DM is a complex disorder, with defects in insulin secretion and insulin sensitivity. It often has an insidious onset and develops due to hormonal, genetic, or environmental influences. T2DM is a progressive disease, which starts with a period of insulin resistance. Insulin resistance itself does not necessarily lead to diabetes unless beta cell secretion of insulin is decreased. T2DM starts with a period of hyperinsulinemia and normal glucose levels. As insulin resistance increases, hyperglycemia is present along with hyperinsulinemia.

Insulin is released in response to beta cell stimulation and mediates the uptake of glucose, amino acids, and fatty acids by insulin-sensitive tissues. These tissues then provide feedback to the islet cells regarding the need for insulin. When insulin resistance is present, the beta cell must increase insulin output to maintain normal glucose levels. When the beta cell loses the ability to perform this task, the result is an elevation in plasma glucose.When beta cell function decreases to 50% or less, overt diabetes develops. Beta cell failure develops in the setting of genetic predisposition, environment, and lifestyle influences.

Impaired beta cell function is already present in those known to be at risk for diabetes: first-degree relatives of those with T2DM, women with gestational diabetes mellitus, women with polycystic ovary syndrome (PCOS), and older individuals. Additionally, decreased beta cell function may be passed genetically and determines glucose intolerance in different racial and ethnic groups.[53]

Beta cell dysfunction, however, is not the only culprit in the development of diabetes. The "ominous octet"—the beta cell along with the brain, adipocytes, muscle tissue, the liver, kidneys, GI tissues, and pancreatic alpha cell—all play a role in the pathogenesis of T2DM[54]

LIVER

In the liver, gradual loss in signaling factors that influence insulin action results from a breakdown in insulin's ability to suppress hepatic gluconeogenesis. As a result, increased free fatty acids in the liver increase gluconeogenesis, playing a role in increased hepatic glucose production.[55]

MUSCLE

Insulin resistance in muscle tissue is displayed in defects in intracellular phosphorylation and glucose transport. Insulin access is impaired and signaling in the muscle microvasculature is responsible for these deficits. In the muscles, insulin directly affects the action of hexokinase, glucose synthase, and pyruvate dehydrogenase and its deficit—either via insulin deficiency or due to resistance—reduces glycogen synthesis and glycolysis in the muscle cell leaving plasma glucose levels to rise.[55]

ADIPOCYTES

"Lipotoxicity" refers to excessive free-floating fatty acids on insulin action and secretion. Lipotoxicity is detrimental to the body, causing insulin resistance in the liver, muscles, brain, and pancreas. It presents as hypertriglyceridemia and nonalcoholic fatty liver disease (NAFLD), both common comorbidities to T2DM. In the liver, hyperinsulinemia activates lipogenesis and leads to excessive free fatty acid production. BMI is a known leading risk factor for T2DM, with the risk increasing 50 to 80 times with a BMI >35.[55]

KIDNEYS

In the kidneys, two manifestations of diabetes are increased gluconeogenesis and increased glucose reabsorption. These two factors impact glucose levels to directly exacerbate hyperglycemia. In T2DM, the kidneys increase glucogenesis, generating more glucose. As glucose levels remain elevated over time in the body, the glucose reabsorption threshold increases.[55]

GASTROINTESTINAL TRACT

In the GI tract, incretin hormones include glucose dependent insulinotropic polypeptide (GIP) and glucagon-like peptide (GLP-1). These hormones are secreted in the gut, regulating glucose homeostasis due to enhanced insulin secretion from pancreatic beta cells and suppression of glucagon secretion. Oral glucose intake and the rise in glucose that follows stimulates GIP and GLP-1, known as the "incretin effect." GIP and GLP-1 hormones may contribute between 25% and 75% of insulin secretory response after oral glucose load. Studies to assess GIP and GLP-1 in patients with T2DM have not consistently shown decreased secretion of hormones in response to oral glucose tolerance test (OGTT) and mixed meal tests when compared to healthy subjects. Evidence supports decreased incretin function and possible development of incretin resistance in patients with T2DM, especially those patients with long-standing disease.[55]

PANCREAS (BETA AND ALPHA CELLS)

Hyperglycemia and dyslipidemia reduce the expression of key regulating factors and lead to dedifferentiation of the beta cell, or regression in their functional status. In patients with overnutrition and obesity, increased metabolic demands lead to stress and exhaustion of the endoplasmic reticulum within the beta cells. Over time, these stressed out cells may dedifferentiate to alpha cells and produce glucagon, further exacerbating hyperglycemia, or they may continue and proceed to apoptosis.[55]

Alpha cells in the pancreas release glucagon, which is regulated by glucose levels. Glucagon is secreted in healthy individuals when circulating insulin levels are low. Glucagon is secreted through the portal vein into the liver to stimulate gluconeogenesis, which allows glucose to be secreted by the liver.[55] In patients with hyperglycemia, high levels of glucagon are observed throughout the day, even when they are already hyperglycemic. Glucagon is inappropriately released in response to a meal, which may explain the postprandial rise in glucose levels seen in T2DM.

BRAIN

The hypothalamus and pituitary gland coordinate numerous peripherally released hormones to influence appetite, energy balance, and metabolism. Insulin, leptin, glucagon, GLP-1, and ghrelin influence glucose level via the CNS. These hormones communicate with the hypothalamus through numerous mechanisms, including direct sensing in the gut. In the healthy hypothalamus, insulin suppresses the appetite. Obesity is associated with CNS hormonal dysfunction. Overnutrition, high fat feeding, and obesity promote insulin resistance in both the medial basal hypothalamus and the dorsal vagal complex, increasing glucose production and hyperphagia. The ratio of insulin present in the CSF to plasma is inversely related to BMI, indicating potential problems with insulin transport to the hypothalamus as cause for hypothalamic insulin resistance.[55]

Disturbances in HPA axis and the autonomic nervous system are also seen in the pathogenesis of T2DM. Chronic overaction of the HPA axis and the autonomic nervous system are seen in psychiatric diseases and neurogenerative diseases, which have ties to metabolic syndrome, insulin resistance, and T2DM.[55]

MEDICAL HISTORY AND CLINICAL PRESENTATION

Type 1 Diabetes Mellitus

These patients may report noticing polyphagia, polyuria, or polydipsia. Often, there is unexplained weight loss, weakness, and/or fatigue. It is important to ask if there are any family members who also have T1DM. Children may not be diagnosed until they end up presenting urgently or emergently for care when they are experiencing diabetic ketoacidosis (DKA).

Type 2 Diabetes Mellitus

Often T2DM has an insidious onset and is found when routine lab work returns with hyperglycemia or glycosuria noted. Some patients may notice they have felt more tired, thirsty, or hungry than usual. They may feel tired or report visual disturbances, primarily blurred vision. Diabetes is a heterogeneous disease; there is often a first-degree relative with T2DM.

SIGNS AND SYMPTOMS

Signs and symptoms for both T1DM and T2DM are similar, although typically patients with T1DM are not obese.

T1DM is identified in children and adults as they show signs of the following symptoms:

- Headaches
- Weight loss
- Blurry vision
- Extreme thirst
- Frequent urination
- Increased appetite
- Fruity breath odor
- Fatigue and weakness
- Rapid deep breathing

All patients may be asymptomatic or present with complaints of polyuria, polydipsia, or polyphagia. Often patients complain of unexplained fatigue and may have complaints of blurred vision. Acanthosis nigricans may be noted in the axilla, on the neck, or in the groin in patients with T2DM. If diabetes has been present for some time, patients may have neurologic, renal, or cardiovascular complications. Diabetes may be suspected in those who have frequent skin infections, frequent fungal infections, or mild hypertension on exam. In women who have chronic *Candida* infections, who delivered a baby larger than 9 lb, or who have had polyhydramnios or preeclampsia, diabetes may be suspected. In men, balanoposthitis may occur.

Typically, in obese patients, fat distribution will be central, occurring on the face, neck, chest, and abdomen. The appendages are often leaner and sometimes muscular. Waist circumference of >40 inches in men and >35 inches in women carries an increased risk of diabetes.

At the extreme, the patient with T2DM may present with HHNK or hyperglycemic hyperosmolar nonketotic coma. With T1DM, patients may present in DKA. These patients are profoundly dehydrated, hypotensive, lethargic, or comatose and are profoundly hyperglycemic.

PHYSICAL EXAMINATION

For patients presenting with hyperglycemia, dehydration may be present. Check skin turgor and mucous membranes, and evaluate the eyes for signs of dehydration. Fruity breath may be present in a diabetic patient presenting with ketosis.

Patients may not demonstrate any physical findings in T2DM or there may be central obesity with fat deposits primarily on the face, neck, chest, and abdomen. Some patients with long undiagnosed diabetes may have acanthosis nigricans or skin infections. Patients may have eye hemorrhages, exudates, or neovascularization. Patients with long-standing undiagnosed diabetes may have decreased or absent sensation of light touch, loss of DTRs in the ankles, dry skin (especially on the feet), and/or diabetic ulcers.

DIFFERENTIAL DIAGNOSIS

Type 1 Diabetes

Disorders of target tissues (liver, muscles, adipose tissue), T2DM, nondiabetic glycosuria, cystic fibrosis, chronic pancreatitis, monogenic diabetes (MODY), endocrine disorders, drug affect (thiazide diuretics, glucocorticoids, and phenytoin), Prader-Willi syndrome, and renal glycosuria are considered in the differential diagnosis.

Type 2 Diabetes

The differential diagnosis includes T1DM and DI.

DIAGNOSTIC STUDIES

Type 1 Diabetes Mellitus

If there is a high suspicion of T1DM, checking a POCT glucose is a specific, convenient method for determining if the patient is spilling both glucose and ketones into the urine. Serum glucose may be checked as well to determine the blood glucose level. Hemoglobin A1c (HbA1c) may be performed or deferred for follow-up visits. In patients (with either T1DM or T2DM) with recent acute blood loss, who are pregnant, or who have sickle cell anemia or hemoglobin variants, the fructosamine test may be a more reliable indicator since it gives an average of glucose levels for the past 2 to 3 weeks. Additionally, a complete blood count and blood and urine cultures may be indicated if it is necessary to rule out infection. If it may be necessary to determine if the patient has T1DM or T2DM, C-peptide, anti-insulin antibodies, and anti-GAD may also be ordered to obtain a definitive diagnosis.

Type 2 Diabetes Mellitus

Testing should be considered in patients 45 years of age and older, and if normal should be repeated every 3 years. Testing should be considered in younger individuals or more frequently if any of the following is evident:

- Overweight with a BMI ≥25 kg/m^2
- A first-degree relative with diabetes mellitus
- High-risk population (e.g., African Americans, Hispanic American, Native American, Asian Americans, and Pacific Islanders)
- History or current gestational diabetes mellitus (should be tested every 3 years for life)
- Hypertensive ≥140/90 mm Hg
- High-density cholesterol <35 mg/dL, TGs >250 mg/dL
- Prior impaired glucose tolerance or impaired fasting glucose (tested yearly)
- PCOS
- CVD
- Signs of insulin resistance (acanthosis nigricans, severe obesity, BMI >40 kg/m^2)

EVALUATION

For all patients, a comprehensive medical history and evaluation should be performed. The diagnosis of diabetes, whether type 1 or 2 must be made and confirmed via testing.

Patients should be evaluated for diabetes at age 45 and above. If fasting glucose is normal, repeat testing every 3 years after that. Testing should be considered at a younger age or be carried out more frequently in individuals who demonstrate any of the items listed in the preceding section.

HbA1c should be repeated twice a year in those patients meeting their treatment goals and who have stable glycemic control. In patients who are not or whose diabetes therapy has changed, check HbA1c quarterly.

TREATMENT

T1DM is often very difficult to manage; patients should be referred to pediatric endocrinology if under the age of 18 or, for adults, to endocrinology for optimal management and evaluation for insulin pump.

In managing T2DM, lifestyle management and changes are key. Whether the patient has prediabetes or has an elevated HbA1c, the first recommendation to patients needs to be a change to their current habits. Overnutrition and having a sedentary lifestyle are the two most detrimental factors to a patient's health. Additionally, tobacco users should be counseled about quitting. Patients must be encouraged to make changes to their diet, choosing a well-balanced and nutritious diet limiting carbohydrate intake to 45 to 60 g/meal with three meals per day. Exercise should be encouraged and should include of 30 minutes of cardiovascular exercise daily and weight-bearing exercise as tolerated, 5 days of the week. Target HbA1c goals should be set with the patient and discussed during follow-up visits.

ADA Standards of Care 2020 recommends an A1c of <7.0% for most nonpregnant adults. If the patient is newly diagnosed with diabetes, has an expected long life span, and no CVD, the goal may be set for <6.5%. In the elderly, those with extensive comorbidities or those with a history of extreme hypoglycemia, a less stringent goal of 8.0% to 8.5% may be set.[56]

Treatment starts with metformin, which is the first-line treatment for T2DM. It should be started at the lowest dose and slowly titrated up to avoid unpleasant GI side effects. Start with 500 mg daily with breakfast and have the patient increase to 500 mg with breakfast and dinner after 1 week. Metformin may be dosed up to a total of 2,000 mg daily over 1 to 2 months. Patients with GFR <38 cannot take metformin. It is also important to remind patients to stop metformin prior to any imaging they will receive when contrast agent may be used.

If the patient's A1c does not improve, a second therapy may be needed. The second therapy should be added based on any comorbidities. If the patient has atherosclerotic CVD with an increased risk for heart failure, a sodium-glucose co-transporter 2 (SGLT-2) inhibitor is preferred. For the patient with CKD, choose an SGLT-2 inhibitor or GLP-1 to reduce risk of CKD progression, reduce risk of CVD events, or both. For patients on a fixed income who don't have a history of severe hypoglycemia and are not elderly and at higher risk of hypoglycemia, a sulfonylurea or thiazolinedione may be added. Patients with a compelling need to promote weight loss may try an SGLT-2 inhibitor or GLP-1.

The patient should be seen every 3 to 6 months and therapy should be intensified when the patient is not meeting A1c goals; treatment should not be delayed. Early introduction of insulin should be considered if the patient is experiencing weight loss or symptoms of hyperglycemia or when glucose is >300 mg/dL or A1c is >10.0%.

In addition to managing the patient's insulin, monitoring the patient's blood pressure and cholesterol must be done. Patients with elevated blood pressure should be started on an angiotensin-converting enzyme (ACE) inhibitor or an angiotensin-receptor blocker (ARB) for renal protection and blood pressure management. Cholesterol management is more aggressive in patients with diabetes due to their risk of comorbid heart disease.

TABLE 16.30 Criteria for Prediabetes

Testing	Prediabetes	Diabetes
Hemoglobin A1c	5.7 to 6.4%	≥6.5%
FPG	100–125 mg/dL	≥126 mg/dL
OGTT	140–199 mg/dL	≥200 mg/dL
RPG		≥200 mg/dL AND clinical symptoms present

FPG, fasting plasma glucose; OGTT, oral glucose tolerance test; RPG, random plasma glucose.With RPG, patient must have clinical symptoms (i.e. fatigue, polydipsia, or polyuria with elevated glucose levels).

PATIENT EDUCATION

Patient education for patients with type 1 and type 2 diabetes is the same. Educate patients on the importance of lifestyle changes. Encourage healthy diets such as the DASH (Dietary Approaches to Stop Hypertension) diet or Mediterranean diet to promote weight loss, lower blood pressure, and lower blood sugars. Patients should meet with a certfied diabetic educator (CDE) to learn how to count carbohydrates, how to design an appropriate diet and intake for their age and activity level, and how they can modify their current lifestyle to achieve better controlled glucose levels. Additionally, CDEs are able to teach patients how to use insulin pumps and continuous glucose monitors (CGMs).

Always offer assistance with tobacco cessation for patients who smoke. It is vitally important to educate the patient on the microvascular complications involved with smoking and diabetes. Discuss healthy weight loss and weight management, exercise, and the importance of avoiding being sedentary.

Emphasize the importance of regular follow-up visits (every 3 months) to manage diabetes, yearly diabetic eye exams to avoid diabetic eye complications, and dental exams every 6 months. Encourage patients to always get their scheduled immunizations. Teach patients how to examine their feet daily and the importance of wearing shoes always, especially in those patients who have experienced some loss of sensation.

DIABETIC COMPLICATIONS

Patients with both type 1 and type 2 diabetes are at risk of many complications. From infections to comorbid chronic disease, it is important to consider and evaluate the patient at each visit for complications arising from diabetes.

- **Infection:** Patients with diabetes are susceptible to infection, the most common being:
  - Malignant otitis externa
  - Rhinocerebral mucormycosis
  - Bacteriuria
  - Pyuria
  - Cystitis
  - Upper urinary tract infection
  - Intrarenal bacterial infection
  - Skin and soft tissue infections
  - Osteomyelitis
- **Ophthalmologic complications:** Patients with diabetes may report seeing "floaters," which may be signs of retinal hemorrhage. They should be referred to ophthalmology immediately for evaluation and followed yearly (or per the ophthalmologist's recommendations) for laser treatment.
- **Diabetic nephropathy:** Patients with diabetes should have renal function monitored annually. In patients with T1DM for >5 years, check urine albumin excretion as well. Monitor all patients' list of prescriptions for nephrotoxic medications and discontinue them when possible. If patients have reduced creatinine, be sure to renally dose prescriptions as necessary. Exercise caution when ordering contrast studies in a patient with a creatinine above 2 mg/dL and patients with a creatinine level above 3 mg/dL should not be given contrast for any radiologic procedure.
- **Diabetic neuropathy:** Diabetic neuropathy is the most common complication of diabetes, affecting 50% of patient with both T1DM and T2DM. Diabetic peripheral neuropathy is the presence of symptoms when all other causes have been ruled out. In patients with T1DM, it typically takes many years of hyperglycemia before symptoms of neuropathy are noticed. In T2DM, only a few years of uncontrolled glucose may cause neuropathic symptoms. Symptoms are found in the sensory, motor, or autonomic systems. Patients with sensory symptoms typically have an insidious onset of symptoms and notice a "stocking glove" distribution; the neuropathy affects their hands and feet first. Autonomic neuropathy is also common, causing problems with urinary function, gastroparesis, cardiovascular system, and sweat glands.
- **Diabetic foot disease:** Diabetic foot disease is common among patients with diabetes. It is important to perform diabetic foot exams on patients every year and more frequently in patients with active diabetic foot disease. Patient should be taught how to check their feet at home daily and be reminded to wear shoes and to take care of any injuries immediately. Monitor patients for cuts, callouses, fungal and skin infections, and diabetic foot ulcers. Treat diabetic foot disease aggressively, prescribing antibiotics for any suspected infections. Order crutches or bedrest as necessary when the patient needs to avoid weight bearing. Patients with diabetic foot disease should be seen by podiatry for care of callouses and nails to avoid potential skin injuries, which contribute to diabetic wounds. Any patient with a diabetic ulcer where tendon or bone is exposed will probably require hospitalization for IV antibiotic treatment. Charcot foot disease occurs when the tendons of the foot progressively degrade due to diabetic neuropathy. These patients are at high risk of diabetic ulcer due to the collapse of the arch of their foot.
- **Macrovascular disease:** Diabetes contributes to ischemic heart disease, peripheral vascular disease, and cerebrovascular disease, which results in damage to tissues and organs. Chronic hyperglycemia contributes to the development of these complications. When treating patients with diabetes, clinicians must also evaluate for CVD, cerebrovascular disease, and peripheral artery disease. Check blood pressure at every visit. Patients with diabetes and hypertension with a higher 10-year atherosclerotic cardiovascular disease (ASCVD) risk of >15% should be treated to a blood pressure target of <130/80 mm Hg. Individuals with diabetes, hypertension, and a 10-year ASCVD risk of <15% should be treated with medication to a blood pressure target of <140/90 mm Hg. Pregnant patients with diabetes and preexisting hypertension should have a target of 135/85 mm Hg to reduce risk of accelerated maternal hypertension, minimizing impaired fetal growth. Patients should be educated on monitoring their blood pressure at home between office visits. Lipid management is also important, and patients should be counseled on lifestyle modifications, to include a diet and exercise plan that focuses on weight loss. Clinicians should recommend a Mediterranean style diet or the DASH diet to reduce saturated and trans-fat intake. Monitor lipid panel and initiate statins per recommendations under Hyperlipidemia later in this chapter. Antiplatelet therapy may be necessary to reduce cardiovascular morbidity and mortality in high-risk patients with previous myocardial infarction (MI) or stroke and is strongly recommended in those patients with diabetes and a history of ASCVD. Use aspirin (75–162 mg daily) or in patients with intolerance or allergy to aspirin, clopidogrel 75 mg daily should be used. Clinicians should recognize that patients with diabetes may have atypical cardiac symptoms such as unexplained dyspnea or chest discomfort, signs/symptoms of associated vascular disease (including carotid bruits, transient ischemic strokes, stroke, claudication, peripheral artery disease or EKG abnormalities).

16.8 HYPOGLYCEMIA

OVERVIEW

Hypoglycemia is defined by low blood sugar, with the cutoff usually hovering near 70 mg/dL and symptoms presenting around 55 mg/dL. While most of the conversation surrounding diabetes mellitus revolves around hyperglycemia, hypoglycemia is a very serious and sometimes fatal complication.

EPIDEMIOLOGY

Hypoglycemia is most commonly the result of injecting too much exogenous insulin (accidentally or intentionally), delayed or inadequate carbohydrate intake following insulin injection, or the presence of an insulinoma. Hypoglycemia is very uncommon in individuals who do not have a history of diabetes mellitus; however, it can be also be seen in adrenal insufficiency and insulin autoimmune hypoglycemia.

PATHOPHYSIOLOGY

The pathophysiology of hypoglycemia is dependent on the cause. Insulin is produced by the beta cells of islets of Langerhans in the pancreas. Insulin is released in response to carbohydrate ingestion to facilitate glucose uptake. In all individuals with T1DM, and some with other variations of diabetes, there is beta cell dysfunction, and exogenous insulin administration is necessary to maintain normal glucose concentration. While the amount of insulin to be injected daily is usually discussed with the prescribing clinician, individuals may mistakenly or intentionally inject too much insulin, which results in excessive cellular glucose uptake and subsequent hypoglycemia. Additionally, delays in meals after insulin is injected can also cause hypoglycemia.

An insulinoma is a small, benign pancreatic tumor, usually <2 cm across, that produces excessive amounts of insulin. Insulin production from an insulinoma is not in response to circulating glucose levels and therefore results in increased glucose uptake leading to hypoglycemia.

MEDICAL HISTORY AND CLINICAL PRESENTATION

The vast majority of individuals experiencing hypoglycemia have a known history of diabetes mellitus. It is important to gather a detailed history, especially in relationship to exogenous insulin injection (if applicable) and timing of meals. Additionally, detailed medication, medical, and family histories should be obtained. Sulfonylureas and meglitinides are oral medications that can often result in hypoglycemia. If a likely cause is not readily apparent, further evaluation for adrenal insufficiency or insulinoma should begin. If a patient reports hypoglycemia but it is not witnessed by the clinician, controlled and monitored replication of the scenario that resulted in hypoglycemia may be performed in order to obtain more official lab values.

SIGNS AND SYMPTOMS

While some patients may remain asymptomatic during a hypoglycemic episode, most present with anxiousness, clamminess, shaking, sweating and/or chills, and/or nausea. As the blood glucose level continues to drop, patients may complain of confusion, extreme lethargy, and impaired vision. If left untreated, it can result in coma or death. Patients who typically have very high blood glucose may begin to experience these symptoms with glucose levels much higher than the traditional cutoff for hypoglycemia. For example, a patient who has a usual daily blood glucose average in the 300s may feel symptomatic for hypoglycemia in the low to mid 100s.

PHYSICAL EXAMINATION

If the patient is hypoglycemic at the time of evaluation, physical exam may reveal tremors, diaphoresis, tachycardia, confusion, pallor, and lethargy. Depending on the level of blood glucose, the patient may be unresponsive.

DIFFERENTIAL DIAGNOSIS

In addition to the multiple causes of hypoglycemia, differential diagnosis includes adrenal insufficiency and substance abuse.

DIAGNOSTIC STUDIES AND EVALUATION

If the patient has a known history of diabetes, laboratory testing may not be necessary as exogenous insulin dosing adjustments will usually suffice for resolving associated symptoms. If a patient without a known history of diabetes or a patient with a history of diabetes that has an irregular pattern of hypoglycemic events presents with symptoms, prompt measurement of glucose, c-peptide, and antibodies to insulin should be obtained. Patients with glucose <55 mg/dL and decreased or normal C-peptide, and negative antibodies should be evaluated for possible overadministration of exogenous insulin. If C-peptide is elevated, an insulinoma should be suspected. If beta-hydroxybutyrate is elevated in the presence of hypoglycemia, decreased C-peptide, and absent antibodies, the patient should be evaluated for IGF-mediated hypoglycemia. If antibodies to insulin are present, the patient likely has an insulin autoimmune disorder.

If symptoms typically occur after fasting or after meals, these scenarios should be reproduced with frequent serum glucose checks to monitor for the development of hypoglycemia. In more extreme cases, a patient may need to undergo a monitored 72-hour fast to distinguish hyperinsulinemia from other possible causes of the patient's hypoglycemia.

TREATMENT

- If the cause is exogenous insulin administration, insulin regimen should be titrated accordingly. Sometimes something as simple as adding a snack before bedtime may help to reduce nocturnal hypoglycemic events.
- In the event of an acute episode, oral glucose tablets should be administered with frequent glucose monitoring. If the blood glucose level continues to drop, IM glucagon may be necessary.
- If an insulinoma is the cause, surgical resection is required.

PATIENT EDUCATION

- Hypoglycemia is a potentially life-threatening complication of diabetes mellitus. Close monitoring of symptoms and proper education of family members and friends are essential.

- While hypoglycemia is most often secondary to complications with diabetes mellitus management, there are other possible causes.
- Patients and family members should always carry glucose tablets or hard candies that can administer glucose rapidly at the onset of hypoglycemia.

16.9 HYPOGONADISM

OVERVIEW

Hypogonadism is the result of decreased production of sex hormones from the testes in males and the ovaries in females. At 5 weeks' gestation, sexual differentiation occurs resulting in the eventual development of testes or ovaries (gonads). The gonads become part of a hormone feedback loop; collectively, the hormone feedback loops in males and females are referred to at the hypothalamic-pituitary-gonadal axis. In both sexes, the hypothalamus releases GnRH, which stimulates the anterior pituitary to release LH and FSH. In males, LH and FSH trigger testosterone production in testes. In females, LH and FSH trigger estrogen and progesterone production in the ovaries. Testosterone is responsible for regulating spermatogenesis as well as the development of secondary sex characteristics in males, while estrogen is responsible for the development of secondary sex characteristics in females (Table 16.30). Dysfunction at any point in this axis can result in hypogonadism; when dysfunction occurs at either the testes or the ovaries, it is classified as primary (hypogonadotropic) hypogonadism and when dysfunction occurs at the hypothalamus or pituitary gland, it is classified as secondary (central; hypergonadotropic) hypogonadism.

There are many causes of hypogonadism in both males and females. Causes of primary hypogonadism include genetic disorders (Turner syndrome, Klinefelter syndrome), autoimmune disorders (Addison's disease, hypoparathyroidism), childhood infections (mumps), varicocele, and radiation exposure. Likewise, secondary hypogonadism can also have many different causes including genetic disorders (Kallmann syndrome), infections (HIV), pituitary adenomas, nutritional deficiencies or obesity, and radiation exposure. Both primary and secondary hypogonadism can be further classified as congenital or acquired. Drugs that may disrupt testosterone secretion, such as spironolactone, or gonadotropin secretion, such as marijuana and heroin, should also be considered.

TABLE 16.30 Normal Primary and Secondary Sex Characteristics by Sex

Male	Female
Primary	
Penis and scrotum enlargement	Increased size of vagina and uterus
Hormone production leading to spermatogenesis	Hormone production leading to menstruation
Secondary	
Hair growth (face, chest, axilla, pubic)	Hair growth (axilla, pubic)
Increased muscle mass	Broadening of pelvis
Voice deepens	Increase adipose tissue
	Breast enlargement, increased areola size

EPIDEMIOLOGY

Prevalence of hypogonadism is known to increase with comorbidities of obesity, T2DM, and metabolic syndrome. Additionally, prevalence has been shown to increase with age.

PATHOPHYSIOLOGY

The hypothalamic-pituitary-gonadal axis is responsible for maintaining the intricate balance of sex hormones. GnRH is released from the hypothalamus, triggering the release of LH and FSH from the pituitary gland. In males, this stimulates testosterone production in the testes and in females, estrogen and progesterone production in the ovaries.

Release of GnRH from the hypothalamus begins to increase around age 8. During puberty, the hypothalamus and pituitary gland become less sensitive to the negative feedback signals of testosterone and estrogen, allowing for increased production of both sex hormones. Prior to puberty, the hypothalamus and pituitary glands are very sensitive to this negative feedback in order to maintain low circulating levels. Disruption in the hypothalamus or pituitary gland results in hypergonadotropic hypogonadism whereas disruption in the gonads results in hypogonadotropic hypogonadism.

MEDICAL HISTORY AND CLINICAL PRESENTATION

The medical history and clinical presentation of a patient with hypogonadism will vary highly based on the type (hypogonadotropic hypogonadism vs. hypogonadotropic hypogonadism) and the age of onset (prepubertal vs. postpubertal). In young children who have not yet reached puberty, signs and symptoms of hypogonadism are frequently absent. Individuals with Klinefelter syndrome (karyotype XXY) will typically present with gynecomastia alongside the cessation of puberty. Patients with Turner syndrome (karyotype XO) typically have no development of sex characteristics and are short in stature. Patients with Kallmann syndrome will also complain of anosmia.

SIGNS AND SYMPTOMS

Signs and symptoms of hypogonadism in males are dependent on whether onset occurs before or after puberty (Table 16.31).

Females may present with delayed onset of menstruation (primary amenorrhea), absence of pubic or axillary hair growth, or signs and symptoms associated with Turner syndrome, including lymphedema, short stature, webbed neck, and hypertension. Signs and symptoms of hypogonadism that occur after puberty include cessation of menses (secondary amenorrhea) and perimenopause.

TABLE 16.31 Signs and Symptoms of Hypogonadism in Males

Prepubertal Hypogonadism	Postpubertal Hypogonadism
Small testes and penis	Normally developed testes and penis
Limited hair growth (axilla, face, pubic, chest)	Thinning of hair (axilla, face, pubic, chest)
High-pitched voice	Normal voice
Decreased libido	Loss of libido, erectile dysfunction
Low muscle mass	Loss of muscle mass
Gynecomastia	Gynecomastia

PHYSICAL EXAMINATION

Physical exam for males with suspected hypogonadism should include evaluation of the testes for size and position. The size of the penis should be evaluated, along with any malformations such as hypospadias. The evaluation of secondary sex characteristics and gynecomastica and Tanner staging should be performed. In females, evaluation of external genitalia should be performed along with the assessment for androgenization. Tanner staging should be performed.

DIFFERENTIAL DIAGNOSIS

Differential diagnosis for hypogonadism includes constitutional delay of puberty, which is a temporary delay in growth with no diagnosis accounting for the delay.

DIAGNOSTIC STUDIES

The first step in diagnosing hypogonadism is two morning labvalues for testosterone, both of which will be low. Once established, differentiation between primary and secondary hypogonadism can be made through lab measurements of serum concentrations of two hormones secreted from the anterior pituitary gland: LH and FSH. For males, serum concentrations of testosterone and sperm count will be subnormal in both conditions. However, in primary hypogonadism FSH and LH will be elevated in attempts to stimulate the testes, whereas in secondary hypogonadism FSH and LH will be either normal or reduced. If primary hypogonadism is established, further diagnostic studies, such as karyotyping, should be completed to confirm a cause. If secondary hypogonadism is established, the function of the anterior pituitary should be further assessed.

In females, estrogen levels will be decreased; in primary hypogonadism, FSH and LH will be elevated, while in secondary hypogonadism, FSH and LH levels will be decreased. Once deficiency is established, further testing should be performed to determine a cause. This may include karyotyping for the diagnosis of Turner syndrome and MRI to rule out a pituitary tumor in addition to a pelvic ultrasound examination to assess the ovaries.

EVALUATION

Once the presence of hypogonadism is suspected or established, a referral to an endocrinologist for further evaluation and treatment is warranted. Additionally, patients should be evaluated for CVD and osteoporosis because hypogonadism can increase risks of both conditions.

TREATMENT

- Treatment for hypogonadism is directed by the cause; in the case of a pituitary adenoma, resection of the mass is indicated.
- Hormone replacement therapy (estrogen and progesterone in females, testosterone in males) is often indicated. If decreased libido persists for women, low-dose testosterone may be used.

PATIENT EDUCATION

- Hypogonadism is a general term that refers to decreased sex hormone production from either the testes or ovaries.
- With proper management, the common concerns of energy, libido, muscle mass, and fertility may be restored.

KEY POINTS

- Patients with a delayed onset of secondary sex characteristics should be evaluated for hypogonadism; population-based screening is not recommended.
- Morning serum total testosterone concentration should be measured between 8 and 10 am for accurate testing, and must be repeated.
- Hypogonadotropic hypogonadism will have normal or decreased LH and FSH, whereas hypergonadotropic hypogonadism will have elevated LH and FSH.
- Once hypogonadism is established, further testing is needed to determine the cause.

16.10 HYPERLIPIDEMIA

OVERVIEW

CVD is the leading cause of death in the United States. Patients with elevated cholesterol are at nearly double the risk of developing CVD as those with normal levels of cholesterol. Additionally, they are at increased risk of myocardial infarction and stroke. Hyperlipidemia is an all-encompassing term that refers to elevated lipids, which can be cholesterol or TGs in the blood. Lipoproteins transport fat in the blood; there are two types: high-density lipoproteins (HDLs) and LDLs. Lipoproteins transport cholesterol from the liver, where it is produced, to the cells. HDL, or "good cholesterol" is favorable as it transports cholesterol back to the liver where it is excreted. LDL, or "bad cholesterol," that remains in the bloodstream has a negative impact on health, as it allows excess cholesterol to remain in circulation. Elevated LDL may lead to a buildup of plaques in the arteries, increasing the risk of atherosclerotic vascular disease as well. Hyperlipidemia is the imbalance of HDL and LDL in the bloodstream.

In patients with hyperlipidemia, lifestyle modification is important in improving lipid levels and life expectancy.

EPIDEMIOLOGY

According to the CDC, 71 million Americans have high LDL cholesterol. Less than half of those with high LDL cholesterol are getting treatment.[57] Those patients with familial hypercholesterolemia (FH) are at greater risk of developing CVD; therefore, it is imperative to screen at an early age in this population.[58] Approximately 31 million American adults have total cholesterol levels that exceed 240 mg/dL, placing them at about twice the risk for ASCVD compared to those with total cholesterol levels that are at goal.[58]

PATHOPHYSIOLOGY

Blood lipids are transported as lipoproteins. Cholesterol esters and TGs are located in the hydrophobic core, while free cholesterol, phospholipids, and apolipoproteins are on the hydrophilic surface. There are five major categories of lipoproteins (from largest to smallest): chylomicrons, very LDLs (VLDLs), intermediate density lipoproteins (IDLs), LDLs, and HDLs.

Chylomicrons are very large lipoproteins that consist mainly of TGs and minor amounts of cholesterol and phospholipids. Chylomicrons are formed by the intestinal epithelial cells postprandially. They are derived from dietary fats and are secreted into the intestinal lymph and released into the blood. Upon delivery to the endothelial cells, TGs are rapidly broken down into free fatty acids by lipoprotein lipase and taken up by the tissues. The resulting particle, known as a chylomicron remnant, is removed from circulation by hepatic receptors.[59]

VLDLs comprise a large quantity of TGs, smaller amounts of cholesterol, and phospholipids. VLDLs are produced by hepatocytes and carry endogenously synthesized lipids, especially TGs, to the liver. In the blood, lipoprotein lipase hydrolyzes TGs and the size of the particles diminishes forming IDLs. After further hydrolysis of TGs by hepatic lipase, LDLs are formed. LDL is the main transporter of cholesterol in the bloodstream, transporting cholesterol to tissues. LDL comprises a single apolipoprotein B-100 molecule (apo B), large amounts of cholesterol esters, and small amounts of free cholesterol, TGs, and phospholipids. Apo B interacts with specific LDL receptors located on cell surfaces in tissues, resulting in the removal of LDL particles from circulation. LDL particles with more TGs are larger, less dense, and less atherogenic versus small, dense LDLs, which are more atherogenic.[59]

HDL is formed as a precursor in the liver and the intestine. It contains protein and phospholipids released from the tissues. HDL gains phospholipids and free cholesterol from the tissues and cholesterol esters from VLDL to become mature HDL. HDL has an important role in reverse cholesterol transport. It carries cholesterol from peripheral tissues back to the liver for excretion as bile acids and bile cholesterol.

MEDICAL HISTORY AND CLINICAL PRESENTATION

Generally, patients do not present with any significant symptoms or signs. Most patients are discovered to have high cholesterol on routine screening labtests as part of the workup for CVD or with routine preventive care screenings. It is important to take a full medical and family medical history from the patient.

SIGNS AND SYMPTOMS

Patients with high cholesterol generally do not have any signs or symptoms. Extremely high levels of chylomicrons or VLDL result in the formation of eruptive xanthomas, red-yellow papules typically found on the buttocks. High LDL concentrations may cause tendinous xanthomas on certain tendons—usually the Achilles, patella, or back of the hand. These findings are generally consistent in patients with one of the FH types.

When TGs are greatly elevated to levels above 1,000 to 2,000 mg/dL, the patient may have pain—usually epigastric or in the back. They may present with pain, nausea, vomiting, and/or dyspnea. Patients with TGs that are out of control, usually above 5,000 mg/dL, may develop pancreatitis, although usually high-risk alcohol use, diabetes, or obesity is present.

PHYSICAL EXAMINATION

With hypercholesterolemia, patients may report xanthomas. Lipemia retinalis, or cream-colored blood vessels, may be found in the fundus with extremely high TG levels (above 2,000 mg/dL). Patients do not always have any positive exam findings with hyperlipidemia.

DIFFERENTIAL DIAGNOSIS

- Alcohol abuse
- Renal failure
- Pancreatitis
- Chylomicronemia
- T1DM
- T2DM
- Hormone replacement therapy

DIAGNOSTIC STUDIES

The only test necessary to assess for hyperlipidemia is a fasting lipid panel. The lipid profile/panel will evaluate total cholesterol, TGs, and the lipoproteins (HDL, LDL, and VLDL). The fasting lipid panel is more important for evaluating the level of TGs and has minor effects on cholesterol measurement. Advise the patient to fast for 12 hours prior to getting their lipid panel drawn. An accurate TG level is a good indicator of metabolic syndrome. Patients are at increased risk for pancreatitis with a TG level >400. It is important to note that an elevated TG level will reduce the accuracy of cholesterol measurement.

Low HDL-cholesterol is caused by elevated TGs, overweight/obesity, being sedentary, cigarette smoking, very high cholesterol intake, T2DM, and certain medications (i.e., beta blockers, anabolic steroids).

EVALUATION

Hyperlipidemia may have primary or secondary causes. Primary hyperlipidemia is genetic; patients may have lipoprotein lipase deficiency, apo C2 deficiency, FH, polygenic hypercholesterolemia, familial combined hyperlipidemia, familial dysbetalipoproteinemia, familial hypertriglyceridemia, or sporadic hypertriglyceridemia. Secondary causes include obesity, high caloric intake, high TGs, saturated fat diets, increased VLDL production (high refined carbohydrate diet), sedentary lifestyle, or diabetes.[60]

In patients without a familial history of a lipid disorder, it may be necessary to evaluate the patient for other disorders that may increase their LDLs: hypothyroidism, obstructive liver disease, nephrotic syndrome, pregnancy, GH deficiency, anorexia nervosa, monoclonal gammopathy, Cushing syndrome, acute intermittent porphyria (AIP), hepatoma. Additionally, be aware that several drugs can cause increases in LDL-cholesterol (LDL-C): cyclosporine and tacrolimus, amiodarone, glucocorticoids, danazol, some progestins, protease inhibitors, antipsychotics, bile acid sequestrants, L-asparaginase, and cyclophosphamide. One should always consider the possibility of genetic causes, and specialized genetic testing may be ordered if necessary.[61]

TREATMENT

The 2019 American College of Cardiology/American Heart Association (AHA) guidelines on treating hyperlipidemia[62] (see Table 16.32):

- Patients age 20 to 75 years and LDL-C ≥190 mg/dL, the clinician may use high-intensity statin without ASCVD risk assessment.
- T2DM and age 40–75 years, use moderate-intensity statin and risk estimate to consider high-intensity statins. Risk-enhancers in diabetics include ≥10 years for T2DM and 20 years for T1DM, ≥30 mcg albumin/mg creatinine, eGFR <60 mL/min/1.73 m^2, retinopathy, neuropathy, ankle-brachial index (ABI) <0.9. In those with multiple ASCVD risk factors, consider high-intensity statin with aim of lowering LDL-C by 50% or more.
- Patients age >75 years, clinical assessment, and risk discussion—shared decision-making with the patient.
- Patients age 40 to 75 years and LDL-C ≥70 mg/dL and <190 mg/dL without diabetes, use the risk estimator that best fits the patient and risk-enhancing factors to decide intensity of statin.
  - Risk 5% to <7.5% (borderline risk). Risk discussion: If risk-enhancing factors are present, discuss moderate-intensity statin and consider CACS (coronary artery calcium score) in select cases.
  - Risk ≥7.5–20% (intermediate risk). Risk discussion: Use moderate-intensity statins and increase to high-intensity with risk enhancers. Option of CACS to risk stratify if there is uncertainty about risk. If CACS = 0, can avoid statins and repeat CAC test in the future (5–10 years), the exceptions being high-risk conditions such as diabetes, family history of premature CHD, and smoking. If CACS 1–100, it is reasonable to initiate moderate-intensity statin for persons ≥55 years old. If CACS >100 or 75th percentile or higher, use statin at any age.
  - Risk ≥20% (high risk). Risk discussion: Initiate high-intensity statin to reduce LDL-C by ≥50%.[62]
  - In highest risk patients who cannot tolerate statins, start a PCSK9 inhibitor or ezetimibe after assessing statin myopathy.

TABLE 16.32 Statin Treatment of Hyperlipidemia

Statins by Name	Low—Moderate Intensity	Moderate Intensity	High Intensity
Pravastatin	40 mg	40 mg	
Lovastatin	20–40 mg	40 mg	
Atorvastatin	10 mg	40 mg	40–80 mg
Rosuvastatin	10 mg	20 mg	20–40 mg
Simvastatin		40 mg	

The AHA recommends patients pursue "a healthy lifestyle throughout life," have a 10-year ASCVD risk assessment, and shared clinician-patient decision-making prior to starting any antihypertensives, statins, or aspirin. A healthy diet is recommended, which includes decreasing trans-fat, meat, refined carbohydrate, and sweetened drink intake. Plant-based, Mediterranean diets or other diets high in vegetables, fruits, nuts, whole grains, lean vegetable or animal protein (preferably fish), and vegetable fiber have been shown to lower the risk of all-cause mortality compared to control or standard American diet.[62]

Counseling should be given to overweight and obese patients for calorie-restricted diets. All patients should strive for 150 minutes of moderate intensity or 75 minutes of vigorous intensity exercise.

Adherence to statin therapy should be assessed 6 to 8 weeks after starting therapy by rechecking the lipid panel. Discuss patient's compliance with the medication and ask about missed doses. Discuss and assess patient's lifestyle at each visit for tobacco use, and those who use tobacco should be assisted and strongly advised to quit on every visit. Referral may be made to specialists for behavioral modification, nicotine replacement, and drug treatments.[62]

COMMON CHIEF COMPLAINTS

APPROACH TO POLYURIA IN AN ADULT

There are many possible causes of polyuria, which is defined as a urine output >3 L/day in adults (Figure 16.13). First, rule out perceived polyuria, which is often increased urinary frequency rather than increased daily volume and seen with conditions such as benign prostatic hyperplasia (BPH) or nocturia, a common condition in childhood that may persist into adolescence. Evaluation of suspected polyuria is driven by the patient's history, age, and known comorbidities. Once the use of polyuria-inducing medications (large volumes of saline, exogenous glucocorticoids, mannitol, and SGLT2 inhibitor) have been ruled out, a reasonable first step in evaluation is a basic metabolic panel. In patients with severe hyperglycemia, further diagnostic testing of diabetes mellitus, including hemoglobin A1c, should be performed and polyuria can be attributed to osmotic diuresis that results from glucosuria.

When hyperglycemia is not found, the next step is confirming the presence of polyuria through a 24-hour urine specimen and measuring urine osmolality, which can be used in conjunction with the serum sodium concentration to help differentiate solute and water diuresis. In solute diuresis, an increased amount of concentrated urine will be appreciated. In water diuresis, an increased amount of dilute urine will be appreciated. Low plasma sodium concentration with low urine osmolality is attributed to primary polydipsia. Normal plasma sodium concentration with increased urine osmolality (>600 mOsm/kg) is indicative of an osmotic diuresis. High plasma sodium concentration with decreased urine osmolality is suggestive of DI.

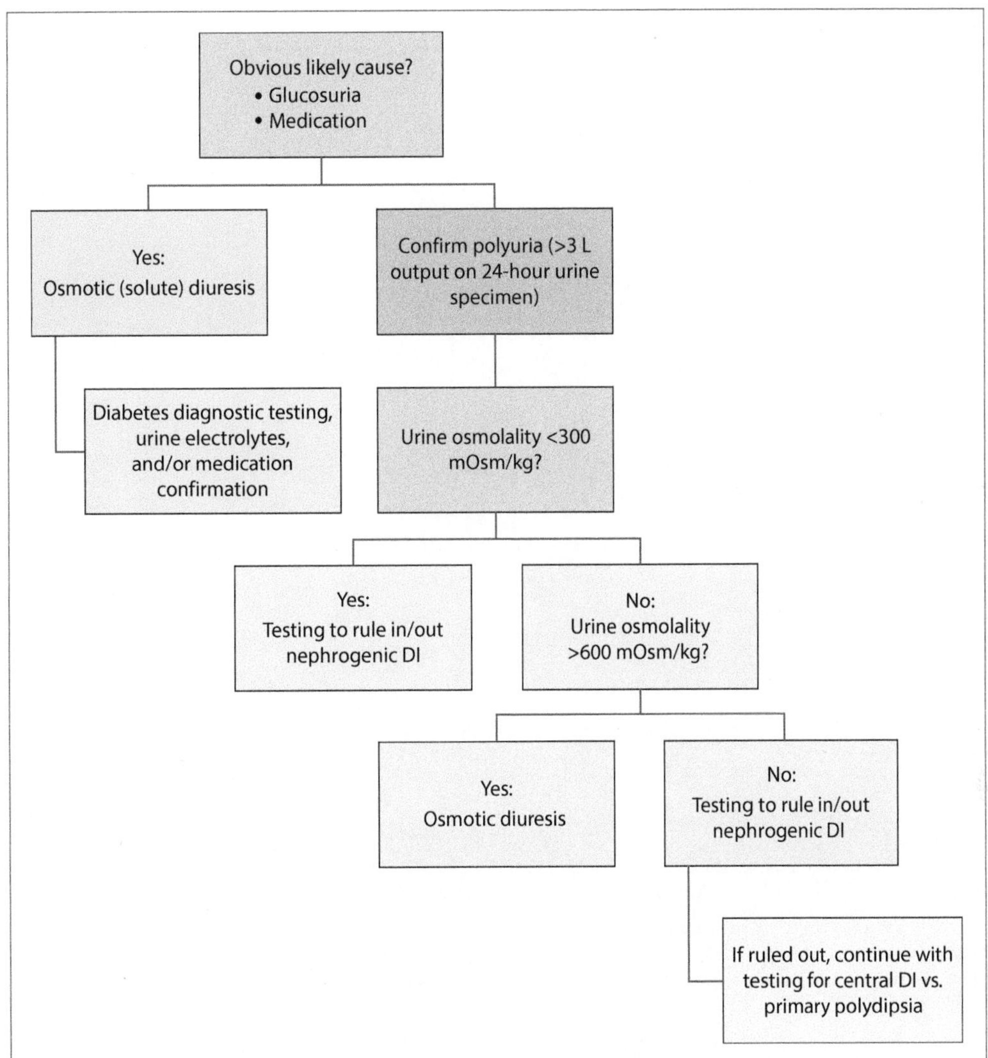

Figure 16.13 Approach to polyuria. DI, diabetes insipidus.

KNOWLEDGE CHECKS

1. Hypothyroidism and hyperthyroidism present with primarily contrasting symptoms. Contrast the symptoms that present with each condition, making note of any symptoms that overlap.
2. Understanding the relationship between hypothalamic, pituitary, and target gland hormones is key to understanding the endocrine system. Create a table outlining the hormones released from each of these locations.
3. Negative and positive feedback loops are common throughout the body. Draw a diagram representing both a negative and a positive feedback loop.

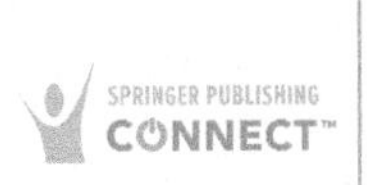

A robust set of instructor resources designed to supplement this text is located at **https://connect.springerpub.com/content/book/978-0-8261-8243-2**. Qualifying instructors may request access by emailing **textbook@springerpub.com.**

REFERENCES

The complete reference list for this chapter appears in the digital version of the chapter, accessible at https://connect.springerpub.com/content/book/978-0-8261-8243-2/chapter/ch16.

CHAPTER 17

INFECTIOUS DISEASES

JAMES VAN RHEE AND SAMPATH WIJESINGHE

LEARNING OBJECTIVES

- Discuss the microbiology, epidemiology, clinical syndromes, and treatment of the various bacterial infections.
- Discuss the microbiology, epidemiology, clinical syndromes, and treatment of the various chlamydial infections.
- Discuss the microbiology, epidemiology, clinical syndromes, and treatment of the various viral infections.
- Discuss the microbiology, epidemiology, clinical syndromes, and treatment of the various rickettsial and spirochetal infections.
- Discuss the microbiology, epidemiology, clinical syndromes, and treatment of the various parasitic infections.
- Discuss the microbiology, epidemiology, clinical syndromes, and treatment of the various mycotic infections.
- Discuss the microbiology, epidemiology, clinical syndromes, and treatment of the various HIV infections.
- Describe the various opportunistic infections noted in patients with HIV infection.
- Describe the various etiologies and evaluation of the patient with fever of unknown origin.
- Discuss the etiology, presentation, and treatment of animal and human bites.
- Discuss the evaluation, diagnostic criteria, and treatment of the septic patient.
- Discuss the indications, side effects, and contraindications to various vaccines and immunizations.

INTRODUCTION

Infectious diseases are the world's greatest killers. In the United States alone, 15.5 million physician office visits[1] and 4.1 million visits to the ED[2] are due to infectious and parasitic disease in a given year. Most deaths from infectious diseases occur in developing countries.

Infectious diseases are disorders caused by organisms such as bacteria, viruses, fungi, or parasites. Infections may be localized or systemic. Infectious diseases are spread via various routes, including person to person, through insects or animals, by contaminated food or water, or from environmental factors.

Signs and symptoms vary depending on the organism causing the infection, but often include fever and fatigue. Mild infections may respond to rest and home remedies, while some life-threatening infections require hospitalization.

Treatment of infectious diseases consists mainly of antimicrobial medications. Prevention of many infectious diseases can be accomplished via vaccines and immunizations. Frequent handwashing also helps protect from most infectious diseases.

17.1 BACTERIAL INFECTIONS

OVERVIEW

Bacteria are microorganisms that have circular double-stranded DNA and cell walls, except for mycoplasmas. Most bacteria live extracellularly. Some bacteria, such as *Salmonella typhi, Neisseria gonorrhoeae, Legionella, Mycobacterium*, and *Rickettsia* prefer to live and multiply intracellularly. Some bacteria, such as *chlamydia*, are obligate intracellular pathogens; they grow, reproduce, and cause disease only in the host cells. Others, such as *Salmonella, Brucella* sp., *N. gonorrhoeae, N. meningitidis, Legionella*, and *Mycobacterium tuberculosis*, are facultative intracellular pathogens.

Many bacteria are present as normal flora, often in large numbers, and only a few bacterial species are human pathogens.

EPIDEMIOLOGY

One way to separate out the various types of bacteria is via their Gram stain results, gram-positive or gram-negative, and the bacteria's morphology, either cocci or bacilli. See Table 17.1 for the Gram stain results of the more common bacteria that cause human disease.

TABLE 17.1 Gram Stain for the Common Bacterial Pathogens

Gram-Positive Cocci	Gram-Negative Cocci	Gram-Positive Bacilli	Gram-Negative Bacilli
Staphylococcus	*Neisseria*	*Corynebacterium*	*Acinetobacter*
Streptococcus	*Brucella* (coccobacilli)	*Listeria*	*Moraxella*
Enterococcus	*Bordetella* (coccobacilli)	*Erysipelothrix*	*Bacteroides*
Peptostreptococcus		*Propionibacterium*	*Haemophilus*
		Bacillus	*Pasteurella*
		Clostridium	*Francisella*
		Lactobacillus	*Eikenella*
		Mycobacterium (acid-fast)	*Fusobacterium*
		Actinomyces	*Vibrio*
		Nocardia	*Campylobacter*
		Streptomyces	*Spirillum*
			Enterobacteriaceae
			Pseudomonas
			Aeromonas

PATHOPHYSIOLOGY

The development of an infection depends on multiple factors: interaction of host susceptibility to infection, organism virulence, and the opportunity for interaction between host and organism. Not all bacteria cause disease; however, some always cause disease. The human body is colonized with numerous microbes. Normal flora bacteria aid in the digestion of food, produce vitamins, protect the host from colonization with pathogenic microbes, and activate the host immune response. These normal flora bacteria reside in locations such as the gastrointestinal (GI) tract, mouth, skin, and upper respiratory tract. The presence and distribution of the normal flora can be disrupted by antibiotic treatment, diet, stress, and changes in the host response to the flora. An altered normal flora can lead to inappropriate immune responses, causing inflammatory bowel diseases.

Normal flora bacteria cause disease if they enter normally sterile sites of the body. Virulent bacteria have mechanisms that promote their growth in the host at the expense of the host's tissue or organ function. Opportunistic bacteria take advantage of preexisting conditions, such as immunosuppression, to cause serious disease. For example, patients with cystic fibrosis are at higher risk of *Pseudomonas aeruginosa* infection, and patients with AIDS are very susceptible to infection by intracellular bacteria, such as the mycobacteria.

The signs and symptoms of infection are determined by change to the affected tissue. There may be a systemic response due to toxins and cytokines produced in response to the infection. The strain of bacteria and the inoculum size also are major factors in determining whether infection occurs. The threshold for the development of disease is different for different bacteria; for example, <100 *Shigella* organisms are necessary to cause disease.[3]

Host factors also play a role in infection. For example, while over a million *Salmonella* organisms are needed to cause gastroenteritis in a healthy person, only a few thousand are needed in a person whose gastric pH has been neutralized. Congenital defects, immunodeficiency states, and other disease-related conditions, such as diabetes, increase infection susceptibility.

For infection to become established, bacteria must first enter the body. There are several natural defense mechanisms and barriers, such as the skin, mucus, ciliated epithelium, and secretions containing antibacterial substances that make it difficult for bacteria to enter the body. When these barriers are broken this provides a portal of entry for the bacteria, or the bacteria may have the means to compromise the barrier and invade the body. Once inside the body, the bacteria can travel in the bloodstream to other sites in the body. Methods of entry include ingestion, inhalation, trauma, needlestick, arthropod bite, and sexual transmission.

17.1A STREPTOCOCCAL INFECTIONS

Streptococci are a large heterogeneous group of gram-positive cocci bacteria that are widely distributed in nature. Some of the most important agents of human disease as well as members of the normal human flora are in this group. The species known to cause human disease are from two broad categories: pyogenic streptococci and enteric and oral streptococci. Pyogenic streptococci, including β-hemolytic streptococci and pneumococcus, are not generally part of the normal flora but cause acute infections in normal hosts. Enteric and oral streptococci are typically part of the normal flora and are more frequently associated with opportunistic infections (OIs).

Streptococci are characterized by the type of hemolytic reaction displayed on the blood agar on which they are grown: complete (β), incomplete (α), or no (γ) hemolysis. Hemolytic streptococci can be classified into Lancefield groups A, B, C, F, G, and L based on carbohydrate antigens of the cell wall. *Streptococcus pyogenes* contains the Lancefield group A antigen on their cell surface and is therefore referred to as group A streptococcus (GAS). The GAS cell surface M proteins contain antigenic targets of the major serologic typing scheme

S. pyogenes causes several diseases in humans, including pharyngitis, skin infections, acute rheumatic fever, scarlet fever, poststreptococcal glomerulonephritis, a toxic shock–like syndrome, and necrotizing fasciitis. Environmental factors that predispose to GAS infections are inadequate hygiene and overcrowding.

Streptococcus agalactiae, group B streptococcus (GBS), is a β-hemolytic organism that carries the Lancefield group B antigen. GBS are encapsulated organisms and 10 antigenically distinct capsular serotypes have been described

Enterococci are gram-positive cocci from the family Enterococcaceae. These organisms were previously classified as belonging to the genus *Streptococcus* but were placed in their own genus, *Enterococcus*. Although there are several species associated with human infections, most infections are caused by two species: *Enterococcus faecalis* and *E. faecium*.

Streptococcus pneumoniae, or pneumococcus, is an α-hemolytic organism and is an important pathogen as the major cause of pneumonia. The organisms can reside asymptomatically in the nasopharynx of healthy carriers and are transmitted by sneezing, coughing, and direct contact with an infected person. *S. pneumoniae* is one of the most common causes of meningitis and acute otitis media. The organism is also the etiologic agent of bronchitis, rhinitis, sinusitis, bacteremia, sepsis, osteomyelitis, septic arthritis, cellulitis, and brain abscess.

MEDICAL HISTORY AND CLINICAL PRESENTATION

Pharyngitis and impetigo are associated with crowding—increased incidence is noted in schools, childcare centers, and military installations. Pharyngitis results from contact with respiratory secretions in a person who has GAS pharyngitis. GAS pharyngitis and invasive infections are more common during late autumn, winter, and spring in temperate climates, because of close person-to-person contact and predisposing viral infections. Impetigo is more common in tropical climates and warm seasons because of insect bites and other minor skin trauma.

Intrapartum antibiotic prophylaxis is used to prevent GBS infections in newborn infants; 80% of invasive GBS disease now occurs in nonpregnant adolescents and adults. Invasive GBS disease can occur in adults of all ages. The rate of infection increases with advancing age and is twice as high in Black people as in Whites in the United States. The fatality rate is 6.5% in the United States[4]; this rate is highest in the elderly.

GBS disease in pregnant women is associated with upper genital tract disease that can lead to fetal death. Most cases occur in healthy pregnant women.

The majority of enterococcal infections occur in the hospital environment. Infections that originate in the community usually include urinary tract infections (UTIs) and endocarditis. Enterococci are normal flora of the GI tract.

SIGNS AND SYMPTOMS

The signs and symptoms vary with the site and severity of the infection (Table 17.2).

PHYSICAL EXAMINATION

See Table 17.2 for the common physical examination findings of the various infections cause by streptococcal organisms.

TABLE 17.2 Signs and Symptoms and Physical Examination Findings of *Streptococcus* Infections

Type of Infection	Signs and Symptoms	Physical Examination Findings
Pharyngitis	Sore throat, fever, odynophagia	Erythematous pharynx with purulent tonsillar exudate, cervical lymphadenopathy
Otitis media	Otalgia, fever	Erythematous tympanic membrane, regional lymphadenopathy
Rhinosinusitis	Nasal congestion, nasal drainage, facial pain, headache	Sinus tenderness, purulent nasal drainage
Pneumonia	Fever, productive cough with rusty-colored sputum, dyspnea	Signs of consolidation on pulmonary examination
Urinary tract infection	Dysuria, hematuria, cloudy urine	Hematuria and pyuria on urinalysis
Scarlet fever	Fever, pharyngitis, dysphagia, headache	Diffuse pink-red rash that blanches with pressure, noted on abdomen and chest; strawberry tongue
Impetigo	Rash, mild discomfort, pruritus	Vesicles or pustules, honey-crusted lesions
Erysipelas	Fever, rash	Shiny, red, raised, indurated lesions with distinct margins
Cellulitis	Fever, chill, tachycardia, rash	Local erythema, tender, indistinct rash borders, regional lymphadenopathy
Meningitis	Fever, headache, nuchal rigidity	Positive Brudzinski and Kernig signs

DIAGNOSTIC STUDIES

Gram stain of infections due to streptococcal organisms reveal gram-positive cocci in chains; *Streptococcus pneumoniae* will appear as gram-positive cocci in pairs, described as lancet-shaped. Culture results vary with the type of streptococcus species. GAS presents with beta hemolysis on blood agar plates, alpha hemolysis is noted with *Streptococcus pneumoniae* and *Streptococcus viridans*, and gamma hemolysis is noted with enterococcus.

There are several rapid tests available for the diagnosis of GAS and pneumococcus. For GAS the rapid test specificity is generally high, but the sensitivity varies considerably. Because of the sensitivity and specificity, when a patient suspected of having GAS pharyngitis has a negative rapid streptococcal test, a throat culture should be obtained to ensure that the patient is not infected. Because of the high specificity, a positive test result does not require culture confirmation. Pneumococcal antigen may be detected in various body fluids, including urine samples. Methods using immunochromatography have a very good sensitivity and specificity.

Serologic studies targeting nonspecific streptococcal extracellular products, such as streptolysin O and DNase B, may be useful in differentiating a patient with a carrier state of GAS from acute infection or identifying past infection. Both acute and convalescent titers are needed to determine whether there is a new exposure to a pathogen. A single elevated antibody titer may simply reflect antibody persistence from an infection that occurred months earlier. Serologic studies performed on at least two occasions, 2 to 4 weeks apart, can perhaps separate the patient with acute GAS pharyngitis from the chronic carrier of this pathogen.

TREATMENT

Penicillin remains the treatment of choice for infections due to GAS. For mild to moderate infections including pharyngitis and skin and soft tissue infections, oral penicillin V for 10 days is recommended. A first-generation cephalosporin is an alternative unless there is a history of immediate hypersensitivity to a beta-lactam antibiotic. Erythromycin, clarithromycin, azithromycin, and clindamycin are commonly used first-line drugs against GAS infections in patients with beta-lactam allergies. Alternative antimicrobials for treatment include the fluoroquinolones: levofloxacin and moxifloxacin, tetracycline or doxycycline, linezolid oral or parenteral, and vancomycin.

Streptococcal pharyngitis due to GBS is treated with penicillin V or amoxicillin for 10 days. Cephalosporins, cefazolin for nonmeningitis and ceftriaxone or cefotaxime for meningitis, can be used in penicillin-allergic individuals who are not at high risk for anaphylaxis. Erythromycin and clindamycin can be used, but only after checking susceptibility via antimicrobial susceptibility testing. Aminoglycosides work synergistically with penicillin killing GBS; this combination can be used the first 2 weeks of the 4- to 6-week antibiotic course for GBS endocarditis.

For enterococcal infections caused by *E. faecalis* and ampicillin-susceptible *E. faecium*, monotherapy with ampicillin is not recommended; but the addition of an aminoglycoside, such as gentamicin, can achieve synergistic bactericidal therapy if the organism does not exhibit high-level resistance to the aminoglycoside.

Vancomycin has good activity against many enterococci and is the usual alternative to ampicillin to treat enterococcal infections. Synergistic therapy is also achieved with aminoglycosides, and the combination could be used for the treatment of severe infections, including endocarditis and other endovascular infections, when ampicillin cannot be used.

The treatment for vancomycin-resistant *E. faecium* includes quinupristin-dalfopristin (Q/D) and linezolid. Linezolid is not bactericidal against enterococci and use as first-line therapy in severe endovascular infections is not recommended. Linezolid may be used in the treatment of enterococcal meningitis. Q/D is a mixture of streptogramin antibiotics with bactericidal activity against many *E. faecium* (but not *E. faecalis*).

Daptomycin is bactericidal against ampicillin- and vancomycin-resistant *E. faecalis* and *E. faecium* and is frequently used to treat vancomycin-resistant enterococci (VRE). Treatment failures have been noted at normal dosage, so higher doses may be required.

Nitrofurantoin and fosfomycin are good alternatives for the treatment of uncomplicated UTIs. Fosfomycin is approved for vancomycin-susceptible *E. faecalis*. High-dose ampicillin may be useful in the treatment of uncomplicated UTI since concentrations of ampicillin in the urine are usually high enough to achieve a therapeutic effect.

The treatment of *S. pneumoniae* varies with the location of the infection. For community-acquired pneumonia (CAP) the preferred treatment is penicillin G or amoxicillin. Alternative treatment options include the macrolides, azithromycin, or clarithromycin; the oral cephalosporins, cefpodoxime, cefprozil or cefdinir; the parenteral cephalosporins, ceftriaxone or cefotaxime; clindamycin, doxycycline, or the respiratory fluoroquinolones.

For endocarditis the first-line treatment is penicillin G or vancomycin if penicillin allergic. Other options include cefotaxime and vancomycin or cefazolin or ceftriaxone.

Sinusitis is treated first line with amoxicillin/clavulanate or doxycycline. Alternative treatment includes the respiratory fluoroquinolones, levofloxacin, or moxifloxacin.

Meningitis due to GBS is best treated with vancomycin and a third-generation cephalosporin, such as ceftriaxone or cefotaxime and rifampin. Other options include meropenem and fluoroquinolones.

PATIENT EDUCATION

The pneumococcal vaccine is recommended for all children and adults over age 65 years. For all children under the age of 2 years the following is recommended[5]:

- Pneumococcal conjugate vaccine (PCV13) is given to infants as a series of four doses, one dose at 2 months, 4 months, 6 months, and 12 through 15 months of age.
- Children who miss their shots or start the series later should still get the vaccine. The number of doses recommended and the intervals between doses will depend on the child's age when vaccination begins.

Pneumococcal polysaccharide vaccine (PPSV23) is recommended for all adults 65 years or older. It is recommended that PCV13 be offered to patients based on shared clinical decision-making for adults 65 years or older who do not have an immunocompromising condition, cerebrospinal fluid (CSF) leak, or cochlear implant and have never received a dose of PCV13.[6]

- For immunocompetent adults 65 years or older who only want to receive PPSV23:
  - Administer one dose of PPSV23.

    - Anyone who received any doses of PPSV23 before age 65 should receive one final dose of the vaccine at age 65 or older. Administer this last dose at least 5 years after the prior PPSV23 dose.
- For immunocompetent adults 65 years or older who want to receive PCV13 and PPSV23:
  - Administer one dose of PCV13 first then give one dose of PPSV23 at least 1 year later.
    - If the patient already received PPSV23, give the dose of PCV13 at least 1 year after they received the most recent dose of PPSV23.
    - Anyone who received any doses of PPSV23 before age 65 should receive one final dose of the vaccine at age 65 or older. Administer this last dose at least 5 years after the prior PPSV23 dose.

17.1B STAPHYLOCOCCAL INFECTIONS

Staphylococci are gram-positive aerobic cocci. *Staphylococcus aureus* is the most pathogenic and is the cause of skin infections, pneumonia, endocarditis, and osteomyelitis. Some strains of *S. aureus* produce a toxin that causes gastroenteritis, scalded skin syndrome, and toxic shock syndrome (TSS).

The presence of coagulase separates the coagulase-positive *S. aureus* from the coagulase-negative species, *S. epidermidis* and *S. saprophyticus*.

Pathogenic staphylococcus can be carried in the anterior nares and on the skin in healthy people. Patients predisposed to staphylococcal infection include:

- Neonates and breastfeeding mothers
- Patients with influenza, chronic bronchopulmonary disorders, leukemia, cancer, chronic skin disorders, or diabetes mellitus
- Patients with implanted prosthesis, foreign bodies, or an indwelling intravascular catheter
- Patients receiving steroids, irradiation, immunosuppressants, or chemotherapy
- Intravenous (IV) drug users
- Patients with chronic kidney disease on dialysis
- Patients with surgical incisions, open wounds, or burns

Transmission via the hands of personnel is the most common means of spread; airborne spread can also occur.

Staphylococci cause disease by direct invasion or exotoxin production. Direct invasion is the most common method and is the cause of skin infections, pneumonia, endocarditis, and osteomyelitis. Multiple exotoxins can be produced by staphylococci. Some toxins have a local effect and others cause systemic effects through the release of cytokines. Toxin-mediated infections include TSS, staphylococcal scalded skin syndrome, and staphylococcal food poisoning.

MEDICAL HISTORY AND CLINICAL PRESENTATION

Staphylococcal bacteremia can develop from infection related to intravascular catheters or foreign bodies and can cause metastatic foci of infection. Staphylococcal bacteremia is an important cause of morbidity and death in debilitated patients.

Skin infections are the most common form of staphylococcal disease. Superficial infections include impetigo, cellulitis, or furuncles and carbuncles. Staphylococci are also implicated in wound and burn infections, postoperative incision infections, and mastitis or breast abscess in breastfeeding mothers.

Staphylococcal pneumonia is rare but may develop in patients who are postinfluenza, are taking corticosteroids or immunosuppressants, or have chronic pulmonary disease. *S. aureus* is a common cause of hospital- and ventilator-acquired pneumonia. Lung abscesses may develop along with empyema.

Staphylococcal endocarditis develops most often in IV drug abusers and patients with prosthetic heart valves.

Staphylococcal osteomyelitis occurs more often in children. Articular infection may occur leading to septic arthritis rather than osteomyelitis. Most infections of the vertebrae and intervertebral discs in adults involve *S. aureus*.

Staphylococcal TSS may result from the use of vaginal tampons or complicate any type of *S. aureus* infection.

Staphylococcal scalded skin syndrome, due to exfoliatin toxins, is an exfoliative dermatitis of childhood that starts with large bullae and peeling of the upper layer of skin. Scalded skin syndrome most commonly occurs in infants and children <5 years of age.

Staphylococcal food poisoning is due to the ingestion of a heat-stable staphylococcal enterotoxin. The toxin is noted in incompletely cooked food or food left at room temperature. Symptoms begin 2 to 8 hours after ingestion and last <12 hours.

SIGNS AND SYMPTOMS

Skin and soft tissue infections have a wide range of manifestations, including furuncles, abscesses, cellulitis, surgical wound infections, and necrotizing fasciitis. Signs and symptoms range from tender nodules or pustules noted with furuncles to clusters of vesicles, pustules, or bullous lesions with honey-crusted lesions of impetigo, to the red, warm, tender lesions of cellulitis.

Bacteremia requires evaluation of primary or metastatic sites of infection, including IV catheter sites, any areas containing prosthetic material, bones and joints, epidural space and intervertebral discs, heart valves, the liver, kidney, and spleen. Signs and symptoms may include focal pain, point tenderness, joint effusions, murmurs, or peripheral stigmata of endocarditis.

S. aureus is common cause of bacterial endocarditis and a leading cause of prosthetic valve endocarditis. Infection presents as an acute febrile illness often accompanied by visceral abscesses, subungual petechiae, subconjunctival hemorrhage, purpuric lesions, heart murmurs, and heart failure.

Staphylococcus is an uncommon cause of CAP but has been associated with a preceding/concurrent influenza-like illness, necrotizing/cavitary infiltrates, and empyema.

Bone and joint infections, including osteomyelitis, septic arthritis, and prosthetic joint infections, can arise from direct inoculation due to trauma, a medical procedure, or a contiguous focus of infection, or hematogenous seeding. Staphylococcal osteomyelitis presents with chills, fever, and pain over the involved bone.

Central nervous system (CNS) infections, including meningitis and brain abscess, can occur as a complication of a neurosurgical procedure, contiguous focus of infection, or hematologic spread.

Staphylococcal TSS presents with the isolation of *S. aureus* from a mucosal or normally sterile site, fever, hypotension, diffuse macular rash with desquamation, mainly of the palms and soles, 1 to 2 weeks after onset of illness, and multiorgan involvement.

Staphylococcal scalded skin syndrome is a superficial skin disorder that manifests as a local blistering to generalized desquamation It is typically due to mucosal or skin colonization with a toxin-producing strain of *S. aureus*.

Staphylococcal food poisoning occurs because of ingestion of preformed enterotoxin that has been released into contaminated food. Disease occurs 2 to 6 hours after ingestion with nausea, vomiting, abdominal pain, and diarrhea. It is self-limited with resolution of symptoms within 6 to 12 hours.

PHYSICAL EXAMINATION

Physical examination findings vary with the infection location.

DIAGNOSTIC STUDIES

Diagnosis of staphylococcal infections is by Gram stain and culture of infected material. Gram stain reveals gram-positive cocci that can occur singly, in pairs, tetrads, and irregular grapelike clusters

Susceptibility tests should be completed to determine possible antimicrobial therapy.

When staphylococcal scalded skin syndrome is suspected, cultures should be obtained from blood, urine, nasopharynx, or any suspected focus of infection, as the intact bullae are sterile.

Staphylococcal food poisoning is usually suspected because of case clustering and is confirmed by isolating staphylococci from suspect food and testing for enterotoxins.

In osteomyelitis, x-ray changes such as periosteal reaction may be noted. Abnormalities in MRI, CT, or radionuclide bone scans may be noted before x-ray changes. Bone biopsy should be done for pathogen identification and susceptibility testing.

TREATMENT

Management of staphylococcal infections includes local measures such as abscess drainage, debridement of necrotic tissue, removal of foreign bodies, and antibiotic use.

Treatment of toxin-mediated staphylococcal disease involves decontamination of the toxin-producing area, IV fluid supports, vasopressors, respiratory assistance, and antimicrobials. Antibiotic options include the combination of beta-lactamase–resistant, antistaphylococcal antimicrobial agent, such as nafcillin, oxacillin, or vancomycin; plus a protein synthesis inhibitor, such as clindamycin or linezolid.

For staphylococcal strains that produce penicillinase treatment options include penicillinase-resistant penicillins (oxacillin, nafcillin, dicloxacillin), cephalosporins, carbapenems (imipenem, meropenem), tetracyclines, macrolides, fluoroquinolones, trimethoprim/sulfamethoxazole (TMP-SMX), gentamicin, and vancomycin.

Community-associated methicillin-resistant *S. aureus* (MRSA) is resistant to most beta-lactams but is usually susceptible to TMP-SMX and tetracyclines and is often susceptible to clindamycin. Vancomycin is effective against most MRSA, with rifampin and an aminoglycoside added for serious infections. Vancomycin-resistant *S. aureus* requires treatment with linezolid, daptomycin, TMP-SMX, or ceftaroline.

Because of an increase in the incidence of MRSA, initial empiric treatment for staphylococcal infections should include a drug with reliable activity against MRSA. Options include vancomycin, daptomycin, or linezolid.

Staphylococcal food poisoning can be prevented by appropriate food preparation.

17.1C CLOSTRIDIAL INFECTIONS

17.1CA GANGRENE

OVERVIEW

Clostridium perfringens is associated with three clinical conditions: necrotizing or gangrenous soft tissue infections, endometritis following childbirth or abortion, and foodborne gastroenteritis. Necrotizing soft tissue infections caused by *C. perfringens* are also called "gas gangrene" or clostridial myonecrosis when muscle is involved.

Other *Clostridium* species can cause soft tissue infection and include *C. septicum*, *C. sordellii*, *C. histolyticum*, and *C. novyi*. Because antimicrobial sensitivities are similar among these clostridia, the same antibiotics can be used treat the infection.

Clostridia are spore-forming anaerobes that survive in the environment. Clostridia are soil organisms, but also colonize or contaminate the enteric tracts of animals and humans.

C. perfringens or *C. sordellii* endometritis can develop in previously well, reproductive age patients and usually follows within 1 week of childbirth or abortion and may also develop after simple obstetric or gynecologic procedures, such as amniocentesis or cervical excisions.

All patients who survive an episode of spontaneous clostridial gangrene should be investigated for occult GI sources, particularly colonic tumors, diverticula, or ulcers.

Gastroenteritis is acquired by ingesting vegetative *C. perfringens* organisms, which may contaminate improperly handled foods. Improperly cooked or stored meat products are commonly implicated. Cooked food that sits out at room temperature for long periods of time can allow heat-resistant spores of *C. perfringens* to germinate and reproduce in large numbers. After ingestion, these bacteria produce an enterotoxin, which causes symptoms.

Clostridial infections primarily cause signs and symptoms through the actions of their toxins. One of these toxins is a lecithinase (phospholipase C or in *C. perfringens*, alpha toxin). The alpha toxin of *C. perfringens* produces myonecrosis by inducing platelet activation, microvascular thrombosis, and local ischemia. Other toxins include a theta toxin (perfringolysin O), which is a cholesterol-dependent cytolysin that contributes to infection; hemolysins; proteases; collagenase; hyaluronidase; DNase; and neuraminidase.

The incidence of clostridial infection varies.

- There are <1,000 cases per year of gas gangrene in the United States.[7]
- Clostridial toxic shock in women of reproductive age is rare.
- There are nearly 1 million cases of foodborne illness secondary to *C. perfringens* each year in the United States.[8]

MEDICAL HISTORY AND CLINICAL PRESENTATION

Clostridial tissue infections may be secondary to trauma, surgery, frostbite, electrical burns, or pressure sores. Injection drug users may inject contaminated heroin into their skin or soft tissues and develop sepsis, bacteremia, and necrotizing infections caused by clostridia, including *C. perfringens*, *C. sordellii*, and *C. novyi*.

Endometritis may present with fulminant shock, weakness, nausea, vomiting, and abdominal or pelvic pain. A recent history of childbirth, medical abortion, surgical abortion, spontaneous abortion, or amniocentesis should be noted. This syndrome can be caused by either *C. perfringens* or *C. sordellii.*

Clostridial TSS associated with endometritis can occur in otherwise healthy women and is noted after recent childbirth, abortion, or gynecologic procedure.

Gastroenteritis may develop within 6 to 12 hours after eating meat that was improperly stored.

C. perfringens food poisoning is common and is acquired by the oral ingestion of large numbers of vegetative bacteria, from red meat or poultry that has been sitting at room temperature for a long period of time. When gastroenteritis occurs, it is typically part of an outbreak and not an isolated event.

Clostridial gangrene is uncommon. Contaminated wounds are a risk factor and clostridial gangrene should be considered in patients who present with toxic shock, with necrotizing soft tissue infection or an obstetric/gynecologic infection. It should also be considered in patients who are active injection drug users.

Spontaneous gas gangrene, due to *C. septicum*, has an increased incidence in patients with GI malignancies, recent GI surgery, profound immunosuppression, and diverticulitis.

SIGNS AND SYMPTOMS

The major symptom of *C. perfringens* soft tissue infection is severe pain, out of proportion to the physical examination, at a site of recent trauma or surgery. Onset is within 1 to 3 days of the incident. The triad of severe pain at a site, signs of systemic toxicity, and gas in the involved soft tissues accounts for the major presenting signs and symptoms. Rapid progression is possible.

Most patients with *C. perfringens* gastroenteritis present with profuse, watery diarrhea, and a smaller number of patients present with vomiting. Other symptoms include abdominal cramps and fever. Symptoms are self-limiting and resolve within 24 to 48 hours.

PHYSICAL EXAMINATION

The physical examination findings of *C. perfringens* gangrene include tachycardia, hypotension, and minimal or no fever. Examination of the skin reveals a surgical wound or trauma with ischemic skin changes, including pallor or cyanosis. Hemorrhagic bullae may be present. The fluid in the necrotic tissues is described as having a sweet putrid odor thinner than normal pus. Air in the tissue may present as crepitus on physical examination.

In *C. perfringens* endometritis, a TSS may be present and is characterized by tachycardia, hypotension, and lack of fever. Diffuse edema may occur with nonpurulent vaginal discharge.

DIFFERENTIAL DIAGNOSIS

Necrotizing soft tissue infections can be caused by many different bacteria. It is difficult to distinguish clostridial gangrene from other microbial etiologies without cultures results.

Toxic shock in women of reproductive age suggests infection of the female reproductive tract. Possible etiologies, other than *C. perfringens,* include GAS and *Staphylococcus aureus*. GAS complicates childbirth and *S. aureus* is tampon-associated.

Staphylococcal food poisoning has a rapid onset, 2 to 8 hours after ingestion, and the primary symptom is vomiting, not diarrhea.

DIAGNOSTIC STUDIES

Peripheral white blood cell (WBC) count is elevated with a left shift. *C. perfringens* produces a hemolysin that can cause a hemolytic anemia. Women with clostridial endometritis and toxic shock can have a markedly elevated leukocyte count or leukemoid reaction, with WBC counts above 50,000/μL.

Blood cultures are positive in 15% of patients with soft tissue infection or suspected endometritis.

Metabolic profile may reveal hyperbilirubinemia, elevated transaminases, and acute kidney injury.

Creatine kinase (CK) is elevated when myonecrosis is present.

Culture is the definitive diagnostic test. A positive culture from a deep tissue culture in a patient with clinical illness should be considered a true positive. However, clostridial spores can contaminate the skin or feces, so isolating clostridia from superficial sites without necrotic or gangrenous soft tissues should be considered contamination.

Blood cultures—though not often positive in gangrene TSS—are diagnostic. Isolating *C. septicum* from the bloodstream suggests a colorectal source.

TREATMENT

Preventing foodborne *C. perfringens* infection is best accomplished by keeping meat at the proper temperature. Cooked meats should be served hot (>140 °F) as soon as possible and any leftover should be refrigerated. Reheating cold meats should achieve an internal temperature of 165 °F or higher to kill bacteria that may have grown during cooling.

Treatment of gas gangrene should be started immediately. High-dose penicillin or clindamycin should be started, and all dead and infected tissue removed surgically. Amputation may be required in patients with gas gangrene in a limb. Treatment with high-pressure oxygen, hyperbaric oxygen, may be helpful.

PATIENT EDUCATION

- The mortality rate of clostridial gangrene without TSS is around 10% to 30%.[9]
- Women with reproductive tract TSS caused by *C. sordellii* or *C. perfringens* have a very high mortality risk.
- *C. perfringens* food poisoning is a self-limited illness.

17.1CB TETANUS

OVERVIEW

Tetanus is caused by toxins produced by *Clostridium tetani.* Patients will have a well-defined wound or other portal of entry for the spores. Tetanus is preventable with adequate immunization and appropriate wound care.

Tetanus toxin, a metalloproteinase, is synthesized as a single chain and divides into a heavy and light chain. The heavy chain enables the toxin to bind to its receptor on the presynaptic neuron of the neuromuscular junction. The toxin is internalized via endocytosis, and then released into the cytoplasm. The light chain interacts with synaptic vesicle release that is responsible for depolarization of the presynaptic neuron, inhibiting one of the several proteins involved in transmitter release.

The manifestations of botulism result from this this effect, with the motor manifestations due to inhibition of transmitter release at the neuromuscular junction, and the ocular and GI effects are a result of muscarinic synaptic inhibition.

The toxin also moves via the neuronal retrograde transport system into the central nervous system, where it has a high affinity for cells responsible for inhibition. The combined effect on the inhibitory neurons results in the widespread, sustained contractions of muscles whenever a muscle contracts.

MEDICAL HISTORY AND CLINICAL PRESENTATION

Certain portals of entry are more prone to cause tetanus than others; these include puncture wounds, burns, surgical procedures, compound fractures, abortions performed outside of medical facilities, and nonsterile intramuscular injections.

The initial complaints of generalized tetanus are muscle rigidity and trismus. Later spasms develop that progress to posturing whereby the back becomes arched; this can cause airway compromise and death. Patients with local tetanus have weakness near the site of infection, then unilateral weakness before the onset of diffuse stiffness and spasms. Patients with local forms of tetanus have lower motor neuron muscle weakness near the site of toxin production.

SIGNS AND SYMPTOMS

Incubation period is about 10 days. The further the injury site is from the central nervous system, the longer the incubation period. A shorter incubation period is associated with more severe disease, complications, and a higher chance of death. There are three clinical forms of tetanus: generalized, localized, and cephalic.

Generalized tetanus is the most common and severe form. The initial finding is trismus or "lockjaw." Other signs and symptoms are painful spasms in muscle of the neck, trunk, and extremities and generalized, seizure-like activity or convulsions in severe cases.

Localized tetanus is an unusual form of the disease consisting of muscle spasms in a confined area close to the site of the injury. Localized tetanus often occurs in people with partial immunity and is typically mild, but progression to generalized tetanus can occur.

Cephalic tetanus, the rarest form, is associated with lesions of the head or face and may be associated with otitis media. The incubation period is typically 1 to 2 days. Unlike generalized and localized tetanus, cephalic tetanus results in flaccid cranial nerve palsies rather than spasm. Cephalic tetanus can progress to the generalized form.

PHYSICAL EXAMINATION

Physical examination findings vary with the form of disease and are consistent with signs and symptoms for traumatic, localized, and cephalic tetanus described above

DIFFERENTIAL DIAGNOSIS

The differential diagnosis includes strychnine intoxication and the stiff-person syndrome. Strychnine poisoning presents with relaxation of the abdominal musculature between spasms. Patients with stiff-person syndrome have a long history of complaints related to muscle stiffness before they develop spasms. Dental infections may also cause trismus, and be confused with cephalic tetanus.

A dystonic reaction to a dopamine antagonist can mimic tetanus. Dystonic reactions involve sustained lateral head movement that is not noted in tetanus. A dose of diphenhydramine or benztropine will relieve a dystonic reaction but will not affect tetanus.

DIAGNOSTIC STUDIES

There is no diagnostic test for tetanus. The presence of anti-tetanus antibodies may be tested for before giving human tetanus immune globulin.

TREATMENT

The initial therapy for generalized tetanus is airway maintenance, done with IV benzodiazepines or possible endotracheal intubation.

The antibiotics used in the treatment of tetanus include metronidazole, penicillin G, and doxycycline.

Human tetanus immune globulin should be administered intramuscularly as soon as possible. At a different site, the first dose of the age-appropriate form of tetanus toxoid vaccine should be administered. A complete series of toxoid injections should be given since the amount of toxin produced during an episode of severe tetanus is not adequate to induce immunity.

Tetanus is completely preventable with immunization. There are four types of vaccines used to protect against tetanus, all of which also protect against other diseases:

- Diphtheria and tetanus (DT) vaccines
- Diphtheria, tetanus, and pertussis (DTaP) vaccines
- Tetanus and diphtheria (Td) vaccines
- Tetanus, diphtheria, and pertussis (Tdap) vaccines

Babies and children younger than 7 years receive DTaP or DT, while older children and adults receive Tdap and Td.

According to the Centers for Disease Control and Prevention (CDC) the following schedule should be followed[10]:

- Infants and children receive five doses of DTaP. One dose is given at the following ages: 2 months, 4 months, 6 months, 15 through 18 months, and 4 through 6 years.
  - Use DT for infants and children who should not receive acellular pertussis-containing vaccines.
- Adolescents receive a single dose of Tdap, preferably at 11 to 12 years.
- Pregnant women should receive a single dose of Tdap during every pregnancy, preferably during the early part of gestational weeks 27 through 36. If a woman did not receive Tdap during her current pregnancy but did receive a prior dose of Tdap, then she should not receive a dose of Tdap postpartum.
- Adults should receive a single dose of Td every 10 years. For adults who have never received Tdap, a dose of Tdap can replace one of the 10-year Td booster doses. Clinicians can give Tdap regardless of the time since the patient's most recent Td vaccination.

After an injury, the toxoid and human tetanus immunoglobulin (HTIG) should be given based on the following (see Table 17.3)[11]:

- Clean minor wounds in patient with documented primary vaccination: HTIG not needed; toxoid not needed unless more than 10 years since last booster vaccination.
- Clean minor wounds in patient with no or unknown primary vaccination: HTIG not needed; give toxoid and follow with basic immunization series.

TABLE 17.3 Guide to Tetanus Prophylaxis With Tig in Routine Wound Management

	Clean, Minor Wound		All Other Wounds*	
History of adsorbed tetanus toxoid-containing vaccines	**DTap, Tdap, or Td †**	**TIG ‡**	**DTap, Tdap, or Td †**	**TIG ‡**
Unknown or <3 doses	Yes	No	Yes	Yes
≥3 doses	No	No	No	No

*Such as wounds contaminated with dirt, feces, soil, or saliva; puncture wounds; crush injuries; avulsions; and wounds resulting from missiles, burns, or frostbite.
† For patients ≥10 years old who have not previously received a dose of Tdap, a single dose of Tdap should be given instead of one Td booster. Children <7 years should be given DTaP or, if pertussis vaccine is contraindicated, DT. Children age 7–9 years should be given Td.
‡ People with HIV infection or severe immunodeficiency who have contaminated wounds should also receive TIG, regardless of their history of tetanus immunizations.
DT, diphtheria and tetanus toxoids (for children); DTaP, diphtheria and tetanus toxoids, acellular pertussis (for children); Td, tetanus and diphtheria toxoids adsorbed (for adults); Tdap, tetanus and diphtheria toxoids, acellular pertussis (for adults); TIG, tetanus immune globulin (human).
Source: Data from Havers FP, Moro PL, Hunter P, Hariri S, Bernstein H. Use of tetanus toxoid, reduced diphtheria toxoid, and acellular pertussis vaccines: Updated Recommendations of the Advisory Committee on Immunization Practices—United States, 2019. MMWR Morb Mortal Wkly Rep. 2020;69:77–83. doi:10.15585/mmwr.mm6903a5

- All other wounds in patient with documented primary vaccination: No need for HTIG; give toxoid if >5 years since last booster vaccination.
- All other wounds in patient with no or unknown primary vaccination: Give HTIG and toxoid followed with basic immunization series.

PATIENT EDUCATION

- The complications of tetanus arise from autonomic instability causing respiratory and cardiovascular dysfunction.
- The prognosis depends on several factors including time from the first symptom to the first spasm. In general, with a short time to symptom manifestation, the prognosis is poor. Neonatal and cephalic tetanus have a poor prognosis.
- Recovery can take months.

17.1CC BOTULISM

OVERVIEW

Botulism is caused by a toxin produced by *C. botulinum*. In the United States, there were 182 confirmed cases of botulism in 2017.[12]

Botulinum toxin is a neurotoxin. The toxin prevents the release of acetylcholine from axon endings at the neuromuscular junction. There are several types of botulinum toxin; types A, B, E and F can cause human disease.

Each toxin type targets an individual component of the release mechanism. All the manifestations of botulism are from this effect, with the motor manifestations resulting from inhibition of transmitter release at the neuromuscular junction, and the ocular and GI effects a consequence of muscarinic synaptic inhibition.

Recovery from botulism involves the development of new neuromuscular junctions and synapses. Each form of botulism has a different source of toxin. Infant botulism and adult GI botulism follow ingestion of the spores of *C. botulinum*, which germinate and produce a toxin within the gut. Wound botulism follows inoculation of spores into tissues. Patients who have received therapeutic injections of botulinum toxin can develop systemic signs of botulism.

MEDICAL HISTORY AND CLINICAL PRESENTATION

There is no immunization against botulism. Infants and adults who lack or suppress gastric acid production are at risk of GI colonization and local toxin production. Raw honey is a common source of infection in infants; in adults, poorly canned or vacuum-packed foods are a common source. Wound botulism typically occurs with trauma or open fracture contaminated by soil, but most cases are seen with injection drug users who inject the spores into tissues.

SIGNS AND SYMPTOMS

Botulism presents early with bilateral cranial nerve dysfunction, difficulty swallowing, dysarthria, blurred vision, and diplopia. Symmetric weakness of the upper extremities follows, then lower extremity weakness. Respiratory failure may occur due to upper airway weakness, difficulty handling secretions, or weakness of the diaphragm or parasternal intercostal muscles. Botulism produces constipation, but the patient may initially complain of diarrhea, nausea, and vomiting after ingestion of improperly prepared or preserved food.

PHYSICAL EXAMINATION

The most common physical findings on presentation include ptosis, ophthalmoparesis, tongue weakness, symmetric facial paresis, and weakness of the extremities. Infants with botulism are floppy and have weak cries and difficulty feeding. Dilated pupils and diminished deep tendon reflexes are noted in botulism.

DIFFERENTIAL DIAGNOSIS

The differential diagnosis includes myasthenia gravis and Lambert-Eaton syndrome. A variant of Guillain-Barré syndrome may present with similar cranial nerve findings as noted in botulism. Tick paralysis has a similar presentation.

Myasthenia gravis presents with a long history of moderate weakness and diplopia. Myasthenia does not present with pupillary dilation, so blurred vision is not noted. Myasthenic patients do not have GI complaints. Patients with the Lambert-Eaton syndrome tend to have small, poorly reactive pupils.

DIAGNOSTIC STUDIES

There are no routine laboratory tests that assist with the diagnosis of botulism.

Repetitive nerve stimulation at high frequency can aid in the diagnosis. Botulism and Lambert-Eaton syndrome will have an incremental muscle response to high frequency stimulation. At lower frequencies patients with botulism may show no change, or even a decrease.

The diagnosis is confirmed by recovery of the toxin from the serum or stool. Anaerobic cultures of food or stool positive for *C. botulinum* are supportive of the diagnosis but are not diagnostic. Positive anaerobic cultures of wound tissue are diagnostic.

TREATMENT

Adult-type botulism—food-borne or existing in a wound—require treatment with heptavalent botulism antitoxin. The antitoxin prevents progression of disease by binding with circulating toxin. Antitoxin does not reverse signs or symptoms that are already present.

Infants with suspected or proven infant botulism require treatment with human botulism immune globulin. Botulism immune globulin prevents progression of neuromuscular paralysis by binding with circulating toxin.

Antibiotics are not indicated for patients with botulism; aminoglycosides can worsen neuromuscular paralysis.

PATIENT EDUCATION

- Proper food handling is the most important preventive measure.
- Botulinum spores are relatively resistant to heat, including boiling, but will be destroyed in a properly operated pressure cooker. The toxin is denatured by cooking at 85 °C.
- Avoiding honey has decreased cases of infant botulism by half.
- The mortality rate for adults with botulism is about 5%.[13] The mortality rate of infant botulism is <1%.[14]

17.1CD COLITIS

OVERVIEW

Clostridioides difficile is a spore-forming, gram-positive anaerobic bacillus that produces two major toxins, toxin A and toxin B, which are important in disease pathogenesis. Some strains of *C. difficile* do not produce toxins; these strains do not cause infection.

C. difficile, an obligate anaerobe, will die within minutes of exposure to air in its vegetative state. *C. difficile* forms spores that enable the bacteria to survive in the physical environment for long periods, thus facilitating transmission. It is the most common cause of healthcare-associated diarrhea among adults in the United States and is associated with significant morbidity and mortality.

Previous antibiotic exposure is the single most important risk factor for the development of *C. difficile* infection. Although clindamycin and cephalosporins have been implicated most often in infection, nearly all antimicrobials have been associated with the development of the disease. The antibiotics predisposing patients to *C. difficile* are noted in Table 17.4.

Three major factors are linked to the development of *C. difficile* infection:

TABLE 17.4 Antimicrobial Agents Predisposing Patients to *Clostridioides difficile* Infection

Frequently Related	Less Commonly Related	Uncommonly Related
Clindamycin	Other penicillins	Aminoglycosides
Ampicillin/amoxicillin	Sulfonamides	Metronidazole
Cephalosporins	Trimethoprim	Rifampin
Fluoroquinolones	Cotrimoxazole	Tetracycline
	Macrolides	
	Carbapenems	

- Host factors, including age, severity of illness, and immune status
- Increased exposure to *C. difficile* spores through prolonged hospital stays, contact with contaminated health-care environments, or poor hand hygiene by healthcare workers
- Exposure to antimicrobial agents and previous hospitalization

MEDICAL HISTORY AND CLINICAL PRESENTATION

C. difficile is a common cause of antibiotic-associated diarrhea among adults.

Infection can occur in both endemic and epidemic settings and often appears in clusters or outbreaks within institutions. A detailed medication history, including recent antibiotic or chemotherapy use, should be obtained.

Transmission occurs mainly through the fecal-oral route through contact with *C. difficile* spores in the healthcare environments. Hand contamination of healthcare workers caring for patients with *C. difficile* infection is a primary mode of transmission.

SIGNS AND SYMPTOMS

The most common manifestation of *C. difficile* disease is watery diarrhea, rarely with blood or mucus. Other signs and symptoms include fever, abdominal pain, and lower quadrant tenderness. The formation of pseudomembranes in the colon may be present in up to half of the cases. Less common but severe presentations may include fulminant or complicated colitis (including toxic megacolon, ileus, or bowel perforation), renal failure, and hypotension/shock. Death may also occur.

PHYSICAL EXAMINATION

C. difficile infection presents with a low-grade fever and abdominal tenderness. Additional signs on physical examination, such as high-grade fever, hypotension, and tachycardia, may be suggestive of worsening infection, complicated disease, or failure of antimicrobial therapy. Worsening abdominal tenderness, distention, palpable masses, or inactive bowel sounds, may suggest the development of toxic megacolon, abscess development, or ileus.

DIFFERENTIAL DIAGNOSIS

Mild forms of *C. difficile* infections mimic viral gastroenteritis. *C. difficile* colitis should be differentiated from other infectious causes of diarrheal disease, including *Salmonella, Shigella, Campylobacter*, and *Yersinia*.

The abdominal pain and tenderness associated with *C. difficile* colitis may mimic peritonitis and overlap with appendicitis, intussusception, and ischemic bowel. The presence of toxic megacolon in an ill patient should raise the possibility of Hirschsprung disease.

DIAGNOSTIC STUDIES

C. difficile is a clinical diagnosis. Stool testing should be performed on unformed stool specimens from symptomatic patients. There are two major categories of *C. difficile* testing:

- Toxin testing: enzyme-linked immunoassay (EIA) and tissue culture cytotoxicity
- Organism identification: glutamate dehydrogenase (GDH) EIA, stool culture, and nucleic acid amplification tests (NAATs; polymerase chain reaction [PCR])

The most commonly used test is EIA performed on stool specimens for detecting *C. difficile* toxins A and B. The test is rapid, specific, and inexpensive. Assays that identify both toxins are preferable.

Cytotoxicity assays were the gold standard before the more widespread introduction of EIA testing. The assay is expensive, requires special equipment, and has a slow turnaround time.

EIA testing for *C. difficile* GDH is used for organism identification and is both rapid and sensitive. The tests are not specific for toxigenic strains so confirmatory testing with toxigenic culture or cytotoxicity assay is required.

Stool culture remains the most sensitive method but is not clinically practical because of its slow turnaround time.

TREATMENT

Oral vancomycin and fidaxomicin are first-line options for both nonsevere and severe initial episodes of *C. difficile* infection. Metronidazole is only recommended for nonsevere initial episodes when patients are unable to obtain or be treated with oral vancomycin or fidaxomicin. Repeated or prolonged treatment courses with metronidazole should be avoided owing to the risk of neurotoxicity.

For recurrent infection, metronidazole should not be used. If metronidazole was used for initial treatment, patients should receive oral vancomycin. If vancomycin was used as initial treatment, vancomycin can be administered again but as a tapered and pulsed regimen, or fidaxomicin can be used.

PATIENT EDUCATION

- The estimated number of *C. difficile* infections per year in the United States is estimated to be around 223,900.[15]
- Approximately 12,800 deaths per year are attributed to *C. difficile* infection in the United States.[15]

17.1D ANTHRAX

Bacillus anthracis is a gram-positive, spore-forming rod in the *Bacillus cereus* group. The main risk factor for infection is the presence of *B. anthracis* spores in the host's environment. The type of disease and route of exposure are based on the patient's interaction with the environment. Aerosol exposure leads to inhalation anthrax, contact exposure leads to cutaneous anthrax, ingestion leads to GI anthrax, and injection leads to skin or soft tissue anthrax.

Anthrax is mostly a zoonotic infection in areas of the world with an agriculture-based economy.

Anthrax is endemic in many areas of the world, including East, Central, and Southeast Asia; the Indian subcontinent; Indonesia; sub-Saharan Africa; Mexico; and parts of Central and South America. Rare cases occur in the United States, particularly in New Mexico, southwestern Texas, and the Midwest.

Both the innate and adaptive arms of the immune system participate in the protection from infection. *B. anthracis* has several ways to overcome these protective responses and cause disease. One mechanism is the production of anthrax toxin, leading to a paralysis of both innate and adaptive immune responses. Administration or natural production of antibodies directed against protective antigen, a component of anthrax toxin, provides a significant measure of protection against anthrax.

People with increased exposure to *B. anthracis* spores have a higher risk for contracting the disease. Patients who are immunocompromised, such as those with organ transplants, HIV/AIDS, or hematologic malignancies, are at increased risk for infection.

The pathophysiology of inhalational anthrax begins with the phagocytosis of the spores by alveolar macrophages and dendritic cells in the lung. The spores are transported to regional mediastinal lymph nodes and undergo germination into the bacillary form. After germination, the organism encapsulates and begins producing anthrax toxin. *B. anthracis* has several virulence factors that aid in escape from the phagocytes. These factors include a cholesterol-dependent cytolysin, anthrolysin O, and phospholipases. Once the organism has escaped from phagocytes, replication begins, and they enter the circulation, disseminating to other organs. The bacilli multiply in the blood and produce anthrax toxin. The toxin components, protective antigen, edema factor (EF), and lethal factor (LF), work to interfere with the host immune response, damage host tissues, and promote survival and dissemination of *B. anthracis*.

MEDICAL HISTORY AND CLINICAL PRESENTATION

The main forms of anthrax are cutaneous, GI, inhalational, injection-related, and meningeal. Cutaneous anthrax is the most common and associated with the lowest mortality rate, and anthrax meningitis is almost always fatal.

Cutaneous anthrax manifests on skin surfaces as a painless, ulcerating papule. The lesions begin as a papule, but evolve with central ulceration, eschar formation, and edema around the lesion. The eschar is usually very dark. In severe disease, systemic signs and symptoms, such as fever, leukocytosis, and hypotension, may be present. Untreated cutaneous anthrax may lead to dissemination, septic shock, and death.

GI anthrax is usually acquired by eating the meat from an animal that is undercooked and contaminated with anthrax spores. There are two main forms of GI anthrax: oropharyngeal and intestinal.

Oropharyngeal anthrax may present as a severe ulcerative pharyngitis. This disease presents with pseudomembrane formation and systemic toxicity. GI anthrax presents as gastroenteritis, with nausea, vomiting, typically bloody diarrhea, abdominal pain, fevers, chills, and malaise. Severe ascites may develop.

Inhalational anthrax is a biphasic illness; the initial phase presents like an influenza-like illness with malaise, cough, fever, and chills, followed by rapid progression to acute respiratory failure, hypotension, change in mental status, multisystem organ failure, and death.

Injection-related anthrax is due to inoculation of spores into the subcutaneous tissues or muscle during intramuscular drug use. This results in the development of severe soft tissue infections. Clinical features include soft tissue edema, local excessive bruising or hemorrhage and pain at the injection site. Injection-related anthrax may be mistaken for necrotizing fasciitis.

Anthrax meningitis is a complication of systemic anthrax cases and may occur as the sole presentation of anthrax. This form carries a very high mortality rate. Clinical presentation includes fever, headache, confusion, neck stiffness, seizures, and focal motor deficits. Signs of meningismus may be absent. A petechial rash may be noted and mistaken for meningococcemia.

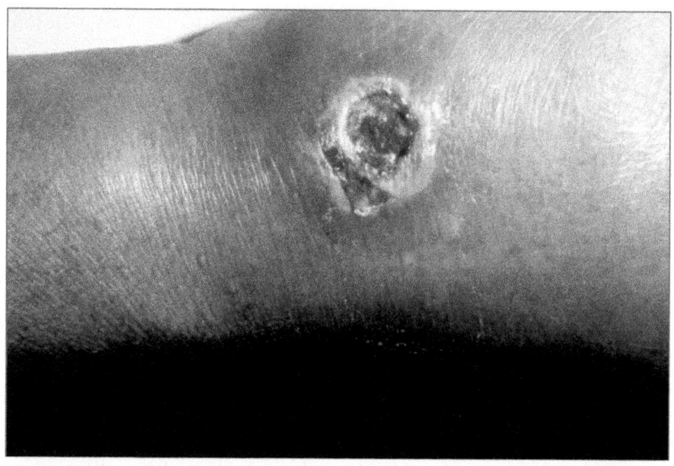

Figure 17.1 **This anthrax lesion shows the classic central depression with black scabs. The surrounding tissue is red and edematous.** *(Source: Centers for Disease Control and Prevention/F. Marc LaForce, MD. https://phil.cdc.gov/details_linked.aspx?pid=21741)*

SIGNS AND SYMPTOMS

The symptoms of anthrax infection depend on the mode of anthrax exposure in the patient. Cutaneous anthrax is characterized by a skin blister that ulcerates with a black center, myalgias, fever, and vomiting. The ingestion or GI type may include symptoms of fever, chills, pharyngitis, odynophagia, and abdominal pain. Inhalation anthrax presents with fever, chills, fatigue, pharyngitis, and dyspnea. Injection anthrax presents with symptoms like cutaneous anthrax. The symptoms of the injection type of anthrax include fever, chills, skin ulcer, and subcutaneous abscesses. When anthrax is considered as a possible diagnosis, a history of exposure to contaminated animal materials, occupational exposure, and living in an endemic area should be noted.

PHYSICAL EXAMINATION

The physical findings of anthrax infection depend on the mode of exposure. Common findings noted with cutaneous anthrax include fever, tachycardia, and skin changes including blister that becomes an eschar, edema, and lymphadenopathy (Figure 17.1).

Ingestion or GI anthrax findings include fever, tachycardia, and oropharyngeal ulcers with edema. Inhalation anthrax presents with fever, tachycardia, decreased respirations, pallor with cyanosis, decreased breath sounds, and signs of pleural effusion. Injection anthrax presents with fever, localized skin changes with edema and abscesses.

DIFFERENTIAL DIAGNOSIS

The differential diagnosis of anthrax includes a wide range of conditions and varies depending on the mode of anthrax exposure in the patient. A history of exposure to contaminated animal materials, occupational exposure, and living in an endemic area should be noted. See Table 17.5 for the differential diagnosis of anthrax

DIAGNOSTIC STUDIES

Systemic anthrax presents with several nonspecific laboratory abnormalities. These include anemia, thrombocytopenia, and leukocytosis. Other laboratory findings include hyponatremia, elevated blood urea nitrogen, increased transaminase levels, and hypoalbuminemia.

TABLE 17.5 Differential Diagnosis for Various Types of Anthrax

Cutaneous	Oropharyngeal	Gastrointestinal	Inhalational
Erysipelas	Diphtheria	Food poisoning	*Mycoplasma pneumoniae*
Glanders	Streptococcal infection	Acute abdomen	Legionnaires disease
Plague	Vincent angina	Hemorrhagic gastroenteritis	Psittacosis
Syphilis chancre	Ludwig, angina	Necrotizing enteritis	Tularemia
Rickettsial diseases	Parapharyngeal abscess	Dysentery	Q fever
Rat bite fever	Deep-tissue neck infection		Viral pneumonia
Leishmaniasis			Histoplasmosis
Ecthyma gangrenosum			Coccidioidomycosis
Herpes			Malignancy

Cultures from the initial skin lesion, blood, CSF, or pleural fluid can be used to identify the organism and are the gold standard for the routine isolation and identification of *B. anthracis*.

Gram staining is the best staining technique. Gram-positive rods, commonly described as boxcar-shaped, growing in chains of varying length are noted with microscopic examination. Under certain growth conditions, terminal spores may be seen (Figure 17.2).

Chest x-ray is used in the evaluation of inhalation anthrax. Abnormalities include mediastinal widening, paratracheal fullness, pleural effusions, parenchymal infiltrates, and mediastinal lymphadenopathy. Chest CT scan findings include mediastinal widening, hyperdense lymph nodes, and edema of the mediastinal fat.

The CSF in anthrax meningitis reveals an increase in neutrophils, elevated total protein, and decreased glucose.

Biochemical assays have limited utility when trying to differentiate *B. anthracis* from other *Bacillus* species and may not be needed at all when other techniques are employed. A direct fluorescence assay for both capsule and cell wall polysaccharide is used as a confirmatory test.

PCR-based techniques are helpful for the rapid detection of *B. anthracis* in both clinical and environmental samples.

TREATMENT

Treatment of localized cutaneous anthrax with no evidence of systemic illness or dissemination is oral ciprofloxacin or doxycycline for 7 to 10 days.

Systemic anthrax, including inhalational, GI, meningeal, and injectional, is treated with IV ciprofloxacin, levofloxacin, or doxycycline. This can be changed to oral medications when clinically indicated. Linezolid or other protein synthesis inhibitors, such as clindamycin, may be added to impair toxin synthesis. In cases of anthrax meningitis at least one agent with effective central nervous system penetration and activity against *B. anthracis* should be used, such as ciprofloxacin; other options include meropenem and penicillin. Antitoxin should also be given. Antitoxins inhibit binding to anthrax toxin receptors and translocation of the two primary toxins into cells. The two antitoxins are raxibacumab and anthrax immune globulin. Any person with anthrax should be considered contagious until appropriately evaluated.

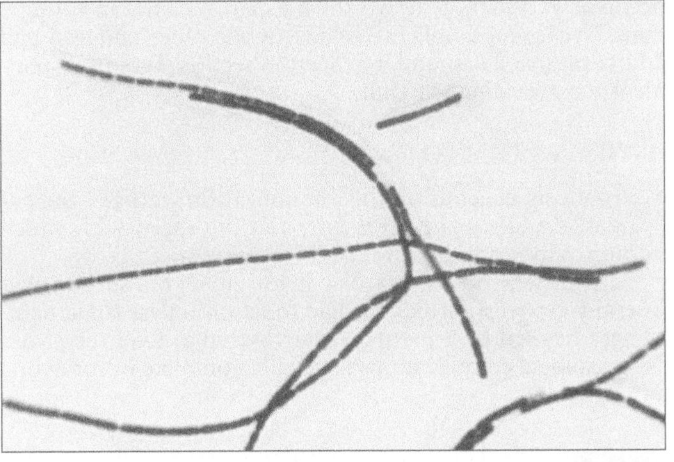

Figure 17.2 **Under a magnification of 1150×, this Gram-stained photomicrograph depicted numerous, gram-positive, rod-shaped, *Bacillus anthracis* bacteria, which were arranged in long filamentous strands.**

(Source: Centers for Disease Control and Prevention/Dr. Brodsky. https://phil.cdc.gov/details_linked.aspx?pid=20496)

Postexposure anti-infective prophylaxis is recommended for anyone with potential aerosol exposure to *B. anthracis* spores. The current recommendation regarding duration of therapy is 60 days with one of the following agents:

- Ciprofloxacin or doxycycline are first-line therapy.
- Levofloxacin is second-line therapy.

PATIENT EDUCATION

- The prognosis of anthrax depends on the type of anthrax, how early the disease was diagnosed, bacterial strain, and the patient's age and health status.
- Following recovery, resolution of small to medium-size cutaneous lesions is complete with minimal scarring. Larger lesions may scar and contractures may develop.

17.1E DIPHTHERIA

Corynebacterium diphtheriae is an aerobic, nonencapsulated gram-positive nonmotile pleomorphic rod. Humans are the only known reservoir. There are three phenotypes of *C. diphtheriae* (mitis, intermedius, and gravis), each capable of producing toxin and disease.

Prior to the development of the vaccine there were an estimated 21,053 cases and 1,822 deaths per year in the United States between 1936 and 1945.[16] The disease mainly affected children under 15 years of age. After the development of the vaccine the incidence of the disease dropped, and in 2018 there was one reported case of diphtheria in the United States.[17]

C. diphtheriae is spread by respiratory tract droplets and by contact with exudate from skin lesions. The incubation period is 2 to 7 days and infected individuals shed the organism from the nose and throat or from skin lesions for 2 to 6 weeks following infection, if not treated.

Diphtheria is an infection that usually involves the throat, but the nasal mucosa and/or larynx may be affected. In untreated cases, complications can develop leading to airway compromise. Circulating toxin can precipitate circulatory collapse, respiratory failure, stupor, coma, and death.

There are several presentations. Nasal diphtheria is more common in infants and is less likely to cause serious systemic disease because the toxin is less well absorbed from the nasal mucosa.

Cutaneous diphtheria has been reported among individuals living in crowded and poor hygienic conditions in the United States.

The infecting organism produces and releases a toxin after an incubation period. The B fragment of the toxin attaches to host cell receptors and enters the cell. The A fragment interrupts cellular protein synthesis. The effect of toxin activity is to produce necrosis, edema, and membrane formation. This membrane is made up of epithelial cells, fibrin, inflammatory cells, erythrocytes, and organisms.

Toxin is also distributed through the bloodstream reaching distant organs. Toxin effects include cardiac conduction system abnormalities due to cellular infiltration, pharyngeal and palatal paralysis due to myelin sheaths undergoing fatty degeneration, necrosis of renal tubules and hepatic parenchyma, and thrombocytopenia and adrenal hemorrhage.

MEDICAL HISTORY AND CLINICAL PRESENTATION

Diphtheria is an infection that usually involves the throat, but the nasal mucosa and/or larynx may be affected. The initial symptoms include sore throat and low-grade fever. Two to 4 days later a pseudomembrane forms on the pharyngeal walls, tonsils, uvula, and soft palate. The soft tissue of the neck becomes edematous and enlarged lymph nodes cause swelling of the neck, a "bull-neck" appearance.

Patients with diphtheria may hold the neck in extension to relieve pressure on the throat and larynx. The definition of the angle of the jaw and sternocleidomastoid muscle is "erased" by the brawny edema that is pitting, warm, tender, but not erythematous. Swallowing may be compromised by unilateral or bilateral paralysis of the muscles of the palate.

SIGNS AND SYMPTOMS

Respiratory diphtheria presents initially with clear nasal discharge, followed by serosanguineous and then mucopurulent drainage with excoriation of the upper lip and nares. Pseudomembrane may develop on the nasal septum, and a foul odor may be appreciated. Other symptoms include pharyngitis, cough, rhinorrhea, hoarseness, nasal obstruction, and hemoptysis; systemic symptoms include fever, chills, malaise, palpitations, myalgia, cervical adenopathy, and nausea and vomiting.

Cutaneous diphtheria results in pain, tenderness, and erythema at the site of infection, leading to ulceration and formation of a brownish gray membrane.

PHYSICAL EXAMINATION

With diphtheria the patient is often ill-appearing with fever, tachycardia, and tachypnea. Skin may have ulcerations. The major findings are respiratory and include cervical adenopathy and edema leading to a bull-neck appearance, pseudomembranous tonsillopharyngeal exudate, and rhinorrhea. Respiratory and cardiac findings include cough, dyspnea, stridor, hemoptysis, arrhythmias, and distant heart sounds. Neurologic findings include peripheral neuropathy and cranial nerve palsies.

DIFFERENTIAL DIAGNOSIS

The differential diagnosis includes other causes of exudative pharyngitis including *Streptococcus pyogenes*, adenovirus, and Epstein-Barr virus (EBV). The clinical findings of pharyngeal diphtheria, the pseudomembrane extending beyond the tonsillar area, along with few systemic signs and symptoms, assist in distinguishing diphtheria from other etiologies.

Oral or pharyngeal ulcerations are noted in herpes simplex and hand-foot-mouth disease but not in diphtheria.

Epiglottitis presents with trouble swallowing, drooling, and stridor. Infectious mononucleosis (IM) presents with a nonexudative pharyngitis, lymphadenopathy, splenomegaly, and fatigue.

DIAGNOSTIC STUDIES

Specimens for culture should be obtained from the nose and throat and any mucocutaneous site that is involved. If possible, a portion of the membrane should be submitted for culture. Gram stain and fluorescent antibody staining for identification of *C. diphtheriae* is unreliable. Suspicious isolates should be tested for toxin production.

The WBC count may be normal or slightly elevated. If neurologic involvement is suspected and CSF is obtained, the CSF protein may be elevated with a slight CSF pleocytosis.

If cardiac involvement is suspected an EKG may demonstrate prolonged PR interval, ST-segment elevation, and T-wave changes. Arrhythmias may also be detected.

TREATMENT

Treatment of diphtheria involves both the administration of equine antitoxin and antimicrobial therapy.

A single dose of antitoxin should be administered as soon as possible if the clinical condition is suggestive of diphtheria. While administration of the antitoxin leads to neutralization of circulating toxin, it has no effect on toxin that has already entered cells.

Only horse antidiphtheria antiserum is available in the United States; approximately 10% of individuals have preexisting hypersensitivity to horse serum.[18] A scratch test to the antitoxin should be performed prior to antitoxin administration. If no reaction is seen, the scratch test should be followed by an intradermal test. Even if both tests are negative the antitoxin should be administered carefully.

The dose of IV antitoxin depends upon the degree and duration of illness. Antitoxin is probably not needed for treating cutaneous disease.

Antibiotic therapy should be given along with antiserum; either penicillin G or procaine penicillin for 14 days may be used. Erythromycin is an option if the patient is allergic to penicillin.

Patients with respiratory diphtheria should be isolated and placed on droplet precautions until two cultures from the nose and throat taken 24 hours after antimicrobial therapy are negative. Patients with cutaneous diphtheria should be on contact precautions until cultures from the affected skin taken 24 hours after completion of antibiotics are negative. The disease is not contagious 48 hours after antibiotic treatment begins.

Active immunization with diphtheria toxoid should be undertaken during convalescence, since disease does not necessarily confer immunity.

All household contacts and others with close contact to the patient should be treated with oral erythromycin or with a single intramuscular dose of benzathine penicillin G.

The CDC recommends diphtheria, tetanus, and acellular pertussis vaccination across the lifespan.[11] Children younger than 7 years receive DTaP or DT, while older children and adults receive Tdap and Td. See the section Tetanus: Treatment for a vaccine schedule.

PATIENT EDUCATION

- Prognosis depends on the immunization status of the patient, the site of involvement, and the speed with which antitoxin is administered.
- Patients who develop cardiac involvement but survive generally recover normal cardiac function unless toxic damages has led to a permanent arrhythmia. Recovery from neurologic complications is usually complete in survivors.

17.1F LISTERIOSIS

Listeria monocytogenes is a short, nonbranching, nonspore-forming, anaerobic gram-positive rod. There are several species of *Listeria*, but only *L. monocytogenes* is a cause of human disease. *Listeria* is usually found in soil, water, vegetation, and fecal material. It is transmitted via contaminated food, including uncooked meats and vegetables, unpasteurized raw milk and cheeses, as well as other foods made from unpasteurized milk, and cooked or processed foods (e.g., certain soft cheeses, processed meats, and smoked seafood). In neonates, transmission is vertical from mother to fetus.

Following transmission, *Listeria* encodes a thermoregulated virulence factor, invades intestinal epithelium, and multiples within phagocytic phagolysosomes. The organism evades destruction by producing phospholipases and listeriolysin O, which causes lysis of the vacuole membrane. *Listeria* then migrates between cells.

Protection against infection is mediated by both innate and adaptive immunity; the adaptive response is mediated by the cellular part of the immune system. The role of humoral immunity is unknown, but the incidence of listeriosis is not increased in patients with immunoglobulin disorders, neutropenia, neutrophil dysfunction, splenectomy, or complement deficiency.

Patients at the greatest risk for infection include those with impaired cell-mediated immunity, including pregnancy, lymphoma, AIDS, or the use of corticosteroids and anti-tumor necrosis factor agents. Those at the extremes of age are also at risk, with the highest infection rate noted in neonates (23%) and those >60 years of age (22%).[19]

MEDICAL HISTORY AND CLINICAL PRESENTATION

Listeriosis is a foodborne illness that occurs year-round but is relatively rare causing only 1% of foodborne illness in the United States.[19] Patients often have a history of ingestion of delicatessen style ready-to-eat meats, particularly poultry products, soft cheeses, hot dogs, milk, and smoked fish. Other sources of infection include fresh fruits (cantaloupes) and vegetables (sprouts).

While most foodborne diseases result in GI distress, infection following ingestion of *Listeria* manifests as invasive disease with bacteremia or meningitis. While listeriosis is rare, it is associated with a high rate of death, causing 19% of all foodborne disease-related deaths.[19]

Listeriosis is quite uncommon in the general population, but it is a major cause of bacteremia and CNS infection in those with impaired cell-mediated immunity

Other than transmission from an infected mother to her fetus or newborn at birth, human-to-human transmission does not occur.

SIGNS AND SYMPTOMS

Listeria can cause a variety of infections. In pregnancy, infection is typically noted in the third trimester. The organism proliferates in the placenta and spreads cell-to-cell to facilitate maternal-fetal transmission. Bacteremia develops and presents as an acute febrile illness, accompanied by myalgia, arthralgia, headache, and backache. Outcomes of infection include stillbirth or neonatal deaths; premature labor and spontaneous abortion are common.

Neonatal infection presents in two forms: early-onset sepsis syndrome, acquired in utero and associated with prematurity; and meningitis, occurring at 2 weeks of age in term infants, who acquire the organism from the maternal vagina at birth. Clinical manifestations include fever and myalgias with a prodromal illness with nausea and diarrhea.

CNS infection presents with altered consciousness, seizures, or movement disorders.

Other clinical features of meningitis include headache, nausea, fever, and nuchal rigidity. Focal neurologic deficits are present in about one-third of patients.

Febrile gastroenteritis typically presents in disease outbreaks. Presentation occurs 24 hours after ingestion of the bacteria and symptoms last 1 to 3 days. Symptoms include fever, watery diarrhea, nausea, headache, and pains in joints and muscles.

PHYSICAL EXAMINATION

Physical examination findings vary depending on the type of infection. Common findings include fever, tachycardia, pallor, and abdominal tenderness. Neurologic findings include altered mental status, paralysis, and coma.

DIFFERENTIAL DIAGNOSIS

Differential diagnosis of listeriosis includes leukemia and lymphoma, thyroid disease, drug fever, vasculitis, and rheumatologic disorders. The differential diagnosis varies based on the location of the infection and includes the following:

- Gastroenteritis: *E. coli, Shigella, Salmonella*, and *Campylobacter* infections
- Neonatal meningitis: *E. coli* and GBS
- Meningitis: *N. meningitidis* and *Streptococcus* spp.
- Other locations: *Candida, E. coli, Staphylococcus,* Enterobacteriaceae, and *Haemophilus*

DIAGNOSTIC STUDIES

Listeria is most often isolated from blood culture and CSF culture. On Gram stain, *Listeria* appears as short, nonbranching, gram-positive rods resembling diphtheroids. On microscopic examination, characteristic tumbling motility is noted at room temperature.

CSF findings include an elevated WBC count and elevated total protein.

TREATMENT

The treatment of choice is ampicillin or penicillin. For infections of the CNS and endocarditis or infection in the neonate or immunocompromised patients, gentamicin should be added.

Patients with life-threatening allergies to penicillin should be treated with TMP-SMX. Other options include meropenem and linezolid.

Iron is a virulence factor for *Listeria*. Patients who are iron deficient should have iron supplements held until the infection is cured or under control.

Prevention of infection is best accomplished by thoroughly cooking and appropriately storing foods that transmit disease. Unpasteurized milk should be avoided. Anti-infective prophylaxis is not generally recommended. If foodborne illness develops in immunosuppressed patients, they may be given a short course of oral ampicillin or TMP-SMX to eradicate GI colonization and prevent invasive disease.

PATIENT EDUCATION

- The prognosis of listeriosis depends on the health status of the host:
  - Healthy children and young adults have a good prognosis and are at low-risk of developing complications and long-term sequelae.

- High-risk populations, including pregnant women, neonates, elderly, and those immunosuppressed, have a poorer prognosis with a high death rate.

17.1G PERTUSSIS

Pertussis is caused by a fastidious gram-negative, pleomorphic bacillus, *Bordetella pertussis*. The rate of infection has significantly decreased in developed countries due to the pertussis vaccine, but the incidence has increased in recent years. The increase in pertussis in the United States is due to waning of vaccine-induced and natural immunity in adolescents and adults and disease in infants too young to be immunized or who are incompletely immunized. Humans are the only known hosts of the disease.

Transmission occurs via droplets from a coughing person with attack rates in susceptible household contacts of 80%.[10]

Use of the pertussis vaccine has led to a decline in cases from 175,000 annually in the 1940s to just over 5,000 cases in the 1970s.[10] Since the 1970s, there has been a substantial increase in the number of cases reported. In 2012, the last peak year, the CDC reported 48,277 cases of pertussis in the United States, but many more go undiagnosed and unreported.[10]

Several virulent factors facilitate the invasion and damage of the epithelium of the airway and the alveoli by interfering with ciliary movements. The actions of the toxins have direct effects on the lung parenchyma, including necrotizing bronchitis and bronchiolitis and some affect immune regulation.

Hypoxemia is due to extensive damage to the alveolar and bronchiolar epithelium. The necrotic tissue contributes to the development of thick tenacious secretion of this disease. The combination of hypoxia, tenacious secretion, and the damage of the alveoli epithelium further exacerbates the development of pulmonary hypertension.

MEDICAL HISTORY AND CLINICAL PRESENTATION

Pertussis typically presents with a cough in three distinct phases. After the 6- to 10-day incubation period the following phases occur:

- Catarrhal phase: duration 1 to 2 weeks, most contagious period, indistinguishable from a mild upper respiratory tract infection
- Paroxysmal phase: duration 3 to 6 weeks, increase in cough frequency and severity with spells of coughing, characteristic whoop, vomiting, cyanosis, and apnea
- Convalescent phase: duration up to several months with gradual decrease in symptoms

SIGNS AND SYMPTOMS

Pertussis shares many of the same features as other common viral infections such as respiratory syncytial virus (RSV), influenza, and parainfluenza infections. Common signs and symptoms include a history of exposure to individuals with cough, past medical history of not having received pertussis immunization, mild leukocytosis with moderate lymphocytosis, multilobar consolidation on chest x-ray (CXR), and clinical symptoms including paroxysmal coughing spells, whooping cough, post-tussive emesis, seizures, and encephalopathy.

PHYSICAL EXAMINATION

Physical examination findings are consistent with other causes of upper respiratory infections. Differences noted in pertussis include:

- Restlessness and agitation due to prolonged coughing episode with difficulty catching breath
- Tachycardia or bradycardia (young infants), tachypnea or apnea (young infants)
- Perioral cyanosis
- Subconjunctival hemorrhages
- Coryza
- Paroxysmal cough with inspiratory whoop

Pulmonary examination reveals retractions, rib tenderness, asymmetric or decreased breath sounds, rhonchi, and wheezing or crackles.

DIFFERENTIAL DIAGNOSIS

Pertussis should be considered in the differential diagnosis for all patients who present with upper respiratory symptoms.

- RSV presents with upper respiratory infection symptoms, fever, cough, post-tussive emesis, apnea in infants, and superinfection with bacterial pneumonia.
- Influenza and parainfluenza viruses present with fever, upper respiratory infection symptoms, cough, encephalopathy, and pneumonia.

DIAGNOSTIC STUDIES

Laboratory results noted in pertussis include an increased WBC count with an absolute lymphocytosis of 10,000 or greater in young infants and under- or unimmunized children. Lymphocytosis is uncommon in older children and adolescents.

Cultures, gold standard for diagnosis, should be obtained from the posterior nasopharynx, not the throat or sputum. Culture and PCR testing should be obtained. These tests have their highest yield during the first 3 to 4 weeks of cough and the diagnosis is confirmed if culture and/or PCR are positive.

After 4 weeks of illness, a pertussis serology test can confirm the diagnosis. The enzyme-linked immunosorbent assay (ELISA) measures antibodies to the pertussis toxin. High antibody titers are highly suggestive of a current or recent infection. If the patient has been recently immunized or recently completed a course of antibiotics, the immune response may be blunted.

TREATMENT

The macrolide antibiotics—erythromycin, azithromycin, and clarithromycin—are recommended for both treatment and prophylaxis of pertussis. Azithromycin is the drug of choice for all age groups. Erythromycin therapy is contraindicated in infants under 4 weeks of age due to the risk of hypertrophic pyloric stenosis. For patients unable to tolerate or allergic to the macrolide antibiotics, the second-line choice is TMP-SMX in all age groups.

CDC recommends diphtheria, tetanus, and acellular pertussis vaccination across the lifespan. Children younger than 7 years receive DTaP or DT, while older children and adults receive Tdap and Td.[11] Vaccination protocols are given in the section Tetanus: Treatment.

PATIENT EDUCATION

- Pneumonia is the most frequent complication. Other complications include sinusitis, otitis media, both bacterial and viral superinfection, and neurologic complications.
- Neonatal pertussis disease is more virulent and associated with highest morbidity and mortality rates.

17.1H LEGIONNAIRES DISEASE

Legionellosis is caused by *Legionella pneumophilia*, a pleomorphic, aerobic, non-spore-forming, motile gram-negative bacillus. Most cases are reported between June and October. The incidence of disease is 1.4 to 1.8 per 100,000 persons per year in the United States with a case fatality rate of around 9%.[20] Legionellosis is classified into three types based the organ system affected and the clinical presentation:

- Pulmonary infection or Legionnaires disease
- Extrapulmonary infection
- Pontiac fever

Legionella is transmitted by aerosol droplets when people breathe in contaminated mist or vapor, from whirlpool spa, rivers, cruise ships, cooling towers, air conditioners, or water supply systems. *Legionella* is not contracted through person-person spread.

L. pneumophila invades host cells and replicates intracellularly. In Legionnaires disease, most exposed patients do not develop any symptoms.

L. pneumophilia is the most pathogenic of the species. Serotype 1 is responsible for 90% of infections in humans and is associated with community/hospital outbreaks of infection. Serotypes 1 and 6 most commonly associated with Legionnaires disease.

Legionella infection is transmitted through inhalation from a fresh water source or soil. The bacterium then enters mammalian cells through phagocytosis and multiplies intracellularly within the endoplasmic reticulum, ultimately leading to host cell necrosis. The host response is mainly a cell-mediated immunity response.

MEDICAL HISTORY AND CLINICAL PRESENTATION

Infection is acquired by aspiration of contaminated water or through inhalation of aerosolized fresh water sources or soil. Because of the bacteremia that can develop, patients can develop extrapulmonary infection. Extrapulmonary infections include sinusitis, pyelonephritis, cellulitis, pancreatitis, pericarditis, endocarditis, and myocarditis. Patients with legionellosis often report a recent history of travel, hospitalization, exposure to contaminated water, or exposure to healthcare settings.

There are two clinical syndromes:

- Legionnaires disease: a multiorgan system infection, predominately pneumonia. Onset of symptoms is delayed, typically 2 to 14 days after exposure.
- Pontiac fever: self-limited, influenza-like illness, with fever, headache and myalgias, but no signs of pneumonia. Onset of symptoms is abrupt, typically within 24 to 48 hours of exposure.

SIGNS AND SYMPTOMS

Legionellosis may manifest with either Legionnaires disease or Pontiac fever. Legionnaires disease is more severe while Pontiac fever is a milder form of respiratory flu-like disease that does not result in pneumonia.

Symptoms of Legionnaires disease may include fever, chest pain, nonproductive cough, dyspnea, hemoptysis, headache, myalgia, altered mental status, GI symptoms, and abdominal pain.

PHYSICAL EXAMINATION

No single clinical manifestation distinguishes *Legionella* infection from other types of pneumonia. Symptoms last 2 to 14 days. Physical exam is notable for fever ≥39 °C and signs of lung consolidation on examination and x-ray.

Patients with advanced disease may develop neurologic signs, including change in mental status, weakness, and ataxia. A relative bradycardia may be noted.

DIFFERENTIAL DIAGNOSIS

The differential diagnosis includes other common causes of CAP such as *Mycoplasma pneumoniae* and *Streptococcus pneumoniae.*

DIAGNOSTIC STUDIES

Laboratory results noted in legionellosis include leukocytosis or leukopenia with a left shift, thrombocytosis or thrombocytopenia associated with disseminated intravascular coagulation, hyponatremia, and acute kidney injury.

Diagnosis can be confirmed with respiratory cultures and Gram stain. Gram stain reveals weakly staining gram-negative rods or no microbes in the setting of multiple polymorphonuclear neutrophils. Culture of sputum, pleural fluid, or bronchoalveolar lavage is the gold standard for diagnosis.

Legionella urine antigen test is used to detect *L. pneumophilia*, serotype 1. The test has a sensitivity of 70% to 80% and specificity of 99%.[21]

The CXR, while not diagnostic, reveals a patchy, alveolar infiltrate (Figure 17.3). There are usually no CXR findings in Pontiac fever.

The CT scan may reveal bilateral, multiple affected segments and peripheral lung consolidation with a ground-glass opacity. There are usually no chest CT findings in Pontiac fever.

Other tests include direct fluorescent antibody testing performed on respiratory samples. Results are usually obtained in 2 to 4 hours. This test is less sensitive than culture because it requires more organisms to become positive. To be positive, antibody titers require a fourfold increase in serum titers between acute phase and convalescent phase; single titer in patient with acute pneumonia of ≥1:128 is presumptive evidence of infection. Subsequent titer of ≥1:256 in comparison is definitive evidence of infection.

TREATMENT

The treatment of choice includes the fluoroquinolone (levofloxacin or moxifloxacin) and macrolide (azithromycin).

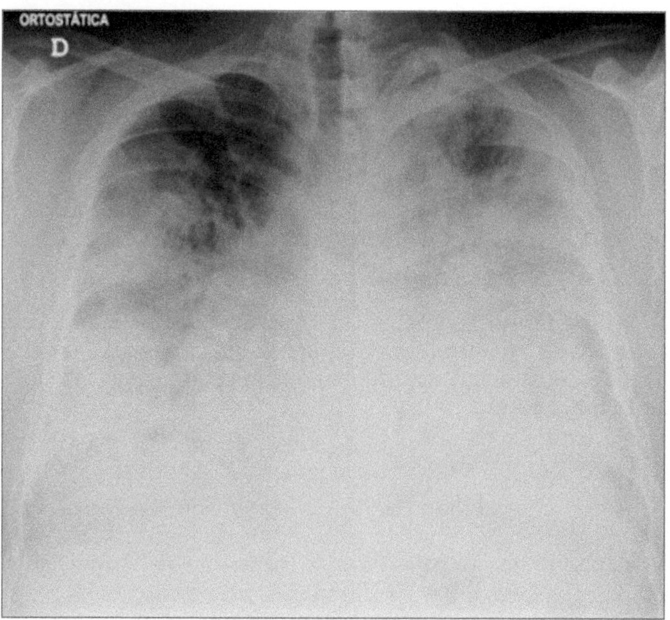

Figure 17.3 **Legionella pneumonia. This chest x-ray reveals multiple bilateral airspace opacities and a right basilar pleural effusion.** *(Source: Radiopaedia.org; courtesy of Dr. Sigmund Stuppner.)*

Alternative regimens include rifampin, TMP-SMX, or doxycycline. The recommended treatment duration is 10 to 14 days for immunocompetent hosts and 21 days for immunosuppressed hosts

PATIENT EDUCATION

- With appropriate and timely treatment patient will improve within 3 to 5 days.
- Poorer outcomes are noted in older patients, those with underlying lung disease, and those patients whose treatment was delayed or inappropriate.
- Mortality rate is reported between 5% and 30%.[22]

17.1I SALMONELLOSIS

Salmonella is a facultative intracellular, gram-negative bacillus. The genus *Salmonella* is a member of the family Enterobacteriaceae. This bacterium is classified into two different species: *Salmonella enterica* and *Salmonella bongori,* based on phenotypic makeup. *Salmonella enterica* is divided in six different subspecies.

Salmonella bacteria are classified as either typhoidal or nontyphoidal, based on their serotype.

Typhoidal *Salmonella* refers to the specific *Salmonella* serotypes that cause typhoid fever or paratyphoid fever, including *typhi, paratyphi A, paratyphi B, and paratyphi* C. Nontyphoidal *Salmonella* refers to all other *Salmonella* serotypes.

Salmonella typhi and *paratyphi* only infect humans and can only be acquired from ill individuals or chronic carriers who fecally contaminate food or water. In the United States, all cases are from travelers or outbreaks related to chronic carriers. Travelers to South-Central and Southeast Asia have the highest risk of infection followed by Mexico and Haiti. The incidence in the United States is low, with <500 cases per year.[23] Risk factors for infection include poor sanitation and lack of access to quality water supplies.

CDC estimates that approximately 1.35 million illnesses and 420 deaths occur due to nontyphoidal *Salmonella* annually in the United States.[24] There is an annual incidence of 15.7 illnesses per 100,000 individuals.[25]

Nontyphoidal *Salmonella* colonize many animals and can be acquired from many food sources, including meat, eggs, poultry, and a variety of fresh and processed foods. The second most common serotype, *Salmonella enteriditis,* can colonize and penetrate the developing chicken oviduct and can be present in the egg yolk of fresh eggs.

Salmonella infection is more common in the summer months. Groups more likely to get a *Salmonella* infection include children under age 5, nonbreastfed infants, those with weakened immune system, and those utilizing medications that reduce gastric acid production.

Both humoral- and cell-mediated immunity are required for protection against *Salmonella.* HIV-infected individuals, those with low stomach acidity, residents of nursing homes, neonates, those treated with tumor necrosis factor-alpha antagonists, persons with sickle cell disease, patients who have lymphoproliferative diseases, and transplant recipients are at higher risk.

MEDICAL HISTORY AND CLINICAL PRESENTATION

Patients with salmonellosis typically present with acute bloody or nonbloody diarrhea, abdominal pain, nausea, vomiting, and fever. A detailed clinical history, particularly the previous 72 hours prior to presentation, should include recent food ingestion, recent travel, and contact with family members and friends with similar symptoms.

The following questions should be asked:

- Recent travel history
- Presence of similar symptoms among close contacts
- Details of recent meals
- Recent farm or zoo visits
- Contact with pets, rodents, reptiles
- Occupation
- Recent antibiotic use
- Daycare attendance
- Medication use

Salmonella typhi and *S. paratyphi* cause enteric fever, a syndrome associated with fever and abdominal pain. Nontyphoidal *Salmonella* cause gastroenteritis. A small percentage of patients with gastroenteritis develop bacteremia. Bacteremia can lead to focal infections, particularly endovascular infections in those with atherosclerotic cardiovascular disease.

SIGNS AND SYMPTOMS

The symptoms of salmonellosis are indistinguishable from those caused by other pathogens. Symptoms usually have an acute onset and include:

- Fever
- Crampy abdominal pain
- Diarrhea, nonbloody or bloody
- Nausea
- Vomiting

PHYSICAL EXAMINATION

Salmonellosis is commonly associated with fever, pallor, abdominal distention, and abdominal tenderness. The appearance of the patient may range from normal to severely dehydrated, hypotensive, and with sunken eyes.

DIFFERENTIAL DIAGNOSIS

The differential diagnosis of salmonellosis includes other infectious agents that can cause an acute inflammatory diarrhea. This includes *Shigella, Campylobacter, C. difficile,* and *Entamoeba histolytica*. See Table 17.6 for the differential diagnosis of acute inflammatory diarrhea.

DIAGNOSTIC STUDIES

Typhoid fever is diagnosed by culture of blood, bone marrow, stool, or intestinal secretions. Bone marrow culture and examination should be performed if the diagnosis is strongly suspected. The duodenal string test is also another noninvasive culture method for isolation of *S. typhi*. Several serologic tests for *S. typhi* have been developed; the most widely used is the Widal test, but they are not recommended due to poor sensitivity and specificity.

Nontyphoidal gastroenteritis is diagnosed by stool culture. Bacteremia and focal infections are diagnosed by blood cultures or direct culture of infected tissue.

Commercially available polyvalent antisera can be used to identify common serotypes or groups. The organism is reportable to public health authorities.

TREATMENT

For typhoid fever, the typical therapy for susceptible strains is an oral fluoroquinolone (ciprofloxacin or ofloxacin for 5 to 7 days). If fluoroquinolone resistance is a concern, a higher dose and longer duration treatment with ciprofloxacin has been successful for these strains.

Alternative therapy options include oral azithromycin, ceftriaxone, cefotaxime, and oral cefixime.

Patients with persistent nausea, vomiting, diarrhea, or altered mental status should be treated with parenteral therapy with a third-generation cephalosporin or fluoroquinolone for at least 10 days or 5 days after fever is resolved.

Chronic carriers, those with positive cultures more than 12 months after original infection, of *S. typhi* should be treated for 4 to 6 weeks with an antibiotic. Antibiotic therapy includes oral amoxicillin, TMP-SMX, ciprofloxacin, or norfloxacin.

Nontyphoidal *Salmonella* gastroenteritis is usually self-limited and does not require antibiotic therapy but does require fluid and electrolyte replacement. Antimicrobial therapy to prevent bacteremia should be considered for those younger than 3 months of age, those over 50 years of age who have atherosclerosis because of the risk for endovascular infection, and those with prosthetic devices, immunosuppression, arthritis, or other endovascular abnormalities.

PATIENT EDUCATION

- The prognosis of salmonellosis is good for most patients.
- It may take several months until a patient's bowel habits become entirely normal.

17.1J SHIGELLOSIS

Shigella, a member of the Enterobacteriaceae family, is a nonmotile gram-negative bacillus. There are four major serologic groups, A through D. *S. sonnei* (group D) is most common followed by *S. flexneri* (group B).

Shigella can survive the acid environment of the stomach; a patient may only need to ingest 50 to 200 bacteria to cause shigellosis. Because disease can develop with a low number

TABLE 17.6 Differential Diagnosis of Acute Inflammatory Diarrhea

Pathogen	Transmission	Clinical Manifestations			
		Fever	Nausea/Vomiting	Abdominal Pain	Bloody Stool
Salmonella	Foodborne transmission, community-acquired	++	+	++	+
Shigella	Community-acquired, person-to-person	++	++	++	+
Campylobacter	Community-acquired, undercooked poultry	++	+	++	+
Escherichia coli	Foodborne transmission, undercooked hamburger	-	+	++	+ (EHEC or EIEC), - (ETEC, EAEC, EPEC)
Clostridioides difficile	Nosocomial spread, antibiotic use	+	±	+	+
Entamoeba histolytica	Travel tropical regions	+	±	+	±
Vibrio cholerae	Travel endemic area	+	+	+	–

-, not noted in cases; ±, may or may not be noted in cases; +, noted in some cases; ++, noted in many cases; EAEC, enteroaggregative Escherichia coli; EHEC, enterohemorrhagic Escherichia coli; EIEC, enteroinvasive Escherichia coli; EPEC, enteropathogenic Escherichia coli; ETEC, enterotoxigenic Escherichia coli.

of organisms, *Shigella* can readily spread from person to person, while *Salmonella* and *Campylobacter* are primarily spread via contaminated foods or water. Secondary cases are common.

Common sources of *Shigella* infection include day care centers, oral-anal contact, and contaminated food and water. *Shigella* can survive in water for 6 months; chlorination kills the organism and eliminates the risk of waterborne disease. Other infection control measures include handwashing with soap and water or with alcohol-based hand sanitizers, control of fly population, and proper handling, refrigeration, and cooking of food.

The localized cell-to-cell spread of the *Shigella* bacterium is via the formation of a large membrane protrusion. This protrusion, with the help of a protein from the host cell, pushes into an adjacent cell. In the adjacent cell the bacterium is ingested and escapes into the cell's cytoplasm. This allows *Shigella* to spread from cell to cell without ever entering the extracellular space. The *Shigella* bacterium also produces toxins that cause premature host cell death and development of necrosis in the bowel wall, leading to neutrophil infiltrated bloody ulcerations. The ability to spread from cell to cell and cause cell necrosis explains the development of bloody diarrhea and the presence of numerous neutrophils in the stools of patients with *Shigella* dysentery.

Complications are rare, but include proctitis or rectal prolapse, intestinal obstruction, toxic megacolon, hemolytic-uremic syndrome (HUS), and reactive arthritis.

MEDICAL HISTORY AND CLINICAL PRESENTATION

Shigella infections present in a typical fashion. In the first 1 to 7 days after ingestion *Shigella* infects the small intestine causing a high-volume watery diarrhea accompanied by cramps. This is accompanied by fever, anorexia, and fatigue. Within days the infection spreads to the lower GI tract causing lower abdominal cramps with bilateral lower quadrant abdominal tenderness and small volume diarrhea. Tenesmus may also be noted. Mucoid diarrhea is most common, but half of patients may have bloody diarrhea.

Disease severity depends on the serotype causing infection. *S. sonnei* usually causes mild disease with watery diarrhea but can cause bacteremia in patients with diabetes or malignancy. *S. dysenteriae* and *S. flexneri* typically cause bloody diarrhea. The disease is usually self-limited, lasting no more than 7 days in the absence of antibiotic treatment.

SIGNS AND SYMPTOMS

Symptoms range from mild abdominal discomfort to severe colicky, diffuse abdominal pain. Small volume diarrhea precedes the large volume dysentery. Most patients report mucoid diarrhea, and up to half of patients report bloody diarrhea. Other common symptoms include fever, nausea, vomiting, and tenesmus.

PHYSICAL EXAMINATION

Patients with shigellosis are usually lethargic. Physical examination reveals diffuse abdominal tenderness and fever. Less common physical examination findings include signs of dehydration, including hypotension, tachycardia, and dry mucous membranes.

A small number of people who are infected with *S. flexneri* experience postinfectious arthritis, causing joint pains, eye irritation, and painful urination. The syndrome occurs in people who have a specific genetic makeup, positive for HLA-B27. Symptoms can last for months or years and lead to chronic arthritis. This postinfectious arthritis does not occur in infections due to *S. sonnei*, *S. boydii*, or *S. dysenteriae*

DIFFERENTIAL DIAGNOSIS

See Table 17.6 for the differential diagnosis of acute inflammatory diarrhea.

DIAGNOSTIC STUDIES

Evaluation of the stool in a patient with *Shigella* infection reveals many neutrophils and red blood cells. The definitive diagnosis is made with stool culture. *Shigella* is a very fastidious organism and stool samples should be promptly cultured. PCR testing can be used to detect as few as 10 organisms.

TREATMENT

Antibiotic resistance is an issue when treating *Shigella*. In most cases the treatments of choice are either ciprofloxacin, levofloxacin, or azithromycin. An alternative option is TMP-SMX, but resistance is high. Ceftriaxone is preferred in very ill patient and patients from Asia.

Antibiotic resistance develops in *Shigella* due to R plasmids carrying resistance genes directed against ampicillin, tetracycline, TMP-SMX, chloramphenicol, and streptomycin. Resistance can also develop via transposons transferring resistance genes or via mobile genes within chromosomes transferring resistance. In the United States resistance to ampicillin and TMP-SMX is extremely common; and resistance to ceftriaxone, ciprofloxacin, and nalidixic acid is increasing. Because of increasing risk of antibiotic resistance, whenever possible the organism should be cultured, and antibiotic sensitivities determined.

Antibiotic treatment shortens symptomatic disease by 2 days and shortens the shedding of *Shigella* in the stools reducing person-to-person spread of the disease.

PATIENT EDUCATION

- Prognosis is excellent, and most patients recover without sequelae.
- A poorer prognosis is associated with duration of disease >7 days, development of complications, and certain patient populations, such as young children, elderly patients, and immunocompromised patients.

17.1K *CAMPYLOBACTER* INFECTION

Campylobacter jejuni subspecies *jejuni* and *Campylobacter fetus* subspecies *fetus* are gram-negative rods in the family Campylobacteraceae. Both organisms are zoonoses. *C. jejuni* infection is often foodborne and affects immunocompetent and immunocompromised persons; *C. fetus* is only seen in immunocompromised patients.

Infection caused by *C. jejuni* is common and is a leading cause of food-borne illness in the United States. The CDC) predicts an incidence rate of *Campylobacter* infection of 19.2 infections per 100,000 persons.[26] The case fatality rate is 0.21%.[25]

Infections occur year-round but peak in July and August.

The animal reservoirs for infection include poultry and cattle. Most sporadic infections are acquired through the improper handling and/or cooking of chicken and turkey or with ingestion of unpasteurized milk. Since infected animals may contaminate water sources, drinking untreated water is another major source of *C. jejuni* infection.

The infective dose is 500 to 800 organisms; the larger the inoculum, the shorter the incubation period.[27] *C. jejuni* adheres to intestinal tissue via adhesions, which leads to tissue injury throughout the small bowel, colon, and rectum.

C. jejuni is directly killed by gastric acid. *C. jejuni* can be opsonized by complement and/or antibody and then phagocytized and killed in the blood as well as in intestinal tissues.

MEDICAL HISTORY AND CLINICAL PRESENTATION

Most children have multiple *Campylobacter* infections by 2 years, and most of the population has been exposed by 5 years. *Campylobacter* infection should be considered as a cause of acute diarrheal illness in travelers.

C. fetus infections are uncommon and typically occur in immunocompromised persons, such as those with diabetes, cirrhosis, alcoholism, asplenia, AIDS, bone marrow transplantation, or chronic steroid therapy. The animal reservoirs include cattle, pigs, sheep, and other farm animals, as well as reptiles; persons in regular contact with these animals are at increased risk for contracting infection.

C. jejuni presents with a self-limited gastroenteritis and cannot be easily distinguished from other common causes of enteritis. The incubation period is 3 days after ingestion of contaminated food or water. Initial symptoms include fever, myalgia, malaise, and/or headache, about 24 hours before the onset of diarrhea and right lower quadrant crampy abdominal pain. The GI symptoms last between 1 and 7 days before resolving. Diarrhea may be severe, and/or bloody, with concomitant tenesmus. The infection can become fulminant, mimicking enteric fever and progressing to toxic megacolon. Bacteremia is rare in immunocompetent persons. In infants, *C. jejuni* disease may present as fever or vomiting only or with grossly bloody stools. Severe disease may mimic necrotizing enterocolitis.

C. fetus has an affinity for the vascular system and has been associated with mycotic aneurysms, septic thrombophlebitis, endocarditis, and infection of the placenta. In pregnant patients, infection leads to increase fetal loss, even with appropriate therapy. Fetal loss can occur even if the mother is only mildly ill.

Meningoencephalitis is the second most common manifestation of *C. fetus* infection. Patients may develop brain abscess, cerebral infarction, or hemorrhage. Reactive arthritis may develop as a late complication of *Campylobacter* infections, more commonly in patients with HLA-B27 phenotype.

SIGNS AND SYMPTOMS

Most people become ill within 2 to 5 days after exposure and present with diarrhea, crampy abdominal pain, and fever. The diarrhea may be bloody and accompanied by nausea and vomiting. The illness lasts about 1 week.

Evaluate for a history of ingestion of inadequately cooked or contaminated meat, unpasteurized milk, or untreated water. After a brief latent period of 1 to 2 days, headache and myalgias develop lasting 24 hours, followed by crampy abdominal pain, fever as high as 40 °C, and up to 10 watery, bloody, bowel movements per day. The abdominal pain and tenderness may be localized, mimicking acute appendicitis.

PHYSICAL EXAMINATION

Physical examination reveals diffuse abdominal tenderness and fever. Less common physical examination findings include dehydration, hypotension, tachycardia, and dry mucous membranes. Abdominal pain may be localized to the right lower quadrant.

DIFFERENTIAL DIAGNOSIS

See Table 17.6 for the differential diagnosis of acute inflammatory diarrhea.

DIAGNOSTIC STUDIES

Campylobacter organisms are motile, non-spore-forming, small, gram-negative curved rods with dipolar flagella. A modified Gram stain is often used to identify the organism.

All *Campylobacter* grow at 37 °C, are fastidious and microaerophilic; special medium is used to culture *Campylobacter* in a carbon dioxide atmosphere of 10% to 15%. Although the sensitivity of a single stool culture is high, two stool samples may be needed to rule out *Campylobacter* disease.

Stool antigen tests are available and have sensitivities between 80% and 96%, and specificity >97%. Molecular testing, including PCR, is also available.

In meningoencephalitis the CSF shows an increase in neutrophils, decreased glucose, and elevated protein.

TREATMENT

The treatment of choice for acute gastroenteritis or colitis in immunocompetent adults is a macrolide, such as azithromycin. While erythromycin is effective, it is not currently first line due to GI side effects and frequent dosing requirements. Clarithromycin is likely to be as effective as azithromycin.

Fluoroquinolones are an alternative to macrolides but should be used only when susceptibility has been established, because resistance rates can be as high. Resistance can develop during treatment.

Alternative treatment options in children include clindamycin and tetracycline in children over 8 years of age.

The preferred treatment for *C. fetus* infection is parenteral ampicillin. In penicillin-allergic patients, gentamicin may be given. Resistance to cephalosporins, macrolides, tetracyclines, and fluoroquinolones is high, and these agents should not be used to treat *C. fetus* infections.

PATIENT EDUCATION

- Infection control issues include the use of contact precautions in patients with diarrhea.

17.1L CHOLERA

Vibrio cholerae, the cause of cholera, is a gram-negative bacillus with a curved-rod shape.

Cholera is an acute, diarrheal illness and causes large epidemics, and pandemics around the globe.

An estimated 3 million cases and over 100,000 deaths occur each year around the world.[28] Infection can vary from asymptomatic or mild to severe disease. Severe disease presents with profuse watery diarrhea, vomiting, and leg cramps. In severe disease, rapid loss of body fluids leads to dehydration and shock. Without fluids and electrolytes, death can occur in hours.

The life cycle enables the organism to survive for years in a water environment, it survives adherent to crustaceans and algae. Under the right conditions, the organism will multiply and reinitiate the free life cycle. If the environment is adverse, the organism can maintain a latent state, inactive, and resistant to chlorine.

The infectious cycle occurs when the bacteria move from the water environment into a human through contaminated water and contaminated food. Those who are infected excrete high numbers of bacteria, creating massive environmental contamination and rapid transmission to others.

Most of *V. cholerae* bacteria cannot survive the highly acidic conditions of the stomach. The bacteria that survive the stomach acidity shut down protein production and restart production in the more favorable environment of the small intestine.

The toxins produced by the organism interact with the host cell and pump chloride ions into the small intestine. This prevents sodium ions from entering the cell. The chloride and sodium ions create an environment that via osmosis can pull up to 6 L of water per day through the intestinal cells. This causes the high frequency diarrhea and dehydration.

MEDICAL HISTORY AND CLINICAL PRESENTATION

Cholera presents with severe watery diarrhea and vomiting with severe dehydration in patients who have recently traveled to a cholera-endemic area. Other presentations include a milder diarrheal illness noted in people returning from cholera-endemic areas or in persons with a recent history of ingestion of raw seafood from a cholera-endemic area. The incubation period of cholera is between 2 hours and 5 days, with most patients developing symptoms within 24 to 48 hours of infection.

Patients present with sudden-onset, painless, odorless, rice-water, large-volume stool; abdominal cramps; vomiting; and fever. If not treated severe dehydration and electrolyte disturbances may develop within hours. Cholera has been called the blue death because of the patient's skin turning bluish gray from the loss of fluids.

SIGNS AND SYMPTOMS

Cholera is a diarrheal disease, easily mistakable for several other diseases, although some clinical features are characteristic of cholera. These characteristics include the presence of watery diarrhea with the appearance of rice water. Other symptoms include abdominal pain, vomiting, tenesmus, change in mental status, and signs of dehydration. Fever is less common.

PHYSICAL EXAMINATION

Physical examination findings depend on the level of dehydration. Findings include tachycardia, hypotension, dry mucous membranes, sunken eyes, and oliguria. With severe dehydration, electrolyte abnormalities may develop. Physical exam findings of hyponatremia and hypokalemia may be noted. See Table 17.7 for assessment criteria for various levels of dehydration.

DIFFERENTIAL DIAGNOSIS

See Table 17.6 for the differential diagnosis of acute inflammatory diarrhea.

DIAGNOSTIC STUDIES

The diagnosis of cholera can be confirmed by stool culture. The culture medium most commonly used is thiosulfate citrate bile salts sucrose agar and taurocholate and tellurite gelatin agar. The serogroup can be identified using antiserum. Identification of *Vibrio cholerae* serogroup O1 or O139 by culture of a stool specimen remains the gold standard for the laboratory diagnosis of cholera.

Rapid direct exam with darkfield microscopy allows a quick identification. Darkfield microscopy reveals numerous bacteria with chaotic movement.

The World Health Organization (WHO) recommends the following clinical definition for suspected cholera cases: cholera should be suspected when a child older than 5 years or an adult develops severe dehydration from acute watery diarrhea (usually with vomiting), or any patient older than 2 years has acute watery diarrhea when cholera is known to be occurring in the area. Younger children also develop cholera, but the illness may be difficult to distinguish from other causes of acute watery diarrhea, especially rotavirus.[29]

TREATMENT

Treatment of cholera should focus on rehydration and antibiotic therapy.

TABLE 17.7 Dehydration Assessment Criteria

Dehydration Level	Skin Turgor	Eyes	Thirst	Mental Status Changes
Mild	Spontaneously	Normal	Normal	Alert
Moderate	<2 seconds	Sunken	Increased	Irritable
Severe	>2 seconds	Sunken	Increased	Severe changes

Hypovolemia can result in lactic acidosis, shock, and renal failure. Oral hydration is effective when initiated early in the disease. Hypo-osmolar solutions, such as the WHO oral rehydration solution, are most effective at replacing volume and reducing the volume of diarrhea. Oral hydration containing rice or cereal as the calorie source rather than glucose is more effective at reducing the volume and duration of diarrhea. Rehydration volumes of 2–4 L are recommended for those over 30 kg in weight. Half the volume should be given within 30 minutes.

IV rehydration, with isotonic solution, is recommended for those who have lost over 10% of their body weight, or unable to take oral fluids because of vomiting or depressed mental status.

Antibiotics are initiated after the patient has been hydrated. Antibiotic treatment shortens the duration and volume of diarrhea and reduces the infectiousness of the stool. *V. cholerae* excretion is usually eliminated after 24 hours of antibiotic treatment

Oral antibiotics are generally recommended, including doxycycline, ciprofloxacin or norfloxacin, or erythromycin or azithromycin.

Prevention of cholera includes sanitary education and water decontamination.

The Food and Drug Administration (FDA) has approved a single-dose live oral cholera vaccine called Vaxchora (lyophilized CVD 103-HgR) in the United States. This vaccine is approved for adults 18 to 64 years old who are traveling to an area of active cholera transmission. Vaxchora has been reported to reduce the chance of severe diarrhea in people by 90% at 10 days after vaccination and by 80% at 3 months after vaccination.[30]

PATIENT EDUCATION

- If cholera is treated quickly, the mortality rate is <1%. If untreated, the mortality rate rises to 50% to 70%.[31]

17.1M BRUCELLOSIS

In humans, brucellosis is a zoonotic infection with a gram-negative intracellular coccobacillus of the genus *Brucella*. *Brucella* species varies by animal. *Brucella melitensis*, the most common pathogen in humans, is found in sheep and goats. *B. suis*, second most common pathogen in humans, is found in pigs. *B. canis* is found in dogs and *B. abortus* is found in cattle; both cause less severe disease in humans.

The organism is typically acquired by inhalation of aerosolized particles, contact with infected animals, or consuming unpasteurized dairy products or undercooked meat products. Others at risk for infection include people involved with animal husbandry and those who encounter sheep, goats, or pigs. Prevalence of infection in the United States is between 100 and 200 cases per year, with most of the cases occurring in California, Texas, Arizona, and Florida.[32]

After ingestion or inhalation, the bacteria replicate in lymph nodes and then move to the spleen, liver, and bone marrow. *Brucella* is an intracellular organism and can exist inside phagocytic cells and avoid destruction by neutrophils. The major virulence factor is smooth lipopolysaccharide (S-LPS), which makes the organism resistant to lysis.

MEDICAL HISTORY AND CLINICAL PRESENTATION

Brucellosis is more common in persons with exposure to infected sheep, goats, or pigs or their secretions.

After an incubation period of several weeks, generalized symptoms develop gradually over 2 to 4 weeks, and include fever, anorexia, fatigue, sweats, arthralgias, myalgias, headache, and GI complaints. Subclinical infections are common.

SIGNS AND SYMPTOMS

Signs and symptoms include fever, generalized lymphadenopathy, and hepatosplenomegaly.

A localized infection can occur in less than half of patients. This results in arthritis with lower extremity joint pain, sacroiliitis, or vertebral osteomyelitis; testicular or scrotal pain of orchitis, epididymitis, or testicular abscess; or abdominal and/or pelvic pain of nephritis, renal disease, or tubo-ovarian abscess.

Other manifestations include endocarditis, myocarditis, pericarditis, mycotic aneurysm, uveitis, keratoconjunctivitis, endophthalmitis, and skin findings, including rashes, ulcerations, petechiae, purpura, and abscesses. A classic symptom is "malodorous sweat."

PHYSICAL EXAMINATION

Patients with brucellosis are usually well appearing. Physical examination usually reveals a combination of several nonspecific findings and varies, as noted above, according to the organ system affected. Fever, generalized lymphadenopathy, and hepatosplenomegaly are common.

DIFFERENTIAL DIAGNOSIS

The differential diagnosis includes tuberculosis, HIV infection, malaria, influenza, tularemia, Q fever, endocarditis, EBV infection, cytomegalovirus (CMV) infection, and occult abscesses. There are also noninfectious etiologies that can mimic brucellosis, including malignancy and connective tissue diseases. Brucellosis can present as a fever of unknown origin.

DIAGNOSTIC STUDIES

General laboratory results are nonspecific and not helpful in diagnosis. The complete blood count (CBC) may be normal or reveal pancytopenia. Liver function tests may be mildly elevated. If neurologic involvement is present the CSF test results are consistent with aseptic meningitis, a mildly elevated, mononuclear WBC count, elevated protein, and mildly decreased glucose.

Blood cultures and bone marrow culture can confirm the diagnosis.

Bone marrow culture is the gold standard for diagnosis but is reserved for patients with fever of unknown origin and evidence of bone marrow involvement.

Serology testing, using the *Brucella* microagglutination test (BMAT) can detect antibodies to the S-LPS of the outer membrane in *Brucella* species—*abortus*, *melitensis* or *suis*. There is no serologic test available to detect antibodies to *B. canis*. Acute and convalescent samples are required. The first sample should be obtained during the acute illness and the second sample obtained 2 to 4 weeks later to check for a fourfold or greater rise in antibodies. This increase indicates a positive test for brucellosis.

The ELISA is commonly used but does not have the same sensitivity as the BMAT.

TREATMENT

If the patient is acutely ill, empirical coverage should be started while completing the patient workup.

Treatment options include oral doxycycline for 6 weeks with IV streptomycin (14 to 21 days) or gentamicin (7 to 10 days); or oral doxycycline and rifampin for 6 weeks. Combination therapy with oral TMP-SMX or fluoroquinolones can be used if tetracyclines are contraindicated.

PATIENT EDUCATION

- Relapsing disease can occur in first 6 to 12 months after completion of treatment.
- Endocarditis is a rare clinical manifestation but is the most common cause of death in brucellosis.
- Prognosis is good with treatment; mortality rate is <1%.

17.1N TULAREMIA

Francisella tularensis is a small aerobic gram-negative coccobacillus. It is a zoonotic pathogen and infects humans through contact with animals, including rabbits (most common), beaver, muskrats, squirrels, and birds. Hunters develop skin infections after skinning, dressing, or eating an infected animal.

Tularemia is most commonly noted in Arkansas, Missouri, Kansas, South Dakota, Oklahoma, and California.[33]

Tularemia begins when the organism gains entry to the body through a break in the skin. The bacterium cell wall capsule has a high fatty acid content that resists serum bactericidal activity. The organism is phagocytosed by monocytes, where they survive intracellularly. The organism moves into the cytoplasm where it multiplies. As the organisms grow, the cells lyse and induce an acute inflammatory reaction; tissue necrosis is followed by granuloma formation. Only a small number of bacteria are required to cause skin and pulmonary infection.

MEDICAL HISTORY AND CLINICAL PRESENTATION

Obtaining an occupational history along with a history of animal exposures and outdoors activities is vital. Hunters are at highest risk, along with sheep herders and shearers, farmers, and landscapers.

Infection presents with the abrupt onset of fever, chills, malaise, myalgias, chest discomfort, vomiting, abdominal pain, and diarrhea. A generalized headache is often present.

There are multiple forms of tularemia. The most common form is ulceroglandular fever. Presentation is a painful ulcer with raised borders at the site where the bacteria first entered the skin. Regional lymph nodes draining this region are swollen and painful. Glandular fever has less lymphadenopathy and no ulcerative skin lesion. Oculoglandular fever develops if the eyes are involved and presents with conjunctival ulcers with lymphadenopathy in the periauricular, submandibular, and cervical areas. Pharyngeal infection is contracted during ingestion of contaminated food. The pharyngitis is exudative, extremely painful, and accompanied by regional lymphadenopathy. Pneumonic tularemia is the most serious form. Symptoms include cough, chest pain, and difficulty breathing. This form results from breathing dusts or aerosols containing the organism. It can also occur when other forms of tularemia are left untreated and the bacteria spread to the lungs. Typhoidal form is characterized by any combination of the general symptoms, without localizing symptoms.

SIGNS AND SYMPTOMS

Signs and symptoms of tularemia include nonspecific flu-like symptoms. These include fever, chills, headache, diarrhea, myalgias, and weakness. Symptoms and clinical manifestations will differentiate according to the type of tularemia infection. These symptoms can include skin ulcers, swollen and painful lymphadenopathy, pharyngitis, and swollen and painful eyes.

PHYSICAL EXAMINATION

Typically signs of tularemia include a fever, tachycardia, and blood pressure changes. Other physical examination findings depend on the mode of transmission and may include skin ulcers, eye infection, and pharyngeal edema.

The skin ulcer is common and noted at the site of infection. With eye infection the eyes will appear irritated and inflamed. Oropharyngeal infection presents with sore, swollen throat and lymphadenopathy.

DIFFERENTIAL DIAGNOSIS

The differential diagnosis varies with the form of tularemia. Table 17.8 summarizes the differential diagnosis for the various forms of tularemia.

DIAGNOSTIC STUDIES

Routine laboratory testing is nonspecific. WBC count can be elevated, normal, or low and thrombocytopenia may be noted. Hyponatremia and abnormal liver function tests may be noted.

TABLE 17.8 Differential Diagnosis of the Various Forms of Tularemia

Tularemia Form	Diagnosis
Ulceroglandular disease	Cat scratch disease, malignancy, mycobacterial infection, toxoplasmosis, fungal infection, herpes simplex infection, syphilis, bubonic plague, anthrax, rat bite fever
Glandular fever	Cat scratch disease, malignancy, mycobacterial infection, toxoplasmosis, fungal infection, herpes simplex infection, syphilis, bubonic plague, anthrax, rat bite fever
Oculoglandular disease	Cat scratch disease, herpes simplex, adenovirus infection, other forms of pyogenic conjunctivitis
Pharyngeal disease	Group A streptococcal pharyngitis, mononucleosis, adenoviral pharyngitis, diphtheria
Typhoidal disease	Salmonella, brucellosis, Q fever, endocarditis
Pulmonic disease	Q fever, psittacosis, tuberculosis, pneumonic plague, pulmonary fungal infection, community-acquired pneumonia

Gram stains of the sputum and skin lesions are unrevealing. Organisms can be identified with silver staining of lymph node biopsies

A presumptive diagnosis of tularemia may be made through testing of specimens using direct fluorescent antibody, immunohistochemical staining, or PCR. Agglutination tests, positive with an elevated initial titer or a fourfold increase between acute and convalescent, requires 2 weeks to become positive. These tests should only be ordered if tularemia is a strong possibility and should not be used for routine screening.

Growth of *F. tularensis* in culture is the definitive means of confirming the diagnosis of tularemia.

TREATMENT

F. tularensis is not sensitive to cephalosporins or penicillins. Aminoglycosides are the treatment of choice; gentamicin is first choice but streptomycin can also be used. For mild disease, oral doxycycline is recommended, but since the organism grows within cells, relapse is quite common following doxycycline treatment. Because of relapse doxycycline should be used for 21 days. Alternative treatment option includes fluoroquinolones.

PATIENT EDUCATION

- The prognosis is good for the common forms of tularemia. Ulceroglandular forms of tularemia usually heal over the course of several months.
- Even when left untreated, ulceroglandular and glandular forms of tularemia are rarely fatal.
- Prevention of disease consists of wearing rubber gloves when handling or skinning rodents or rabbits and avoid ingesting uncooked wild game and untreated water sources.

17.10 *NEISSERIA* INFECTIONS

The genus *Neisseria* has two major species that cause human disease, *N. meningitidis* and *N. gonorrhoeae*. *N. meningitidis* infection causes bacterial meningitis and *N. gonorrhoeae* causes gonorrhea, a sexually transmitted infection (STI).

N. meningitidis is a pleomorphic gram-negative coccus. Thirteen serogroups have been identified; five are commonly associated with human disease. Those include serogroups A, B, C, W-135, and Y. Invasiveness of the organism is enhanced by a polysaccharide capsule, which allows the organism to resist phagocytosis. A variation in the bacterial surface structure leads to invasion across the nasopharyngeal mucosa into the bloodstream, followed by release of an endotoxin. The endotoxin triggers a cascade of inflammatory protein. Invasion of the meninges results in similar release of inflammatory proteins resulting in inflammation and neurologic injury.

Serogroups B, C, and Y account for about a third of meningitis cases, serogroup B is a more common cause among infants, and serogroup C is more common among adolescents. This serogroup distinction is important as the available vaccines provide protection against serogroups A, B, C, Y, and W-135.

Individual susceptibility is increased in situations that lead to crowding, those exposed to tobacco smoke, those with prior respiratory tract infection (especially influenza), and those with a history of contact with a patient with meningococcal disease.

Neisseria gonorrhoeae is a gram-negative coffee bean-shaped diplococcus. *N. gonorrhoeae* is transmitted from person to person during sexual relations. The organism uses hair-like projections called pili to anchor onto cells on the urethra, fallopian tubes, and endocervix, aiding in transmission and infection. Established routes of transmission include vaginal intercourse, rectal intercourse, oral sex, and perinatal.

In pregnancy, *N. gonorrhoeae* can be transmitted to the fetus at delivery. This results in infection of the conjunctiva. This presents 1 to 4 days after birth as severe discharge with marked swelling and redness of the eyelids and conjunctivae.

N. gonorrhoeae can disseminate into the blood due to a variety of predisposing factors such as change in pH, pregnancy, menstruation, and complement deficiencies. This leads to the development of disseminated gonococcal infection (DGI).

MEDICAL HISTORY AND CLINICAL PRESENTATION

The most common clinical findings of meningococcal infection are fever, chills, malaise, and rash. The rash begins as macular or maculopapular, but petechiae and purpura rapidly develop.

Meningitis is the most common focal complication of meningococcemia. Symptoms include headache, photophobia, neck stiffness, and vomiting.

Meningococcal septicemia may progress to fulminant disease, causing shock, coagulopathy, purpura, limb ischemia, and pulmonary edema.

Invasive meningococcal infection is most common in infants <2 years old. Others at risk include adolescents between the ages of 15 and18 years, recruits in military boot camps, and freshman college students living in dormitories. Transmission from asymptomatic carriers to nonimmune individuals is via respiratory droplets.

In patients with gonorrhea obtaining a complete sexual history is key. The following should be noted:

- Number and type of sexual partners
- Previous history of gonococcal infection or other STIs
- Current contraception, if any
- History of sexual assault
- Reproductive history
  - Details of parity including history of ectopic pregnancies
  - Last menstrual period
  - Potential for pregnancy

Gonorrhea presents with purulent urethral or cervical discharge.

SIGNS AND SYMPTOMS

Meningococcal meningitis signs and symptoms include fever, neck stiffness, headache, and altered mental status. Symptoms are similar to other etiologies of bacterial meningitis. A petechial rash can be present and can coalesce and form larger lesions that appear like ecchymoses.

Gonorrhea presents with thick, copious, white, yellow, or green discharge from the penis or cervix. In males, other symptoms include dysuria, urinary urgency, and scrotal pain and swelling. In females, over half of patients are asymptomatic. Symptoms include dyspareunia, vaginal spotting, bleeding after intercourse, dysuria, and urinary urgency and increased frequency. Lower abdominal pain may develop if the infection spreads to the fallopian tubes and endometrium.

PHYSICAL EXAMINATION

The physical examination in meningococcal infection may reveal fever, hypotension, petechial rash, nuchal rigidity, seizures, edema, and dyspnea. The rash is petechial with discrete lesions 1–2 mm in diameter on the trunk and lower extremities. The rash may coalesce and appear ecchymotic (Figure 17.4).

One of four outcomes are possible:

- Meningococcemia without sepsis: blood cultures are positive for *Neisseria meningitidis*.
- Meningococcemia without meningitis: patient is septic with elevated WBC count, generalized malaise, headache, and hypotension.
- Meningitis with or without meningococcemia: patient presents with headache, fever, meningeal signs, with no pathologic reflexes.
- Meningoencephalitis: presents with the patient being obtunded; meningeal signs, altered reflexes, and pathologic reflexes may be present.

Women with gonococcal infection usually appear to be well until complications develop such as pelvic inflammatory disease. Physical examination in women with gonococcal infection reveals a mucopurulent urethral, cervical, or vaginal discharge. Pelvic examination reveals a friable appearing cervix and cervical motion tenderness may be noted. In men the physical examination findings include a mucopurulent urethral discharge, penile edema, and epididymal tenderness and edema.

Physical examination in patients with pharyngeal gonococcal infection reveals mild pharyngeal exudates and rectal gonococcal infection presents with mucopurulent anal discharge.

Physical examination of patients with DGI reveals fever, pustular or vesicular rash, and musculoskeletal findings, such as joint swelling and erythema.

DIFFERENTIAL DIAGNOSIS

Fever and petechial rash are common presentations of many childhood infections. Causes include enterovirus, parvovirus B19, EBV, influenza and other respiratory tract viruses, and CMV.

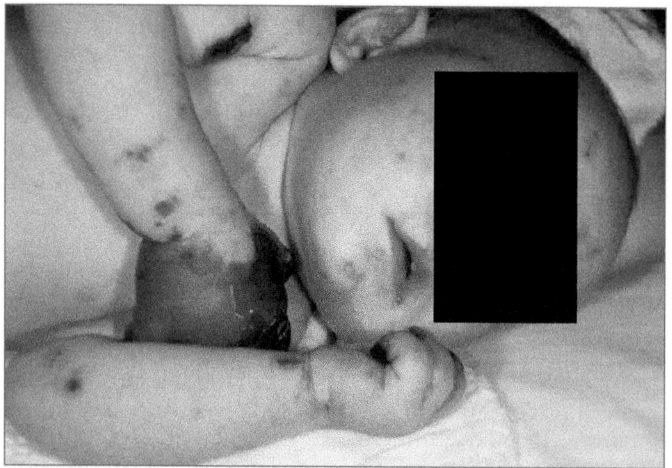

Figure 17.4 *Neisseria meningitidis* infection causing meningococcemia. The ischemic insult and gangrene can develop due to arterial occlusions.

(Source: Centers for Disease Control and Prevention/Mr. Gust. https://phil.cdc.gov/details_linked.aspx?pid=1334)

Petechiae rash with or without fever is also noted the rickettsial infection, Rocky Mountain spotted fever (RMSF), rat bite fever, Henoch-Schönlein purpura, collagen vascular disorders, idiopathic thrombocytopenic purpura and other coagulation abnormalities, and drug reactions.

Meningitis due to *Neisseria meningitidis* cannot be distinguished from those due to other bacterial causes of infectious meningitis without laboratory testing.

Gonorrhea must be differentiated from other sexually transmitted infections, including nongonococcal urethritis, vaginitis, cervicitis, UTI, prostatitis, and orchitis.

DGI must be differentiated from herpes simplex infection, nongonococcal septic arthritis, syphilis, HIV infection, reactive arthritis, and Lyme disease.

DIAGNOSTIC STUDIES

There are several nonspecific laboratory findings in meningococcal meningitis. Hypoglycemia, electrolyte abnormalities, and coagulopathies may be noted in children suspected of *Neisseria meningitidis* septicemia and/or meningitis. CBC may demonstrate anemia and either leukocytosis or leukopenia.

In meningococcal meningitis, cultures of the blood and CSF are most likely to provide a definitive diagnosis. Cultures should be obtained prior to starting antibiotics. Blood cultures are positive in 50% to 60% of untreated patients and CSF is positive in 80% to 90%.[34]

CSF should be sent for cell count, protein, and glucose analysis in addition to culture and Gram stain. In meningococcal meningitis the WBC count is elevated, protein is elevated, and glucose is decreased.

Antigen detection and PCR testing can be used to diagnosis meningococcal meningitis.

In men with gonorrhea, Gram stain of urethral discharge is highly sensitive and specific in men with symptoms. Gram stain of endocervical, pharyngeal, and rectal specimens is not recommended. In symptomatic men, the presence of neutrophils with intracellular gram-negative diplococci is diagnostic of *Neisseria gonorrhoeae*. In female patients, a positive Gram stain is presumptive positive for *Neisseria gonorrhoeae*, a positive culture, utilizing Thayer-martin medium, is needed to confirm the diagnosis.

NAATs are the gold standard for diagnosing gonococcal infections.

These tests include PCR, transcription-mediated amplification (TMA), and strand displacement amplification (SDA).

DGI should be considered in all young, sexually active individuals who present with arthralgias and joint pain. Gonococcal arthritis and DGI present with a mild leukocytosis and elevated erythrocyte sedimentation rate (ESR). Common laboratory findings of DGI may include the following:

- Blood cultures positive for *N. gonorrhoeae*.
- Synovial fluid culture positive for *N. gonorrhoeae* and synovial WBC count is elevated.
  - Synovial fluid glucose, lactate dehydrogenase (LDH), and protein are of limited value.

TREATMENT

Antibiotic therapy for meningococcal meningitis should include a third-generation cephalosporin, usually ceftriaxone. If meningococcal meningitis is confirmed, penicillin G, ampicillin, or an extended-spectrum cephalosporin should be started. Ceftriaxone or cefotaxime are effective options for treatment of invasive *N. meningitidis* disease. Appropriate antimicrobial therapy should be continued for 7 days for patients with meningitis, septicemia, or both.

Meningococcal conjugate vaccine (MenACWY) and serogroup B meningococcal vaccine (MenB) are available in the United States. The recommended vaccination for adolescents is the MenACWY, preferably at 11 or 12 years, with a booster dose at 16 years. If the first dose of MenACWY is given after age 16 a booster is not needed. The two-dose primary series of meningococcal conjugate vaccines (MCV4) is recommended for persons ages 2 to 54 with terminal complement deficiency and persons with functional or anatomic asplenia. A booster dose should be provided every 5 years for these individuals.

The following persons at higher risk of disease should also be vaccinated:

- College freshmen living in a dormitory
- Military recruits
- Travelers to countries in which meningococcal disease is endemic

CDC recommends a MenB vaccine for children 10 years or older and adults if they:

- Have a rare type of immune disorder called complement component deficiency
- Are taking a type of medicine called a complement inhibitor
- Have a damaged spleen or their spleen has been removed
- Are part of a population identified to be at increased risk because of a serogroup B meningococcal disease outbreak

Antibiotic chemoprophylaxis is indicated in close contacts of patients with meningococcal infection and should be given as early as possible following the exposure. Close contact is defined as individuals who have had prolonged (>8 hours) contact while near (<3 feet) the patient or who have been directly exposed to the patient's oral secretions during the 7 days before the onset of the patient's symptoms and until 24 hours after initiation of appropriate antibiotic therapy.

Antibiotic options include ciprofloxacin, ceftriaxone, and rifampin. Rifampin is not recommended in pregnant women and ciprofloxacin is not generally recommended in persons under age 18 and lactating women.

Routine prophylaxis is not recommended for healthcare professionals unless they have intimate contact with respiratory secretions from the infected patient; such would occur during unprotected mouth-to-mouth resuscitation, intubation, or suctioning before or <24 hours after initiation of appropriate antibiotic therapy.

The recommended treatment for gonococcal infection of the urethra, cervix, and rectum is ceftriaxone intramuscular single dose and azithromycin as a single dose. Alternative therapy options include cefixime and azithromycin.

To prevent gonococcal infection of the eye in newborn infants, erythromycin ophthalmic ointment is applied to both eyes at birth.

PATIENT EDUCATION

- Overall case fatality rate for patients with invasive meningococcal infection is 10% to 15% even with appropriate therapy.[35]
- Hearing loss, motor dysfunction, and other neurologic deficits occur in 5% of pediatric survivors of meningococcal meningitis.[36]
- Complications of gonorrhea in women include salpingitis and pelvic inflammatory disease.

17.1P CHANCROID

Chancroid is caused by a gram-negative facultative anaerobic bacillus called *Haemophilus ducreyi*. Chancroid is uncommon with <20 cases per year in the United States; there were only three cases in the United States in 2018.[37] Chancroid is more common in Africa and Southeast Asia and in other parts of the world where HIV is endemic.

Chancroid should be suspected in any patient who presents with a painful genital ulcer, with a congruent sexual history and the proper epidemiologic setting.

The disease is transmitted by sexual contact. *H. ducreyi* enters the skin through breaks in the epithelium. The organism produces fimbria-like proteins that assist the bacteria in adhering to subcutaneous epithelial cells. The organism recruits inflammatory cells to the site of infection and interleukins are produced that induce WBCs to form abscesses. *H. ducreyi* can avoid phagocytosis.

MEDICAL HISTORY AND CLINICAL PRESENTATION

The CDC standard definition for a probable case of chancroid includes[38]:

- Patient has one or more painful genital ulcers with tender or suppurative adenopathy.
- No evidence of *Treponema pallidum* by darkfield examination of ulcer or by serologic testing at least 7 days after the onset of ulcer.
- Clinical presentation is not typical of herpes simplex virus (HSV) or culture results for herpes is negative.

SIGNS AND SYMPTOMS

The characteristic presentation of chancroid is a painful, nonindurated ulcer. Ulcers may have a gray/yellow exudative discharge. Other symptoms include painful inguinal lymphadenitis, called buboes. Buboes are also noted in bubonic plague, gonorrhea, tuberculosis, and syphilis. Other symptoms include dysuria and dyspareunia in females.

PHYSICAL EXAMINATION

Chancroid begins as a small papule that becomes a pustule and then ulcerates. The ulcers are deep, 0.3 to 5 cm in diameter, with an irregular and sharp, violaceous border and the base is covered with a yellow-gray exudate.

In males the chancroid typically occurs on the corona of the penis. Unilateral inguinal adenopathy occurs in half the cases.

DIFFERENTIAL DIAGNOSIS

The differential diagnosis includes syphilis, herpes simplex, Behçet disease, lymphogranuloma venereum, and fixed drug eruption.

DIAGNOSTIC STUDIES

Diagnosis is typically made on clinical grounds alone. A definitive diagnosis can be made by culturing the exudate from the ulcer base or by aspiration and culture of a bubo. Gram stain of the ulcer exudate may show gram-negative coccobacilli in a characteristic "school of fish" appearance (Figure 17.5).

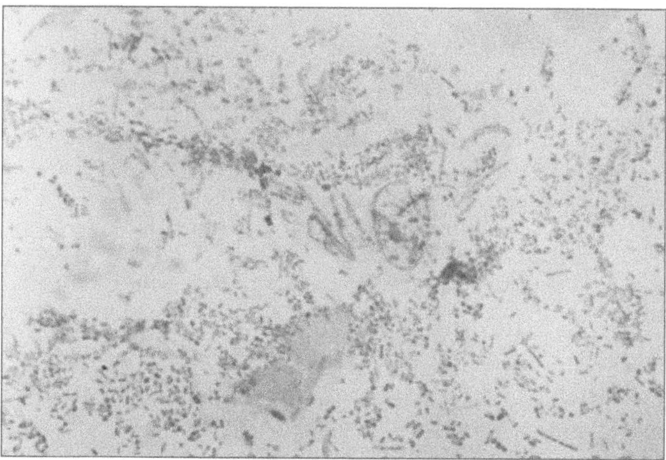

Figure 17.5 Gram-negative, *Haemophilus ducreyi* coccobacilli, indicative of a chancroid infection.

(Source: Centers for Disease Control and Prevention/Joe Miller, Dr. N.J. Fiumara. https://phil.cdc.gov/details_linked.aspx?pid=4420)

H. ducreyi requires special culture medium to grow in the laboratory. PCR testing and indirect immunofluorescence tests for *H. ducreyi* are available.

All patients with suspected chancroid should be tested for other sexually transmitted diseases, including HIV infection, *Chlamydia* infection, gonorrhea, syphilis, and HSV infection.

TREATMENT

Treatment options include azithromycin, erythromycin, ciprofloxacin, and ceftriaxone.

First-line therapy is single-dose ceftriaxone or azithromycin. Single-dose regimens with ciprofloxacin should not be used. Due to a high rate of treatment failures amoxicillin-clavulanic acid should not be used.

Patients should be reexamined 3 to 7 days after initiation of therapy. If treatment is successful, ulcers usually improve symptomatically within 3 days and objectively within 7 days.

PATIENT EDUCATION

- Chancroid is not lethal.
- Prognosis is poor without treatment.

17.1Q *BARTONELLA* INFECTION

Bartonella species are small gram-negative intracellular organisms. There are three species, *Bartonella henselae*, *Bartonella quintana,* and *Bartonella bacilliformis,* that cause a majority of human disease, each with a distinct clinical syndrome.

B. henselae, the cause of cat scratch disease, is associated with exposure to cats, especially kittens, and their fleas. The infection can take a classic cutaneous course or become disseminated.

B. quintana is the cause of trench fever. The vector is the human body louse. There is often a history of homelessness or alcoholism, and the disease presents with fever, malaise, and bone pain in the pretibial region.

B. quintana and B. henselae also cause bacillary angiomatosis. This condition is noted in HIV patients, transplant patients, and other immunosuppressed patients.

B. bacilliformis is the agent of bartonellosis (Carrión disease). The condition has two phases: Oroya fever and verruga peruana. The vector is the sand fly and the disease is endemic in the Andes Mountains in South America.

MEDICAL HISTORY AND CLINICAL PRESENTATION

Cat scratch disease presents as a cutaneous disorder or may become disseminated. The initial skin lesion is a vesicle or pustule. After 1 to 3 weeks tender regional lymphadenopathy with overlying erythema develops. If the initial inoculation site is near the eye, conjunctivitis with preauricular lymphadenopathy may occur. Disseminated infection is more common in children but can be seen in adults. Disseminated *B. henselae* infection can present with ocular findings or CNS infections. Myalgias, arthralgias, arthritis, and osteomyelitis have been described.

Bacillary angiomatosis presents with lesions on the skin, mucous membrane, or subcutaneous region and bone pain. If there is hepatic or splenic disease symptoms include abdominal pain, nausea, and vomiting.

Trench fever presents with recurrent fever, due to the bacteremia. Patients may also have a macular or papular rash and splenomegaly.

Bartonellosis has two phases: Oroya fever and verruga peruana. Within 3 weeks of being bitten by an infected sand fly the patients with Oroya fever may be asymptomatic or develop fever, nausea, malaise, and headache. This phase is due to dissemination of the organism and invasion of erythrocytes and endothelial cells causing significant anemia. If untreated, patients may worsen and develop complications including anasarca, neurologic abnormalities, and superimposed infections with *Staphylococcus*, *Salmonella*, *Shigella*, or *Enterobacter*. In the chronic phase of infection, verruga peruana, patients present with erythematous lesions of the skin and mucous membranes. Most patients with verruga peruana do not recall an earlier, febrile illness and likely were asymptomatic initially.

PHYSICAL EXAMINATION

Physical examination findings in cat scratch disease includes painful lymphadenopathy and vesicular or pustular lesions at the initial site of skin inoculation. In disseminated disease, findings are specific to the organ system involved.

In HIV-infected patients, bacillary angiomatosis presents with cutaneous or mucous membrane lesions. These lesions start out pearly but become red or purple due to vascular proliferation and may ulcerate and bleed.

Physical findings of Oroya fever include pallor, weakness, painless hepatosplenomegaly, and generalized lymphadenopathy. The appearance of the lesions of verruga peruana vary with the stage.

DIFFERENTIAL DIAGNOSIS

The differential diagnosis of cat scratch disease includes other causes of nodular lymphangitis, including infections with *Streptococcus*, *Staphylococcus*, *Mycobacterium marinum*, *Nocardia* species, *Francisella tularensis*, *Yersinia pestis*, *Bacillus anthracis*, *Pseudallescheria boydii*, and *Sporothrix schenckii*.

The differential diagnosis for trench fever includes tick-borne relapsing fever (TBRF), malaria, typhoid fever, leptospirosis, tularemia, and babesiosis. The differential for cutaneous bacillary angiomatosis includes Kaposi sarcoma.

DIAGNOSTIC STUDIES

Routine laboratory testing is not helpful in diagnosing infections due to *Bartonella* species. One exception is that anemia will be seen in patients with Oroya fever.

For cat scratch disease, three of the following criteria are needed to make the diagnosis:

- Exposures to cats or their fleas
- Sterile pus from a lymph node, positive PCR for *Bartonella*, hepatic or splenic lesions on CT
- Positive serology for *B. henselae* via EIA or immunofluorescence assay (IFA)
- Biopsy with a positive Warthin-Starry stain or granulomatous change consistent with cat scratch disease

Blood cultures can be done for *Bartonella* species, but the lab should be alerted since this fastidious organism requires special handling. Cultures should be obtained prior to antibiotics, if possible.

For other *Bartonella* species the diagnosis may be made via:

- Histopathologic findings seen with bacillary angiomatosis or culture
- Serology testing via EIA or IFA
- PCR testing
- Blood culture or Giemsa-stained blood smear

TREATMENT

Most cases of cat scratch disease will resolve without treatment, some may develop complications from disseminated disease. The treatment of choice is azithromycin. Other antibiotics effective against *Bartonella* include penicillins, doxycycline, cephalosporins, and aminoglycosides. First-line treatment for other *Bartonella* infections are the aminoglycosides.

PATIENT EDUCATION

- There are no vaccines for *Bartonella* species.
- Prevention includes avoidance of cats, kittens, and their fleas.

17.1R ACTINOMYCOSIS AND *NOCARDIA* INFECTION

Actinomycosis is caused by any organisms of the genus *Actinomyces*. *Actinomyces* are filamentous gram-positive, facultative anaerobic bacilli that are frequent commensals of the human GI, respiratory, and female genitourinary tract. *A. israelii* is the most common species to cause disease in humans, but disease can be caused by a number of species (e.g., *A. odontolyticus*, *A. viscosus*, *A. naeslundii*). *Actinomyces* cause disease after breakdown of the normal mucosal barriers. Once through the mucosal barriers the organisms have the potential to invade locally and cross fascial planes.

Nocardiosis refers to the disease caused by *Nocardia* species. *Nocardia* are gram-positive, partially acid-fast, branched, filamentous environmentally ubiquitous aerobic rods. The most commonly isolated species in the United States are *N. brasiliensis*, *N. nova*, and *N. farcinica*. These species can colonize the skin or upper respiratory tract. Localized cutaneous and lymphocutaneous forms of *Nocardia* are more common in males and tends to affect older adults. *Nocardia* causes disease after mucosal barriers have been breached. Penetration of tissue planes and then dissemination of disease follow.

MEDICAL HISTORY AND CLINICAL PRESENTATION

The classic presentation of actinomycosis is a firm mass, which develops fistula tracts that drain purulent material or sulfur granules. The masses are extremely firm or have a "woody" texture; they can be confused with malignancy. Clinically, actinomycosis takes one of three forms: cervicofacial, thoracic, or abdominopelvic.

Cervicofacial actinomycosis is most common in pediatrics. It presents with the development of a painless, firm neck or mandibular mass. Sinus tracts may be present. A predisposing factor for cervicofacial actinomycosis is disruption of the gingiva, as a result of dental caries, extractions, or trauma.

Thoracic actinomycosis disease presents with a chest wall mass, chronic cough, pain, fever, weight loss, and chest wall–draining sinuses. It is associated with aspiration of oral secretions or foreign bodies, which disrupt the normal bronchial mucosal barriers

Abdominopelvic actinomycosis presents with intra-abdominal abscesses most commonly in the ileocecal region, but can present in other abdominal locations, and presents as a hard, irregular right lower quadrant mass. It may suppurate with a fistula to the skin. Abscesses develop because of surgical complications or abdominal trauma.

Nocardiosis is a cutaneous infection, occurring after direct inoculation of the organism into the skin. In immunocompromised patients disseminated disease can occur; the most common sites are the lungs and hematogenous dissemination to the brain and other distant sites. Person-to-person transmission of *Nocardia* does not occur.

Localized cutaneous infection following skin trauma, presents as tender abscesses or pustules and cellulitis. Shallow ulcers and satellite lesions are present. The infection can spread to regional lymph nodes and nodules can develop along lymphatic tracts.

Nocardial mycetoma is a chronic infection of the skin and subcutaneous tissues, with a draining sinus tract. It is characterized by a hard, painless lump under the skin; it ulcerates from the center and drains pus with white granules. It can persist for years and involve underlying muscle and bone.

PHYSICAL EXAMINATION

The physical examination findings of actinomycosis vary depending on location of the infection. With cervicofacial actinomycosis the infection presents as a chronic, slowly progressive, nontender, indurated mass, which evolves into multiple abscesses, fistulas, and draining sinus tracts. Characteristic lesions adhere to the skin giving it a bluish or reddish appearance. Any tissue or structure surrounding the upper or lower mandible can be involved. Abdominal actinomycosis presents with constitutional or nonspecific abdominal symptoms and an abdominal mass. Physical examination findings include a palpable mass, visible sinus tracts, or fistulas.

Nocardia infection can disseminate to virtually any organ, particularly the lungs and central nervous system. There are no pathognomonic signs or symptoms and it should be suspected in any patient who presents with brain, soft tissue, or cutaneous lesions and a concurrent or recent pulmonary process. Physical examination findings vary with the system involved and are nonspecific.

DIFFERENTIAL DIAGNOSIS

The differential diagnosis varies with the location of actinomycosis infection. For cervicofacial infection the differential includes lymphoma, extrapulmonary tuberculosis, bacterial adenitis, *Bartonella* infection, and jaw osteomyelitis. With thoracic infection the differential includes malignancy, pulmonary tuberculosis, and rib osteomyelitis. With abdominopelvic infection the differential includes sarcoma, pelvic inflammatory disease, and tubo-ovarian abscess.

The differential diagnosis for *Nocardia* varies with the location of infection. Localized cutaneous disease differential includes other pyogenic organisms such as *Staphylococcus aureus* and *Streptococcus pyogenes.* Lymphocutaneous disease differential includes sporotrichosis. Nocardial mycetoma differential includes infection with *Actinomyces, Aspergillus,* or *Pseudallescheria boydii*; chronic osteomyelitis; leprosy; and syphilis.

DIAGNOSTIC STUDIES

The diagnosis of actinomycosis is based on culture results and histopathologic evaluation of tissue samples. Histologic analysis reveals filamentous clusters of organisms in a mat-like configuration; macroscopic sulfur granules may be noted (Figure 17.6).

Sulfur granules are not pathognomonic for actinomycosis and can be seen with other organisms, such as *Nocardia*; an important distinction is that *Nocardia* are acid-fast and actinomycetes are not.

With *Nocardia*, cultures including blood cultures and Gram stain should be obtained. Special stains, such as modified acid-fast and silver stain, are used to diagnose *Nocardia* infection. With lung involvement the chest x-ray results are variable and include single and multiple nodules, masses with or without cavitation, reticulonodular infiltrates, interstitial infiltrates, lobar consolidation, and pleural effusions (Figure 17.7).

TREATMENT

The cornerstone of treatment of actinomycosis is a combination of extensive surgical debridement and long-term antimicrobial agents. *Actinomyces* is sensitive to penicillin; penicillin and other beta-lactams are the antibiotics of choice. Ceftriaxone, doxycycline, carbapenems, and

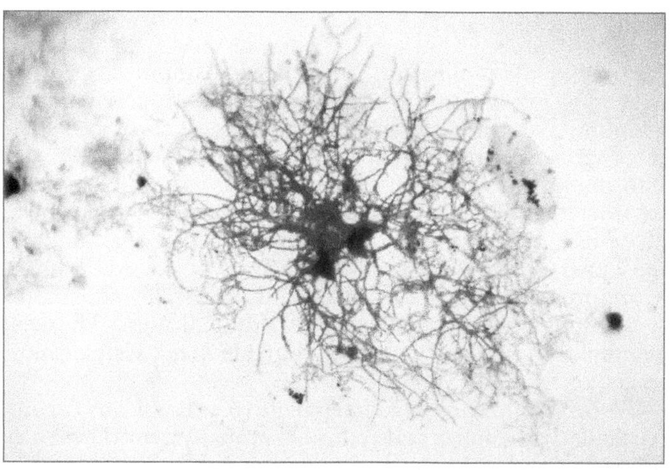

Figure 17.6 **Tissue specimen of *Nocardia* stained using the modified Kinyoun acid-fast staining technique. Magnified 324×.**
(Source: Centers for Disease Control and Prevention/Dr. Kaplan. https://phil.cdc.gov/details_linked.aspx?pid=21741)

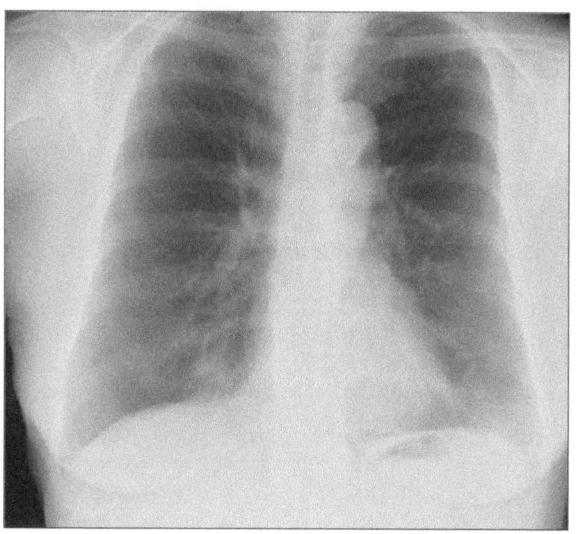

Figure 17.7 **Pulmonary *Nocardia* with right basal consolidation and pleural effusion with nodules throughout the lung.**
(Source: Radiopaedia.org. Courtesy of Dr. Henry Knipe.)

macrolides are possible alternatives. There are high rates of resistance to ciprofloxacin and metronidazole. A prolonged course of antibiotics—6 to 12 months—is recommended.

Because *Nocardia* has variable resistance to antibiotics, treatment should consist of two to three agents in patients with severe infection. Cutaneous disease can be treated with a single agent. First-line therapy consists of TMP-SMX. Alternative treatment options include ceftriaxone, cefotaxime, imipenem, meropenem, minocycline, moxifloxacin, linezolid, and dapsone.

PATIENT EDUCATION

- Most patients do well with treatment, and cure can be achieved in most patients.
- Fistulous tracts are common with all forms of the disease.

17.1S MYCOBACTERIAL INFECTIONS

OVERVIEW

Mycobacteria other than *Mycobacterium tuberculosis* can infect humans. These organisms are nontuberculous mycobacteria (NTM) and are commonly present in soil and water and are much less virulent in humans than is *M. tuberculosis*.

Most exposures to these organisms do not cause disease. Development of disease requires a defect in local or systemic host defenses; the frail elderly and immunocompromised people are at the highest risk.

There are more than 180 recognized species of NTM and some cause human disease. NTM can be divided into two groups based on how long they take to grow in a culture:

- Rapid-growing species: typically grow within 7 to 10 days
- Slow-growing species: need >14 days to grow

Rapid-growing species include *M. abscessus, M. chelonae, M. fortuitum,* and *M. mucogenicum*.

Slow-growing species include *M. avium* complex (includes *M. avium* and *M. intracellulare* species), *M. chimaera, and M. kansasii.*

M. avium complex (MAC), closely related species of *M. avium* and *M. intracellulare*, account for most diseases. Person-to-person transmission has not been documented.

Signs and symptoms can be vague and are dependent on the site of infection. This section will cover *Mycobacterium leprae* and *M. avium* complex. *Mycobacterium tuberculosis* is covered in Chapter 4, Pulmonary System.

17.1SA *MYCOBACTERIUM AVIUM*

Mycobacterium avium complex (MAC) includes many species of nontuberculous mycobacteria. MAC predominately causes pulmonary and disseminated disease. Pulmonary disease is due to inhaling contaminated aerosols from contaminated water. Disseminated disease results from entry of the organism into the bloodstream from a pulmonary infection. HIV infected patients develop disseminated disease in the setting of advanced immunosuppression (CD4 lymphocyte count <50 cells/μL).

MEDICAL HISTORY AND CLINICAL PRESENTATION

The symptoms and signs of MAC lung disease are variable and depend on the presence of underlying lung disease. Symptoms include a productive or dry cough, fatigue, malaise, weakness, dyspnea, chest discomfort, and hemoptysis. Fever and weight loss may occur but are more common in tuberculosis. There are two major pulmonary presentations, in those with underlying pulmonary disease and those without pulmonary disease.

Disease in those with underlying lung disease occurs primarily in older men with a history of smoking and underlying chronic obstructive pulmonary disease. The disease clinically resembles typical tuberculosis, but symptoms are less severe, with cough, weight loss, upper lobe infiltrates, and cavities. Lung destruction may be quite extensive at the time of diagnosis with very large cavities on chest radiograph.

Disease in those without underlying disease occurs mostly in nonsmoking women over age 50 who have abnormal chest x-ray consistent with bronchiectasis. Patients typically have a long history of progressive respiratory symptoms and recurrent respiratory infections due to underlying bronchiectasis. Presentation includes a persistent cough with variable sputum production, without fever or weight loss.

Two other less common forms of MAC disease include solitary pulmonary nodules and hypersensitivity pneumonitis.

Disseminated MAC disease occurs in severely immunocompromised patients and is a complication of MAC pulmonary disease. Clinical presentation includes intermittent or persistent fever, night sweats, weight loss, fatigue, malaise, and anorexia. Other symptoms occur depending on the organ system involved; anemia and neutropenia noted with bone marrow involvement; adenopathy or hepatosplenomegaly with lymphoreticular involvement; diarrhea, abdominal pain, hepatomegaly, and elevations of liver enzymes with GI involvement; and cough and lung infiltrates with pulmonary involvement.

SIGNS AND SYMPTOMS

Pulmonary disease presents with variable signs and symptoms. Chronic or recurring dry or productive cough is the most common symptom. Other symptoms include fatigue, malaise, low-grade fever, night sweats, weight loss, and dyspnea.

Disseminated disease, typically noted in advanced HIV infection, presents with fever, night sweats, and weight loss. Additional symptoms include abdominal pain and diarrhea. In non-HIV infected immunocompromised patients, disseminated disease may present as cutaneous nodules and abscesses.

PHYSICAL EXAMINATION

Physical examination of the lungs is often normal or presents with findings consistent with the underlying lung disease, such as chronic obstructive lung disease or bronchiectasis. Disseminated disease presents with cutaneous nodules, abdominal tenderness, hepatosplenomegaly, and lymphadenopathy.

DIFFERENTIAL DIAGNOSIS

The differential diagnosis for pulmonary disease includes chronic obstructive pulmonary disease, tuberculosis, sarcoidosis, histiocytosis X, and chronic hypersensitivity pneumonitis.

DIAGNOSTIC STUDIES

Diagnosis is based on clinical, x-ray, and microbiologic findings. Three sputum samples or single bronchoalveolar lavage specimens should be obtained for acid-fast smear and mycobacterial culture, as well as bacterial and fungal cultures. A positive acid-fast bacillus (AFB) smear may be due to nontubercular mycobacterial disease; but tuberculosis should be considered as the most likely diagnosis. Chest x-ray reveals nodular or cavitary lesions. Chest CT scan reveals multifocal bronchiectasis with centrilobular nodules.

The diagnosis of disseminated disease is established with blood cultures positive for mycobacteria. Mycobacterial growth can be detected in a few days after obtaining cultures but should not be considered negative until after 6 weeks with no growth.

Specimens from bone marrow, or fluid or tissue from suspected sites of involvement should also be submitted for culture and histopathology. Noncaseating granulomas on pathology are supportive of mycobacterial involvement.

TREATMENT

Treatment of pulmonary disease should be with a multidrug (three or more drugs) regimen to prevent the emergence of resistance. Duration of therapy is 12 months past the point cultures become negative. Surgical resection of the most involved lung segments may be indicated in some patients, particularly those with focal disease who have failed medical therapy.

The antibiotics of choice are an oral macrolide (azithromycin or clarithromycin), rifamycin (rifampin or rifabutin), and ethambutol. With cavitary disease, daily therapy should be given, and use of an IV aminoglycoside is strongly recommended.

The initial treatment of disseminated MAC in HIV infected patients should consist of two or more antimycobacterial drugs to prevent the emergence of resistance. Clarithromycin is the first drug of choice; azithromycin can be substituted if the patient cannot take clarithromycin. Ethambutol is the second drug of choice for the initial treatment of MAC disease, with rifabutin as a third option.

In disseminated disease primary prophylaxis is indicated if the patient is not on fully suppressive antiretroviral therapy (ART) and the CD4 count is <50 cells/mm^3. The preferred therapy is azithromycin or clarithromycin. Rifabutin is an alternative treatment option.

PATIENT EDUCATION

- Treatment success in patients without HIV infection has averaged about 50% to 60% clinical success.[39]
- Patients with more extensive disease have a 90% chance of recovery and a 20% chance of relapse after treatment.[39]

17.1SB LEPROSY

Mycobacterium leprae, an acid-fast bacterium, is the cause of leprosy (Hansen disease). Leprosy presents with various clinical symptoms that involve the skin and peripheral nerves. Transmission is zoonotic, via the nine-banded armadillo, and human-to-human spread via nasal secretions.

There are two classification systems of leprosy. One is the Ridley-Jopling classification, which is based on clinical and biopsy findings (Table 17.9). The second is per WHO and based on clinical categories.

In areas where biopsy is not available, WHO has made broad clinical categories of paucibacillary leprosy (PB), which is defined as five or fewer skin lesions, and multibacillary (MB), in which there are six or more lesions.

Leprosy is most commonly found in developing countries. The highest incidence of new cases is noted in Nigeria, Brazil, Indonesia, Bangladesh, and India. There are about 150 new cases of leprosy diagnosed in the United States each year; 159 new cases were reported in 2020.[40] Most cases are found in Arkansas, California, Florida, Hawaii, Louisiana, New York, and Texas. Risk factors for transmission of leprosy include close contact with an index case, elderly, higher burden of microorganisms in the index case, and immunosuppression in the susceptible individual.

MEDICAL HISTORY AND CLINICAL PRESENTATION

Skin lesions are the most common finding. Skin findings range from a solitary macule to heaped, nodular, and widely distributed lesions.

Peripheral neuropathy is noted and presents as decreased sensation, paresthesia, and motor loss, rather than pain in the nerve distribution. The early skin lesions themselves often demonstrate decreased sensation. Tender or enlarged peripheral nerves may be noted. Late in the disease there can be disfiguring collapse of the nasal septum, loss of eyebrows or eyelashes, foot drop, and claw hand. The organism prefers cooler areas of the body, so the trunk is spared from effects compared to the extremities, ear lobes, and nose.

PHYSICAL EXAMINATION

Skin changes are the major physical examination finding in leprosy. These changes include flat, discolored, or faded skin; nodules, thick, stiff, dry skin; painless ulcers on the soles; painless swellings on the face; and loss of eyebrows and eyelashes. Late in the disease course disfiguring changes can occur. Collapse of the nasal septum can occur (Figure 17.8).

Peripheral neuropathy with decreased sensation, paresthesia, and, eventually, motor weakness or paralysis, rather than pain in the nerve distribution is noted. Depending on nerves involved other findings may be noted. For example, with facial nerve involvement the patient may not be able to close the eyelids completely and have visual difficulty; involvement of the great auricular nerve can lead to facial edema; and a swollen, tender, common peroneal nerve can lead to foot drop.

DIFFERENTIAL DIAGNOSIS

The differential diagnosis includes cutaneous leishmaniasis, lupus vulgaris, sarcoidosis, syphilis, yaws, psoriasis, atypical mycobacterial infections, and cutaneous lymphoma.

DIAGNOSTIC STUDIES

There are no routine laboratory tests that assist in the diagnosis. The diagnosis is confirmed based on classic physical examination findings including chronic skin lesions, sensory changes, or enlarged and tender peripheral nerves; and a biopsy of a cutaneous nerve showing acid-fast bacilli.

TREATMENT

The treatment of choice is a multidrug therapy depending on the form of the disease. Paucibacillary form is treated with dapsone daily and rifampicin once per month. The MB form is treated with dapsone, rifampicin, and daily clofazimine. Treatment lasts 1 to 2 years.

TABLE 17.9 Ridley-Jopling Classification for Leprosy

	Tuberculoid	Borderline Tuberculoid	Mid-Borderline	Borderline Lepromatous	Lepromatous Leprosy
Number of lesions	Single	Single to few	Several	Many	Very many
Lesion size	Variable	Variable	Variable	Variable	Small
Lesion surface	Very dry	Dry	Slightly shiny	Shiny	Shiny
Lesion sensation	Absent	Markedly diminished	Moderately diminished	Slightly diminished	Not affected
Lesion hair growth	Absent	Markedly diminished	Moderately diminished	Slightly diminished	Not affected
# AFB in lesion	None	None or scant	Moderate	Many	Very many
Lepromin skin test	Strong positive	Weak positive	Negative	Negative	Negative

AFB, acid-fast bacilli.

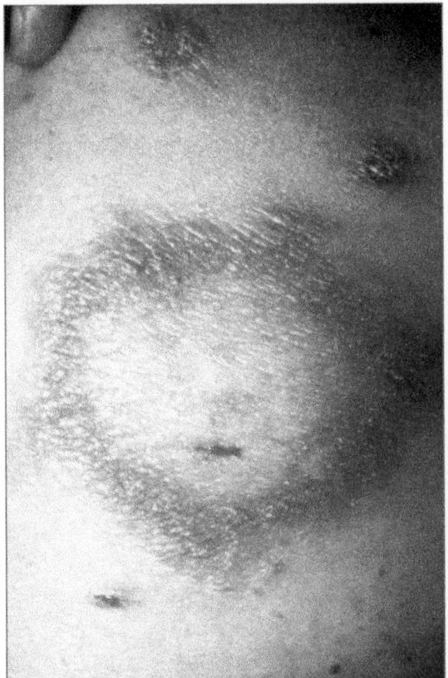

Figure 17.8 **Leprosy skin lesion. A well-demarcated plaque with an elevated border, and a loss of sensitivity in its central region. Classified as paucibacillary leprosy.**

(Source: Centers for Disease Control and Prevention/Arthur E. Kayne. https://phil.cdc.gov/details_linked.aspx?pid=19222)

PATIENT EDUCATION

- Patients become noninfectious after only a few doses of medication and need not be isolated from family and friends.
- Patients can have multiple complications because of leprosy.

17.2 *CHLAMYDIA* INFECTION

OVERVIEW

Chlamydiaceae family consists of three organisms that cause human disease: *Chlamydophila psittaci, Chlamydia pneumoniae,* and *Chlamydia trachomatis*. All are obligate intracellular gram-negative bacteria. These organisms share a unique developmental cycle that is different from all other bacteria. *C. psittaci* is spread by infected avian species and leads to pulmonary symptoms. *C. pneumoniae* is a common cause of pneumonia in young adults and the elderly. *C. trachomatis* is a common cause of STI.

EPIDEMIOLOGY

C. psittaci is rare with about 10 reported cases per year, although the actual number of infections is thought to be much higher.[41]

C. pneumoniae infection has a wide spectrum of clinical symptoms and a 3- to 4-week incubation period. Because of a varied clinical presentation and lack of standardized diagnostic methods making a diagnosis can be difficult. *C. pneumoniae* infection is likely underdiagnosed, with the actual number of cases each year being unknown. Primary infection occurs mainly in school-age children or young adults, while reinfection is most common in older adults.

C. trachomatis is the most common STI, and most commonly noted in young females. In 2018, the CDC reported a total of over 1,758,000 infections in the United States, corresponding to a rate of 539 cases per 100,000 population.[42]

PATHOPHYSIOLOGY

Chlamydia growth consists of two alternating forms, the elementary bodies and the reticulate bodies. Elementary bodies are metabolically inactive. Once infected the cell ingests the organism. Inside the cell the elementary bodies differentiate into reticulate bodies. Reticulate bodies are metabolically active but noninfectious. The reticulate bodies rely on the host for energy, divide by binary fission, and induce a host immune response. After 48 to 72 hours, the reticulate bodies reorganize and condense to form new elementary bodies. These elementary bodies then leave the host cell and start a new infectious cycle. These organisms cannot be grown using typical bacterial culture media.

17.2A PSITTACOSIS

C. psittaci is an obligate intracellular gram-negative bacterium, transmitted by direct contact with infected birds or inhalation of aerosolized organisms in dried feces or respiratory secretions from infected birds. Psittacosis is most common in adults between the ages of 35 and 55 years of age and is uncommon in children. Human-to-human transmission can occur but it is very uncommon.

In humans, following inhalation, the organism spreads via the bloodstream until it finally reaches the alveoli and the reticuloendothelial cells of the liver and spleen. Once it reaches the lungs a lymphocytic inflammatory response occurs, which results in edema of the alveolar walls and interstitial tissues. The alveolar spaces fill with fluid, red blood cells, and lymphocytes. Macrophages may contain Levinthal-Coles-Lille inclusion bodies, which are characteristic of psittacosis. The incubation period is 5 to 15 days.

MEDICAL HISTORY AND CLINICAL PRESENTATION

A history of exposure to birds is the key to the diagnosis of psittacosis; psittacosis can occur in the absence of bird exposure. Exposure to caged pet birds accounts for most of the psittacosis cases. Increased risk of disease is seen in owners of companion birds or bird fanciers, pet shop employees, employees in poultry-processing plants, veterinarians and veterinary technicians, farmers, and zoo workers. Infection can result from transient exposure to infected birds or their contaminated droppings.

SIGNS AND SYMPTOMS

The clinical presentation ranges from a subclinical illness to severe pneumonia. Common symptoms include fever, rigors, sweats, and headache. Cough occurs in most patients, but typically appears late and is nonproductive or productive of mucoid sputum. Hemoptysis is rare. A few patients will have no respiratory symptoms. The extrapulmonary manifestations, such as Horder spots and splenomegaly, may be noted.

PHYSICAL EXAMINATION

Physical examination is remarkable for fever, respiratory distress, Horder spots, and splenomegaly. Respiratory examination will show signs of consolidation, rales, diminished breath sounds, and possible pleural friction rub. Splenomegaly, when present, is typically noted by the end of the first week of infection. Neurologic examination may reveal cranial nerve palsy including cranial nerves II, IV, VI, and VII.

DIFFERENTIAL DIAGNOSIS

Psittacosis may present like other diseases that cause atypical pneumonia and fever. Three diseases must be differentiated from psittacosis: *Chlamydia* pneumonia, *Mycoplasma* pneumonia, and *Legionella* disease. See Table 17.10 for the differential diagnoses.

DIAGNOSTIC STUDIES

Laboratory isolation of *Chlamydia* organisms is difficult; possible specimens include sputum, bronchial washings, biopsy specimens, and blood.

The WBC count is usually normal, and eosinophilia may be present. CXR reveals no distinctive pattern, findings include multilobe involvement and pleural effusion, which may take up to 4 to 12 weeks to show clearing.

Serology testing will reveal a fourfold increase in antibody titer between acute and convalescent serum samples. The most common methods include complement fixation (CF) test or the microimmunofluoresence (MIF) test. A single IgM titer ≥1:32 by MIF is diagnostic. Cross-reactivity between *C. pneumoniae*, *C. trachomatis*, and *C. psittaci* may be noted. PCR testing has been used to diagnose psittacosis.

TREATMENT

There are no vaccines that protect against *C. psittaci*. Treatment consists of tetracycline or doxycycline for 10 to 21 days; response to treatment is prompt. Azithromycin is an alternative treatment but is less effective. Respiratory quinolones, such as moxifloxacin, gatifloxacin, and levofloxacin, are also effective.

PATIENT EDUCATION

- Complications include severe fatigue that may persist for 2 to 3 months following resolution of the acute disease.
- The CDC has the following recommendations for prevention of transmission of *C. psittaci* to persons and birds:[43]
  - Persons at risk should wear protective clothing, gloves, and an N95 respirator for contact with infected birds or when cleaning cages. Use disinfection measures.
  - Avoid birds that have signs of avian chlamydiosis, including ocular or nasal discharge, diarrhea, or low body weight.
  - Isolate new birds for 30 to 45 days and test or prophylactically treat them before adding them to a group.

KEY POINTS

- *Chlamydia psittaci* is a rare cause of pneumonia, acquired from birds, and treated with doxycycline or azithromycin.

17.3 VIRAL INFECTIONS

OVERVIEW

There are several viruses that cause a variety of infections. The most common infections include respiratory, meningitis/encephalitis, skin, and hepatic.

The most common viral causes of pneumonia, in adults, are influenza and parainfluenza; pneumonia typically develops because of bacterial infection in the setting of a viral respiratory infection. Adenovirus and RSV are more common causes of pneumonia in children and infants.

Most viral causes of meningitis do not cause critical disease, except for HSV. West Nile virus (WNV), Eastern and Western equine encephalitis viruses (EEEV and WEEV), St. Louis virus, Colorado tick fever virus, and others are etiologies of neurologic infections. Measles, mumps, varicella, influenza, and rubella can cause both a viral encephalitis and immune-mediated postinfectious encephalitis. Nonpolio enteroviruses are the most common cause of viral meningitis in the United States.[44]

Viral skin infections are most commonly due to HSV and varicella-zoster virus (VZV). These viruses may lie dormant in nerve roots from the time of infection until immunosuppression or stress causes reactivation.

TABLE 17.10 Differential Diagnosis of *Chlamydia psittaci*

	Clinical Manifestations					Laboratory Results		
Disease	**Cough**	**Sputum**	**Dyspnea**	**Pharyngitis**	**Headache**	**Hyponatremia**	**Leukopenia**	**Abnormal LFTs**
Psittacosis	++	–	+	–	+++	–	+	–
Chlamydia pneumonia	+	+	+	+++	++	–	–	–
Mycoplasma pneumonia	++	++	++	–	–	–	–	+
Legionella disease	+	+++	+++	–	+	++	+	++
Influenza	++	++	++	++	++	–	–	–

+, noted in some cases. ++, noted in many cases. +++, noted frequently in cases. LFTs, liver function tests.

Viruses are the most common cause of infectious hepatitis. Chronic hepatitis can be caused by hepatitis B, C, and D viruses. EBV and CMV can cause a mild hepatitis.

EPIDEMIOLOGY

Viruses cause 10% to 30% of CAP in adults with influenza and parainfluenza being the most common; rhinovirus and coronavirus are also possible etiologies. RSV is an important cause of viral pneumonia in pediatric patients and immunocompromised adults. Influenza pneumonia typically occurs in high-risk patients.

The severe acute respiratory syndrome (SARS) outbreak lasted from February to July of 2003 and involved over 8,000 cases in 29 countries. No cases of SARS have been identified since 2004. Another outbreak of SARS-CoV-2 (COVID-19) occurred in 2019.

Hepatitis B is a global issue with transmission occurring perinatally, via sexual contact, via close contact, by percutaneous inoculation, and because of blood transfusion or organ transplantation.

Transmission of herpes simplex is person to person because of contact with infected lesions, while CMV is transmitted person to person through blood, body fluids, and vertical transmission. These viruses remain latent in the body and reactivate in response to immunosuppression or stress.

PATHOPHYSIOLOGY

While viruses vary, they have several common features. Viruses have a protective shell or capsid, DNA or RNA genome inside the capsid, and a membrane layer called the envelope.

The life cycle of a virus consists of several steps:

- Attachment of the virus, via a specific protein on the capsid, to a receptor on the surface of the host cell.
- Viral entry into the cell is via fusion. Other route of entry is via endocytosis and direct fusion of the virus with the cell membrane and release of viral contents into the cell. This is followed by uncoating and replication.
- Once inside the cell the viral genome is copied, and viral proteins are produced. The mRNA encoding viral genes are translated into viral proteins using the host's ribosomes. The viral proteins produced vary from virus to virus and include capsid proteins, envelope proteins, and proteins that can block host defenses or assist with viral replication.
- Viral particles are assembled from the viral proteins and copies of the viral genome. The new capsid proteins form capsomeres that join with other capsomeres to produce a full capsid.
- Completed viral particles are released from the cell and infect other cells. This release can occur via lysis of the host cell, exocytosis, or bud from the plasma membrane.

17.3A HERPES INFECTION

HSVs 1 and 2 are common causes of infection; type 1 affects primarily the oral region and type 2 affects the genital region. While type 2 is the most common cause of genital ulcer, type 1 is a common cause of genital ulcers in young women. Infection may be asymptomatic, and the patient may have asymptomatic shedding of the virus.

HSV type 1 is primarily spread by contact with infected lesions, saliva, or other secretions; HSV type 2 is primarily spread by sexual contact. The virus replicates at the site of infection, then travels to the dorsal root ganglion and establishes latent infection. Recurrent lesions occur with reactivation of latent disease. Triggers for reactivation of latent disease include stress, fever, damage to local tissue, UV light, and being immunocompromised. HSV can spread by infected individuals who are asymptomatic or symptomatic during times of viral shedding.

The presence of HSV type 2 increases the risk of HIV acquisition three-fold, and HSV type 2 reactivated more often in advanced HIV infection.[45]

MEDICAL HISTORY AND CLINICAL PRESENTATION

Oral disease is commonly acquired in childhood and 90% of young adults are HSV-1 antibody positive.

Risk factors for acquiring genital disease include being between the ages of 15 and 30 years, increased number of sexual partners, Black or Hispanic race, and HIV positivity.

SIGNS AND SYMPTOMS

In primary infection, symptoms occur 3 to 7 days after exposure and begin with a prodrome of fever, malaise, loss of appetite, and localized pain and/or burning at the lesion site. The prodrome may occur in patients with recurrent lesions, but the symptoms are decreased in severity and duration. Oral herpes can cause edema and pain, which can lead to dysphagia.

Genital herpes can present with extreme pain, edema, and dysuria. Systemic complaints are more common in women and may manifest with extragenital lesions, urinary retention, or aseptic meningitis. Recurrent lesions may have limited symptoms, and outbreaks occur on average from four to seven times per year.

In immunosuppressed patients, lesions are atypical, occur more frequently, and are less likely to resolve spontaneously.

PHYSICAL EXAMINATION

Skin lesions typically start as a painful cluster of vesicles on an erythematous base, progress to pustules, and then ulcerate. The ulcerations cluster, forming one large ulcer with a scalloped border. Lymphadenopathy may be noted before or during the outbreak. Ulceration and crusting of lesions, with ultimate resolution, occurs in 1 to 3 weeks in immunocompetent patients (Figure 17.9).

In orolabial herpes the buccal and gingival mucosa and lips are the most common sites of infection. Recurrent lesions are commonly noted on the vermilion border, but other possible sites include perioral skin, nasal mucosa, and hard palate.

Primary genital herpes in women can also involve the cervix, buttocks, and perineum. In men the lesions most often occur on the penile shaft or glans; recurrent lesions may occur on the genitals or buttocks (Figure 17.10).

Frequency of recurrent lesions may be related to the severity of the primary infection.

Other locations for infections include the eye causing uveitis, keratitis, blepharitis, and keratoconjunctivitis; central nervous system causing encephalitis; and GI tract causing esophagitis and proctitis. HSV type 1 can also infect the facial nerve leading to Bell palsy.

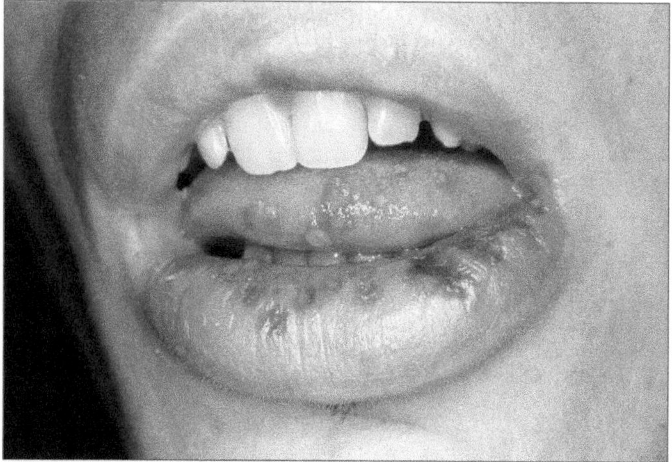

Figure 17.9 Oral herpes simplex virus type 1 lesions.
(Source: CDC/Robert E. Sumpter. Retrieved from https://phil.cdc.gov/Details.aspx?pid=12616)

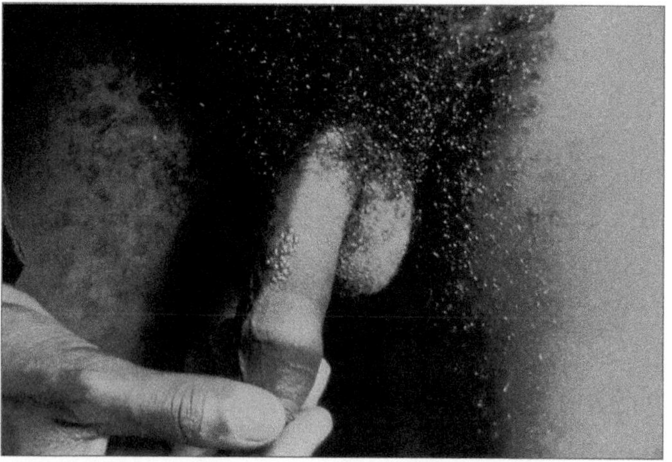

Figure 17.10 Herpetic lesion. Small vesicles on an erythematous base on the shaft of the penis.
(Source: Centers for Disease Control and Prevention/Dr. Paul Wiesner. https://phil.cdc.gov/Details.aspx?pid=5393)

DIFFERENTIAL DIAGNOSIS

The differential diagnosis includes varicella-zoster infection, Stevens-Johnson syndrome, and aphthous ulcers. Other ulcerating genital infections include syphilis, chancroid, and lymphogranuloma venereum.

Table 17.11 summarizes the differential diagnoses for herpes infections.

DIAGNOSTIC STUDIES

Serologic tests can show primary seroconversion for HSV-1 or HSV-2 infection; but they do not definitively diagnose active disease. Active disease can be diagnosed with the following:

- Tzank smear: Scraping of the base of a blister reveals multinucleated epithelial giant cells.
- Tissue biopsy: Tissue sample reveals virally infected multinucleated epithelial giant cells.
- Viral tissue culture: Culture is positive within 48 hours and can allow for resistance testing.
- HSV DNA detection: Gene amplification by PCR can be done on skin lesions or spinal fluid.
- Direct fluorescent antibody: Cells scraped from the base of an early unroofed blister are stained with a direct fluorescent antibody.

TABLE 17.11 Differential Diagnosis for Herpes Infections

Diagnosis	Description
Varicella-zoster	Very similar in appearance to herpes simplex but follows a dermatomal pattern
Stevens-Johnson syndrome/ toxic epidermal necrolysis	Oral and or genital ulcerations, most often presents with ocular involvement, subepidermal blisters, epidermal sloughing, and involvement of the palms and soles
Aphthous ulcers	Most often noted in the mouth as small round ulcers with a yellow ulcer floor, typically heal in 1 week
Syphilis	Single, painless ulcer, not recurrent
Chancroid	Painful single or multiple ulcer with yellow or gray exudate
Lymphogranuloma venereum	Painful papule that may ulcerate

In encephalitis or meningitis, the CSF will reveal a pleocytosis and MRI may demonstrate increased signal in the temporal and frontal lobes.

TREATMENT

Treatment consists of antiviral medications. Most medications work by inhibiting the replication of HSV type 1 and HSV type 2. See Table 17.12 for the treatment option of the various herpes simplex infections.

PATIENT EDUCATION

Chronic suppressive regimens of antiviral medications can be used to prevent outbreaks, reduce viral shedding, and decrease disease transmission. Barrier protection is useful for preventing transmission of genital herpes infection.

TABLE 17.12 Treatment Options for Herpes Simplex Virus Infection

Type of Infection	Antiviral Agent	Notes
Orolabial (recurrent)	Famciclovir Valacyclovir	Treatment should be started at first sign of recurrence
Genital (primary)	Acyclovir Famciclovir Valacyclovir	Duration of treatment is 7–10 days
Genital (recurrent)	Acyclovir Famciclovir Valacyclovir	Treatment should be started at first sign of recurrence
Chronic suppression	Acyclovir Famciclovir Valacyclovir	
Acyclovir resistant	Foscarnet	Nephrotoxicity and electrolyte disturbances can occur

17.3B VARICELLA-ZOSTER INFECTION

Varicella or chickenpox, a human herpesvirus caused by the DNA virus VZV, is spread by airborne contagion. VZV causes the primary infection of chickenpox and the recurrent infection shingles. The symptoms of chickenpox include fever, and a vesicular-pustular, pruritic rash. The vesicular rash presents with lesions in all stages of development, including macules, papules, vesicles, pustules, and scabs. Shingles presents with pain and unilateral localized vesicles, in a dermatomal pattern that evolves from maculopapular to vesicles, pustules, and scabs. Primary infection is acquired by a susceptible individual exposed to someone shedding VZV either immediately prior to the development of the rash or during active infection. Shingles is the consequence of reactivation of latent virus from the sensory ganglia.

Prior to universal immunization, outbreaks occurred in late fall and early winter during the school year. With universal varicella immunization, varicella outbreaks are now rare.

Zoster is more common in women than men, older patients, and those immunocompromised; and incidence is lower in African Americans.

MEDICAL HISTORY AND CLINICAL PRESENTATION

Patients with varicella are contagious for 1 to 2 days before the rash appears and for 4 days after the rash erupts when there are no new lesions or lesions have crusted over. The virus is spread via respiratory secretion and is easily spread to others near the infected patient.

A common complication is secondary bacterial infection of the skin vesicles, due to *Staphylococcus* or *Streptococcus*. Less common complications include spread of the infection to the central nervous system, leading to a meningoencephalitis and varicella pneumonia.

After an asymptomatic period of respiratory tract viral replication, the virus enters the bloodstream and spreads throughout the body. The incubation period ranges from 10 to 20 days, and newly infected patients become contagious in the last 2 days of the incubation period.

SIGNS AND SYMPTOMS

Varicella starts with the prodromal symptoms that include headache, fever, and malaise.

PHYSICAL EXAMINATION

With varicella the characteristic vesicular rash typically begins on the face and then moves over the trunk and extremities within 5 to 7 days. The lesions crust within a week and full recovery is the normal outcome.

With zoster the rash starts out as erythematous plaques and transforms into vesicles and bullae. The rash is usually located in one dermatome unilaterally, but it can include multiple adjacent dermatomes (Figure 17.11).

Rash is most commonly located in the thoracic and lumbar dermatomes but can also be seen in other areas, including the distribution of cranial nerves. Other symptoms include:

- Neuritis: a burning, stabbing pain located in the dermatomal region of the associated rash
- Ramsay Hunt syndrome: ipsilateral facial paralysis, ear pain, and vesicles in the auditory canal
- Hutchinson sign: a herpes lesion located on the tip of the nose, associated with ocular involvement

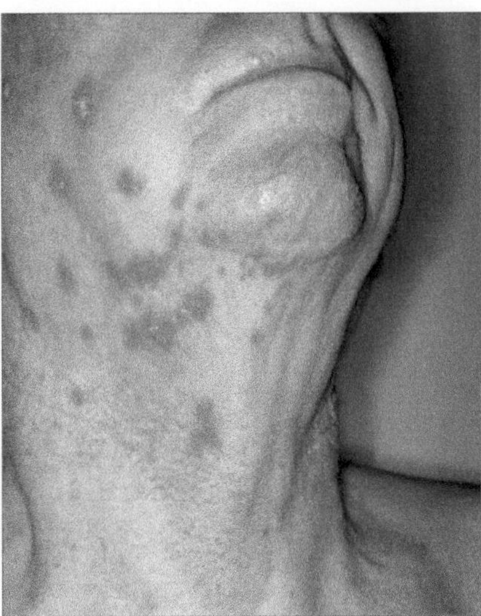

Figure 17.11 Dermatomal pattern of shingles.
(Source: National Institute of Allergy and Infectious Diseases (NIAID). https://phil.cdc.gov/details_linked.aspx?pid=18254)

DIFFERENTIAL DIAGNOSIS

Table 17.11 summarizes the differential diagnosis for various herpes infections.

DIAGNOSTIC STUDIES

Diagnosis is made by the presence of the characteristic vesicular rash. A scraping of a vesicular skin lesion can be sent for viral immunofluorescence diagnosis or evaluated for the presence of giant multiple nucleated cells. Diagnostic testing may be performed on fluid from the vesicles or from CSF. A PCR test, the preferred test in most cases, confirms the presence of VZV DNA. Direct immunofluorescent antibody test has a lower sensitivity and specificity than PCR. Viral culture is rarely used due to low sensitivity and long processing time.

The WBC count will typically be normal in the immunocompetent host. Liver enzymes may be elevated in chickenpox.

TREATMENT

With the development of the varicella vaccine the incidence of disease has been decreasing. Antiviral treatment consists of acyclovir, valaciclovir, or famciclovir. If a case of varicella is diagnosed in a healthy child, treatment can be started with oral acyclovir suspension or tablets. As an alternative to acyclovir, adolescents can be treated with valacyclovir.

If secondary bacterial infection of the skin vesicles develops, initial treatment with an oral antibiotic, such as clindamycin, should be started to treat community-acquired MRSA.

Localized treatment, with conservative options such as sterile saline dressing, may increase the healing of skin lesions, decrease viral shedding, prevent and lessen acute neuritis, and reduce the risk of postherpetic neuralgia.

Postherpetic neuralgia (PHN) is the chronic pain that occurs after resolution of lesions, particularly in the elderly and after ophthalmic zoster. The most effective prevention strategy is treatment of acute zoster with antivirals. Gabapentin has been shown to be effective in PHN but has side effects including somnolence, dizziness, and ataxia. Regional nerve blocks can also be used. Tricyclic antidepressants can be used; due to adverse effects including dry mouth, constipation, and dizziness, it is not commonly utilized.

For immunocompromised patients unable to receive the vaccination, the recommended treatment following exposure to varicella is varicella-zoster immune globulin (VariZIG).

Two live, attenuated virus vaccines are available in the United States: Varivax, a single-antigen varicella vaccine and ProQuad, a combination measles, mumps, rubella, and varicella (MMRV) vaccine. In children 12 months to 12 years of age, two doses of varicella vaccine should be given at least 3 months apart. Single-dose vaccine and MMRV vaccine can be used with the first dose at 12 to 15 months of age and second dose between ages 4 and 6 years. In patients over age 13, two doses of the single-antigen varicella vaccine should be given 4 to 8 weeks apart.

For zoster, the CDC recommends Shingrix, a recombinant zoster vaccine over Zostavax, a live vaccine for the prevention of herpes zoster and related complications. Two doses of Shingrix should be separated by 2 to 6 months in immunocompetent adults age 50 years and older. Zostavax may still be used in healthy adults age 60 years or older, if allergic to Shingrix, prefer Zostavax, or Shingrix is not available. Patients may receive the vaccines regardless of a history of previous episode of herpes zoster or a history of chronic medical conditions.[46]

PATIENT EDUCATION

- Most healthy children who develop varicella will have a complete recovery with no sequelae.
- The most common complication of varicella is secondary bacterial infection. This is treated with the appropriate antibiotics.
- Postherpetic neuralgia may last more than 120 days after appearance of rash; the condition is worse with age and occurs in up to 10% to 15% of patients.[47]

17.3C EPSTEIN-BARR INFECTION

EBV belongs to the family Herpesviridae. EBV is transmitted via saliva, but sexual transmission and transmission via blood and transplanted organs has been noted. In the United States, half of the population contracts primary EBV infection between the ages of 1 to 5 years. Infection is usually subclinical in childhood. Primary EBV infection is rare in the first year of life, due to protective maternal antibodies. In the United States, one-half of adolescents are still susceptible to infectious mononucleosis (IM) in their teens and early adulthood, with the highest incidence in the 15 to 24-year-old age group.

Mononucleosis is known as the “kissing disease” and the primary mode of transmission is by saliva. Long-term shedding of EBV in the saliva has been noted; patients may have low titers of EBV in their saliva up to 18 months after IM.

MEDICAL HISTORY AND CLINICAL PRESENTATION

IM is the most common illness associated with EBV. The incubation period is 4 to 6 weeks. The prodrome lasts 3 to 5 days and presents with headache, malaise, and fatigue. This is followed by fever, which decreases over the next 5 to 6 days. Generalized lymphadenopathy is common and any lymph node group can be involved; the posterior cervical chain and posterior auricular nodes are the most common. Pharyngitis is the cardinal symptom of IM. Tonsils are enlarged, red, tender, and covered with a white exudate. Petechiae at the junction of the hard to soft palate may be present; this is also noted in streptococcal pharyngitis.

Splenomegaly is seen in 50% to 60% of patients by the second and third weeks of illness. Spontaneous or trauma-induced rupture of the spleen can lead to hemorrhage, shock, and death. The triad of lymphadenopathy, splenomegaly, and exudative pharyngitis in a febrile patient is typical but not pathognomonic of IM.

SIGNS AND SYMPTOMS

The classic triad generally seen in IM includes fever, pharyngitis, and lymphadenopathy. Other symptoms include malaise, fatigue, and headache.

PHYSICAL EXAMINATION

Splenomegaly is noted in 50% to 60% of individuals with IM and is caused by the infiltration of the spleen with lymphocytes and atypical lymphoid cells. Splenic rupture can occur as late as 7 weeks after the onset of IM.

Rash may be noted. The rash is generalized and appears during the first few days of illness, lasting 1 to 6 days. It is described as erythematous, maculopapular, urticarial, or petechial. An increased incidence (33%) of rash can occur in patients with EBV IM who are prescribed beta-lactam antibiotics. This rash does not represent hypersensitivity to beta-lactam antibiotics.[48]

Other common physical findings include lymphadenopathy, most often involving the posterior cervical chain and posterior auricular nodes. The lymph nodes are large and can be tender.

Oral findings include tonsillar enlargement, often with an exudate and palatal petechiae.

DIFFERENTIAL DIAGNOSIS

The differential diagnosis is broad. Table 17.13 summarizes the differential diagnosis for IM.

DIAGNOSTIC STUDIES

Diagnosis is based on general laboratory findings. The heterophile antibody or monospot test is a latex agglutination assay. Heterophile antibodies appear within 1 week, peak during the second or third week, and can persist for up to 1 year. False positive results can occur in patients with HIV, lymphoma, systemic lupus erythematosus, rubella, and parvovirus.

CBC with differential reveals a lymphocytosis with at least 10% atypical lymphocytes. Atypical lymphocytes are noted in 70% of patients and peak during the second or third week of illness. Atypical lymphocytes can also be found in toxoplasmosis, rubella, HHV-6, viral hepatitis, mumps, CMV, acute HIV, and certain drug reactions.

Elevated hepatic transaminases are seen in a majority of patients.

The most valuable serologic marker for diagnosing acute IM is the EBV viral capsid antigen (VCA) IgM. Anti-VCA IgM lasts 1 to 3 months. False positive results can be caused by the presence of rheumatoid factor, found in the setting of rheumatoid arthritis or hepatitis C. EBV VCA IgG peaks during acute illness, decreases over the next few weeks to months, and then persists at a low level throughout life. A positive VCA IgG indicates past infection. Epstein-Barr nuclear antigen (EBNA) IgG appears 6 to 12 weeks after initial symptoms, so it is negative in acute infection.

TABLE 17.13 Differential Diagnosis for Infectious Mononucleosis

Diagnosis	Description
Cytomegalovirus (CMV) mononucleosis	CMV usually causes an asymptomatic infection early in life. Spread via saliva. Diagnosis is made via serology or DNA PCR. Microscopic exam may reveal intranuclear inclusions ("owl's eye"). Symptoms include fever, pharyngitis, lymphadenopathy, headaches, and a rash that generally appears after the prodrome period. Atypical lymphocytes can be present. Transaminases are more commonly elevated.
Streptococcus pyogenes pharyngitis	A common cause of sore throat. Diagnosis made via throat culture or rapid antigen testing. Presenting signs and symptoms include pharyngitis often with exudates, severe odynophagia, as well as fever and lymphadenopathy. Splenomegaly and elevated AST/ALT are rare.
HHV-6 (human herpes virus 6)	Cause of roseola infantum. Characterized by a maculopapular rash, prolonged fever, cervical lymphadenopathy, and atypical lymphocytosis. Splenomegaly and elevated AST/ALT are rare.
Herpes simplex virus type 1-primary	Primary infection can present similarly to mononucleosis, as opposed to herpes labialis. Presenting signs and symptoms include fever, pharyngitis with exudates, and prolonged cervical lymphadenopathy. Splenomegaly and elevated AST/ALT are rare.
HIV infection—acute retroviral	Presenting signs and symptoms include pharyngitis, headache, malaise, fevers, lymphadenopathy, and maculopapular rash. Atypical lymphocytes are often present. Mucocutaneous ulceration often occurs and is not seen in EBV mononucleosis. Initial HIV testing may be negative, HIV RNA viral load should be checked.
Adenovirus infection	Causes respiratory tract infections, conjunctivitis, and mononucleosis-like syndrome. Presents with pharyngitis, fever, and cervical lymphadenopathy. Splenomegaly and elevated AST/ALT are rare.

ALT, alanine transaminase; AST, aspartate transaminase; EBV, Epstein-Barr virus; PCR, polymerase chain reaction.

Immunocompromised patients may not produce these antibodies. See Table 17.14 for antibody results in acute and past EBV infection.

EBV DNA PCR is a very sensitive and specific test. EBV DNA can be detected in serum, plasma, and lymphocytes. This test is used to detect the presence of disease in the first few weeks.

TREATMENT

For acute uncomplicated IM management consists of supportive care, including rest, fluids, and antipyretics. Acetaminophen and saline gargles can be used to control the pharyngeal discomfort caused by enlarged lymph nodes and pharyngitis. Antiviral medications provide no benefit to the patient.

PATIENT EDUCATION

- IM can be prevented by limiting oral and sexual contacts. Other methods of prevention include handwashing and avoiding shared utensils or cups.
- Complications include:
  - Splenic rupture: This is rare and typically occurs in the first 21 days of the disease. Conservative management is appropriate.
  - Hepatitis: Elevations in AST/ALT (aspartate transaminase/alanine transaminase) to two to three times normal is common. Treatment is supportive.

TABLE 17.14 Patterns of Acute and Past Epstein-Barr Infection

	VCA IgM	VCA IgG	EBNA IgG
Acute infection	Positive	Positive	Negative
Past infection	Negative	Positive	Positive

EBNA, Epstein-Barr nuclear antigen; IgM, immunoglobulin M; IgG, immunoglobulin G; VCA, viral capsid antigen.

17.3D CYTOMEGALOVIRUS

Human CMV, a member of the Herpesviridae family, causes symptomatic infection in the newborn or in immunocompromised individuals, including those infected with HIV/AIDS, stem cell transplant recipients, and organ transplant recipients. Symptoms of infection are variable. Immunocompetent individuals exhibit symptoms of a mild mononucleosis-like syndrome.

The virus enters through the mucosal surfaces of the upper respiratory tract, GI tract, and urogenital tract. Possible sources of infection include oral secretions, urine, breast milk, semen, and cervical and vaginal secretions. Indirect transmission can occur via contaminated fomites.

The virus uses neutrophils to spread through the body to infect various organs. In the fetus and neonate, CMV infection commonly involves salivary glands and neurons. In immunocompetent individuals, the virus typically infects lymphoid tissues and in immunocompromised patients the targets are the lungs or other organs.

MEDICAL HISTORY AND CLINICAL PRESENTATION

All persons are at risk of developing CMV infection, but those at risk of developing disease include newborns, fetuses, immunocompromised individuals, and HIV/AIDS patients.

Only about 50% of adults have evidence of infection; higher rates are associated with older age, female gender, and lower household income. Most patients exhibit no clinical symptoms.

In the United States, CMV seroprevalence is higher in non-Hispanic Blacks (71%) and Mexican Americans (77%) than non-Hispanic Whites (40%).[49]

Sexual transmission also plays a role in CMV infection, as individuals with sexual risk factors, including multiple partners, men who have sex with men (MSM), and a history of sexually transmitted diseases, are more likely to be infected with CMV.

SIGNS AND SYMPTOMS

CMV infections in childhood are asymptomatic and frequently occur in the day care setting, due to transmission via saliva and other secretions. In immunocompetent adults, the virus is transmitted through secretions, which are more likely to occur during sexual activity or intimate physical interactions. Blood transfusion carries a small risk of CMV transmission; since CMV is carried in polymorphonuclear cells, the use of leukocyte-depleted or cryopreserved blood decreases the risk and is used when transplant recipients require transfusion. Patients with low CD4 counts are more susceptible to CMV disease.

PHYSICAL EXAMINATION

Congenital CMV disease is a common cause of intrauterine infection in humans and is the leading infectious cause of deafness and mental retardation. Since CMV is usually asymptomatic, diagnosis in pregnancy based on clinical findings alone is difficult. CMV infection in the fetus should be considered when certain ultrasound findings are noted, including echogenic bowel, ascites, fetal hydrops, intracranial or liver calcifications, microcephaly, pleural effusion, and early onset intrauterine growth restriction.

From 10% to 15% of congenitally infected infants will have symptoms at birth including intrauterine growth retardation, microcephaly, cerebral atrophy, jaundice, thrombocytopenia, seizures, hepatosplenomegaly, intracranial calcifications, petechiae, and a "blueberry muffin" appearance secondary to extramedullary erythropoiesis.[50] A small number of infants will die, primarily of disseminated intravascular coagulation, hepatic dysfunction, or superinfection. Most survivors will develop long-term neurologic sequelae including sensorineural hearing loss, mental retardation, cerebral palsy, paraparesis, and impaired vision or blindness from chorioretinitis.

CMV infection in immunocompetent patients results from acute primary infection and presents as CMV-induced mononucleosis. CMV infection should be considered in a patient with fever, fatigue, and malaise without any examination findings or history consistent with another diagnosis. CMV infection is indistinguishable from EBV IM and there are no characteristic findings on physical examination that establish or suggest the diagnosis of CMV infection. CMV infected patients develop a maculopapular rash when given penicillins during the illness, the same as with EBV infection. The course of the disease is usually benign and self-limited; complications are rare, but include hemolytic anemia, splenic infarction, interstitial pneumonia, thrombocytopenia, Guillain-Barré syndrome, meningoencephalitis, myocarditis, and arthritis.

CMV retinitis is the most frequent form of CMV disease in AIDS patients followed by infection of the GI tract. The clinical presentation of CMV retinitis includes blurry vision and loss of visual fields. The condition is painless but may progress to blindness if not treated. Fundoscopic examination reveals a yellow-white exudate with hemorrhage.

Infection of the GI tract can result in colitis with symptoms of diarrhea, hematochezia, and abdominal pain. Esophagitis presents with odynophagia.

DIFFERENTIAL DIAGNOSIS

Table 17.13 summarizes the differential diagnosis for CMV infection.

DIAGNOSTIC STUDIES

Typical laboratory findings in patients infected with CMV include the presence of atypical lymphocytes and mild elevations in the liver transaminases, but the heterophile test/monospot is negative.

Tissue diagnosis of CMV infection is specific, but not sensitive. CMV is characterized by the "owl's eye" appearance representing inclusion bodies within infected endothelial cells. These lesions are similar to those seen in HSV and VZV infections.

The test of choice for fetal infection with CMV is amniocentesis after 21 weeks' gestation with CMV PCR amplification; the test is 90% sensitive and specific. Detection cannot predict disease severity. In the newborn, the most accurate test is the isolation of CMV in urine. CMV may be shed in the urine of children infected as newborns for up to 8 years.

Other diagnostic modalities include tissue culture, histologic-cytologic detection, immunologic methods, nucleic acid testing, and antigen detection.

TREATMENT

The major therapeutic approach for CMV infection should include prevention. Prevention of CMV infection in immunocompromised patients who are CMV negative begins with selection of the appropriate CMV antibody-negative blood products.

Prophylactic treatment of immunocompromised and transplant patients with CMV immune globulin (CMVIG) can decrease the rate and severity of CMV disease and complications of infection but does not prevent primary infection.

No antiviral therapy is recommended for the treatment of congenital CMV infection. The medical treatment options for CMV-infected AIDS patients and transplant patients includes IV ganciclovir, foscarnet, or cidofovir; or oral valganciclovir.

CMV retinitis that is life-threatening or threatening to vision is treated with ganciclovir. Ganciclovir suppresses active infection but does not cure CMV infection. Oral ganciclovir is most commonly used for long-term maintenance. Treatment with ganciclovir is recommended in immunocompromised patients infected with CMV and prophylaxis of CMV in transplant recipients. Valganciclovir has been approved for the treatment of CMV retinitis in adult patients with AIDS, as well as for prophylaxis of CMV disease in organ transplant recipients. It is the drug of choice in mild to moderate CMV disease.

Foscarnet is a second-line agent for treatment of CMV infections, mainly CMV retinitis in AIDS patients. It is effective against ganciclovir-resistant CMV strains and is less toxic to bone marrow than ganciclovir.

PATIENT EDUCATION

- Congenital CMV disease is a common cause of intrauterine infection in humans and is the leading infectious cause of deafness and mental retardation.
- IV ganciclovir and valganciclovir are the first-line antiviral agents of choice for treatment of congenital CMV disease.
- In the immunocompetent patient infected with CMV, there are generally no systemic complications.
- In the AIDS patient, systemic complications include CMV retinitis, colitis, and esophagitis.
- In the transplant patient, systemic complications occur because of CMV infection and include severe, life-threatening bacterial, fungal, or OI.

17.3E MUMPS

Mumps, caused by a virus of the Paramyxoviridae family, is an acute viral infection usually seen in childhood. It is transmitted through respiratory secretions with viral replication in the nasopharynx and lymph nodes, followed by viremia and spread to multiple organs, including the CNS and epithelium of salivary glands.

The virus has an affinity for the CNS; infected individuals may have CSF pleocytosis, but meningitis and encephalitis are rare. Complications include orchitis, oophoritis, arthritis, pancreatitis, cerebellar ataxia, transverse myelitis, thrombocytopenia, and hearing impairment.

MEDICAL HISTORY AND CLINICAL PRESENTATION

Mumps is characterized by unilateral or bilateral swelling of the salivary glands, typically the parotid gland. This is preceded for 1 to 2 days by headache and loss of appetite. Approximately one third of infected children have no salivary gland involvement. On average the incubation period is 16 to 18 days. The time of greatest infectivity is 1 to 2 days prior to the onset of parotid swelling.

PHYSICAL EXAMINATION

Physical examination reveals swelling of the parotid area with upward and outward displacement of the earlobe. This swelling also leads to the mandible being obscured (Figure 17.12). Opening of Stensen duct is edematous and erythematous. Pain may also be noted when eating or drinking acidic foods.

Orchitis is uncommon in prepubertal males but complicates mumps in about 15% to 30% of postpubertal teens.[51] Affected boys develop fever, lower abdominal pain, and unilateral testicular pain 4 to 8 days following onset of parotid involvement. Infertility is uncommon and about 50% may have some testicular atrophy.[52]

DIFFERENTIAL DIAGNOSIS

Parotid gland inflammation and swelling can be caused by other viruses, including influenza, enteroviruses, parainfluenza, CMV, lymphocytic choriomeningitis virus, and HIV. Bacterial infection of the parotid gland, due to *Staphylococcus aureus*, may result from hematogenous spread or from ascending infection. Salivary duct stones and metabolic disorders, such as diabetes mellitus, cirrhosis, and malnutrition, can all lead to parotitis. The drugs phenylbutazone, thiouracil, and iodides have also been implicated in parotid gland swelling.

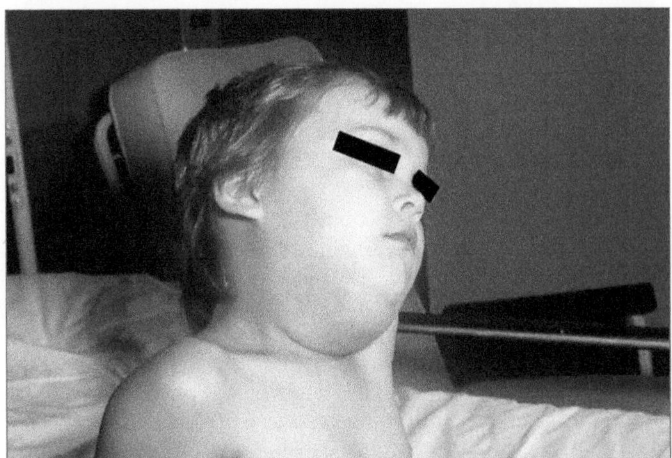

Figure 17.12 Parotid gland enlargement in mumps.
(Source: Centers for Disease Control and Prevention. https://phil.cdc.gov/Details.aspx?pid=130)

DIAGNOSTIC STUDIES

The WBC count is usually low or within the normal range with a relative lymphocytosis. Serum amylase may be elevated during the first week of illness.

The diagnosis can be confirmed by isolation of the virus from Stenson duct exudate, throat washings, saliva, or spinal fluid or by detection of the virus using PCR testing. Virus may be present in saliva as early as a week before symptoms appear.

Detection of virus-specific IgM or a rise in IgG titers from samples collected during the acute illness and again in convalescence confirms the diagnosis.

EVALUATION

Mumps should be suspected in any patient who has acute unilateral or bilateral swelling of the parotid or other salivary glands for more than 2 days without alternative explanation. Cases of mumps should be reported to public health authorities.

TREATMENT

There is no specific treatment for mumps. Supportive treatment involves hydration and avoidance of acidic foods.

Vaccination is key to the prevention of mumps and its complications. The vaccine is included in the combination measles-mumps-rubella (MMR) and MMRV vaccines. The MMR is only licensed for use in children who are 12 months through 12 years. Children should get two doses of MMR vaccine, the first dose at 12 through 15 months, and the second dose at 4 through 6 years.

Two doses of mumps vaccine are 88% effective at preventing the disease; one dose is 78% effective.

The advisory Committee on Immunization Practices recommends that people identified by public health authorities as being part of a group at increased risk for acquiring mumps because of a mumps outbreak should receive a third dose of MMR vaccine.

PATIENT EDUCATION

- The symptoms of mumps usually resolve without complication in 3 to 5 days.

- In cases with central nervous system involvement (meningitis or encephalitis), the infection is usually self-limited, but complications may include ataxia, behavioral problems, and sensorineural hearing loss.
- Infertility is an uncommon complication in boys who develop orchitis due to mumps.

17.3F POLIOMYELITIS

Poliovirus is a single-strand RNA enterovirus, member of the virus family Picornaviridae. The virus enters the body orally and infects the GI tract. The virus replicates and then secreted in the feces, allowing further transmission of the virus, or enters the bloodstream causing a viremia and spreading to other parts of the body. Viremia allows the virus to spread to and replicate in the CNS; this leads to death of the anterior horn motor neurons of the spinal cord. The death of the anterior motor horn cells is responsible for the paralysis noted in poliomyelitis.

There are four categories of poliomyelitis:

- Subclinical poliomyelitis
- Abortive poliomyelitis
- Nonparalytic poliomyelitis
- Paralytic poliomyelitis, is divided into two forms:
  - Spinal poliomyelitis, affects muscles supplied by the spinal nerves.
  - Bulbar poliomyelitis affects muscles supplied by the cranial nerves.

MEDICAL HISTORY AND CLINICAL PRESENTATION

Enteroviruses are more common in temperate climates and the infection rate is highest in the summer and fall. Poliovirus has been mostly eradicated because of a worldwide vaccination campaign. The number of worldwide polio cases has decreased from 350,000 in 1988 to 33 cases in 2018.[53] Four regions of the world are considered polio-free: the Americas, Europe, South East Asia, and Western Pacific. There are only three polio-endemic countries: Afghanistan, Nigeria, and Pakistan.

SIGNS AND SYMPTOMS

Most cases of poliomyelitis are asymptomatic. There are three clinical syndromes of symptomatic disease.

- Abortive poliomyelitis presents with mild symptoms including gastroenteritis, acute respiratory infection, and flu-like illness.
- Nonparalytic poliomyelitis presents with fever, headache, irritability, muscle spasms, and neck, back, abdominal pain.
- Paralytic poliomyelitis presents with the symptoms noted in nonparalytic disease, plus muscle weakness, asymmetric paralysis, muscle atrophy, and tremors.

PHYSICAL EXAMINATION

The most severe clinical manifestation of poliomyelitis is acute flaccid paralysis. Asymmetric muscle weakness is noted with the distribution dependent on the extent of infection. The legs are more commonly affected than arms, and proximal more often than distal muscles. Reflexes are absent or diminished, but sensation is normal.

Most patients with a normal immune system are asymptomatic and have a normal physical examination.

DIFFERENTIAL DIAGNOSIS

Abortive poliomyelitis must be differentiated from other diseases such as gastroenteritis and acute respiratory infection. The differential diagnosis for paralytic poliomyelitis includes Guillain-Barré syndrome, transverse myelitis, and WNV infection.

DIAGNOSTIC STUDIES

Diagnosis of poliomyelitis is made by its classic presentation or via a variety of laboratory methods. The gold standard for confirming the diagnosis is viral isolation from the stool. CSF can be used for culture or PCR testing.

Analysis of the CSF reveals an increased number of WBCs, mainly lymphocytes, and mildly elevated total protein. These findings are like aseptic meningitis due to other viruses.

TREATMENT

Poliovirus is treated with supportive measures, including pain control and mechanical ventilation and intubation if needed.

The CDC recommends that children receive inactivated poliovirus vaccine (IPV) to protect against polio, or poliomyelitis. IPV is given by injection in the leg or arm, depending the person's age. It may be given at the same time as other vaccines. Children receive four doses of IPV at the following ages:

- 2 months
- 4 months
- 6 through 18 months
- 4 through 6 years

Several combination vaccines contain IPV, such as Pentacel (DTaP-IPV/Hib), Pediarix (DTaP-IPV-HepB), or Kinrix (DTaP-IPV). Children getting these vaccines may get one more (fifth) dose of IPV, which is safe.

PATIENT EDUCATION

- Rarely, vaccination with live oral polio vaccine (OPV) can lead to vaccine-related poliomyelitis in the vaccinated individual or a contact. This occurs in only 1 in 2.5 million cases of vaccination. The inactive polio vaccine (IPV) is not associated with this side effect.
- A complication includes postpolio syndrome in which weakness suddenly worsens many years or even decades after the initial illness. This can be accompanied by pain and general fatigue.
  - Management is supportive, with pain control and regular but nonstrenuous exercise or physical therapy.

17.3G MEASLES

Measles is caused by a single-stranded RNA rubeola virus from the family Paramyxoviridae.

Measles is a highly contagious, acute systemic viral infection with fever, respiratory symptoms, and rash. Infection confers lifelong immunity. Until recently, measles was rare in the United States. Due to parental fear of vaccinating children and a decrease in herd immunity (95% immunization rate is required to achieve herd immunity) there has been an increase in the number of reported cases in the United States.

Beginning in 2008, there has been an increase in measles cases in the United States; 1,282 cases were reported in 2019.[54] Many cases were related to travel in European and Asian countries, where there were many unvaccinated individuals. The increase in measles has been attributed to the failure of parents to immunize their healthy infants, mainly from fear that the vaccine may cause autism. Many studies have failed to demonstrate a causal relationship between MMR vaccine and autism.

After exposure, the virus is localized to the epithelial cells of the nasopharynx and conjunctivae, and then spreads to the regional lymph nodes. In a few days viremia develops and the virus spreads to other reticuloendothelial organs, particularly the spleen, appendix, and posterior cervical and mesenteric lymph nodes. After 5 to 7 days a secondary viremia occurs, followed by onset of the prodromal phase. This secondary viremia leads to involvement of skin, respiratory tract, and conjunctivae. Viral replication continues with a peak viral load (VL) by the 14th day; after this the VL falls off rapidly over 2 to 3 days.

MEDICAL HISTORY AND CLINICAL PRESENTATION

Measles typically occurs in winter and early spring in temperate climates with an incubation period of 8 to 12 days.

In the prodromal phase the patient presents with a high fever, up to 105° F; profuse rhinorrhea; harsh, dry cough and a nonpurulent conjunctivitis. This is followed by a skin rash. A history of contact with a case of measles may be noted.

The complication of acute encephalitis occurs in 1 in 1,000 measles patients.[55] Symptoms of encephalitis usually develop during the first week after the onset of the rash. Symptoms range from mild to severe and neurologic complications are common. Because measles encephalitis is thought to result from infection of the CNS, steroids are not recommended for its treatment.

Other complications include pneumonia and otitis media. Bacterial superinfections of the respiratory tract are common complications and can usually be treated successfully with appropriate antimicrobials.

A rare fatal complication, subacute sclerosing panencephalitis (SSPE), with an incubation period of up to 10 years, occurs mainly in children who contracted measles before the age of 2 years. Symptoms include a gradual onset of behavioral and intellectual deterioration, with seizures, eventually progressing to coma and death.

SIGNS AND SYMPTOMS

Measles is spread by the airborne route of respiratory secretions from infected individuals. A prodrome develops with symptoms like the common cold, with some cough, lasting about 3 days. The prodrome is followed by fever and gradual development of rash. The disease is most contagious just before rash onset and during the first few days after the rash appears.

PHYSICAL EXAMINATION

Patients with the prodrome of measles have a 3-day history of nonspecific respiratory symptoms.

Koplik spots, tiny white spots on the buccal mucosa opposite the first or second molar, are pathognomonic of measles. Koplik spots appear during and following the prodrome.

This is followed by influenza-like symptoms, such as fever, cough, conjunctivitis, and coryza. A few days later the typical maculopapular, erythematous, nonpruritic rash begins on the head and face and progresses down the body (Figure 17.13).

Rash first appears behind the ears and on the hairline and then spreads to the trunk and extremities, including palms and soles. The rash blanches on pressure and may become confluent on the face and neck. It clears first on the face and then the body. Desquamation may occur during the healing phase. The rash lasts about 5 days.

DIFFERENTIAL DIAGNOSIS

The differential diagnosis includes:

- Kawasaki disease (KD) is noted in children <2 years of age; presents with fever for more than 5 days, no Koplik spots, history of measles immunization, swollen hands and feet, and prominent cervical lymph nodes.
- Rubella presents with a milder, pink rash and prominent suboccipital lymphadenopathy.
- Parvovirus B19 infection presents with skin rash after the fever subsides, and the child appears well.
- IM, roseola infantum and coxsackie virus and enteroviral infections lack the rhinorrhea and conjunctivitis seen during prodromal phase.

DIAGNOSTIC STUDIES

Measles should be considered in unvaccinated children or with a history of exposure. The CBC reveals leukopenia with a relative lymphocytosis; thrombocytopenia is noted and can be severe. ESR and C-reactive protein are normal.

Confirmation of the diagnosis is made by demonstrating the presence of antimeasles IgM antibodies. The antibodies are detectable 3 days after the onset of the rash and may persist for up to 1 month. Confirmation of diagnosis is made by demonstrating a fourfold or greater rise in the IgM antibody titer in acute and convalescent samples.

Figure 17.13 Skin rash noted in measles.
(Source: Centers for Disease Control and Prevention. https://phil.cdc.gov/Details.aspx?pid=4514)

TREATMENT

Since there is no specific antiviral therapy available, treatment is supportive including antipyretics and fluids.

Bacterial superinfections, such as pneumonia and otitis media, should be treated with appropriate antimicrobials. Children with measles should be administered vitamin A once daily for 2 days.

Prevention is the most successful approach to limiting measles. Measles vaccine is given as the combination MMR vaccine. Two doses are administered, at 12 to 15 months of age (in outbreaks, vaccine can be given after 6 months of age) and the second dose is given at the start of school but can be given sooner. The minimum interval between doses is 1 month. Side effects of the vaccine include a transient measles-like rash, transient thrombocytopenia, and anaphylaxis. Measles vaccine is considered to be extremely safe.

PATIENT EDUCATION

- Measles in hospitalized patients requires strict airborne isolation with proper handwashing, gowns, masks, and gloves. Measles cases should be reported to the local health department.
- During an outbreak, infants as young as 6 months of age can be vaccinated; such children should eventually receive a total of three doses of measles vaccine.

17.3H RUBELLA

Rubella virus is single-stranded RNA virus of the Togaviridae family. Rubella virus infection gives rise to two distinct clinical entities: when acquired postnatally it produces a mild illness with a characteristic rash; when acquired during fetal development it produces the congenital rubella syndrome (CRS).

Humans are the only known host for rubella virus. Infection is more common in late winter and early spring; it is transmitted via respiratory droplets and is present in respiratory sections of infected individuals from 7 days before to 14 days after the onset of rash. The incubation period is 14 days.

In postnatal rubella, virus first infects the nasopharyngeal respiratory epithelium and then spreads to regional lymph nodes. Localized replication occurs for 7 to 10 days before the virus spreads throughout the body. Viremia peaks about 2 weeks following infection and viral shedding in respiratory secretions can occur up to 3 weeks following initial exposure.

Transplacental infection of the fetus occurs during the viremia that accompanies maternal infection. The risk of infection is greatest when maternal infection occurs during the first trimester, decreases during the second trimester, then increases again near term. Following transplacental infection, virus disseminates throughout the fetus and persistently infects a wide range of cell types.

MEDICAL HISTORY AND CLINICAL PRESENTATION

Rubella presents with polyarticular arthralgias and arthritis. Neurologic involvement is less common.

Hemorrhagic complications, such as thrombocytopenic purpura, are unusual.

Congenital rubella occurs when a nonimmune female passes the virus to the fetus in utero during pregnancy. The birth defects include deafness, cataracts, CNS defects such as microcephaly and hydrocephaly, and cardiac disease such as patent ductus arteriosus and ventriculoseptal defect.

Congenital rubella is a cause of the TORCH (Toxoplasmosis, **O**ther agents, **R**ubella, **C**ytomegalovirus, and **H**erpes simplex) syndrome resulting in a "blueberry muffin baby," secondary to extramedullary hematopoiesis. Disseminated erythematous to violaceous papules and nodules are seen in the neonate. Long-term complications may develop over weeks to years, including mental retardation and behavioral disorders, spastic diplegia, endocrinopathies, specifically diabetes, and seizure disorders

SIGNS AND SYMPTOMS

Rubella is characterized by a prodrome of fever, headache, and upper respiratory symptoms, followed 1 to 5 days later by a rash that spreads from the head to the feet. The rash resolves in 2 to 3 days in the direction in which it started.

The prodromal symptoms in young children include mild coryza and diarrhea or they may be asymptomatic until the rash develops. In older patients the prodromal symptoms occur 1 to 5 days prior to the onset of rash. Symptoms include eye pain, primarily with lateral and upward gaze, sore throat, headache, lymphadenopathy, fever, aches, chills, anorexia, and nausea.

PHYSICAL EXAMINATION

The rash in rubella presents about 18 days after exposure. It begins on the face and spreads outward over the rest of the body, including the hands and feet, over the next 24 hours. It is most confluent on the face and upper body and remains patchy on the lower extremities. On the second day the rash fades from the face and by the third day it has resolved completely. The rash is composed of areas of discrete erythematous maculopapular lesions that can be pruritic.

Lymphadenopathy of the postauricular and suboccipital nodes is noted. Lymphadenopathy is noted 1 to 7 days prior to the onset of rash.

Arthralgia is frequently reported in women but is less common in men and children. Frank arthritis, often of fingers, wrists, and knees, can be noted. Joint symptoms typically begin in the first week after the onset of the rash and can take weeks to resolve.

Petechiae of the soft palate, Forchheimer spots, may be seen. These spots are not pathognomonic for rubella.

DIFFERENTIAL DIAGNOSIS

The differential diagnosis for rubella includes measles, viral infections, and toxoplasmosis.

Measles has a similar but more pronounced fever and rash, and children with measles are more ill appearing at the time of presentation.

Other viral infections, such as enterovirus and adenovirus, can present with diffuse rash, fever, and lymphadenopathy.

Toxoplasmosis can cause postauricular and suboccipital lymphadenopathy.

Of the congenital infections, CMV infection is most like CRS.

DIAGNOSTIC STUDIES

Since the presentation of rubella is like other viral exanthems, diagnostic confirmation is achieved by the detection of IgM antibodies or an increase in IgG antibodies. The presence of rubella-specific IgM in acute serum or a fourfold rise in rubella-specific IgG from acute to convalescent samples suggests recent infection.

CBC with differential will reveal leukopenia with lymphopenia; thrombocytopenia may be noted later in the disease.

In CRS the CBC reveals thrombocytopenia and less commonly anemia. With liver involvement the liver transaminases may be elevated.

Virus can be recovered from the nasopharynx and blood during the prodromal phase and up to 4 days following the onset of rash. Rubella-specific IgM can be detected at birth and can persist through the first year of life. Detection of rubella-specific IgG beyond 6 months of age is consistent with congenital infection. PCR is used mainly in prenatal diagnosis.

TREATMENT

Prevention is key. The current immunization schedule for the rubella vaccine, given along with the measles and mumps vaccines, is at 12 to 15 months, and repeated at 4 to 6 years.

Rubella vaccine is a live attenuated virus vaccine. It is currently available combined with MMR or with MMRV. Immunity is noted in over 95% of vaccinated people at least 12 months of age and immunity lasts for 15 years in more than 90%.[56] A second dose of the vaccine is recommended at 4 to 6 years of age to produce immunity in those who failed to respond. The second dose of MMR may be given as soon as 28 days following the first; the minimum interval between MMRV doses is 3 months.

Adults born in 1957 or later should receive at least one dose of MMR, unless they have documentation of previous vaccination or serologic evidence of immunity to MMR.

Rubella vaccine is a live vaccine and should not be given to immunodeficient and immunosuppressed patients.

Supportive therapy should be based on symptoms.

PATIENT EDUCATION

- Pregnant women should not receive rubella vaccine.
- Children receiving vaccine before 12 months of age should be revaccinated when they are at least 12 months of age.
- Infected individuals should be counseled to avoid pregnant, nonimmune individuals.
- Patients with rubella infection have an excellent prognosis. Exceptions include patients with encephalitis in which prognosis is related to the severity and extent of encephalitis.
- CRS prognosis is directly related to the number and severity of organ systems involved. Most common complications include hearing loss, mental retardation, and visual deficits.

17.3I RABIES

Rabies is caused by an RNA virus from the Rhabdoviridae family. Rabies is most commonly transmitted by a canine vector. In developed countries domestic animals only account for 10% of human exposures, while wild animals (skunks, foxes, raccoons, bats, and coyotes) account for the other 90%. In the United States bats represent the most common source of clinical rabies infection.[57]

Rabies is usually transmitted from infected animal bites, but can be transmitted by scratches, mucous membrane contamination, aerosolized virus that enters the respiratory tract, and corneal transplants.

There were 25 cases of human rabies diagnosed in the United States and Puerto Rico from 2009 through 2019.[58]

The virus binds to receptors in the muscle, dermis, or epidermis. After budding from the membrane of the muscle cells, the virus enters the unmyelinated nerve endings at the neuromuscular junction or the muscle spindles. The virus replicates again once it reaches the dorsal root ganglia and anterior horn cells. If the patient's immune system responds to the viral replication at the dorsal root ganglia, neuritis may develop and present as neuropathic pain at the bite site. Once the pain develops, prophylaxis with vaccine and human rabies immunoglobulin will not be able to prevent death.

The virus is transported via retrograde flow to the central nervous system. Once the virus reaches the central nervous system rapid dissemination occurs within the brainstem, thalamus, basal ganglia, and spinal cord. The virus then spreads from the CNS to the rest of the peripheral nervous system and the organs they innervate, especially the salivary glands. This leads to hypersalivation and spasms of the pharyngeal muscles at the sound, sight, or taste of water. The virus will eventually manifest as encephalomyelitis, generalized nervous system failure, and death.

MEDICAL HISTORY AND CLINICAL PRESENTATION

In developed countries, individuals at high risk for exposure to rabies virus include veterinarians, animal handlers, laboratory personnel handling infected specimens, cave explorers, and travelers to areas with endemic canine rabies.

There are two classic forms of rabies: encephalitic and paralytic. Each of these forms evolve through five general stages: incubation, prodromal, acute neurologic, coma, and death.

The incubation state is typically asymptomatic, except for the pain and inflammation at the site of the bite. The prodromal stage presents with systemic, flu-like symptoms including fever, malaise, nausea and vomiting, anorexia, and sore throat. Pain, paresthesia, and pruritus may also be noted at the site of the bite. The paralytic form presents with choreiform movements of the infected limb during the prodromal stage. During the acute neurologic stage, the patient experiences a variety of symptoms depending on the clinical form of rabies.

In the encephalitic form, the acute neurologic stage includes painful pharyngeal spasms after exposure to a gust of air or a drink of water. They may also experience fever, hypersalivation, hyperactivity, fluctuating consciousness, and seizures. In the paralytic form, the acute neurologic stage presents with generalized weakness and quadriparesis. Other symptoms include a lack of sensation disturbances, bladder dysfunction, and fever with the limb weakness.

During the coma stage the patient may become nonresponsive and experience worsening hydrophobia, prolonged apnea, and generalized flaccid paralysis and the development of respiratory and cardiovascular collapse. The ultimate end in the natural history of an untreated rabies infection is death.

PHYSICAL EXAMINATION

Physical examination findings vary with the stage of the disease, but include myoclonus, focal brainstem signs, hemiparesis, hemisensory loss, ataxia, seizures, fever, changes in level of consciousness, autonomic dysfunction including hypersalivation, fixed pupils, and weakness.

DIFFERENTIAL DIAGNOSIS

The differential diagnosis for rabies is summarized in Table 17.15.

DIAGNOSTIC STUDIES

Most routine laboratory tests are nondiagnostic and routine CSF studies reveal a moderate lymphocytosis, normal glucose, and an increase in protein.

Diagnostic laboratory tests include detection of virus RNA by reverse transcriptase PCR, and isolation of infectious virus in cell culture on saliva samples. Skin biopsy, from the posterior region of the neck at the hairline, can be used to detect viral antigen via reverse transcriptase PCR.

MRI scans, while not diagnostic, may reveal hypersignaling in the brainstem, hippocampus, or hypothalamus.

TREATMENT

Rabies infections are almost always fatal unless the vaccine is administered prior to the onset of symptoms. Treatment of symptomatic rabies is largely supportive. The cornerstone to management of rabies infection is exposure prevention, pre-exposure prophylaxis (PrEP), and postexposure prophylaxis.

The CDC recommends postexposure prophylaxis for anyone who has contact with a bat, even if there is no evidence of a bite.

The animal should be captured and undergo testing for rabies. Postexposure prophylaxis should be discontinued if the animal is found to be negative for rabies.

The first step is cleaning the wound with soap and water for a minimum duration of 15 minutes. Antiseptics such as povidone iodine and ethanol may also be used. Closure of bite and scratch wounds should be avoided.

PrEP should be administered to individuals who are at high risk for encountering rabies virus. The vaccine should be given on days 0, 7, and 21 or 28.

For patients not previously vaccinated, those who were vaccinated more than 2 years earlier, or those whose titers have decreased, rabies vaccine should be administered day 0 and on day 3, 7, and 14. Vaccine should be administered at a site distant from the site of administration of human rabies immune globulin (HRIG), which can interfere with the immune action of the vaccine. HRIG should be immediately administered directly into the wound, or intramuscularly in the upper arm or lateral thigh muscle. If HRIG is not given on the same day the first vaccination is given, it can be given up to day 7 of the vaccination series. After day 7 an immune response should have occurred so use of HRIG is no longer warranted.

For patients who have received vaccination within the previous 2 years, the vaccine should be administered immediately, and a second dose should be administered on day 3. No HRIG is warranted as passive antibody administration may interfere with innate antibody production.

When used appropriately, postexposure prophylaxis is nearly 100% effective.

TABLE 17.15 Differential Diagnosis of Rabies

Diseases That Mimic Encephalitic Rabies	Diseases That Mimic Paralytic Rabies
Viral encephalitis	Polio myelitis
Delirium tremens	Guillain-Barré syndrome
Acute substance intoxication	Botulism
Acute psychoses	Diphtheria
Bacterial meningitis	West Nile virus infection
Tetanus	

PATIENT EDUCATION

- Prognosis in patients with potential rabies virus exposure is excellent if timely prophylaxis is provided.
- Rabies has the highest fatality rate of any infectious disease and prevention is the key to management.

17.3J PRION DISEASES

Prion diseases, spongiform encephalopathies, are a family of rare progressive neurodegenerative disorders that affect humans and animals.

A prion is an infectious agent that is transmissible and can induce abnormal folding of cellular proteins called prion proteins that are found mostly in the brain. The abnormal folding of the prion proteins leads to brain damage and the characteristic signs and symptoms of the disease. Prion diseases are rapidly progressive and always fatal.

The major prion disease in humans is Creutzfeldt-Jakob disease (CJD). CJD is a rapidly progressive, fatal neurodegenerative disorder. Infection with this disease leads to death within 1 year of onset of illness.

MEDICAL HISTORY AND CLINICAL PRESENTATION

Individuals over the age of 50 are at higher risk of developing CJD with the most common age at diagnosis being 60 to 65 years. Variant CJD is more common among younger individuals.

SIGNS AND SYMPTOMS

Common symptoms of CJD include progressive dementia, depression, personality changes, sleep disorders, and myoclonus movements.

PHYSICAL EXAMINATION

Physical examination findings include myoclonus, extrapyramidal signs, mutism, and visual or cerebellar signs.

DIFFERENTIAL DIAGNOSIS

CJD must be differentiated from other causes of rapidly progressive dementia, such as other neurodegenerative diseases, infections, Alzheimer disease, vascular dementia, and dementia due to metabolic or toxic etiology.

DIAGNOSTIC STUDIES

CSF studies reveal the presence of 14-3-3 protein and presence of neuron specific enolase and tau protein. Prion protein amplification techniques such as real-time quaking-induced conversion (RT-QuIC) is used to identify a disease-associated prion protein (PrP^{Sc}) which initiates a rapid conformational transition in recombinant prion protein (recPrP), resulting in the formation of amyloid protein.[59]

MRI findings include high signal abnormalities in the caudate nucleus and putamen.

Definitive diagnosis is made by brain biopsy. Biopsy reveals spongiform changes, neuronal loss, and accumulation of abnormal prion proteins.

TREATMENT

Management is directed toward palliative care as there is no effective treatment.

PATIENT EDUCATION

- There is no vaccine against CJD.
- Preventive measures that reduce transmission include sterilizing medical equipment before use, avoiding the use of infected patients as cornea donors, managing infected animals, and not accepting transfusions from individuals with certain travel histories.

17.3K DENGUE FEVER

Dengue virus is a *Flavivirus* and responsible for dengue fever. It is a mosquito-borne, *Aedes* species, viral infection that causes a self-limited febrile illness, but can give rise to a hemorrhagic fever or shock syndrome. Incidence varies with it being the highest in tropical urban areas in the Americas and Asia.

The virus gains entry via the bite of an infected mosquito and infects immature Langerhans cells. Infected cells disseminate through the lymphatic system. Myeloid dendritic cells, monocytes, and splenic and hepatic macrophages are infected. The incubation period from infected mosquito bite to the development of symptoms is 3 to 5 days. In most cases the virus is cleared and controlled within 1 week.

MEDICAL HISTORY AND CLINICAL PRESENTATION

Risk factors for dengue fever are living or traveling in an endemic region, subtropical and tropical regions, and being exposed to mosquito bites. Transmission is more common in urban, crowded settings.

There are several host factors associated with developing severe disease including age <5 years, female gender, certain HLA alleles, and comorbidities, such as asthma, sickle cell disease, and diabetes mellitus.

SIGNS AND SYMPTOMS

According to WHO there are three classifications for dengue: dengue without warning signs, dengue with warning signs, and severe dengue.

The disease course is divided into three phases:

- Febrile phase presents with abrupt-onset fever and two of the following: headache, retro-orbital pain, arthralgia, myalgia, diffuse rash, and mild hemorrhagic manifestations. This phase usually lasts 2 to 7 days.
- Critical phase lasts 1 to 2 days. As the fever subsides, abdominal pain, persistent vomiting, fluid accumulation, lethargy or restlessness, mucosal bleeding, or hepatomegaly may develop. It may progress to shock due to hemorrhage or plasma leakage. The fatality rate is high.
- During the convalescent phase, the patient becomes hemodynamically stable as plasma leakage stops and the reabsorption of fluids commences. A diffuse, erythematous, maculopapular rash may appear.

PHYSICAL EXAMINATION

Physical examination findings include a positive tourniquet sign, or capillary fragility test, with 10 or more petechiae per square inch after inflating a blood pressure cuff between the systolic and diastolic blood pressure for 5 minutes, positive in dengue hemorrhagic fever; petechiae on the lower extremities, a diffuse erythematous maculopapular rash, decreased skin turgor, and evidence of plasma leakage by fluid accumulation in the form of ascites, diminished breath sounds due to pleural effusion, and hepatomegaly.

DIFFERENTIAL DIAGNOSIS

The differential diagnosis of dengue fever includes other hemorrhagic fevers, Zika, malaria, chikungunya, leptospirosis, typhoid fever, parvovirus B19, HIV, viral hepatitis, and rickettsial infection.

DIAGNOSTIC STUDIES

Laboratory findings include thrombocytopenia, leukopenia, elevated hemoglobin (due to hemoconcentration), and elevated transaminases with liver involvement.

Early in the course of disease the reverse transcription PCR (RT-PCR) allows for the serotyping of the strain and is highly sensitive and specific. Late in the course of the disease IgM ELISA with IgG ELISA on acute and convalescent sera can be used to make the diagnosis.

TREATMENT

No dengue-specific therapy is available. Most cases are self-limited and require only oral fluid administration and acetaminophen. Drugs with antiplatelet and anticoagulant effects should be avoided.

No anti-infective agents are available for dengue.

Infection with dengue provides long-term protection against reinfection with the same type. One vaccine (CYD-TDV) has been approved for use in dengue-endemic territories in children of middle-school age.

PATIENT EDUCATION

- Patients typically recover without any complications, but complications, such as multiorgan failure, associated with hemorrhage and shock can occur.
- Mortality rate due to dengue ranges from 1% to 5% without adequate treatment; with prompt and appropriate treatment, mortality rate is <1%.

17.3L HANTAVIRUS

Hantavirus cardiopulmonary syndrome (HCPS) is caused by zoonotic RNA viruses from the Bunyaviridae family. Sin Nombre virus (SNV), a member of the hantavirus genus, is the major cause of HCPS in North America.

MEDICAL HISTORY AND CLINICAL PRESENTATION

Hantavirus infection occurs by inhalation of dust contaminated by droppings, urine, or saliva from infected rodents, the deer mice. HCPS is a rural disease associated with the risk factors of farming, hunting, and camping. As of January 2017, there have been over 720 cases of hantavirus disease in the United States since reporting started in 1993.[60]

SIGNS AND SYMPTOMS

The incubation period averages from 14 to 17 days. The prodromal phase presents with flu-like symptoms, including fever, headache, chills, and muscle pain in large muscle groups and lasts 2 to 8 days. Other symptoms include abdominal pain, nausea, vomiting, and dizziness. This phase may progress rapidly to severe respiratory disease characterized by nonproductive cough and dyspnea.

PHYSICAL EXAMINATION

Almost 40% of cases will have rapid deterioration, cardiac insufficiency, and respiratory failure caused by edema and hypotension, shock, and death within 2 to 10 days after the onset of illness.[61]

DIAGNOSTIC STUDIES

CXR reveals bilateral pulmonary edema. Hematologic findings include thrombocytopenia and leukocytosis with a left shift. Diagnosis relies on a history of rodent exposure, symptoms of respiratory involvement, severe thrombocytopenia, and positive serologic tests. High titers of IgM and IgG antibodies are detectable in the sera of patients during the acute phase of the disease. PCR will detect viral RNA in blood samples collected during the acute phase.

TREATMENT

No specific antiviral therapies are available. Treatment is hospitalization and supportive care until the virus is cleared. Extracorporeal membrane oxygenation has been successful in a number of severely ill patients.

17.3M YELLOW FEVER

Yellow fever is caused by a single-stranded RNA virus in the genus *Flavivirus*. Vector-borne transmission occurs via the bite of an infected mosquito, *Aedes* or *Haemagogus* species. Human primates are a major reservoir for the virus, with human-to-vector-to-human transmission occurring. Humans infected with the yellow fever virus experience a high level of viremia and can transmit the virus to mosquitoes from just before the onset of fever through the first 3 to 5 days of symptoms.

MEDICAL HISTORY AND CLINICAL PRESENTATION

Yellow fever is endemic and occasionally epidemic in sub-Saharan Africa and tropical South America. Initial symptoms of yellow fever start 3 to 6 days after the mosquito bite. While most patients improve after these initial symptoms, 15% of people will have a period without symptoms and then develop a severe form of yellow fever disease. Possible complications include coma, disseminated intravascular coagulation, renal failure, hepatic failure, and shock. For most patients with mild disease the prognosis is good with a complete recovery.

SIGNS AND SYMPTOMS

Infected patients may have no symptoms; if symptoms develop they include fever, muscle pain (with severe backache), headache, rigors, anorexia, and nausea or vomiting. After 3 to 4 days most patients improve, and symptoms disappear. About 15% of patients will enter the toxic phase in the first 24 hours. In the toxic phase the patient redevelops fever, along with jaundice, abdominal pain with vomiting, bleeding, and renal failure.

PHYSICAL EXAMINATION

Physical findings include fever, jaundice, bleeding in the form of melena, hematemesis, petechiae or ecchymoses, abdominal pain, and hepatomegaly.

DIFFERENTIAL DIAGNOSIS

The differential diagnosis includes Ebola, typhoid fever, malaria, Zika virus, and Lassa fever.

DIAGNOSTIC STUDIES

Abnormal laboratory findings include leukopenia or leukocytosis, bleeding abnormalities, thrombocytopenia, and elevated liver transaminases. Laboratory diagnosis of yellow fever is done via the detection of virus-specific IgM and neutralizing antibodies. PCR can be used to detect viral genome in blood or tissue.

TREATMENT

There are no antivirals approved for the treatment of yellow fever, so vaccination is vital. Treatment is symptomatic and supportive. There is no specific antiviral therapy available. Hypotension is treated with fluid replacement and dialysis may be needed in cases of renal failure.

Vaccination and vector control are the major methods used in the prevention of yellow fever. The yellow fever vaccine is recommended for persons over 9 months of age who are traveling to or living in South America and Africa, in areas at risk for yellow fever.

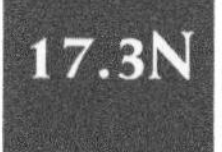

17.3N RESPIRATORY VIRAL INFECTIONS

OVERVIEW

Viral infections commonly affect the upper or lower respiratory tract. Respiratory infections can be classified by viral agent or by the syndrome produced. While specific pathogens commonly cause characteristic clinical manifestations, such as the rhinovirus causes the common cold and RSV causes bronchiolitis, each can cause many of the viral respiratory syndromes. See Table 17.16 for causes of common viral respiratory infections.

EPIDEMIOLOGY

Acute viral respiratory illnesses are one of the most common, accounting for more than one-half of all acute illnesses. The incidence of acute respiratory disease in the United States is 3 to 5.6 cases per person per year.[62] The rates are highest among children <1 year old and remain high until age 6, when a progressive decrease begins. Adults have 3 to 4 cases per person per year.[63] Over 66% of acute respiratory illness are caused by viruses.

TABLE 17.16 Causes of Common Viral Respiratory Infections

Syndrome	Common Etiologies	Uncommon Etiologies
Common cold	Rhinovirus Coronavirus	Influenza virus Parainfluenza virus Adenovirus Enterovirus Human metapneumovirus
Croup	Parainfluenza virus	Influenza virus Respiratory syncytial virus
Bronchiolitis	Respiratory syncytial virus	Influenza virus Parainfluenza virus Adenovirus Rhinovirus
Influenza-like	Influenza virus	Parainfluenza virus Adenovirus
Pneumonia	Influenza virus Adenovirus	Parainfluenza virus Enterovirus Rhinovirus Human metapneumovirus

17.3NA RESPIRATORY SYNCYTIAL VIRUS INFECTION

Human RSV is a single-stranded RNA virus of the family Paramyxoviridae.

In the United States, most infants are infected during their first year of life and almost all children will have been infected by 2 to 3 years of age. RSV causes respiratory tract infections in patients of all ages and is the major cause of lower respiratory tract infection during infancy and childhood. RSV is the most common cause of bronchiolitis and pneumonia in children under the age of 1.

SIGNS AND SYMPTOMS

Symptoms include those of the common cold with rhinorrhea, nasal congestion, and cough. A low-grade fever is possible. In infants the onset of symptoms includes apnea and may be rapid and lead to respiratory failure. Other RSV symptoms noted include listlessness, anorexia, and fever.

PHYSICAL EXAMINATION

The most common symptoms of lower respiratory involvement include cough, retractions, and wheeze.

Wheezing may be dominant; crackles will be noted if pneumonia develops.

DIAGNOSTIC STUDIES

The most common test used to diagnosis RSV is the rapid viral antigen test of nasal washings using PCR or rapid antigen detection test. PCR is highly specific and sensitive and its use is increasing.

Bronchoscopy with bronchoalveolar lavage may be indicated in patients with lower respiratory tract infection.

CXR is typically not indicated but may be indicated in immunocompromised patients with possible pneumonia. Findings vary depending on the clinical syndrome.

TREATMENT

Supportive treatment is the mainstay of therapy for infections due to human RSV. Supportive care includes adequate hydration and supplemental oxygen therapy. Routine use of ribavirin is not recommended.

Supportive care is the mainstay of treatment for bronchiolitis. Clearance of the upper airway using suction can improve respiratory distress, particularly in young infants who are obligate nasal breathers.

If wheezing is assessed on physical examination after suctioning, a trial of bronchodilators is an option. Epinephrine may be more effective but is limited to the hospital setting.

Ribavirin is approved for treatment of lower respiratory infection in high-risk infants and children when delivered in the aerosol form. Ribavirin is useful in preventing the progression from upper respiratory infection associated with RSV to a lower respiratory tract infection in the patients who are immunosuppressed.

Preventive therapy available to prevent severe RSV disease is the monoclonal antibody palivizumab. It is approved for high-risk infants, including preterm babies, and infants with chronic lung disease or hemodynamically significant congenital heart disease.

Outcomes for infants with bronchiolitis are good.

PATIENT EDUCATION

- RSV is a major cause of morbidity in neonates/infants.

17.3NB INFLUENZA

Influenza viruses are orthomyxoviruses. There are three types, A, B and C, with type C causing sporadic mild influenza-like illness in children. Influenza type A is subcategorized by the presence of two surface antigens, hemagglutinin antigen (HA) and neuraminidase antigen (NA). The type A subtypes currently include the H1N1, H1N2, and H3N2 viruses. Influenza B viruses are not separated into subtypes.

Influenza is a contagious airborne disease, affecting the upper respiratory system. Peak influenza activity in the United States is between November and May, with peak incidence in January and February.

Antigenic drift is responsible for the production of new strains of influenza A and B. This antigenic shift or major changes in the influenza A virus lead to pandemics. These changes lead to the creation of new HA or NA components of the influenza A virus.

MEDICAL HISTORY AND CLINICAL PRESENTATION

The influenza virus is transmitted when a person comes in contact with infectious respiratory droplets from coughing or sneezing or from contact with droplet-contaminated surfaces. The incubation period is 1 to 3 days. Shedding of the virus in nasal secretions peaks during the first 3 days of illness and ends in 7 days and is correlated with the degree of fever. Patients are considered infectious during the 24 hours prior to onset of symptoms.

SIGNS AND SYMPTOMS

Influenza virus infection presents with acute onset of fever and chills, rigors, malaise, headache, diffuse myalgia, and nonproductive cough. Other signs and symptoms include nasal congestion, rhinitis, sore throat, and persistent cough. Less common symptoms include abdominal pain, nausea and vomiting, diarrhea, and conjunctival injection.

PHYSICAL EXAMINATION

Physical examination reveals fever, tachycardia, tachypnea, and fatigue. Examination of the upper respiratory tract reveals eye redness and excessive tearing, nasal discharge, and pharyngeal erythema. Lung examination may be normal or present with focal wheezing or rales.

DIFFERENTIAL DIAGNOSIS

The differential diagnosis includes several other respiratory viruses. These include rhinovirus, adenovirus, RSV, parainfluenza virus, and human metapneumovirus. Several atypical bacteria can lead to similar symptoms, and these include *Bordetella pertussis, Mycoplasma pneumoniae,* and *Chlamydia pneumoniae*.

Influenza infection generally presents with a greater severity of symptoms than the more common upper respiratory tract infections. See Table 17.16 for the differential diagnosis of upper respiratory tract infections.

DIAGNOSTIC STUDIES

Diagnostic study samples should be obtained within the first 72 hours of illness. Treatment should not be delayed while awaiting definitive influenza test result.

Tests available for identifying the influenza virus include viral culture, RT-PCR, immunofluorescence, and rapid influenza diagnostic testing (RIDT).

Viral cultures have moderate sensitivity and high specificity but are not recommended due to delay in obtaining test results.

RT-PCR testing is the most sensitive and specific test, used as a confirmatory test, and can be used to differentiate between influenza types and subtypes.

Immunofluorescence, either direct or indirect fluorescent antibody staining for influenza antigen detection, has a lower sensitivity and specificity than viral cell culture and is used as a screening test. Immunofluorescence testing does distinguish between influenza A and B.

RIDT is used as a screening test and has a sensitivity of 50% to 70% and a specificity of 90% to 95%.[64] Results must be interpreted with caution and must consider the disease prevalence.

Other laboratory tests are not needed to confirm the diagnosis of influenza disease. A CBC and blood culture may be indicated if bacterial disease is a concern.

TREATMENT

Antiviral medication should be started within 48 hours from onset of symptoms to reduce the severity and duration of symptoms. In moderate to severe disease, treatment started after 48 hours from the onset of symptoms may still prove beneficial. Antivirals can be effective in preventing influenza but should never be used as a replacement for influenza vaccine.

The antiviral medication available for treatment or prophylaxis of influenza infections includes the neuraminidase inhibitors (oseltamivir and zanamivir), baloxavir, and the adamantanes (amantadine and rimantadine).

The adamantanes (amantadine and rimantadine) block the M2 proton ion channel of the virus and inhibit uncoating of viral RNA in the infected host cell, preventing viral replication in regard to influenza A only. Side effects are numerous and include central nervous system side effects such as nervousness, anxiety, lightheadedness, seizures, and hallucinations. GI side effects include nausea and anorexia. The Advisory Committee on Immunization Practices recommends not using adamantanes for the treatment of influenza.[65]

Oseltamivir and zanamivir are neuraminidase inhibitors that interfere with release of influenza virus from infected host cells preventing spread of infection with in the respiratory tract. Oseltamivir is given orally, and side effects include GI side effects including nausea and vomiting. Transient neuropsychiatric events, such as delirium, have been reported. Zanamivir is inhaled and side effects include cough and bronchospasm. Because of these respiratory side effects, the drug is not indicated in patients with underlying lung disease.

Baloxavir marboxil is a novel selective inhibitor of influenza cap-dependent endonuclease that blocks influenza proliferation by inhibiting the initiation of mRNA synthesis. Baloxavir is approved in the United States for the treatment of acute uncomplicated influenza in adults and children over the age of 12 who have been symptomatic for 48 hours.

Children and adolescents with influenza should never receive aspirin or any salicylate-containing products secondary to the risk of developing Reye syndrome.

Vaccination is the method of choice for prevention of disease. Routine annual influenza vaccination is recommended for all persons age ≥6 months who do not have contraindications. High-risk groups and their contacts should be strongly encouraged to receive the vaccine. These high-risk groups include:

- Children ages 6 through 59 months
- Adults age ≥50 years
- Persons with chronic pulmonary (including asthma), cardiovascular (excluding isolated hypertension), renal, hepatic, neurologic, hematologic, or metabolic disorders (including diabetes mellitus)
- Persons who are immunocompromised due to any cause, including medications or HIV infection
- Women who are or will be pregnant during the influenza season
- Children and adolescents (ages 6 months through 18 years) receiving aspirin- or salicylate-containing medications who might be at risk for Reye syndrome after influenza infection
- Residents of nursing homes and other long-term care facilities
- American Indians/Alaska Natives
- Persons who are extremely obese (BMI ≥40 for adults)
- Caregivers and contacts of those at risk:
  - Healthcare personnel, working in healthcare settings who have potential for exposure to patients and/or to infectious materials
  - Household contacts and caregivers of children age <59 months, particularly contacts of children age <6 months, and adults over age 50 years
  - Household contacts and caregivers of persons with medical conditions associated with increased risk of severe complications from influenza

PATIENT EDUCATION

- Influenza causes significant morbidity and mortality every season. In the 2018 to 2019 influenza season, there were 35.5 million cases in the United States, resulting in 16.5 million medical visits, 490,600 hospitalizations, and 43,200 deaths.[66]
- Most cases of influenza resolve without serious complications for healthy persons between the ages of 2 and 65.
- High-risk groups include patients with hemoglobinopathies, bronchopulmonary dysplasia, asthma, cystic fibrosis, malignancy, diabetes mellitus, chronic renal disease, and congenital heart disease.

17.3NC AVIAN INFLUENZA

Avian influenza is caused by influenza A virus in the Orthomyxoviridae family. Birds are the natural host and multiple genetic changes are required for the virus to be transmitted and infect humans. Illness in humans ranges from mild disease to rapidly progressive respiratory disease and death.

MEDICAL HISTORY AND CLINICAL PRESENTATION

The major risk factor for infection in humans is exposure to infected poultry live or dead, or contaminated avian environments. The major types are H5N1, which has an aggressive clinical course; and H7N9, first reported in China. Travel history is key to making the diagnosis. The incubation period for H5N1 avian influenza is 2 to 8 days.

SIGNS AND SYMPTOMS

Distinguishing avian influenza from seasonal influenza is difficult. The signs and symptoms of avian influenza A virus infections range from mild to severe and include high fever, cough, pharyngitis, and myalgias. Other symptoms include conjunctivitis, nausea and vomiting, abdominal pain, and diarrhea. Severe respiratory symptoms, such as dyspnea, acute respiratory distress, and respiratory failure, can develop.

PHYSICAL EXAMINATION

Physical examination may reveal fever, tachycardia, tachypnea, and other symptoms that may indicate organ failure. Other physical examination findings are consistent with seasonal influenza.

DIFFERENTIAL DIAGNOSIS

Avian influenza should be differentiated from other diseases that cause respiratory tract infections or flu-like illness. This includes other influenza viruses; viral, bacterial, and fungal causes of pneumonia; and other pulmonary diseases such as asthma or chronic obstructive pulmonary disease.

DIAGNOSTIC STUDIES

Current rapid antigen tests are not sensitive or specific for the detection of H5N1 influenza. RT-PCR testing is the test of choice.

TREATMENT

Patients with severe disease and confirmed and probable cases with mild disease should be treated as soon as possible. First-line treatment is the neuraminidase inhibitors, oseltamivir or zanamivir, for 5 days. Longer treatment may be needed in severe disease. In most areas the H5N1 strains are resistant to amantadine and rimantadine.

PATIENT EDUCATION

- Avoidance is the key to preventing avian influenza. Precautions should be taken in patients exposed to poultry.
- Postexposure prophylaxis is recommended for close contacts exposed to patients with proven disease. Treatment consists of oseltamivir or zanamivir.
- Current vaccines do not provide cross protection against strains of H5, H7, or H9 influenza viruses.

17.3ND CORONAVIRUSES

There are several coronaviruses, but only seven are known to cause disease in humans. Four of the seven coronaviruses frequently cause symptoms of the common cold. Coronaviruses 229E, OC43, and serotypes NL63 and HUK1 are associated with the common cold.

Three of the seven coronaviruses cause much more severe, sometimes fatal, respiratory infections in humans and have caused major outbreaks of deadly pneumonia. These include:

- **SARS-CoV-2:** identified as the etiology of coronavirus disease 2019 (COVID-19) that began in Wuhan, China in late 2019 and spread worldwide
- **MERS-CoV:** identified in 2012 as the cause of Middle East respiratory syndrome (MERS)
- **SARS-CoV:** identified in 2002 as the cause of an outbreak of SARS

All are spread via person-to-person contact and respiratory droplets. These coronaviruses that cause severe respiratory infections are zoonotic pathogens. See Table 17.17 for a comparison of COVID-19, MERS, and SARS.

17.3O COXSACKIE VIRUS

Coxsackie virus is an enterovirus in the Picornaviridae family. There are 23 coxsackie A viruses and 6 coxsackie B viruses. The mode of transmission is typically via the fecal-oral route. Enteroviruses can also spread through contact with virus-contaminated oral secretions, vesicular fluid, contaminated surfaces or fomites, and viral respiratory droplets.

This group of viruses leads to several disorders; see Table 17.18 for a summary of the various disorders.

This section focuses on hand, foot, and mouth disease and herpangina.

Hand, foot, and mouth disease is a common, highly contagious disease of children and infants, most common in the summer and fall months. The etiology is coxsackie virus A16 and patients presents with fever and sores on the hands and feet. It is spread via direct contact with oral secretion and feces of infected people.

Herpangina is a self-limited infection of the upper respiratory tract, most often in the pediatric age group and most common in the summer. Herpangina begins with a sudden fever, pharyngitis, dysphagia, and the appearance of a rash.

TABLE 17.17 Disorders Due to Coronaviruses

Feature	SARS	MERS	COVID-19
Clinical Findings			
Fever or chills	+	+	+
Dyspnea	+	+	+
Malaise	+	+	+
Headache	+	+	+
Cough	Dry	Dry or productive	Dry
Diarrhea	+	+	Uncommon
Nausea/vomiting	+	+	Uncommon
Sore throat	+	Uncommon	Uncommon
Arthralgia	+	Uncommon	
Diagnosis			
Imaging normal	15%–20%	17%	15%–20%
Imaging common	Peripheral multifocal airspace opacities on CXR and CT	Peripheral multifocal airspace opacities on CXR and CT	Peripheral multifocal airspace opacities on CXR and CT
Laboratory testing		rRT-PCR	
Treatment	Supportive	Supportive	Supportive
Mortality	9.6%	34.3%	3.4%

+, present; COVID-19, coronavirus disease 2019; CXR, chest x-ray; MERS, Middle East respiratory syndrome; rRT-PCR, real-time reverse transcriptase-polymerase chain reaction; SARS, severe acute respiratory syndrome.

TABLE 17.18 Disorders Due to Coxsackie Viruses

Coxsackie A Virus	Coxsackie B Virus
Hand, foot, and mouth disease	Pericarditis
Herpangina	Myocarditis
Acute hemorrhagic conjunctivitis	Hepatitis
Aseptic meningitis	Acute flaccid paralysis (coxsackie B4 virus)

MEDICAL HISTORY AND CLINICAL PRESENTATION

Hand, foot, and mouth disease presents with fever, headache, anorexia, pharyngitis, ulcerations on the throat, mouth, and tongue, and a tender or painful vesicular rash with small blisters on the hands, feet, and diaper area. Hand, foot, and mouth disease starts with fever and 1 to 2 days later sores develop in the mouth. These sores blister and become ulcers.

Herpangina presents with fever, pharyngitis, dysphagia, myalgia, headache, vomiting, and abdominal pain. The pharyngitis and dysphagia occur 24 hours before the rash appears.

PHYSICAL EXAMINATION

Patients with hand, foot, and mouth disease will appear ill with fever. The lesions in the mouth are irregularly shaped shallow ulcers with a yellow-gray base and red margin. The lesions are noted on the tongue, buccal mucosa, soft palate, and pharynx. Skin lesions are vesicles on the hands, feet, and buttocks.

Herpangina presents with sudden onset of fever, and on physical examination the rash presents with punctate macules that evolve into 2- to 4-mm erythematous papules that become vesicles and then centrally ulcerate. The lesions are noted on the soft palate and uvula, tonsils, posterior pharyngeal wall, and buccal mucosa.

DIFFERENTIAL DIAGNOSIS

The differential diagnosis includes herpes simplex, chickenpox, and measles (Table 17.19).

DIAGNOSTIC STUDIES

Physical examination is typically diagnostic for hand, foot, and mouth disease. Laboratory studies may be needed to rule out other possible disorders.

TREATMENT

No specific treatment is available for the management of hand, foot, and mouth disease or herpangina. Symptomatic

TABLE 17.19 Differential Diagnosis for Coxsackie Virus Infection

Diagnosis	Description
Coxsackie virus infection	Presents with fever, headache, anorexia, pharyngitis, ulcerations on the throat, mouth and tongue, and a tender or painful vesicular rash with small blisters on the hands, feet and buttocks.
Chickenpox	Prodrome of headache, fever, and malaise. The vesicular rash typically begins on the face and then moves over the trunk and extremities.
Measles	The prodrome consists of nonspecific respiratory symptoms. Koplik spots on the buccal mucosa is pathognomonic. Develop fever, cough, conjunctivitis, and coryza. Later the typical maculopapular, erythematous, nonpruritic rash begins on the head and face and progresses down the body.
Herpangina	Presents with sudden onset of fever, on examination the rash is punctate macules that over 24 hours evolve into 2–4 mm erythematous papules that become vesicles and then centrally ulcerate. Lesions noted on the soft palate and uvula.
Herpes simplex	Presents with vesicles on the buccal mucosa, tongue, pharynx, and palate. Vesicles rupture to form ulcerations.

treatment includes antipyretics, hydration, analgesics, and topical oral anesthetic.

17.3P ECHOVIRUS

Echovirus is an RNA virus from the genus *Enterovirus* of the family Picornaviridae. Echoviruses are found in the GI tract and infection with the virus causes OI and severe systemic disease. The "echo-" prefix originally was an acronym for "enteric cytopathic human orphan."

MEDICAL HISTORY AND CLINICAL PRESENTATION

Echovirus is very infectious and primarily causes infection in children. The echovirus is one of the leading causes of acute febrile illness in infants and young children and is the most common cause of aseptic meningitis. Infection of an infant with this virus following birth can cause severe systemic disease and is associated with a high infant mortality rate.

SIGNS AND SYMPTOMS

Symptoms depend on the site of infection and include difficulty breathing with a harsh cough, mouth sores, rashes, and pharyngitis. Chest pain can be noted if the infection affects the heart muscle or pericardial sac leading to pericarditis. Severe headache, mental status changes, fever and chills, nausea and vomiting can be noted if the virus infects the central nervous system leading to meningitis.

PHYSICAL EXAMINATION

Physical examination findings depend on the location of the infection.

DIAGNOSTIC STUDIES

Because the illness is often mild and has no specific treatment, testing for echovirus is not done.

TREATMENT

Treatment is directed at symptomatic care. There is no specific treatment for echovirus infection.

PATIENT EDUCATION

- Patients with mild disease should recover completely without treatment.

17.3Q ZIKA VIRUS

Zika virus, an arthropod-borne virus, is a member of the family Flaviviridae. The primary vectors are the *Aedes* species mosquitoes. Sexual transmission of Zika has also been reported, and the virus can persist for weeks to months in semen. Zika virus is found in other body fluids such as saliva and urine.

Zika virus was associated with only sporadic human cases until 2007, when it caused an outbreak on the Micronesian island of Yap. It then spread to French Polynesia and Easter Island and then the Americas in early 2015. Indigenous transmission has been reported in most countries in the Caribbean and Central and South America. As a result of herd immunity, transmission has died down on many of the islands that were initially affected.

The Zika virus infects human embryonic neural progenitor cells. Once infected the cells experience increased cell death, cell cycle and transcription dysregulation, and produce infectious viral particles.

MEDICAL HISTORY AND CLINICAL PRESENTATION

A vast majority of people infected are asymptomatic. The patients who present with symptoms typically have a mild self-limited illness lasting 2 to 7 days. Congenital infections are linked to microcephaly and other neurologic abnormalities in the neonate. Death due to Zika is very rare but has been noted in patients with sickle cell disease, congenital Zika infection, and post-Zika Guillain-Barré syndrome.

SIGNS AND SYMPTOMS

Most patients are asymptomatic. Other symptoms include fever, arthralgias, myalgias, headache, macular or papular rash, conjunctivitis, and edema.

PHYSICAL EXAMINATION

Physical examination is usually remarkable for fever and a maculopapular rash that involves the face, trunk, and extremities. It may involve the palms and soles. Other physical examination findings include nonpurulent conjunctivitis and edema.

DIFFERENTIAL DIAGNOSIS

The differential diagnosis for Zika infection includes dengue fever, chikungunya, malaria, WNV infection, Venezuelan equine encephalitis, Epstein-Barr infection, parvovirus infection, acute HIV infection, and influenza.

DIAGNOSTIC STUDIES

Laboratory results include a normal CBC, but a mild thrombocytopenia may be noted.

The diagnosis of Zika infection can be confirmed with a positive Zika-specific RT-PCR. The serum, urine or whole blood test may be positive within the first week of symptom onset. After 1 week onset, Zika can be diagnosed by IgM ELISA, but *Flavivirus* cross-reactivity to related flaviviruses may occur and ELISAs should be confirmed by plaque reduction neutralization testing. Zika is a nationally notifiable condition in the United States.

For mild disease in a nonpregnant individual, no imaging is indicated. If Zika exposure is suspected in a pregnant woman, serial fetal ultrasounds are recommended to assess for microcephaly and other intracranial abnormalities.

EVALUATION

There is an association between Zika virus and microcephaly. Other abnormalities include intrauterine growth restriction with and without microcephaly, cerebral calcifications, cerebral atrophy, agenesis vermis, abnormal arterial flow in cerebral or umbilical arteries, oligohydramnios, and anhydramnios.

The CDC recommends the following management plan for pregnant women with a history of travel to an area with ongoing Zika transmission[63]:

- Zika virus NAAT testing should be obtained in symptomatic patients up to 12 weeks after onset of symptoms and should be considered in asymptomatic patients up to 12 weeks after travel to Zika infection risk area.
- Zika virus IgM antibody testing is not recommended because IgM can persist for months after infection; therefore, IgM results cannot reliably determine whether an infection occurred during the current pregnancy.

For pregnant women with a clinically compatible illness and recent possible exposure to dengue and Zika virus with a specimen collected within 12 weeks of symptom onset:

- Specimens should be collected as soon as possible after onset.
- The following diagnostic testing should be performed at the same time:
  - Dengue and Zika virus NAAT and dengue IgM antibody testing on a serum specimen, and
  - Zika virus NAAT on a urine specimen
- A positive NAAT result on any specimen typically provides adequate evidence of recent infection. However, if NAAT is only positive for Zika virus on a single specimen and IgM antibody testing is negative, the NAAT should be repeated on newly extracted RNA from the same specimen to rule out false positive NAAT results.
- If both dengue and Zika virus NAATs are negative but either IgM antibody test is positive, confirmatory PRNTs should be performed against dengue, Zika, and other flaviviruses endemic to the region where exposure occurred.

TREATMENT

No specific therapies or vaccines currently exist. Treatment is supportive. For mild disease, symptoms can be alleviated with analgesics and antipyretics. There is no postexposure prophylaxis or vaccine available.

Infection control is best accomplished by avoiding mosquito bites. Precautions should include applying insect repellant, wearing permethrin-impregnated clothing, staying in screened environments, and using mosquito netting.

SPECIAL CONSIDERATIONS

- According to CDC guidelines Zika testing should be offered to pregnant women with exposure history with or without clinical symptoms of Zika. If the ultrasound is positive, serial ultrasounds every 3 to 4 weeks should be considered to evaluate for brain anomalies. At the time of delivery, the placental tissue should undergo histopathologic examination.[63]
- If the woman tests negative for Zika, she should receive routine prenatal care including a fetal anatomy ultrasound at 18 to 20 weeks of gestation. The ultrasound should be used to evaluate for the presence of microcephaly or intracranial calcifications; if any abnormalities exist, additional ultrasounds should be considered as the pregnancy progresses. Referral to a fetal-maternal specialist is recommended for pregnant women testing positive or inconclusive for Zika.

17.3R WEST NILE VIRUS INFECTION

WNV is a mosquito-transmitted arbovirus of the family Flaviviridae. Several bird species are normal reservoirs for the virus, with incidental human transmission mediated by the *Culex* genus of mosquitoes.

WNV disease should be part of the differential diagnosis in any patient with a febrile or acute neurologic illness with a history of recent exposure to mosquitoes, blood transfusion, or organ transplantation, especially during the summer months in areas where virus activity has been reported.

WNV is widely distributed across North America. Peak transmission occurs between June and September. In 2019, there were 958 cases of WNV disease, 626 classified as neuroinvasive and 332 as non-neuroinvasive; more than 2,600 West Nile diagnoses were recorded. In 2019, 54 people died from the disease.[67]

MEDICAL HISTORY AND CLINICAL PRESENTATION

Most cases are transmitted by mosquito bite, but can be transmitted by organ transplantation, blood transfusion, and from mother to infant during pregnancy, delivery, or breastfeeding. Human-to-human transmission and sexual transmission has not been noted. The incubation period is 2 to 6 days, but it may extend to 14 days.

West Nile fever presents as a systemic febrile illness with headache, retro-orbital and back pain, arthralgias, and myalgias. Other signs and symptoms include vomiting, diarrhea, cough, and sore throat. A maculopapular rash on the chest, back, and arms may be noted.

Most patients recover, though fatigue can persist for weeks. A small percentage of patients, typically those over age 60 or immunocompromised, develop neuroinvasive disease, with headache, fever, neck stiffness, altered mental status, tremors, seizures, or paralysis.

Neuroinvasive disease presents with up to a week of prodrome symptoms including fever, followed by neurologic symptoms. Manifestations of WNV encephalitis range from mild confusion to coma and death.

SIGNS AND SYMPTOMS

A majority of human WNV infections are subclinical or asymptomatic. Symptomatic patients present with an acute febrile illness with headache, weakness, myalgia, or arthralgia; GI symptoms and a transient maculopapular rash are common. Neuroinvasive disease presents with meningitis, encephalitis, or acute flaccid paralysis. WNV acute flaccid paralysis is usually clinically identical to poliovirus-associated poliomyelitis, with damage of anterior horn cells, and may result to respiratory paralysis.

PHYSICAL EXAMINATION

Physical examination may reveal ophthalmologic manifestations such as uveitis, vitritis, vasculitis, and vitreal hemorrhage. Neurologic findings include signs of basal ganglia damage, such as increased tone, rigidity, resting tremor, and bradykinesia. Cases of myelitis present with an asymmetric polio-like flaccid paralysis. Skin findings include an erythematous maculopapular rash.

DIFFERENTIAL DIAGNOSIS

The differential diagnosis includes other causes of encephalitis and aseptic meningitis, such as HSV and enteroviruses, and other arboviruses, such as La Crosse, St. Louis encephalitis, Eastern equine encephalitis, and Powassan viruses.

DIAGNOSTIC STUDIES

Routine clinical laboratory studies are nonspecific. The WBC count may vary, and hyponatremia may be present. With neuroinvasive disease the CSF will reveal an increase in total WBCs with an increase in lymphocytes and an elevated total protein. MRI of the brain is frequently normal, but signal abnormalities in the basal ganglia, thalamus, and brainstem may be seen in patients with encephalitis, and in the anterior spinal cord in patients with poliomyelitis.

Laboratory tests used to confirm the diagnosis include presence of WNV in the CSF by PCR. Serum IgM antibody testing is positive in most patients 7 to 10 days after illness onset. CSF IgM antibody should also be tested as it may appear before serum IgM.

Meningitis or encephalitis is diagnosed by the detection of WNV ribonucleic acid by PCR or WNV IgM in CSF.

TREATMENT

There is no proven antiviral therapy for WNV encephalitis and no vaccines. Treatment is supportive.

PATIENT EDUCATION

- WNV encephalitis is associated with a poor prognosis.
- With myelitis and flaccid paralysis, incomplete recovery is typical. Improvement may occur, but residual deficits are typical.

17.3S ROTAVIRUS

Rotavirus is a nonenveloped, double-stranded, RNA virus of the Reoviridae family. Considered a single pathogen, the rotavirus genus includes several distinct groups, each causing diarrheal disease. The virus is stable in the environment.

Infants between 6 months and 3 years of age are at greatest risk for infection and severe gastroenteritis. This increased risk is due to weakening of the passive maternal immunity and that active host immunity has not matured. A very small inoculum is needed for transmission.

Fecal-oral contact is the most likely etiology for spread of the disease. In northern latitudes the incidence peaks in the autumn and winter months and spreads geographically from west to east.

Infection causes a structural protein change that enables rotavirus fusion and entry into the cell. The virus induces diarrhea by the destruction of intestinal villi reducing overall surface area and the total number of functioning epithelial cells needed for adequate absorption of sodium, glucose, and water.

MEDICAL HISTORY AND CLINICAL PRESENTATION

Symptoms present within 1 to 3 days of infection. Clinical disease starts with low-grade fever and emesis followed by profuse, nonbloody diarrhea. In children, most cases are self-limited, but a small percentage will develop severe volume depletion with hypotension, tachycardia, and metabolic acidosis. Adults present with similar signs and symptoms but are less likely to develop serious complications.

SIGNS AND SYMPTOMS

Rotavirus disease is characterized by vomiting, more prolonged than other GI virus infections, and watery diarrhea. Presence of bloody diarrhea excludes rotavirus as the diagnosis. Other symptoms include fever, abdominal pain, and anorexia. Symptoms of dehydration may develop and include decreased urine output, dry mucous membranes, and sleepiness or increased irritability.

Rotavirus infection can recur due to full immunity not developing after vaccination or natural infection.

PHYSICAL EXAMINATION

Patients infected with rotavirus infection appear lethargic and pale in severe cases. Patients will be hypotensive and have an elevated temperature. Signs of dehydration in infants includes sunken eye and depressed fontanelles.

DIFFERENTIAL DIAGNOSIS

The differential diagnosis includes infection with viruses, such as coronavirus, enterovirus, adenovirus, hepatitis A, or bacteria, such as enterotoxigenic *Escherichia coli*, *Salmonella* species, and *Campylobacter* strains.

DIAGNOSTIC STUDIES

Laboratory abnormalities are nonspecific. The most common abnormalities include electrolyte disturbances in cases of severe dehydration. The liver transaminases and uric acid levels can also be elevated during infection. There is no elevation in WBC count in the blood or stool.

Laboratory confirmation of rotavirus infection is rarely needed. Antigen testing is the test of choice. Both EIA and latex agglutination have high sensitivity but require a very large viral burden to detect infection. There is also a high rate of false positives in neonates. PCR assays are also used and have an enhanced sensitivity and specificity.

TREATMENT

Since the major cause of morbidity and mortality are dehydration and electrolyte abnormalities, oral rehydration is the mainstay of therapy. WHO recommends that those who can tolerate oral intake should be given a rehydration formula of low osmolarity sodium, potassium, chloride, glucose, and bicarbonate or citrate. In severe gastroenteritis or hypotension, IV rehydration should be used.

Anti-infectives are not recommended for the treatment of rotavirus gastroenteritis. With rotavirus, only one agent, nitazoxanide, an antiprotozoal, has demonstrated some benefit.

Rotavirus spreads easily among infants and young children. Good hygiene measures like handwashing are important but are not enough to control the spread of the disease. Rotavirus vaccine is the best way to protect children against rotavirus disease. With RotaTeg 94% of children who get the vaccine are protected from severe rotavirus disease and 74% are protected from rotavirus disease of any severity.[68]

Currently there are two rotavirus vaccines licensed for infants in the United States:

- RotaTeq (RV5) is given in three doses at ages 2 months, 4 months, and 6 months.
- Rotarix (RV1) is given in two doses at ages 2 months and 4 months.

The first dose of either vaccine should be given before a child is 15 weeks of age and all doses of the rotavirus vaccine should be given before 8 months of age.

PATIENT EDUCATION

- The most common complications of rotaviral infection occur because of dehydration and associated electrolyte abnormalities.
- There is an association with lactose intolerance in young children and this may persist.
- The prognosis for rotavirus gastroenteritis is generally excellent in settings in which the infected have access to clean, potable water supplies and nutrients that can act as rehydration solutes.

SPECIAL CONSIDERATIONS

- Mumps infection during the first trimester of pregnancy has been associated with spontaneous abortion, though there is no demonstrated risk of congenital anomalies to infants born following maternal infection.

KEY POINTS

- Respiratory viral infections are typically spread via respiratory droplets person-to-person.
- The main symptoms of viral GI infections are vomiting and diarrhea.
- The mainstay of therapy for viral GI infections is supportive care. Disease spread can be prevented via hand-washing and good sanitation measures.

17.4 *RICKETTSIA* INFECTION

OVERVIEW

Rickettsial infection and related diseases are due to a group of gram-negative, obligately intracellular coccobacilli. All have an arthropod vector, except for *Coxiella burnetii*. Symptoms include fever with severe headache, malaise, and a characteristic rash. The diagnosis is made clinically and confirmed by IFA or PCR. See Table 17.20 for summary of diseases caused by *Rickettsia*, *Orientia*, *Ehrlichia*, *Anaplasma*, and *Coxiella*.

Rickettsial and related diseases may be confused with other acute infections including rubeola, rubella, and meningococcemia. A history of vector contact can be helpful. Rubeola rash begins on the face, spreads to the trunk and arms, and then becomes confluent. Rubella rash usually remains discrete, and the presence of postauricular lymph

TABLE 17.20 Diseases Caused by *Rickettsia, Orientia, Ehrlichia, Anaplasma*, and *Coxiella*

Disease	Organism	Rash/Eschar	Vector	Location
Epidemic typhus	*Rickettsia prowazekii*	Trunk to extremities No eschar	Body lice	Worldwide
Murine typhus	*Rickettsia typhi*	Trunk to extremities No eschar	Rat flea	Worldwide
Scrub typhus	*Orientia tsutsugamushi*	Trunk to extremities Eschar present	Chiggers	Asia-Pacific
Rocky Mountain spotted fever	*Rickettsia rickettsii*	Extremities to trunk No eschar	Wood tick Dog tick	Western Hemisphere
Rickettsialpox	*Rickettsia akari*	Trunk, extremities, face Eschar present	Mites	United States, Russia, Korea
Ehrlichiosis	*Ehrlichia chaffeensis*	Rash rare No eschar	Lone star tick	Southeast/South central United States
Anaplasmosis	*Anaplasma phagocytophilum*	No rash No eschar	Deer tick	Northeast, Mid-Atlantic, Upper Midwest, West Coast United States
Q fever	*Coxiella burnetii*	Rash rare No eschar	No vector	Worldwide

node enlargement and lack of toxicity suggest rubella. Meningococcemia presents with a rapidly developing, petechial rash that may become confluent.

EPIDEMIOLOGY

Rickettsia infections are mostly vector-borne, transmitted by ticks, body lice, and fleas. In most cases humans are an accidental hosts. Cases are reported year round, but most cases are noted between April and September, same time as peak levels of tick host-seeking activity.

PATHOPHYSIOLOGY

Rickettsia infect vascular endothelial cells lining the small and medium vessels throughout the body. The infection of endothelial cells leads to disseminated inflammation, loss of barrier function, and altered vascular permeability. This leads to the fever, myalgias, central nervous system symptoms such as a headache and confusion, rash, and cardiovascular instability.

17.4A TYPHUS INFECTION

The typhus group of *Rickettsia* organisms includes *R. prowazekii*, the agent of epidemic typhus, and *R. typhi*, the agent of endemic or murine typhus. This group of organisms are transmitted by insects, lice or fleas. *R. prowazekii* is maintained by horizontal transmission, while *R. typhi* is acquired and maintained by both horizontal and vertical transmission. Epidemic typhus is a disease of the colder months, while endemic typhus occurs in warm climates.

After infection the organisms spread directly to the blood-stream and target endothelial cells. The bacteria bind to the target cell and phagocytosis is induced. The bacteria escape the phagosomes into the cytosol and multiply within the cytosol until mechanical lysis occurs. This causes infection of additional cells, inducing a vasculitis and vascular dysfunction. Inflammatory mediators are released, increasing microvascular permeability. Passage of fluids into surrounding tissues and lesions occurs, leading to rash, edema, and hemorrhage.

In the case of epidemic typhus, after cure, bacteria are not totally cleared and years later may recur in susceptible hosts; this is called Brill-Zinsser disease.

MEDICAL HISTORY AND CLINICAL PRESENTATION

Epidemic typhus is transmitted to humans by the infected body louse, *Pediculus humanus corporis*. The transmission of *R. prowazekii* occurs via contamination of broken skin, conjunctivae, or mucous membranes by the feces or crushed bodies of infected lice. *R. prowazekii* can persist for 100 days in the feces of lice.

Endemic typhus is transmitted to humans via the rat flea, *Xenopsylla cheopis*. Human beings are contaminated either by infected flea feces into damaged skin or the respiratory tract, or by direct flea bite.

SIGNS AND SYMPTOMS

The clinical manifestations of endemic typhus and epidemic typhus are similar, except that endemic typhus is less severe. Both begin with abrupt onset, typically 8 to 16 days following exposure. Signs and symptoms include fever, chills, severe headaches, myalgias, arthralgias, dry cough, nausea, and vomiting.

PHYSICAL EXAMINATION

Typhus presents with high-grade fever and a maculopapular rash. The rash develops 7 days after the onset of fever. In the early stages the rash is discrete, pink macular lesions that become maculopapular. The rash starts on the trunk and spreads outward. The rash spares the face, palms, and soles. Eschars are absent in typhus group rickettsial disease.

Generalized lymphadenopathy is present in the majority of the patients.

DIFFERENTIAL DIAGNOSIS

The differential diagnosis of epidemic and endemic typhus includes RMSF, meningococcemia, measles, typhoid fever, meningitis, secondary syphilis, leptospirosis, IM, and rubella.

DIAGNOSTIC STUDIES

Laboratory abnormalities include anemia, thrombocytopenia, increased ESR, increased hepatic transaminases, and hypoalbuminemia.

Diagnosis is made by immunofluorescence. Testing a sample obtained from the convalescent phase is required to confirm the initial diagnosis.

Separation of epidemic typhus from endemic typhus is based on a fourfold increase of specific antibody titer in the case of epidemic typhus. The two diseases can also be distinguished by Western blot combined with cross-adsorption tests.

TREATMENT

The treatment of choice is doxycycline, which should be started in any suspected case without waiting for laboratory confirmation. Treatment should continue until 3 days after the patient becomes afebrile. In doxycycline-hypersensitive patients or pregnant women, chloramphenicol can be used as an alternative treatment. Ciprofloxacin does not protect a patient with epidemic typhus from death, but it may be used as an alternative treatment for endemic typhus.

Preventing spread of epidemic and endemic typhus is by limiting the spread of lice and fleas and to eliminate conditions that facilitate their spread. Delousing measures such as changing and washing clothes and bathing patients should be considered. Insecticides are also effective louse-eradication measures. Prevention of endemic typhus can be accomplished by controlling vectors and the reservoirs.

PATIENT EDUCATION

- Death is rare in endemic typhus if the appropriate antibiotics are given.

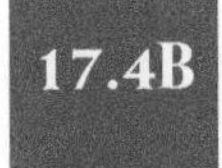

17.4B ROCKY MOUNTAIN SPOTTED FEVER

RMSF is caused by infection with the obligate intracellular bacterium, *Rickettsia rickettsii*. The bacterium life cycles between ticks and small mammal hosts, like field mice. When an infected tick bites a human and transmits the organism, it disseminates to infect endothelial cells in all tissues and organs, compromising vascular function, increased vascular permeability, and leading to end-organ ischemia and damage.

Infection occurs in all states in the United States except Alaska and Vermont; the incidence is much higher in the South Central, Southeast, and Mountain states. Most cases in the United States occur in the summer months of June to August.

The ticks involved include the American dog tick (*Dermacentor variabilis*) in eastern and south central United States and the wood tick (*Dermacentor andersoni*) in the mountain states west of the Mississippi River.

Tick attachment for approximately 6 to 10 hours is needed to reactivate rickettsial virulence, providing a short window for tick removal and transmission prevention. RMSF virtually only occurs after tick bites; thus, a history of tick bite or exposure to tick habitats is an important feature, typically in the prior 10 days since the incubation period is 1 week.

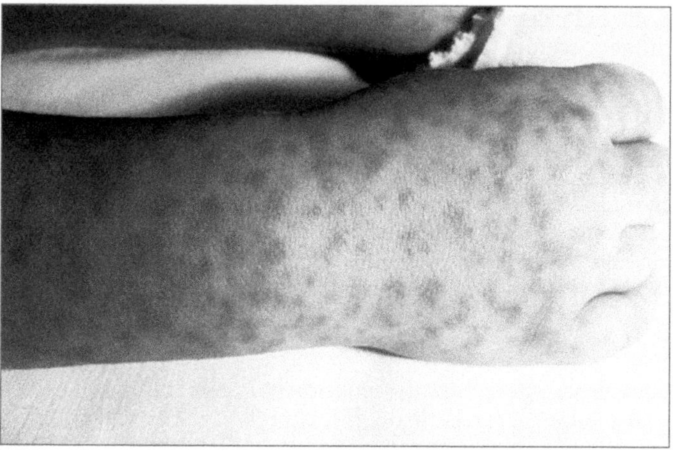

Figure 17.14 Skin rash noted in Rocky mountain spotted fever. *(Source: Centers for Disease Control and Prevention. https://phil.cdc.gov/Details.aspx?pid=1962)*

MEDICAL HISTORY AND CLINICAL PRESENTATION

RMSF is the only rickettsial disease in which the rash starts peripherally and there is no eschar identifying the initial bite site of the vector. Patients will give a history of a tick bite, or a history of a possible exposure to ticks.

The disease presents with nonspecific symptoms of fever, headache, and myalgias. Only a small percentage of patients will have a rash at the time of presentation; the rash typically develops on the third or fourth day of illness.

SIGNS AND SYMPTOMS

Early diagnosis is typically based on clinical grounds alone, and rapid diagnosis is critical to avoid adverse outcomes. The most common symptoms include fever, a macular, maculopapular, or petechial rash, and nausea or vomiting. Other signs and symptoms include headache, myalgia, and abdominal pain. The rash is petechial in nature and begins on the wrists and ankles with spread to the rest of the body.

RMSF is an acute, sudden onset disease, escalating over days. The illness lasts generally <2 weeks if untreated. The fever resolves around 9 days after onset.

PHYSICAL EXAMINATION

The diagnosis of RMSF is made based on clinical signs and symptoms, and later confirmed using laboratory tests. Treatment should never be delayed pending laboratory test results, or withheld on the basis of an initial negative finding for *R. rickettsii*.

Initial physical examination findings include fever, muscle tenderness, and anorexia. Later findings are development of the maculopapular or petechial rash, abdominal tenderness, and joint pain.

Rash is very common during the course of the disease. The classic rash of RMSF first appears 2 to 5 days after the onset of fever and appears as small, flat, pink, nonpruritic macules on the wrists, forearm, and ankles and then spreads to the trunk and palms and soles. The transition of red to purple discoloration indicates a progression to severe disease (Figure 17.14).

DIFFERENTIAL DIAGNOSIS

The differential diagnosis includes other rickettsial infections, such as ehrlichiosis, anaplasmosis, and murine typhus. Rash and septic-like presentations can occur with meningococcemia. Other disorders to consider in the differential diagnosis include enteroviruses, typhoid fever, secondary syphilis, Lyme disease, leptospirosis, scarlet and rheumatic fever, rubella, parvovirus infection, KD, idiopathic thrombocytopenic purpura, thrombotic thrombocytopenic purpura, and Henoch-Schönlein purpura/HUS.

DIAGNOSTIC STUDIES

The diagnosis of RMSF depends on clinical, historical, and laboratory findings. The WBC count is often normal but can be elevated and thrombocytopenia is common. Hyponatremia is typical and as the disease progresses, acute kidney injury and hepatic involvement appear and may progress to multiorgan failure.

The standard serologic test for diagnosis of RMSF is the IFA assay for IgG using *R. rickettsii* antigen. The IgG IFA assays should be performed on paired acute and convalescent serum samples collected 2 to 4 weeks apart to demonstrate evidence of a fourfold seroconversion. RMSF cannot be confirmed using single acute antibody results. Most tests are unable to differentiate one spotted fever infection from another using these serologic methods.

Antibodies to *R. rickettsii* may remain elevated for many months after the disease has resolved. In certain people, high titers of antibodies against *R. rickettsii* have been observed up to 4 years after the acute illness. Comparison of paired, and appropriately timed, serologic assays provides the best evidence of recent infection.

PCR amplification is performed on DNA extracted from whole blood. Although a positive PCR result is helpful, a negative result does not rule out the diagnosis, and treatment should not be withheld because of a negative result.

TREATMENT

Most RMSF infections are severe enough to require hospitalization. Long-term complications, especially neurologic sequelae, include speech/swallowing dysfunction, encephalopathy, ataxia, cortical blindness, and behavioral and learning disabilities. Ischemic injury can result in autoamputation of digits, even limbs, and can cause long-term disability.

The treatment of choice is doxycycline. This should be given even to children and pregnant women since it is the only proven effective therapy and the diseases have high mortality and morbidity rates. Chloramphenicol is the alternative but is associated with rare serious adverse effects. Early treatment, before day 5 of illness, increases the likelihood of a good outcome. Treatment should be continued until 3 days after fever resolves and clinical improvement is observed. The typical treatment duration is 7 to 10 days.

PATIENT EDUCATION

- RMSF is a nationally reportable condition.
- Prophylactic doxycycline for tick bites is considered contraindicated because it is only bacteriostatic for *R. rickettsii* and only a few ticks in endemic areas are infected.
- No effective vaccine is available.
- Preventive measures include avoiding tick-infested environments; "tick checks" with prompt removal of any attached ticks; use of long pants and long-sleeve shirts; and tick repellants.

17.4C EHRLICHIOSIS

Four primary illnesses are linked to an *Ehrlichia* infection: human ehrlichiosis ewingii (HEE), human monocytotropic ehrlichiosis, ehrlichiosis muris-like (EML), human granulocytotropic anaplasmosis. ehrlichiosis is caused by the bacteria *Ehrlichia chaffeensis*, *E. ewingii*, or *E. muris eauclairensis*. The disease is spread by infected tick bites from the lone star tick (*Amblyomma americanum*) and the blacklegged tick (*Ixodes scapularis*).

The type of ehrlichiosis depends on the geographic location of the species causing disease. *E. chaffeensis* and *E. ewingii* infections occur primarily in south-central, southeastern, and mid-Atlantic states, while *E. muris eauclairensis* infection has only been reported from Wisconsin and Minnesota and travelers to those states. Anaplasmosis is a tickborne disease caused by *Anaplasma phagocytophilum*. This bacteria is carried by blacklegged tick (*Ixodes scapularis*) in the Northeast and Midwest United States and by the western blacklegged tick (*Ixodes pacificus*) on the West coast.

The majority of cases occur during the summer months with a peak incidence in June and July.

Ehrlichiosis is a reportable disease. In 2018, there were more than 1,799 cases.[69] Most cases are reported in Oklahoma, Missouri, and Arkansas. Incidence is highest among males and adults between the ages of 60 to 69 years of age. Case-fatality is highest among children <10 years of age, adults over age 70 years, and patients who are immunosuppressed.

The pathophysiologic process of ehrlichiosis begins with a bite from an infected tick. Following inoculation, the organism enters the circulatory system infecting target cells. The infectious agent then enters the cell via endocytosis. The organism completes its reproduction process within the host cell. The agent then reprograms the host cell's defense mechanisms to silently proliferate.

MEDICAL HISTORY AND CLINICAL PRESENTATION

Ehrlichiosis clinical manifestations will present differently depending on the infectious agent. All infections will include symptoms of fever, headache, and nausea. Rash is also common.

Anaplasmosis signs and symptoms include fever, headache, and myalgia, with GI symptoms occurring in less than half of the patients and a skin rash in <10% of patients.

SIGNS AND SYMPTOMS

Signs and symptoms noted the early days of infection include fever, chills, rigors, headache, malaise, myalgia, confusion, and GI symptoms of nausea, vomiting, diarrhea, anorexia. Rash is more common in children and begins 5 days after onset of symptoms. The rash spares the face but may spread to the palms and soles. Rash is rare in patients with anaplasmosis.

PHYSICAL EXAMINATION

Patients with ehrlichiosis will often display a fever, lymphadenopathy, myalgias, hypertension, and tachycardia. A maculopapular or petechial rash may be noted on the body including palms and soles; the face is typically spared. In anaplasmosis, rash is noted in <10% of patients.

DIFFERENTIAL DIAGNOSIS

Ehrlichiosis infections must also be differentiated from other tick-borne diseases that cause fever, chills, headaches, body ache, and rash (Table 17.21).

DIAGNOSTIC STUDIES

Basic laboratory findings include normal or elevated WBC count and thrombocytopenia. As the disease progresses renal insufficiency and hepatic involvement can develop.

PCR, peripheral blood smear, and an IFA are the three primary laboratory methods to diagnose ehrlichiosis.

PCR and peripheral blood smear examinations are most effective in the first week of the illness. Microscopic examination of a peripheral blood smear might reveal morulae; microcolonies of *Ehrlichia*, in the cytoplasm of WBCs is highly suggestive of a diagnosis. *E. chaffeensis* most commonly infects monocytes. *E. ewingii* more commonly infects granulocytes. Blood smear examination is relatively insensitive and should not be relied upon alone to diagnose ehrlichiosis.

TABLE 17.21 Differential Diagnosis for *Ehrlichia* Infections

Diagnosis	Description
Lyme disease	Presents with erythema migrans rash, fatigue, fever, and arthritis.
Relapsing fever	Presents with high fevers, rigors, flu-like symptoms, headaches, myalgias, and rash.
Rocky Mountain spotted fever	Presents with fever, change in mental status, myalgias, headaches, and a petechial rash.
Anaplasmosis	Presents with fever, headache, chills, malaise, and myalgias, rash is rare.
Tularemia	Presentation varies based on site of infection, high fever is common in all. Main forms include ulceroglandular (skin ulcer at site infections), glandular (skin infection, no ulcer), oculoglandular (eye inflammation, lymphadenopathy), oropharyngeal (pharyngitis, lymphadenopathy), pneumonic (cough, dyspnea), and typhoidal (general symptoms).

The gold standard test is the indirect IFA assay for IgG. This test is performed on paired acute and convalescent serum samples collected 2 to 4 weeks apart to demonstrate evidence of a fourfold seroconversion. There may be some cross-reaction with other *Ehrlichia* and *Anaplasma* species.

TREATMENT

The treatment of choice for *Ehrlichia* and *Anaplasma* infections is doxycycline. Doxycycline should be started within the first week of the illness and should be given even to children and pregnant women since it is the only proven therapy. Rifampin and chloramphenicol are alternative choices. When treated with doxycycline, fever generally subsides within 24 to 48 hours and treatment should continue until 3 days after improvement in fever and until evidence of clinical improvement.

PATIENT EDUCATION

- Post-tick bite antibiotic prophylaxis is not recommended to prevent ehrlichiosis.
- Estimated mortality rate is between 2% and 10%.[70]

17.4D Q FEVER

Q fever is caused by *Coxiella burnetii*, an intracellular gram-negative bacterium that can form spores. This organism is found in cattle, sheep, goats, and domestic mammals, including cats and dogs. The infection is due to inhalation of contaminated particles or from contact with the infected animal secretions, milk, feces, urine, and placenta. The incubation period is 2 to 3 weeks. Humans can be infected by a single bacterium.

Most cases of illness occur in spring and early summer months, peaking in April and May, the same time frame as peak birthing season for cattle, sheep, and goats. Q fever is a notifiable disease in the United States. In 2017, 153 acute Q fever cases were reported, as well as 40 chronic Q fever cases.[71]

MEDICAL HISTORY AND CLINICAL PRESENTATION

The clinical manifestations of Q fever include a wide variety of conditions. These include a self-limited fever; pneumonia; hepatitis; endocarditis; and possibly, aseptic meningitis, encephalitis, optic neuritis, pericarditis, myocarditis, and hemolytic anemia.

SIGNS AND SYMPTOMS

Q fever can present with a wide variety of symptoms based on the organs involved. Q fever can be classified as acute or chronic based on the onset of symptoms. Acute Q fever presents with flu-like symptoms (high fever, chills, headaches, and arthralgias), pneumonia (cough, dyspnea, pleuritic chest pain), endocarditis, and hepatitis (right upper quadrant pain, jaundice, nausea and vomiting, and diarrhea). Chronic Q fever presents with endocarditis and occasional musculoskeletal and vascular manifestations. Up to 50% of patients are asymptomatic.

PHYSICAL EXAMINATION

Patients with Q fever appear ill and show findings of fever, pneumonia, and hepatomegaly.

Physical examination may reveal high-grade fevers with chills and sweats, tachycardia, and tachypnea.

Skin reveals a maculopapular or punctate rash, erythema nodosum, or jaundice. Lung exam may reveal crackles in the lower lung fields or be normal. Cardiac examination may reveal a new murmur consistent with endocarditis or a pericardial friction rub if pericarditis is present.

DIFFERENTIAL DIAGNOSIS

The differential diagnosis for Q fever includes the atypical pneumonias, *Mycoplasma pneumoniae*, legionellosis, and *Chlamydia pneumoniae* (Table 17.22).

DIAGNOSTIC STUDIES

The diagnosis of Q fever is made by serologic testing. The best test is the microimmunofluorescence test. Acute Q fever is best diagnosed using acute and convalescent serum samples, looking for a fourfold rise in titer; a single titer of 1:512 or greater with a compatible clinical picture may also provide strong evidence of acute Q fever. *C. burnetii* does not grow in blood cultures.

PCR is diagnostically useful and is most sensitive during the first week of the illness. A negative PCR does not rule out the diagnosis.

TREATMENT

Doxycycline is the treatment of choice for acute Q fever. Second-line treatment options include a macrolide or TMP-SMX. A respiratory fluoroquinolone, such as levofloxacin or moxifloxacin, can be used in patients who cannot be treated with doxycycline.

For persistent localized disease, the treatment option includes a combination of doxycycline and hydroxychloroquine. Hydroxychloroquine has no activity against *C. burnetii*, but

TABLE 17.22 Differential Diagnosis for Q Fever

Diagnosis	Description
Q fever	Characterized by abrupt onset of fever, myalgia, and headache. Dry cough is the major respiratory symptom with dyspnea and pleuritic chest pain.
Mycoplasma pneumonia	Patients can be asymptomatic or present with headache, nausea, and malaise. Intractable cough is present and is nonproductive.
Legionellosis	Characterized by mildly productive cough, chills, myalgias, and arthralgias. Gastrointestinal symptoms include diarrhea, nausea and vomiting.
Chlamydia pneumonia	There are no specific features and symptoms appear gradually.
Epstein-Barr virus	Presents with fatigue, lymphadenopathy, splenomegaly, and rash.
Leptospirosis	Patients present with dyspnea, cough, and change in mental status. Hyponatremia is common.
Brucellosis	Presents with cough and headache.

because it alkalinizes the phagolysosome, it renders doxycycline bactericidal against *C. burnetii.*

Treatment is monitored by following the antibody titers to *C. burnetii*. Antibody titers should be done every 2 months for the first 6 months, and if falling titers are noted this indicates treatment success; titers should then be measured every 3 to 4 months.

PATIENT EDUCATION

- Q fever vaccines are not available in the United States.
- The risk of Q fever can be reduced by avoiding contact with animals, especially while animals are giving birth.
- Consuming raw milk or raw milk products should be avoided.

17.4E KAWASAKI DISEASE

KD is a self-limited vasculitis that affects many organs, including the skin, mucous membranes, lymph nodes, blood vessels, and heart. KD is not a contagious disease and is predominantly a disease of young children, with 80% of patients <5 years of age. KD can cause vasculitis changes in the coronary arteries and subsequent coronary artery aneurysms.

KD is the most common cause of acquired heart disease in children. There are approximately 5,000 new cases per year of KD diagnosed and treated in the United States. The overall incidence in the United States is 20 per 100,000 children under 5 years of age.[72]

The etiology of KD is unknown; one theory is that an infectious agent triggers an immunologic response in genetically susceptible hosts. KD is a self-limited vasculitis of medium-sized arteries with the coronary arteries as the principal target; this weakening of the arterial wall can lead to coronary artery dilatation and aneurysm development.

MEDICAL HISTORY AND CLINICAL PRESENTATION

KD is diagnosed based on clinical criteria with supporting laboratory data. The diagnosis should be suspected in a child who has had a fever for at least 5 days and fits four or more of the following criteria:

- Bilateral conjunctival injection
- Oropharynx changes: erythema and fissuring of the lips, "strawberry" tongue, or erythema of oropharyngeal mucosa
- Extremity changes: edema of the hands and feet, palm and sole erythema, or periungual desquamation in the convalescent phase
- Polymorphous exanthema
- Cervical lymph node mass ≥1.5 cm

SIGNS AND SYMPTOMS

Common symptoms of KD include high-grade fever, red eyes, bright red and cracked lips, red oral mucous membranes, strawberry tongue, white coating on the tongue or prominent red papillae on the back of the tongue, red palms and soles, swollen hands and feet, and rash. KD often begins with a high and persistent fever that is nonresponsive to normal doses of ibuprofen or acetaminophen. The fever may rise steadily for up to 2 weeks and is accompanied by irritability. The skin rash occurs early in the disease, and peeling of the skin in the genital region, hands, and feet may occur in later phases. Symptoms may come and go during the course of the illness.

PHYSICAL EXAMINATION

Findings on physical examination include fever and irritability. Tachycardia will be present out of proportion to the fever. Bilateral conjunctival injection is seen, with sparing of the limbus with no exudate or excessive tearing. Oral examination reveals erythema with chapping or fissuring; erythema of oropharyngeal mucosa without lesions, ulcerations, or exudates; a strawberry tongue with loss of filiform papillae. Abdominal examination may note some right upper quadrant tenderness; the spleen is never enlarged.

Skin examination reveals nonspecific skin changes that may be maculopapular, raised edematous plaques, target-like lesions, or urticarial lesions and is never bullous or vesicular. The rash is typically noted over the trunk and extremities. Rash spares the scalp, palms, and soles.

Edema of the dorsal hands/feet; erythema of palms/soles; and arthritis of the proximal interphalangeal (PIP) joints or large joints are seen.

DIFFERENTIAL DIAGNOSIS

Differential diagnosis includes adenovirus infection, enterovirus infection, measles infection, scarlet fever, and early Stevens-Johnson syndrome.

DIAGNOSTIC STUDIES

Laboratory findings include leukocytosis, thrombocytosis, elevated sedimentation rate and C-reactive protein, and elevated alanine transaminase (ALT) and gamma-glutamyl transpeptidase. Skin biopsy reveals nonspecific edema with no evidence of small vessel vasculitis. Echocardiogram is recommended to evaluate for cardiac findings.

Diagnosis is established by history, physical examination, and supporting lab results.

EVALUATION

The illness is self-limited and will resolve, even in the absence of treatment; cardiac complications are the greatest concern. Other complications include small and large joint arthritis that can impede walking.

TREATMENT

IV immunoglobulin and aspirin are indicated in the treatment of KD. Treatment should be started as soon as the diagnosis is made to prevent damage to the coronary arteries. KD is one of the exceptions to the use of aspirin in children; aspirin is typically not recommended for children due to its association with Reye syndrome.

PATIENT EDUCATION

- With early treatment, rapid recovery from the acute symptoms can be expected and the risk of coronary artery aneurysms greatly reduced.
- Untreated, the acute symptoms of KD are self-limited, but the risk of coronary artery involvement is much greater.

SPECIAL CONSIDERATIONS

- Treatment of Q fever in children is doxycycline for children over the age of 8 and TMP-SMX for children <8 years of age.
- In pregnant women the treatment of choice for Q fever is TMP-SMX. The drug is discontinued at the eighth month of pregnancy. Folate should be given to pregnant women taking TMP-SMX.

KEY POINTS

- Rickettsial diseases and related diseases are caused by a group of gram-negative, obligately intracellular coccobacilli.
- All rickettsial diseases have an arthropod vector except for *Coxiella burnetii.*
- Rickettsial diseases cause fever, a local eschar, petechial rash, lymphadenopathy, encephalitis, vasculitis, gangrene of skin, and organ dysfunction.
- Treat with antibiotics; tetracyclines are the drug of choice.

17.5 SPIROCHETAL INFECTIONS

Overview

Spirochetes are bacteria with a spiral morphology. The organisms are found in the human oral cavity and GI tracts of humans. Three spirochetes cause human infection: (1) *Treponema*, which causes syphilis; (2) *Borrelia*, which causes Lyme disease and relapsing fever; and (3) *Leptospira*, which causes leptospirosis.

EPIDEMIOLOGY

Syphilis and Lyme disease are common disorders, with 35,063 cases of primary and secondary syphilis in 2018 and 33,666 cases of Lyme disease in 2018.[73] Leptospirosis, rat bite fever, and relapsing fever are rare.

PATHOPHYSIOLOGY

All spirochetal diseases have a number of similarities. The portal of entry involves skin or mucus membranes. They disseminate via blood, tissue, and body fluids, especially to cardiovascular, neurologic, and skin tissues. Because of their lack of surface proteins on their outer membrane they can evade the immune system.

Neurotropic spirochetes enter the central nervous system early in the course of disease. *T. pallidum* and *B. burgdoferi* lay dormant in the central nervous system until they activate; this makes therapy difficult. Leptospiral and recurrent fever organisms do not lay dormant in the central nervous system, and their therapy is more straightforward.

Spirochetal diseases occur in stages, with intervening latent periods. Untreated infection may last in hosts from months to years.

17.5A SYPHILIS

Treponema pallidum is a member of the family Spirochaetaceae. Treponemas have helical coiled shape and are motile because of the corkscrew motion from the actions of endoflagella. *Treponema* cannot be cultured directly in vitro.

Syphilis is primarily sustained in the population through sexual contact with infected persons.

Since 2001 the rate of syphilis has increased every year. This increase has been attributed to increased cases among MSM. There has recently been an increase in syphilis among women, which is associated with an increase in congenital syphilis.

Recent trends in the United States show the highest incidence of infection in the South and in urban areas in the rest of country. Many new cases have occurred among persons with HIV infection.

Pathologically syphilis is a systemic vasculitis. The organism induces a perivascular cellular immune infiltration as the organism invades tissues. In congenital syphilis, the placenta is thickened, and the villi are hypercellular. Spirochetes may be found in the walls of umbilical vessels. Humans are the only natural reservoir of *T. pallidum.*

MEDICAL HISTORY AND CLINICAL PRESENTATION

Acquired syphilis is transmitted by any type of sexual activity that leads to direct skin or mucous membrane contact with an infectious skin lesion of an infected person. Transmission of the infection is at the site of contact. Transmission from contact is not universal but occurs in about one third of episodes.

The incubation period for syphilis ranges from 3 to 90 days, with an average of 3 weeks. Once an immunocompetent person has been infected for more than 4 years, they are unlikely to spread infection by sexual contact even if never treated.

SIGNS AND SYMPTOMS

Primary syphilis occurs in sexually active patients. The characteristic lesion is the chancre, which begins as a papule that progresses to central ulceration with raised, firm borders. Chancres are painless unless secondarily infected. Most infected patients have only a single chancre, but multiple lesions can be present. In females, primary lesions on the cervix or vaginal walls are common and often go unrecognized. The other sign of primary infection includes nontender, regional adenopathy. Systemic signs are absent. Spontaneous healing of primary lesions occurs in 3 to 12 weeks.

In secondary syphilis any organ system can be involved. Signs and symptoms of secondary syphilis appear 2 to 10 weeks after primary lesions develop and include rash, fever, and lymphadenopathy. Primary lesions may still be present at the time. Secondary syphilis is a time of systemic dissemination of the microbes and it is during this period there is the highest microbial burden. Manifestations of secondary syphilis disappear without treatment in 3 to 12 weeks, and the infection then enters a latent period.

Neurosyphilis develops in about 30% of patients during the early stages of primary and secondary syphilis. It may be asymptomatic or cause symptoms and signs of meningitis and cranial or spinal nerve involvement. Early neurosyphilis resolves in about half of cases but can progress to late neurosyphilis over 5 or more years. Classic manifestations of late neurosyphilis are dementia, tabes dorsalis, optic atrophy, and seizures.

Tertiary syphilis occurs in about 40% of untreated persons and patients can develop nonprogressive localized nodules, gummata, in the skin and supporting structures of the body. Gummata are granulomatous and fibrotic with central necrosis and represent an immune response of the host. Gummata appear 15 to 30 years after initial infection or 3 to 10 years after the last evidence of secondary syphilis.

PHYSICAL EXAMINATION

The clinical presentation of syphilis can be divided into early syphilis and late syphilis.

Early syphilis includes primary and secondary syphilis. In primary syphilis the primary ulcer or chancre may be located on the genitals, perianal skin, within the rectum, oral cavity, and any other skin or mucous membrane surface exposed to an infectious lesion that was present on the source sexual partner (Figure 17.15).

These lesions are few, typically one, clean based, indurated, and painless to palpation. In secondary syphilis cutaneous and/or mucous membrane lesions are the most common clinical manifestations. The erythematous macules evolve into hyperpigmented papules, with a thin rim of scaly hyperkeratosis. These lesions are usually present on both the palms and soles. Individual lesions are pink to red and range from 3 to 10 mm in size. Generalized painless lymphadenopathy and mucous membrane lesions are common. Epitrochlear node enlargement is common and should raise suspicion for secondary syphilis (Figure 17.16).

Late syphilis includes neurosyphilis. Neurosyphilis findings are consistent with meningitis. Cranial nerve palsies, nerves III, VI, VII, and VIII, occur in just under one-half of the cases along with symptoms of increased intracranial pressure. Deafness is present in 20% of patients and may be the single presenting complaint.

DIFFERENTIAL DIAGNOSIS

The presentations of primary syphilis can have overlap with other ulcerative STIs such as genital herpes, chancroid, and granuloma inguinale. Primary genital herpes has clusters of painful vesicles, systemic symptoms, and regional adenopathy. Chancroid presents as a painful genital ulcer with associated tender, suppurative inguinal adenitis. Donovanosis is extremely rare in the United States and presents as slowly progressive, painless genital ulceration without associated adenopathy.

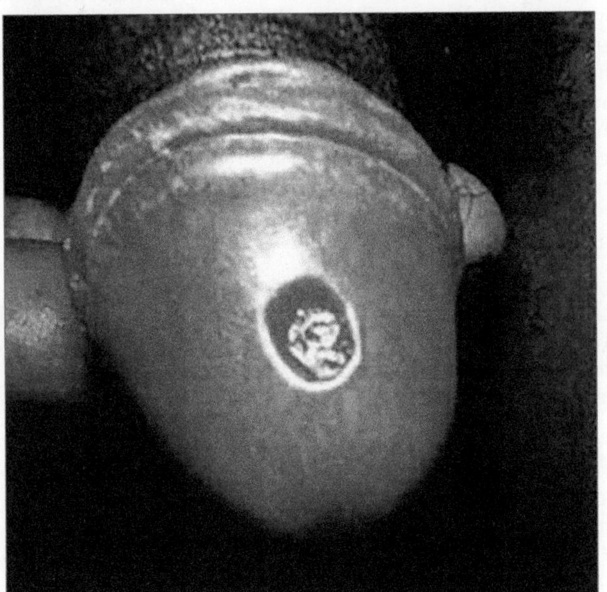

Figure 17.15 **Syphilis chancre.**

(Source: Centers for Disease Control and Prevention. https://phil.cdc.gov/Details.aspx?pid=2359)

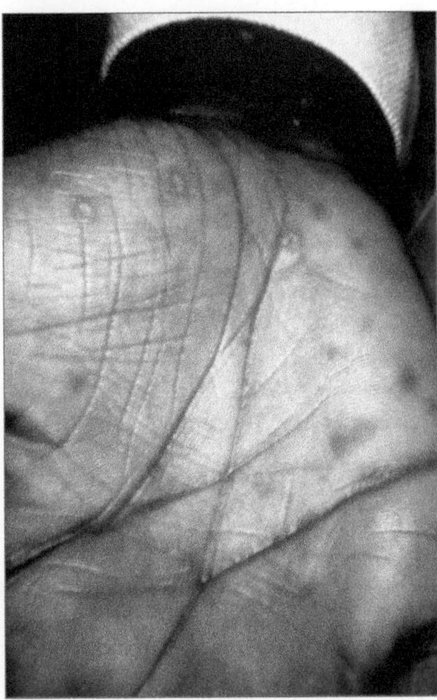

Figure 17.16 **Skin rash noted in syphilis.**

Secondary syphilis can mimic many systemic diseases, including IM, subacute or chronic bacterial infections, rheumatologic conditions, and malignancies.

DIAGNOSTIC STUDIES

Definitive diagnosis of syphilis is made by darkfield microscopy or tests that detect *T. pallidum* in lesion exudates or tissue specimens. Presumptive diagnosis of syphilis is made by two types of serologic tests: (1) nontreponemal tests and (2) specific treponemal tests.

Nontreponemal tests traditionally have been used as the initial serologic test for diagnosis of syphilis, followed by treponemal tests when the nontreponemal test is positive. Positive results of both tests at the same time support the presumptive diagnosis of active syphilis infection.

Nontreponemal tests detect antibodies that react with cardiolipin embedded in lecithin-cholesterol liposomes. The titers of these antibodies rise as the spirochetal infection progresses and then fall with treatment of the infection or immunologic control when untreated. The two available nontreponemal assays are the Venereal Disease Research Laboratory (VDRL) and rapid plasma reagin (RPR) tests. Most patients become nonreactive by these tests after successful treatment or spontaneous resolution of the infection.

False positive nontreponemal test results occur in about 1% to 2% of adults.[74] False positive results can occur with EBV infection, hepatitis, varicella, measles, tuberculosis, malaria, HIV infection, and endocarditis. Lymphoma, rheumatologic conditions, especially systemic lupus erythematosus, pregnancy, and immunizations, including MMR, influenza, and smallpox, can cause false positive results. Lyme disease does not cause positive nontreponemal tests.

Several specific treponemal tests are available: (1) fluorescent treponemal antibody absorbed (FTA-ABS) tests; (2) *T. pallidum* passive particle agglutination (TP-PA); and (3) various *T. pallidum* enzyme immunofluorescence assays (TP-EIAs). A positive specific test indicates current or past infection. Most patients infected with syphilis remain seropositive for life.

False positive treponemal tests can occur in patients with other treponemal infections, including Lyme disease.[75]

Patients with a positive nontreponemal test followed by a positive treponemal test result have presumptive syphilis. Those with a positive nontreponemal test and negative treponemal test likely have a false positive nontreponemal result.

Diagnosis of neurosyphilis requires CSF analysis. CSF protein is elevated and pleocytosis is usually present. The VDRL test is the nontreponemal test used for spinal fluid. The VDRL can be falsely positive in neonates born to mothers with syphilis due to transplacental and blood-CSF barrier passage of maternal antibodies. The FTA-ABS test on CSF is highly sensitive but less specific. A negative CSF FTA-ABS makes neurosyphilis unlikely. The RPR test cannot be utilized with spinal fluid.

TREATMENT

Penicillin G is the preferred agent for treating all stages and types of syphilis. The stage of disease and clinical manifestations determine the preparation, dosage, and length of treatment. Occasionally a Jarisch–Herxheimer reaction may be induced (fever, chills, and myalgias). Patients should be notified of this possibility and over-the-counter antipyretics can be used to reduce the fever.

In patients with penicillin allergy, desensitization, and treatment with benzathine penicillin is always an option to consider. Pregnant females and young children with penicillin allergy should be desensitized and treated with the penicillin.

Alternatives for early syphilis include doxycycline, tetracycline, ceftriaxone, and azithromycin. Azithromycin-resistant strains of *T. pallidum* have been seen in the United States. Azithromycin should not be used in MSM or in pregnant females.

The only alternatives to penicillin for treatment of latent syphilis are doxycycline and tetracycline.

The primary method for the prevention of syphilis includes screening at-risk groups for infection and treatment of sexual partners of persons with syphilis. All recent sexual contacts should be identified. Patients with evidence of any STI or HIV infection should be tested for syphilis.

Asymptomatic persons with contact with an infected person within the past 3 months may still be seronegative and should be treated for possible early primary syphilis. In any patient, if test results are not immediately available or follow-up is not assured, treatment should be administered.

All cases of confirmed or suspected syphilis should be reported to local health authorities to allow for follow-up of patients and appropriate contact investigations.

PATIENT EDUCATION

- Allergic reactions are the primary side effects that occur with administration of antibiotics to treat syphilis.
- The Jarisch-Herxheimer reaction is an acute febrile event that usually occurs within 2 to 12 hours after initiation of any therapy for any spirochetal infections, including syphilis. It is characterized by headache, fever, myalgia, and diaphoresis. It is due to release of treponemal endotoxin-like compounds as the microbes lyse.

17.5B RELAPSING FEVER

Relapsing fever is due to *Borrelia hermsii, B. parkerii,* and *B. turicatae*. *Borrelia* is a gram-negative bacterium that has a corkscrew shape.

TBRF is endemic in the Americas, Africa, Asia, and Europe. In the United States, it is confined to the western states, with occurrence highest from May to September.

Rodents are the reservoir for the bacteria. Ticks transmit the organism to humans via the tick's saliva or excreta. Infection is acquired by people sleeping in rodent-infested cabins in the mountains and has been associated with spelunking

Louse-borne relapsing fever (LBRF) is caused by *Borrelia recurrentis*, which is transmitted from human to human by the body louse. LBRF outbreaks most commonly occur in conditions of overcrowding and social disruption. LBRF causes sporadic illness and outbreaks in sub-Saharan Africa, particularly in regions affected by war and in refugee camps. A mortality rate of 30% to 70% is noted in outbreaks.

MEDICAL HISTORY AND CLINICAL PRESENTATION

Most patients do not report a history of tick bite but may report an overnight exposure to caves or rustic dwellings. When present, louse infestation is usually obvious.

TBRF is characterized by febrile episodes that last 3 days, separated by afebrile periods of 7 days. During the chill phase of the crisis, a very high fever (up to 106.7 °F or 41.5 °C) is noted along with delirium, agitation, tachycardia, and tachypnea. This is followed by the flush phase, which is characterized by drenching sweats and a rapid decrease in body temperature. During this phase hypotension may be noted transiently. If not treated, these phases will recur before illness resolves.

SIGNS AND SYMPTOMS

Symptoms vary depending on the bacterial infection load and after a number of days resolve when the organism is cleared from the blood. Bacteremia and symptoms then return after about a 1-week afebrile period. When symptoms return they are less severe. A single relapse characterizes LBRF, and up to 10 relapses can occur in TBRF.

Sudden chills are noted at the onset, followed by high fever, tachycardia, severe headache, nausea, vomiting, muscle and joint pain, and often delirium. An erythematous macular or purpuric rash may appear early over the trunk and extremities, with an eschar at the site of the tick bite. Conjunctival, subcutaneous, or submucous hemorrhages may be present. After 3 to 5 days the fever abruptly stops. Later in the disease course, jaundice, hepatomegaly, splenomegaly, myocarditis, and heart failure may occur, typically in louse-borne disease. Neurologic complications are more common in TBRF.

PHYSICAL EXAMINATION

Physical examination findings vary depending on the severity of illness. There are no specific findings for TBRF. Patients appear moderately ill and possibly dehydrated. Occasionally a macular rash or scattered petechiae may be present on the trunk and extremities.

DIFFERENTIAL DIAGNOSIS

The differential diagnosis includes Lyme disease, malaria, dengue fever, yellow fever, leptospirosis, and influenza.

DIAGNOSTIC STUDIES

The diagnosis of relapsing fever is suggested by recurrent fever and confirmed by visualization of spirochetes in the blood during a febrile episode. The spirochetes may be seen on darkfield examination or Wright- or Giemsa-stained thick and thin blood smears. Serologic tests are unreliable. Serologic tests for syphilis and Lyme disease may be falsely positive.

TREATMENT

In TBRF or LBRF the treatment of choice is tetracycline or erythromycin.

If not able to use oral medications or if the central nervous system is involved IV ceftriaxone or doxycycline is indicated; in children under age 8 IV penicillin is indicated.

PATIENT EDUCATION

- Given appropriate treatment, most patients recover within a few days. Long-term sequelae of TBRF are rare.
- TBRF contracted during pregnancy can cause spontaneous abortion, premature birth, and neonatal death.

17.5C RAT BITE FEVER

Rat bite fever is a zoonosis due to *Streptobacillus moniliformis*; there are only several cases reported in the United States each year. Children account for more than 50% of cases in the United States, followed by laboratory personnel and pet shop employees.[76] *S. moniliformis* is a pleomorphic, filamentous, gram-negative, nonmotile, and non-acid-fast rod.

S. moniliformis is a found in the nasopharyngeal area of rats and is excreted in their urine. Rat bites are the most common source of inoculation; transmission can occur following scratches or handling of rats. The risk of disease following a documented rat bite is about 10%.[77] Haverhill fever (epidemic arthritic erythema) occurs following transmission of *S. moniliformis* by ingestion of food or water contaminated by rats.

MEDICAL HISTORY AND CLINICAL PRESENTATION

Symptoms of rat bite fever manifest within 3 to 10 days of inoculation with *S. moniliformis*. Symptoms include acute onset of fever, shaking chills, headache, and vomiting. Other symptoms include maculopapular rash involving the palms and soles; rash may be petechial, pustular, or purpuric. Migratory arthralgias or arthritis with or without joint effusions is noted in half the cases. No lymphadenopathy is noted.

Haverhill fever, associated with ingestion of the organism, presents with acute onset of fever, chills, rash, and arthritis. Rash is smaller in distribution and more uniform than with parenteral inoculation. Upper respiratory and GI symptoms are common.

SIGNS AND SYMPTOMS

Initial symptoms are nonspecific and include fever, chills, arthralgia, myalgias, headache, and vomiting. A maculopapular rash on the extremities may develop 2 to 4 days after onset of the fever. If not treated the patient may develop endocarditis, myocarditis, meningitis, pneumonia, and sepsis.

PHYSICAL EXAMINATION

The findings of a maculopapular rash, fever, and arthritis in a patient with a history of exposure to rats suggests the diagnosis of rat bite fever.

DIFFERENTIAL DIAGNOSIS

The differential diagnosis includes meningococcemia, DGI, RMSF, ehrlichiosis, leptospirosis, Lyme disease, relapsing fever, syphilis, brucellosis, viral infections, such as parvovirus, chikungunya, and dengue; and juvenile arthritis and collagen vascular disease.

DIAGNOSTIC STUDIES

Laboratory abnormalities include leukocytosis with a left shift and mild anemia. The definitive diagnosis requires direct detection of the organism in blood or other body fluid.

S. moniliformis is a fastidious organism that has special growth requirements. The organism grows best in anaerobic culture bottles. *S. minus* does not grow well in any artificial medium and requires nonculture methods to confirm infection. PCR-based methods are not available for diagnosis.

S. moniliformis may be seen on Giemsa stain of blood or body fluid. *S. minus* spirochetes are rarely seen on examination of the peripheral blood smear or darkfield examination of ulcer exudate.

TREATMENT

The treatment of choice for rate bite fever is penicillin. Alternative treatment options include doxycycline or streptomycin. If endocarditis is present first-line therapy includes penicillin in combination with gentamicin. Alternative treatment includes ceftriaxone and gentamicin.

PATIENT EDUCATION

- Rat bite fever is best prevented by limiting exposure to rats, precautions to avoid bites and scratches, and avoiding consumption of unpasteurized milk.
- Antibiotic prophylaxis with amoxicillin or amoxicillin-clavulanic acid may be considered following documented bites in young infants, who are at increased risk of severe disease and death.

17.5D LEPTOSPIROSIS

Leptospirosis is a zoonosis caused by spirochetes from the genus *Leptospira,* spread by direct or indirect contact with urine from infected animals. It occurs occasionally in temperate climates and is endemic in tropical countries. Leptospirosis has been traditionally considered an occupational disease, but it is also linked to poor sanitary conditions and from recreational exposures. Most cases are subclinical or self-limiting. In the United States the disease is rare with a majority of cases noted southern and pacific costal states and Hawaii.

Leptospira bacteria are spread through direct or indirect contact between urine from infected animals and breaks in human skin or mucous membranes. The most common means of indirect contact is contaminated water, soil, or contaminated fomite.

Occupations at risk for developing disease include work involving irrigation, sewage, farming, or animal husbandry, which are potential sources of exposure. Recreational activities putting patients at risk include those involving close contact with animals or exposure to nonsanitary water, including natural rivers or lakes.

MEDICAL HISTORY AND CLINICAL PRESENTATION

The clinical manifestations of leptospirosis are nonspecific. The disease course is typically biphasic; the initial period consists of fever, myalgias, and mild symptoms lasting about 1 week. During this initial phase, the patient has bacteremia. After the initial phase the patient will improve for 3 to 4 days. Then the patient may progress to the second phase, with return of symptoms, presence of the organism in urine, and possible progression to meningitis, myocarditis, renal failure, and respiratory failure.

An estimated 90% of cases are subclinical. Because of an incubation period of days to weeks, initial presentation may be removed from original exposure.

SIGNS AND SYMPTOMS

Common symptoms of leptospirosis are fever, myalgias, respiratory symptoms and GI complaints, including nausea and vomiting.

Patient may develop renal failure, due to impaired proximal tubule sodium reabsorption. This causes decreased sodium delivery to the distal tubule, potassium wasting, and polyuria or nonoliguric renal failure. Renal failure may lead to volume depletion and oliguric renal failure by acute tubular necrosis.

PHYSICAL EXAMINATION

Physical examination findings include icterus, fever, tachycardia, and conjunctival redness without inflammatory exudates.

DIFFERENTIAL DIAGNOSIS

The differential diagnosis includes dengue fever, malaria, typhoid, typhus, influenza, Q fever, brucellosis, and ehrlichiosis.

DIAGNOSTIC STUDIES

Basic laboratory findings include a normal WBC count and thrombocytopenia. Blood chemistry reveals an elevated creatinine level, potassium abnormalities, elevated transaminases, and elevated bilirubin. Urinalysis may be abnormal including pyuria, hematuria, and proteinuria.

To confirm the diagnosis culture may be needed. *Leptospira* can be grown from blood, urine, and spinal fluid. Special media is required, and growth may take several weeks. *Leptospira* stain poorly with typical stains and is best seen by darkfield microscopy, fluorescent microscopy, or silver stain.

Diagnosis of leptospirosis requires a high index of suspicion. Identification of IgM and IgG antibodies may be useful for diagnosis. IgM antibodies appear as early as 2 days after infection, and IgG may appear by day 7.

Current preferred reference test is the microscopic agglutination test (MAT), which is limited by test availability and clinical factors. PCR is most accurate when taken during the acute phase of illness, as these samples are more likely to contain organisms.

TREATMENT

The recommended treatment is oral doxycycline or azithromycin for mild to moderate leptospirosis. Both have been shown to reduce length of illness and decrease shedding in the urine. For severe disease, the recommended treatment is IV penicillin G, ceftriaxone, cefotaxime, or doxycycline.

PATIENT EDUCATION

- Doxycycline is the only currently recommended prophylactic medication.
- Because of the increasing incidence of recreational acquisition, doxycycline prior to high-risk recreational activity and continuing through duration of potential exposure is recommended.

17.5E LYME DISEASE

Lyme disease is the most common tick-borne illness in North America and Europe. Lyme disease is caused by the spirochete *Borrelia burgdorferi*, transmitted by *Ixodes scapularis* (deer tick) in the eastern and northern midwestern states and by *Ixodes pacificus* ticks in the western states.

Typical symptoms include fever, headache, fatigue, and a skin rash called erythema migrans (EM). If not treated the infection can spread to the joints, heart, and nervous system.

Lyme disease can be treated successfully with antibiotics. Prevention of Lyme disease includes using insect repellent, removing ticks promptly, applying pesticides, and reducing tick habitat.

MEDICAL HISTORY AND CLINICAL PRESENTATION

Patient history will include presence in a Lyme endemic area within 30 days of the rash development. The highest incidence is in the coastal areas of Northeast, northwest California, and the Great Lakes region of the United States. The disease typically presents between April and November.

In early disease, 30 days after tick bite, the most common finding is the rash EM. Other symptoms include intermittent arthralgia, myalgia, headache, fatigue, and occasional fever.

In early disseminated disease, weeks to months after tick bite, manifestations include neurologic symptoms, cardiac disease, and conjunctivitis.

Late disease, weeks to years after tick bite, manifestations include arthritis and peripheral neuropathy or encephalopathy.

SIGNS AND SYMPTOMS

Early in the disease the most common finding is EM, a painless, round, expanding erythematous macule or papule. Other symptoms include arthralgia, myalgia, headache, fatigue, and fever.

Early disseminated disease presents with neurologic findings including cranial nerve palsies, including facial nerve palsy, aseptic meningitis, peripheral neuropathy, radiculopathy, and encephalitis; cardiac findings include acute onset atrioventricular (AV) block and myocarditis; and conjunctivitis.

Late disease presents with arthritis, typically involving the knees, and neurologic signs including peripheral neuropathy or encephalopathy, which may present as memory loss, mood changes, or sleep disturbance.

PHYSICAL EXAMINATION

The classic finding is the rash of EM, which presents as a red macule or papule that expands, forming a red lesion at least 5 cm in size, with partial central clearing. Secondary lesions may develop. The rash can reach 5 to 20 cm. Regional lymphadenopathy is noted in area of tick bite.

Facial nerve or other cranial nerve palsy can be noted (Figure 17.17).

DIFFERENTIAL DIAGNOSIS

Differential diagnosis varies depending on the presenting signs and symptoms (Table 17.23).

DIAGNOSTIC STUDIES

A two-step testing process is recommended for making the diagnosis. Serologic testing is done for antibodies to *Borrelia burgdorferi* with ELISA or IFA, with confirmation of a positive test by Western blot. Presence of IgM or IgG antibodies indicates previous exposure and not always active infection. A fourfold increase in titers from acute to convalescent samples may be noted.

For Lyme meningitis, CSF reveals a lymphocyte-predominant leukocytosis, elevated total protein, normal to low glucose, and diagnostic titers of IgG or IgM in spinal fluid.

EKG may demonstrate varying degrees of AV block; complete heart block is rare.

TREATMENT

Treatment of choice includes doxycycline, amoxicillin, or cefuroxime axetil. Treatment duration is 10 to 21 days. If neurologic or cardiac forms of the disease are present, IV ceftriaxone or penicillin should be used.

People treated with appropriate antibiotics in the early stages of Lyme disease usually recover rapidly and completely.

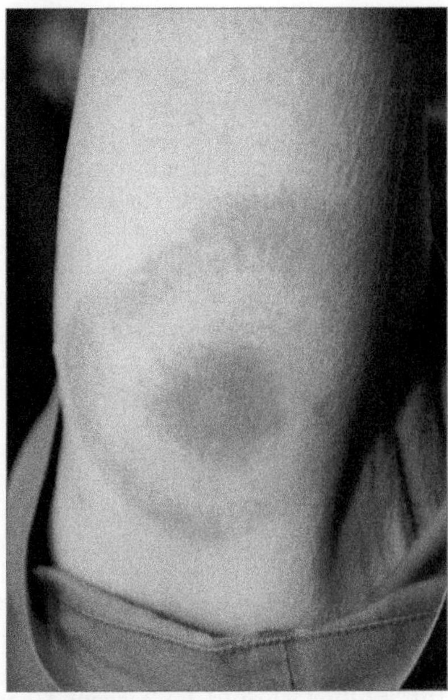

Figure 17.17 **Erythema migrans of Lyme disease.**
(Source: Centers for Disease Control and Prevention/James Gathany. https://phil.cdc.gov/Details.aspx?pid=9874)

In rare cases, symptoms of fatigue and muscle aches may last for more than 6 months; this is post-treatment Lyme disease syndrome. There is no evidence of symptomatic post-treatment Lyme disease syndrome after recommended therapy, and antibiotic therapy has not been proved to be useful in patients with symptoms lasting more than 6 months after appropriate therapy.[78]

TABLE 17.23 Differential Diagnosis for Lyme Disease

Presentation	Diagnosis	Description
Tick bite	Nondeer tick bite	
	Brown recluse spider bite	Pain, swelling, erythema around bite
Erythema migrans	Erythema multiforme	Multiple lesions, mucosal lesions, due to drugs/infections
	Spider bite	Often painful
Fever/myalgias/arthralgias	Babesiosis	Red blood cell parasite, anemia
	Anaplasmosis	Fever, headache, chills, and muscle aches
	Viral infection	Respiratory or gastrointestinal symptoms
Cranial nerve palsies	Herpes simplex/varicella-zoster	Vesicular rash, dermatomal pattern of rash
	Idiopathic facial nerve palsy	Postauricular pain, unilateral facial numbness, flat and expressionless Pain in external auditory canal and a small patch behind the ear
Myocarditis	Rheumatic fever	Severe, valvular disease
Post-Lyme disease syndrome	Chronic fatigue syndrome	Reduction in the ability to engage in needed levels of normal activities for >6 months, postexertional malaise, unrefreshing sleep
	Fibromyalgia	Generalized aching, muscle tenderness, fatigue, poor sleep
Arthritis	Reactive arthritis	Sausage fingers/toes, mucocutaneous ulcers
	Juvenile idiopathic arthritis	Arthritis, fever, rash, adenopathy, and splenomegaly

PATIENT EDUCATION

- A rash that develops while the tick is attached, or in <48 hours after the tick is removed, is most likely a hypersensitivity reaction to the tick bite and not EM.
- Palpitations, bundle branch block, bradycardia, or myocarditis alone are not sufficient for the diagnosis of cardiac Lyme disease.
- Headache, paresthesia, fatigue or a stiff neck alone are not sufficient for diagnosis of neurologic Lyme disease.
- Tick prevention includes protective clothing, tick repellents, inspecting the body daily for ticks and prompt removal.

SPECIAL CONSIDERATIONS

- Lyme disease treatment for pregnant women consists of amoxicillin or cefuroxime axetil.
- Lyme disease is not transmitted via breast milk.
- In the treatment of syphilis in pregnant patients who have a history of penicillin allergy, should be desensitized and treated with penicillin.
- All pregnant women should be screened early in pregnancy for syphilis. Maternal syphilis testing should be performed at delivery. In high-risk populations, pregnant women should be tested at 28 to 32 weeks of gestation.
- Leptospirosis in pregnancy is treated with azithromycin or amoxicillin.

KEY POINTS

- The primary skin lesion of syphilis is the chancre and is located at the site of the primary infection.
- The treatment of choice for syphilis is benzathine penicillin.
- Leptospirosis is a zoonosis; human infections are acquired by contact with infected urine or contaminated water/soil.
- Lyme disease is caused by *Borrelia burgdorferi* and the primary vector is the deer tick.
- EM is noted in a majority of Lyme disease cases.

17.6 PARASITIC INFECTIONS

OVERVIEW

Parasite infections are organisms that infect a human host and cause symptomatic or asymptomatic diseases. There are three main classes of parasites that cause disease in humans:

- **Protozoa:** microscopic organisms that live in the blood or stool
- **Helminths:** multicellular organisms that can cause systemic tissue invasive infection or infection in the gut
- **Ectoparasites:** organisms that burrow in the skin causing prolonged infections

The prevalence of parasitic infections in the United States is not as widespread as the rest of the world, but there are areas in the United States that have an increased incidence of parasite infections; typically these are areas of poverty and poor sanitation. Travel history should be considered when symptoms appear in immigrants/travelers from areas of the world that are endemic for these infections.

17.6A PROTOZOAL INFECTIONS

OVERVIEW

Protozoa are microscopic, one-celled organisms that can be free-living or parasitic in nature. They multiply in humans, which aids in their survival and permits serious infections to develop from just a single organism. Transmission typically occurs via a fecal-oral route. Protozoa that live in the blood or tissue of humans are transmitted to other humans by an arthropod vector. See Table 17.24 for a list of the more common protozoa that infect humans.

TABLE 17.24 Common Protozoan Infections in Humans

Location	Organism	Transmission	Disease State
Blood and tissue	*Trypanosoma* species *T. cruzi* *T. gambiense*	Triatomine bug Tsetse fly	Trypanosomiasis Chagas disease Sleeping sickness
	Leishmaniasis species *L. donovani* *L. tropica*	Sand fly Sand fly	Visceral leishmaniasis Cutaneous leishmaniasis
	Plasmodium species *P. vivax, P. ovale, P. malariae, P. falciparum*	Anopheles mosquito	Malaria
	Toxoplasma gondii	Ingestion of cysts	Toxoplasmosis
Intestinal	*Entamoeba histolytica* *Giardia lamblia* *Cryptosporidium* species	Ingestion of cysts Ingestion of cysts Ingestion of cysts	Amebiasis Giardiasis Cryptosporidiosis
Urogenital	*Trichomonas vaginalis*	Sexual	Trichomoniasis

PATHOPHYSIOLOGY

Protozoa infect various parts of the body. Intracellular protozoa infect a number of cells, including red blood cells, macrophages, brain, and muscle. Extracellular protozoa are located in the blood, intestine, and urogenital tract.

In humans the reproduction of protozoa is usually asexual, by binary or multiple division of growing stages (i.e., trophozoites). Sexual reproduction is normally absent or occurs in the insect vector phase of the life cycle. Asexual reproduction allows for a rapid rise in organisms, particularly where host defenses are impaired. An individual protozoan is both male and female.

Some protozoa can develop a cyst form to protect it from harsh conditions, such as extreme temperatures, harmful chemicals, or a period without food, water, or oxygen. The cyst form enables the protozoa to survive outside the host, allowing transfer from one host to another.

17.6AA TRYPANOSOMIASIS

There are two types of trypanosomiasis:

- Chagas disease (Trypanosoma American) due to *Trypanosoma cruzi*
- Human African trypanosomiasis (sleeping sickness) due to *Trypanosoma brucei rhodesiense* in East Africa, and *Trypanosoma brucei gambiense* in West and Central Africa.

In Chagas disease infection is caused by the bite of the triatomine or kissing bug. Infection can also occur by ingestion of contaminated food or congenital transmission. Sleeping sickness is caused by the bite of the tsetse fly.

The life cycle for both diseases is similar. The trypanomastigote form is present in the feces of the vector bug. During a blood meal, the bug defecates, and the organism enters via the bite wound; entry through mucus membranes or the conjunctivae can occur.

An uninfected bug may then bite an infected host for a blood meal; in acute infection there are large numbers of parasites in the host blood in the trypanomastigote form. These then migrate to the bug's midgut where they multiply as epimastigotes, and then in the hindgut become infectious trypanomastigotes, completing the cycle.

In the patient the amastigotes multiply and differentiate into trypomastigotes and are released into the bloodstream. Trypomastigotes infect tissue cells and other sites. The bloodstream trypomastigotes do not replicate, which is different from the African trypanosomes. Replication resumes when the parasites enter another cell or are ingested by another vector. The vector becomes infected by feeding on human or animal blood that contains circulating parasites

For Chagas disease the distribution of disease is due to distribution of the vector. This includes the southern United States through southern Argentina. Old or poor housing in rural, impoverished areas are a major risk factor for infection. An estimated 8 to 10 million people are infected.

Sleeping sickness is rare in the United States and is more frequent is East or West Africa. Travelers to these areas can become infected if bitten by an infected vector.

MEDICAL HISTORY AND CLINICAL PRESENTATION

The acute phase of Chagas disease starts 1 to 2 weeks after the initial infection. Patients may be asymptomatic or have mild symptoms consisting of fever and malaise. Most cases resolve in a few weeks. Very few patients develop severe acute disease, including myocarditis, pericarditis, and meningoencephalitis.

The chronic phase begins weeks or months after the initial infection, but symptoms may not appear for decades. Symptoms most commonly involve the cardiac or GI systems. Cardiac symptoms of Chagas disease include heart failure, arrhythmias, and thromboembolism due to cardiac mural thrombi.

Esophageal disease is more common, followed by colonic disease; symptoms are due to destruction of submucosal and myenteric nerves that lead to progressive dilation. Symptoms include dysphagia, regurgitation, malnutrition, constipation, abdominal pain, and volvulus.

Sleeping sickness presents acutely with intermittent fever, headaches, malaise, weight loss, and rash.

Symptoms may present years after exposure. In the late stages of the disease patients note headache, sensorineural disorders, personality changes, tremor, and frank psychosis. Disruption of the normal circadian rhythm causes daytime somnolence leading to the name "sleeping sickness." Patients become less arousable with progressive disease, leading to coma and death.

SIGNS AND SYMPTOMS

Acute Chagas disease starts immediately after infection and may last for a few weeks or months. During the acute phase patients are asymptomatic or symptoms are mild. Acute infection rarely results in severe inflammation of the heart muscle or the brain.

Following the acute phase, infected people may have a prolonged asymptomatic form of disease during which few or no parasites are noted in the blood. Many people may remain asymptomatic for life and never develop Chagas-related symptoms. If chronic disease does develop complications can develop and include heart rhythm abnormalities that can cause sudden death, cardiomyopathy leading to heart failure, or a dilated esophagus or colon leading to dysphagia and bowel obstruction.

Sleeping sickness has two stages. In the first stage, the parasite is found in the peripheral circulation, but has not invaded the nervous system. Patients develop fever, headache, and muscle and joint aches within 1–2 weeks of the infective bite. Once the blood-brain barrier is crossed and the central nervous system infected the disease enters the second phase. Phase two leads to mental deterioration and other neurologic problems. If not treated the infection will lead to coma and death.

PHYSICAL EXAMINATION

In Chagas disease the classic physical examination finding is the chagoma. A chagoma is swelling at the site of inoculation. A chagoma near the eye after conjunctival inoculation is called Romana sign. If there is cardiac involvement a cardiac heave, mitral or tricuspid regurgitation, elevated jugular venous pulses, peripheral edema, and tachycardia may be noted.

Physical exam of patients with chronic GI disease secondary to Chagas may show cachexia, abdominal distention and tenderness, and impacted stool.

Sleeping sickness presents with a chancre at the initial inoculation site followed by lymph node infection and parasitemia. The chancre is a painful, red, papule 2–4 cm in diameter. Lymphadenopathy may be noted. Splenomegaly and lymphadenopathy may be noted early in the disease.

DIFFERENTIAL DIAGNOSIS

Chagas infection differential diagnosis includes malaria, typhoid, tuberculosis, influenza, and noninfectious causes of fever and malaise including connective tissue disease and malignancy.

Sleeping sickness differential diagnosis includes HIV infection, miliary tuberculosis, cerebral malaria, lymphoma, and connective tissue disease.

Preseptal cellulitis presents with eyelid edema, fever, and erythema.

DIAGNOSTIC STUDIES

There is no standard laboratory test that is helpful in making the diagnosis of Chagas disease. EKG may reveal cardiac abnormalities such as bundle branch block, nonspecific ST segment changes, AV block, and prolonged QT intervals.

Acute infection can be confirmed by identifying trypomastigotes on blood smears. In the chronic phase smears may be negative as the parasite load decreases. A PCR assay is the test of choice; it has a higher sensitivity than blood smears to detect parasitemia in early acute infection. For congenital cases, the test of choice is PCR.

Serologic testing for IgG to *T. cruzi* is the test of choice for indeterminate or chronic Chagas disease. Two different types of tests must be used, and if there are discordant results, a third serologic test must be used.

In chronic infection the role of PCR is clear, and diagnosis should be based on serology, epidemiology, and clinical picture.

TREATMENT

Treatment is indicated for all cases of acute, reactivated, or congenital Chagas disease and for chronic infection in children up to age 18. In adults up to age 50, with chronic infection and no signs of advanced cardiomyopathy, treatment is strongly recommended. For adults older than 50 years with chronic infection the decision to treat should be determined on a case-by-case basis.

The antiparasitic drugs of choice are benznidazole and nifurtimox. Benznidazole is approved by for use in children over 2 years of age. Nifurtimox is not commercially available in the United States. It is available under investigational protocols from CDC and is available in other parts of the world where the disease is endemic. Side effects are common with both drugs. Contraindications for treatment include severe hepatic and/or renal disease.

Treatment is indicated for all persons diagnosed with African trypanosomiasis or sleeping sickness. The choice of therapy depends on the infecting subspecies and the disease stage. The first-line drugs for first and second stage disease include the following:

- Pentamidine: IV or intramuscular injection for first stage infections with *T. b. gambiense* Well tolerated, but adverse reactions include hypoglycemia, injection site pain, diarrhea, nausea and vomiting.
- Suramin: for first stage of infection with *T. b. rhodesiense*. Does not cross blood-brain barrier. Adverse reactions include drug rash, nephrotoxicity, and peripheral neuropathy.
- Eflornithine: IV for second stage infection with *T. b. gambiense*. Adverse effects include bone marrow suppression, GI symptoms, and seizures. Contraindicated in pregnancy.
- Melarsoprol is used to treat the second stage *T. b. rhodesiense*. Adverse reactions include a life-threatening encephalopathic reaction, skin reactions, GI upset, and peripheral neuropathy.

There is no test of cure for African trypanosomiasis. Patients should be followed with a lumbar puncture every 6 month for 2 years after treatment to detect a relapse.

PATIENT EDUCATION

- Spread of disease can be limited by vector control measures in endemic countries. This includes spraying insecticides.

17.6AB LEISHMANIASIS

Leishmaniasis is due to protozoan parasites of the genus *Leishmania*. There are multiple clinical syndromes: cutaneous, due to infection in macrophages in the dermis; mucosal, due to infection in the naso-oropharyngeal mucosa; and visceral, due to infection throughout the reticuloendothelial system. The various infections range from asymptomatic to severe. Cutaneous and mucosal leishmaniasis can cause substantial morbidity, whereas visceral leishmaniasis can be life threatening.

The transmission vector is the female sand fly. The organism exists in two forms, an extracellular promastigote in the gut of the sand fly is injected via bite into the host where they are taken up by macrophages and transform into intracellular amastigotes. They can then either multiply locally or disseminate throughout the reticuloendothelial system.

MEDICAL HISTORY AND CLINICAL PRESENTATION

The various types of leishmaniasis have various presentations. Cutaneous leishmaniasis primary symptoms are single or multiple skin lesions. Mucosal leishmaniasis primarily affects the nose and mouth. The nasal septum can be destroyed leading to disfigurement. Visceral leishmaniasis has two clinical manifestations:

- Kala-azar (black fever) has gradual onset of malaise, fever, weight loss, abdominal pain, and left upper quadrant fullness. In late stages of the disease hepatic dysfunction, cachexia, ascites, and bleeding complications can occur.
- Viscerotropic disease is a systemic illness that is milder than kala-azar and presents with fever, abdominal pain, adenopathy, malaise, and lymphadenopathy.

SIGNS AND SYMPTOMS

Cutaneous leishmaniasis is the most common form of leishmaniasis. Different *Leishmania* species cause disease in different regions; those that cause leishmaniasis in the Eastern Hemisphere are *Leishmania tropica*, *L. major*, *L. aethiopica*, *L. infantum*, and *L. donovani* and for the Western hemisphere the species are *L. mexicana* species complex or the subgenus *Viannia*.

Cutaneous leishmaniasis causes skin lesions that develop within weeks or months after the exposure and can persist for years. The lesions start as papules then evolve to nodular plaques and ulcerative lesions, with a raised border and central depression. The lesions are typically painless.

Mucosal leishmaniasis is due to dissemination of parasites from the skin to the naso-oropharyngeal mucosa. Mucosal leishmaniasis is caused by species in the *Viannia* subgenus or *L.L. amazonensis*.

Mucosal disease typically becomes clinically evident within several years of the original cutaneous lesions, which were not treated or received suboptimal treatment. The initial manifestations include persistent, unusual nasal symptoms or oropharyngeal symptoms. The disease can progress to destruction of the naso-oropharyngeal mucosa.

Visceral leishmaniasis has an incubation period of weeks to months; symptoms may not be noted for years. Visceral leishmaniasis is caused by the species *L. donovani* and *L. infantum* and affects internal organs, such as the spleen, liver, and bone marrow. Systemic symptoms include fever and cachexia.

PHYSICAL EXAMINATION

Physical examination reveals painless papules then evolve into nodular plaques and then ulcerative lesions, with a raised border and central depression. With visceral disease hepatosplenomegaly and lymphadenopathy are noted.

DIFFERENTIAL DIAGNOSIS

The differential diagnosis for cutaneous disease includes sporotrichosis, blastomycosis, cutaneous tuberculosis, atypical mycobacterial infections, syphilis, yaws, leprosy, sarcoidosis, discoid lupus, and neoplasms.

The differential diagnosis for mucosal disease includes paracoccidioidomycosis, sarcoidosis, malignancy, yaws, syphilis, and histoplasmosis.

The differential diagnosis for acute visceral disease includes malaria, schistosomiasis, acute Chagas disease, tuberculosis, and typhoid fever. The differential diagnosis for chronic visceral disease includes brucellosis, hepatosplenic schistosomiasis, hematologic malignancy, and chronic malaria.

DIAGNOSTIC STUDIES

For cutaneous and mucosal disease, the CBC is normal, in visceral disease there is a pancytopenia and eosinophilia. Visceral disease also reveals elevated liver function tests, hyperbilirubinemia, and decreased serum albumin and gamma globulins.

To confirm the diagnosis of cutaneous and mucosal disease, a scraping or biopsy of the lesion should be obtained. The sample should be examined for parasites with the Giemsa or Wright stains. It is not possible to distinguish *Leishmania* species by morphology.

Culture can be performed but it may take up to 4 weeks for growth to appear. Serology is not helpful in cutaneous disease.

In visceral disease a bone marrow sample to be obtained and stained to identify the organism or cultured.

Serology can be helpful in visceral disease but must be interpreted in context of the clinical presentation and history. IFA and ELISA are useful.

TREATMENT

Wound care is an important part of cutaneous leishmaniasis treatment. Specific treatments are as follows: local treatment includes topical paromomycin and paromomycin-gentamicin, intralesional antimony, cryotherapy, thermotherapy, and selective irradiation; oral treatment involves miltefosine and azoles; parenteral treatments include pentavalent antimony compounds, such as sodium antimony gluconate, which is available from the CDC; parenteral amphotericin B, liposomal amphotericin B, or pentamidine can be used if antimony treatment is not tolerated.

For mucosal leishmaniasis the recommended treatment is pentavalent antimony compounds, miltefosine, amphotericin or pentamidine

The preferred treatment for visceral leishmaniasis is liposomal amphotericin, conventional amphotericin B, and pentavalent antimony compounds. Second-line agents include miltefosine and paromomycin.

PATIENT EDUCATION

- Congenital infections can occur with visceral leishmaniasis infections in pregnancy.
- Severe deformities can result from cutaneous or mucosal lesions of the face and oral or nasal mucosa.
- No vaccines or drugs to prevent infection are available.
- Prevention is best done by providing protection from sand fly bites. Protective measures include limiting nighttime outdoor activities, wearing protective clothing, and applying insect repellent.

17.6AC MALARIA

Malaria is one of the most important tropical diseases affecting humans. The condition is caused by protozoa of the genus *Plasmodium* and transmitted to humans by the female anopheline mosquito.

There are four *Plasmodium* species known to cause malaria in humans: *P. falciparum*, *P. vivax*, *P. ovale*, and *P. malariae*.

According to WHO estimates, malaria infected over 228 million people worldwide and caused 405,000 deaths in 2018.[79] Most of the deaths and serious complications of malaria are caused by *P. falciparum*.

Malaria is widely distributed in sub-Saharan Africa, Central America and the Caribbean, South America, the Middle East, Far East, and Indonesia. *P. falciparum* is predominant in Africa, New Guinea, Haiti, and the Dominican Republic. *P. falciparum* and *P. vivax* are predominant in South America and the Indian subcontinent. *P. malariae* is predominant in sub-Saharan Africa (Figure 17.18).

P. vivax and *P. ovale* generally infect young erythrocytes, while *P. malariae* infects old red blood cells. *P. falciparum* infects erythrocytes of all ages.

Malaria has two life cycles, one in humans and one in the *Anopheles* mosquito. Sporozoites, the infectious form of the parasite, are injected into the bloodstream of a human when the *Anopheles* mosquito is taking a blood meal, initiating the start of the human cycle. Sporozoites in the bloodstream are removed by the body's defense systems; those not eliminated develop into liver schizonts. After several days, the liver schizont ruptures and merozoites are released into the bloodstream. For *P. vivax* and *P.ovale*, the sporozoites may develop into hypnozoites, a latent form that remains in the liver.

Once in the bloodstream, the merozoites infect red blood cells; they go through several stages of trophozoite development before developing into erythrocytic schizonts. The erythrocytic schizonts rupture releasing merozoites into the

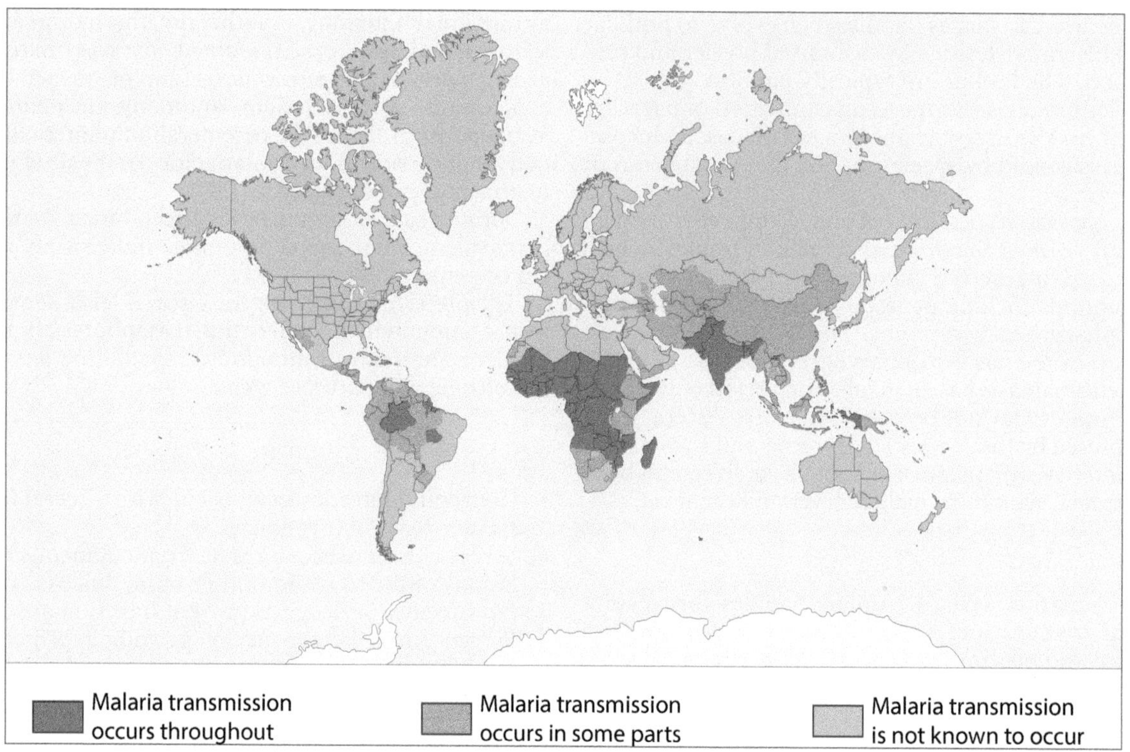

Figure 17.18 **Global distribution of malaria.**
(Source: Centers for Disease Control and Prevention.)

circulation. The time from initial inoculation of sporozoites to release of merozoites varies by *Plasmodium* species.

Some of the merozoites develop into sexual forms known as gametocytes; only mature gametocytes are found in the peripheral blood. The patient is infective during this stage.

MEDICAL HISTORY AND CLINICAL PRESENTATION

The symptoms of uncomplicated malaria, the blood stage of infection, include fever, rigors, headache, malaise, anorexia, and cough.

The classic fever cycles of 48 hours for *P. falciparum*, *P. vivax*, and *P. ovale* and 72 hours for *P. malariae* are not frequently noted in clinical settings and should not be used for making or ruling out a diagnosis of malaria.

Complicated malaria presents with symptoms of acute renal failure, pulmonary edema, disseminated intravascular coagulation, intravascular hemolysis, fever, shock, delirium, stupor, and coma.

P. falciparum malaria has an insidious onset and patients present with flu-like symptoms such as fever, headache, malaise, aches and pains, and jaundice resulting in an initial diagnosis of IM or viral hepatitis.

P. vivax malaria onset is abrupt with chills and rigors. This "cold stage" lasts an hour and is usually followed by a "hot stage" that lasts 4 to 6 hours, during which the patient develops high fever, headache, malaise, vomiting, abdominal pain, thirst, and polyuria. The "hot stage" is followed by the "sweating stage," which lasts 1 hour during which the fever breaks and the symptoms resolve.

SIGNS AND SYMPTOMS

Symptoms of malaria are generally nonspecific and most commonly consist of fever, headache, malaise, weakness, GI complaints, neurologic complaints, back pain, myalgia, chills, and/or cough. The diagnosis of malaria should also be considered in any person with fever of unknown origin regardless of travel history.

PHYSICAL EXAMINATION

Physical examination findings vary with the stage of disease. Findings include tachycardia, tachypnea, splenomegaly, and hepatomegaly. The patient may appear ill with fever, chills, and sweating. With hemolysis and anemia the patient may be pale and cyanotic, and sclerae may be icteric.

With cerebral malaria mental status will be altered, seizures may develop, and coma may be present.

DIFFERENTIAL DIAGNOSIS

The differential diagnosis for malaria includes dengue, typhoid fever, pneumonia, influenza, viral hepatitis, leptospirosis, rickettsial infections, meningococcal meningitis, and viral encephalitis.

DIAGNOSTIC STUDIES

The diagnosis of malaria is made by examining the peripheral blood. Thick and thin blood smears remain the major laboratory diagnostic test for malaria. Rapid diagnostic testing for the detection of malaria based on lateral-flow immunochromatography is available (Figure 17.19).

Other laboratory findings include a normochromic normocytic anemia, thrombocytopenia, and leukopenia. ESR and C-reactive protein levels are elevated.

Chemistry profile reveals mild hyponatremia, and metabolic acidosis with an elevated anion gap is possible. Liver enzyme tests may show elevated levels of bilirubin, ALT and AST. CSF testing is usually normal in cerebral malaria although total protein may be elevated.

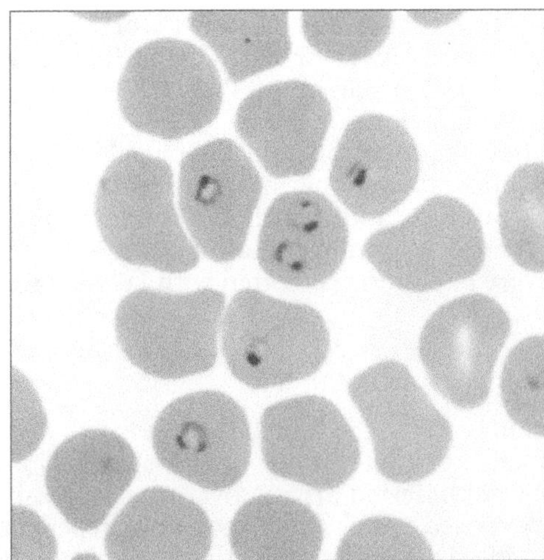

Figure 17.19 **Thin blood smear of *Plasmodium falciparum* ring forms.**

Thick and thin blood smears are the gold standard for diagnosis in endemic countries. Typically, 2 to 3 blood smears done daily for 3 to 4 days must be negative to rule out the diagnosis of malaria.

Serology testing is of no use for the diagnosis of an acute attack of malaria.

TREATMENT

The CDC guidelines provide a general approach to the treatment of malaria.[80] Treatment is based on the *Plasmodium* species and where in the world the infection was acquired.

P. falciparum or Species Not Identified—Acquired in Areas With Chloroquine Resistance

For *P. falciparum* infections acquired in areas with chloroquine resistance there are four treatment options:

- Artemether-lumefantrine
  - The preferred option if available.
- Atovaquone-proguanil
- Quinine sulfate plus doxycycline, tetracycline, or clindamycin
  - Quinine sulfate plus either doxycycline or tetracycline is preferred to quinine sulfate plus clindamycin.
- Mefloquine
  - Associated with rare but potentially severe neuropsychiatric reactions when used at treatment dose.
  - Recommended only when the other options cannot be used.
  - Due to drug resistance mefloquine is not recommended for infections acquired in certain parts of Southeast Asia.

For pediatric patients, the treatment options are the same as for adults except the doses are adjusted by patient weight; artemether-lumefantrine and atovaquone-proguanil can only be used in children who weigh ≥5 kg.

P. falciparum or Species Not Identified—Acquired in Areas Without Chloroquine Resistance

- *P. falciparum* infections acquired in areas without chloroquine-resistant strains is treated with oral chloroquine, or as a second option hydroxychloroquine.
- Any of the regimens listed for the treatment of chloroquine-resistant malaria may be used for the treatment of chloroquine-sensitive *P. falciparum* malaria.
- If infections initially due to an unidentified species are identified as *P. vivax* or *P. ovale*, additional treatment with primaquine or tafenoquine should be administered.

P. malariae

- There is no chloroquine resistance in *P. malariae* so chloroquine or hydroxychloroquine can still be used to treat this infection. Also any of the regimens listed above for the treatment of chloroquine-resistant *P. falciparum* may be used for the treatment of *P. malariae* infection.

P. vivax and *P. ovale*

- Chloroquine or hydroxychloroquine remain effective choices for *P. vivax* and *P. ovale* infections except for *P. vivax* infections acquired in Papua New Guinea or Indonesia where there is a high prevalence of chloroquine-resistant *P. vivax*. Rare chloroquine-resistant *P. vivax* has been documented in Myanmar, India, and Central and South America. Infections due to *P. vivax* infections from these regions can be treated with artemether-lumefantrine, atovaquone-proguanil, quinine sulfate plus doxycycline or tetracycline or clindamycin, or mefloquine. Persons acquiring *P. vivax* infections in Papua New Guinea or Indonesia should initially be treated with a regimen recommended for chloroquine-resistant *P. vivax* infections.
- Infections with *P. vivax* and *P. ovale* can relapse due to hypnozoites that remain dormant in the liver. To eradicate the hypnozoites, patients should be treated with either primaquine phosphate or tafenoquine

PATIENT EDUCATION

- Vector control, including insecticide-treated mosquito nets and indoor residual spraying, is the main method for the prevention and reduction of malaria transmission.
- Recommendations for drugs to prevent malaria differ by country of travel and the CDC should be contacted for the appropriate medication options.
- No antimalarial drug is 100% protective and must be combined with the use of personal protective measures.

17.6AD BABESIOSIS

Babesiosis caused by *Babesia microti,* a blood protozoan, is highly endemic in the U.S. areas of southern Massachusetts, southern Rhode Island, coastal Connecticut and offshore islands, the Lower Hudson Valley, and central New Jersey. Other highly endemic areas are found in Wisconsin and Minnesota.

Tick bite is the primary mode of transmission to humans. *Ixodes scapularis* nymphs are the primary vector. The incubation period is 1 to 6 weeks. Transfusion of blood products obtained from asymptomatic carriers is the second most frequent mode of transmission.

B. microti is a parasite of small rodents, including the white footed mouse, shrews, chipmunks, voles, and rats. The white-tailed deer are not competent reservoirs for *B. microti* but are required for the survival, by providing a blood meal for the adult tick and mating of adult ticks.

In humans the *B. microti* protozoan invades red blood cells only. Following entry, parasites mature into trophozoites that move in the cytoplasm. Asexual replication yields four merozoites. As merozoites leave the cell the cell lyses. Free merozoites attach to nearby red blood cells and invade these host cells.

MEDICAL HISTORY AND CLINICAL PRESENTATION

Most cases of babesiosis occur in May through September, with most cases in July and August. Certain environmental conditions predispose a patient to infection; this includes a large deer population and areas with tall grass, brushes, and foliage. Presentation includes fatigue, malaise, and weakness.

SIGNS AND SYMPTOMS

At the time of presentation patients present with onset of fatigue, malaise, and weakness. Fever is intermittent or sustained and is typically accompanied by chills, sweats, headache, myalgia, arthralgia, or anorexia. Other symptoms include sore throat, dry cough, neck stiffness, shortness of breath, left upper quadrant pain, nausea, vomiting, weight loss, and diarrhea.

PHYSICAL EXAMINATION

Patients may have no physical examination findings. Physical examination findings will vary depending on the severity of the infection and patient's underlying medical condition and medical history. The main physical examination finding is fever. Occasionally mild splenomegaly and hepatomegaly may be noted; lymphadenopathy is absent.

DIFFERENTIAL DIAGNOSIS

Because of the nonspecific symptoms the infection may be mistaken for a viral illness. Other disorders in the differential diagnosis include Lyme disease, anaplasmosis, rickettsial disease, and bacterial endocarditis.

DIAGNOSTIC STUDIES

Because of the hemolytic process, patients present with anemia, decreased haptoglobin, and elevated LDH. Increased reticulocytes will be noted and schistocytes and helmet cells may be noted on peripheral blood smear. Thrombocytopenia is common and WBC count is normal or slightly elevated.

On peripheral blood smear, *B. microti* trophozoites appear as rings with a pale blue cytoplasm and one or two red chromatic dots and merozoites are arranged in tetrads, also called a "Maltese cross." *B. microti* rings may be mistaken for *Plasmodium falciparum* early stage trophozoites, but malaria can be ruled out by travel history and careful microscopic examination of the blood.

PCR is useful to diagnose babesiosis when the parasite burden is low. Indirect immunofluorescent antibody testing is used to detect antibodies against *Babesia* species. IgG titers ≥1,024 indicate active or recent infection and titers will decline over time and are considered negative when titer levels are <64.

TREATMENT

Therapy should be given to symptomatic patients if *Babesia* is detected on blood smear or by PCR for longer than 3 months. Treatment is not indicated when *Babesia* is not detected on blood smear or by PCR or *Babesia* has been detected on blood smear or by PCR for <3 months in an asymptomatic individual.

The initial treatment of mild babesiosis consists of azithromycin plus atovaquone in adults and children. Other treatment option in adults includes clindamycin plus quinine; this treatment option has a high incidence of adverse effects. Severe babesiosis is treated with IV clindamycin and quinine.

PATIENT EDUCATION

- There is no vaccine for human babesiosis.
- Avoidance of tick bites is key to prevention. This includes avoiding tick-infested areas; covering parts of body that may be exposed to ticks; and use of tick repellents, diethyltoluamide (DEET), or permethrin.

17.6AE TOXOPLASMOSIS

Toxoplasma gondii is an obligate intracellular parasite found worldwide. Cats are the definitive host with humans as intermediate host. Humans harbor the parasite in the brain, eye, heart, and skeletal muscle.

T. gondii primarily exists in three infectious forms:

- **Tachyzoite:** rapidly replicating form responsible for the clinical manifestations and dissemination of the parasite in patients
- **Bradyzoite:** hibernating form contained in tissue cysts and responsible for the chronic state of the infection
- **Oocyst:** form excreted by infected cats and responsible for its wide dissemination in nature

In North America, the major risk factor for transmission of the parasite is through contaminated and undercooked meat. There is no evidence for person-to-person transmission of *T. gondii*.

After oral infection of tissue cysts or oocysts, the cyst walls are disrupted by digestive enzymes. The bradyzoites and sporozoites are released and converted to the tachyzoite form. The tachyzoites spread via hematogenous or lymphatic spread and infect other tissues. This leads to necrosis and surrounding inflammation of the infected tissue.

In the immunocompetent patient, the immune system controls the proliferation of the tachyzoite and it reverts back to the bradyzoite form; this leads to the formation of tissue cysts, noted in chronic infections. Tissue cysts persist for life. An intact immune system is required for successful resistance against *T. gondii*.

In immunocompromised patients previously infected, decreased T-cell-mediated immune responses facilitate the reactivation of their infection.

MEDICAL HISTORY AND CLINICAL PRESENTATION

Primary or acute infection is defined as the first encounter of the individual with the parasite. Chronic infection follows the acute infection by 6 months after the initial infection. The possibility of a toxoplasmosis infection cannot be ruled out because the patient did not consume undercooked meat or does not own cats, as up to half of infected patients do not recall having been exposed to any known risk factor.

Immunocompetent patients with primary or acute infection present asymptomatic or present with a wide variety of symptoms. See Box 17.1 for toxoplasmosis signs and symptoms.

Chronic infection in immunocompetent patients is asymptomatic except for chorioretinitis, which can develop because of reactivation of chronic infection.

In pregnancy the main concern is infection in the fetus. Mother-to-child transmission can occur through the placenta in immunocompetent women who acquire primary infection during gestation or in immunocompromised women who reactivate their chronic infection during gestation.

Congenital toxoplasmosis can result in a wide spectrum of clinical manifestations, ranging from no clinical manifestations to serious neurologic signs. The fetus may present with hydrocephalus, brain or hepatic calcifications, or splenomegaly. The newborn may present with failure to thrive, diarrhea, hypothermia, petechiae, rash, blindness, seizures, microcephaly or hydrocephalus, mental retardation, hepatosplenomegaly, and jaundice.

In the immunocompromised patient, toxoplasmosis can result in significant morbidity and mortality; this includes patients with AIDS, transplant patients, those with a history of hematologic malignancies, or those on immunosuppressive drugs.

Primary infection in immunocompromised patients has been rarely described, except for solid organ transplant patients. Toxoplasmosis can develop in AIDS patients infected with *T. gondii* whose CD4 T cell counts are below 200 cells/mm^3 and who are not taking effective antitoxoplasma prophylaxis. Multiple brain abscesses are commonly described in AIDS patients with toxoplasmosis encephalitis.

SIGNS AND SYMPTOMS

Acquired infection in immunocompetent patients is generally asymptomatic. A small number of patients with acute infection will develop cervical lymphadenopathy and a flu-like illness. The disease course is usually benign and self-limited, resolving within a few months to a year. Immunocompromised patients present with central nervous system disease, retinochoroiditis, or pneumonia. In AIDS patients, toxoplasmosis encephalitis is the most common cause of intracerebral mass lesions and is typically due to reactivation of chronic infection.

PHYSICAL EXAMINATION

Physical examination findings include painless lymphadenopathy in immunocompetent individuals. Other findings include fever, malaise, myalgias, and a maculopapular skin rash that spares the palms and the soles. If retinochoroiditis is present, examination reveals multiple yellow-white cotton-like patches with indistinct margins located in small clusters.

BOX 17.1 Signs and Symptoms of Toxoplasmosis Infection in Immunocompetent Hosts

Chorioretinitis	Lymphadenopathy
Fever	Headache
Myalgias/arthralgias	Sore throat
Stiff neck	Nausea
Abdominal pain	Diarrhea
Anorexia	Rash
Mental status changes	General malaise/fatigue

DIFFERENTIAL DIAGNOSIS

In immunocompetent patients the differential diagnosis varies with symptoms.

Chorioretinitis with can mimic chorioretinitis due to herpes simplex, VZV infection, or CMV infection.

If systemic symptoms are present the differential includes upper respiratory viral infections, streptococcal pharyngitis, HIV, and IM-like syndrome.

If lymphadenopathy is present the differential includes lymphadenitis; infection due to *Bartonella*, mycobacteria, or fungi; and lymphoma.

In immunocompromised patients the differential diagnosis includes:

- Pneumonia due *Pneumocystis jirovecii*, *Mycoplasma pneumoniae*, *Chlamydia pneumoniae*, *Legionella pneumophila*, or viruses.
- Central nervous system disorder such as central nervous system lymphoma, progressive multifocal leukoencephalopathy, and Chagas disease.

DIAGNOSTIC STUDIES

Serologic tests, including *T. gondii*-specific IgG and IgM, PCR, and visualization of the parasite in cytologic and histologic slides, are used for the diagnosis of *T. gondii* infection and toxoplasmosis.

To diagnosis reactivation of chronic infection in immunocompromised patients the following are required:

- The visualization of tachyzoites in body fluid or tissue
- A successful amplification of the parasite DNA in body fluid
- *T. gondii*-specific immunohistochemistry that reveals the presence of parasite antigens surrounded by an inflammatory response

In immunocompetent individuals and during pregnancy and congenital infection diagnosis requires:

- *Toxoplasma*-specific IgG and IgM: Initial serologic screening should be performed to determine whether the patient has ever been infected or is acutely or chronically infected.
  - Negative IgG and negative IgM: If the patient is able to produce IgG and IgM, these negative results would indicate no serologic evidence of *T. gondii* infection.
  - Positive IgG and negative IgM: The patient has been infected with *T. gondii* for some time, probably more than 3–6 months.
  - Positive IgM, regardless of the IgG test result: A positive IgM test result can be observed in acute or chronic infections.

In immunocompromised patients initial screening with a *Toxoplasma*-specific IgG test should be performed in all individuals before or shortly after they become immunosuppressed. A positive IgG antibody test establishes that the patient has been infected and is at risk of reactivation of disease.

For immunocompromised patients who present with symptom and signs that suggest infection, a PCR, direct visualization of tachyzoites in body fluids or tissues, or histologic examination can be completed to aid in the diagnosis of toxoplasmosis.

Brain and spinal cord imaging studies, such as MRI, should be obtained in immunocompromised patients who present with CNS symptoms or signs. In HIV-infected individuals, the diagnosis of toxoplasmosis encephalitis can be established as probable in those who present with multiple ring-enhancing brain-occupying lesions, often involving the basal ganglia.

Toxoplasmosis pneumonia is associated with bilateral interstitial pulmonary infiltrates.

TREATMENT

In the immunocompetent patient treatment is indicated in those with severe or ongoing clinical manifestations in the setting of acute infection. Treatment is also indicated for patients with active chorioretinitis due to primary infection or reactivation of a latent infection. The duration of treatment is typically 3–4 weeks or until symptoms have resolved.

Currently recommended treatment for toxoplasmosis targets the tachyzoite stage and does not eradicate encysted parasites in the tissues. Pyrimethamine, the most effective medication against toxoplasmosis, is a folic acid antagonist with the side effect of bone marrow suppression; this side effect can be controlled with the concurrent administration of folinic acid. A second drug, such as sulfadiazine or clindamycin, should be included. The fixed combination of trimethoprim with sulfamethoxazole has been used as an alternative.

Treatment for ocular diseases, in adults and pediatric patients, consists of pyrimethamine plus sulfadiazine plus folinic acid. Therapy should be for 4 to 6 weeks followed by reevaluation. Corticosteroids can be prescribed in addition to antiparasitic agents.

Management of maternal and fetal infection varies; spiramycin is recommended for women whose infections were acquired and diagnosed before 18 weeks gestation and infection of the fetus is not documented or suspected. Pyrimethamine, sulfadiazine and leucovorin are recommended for infections acquired at or after 18 weeks gestation or infection in the fetus is documented or suspected. PCR is used on amniotic fluid at 18 gestation weeks to determine if the infant is infected. Congenitally infected newborns are generally treated with pyrimethamine, a sulfonamide, and leucovorin for 12 months.

Toxoplasmosis in immunocompromised patients is often fatal if not treated. Standard treatment consists of pyrimethamine, folinic acid, and sulfadiazine. Treatment is recommended for 4 to 6 weeks beyond resolution of all clinical signs and symptoms but may be required for 6 months or longer. Relapses can occur in AIDS patients and maintenance therapy is recommended until a significant immunologic improvement is achieved in response to ART.

PATIENT EDUCATION

- Immunocompetent patients with ocular disease can be left with serious visual sequelae or blind.
- An infected newborn can be born normal but develop new lesions later in life. They can develop hydrocephalus, intracranial calcifications, chorioretinitis, hearing deficits, neurologic complications, or hematologic abnormalities.

17.6AF AMEBIASIS

Amebiasis is caused by *Entamoeba histolytica*. *E. histolytica* has two forms, the infectious cyst and the invasive trophozoite; both can be found in the stool of infected patients.

Infection occurs via the fecal-oral route; cysts are ingested in fecal-contaminated food, water, or by hands. Cysts are environmentally resistant and can survive for days to weeks in the external environment.

E. histolytica is found worldwide, but is endemic in Mexico, India, Bangladesh, South Africa, some Central and South American countries, and Asian Pacific countries.

In developed countries, high-risk groups include travelers, immigrants from endemic areas, and MSM.

E. histolytica is the cause of amebic liver abscesses, which are 10 times more common in men than women and are rare in children. Liver abscesses are more common in the fourth and fifth decade of life. Risk factors include travel to endemic areas and a history of alcohol abuse.

Infection control and prevention in travelers includes limiting parasite exposure by avoiding the drinking local water and eating only cooked or peeled food. If bottled water is not available, the water should be boiled before being consumed.

Once the parasite is ingested, excystation occurs in the small intestine, and trophozoites are released. The trophozoites migrate to the large intestine where they multiply by binary fission. In the asymptomatic patient who is a carrier, the trophozoites remain confined to the intestinal lumen and cysts are passed in stools.

When the trophozoites invade the intestinal mucosa, the patient presents with colitis. *E. histolytica* trophozoites are cytolytic and can kill both epithelial cells and inflammatory cells. If the trophozoites spread through the bloodstream to extraintestinal sites, infection of the liver, brain, and lungs can occur.

MEDICAL HISTORY AND CLINICAL PRESENTATION

Predisposing factors include foreign travel or immigration from an area of endemic transmission. Steroids or other immunosuppressive medications can activate a latent infection.

Amebiasis should be considered in the differential diagnosis of diarrhea, dysentery, colitis, liver abscess, or brain abscess.

Most infected people are asymptomatic. Symptoms can range from mild diarrhea to dysentery with blood and mucus. Other symptoms include fever, fatigue, tenesmus, vomiting, abdominal tenderness, and weight loss.

SIGNS AND SYMPTOMS

Most patients are asymptomatic. Amebic colitis presents with symptoms ranging from mild diarrhea to fulminant colitis. The onset is often gradual, and patients frequently report several weeks of symptoms.

Presenting features of amebic colitis include bloody diarrhea, abdominal pain, weight loss, and fever.

Amebic liver abscess is the most common extraintestinal manifestation of amebiasis and is due to spread via the portal venous system. Symptoms include fever, right upper quadrant pain, hepatomegaly, diarrhea, and cough.

Jaundice is uncommon, and its presence indicates large or multiple abscesses, bacterial superinfection, or hepatic dysfunction.

PHYSICAL EXAMINATION

Physical examination findings vary depending on severity of disease. Findings can include signs of tachycardia, hypotension due to dehydration, weight loss signs of malnourishment, abdominal tenderness, and stool positive for the presence of blood.

With liver abscess there are right upper quadrant tenderness, hepatomegaly, and if there is rupture of the abscess signs of sepsis.

DIFFERENTIAL DIAGNOSIS

The differential diagnosis includes infection due to *Salmonella, Shigella, Campylobacter* species, amebic liver abscess, and enterohemorrhagic *Escherichia coli.*

DIAGNOSTIC STUDIES

Common laboratory findings in amebic liver abscess include leukocytosis without eosinophilia, mild anemia, increased bilirubin, and increased alkaline phosphatase. Positive fecal occult blood test may be seen in patients with amebic colitis.

Stool microscopy may be difficult to interpret because of the difficulty in differentiating between different species of *Entamoeba.* In the presence of acute colitis and positive stool microscopy it can be presumed there is infection with *E. histolytica.* Examination of a minimum of three stool samples is recommended. Finding trophozoites containing ingested red blood cells is not diagnostic, as this can also be noted with *E. dispar* (Figure 17.20).

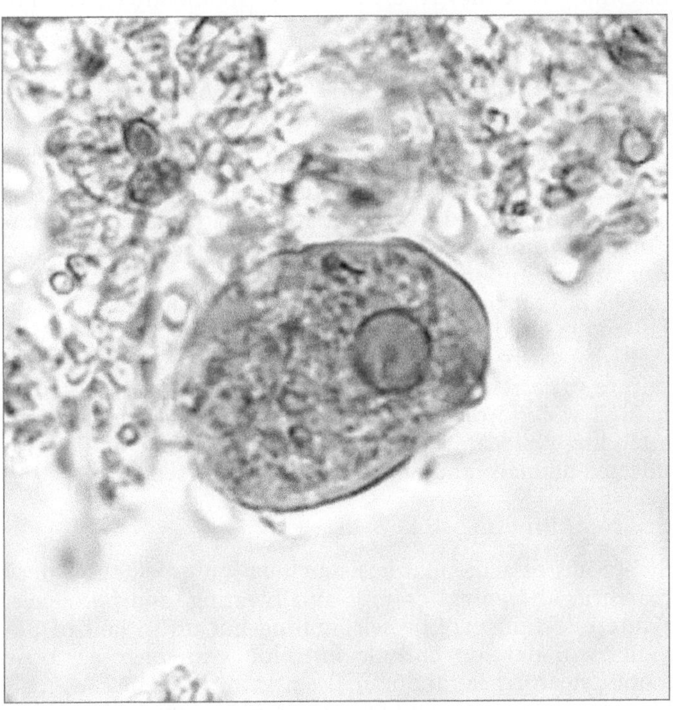

Figure 17.20 ***Entamoeba histolytica*** **trophozoite on wet prep.**

Stool antigen tests are increasingly used for diagnosis. Stool antigen detection is performed using antigen-based ELISA kits. The advantages of antigen detection tests include ability to differentiate between species of *Entamoeba*, rapid testing, and increased sensitivity.

Other tests such as serology have limitations in differentiating between acute and past infection with *E. histolytica.* Colon biopsy may be needed to diagnose amebic colitis if other diagnostic tests are negative.

PCR based approaches are generally considered the method of choice in developed countries. PCR can identify *E. histolytica* in a variety of clinical specimens, including feces, tissues, and liver abscess aspirates and is shown to be specific.

TREATMENT

The drug of choice for amebiasis, amebic colitis or amebic hepatic abscess, is metronidazole. Other options include tinidazole. Since these drugs do not eliminate intestinal carriage, they must be followed with either iodoquinol or paromomycin.

Asymptomatic infection should be treated because of the potential risk of developing invasive disease and the risk of spread to family members. Current treatment guidelines for asymptomatic infection include iodoquinol or paromomycin or diloxanide furoate.

PATIENT EDUCATION

- The most feared outcome is development of an amebic liver abscess. An amebic liver abscess can extend to the pleural or pericardial spaces.

17.6AG CRYPTOSPORIDIUM

Cryptosporidiosis is caused by an intracellular protozoan from the genus *Cryptosporidium*, and the most common are *C. parvum* and *C. hominis*. The parasite affects both immunocompetent and immunocompromised hosts; immunocompromised patients are predisposed to life-threatening disease.

Cryptosporidiosis is a public health concern due to a number of factors, including oocyst resistance to disinfectants and conventional water treatments, no effective treatment, low infective dose (10–100 oocysts), and person-person fecal-oral transmission. Cryptosporidiosis is noted worldwide, with the highest risk groups being children and AIDS patients.

Infection is acquired when the patient ingests the oocysts. In the GI tract the oocyst releases infective sporozoites that infect the host cell after being internalized. The sporozoite then matures into a schizogont, using asexual reproduction, to produce merozoites. Merozoites are released into the intestinal lumen where they infect new cells or undergo sexual reproduction into gametocytes. Gametocytes produce new oocysts that are excreted in the feces or release more sporozoites to infect other cells. This life cycle is repeated in the intestinal lumen leading to autoinfection and heavy persistent infections, with shedding of oocysts in the feces. The infection of the GI epithelium produces watery diarrhea.

MEDICAL HISTORY AND CLINICAL PRESENTATION

The clinical presentation of cryptosporidiosis varies depending on the patient's immunologic status. The infection can be asymptomatic, but most develop watery diarrhea containing mucus and rarely red blood cells or WBCs; intestinal malabsorption is also noted.

In immunocompetent patients cryptosporidiosis presents as an asymptomatic carrier or self-limited acute or persistent diarrhea. The incubation period is 7 to 10 days with symptoms lasting about 2 weeks with acute diarrhea, and about 2.5 months with persistent diarrhea.

In immunocompromised patients there is a wider spectrum of symptoms. Symptoms vary from asymptomatic infection, subacute diarrhea, chronic diarrhea, or fulminant diarrhea. The most common is chronic diarrhea lasting longer than 2 months. The fulminant form occurs in patients with CD4 counts <50/mm^3.

Extraintestinal manifestations are noted in AIDS patients who are not be treated with highly active ART. Biliary tract is the most common site, but other sites include the pancreas, liver, stomach, and lung.

SIGNS AND SYMPTOMS

Cryptosporidium patients present with diarrhea with an average of 10 watery stools per day, cramping abdominal pain, fever, nausea and vomiting, and weight loss. Biliary cryptosporidiosis presents with right upper quadrant pain, nausea, vomiting, fever, and elevated alkaline phosphatase.

PHYSICAL EXAMINATION

There are no characteristic physical examination findings. The hallmark of cryptosporidiosis is diarrhea.

DIFFERENTIAL DIAGNOSIS

Differential diagnosis for cryptosporidiosis, in HIV patients, includes other causes of diarrhea, including the bacteria *Shigella, Salmonella, Campylobacter, Clostridium difficile*; parasites *Giardia lamblia, Isospora belli, Cyclospora, Entamoeba histolytica;* and others such as *Mycobacterium avium, Microspora,* and CMV. Biliary cryptosporidiosis may mimic acute cholecystitis.

DIAGNOSTIC STUDIES

Microscopy is the preferred method to diagnose cryptosporidiosis. A modified Ziehl-Neelsen acid-based staining method is used to identify oocysts in stool. Due to intermittent shedding of oocysts multiple stool samples may be needed. Serology tests are of limited value as many healthy patients have antibodies.

Liver function tests or lipase may be abnormal if the biliary tract, liver, and pancreas are affected.

In biliary cryptosporidiosis endoscopic retrograde cholangiopancreatographic (ERCP) findings include papillary stenosis plus intrahepatic sclerosing cholangitis, and stenosis or sclerosing cholangitis alone.

TREATMENT

Most patients with *Cryptosporidium* infection have mild to moderate symptoms and can maintain their fluid status without additional treatment. Those with severe disease may require supportive care with antidiarrheal agents, such as loperamide, and oral or IV hydration or nutrition support.

The treatment of choice is nitazoxanide, for all patients over the age of 1. Nitazoxanide is well tolerated with minimal GI side effects. Second-line therapy consists of paromomycin.

In HIV-positive immunocompromised patients ART should be started to restore immune function, nitazoxanide should be started while waiting for the CD4 count to improve, and supportive care is administered.

PATIENT EDUCATION

- Prognosis will vary with immune status as described above.
- Counseling is focused on prevention. Enteric precautions and good hygiene are essential to prevent transmission and reinfection.
- Patients are to avoid drinking water from rivers or lakes and use water filters that remove particles.

17.6AH GIARDIASIS

Giardiasis is due to the flagellated protozoan *Giardia duodenalis* and is the most common diarrheal parasite in the United States. *Giardia* is found worldwide and is found in several mammals, including beavers, dogs, cattle, and sheep.

The organism is shed in feces and can survive in freshwater mountain streams or lakes. Untreated well water and fecal contaminated food and water are the most common sources of infection. In 2018, there were 15,548 cases of giardiasis in the United States.[17]

Giardia is a noninvasive organism; the cysts can attach to the duodenum and jejunum and release trophozoites. The trophozoites divide by binary fission, then move to the large intestine where they revert to cyst forms and are excreted in the feces.

MEDICAL HISTORY AND CLINICAL PRESENTATION

Giardia infection presents with symptoms that develop over 1 to 2 weeks. Symptoms include watery diarrhea, steatorrhea, abdominal pain and bloating, flatulence, and vomiting. Symptoms of chronic giardiasis include anorexia, weight loss, and malaise.

The peak incidence of giardiasis is early summer through fall and in children younger than 5 years of age.

Risk factors for acquiring *Giardia* infection include exposure to recreational water, swimming in or drinking untreated water from streams or lakes; international travel; attending childcare facility or nursing home; contact with infected animals; and unprotected anal intercourse.

SIGNS AND SYMPTOMS

Symptoms of acute giardiasis include foul-smelling, watery diarrhea, abdominal cramps and bloating, and flatulence. Acute infection may be self-limiting but up to half of patients will develop chronic infection with ongoing loose stools, steatorrhea, abdominal cramping, weight loss, malabsorption, malaise, and fatigue lasting months.

If untreated, symptoms persist for 2 to 4 weeks or more and significant weight loss may occur. Many patients experience acquired lactose intolerance, which can persist for months, even after the infection resolves.

PHYSICAL EXAMINATION

Physical examination is usually unremarkable. In acute infection patients appear sick and in chronic infection they appear malnourished with significant weight loss. Other findings include low-grade fever, dehydration, and abdominal tenderness.

DIFFERENTIAL DIAGNOSIS

The differential diagnosis includes other protozoan infections, including *Cryptosporidium* and *Cyclospora*; malabsorption syndrome, lactose intolerance, and inflammatory bowel disease.

DIAGNOSTIC STUDIES

Giardia is noninvasive, so eosinophilia or leukocytosis are not noted in the peripheral blood and no WBCs are noted on examination of the stool.

Examination of fresh stool may reveal *Giardia* cysts and trophozoites (Figure 17.21).

Giardia antigen detection assays, ELISA or direct-fluorescent antibody assay, are available and have increased sensitivity compared with microscopic examination.

Duodenal biopsy may be needed to make the diagnosis if noninvasive tests do not reveal the diagnosis.

TREATMENT

Antiparasitic treatment options for giardiasis includes metronidazole, albendazole, or nitazoxanide. In pediatric patients furazolidone or nitazoxanide may be used. Side effects of metronidazole include metallic taste, nausea, vomiting, dizziness, headache, disulfiram-like effect, and neutropenia.

PATIENT EDUCATION

- Treatment of asymptomatic individuals should be considered in an outbreak to help control spread.

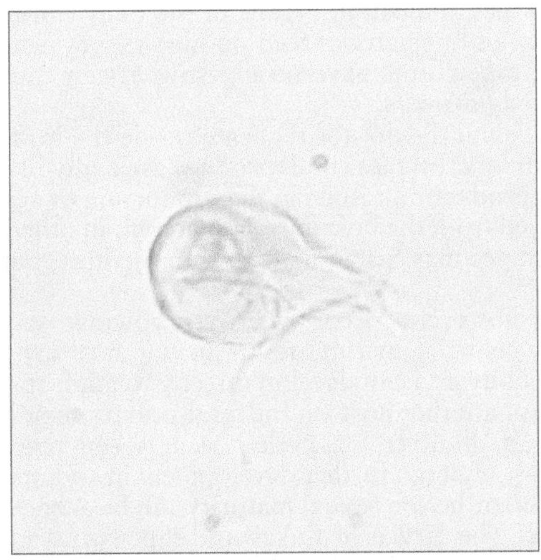

Figure 17.21 ***Giardia duodenalis*** **trophozoite on wet prep.**

17.6AI TRICHOMONIASIS

Trichomoniasis is due to the flagellated protozoan, *Trichomonas vaginalis*. Humans are the only known host. The organism resides in the female lower genital tract and the male prostate and urethra. Transmission is primarily sexual. There are an estimated 3.7 million people with disease in the United States; the prevalence increases with age and is more common in African American females, and more commonly noted in females between 13 and 49 years of age,[81] with 11% of cases noted in females over age 40.[82]

T. vaginalis divides by binary fission and does not have a cyst form. The organism causes damage to host epithelium by direct contact with surface proteins, which result in microulcerations. Adhesins aid in the attachment to vaginal epithelial cells, and glycoproteins and proteinases mediate cytotoxicity and apoptosis as well as degrade immunoglobulins and complement to evade the immune response.

MEDICAL HISTORY AND CLINICAL PRESENTATION

Medical history should evaluate for risk factors in the development of trichomoniasis including multiple sexual partners, unprotected sexual activity, IV drug use, and coexisting venereal disease.

Most patients with trichomoniasis are asymptomatic. One-third of asymptomatic women become symptomatic. Common symptoms in women include a diffuse, malodorous, yellow-green or gray vaginal discharge; dysuria, lower abdominal pain, and dyspareunia. Symptoms in men include clear or mucopurulent urethral discharge, dysuria, and itching or burning pain after intercourse.

SIGNS AND SYMPTOMS

Trichomoniasis is typically asymptomatic in women and men. The most common symptoms in women are vaginitis and include malodorous discharge, dysuria, dyspareunia, and pruritus. Findings in men are usually absent, but men may note dysuria, urethral discomfort, and clear or mucopurulent discharge.

PHYSICAL EXAMINATION

Patients with trichomoniasis usually appear well. Common physical examination findings on pelvic examination include a strawberry cervix, due to petechial hemorrhages on the ectocervix, and fishy, foul-smelling, frothy, and mucopurulent green or gray vaginal discharge (Figure 17.22). In males, there may be scanty, mucopurulent urethral discharge.

DIFFERENTIAL DIAGNOSIS

The differential diagnosis includes candidal vaginitis and bacterial vaginosis. Other STIs including *Chlamydia* infection and gonorrhea may present in a similar fashion. Other causes of urethritis in men include *Chlamydia*, gonorrhea, and *Mycoplasma genitalium.*

DIAGNOSTIC STUDIES

The diagnosis is confirmed by vaginal wet prep microscopy that reveals motile, pear-shaped organisms (Figure 17.23). Wet mount has a 60% to 70% sensitivity for diagnosing infection.[83] *T. vaginalis* can also be cultured in liquid medium

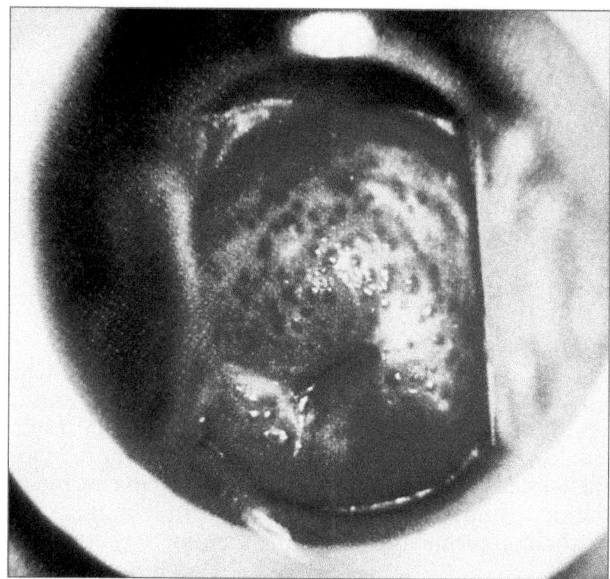

Figure 17.22 **Strawberry cervix from trichomoniasis. Note the cervical erythema with petechiae.**
(Source: Centers for Disease Control and Prevention. https://phil.cdc.gov/Details.aspx?pid=5240)

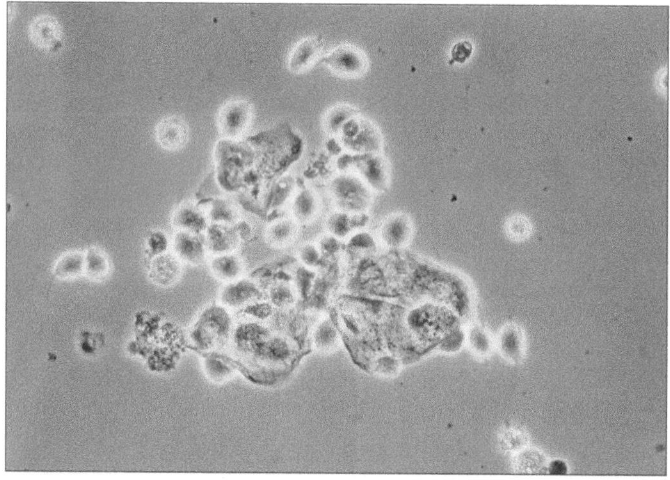

Figure 17.23 ***Trichomonas vaginalis* protozoan on wet prep.**

called Diamond medium. There are point of care tests, which detect *T. vaginalis* antigen, and a NAAT. The NAAT test is the test of choice for *T. vaginalis* infections.

TREATMENT

Treatment options include daily oral metronidazole, daily oral tinidazole, or twice daily metronidazole for 7 days. In most cases the one daily dose is as effective and compliance is greater than longer treatment courses. Topical metronidazole is less effective than oral treatment.

In HIV-infected women a longer treatment course is more effective at eradicating the infection. Male partners of infected women should be treated with one of the single-dose regimens. Recurrent disease is treated with metronidazole or tinidazole daily for 5 days.

Primary prevention is key in preventing trichomoniasis. Primary preventive measures include abstinence from sexual contact, use of male condoms, and prompt notification and treatment of recent sex partners.

PATIENT EDUCATION

- Trichomoniasis is associated with an increased risk of HIV infection, pelvic inflammatory disease in HIV-infected women, epididymitis and prostatitis in men, and premature rupture of membranes and low infant birth weight in pregnant women.

17.6B HELMINTHIC INFECTIONS

OVERVIEW

Helminths are large, multicellular organisms that can be seen with the naked eye, in their adult form. There are three major groups that cause human disease (see Table 17.25).

- **Tapeworms (Cestoda):** Flat bodies with muscular suckers and/or hooks for host attachment
- **Flukes (Trematoda):** Flat bodies with muscular suckers and/or hooks for host attachment
- **Roundworms (Nematoda):** Long cylindrical bodies and no attachment organs

EPIDEMIOLOGY

Helminth infections are one of the most common infectious diseases in the world. The prevalence of helminth disease is highest in warm, developing areas where the environment is favorable to the life cycle of the organism.

PATHOPHYSIOLOGY

Transmission of helminth infections occurs four ways:

- Ingestion of eggs or larvae through the oral-fecal route
- Ingestion the larvae in the tissue of another host
- Penetration of the skin by a larva
- Bite of insect vector

Many helminths live in the intestine and others live in the deeper tissues; almost all organs of the body can be infected. Flukes and nematodes feed on host tissues or intestinal contents; tapeworms have no digestive system and absorb predigested nutrients.

Most helminths do not replicate inside the host; certain tapeworm larval stages can reproduce asexually in humans. Sexual reproduction results in the production of eggs which are released from the host in fecal material. In others, reproductive stages may accumulate within the host, but do not mature.

Direct life cycles occur when reproductive stages produced by sexually mature adults in one host are released from the body and can develop directly to adult stages after infection of another host via the fecal-oral route or by direct penetration. Indirect life cycles occur when reproductive stages must undergo further development in an intermediate host or vector before sexual maturity can be achieved in the final host. The larvae of flukes and tapeworms must pass through one or more intermediate hosts, but nematodes can develop to maturity within a single host.

TABLE 17.25 Common Tapeworms, Flukes, and Roundworms Causing Human Disease

Species	Acquired From	Human Sites
Tapeworms		
Adult worms		
Taenia saginata	Larvae in beef	Intestine
Taenia solium	Larvae in pork	Intestine
Diphyllobothrium latum	Larvae in fish	Intestine
Larval worms		
Taenia solium (cysticercosis)	Eggs in food or water contaminated with human feces	
Echinococcus granulosus (cystic echinococcosis)	Eggs passed by dogs	
Flukes		
Schistosoma haematobium *S. japonicum* *S. mansoni*	Released from snails, larval stage penetrates skin	Blood vessels of bladder Blood vessels of intestine Blood vessels of intestine
Paragonimus westermani	Ingest larval stage in freshwater crabs	Lungs
Nematodes		
Ascaris lumbricoides	Ingestion of eggs	Small intestine
Enterobius vermicularis	Ingestion of eggs	Large intestine
Ancylostoma duodenale	Skin penetration by infective larvae	Small intestine
Necator americanus	Skin penetration by infective larvae	Small intestine
Strongyloides stercoralis	Skin penetration by infective larvae Autoinfection	Small intestine and general tissue
Trichuris trichiura	Ingestion of eggs	Large intestine
Brugia malayi	Mosquito bite with infective larvae	Lymphatics and blood
Onchocerca volvulus	*Simulium* fly bite with infective larvae	Skin and eye
Wuchereria bancrofti	Mosquito bite with infective larvae	Lymphatics and blood
Loa	Deer fly bite with infective larvae	Subcutaneous tissue and blood
Toxocara canis	Ingestion of eggs passed by dogs	Tissue, eye, central nervous system
Trichinella spiralis	Ingestion of larvae in pork, wild mammals	Small intestine and muscle

Adult tapeworms are acquired by eating undercooked or raw meat containing larval stages. Adult tapeworms are relatively harmless despite reaching a large size.

Flukes have an indirect life cycle involving stages of larval development in the body of an intermediate host. Humans become infected when they encounter water containing infective larvae released from the intermediate host or consume the intermediate host.

Many helminth infections are long lived, worms surviving in the host for many years, despite living in parts of the body where there are effective immune defenses.

17.6BA SCHISTOSOMIASIS

Schistosomiasis is secondary to infection with *Schistosoma haematobium, S. japonicum,* or *S. mansoni.*

The intermediate host vector for transmission to humans are snails. Infection peaks in the summer season and with activities that lead to contact with infested or contaminated water, including wading, bathing and swimming to scuba diving, water skiing and rafting. The geographic distribution varies based on the species with *Schistosoma mansoni* found in South America and the Caribbean, Africa and the Middle East; *S. haematobium* found in Africa and the Middle East; and *S. japonicum* found in the Far East.

There are two stages in the life cycle. In the diagnostic stage eggs exit the human body in feces or urine. The eggs hatch and release miracidia, which swim and penetrate the snail intermediate host. The stages in the snail includes two generations of sporocysts and the production of cercariae. In the infective stage the cercariae are released from the snail, swim and penetrate human skin. Over several weeks, the parasites migrate through host tissue and develop into adult worms inside the blood vessels. Once mature, the worms mate and the females produce eggs. The eggs are deposited in the capillaries of the target organ. With *S. haematobium*, the target organ is the urinary tract and the sacral and pelvic vessels; with *S. mansoni* and *S. japonicum* the target is the intestinal mucosa. Once deposited, a proportion of the eggs then enter the lumen of the bladder or intestines.

MEDICAL HISTORY AND CLINICAL PRESENTATION

Symptoms of schistosomiasis are not caused by the worms, but by the patient's reaction to the eggs. Incubation period for acute schistosomiasis is several weeks and most patients have no symptoms when first infected. Acute infection is due to a systemic hypersensitivity reaction against the migrating schistosomula and eggs. Eggs shed by the adult worms that do not pass out of the body can become lodged in the intestine or bladder, causing inflammation or scarring. With years of infection, the parasite can also damage the liver, intestine, spleen, lungs, and bladder. A detailed travel history should be obtained.

SIGNS AND SYMPTOMS

While the incubation period is long, within days of becoming infected, the patient may develop a limited rash or itchy skin. Within a few months, acute infection may present with fever, rash, headache, myalgias, abdominal discomfort, and respiratory symptoms. Without treatment, schistosomiasis can persist for years and manifest with abdominal pain, hepatomegaly, blood in the stool or the urine, and problems passing urine. Chronic infection can also lead to an increased risk of bladder cancer.

PHYSICAL EXAMINATION

In acute infection, physical examination may reveal a rash, hepatomegaly, and possible splenomegaly. In chronic infection physical examination findings are related to chronic blood loss including pallor due to anemia; bladder inflammation with hematuria, hydronephrosis; hepatic inflammation with ascites; and/or splenomegaly secondary to portal hypertension.

DIFFERENTIAL DIAGNOSIS

The differential diagnosis includes other invasive parasitic infections.

DIAGNOSTIC STUDIES

CBC reveals an elevated WBC count with eosinophilia. Anemia can be seen in chronic infection, either anemia of chronic disease or iron deficiency secondary to blood loss. Urinalysis may show microscopic or macroscopic hematuria in *S. haematobium* infection.

The gold standard for making the diagnosis is the presence of eggs in the stool or urine. The choice of sample depends on the species of parasite. The adult stages of *S. mansoni* and *S. japonicum* are shed in stool; *S. haematobium* adult worms are shed in urine. The eggs are passed intermittently and in small amounts and may not be detected. To increase the diagnostic yield of stool and urine examination, three samples should be collected on different days.

Serologic testing for antischistosomal antibody is indicated in the diagnosis of travelers or immigrants from endemic areas who have not been treated for schistosomiasis in the past. Commonly used serologic tests detect antibody to the adult worm. Testing should be done 6 to 8 weeks after exposure to allow for full development of the parasite and antibody. Serologic testing may not be appropriate in patients who have been repeatedly infected and treated in the past because antibodies can persist despite cure.

Ultrasound or abdominal CT scan can be used for *S. mansoni* and *S. japonicum* infection. Ultrasound of the kidneys and bladder can be used in *S. haematobium* infection.

TREATMENT

Praziquantel is the drug of choice for infections caused by all *Schistosoma* species. Praziquantel directly kills susceptible adult schistosomes; the dead worms are dislodged from their site of residence in the mesenteric or pelvic veins to the liver where they undergo phagocytosis. The timing of treatment is important since praziquantel is most effective against the adult worm and requires the presence of a mature antibody response to the parasite. For travelers, treatment should be at least 6–8 weeks after last exposure. If initially positive, reexamination of feces or urine 1 month after treatment is recommended to assess clearance.

PATIENT EDUCATION

- Anti-infective prophylaxis is currently not recommended.
- No vaccine is currently available.
- Strategies for avoiding exposure when in endemic regions include:
  - Avoid swimming or wading in fresh water.
  - Drink safe water; water directly from canals, lakes, rivers, streams and springs should be filtered or brought to a boil for 1 minute.
  - Use precautions for water used for bathing or using water held in a storage tank.

17.6BB TAPEWORM

Tapeworms, or cestodes, include species of flatworms that reside in the GI tract. The most common species include *Taenia saginatum*, *Taenia solium*, and *Diphyllobothrium latum*.

Taenia infections are found worldwide and increased in regions where the animal hosts are kept near human waste. In the parasite life cycle, humans are the only definitive hosts in which *T. saginatum* and *T. solium* can complete their life cycle. The eggs passed by infected humans can be ingested by cattle (*T. saginatum*) or swine (*T. solium*). In the animals the eggs hatch and the organism migrate through the intestinal wall and via the bloodstream to the muscles, forming cysticerci. Humans become infected by eating undercooked meat that contains cysticerci. In the human intestine, protoscolices are released from the cysts and attach to the intestinal wall and they gradually add proglottids over time that contain eggs. The proglottids break off and are passed in the stool, releasing eggs.

D. latum is predominately seen in northern Europe and Japan and produce infection from the eating of raw or undercooked freshwater fish. The adult parasite lives in the intestinal tract and sheds eggs and proglottids in the stool. Once in water, coracidia hatch from the eggs and enter small crustaceans. The coracidia develop into larvae in the crustacean, which in turn is ingested by a small freshwater fish. The larvae migrate to the muscles. After humans ingest the raw or undercooked fish the parasite matures into the adult tapeworm in the intestine.

Adult tapeworms in the intestine cause minimal inflammatory response. This may lead to mild elevations in peripheral eosinophils or intraluminal IgE, but this response is not sufficient to clear the organism or stimulate an immune response.

MEDICAL HISTORY AND CLINICAL PRESENTATION

Tapeworms produce only mild abdominal discomfort or are asymptomatic. The main symptom is the passage of proglottids. *T. saginatum* is more asymptomatic than *T. solium*. Infection is noted by patients when they pass segments of the worm in their stool. If the eggs of *T. solium* are ingested, cysticercosis may develop as calcified cysts in the muscle and other tissues, including the central nervous system.

SIGNS AND SYMPTOMS

Many infected patients are asymptomatic. The most common GI symptoms include nausea, diarrhea, epigastric discomfort, or decreased appetite. There may be nonspecific complaints including anxiety, fatigue, or dizziness.

A rare manifestation of *D. latum* infection is vitamin B12 deficiency and megaloblastic anemia. Fatigue and neuropathy including paresthesia and ataxia may develop.

PHYSICAL EXAMINATION

In tapeworm infections there are typically no physical examination findings. Patients may appear fatigued or have mild to moderate abdominal pain on palpation. In patients who develop megaloblastic anemia, glossitis, ataxia, and decreased sensation may be present.

DIFFERENTIAL DIAGNOSIS

The differential diagnosis includes other infectious causes of gastroenteritis, including viral or mild bacterial infections.

DIAGNOSTIC STUDIES

Mild eosinophilia may be noted in some cases and in infection due to *D. latum* vitamin B12 deficiency may be noted.

Confirmation of the diagnosis is made by identifying proglottids or eggs in the stool. Because shedding of proglottids and eggs is intermittent, repeat sampling is often needed to increase sensitivity. The various species of *Taenia* can be distinguished by proglottid morphology.

TREATMENT

The treatment of choice for tapeworms is praziquantel. Stools should be reexamined for *Taenia* eggs 1 and 3 months after treatment to be sure the infection is cleared.

PATIENT EDUCATION

- For tapeworm infections there is no effective prophylactic treatment or vaccine.
- Good sanitation and thorough cooking of meat and fish are the primary prevention measures.

17.6BC CYSTICERCOSIS

Cysticercosis is an infection caused by the larval stages of *Taenia solium*. After ingestion the tapeworm eggs and larvae enter muscle and brain tissue forming cysts. During the viable phase, cysts do not cause inflammation or symptoms. As the cysts degenerate, an immune response develops that leads to tissue injury and edema. The cysts either resolve or form a calcified granuloma, which can cause seizures if the cysts are in the brain. Cysticercosis is classified according to the site of cysticerci into neurocysticercosis and extraneural cysticercosis.

MEDICAL HISTORY AND CLINICAL PRESENTATION

Presenting symptoms differ according to the site of the cysticerci. Parenchymal neurocysticercosis causes the symptoms and signs of a space-occupying lesion. Extraparenchymal neurocysticercosis causes signs and symptoms of increased intracranial pressure with cysts in the subarachnoid space or ventricles; signs and symptoms of spinal cord compression if present in the spinal cord; or sign and symptoms of eye disease if present in the eye.

SIGNS AND SYMPTOMS

Signs and symptoms vary depending on the site of the infection. Parenchymal infection will be asymptomatic in a majority of cases. If symptoms are present they include focal, generalized seizures; headache; nausea and vomiting; and psychiatric disorders. Extraparenchymal infection symptoms vary. Ocular disease symptoms vary depending on location in the eye, including decreased visual acuity; in the brain or subarachnoid space there can be obstruction of CSF flow leading to increased intracranial pressure causing headache, nausea and vomiting, seizures, and hydrocephalus; in the spinal cord symptoms include low back pain, weakness, paresthesia, and reflex abnormalities.

PHYSICAL EXAMINATION

Physical examination findings vary depending on the site of the infection. With parenchymal infection physical examination findings include motor impairment in the form of hemiparesis or focal motor deficit, sensory deficit, decreased level of consciousness, speech and language deficits, and cerebellar and extrapyramidal deficits.

Extraparenchymal physical examination findings in ocular infection include decreased visual acuity; in the brain or subarachnoid space infection examination findings include papilledema; and in the spinal cord physical examination findings include paralysis and sensory loss below the level of the compression, Lhermitte sign, and positive Babinski sign.

DIFFERENTIAL DIAGNOSIS

The differential diagnosis of cysticercosis includes other brain cystic lesions, such as brain abscess and brain tumors; or ocular lesions, such as retinal detachment.

DIAGNOSTIC STUDIES

Diagnosis of cysticercosis often requires both CNS imaging and serologic testing. A patient may have clinical disease from a single or very few cysticerci. The serologic results may be negative, but the lesions may be visible on imaging. A patient may have cysticerci in locations other than the brain. In this case, CNS imaging is negative but serologic results might be positive, indicating an antibody response to lesions. The location and characteristics of lesions on MRI are needed to determine the best treatment modalities.

There are two available serologic tests to detect cysticercosis, the enzyme-linked immunoelectrotransfer blot or EITB, and commercial enzyme-linked immunoassays. The immunoblot is the test preferred because its sensitivity and specificity have been well characterized in published analyses.

TREATMENT

Cysticercosis is treated with antiparasitic and anti-inflammatory drug combination.

Neurocysticercosis often presents with headaches and new-onset seizures. Anticonvulsant therapy should be started immediately and once seizures are under control, antihelminthic therapy should be started.

Antihelminthic therapy is based on the stage and number of cysts present, their location, and the patient's specific clinical presentation. Antihelminthic therapy should be given in combination with corticosteroids and anticonvulsants to reduce inflammation surrounding the cysts and lower the risk of seizures. Albendazole is preferred over praziquantel due to cost and fewer drug interactions.

Asymptomatic cysts, discovered incidentally on imaging, may never develop symptomatic disease and in most cases do not require therapy. If the cysts are calcified they are already dead and antihelminthic treatment is not needed.

In ocular cysticercosis, surgical removal is necessary for cysts within the eye and cysts outside the globe are treated with antihelminthic drugs. Subcutaneous cysticercosis does not require therapy; if the cysts are painful they can be surgically removed.

Cysticercal encephalitis should not be treated with antiparasitic therapy. Treatment can exacerbate the host inflammatory response and lead to cerebral edema and herniation. Encephalitis will improve with corticosteroid therapy.

PATIENT EDUCATION

- Prevention of disease can be achieved with washing of hands after fecal exposure and before handling food.
- When traveling to areas with poor sanitation, persons should be particularly careful to avoid food and water that may be contaminated by human feces.

17.6BD ECHINOCOCCOSIS

Echinococcal disease of the liver is caused by the parasites of the *Echinococcus* species. These organisms are found worldwide, the most common being *Echinococcus granulosus* and *Echinococcus multilocularis*. These organisms are found in China, the Middle East, Africa, and Central/South America; a history of travel to any of these regions is a sufficient risk factor to acquire the infection. Dogs, cats, and foxes are primary hosts, with humans as accidental hosts. The infection is acquired through fecal-oral contamination.

Infection occurs when the echinococcal oncospheres penetrate the intestines and then lodge in the liver and the lungs. Infection can also occur in the kidneys, bone, spleen, and brain.

There are two forms of echinococcosis; cystic echinococcosis disease, also called hydatid disease, results from being infected with the larval stage of *E. granulosus*. These infections are typically asymptomatic, but can cause slowly enlarging masses in the liver and the lungs. The other form is alveolar echinococcosis. This infection results from infection with the larval stage of *E. multilocularis*. Human cases are rare; infection in humans causes parasitic tumors to form in the liver, lungs, brain, and other organs.

MEDICAL HISTORY AND CLINICAL PRESENTATION

Echinococcal infection has a slow course of progression; patients are diagnosed with the disease incidentally. Patients most commonly present with right upper quadrant abdominal pain; jaundice may be the presenting sign if the infectious cyst obstructs the biliary tree.

The medical history should be evaluated for exposure to cattle, deer, pigs, sheep and feces of dogs, wolves, or coyotes. Travel history to endemic areas, such as eastern part of the Mediterranean region, Northern Africa, southern and eastern Europe, at the southern tip of South America, in Central Asia, Siberia and Western China, should be assessed.

SIGNS AND SYMPTOMS

Persons with echinococcosis are often asymptomatic. The clinical presentation varies depending on the location and size of the cysts. Cyst rupture may be caused by trauma and lead to mild to severe anaphylactic reactions.

Common presentation includes GI complaints of right upper quadrant pain, nausea and vomiting, jaundice; pulmonary symptoms of cough, chest pain, dyspnea, and hemoptysis; renal symptoms of hematuria and flank pain; and central nervous system symptoms including seizures.

PHYSICAL EXAMINATION

In noncomplicated cases, the patient appears well and may not feel ill until the case becomes more complicated. Physical examination may reveal hypotension, fever, jaundice, hepatomegaly, and abdominal tenderness.

DIFFERENTIAL DIAGNOSIS

The differential diagnosis for cystic echinococcosis includes liver abscess, either pyogenic or amebic, liver hemangioma, liver metastases, and fungal liver disease.

DIAGNOSTIC STUDIES

Serology testing, such as ELISA and immunoelectrophoresis, serve as confirmatory tests. If ELISA is positive and there is a high degree of clinical suspicion of disease, radiologic testing can be done next to confirm the diagnosis. Both ultrasound and CT scans are used to identify parasitic cysts. Ultrasound can classify the cyst stage.

TREATMENT

There are three options for the management of an echinococcal cyst: medical, surgical, and percutaneous intervention.

Albendazole is the antiparasitic agent of choice. It is used to treat small cysts, inoperable cysts, cysts present in multiple organs, and for preoperative prophylaxis. Preoperative use can reduce cyst viability and reduces the potential for complications that may occur with accidental spillage during surgery.

Excision of cysts through pericystectomy is an effective treatment. Surgical excision has a higher rate of morbidity and mortality compared to other treatment options. Laparoscopic approach is also effective and is associated with low intraoperative and perioperative complications.

PAIR (percutaneous-aspiration-injection-reaspiration) is an ideal first treatment in a select group of patients. The presence of cystobiliary fistulas must be ruled out for its use.

PATIENT EDUCATION

- Disease control includes limiting dog exposure in endemic regions and preventing animals from consuming meat infected with cysts.
- Prevention should also focus on deworming of dogs, the definitive host.

17.6BE ASCARIASIS

Nematodes (roundworms) are nonsegmented helminths with elongate cylindrical bodies. There are six intestinal nematodes that infect humans: *Ascaris lumbricoides*; *Trichuris trichiura* (whipworm); *Ancylostoma duodenale* and *Necator americanus* (hookworms); *Enterobius vermicularis* (pinworm); and *Strongyloides stercoralis*.

Ascaris is a soil-transmitted helminth. The geographic distribution is determined by sanitation and climate. In developing countries areas of poor sanitation and hygiene, with warm, moist soil are well suited for transmission. Children, typically under the age of 10, in impoverished rural areas are at high risk because of exposure to contaminated soil and by hand-to-mouth behaviors. Children account for most of the worms in a community and most of the eggs that are shed into the environment.

Infected patients pass the eggs in the feces and in a favorable environment, warm, moist soil, they become infectious. Humans acquire the infection by ingesting eggs via contaminated food or water. The eggs hatch in the small intestine and release larvae that penetrate the intestine and later migrate to the lungs. The larvae ascend the tracheobronchial tree or are coughed up, swallowed, and return to the intestines where they mature into adult worms. Egg production begins 2 months after infection, and adult worms live 1 to 2 years.

The symptoms are secondary to the host response and the parasite. During larval migration, the host cells suffer trauma and lysis due to larval enzymes. The larvae induce granuloma formation and a hypersensitivity reaction in the pulmonary parenchyma. The pathologic outcome in the GI tract is due to the presence of worms in the lumen. The severity of symptoms is proportional to the worm burden.

MEDICAL HISTORY AND CLINICAL PRESENTATION

Most people infected with *Ascaris* are asymptomatic, but a small number develop cough during the initial phase of infection, when the larvae are migrating through the lungs. Eosinophilia and eosinophilic pneumonia may be noted during the lung migration phase. During chronic infection, worms in the small intestine often provoke no symptoms or produce only mild abdominal pain or nausea. Heavier infections can adversely affect the nutritional status, intellectual development, and growth of children.

SIGNS AND SYMPTOMS

Infection with *Ascaris* is often asymptomatic. It may present with mild pulmonary and abdominal symptoms, but severe cases can occur following mechanical obstruction of the intestine. The clinical symptoms are usually dependent on the worm burden and the involved organ.

Typical signs and symptoms include low-grade fever, nonproductive cough, chest pain, dyspnea, abdominal discomfort, anorexia, nausea, signs of biliary and intestinal obstruction, and the passage of worms in the stool.

PHYSICAL EXAMINATION

The physical examination findings in ascariasis vary and depend on the worm burden and involved organ. Most patients appear well with minimal or no symptoms on physical examination.

A fever may be present. Icteric sclerae due to obstructive jaundice from biliary involvement may be noted. With lung involvement wheezing or dry rales may be noted. With intestinal involvement there may be abdominal tenderness and distention. Signs of bowel obstruction may be noted. Occasionally, adult worms can pass per rectum or through the nose.

DIFFERENTIAL DIAGNOSIS

The differential diagnosis includes other intestinal parasitic diseases, including the tapeworms and flatworms. Other diseases in the differential include peptic ulcer disease, intussusception, and biliary obstruction.

DIAGNOSTIC STUDIES

The diagnosis of intestinal helminth infections is made primarily by microscopic identification of the eggs. Adult *Ascaris* worms are typically white or pink, nonsegmented, 15–45 cm long, and live in the small intestine. Eggs are thick-shelled and oval (Figure 17.24).

Stool examination is very sensitive for the detection of *Ascaris*, given the high daily egg output of this parasite. Stool samples may be negative until a few months after infection occurs. Larvae can sometimes be found in respiratory secretions of patients infected during the early migratory phase.

Ascaris worms may be seen radiographically, in contrast radiographs of the bowel.

TREATMENT

The treatment of choice for intestinal nematodes is albendazole or mebendazole, with a single dose or short-course regimens.

Alternative antiparasitic drugs are available but are second-line treatment options. These include pyrantel pamoate and ivermectin.

PATIENT EDUCATION

- The prognosis is good, and most cases of ascariasis are asymptomatic.

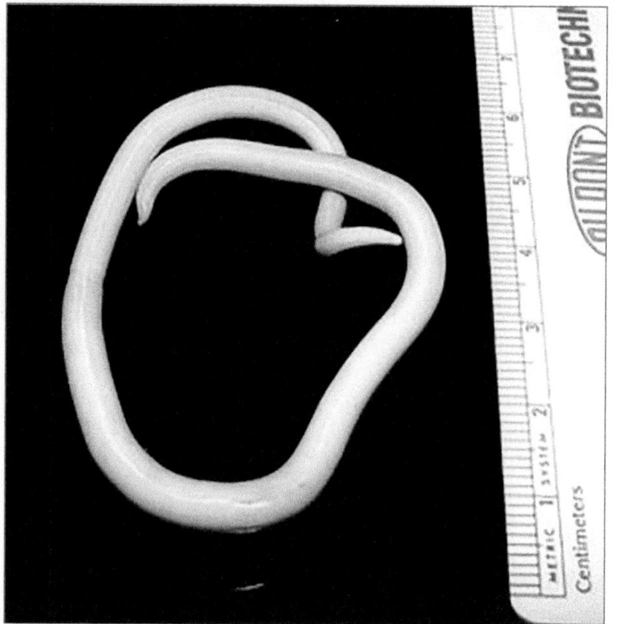

Figure 17.24 ***Ascaris lumbricoides*** **female worm.**

- Prevention is best achieved through improvements in personal hygiene and environmental sanitation.
- Complications of chronic ascariasis are mostly mechanical: intestinal, biliary, or pancreatic obstruction; appendicitis; and intestinal perforation.

17.6BF TRICHURIASIS

Nematodes are nonsegmented worms (helminths) with elongate cylindrical bodies. Many nematodes infect humans with six spending a majority of their life cycle in the bowel lumen and are intestinal nematodes. These include *Ascaris lumbricoides*; *Trichuris trichiura* (whipworm); *Ancylostoma duodenale* and *Necator americanus; Enterobius vermicularis*; and *Strongyloides stercoralis*. *Trichuris* is a soil-transmitted helminth.

T. trichiura is known as whipworm with its long, whip-like head that embeds into the intestinal mucosa. Adult worms are gray-pink and 3–5 cm long and reside in the proximal colon; with heavy infections the worms can be present throughout the entire colon. The eggs have a distinctive barrel-shaped appearance with a thick shell, bipolar plugs. Eggs shed in the feces become infective under moist and shady conditions. After ingestion by humans, larvae emerge from the eggs and move to the cecum. The larvae molt, embed in the epithelium, and mature into adults. Female worms can produce up to 20,000 eggs per day. *T. trichiura* does not appear to occur in areas where temperatures exceed 37 °C–40 °C.

Most cases of *Trichuris* infections occur in nonendemic regions among immigrants and travelers. Infections typically resolve within a few years even without treatment when the adult worms die. Because of the requirement that *Trichuris* eggs or larvae develop on soil before becoming infectious, these parasites cannot be transmitted directly from person-to-person and cannot multiply in the host.

MEDICAL HISTORY AND CLINICAL PRESENTATION

History of patients with whipworm infection may include recent travel to or currently living in an area of known to be endemic for infection, living near water sources, poor personal hygiene, or low socioeconomic status.

Trichuris infection is usually asymptomatic. With heavy infections, chronic abdominal pain and diarrhea can result, and stools may have a strong smell. Infected children may present with anemia, growth retardation, and clubbing.

Complications include dysentery syndrome, characterized by tenesmus and frequent stools containing mucus and blood. Recurrent rectal prolapse is a classic complication of whipworm, with worms often visible.

SIGNS AND SYMPTOMS

The majority of patients with light whipworm infection are asymptomatic. Symptoms of moderate to heavy infection include weight loss, bloody diarrhea, abdominal pain, tenesmus, and rectal prolapse.

PHYSICAL EXAMINATION

There are no specific physical examination findings associated with whipworm infection. Patients with heavy infection may present with pallor, nail clubbing, rectal prolapse, and abdominal tenderness.

DIFFERENTIAL DIAGNOSIS

The differential diagnosis of *Trichuris* infection includes other nematode infections, ascariasis, hookworms, and strongyloidiasis.

DIAGNOSTIC STUDIES

The diagnosis of whipworm infection is made primarily by microscopic identification of eggs in stool. Stool samples may be negative until a few months after infection occurs. Some patients may have eosinophilia.

TREATMENT

The treatment of choice for trichuriasis is albendazole or mebendazole. For *Trichuris* infections, at least 3 to 7 days of albendazole or mebendazole should be used as single-dose cure rates are low.

Alternative antiparasitic drugs are available, including pyrantel pamoate, ivermectin, and nitazoxanide.

PATIENT EDUCATION

- Prognosis is excellent with all patients recovering completely with treatment.

17.6BG HOOKWORM

Nematodes (roundworms) are nonsegmented worms with elongate cylindrical bodies. There are six major nematodes that infect humans, spend most of their life cycle in the bowel lumen, and are therefore classified as intestinal nematodes. These are *Ancylostoma duodenale* and

Necator americanus (human hookworms); *Ascaris lumbricoides*; *Trichuris trichiura*; *Enterobius vermicularis*; and *Strongyloides stercoralis*. Hookworms are known as soil-transmitted helminths. Hookworm prevalence most commonly increases throughout childhood and then plateaus in young adulthood.

The hookworms, *A. duodenale* and *N. americanus,* are small, gray-white worms that live in the upper small intestine. The ovoid, thin-shelled eggs of the two hookworms are identical. The eggs are passed in the stool and develop in soil; they hatch in the soil, becoming larvae in 1 to 2 days. Larvae molt becoming infectious. With contact with human skin, larvae enter the body and are carried to the lungs. They move up the trachea, are swallowed, and migrate to the small intestine. The females start depositing egg about 1 month after infection. *N. americanus* are only transmitted via this percutaneous route; *A. duodenale* can also be transmitted orally.

N. americanus is the predominant hookworm worldwide. Hookworm infections occur in tropical and subtropical areas.

Hookworms' primary pathologic effect is via blood loss. They attach to the intestinal mucosa via teeth and secrete anticoagulants allowing continuous blood ingestion; this can lead chronic iron deficiency.

MEDICAL HISTORY AND CLINICAL PRESENTATION

Most patients infected with hookworm have mild infections and are asymptomatic. Initial infection may present with a pruritic maculopapular rash at the site of larval skin penetration. When the larvae migrate through the lungs it may cause pneumonitis. Epigastric pain, diarrhea, and anorexia may occur a few months after skin penetration, as larvae begin attaching to the small bowel mucosa.

Patients infected with adult hookworms may develop chronic abdominal pain and eosinophilia; other manifestations include iron deficiency anemia and malnutrition.

SIGNS AND SYMPTOMS

There are no specific symptoms or signs of hookworm infection. Larvae present in the skin can cause intense, local itching, usually on the foot or lower leg, described as ground itch. The lesions can blister and last for a week. If infected with numerous larvae patients may experience coughing, chest pain, wheezing. GI complaints such as epigastric pains, indigestion, nausea and vomiting, and change in bowel habits may be noted with infection. With advanced disease the signs of anemia and protein deficiency including weight loss, cardiac failure, and ascites may be noted.

PHYSICAL EXAMINATION

On physical examination an urticarial dermal reaction ("ground itch") due to larvae penetration, and respiratory involvement including eosinophilic pneumonia may be observed. Occult blood in the stool may also be seen in heavy infections (Figure 17.25).

DIFFERENTIAL DIAGNOSIS

The differential diagnosis includes other intestinal parasitic diseases, including intestinal cestodes (tapeworms) and trematodes (flatworms).

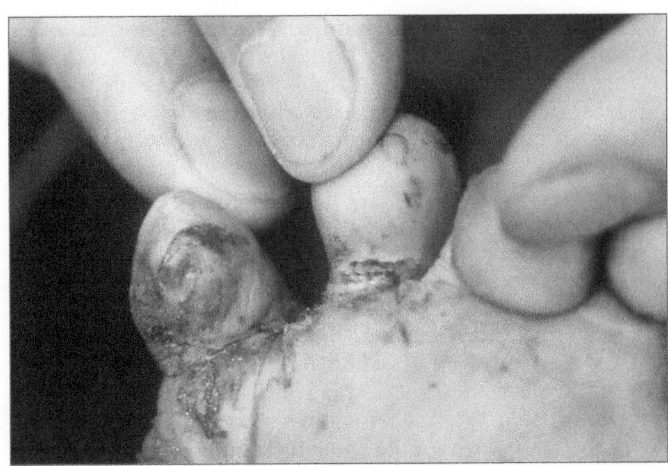

Figure 17.25 **Urticarial dermal reaction or ground itch noted in hookworm infections.**

DIAGNOSTIC STUDIES

The diagnosis is made by the microscopic identification of eggs in the stool. Stool samples may be negative for a few months after infection. Occasionally larvae can be found in respiratory secretions of patients infected with hookworm during the early migratory phase of infection.

TREATMENT

The treatment of choice for intestinal nematodes is albendazole or mebendazole. Single-dose albendazole is preferred over single-dose mebendazole. Pyrantel pamoate is an alternative antiparasitic drug that is available.

PATIENT EDUCATION

- Prevention involves fecal-oral hygiene, provision of clean food and water, good community-wide sanitation, and use of adequate footwear in endemic areas.
- WHO advocates treatment with antihelminthic drugs, such as albendazole, at regular intervals to populations at risk.

17.6BH STRONGYLOIDIASIS

Nematodes (roundworms) are nonsegmented worms (helminths) with elongate cylindrical bodies. Although numerous nematodes infect humans, six spend the majority of their life cycle in the bowel lumen and are classified as intestinal nematodes: *Strongyloides stercoralis, Ascaris lumbricoides*; *Trichuris trichiura*; *Ancylostoma duodenale* and *Necator americanus;* and *Enterobius vermicularis.*

The life cycle of *S. stercoralis* alternates between free-living and parasitic cycles, and includes adult worms, two different larval stages, and eggs.

Infection with *S. stercoralis* is less common than other intestinal nematodes. Strongyloidiasis is found throughout the tropics and subtropics and in limited areas of the United States, the Appalachia region, and Europe. In developing countries, strongyloidiasis prevalence rates can be high; most infections in developed countries are imported.

The highest rates of infection are seen in the institutionalized, those living in poverty, or in rural areas. In developed settings, *Strongyloides* infection is most commonly seen in immigrants from highly endemic countries. In patients with chronic strongyloidiasis, autoinfection is well controlled by cell-mediated immunity, and the number of adult worms remains low and stable. With immunosuppression, more autoinfective larvae complete the cycle, and the population of parasitic adult worms increases, causing hyperinfection.

In the life cycle of *Strongyloides*, filariform larvae in contaminated soil penetrate the human skin and by various routes migrate into the small intestine. The larvae migrate via the blood to the lungs, where they are eventually coughed up and swallowed. In the small intestine the larvae molt twice and become adult female worms. The female worms live in the epithelium of the small intestine and produce eggs that hatch into rhabditiform larvae. The rhabditiform larvae can be passed in the stool or cause autoinfection.

MEDICAL HISTORY AND CLINICAL PRESENTATION

Significant information from the patient's history includes history of travel to the endemic areas and history of exposure to individuals with similar complaints.

Heavy infections can rarely cause bowel obstruction. Hyperinfection syndrome is a possible complication; with this the intestines and lungs contain numerous larvae and diarrhea is common. Other GI manifestations include abdominal pain, vomiting, and intestinal obstruction. Pneumonitis is common, with cough and respiratory failure. Central nervous system invasion may cause meningitis and brain abscesses, with larvae in the CSF or tissue.

SIGNS AND SYMPTOMS

Most people infected with *Strongyloides* are asymptomatic. The symptoms range from subclinical in acute and chronic infection to severe and fatal hyperinfection syndrome and disseminated disease, with high fatality rates. After infection, patients can develop a localized, erythematous, pruritic rash. Pulmonary symptoms may develop days later, followed by diarrhea and abdominal pain. Migrating larvae may produce a serpiginous, erythematous, track-like rash. Chronically infected patients may develop nausea, diarrhea, epigastric pain, and possibly malabsorption.

PHYSICAL EXAMINATION

The physical examination findings in strongyloidiasis vary and are usually dependent on the worm burden and the involved organ. Most patients appear well with few or no physical examination findings. Fever may be present; icteric sclerae are seen if obstructive jaundice is present; signs of eosinophilic pneumonia include dyspnea, rales, or wheezing; abdominal examination reveals tenderness secondary to obstruction; and skin reveals a localized, erythematous, pruritic rash.

DIFFERENTIAL DIAGNOSIS

The differential diagnosis includes other intestinal parasitic diseases such as the intestinal cestodes (tapeworms) and trematodes (flatworms). Strongyloidiasis can mimic other GI disorders like peptic ulcer disease, intussusception, and bile duct stones.

DIAGNOSTIC STUDIES

The diagnosis of strongyloidiasis is confirmed by finding rhabditiform larvae in microscopic stool examination; finding eggs in the stool is uncommon.

Because of microscopic limitations, serologic tests, such as the enzyme-linked immunoassay, are more sensitive and favored for the diagnosis of acute strongyloidiasis. The titer of *Strongyloides* antibodies starts to decline 12 months after cure, as does the peripheral eosinophil count. Chronic and hyperinfection/disseminated strongyloidiasis is diagnosed by microscopic examination of stool or respiratory specimens.

Many patients chronically infected with *Strongyloides* will have low-grade eosinophilia, 5% to 15% of the differential, and if respiratory infection is present diffuse interstitial infiltrates or consolidation are noted on CXR.

TREATMENT

The preferred treatment for uncomplicated strongyloidiasis is oral ivermectin, with high cure rates in chronically infected patients. Ivermectin is the preferred treatment for hyperinfection and disseminated strongyloidiasis; treatment should extend to 1 to 2 weeks after clearance of the parasite.

Alternative treatments for chronic strongyloidiasis include albendazole or thiabendazole; both are generally not used due to low efficacy.

PATIENT EDUCATION

- There are no accepted guidelines regarding chemoprophylaxis for *Strongyloides* infections.

17.6BI ENTEROBIASIS

Nematodes are nonsegmented helminths with elongate cylindrical bodies. There are many nematodes that infect humans. Six major nematodes spend their life cycle in the bowel lumen and are classified as intestinal nematodes: *Enterobius vermicularis* (pinworm); *Ascaris lumbricoides*; *Trichuris trichiura*; *Ancylostoma duodenale* and *Necator americanus;* and *Strongyloides stercoralis*. Pinworm is the most common helminth infection in the United States.

E. vermicularis adult females are small, white roundworms. The eggs are flattened on one side and bean-shaped. *Enterobius* adults live in the proximal colon of infected patients; the females migrate to the perianal region and lay eggs. The eggs stick to the skin and cause severe pruritus. Pruritus facilitates fecal-oral transfer of eggs. Transmission occurs person-to-person, via fecal-oral contamination of hands, and sexually or through fomites, such as bedding. The lifespan of adult females is 4 to 10 weeks. *Enterobius* transmission is favored wherever there is poor sanitation, overcrowding, and lack of water for bathing and washing of hands and clothes.

MEDICAL HISTORY AND CLINICAL PRESENTATION

Most individuals with pinworm infection are asymptomatic. When present symptoms include painful itching around the anus and perineum, restless sleep, poor appetite, and failure to gain weight. The itching occurs mainly during the night.

SIGNS AND SYMPTOMS

Although most pinworm infections are asymptomatic, perianal pruritus can be severe. Other symptoms sometimes associated with pinworm infection include insomnia, nausea, vomiting, and abdominal pain.

PHYSICAL EXAMINATION

Patients with enterobiasis often appear restless. Physical examination is remarkable for skin excoriations as a result of scratching, secondary to perianal itching; perianal skin infections; and visualization at night of adult worms in the perianal region.

DIFFERENTIAL DIAGNOSIS

Enterobiasis must be differentiated from other causes of perianal pruritus and nematode infections.

DIAGNOSTIC STUDIES

Diagnosis is often made clinically by observing the female worms in the perianal region. *Enterobius* eggs are best identified by microscopic examination of adhesive cellophane tape applied to the perianal region. The tape test is best done early in the morning before washing or defecation. The test may be repeated for consecutive mornings to increase the sensitivity. The diagnostic characteristics of egg include typical elongated shape, with one convex side and one flattened side and colorless shell (Figure 17.26).

Ova and parasite studies on stool have a very low yield, but the worms may be noted in the patient's feces. Serologic assays are rarely used to diagnose pinworms.

TREATMENT

The treatment of choice is single-dose therapy with albendazole mebendazole. Household and other close contacts should also be treated, and a second treatment is recommended 2 weeks after the first dose because of high reinfection rates and the frequent occurrence of autoinfection.

Alternative treatment options include single-dose ivermectin or pyrantel pamoate. None are superior to albendazole or mebendazole

PATIENT EDUCATION

- If left untreated, patients with pinworms may develop secondary skin infections.
- Common complications of pinworm infections include bacterial dermatitis, folliculitis, vulvovaginitis, and cystitis.
- Overall prognosis is excellent.

17.6BJ TRICHINOSIS

Nematodes, or roundworms, are a category of helminths. There are three groups of nematodes: *Trichinella*, *Dracuncula*, and filaria. *Trichinella* are tissue nematodes that cause trichinosis. The species that infect humans are *T. spiralis*, *T. pseudospiralis*, *T. nativa*, *T. nelsoni*, *T. bitovi*, *T. murelli*, and *T. papuae*.

Unlike other nematodes, there is no arthropod vector for *Trichinella* species.

The *Trichinella* larvae can be found in the muscles of many animals including rodents, bears, pigs, and moose. Humans often get the infection from eating infected meat from swine or wild game that carry trichinosis. The infection is spread in animals that eat the meat of other infected animals.

According to the CDC, between 2010 and 2015 there were 80 cases of trichinosis in the United States.[84]

Trichinella is usually transmitted to the human host by eating undercooked meat containing *Trichinella* cysts. Following ingestion, the larvae from the cysts are released upon exposure to gastric acid and invade the small intestine mucosa. The cysts break open in the intestine and grow to adult worms. After 1 week, the female worms release more larvae that migrate through the blood to the voluntary muscles where they encyst. On microscopic analysis of the muscle, the encysted cell has a collagen capsule with larvae inside and is surrounded by cellular infiltrates (Figure 17.27).

MEDICAL HISTORY AND CLINICAL PRESENTATION

The patient's history may contain a history of eating undercooked meat such as pork, wild boar, and bear.

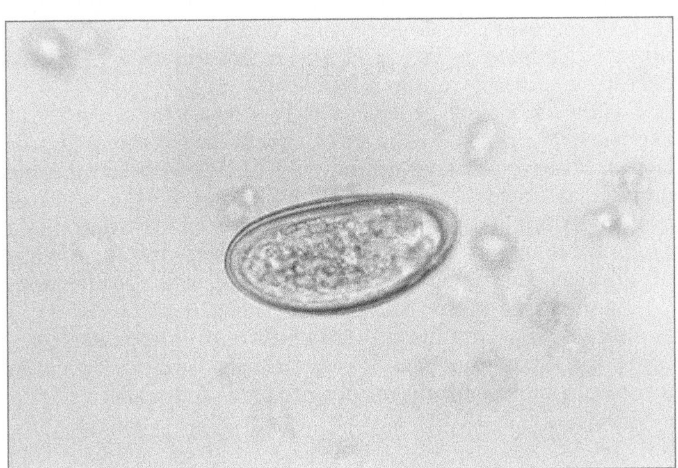

Figure 17.26 ***Enterobius vermicularis* egg.**

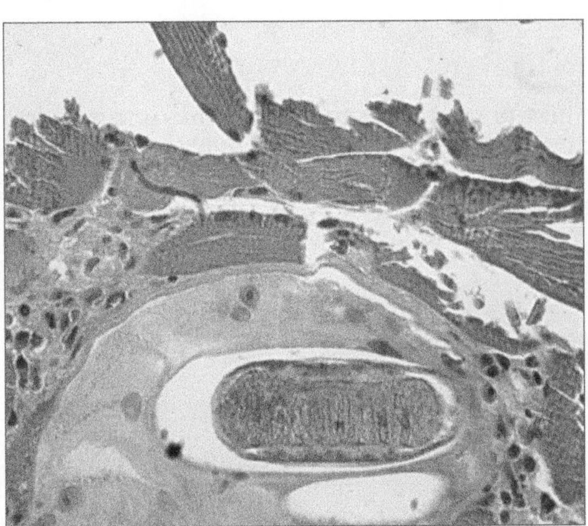

Figure 17.27 ***Trichinella spiralis* cyst, muscle biopsy.**
(Source: James Van Rhee.)

Symptoms depend on the parasite burden and their stage of infection. After ingestion the initial intestinal phase is associated with nausea, abdominal pain, and diarrhea. The muscle encysting phase is associated with myalgias, muscle swelling, and weakness. Fever may be present throughout.

SIGNS AND SYMPTOMS

Trichinosis initially involves the intestines. Symptoms include nausea, dyspepsia, and diarrhea. As the worms encyst in different parts of the human body, other manifestations may occur, including headache, fever, chills, periorbital edema, joint pain, and muscle pain. A history of gastroenteritis, muscle pain, and fever, with a history of recent ingestion of undercooked meat, pork, wild boar, or bear, suggests trichinosis.

PHYSICAL EXAMINATION

Physical examination findings include point muscle tenderness, swelling, and periorbital edema. Rash, splinter hemorrhages of the nails, conjunctival hemorrhages, or hepatosplenomegaly can occur.

DIFFERENTIAL DIAGNOSIS

The differential diagnosis for the severe myalgias associated with trichinosis includes infectious myositis and drug-induced rhabdomyolysis. Cardiac manifestations must be distinguished from myocarditis. Neurotrichinosis can be mistaken for viral, fungal, or other parasitic causes of encephalitis.

DIAGNOSTIC STUDIES

In the muscle stage, trichinosis presents with several laboratory abnormalities. Leukocytosis with marked eosinophilia, elevated CK, and elevated LDH are noted.

The definitive diagnosis is made with muscle biopsy identifying larvae. EIA can aid in the diagnosis, but there is some cross-reactivity with other helminths.

TREATMENT

Most infections are mild and self-limited and require only symptomatic treatment for fever and myalgia. For severe infections, the combination of the antiparasitic drug albendazole and prednisone are used.

PATIENT EDUCATION

- The best prevention is to avoid eating undercooked pork or any meat from a predator, such as cougar, bear, or wild hog.
- Thoroughly cooking meat to a temperature of 77 °C or freezing at –15 °C for 3 weeks typically kills the larvae.

17.6BK TOXOCARIASIS

The roundworms, *Toxocara canis* and *Toxocara cati,* normally infect dogs and cats; but humans can be accidental hosts. Infection with these organisms results in visceral or ocular larva migrans.

Toxocariasis occurs around the world and is most often noted in children age 2 to 7 years.

The adult worms live in the small intestine of dogs and cats. Most puppies are infected at or soon after birth. During the summer, infective eggs are shed and can survive for years in the environment. Humans ingest the eggs orally by eating with contaminated hands. Once they are in the human intestine, the eggs develop into larvae. The larvae penetrate the bowel wall and spread to the liver, muscles, and lungs via the bloodstream. Sometimes the parasite penetrates into the eye and brain. The severity of disease is related to the number of eggs ingested, duration of infection, tissue location of larvae, and the patient's immune response.

MEDICAL HISTORY AND CLINICAL PRESENTATION

The patient will have a history of exposure to contaminated soil, presence of unwormed puppies, unhygienic conditions, and/or pica.

In heavy infections, larvae may migrate through liver and lungs or other internal organs, causing inflammation and symptomatic disease. While rare, larvae may migrate to the central nervous system causing eosinophilic meningoencephalitis or granuloma formation.

SIGNS AND SYMPTOMS

Many infections are asymptomatic. Signs and symptoms are nonspecific and include fever, weakness, cough, pruritus, rash, dyspnea, and abdominal pain.

PHYSICAL EXAMINATION

Visceral toxocariasis may develop hepatomegaly. Ocular toxocariasis is usually unilateral and presents with leukocoria and decreased vision in the affected eye that may be confused with retinoblastoma.

DIFFERENTIAL DIAGNOSIS

The differential diagnosis for visceral disease, with lung involvement, includes asthma. If pulmonary infiltrates are present it may resemble tumor metastases. Ocular disease can result in eye findings similar to other infectious causes of retinoblastoma. The presentation of cutaneous disease can be confused with *Strongyloides* infection.

DIAGNOSTIC STUDIES

In patients with suspected toxocariasis, there is often a history of exposure to dogs or cats, eosinophilia, hyperglobulinemia, hepatomegaly, and an increase in anti-*Toxocara* excretory-secretory antigen IgG level.

Diagnosis of visceral toxocariasis is based on a history of exposure to a potential source of infectious *Toxocara* eggs or larvae. Positive serology testing with ELISA with larval stage antigens is noted. Detectable antibody may be the result of past infection. Seropositivity can be present in asymptomatic *Toxocara* infection. Paired serum samples showing a rise in antibody level over time may be used to confirm active infection.

Diagnosis of ocular toxocariasis is based on physical examination signs and history of exposure to infectious *Toxocara* eggs or larvae. Ocular toxocariasis antibody levels in serum can be low or absent despite clinical disease.

TREATMENT

The treatment of choice for both visceral and ocular toxocariasis is albendazole or the alternative mebendazole. Treatment is indicated for moderate-severe visceral cases. Patients with mild symptoms of toxocariasis may not require anthelminthic therapy. In ocular disease the use of corticosteroids may be needed to suppress the allergic manifestations of the infection. Vitrectomy may also be needed for ocular disease along with antihelminthic therapy and corticosteroids.

PATIENT EDUCATION

- Toxocariasis is often a benign, asymptomatic, and self-limiting disease.
- Ocular involvement, ocular larvae migrans, may cause loss of visual acuity or unilateral blindness.
- Prevention of disease depends on proper hygiene, including handwashing after contact with pets.

17.6BL CUTANEOUS LARVA MIGRANS

Cutaneous larva migrans is a skin disease in humans, caused by the larvae of various nematodes, including *Ancyclostoma braziliense*.

The parasites are found in dog and cat feces. In humans the parasite is only able to penetrate the outer layers of the skin and cause typical wormlike burrows visible underneath the skin. The parasites lack the collagenase enzymes that are needed to penetrate deeper into the skin through the basement membrane.

MEDICAL HISTORY AND CLINICAL PRESENTATION

Intensely pruritic erythematous papules develop, typically on the feet or hands. This is followed in a few days by serpiginous tracks marking the course of the parasite. Several tracks may be present, and the organism can travel millimeters per day. Over time the lesions may become vesiculated, encrusted, or infected. Systemic symptoms and eosinophilia are uncommon.

PHYSICAL EXAMINATION

The infection presents with a red, intense itching eruption. The itching may be very painful and a secondary bacterial infection can develop with scratching.

DIAGNOSTIC STUDIES

The diagnosis is based on the characteristic appearance of the lesions. Biopsy is typically not indicated.

TREATMENT

Without treatment, the larvae will die and be absorbed. Mild cases do not require treatment. Topical thiabendazole can be applied and systemic therapy with albendazole or ivermectin is effective.

Topical freezing agents, with ethyl chloride or liquid nitrogen, can kill the larvae, with some success.

17.6BM FILARIASIS

Filariasis is a parasitic disease caused by infection with filarial nematodes. Filariasis is spread by blood-feeding insects such as black flies and mosquitoes.

Eight filarial nematodes use humans as their definitive hosts and they are divided into three groups. See Table 17.26 for a list of filarial nematodes.

The adult worms release larval forms known as microfilariae into the host's bloodstream. These circulating microfilariae are taken up by the arthropod vector during a blood meal. In the vector they develop into infective larvae that can be transmitted to a new host.

Elephantiasis is due to lymphatic damage secondary to the nematode infection. The infection leads to permanent lymphatic dilatation and dysfunction. This causes swelling and secondary infections resulting in chronic skin changes and continued risk of infection.

MEDICAL HISTORY AND CLINICAL PRESENTATION

Patients with filariasis will have a history of living in an area where the disease is endemic.

There is a history of asymmetric swelling: the legs are most commonly affected; arms along with breasts and genitals can also be affected. Genital symptoms include scrotal elephantiasis or a hydrocele. Swelling is initially reversible but then can become permanent, with associated skin changes.

SIGNS AND SYMPTOMS

The major symptom of lymphatic filariasis is elephantiasis, edema with thickening of the skin and underlying tissues. It is most commonly noted in the lower extremities.

Location of symptoms varies with the filarial worm. *Wuchereria bancroft* affects the legs, arms, breasts, vulva, and scrotum. Patients with subcutaneous worms present with rashes, urticarial papules, pigmentated macules, and arthritis.

TABLE 17.26 Diseases Caused by Filarial Nematodes

Disease	Organism	Location	Syndrome
Lymphatic filariasis	*Wuchereria bancrofti* *Brugia malayi* *Brugia timori*	Lymphatics Lymphatics Lymphatics	Elephantiasis Elephantiasis Elephantiasis
Subcutaneous filariasis	*Loa* *Mansonella streptocerca* *Onchocerca volvulus*	Subcutaneous skin layer Subcutaneous skin layer Subcutaneous skin layer	Loa filariasis River blindness
Serous cavity filariasis	*Mansonella perstans* *Mansonella ozzardi*	Abdominal serous cavity Abdominal serous cavity	

Onchocerca volvulus presents in the eyes, causing river blindness. Serous cavity filariasis presents with symptoms similar to subcutaneous filariasis, plus abdominal pain.

PHYSICAL EXAMINATION

Physical examination findings include asymmetric lymphedema, intermittent fevers, and chyluria. Skin changes include hyperpigmentation and hyperkeratosis.

DIFFERENTIAL DIAGNOSIS

The differential diagnosis for cutaneous larva migrans includes other causes of lymphedema and pelvic pathology and malignancy.

DIAGNOSTIC STUDIES

Diagnosis of active infection is via the identification of microfilariae in a blood smear by microscopic examination. Microfilariae can be detected microscopically on blood smears obtained at night and a thick smear should be made and stained with Giemsa or hematoxylin and eosin.

Serologic EIA tests, including antifilarial IgG1 and IgG4, are an alternative to microscopic detection. Patients with active filarial infection typically have elevated levels of antifilarial IgG4 in the blood.

Other methods of diagnosis include tissue specimens to visualize adult worms or microfilariae as well as ultrasonographic visualization of adult worms.

TREATMENT

Conservative management is important for all disease stages and can prevent disease progression.

Washing the skin with soap and water can reduce acute attacks and reduce progression of the disease.

Leg exercise, elevation, and compression can be helpful to reduce lymphedema.

The treatment of choice is diethylcarbamazine citrate (DEC), which is both microfilaricidal and active against the adult worm. The late phase of chronic disease is not affected by antiparasitic therapy. Ivermectin is effective against the microfilariae of *W. bancrofti*, but has no effect on the adult parasite.

Because lymphatic filariasis is rare in the United States, DEC is not approved by the FDA. Ivermectin treatment can be used but kills only microfilariae and not adult worms.

17.6BN LOA LOA FILARIASIS

Loa filariasis is caused by the nematode worm *Loa loa*. Humans contract the disease through the bite of a horsefly, deer fly, and mango fly. The vectors are blood-sucking and day-biting and are found in high-canopied rain forests of West and Central Africa. Humans are the primary reservoir.

The infected fly introduces third-stage filarial larvae onto the skin of the human host during the blood meal. The larvae develop into adults that reside in the subcutaneous tissue. During the day the microfilariae are found in peripheral blood; during the noncirculation phase they are found in the lungs. The fly ingests microfilariae during a blood meal and after ingestion, the microfilariae lose their sheaths. The microfilariae develop into first-stage larvae and later into third-stage infective larvae. The third-stage infective larvae migrate to the fly's proboscis and can infect another human when the fly takes a blood meal.

MEDICAL HISTORY AND CLINICAL PRESENTATION

The flies that transmit the parasite typically bite during the day and are more common during the rainy season. Travelers to at-risk areas who stay for long periods of time, >1 month, are more likely to become infected than short-term travelers. A traveler's risk for infection depends on the number of bites received and the number of infected flies in the area.

Symptoms include itchy, nonpainful swelling, Calabar swellings, anywhere on the body. Calabar swelling is due to a transient allergic response to microfilariasis. Other symptoms include generalized itching, muscle and joint pain, and fatigue. Infected persons may not have any symptoms at all.

PHYSICAL EXAMINATION

Adult worms may be visibly migrating under the surface of the skin. The eye worm is the visible migration of the adult worm across the surface of the eye.

Calabar swellings are localized, nontender swellings usually found on the extremities and near joints.

Genitals may show edema.

DIAGNOSTIC STUDIES

The diagnosis can be made by identifying the adult worm after removal from under the skin or eye, identification of the larvae on blood smear taken midday, or the identification of antibodies against *L. loa*.

TREATMENT

Treatment involves antiparasitic therapy and possible surgical removal of adult worms followed by systemic treatment. The current treatment of choice in patients without detectable microfilariae is DEC. If there is a high microfilaria load treatment with DEC may be contraindicated, as rapid microfilaricidal actions of the drug can provoke encephalopathy. Albendazole administration has proved helpful as well.

Cure is defined as resolution of symptoms, disappearance of eosinophilia, and decreasing antifilarial antibody titers. Some patients may require additional treatment.

PATIENT EDUCATION

- DEC taken once a week is effective at preventing loiasis in long-term travelers to affected areas.
- Prevention includes avoiding areas where the fly vector breeds. Other prevention efforts include personal protection measures against biting insects.

SPECIAL CONSIDERATIONS

- Infection with toxoplasmosis can cause infection of the brain and eyes in the fetus when a pregnant woman becomes infected.
- Chagas disease can spread via congenital transmission.
- Enterobiasis infection, pinworms, most commonly occurs in school-age children.

KEY POINTS

- Prevention is the key to preventing transmission of various parasitic infections. This includes proper sanitation, handwashing, adequate cooking of food, and clean water.
- *Entamoeba histolytica* and *Giardia lamblia* cause intestinal infections, diagnosed with EIA testing and treated with metronidazole or tinidazole.
- Adult tapeworm infections are best diagnosed by microscopic examination of the stool.

17.7 MYCOTIC INFECTIONS

Overview

Mycotic or fungal infections are classified as either primary or OI. Primary infections are those that develop in immunocompetent hosts and OIs develop in immunocompromised hosts.

Fungal infections can also be local or systemic. Local infections involve one part of the body including the skin, oral cavity, and vaginal and occur in immunocompetent or immunocompromised hosts. Systemic infections are infections that are noted in more than one area of the body and spread in the bloodstream.

Most fungi are opportunists and are typically not pathogenic except in an immunocompromised host.

Opportunistic systemic fungal infections include candidiasis, aspergillosis, and mucormycosis.

Primary fungal infections typically result from inhalation of fungal spores, causing a localized pneumonia as the primary manifestation.

In immunocompetent patients, systemic mycoses have a chronic course and months may go by before seeking medical attention and a diagnosis is made.

Many primary fungal infections have a characteristic geographic distribution; this is noted with the dimorphic fungi. Examples include:

- **Coccidioidomycosis:** Noted in the southwest United States, northern Mexico, and Central and South America
- **Histoplasmosis:** Noted in the Midwestern United States and areas of Central and South America, Africa, Asia, and Australia
- **Blastomycosis:** Noted in North America and Africa
- **Paracoccidioidomycosis:** Noted in South America

A detailed travel and residential history should be obtained if an acute or a chronic primary fungal infection is suspected to determine whether patients may have been exposed to certain endemic mycoses.

Fungi can disseminate from a primary focus in the lung; this leads to manifestations and disease in other areas of the body. For example:

- Cryptococcosis can lead to chronic meningitis.
- Histoplasmosis can disseminate involving the reticuloendothelial system.
- Blastomycosis can lead to skin lesions or involve the central nervous system and bone.
- Coccidioidomycosis can cause bone and joint infections, skin lesions, and meningitis.

EPIDEMIOLOGY

Fungal infections are acquired through two major routes: inhalation of fungal spores into the lungs and paranasal sinuses, or direct contact. Some fungal organisms are normal flora, for example *Malassezia* spp. is acquired during infancy through contact with humans carrying the organism and *Candida albicans* is acquired as intestinal and mucosal flora from passage through the birth canal or later in life by contact with humans carrying the organism.

Other fungal organisms cause disease via various infectious processes including:

- Dermatophytosis (ringworm) is acquired by contact with infected animals, infected persons, or soil.
- Sporotrichosis or mycetoma is acquired through inoculation of saprophytic fungi on vegetation or soil through minor trauma.
- Rhinosporidiosis is acquired through contact with water.
- Histoplasmosis, blastomycosis, coccidioidomycosis, and cryptococcosis are acquired through inhalation and cause a lung infection.
- Ingestion has not proved to be a portal for pathogenic fungi.

PATHOPHYSIOLOGY

Yeasts are generally round or oval and reproduce by budding. Molds are composed of tubular structures called hyphae and grow by branching and longitudinal extension. Some species, such as *Coccidioides* species and *Pneumocystis jirovecii*, are round in tissue and do not bud; instead the cytoplasm divides to form numerous internal spores that are released to form new spherical structures.

Dimorphic fungi can grow either as a yeast or as a mold. They grow in the host as yeast-like forms but grow as molds at room temperature. These fungi include the agents of histoplasmosis, blastomycosis, sporotrichosis, coccidioidomycosis, and paracoccidioidomycosis.

17.7A CANDIDIASIS

Candida is part of the normal flora of the skin and mucous membranes. *Candida albicans* is responsible for a majority of *Candida* infections. Other *Candida* species causing human disease include *C. krusei*, *C. glabrata*, *C. tropicalis*, and *C. auris*. *C. auris* is very drug-resistant, causes invasive infections associated with high mortality rate, and spreads easily among patients in healthcare settings.

Infection is avoided in most patients because of the balance between the organism virulence factors and a patient's immune system. Risk factors for developing candidiasis are a deficiency in cell-mediated immunity and overall poor health of the patient. Candidiasis is usually localized to skin and mucous membranes. Candidiasis can spread causing candidemia and distant infection but is rare. *Candida* infections can be localized, such as oral and esophageal disease and vulvovaginitis; or invasive, such as endocarditis and osteoarticular infection.

MEDICAL HISTORY AND CLINICAL PRESENTATION

Medical history and presentation vary depending on the site of the *Candida* infection. Candidiasis of the mouth, throat, or esophagus is uncommon in healthy adults. People at higher risk for getting candidiasis in the mouth and throat include babies, those younger than 1 month of age, denture wearers; those with a history of diabetes, history of cancer, and history of HIV/AIDS; smokers; those taking antibiotics or corticosteroids or have medical disorders or are on medications that cause dry mouth.

Most people who get esophageal candidiasis have weakened immune systems, including patients with HIV/AIDS or a history of leukemia or lymphoma. Patients with esophageal candidiasis often have oral candidiasis.

Vaginal candidiasis is common. Women who are more likely to get vaginal candidiasis include those who are pregnant, using hormonal contraceptives, with a history of diabetes, wirh a history of HIV, with current or recent use of antibiotics, or on immunosuppressive medications.

Common risk factors for invasive candidiasis include those with the following: ICU stay, presence of central venous catheters, recent use of broad-spectrum antibiotics, current use of total parenteral nutrition, history of renal failure or on dialysis, history of hematologic or solid organ malignancy, and history of IV drug usage.

SIGNS AND SYMPTOMS

Oral cavity candidiasis can present with many different symptoms, including white patches on the buccal mucosa, tongue, roof of the mouth, and throat; redness or soreness; loss of taste; pain while eating or swallowing; and cracking and redness at the corners of the mouth.

Symptoms of esophageal candidiasis include dysphagia and odynophagia.

Most cases of vaginal candidiasis are mild, and symptoms include vaginal itching or soreness, dyspareunia, dysuria, and abnormal vaginal discharge (Figure 17.28).

Signs and symptoms of invasive candidiasis are nonspecific and include fever and chills. Candidemia is the most common form of invasive candidiasis; other forms include endocarditis, peritonitis, meningitis, osteomyelitis, arthritis, and endophthalmitis.

PHYSICAL EXAMINATION

Physical examination findings vary with the location of the infection. Oral candidiasis appears as thick, white curd-like deposits. Underlying mucosa may appear erythematous

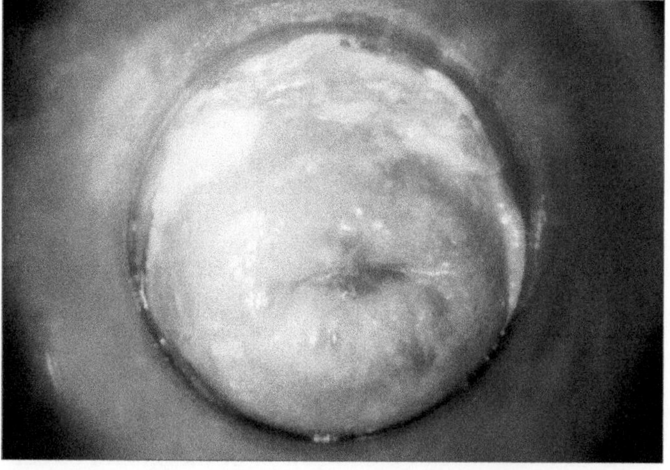

Figure 17.28 Vulvovaginitis secondary to *Candida albicans*.

and slightly raised. *Candida* vulvovaginitis presents with vulvar edema, excoriations, and a thick, curd-like vaginal discharge. Systemic candidiasis may present with fever and hepatosplenomegaly.

DIFFERENTIAL DIAGNOSIS

The differential diagnosis for superficial *Candida* infection includes tinea infections and tinea versicolor. The differential for vulvovaginitis includes bacterial vaginosis, trichomoniasis, and trophic vaginitis.

DIAGNOSTIC STUDIES

Diagnosis of oral candidiasis is typically made on history and physical examination. A wet prep may be obtained and reveal yeast and pseudohyphae.

Candida esophagitis is diagnosed by endoscopy. Visual inspection will reveal white patches and the diagnosis can be confirmed by biopsy. Biopsy will also assist in ruling out other causes of esophagitis including herpesvirus and CMV.

Vaginal candidiasis is diagnosed by wet prep revealing hyphae and pseudohyphae. Culture is the definitive diagnostic test.

Invasive or systemic candidiasis is diagnosed with blood culture. The beta-D-glucan assay is approved as an adjunctive diagnostic tool but is not a very specific test for *Candida*.

TREATMENT

Oral candidiasis is treated with several antifungal medications. These medications are clotrimazole, miconazole, and nystatin. For severe infections, fluconazole can be used orally or IV.

Esophageal candidiasis is treated with fluconazole. Other treatment options include amphotericin B, itraconazole, and voriconazole.

Uncomplicated vaginal candidiasis is treated with nystatin and the topical azoles, including miconazole and clotrimazole. Complicated infections are treated with fluconazole.

For most adult patients with candidemia, the initial treatment is an echinocandin, including micafungin and caspofungin, with transition to fluconazole, if the organism is susceptible, once the specific organism is identified and blood cultures have cleared. Alternative treatments include voriconazole and amphotericin B formulations.

PATIENT EDUCATION

- Antifungal prophylaxis may be indicated in some solid organ transplant recipients, high-risk ICU patients, chemotherapy-induced neutropenia, and stem cell transplant recipients with neutropenia.

17.7B HISTOPLASMOSIS

Histoplasmosis is the most common endemic mycosis in the United States, typically presents as a community-acquired respiratory infection, but may present as a progressive disseminated disease.

Histoplasma capsulatum is a dimorphic fungus in the class Ascomycetes.

Histoplasmosis is typically acquired via inhalation of airborne microconidia, often after disturbance of soil that is contaminated with bird and bat droppings. Increase risk of exposure includes farming and exposure to chicken coops or caves. Histoplasmosis occurs in North, Central, and South America and parts of Asia and Africa.

In most patients, the infection is asymptomatic and resolves. In a few patients acute pulmonary infection can develop with the inhalation of a large amount of the organism. The cell-mediated immune response, by the T-lymphocytes, is responsible for the response to the infection. T-lymphocytes induce the release of cytokines that provide protection from reinfection and activate macrophages, which inhibits the growth and spread of the organism. This results in the formation of a granuloma in which the fungus is present in a nonviable state. Immunosuppressed patients are unable to mount an adequate T-lymphocyte response resulting in uncontrolled growth and spread, increasing the risk of mortality and morbidity.

MEDICAL HISTORY AND CLINICAL PRESENTATION

Histoplasmosis should be considered in patients who reside in or have recently visited endemic areas and those who tested positive for CAP.

Clinical clues that suggest histoplasmosis include failure to respond to appropriate treatment for CAP; diffuse reticular, nodular, or miliary infiltrates; mediastinal or hilar lymphadenopathy; or cavitary lung disease that tests negative for tuberculosis.

Healthy patients exposed to low inoculum are typically asymptomatic. Heavy inoculum may produce mild flu-like symptoms associated with mediastinal lymphadenopathy and/or focal pulmonary infiltrates.

Large inoculum leads to acute pulmonary symptoms within 1 to 2 weeks of exposure and diffuse or miliary infiltrates. Symptoms are moderately severe, and recovery is slow. Severe cases may develop respiratory failure or progressive disseminated disease.

SIGNS AND SYMPTOMS

Most patients are asymptomatic. Acute pulmonary histoplasmosis has an incubation period of 3 to 17 days and presents with fever, dry cough, and dyspnea. Some patients develop rheumatologic symptoms such as erythema nodosum and symmetric joint pain. Disseminated disease presents with fever, malaise, weight loss, and abdominal distention; severe form of the disease presents with the features of sepsis, acute respiratory distress syndrome (ARDS), and disseminated intravascular coagulation.

PHYSICAL EXAMINATION

Physical examination findings in pulmonary disease include erythema nodosum and rales on auscultation. In patients with disseminated disease the physical examination findings are similar to sepsis, including hypotension and altered mental status.

DIFFERENTIAL DIAGNOSIS

Patients with acute and chronic pulmonary histoplasmosis present similar to pneumonia. The differential diagnosis is noted in Table 17.27.

DIAGNOSTIC STUDIES

Skin testing can be used to determine exposure to histoplasmosis.

Culture is the gold standard for diagnosis; cultures are negative in milder cases and in patients with inflammatory complications of the infection. Visualization of yeast in the tissues and respiratory secretions of patients with histoplasmosis may provide a rapid diagnosis; but direct examination may be negative in half of patients with disseminated or chronic pulmonary histoplasmosis and in most with other manifestations of histoplasmosis. Culture sensitivity is highest in respiratory specimens from patients with chronic pulmonary histoplasmosis or progressive disseminated histoplasmosis.

Direct examination of the patient's specimen is not 100% specific, as staining artifacts may be misinterpreted as yeast, and, in some cases, other fungi may be mistaken as *Histoplasma*. Direct examination often involves an invasive

TABLE 17.27 Differential Diagnosis for Histoplasmosis

Diagnosis	Distribution	High-Risk Patients	Clinical Findings
Histoplasmosis	Mississippi and Ohio River valleys, Central and South America	Cave spelunkers	Splenomegaly, positive urine antigen test
Coccidioidomycosis	Southwest United States, Central and South America	AIDS	Night sweats, rash
Paracoccidioidomycosis	Central and South America	AIDS	Lymphadenopathy, hepatosplenomegaly
Aspergillosis	Ubiquitous	Immunocompromised Cystic fibrosis	Weight loss, hemoptysis
Anthrax	Ubiquitous	Livestock handlers	Painless skin ulcer, diarrhea
Legionellosis	Ubiquitous	Chronic lung disease Older patients	Cough, diarrhea, confusion Water exposure, hyponatremia
Tuberculosis		Immunocompromised	Fever, night sweats, hemoptysis, positive acid-fast bacillus smears
Primary lung cancer		Patients over age 65	History of smoking, weight loss, hemoptysis, chest x-ray mass

procedure to obtain tissue. Detection of antigen in bodily fluids is most useful for diagnosis of disseminated and acute pulmonary histoplasmosis. Serologic test for antibodies is useful for diagnosing milder forms of histoplasmosis in which tests for antigens, direct examination, and culture are negative

Detection of antigen in blood, and urine provides the highest diagnostic yield in patients with acute pulmonary infection with over 80% positive and progressive disseminated histoplasmosis infection with over 90% positive. The highest sensitivity is noted in urine and serum testing, bronchial washings, and CSF.

Histoplasma yeasts are oval and show narrow necked budding. Yeasts may be seen on Wright stain of peripheral blood in patients with severe disseminated histoplasmosis. Gomori methenamine silver stain is the most sensitive method for visualization of the yeast.

Serologic testing for antibodies is used in the diagnosis of histoplasmosis. Antibodies develop 1 to 3 months following primary infection and may be falsely negative early. Antibodies may not distinguish active from past infection. Two common methods include immunodiffusion (IDF) and CF.

Chest x-ray may be normal but typically displays small, diffuse, nodular opacities; diffuse, interstitial infiltrates; or diffuse airspace disease and adenopathy (Figure 17.29).

TREATMENT

A lipid formulation of amphotericin B, liposomal amphotericin B, is the treatment of choice for moderately severe and severe cases. Itraconazole is recommended for mild cases and after patients have improved in response to amphotericin B.

Fluconazole is an alternative to itraconazole but is less effective. The echinocandins are not active against histoplasmosis.

PATIENT EDUCATION

- Immunocompetent hosts have an excellent prognosis with resolution in 2 to 3 weeks.
- Immunocompromised patients can have extensive disease and a poor prognosis. Mortality rate is high in HIV patients.

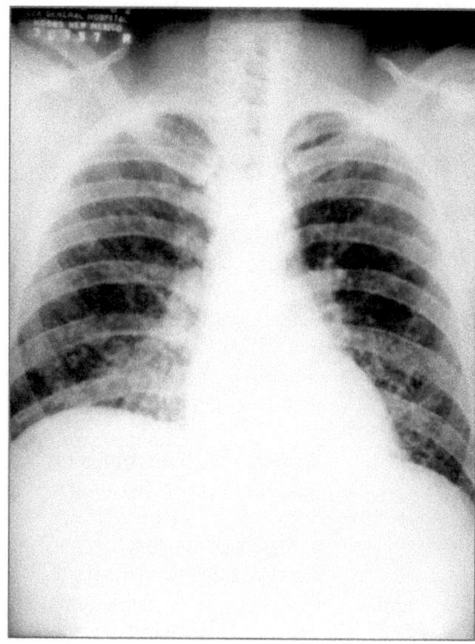

Figure 17.29 **Pulmonary histoplasmosis, chest x-ray.**

17.7C COCCIDIOIDOMYCOSIS

Coccidioidomycosis, or valley fever, is caused by the fungi *Coccidioides immitis* and *Coccidioides posadasii.* The fungi live in the desert soil of the southwestern United States, Arizona and California, Nevada, New Mexico, Texas, and Utah. It was first noted in the San Joaquin Valley of California. In 2018, there were 15,611 cases of Valley fever reported to CDC.[17] Ninety-six percent of these cases were in Arizona or California.[17] Rates of Valley fever are highest among people age 60 and older.

The fungus is dimorphic and only the spore-forming phase causes infection by inhalation. Manifestations of coccidioidomycosis range from clinically asymptomatic to life threatening.

Coccidioidomycosis is an infection caused by inhaling the spores. Spores are found in the soil in certain geographic areas and get into the air when the soil is disturbed by construction, gardening, farming, windy weather, and driving all-terrain vehicles. Coccidioidomycosis cannot be passed from person-to-person. Following transmission, the organisms are deposited into the terminal bronchioles, enlarge, and develop internal septations to form spherules. It then disseminates to the bloodstream and lymphatic system and spread throughout the body.

MEDICAL HISTORY AND CLINICAL PRESENTATION

Obtaining a travel history is critical to making the diagnosis.

Coccidiosis pneumonia presents with fever, cough, fatigue, and headache, and is clinically indistinguishable from bacterial causes of CAP. In endemic areas, coccidiosis may make up about a fourth of CAPs.

Complex infections may develop exudative pleural effusions or pulmonary cavities and nodules.

Skin manifestations such as erythema nodosum or erythema multiforme may be present and do not mean there has been dissemination of disease. The rashes are secondary to an immune response to the fungus and are a favorable prognostic sign. Patients may present with supraclavicular lymphadenopathy.

The presentation of disseminated disease will depend on the location of infection. In the central nervous system, it presents as a meningitis with headache, with or without neurologic deficit; if present the deficits are typically cranial nerve palsies. Bone and joint infection presents with pain and swelling at the site of infection. Vertebral infection will present with localized back pain, with or without fever, and possible neurologic deficit.

Dissemination occurs in approximately in a small number of cases and is more common in African Americans, pregnant women in the third trimester, and patients who are immunocompromised, including HIV, post-transplant, and immunosuppressant patients, including those on steroids or tumor necrosis factor (TNF) blockers.

SIGNS AND SYMPTOMS

Clinical manifestations of coccidioidomycosis can range from subclinical to fatal disseminated disease. Medical history should include any history of travel to endemic areas or contact with people with similar complaints. The most common symptoms of pulmonary coccidioidomycosis include fever, chills, cough, and pleuritic chest pain. Other common symptoms include arthralgias, fatigue, and erythema nodosum. Less common symptoms include weight loss, night sweats, and hemoptysis.

PHYSICAL EXAMINATION

The physical manifestations of the disease depend on the organ of involvement. The most commonly involved organ is the lungs, followed by skin, bones, and genitourinary tract.

Physical examination findings on lung exam include parenchymal consolidation, dullness to percussion, increased tactile fremitus, rales, and rhonchi. Exam of the skin reveals erythema nodosum, tender, red, smooth nodules on the shins; and erythema multiforme, target lesions on the skin.

Other physical examination findings include fever, tachypnea, and regional lymphadenopathy.

DIFFERENTIAL DIAGNOSIS

The differential diagnosis varies based on the organ system involved. With lung involvement the differential includes CAP. With skin and bone involvement the differential includes syphilis, tuberculosis, and cancer.

DIAGNOSTIC STUDIES

Common laboratory findings include eosinophilia and if there is neurologic involvement the CSF will reveal a high protein, low glucose, and eosinophilic pleocytosis.

Laboratory diagnosis can be made several different ways:

- Direct microscopy to visualization the *Coccidioides* spherules in body fluid or tissue
- Serology testing includes many options:
    - EIA for the detection of IgM and IgG
    - IDF also detects IgG and IgM antibodies
    - CF titer of 1:16 increases risk of dissemination
- Fungal culture
- PCR

TREATMENT

Treatment is not needed for clinically insignificant disease, diagnosed only by serologic testing.

Treat of coccidioidomycosis pneumonia should be based on clinical features. Treatment of choice is fluconazole or itraconazole for 3 to 6 months. Longer treatment with higher doses may be needed if there is an increased severity and the presence of risk factors for dissemination.

Treatment of disseminated disease is required with oral azole antifungals, such as fluconazole and itraconazole. If disease is refractory to initial treatment, voriconazole and posaconazole can be used, but side effects are common.

Amphotericin B is widely used to treat complicated patients, HIV infection, pregnancy, or in case of azole failure.

PATIENT EDUCATION

- The prognosis of coccidioidomycosis is excellent in immunocompetent patients.
- Poor prognosis is associated with HIV, pregnancy third trimester, organ transplantation, and immunosuppressant therapy.

17.7D PNEUMOCYSTIS

Pneumocystis pneumonia (PCP) is caused by *Pneumocystis jirovecii*. In the past this disease was thought to be due to a different species, *P. carinii*. Studies have shown that *P. carinii* is a rodent pathogen.

Formerly thought to be a protozoan, studies show that *Pneumocystis* is a unicellular fungus acquired by the airborne route. It is an opportunistic pathogen and noted in patients with depressed cell-mediated immunity.

In immunocompetent patients, the presence of *Pneumocystis* organisms triggers the release of proinflammatory cytokines and the activation of alveolar macrophages, leading to clearance of the organisms and absence of disease. In immunocompromised hosts, alveolar macrophages are not activated by CD4 cells, allowing *P. jirovecii* organisms to proliferate. With infection interstitial fibrosis occurs, compliance decreases, diffusion capacity is impaired, and hypoxia and dyspnea develop.

The risk of pneumonia due to *P. jirovecii* increases when the CD4 count is <200 cells/µL.

The life cycle of *Pneumocystis* is not known. All stages are found in the lungs.

MEDICAL HISTORY AND CLINICAL PRESENTATION

A history of HIV or severe immunosuppression is noted in patients with PCP. Symptoms of PCP include fever, nonproductive cough, shortness of breath, weight loss, and night sweats.

In patients with HIV, the most common manifestations of PCP are subacute onset of progressive dyspnea, fever, nonproductive cough, and chest discomfort that worsens within days to weeks.

In mild cases, pulmonary examination while the patient is at rest is usually normal. Fever is apparent in most cases and can be the predominant symptom.

SIGNS AND SYMPTOMS

Signs and symptoms in HIV-infected patients include subacute onset of a nonproductive cough, progressive exertional dyspnea, and fever.

In non-HIV patients and those on steroids and other immunosuppressive agents, with a history of primary immunodeficiencies, with hematologic/nonhematologic malignancies, and who are severely malnourished symptoms include acute onset of nonproductive cough, dyspnea, and fever.

PHYSICAL EXAMINATION

Physical examination findings include fever, tachypnea, and tachycardia, fine rales on lung exam, and possibly cyanosis.

DIFFERENTIAL DIAGNOSIS

The differential diagnosis includes infectious etiologies of pneumonia due to *Mycoplasma*, *Legionella*, CMV and other viruses, *Mycobacterium tuberculosis,* and *M. avium* complex. Noninfectious etiologies include ARDS, pulmonary embolism, and lymphocytic interstitial pneumonia.

DIAGNOSTIC STUDIES

General laboratory findings include an elevated LDH level and hypoxemia (Pao_2 ≤70 mm Hg or O_2 saturation <90%) and/or an increased A-a gradient. The peripheral WBC count with differential is not helpful in the evaluation of PCP.

The diagnosis can be confirmed by demonstrating the *P. jirovecii* organism in the tissue, sputum specimen, or bronchoalveolar lavage.

With chest x-ray there is no distinct finding pathognomonic for PCP, but a diffuse, patchy infiltrate extending from the perihilar area is common. In patients with a clinically compatible syndrome and an abnormal CXR, no further imaging is required (Figure 17.30).

If the clinical suspicion is high but the chest x-ray is normal, a high-resolution chest CT scan should be obtained. The characteristic finding of patchy, ground-glass opacities is seen.

Numerous stains are used to identify *P. jirovecii*. These include methenamine silver and toluidine blue that stain the wall of organisms and Wright–Giemsa stain stains the organism as well as host cells.

Immunofluorescence using monoclonal antibodies against *P. jirovecii* is the most widely used technique to definitively identify the organism.

TREATMENT

The treatment of choice is TMP-SMX for all severities of PCP, including in pregnancy, and should be given intravenously in severe cases. If mild rash or low-grade fever develop while on TMP-SMX, treatment with antihistamines and antipyretics should be started before changing therapy, since TMP-SMX is the preferred treatment for PCP. The usual course of treatment is 21 days in HIV patients and 14 days for all others.

For HIV patients with severe PCP, defined as a Pao_2 of <70 mm Hg or an A-a gradient >35, corticosteroids should be started within 72 hours of PCP treatment.

For patients with mild to moderate disease and with a sulfa allergy, TMP with dapsone or clindamycin with primaquine are an acceptable regimens once glucose-6-phosphate dehydrogenase (G-6-PD) deficiency has been ruled out.

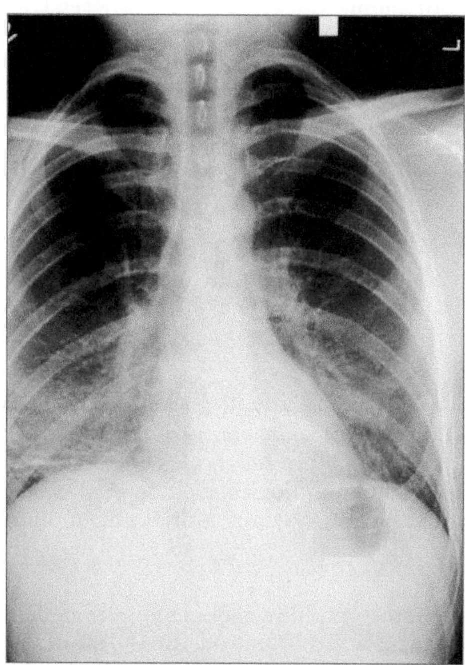

Figure 17.30 **Chest x-ray *Pneumocystis* pneumonia**

For patients with moderate to severe disease who are sulfa allergic and G-6-PD deficient, clindamycin and primaquine are the treatment of choice.

IV pentamidine is as effective as TMP-SMX but its use is limited secondary to toxicity and aerosolized pentamidine is inferior to TMP-SMX and should not be used for the treatment of PCP.

PATIENT EDUCATION

- Most patients with mild PCP recover fully, but if they remain immunosuppressed they are at risk for recurrent disease.
- Prognosis is directly related to the degree of hypoxemia; those who present with an A-a gradient >45 have a mortality rate near 50%.

17.7E CRYPTOCOCCOSIS

Although the *Cryptococcus* genus contains several species, *Cryptococcus neoformans* is the species that causes disease in humans. *C. neoformans* is an encapsulated yeast found in the soil, bird excreta, and other decaying organic matter.

Most cryptococcal infections are in patients with compromised cell-mediated immunity. A strong cellular immune response leading to granulomatous inflammation is essential for control of the infection. Natural killer cells have been shown to have anticryptococcal effects, as well as CD4 and CD8 lymphocytes. The number of CD4 cells influences the risk of developing disease with CD4 lymphocyte counts less than 100 cells/μL associated with an increase in infections among patients with HIV. Humoral immunity is also important in an effective immune response to *Cryptococcus*. Antibodies enhance phagocytosis, natural killer cell function, and improve clearing of capsular polysaccharides.

The life cycle of *Cryptococcus* is not well known. The fungus exists in the soil in a variety of environments. Primary infection with *C. neoformans* and *C. gattii* occur through inhalation of aerosolized spores, which are rapidly converted to their yeast from within the macrophage at body temperature. Dissemination occurs via circulating macrophages. Person-to-person transmission does not occur, except by contaminated transplanted donor tissue or organs.

MEDICAL HISTORY AND CLINICAL PRESENTATION

The symptoms of cryptococcosis depend on the site of infection, virulence of the organism, and the patient's immune status. The two most common sites of infection are the lungs and the central nervous system.

Pulmonary infection ranges from asymptomatic infection to severe pneumonia with ARDS. Pulmonary infection can manifest as a solitary pulmonary nodule or multiple nodules. Lobar involvement, mass-like infiltrates, hilar lymphadenopathy, and lung cavitation may occur.

The central nervous system, with meningitis, is the most common extrapulmonary site of infection. Patients present with headache, confusion, with or without fever. Symptoms are often subacute with onset over 1 to 2 weeks.

Cutaneous cryptococcosis is classified as a primary, usually from direct inoculation into the skin via trauma, or secondary skin infection due to dissemination.

SIGNS AND SYMPTOMS

Patients may be asymptomatic, have latent infection, or have symptomatic disease. Infection can present as a pneumonia-like illness with fever, productive cough, and chest pain. If dissemination occurs to the central nervous system, presenting symptoms include headache, nausea and vomiting, change in mental status, and focal neurologic deficits. Cutaneous cryptococcosis presents with an ulcer or a raised skin rash.

PHYSICAL EXAMINATION

Physical examination findings include fever and signs of distress. The physical examination findings in pulmonary disease include rales on auscultation. Physical examination findings in patients with cryptococcal meningitis include includes nuchal rigidity, nystagmus, papilledema, and cranial nerve deficits. A positive Kernig and Brudzinski sign may be noted; these signs are typically not seen in fungal meningitis. Cranial nerve deficits present with decreased visual acuity, facial weakness, diplopia, and decreased hearing.

Cutaneous cryptococcal infection presents with erythematous papules, pustules, nodules, and ulcers. The infection can spread to deeper tissue and disseminate to the lymph nodes and blood; it occurs most often in immunocompromised hosts.

DIFFERENTIAL DIAGNOSIS

Cryptococcosis is most common in immunocompromised patients. Cutaneous cryptococcal disease differential includes molluscum contagiosum and Kaposi sarcoma. Cryptococcal meningitis must be differentiated from bacterial and viral meningitis. Cryptococcal pneumonia differential includes coccidioidomycosis, histoplasmosis, tuberculosis, and CAP.

DIAGNOSTIC STUDIES

CSF and bronchoalveolar lavage samples are easily obtained and provide the highest yield among patients with central nervous system and pulmonary disease. In patients with disseminated disease and significant immunosuppression, blood cultures may be positive.

Several stains can be used to identify the organism. Alcian blue, mucicarmine stains, periodic acid-schiff and hematoxylin-eosin are used and reveal narrow-based budding yeast. India ink is a preparation used for examination of CSF samples and reveals encapsulated yeasts with narrow-based budding on direct examination (Figure 17.31).

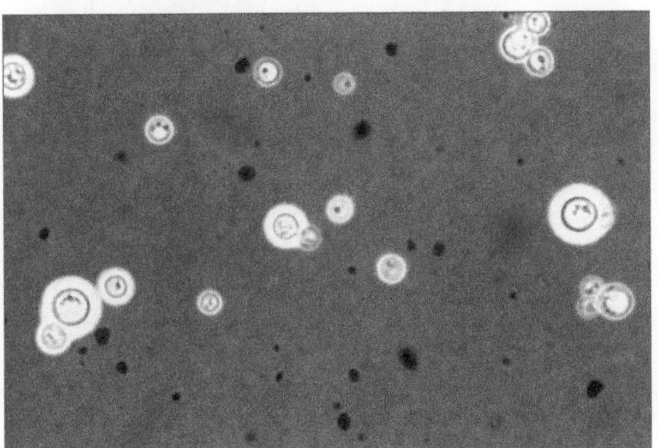

Figure 17.31 India ink prep positive for *Cryptococcus neoformans*.

Culture can also be used to identify *Cryptococcus*. The organism grows on a wide variety of culture media, including blood agar and Saboraud media. *C. neoformans* and *C. gattii* can be separated by use of special media.

Serum or CSF cryptococcal antigen testing using latex agglutination and EIA methodology are more sensitive than culture.

PCR is not routinely available for the diagnosis of cryptococcosis.

TREATMENT

The preferred therapy for cryptococcosis is dependent on the site and severity of infection and the underlying host disorder.

Most infections that are limited to the lungs can be managed with fluconazole for non-life-threatening, mild to moderate disease. If more severe disease is present or extrapulmonary disease is present, such as central nervous system involvement, amphotericin B, either in its conventional or a lipid formulation, is the treatment of choice. If central nervous system disease or severe extraneural disease is present, flucytosine should be added. Once the patient is stable they can be switched to fluconazole.

Cryptococcal meningoencephalitis in HIV-infected patients is best treated with amphotericin B with or without flucytosine for 2 weeks followed by fluconazole for at least 8 weeks. Maintenance therapy with fluconazole is generally advised for patients until their CD4 cell count is consistently >100 cells/mm^3 and there is a low or undetectable HIV viral RNA for at least 3 months.

PATIENT EDUCATION

- Mortality rate of cryptococcal meningitis in HIV patients is around 15%.[85]

17.7F ASPERGILLOSIS

There are many medically important *Aspergillus* species. The most common cause of human infection is *A. fumigatus*. *Aspergillus* species are ubiquitous in the environment and acquired most frequently through inhalation of airborne spores.

The patients at high risk for invasive aspergillosis are those who are neutropenic, have long-term use of corticosteroids leading to neutrophil dysfunction, or have altered immune systems.

Aspergillus species produce many different microbial factors that allow it to cause disease in immunosuppressed people. The organism secretes multiple toxins and metabolites that protect it from host defenses, and it has specific cell wall components that promote survival in the host.

There are several different types of *Aspergillus* diseases. These include:

- **Allergic bronchopulmonary aspergillosis (ABPA):** Causes lung inflammation and allergy symptoms such as coughing and wheezing but does not cause an infection.
- **Allergic *Aspergillus* sinusitis:** Causes sinus inflammation and symptoms of a sinus infection such as drainage, stuffiness, headache but doesn't cause an infection.
- **Aspergilloma:** A ball of *Aspergillus* grows in the lungs or sinuses, but typically does not spread to other parts of the body. Is also called a "fungus ball."

- **Chronic pulmonary aspergillosis:** Infection causes cavities in the lungs and can be a long-term illness with one or more aspergillomas present in the lungs.
- **Invasive aspergillosis:** Causes a serious infection often in the lungs in immunocompromised patients.
- **Cutaneous aspergillosis:** Enters through a break in the skin and causes infection, most often in immunocompromised patients.

MEDICAL HISTORY AND CLINICAL PRESENTATION

The history is vital in the evaluation of the patient with possible aspergillosis. Occupational history and other areas to focus on include any history of immunodeficiency, such as AIDS, cancer, or cystic fibrosis; previous history of cavitary lung disease, such as tuberculosis or sarcoidosis; history of transplantation; and use of immunosuppressive medications, such as chemotherapy and corticosteroids.

Symptoms of aspergillosis depend on the clinical syndrome and extent of disease. ABPA and sinusitis present with signs and symptoms typical of asthma and sinusitis. Symptoms of invasive pulmonary aspergillosis include fever, pleuritic chest pain, productive cough, dyspnea, and hemoptysis. Chronic pulmonary aspergillosis presents with fever, weight loss, productive cough, and hemoptysis.

SIGNS AND SYMPTOMS

Signs and symptoms depend on the specific subtype of disease. ABPA presents with wheezing and cough, and rarely fever. Allergic aspergillus sinusitis presents with sinus drainage, nasal congestion, headache, and facial pain. Aspergilloma patients may be asymptomatic, or present with hemoptysis, cough, and dyspnea. Chronic pulmonary aspergillosis presents with fever, fatigue, weight loss, chronic productive cough, dyspnea, and possibly severe hemoptysis. Invasive pulmonary aspergillosis presents with fever pleuritic chest pain, cough, dyspnea, and hemoptysis. Cutaneous aspergillosis presents with fever and cutaneous lesions with central ulcerations.

PHYSICAL EXAMINATION

On physical examination invasive pulmonary aspergillosis patients are ill-appearing, while patients with pulmonary aspergilloma, ABPA, or allergic sinusitis often appear healthy. Physical examination findings in pulmonary or invasive aspergillosis include decreased breath sounds with wheezes, rales, and increased tactile fremitus. Physical examination findings in cutaneous aspergillosis include single or multiple erythematous-to-violaceous papules, macules, nodules, or plaques.

DIFFERENTIAL DIAGNOSIS

The differential diagnosis includes other infections from fungal, bacterial, viral, and parasitic sources. Additional possibilities are noninfectious pulmonary diseases such as asthma, chronic obstructive pulmonary disease, interstitial lung disease, bronchiectasis, and lung cancer; cardiac diseases such as pericarditis, endocarditis, and myocarditis; sinus diseases such as infectious sinusitis, tumors, and nasal polyps; skin disorders such as eczema, scabies, and cellulitis; and systemic diseases such as Churg-Strauss syndrome, Goodpasture disease, cystic fibrosis, and ciliary dyskinesia.

DIAGNOSTIC STUDIES

The definitive diagnosis of aspergillosis requires a positive culture from a normally sterile site and histopathologic evidence of infection. Other diagnostic tools include radiology, galactomannan antigen detection, beta-D-glucan detection, and PCR.

Microscopic and histopathologic evaluation of respiratory samples with silver stains, such as Gomori methenamine-silver, allows for direct visualization.

Aspergillus species on culture present as rapidly growing molds, but invasive aspergillosis may have negative cultures.

The galactomannan antigen test detects the polysaccharide that makes up part of the cell wall of *Aspergillus* spp. and other fungi. Serum and bronchoalveolar lavage fluid can be tested. There is some cross-reactivity with other fungal infections, such as *Fusarium* spp. or *Histoplasma capsulatum*.

The beta-D-glucan assay detects a component in the cell wall of *Aspergillus* spp., as well as other fungi. It is used to diagnose invasive fungal infections, including those due to *Aspergillus, Candida,* and *Pneumocystis*.

PCR testing can be used to detect *Aspergillus* spp. from clinical specimens, including tissue and bronchoalveolar lavage fluid.

On chest x-ray pulmonary aspergillosis presents with nodular infiltrates with or without a halo sign, and subsequent cavitation (Figure 17.32).

TREATMENT

Treatment of invasive aspergillosis, regardless of the location, requires use of amphotericin B or a broad-acting azole antifungal. The treatment of choice is voriconazole. Alternatives include lipid formulations of amphotericin B and echinocandins. Combination treatment using voriconazole and an echinocandin is better than voriconazole alone.

The treatment protocol of allergic bronchopulmonary includes antifungal medications, oral steroids, and optimization of asthma control. Patients with allergic *Aspergillus* rhinosinusitis require nasal drainage, oral steroids, immunotherapy

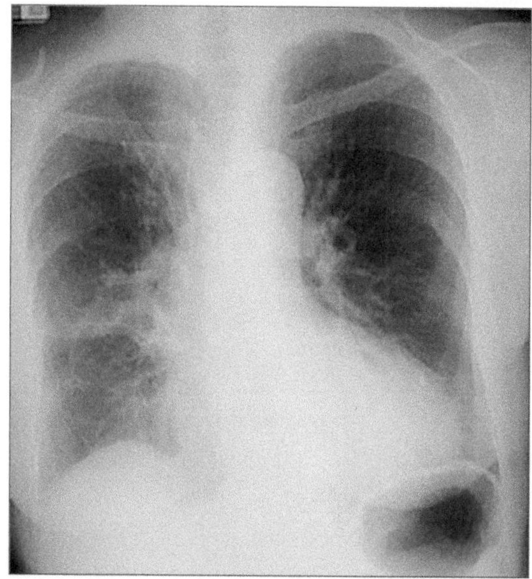

Figure 17.32 **Pulmonary aspergillosis. Widespread rounded lung nodules throughout both lungs, some with cavitation.**
(Source: https://radiopaedia.org/cases/aspergillosis-1?lang=us)

against allergens, and allergy control. Aspergilloma fungus ball requires surgical resection. Chronic pulmonary aspergillosis, invasive aspergillosis, and cutaneous aspergillosis are treated with antifungal medications. Surgery may be required in severe cases of cutaneous aspergillosis.

The preferred antifungal therapy for acute infection is voriconazole. Alternative therapies include liposomal amphotericin B, caspofungin, posaconazole, itraconazole, and micafungin. Prophylaxis against invasive aspergillosis includes posaconazole as the first-line option followed by itraconazole or micafungin. First-line treatment of aspergilloma is voriconazole or itraconazole. The preferred treatment for allergic aspergillus sinusitis is itraconazole.

PATIENT EDUCATION

- ABPA and allergic *Aspergillus* sinusitis generally have a good prognosis and rarely result in death.
- Invasive aspergillosis or chronic necrotizing pulmonary aspergillosis has a poor prognosis, with mortality rate of 29% to 58%.[86]
- Poor prognostic factors include invasive disease, extremes of age, and severe immunosuppression.

17.7G BLASTOMYCOSIS

Blastomycosis is a dimorphic fungal infection caused by *Blastomyces dermatitidis*. The organism is endemic in the Mississippi and Ohio river valleys and around the Great Lakes. Majority of the cases are self-limiting without any progression.

The infection occurs by inhalation of the conidia from the soil. The average incubation period is 3 weeks to 3 months. Once the organisms are inhaled, they multiply in the lungs and initiate a neutrophil response and cell-mediated response that leads to tissue destruction in the lungs, and dissemination to other organs via the bloodstream and lymphatics. It is not spread person to person.

MEDICAL HISTORY AND CLINICAL PRESENTATION

The history should focus on any travel to endemic areas or contact with patients with similar complaints.

The symptoms of blastomycosis depends on the immune status of the individual. In immunocompetent patients it presents as a flu-like illness with fever, chills, myalgias, headache, and a nonproductive cough. In immunocompromised patients it presents as an acute illness with symptoms including high fever, chills, productive cough, and pleuritic chest pain.

SIGNS AND SYMPTOMS

Clinical signs and symptoms range from subclinical to fatal disseminated disease.

Pulmonary blastomycosis can be acute or chronic. Symptoms include fever and chills, night sweats, productive cough, hemoptysis, weight loss, and chest pain. ARDS can develop with spread of the infection.

Extrapulmonary blastomycosis involves the skin, bone, genitourinary tract, and central nervous system. Cutaneous blastomycosis manifests as either verrucous or ulcerative. Osseous blastomycosis presents as an osteomyelitis. Commonly involved bones are the vertebrae, ribs, skull, and long bones. Genitourinary blastomycosis is common in men and involves the prostate, testicles, and epididymis. In men symptoms include pain, swelling, dysuria, and signs of obstruction. In women infection involves the endometrium, fallopian tubes, and ovaries. Central nervous system blastomycosis presents as meningitis or a mass effect.

PHYSICAL EXAMINATION

The physical manifestations of the disease depend on the organ of involvement. General findings include fever and tachypnea. With skin involvement bleeding ulcerative lesions or verrucous lesions, regional lymphadenopathy may be noted. With pulmonary disease there are signs consistent with consolidation, such as dullness to percussion, increased tactile fremitus, and possible pleuritic rub. Central nervous system blastomycosis presents with signs of meningitis including fever and nuchal rigidity.

DIFFERENTIAL DIAGNOSIS

The differential diagnosis of blastomycosis includes other fungal and bacterial diseases, including CAP.

Fungal disorders in the differential include coccidioidomycosis, histoplasmosis, aspergillosis, pneumocystis, and sporotrichosis. Bacterial disorders include anthrax, legionella, listeriosis, brucellosis, and tuberculosis. The differential diagnosis for cutaneous blastomycosis includes basal cell or squamous cell carcinoma and pyoderma gangrenosum.

DIAGNOSTIC STUDIES

Culture of the organism is the definitive diagnosis, but growth is slow and may delay diagnosis. DNA probe can be used to confirm. The diagnosis of blastomycosis is also confirmed by demonstration of the characteristic broad-based budding yeast in sputum or tissues (Figure 17.33).

KOH preparation reveals a broad-based budding yeast multinucleate yeast cell. Special stains include periodic acid-Schiff stain (PAS), PAS with hematoxylin, and Gomori methenamine silver stain for identifying the organism.

Antigen detection for blastomycosis with the EIA is performed on urine or serum. Cross-reactions can occur with histoplasmosis and other fungal diseases.

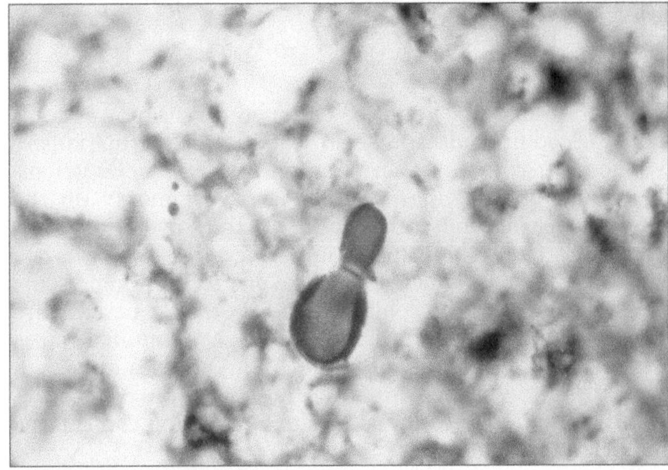

Figure 17.33 Silver stain of blastomycosis. Note the broad-based budding.

(Source: Centers for Disease Control and Prevention/Dr. Libero Ajello. https://phil.cdc.gov/details_linked.aspx?pid=494)

PCR can be used to confirm culture or histopathologic identification and on blood to detect disseminated disease.

Chest x-ray findings in blastomycosis are highly variable. The major CXR findings include airspace consolidation, masses, intermediate-sized nodules, interstitial disease, miliary disease, and cavitary lesions. The disease may be unilateral, or bilateral and multifocal or solitary; upper lobes are preferred.

TREATMENT

Amphotericin B is the treatment of choice for moderate to severe disease, central nervous system disease, and infection in immunosuppressed or pregnant patients. Itraconazole is recommended for mild to moderate disease and step-down therapy.

PATIENT EDUCATION

- Several complications can develop because of blastomycosis. These include pulmonary fibrosis, abscesses, and osteomyelitis.

17.7H SPOROTRICHOSIS

Sporothrix schenckii, a dimorphic fungus, causes sporotrichosis. The organism is found worldwide with the greatest number of cases being reported in South America, North America, and Japan. The fungus is found in soil, moss, and decaying wood. Infection occurs with inoculation of the fungal spores into the skin by a sharp object, such as a thorn, pine needle, or splinter.

S. schenckii can be transmitted as a zoonosis, primarily from cats that have active infection, and from other animal scratches that allow soil to be inoculated. It is not transmitted from person to person.

The primary host defense mechanisms are primarily neutrophils, monocytes, and macrophages that ingest and kill the yeast phase. Antibodies are not protective. The organism is not considered a highly virulent organism, causing mostly localized skin infections.

MEDICAL HISTORY AND CLINICAL PRESENTATION

Occupation history should be obtained as infection is commonly noted in landscapers, gardeners, and veterinarians.

The most common manifestation of *S. schenckii* is lymphocutaneous infection. Lesions occur commonly on the hands and arms, but can appear on the lower extremity, trunk, and face. The primary lesion develops within a few weeks at the site of inoculation. The primary lesion presents as a small nodule that enlarges and ulcerates. Lesions are mildly painful and nonpruritic. Drainage is minimal but is serous and nonodorous. Over time new nodules appear in the distribution of the lymphatic drainage of the primary lesion. Lymph nodes draining the site of infection can enlarge and become painful.

Pulmonary sporotrichosis is a subacute to chronic infection. It occurs in patients with chronic obstructive pulmonary disease and is due to inhalation of the conidia of *S. schenckii.* Symptoms include fever, fatigue, weight loss, productive cough, and hemoptysis.

SIGNS AND SYMPTOMS

Symptoms of cutaneous infection include nodular lesions on the skin at the point of inoculation, as well as along the lymphatic drainage and vessels in the location of the infection site. Initially the lesion is small and painless, and ranges from pink to purple in color. If untreated the lesion becomes larger, ulcerates, and drainage is noted. Lesions are typically noted on the upper extremities, arm, hand, and fingers. Systematic symptoms are rare.

A common extracutaneous form of sporotrichosis is the osteoarticular form. Development is due to contiguity or hematogenous spread of the infection or direct inoculation. It begins as monoarticular disease without systemic symptoms, presenting as a tenosynovitis or bursitis in the knee, wrist, elbow, and ankle.

PHYSICAL EXAMINATION

Common physical examination findings of cutaneous sporotrichosis include small, painless, pink to purple nodular lesions or erythematous plaque on the skin. The lesion may grow, ulcerate, and start to drain. Noncutaneous forms are not generally associated with distinctive physical findings.

DIFFERENTIAL DIAGNOSIS

The differential diagnosis for cutaneous sporotrichosis includes the lesions noted in cutaneous leishmaniasis and mycobacterial infection. Extracutaneous sporotrichosis, such as pulmonary sporotrichosis, must be differentiated from coccidioidomycosis, histoplasmosis, and tuberculosis; osteoarticular sporotrichosis must be distinguished from diseases such as chronic bacterial osteomyelitis and rheumatoid arthritis.

DIAGNOSTIC STUDIES

In most cases *S. schenckii* is diagnosed by biopsy of a skin lesion. Sputum and synovial fluid can be cultured in pulmonary and articular sporotrichosis.

The yeast forms are small, oval, or round budding yeasts that are best stained with methenamine silver. Yeasts are often difficult to see in tissues, so culture is more sensitive.

Serology and PCR assay are not useful for diagnosis or are not available.

Chest radiographs reveal upper lobe cavitary infiltrates.

TREATMENT

All forms of sporotrichosis require antifungal therapy. The treatment of choice is itraconazole for fixed cutaneous, lymphocutaneous, osteoarticular, and less severe pulmonary sporotrichosis. Amphotericin B is the treatment for disseminated infection, meningitis, and severe pulmonary infection. *S. schenckii* is resistant to echinocandins and voriconazole.

Alternative therapy includes saturated solution of potassium iodide (SSKI) and terbinafine. SSKI is difficult to administer, poorly tolerated, causing nausea, metallic taste, and salivary gland swelling.

Osteoarticular sporotrichosis is best treated with itraconazole. The outcome is typically poor with loss of joint function. Fluconazole, SSKI, and terbinafine are not effective.

In the seriously ill patient with pulmonary sporotrichosis, disseminated disease, and meningitis the initial therapy should be amphotericin B.

PATIENT EDUCATION

- Pulmonary sporotrichosis does not respond well to therapy and relapse is common.
- The prognosis for disseminated sporotrichosis in immunocompromised patients is poor.

17.7I PARACOCCIDIOIDOMYCOSIS

Paracoccidioidomycosis is caused by *Paracoccidioides brasiliensis,* a dimorphic fungus most commonly located in Central and South America, mainly Brazil, Argentina, Venezuela, Colombia, and Ecuador.

The initial infection is caused by inhalation; it may be asymptomatic or present with mild symptoms. A progressive disease may occur after the pulmonary infection and tends to be chronic, systemic, and progressive. Human-to-human transmission does not occur.

Most infections occur in men and mainly workers in agricultural occupations.

The fungus may lay dormant for many years only to reactivate as the immune system declines from HIV/AIDS or malnutrition. The immune system has an impact on disease severity and clearance of the fungus. Innate immunity inhibits fungal growth and can control the initial infection. Macrophages act as the key cell to kill the organism.

MEDICAL HISTORY AND CLINICAL PRESENTATION

Paracoccidioidomycosis tends to affect agriculture workers from southern Mexico to northern Argentina and is associated with individuals from rural areas. History of travel to these endemic areas is important to note.

Primary infection is limited and mostly asymptomatic. The progressive form presents with high fever, generalized lymphadenopathy, and pulmonary involvement with miliary lesions. Chronic disease has mostly pulmonary symptoms.

SIGNS AND SYMPTOMS

Signs and symptoms are dependent on the location of the infection. Pulmonary disease presents with dry cough, dyspnea, and possible hemoptysis. Mucocutaneous findings include lesions near mucocutaneous borders and painful ulcers. Mucocutaneous findings typically indicate disseminated disease. Other symptoms include dysphagia, oral mucosa ulcers, dysphonia, weakness, fatigue, and weight loss.

PHYSICAL EXAMINATION

Patients with acute infection typically appear ill. Patients with chronic disease can appear healthy in the early stages of the disease. Physical examination findings can include lymphadenopathy, hepatosplenomegaly, pulmonary findings, and skin lesions.

The oral mucosa is often the first site of involvement in disseminated disease. Small papules, ulcerations on gingivae, tongue, and lips are noted and can destroy surrounding structures.

Skin findings include ulcerated or verrucous indurated papules/plaques near mucocutaneous borders, trunk, or limbs. Ulceration may be noted over enlarged cervical or supraclavicular lymph nodes.

DIFFERENTIAL DIAGNOSIS

The differential diagnosis includes mucocutaneous leishmaniasis, tuberculosis, syphilis, lymphoma, Wegener granulomatosis disease, and other disseminated fungal infections.

DIAGNOSTIC STUDIES

Direct observation of the yeast in tissue via special fungal stains can make a preliminary diagnosis. Typical findings include granulomatous infiltrate with lymphocytes, histiocytes, and Langerhans giant cells and characteristic yeast cells (Mariner wheel) are seen within giant cells.

Antibody tests, CF or IDF, can be used to make the diagnosis and monitor response to therapy. Antigen testing is helpful in making an early diagnosis and when testing for antibodies is indeterminate.

The diagnosis is confirmed by detected growth on culture material.

TREATMENT

The treatment of choice for mild and moderate-to-severe infection include the azoles (itraconazole, ketoconazole, or voriconazole), amphotericin B, or the antibiotic TMP-SMX.

PATIENT EDUCATION

- The prognosis of paracoccidioidomycosis is good with adequate treatment.

SPECIAL CONSIDERATIONS

- The treatment of vulvovaginitis candidiasis in pregnancy consists of topical azole therapy for 1 week.

KEY POINTS

- Invasive candidiasis is typically due to endogenous organisms.
- Aspergillosis is most common in immunocompromised patients and due to inhaling mold spores.
- Histoplasmosis is acquired by inhaling spores and is endemic to the Ohio and Mississippi River valleys; acute primary infection is typically self-limited.
- Coccidioidomycosis is acquired by inhaling spores and is endemic in the southwestern United States and northern Mexico. Treatment consists of fluconazole or itraconazole for mild to moderate disease.

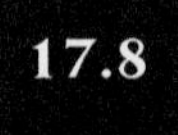

17.8 HUMAN IMMUNODEFICIENCY VIRUS INFECTION

OVERVIEW

HIV causes one of the most challenging infectious diseases affecting humankind in the world. The development of ART has overcome some of the challenge allowing HIV to be a chronic and a manageable condition. However, there are not enough clinicians to manage patients with HIV and so the challenge continues. PAs, nurse practitioners (NPs), and physicians should team up and be part of the solution by managing patients with HIV. The pathophysiology of HIV can be explained by studying the disease life cycle and has led to the discovery of ARV medications. Patients with HIV have a variety of medical histories and clinical presentations. Therefore, clinicians need to evaluate each patient individually, giving personalized attention to each unique patient situation. That stated, understanding the population risk factors can be helpful during a patient evaluation. Also, knowing the symptoms associated with acute retroviral syndrome (ARS) may help detect cases early. While understanding risk factors and knowing symptoms of ARS are important, universal HIV screening should be performed on all persons of ages 13 and 65 even if they appear free of risk factors and asymptomatic.[87] During ARS, patients may develop symptoms that mimic the flu, mononucleosis, nonspecific viral symptoms, or severe symptoms. A physical exam may not suggest a diagnosis; however, clinicians should be knowledgeable about what organ systems and what findings suggest ARS or HIV advanced disease. A differential diagnosis includes a number of conditions, explained later in this chapter. To diagnose the infection, nucleic acid tests (NAT), antibody, or antigen/antibody can be used. Once a patient is diagnosed, performing comprehensive baseline labs and starting ARV as soon as possible are vital. In general, starting ARV medication immediately despite the CD4 count is the current recommendation as it helps the patient and reduces the likelihood of transmission. There are several FDA-approved oral ARV regimens available to treat HIV that come as a once-a-day pill. It appears there will be injectable treatment available soon. Currently, there are two FDA-approved ARV medications available as HIV PrEP. Though HIV is a manageable condition, it is still a difficult diagnosis for many patients to accept. Therefore, providing reassurance and education at the beginning of the diagnosis and partnering with these patients will help viral suppression and disease management.

EPIDEMIOLOGY

Globally, an estimated 37.9 million individuals including 36.2 million adults and 1.7 million children have HIV/AIDS.[88] In the United States over 1.1 million individuals live with HIV today.[89] According to 2016 data, for every 100 people diagnosed with HIV, 64 received medical care and 53 had viral suppression.[89] In the United States, the highest risk of HIV infection is in homosexual men and African Americans. African American MSM risk is higher due to community infection prevalence and other factors such as stigma and access to care.[90] Recently, a significant rise of newly diagnosed cases has been noted in Hispanic/Latino gay or bisexual men. In 2018, 37,968 individuals received an HIV diagnosis in the United States and dependent areas. Of those, 69% of new diagnoses were gay or bisexual men and 86% of all men diagnosed were gay or bisexual. In the same report, heterosexuals accounted for 24% of all diagnoses and people who inject drugs (PWID) accounted for 7% of the 37,832 new HIV diagnoses.[89] Blacks/African Americans account for 42% and Hispanics/Latinos account for 27% of new HIV diagnoses while these populations are respectively 13% and 18% of the U.S. population.[89] HIV diagnoses are unequally distributed regionally in the United States. In 2018, 15.6% cases were in the South; 12.6% were in the U.S. dependent areas; 9.9% in the Northeast; 9.7% in the West; and 7.2% in the Midwest.[89] In 2018, there were 15,820 HIV-related deaths in adults and adolescents in the United States.[89] Overall, since the beginning of the epidemic, there have been more than 650,000 deaths from AIDS in the United States.[91]

The significant developments of ART allows HIV-positive patients an improved quality of life and increased life expectancy. As HIV/AIDS becomes a chronic disease, research recommends using a chronic disease management model.[92] This model requires a multidisciplinary team of HIV specialists, counselors, and primary care clinicians. The Mathematica Policy Research organization investigated HIV clinician shortages in 2016 and concluded "we have a reason to believe HIV provider shortage is continuing and will likely have long-term adverse consequences for public health if not addressed."[93]

Collectively, while the number of HIV clinicians is decreasing, the number of individuals with HIV is increasing because of new HIV infections and greater HIV survival rates due to advanced ART.[94]

Recently it was concluded that primary care clinicians including PAs, NPs, and physicians may be the solution to treat and manage patients with HIV.[95]

PATHOPHYSIOLOGY

After identifying the virus in 1983,[96] it was established that loss of $CD4^+$ cells (T-cells) was the main cause of immunodeficiency (Figure 17.34).[97] After identification of HIV virus, its structure, virulence, and pathogenesis, early HIV drugs emerged. The HIV virus (it is an RNA virus) life cycle permits several treatment options for ART.

HIV Life Cycle

- The HIV binds to a CD4 surface molecule and a chemokine receptor, both present on activated CD4 cells (also known as T cells or helper cells) (Step 1, Figure 17.35).[98]
- After cell entry, the enzyme, reverse transcriptase, transcribes the viral RNA into a DNA copy (Steps 2 and 3).
- This viral DNA fragment integrates into the host's CD4 cell chromosomal DNA (Step 4).
- The integrated viral DNA is transcribed under the host's cell transcription process to produce mRNA, which is then translated into viral proteins (Step 5).
- Finally, the HIV protease cleaves the newly synthesized polypeptides into individual HIV proteins that allow the virus to assemble itself and bud from the host cells[99] (Steps 6 and 7).
- Over time, the HIV infection will deplete the host CD4 cells causing immunodeficiency.

The chronic immune activation is recognized as an etiology causing immune exhaustion.[100] HIV infection causes significant chronic systemic inflammation and OI due to persistent exposure of viral antigens.[101] Loss of gut associated lymphoid tissue has been shown to occur early in HIV infection leading to chronic systemic exposure to highly inflammatory bacterial lipopolysaccharides (LPS).[102–104] This chronic inflammation and depletion of CD4 cells stresses naive T cells and creates short-lived activated CD4 cells. In most patients with HIV, CD4 cells decrease from a normal value of near 1,000 cells/µL to below 200 cells/µL over time.[105] The cell-mediated immunity of a host is significantly weakened when these CD4 cell counts fall below the threshold (i.e., 200 cells/µL, an AIDS-defining event). Because of the immunodeficiency, a host becomes susceptible to OI.

Although ART may end viral replication and regenerate CD4 cell count, inflammation continues despite

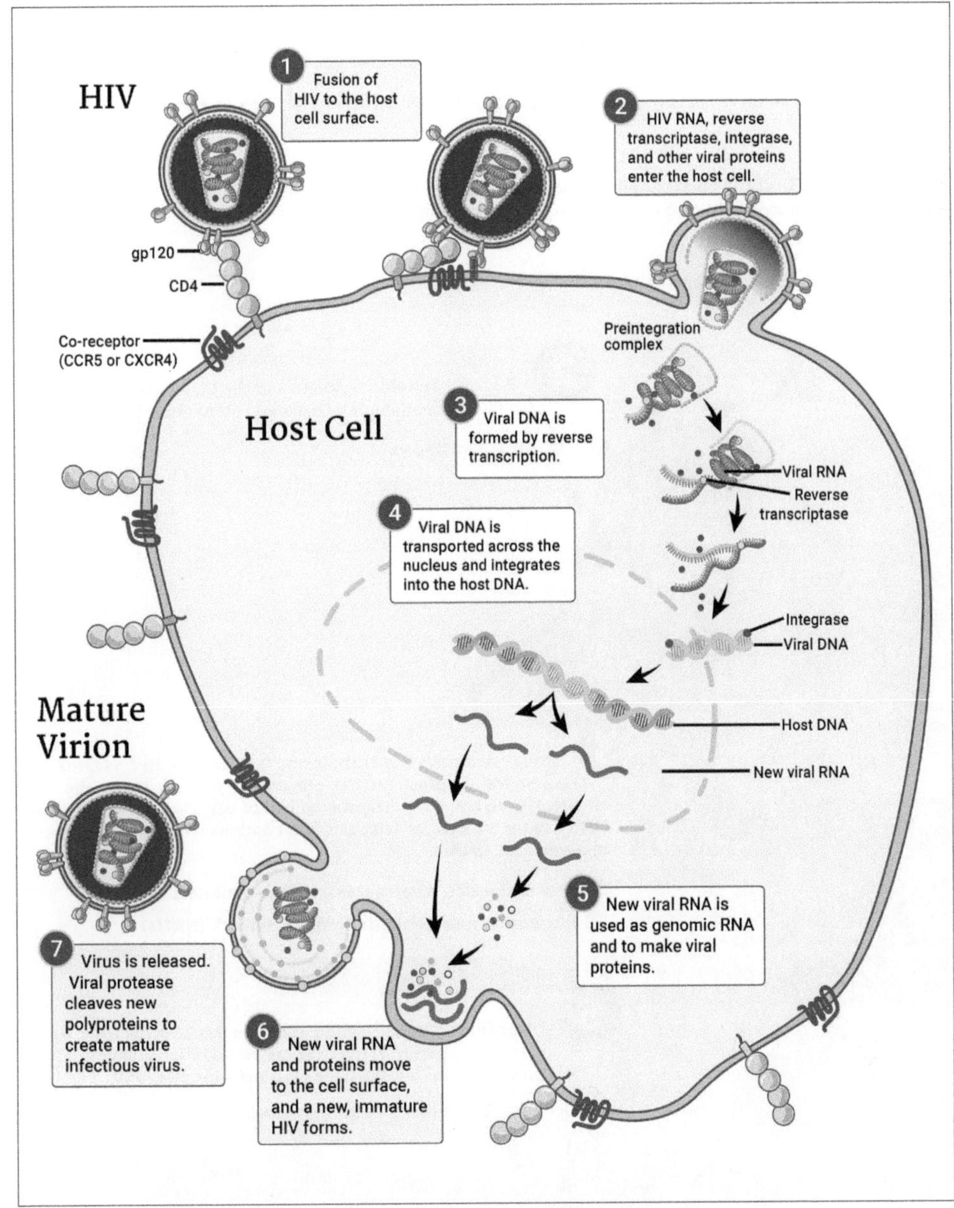

Figure 17.34 HIV replication cycle.
(Source: National Institute of Allergy and Infectious Disease.)

treatment.[106] Chronic inflammation may contribute to renal and cardiac diseases currently seen in patients who have been on ART for many years.[107] The failure to cure HIV infection with ART is partially due to infected long-lived memory T-cells. Although HIV does not infect these quiescent memory cells directly, it may infect active T-cells just as they become inactivated to remain as long-lived memory CD4 cells.[108,109] The integrated HIV DNA is not copied while these cells remain latent. However, if latent HIV-infected memory cells are activated, the HIV genes will be copied. It has been estimated the reservoir of infected quiescent cells slowly decays with a half-life of 40–44 months.[110,111] Researchers are exploring how to target and eradicate these long-lived quiescent cells. However, even with maximum suppression of viral replication using current ART, these memory cells will allow for reappearance of viremia if treatment is stopped.[112]

There are three stages of HIV infection described below. Figure 17.36 illustrates disease progression.

- **Stage 1/Acute HIV Infection:** After contracting the virus, a patient will enter this stage within 2–4 weeks. At this stage, due to elevated VL, the risk of transmission is extremely high. If a person is diagnosed during this stage and initiates ARV immediately, the benefits are significant.
- **Stage 2/Chronic HIV Infection:** Patients may be asymptomatic. This stage is also known as clinical latency. During this period, VL can be relatively stable, with progressive decline in CD4 cell count. Because many individuals with chronic HIV infection have no HIV-related symptoms, this is why universal HIV screening is recommended. Without ARV, chronic HIV infection typically advances to AIDS in approximately 10 years. Some patients progress from HIV to AIDS earlier.

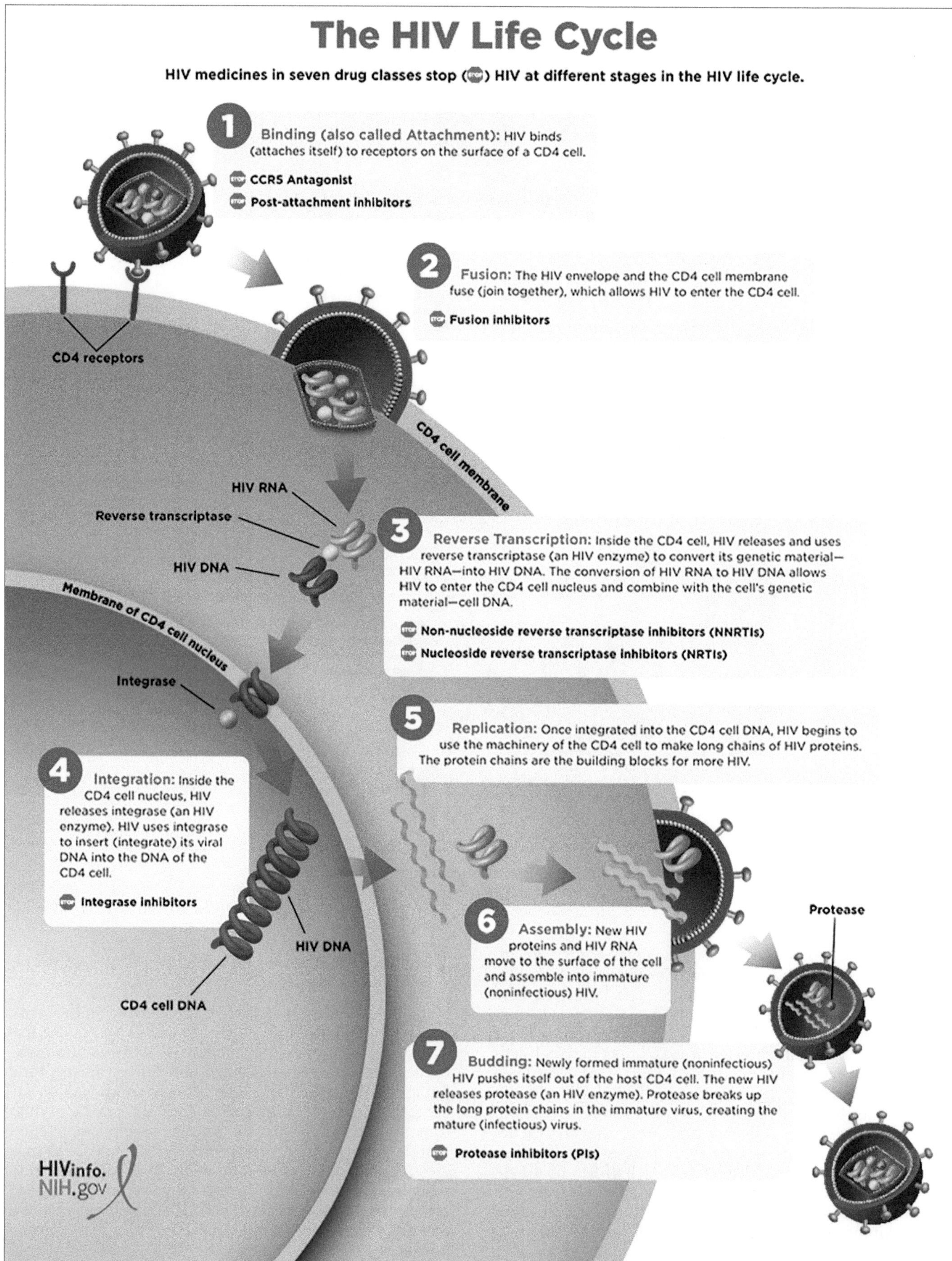

Figure 17.35 **HIV life cycle and antiretroviral therapy development. The illustration demonstrates the HIV life cycle and how each step leads to antiretroviral therapy.**
(Source: HIVInfo. The HIV life cycle. U.S. National Library of Medicine. https://hivinfo.nih.gov/understanding-hiv/fact-sheets/hiv-life-cycle)

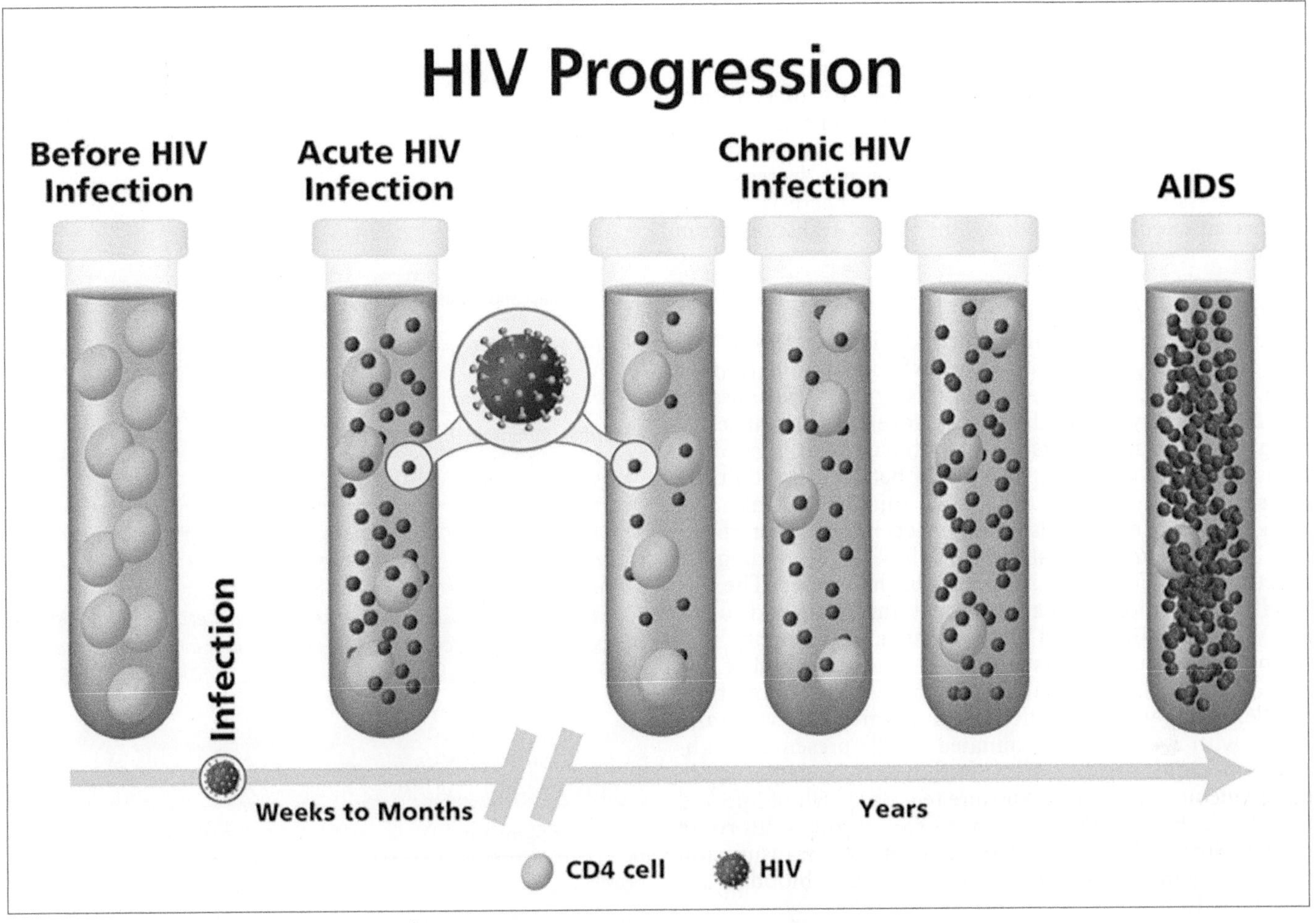

Figure 17.36 **From HIV to AIDS.**
(Source: U.S. National Library of Medicine)

- **Stage 3/AIDS:** Final and most severe stage of HIV infection. By this time, HIV has severely damaged the immune system, so a patient is incapable of fighting off OIs. If a patient's CD4 count is <200 cells/mm^3 or if a patient has an OI (regardless CD4 count), they may be diagnosed as having AIDS. During this stage, patients can have a high VL and can easily transmit the disease to others. Without ARV, individuals with AIDS generally die within 3 years.

MEDICAL HISTORY AND CLINICAL PRESENTATION

Patients' medical histories and clinical presentations vary immensely: some are symptomatic; others are asymptomatic. Once a patient has contracted HIV, they experience acute HIV infection and may present with flu-like symptoms, also known as ARS. Post ARS, patients become asymptomatic. According to the CDC, 1 of 7 HIV-positive individuals are unaware of their status because they are asymptomatic.[89] When evaluating asymptomatic patients, a careful medical/social history can be the key to uncover risk factors. For an example, a gay man who engages in receptive anal intercourse is at higher risk for contracting HIV compared to a gay man who engages in insertive anal intercourse. While anal intercourse is the highest-risk sexual behavior for HIV transmission, knowing that receptive anal intercourse transmission is 13 times higher than insertive anal intercourse transmission can help understand an individual's risk factors.[113] If a gay man is on HIV PrEP, uses condoms, and his HIV-positive partner has an undetectable VL, the risk of transmission is extremely low. Consequently, asking relevant questions is vital during an evaluation. When gathering personal and detailed information from patients, clinicians should begin the conversation by explaining why the information is helpful, being careful to be nonjudgmental and respectful. While some patients are comfortable sharing such personal information, others may find it uncomfortable. Therefore, clinicians need to adjust their approach to a patient's unique personality and situation. Some at-risk individuals may present to request an HIV screening because of the risky sexual behavior without providing detail. This is a straightforward case, so a clinician can order HIV screening while using this as an opportunity for safe sex education and promoting condom use and PrEP.

Sexual Transmission

The incidence of sexual transmission of HIV varies by behavior and exposure. Generally, sexual activities that rupture the mucosa and cause bleeding are linked to higher risk compared to sexual activities that do not rupture mucosa. HIV transmission between MSM is generally higher than transmission between heterosexual partners. In heterosexual transmission, male-to-female transmission is believed to be slightly higher than female-to-male transmission. Female-to-female sexual transmission of HIV is seldom encountered.[114]

STIs may contribute to the risk of HIV infection. The concomitant genital ulcer disease (e.g., HSV, primary syphilis), and other STIs that cause significant urethral irritation (e.g., gonococcal urethritis) increase the risk of transmission. HIV transmission rates may be higher in men who are uncircumcised. While circumcision may decrease the risk of female-to-male HIV transmission, it may not decrease risk of transmission to a female partner.[115,116] There is no evidence that circumcision reduces the risk of transmission in MSM.

Bloodborne Transmission

Prior to effective screening methods in the 1980s, the risk of transmission via blood transfusion was extremely high. Currently, the frequency of this type of transmission has dramatically reduced in most developed countries.[117] Today, the greatest risks of bloodborne transmission is through needle sharing (particularly between the IV drug users) and percutaneous needlestick injuries in healthcare workers.[118,119] Individuals who inject illegal/street drugs tend to engage in high-risk sexual behaviors, so finding the exact transmission mode is difficult in these cases. The risk of HIV acquisition from a needlestick injury depends upon the VL of the source and characteristics of the injury.[120] If an individual (source) has a high VL, it leads to higher risk of transmission. Deep injuries, injury with a hollow-bore needle, injury with a needle used in an artery or vein, and injury with a visibly contaminated needle presents a higher risk of transmission. HIV infection may be acquired via large mucous membrane exposure (e.g., a splash of infected blood into the eye), though transmission through this route is rare. Studies have shown the risk of HIV transmission related to percutaneous exposure of infected blood is approximately at 0.3%.[121]

Perinatal Transmission

The risk of perinatal HIV transmission depends on maternal risk factors and if a mother breastfeeds.[122] The transmission of HIV may occur during pregnancy, at delivery, or after delivery. High VLs of maternal plasma and breast milk are associated with an increased risk of transmission.[123] Also, microtransfusions of maternal blood across the placenta to a fetus are also thought to be a source of perinatal infection, because the majority of in utero exposure of HIV occurs during the third trimester.[124] Placental inflammation (particularly chorioamnionitis) is also thought to increase in utero transmission.[125] Intrapartum transmission occurs from contact of infant mucosal membranes with the HIV in blood and secretions in the vaginal canal. Further, a 4 hours or longer duration of membrane rupture may be linked with an increased risk of transmission.[126] The exact mechanism of transmission during breastfeeding is unknown; however, HIV has been detected in both colostrum and breast milk.[127]

During ARS, while most of the patients present with mild symptoms, some patients may present with more severe symptoms. These include more severe forms of OI,[128] neurologic involvement,[129] and other serious conditions.[130] Recent study concluded that up to 33% of patients had severe symptoms. In severe cases, VL was significantly higher and required more hospital admissions. Those severe acute HIV infections conditions are indicated in Table 17.28.[130]

TABLE 17.28 Characteristics of Patients With Severe Acute HIV Infection (*N* = 74)

Characteristics	Number of Cases (%)
Hepatitis	6 (2.9)
Bacterial pneumonia	3 (1.3)
Oral candidiasis	14 (6.3)
Esophageal candidiasis	7 (3.1)
Esophageal herpes	2 (0.9)
Fever >1 month	1 (0.4)
Diarrhea >1 month	1 (0.4)
Meningoencephalitis	11 (4.9)

This study looked at clinical, biochemical, and immunologic characteristics of severely ill patients. This data represent only some of the data, which is helpful and relevant for clinical presentation.

Source: Data from Nicolás D, Suárez A, Ambrosioni J, et al. Prevalence, clinical characteristics and outcome of severe primary HIV-1 infection: a prospective cohort study. Int J Infect Dis. *2019;88:73–79. doi:10.1016/j.ijid.2019.08.001*

SIGNS AND SYMPTOMS

Several signs and symptoms (Table 17.29) may occur during the acute phase. Those listed in Table 17.29 were observed in a sample of 69 patients experiencing ARS.[131] ARS is the phase typically characterized by viremia as detected by the presence of HIV RNA or p24 antigen. During this time, individuals with HIV typically have a higher VL than those with chronic HIV, and therefore are at a higher risk of sexual transmission to others. Therefore, detecting people with ARS and educating them and initiating ART will help control the disease effectively in them and reduce transmission to others.

TABLE 17.29 Signs or Symptoms Compatible With Acute HIV Infection in 69 Patients

Signs or Symptom	Number (%)
Fever	53 (77)
Myalgia	48 (70)
Fatigue	48 (70)
Headache	42 (61)
Night sweats	38 (55)
Pharyngitis	34 (49)
Gastrointestinal symptoms (nausea, vomiting, or diarrhea)	29 (42)
Rash	19 (28)
Weight loss >2.5 kg	15 (22)
Arthralgia	14 (20)

The duration of signs and symptoms ranged from 5 days to 14 days (median of 8 days). The same researchers pointed out[129] 52% of the study population had ongoing signs or symptoms at the time of testing, 28% had resolved by the time of testing, 13% reported signs or symptoms starting after testing, and 7% reported the absence of signs or symptoms. These data suggest over half of the individuals present with signs at symptoms during ARS. This suggests when patient presents with influenza or mononucleosis-like symptoms, clinicians should keep ARS in the differential. Screening should always be recommended when a patient's social history/behavior suggests high risk for infection.

PHYSICAL EXAMINATION

A complete physical examination, including weight and height, should be performed on patients who are at risk, present with ARS symptoms, have an existing diagnosis of HIV, or AIDS is suspected or established.

During ARS, some individuals may have a completely normal physical exam; others may have the following findings.

- **Vitals:** Febrile, weight loss, tachycardia
- **General:** Mild distress, anxious, ill appearing
- **Psychiatric:** Anxious
- **Skin:** Erythematous maculopapular lesions on face, trunk, and sometimes extremities
- **ENT/Mouth:** Pharyngeal erythema, oral candidiasis, mucocutaneous ulcers
- **Lymphatic:** Generalized lymphadenopathy
- **Abdomen:** Hyperactive bowel sounds due to diarrhea
- **Musculoskeletal:** Myalgia

There are some specific physical exam findings (listed below) not common but important when assessing patients with advanced HIV disease or AIDS. For example, seborrheic dermatitis (listed below) may be associated with HIV disease. This condition is more prevalent in individuals living with HIV compared to individuals without the disease.[132] In addition, if the disease is progressing to advanced disease (e.g., AIDS), patients are at even higher risk of getting seborrheic dermatitis. Seborrheic dermatitis is associated with a worsening immune system. All the other conditions listed below are associated with HIV/AIDS as well.

- **Skin:** Know the findings linked with seborrheic dermatitis, eosinophilic folliculitis, psoriasis, superficial fungal disease, molluscum contagiosum, herpes simplex, herpes zoster, or Kaposi sarcoma.[132]
- **Eyes:** A dilated funduscopic exam may be needed to screen for CMV retinitis in patients with AIDS.[133]
- **Mouth/oral:** Evaluate for candidiasis, oral hairy leukoplakia, aphthous ulcerations, HSV infection, mucosal Kaposi sarcoma, angular cheilitis, and periodontal disease.[134]
- **Lymphatic:** Generalized lymphadenopathy, asymmetric, bulky, or rapidly enlarging adenopathy may be associated with acute HIV infection or advanced HIV (AIDS).[135]
- **Genitourinary:** Recommended to look for other STIs on suspected/established HIV patients. These include syphilis, gonorrhea, *Chlamydia*, HSV, HPV, chancroid, and lymphogranuloma venereum. In women, vaginitis (candida), bacterial vaginosis, and trichomonas infections may be linked with HIV.[136–138]
- **Musculoskeletal:** Areas of fat atrophy (e.g., malar atrophy, thinning of extremities or buttocks) or fat deposition (e.g., prominent cervicodorsal fat pad, visceral adiposity) may be appreciated in patients with HIV. Body fat maldistribution may be appreciated as well (skin fold, waist, and hip).[139,140]
- **Neurologic:** Evaluate for peripheral neuropathy, asymptomatic muscle weakness, or other abnormalities. Also, cognitive function (e.g., mini-mental status exam) may be indicated. With any significant impairment, formal neuropsychologic testing should be ordered.[141,142]

DIFFERENTIAL DIAGNOSIS

During ARS, 40% to 90% patients develop nonspecific symptoms.[128] At this time, acute HIV infection often mimics other medical diagnosis. Table 17.30 summarizes the differential diagnoses for ARS.[143-155]

DIAGNOSTIC STUDIES

In 2006, the CDC revised HIV testing guidelines recommending routine, voluntary testing for everyone between ages 13 and 64.[156,157] In addition, the United States Preventive Service Task Force[158] recommended routine HIV screening for all individuals ages 15 to 65. HIV screening no longer requires an individualized risk factor assessment, special counseling, or signed consent.[157,159] Although universal HIV testing was established over a decade ago, 14% of HIV-positive individuals remain unaware of their status.[89] In 2014, 23% of people newly diagnosed with HIV already had AIDS, underscoring the disparity of the screening process.[159] It has been clearly documented that individuals with HIV who are under consistent medical care and have viral suppression are less likely to transmit HIV.[160] These findings support the need to maximize early screening, testing, and treatment. Timely diagnosis is critical.

When trying to determine the most appropriate testing, it is helpful to understand four stages associated with HIV infection. The eclipse stage is the first 10 to 12 days post-infection. The eclipse stage is without consistently detectable laboratory markers making diagnosis unlikely. The next stage is the seroconversion window, a period between infection and the first antibody detection (IgG). This is followed by acute HIV infection (ARS), the stage of HIV acquisition and detectable HIV RNA or p24 antigen and an absent antibody. It is at this stage that a person is highly infectious. The final stage is established HIV infection/seroconversion, during which time there is detectable IgG antibody test.[161]

The period of acute HIV infection is the first 6 months of virus acquisition. During this period individuals are highly infectious due to high viremia and lack of awareness of their HIV status.[162] The acute infection is marked by a high HIV RNA level and presence of p24 antigen along with a negative or indeterminate antibody testing. When an acute HIV infection is suspected, an HIV RNA and subsequent confirmatory HIV antibody test should be used for diagnosis.[163]

Types of Screening

According to the CDC,[163] the common HIV diagnostic tests (Table 17.31) are NAT, antibody tests, and antigen/antibody tests.[163] The HIV-1 Western blot is no longer recommended as a confirmatory test because the HIV-1/HIV-2 antibody test has greater sensitivity to detect early infection, is performed rapidly, and accurately differentiates HIV-1 from HIV-2.[164,165]

EVALUATION

Whether a patient is diagnosed with HIV (early in the disease or later in the disease), acute HIV infection, AIDS, OI, or pregnant, the recommendation is to initiate ARV as soon as possible if a patient consents.[166] Clinicians should prescribe ART immediately and educate patients. Education should explain about treatment barriers and the importance of treatment adherence. It is recommended to start ART within 2 weeks in most patients with OI. If pregnant,

TABLE 17.30 Differential Diagnosis of Acute Retroviral Syndrome

Diagnosis	Description
Epstein–Barr virus (EBV)	This is a herpes virus spread by intimate contact. EBV commonly causes infectious mononucleosis (IM). Acute infections tend to resolve with supportive care. Symptoms include extreme fatigue fever, sore throat, headaches, myalgia, lymphadenopathy, splenomegaly, hepatomegaly, and/or rash.[143,144]
Cytomegalovirus	This is a common virus that infects people of all ages. More than 50% of adults have been infected with CMV by age 40. Most people infected with CMV are asymptomatic.[145] However, CMV may cause mononucleosis in some people. Therefore, symptoms are similar to those described above.
Viral hepatitis	During the acute infection, symptoms of all types of viral hepatitis (A, B, or C) are similar and can include one or more of the following symptoms: jaundice, fever, fatigue, loss of appetite, nausea, vomiting, abdominal pain, arthralgia, dark urine, clay-colored stool, and diarrhea (hepatitis A virus only).[146]
Non-polio enteroviral infection	Most people are asymptomatic or develop mild symptoms like the common cold. While anyone is susceptible, infants, children, and teenagers are more susceptible than adults as they have not developed immunity. Symptoms of mild illness may include fever, rhinorrhea, sneezing, cough, rash, oral blisters, and/or myalgia.[147]
Secondary syphilis	Patient may present with skin rashes and/or mucous membrane lesions. Mucous membrane lesions may locate in the mouth, vagina, or anus. The rash may appear when the primary sore is healing or several weeks after the sore has healed. The rash may appear on the palms of the hands and/or the plantar surface of the feet. The rash usually is not pruritic. Other symptoms may include fever, lymphadenopathy, sore throat, patchy hair loss, headaches, weight loss, myalgia, and/or fatigue.[148]
Toxoplasmosis	Of infected patients, only very few have symptoms (immunocompetent patients may be asymptomatic as the immune system usually keeps the parasite from causing illness). Symptoms may include flu-like symptoms, lymphadenopathy, and/or myalgia. (Severe toxoplasmosis may cause damage to the brain, eyes, or other organs from an acute *Toxoplasma* infection or from reactivation).[149]
Herpes simplex virus (HSV) with erythema multiforme	HSV type 1 is the most commonly identified etiology, but HSV-2 cause erythema multiforme as well. Erythema multiforme lesions typically begin as pink or red papules that can then become plaques. These skin lesions may be pruritic or painful. The classic lesion of erythema multiforme is called the target or iris lesion. Other symptoms may include fatigue, fever, and malaise. These symptoms usually occur at least 1 week before skin lesions occur. While oral mucosa is the most commonly involved, genital and ocular mucosa also may develop lesions.[150]
Behçet disease (BD)	BD is a systemic autoimmune disease that affects multiple organ systems. Symptoms may include oral aphthous ulcers, genital aphthous ulcers, erythema nodosum, neck pain, headache, abdominal pain, arthralgias, or diarrhea.[151]
Active systemic lupus erythematosus (SLE)	People with SLE may experience a variety of symptoms that include fatigue, rashes, fevers, edema, or arthralgia.[152]
Influenza	Patients with influenza may develop fever, chills, cough, sore throat, rhinorrhea, myalgia, headaches, and/or fatigue. Some patients may present with vomiting and diarrhea, which is more common in pediatric patients compared to adults.[153]
Drug reaction	Some patients who experience drug reactions may present with fever, rash, and/or lymphadenopathy.[154] Also, some patients may present with shortness of breath, wheezing, and/or rhinorrhea.
COVID-19	People may present with the following symptoms such as cough, shortness of breath, fever, chills, myalgia, sore throat, and loss of taste or smell.[155]

it is recommended to start ART immediately for a mother's benefit, as well as to reduce the risk of transmission to the fetus. Before starting treatment in any patient, HIV-1 RNA measurement; CD4 cell count; HIV genotyping for nucleoside reverse transcriptase inhibitors (NRTIs), non-NRTIs, and protease inhibitors (PI); laboratory testing to identify active viral hepatitis; and blood chemistry testing should be performed. While waiting for lab results, treatments may be initiated. If planning to prescribe abacavir (Ziagen), testing for HLA-B *5701 allele should be included with initial labtests. If a patient has a CD4 count lower than 200 cells/µL, they should receive prophylaxis for PCP.[166]

With a newly diagnosed patient, it is important to ask if they were on any HIV PrEP. Box 17.2 summarizes the recommended baseline tests for all individuals with newlydiagnosed HIV.[167]

After years of debate in regard to the optimum time to start ART, the answer is now straightforward. According to the evidence from the NLM, ART should be started as soon as possible regardless of CD4 count.[167] The evidence shows early initiation of ARV reduces risk of progression to AIDS, reduces T-cell activation, and increases the efficacy of vaccines.[168,169]

Prior to starting ART, a drug resistance test (HIV genotype) is done to determine if a patient's virus is resistant to any ARV agents. Up to 10% to 15% of patients may be infected with a drug-resistant virus[170]; however, usually transmitted resistance is more common for older medicines in the NRTI class only, occasionally to the NNRTI class,

TABLE 17.31 Diagnostic Testing for HIV

Type of Test	Description
Nucleic acid test (NAT)	NATs can detect HIV RNA within 10–33 days after infection. These tests are expensive and are generally reserved for acute infection or recent high-risk exposure.
Antibody	Antibody tests are reliable but do not detect early infection or effectively differentiate HIV-1 from HIV-2. Because the test relies on antibody formation the diagnostic capacity varies from 23–90 days.
Antigen/Antibody	Antigen/antibody tests were approved by the FDA in 2010 and are the fourth generation of HIV immunoassay. These tests screen for both antigen p24 and the IgM and IgG antibodies. They have a diagnostic capacity of 18–45 days after infection. The HIV fourth generation (antigen/antibody) assays have >99.7% sensitivity and 99.3% specificity. Positive results from a fourth-generation screening test requires a supplemental HIV-1/HIV-2 differ entiation assay.[164] The differentiation between HIV-1 and HIV-2 is crucial as HIV-2 is genetically different and prone to develop resistance to some of the recommended ART agents.[165]

ART, antiretroviral therapy; FDA, Food and Drug Administration; IgG, immunoglobulin G; IgM, immunoglobulin M.
Source: Data from Centers for Disease Control and Prevention. HIV: diagnostic tests. 2019. https://www.cdc.gov/hiv/clinicians/screening/diagnostic-tests.html

BOX 17.2 Baseline Evaluation in New HIV Infection

- HIV antibody testing (if no documentation available or HIV RNA is below the assay's limit)
- CD4 lymphocyte cell count[a]
- Plasma HIV RNA (viral load)[a]
- Complete blood count (CBC)
- Complete metabolic panel (CMP)
- Fasting blood sugar
- Fasting lipids
- Urinalysis
- Pregnancy test (women of childbearing potential)
- Hepatitis A, B, and C serologies
- Genotypic resistance testing[b]
- Testing for gonorrhea, *Chlamydia*, syphilis, and other sexually transmitted infections
- Viral tropism assay[c]
- HLA-B*5701[d]
- Tuberculosis screening
- Immunizations

[a] CD4 count and plasma HIV RNA are two surrogate markers routinely used to monitor patients with HIV.
[b] If patient's viral load is <500–1,000 copies/mL, viral amplification for resistance may fail.
[c] Prior to initiation of CCR5 antagonist or if there is a virologic failure while patient is on CCR5 antagonist.
[d] Prior to initiation of abacavir (ABC). Baseline assessment allows rapid response if ABC is needed.
Source: Data from Panel on Antiretroviral Guidelines for Adults and Adolescents. Guidelines for the Use of Antiretroviral Agents in Adults and Adolescents with HIV. U.S. *Department of Health and Human Services; 2020. https://aidsinfo.nih.gov/contentfiles/lvguidelines/adultandadolescentgl.pdf*

and the presence of most baseline drug resistance does not prevent the selection of an effective regimen given the presently available ARV medication classes.

TREATMENT

Basic Principles of Treatment

- For patients previously diagnosed with HIV/AIDS, it is vital to obtain history of prior ARV treatment and the results of resistance testing.
- For a newly diagnosed patient with HIV, the Guidelines for the Use of Antiretroviral Agents in Adults and Adolescents with HIV[161] should be followed.
- The development of effective ART has changed HIV to a chronic disease that can be effectively managed. The goal of ART is to reduce HIV-related morbidity and mortality and prevent transmission.
- When managing HIV infection, ART should be initiated as soon as possible regardless of CD4 count.[161]
- Evidence shows early initiation of ART reduces risk of progression to AIDS, reduces T-cell activation, and increases host immune response to vaccines.[168,169,171]
- The primary goal of ART is HIV VL suppression. Changing the ART regimen is not indicated in patients with an undetectable VL even if the CD4 count does not increase.
- Up to 10% to 15% of patients may be infected with a drug-resistant virus.[170] Cross resistance is more common with older drug classes such as nucleoside/nucleotide reverse transcriptase inhibitors (NRTI). Therefore, a drug resistance test (HIV genotype) should be completed to determine if a viral strain is resistant to any ARV agent prior to starting ART.

Pharmacologic Therapy

- Currently, there are over 30 different ARV agents in seven drug classes used for treatment of HIV infection. Each ARV class generally targets a unique step in the life cycle of HIV. FDA-approved HIV medications in the United States can be found on the following link: aidsinfo.nih.gov/understanding-hiv-aids/fact-sheets/21/58/fda-approved-hiv-medicines.[172]
  - NRTIs
  - Non-nucleoside/nucleotide reverse transcriptase inhibitors (NNRTIs)
  - PI

  - Fusion inhibitors (FIs)
  - CCR5 receptor antagonists
  - Integrase strand transfer inhibitors (INSTIs)
  - Postattachment inhibitors
- To maximize the effectiveness, an ARV regimen for a treatment-naive patient consists of two NRTIs in combination with a third active ARV drug from one of three drug classes: INSTI, a NNRTI, or a PI with a pharmacokinetic enhancer (e.g., cobicistat and ritonavir).
- Two-drug regimen, dolutegravir plus lamivudine, also recommended as initial treatment.
- Injectable treatment for HIV is currently under investigation. One injectable was rejected by FDA in December 2019. However, it is anticipated injectable forms (once a month injection) may be available in the future.
- According to the recommendations, the first-line regimen for antiretroviral naïve patients typically includes two NRTIs plus an INSTI.[161] A combination of one NRTI plus an INSTI may be considered ***except*** for individuals with HIV RNA >500,000 copies/mL, HBV coinfection, or in whom ART is to be started before the results of HIV genotypic resistance testing for reverse transcriptase or HBV testing are available.[161]
- Table 17.32 presents typical initial combination regimens for ARV naïve HIV-positive patients. The combination of tenofovir disoproxil and emtricitabine (TDF/FTC) is commonly used as PrEP in HIV-negative persons. Recently, the combination of tenofovir alafenamide and emtricitabine (TAF/FTC) was approved by the FDA for the same purpose. In the setting of a new HIV diagnosis in patients who are taking or have previously taken PrEP, drug resistance results are particularly important. However, one of the regimens listed in Table 17.33 may be initiated pending resistance testing results.[161]
- Additionally, clinicians should adjust drug regimens based on patient-specific factors such as age, pregnancy, and comorbidities. For further information, please also refer to population-specific guidelines available on the AIDSinfo website at www.AIDSinfo.nih.gov.[172]
  - While ART is recommended for all patients, the Panel on Antiretroviral Guidelines for Adults and Adolescents advises urgent initiation of therapies in the following conditions: pregnancy, AIDS-defining conditions, CD4 count below <200 cells/µL, HIV-associated nephropathy, acute/early infection, HIV/hepatitis B virus coinfection, or HIV/hepatitis C virus coinfection.
  - Currently, drugs used in ART can be combined for almost all patients. These drugs have long half-lives allowing once daily dosing and a relatively low viral resistance rate. In addition, disease response can be monitored by clinicians with sensitive HIV RNA assays.
  - Typically, viral suppression can be achieved in 12 to 24 weeks after initiating ART. VL rebound can also be monitored for HIV drug(s) resistance. If drug resistance develops, a different regimen without cross resistant pattern should be implemented. In general, the predictors of virologic success are based on low baseline viremia, high potency of the ARV regimen, regimen tolerability, convenience, and patient adherence.[161]
  - Many of the available HIV medications are small molecules that target viral replication by binding to the active site of a viral protein or structure or enzyme. However, maraviroc, a CCR5 antagonist, targets a human protein, the chemokine receptor on the surface of T-cells that HIV uses for binding and entry to the host cells. The NRTIs are DNA nucleoside analogues that lack the hydroxyl group required to add the next base to the growing DNA chain. As the HIV reverse transcriptase transcribes the viral RNA into a DNA copy, NRTIs are incorporated to prevent the elongation of the DNA copy. NRTI is one of the original drug classes of ARV agents. Zidovudine or AZT was the first clinically effective drug available for HIV treatment.[173] Finally, the NNRTI drug class inhibits HIV reverse transcriptase by binding to its active site.[161]
  - HIV resistance to ARV medications often results from a more traditional mechanism of viral mutations leading to amino acid changes that reduce the ability of the drug to bind and effectively inhibit the enzymes. However, in the case of a drug that targets the human chemokine receptor CCR5 (e.g., maraviroc), resistance does not occur by changing the chemokine receptor; instead, the HIV develops the ability to bind an alternate chemokine receptor, CXCR4, on which this drug has no effect.[161]
  - The viral burden of HIV is commonly expressed as log VL. Using this method of reporting, clinicians track the viral burden. With effective ART, the HIV VL may be suppressed to levels below detection by the currently available HIV RNA assays at 20 copies RNA/µL or less. The use of the log VL allows comparison of drug effectiveness in patients with widely varying baseline VL. The baseline log VL is usually >4, and may be as high as 6–7. Most single ART agents can lower the HIV log VL by 1–2 units; Therefore, monotherapy is ***not*** recommended to treat HIV; a three-drug regimen from two or more drug classes is usually required to lower the log VL to <1.[161]
  - The high mutation rate of the HIV also necessitates the use of combination ART. HIV reverse transcriptase has poor accuracy, which introduces multiple mutations with every transcript.[174] Based on the number of HIV virions present in an average person infected with the virus and the number of mutations introduced while generating this number of virions, it has been estimated that even prior to ART every possible amino acid mutation already exists in the viral population.[175] Thus, if the HIV only requires a single amino acid mutation to become resistant to an ARV medication, that mutant virus already exists in a patient's viral population and will be selected immediately if that ARV agent is given as a single treatment. If multiple ARV medications are given, and especially if medications require more than two or three viral mutations for resistance, there will be adequate effectiveness to stop viral replication and prevent ongoing mutation. It should be noted that there is no pharmacologic agent (i.e., ART) to date that completely eradicates the virus from the host.[176]
  - Current trends in medication development focus on potency, longer durations of action, and intramuscular route of administration. One of the newer developments includes the use of broadly neutralizing antibodies that bind to the viral protein gp120, a CD4 binding molecule.[177,178] Antibodies that bind to almost all clinical isolates of HIV gp120 have been isolated. Infusion of these antibodies can prevent HIV virions from infecting T-cells and may have prolonged effectiveness.[177,178] Despite the various developments in the field of HIV treatment, most ART stops viral replication but has no direct effect on CD4 cell replication. A meta-analysis of interleukin 2 infusion as a strategy to increase CD4 count showed transient increases

TABLE 17.32 Recommended Initial Combination Regimens in the Antiretroviral Naïve Patient for Most People with HIV (Current as of December 18, 2019)

INSTI plus Two NRTIs (in alphabetical order)

INSTI	NRTI combinations	Level of Evidence
Bictegravir (BIC)	Tenofovir alafenamide (TAF) plus emtricitabine (FTC)	AI
Dolutegravir (DTG)	Abacavir (ABC) plus lamivudine (3TC)[a]	AI
DTG	Tenofovir (TAF or TDF)[b] plus (FTC or 3TC)	AI
Raltegravir (RAL)	(TAF or TDF)[b] plus (FTC or 3TC)	BI for TDF/FTC or 3TC BII for TAF/FTC

INSTI plus ONE NRTI

INSTI	NRTI	Level of Evidence
DTG	3TC	AI

[a] Only for individuals who are HLA-B*5701 negative and without chronic hepatitis B virus (HBV) coinfection.
[b] Tenofovir alafenamide (TAF) and tenofovir disoproxil fumarate (TDF) are two forms of tenofovir that are approved by the FDA. TAF has fewer bone and kidney toxicities than TDF, while TDF is associated with lower lipid levels. Safety, cost, and access are among the factors to consider when choosing between these drugs.

Rating of Recommendations: *A = Strong; B = Moderate; C = Optional*
Rating of Evidence: *I = Data from randomized controlled trials; II = Data from well-designed nonrandomized trials, observational cohort studies with long-term clinical outcomes, relative bioavailability/bioequivalence studies, or regimen comparisons from randomized switch studies; III = Expert opinion.*

FDA, Food and Drug Administration; INSTI, integrase strand transfer inhibitor; NRTI, nucleoside reverse transcriptase inhibitor.
Source: Data from Panel on Antiretroviral Guidelines for Adults and Adolescents. Guidelines for the Use of Antiretroviral Agents in Adults and Adolescents with HIV. *U.S. Department of Health and Human Services; 2020. https://aidsinfo.nih.gov/contentfiles/lvguidelines/adultandadolescentgl.pdf*

TABLE 17.33 Prophylaxis to Prevent Opportunistic Infection

Opportunistic Infection	Indication	Preferred	Alternative
Pneumocystis pneumonia (PCP)	CD4 count <200 cells/mm³ **(AI)**, *or* CD4 <14% **(BII)**, *or* CD4 count >200 but <250 cells/mm³ if monitoring CD4 cell count every 3 months is not possible **(BII)**	TMP-SMX[a] 1 PO daily **(AI)**, *or* TMP-SMX[a] 1 daily **(AI)**	TMP-SMX[a] 1 DS PO three times weekly **(BI)**, *or* Dapsone[b] 100 mg PO daily or 50 mg PO BID **(BI)**, *or* Dapsone[b] 50 mg PO daily + (pyrimethamine 50 mg + leucovorin 25 mg) PO weekly **(BI)**, *or* (Dapsone[b] 200 mg + pyrimethamine[c] 75 mg + leucovorin 25 mg) PO weekly **(BI)**; *or* Aerosolized pentamidine 300 mg via Respirgard II nebulizer every month **(BI)**, *or,* *for patients who cannot tolerate TMP-SMX and are also seropositive for Toxoplasma gondii:* Atovaquone 1,500 mg PO daily **(BI)**, *or* (Atovaquone 1,500 mg + pyrimethamine[c] 25 mg + leucovorin 10 mg) PO daily **(CIII)**
Toxoplasma gondii encephalitis	Toxoplasma IgG-positive patients with CD4 count <100 cells/μL **(AII)**	TMP-SMX[a] 1 DS PO daily **(AII)**	TMP-SMX[a] 1 DS PO three times weekly **(BIII)**, *or* TMP-SMX[a] 1 SS PO daily **(BIII)**, *or* Dapsone[b] 50 mg PO daily + (pyrimethamine[c] 50 mg + leucovorin 25 mg) PO weekly **(BI)**, *or* (Dapsone[b] 200 mg + pyrimethamine[c] 75 mg + leucovorin 25 mg) PO weekly **(BI)**; *or* Atovaquone 1,500 mg PO daily **(CIII)**; *or* (Atovaquone 1,500 mg + pyrimethamine[c] 25 mg + leucovorin 10 mg) PO daily **(CIII)**
Mycobacterium tuberculosis infection (TB) (i.e., treatment of LTBI)	(+) screening test for LTBI, with no evidence of active TB, and no prior treatment for active TB or LTBI (AI), or Close contact with a person with infectious TB, with no evidence of active TB, regardless of screening test results (AII).	(INH 300 mg + pyridoxine 25–50 mg) PO daily × 9 months **(AII)**, *or* INH 900 mg PO BIW (by DOT) + pyridoxine 25–50 mg PO daily × 9 months **(BII)**	Rifampin 600 mg PO daily × 4 months **(BIII)**, *or* Rifabutin (dose adjusted based on concomitant ART)[e] × 4 months **(BIII)**, *or* [Rifapentine (see dose below) PO + INH 900 mg PO + pyridoxine 50 mg PO] once weekly × 12 weeks *Rifapentine dose:* 32.1 to 49.9 kg: 750 mg 50 kg: 900 mg Rifapentine only recommended for patients receiving raltegravir or efavirenz-based ART regimen For persons exposed to drug-resistant TB, select anti-TB drugs after consultation with experts or public health authorities **(AII)**.

(continued)

TABLE 17.33 Prophylaxis to Prevent Opportunistic Infection *(continued)*

Opportunistic Infection	Indication	Preferred	Alternative
Disseminated *Mycobacterium avium* complex (MAC) disease	CD4 count <50 cells/µL—after ruling out active disseminated MAC disease based on clinical assessment (**AI**)	Azithromycin 1,200 mg PO once weekly (**AI**), *or* Clarithromycin 500 mg PO BID (**AI**), *or* Azithromycin 600 mg PO twice weekly (**BIII**)	Rifabutin (dose adjusted based on concomitant ART)[e] (**BI**); rule out active TB before starting rifabutin.
Histoplasma capsulatum infection	CD4 count ≤150 cells/µL and at high risk because of occupational exposure or live in a community with a hyperendemic rate of histoplasmosis (>10 cases/100 patient-years) (**BI**)	Itraconazole 200 mg PO daily (**BI**)	
Coccidioido-mycosis	A new positive IgM or IgG serologic test in patients who live in a disease-endemic area and with CD4 count <250 cells/µL (**BIII**)	Fluconazole 400 mg PO daily (**BIII**)	
Penicilliosis	Patients with CD4 cell counts <100 cells/µL who live or stay for a long period in rural areas in northern Thailand, Vietnam, or Southern China (**BI**)	Itraconazole 200 mg once daily (**BI**)	Fluconazole 400 mg PO once weekly (**BII**)

Key to Acronyms: anti-HBc, hepatitis B core antibody; anti-HBs, hepatitis B surface antibody; ART, antiretroviral therapy; BID, twice daily; BIW, twice a week; CD4, CD4 T lymphocyte cell; DOT, directly observed therapy; DS, double strength; HAV, hepatitis A virus; HBV, hepatitis B virus; HPV, human papillomavirus; IgG, immunoglobulin G; IgM, immunoglobulin M; IM, intramuscular; INH, isoniazid; IV, intravenously; IVIG, intravenous immunoglobulin; LTBI, latent tuberculosis infection; MAC, *Mycobacterium avium* complex; PCP, *Pneumocystis* pneumonia; PCV13, 13-valent pneumococcal conjugate vaccine; PO, orally; PPV23, 23-valent pneumococcal polysaccharides vaccine; SQ, subcutaneous; SS, single strength; TB, tuberculosis; TMP-SMX, trimethoprim-sulfamethoxazole; VZV, varicella-zoster virus.

[a] TMP-SMX DS once daily also confers protection against toxoplasmosis and many respiratory bacterial infections; lower dose also likely confers protection.

[b] Patients should be tested for glucose-6-phosphate dehydrogenase (G6PD) before administration of dapsone or primaquine. Alternative agent should be used in patients found to have G6PD deficiency.

[c] Screening tests for LTBI include tuberculin skin test (TST) or interferon-gamma release assays (IGRA).

[d] Refer to Drug Interactions section in the Adult and Adolescent ARV Guidelines for dosing recommendation.

Evidence Rating:
Strength of Recommendation:
A: Strong recommendation for the statement
B: Moderate recommendation for the statement
C: Optional recommendation for the statement
Quality of Evidence for the Recommendation:
I: One or more randomized trials with clinical outcomes and/or validated laboratory endpoints
II: One or more well-designed, nonrandomized trials or observational cohort studies with long-term clinical outcomes
III: Expert opinion
In cases where there are no data for the prevention or treatment of an opportunistic infection based on studies conducted in HIV-infected populations, but data derived from HIV-uninfected patients exist that can plausibly guide management decisions for patients with HIV/AIDS, the data will be rated as III but will be assigned recommendations of A, B, C depending on the strength of recommendation.

Source: NLM AIDSInfo. https://clinicalinfo.hiv.gov/en/guidelines/adult-and-adolescent-opportunistic-infection/whats-new-guidelines

in CD4 cell count but no clinically significant benefit such as reductions in mortality, VL, or OI.[179]

- An international collaboration (the HIV Trials Network) is currently focused on the development of vaccines to prevent HIV/AIDS; however no vaccine is available to prevent HIV infection as of this time.[180]

- NONPHARMACOLOGIC THERAPY
  - Many studies have found associations between disease progression, wasting, and one or more nutrients deficiencies in HIV-positive persons, and poor outcomes.[181,182] To date, routine supplementation of multiple micronutrients has not shown consistent beneficial outcomes on disease progression or mortality. However, these observations should not exclude or deny supplementation of nutrients that have been shown to be deficient in specific cases. Therefore, daily multivitamin with minerals supplementation may still be beneficial and appropriate for HIV-positive patients with minimal risk.[183]
  - Researchers have demonstrated 53%–89.7% of persons with HIV use one or more nonpharmacologic therapies.[184,185] The most common indications for using nonpharmacologic therapies include improving general health, increasing overall sense of well-being and energy (61.4%), preventing or alleviating side effects of ART (50%), or relieving HIV-related conditions

such as dermatologic problems, nausea, depression, insomnia, and weakness.[186–188]
  - Despite various benefits reported such as improved quality of life (70%), improvement of general malaise (62%), and improvement in neuropathy (54.7%), nonpharmacologic therapies are not without risk.[189] This is particularly true when ART is taken together with St. John's Wort or garlic supplements, which reduce the ART therapeutic drug levels. Additionally, echinacea, milk thistle, ginseng, cat's claw, and grapefruit can reduce concentrations of indinavir and saquinavir.[190] It is important to note that interactions between herbal remedies and ARV drugs have not been subjected to robust controlled trials, though patients should be advised about combining herbal remedies with ART and the potential safety implications.[190]

- PROPHYLAXIS AND TREATMENT OF OI
  - The compromised immune system of HIV-positive patients makes them susceptible to a wide spectrum of OIs. Effective ART has reduced the risk of OIs in this population. When a CD4 count is lower than 200 cells/µL, various recommended prophylactic regimens should be initiated. The indications for prophylaxis and preferred treatments for OI are summarized in Tables 17.33 and 17.34.

PATIENT EDUCATION

- Prior to initiating ART, patient's willingness to initiate is important. The patient education should include benefits, risks, and side effects of ART before initiating treatments.
- Clinicians should have a conversation regarding patients' high-risk behaviors including substance use, high-risk sexual behavior, social support, mental illness, comorbidities, and economic factors (i.e. housing, transportation, and medical insurance).
- Patients should be educated about the partner notification. They should be encouraged to share the HIV status with both sexual and/or needle-sharing partners. Patients should also be educated on HIV risk behaviors and strategies to prevent transmission.
- HIV specialists, primary care clinicians, pharmacists, case/social workers, psychologists/psychiatrists, dentists, registered dietitians, dermatologists, and all other necessary medical and support professionals should team up and manage patients with HIV.[191] When taking care of these patients, having multidisciplinary approach, evidence-based practices, and patient-centered care will lead to favorable outcome.
- Clinician-patient communication plays a vital role in influencing new patients' perception of care involvement of HIV. When clinicians make patients feel involved even when patients do not actively make medical decisions, they feel involved and want to take care of themselves.[192]
- HIV is a chronic illness. Therefore, regular exercise, healthy weight, tobacco cessation, and adherence with other age-related healthcare maintenance such as cervical cancer screening, mammography, colonoscopy, and immunizations are important.[193]
- HIV transmission prevention is important. One of the best ways to prevent or minimize risk of transmission is to achieve undetectable VL.[194]
- It is vital to protect self from other infections that may complicate or exacerbate HIV infection, such as infection with chronic viral hepatitis.[195]
- If the partner is HIV-uninfected, there are two interventions available for the partner to prevent or reduce the risk of HIV infection: nonoccupational postexposure prophylaxis (nPEP) and PrEP. For nPEP, individuals who experience a high-risk exposure are started on ART for a time-limited period and must start within 72 hours following a high-risk exposure. Persons remain on nPEP for 28 days and are monitored for HIV infection for several months following completion of therapy. For HIV-uninfected persons at ongoing risk, such as persons who are in an ongoing sexual relationship with a person living with hepatitis, the CDC now recommends HIV PrEP. This is a strategy where HIV-uninfected individuals take ART on a daily basis to prevent infection. Emtricitabine/tenofovir disoproxil (Truvada) and emtricitabine/tenofovir alafenamide (Descovy) are FDA approved for use as PrEP.[196]
- Linkage to services, ARV adherence, self-acceptance of HIV status, healthy and positive living, understanding of what it means to be living with HIV, HIV status disclosure, and family and occupational strengthening are some helpful topics for education.[197]

SPECIAL CONSIDERATIONS

- Mother-to-child transmission is the most common etiology of HIV in infants and children.
- Maternal ART can reduce the incidence of mother-to-child transmission.
- Diagnosis in children under 18 months of age is via qualitative RNA assays or DNA PCR assays; for children over age 18 months diagnosis is a fourth generation HIV-1/2 antigen/antibody immunoassay followed by a second-generation assay.

KEY POINTS

- HIV infects $CD4^+$ lymphocytes and interferes with cell-mediated and humoral immunity.
- HIV is spread by sexual contact, parenteral exposure to contaminated blood, and prenatal and perinatal maternal transmission.
- Treatment with a combination of antiretroviral drugs can restore immune function to nearly normal in most patients.
- Counseling of patients living with HIV about safe sex, the importance of regular physical activity and a healthy diet, and stress management should be done periodically.
- Primary prophylaxis against OI is based on the CD4 count.

ADDITIONAL RESOURCES

For additional information, please refer to the following sites:

- AIDS*info* (HIV Guidelines): https://www.aidsinfo.nih.gov/guidelines
- CDC: https://www.cdc.gov/hiv
- UNAIDS (United Nations): http://www.unaids.org/en
- University of California, San Francisco (UCSF) Clinician Consultation Center: https://nccc.ucsf.edu

TABLE 17.34 Treatment for Common Opportunistic Infections

Opportunistic Infection	Preferred Therapy
***Pneumocystis* pneumonia (PCP)**	Patients who develop PCP despite TMP-SMX prophylaxis can usually be treated with standard doses of TMP-SMX **(BIII)**. Duration of PCP treatment: 21 days **(AII)** *For Moderate-to-Severe PCP*: TMP-SMX: [TMP 15–20 mg and SMX 75–100 mg]/kg/day IV given q6h or q8h **(AI)**, may switch to PO after clinical improvement **(AI)** *For Mild-to-Moderate PCP*: TMP-SMX: [TMP 15–20 mg and SMX 75–100 mg]/kg/day, given PO in 3 divided doses **(AI)**, *or* TMP-SMX: (160 mg/800 mg or DS) 2 tablets PO TID **(AI)** *Secondary Prophylaxis, after completion of PCP treatment*: TMP-SMX DS: 1 tablet PO daily **(AI)**, *or* TMP-SMX (80 mg/400 mg or SS): 1 tablet PO daily **(AI)**
***Toxoplasma gondii* encephalitis**	*Treatment of Acute Infection **(AI)***: Pyrimethamine[a] 200 mg PO 1 time, followed by weight-based therapy: If <60 kg, pyrimethamine[a] 50 mg PO once daily + sulfadiazine 1,000 mg PO q6h + leucovorin 10–25 mg PO once daily If ≥60 kg, pyrimethamine[a] 75 mg PO once daily + sulfadiazine 1,500 mg PO q6h + leucovorin 10–25 mg PO once daily Leucovorin dose can be increased to 50 mg daily or BID. *Duration for Acute Therapy*: At least 6 weeks **(BII)**; longer duration if clinical or radiologic disease is extensive or response is incomplete at 6 weeks After completion of acute therapy, all patients should be initiated on chronic maintenance therapy *Chronic Maintenance Therapy*: Pyrimethamine[a] 25–50 mg PO daily + sulfadiazine 2,000–4,000 mg PO daily (in 2–4 divided doses) + leucovorin 10–25 mg PO daily **(AI)**
Cryptosporidiosis	Initiate or optimize ART for immune restoration to CD4 count >100 cells/µL **(AII)**, *and* Aggressive oral or IV rehydration and replacement of electrolyte loss **(AIII)**, *and* Symptomatic treatment of diarrhea with antimotility agents **(AIII)**.
***Mycobacterium tuberculosis* (TB) disease**	After collecting specimen for culture and molecular diagnostic tests, empiric TB treatment should be started in individuals with clinical and radiographic presentation suggestive of TB **(AIII)**. *Refer AIDSinfo.gov for dosing recommendations.* *Initial Phase (2 Months, Given Daily, 5–7 Times/Week by DOT) **(AI)***: INH + [RIF or RFB] + PZA + EMB **(AI)**, *Continuation Phase*: INH + (RIF or RFB) daily (5–7 times/week) *Total Duration of Therapy (For Drug-Susceptible TB)*: Pulmonary, drug-susceptible TB: 6 months **(BII)** Pulmonary TB and culture-positive after 2 months of TB treatment: 9 months **(BII)** Extrapulmonary TB w/CNS infection: 9–12 months **(BII)**; Extrapulmonary TB w/bone or joint involvement: 6 to 9 months **(BII)**; Extrapulmonary TB in other sites: 6 months **(BII)** Total duration of therapy should be based on number of doses received, not on calendar time
Disseminated *Mycobacterium avium* complex (MAC) disease	*At Least 2 Drugs as Initial Therapy With*: Clarithromycin 500 mg PO BID **(AI)** + ethambutol 15 mg/kg PO daily **(AI)**, *or* (Azithromycin 500–600 mg + ethambutol 15 mg/kg) PO daily **(AII)** if drug interaction or intolerance precludes the use of clarithromycin *Duration*: At least 12 months of therapy, can discontinue if no signs and symptoms of MAC disease and sustained >6 months) CD4 count >100 cells/µL in response to ART
Mucocutaneous candidiasis	*For Oropharyngeal Candidiasis; Initial Episodes (For 7–14 Days)*: *Oral Therapy*: Fluconazole 100 mg PO daily **(AI)** *For Esophageal Candidiasis (For 14–21 Days)*: Fluconazole 100 mg (up to 400 mg) PO or IV daily **(AI)**, *or* Itraconazole oral solution 200 mg PO daily **(AI)** *For Uncomplicated Vulvo-Vaginal Candidiasis*: Oral fluconazole 150 mg for 1 dose **(AII)**, *or* Topical azoles (clotrimazole, butoconazole, miconazole, tioconazole, or terconazole) for 3–7 days **(AII)** *For Severe or Recurrent Vulvo-Vaginal Candidiasis*: Fluconazole 100–200 mg PO daily for ≥7 days **(AII)**, *or* Topical antifungal ≥7 days **(AII)**

TABLE 17.34 Treatment for Common Opportunistic Infections *(continued)*

Opportunistic Infection	Preferred Therapy
Cryptococcosis	*Cryptococcal Meningitis* *Induction Therapy (for at least 2 weeks, followed by consolidation therapy):* Liposomal amphotericin B 3–4 mg/kg IV daily + flucytosine 25 mg/kg PO QID **(AI)** (Note: Flucytosine dose should be adjusted in patients with renal dysfunction.) *Consolidation Therapy (for at least 8 weeks **(AI)**, followed by maintenance therapy):* Fluconazole 400 mg PO (or IV) daily **(AI)** *Maintenance Therapy:* Fluconazole 200 mg PO daily for at least 12 months **(AI)** *For Non-CNS, Extrapulmonary Cryptococcosis and Diffuse Pulmonary Disease:* Treatment same as for cryptococcal meningitis **(BIII)** *Non-CNS Cryptococcosis with Mild-to-Moderate Symptoms and Focal Pulmonary Infiltrates:* Fluconazole, 400 mg PO daily for 12 months **(BIII)**
Coccidioidomycosis	*Clinically Mild Infections (e.g., Focal Pneumonia):* Fluconazole 400 mg* PO daily **(AII)**, *or* Itraconazole 200 mg* PO BID **(BII)** *Bone or Joint Infections:* Itraconazole 200 mg* PO BID **(AI)** *Severe, Non-Meningeal Infection (Diffuse Pulmonary Infection or Severely Ill Patients with Extrathoracic, Disseminated Disease):* Lipid formulation amphotericin B 3–5 mg/kg IV daily **(AIII)**, *or* Amphotericin B deoxycholate 0.7–1.0 mg/kg IV daily **(AII)** Duration of therapy: continue until clinical improvement, then switch to a triazole **(BIII)** *Meningeal Infections:* Fluconazole 400–800 mg* IV or PO daily **(AII)**
ART cytomegalovirus (CMV) disease	*CMV Retinitis* *Induction Therapy (followed by Chronic Maintenance Therapy)* *For Immediate Sight-Threatening Lesions (within 1,500 microns of the fovea):* Intravitreal injections of ganciclovir (2 mg) or foscarnet (2.4 mg) for 1–4 doses over a period of 7–10 days to achieve high intraocular concentration faster **(AIII)**; plus Valganciclovir 900 mg PO BID for 14– 21 days, then 900 mg once daily **(AI)** *For Peripheral Lesions* Valganciclovir 900 mg PO BID for 14– 21 days, then 900 mg once daily **(AI)** *Chronic Maintenance* Valganciclovir 900 mg PO daily **(AI)** for 3–6 months until ART induced immune recovery *CMV Esophagitis or Colitis:* Ganciclovir 5 mg/kg IV q12h; may switch to valganciclovir 900 mg PO q12h once the patient can tolerate oral therapy **(BI)** Duration: 21–42 days or until symptoms have resolved **(CII)** Maintenance therapy is usually not necessary but should be considered after relapses **(BII)**. *Well-Documented, Histologically Confirmed CMV Pneumonia:* Experience for treating CMV pneumonitis in HIV patients is limited. Use of IV ganciclovir or IV foscarnet is reasonable (doses same as for CMV retinitis) **(CIII)**. The optimal duration of therapy and the role of oral valganciclovir have not been established. *CMV Neurological Disease* ***Note: Treatment should be initiated promptly.*** Ganciclovir 5 mg/kg IV q12h + (foscarnet 90 mg/kg IV q12h or 60 mg/kg IV q8h) to stabilize disease and maximize response, continue until symptomatic improvement and resolution of neurologic symptoms **(CIII)** The optimal duration of therapy and the role of oral valganciclovir have not been established. Optimize ART to achieve viral suppression and immune reconstitution **(BIII)**
Herpes simplex virus (HSV) disease	*Orolabial Lesions (For 5–10 Days):* Valacyclovir 1 g PO BID **(AIII)**, *or* Famciclovir 500 mg PO BID **(AIII)**, *or* Acyclovir 400 mg PO TID **(AIII)** *Initial or Recurrent Genital HSV (For 5–14 Days):* Valacyclovir 1 g PO BID **(AI)**, *or* Famciclovir 500 mg PO BID **(AI)**, *or* Acyclovir 400 mg PO TID **(AI)** *Severe Mucocutaneous HSV:* Initial therapy acyclovir 5 mg/kg IV q8h **(AIII)** After lesions begin to regress, change to PO therapy as above. Continue until lesions are completely healed. *Chronic Suppressive Therapy* *For patients with severe recurrences of genital herpes **(AI)** or patients who want to minimize frequency of recurrences **(AI)**:* Valacyclovir 500 mg PO BID **(AI)** Famciclovir 500 mg PO BID **(AI)** Acyclovir 400 mg PO BID **(AI)** Continue indefinitely regardless of CD4 cell count.

(continued)

TABLE 17.34 Treatment for Common Opportunistic Infections *(continued)*

Opportunistic Infection	Preferred Therapy
HHV-8 Diseases *(Kaposi sarcoma Primary effusion lymphoma [PEL], Multicentric Castleman disease [MCD])*	*Mild To Moderate KS (localized involvement of skin and/or lymph nodes)*: Initiate or optimize ART **(AII)** *Advanced KS [visceral **(AI)** or disseminated cutaneous KS **(BIII)**]*: Chemotherapy (per oncology consult) + ART Liposomal doxorubicin first line chemotherapy **(AI)** *Primary Effusion Lymphoma*: Chemotherapy (per oncology consult) + ART **(AIII)** PO valganciclovir or IV ganciclovir can be used as adjunctive therapy **(CIII)**. *MCD Therapy Options (in consultation with specialist, depending on HIV/HHV-8 status, presence of organ failure, and refractory nature of disease)*: ART **(AIII)** along with one of the following: Valganciclovir 900 mg PO BID for 3 weeks **(CII)**, *or* Ganciclovir 5 mg/kg IV q12h for 3 weeks **(CII)**, *or* Valganciclovir PO or ganciclovir IV + zidovudine 600 mg PO q6h for 7–21 days **(CII)** Rituximab +/- prednisone **(CII)** Monoclonal antibody targeting IL-6 or IL-6 receptor **(BII)** *Concurrent KS and MCD* Rituximab + liposomal doxorubicin **(BII)**
Malaria	Because *Plasmodium falciparum* malaria can progress in hours from mild symptoms or low-grade fever to severe disease or death, all HIV-infected patients with confirmed or suspected *P. falciparum* infection should be hospitalized for evaluation, initiation of treatment, and observation **(AIII)**. Treatment recommendations for HIV-infected patients are the same as HIV-uninfected patients **(AIII)**. Choice of therapy is guided by the degree of parasitemia, the species of *Plasmodium*, a patient's clinical status, region of infection, and the likely drug susceptibility of the infected species, and can be found at http://www.cdc.gov/malaria.

Key to Acronyms: ACTG, AIDS Clinical Trials Group; ART, antiretroviral therapy; ARV, antiretroviral; ATV/r, ritonavir-boosted atazanavir; BID, twice a day; BIW, twice weekly; BOC, boceprevir; CD4, CD4 T lymphocyte cell; CDC, Centers for Disease Control and Prevention; CFU, colony-forming unit; CNS, central nervous system; CSF, cerebrospinal fluid; CYP3A4, cytochrome P450 3A4; ddI, didanosine; DOT, directly observed therapy; DS, double strength; EFV, efavirenz; EMB, ethambutol; G6PD, glucose-6-phosphate dehydrogenase; GI, gastrointestinal; ICP, intracranial pressure; IM, intramuscular; IND, investigational new drug; INH, isoniazid; IRIS, immune reconstitution inflammatory syndrome; IV, intravenous; LP, lumbar puncture; NNRTI, nonnucleoside reverse transcriptase inhibitor; NRTI, nucleoside reverse transcriptase inhibitor; NSAID, non steroidal anti-inflammatory drug; PegIFN, pegylated interferon; PI, protease inhibitor; PO, oral; PORN, progressive outer retinal necrosis; PZA, pyrazinamide; qAM, every morning; QID, four times a day; q(n)h, every "n" hours; qPM, every evening; RBV, ribavirin; RFB, rifabutin; RIF, rifampin; SQ, subcutaneous; SS, single strength; TID, three times daily; TVR, telaprevir; TMP-SMX, trimethoprim-sulfamethoxazole; ZDV, zidovudine.

[a] Refer to http://www.daraprimdirect.com for information regarding how to access pyrimethamine.

Evidence Rating:
Strength of Recommendation:
A: Strong recommendation for the statement
B: Moderate recommendation for the statement
C: Optional recommendation for the statement
Quality of Evidence for the Recommendation:
I: One or more randomized trials with clinical outcomes and/or validated laboratory endpoints
II: One or more well-designed, nonrandomized trials or observational cohort studies with long-term clinical outcomes
III: Expert opinion

In cases where there are no data for the prevention or treatment of an opportunistic infection based on studies conducted in HIV-infected populations, but data derived from HIV-uninfected patients exist that can plausibly guide management decisions for patients with HIV/AIDS, the data will be rated as III but will be assigned recommendations of A, B, C depending on the strength of recommendation.

Source: Data from NLM AIDSInfo. https://clinicalinfo.hiv.gov/sites/default/files/guidelines/documents/AdultOITablesOnly.pdf

17.9 FEVER OF UNKNOWN ORIGIN

OVERVIEW

Fever of unknown origin can be a difficult diagnostic evaluation because of the wide differential diagnosis. There is no standard diagnostic approach to fever of unknown origin. Evaluation requires a focused history, physical examination, and selective nonspecific laboratory tests. Fever of unknown origin is defined as fever >38.3 °C (101 °F) for >3 weeks that remains undiagnosed after a hospital workup. Fever on unknown origin can be divided by category: infectious, malignancy/neoplastic, rheumatic/inflammatory, and miscellaneous disorders.

APPROACH

The first step in the approach to the patient is to verify the prolonged fever meets the fever of unknown origin definition. The workup should be driven by history, signs and symptoms, or physical examination. The second step is to determine the category based on the findings in step one. For example, in infectious etiologies chills are common but weight loss is less common. The third step is to determine the pattern of organ involvement that suggests or limits the possible etiologies. For example, systemic lupus erythematosus involves multiple organs, but spares the liver.

DIFFERENTIAL DIAGNOSIS

There are over 200 disorders in the differential diagnosis. See Table 17.35 for the differential diagnosis for fever of unknown origin.

TABLE 17.35 Differential Diagnosis for Fever of Unknown Origin

Category	Common Etiologies	Rare Etiologies
Malignancy/neoplastic	Lymphoma Renal cell carcinoma Preleukemia Myelodysplastic disorders	Multiple myeloma Colon cancer Pancreatic cancer CNS or liver metastases Systemic mastocytosis
Infectious	Tuberculosis, miliary Intra-abdominal/pelvic abscess Nephric abscess Typhoid/enteric fever Cat scratch disease EBV/CMV/HIV Extrapulmonary tuberculosis	Subacute bacterial endocarditis Chronic sinusitis/mastoiditis Vertebral osteomyelitis Relapsing fever Rat bite fever Leptospirosis Histoplasmosis Coccidioidomycosis Malaria Babesiosis Brucellosis Q fever Toxoplasmosis
Rheumatologic/inflammatory	Adult Still disease Giant cell arteritis Polyarteritis nodosa SLE	Takayasu arteritis Sarcoidosis Gaucher disease Pseudogout Behcet disease
Miscellaneous	Drug fever Cirrhosis Subacute thyroiditis Crohn disease	Pulmonary emboli Hypertriglyceridemia Factitious fever

CMV, cytomegalovirus; CNS, central nervous system; EBV, Epstein-Barr virus; SLE, systemic lupus erythematosus.

MEDICAL HISTORY AND CLINICAL PRESENTATION

The medical history and presentation help with placing the patient in one of the various categories. Patients with significant weight loss, >2 pounds per week, with early anorexia is noted in malignant and neoplastic fevers of unknown origin. Post-hot bath pruritus suggests a malignant disorder as well.

For possible infectious disease etiologies, consider a history of prior invasive procedures or surgeries for possible abscesses, and dental procedures for possible subacute bacterial endocarditis. Animal or pet contacts suggests Q fever, brucellosis, toxoplasmosis, cat scratch disease, or trichinosis. Mosquito or tick bites suggest ehrlichiosis or anaplasmosis, babesiosis, Lyme disease, and malaria. Rat exposure suggests rat bite fever, relapsing fever, or leptospirosis. A history of blood transfusions suggests bloodborne pathogens including *Ehrlichia*, *Babesia*, CMV, and HIV. Use of immunosuppressive medications could indicate CMV and tuberculosis.

Rheumatic etiologies typically present with arthralgias or myalgias and the presence of chills decrease the possibility of a rheumatologic etiology. Presence of a dry cough could indicate giant cell arteritis. Oral ulcers indicate Behçet syndrome or systemic lupus erythematosus.

If the history does not suggest a category, the miscellaneous causes, as noted in Table 17.36, should be considered.

PHYSICAL EXAMINATION

Several physical examination findings can direct the clinician to a specific category and possible diagnosis. See Table 17.36 for a list of physical exam findings and most likely diagnosis.

DIAGNOSTIC STUDIES

Laboratory tests should be selected based on the history and physical examination. There are several nonspecific laboratory tests that can aid in the evaluation of the patient. Abnormalities in ESR, serum ferritin, alkaline phosphatase, and rheumatoid factor can focus in on the diagnosis.

A markedly elevated sedimentation rate narrows down the differential diagnosis. The CBC should be obtained to evaluate for an increase or decrease in the various cellular elements. For example, a mild elevation in atypical lymphocytes could indicate drug fever or toxoplasmosis, a marked elevation may indicate EBV or CMV infection.

An isolated increase in alkaline phosphatase could be due to lymphoma. Serum protein electrophoresis may provide clues to the diagnosis; elevated alpha globulin may indicate lymphoma or systemic lupus erythematosus; monoclonal gammopathy may indicate multiple myeloma; and a polyclonal gammopathy could indicate HIV, cirrhosis, sarcoidosis, or malaria. The finding of microscopic hematuria on urinalysis could indicate renal tuberculosis, brucellosis, lymphoma, or renal cell carcinoma.

Imaging studies should be selected based on the fever of unknown origin category and most likely organ involved. One of the most frequent invasive tests obtained is the lymph node biopsy. Biopsy of the posterior cervical, supra-or infraclavicular, or epitrochlear nodes is most likely to be diagnostic. If bone involvement is likely, then a bone marrow biopsy and aspiration should be obtained.

TABLE 17.36 Differential Diagnosis for Fever of Unknown Origin Based on Physical Exam Findings

Physical Examination Finding	Diagnosis
Malignant/Neoplastic Disorders	
Relative bradycardia	Lymphoma, central nervous system malignancy
Roth spots	Lymphoma, atrial myxoma
Retinal hemorrhage	Myelodysplastic syndrome (MDS)
Sternal tenderness	Preleukemia, myeloproliferative disorder
Hepatomegaly, isolated	Hepatoma, renal cell carcinoma, liver metastases
Infectious Diseases	
Cardiac murmur	Subacute bacterial endocarditis
Morning temperature spikes	Miliary tuberculosis, typhoid/enteric fever, Whipple disease
Relative bradycardia	Typhoid/enteric fever, malaria, babesiosis, leptospirosis, Q fever, ehrlichiosis/anaplasmosis
Two daily fever spikes	Malaria, miliary tuberculosis, visceral leishmaniasis
Two fever peaks per week	Ehrlichiosis/anaplasmosis, leptospirosis, brucellosis, rat bite fever
Spinal tenderness	Subacute vertebral osteomyelitis, typhoid/enteric fever, spinal tuberculosis, brucellosis
Hepatomegaly, isolated	Q fever, typhoid/enteric fever, visceral leishmaniasis, rat bite fever, brucellosis
Splenomegaly	Miliary tuberculosis, Epstein-Barr virus, cytomegalovirus, typhoid/enteric fever, brucellosis, histoplasmosis, malaria, Q fever, cat scratch disease, ehrlichiosis/anaplasmosis, rat bite fever
Rheumatic/inflammatory Disorders	
Morning temperature spikes	Periarteritis nodosa
Rash	Sarcoidosis, systemic lupus erythematous, adult Still disease
Unequal pulses	Takayasu arteritis
Oral ulcers	Behcet disease, systemic lupus erythematosus
Lymphadenopathy	Systemic lupus erythematosus, sarcoidosis, late-onset rheumatoid arthritis
Cardiac murmur	Libman-Sacks endocarditis
Miscellaneous Disorders	
Relative bradycardia	Drug fever/factitious fever
Splenomegaly	Crohn disease, cirrhosis

KEY POINTS

- Classic fever of unknown origin is body temperature ≥38.3° C >3 weeks with no identified cause after 3 days of hospital investigation or more than three outpatient visits.
- Identified causes can be categorized as infectious, connective tissue, neoplastic, or miscellaneous.

17.10 ANIMAL AND HUMAN BITES

OVERVIEW

Human and animal bites are a common cause of primary care and ED visits per year. There are an estimated 400,000 cat bites and 4.5 million dog bites per year in the United States.[198] A very small number of cases are due to rodents. There are about 250,000 human bites per year in the United States.[198]

MEDICAL HISTORY AND CLINICAL PRESENTATION

The following history should be obtained in all bite cases.

- How did the bite occur?
- How long ago was the bite incident?
- If an animal bite, was the animal provoked, has the animal bitten before, and what is the animal's vaccination history?

The patient history to be obtained includes presence of comorbid conditions and the tetanus status.

Human bites may be the result of sexual crimes, child abuse, physical altercations, and consensual sexual activity and this should be investigated.

PHYSICAL EXAMINATION

A complete evaluation of the wound should be completed. Aggressive irrigation should be performed with sodium chloride solution or povidone-iodine solution. A neurologic examination should be completed to assess for underlying nerve injury. If the wound is complicated and involves the muscle, tendons, or joints, surgical evaluation should be considered.

An oval or semilunar hematoma and abrasion are noted in human bites.

DIAGNOSTIC STUDIES

Culture may be needed to identify any possible source of infection. X-ray may be needed to determine the presence of foreign bodies, such as broken teeth.

TREATMENT

Closure of the wound depends on the type of animal and the severity of the bite. Primary closure of the wound is appropriate in bites with no underlying injury, patient is immunocompetent, bites on the face and scalp, or simple wounds.

Treatment of high-risk bites is complicated. High-risk bites are noted in Box 17.3.

Most animal bites are polymicrobial and include aerobic and anaerobic bacteria. The most common aerobic organisms include *Streptococcus, Staphylococcus, Moraxella,* and *Neisseria*; the most common anaerobic organisms include *Fusobacterium, Bacteroides, Prevotella,* and *Pasteurella. Pasteurella* spp. is the most common organism isolated from dog and cat bites. Rat bite infections are typically due to *Spirillum minus*. The most common organisms noted in human bites include *Streptococcus*, *Staphylococcus aureus*, and *Eikenella corrodens*.

Prophylactic antibiotic postexposure is indicated for bites involving the hand and for high-risk bites. The treatment of choice is amoxicillin-clavulanate for prophylactic treatment. If the patient is allergic to penicillin, doxycycline, TMP-SMX, or a fluoroquinolone plus clindamycin or metronidazole can be used. Rodent bites should be treated with IV penicillin; doxycycline or tetracycline can be used if penicillin allergic.

Tetanus vaccination should be given if it is more than 5 years since the patient has been immunized.

BOX 17.3 Examples of High-Risk Bites

Cat bites
Human bites
Livestock bites
Monkey bites
Dog bites >8 hours old and those that involve muscle, tendon, or joints
Heavily contaminated bites
Bites in patients with diabetes
Bites in immunosuppressed patients

TABLE 17.37 CDC Recommendations for Rabies Postexposure Treatment

Animal	Rabies Status	Recommended Treatment
Cats, dogs, ferrets	Healthy animal	No vaccination needed unless animal develops symptoms of rabies
	Suspected rabies or unknown	Vaccinate
Raccoons, skunks, foxes, bats	Regard as positive for rabies	Vaccinate
Rabbits, rodents, other	Case by case basis	Vaccination typically not required

Source: Data from Centers for Disease Control and Prevention. https://www.cdc.gov/rabies/exposure/animals/domestic.html

Rabies infections are rare, but postexposure rabies prophylaxis should be considered in select patients. See Table 17.37 for bites from bats or dogs.

If treatment for rabies is needed, administer rabies immune globulin around the borders of the wound and intramuscularly distal to the site. In this group, rabies vaccine series should be given with vaccinations on days 0, 3, 7, and 14. If the patient has received the rabies vaccine previously, they do not require the rabies immunoglobulin and only need a vaccine booster on days 0 and 3.

KEY POINTS

- Wounds cleaning and debridement are key to reducing the risk of infection.
- Patients may need rabies postexposure prophylaxis.
- Wounds at risk for infection should not be closed by primary intention.

17.11 SEPSIS

OVERVIEW

Sepsis is defined as "life threatening organ dysfunction caused by dysregulated host response to infection."[199] The clinical diagnosis is based on a patient having infection and an elevated Sequential (Sepsis-related) Organ Failure Assessment Score (SOFA), with a change in score of 2 or greater from baseline being diagnostic (Table 17.38).[199, 200]

Septic shock is defined as a "subset of sepsis with particularly profound circulatory, cellular and metabolic abnormalities associated with a greater risk of mortality than sepsis alone."[199] The diagnostic criteria of septic shock are a "vasopressor requirement required to maintain a MAP of >65 mmHg and a serum lactate level >2 mmol/L in absence of hypovolemia."[199]

The SOFA score is complex, and all information required to make the calculation may not be available. The qSOFA (quick SOFA) is used as a bedside tool to rapidly identify patients with infection who are likely to have poor outcomes. The qSOFA is positive if at least two of the following are positive:

TABLE 17.38 Sequential (Sepsis-Related) Organ Failure Assessment Score

	Score				
System	**0**	**1**	**2**	**3**	**4**
Respiratory $Pa{O_2}/Fi{O_2}$ (kPa)	≥53.3	<53.3	<40	<26.7 with respiratory support	<13.3 with respiratory support
Coagulation Platelets (×10⁹/L)	≥150	<150	<100	<50	<20
Liver Bilirubin (mg/dL)	<1.2	1.2–1.9	2.0–5.9	6.0–11.9	>12.0
Cardiovascular MAP (mm Hg) Dose (µg/kg/min)	≥70	<70	Dopamine <5 or dobutamine (any dose)	Dopamine >5 or epinephrine ≤0.1 or norepinephrine ≤0.1	Dopamine >15 or epinephrine >0.1 or norepinephrine >0.1
Central nervous system (GCS score)	15	13–14	10–12	6–9	<6
Renal Creatinine (mg/dL) Urine output (mL/day)	<1.2	1.2–1.9	2.0–3.4	3.5–4.9 or <500 mL/day	≥5.0 <200 mL/day

GCS, Glasgow Coma Scale; MAP, mean arterial pressure.

Source: Adapted from Keeley A, Hine P, Nsutebu E. The recognition and management of sepsis and septic shock: a guide for non-intensivists. Postgrad Med J. *2017;94:626–634.*

- Respiratory rate of 22/minute or greater
- Altered mental status (Glasgow Coma Scale score <15)
- Systolic blood pressure of 100 mm Hg or less

The qSOFA should be used to evaluate the patient for organ dysfunction, start or enhance therapy as appropriate, and consider referral to critical care or increase the frequency of monitoring.

Systemic inflammatory response syndrome (SIRS) is a proinflammatory state that may or may not be caused by infection. SIRS is no longer required for the diagnosis of sepsis.

EPIDEMIOLOGY

Sepsis is common and often fatal. The incidence of sepsis varies, ranging from 66 to 300 per 100,000 population in the developed world.[200] The incidence is increasing secondary to an aging population, increasing comorbid conditions, increased use of immunosuppressive medications, and high-risk interventions. Mortality rate of sepsis ranges from 27% to 36%.[200]

PATHOPHYSIOLOGY

The pathophysiology of sepsis in not completely understood. Sepsis is characterized by changes in endothelial tissue, activation of the coagulation cascade, and a change in blood flow. Infectious microorganisms cause the release of proinflammatory substances. These substances, called cytokines, cause damage to endothelial cells that leads to activation of the coagulation cascade. The damage to small blood vessels and activation of the coagulation cascade impede blood flow leading to tissue hypoxia and cell death. The cytokines also lead to cardiovascular dysfunction and tissue leakage leading to pulmonary edema. The pulmonary edema leads to shortness of breath. Cytokines also causes dilatation of blood vessels leading to hypotension.

See Figure 17.37 for a summary of the pathophysiology of sepsis.

MEDICAL HISTORY AND CLINICAL PRESENTATION

Rapid recognition and treatment are key to the effective management of sepsis. History and physical examination will vary with the various etiologies of the infection. Common signs and symptoms include hypotension, tachycardia, altered mental status, and symptoms related to the source of infection.

EVALUATION

The initial evaluation steps should aid in the identification of end-organ hypoperfusion and identify the source of infection. The workup should include a CBC, prothrombin time, electrolytes and renal function, liver function tests, serum lactate, and arterial blood gas.

Lactate level is used as a predictor of outcome. Lactate levels >4 mmol/L were linked to a significant increase in mortality. The clearance of lactate is a good prognostic indicator.

The collection of appropriate cultures before beginning antibiotics is key. Two sets of blood cultures should be obtained, and other cultures should be collected depending on what is clinically indicated.

TREATMENT

The goal of treatment is to improve tissue oxygenation and perfusion, and to provide the appropriate antimicrobial therapy.

Early antibiotics is one of the keys to treatment of sepsis. It is recommended that IV antibiotics be started within 1 hour of recognizing sepsis. The selection of the antibiotics

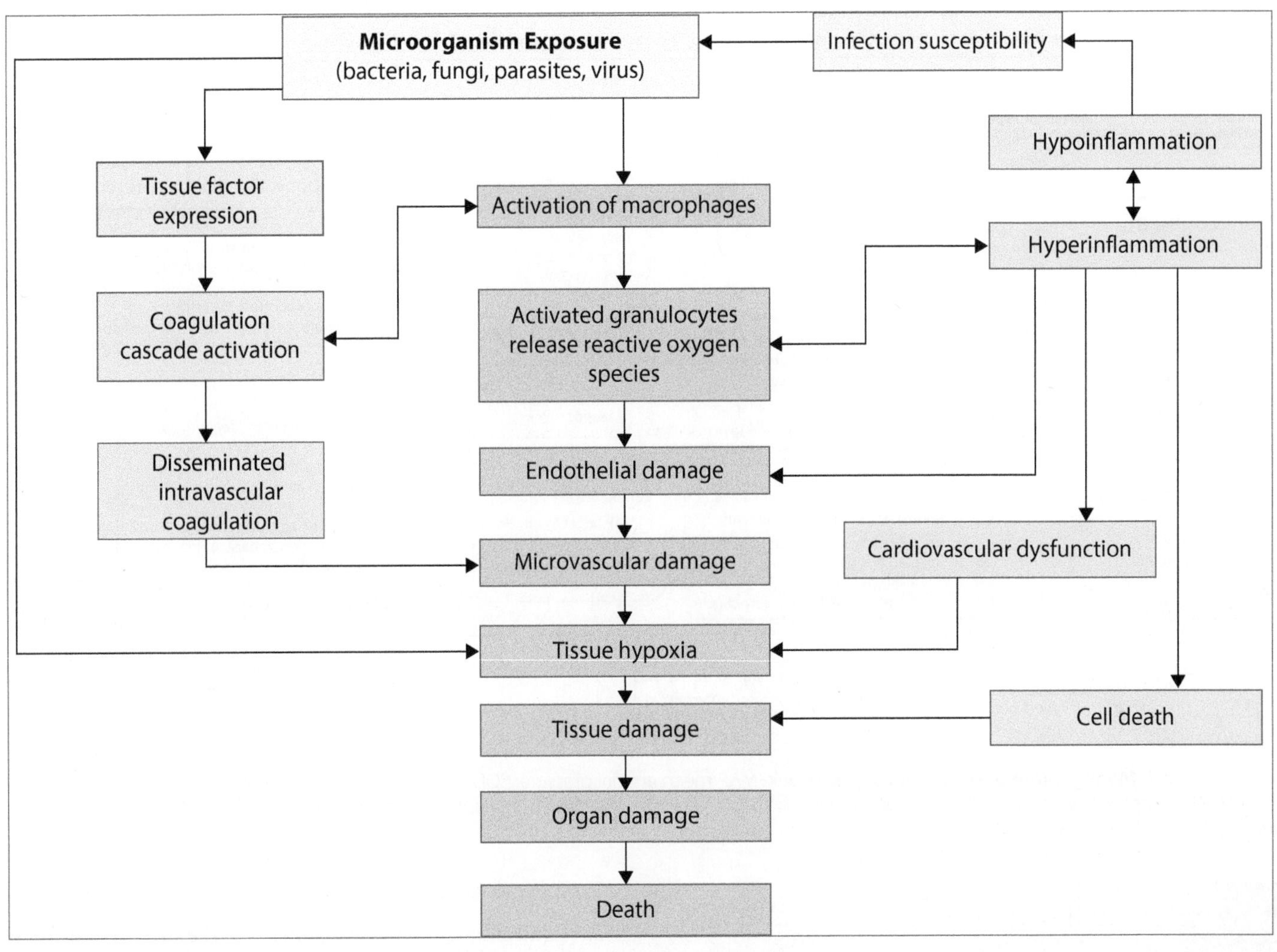

Figure 17.37 **Pathophysiology of sepsis.**

should be based on local antimicrobial resistance patterns and be broad enough to treat all likely causative organisms. Empiric treatment should cover several resistant organisms such as MRSA, VRE, and carbapenemase-producing Enterobacteriaceae.

Fluid resuscitation should be with crystalloids. In patients with hypoperfusion, a minimum of 30 mL/kg of IV crystalloid fluid should be given as a fluid challenge over 3 hours. Caution should be taken in patients with pulmonary edema, from sepsis-induced lung injury, as too much fluid could worsen the patient's condition.

Elimination of the possible infectious source should be undertaken. This may include drainage of fluid collections, debridement of infected tissue, and removal of foreign bodies and vascular access devices.

Frequent patient monitoring is important. Monitoring hourly urine output and blood pressure response to fluids is essential in the management of septic patients. Lactate monitoring should be done; clearing of lactate improves outcomes and can identify patients not responding to fluid resuscitation.

Oxygen should be provided to maintain oxygen saturations at >94% unless there is a history of chronic obstructive pulmonary disease and type II respiratory failure; in those patients a lower oxygen saturation target should be used.

Other treatment options include vasopressors, corticosteroids, and blood transfusions. Vasopressors increase blood pressure by increasing peripheral vascular resistance. Vasopressors are used in patients who remain hypotensive despite adequate fluid resuscitation or in patients who develop cardiogenic pulmonary edema. Norepinephrine is the treatment of choice in patients who need vasopressors. If no improvement, dobutamine can be started. Corticosteroids can be used in patients with septic shock who fail to maintain adequate mean arterial pressure despite adequate fluid hydration and vasopressors. Transfusion of red blood cells is indicated in patients with sepsis when the hemoglobin is below 7 g/dL (Figure 17.38).

KEY POINTS

- qSOFA is used to identify patients with infection who may have sepsis.
- Treatment should focus on restoring tissue hypoperfusion.
- Early antibiotics and fluid hydration are key to treatment.

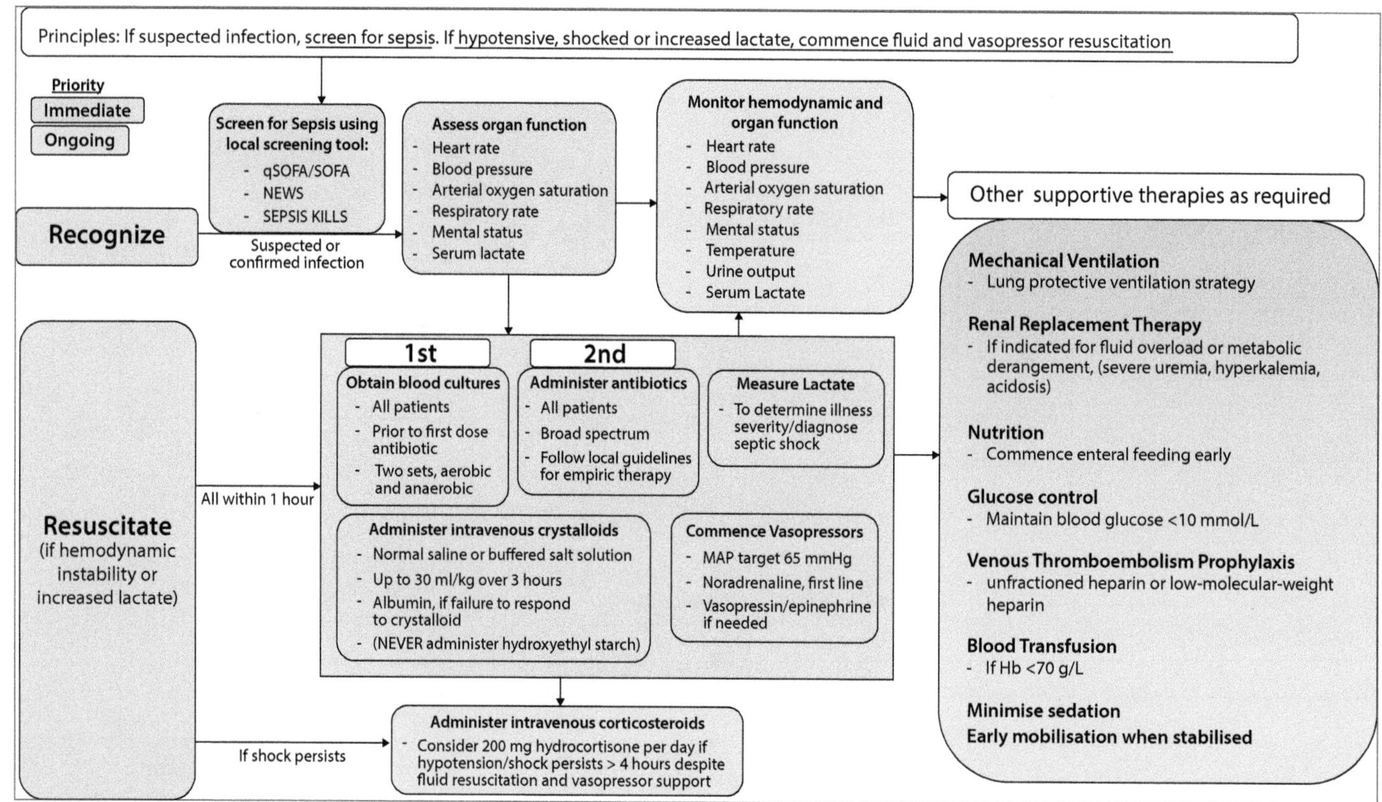

Figure 17.38 Management of sepsis and septic shock. MAP, mean arterial pressure; SOFA, Organ Failure Assessment Score. *(Source: Thompson K, Venkatesh B, Finfer S. Sepsis and septic shock: current approaches to management.* Intern Med J. *2019;49(2):160–170. doi:10.1111/imj.14199)*

17.12 IMMUNIZATIONS AND VACCINES

OVERVIEW

Immunization enables the body to defend itself against diseases caused by certain bacteria or viruses. Immunity may occur naturally or through vaccination. Vaccines available are highly reliable and well tolerated. Side effects are rare.

Active immunization is defined as using vaccines to stimulate the body's natural defense mechanisms. Vaccines are prepared by using noninfectious fragments of bacteria or viruses, either a toxin produced by bacteria that has been modified to be harmless (a toxoid), or weakened (attenuated) live whole organisms that do not cause illness. The body's response to the vaccine is to produce antibodies that will recognize and attack the specific bacteria or virus contained in the vaccine when exposed again in the future.

In passive immunization, antibodies against a specific infectious organism are given directly to the patient. These antibodies are obtained from several sources; the serum of animals that have been exposed to a certain organism or toxin and has developed immunity, pooled human immune globulin, hyperimmune globulin, or antibody-producing cells. Passive immunization is used for people who have not responded adequately to an infection or people who acquire an infection before they can be vaccinated. Passive immunization is also used to prevent disease when people are likely to be exposed and do not have time to get or complete a vaccination series. Passive immunization lasts for only a few weeks, until the body eliminates the injected antibodies.

Four types of vaccines are currently available:

- **Live (attenuated) virus vaccines** use the attenuated form of the virus. Examples include the MMR vaccine and the varicella (chickenpox) vaccine.
- **Killed (inactivated) vaccines** are made from a protein from a virus or bacteria. An example is the polio vaccine.
- **Toxoid vaccines** contain a toxin or chemical made by the bacteria or virus. Examples include the DT vaccines.
- **Biosynthetic vaccines** contain human-made substances that are like pieces of the virus or bacteria. An example is the hepatitis B vaccine.

See Figure 17.39 for immunization schedules for children and adults.

17.13 ANTIMICROBIAL THERAPY

OVERVIEW

Antibacterial drugs are derived from bacteria or molds or are synthesized de novo. Antibiotics have many mechanisms of action, including:

- Inhibiting cell wall synthesis
- Increasing cell membrane permeability
- Interfering with protein synthesis, nucleic acid metabolism, and other metabolic processes

Many antibiotics are chemically related and are grouped into classes. Although drugs within each class share structural and functional similarities, they often have different pharmacology and spectrum of activity.

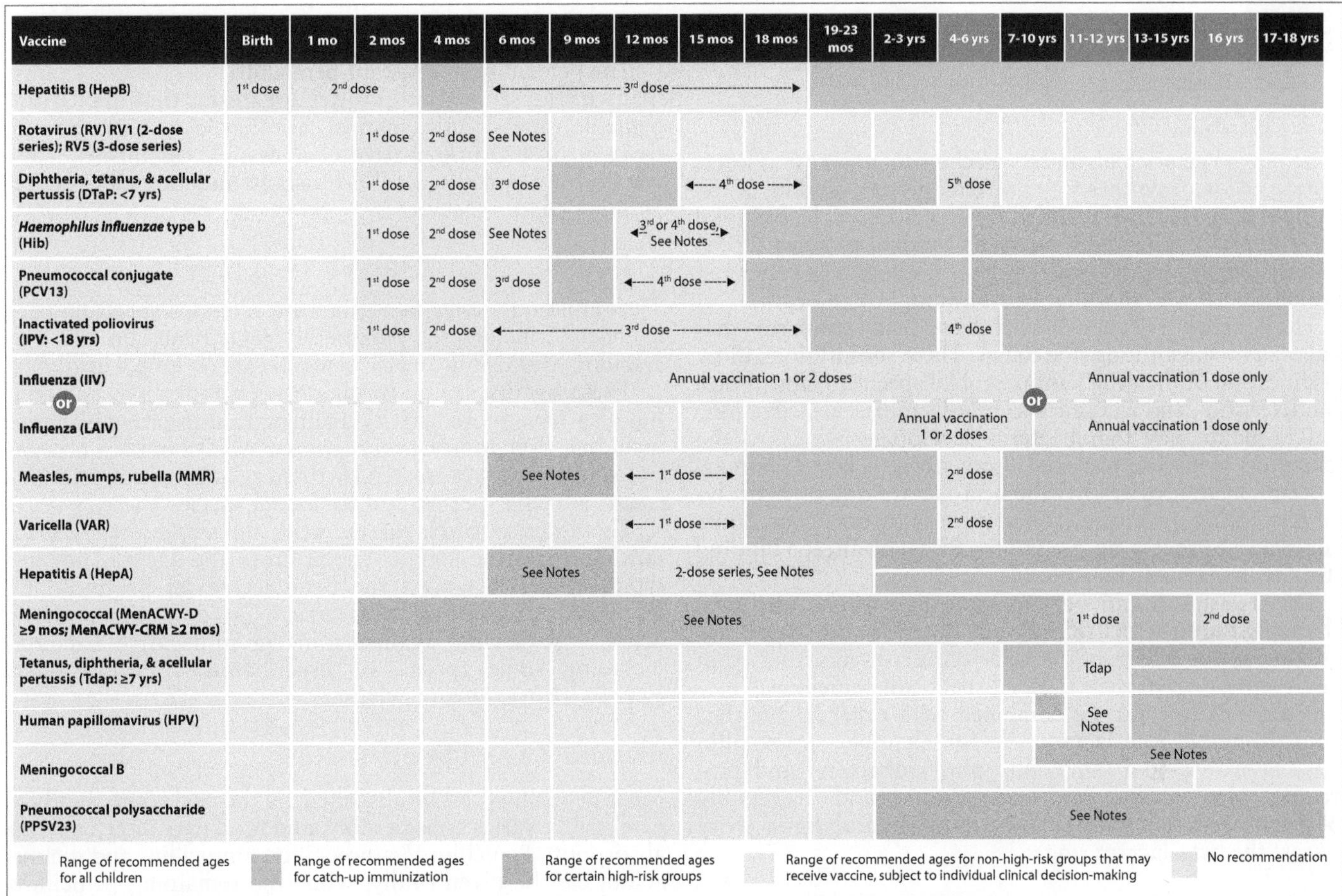

Vaccine	Birth	1 mo	2 mos	4 mos	6 mos	9 mos	12 mos	15 mos	18 mos	19-23 mos	2-3 yrs	4-6 yrs	7-10 yrs	11-12 yrs	13-15 yrs	16 yrs	17-18 yrs
Hepatitis B (HepB)	1st dose	2nd dose					←3rd dose→										
Rotavirus (RV) RV1 (2-dose series); RV5 (3-dose series)			1st dose	2nd dose	See Notes												
Diphtheria, tetanus, & acellular pertussis (DTaP: <7 yrs)			1st dose	2nd dose	3rd dose			←4th dose→				5th dose					
Haemophilus influenzae type b (Hib)			1st dose	2nd dose	See Notes		←3rd or 4th dose, See Notes→										
Pneumococcal conjugate (PCV13)			1st dose	2nd dose	3rd dose		←4th dose→										
Inactivated poliovirus (IPV: <18 yrs)			1st dose	2nd dose			←3rd dose→					4th dose					
Influenza (IIV)									Annual vaccination 1 or 2 doses						Annual vaccination 1 dose only		
or																	
Influenza (LAIV)												Annual vaccination 1 or 2 doses			Annual vaccination 1 dose only		
Measles, mumps, rubella (MMR)					See Notes		←1st dose→					2nd dose					
Varicella (VAR)							←1st dose→					2nd dose					
Hepatitis A (HepA)					See Notes			2-dose series, See Notes									
Meningococcal (MenACWY-D ≥9 mos; MenACWY-CRM ≥2 mos)								See Notes						1st dose		2nd dose	
Tetanus, diphtheria, & acellular pertussis (Tdap: ≥7 yrs)														Tdap			
Human papillomavirus (HPV)														See Notes			
Meningococcal B															See Notes		
Pneumococcal polysaccharide (PPSV23)														See Notes			

Range of recommended ages for all children

Range of recommended ages for catch-up immunization

Range of recommended ages for certain high-risk groups

Range of recommended ages for non-high-risk groups that may receive vaccine, subject to individual clinical decision-making

No recommendation

Figure 17.39 **Immunization schedule for children and adolescents for ages 18 years and younger.**
(Source: https://www.cdc.gov/vaccines/schedules https://www.cdc.gov/vaccines/schedules/hcp/imz/child-adolescent.html)

Antibiotics should be used only if clinical or laboratory evidence suggests bacterial infection. Use for viral illness or undifferentiated fever is inappropriate in most cases; it exposes patients to drug complications without any benefit and contributes to bacterial resistance.

Certain bacterial infections require surgical intervention and do not respond to antibiotics alone.

There are some characteristics that all antibiotics share. All antibiotics can elicit allergic response that can range from mild rashes to life-threatening anaphylaxis and Stevens-Johnson syndrome.

All antibiotics affect normal body flora as well as pathogens; this can cause an overgrowth of *Candida* and pathogenic bacteria such as *Clostridioides difficile*.

SPECTRUM OF ACTIVITY

Cultures and antibiotic sensitivity testing are essential for selecting a drug for serious infections. Treatment must often begin before culture results are available, necessitating selection of empiric antibiotic selection, according to the most likely pathogens.

Drugs with the narrowest spectrum of activity that can control the infection should be used. For empiric treatment of serious infections that may involve any one of several pathogens or that may be due to multiple pathogens, a broad spectrum of activity is desirable. The most likely pathogens and their susceptibility to antibiotics vary according to geographic location and can change over time.

ANTIBIOTIC RESISTANCE

Repeated exposure to an antibiotic may lead to the emergence of selective subpopulations of the same or related bacteria now resistant to the therapeutic agent. The CDC notes that approximately 2.8 million people become infected with bacteria that are resistant to antibiotics, and approximately 35,000 people die annually because of these infections.[201] Mechanisms of microbial resistance include:

- Altered cell permeability causing the intracellular concentration of the drug to be decreased, noted in resistance to the beta-lactams, quinolones, and vancomycin.
- Increased efflux of the antibiotic from the cell, noted in the resistance to the tetracyclines and quinolones.
- Release of enzymes that alter the antibiotic's interaction with binding sites within the cell wall or cytoplasm, noted in the resistance to penicillins and cephalosporins.

Bacterial resistance can be transferred from one bacterium to another, or from one bacterial species to related group, by means of plasmids or transposons that gain entry to the cell.

Methods to counter the resistance that bacteria have developed include the addition of beta-lactamase inhibitors to extended-spectrum penicillins, alteration of cephalosporin side chains to produce new generations of the drug with broader activity, and pairing two drugs to enhance the antimicrobial effect (e.g., sulfamethoxazole with trimethoprim).

17.13A PENICILLINS

MECHANISM OF ACTION

Penicillin is bactericidal, and its mechanism of action is interrupting cell wall synthesis by preventing cross-binding of the peptidoglycan polymers needed for formation of the bacterial cell wall and binding with penicillin-binding proteins (PBPs) that are part of the cell wall synthesis process. The result is a weakened cell wall that that lyses, leading to cell death.

The basic form of penicillin involves a beta-lactam ring that is altered by substituting side chains. These substitutions allow modification of the drug's antimicrobial spectrum, absorption characteristics, and resistance to beta-lactamase deactivation.

The major way that bacteria develop resistance to the penicillins is via the bacterial production of beta-lactamases. Beta-lactamases destroy the beta-lactam ring by hydrolysis, preventing the antimicrobial activity by the agent. Some bacteria can prevent binding to the PBPs, by altered binding sites for the penicillins.

This resistance can be overcome by various methods. Changing the structure of the penicillin molecule so they are resistant to the effects of the beta-lactamases has resulted in the development of the extended-spectrum penicillins.

Penicillins can also be combined with other agents that block bacterial beta-lactamases, for example, amoxicillin plus clavulanic acid, ampicillin plus sulbactam, and piperacillin plus tazobactam. These agents bind irreversibly to many beta-lactamases, preventing hydrolytic activity against the beta-lactam ring.

NATURAL PENICILLINS

The natural penicillins include penicillin G and penicillin V potassium. Penicillin G is very unstable in stomach acid and must be given parenterally. Penicillin V potassium is more acid-stable and can be given orally.

The natural penicillins are active against gram-positive organisms such as streptococci, *Enterococcus faecalis*, and *Listeria monocytogenes*; and active against oral anaerobic species and *Fusobacterium* species. Most *S. aureus* isolates are resistant. With parenteral administration, the natural penicillins are effective against some gram-negative bacteria, such as *H. influenzae*, *Neisseria gonorrhoeae*, and *Treponema pallidum*.

AMINOPENICILLINS

The aminopenicillins include ampicillin and amoxicillin and have the same activity as the natural penicillins against susceptible gram-positive organisms, plus coverage of selected gram-negative bacilli, including Enterobacteriaceae. Amoxicillin/clavulanic acid and ampicillin/sulbactam have better coverage against *H. influenzae* and *Klebsiella* species than the natural penicillins and the aminopenicillins alone.

Ampicillin can be given parenterally or orally. Amoxicillin is the best absorbed of the oral penicillins. They are useful for the management of sinusitis/bronchitis, endocarditis, meningitis, susceptible UTI, and salmonellosis. Amoxicillin is acid-stable and its absorption, unlike ampicillin, is not affected by food.

PENICILLINASE-RESISTANT PENICILLINS

The penicillinase-resistant penicillins are resistant to hydrolysis by the lactamase produced by the staphylococci, and include nafcillin and oxacillin, which are parenteral formulations, and dicloxacillin, which is given orally. Methicillin is no longer available.

The penicillinase-resistant penicillins are effective against many of the same gram-positive organisms that the natural penicillins are effective against, but they lack significant activity against gram-negative or anaerobic organisms. They are useful against penicillin-resistant (methicillin-sensitive) *Staphylococcus* species.

ANTIPSEUDOMONAL PENICILLINS

The antipseudomonal penicillins are extended-spectrum penicillins and include the parenteral agents ticarcillin and piperacillin. Mezlocillin and carbenicillin are no longer available.

These agents are active against gram-positive bacteria, but also have more activity against gram-negative bacteria, including *Pseudomonas aeruginosa*. Additional gram-negative species that are treated by these agents include *H. influenzae*, *Serratia* species, and *Klebsiella* species.

The addition of clavulanic acid, sulbactam, or tazobactam increases the activity spectrum of the agent. They are typically active against the beta-lactamases produced by *H. influenzae*, *Moraxella catarrhalis*, and *S. aureus*. Their activity is variable against some gram-negative bacteria, including some species of *Pseudomonas*, *Enterobacter*, *E. coli*, *Klebsiella*, and *Serratia*.

ABSORPTION/ELIMINATION

Most penicillins can be absorbed via the oral route, but bioavailability varies considerably, and food may interfere with absorption. Penicillin V, amoxicillin, ampicillin, and dicloxacillin can be given orally, while the remaining penicillins are given intravenously due to instability in the acidic stomach environment or to achieve sustained therapeutic levels. Amoxicillin is the best absorbed of the oral penicillins and the least affected by a recent meal.

Penicillins are widely distributed throughout the body and therapeutic concentrations are achieved in tissues and secretions (e.g., joint, pleural, and pericardial fluids, and bile). Low concentrations are found in prostatic secretions, brain tissue, and intraocular fluid. CSF concentrations are very low when the meninges are normal, but with inflammation of the meninges may raise and can be increased even more with the coadministration of probenecid. Urine concentration is high due to renal clearance mechanisms.

Penicillins are excreted in the kidney by means of glomerular filtration and renal tubular secretion. Concurrent use of probenecid reduces the tubular secretion of the penicillins and decreases the volume of distribution, resulting in higher serum levels. While biliary excretion is most important for antipseudomonal penicillins and nafcillin, all penicillins are excreted to some degree in the bile.

Dose adjustment is not needed with mild renal insufficiency, except with ticarcillin. If the creatinine clearance is <50 mL/min, then dosage adjustments of parenteral penicillins should be made to avoid excess serum levels. Nafcillin undergoes extensive hepatic metabolism, and the dosage must be adjusted for severe renal and hepatic insufficiency.

SIDE EFFECTS

These drugs are usually well tolerated, but GI disturbances may occur with all oral penicillins.

Allergy to any of the penicillins is the only absolute contraindication to its use. The percentage of individuals with an IgE-mediated allergic reaction is around 10%, with penicillin-induced anaphylaxis death rate estimates very low at 0.002% of the general population.[202]

Other rare reactions include serum sickness, exfoliative dermatitis, and Stevens-Johnson syndrome. The major determinant of the immunologic reaction is the similarity in the side chain of first-generation cephalosporins and penicillins, not the beta-lactam structure, with the reaction nearing zero in third-generation cephalosporins.

Penicillins may cause rare hematologic reactions such as neutropenia due to reversible bone marrow suppression and abnormal platelet aggregation, particularly with ticarcillin. Other rare reactions include hepatitis, seizures, interstitial nephritis, and hypokalemia due to local effects in the renal tubules.

DRUG INTERACTIONS

The penicillins should not be given concurrently with tetracycline or other bacteriostatic agents. Penicillin works in cells that are actively synthesizing cell wall components, and if metabolism is prevented by a bacteriostatic agent, then the actions of penicillin may be impaired. The antipseudomonal penicillins also may affect warfarin metabolism. Therefore, the prothrombin time and international normalized ratio (INR) should be monitored.

17.13B CEPHALOSPORINS

MECHANISM OF ACTION

The cephalosporins are beta-lactams in which the beta-lactam ring is joined to a dihydrothiazine ring. The mechanism of action is through inhibition of bacterial cell wall synthesis by blocking the transpeptidases and other penicillin-binding proteins involved in the synthesis and cross-linking of peptidoglycan.

Resistance to cephalosporins results from changes in the penicillin-binding proteins that prevent cephalosporins from binding to them, and from the production of extended-spectrum beta-lactamases that deactivate the drug. An additional source of resistance noted in gram-negative bacteria is the alteration in the cell-membrane porins that normally allow passage of the cephalosporins.

PHARMACOKINETICS

The cephalosporins are classified based on chemical structure and pharmacologic activities. The most common classification system groups the cephalosporins into generations based on antimicrobial coverage.

FIRST-GENERATION CEPHALOSPORINS

The first-generation cephalosporins, including cefazolin, cephalexin, and cefadroxil, are most active against aerobic gram-positive cocci. They are often used for skin infections caused by *S. aureus* and *Streptococcus* and for susceptible UTIs. They have activity against *E. coli* and some activity against *H. influenzae* and *Klebsiella* species. Because of limited gram-negative coverage they are not first-line agents for infections that are caused by gram-negative bacteria.

SECOND-GENERATION CEPHALOSPORINS

The second-generation cephalosporins, cefprozil, cefuroxime, cefaclor, cefoxitin, and cefotetan, have increased activity against gram-negative organisms *Moraxella*, *Neisseria*, and *Shigella*. These drugs are used primarily for respiratory tract infections because they are better against some strains of beta-lactamase-producing *H. influenzae*. Cefoxitin and cefotetan, which are included in this group although they are technically cephamycins, also have more coverage against anaerobic bacteria.

THIRD-GENERATION CEPHALOSPORINS

The third-generation cephalosporins, cefdinir, cefditoren, cefixime, cefotaxime, ceftazidime, ceftibuten, cefpodoxime, and ceftriaxone, have increased activity and broader spectrum activity against gram-negative organisms, including *Neisseria* species, *M. catarrhalis*, *Klebsiella*, and other Enterobacteriaceae. Ceftriaxone has the best activity against gram-positive cocci, specifically *S. pneumoniae* and methicillin-sensitive *S. aureus*. Ceftazidime is active against *P. aeruginosa*. These drugs are useful for more severe community-acquired respiratory, intra-abdominal, and UTIs and for nosocomial infections.

FOURTH-GENERATION CEPHALOSPORINS

Cefepime is a fourth-generation cephalosporin because it has good activity against both gram-positive and gram-negative bacteria, including *P. aeruginosa* and many Enterobacteriaceae. The gram-negative and anaerobic coverage makes cefepime useful for intra-abdominal infections, respiratory tract infections, and skin infections.

FIFTH-GENERATION CEPHALOSPORINS

Ceftaroline is an advanced-generation cephalosporin used in the treatment of community-acquired bacterial pneumonia and bacterial skin and soft-tissue infections. It exerts its antimicrobial effect by binding to PCP and inhibiting cell wall synthesis. It also has a high affinity for the penicillin-binding protein 2a, which is associated with resistance to methicillin. Because of this it is highly active against methicillin-sensitive and resistant strains of *S. aureus* and against multidrug-resistant *S. pneumoniae*. It is ineffective for *P. aeruginosa*, and its activity against Enterobacteriaceae is variable.

ABSORPTION/ELIMINATION

The orally administered cephalosporins include cefaclor, cefadroxil, cephalexin, cefprozil, cefuroxime axetil, cefixime, cefpodoxime proxetil, ceftibuten, and cefdinir, and are absorbed rapidly. Cephalexin, cefadroxil, cefaclor, cefixime, ceftibuten, and cefdinir are absorbed from the GI tract by active transport in the small intestine. Cefuroxime and cefpodoxime are passively absorbed. Once absorbed into the cells lining the small intestine, they are hydrolyzed and then excreted into the bloodstream as active cephalosporins.

Depending on the drugs the presence of food or antacids may increase or decrease the absorption. Cefuroxime and cefpodoxime have increased absorption when taken with food, while cefaclor, cefadroxil, and cephalexin have slowed absorption when taken with food. Cefixime, cefprozil, and ceftibuten are not affected by the presence of food.

There is extensive distribution of the cephalosporins into body tissues and fluids. Cephalosporins cross the placenta, found in synovial fluid, bile, and urine. Most cephalosporins do not cross into the CSF in sufficient concentration to be used in the treatment of meningitis, except cefuroxime, cefotaxime, ceftriaxone, cefepime, and ceftaroline, which all have good penetration into the CSF.

Most cephalosporins are eliminated by the kidney, except for cefixime, half of which is excreted in the urine and the other half excreted in the bile.

SIDE EFFECTS

Cephalosporins are relatively well tolerated. The most common complaints are GI upset, including nausea, vomiting, or diarrhea. Thrombophlebitis can occur with IV administration. Allergic reaction is uncommon with anaphylaxis being rare. Cross-sensitivity with true penicillin allergy is infrequent and occurs most often with the first-generation cephalosporins. If a patient develops urticaria, anaphylaxis, or angioedema with a penicillin or cephalosporin, use of any cephalosporin should be avoided.

Nephrotoxicity is uncommon. Some cephalosporins, such as cefotetan, contain the methylthiotetrazole (MTT) side chain and may induce a disulfiram-like reaction with alcohol ingestion. Symptoms include flushing, tachycardia, nausea and vomiting, diaphoresis, dyspnea, hypotension, and confusion.

Ceftriaxone has been associated with cholelithiasis and cholestatic hepatitis due to precipitation in the bile. Rare reactions include hematologic toxicity with resultant eosinophilia, thrombocytopenia, and leukopenia, all of which resolve after stopping treatment. Hypoprothrombinemia may occur with cephalosporins with the MTT side chain because of interference with the synthesis of vitamin-K-dependent clotting factors. False positive glucosuria testing with a copper reduction test (Clinitest) may occur with many cephalosporins.

17.13C CARBAPENEMS

MECHANISM OF ACTION

Carbapenems, bactericidal beta-lactam antibiotics, inhibit mucopeptide synthesis in the bacterial cell wall by binding to penicillin-binding proteins, leading to lysis and cell death. Bacterial resistance may occur due to a specific beta-lactamase that affects carbapenems and through a mutation that results in the absence of the outer membrane porin, thus not allowing transport of the drug into the cell.

PHARMACOKINETICS

Imipenem and ertapenem have a wide antimicrobial spectrum with excellent activity against anaerobic bacteria, including *Bacteroides* species; cover many gram-positive cocci, such as *Staphyloccus species* that are methicillin-susceptible and *Streptococcus*; as well as many gram-negative bacteria. Meropenem has greater activity against gram-negative bacteria, which are not affected by most beta-lactamases.

Imipenem and ertapenem are used in UTIs, pneumonia, intra-abdominal infections, and skin and soft-tissue infections. Meropenem is used for the treatment of intra-abdominal infections, skin and skin structure infections, and meningitis in patients older than 3 months of age.

ABSORPTION/ELIMINATION

Due to instability in stomach acid, imipenem/cilastatin, meropenem, and ertapenem are given parenterally. Imipenem is combined with cilastatin, which inhibits dehydropeptidase I in the proximal renal tubular cells. Dehydropeptidase I inactivates imipenem by hydrolysing the beta-lactam ring, so the addition of cilastatin allows increased levels of imipenem in the urine and prevents the production of nephrotoxic metabolites.

Meropenem is well distributed in body tissues and fluids, including the CSF. Imipenem/cilastatin and ertapenem are distributed throughout body tissues, but with only low concentrations in the CSF.

Imipenem/cilastatin is mainly excreted in the urine. Meropenem is excreted unchanged into the urine by means of glomerular filtration and tubular secretion. Ertapenem is metabolized by hydrolysis of the beta-lactam ring, and both the metabolite and parent drug are excreted in the urine.

The carbapenems require dosage adjustment in patients with renal insufficiency, but no change in dose is necessary for patients with hepatic insufficiency.

SIDE EFFECTS

The carbapenems are generally well tolerated. Occasional reactions include nausea and vomiting, phlebitis at the infusion site, elevation of liver enzymes, leukopenia, and seizures. The risk of seizures is higher in patients with underlying central nervous system disease and in patients with renal disease. Hypersensitivity reactions may occur, and the degree of cross-sensitivity with penicillins is low. Carbapenems should be used with caution in patients allergic to the carbapenems or penicillins.

DRUG INTERACTIONS

There are few drug interactions associated with the carbapenems. Ertapenem cannot be infused with dextrose or other medications. Meropenem reduces valproic acid levels.

17.13D MONOBACTAMS

MECHANISM OF ACTION

Aztreonam inhibits mucopeptide synthesis in the bacterial cell wall by binding to the penicillin-binding proteins of gram-negative bacteria, leading to cell lysis and death. Aztreonam is resistant to most beta-lactamases.

PHARMACOKINETICS

Aztreonam does not have activity against gram-positive or anaerobic bacteria and is used as an alternative therapy for gram-negative bacterial infections, including *P. aeruginosa* and *Klebsiella*, that are resistant to the first-line beta-lactams or carbapenems. Aztreonam is used in pneumonia, soft-tissue infections, UTIs, and intra-abdominal and pelvic infections caused by gram-negative aerobic bacteria.

Parenteral administration is the only route of delivery and IV. The drug is widely distributed in body tissues and fluids, including inflamed meningeal tissue. Aztreonam is mainly excreted in the urine as an unchanged drug. Doses must be adjusted for renal insufficiency based on glomerular filtration rate.

SIDE EFFECTS

Adverse reactions include elevated liver enzymes and transient eosinophilia. Less common reactions include phlebitis at the infusion site, rash, diarrhea, and nausea.

Patients with penicillin and cephalosporin allergy can typically tolerate aztreonam. Aztreonam is contraindicated in patients with prior allergic reactions to it or to any component of the formulation, such as with ceftazidime.

17.13E AMINOGLYCOSIDES

MECHANISM OF ACTION

The basic structure of the aminoglycosides is an aminocyclitol ring and the various members of this group vary based on the glycosidic linkages and side groups.

The aminoglycosides have two effects on the bacterial cell that result in cell death. They inhibit protein synthesis by binding to the 30S subunit of the ribosome, causing miscoding and termination. These medications also bind negative charges in the outer phospholipid membrane, displacing the cations that link the phospholipids causing cell wall disruption and leakage of cell contents.

While aminoglycoside resistance is rare, it can develop due to three mechanisms. First, involves modification of the aminoglycoside molecule by enzymes produced by some bacteria. After the aminoglycoside is altered, it cannot bind as well to the ribosomes. The genes that encode for these enzymes are carried on plasmids, allowing rapid transfer of resistance between bacteria. Second, the binding site for aminoglycosides on the rRNA of the ribosome may also be altered, reducing binding. Third, mutations that cause reduced uptake of aminoglycosides have been documented.

PHARMACOKINETICS

The aminoglycosides, gentamicin, tobramycin, and amikacin, are used in the treatment of aerobic gram-negative bacilli, such as *Klebsiella* species, *Enterobacter*, and *P. aeruginosa*. There is no activity against anaerobes and gram-positive organisms, so combination therapy with a beta-lactam, vancomycin, or other agents active against gram-positive organisms and anaerobes is needed. Aminoglycosides are indicated for infections caused by susceptible organisms of the urinary tract, respiratory tract, skin and soft tissues, and sepsis due to gram-negative aerobic bacilli.

Aminoglycosides have no oral absorption and require parenteral administration. They can be given directly into pleural and peritoneal cavities are used to treat infections in these locations. Tobramycin is particularly useful for treatment of recurrent *Pseudomonas* infection in patients with cystic fibrosis and can be administered by aerosolized inhalation to facilitate optimal local antimicrobial effect.

Aminoglycosides are relatively insoluble in lipid, so the volume of distribution is lower in obese patients. They have poor distribution in bile, aqueous humor, bronchial secretions, sputum, and the CSF.

Aminoglycosides are excreted unchanged by the kidneys. In renal failure, the dosage must be carefully adjusted based on glomerular filtration rate and measured serum levels. Serum drug levels should be monitored in all patients with reduced renal function. There is no dose reduction needed in liver failure, as there is no hepatic metabolism of these agents.

SIDE EFFECTS

The most common adverse effect is renal failure, which is typically reversible when the drug is stopped. Renal tubular toxicity decreases blood flow to the kidneys and reducing glomerular filtration rate. While there is no hepatic metabolism, concurrent liver disease increases the likelihood of the development of renal failure.

Vestibular and auditory impairment may develop during treatment with aminoglycosides, but there are rare. These effects are usually reversible. If aminoglycoside therapy is to be >5 to 7 days, baseline testing of auditory function should be performed and monitored during treatment.

Due to curare-like effect, neuromuscular blockage has also been observed. Aminoglycosides may aggravate muscle weakness in patients with disorders, such as myasthenia gravis and Parkinson disease.

Hypersensitivity reactions are rare, but rash, fever, urticaria, angioneurotic edema, and eosinophilia may occur. Bronchospasm has been noted with tobramycin inhalation solution.

The aminoglycosides are contraindicated in patients with hypersensitivity to the drug. Streptomycin also contains metabisulfite and should be avoided if the patient is allergic to sulfites.

DRUG INTERACTIONS

There are numerous drug interactions with aminoglycosides. Nephrotoxicity may increase with administration of other drugs that are nephrotoxic or in patients receiving loop diuretics. Respiratory depression may occur if aminoglycosides are given with nondepolarizing muscle relaxants. Gentamicin may also cause increased serum digoxin levels.

17.13F MACROLIDES

MECHANISM OF ACTION

The macrolides are bacteriostatic, inhibiting protein synthesis by binding at the 50S ribosomal unit and by blocking transpeptidation and translocation.

Many bacteria resistant to the penicillins are resistant to erythromycin. Resistance may result from decreased permeability of the cell membrane or from an increase in active efflux of the drug by incorporating a transporter protein into the cell wall; mutations of the 50S ribosomal receptor site may also develop preventing binding of the erythromycin; and bacterial enzymes have been described that may deactivate erythromycin.

Many strains of *H. influenzae* are resistant to erythromycin but are susceptible to a combination of erythromycin plus a sulfonamide. The combination of erythromycin ethylsuccinate and sulfisoxazole is useful in treating acute otitis media in children older than 2 months of age.

PHARMACOKINETICS

Erythromycin has a wide spectrum of activity against gram-positive bacteria including the *Streptococcus* species. Erythromycin is a second-line agent for gram-negative bacteria, such as *H. influenzae* and *M. catarrhalis*. Macrolides provide coverage of atypical bacteria, such as *Mycoplasma* and *Chlamydia*, and some spirochetes and mycobacteria. Macrolides are indicated for upper respiratory tract infections, such as sinusitis, otitis media, pharyngitis, and bronchitis. They are also useful in the treatment of pertussis, Legionnaires, disease, and diphtheria.

Erythromycin base is placed in enteric-coated tablets or capsules to protect the drug since it is deactivated by gastric acid. The drug is absorbed in the duodenum. Eating may slow absorption. Erythromycin may also be given intravenously.

Clarithromycin and azithromycin have excellent absorption after oral dosing. Clarithromycin may be given with food, but azithromycin absorption may be delayed in the presence of food in the stomach.

All macrolides have extensive tissue distribution, with decreased penetration into the brain tissue and the CSF. Erythromycin and azithromycin are primarily excreted unchanged into the bile. Clarithromycin is excreted in the bile and in the urine.

Macrolide doses may need to be reduced in the presence of severe hepatic insufficiency. Azithromycin and clarithromycin doses may have to be reduced in severe renal failure.

SIDE EFFECTS

Serious side effects are rare, and milder side effects are common. Erythromycin stimulates GI motility and may cause abdominal cramping, diarrhea, nausea, and vomiting. Other side effects include hepatic dysfunction with or without jaundice, reversible hearing loss when given in high doses or in the presence of renal insufficiency, and IV erythromycin may prolong the QT interval and ventricular tachycardia may occur.

Clarithromycin may cause nausea, diarrhea, abnormal taste, dyspepsia, and headache.

Allergic reactions to macrolides are rare but may include rash and eosinophilia. The drugs are contraindicated in patients with known hypersensitivity to the macrolides.

DRUG INTERACTIONS

Drug interactions are numerous. Erythromycin and clarithromycin are inhibitors of the cytochrome P450 enzyme system (CYP3A4). If given with a drug that is primarily metabolized by CYP3A, the drug serum levels may be increased and/or prolonged. Erythromycin and clarithromycin are contraindicated with concurrent use of cisapride, pimozide, astemizole, or terfenadine. Serum levels of theophylline, cyclosporine, digoxin, ergotamine, carbamazepine, benzodiazepines, warfarin, amiodarone, and tacrolimus may also be affected by concurrent administration with erythromycin and clarithromycin.

Azithromycin is not likely to interact with drugs metabolized by CYP3A4.

17.13G QUINOLONES

MECHANISM OF ACTION

Quinolones cause bacterial cell death by inhibiting DNA synthesis by inhibiting DNA gyrase and DNA topoisomerase, enzymes that mediate DNA supercoiling, transcription, and repair.

Bacterial resistance develops because of spontaneous mutations that change the binding sites for quinolones on the DNA gyrase and the DNA topoisomerase and mutations that decrease the ability of quinolones to cross the cell membrane.

PHARMACOKINETICS

The quinolones are active against many gram-positive cocci, gram-negative bacilli, and atypical bacteria, such as *Legionella* and *Mycoplasma*. Quinolone activity against streptococci and anaerobes is poor, except for moxifloxacin, which has better coverage for anaerobes. Gram-negative coverage includes *Campylobacter*, *Enterobacter*, *E. coli*, *H. influenzae*, *Klebsiella*, *Salmonella typhi*, *Shigella*, and *Vibrio cholerae*. Indications include UTIs, nongonococcal infections of the urethra and cervix, pneumonia, sinusitis, soft tissue infections, and prostatitis. Ciprofloxacin is indicated for postexposure prophylaxis for anthrax, and levofloxacin can be used in the treatment of inhalation anthrax infection. Absorption of quinolones is excellent with oral administration and serum levels are equal to those achieved with IV usage. They are distributed well throughout all tissues, including the prostate.

Clearance mechanisms vary with the quinolones. Levofloxacin and ofloxacin are cleared by renal excretion with minimal hepatic clearance. Moxifloxacin is mainly excreted nonrenally and is metabolized in the liver to an inactive metabolite. Norfloxacin, ciprofloxacin, and gemifloxacin have mixed routes of elimination. Norfloxacin has some hepatic metabolism to active metabolites; the metabolites and parent drug are excreted by the kidney. Ciprofloxacin dose is excreted renally and in the bile after hepatic metabolism. Gemifloxacin is excreted in the feces and in the urine.

SIDE EFFECTS

The most common side effect with the quinolones is GI upset. Less common side effects include headache, insomnia, dizziness, peripheral neuropathy, tendon rupture, elevated liver enzymes, and interstitial nephritis. Hematologic toxicities have occurred rarely, including hemolytic anemia, aplastic anemia, and agranulocytosis.

Allergic reactions are not common; they range from a rash to severe reactions, such as Stevens-Johnson syndrome. Severe hypoglycemia has been reported with concurrent treatment with glyburide and ciprofloxacin. Peripheral neuropathy is associated with the use of oral or injectable fluoroquinolones.

DRUG INTERACTIONS

Drug interactions are common. Antacids decrease the absorption of these agents. Iron and other cation supplements cause quinolone-cation complexes and impair absorption. Concurrent use of nonsteroidal anti-inflammatory drugs appears to increase the risk of seizures.

Theophylline, phenytoin, warfarin, and mexiletine levels may be elevated in patients concurrently treated with ciprofloxacin.

17.13H SULFONAMIDES

MECHANISM OF ACTION

Sulfonamides are bacteriostatic and competitive antagonists of para-aminobenzoic acid (PABA). The sulfonamides inhibit dihydropteroate synthase from using PABA to synthesize dihydropteroic acid, a precursor of folic acid. This lack of folic acid intermediates results in impaired synthesis of nucleotides. Bacteria that use preformed folate are not susceptible to the bacteriostatic action.

Bacterial resistance to sulfonamides is common. Resistance is due to mutations that result in additional production of PABA or changes in the enzyme binding sites for sulfonamides.

Bacterial activity against potentially resistant strains is improved with the addition of trimethoprim. Trimethoprim is a competitive inhibitor of dihydrofolate reductase, another enzyme active in the synthesis of folate.

PHARMACOKINETICS

The sulfonamides can be divided into groups based on absorption and excretion characteristics. They are classified as short to medium-acting agents, agents limited to activity in the GI tract, and topical agents.

SHORT-TO MEDIUM-ACTING SULFONAMIDES

The short-to medium-acting agents include sulfisoxazole, sulfamethoxazole, and sulfadiazine. Sulfisoxazole is metabolized to *N*-acetylsulfisoxazole and both are excreted in the urine. Sulfisoxazole is indicated for uncomplicated UTI and chloroquine-resistant malaria. Sulfamethoxazole is combined with trimethoprim and used for *Pneumocystis jirovecii* prophylaxis and treatment, upper respiratory tract infections, and UTIs. The only indication for sulfadiazine is toxoplasmosis.

LIMITED TO GASTROINTESTINAL TRACT ACTIVITY

The agents limited to the GI tract are poorly absorbed and are used for reducing bacterial flora in the bowel before surgery. The only agent in this class is sulfasalazine, which is used in the treatment of ulcerative colitis.

TOPICAL AGENTS

The topical sulfonamides include mafenide acetate and silver sulfadiazine, which are used in the treatment of burns. Mafenide is used less often because it may cause a metabolic acidosis because of carbonic anhydrase inhibition. Another topical agent is sulfacetamide, used in ophthalmic and lotion formulations. Topical sulfonamides may be absorbed systemically, and if large burn areas are treated, absorption may be significant.

ABSORPTION/ELIMINATION

The sulfonamides are quickly absorbed after administration unless they have been altered to stay in the lumen of the intestine. After absorption, they are acetylated in the liver into a toxic but inactive form. This acetylated form is excreted in the urine, with a small amount excreted in bile. These drugs are widely distributed throughout body tissue and fluids, including the CSF and peritoneal fluid.

The sulfonamides undergo acetylation and glucuronidation in the liver. Both the unchanged and metabolized forms are excreted in the urine through glomerular filtration and renal tubular secretion. Dosage and frequency of administration must be adjusted in renal failure.

SIDE EFFECTS

Allergic reactions are common, and symptoms include rash and itching. Other side effects include nausea, vomiting, diarrhea, headache, and photosensitivity. Severe hypersensitivity reactions, including vasculitis, anaphylaxis, serum sickness, and Stevens-Johnson syndrome, may occur but are rare.

Sulfonamide ophthalmic preparations may cause local irritation. Systemic reactions may develop during treatment with ophthalmic and topical preparations of sulfonamides due to systemic absorption.

Very rare blood dyscrasias can occur and include agranulocytosis, aplastic anemia, thrombocytopenia, and hemolytic anemia.

Sulfonamides are contraindicated in patients who are known to be allergic to sulfa drugs.

DRUG INTERACTIONS

Warfarin, phenytoin, and sulfonylureas may be potentiated due to displacement of the drugs from serum albumin by the sulfonamides. Cyclosporine levels may be decreased.

17.13I TETRACYCLINES

MECHANISM OF ACTION

Tetracyclines bind to the 30S ribosomal subunit, blocking the binding of aminoacyl transfer-RNA, which results in the inhibition of protein synthesis.

Bacterial resistance results from mutations that either prevent entrance of tetracyclines into the cell or increase the export of tetracycline out of the cell.

The tetracyclines have a broad spectrum of activity including aerobic gram-positive and gram-negative bacilli; atypical bacteria such as *Chlamydia trachomatis*, *Chlamydia psittaci*, and *Mycoplasma pneumoniae*; and spirochetes, such as *Borrelia burgdorferi*. Tetracycline is second-line for *T. pallidum*. It is used in the treatment of rickettsial infections, typhus, RMSF, trachoma, nongonococcal urethritis, and lymphogranuloma venereum.

Resistance to tetracyclines is high among common gram-positive and gram-negative pathogens. Because of this the use of tetracyclines is limited. The primary indication is for atypical infections and zoonoses.

The tetracyclines may be divided into three groups, short-acting group, intermediate-acting group, and long-acting group, based on their pharmacokinetic traits. The varying half-lives are the result of different rates of renal excretion.

SHORT-ACTING TETRACYCLINES

Tetracycline is the only short-acting tetracycline. Because of the short half-life frequent dosing, every 6 hours for most indications, is needed.

INTERMEDIATE-ACTING TETRACYCLINES

The only intermediate-acting agent available in the United States is demeclocycline. Demeclocycline is no longer used as an antibiotic but rather has been used as an off-label drug to treat the syndrome of inappropriate antidiuretic hormone secretion (SIADH).

LONG-ACTING TETRACYCLINES

The long-acting tetracycline agents are doxycycline and minocycline. The major difference between the long-acting and the short-acting agents is the dosing frequency. The spectrum of bacterial coverage and indications are basically the same.

ABSORPTION/ELIMINATION

All tetracyclines are well absorbed after an oral dose in the fasting state. Doxycycline and minocycline are also well absorbed when taken with food.

The tetracyclines are well distributed throughout body tissues and fluids; distribution in the CSF is adequate for the treatment of some infections. Because of this excellent tissue penetration, the drugs crosses into the dentin, where the drug permanently chelates with the calcium.

Most of a tetracycline dose is excreted unchanged into the urine by glomerular filtration, with some biliary excretion.

TABLE 17.39 Antibiotic Selection for Common Bacterial Pathogens—Gram-Positive Cocci and Anaerobes

	Gram-Positive Cocci						Anaerobes		
	Streptococci		Staphylococci						
	S. pneumoniae *S. pyogenes* *S. virdans*	*Entercocci* (Group D strep)	*S. aureus*	*S. epidermidis*	MRSA Community-Acquired	MRSA Hospital-Acquired	Above Diaphragm (Peptostreptoccal)	Below Diaphragm (*Bacteroides*)	*Clostridioides difficile*
Penicillin									
Penicillin V/G	X	X					X		
Amoxicillin/ampicillin	X	X					X		
Ampicillin									
Amoxicillin-clavulanate	X	X	X				X		
Piperacillin-tazobactam	X	X	X				X	X	
Cloxacillin			X	X					
Penicillin G									
Cephalosporins									
Cefazolin/cephalexin	X		X				X		
Cefuroxime	X		X				X		
Cefoxitin/cefotetan	X		X				X	X	
Ceftriaxone/cefotaxime	X		X				X		
Cefixime	X								
Cefepime	X		X				X		
Ceftazidime									
Carbapenems									
Ertapenem	X						X	X	
Meropenem/imipenem							X	X	
Macrolides									
Clarithromycin/ azithromycin	X		X						
Erythromycin	X		X						
Azithromycin									

Tetracyclines									
Tetracycline/doxycycline	X		X		X		X		
Tigecycline	X	X	X	X	X	X	X	X	
Quinolones									
Levofloxacin/ moxifloxacin	X						X		
Ciprofloxacin/ norfloxacin									
Moxifloxacin								X	
Ciprofloxacin									
Aminoglycosides									
Gentamicin/tobramycin/ amikacin/colistin									
Glycopeptides									
Vancomycin/linezolid/ daptomycin	X	X	X	X	X	X	X		
Vancomycin									X
Clindamycin	X		X	X	X		X	X	
Trimethoprim-sulfamethoxazole			X		X				
Chloramphenicol	X						X	X	
Metronidazole							X	X	X
Nitrofurantoin/ frosfomycin (bladder infection)		X							
Rifampin			X	X	X	X			
Fidaxomicin									X

TABLE 17.40 Antibiotic Selection for Common Bacterial Pathogens—Gram Negative Bacilli, Gram-Negative Cocci, and Atypicals

	Gram-Negative Bacilli				Gram-Negative Cocci		Atypicals		
	Non-Beta-lactamase *Escherichia coli Klebsiella Haemophilus*	Beta-lactamase *Escherichia coli Klebsiella Haemophilus*	*Serratia Proteus Acinetobacter Citrobacter Enterobacter*	*Pseudomonas aeruginosa*	*Neisseria meningitidis*	*Neisseria gonorrhoeae*	*Mycoplasma*	*Legionella*	*Chlamydia*
Penicillin									
Penicillin V/G									
Amoxicillin/ampicillin	X								
Ampicillin					X				
Amoxicillin-clavulanate	X	X	X						
Piperacillin-tazobactam	X	X	X	X	X				
Cloxacillin									
Penicillin G					X				
Cephalosporins									
Cefazolin/cephalexin	X								
Cefuroxime	X	X	X						
Cefoxitin/cefotetan	X	X	X						
Ceftriaxone/cefotaxime	X	X	X		X	X			
Cefixime	X	X	X			X			
Cefepime	X	X	X	X	X				
Ceftazidime	X	X	X	X	X				
Carbapenems									
Ertapenem	X	X	X						
Meropenem/imipenem	X	X	X	X	X				
Macrolides									
Clarithromycin/azithromycin	X*						X	X	
Erythromycin							X	X	X
Azithromycin						X			X

Tetracyclines									
Tetracycline/doxycycline	X*						X	X	X
Tigecycline	X	X	X				X	X	
Quinolones									
Levofloxacin/moxifloxacin	X	X	X				X	X	
Ciprofloxacin/norfloxacin	X	X	X	X	X				
Moxifloxacin									
Ciprofloxacin								X	
Aminoglycosides									
Gentamicin/tobramycin/ amikacin/colistin	X	X	X	X					
Glycopeptides									
Vancomycin/linezolid/ daptomycin									
Vancomycin									
Clindamycin									
Trimethoprim-sulfamethoxazole	X	X	X						
Chloramphenicol	X	X			X	X			
Metronidazole									
Nitrofurantoin/fosfomycin (bladder infection)	X	X							
Rifampin					X				
Fidaxomicin									

*only *H. influenzae*

Tetracycline should be avoided in the presence of renal insufficiency, because it accumulates rapidly in the serum in the presence of decreased renal function. Nonrenal mechanisms account in large part for excretion of doxycycline and minocycline. Doxycycline may be used in renal failure, as it will be excreted into the bile. Because tetracyclines have been known to cause hepatic toxicity, they should not be used in patients with hepatic insufficiency.

SIDE EFFECTS

Tetracyclines cause nausea, vomiting, and diarrhea. They cross into dentin leading to staining and deformity of the teeth in children younger than 8 years of age. Tetracyclines should not be used in children younger than 8 years of age because of the risk for tooth deformity. Rare side effects include photosensitivity, idiopathic intracranial hypertension, esophageal ulceration, and hepatotoxicity.

Minocycline is associated with vertigo, nausea, and vomiting. Prolonged use of minocycline may cause reversible discoloration of the fingernails, the sclerae, and the skin; and has been associated with a lupus-like reaction.

Allergic reactions to tetracyclines are not common but may range from mild rashes to anaphylaxis. Tetracyclines are contraindicated in patients with known hypersensitivity to any tetracyclines.

DRUG INTERACTIONS

There are many drug interactions with tetracyclines. Agents that alkalinize the urine will increase excretion of the tetracyclines. Metal cations, calcium, aluminum, zinc, magnesium, and iron, and bismuth decrease absorption. Drugs that induce hepatic enzymes decrease the half-life of doxycycline.

Concurrent use of oral contraceptives may make the contraceptive less effective. The effects of warfarin are increased. Digoxin effects may be increased because of changes in the bowel flora that are responsible for digoxin metabolism.

17.13J VANCOMYCIN

MECHANISM OF ACTION

Vancomycin is a glycopeptide antibiotic. Glycopeptides bind to peptides found in bacterial cell walls and disrupt peptidoglycan polymerization, imparting rigidity to the cell wall. Both gram-positive cocci and bacilli are highly susceptible to glycopeptides.

Vancomycin is used in the treatment of infections caused by MRSA, methicillin-resistant *S. epidermidis* (MRSE), and ampicillin-resistant enterococci. Oral vancomycin is used for the treatment of *C. difficile*-associated diarrhea/colitis.

Vancomycin is not absorbed by the intestinal tract and must be administered by IV infusion, except for the oral form used to treat *C. difficile*-associated diarrhea/colitis. Close monitoring of therapy is required to determine a safe, effective dosage regimen. A rapid infusion causes an uncomfortable generalized erythroderma called red man syndrome. The red man syndrome is a histamine-mediated flushing that occurs during or immediately following infusion and does not mandate discontinuation unless slowing the infusion rate fails to mitigate the reaction.

ABSORPTION/ELIMINATION

Vancomycin is cleared by the kidneys. Prolonged usage at high therapeutic serum levels is associated with nephrotoxicity and ototoxicity.

SIDE EFFECTS

Apart from the red man syndrome, vancomycin administration is well tolerated, and side effects are uncommon. Vancomycin is a good sensitizing agent and drug eruptions and drug fever are common. The incidence of vancomycin nephrotoxicity is low, and the exact mechanism is poorly understood. The nephrotoxicity is usually reversible when the drug is discontinued. Risk factors for nephrotoxicity include total daily dose more than 3–4 g, elevated trough serum vancomycin levels, preexisting renal disease, concomitant use of other nephrotoxic drugs, and duration of therapy longer than 1 week.

Reversible neutropenia, presumably from bone marrow toxicity, is sometimes seen in patients receiving prolonged vancomycin therapy. Oral vancomycin is not absorbed and thus imposes no risk of nephrotoxicity or ototoxicity.

17.13K LIPOGLYCOPEPTIDES

The glycopeptide analogues, lipoglycopeptides, have a greater potency against gram-positive bacteria with activity against vancomycin-resistant strains. Lipoglycopeptides must be administered intravenously. A lipophilic side chain prolongs the drug half-life and helps anchor them to the outer structure of the bacterial cell.

There are three lipoglycopeptides, telavancin, dalbavancin, and oritavancin, which are used in the treatment of acute bacterial skin and soft tissue infection. The side effect profile is mild and includes headache, nausea, pruritus, pain at injection site, and fever.

Antibiotic Selection

Tables 17.39 and 17.40 summarize antibiotic selection for common bacterial pathogens.

KNOWLEDGE CHECKS

1. Infections due to staphylococcal and streptococcal species often present with similar signs and symptoms. Compare and contrast staphylococcal and streptococcal infections.
2. Infectious diarrhea can be due to numerous bacterial, viral, and parasitic organisms. Develop a focused approach based on an understanding of the pathophysiology and presentation of the various diseases.
3. Compare and contrast the various viral exanthems.
4. Syphilis is known as the great imitator. Describe the various stages of syphilis including presentation, diagnosis, differential, diagnosis, and treatment.

5. *Candida* species are a common cause of infection in several areas of the body. Create a table outlining various sites of infection including presentation and treatment.
6. Compare and contrast the various dimorphic fungal infections.
7. OI are common in HIV-positive patients. Create a table outlining the various OI including presentation and treatment.

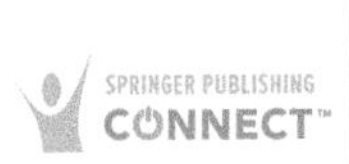

A robust set of instructor resources designed to supplement this text is located at **https://connect.springerpub.com/content/book/978-0-8261-8243-2.** Qualifying instructors may request access by emailing **textbook@springerpub.com.**

REFERENCES

The complete reference list for this chapter appears in the digital version of the chapter, accessible at https://connect.springerpub.com/content/book/978-0-8261-8243-2/chapter/ch17.

CHAPTER 18

PSYCHIATRY

STEPHANIE NEARY

LEARNING OBJECTIVES

- Describe the role of the *Diagnostic and Statistical Manual of Mental Disorders*, 5th edition (*DSM-5*) in recognizing, diagnosing, and treating medical health conditions. Use its criteria, along with clinical judgment, to diagnose psychiatric disorders in pediatric and adult patients.
- Compare and contrast the most common psychiatric disorders with regard to epidemiology, clinical presentation, diagnosis, and management.
- Create a treatment plan for a patient with a psychiatric disorder, including potentially further medical workup, therapy, medication management, and/or specialist referral.

INTRODUCTION

RACHEL BYRNE

Psychiatry is the branch of medicine focused on the diagnosis, treatment, and prevention of mental, emotional, and behavioral disorders.[1] People often associate *psychiatry* with a patient lying on a couch talking about their childhood. For much of the 20th century, the most common treatment of psychiatry disorders was via psychoanalysis (developed by Sigmund Freud), which stressed revealing a patient's unconscious thoughts and involved intensive, couch-based therapy.[2] In 1952, chlorpromazine was first used on a patient with mania, which paved the way for the "neurobiologic" basis of psychiatric illnesses. The field has greatly evolved and the psychiatric community now recognizes that mental health is influenced by a variety of factors including environmental experiences, genetics, epigenetics, and physical conditions.

Regardless of a PA's area of practice, they will encounter patients with mental health concerns, patients taking psychotropic medications, or patients with substance use disorders (SUDs). Depression is the number one cause of disability worldwide and suicide the second leading cause of death in 18- to 29-year-olds.[3] It is estimated that 20% to 40% of primary care office visits are related to mental health concerns.[4] Frequent users of the healthcare system are highly likely to have a comorbid or primary psychiatric diagnosis.[5] The opioid epidemic has surpassed motor vehicle collisions as a cause of death and alcohol-related deaths have doubled in the past 20 years.[6]

As a result of the lack of specialists in psychiatry, PAs are often tasked with treating their patients' conditions long term, or at least initiating treatment until a referral can happen. Options include medications, therapy, lifestyle modifications, and treatment of comorbid physical conditions.

18.1 ANXIETY DISORDERS

MICHAEL HIGBEE

OVERVIEW

Anxiety disorders are the most common mental illness in the United States, affecting over 40 million adults. In general, anxiety disorders are characterized by excessive worry and other related symptoms that occur on most days. An important distinction to note is the difference between anxiety and fear, a theme that will inevitably arise in clinical practice. Fear is elicited by a known threat that can potentially be harmful to an organism whereas anxiety is a response to a vague or unknown threat. Educating patients on this distinction can assist with their decision as to whether to pursue treatment. Anxiety disorders cause immense suffering in afflicted individuals and clinicians can have a significant impact on the lives of patients by providing proper treatment.

EPIDEMIOLOGY

Despite headlines in popular media, there is no convincing evidence to date that the prevalence of anxiety disorders is increasing. As hereditability of anxiety disorders is estimated at 30% to 50%, it is unlikely that rapid changes in prevalence would occur over a short time frame; however, increased acknowledgment and acceptance of anxiety disorders can lead to increased awareness and diagnosis. The female-male ratio of anxiety disorders is approximately 2:1. The peak age of onset is 11 years old; however, different subtypes of anxiety tend to manifest at different ages.[7] Up to 50% of people diagnosed with depression suffer from comorbid anxiety and a there is a high prevalence of comorbid SUD. The typical course of anxiety disorder consists of onset in childhood, adolescence, or early adulthood, followed by a peak during middle age with a gradual tapering off during older age.

It is estimated that only 50% of cases of anxiety are recognized and only one-third of recognized patients receive medical treatment.[8] One reason for lack of care is that patients with anxiety disorders feel a sense of shame and embarrassment and avoid seeking treatment. An exception to this is panic attacks, in which the patient may be convinced that they are suffering a myocardial infarction (MI) or other medical emergency and, as a result, are likely to be encountered in a medical setting or ED.

PATHOPHYSIOLOGY

The psychological concept of fear extinction is essential to understanding anxiety disorders. Known as Pavlovian fear extinction, this psychological principle has been demonstrated in both humans and animals. The more popularized example is that of a rat hearing a tone followed by receiving a shock, which subsequently conditions a fear response at the sound of the tone by itself. A lesser-known demonstration of this concept involves an infant and a rat in the 1920s. The infant was allowed to play with an innocent looking white rat, which the child can be seen enjoying. Afterward, the rat—which served as the conditioned stimulus—was taken away and multiple times reintroduced paired with a loud noise—which served as the unconditioned stimulus—causing the infant to cry. Eventually, the rat was again introduced without the loud noise; however, at the sight of the rat alone, the infant began to cry even in the absence of the loud noise.

In adults, a process of fear extinction should typically occur whereby a process of unlearning a fear gradually takes place (Figure 18.1). In the above example, the rat being reintroduced without the loud noise would cease to induce a fear response over time. This is thought to be mediated by the frontal lobe, which may inhibit the fight or flight structures in the deeper limbic system.[9] In anxiety disorder, it is as though the evolutionarily newer frontal cortex "screams" at the older limbic system that a given stimulus is harmless, but this latter system does not "hear" the scream (Figures 18.2). The malfunctioning of frontolimbic circuitry may underlie the pathogenesis of anxiety disorders.

The amygdala has received a lot of attention as the "seat" of fear and anxiety. As part of the limbic system, this structure seems to direct the fear response via outputs to other structures including the thalamus, hypothalamus, and

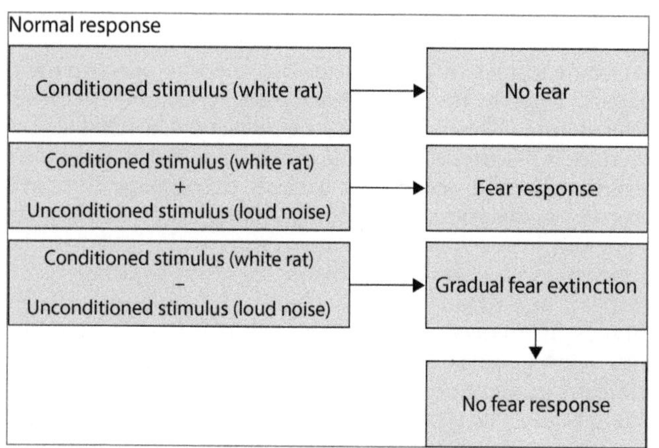

Figure 18.1 **Normal process of fear extinction.**

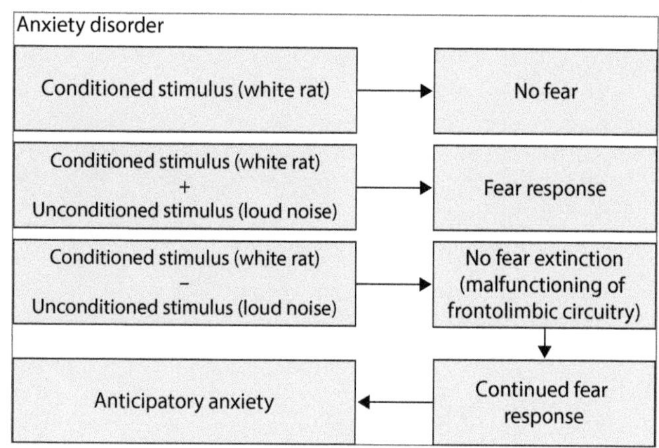

Figure 18.2 **Absence of fear extinction in anxiety disorder.**

sympathetic nervous system. This is akin to a dispatcher relaying the emergency details to the police, firefighters, and other relevant personnel so that they may respond. Under the direction of the amygdala via neuronal projections, the thalamus stimulates the brainstem to release norepinephrine and the sympathetic nervous system releases both epinephrine and norepinephrine. On the other hand, also under the direction of the amygdala, the hypothalamus secretes releasing hormones, eventually leading the adrenal glands to release epinephrine. Within milliseconds, this cascade results in increased heart rate, increased respiratory rate, vasoconstriction, decreased digestion, dilated pupils, muscle tension, urinary retention, sweating, tremor, and pallor or flushing (Figure 18.3).

Regarding anatomic differences in brain structures, decreases in the volume of the amygdala as well as gray matter changes have been found.[10]

Various neurotransmitters that have been implicated in anxiety disorders include gamma-aminobutyric acid (GABA), serotonin, epinephrine, and norepinephrine. The action of these neurotransmitters and their contribution to anxiety are listed below.

- **GABA:** Known as gamma-aminobutyric acid, GABA is the principal inhibitory neurotransmitter. GABA release slows down the firing of neurons and causes feelings of relaxation. GABA receptors are the target of benzodiazepines, such as Xanax and Valium, among others. Because of the effectiveness of benzodiazepines in the treatment of anxiety, it has been postulated that an abnormality of the GABA receptor contributes to the disorder.
- **Serotonin:** Known as 5-hydroxytryptamine or 5-HT, serotonin leads to feelings of calm and well-being. 5-HT may be stimulatory or inhibitory dependent upon type and location of actions. The amygdala is normally rich in 5-HT receptors. Serotonin action is the target of selective serotonin reuptake inhibitors (SSRIs), monoamine oxidase (MAO) inhibitors, tricyclic antidepressants (TCAs), and buspirone.
- **Epinephrine:** As both a neurotransmitter and a hormone, epinephrine is excitatory. Epinephrine is responsible for the fight or flight response. This action can be blocked by the use of beta blockers such as propranolol.
- **Norepinephrine:** As with epinephrine, norepinephrine is both a neurotransmitter and a hormone. Norepinephrine is excitatory and is involved with fear memory formation. This is the target of serotonin-norepinephrine reuptake inhibitors (SNRIs). As with epinephrine, the action of norepinephrine can also be blocked by beta blockers.

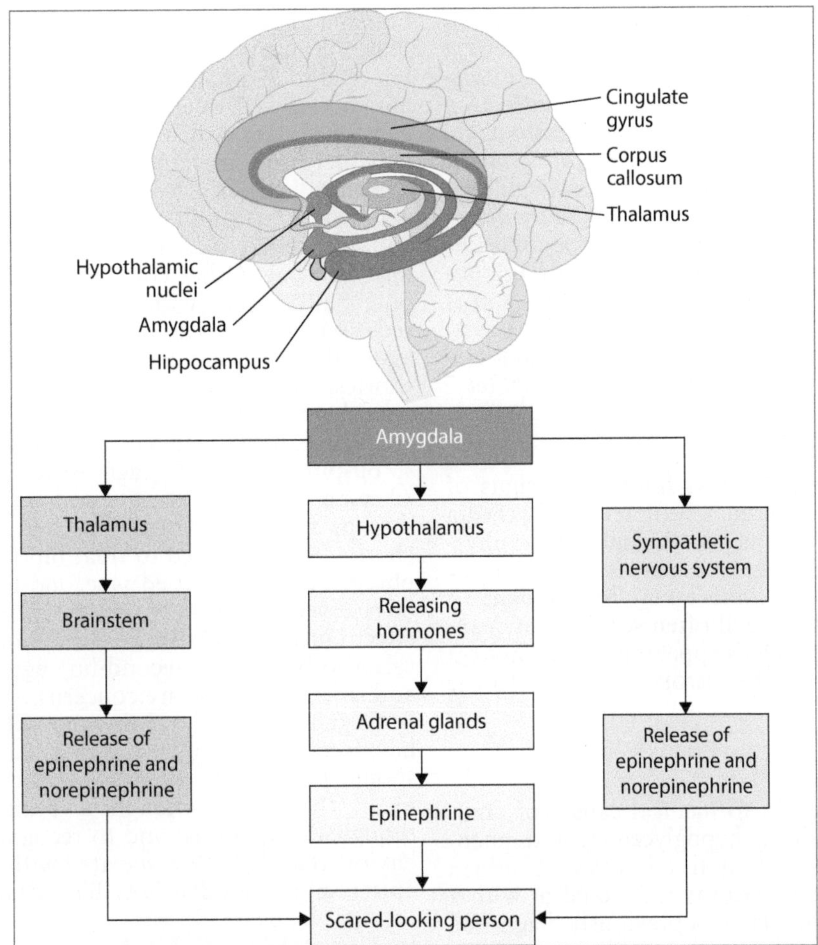

Figure 18.3 Diagram of brain structures resulting in scared-looking person.
(Source: Tkacs, NC, Compton PA, Pavone K. Nervous system. In: Tkacs, NC, Hermann LL, Johnson RL, eds. Advanced Physiology and Pathophysiology: Essentials for Clinical Practice. *Springer Publishing Company; 2021:543.)*

The root cause of anxiety disorders appears to be the result of complex genetic and environmental interactions, though the mechanisms are still poorly understood. The proper genetic blueprint for anxiety combined with early life stressors can result in a constant state of hypervigilance and physiologic arousal in the case of generalized anxiety disorder (GAD) or context dependent anxiety (e.g., social phobia).

The causes of anxiety can be best summarized to patients as having inherited a nervous system that seems to be easier to trigger through external stimuli and/or thoughts.

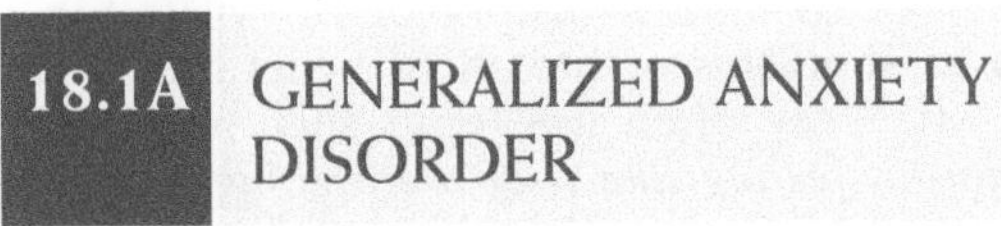

18.1A GENERALIZED ANXIETY DISORDER

MEDICAL HISTORY AND CLINICAL PRESENTATION

Patients with GAD tend to present in their late teens to early 30s. The patient will typically describe an underlying worry that occurs most of the day and is extremely difficult to control. The source of the worry may be difficult to pinpoint as opposed to specific phobias (SPs) for which the trigger is often easily identified. The patient may have a history of seeing a primary care clinician or specialist for a somatic complaint such as headaches, diarrhea, or abdominal pain. They are frequently told that their symptoms are that of an anxiety disorder; however, they may be reluctant to accept it as a diagnosis. Patients are more often female and family history is usually positive for an anxiety disorder in a first-degree relative.

SIGNS AND SYMPTOMS

GAD presents as excessive anxiety that occurs most days and is usually accompanied by physical symptoms such as frequent headaches, diarrhea, acid reflux/heartburn, muscle tension, tremor, increased heart rate, frequent urination, and sweating. Patients will describe subjective symptoms including irritability, fatigue, restlessness, poor concentration, and difficulty with sleep onset or maintenance. They will often show a preference or a cognitive bias toward seemingly threatening stimuli in the environment. A thorough history will often reveal that the anxiety interferes with multiple aspects of life.

Clinical Vignette

Mr. H is a 28-year-old male with no significant medical history who presents to his primary care clinician with a complaint of "heart palpitations" that have been ongoing several times a day for the last year. He has been to a cardiologist who performed a full workup that was negative for any cardiac disease. He has also been to a gastroenterologist for evaluation of loose bowel movements that were occurring multiple times throughout the day. He is convinced that a medical cause is the root of these symptoms. A careful history reveals that Mr. H has been having trouble with sleep onset, is often fatigued, and has difficulty concentrating. He describes worrying frequently about finances, job security, and having severe health problem despite no evidence that any of these aspects of his life are in danger. Mr. H's wife often complains that he is irritable. He tries to cope with this worry by playing sports and reading; however, he has trouble focusing during these leisurely activities and instead is overcome with anxious rumination. He reluctantly agrees to a trial of fluoxetine 5 mg stating that "I'll only start at a low dose because I usually get every side effect in the pamphlet."

PHYSICAL EXAMINATION

Patients with anxiety may present as fidgety and signs of muscle tension such as a tremor may be noted. Tachycardia and diaphoresis may also be clues to the underlying physiologic arousal. Pallor, flushing, and increased respiratory rate may also be found. Eye contact may be avoidant or shifty as patients with anxiety will often scan the environment for threats. Often, a patient's appearance and physical examination are normal and the history is the key to the diagnosis.

DIFFERENTIAL DIAGNOSIS

Consideration should be given to medical causes of anxiety including hyperthyroidism, hypoglycemia, and pheochromocytoma. This is particularly true in cases of sudden onset in a previously mentally healthy individual or with a change in character of the anxiety in a previously diagnosed patient. Substance use or withdrawal should also be ruled out. Common substances that can induce anxiety include steroids, thyroid replacement, asthma medications, stimulants, and caffeine.

DIAGNOSTIC STUDIES

No specific diagnostic studies are available to confirm GAD; however, a basic workup including complete blood count (CBC), comprehensive metabolic panel (CMP), and thyroid function tests can be considered to rule out alternative causes. Care should be taken to avoid ordering too many diagnostic studies as this can reinforce the patient's concern that an underlying medical cause is to blame.

EVALUATION

Multiple questionnaires are available to evaluate anxiety. The GAD-7 is a user friendly, widely available, and frequently used survey. The PHQ-9, a commonly used questionnaire for depression risk, should also be considered due to the common association of anxiety with depression.[11]

TREATMENT

Treatment of GAD should typically involve a combination of pharmacotherapy and psychotherapy. SSRIs and SNRIs are considered first-line treatments. SSRIs are recommended as initial medication because studies suggest that SSRIs are tolerated better than SNRIs.[12] Since efficacy has not been shown to be more favorable between one versus another medicine within the class of SSRIs, tolerability should be the first consideration. A "start low, go slow" approach works best and improves compliance. Patients should be counseled that side effects typically occur within the first 1 to 2 weeks but tend to dissipate after this time. Conversely, the benefits may take 2 to 4 weeks and sometimes up to 6 weeks to occur. Scheduling visits every 2 weeks during this time period may increase compliance.

Benzodiazepines, while very effective for anxiety, are best avoided or used minimally due to the addictive properties and long-term concerns such as potentially irreversible cognitive decline. Other concerns include increased tolerance, potentially severe withdrawal, and side effects including sedation and decreased reaction times. If use cannot be avoided, the lowest possible dose should be used for the shortest amount of time. Other medications that can be considered for as-needed use in place of benzodiazepines include pregabalin, beta blockers, hydroxyzine, and clonidine.

Buspirone, a 5-HT_{1A} agonist, can be tried alone or added to an existing treatment, and is considered a second-line therapy for GAD. Quetiapine and other atypical antipsychotics, typically used to treat bipolar disorder and schizophrenia, can also be used as second-line agents. These should be reserved for severe or refractory cases due to the high side effect burden. TCAs such as imipramine and clomipramine can also be used as second-line agents, though side effects and risk of overdose are concerns.

Cognitive behavioral therapy (CBT) has been shown to be effective in multiple studies as a treatment for GAD and should be used in conjunction with pharmacologic treatment. The patient is taught to evaluate and question their thoughts (cognitions) and to recognize and modify the behaviors that they are associated with. A list of certified therapists can be found at NACBT.ORG.

PATIENT EDUCATION

Patients should be educated on the causes and course of GAD. Helping patients understand the biologic roots of anxiety can assist in alleviating shame and increasing collaboration on a comprehensive treatment plan. Stress reduction, including regular exercise, meditation, journaling, and other activities tailored toward each patient, should be discussed.

18.1B PANIC DISORDER

MEDICAL HISTORY AND CLINICAL PRESENTATION

Patients with panic disorder tend to present in their early to mid-20s. They often have a history of ED visits for a complaint such as shortness of breath or belief they were experiencing a MI. They often use terms such as *a sense of impending doom, feeling like they were going crazy* or *having a heart attack*. Typically, they are unable to identify a specific trigger, although panic attacks can occasionally follow physical exertion, excitement, decreased sleep, or stimulant use (e.g., caffeine). The signs and symptoms of the panic attack will have a sudden onset with increasing intensity over several minutes, a peak within minutes to up to an hour, and a slow taper. Females are more likely to have panic disorder and a family history of panic attacks may be present. Life stressors, while not directly causing the panic attacks, may increase the risk of having one.

SIGNS AND SYMPTOMS

Patients with panic disorder describe some of the following symptoms, usually occurring spontaneously:

- Sense of impending doom
- Pounding feeling in the chest
- Shortness of breath
- Fear of death or loss of control
- Sweating
- Tremor
- Chills
- Chest pain or palpitations
- Headache
- Abdominal pain
- Nausea
- Dizziness, lightheadedness, or faintness
- A feeling of unreality
- Numbness and/or tingling, particularly around the mouth

Patients typically develop an anticipatory anxiety based on the fear of having another panic attack, which results in maladaptive patterns of avoidance or other behaviors thought to reduce the possibility of having another attack. For instance, patients may develop agoraphobia due to the constant worry of having a panic attack and not being able to escape to somewhere safe or familiar. Patients may also develop comorbid depression.

PHYSICAL EXAMINATION

In the midst of a panic attack, tachycardia, dyspnea, diaphoresis, tremor, and other signs of sympathetic activation may be seen in an otherwise healthy patient. A mental status examination (MSE) may show difficulty speaking and/or preoccupation with the fear of dying or "going crazy." Syncopal episodes may occur as well. It should be noted, however, that the clinician will more likely encounter the patient at a time when the panic attack has already occurred in the recent or remote past. As such, the diagnosis of panic disorder is usually based on history.

DIFFERENTIAL DIAGNOSIS

The symptoms of a panic attack can mimic those of a serious acute and life-threatening cause. As such, care should be taken to rule out a cardiovascular or pulmonary event such as an MI or exacerbation of asthma. Other common considerations include hypoglycemia, hyperthyroidism, substance intoxication, and substance withdrawal (alcohol, opiates/opioids, sedative-hypnotics). Other psychiatric conditions such as social or SPs and posttraumatic stress disorder (PTSD) should be considered.

DIAGNOSTIC STUDIES

While no specific biomarkers or diagnostic studies are available to diagnose panic disorder, diagnostic studies may be indicated to rule out an underlying cause. Because of ease of use and low cost, EKG should be done. If accompanied by syncope or near-syncope, consideration should be given to a Holter monitor. CBC, CMP, and thyroid function tests should also be considered.

EVALUATION

The diagnosis of panic disorder is typically history-based, but the Panic Disorder Severity Scale (PDSS) can be used to assess the effectiveness of treatment. Other instruments such as the GAD-7 and PHQ-9 can help identify comorbid GAD and MDD risk.

TREATMENT

Similar to GAD, the first line of treatment is SSRIs or SNRIs, with preference given to SSRIs due to potentially better tolerance. Again, follow the "start low and go slow" approach. Consideration can be given to concomitant treatment with benzodiazepines, specifically clonazepam, for several weeks until the effects of the SSRI or SNRI have been noted at which time a tapering of the benzodiazepine takes place. As-needed alternatives to benzodiazepines are similar to the ones used for GAD. CBT should also be incorporated.

PATIENT EDUCATION

Patients should be counseled that while panic attacks occur from a spontaneous, complicated, and not yet fully understood mechanism, increased stress may lead to easier activation of this mechanism. As such, stress reduction strategies should be discussed with the patient. They should also be educated to avoid caffeine and alcohol.

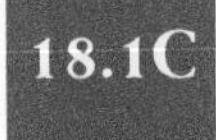

18.1C SOCIAL ANXIETY DISORDER AND SPECIFIC PHOBIAS

MEDICAL HISTORY AND CLINICAL PRESENTATION

Symptoms of social anxiety disorder usually appear in the early to mid-teens and patients present for treatment around the mid-20s. The symptoms last a mean of 16.3 years.[13] Symptoms of SP have a mean age of onset of 9.7 years with a duration of 20 years.[14] Social anxiety affects males and females equally; however, males are less likely to seek help. SP shows a 2:1 female prevalence. With both disorders, patients describe intense anxiety when exposed to a specific object or situation. To cope, they will typically avoid triggering situations, although some patients will endure the symptoms in the presence of the situation or object. With social anxiety disorder, the anxiety is related to how other people perceive them. Patients will describe feeling negatively evaluated by others and fearing that they will somehow greatly embarrass themselves. Common areas for social anxiety include conversations, eating or drinking in front of others, and public speaking. Social anxiety disorder can be broken down into a generalized type and performance only type. With SP, the anxiety centers around an object or situation. Individuals recognize that their phobia is excessive to any real threat caused by the situation but still work to avoid exposure. This is different from fear, which is a normal psychological real or threatened danger. Common themes include injections, blood, flying, heights, animals (e.g., snakes), and open spaces. With both disorders, patients usually describe anticipatory anxiety about encountering the specific situation or being in the presence of the specific object that triggers the cascade of symptoms (Figure 18.4).

SIGNS AND SYMPTOMS

When thinking about exposure to the triggering situation or object, patients with social anxiety and SP usually describe the following symptoms:

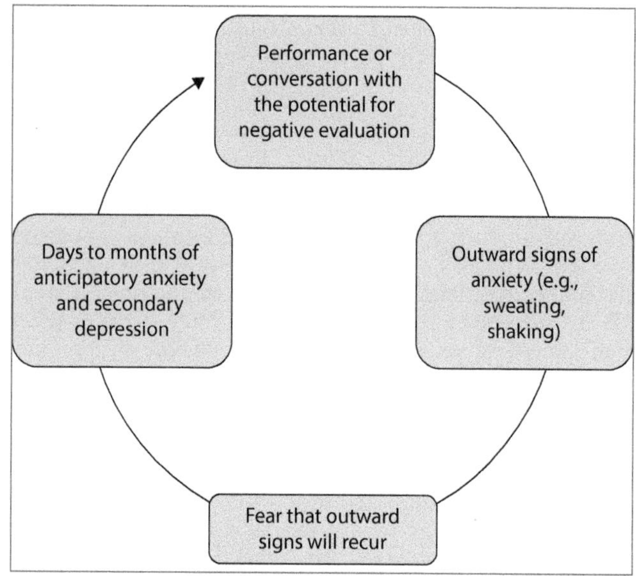

Figure 18.4 Social anxiety circle.

- Anticipatory anxiety
- Thoughts of how to avoid the object or situation
- Stuttering or recurrent throat clearing with public speaking
- Poor concentration
- Catastrophizing or a constant rumination about the worst-case scenario

Upon exposure to the feared stimulus, signs of anxiety include:

- Increased heart rate
- Poor concentration
- Blushing
- Diaphoresis
- Trembling
- Gastrointestinal (GI) discomfort
- Muscle tension
- Dizziness or lightheadedness
- Bradycardia and/or hypotension in the case of SP

PHYSICAL EXAMINATION

Unless exposed to the feared stimulus at the time of assessment, physical examination is likely to be normal. Care should be taken to evaluate for the presence of comorbid depression. In addition to symptoms discussed above, patients will describe being intensely troubled by their anxiety.

DIFFERENTIAL DIAGNOSIS

Differential diagnosis of social anxiety disorder should include other psychiatric disorders such as panic disorder, agoraphobia, major depressive disorder (MDD), avoidant personality disorder, and schizoid personality disorder. Unlike shyness, patients with social anxiety avoid situations likely to trigger symptoms and describe impairment across multiple aspects of life; on the other hand, people who are shy will continue to attend social events. Differential diagnoses for SP include panic disorder, obsessive-compulsive disorder (OCD), and substance intoxication.

DIAGNOSTIC STUDIES

Diagnosis is based on an MSE and history. Otherwise, no specific diagnostic studies are available. Care should be taken in the case of social anxiety disorder to delineate between generalized and performance only subtypes as this will influence treatment choice.

EVALUATION

Several tools to evaluate social anxiety are available and include the Social Phobia Inventory (SPIN) and the Social Anxiety Questionnaire (SAQ-A30). It is recommended that patients take the time to complete these questionnaires prior to their visit because they can often be time consuming. For SPs, the Severity Measure for SP is a 10-question tool that can be used.

TREATMENT

The treatment of choice for SPs is CBT with a focus on exposure. Pharmacologic treatment of SPs is limited to benzodiazepines or beta blockers on an as needed basis. These should be used only in the case of infrequent exposure to the provoking stimulus. Trials of SSRIs have shown mixed evidence in studies and as such, they are not typically recommended.

For performance-type social anxiety, treatment generally consists of PRN (as needed) 20 to 40 mg propranolol or benzodiazepines. For generalized social anxiety, SSRIs are the first-line pharmacologic treatment. Prescribers should follow the previously mentioned guidelines for choosing the SSRI based on tolerability and safety first as well as a “start low, go slow” approach. Subsequent treatment choices are similar to those for other anxiety disorders. Nonpharmacologic treatment of social anxiety should include referral to a certified cognitive behavioral therapist.

PATIENT EDUCATION

Patients with SP or social anxiety should be counseled about the biopsychosocial aspects of the disorders. Specifically, they should be educated about how their nervous system has a propensity to form a sympathetic response more easily and how, through proper treatment, they should be able to decrease this sensitivity. Information should be given to the patient to assist them on finding a certified cognitive behavioral therapist (NACBT.ORG).

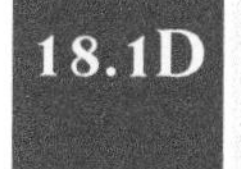

18.1D OBSESSIVE-COMPULSIVE DISORDER

MEDICAL HISTORY AND CLINICAL PRESENTATION

Patients with OCD usually present in their late teens to early 20s. Men and women are equally affected as adults, but males tend to have an earlier onset, often in childhood or adolescence. Unlike patients with psychotic disorders, patients with OCD often have preserved insight and are able to both recognize the irrationality of their thoughts and behaviors and be very troubled by them (*ego-dystonic*). The *obsessions* are intrusive, repetitive thoughts and the patient will express frustration at being unable to control them. Some of the more common obsessions relate to contamination (germs), doubt (“I forgot to lock the door”), symmetry (“things are out of balance”), or unacceptable sexual or violent urges. The *compulsions* are the behaviors patients perform in attempts to relieve the anxiety associated with the obsessions. Common compulsions include checking, frequent handwashing, counting, or making things symmetrical. Compulsions may also be mental acts such as repeating a mantra. Compulsions may only relieve anxiety for a short time, if at all, and must therefore be repeated.

Earlier onset OCD cases are more likely to present with positive family history.[15] History may also be significant for tic disorder.

SIGNS AND SYMPTOMS

Patients with OCD will describe unwelcome, unacceptable thoughts and their behavioral efforts to relieve them. They are often hesitant to discuss these thoughts due to associated shame (e.g., a patient may have intrusive thoughts about molesting someone). Patients with OCD frequently present with comorbid depression.

PHYSICAL EXAMINATION

Physical examination in patients with OCD is usually normal and, as mentioned above, patients often recognize their thoughts and behaviors are not "normal." Attention should be paid for the presence of tics due to the relatively common association.

DIFFERENTIAL DIAGNOSIS

Neurologic conditions including Sydenham chorea, Huntington disease, and Tourette disorder should be included in the differential diagnosis. Other psychiatric conditions need to be included as well including psychotic disorders and depression. OCD is commonly confused with obsessive-compulsive personality disorder, which is a constellation of personality traits (rigidity and perfectionism) and does not involve obsessions and compulsions.

DIAGNOSTIC STUDIES

Neuroimaging studies have shown increased activity in the frontal lobe and basal ganglia. Despite this, no diagnostic studies are recommended for diagnosis.

EVALUATION

Two commonly used tools for evaluation of OCD include the Yale-Brown Obsessive-Compulsive Scale (Y-BOCS) and the Obsessive-Compulsive Inventory-Revised (OCI-R). In addition, the PHQ-9 can help identify the common occurrence of comorbid depression.

TREATMENT

First-line pharmacologic treatment of OCD is SSRIs. Frequently, the dose of SSRIs needs to be higher than that used to treat depression or anxiety.[16] Also, a longer trial of 8 to 12 weeks is needed before augmentation or switching to another agent.[17] While used, SNRIs do not have good evidence backing their use. If no response is seen in 8 to 12 weeks, a trial of a different SSRI should be considered. Failing this, consideration should then be given to switching to clomipramine, a TCA. As mentioned in previous sections, side effects and overdose potential limit the use of this medication.

Medications used to augment a primary treatment may include mood stabilizers or an atypical antipsychotic. Risperidone is a good choice for patients with OCD with comorbid tic disorders.[18]

Nonpharmacologic treatment should include CBT with a focus on exposure and ritual and response prevention.[19]

PATIENT EDUCATION

Patients should be educated that the course of OCD is usually chronic with periods of waxing and waning. They should be educated that CBT for a period of fourteen to sixteen 1-hour sessions is typical and compliance is paramount for successful treatment. Another important part of psychoeducation should be the expectation that even with successful treatment, symptoms—although less severe in intensity—will likely remain.

18.2 POSTTRAUMATIC STRESS DISORDER

Marci Contreras

OVERVIEW

PTSD is a mental health condition in which a person is exposed to a severe traumatic event (i.e., serious injury, physical or sexual assault, threatened death, or after a critical illness). It is important to point out that the person with PTSD does not have to directly experience the traumatic event but might have witnessed the event or learned that the event happened to a close friend or family member.

EPIDEMIOLOGY

The prevalence of PTSD among adults in the United States is approximately 7%.[20] Women are twice as likely to develop PTSD even though men may be exposed to more trauma. Certain groups are at higher risk for developing PTSD, including:

- First responders (e.g., firefighters, police officers, healthcare workers)
- Survivors of motor vehicle collisions
- Female rape victims
- Military service
- Lower socioeconomic status
- Exposure to natural disasters, mass casualty, or terrorism

One should note that not everyone who experiences a traumatic event develops PTSD. It remains unclear why some people develop PTSD after a traumatic experience while others do not.

PATHOPHYSIOLOGY

The hippocampus, amygdala, and prefrontal cortex are involved in the pathophysiology of PTSD. Impairment to these areas that are important in emotion (e.g., fear and anger), memory, and executive function can lead to a higher predisposition to PTSD. There may also be implication of a genetic predisposition to the development of PTSD.

MEDICAL HISTORY AND CLINICAL PRESENTATION

In addition to performing a complete medical history, the PA should gather information specific to the stressful event that is considered to be traumatic. The clinician should also explore substance use, family history of mental health conditions, as well as quality of relationships and social activities. Patients with PTSD may have difficulty remembering parts of the traumatic event and feel as though they are always "on guard"; because of this, detailed questioning should be avoided as it may trigger severe symptoms. Patients with PTSD may also describe feeling numb or detached from others, activities, or surroundings.

SIGNS AND SYMPTOMS

- Intrusive memories/flashbacks
- Avoidance of people or activities for fear of triggering an event
- Heightened startle response
- Difficulty sleeping/nightmares
- Negative view of self, negative view of the world, or distorted belief that the world is dangerous
- Paranoia/social phobia
- Blunt affect, anger or aggression, or other mood changes
- Cognitive changes, memory loss, or decreased cognitive functioning
- Feeling detached or dissociation
- Suicidal ideation

Symptoms usually begin within 1 year following a traumatic event and persist beyond 1 month for a diagnosis of PTSD. Symptoms typically interfere with the patient's relationships, sleep, self-care, ability to concentrate, and overall quality of life. It is possible for PTSD to develop years after the trauma such as in the case with exposure to domestic violence during childhood or with veterans years after military service.

DIFFERENTIAL DIAGNOSIS

- Acute stress disorder
- Dissociative disorders
- Depression
- Generalized anxiety
- Panic disorder
- Phobias
- Substance abuse

EVALUATION

It is important to keep in mind that avoiding trauma triggers is a notable symptom of PTSD. Therefore, it is unlikely that patients will spontaneously report their symptoms. The PA should identify any signs or symptoms of PTSD and explore whether patients have any feelings of fear, horror, guilt, or shame. A thorough MSE should be performed. Clinicians should screen patients for suicide risk. Common comorbidities in patients with PTSD include depression, anxiety, panic attacks, and substance use disorder.

TREATMENT

It is important to validate the patient's feelings and let them know that it is *not their fault*. Many patients with PTSD have self-blame and shame. As part of recovery it is necessary to help the patient change their view of self and the rest of the world. There is no cure for PTSD.

- A team of healthcare workers may be helpful and include:
  - Primary care clinician/PA
  - Psychiatrist/mental health clinician
  - Social worker
- Counseling may include:
  - Group therapy (veterans, addiction, abuse survivors)
  - CBT is the treatment of choice. This often involves guiding the patient to "process" the trauma and desensitizing them to the memories.
- Medications such as SSRIs can help reduce depression, anxiety, and insomnia. Currently there is no recommended pharmacotherapy for the treatment of posttraumatic nightmares.
- Alternative therapies include:
  - Mindfulness or mindfulness-based stress reduction (MBSR)
  - Meditation
  - Yoga
  - Art therapy
  - Creative writing
  - Biofeedback
  - Acupuncture
  - Hypnosis

Good predictors for recovery include those patients with increased social support, improved coping strategies, and positive stress reduction techniques. Self-compassion is also a good predictor for recovery and may help to reduce social isolation and negative emotions such as guilt and shame. Avoidance and denial can impede recovery. Virtual reality exposure (VRE) therapy and noninvasive brain stimulation have both been studied as treatments for PTSD but further research is required regarding effectiveness. There is some evidence to support that prazosin can help with nightmares associated with PTSD but does not resolve them completely. Eye movement desensitization and reprocessing (EMDR) is also highly recommended as a treatment option.

PATIENT EDUCATION

- National Center for PTSD: www.ptsd.va.gov/apps/decisionaid
- American Psychological Association: www.apa.org/ptsd-guideline/patients-and-families

18.3 MOOD DISORDERS

Jeniece Wert

OVERVIEW

Mood disorders are pervasive psychiatric disorders that affect all aspects of a patient's life and can drastically decrease a patient's quality of life.[21,22] Mood disorders have been positively linked to an increased risk of suicide and substance abuse and increased mortality.[23–25] The importance of screening patients for mood disorders is demonstrated by these increased risk factors and should be evaluated by all clinicians. MDD, persistent depressive disorder (PDD), and premenstrual dysphoric disorder (PMDD) will be discussed in Sections 18.3A, 18.3B, and 18.3C, respectively.

EPIDEMIOLOGY

An estimated 9.7% of adults in the United States experienced a mood disorder in the past year with a prevalence of 21.4% adults experiencing a mood disorder over their lifetime.[26] MDD affects an estimated 6% of the United States adult population.[27] The World Health Organization (WHO) lists MDD as the 11th leading cause of disability and death worldwide with a lifetime prevalence of 10.8% in adults.[28]

By the year 2030, WHO estimates that MDD will be ranked as the leading cause of burden of disease.[29] As adults in the United States age, the prevalence of depression decreases compared to the younger population, with adults older than 65 years of age reporting the lowest rates of MDD.[30,31] Persistent and severe MDD is classified as PDD. The yearly prevalence of PDD in the Unites States is an estimated 2%.[27] Though mood disorders affect many adults, many women experience at least one psychiatric and/or physical symptoms during the luteal phase of the menstrual cycle.[32] However, an estimated 5% of women of childbearing age experience symptoms severe enough to interfere with their life and meet the criteria for PMDD.[33]

PATHOPHYSIOLOGY

While the exact pathogenesis of mood disorders is unknown, it is hypothesized to be a combination of three sets of factors: internalizing factors, externalizing factors, and adversity.[34] These three sets of factors contribute to the likelihood of an individual developing illness (Table 18.1). Many of these factors carry cross-influences with each other and contribute to the development of MDD and other depressive type mood disorders.

Genetics play a major role to the development of depressive-type mood disorders and several genetic associations contribute to the development of depression.[35] The heritability of mood disorders is estimated at 50%, which supports the contribution of genetics as well as other factors toward the development of mood disorders.[36]

Though the pathogenesis of mood disorders is generally accepted to be a cross-sectional design incorporating a multitude of factors as described above, there are neurobiologic abnormalities seen with mood disorders. These abnormalities may signify etiologic cause of mood disorders, sequelae due to mood disorders, or a combination of both. A corticotropin-releasing hormone (CRH) overproduction increases the activity of the hypothalamic-pituitary-adrenal (HPA) cortex axis in patients with mood disorders.[37] Patients with prolonged and recurrent depressive symptoms have an increased morning serum cortisol compared to individuals without depressive symptoms.[37] Chronic stress also contributes to a permanent decreased glucocorticoid receptor signaling in mood disorders[38] and may increase susceptibility to psychopathology.[39] Glucocorticoid receptors are responsible for maintaining homeostasis by regulating physiologic adaptations to stress[40] and without the function of these receptors, glucocorticoid levels with remain elevated leading to increased risk of neuro- and psychopathology.[41] The relationship between mood disorders and the HPA axis is depicted in Figure 18.5 below.

In Figure 18.5, the brain cortex and amygdala interpreted stress and transmit to the hypothalamus that releases CRH. Corticotropin causes the adrenal cortexes to secrete cortisol.[42] The red arrow in Figure 18.5 indicates the negative feedback that cortisol exhibits on the hypothalamus and pituitary to suppress CRH and corticotropin, leading to the physical changes depicted in the illustration. It is important to point out that the relationship between elevated cortisol and depressive symptoms does not indicate whether depressive symptoms lead to elevated cortisol or vice versa, further emphasizing a multifactorial approach to the development of mood disorders. Disturbances in sleep and circadian rhythm, inflammation and substance abuse are positively associated with the neurobiologic changes associated with mood disorders.[43–48]

Neurochemical imbalances can also contribute to the occurrence of mood disorders and it is necessary to understand the role of neurotransmitters in the treatment of mood disorders. At a neurobiologic level, neurotransmitters are released from presynaptic neural cells to postsynaptic receptors to control everyday functions. Dopamine, serotonin, and norepinephrine are neurotransmitters responsible for regulating stress, emotion, and sleep cycles and are associated with feelings of happiness.[45,49,50] Decreased levels

TABLE 18.1 Pathogenetic Factors of Mood Disorders

Internalizing Factors	Externalizing Factors	Adversity
• Neuroticism • Low self-esteem • Early-onset anxiety • Past history of major depression	• Genetic risk factors • Conduct disorder • Substance misuse	• Low parental warmth • Childhood abuse • Parental loss • Low education • Lifetime trauma • Low social support • History of divorce • Past history of major depression • Marital problems • Stressful life events

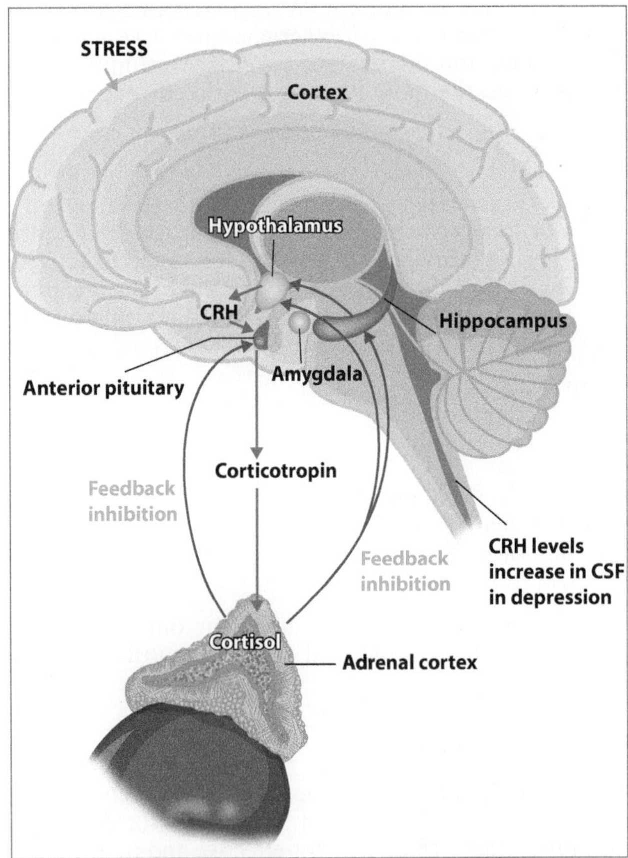

Figure 18.5 **The hypothalamic-pituitary-adrenal axis in depression. In depression, hippocampus size decreases and anterior pituitary and adrenal cortex size increases. Cortisol levels may also increase.** CRH, corticotropin-releasing hormone; CSF, cerebrospinal fluid.

of these three neurotransmitters are associated with mood disorders and increasing the availability of these neurotransmitters is the mainstay of pharmacologic treatment.[51]

18.3A MAJOR DEPRESSIVE DISORDER

MEDICAL HISTORY AND CLINICAL PRESENTATION

MDD is characterized by loss of interest in once enjoyed activities; 4% of women of childbearing age screen positive for MDD.[52] A patient presenting with MDD may also complain of vague symptoms such as insomnia, fatigue, and/or impaired memory and concentration. When obtaining a history from a patient with depressive symptoms, it is important to inquire about suicidal ideation; 80% of individuals who successfully complete suicide were seen by a clinician in the year prior and about 44% saw a clinician within the 1 month prior to death by suicide. When inquiring about suicidal ideation, ask straightforward questions regarding the patient's intent to attempt suicide and if the patient has a plan to die by suicide. Of note is recognizing the risk factors for the onset of depressive disorders. Risk factors for initial onset of MDD include female sex, substance abuse, conflictual interpersonal relationships (divorce, intimate partner violence, etc.), poor physical health, stressful life events, comorbid psychiatric disorders, and family history of MDD.[53] Risk of recurrence of MDD episodes include comorbid anxiety, negative emotionality (the tendency to experience negative emotional states), rumination, and age of onset (the younger the age of initial onset, the more likely it is for recurrence).

SIGNS AND SYMPTOMS

MDD is characterized as depressive mood for a period of 2 weeks or longer with symptoms present for the majority of each day. Key findings are a loss of interested in activities (anhedonia) and a depressed or down mood. The pneumonic SIG E CAPS is frequently used to describe common findings in patients with depression:

- Sleep
- Interest (diminished)
- Guilt
- Energy loss
- Concentration (diminished)
- Appetite change
- Psychomotor changes
- Suicidal thoughts

Patients must also not have any symptoms of mania or hypomania, as this would lead to the diagnosis of bipolar disorder.

PHYSICAL EXAMINATION

There are no specific physical examination findings for depression, but all patients should be screened for depression. The PHQ-9 (Table 18.2) is a cost-effective and time-effective screening method consisting of 9 questions for which a patient rates on a scale of 0 to 3 (max score 27). A positive PHQ-9 should warrant further investigation by way of psychiatric interviewing described below. The shorter PHQ-2 can be used as an initial screening if needed.

DIFFERENTIAL DIAGNOSIS

Differential diagnosis for MDD is summarized in Table 18.3.

DIAGNOSTIC STUDIES

A number of general medical disorders are associated with MDD and warrant further investigation based on the presenting features of the patient. A patient presenting with signs and symptoms of MDD should be evaluated for thyroid disease and vitamin D deficiency as these are common causes of symptoms mimicking MDD.[54–56] The following lab tests are recommended for new-onset depression, severe depression, and treatment-resistant depression: CBC, serum chemistry panel, urinalysis, thyroid-stimulating hormone (TSH),[60] rapid plasma regain, vitamin D level,[55] human chorionic gonadotropin (to rule out pregnancy), and urine toxicology screen for drug abuse.

EVALUATION

Screening with the PHQ-9 is the initial step in evaluating patients for MDD and patients with a positive screen would warrant further investigation. In primary care, this may warrant a referral to psychiatry and counseling and the initiation of antidepressant pharmacotherapy. A complete psychiatric interview is shown in Table 18.4.

TREATMENT

- The mainstay of treatment for MDD with the greatest efficacy is the combination of antidepressant medication and psychotherapy.[57]
- SSRIs are the most widely prescribed class of antidepressants. Alternatively, SNRIs, atypical antidepressants, and serotonin modulators can be used to treat MDD.
- Pharmacologic treatment takes 2 to 6 weeks to be effective.

PATIENT EDUCATION

- It is imperative to discuss a plan with patients should they experience suicidal ideation. This plan can include presenting to the ED, calling the National Suicide Prevention Lifeline, and/or calling the local crisis center.
- Some antidepressant medications are contraindicated during pregnancy and breastfeeding. Female patients of childbearing age should be counseled to present to a clinician if they become pregnant or are thinking of becoming pregnant.

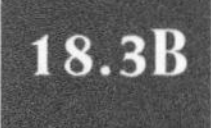

18.3B PERSISTENT DEPRESSIVE DISORDER

MEDICAL HISTORY AND CLINICAL PRESENTATION

PDD, previously known as dysthymic disorder, is characterized by long-term depressed mood. A patient with PDD may have experienced depressive symptoms for years whether diagnosed with MDD or not. The persistence of depressive symptoms for 2 years or longer is the classic presentation of PDD. These patients may be considered a "downer" or a person with a gloomy personality.

TABLE 18.2 PHQ-9 Depression Questionnaire

Name:	**Date:**			
Over the last 2 weeks, how often have you been bothered by any of the following problems?	**Not at all**	**Several days**	**More than half the days**	**Nearly every day**
Little interest or pleasure in doing things	0	1	2	3
Feeling down, depressed, or hopeless	0	1	2	3
Trouble falling or staying asleep, or sleeping too much	0	1	2	3
Feeling tired or having little energy	0	1	2	3
Poor appetite or overeating	0	1	2	3
Feeling bad about yourself, or that you are a failure, or that you have let yourself or your family down	0	1	2	3
Trouble concentrating on things, such as reading the newspaper or watching television	0	1	2	3
Moving or speaking so slowly that other people could have noticed? Or the opposite, being so fidgety or restless that you have been moving around a lot more than usual.	0	1	2	3
Thoughts that you would be better off dead, or of hurting yourself in some way	0	1	2	3
Total ___ =	___	+___	+___	+___
PHQ-9 score ≥10: Likely major depression				
Depression score ranges:				
5 to 9: mild				
10 to 14: moderate				
15 to 19: moderately severe				
≥20: severe				
If you checked off any problems, how difficult have these problems made it for you to do your work, take care of things at home, or get along with other people?	Not difficult at all ___	Somewhat difficult ___	Very difficult ___	Extremely difficult ___

PHQ, Patient Health Questionnaire.
Source: Developed by Drs. Robert L Spitzer, Janet BW Williams, Kurt Kroenke, and colleagues, with an educational grant from Pfizer, Inc. No permission required to reproduce, translate, display or distribute. https://www.uptodate.com/contents/image?imageKey=PSYCH%2F59307

TABLE 18.3 Differential Diagnosis for Major Depressive Disorder

Diagnosis	**Description**
Hypothyroidism	Weight changes, bowel changes, anxiety, fatigue, and agitation are common symptoms; characterized by an elevated TSH
Anemia	Fatigue, pallor, dizziness, and muscle cramps; characterized by a decreased hemoglobin
Hypercortisolism	Insomnia, memory loss, sadness, hypertension, proximal muscle weakness, progressive truncal obesity, and sleep apnea; characterized by elevated 24-hour urinary free cortisol excretion level
Obstructive sleep apnea	Poor concentration, insomnia, daytime sleepiness, and morning headaches; diagnosed by polysomnography (sleep study)

TSH, thyroid-stimulating hormone.

SIGNS AND SYMPTOMS

Symptoms of PDD are same as those of MDD with a longer period of constant symptoms (one of which must be depressed mood) of 2 years or more. During this period, symptom-free periods must not be >2 consecutive months without clearly demarcated episodes.[58] The defining feature of PDD is pervasive depressed mood that is present all day for the majority of the 2-year period with two other symptoms consistent with MDD.[59] These symptoms must interfere with the patient's quality of life and impair their daily function.

TABLE 18.4 Psychiatric Interview

Elements of Psychiatric Interview	Information to Inquire About
Symptoms	• Depressive symptoms • Mania • Psychosis (hallucinations: visual and auditory) • Suicidal ideation • Homicidal ideations
Past psychiatric health history	• Similar symptoms in the past • Previous diagnoses • Childhood mental health • Past trauma • Previous hospitalizations • Past treatments
Psychosocial history	• Family history (e.g., spouse, kids, parents, siblings) • Stressors (acute and chronic) • Education • Employment • Legal issues • Habits (e.g., diet, sleep, exercise)

PHYSICAL EXAMINATION

While there are no physical examination findings consistent with PDD, if a clinician has followed the patient for an extended period of time, the clinician may note a gloomy personality present in the patient. If a patient complains of any somatic symptoms associated with PDD such as fatigue or stomach upset, it may be necessary to investigate these symptoms to rule out other causes.

DIFFERENTIAL DIAGNOSIS

The differential diagnosis for PDD is summarized in Table 18.5.

DIAGNOSTIC STUDIES

Lab studies in the presence of PDD are only used to rule out other causes of depressive symptoms. The studies obtained will be driven by the presenting symptoms of the patient.

EVALUATION

In-depth psychiatric interviewing is helpful in establishing the etiology and manifestations of the patient's PDD. PDD has a high-risk estimate for suicidal attempt and interviewing should focus on suicidal ideation and intent as a prevention of death by suicide.[60,61]

TREATMENT

- Pharmacotherapy in addition to psychotherapy is the most effective treatment option and show greater improvement of symptoms than either option alone.
- SSRIs are the most widely accepted treatment for PDD.
- CBT and interpersonal psychotherapy are therapy types used for PDD.

PATIENT EDUCATION

- As with MDD, patients should have a crisis plan should they experience suicidal ideation or self-harming thoughts.

TABLE 18.5 Differential Diagnosis for Persistent Depressive Disorders

Diagnosis	Description
Complicated grief	Prolonged period of intense sadness following loss
Adjustment disorder	Low mood, hopelessness, and stress occurring within 3 months of a stressor and resolves within 6 months after resolution of stressor
Substance abuse	Mood disturbance before intoxication or withdrawal particularly with alcohol, cannabis, cocaine, amphetamines, and stimulants
Chronic fatigue syndrome	Overwhelming fatigue exacerbated by physical activity present for 6 months or longer without a history of multiple somatic symptoms; characterized by severe intensity of symptoms

- Treatment can take 2 to 8 weeks to reach full effect. Patients should be told that it may take several weeks to feel the effects of the medication and to allow for enough time for medication to reach full potential.

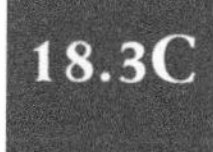

18.3C PREMENSTRUAL DYSPHORIC DISORDER

MEDICAL HISTORY AND CLINICAL PRESENTATION

A female patient of childbearing age will present with a complaint of severe affective and/or somatic symptoms before menstruation that resolve within a few days of onset of menses. These patients may complain of mood changes, weight gain, changes in sleep patterns, depressed mood, and/or increased anger. Onset of symptoms of PMDD usually occur in patients in their adolescence or early 20s.[62] These symptoms cannot be explained by any other medical diagnosis. It is important to note that this can also occur in women who have had a hysterectomy but maintain normal ovarian function.

SIGNS AND SYMPTOMS

To meet criteria for PMDD, a patient must have five symptoms divided into the categories of somatic symptoms and mood symptoms.[62] These symptoms must occur during the second half of the menstrual cycle and must occur for several months and interfere with patient's normal activity. Typically, symptoms will onset 2 or 3 days before menstruation and last an average of 6 days. In addition, the symptoms cannot be attributed to other medical or psychiatric diagnoses.

Patients with PMDD present with a combination of somatic and mood symptoms such as:[32]

- Decreased ability to concentrate
- Appetite changes/food cravings
- Decreased interest in activities
- Fatigue
- Breast tenderness, bloating, weight gain, or muscle aches
- Changes in sleep
- Hot flashes

- Dizziness
- Headaches
- Rapid changes in mood
- Anger
- Increased irritability
- Depressed mood
- Increased hopelessness
- Anxiety
- Increased critical thoughts

Of note, suicidal ideation is not typically associated with PMDD.[63]

PHYSICAL EXAMINATION

There are no specific physical exam abnormalities associated with PMDD. However, a full physical examination would eliminate other causes for physical manifestations of PMDD. Physical examination should be guided by the presenting symptoms of PMDD. For example, a comprehensive abdominal exam would eliminate other causes for abdominal bloating, pain, and other abdominal manifestations.

DIFFERENTIAL DIAGNOSIS

The differential diagnosis for PMDD is summarized in Table 18.6.

DIAGNOSTIC STUDIES

There are no specific laboratory findings to diagnose PMDD. As with physical examination, the diagnostic studies chosen should be driven by the presenting symptoms of the patient. For example, complaints of fatigue should be evaluated with a CBC to rule out anemia and TSH to rule out hypothyroidism. If menopause is suspected as a cause of these presenting symptoms, an elevated FSH level would point toward menopausal disorder rather than PMDD.

EVALUATION

Female patients with major complaints associated with menstruation should be asked comprehensive questioning regarding all symptoms and timing of symptoms. It is helpful to have patients keep a diary of symptoms and menstrual cycle to analyze for trends. Untreated PMDD is associated with a loss of quality-adjusted life years of around 3 years indicating a need to treat these patients as soon as possible to prevent a decreased quality of life.[64]

TABLE 18.6 Differential Diagnosis of Premenstrual Dysphoric Disorder

Diagnosis	Description
Endometriosis	Dyschezia, bowel changes, dyspareunia, dysmenorrhea, and fatigue; diagnosed by laparoscopy and biopsy
Anemia	Fatigue, pallor, dizziness, and muscle cramps; characterized by a decreased hemoglobin
Hypothyroidism	Weight changes, bowel changes, fatigue, anxiety, and agitation are common symptoms; characterized by an elevated TSH
Menopause	Anxiety, hot flashes, irregular menstruation, and weight changes; onset is 40s or 50s unlike PMDD, which has a usual onset of early 20s; characterized by an elevated FSH

FSH, follicle-stimulating hormone; PMDD, premenstrual dysphoric disorder; TSH, thyroid-stimulating hormone.

TREATMENT

- Treatment for PMDD involves the use of combined estrogen-progestin oral contraceptives (COCs) and/or SSRIs.

PATIENT EDUCATION

- Record symptoms in a diary with the dates in relation to menstrual cycle will help clinicians properly diagnose and treat PMDD symptoms.
- Regular exercise and having a relaxation routine help to decrease mood symptoms.
- If patients have bloating symptoms, they should avoid salty foods and large meals.
- Nonsteroidal anti-inflammatory drugs (NSAIDs) can be used for pain and/or headaches.

SPECIAL CONSIDERATIONS

- MDD in pregnancy is associated with poor nutrition, increased risk of suicide, and impaired mother/baby relationships.[65] If the pregnant mother was taking an antidepressant at conception, the medication can usually remain the same unless the patient prefers otherwise.[66]
- With the exception of the MAO inhibitors (MAOIs), there has not been compelling evidence to indicate severe fetal side effects of taking antidepressants during the antenatal period.[66]
- Successful treatment of teens and adolescents with MDD requires the cooperation and collaboration between patient, family, and clinician.[67] Typically, psychotherapy alone is the initial treatment with the addition of an SSRI at a later date.[68]

18.4 SUBSTANCE USE DISORDERS

Richard Bottner

OVERVIEW

Addiction is a chronic, complicated, and treatable waxing and waning disease with clear genetic and environmental predisposition.[69]

EPIDEMIOLOGY

The misuse of substances is a major public health crisis of our time. Over 20 million U.S. adults have a diagnosed SUD.[70] Misuse of alcohol, tobacco, prescription opioids, and illicit drugs costs the U.S. economy over $740 billion annually when taking into account expenses related to healthcare, lost wages, and the criminal justice system.[71] The National Survey of Drug Use and Health found that the vast majority of individuals have consumed alcohol at some point (>80%), 57% identifying as having used tobacco, and just under half of respondents having used an illicit drug at some point which may include stimulants, sedatives, opioids, hallucinogens, or marijuana, among others.[72] Over 25% of Americans report binge drinking in the past year.[73] Over 67,000 Americans lost their lives to drug-involved poisonings in 2018 alone (Figure 18.6).[74] Ten percent of adults in the United States

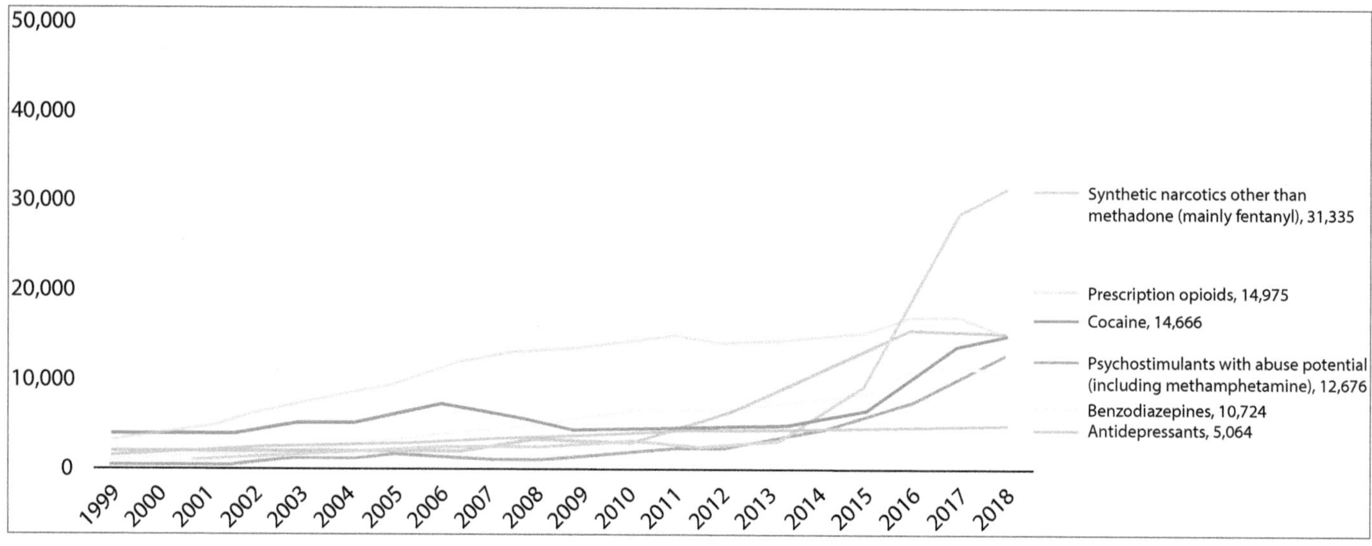

Figure 18.6 **National drug overdose deaths involving select prescription and illicit drugs.**
(Source: National Institute on Drug Abuse. Overdose death rates. United States Department of Health and Human Services. https://www.drugabuse.gov/drug-topics/trends-statistics/overdose-death-rates)

endorse having a SUD in their lifetime and three-quarters of these individuals describe never receiving treatment.[75] Poisonings from substance misuse generates over 1 million ED visits annually.[76] Importantly, many patients have co-occurring SUD. For example, over 2 million U.S. adults have an alcohol use disorder and a drug use disorder (Figure 18.7).[70] Co-occurring SUDs may be more common among males and influenced by age (especially young adults between the ages of 26 and 34), education level, and employment status.[77] It has been suggested that over 50% of patients in the primary care setting who identify substance use of any kind may qualify for a SUD diagnosis.[78] Feelings of loneliness and decreased social connectedness are commonly reported by people with SUDs.[79] Approximately one in five individuals who use cannabis qualify for a cannabis use disorder.[80]

MEDICAL HISTORY AND CLINICAL PRESENTATION

The U.S. Preventive Services Task Force recommends screening all adults (age 18 and older) for unhealthy drug use.[81] Clinicians must be comfortable and empowered to have conversations with patients about substance use. In fact, such discussions lead to an increased likelihood that patients receive treatment for underlying addiction.[82] There may be an increased likelihood of developing a SUD in the presence of comorbid psychiatric diagnoses including GAD, MDD, bipolar disorder, or PTSD in addition to antisocial, borderline, and schizotypal personality disorders.[81] Patients should be screened for suicidal ideation as SUD may increase the risk of self-harm.[83] It is critically important to ask about and document which substances a patient is using, how frequently the substances are used, how much is used, and time of last use. Psychosocial manifestations of SUD may include marital issues, isolation from friends and family, worsening job or school performance, encounters with law enforcement, or financial troubles.[84]

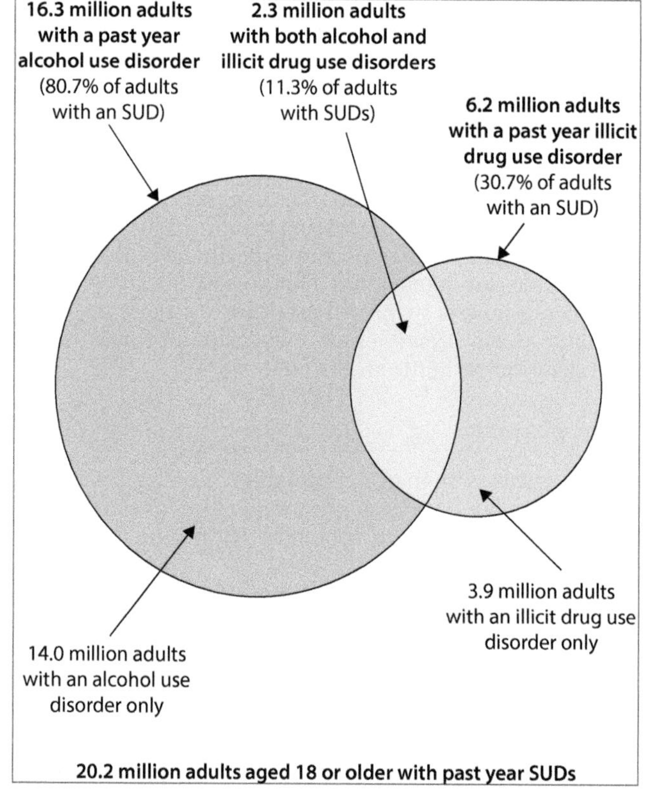

Figure 18.7 **Substance use disorders (SUDs) in 2014 among adults age 18 or older.**
(Source: Substance Abuse and Mental Health Services Administration. Trends in substance use disorders among adults aged 18 or older. United States Department of Health and Human Services. https://www.samhsa.gov/data/sites/default/files/report_2790/ShortReport-2790.pdf)

SIGNS AND SYMPTOMS

SUD comprises several categories. Generally, patients may experience loss of control, consequences of substance use such as loss of employment or housing, development of directly related medical complications, and the development of physiologic tolerance or withdrawal with abrupt cessation.[85] Importantly, tolerance and withdrawal alone are not enough to make the diagnosis of a SUD.[85] For example, patients with malignancy or chronic pain may be receiving relatively high doses of opioid analgesia while under appropriate medical supervision. Such patients will certainly develop tolerance requiring increased doses over time and withdrawal with abrupt cessation; however, these physiologic phenomena do not necessarily qualify for a SUD.

PHYSICAL EXAMINATION

In its early stages, substance use is extremely challenging to diagnose with physical examination alone. However, certain exam findings may offer clues into recent substance use. These include damage to nasal mucosa for drugs used intranasally and pupillary findings such as nystagmus, miosis, and mydriasis may be present with use of variety of substances such as hallucinogens, stimulants, and opioids.[84]

DIAGNOSTIC STUDIES

The urine drug screen (UDS) is commonly used to assess for drug use. Alcohol can be assessed in the urine or breath.[84] It is important to recognize that false positives may occur in a UDS obtained from a patient taking certain prescription medications. For example, trazodone and bupropion may cause a positive amphetamine test, verapamil and quetiapine may cause a positive methadone test, and sertraline may cause a positive benzodiazepine test.[86] Laboratory testing may reveal abnormalities, for example, macrocytic anemia or elevated transaminases in the setting of alcohol use disorder.[84]

EVALUATION

Patients with a history of intravenous (IV) drug use should be screened for viral hepatitis and HIV.[69] Consideration should be given toward screening for sexually transmitted infections (STIs) as drug use may lead to risky sexual activity.

TREATMENT

The Screening, Brief Intervention, and Referral to Treatment (SBIRT) model of providing care has been widely used since the 1990s. While initially developed for alcohol and tobacco use disorders, its many principles have now been applied to additional SUDs.[87] The SBIRT model has been shown to be effective for addressing SUDs across the care continuum.[88] Several screening tools can be applied in the primary care setting including the CAGE and AUDIT (Alcohol Use Disorders Identification Test) assessments; these screening tools gauge risky behaviors surrounding alcohol use including guilt associated with drinking, continuation of drinking despite harm to others, and the need for alcohol upon waking in the morning. When a patient's screen is positive, motivational interviewing techniques may be used to raise awareness and promote change talk, which may increase the chances for clinical improvement.[89] Patients can then be referred to the appropriate level of care for treatment.[88]

Integrating behavioral-based strategies including mindfulness and counseling directly into the primary care environment may improve outcomes for patients with SUDs, especially those with co-occurring chronic pain or depression.[90]

Like other chronic medical conditions, treatment plans and outcomes must be tailored to the patient through shared decision-making.[91] Patient-centered outcomes are paramount. While many believe that abstinence or substance-free days define successful treatment there are other important measures to follow as well including substance cravings and overall quality of life as perceived and reported by the patient.[92] In addition, recurrence of the disease over the course of treatment, similar to treatment of other chronic medical conditions such as diabetes and hypertension, is expected.[69]

Some patients may require long-term or short-term residential treatment, intensive outpatient treatment programs, or behavioral health counseling in a group setting or individually.[69]

Pharmacotherapy is an option for certain SUDs. For opioid use disorder, patients may receive buprenorphine, methadone, or naltrexone. Each of these medications function primarily at the mu opioid receptor. This receptor is responsible for analgesic effects but can also cause euphoria and respiratory depression, which can lead to respiratory arrest if not monitored closely. Full agonist opioids include typical opioid analgesics such as hydrocodone and oxycodone, as well as illicit opioids such as heroin. These fully activate the mu receptor and act synergistically with each other. Methadone is a full agonist opioid, which can be used to treat opioid use disorder, but must be administered through a federally and state regulated opioid treatment program.[93] Buprenorphine is a partial agonist opioid that controls cravings and treats withdrawal with less risk of adverse side effects.[94] Naltrexone is an antagonist that blocks all opioid activity at the mu receptor.[95] Each of these treatment options offer unique benefits to the patient with opioid use disorder. However, in the primary care setting, buprenorphine may be particularly advantageous in initiating treatment in the Office Based Opioid Treatment model.[96]

For tobacco use disorder, patients may be offered treatment with bupropion or varenicline. Bupropion is typically started 1 week prior to the quit date, then continued for an additional 11 weeks; bupropion is contraindicated in individuals with seizure disorders. Bupropion was initially promoted as an antidepressant that limited reuptake of norepinephrine and dopamine, thus reducing tobacco cravings without weight gain. Varenicline operates directly at the nicotine receptors where it activates the receptor without the release of dopamine.[75] The use of nicotine replacement therapies, either individually or as combination therapy, should also be considered.

There are several pharmacologic interventions for alcohol use disorder. Acamprosate affects the GABA systems and reduces the symptoms of prolonged withdrawal, which make it particularly suitable for patients with severe alcohol use disorder. Disulfiram inhibits the metabolism of alcohol and results in the buildup of acetaldehyde, which results in highly unpleasant GI side effects.[69] Naltrexone works at the endorphin receptors and decreases cravings for alcohol and feelings of euphoria alcohol generates for many individuals.[95] For acute alcohol withdrawal, benzodiazepines are considered first-line therapy in addition to folic acid, thiamine, and vitamin B12 supplementation as needed. Underlying electrolyte abnormalities should be screened for and corrected.

Twelve-step programs provide active engagement in a self-help group setting.[69] Such groups provide an effective social structure for many patients, but may also shun the evidence-based use of pharmacologic interventions by sharing myths such as treatment "replaces one addiction for another."[97,98]

Any patient with an opioid use disorder or any IV drug use history should be prescribed rescue naloxone and provided counseling on its appropriate administration. Naloxone should also be co-prescribed with opioid prescriptions totaling >50 MMEs daily, for patients prescribed opioids who have chronic respiratory conditions, and for patients using benzodiazepines.[99]

PATIENT EDUCATION

Stigma of patients with SUD is widespread among clinicians and directly contributes to decreased access to care.[100] There are three main types of stigma that exist among patients with SUD. Social stigma encompasses the stereotypes and prejudices and resulting discrimination that occurs against people with SUD.[101] Meaningful interventions to reduce social stigma include motivational interviewing techniques and the sharing of patient stories.[102] Structural stigma represents the intentional or unintentional constraints placed within healthcare organizations and by policymakers at the local, state, and federal level that may limit access to care for patients with SUD.[101] Such stigma can be reduced through widespread educational initiatives.[102] Lastly, self-stigma is a feeling of worthlessness experienced by patients as a result of structural and social stigma.[102] It results in the "why try" effect wherein patients internalize the perceived messages of society and the healthcare system that they may not be worthy of receiving addiction-related treatment.[103] Self-stigma may be overcome with counseling and group-based behavioral therapies.[102]

Decreasing stigma starts with using appropriate terminology. Never use the words "addict," "user," "abuser," "junkie," or "alcoholic." Always use patient-first recovery-centered language such as "person with an SUD" or "patient with harmful alcohol use" or "individual misusing opioids."

18.5 DISSOCIATIVE DISORDERS

Elesea Villegas

OVERVIEW

Dissociative disorders are a group of disorders that can be characterized by a partial or complete loss of the normal integration between memories of the past, awareness of identity, immediate sensations, and control of bodily movement.[104] This disorder can be further divided into subcategories, including dissociative identity disorder (DID), dissociative amnesia, depersonalization/derealization disorder, other specified dissociative disorder, and unspecified dissociative disorder (Box 18.1).

Often, this group of disorders will follow a tragic event in the patient's early life, such as physical and/or sexual abuse and neglect. It is for this reason that dissociative disorders can be seen in patients with PTSD. It is believed that dissociation acts as a regulatory strategy to restrain extreme arousal in PTSD through hyperinhibition of limbic regions.[105] This dissociation can occur in various ways, including alternative personalities, loss of memory of experienced events and/or self, and the dissociation of self and/or surrounding environment.

EPIDEMIOLOGY

Dissociative disorders are uncommon among the general population. DID is the most common subcategory among the dissociative disorders, and it is estimated that approximately 1% of the general population has DID.[106] This estimate increases in both the inpatient and outpatient psychiatric settings. Overall, the prevalence of dissociative disorders in this setting seems to be around 10%, with approximately 5% having DID.[106] It was also previously believed that dissociative disorders were more common in females than males; however, recent studies are showing that the sex differences in the prevalence of dissociative disorders are not statistically significant[107] making dissociative disorders equally common among men and women. In addition, there appears to be a link to early-life abuse and neglect and dissociative disorders. It is for this reason that childhood trauma should be viewed as a risk factor for dissociative disorders.[108,109]

BOX 18.1 Subcategories of Dissociative Disorders
Dissociative identity disorders
Dissociative amnesia
Depersonalization/derealization disorder
Other specified dissociative disorder
Unspecified dissociative disorder

PATHOPHYSIOLOGY

The pathogenesis of dissociative disorders is not well understood. We know that there is a positive correlation between patients who have suffered childhood traumas and are subsequently diagnosed with PTSD, and those who go on to develop dissociative disorders. Patients with DID have been found to have significantly smaller hippocampal and amygdala volumes, as compared with healthy subjects. The same findings can be seen in patients who suffer from PTSD. However, the neurobiologic relationship between these two disorders has not been well studied.

MEDICAL HISTORY AND CLINICAL PRESENTATION OF DISSOCIATIVE DISORDERS

Dissociative disorders are a group of disorders that can be characterized by a partial or complete loss of the normal integration between memories of the past, awareness of identity, immediate sensations, and control of bodily movement. They can be further subcategorized into DID, dissociative amnesia, depersonalization/derealization disorder, other specified dissociative disorder, and unspecified dissociative disorder. DID, dissociative amnesia, and depersonalization/derealization disorder will be discussed further.

Dissociative Identity Disorder

DID is considered the most severe subcategory of dissociative disorders. Patients will present with a disruption of their own identity, which manifests as two or more distinct personalities. Each personality state has its own way of thinking and perceiving both self and environment.[110] The different personality states may differ in age, gender, behavior, and have different demeanors. The primary personality usually has no recollection of alternate identities; the alternate identities or personalities may have some awareness of each other. It is also common for one alter personality to hold a central role and be aware of and familiar with all the others.[111]

Dissociative Amnesia

In dissociative amnesia, patients will experience loss of recent and/or remote autobiographical memory. This autobiographical memory can involve a specific period of time or a specific event (localized amnesia), or it can involve forgetting one's entire life, including memory for personal identity (generalized amnesia). Often, the loss of memory is associated with traumatic or stressful events of the patient's past.

Most everyone has moments when they are forgetful and may even forget events in their past. Dissociative amnesia goes beyond "normal" forgetfulness. A "normal" person may forget what shirt they were wearing when they were involved in a traumatic or stressful event, such as a car crash. A person with dissociative amnesia may forget the entire event (localized amnesia) or even their own personal identity (generalized amnesia) when presented in the same situation or when reminded of the situation.[112]

TABLE 18.7 Differential Diagnosis for Dissociative Disorder

Diagnosis	Description
Posttraumatic stress disorder (PTSD)	Occurs when a person experiences or witnesses a traumatic event. They often experience intrusive symptoms such as distressing memories, flashbacks, and intense psychological distress.
Bipolar disorder	Occurs when a patient has experienced at least one episode of mania. Is most often alternated with depressive episode(s). A person in a manic phase may have altered personality and behavior, including increased self-esteem and risk taking.
Neurologic disorders (e.g., brain injury, brain tumor)	Traumatic injury to the brain may result in memory loss. Depending on the location of the defect/injury, could also result in personality change.
Substance use disorders	Can result in change in patient's normal behavior as well as loss of memory. When symptoms are exhibited in the presence of a substance, dissociative disorders should not be considered.

Depersonalization/Derealization Disorder

In depersonalization/derealization disorder, the patient feels detached from themselves and their own feelings (depersonalization) or from their surroundings (derealization). The patient may feel that their feelings and experiences are not their own—almost as if they are living in a dream or having an out-of-body experience. With derealization, the patient may present with the idea that their surroundings (e.g., objects, people, events) are not real. As with the other subcategories of dissociative disorder, this is often seen in individuals with a history of trauma and abuse.[112]

SIGNS AND SYMPTOMS

Signs and symptoms of dissociative disorder can vary depending on the subcategory. Patients have found strange occurrences in their home or their surroundings and have no memory of how this happened. For example, one patient with DID came home and found "someone had decided to paint the bedroom" but she had no recollection of this. Other individuals report strange cuts or bruises on themselves with no memory of how they happened.[111] Others have found themselves in strange places with no knowledge of who they are or why they are there.

PHYSICAL EXAMINATION

Physical examination of the patient should be grossly normal with the exception of the MSE. If dissociative disorder is the suspected diagnosis, it is essential to perform a thorough neurologic examination, including the cranial nerves, to rule out possible neurologic causes such as head injury or brain tumor. It is also important to note that the patients' symptoms are typically present or worsened during states of high stress or when presented with reminders of the traumatic events of their past. This means that the patient's MSE may be normal if they are presenting in the absence of stressors or reminders. Potential abnormal MSE findings can include abnormal appearance and behavior depending on the patient's personality. They may express feeling of anxiety or irritability about not being able to remember an event or even remember who they are. There might also be alteration in their thought process and thought content and they may express poor insight and judgment.

DIFFERENTIAL DIAGNOSIS

The differential diagnosis for dissociative disorders is summarized in Table 18.7.

DIAGNOSTIC STUDIES

Diagnostic studies should be used to rule out other organic causes that may be contributing to the patient's symptoms but should not be used to confirm diagnosis. These tests can be found in Table 18.8. No tests are used to confirm dissociative disorders as a diagnosis.

TABLE 18.8 Diagnostic Tests to Rule Our Other Organic Causes of Dissociative Symptoms

Test	Results
Head MRI	May demonstrate smaller hippocampus/ amygdala but should appear otherwise normal.
Urine drug screen	Normal

EVALUATION

It is important to rule out other organic causes of the patient's symptoms before making the diagnosis of a dissociative disorder. Further diagnostic information can be found in Table 18.9.

TREATMENT

- Psychotherapy is the mainstay of treatment for dissociative disorders. It is important to establish a level of trust in the therapeutic alliance to prevent the patient from quitting therapy. Express empathy, compassion, and nonjudgment when speaking with the patient.
- There are no medications that specifically treat dissociation. Pharmacotherapy such as SSRIs, should be used to treat comorbid symptoms, including depression, anxiety, mood lability and hyperarousal (see Section 18.15 Psychopharmacology).
- It is important to note that, as always, benzodiazepines should be used with caution to decrease anxiety; this medication class may exacerbate dissociation.[111]

PATIENT EDUCATION

- There are higher rates of suicidal and self-injurious behaviors among patients with dissociative disorders compared to patients with other psychiatric disorders, often leading to long courses of treatment in outpatient psychiatric clinics.[111]

18.6 CONDUCT DISORDER

Jennifer Simms Zorn

OVERVIEW

Conduct disorder is categorized with other mental health disorders related to conduct, issues with impulse control, and disruptive behavior. Additional examples of the disorders

TABLE 18.9 Diagnostic Evaluation for Dissociative Disorders

Dissociative Disorder Subcategory	Criteria
Dissociative identity disorder	Patients experience a disruption of their own identity which manifests as two or more distinct personalities. Each personality state has its own way of thinking and perceiving both self and environment.
Dissociative amnesia	Patients experience loss of recent and/or remote autobiographical memory. This autobiographical memory can involve a specific period of time or a specific event (localized amnesia), or it can involve forgetting one's entire life, including memory for personal identity (generalized amnesia).
Depersonalization/derealization disorder	The patient experiences feelings of detachment from themselves and their own feelings (depersonalization) or from their surroundings (derealization). The patient may feel that their feelings and experiences are not their own or the patient may present with the idea that their surroundings (objects, people, events, etc.) are not real.

Source: Data from Hartmann E, Benum K. Rorschach assessment of two distinctive personality states of a person with dissociative identity disorder. J Pers Assess. *2019;101(2):213–228. doi:10.1080/00223891.2017.1391273; Spiegel D, Lowenstein R, Lewis-Fernandez R, et al. Dissociative disorders in DSM-5.* Depress Anxiety. *2011;28(9):824–852. doi:10.1002/da.20874*

grouped with conduct disorder include oppositional defiant disorder and intermittent explosive disorder. It does not include attention-deficit/hyperactivity disorder.[113]

Conduct disorder is described as a patient's behavior violating norms within society, violating age-appropriate norms, and/or violating others' rights in a consistent and persistent pattern of behavior. Conduct disorder symptoms can be classified into four categories: aggression to both humans and animals, lying or stealing, property destruction, and significant violation of rules to include running away or truancy.[114]

Patients with conduct disorder have varied outcomes, but there exists significant risk for patients to have undesirable lifetime outcomes. These patients are at risk for concurrent as well as future mental health disorders. As an individual progresses from adolescence to adulthood, there is a likelihood of increasing severity of behavior and criminality, possibly leading to a diagnosis of antisocial personality disorder (not diagnosable prior to age 18).[113] Considering the impairment and potential societal burdens with this diagnosis, there is research to understand the causes and risks as well as consideration of how to assess and treat.[114]

EPIDEMIOLOGY

Lifetime prevalence of conduct disorder in the United States is estimated at 9.5% overall with an increased prevalence in males at a rate of 12.5% over females at 7.1%.[115] Additional studies note males are two to four times more likely to develop a conduct disorder over females, with males being 10 to 15 times more likely than females to develop persistent conduct disorder.[116] Onset of conduct disorder can be in childhood (<10 years old) or in adolescence. Knowing the age at onset is important since a conduct disorder diagnosis with childhood onset is considered to have increased risk for persistent disorder. The median age of onset has been noted at 11.6 years of age, but symptoms can be present as early as preschool.[115]

The risk factors and development of conduct disorder are considered to be multicausal. Risk factors identified through research include neurocognitive deficits, neurochemical irregularities, and autonomic irregularities, in addition to environmental and relationship issues. The environmental/relationship concerns can relate to prenatal care including exposure to toxins, poor quality early childcare, family issues including instability, abuse, low socioeconomic status or inconsistent discipline, peers influencing behavior negatively, and increased exposure to violence.[114] It is important to consider circumstances related to relationships and environments in evaluating a patient for a potential diagnosis of conduct disorder. Studies have noted the possibility of diagnosis bias related to overdiagnosis of adolescents that are Latinx or African American and may occur when clinicians are not considering the influence of socioeconomic status and exposure to violence and racism.[117]

PATHOPHYSIOLOGY

The etiology of conduct disorder, as previously noted, is influenced by both environmental and biologic factors. Biologic factors include low serotonin or neurochemical changes, and a low resting heart rate or autonomic irregularity as well as anatomic differences.[114]

In her dual taxonomy theory, Dr. Terrie Moffitt proposes that early-onset conduct disorder is a neurodevelopmental condition whereas adolescent onset is a result of societal influences and the patient copying poor behaviors.[118] However, a study by Fairchild et al., evaluating brain structure abnormalities in conduct disorder, demonstrates reduction of the amygdala gray matter volume in both early and adolescent onset conduct disorder. This study would support that both forms of conduct disorder may relate to the dysfunction of emotional processing in the brain.[119]

Conduct disorder is considered transmissible through the family by both genetic and environmental influences. Twin studies support that conduct disorder and antisocial behavior are related to genetic factors. However, the genetic studies thus far demonstrate more of a probability of development of conduct disorder than directly heritable disease. The genetic predisposition can be altered by the environmental factors, which can also be influenced by the family. This research continues to support the complexity of genetic and environmental factors influencing the development of conduct disorder, and further research is necessary to better understand the genetic and environmental influences.[120]

MEDICAL HISTORY AND CLINICAL PRESENTATION

When obtaining a history to evaluate a patient for conduct disorder, it is beneficial to involve parents or caregivers and teachers in the collection of information. It is also important to specifically inquire about behaviors specific to conduct disorder in that they may have a low frequency and potentially be underreported.[121]

The individual with conduct disorder will have a persistent history of behavior that violates others' rights and societal and age-related norms. This behavior has a negative impact on the functioning of the patient in academic, social, and occupational functioning. The patient will have at least three of a possible 15 criteria described in the *DSM-5* within the last 12 months, including one within the last 6 months.[121]

SIGNS AND SYMPTOMS

The 15 possible symptoms for patient with conduct disorder can be placed into four groups of behaviors: significant violation of rules, damage to property, lying and theft, and aggressive behavior toward humans and animals.[121] The behaviors utilized to diagnose an individual with conduct disorder are provided in Box 18.2.

PHYSICAL EXAMINATION

The patient should have a complete evaluation, including an MSE. The physical examination itself will be unremarkable related specifically to conduct disorder.

DIFFERENTIAL DIAGNOSIS

The differential diagnosis for conduct disorder is summarized in Table 18.10.

DIAGNOSTIC STUDIES

There are several assessments or rating scales that may be helpful, including the Vanderbilt Assessment Scale, Strengths and Difficulties Questionnaire as well as evaluation of callous-unemotional traits. These rating assessments are utilized by the parent and teacher or even by the individual (depending on age) to answer a series of questions. The Strengths and Difficulties Questionnaire rating scale is 25 items designed for evaluation of 4- to 17-year-olds and completed by both the parent and teacher. It has been shown to have a specificity of 90% in the parent score and 95% specificity in the teacher evaluation. However, the sensitivity is only 67% and 33%, respectively, related to conduct disorder.[122]

Despite the changes noted in neuroimaging, brain imaging is not currently considered diagnostic.

EVALUATION

In evaluation of the patient, the age of onset is important to determine the specifier. If at least one symptom is exhibited prior to age 10, then the patient can be diagnosed with childhood-onset. If no symptoms existed prior to age 10, the individual is considered to have the adolescent-onset. An individual can also be given the specifier of *limited prosocial emotions* if the patient demonstrates two of the following consistently over the past 12 months: does not demonstrate concern over one's performance, lack of guilt or remorse, lack of empathy, lack of emotion, or superficial emotion shared with others. Severity of the disorder is specified and ranges from mild to severe in relation to the conduct issues exhibited.[113]

TREATMENT

- Psychosocial interventions are considered first-line treatment for conduct disorder and include interventions focused on the individual and the family.[123]
    - Interventions for the patient include anger management, problem-solving skills, and development of social skills.
    - Intervention with the family include teaching consistent parenting, modeling empathy and emotional expression to the child, developing a supportive home environment with positive feedback, and encouraging parents to seek treatment for their own mental health disorders if relevant.

BOX 18.2 Groups of Behavior Utilized to Diagnose Conduct Disorder

Violating rules
Truancy in school begins before 13 years old
Despite parent objection, is out at night beginning prior to 13 years old
Runs away from home overnight on either two occasions or for an extended time while living with parents or an equivalent home
Property destruction
Sets fire intentionally to cause significant damage
Damages other property intentionally without setting fire
Lying and stealing
Lies in order to avoid responsibility or to gain commodities or favors
Steals items that have significant value without confronting victim
Breaks into another's car, home, or building
Human and animal aggression
Physically cruel to animals
Physically cruel to other humans
Initiates physical altercations often
Often engages in intimidation, threats or bullying of others
Utilizes a weapon that can result in serious harm to others
Steals from another while confronting them
Forces another to engage in sexual activity

Source: Data from Johnson S, Hollis C, Marlow N, Simms V, Wolke D. Screening for childhood mental health disorders using strengths and difficulties questionnaire: the validity of multi-informant reports. Dev Med Child Neurol. *2014;56(5):453–459. doi:10.1111/dmcn.12360*

TABLE 18.10 Differential Diagnosis for Conduct Disorder

Diagnosis	Description
Adjustment disorder	Behavior in response to a stressor can be irritable or disruptive, but this resolves within 6 months after stressor removed.
Attention-deficit/hyperactivity disorder	Symptoms include impulsivity and disruptive behavior, but not at the expense of others' rights. Individuals do not violate the social or age-related norms.
Depression	Irritable mood or aggression related to depressed mood are primary symptoms. Conduct disorder if present would have problems with behavior outside of any mood disturbance
Intermittent explosive disorder	Symptoms include aggressive and impulsive behavior, but not premeditated or for one's own gain.
Oppositional defiant disorder	Symptoms include conflict with adults and authority. Individuals often irritable or have an angry mood, but not violating norms or rights of others.

- Patients should be treated for any other comorbid diagnosis.
- Pharmacologic agents are not currently approved by the Food and Drug Administration (FDA) in the United States for treatment of conduct disorder, but risperidone and valproate have conditional recommendations and have been studied.[123]

PATIENT EDUCATION

- Conduct disorder diagnosis places patient at risk of developing antisocial personality disorder.
- Those with childhood onset of disease or an early onset have poorer prognosis with increased risk of criminal activities. The earlier the onset, the poorer the prognosis.

18.7 CHRONIC PAIN SYNDROMES

MARCI CONTRERAS

OVERVIEW

Chronic pain syndrome is a complex neurologic problem with devastating effects. In most circumstances acute pain may be considered useful as it helps one identify injury or illness. Pain lasting >12 weeks is considered *chronic*. In chronic pain syndromes, often the cause is unknown and can be complicated by biologic, psychological, and social factors. Chronic pain syndromes can stem from several different areas and might involve more than one organ system. Some types of chronic pain syndromes include:

- Musculoskeletal disorders such as low back pain, neck pain, or fibromyalgia
- Chronic visceral disorders such as inflammatory bowel disease, endometriosis, or interstitial cystitis
- Peripheral neuropathy
- Trigeminal neuralgia
- Lesions of the central nervous system (CNS) such as a spinal cord injury, stroke, or multiple sclerosis
- Cancer pain
- Headache
- Psychogenic pain

EPIDEMIOLOGY

Approximately 20% of adults live with chronic pain in the United States.[124] Chronic pain syndromes occur more commonly in women. There is higher prevalence in adults with advancing age.

PATHOPHYSIOLOGY

It is possible that an acute injury could turn into a chronic pain syndrome in which pain signals continue to fire for weeks, months, or even years. Some patients suffer from chronic pain without ever having a previous injury or concomitant disease. For reasons poorly understood, there is a disruption of nociception and how the nerves transmit signals. Persistent pain signals eventually cause the nervous system to undergo "remodeling" in which pain receptors become hypersensitive.[125] This altered state leads to an amplified or dysfunctional perception of pain even in the absence of a stimulus. This pain continues beyond a certain threshold and becomes a vicious cycle.

MEDICAL HISTORY AND CLINICAL PRESENTATION

The approach to the patient with chronic pain should be one of compassion while trying to build a good rapport. The clinician should have good communication skills and respect the patient's situation. Without validation, the patient is not likely to trust their clinician nor are they likely to feel heard.

Questions to ask patients:

- Where does the pain occur?
- How often do you have pain?
- How long does the pain last?
- Does the pain occur at a certain time of day? Are there other associations?
- Rate the pain on a scale of 0–10 with 0 having no pain at all and 10 having the "worst pain ever."
- Describe the characteristic(s) of the pain (e.g., dull, aching, sharp, shooting, tingling, burning, throbbing).
- Does the pain prohibit you from daily activities? Work? Sex? Hobbies?
- Does the pain interfere with your sleep?
- How do others who are close to you respond when you are in pain?
- Does anything help to alleviate the pain? Does anything exacerbate the pain?

Chronic pain is commonly associated with depression. Often these patients will present with anxiety, frustration, or even anger. Because of their chronic pain condition, patients will have difficulty falling asleep or staying asleep. This disruption in sleep patterns only adds to the patient's fatigue and mood abnormalities. Social isolation can be common, as the patient may feel as though they are always complaining to others and do not want to be viewed as a burden.

SIGNS AND SYMPTOMS

Depending on the location of the pain, patients may have symptoms of low back pain, headaches, pelvic pain, myofascial pain, or other. It is important to understand that physical symptoms may not be fully explained by an established underlying diagnosis. Chronic pain can occur without ever knowing of a root cause. Discover what type of behaviors the patient exhibits when they are in pain (e.g., grimace, moan, limp, or guarding).

PHYSICAL EXAMINATION

It is possible that a patient's chronic pain syndrome may have originated with an acute injury, inflammation, or neuropathy. However, the more typical scenario is that there are no physical signs or evidence of a noxious stimulus. A complete neurologic examination and musculoskeletal examination should be performed.

DIFFERENTIAL DIAGNOSIS

The differential diagnosis for chronic pain syndrome is summarized in Table 18.11.

At this stage, all necessary "rule-outs" should be determined to identify an underlying cause or possible trigger for the chronic pain. Some examples of these conditions might include osteoarthritis, herniated disc, peripheral neuropathy, multiple sclerosis, inflammatory bowel disease, and interstitial cystitis.

TABLE 18.11 Differential Diagnosis for Chronic Pain Syndrome

Diagnosis	Description
Complex regional pain syndrome	Usually affects one limb long after an initial injury (>6 months)
Autoimmune disorders	Rheumatoid arthritis, systemic lupus erythematosus, Sjögren disease

DIAGNOSTIC STUDIES

Appropriate laboratory studies should be performed to rule out autoimmune disorders or other inflammatory markers as discussed. Imaging the target area should include x-rays, CT scans, or MRIs. Diagnostic procedures might include electromyography (EMG) or nerve conduction studies.

EVALUATION

The patient-clinician relationship should be built on trust and collaboration. The compassionate clinician acknowledges the patient's problem and understands the patient's goals for treatment. It is not the clinician's job to decide whether the pain is "inappropriate" but rather should be focused on the patient's *response to pain and ability to function*. The clinician should respond with empathy to the patient's emotions. What does the pain keep the patient from doing? What are the social consequences? How does the pain affect productivity or quality of life?

Chronic pain syndromes may be complicated by an SUD as some patients tend to self-medicate with alcohol or drugs in an effort to reduce the pain.

TREATMENT

Treatment for chronic pain syndromes can be challenging for the clinician and frustrating for the patient. Treatment should be individualized as what works for one person may not work for another. The clinician should avoid the use of opioid medications. Analgesics and antianxiety medications are typically not helpful and may lead to misuse. Antidepressants tend to be the most effective pharmacologic therapy as well as antiepileptic medications.

A goal in management should be to improve quality of life and functionality rather than completely eradicating the pain, as this is not always realistic. It is extremely important to discuss the patient's goal in treatment. Some patients think they should "tough it out" while others want the pain to be treated aggressively to eliminate the pain.

Having negative emotions and little sleep certainly does not help to improve the patient's condition. Some strategies to help cope with chronic pain conditions and to be used in therapeutic management include:

- Mindfulness/meditation
  - Allows for a positive distraction
- Sleep hygiene
- Stress reduction/relaxation techniques
- Physical therapy/exercise
  - Low-impact exercise such as walking, bicycling, or swimming
  - Yoga, stretching
  - Improves mood
  - Increases function
  - Inactivity and isolation are not helpful
- Massage/muscle relaxation
- Biofeedback
- Psychotherapy/CBT
- Acupuncture
- Hypnosis
- Transcutaneous electrical nerve stimulation (TENS)
- Journaling
  - Keeping a diary of thoughts and events but then destroying what was written allows the patient to "let go" and avoid holding on to the negativity or pain.

PATIENT EDUCATION

What is the patient's goal for treatment? Consider whether the patient has unrealistic expectations, as there may be no "cure." It is important that the patient understand their role in management (e.g., improve sleep patterns, stress reduction, physical activity). How might the clinician help the patient "live" with this condition? Does the patient have support from family? Friends? Are certain accommodations needed at work?

Patients have a better prognosis and need less pain medication if they are willing to participate in the above suggested therapies. Patients with poor coping skills, noncompliance, and those with a negative outlook tend to have a poor prognosis. These patients may feel defeated, continually ruminate, or catastrophize their pain (e.g., "end up in a wheelchair," or their "life is over"). It is important that the PA provide hope.

Pearls

- *The pain is real.* It is important that the clinician acknowledge this to establish a therapeutic relationship with the patient.
- Patients with chronic pain may present with anger or other mood abnormality.
- Consider cultural influences.
- Distressing symptoms from other comorbid conditions may lower pain threshold (or decrease pain tolerance.)

18.8 PERSONALITY DISORDERS

Jill Cavalet

OVERVIEW

Personality disorders are common and are seen in a variety of clinical settings. Individuals with a personality disorder display persistent unhealthy and inappropriate thoughts or behaviors that may disrupt the clinician-patient relationship. Additionally, clinicians should realize that patients may exhibit traits of personality disorders that are below the threshold for a diagnosis, but these can still influence the patient's functioning and the patient encounter.

There are currently 10 personality disorders, which are categorized into three clusters. Each cluster comprises disorders that share similar symptoms. Cluster A is characterized by odd and eccentric behaviors and includes paranoid, schizoid, and schizotypal personality disorders. Cluster B disorders exhibit dramatic, emotional, erratic, and impulsive symptoms and include antisocial, borderline, histrionic, and narcissistic personality disorders. Cluster C is characterized by anxious and fearful symptoms and includes avoidant, dependent, and obsessive-compulsive personality disorders. Some individuals may display traits of several disorders within a cluster because of the overlap of symptoms.[122]

Personality disorders are lasting and fixed; symptoms can be traced back at least to adolescence or early adulthood. The symptoms are present in a variety of settings and behaviors do not align with those expected within cultural norms.[122] The use of immature defense mechanisms is largely seen in personality disorders. These mechanisms are used frequently and become a maladaptive way of coping.[126]

EPIDEMIOLOGY

Personality disorders are common. The prevalence of personality disorders ranges from 10% to 20%.[122,126] Approximately 15% of U.S. adults have at least one personality disorder.[122] Approximately half of patients with another psychiatric disorder also have a personality disorder.[126] Obsessive-compulsive personality disorder is one of the most common, with prevalence estimated as high as 7%.[122]

There are gender differences seen in the prevalence of personality disorders. Borderline, histrionic, and dependent personality disorders are diagnosed more frequently in females. Antisocial and narcissistic personality disorders are diagnosed more frequently in males.[122]

PATHOPHYSIOLOGY

Like most other psychiatric illnesses, the exact etiology of personality disorders is unknown. Familial and genetic risks have been noted. Environmental influences may play a role as well. Biologic factors such as the role of neurotransmitters or hormones continue to be explored.[122,126] As noted above, the use of defense mechanisms in personality disorders must also be appreciated.

There are several other known risks for personality disorders. Schizoid and schizotypal personality disorders may be more prevalent in those with a positive family history of schizophrenia. Risks for antisocial personality disorder include child abuse, unstable parenting, inconsistent discipline, and a personal history of conduct disorder. Patients with borderline personality disorder often have histories of physical and sexual abuse, neglect, early parental loss, and hostile conflict. A history of harsh discipline is seen in patients with obsessive-compulsive personality disorder.[122,126]

A personality *change* from the individual's baseline (which is more abrupt and not as long-standing as a personality disorder) should prompt a medical evaluation to rule out any organic cause of that symptom. An abrupt personality or behavioral change from baseline is not typical of a personality disorder.

MEDICAL HISTORY AND CLINICAL PRESENTATION

Most patients with personality disorders will not self-present with a complaint or concern due to the ego-syntonic nature of the disorder. The thoughts and behaviors that occur as part of the disorder are acceptable to the ego, and do not cause distress for the patient despite negatively affecting others. Individuals have limited to no insight into their behavior and are often brought for evaluation by a family member or other loved one. Comorbid psychiatric complaints such as depression or anxiety might be reasons for self-referral. Additionally, consequences of the patient's behavior, such as a job loss or ending of a relationship, might also prompt an evaluation.[127]

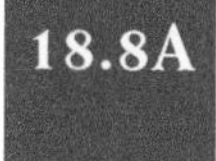

18.8A CLUSTER A PERSONALITY DISORDERS

SIGNS AND SYMPTOMS

Paranoid personality disorder is characterized by symptoms of mistrust and suspiciousness. Individuals feel that others will harm, exploit, or deceive them. They will not readily confide in others and often bear grudges. Patients with this disorder frequently do not get along well with others, although they may feel comfortable with groups that share common paranoid beliefs. They are often guarded and secretive, and may also be argumentative or aloof.[122,126]

Schizoid personality disorder exhibits a disinterest in close relationships and a diminished range of emotional expression. Those with schizoid personality disorder are "loners" and prefer it that way, appearing cold and aloof. They will have few friends, are often unmarried, and participate in solitary activities. They may be employed in positions with little contact with others, such as preferring the night shift. If they do seek medical care, they may appear uncomfortable, emotionally detached, and display poor eye contact.[122,126]

Schizotypal personality disorder presents with eccentric behavior, discomfort in close relationships, and cognitive or perceptual distortions. Individuals are noticeably odd or strange and are uncomfortable relating to others, with possible signs of social anxiety. Gathering a history might be challenging. Those with schizotypal personality disorder typically lack close friends. They may exhibit ideas of reference, feel that they have magical control, or believe they have special powers such as reading minds or predicting the future. Patients' affect may be inappropriate to the situation and speech may be unusual and/or vague. Individuals may also display suspiciousness or paranoia, especially when under stress.[122,126] Patients with schizotypal personality disorder are at risk for developing schizophrenia.

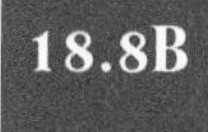

18.8B CLUSTER B PERSONALITY DISORDERS

SIGNS AND SYMPTOMS

Antisocial personality disorder exhibits a disregard for the rights of others; individuals generally lack empathy and are deceitful and manipulative. Those with antisocial personality disorder are also referred to as "psychopaths" or "sociopaths." They will repeatedly engage in activities that are grounds for arrest and can be aggressive and reckless. They may display inflated self-esteem and can also be charming. Histories of truancy, thefts, fights, and comorbid substance use are common.[122,126] The diagnosis of antisocial personality disorder is given to individuals 18 years of age or older, and is given only if there is a history of conduct disorder symptoms prior to age 15.[122]

Borderline personality disorder is characterized by impulsive behaviors and unstable relationships, self-image, and affect. Individuals are often in a state of crisis and will have labile moods and/or angry outbursts. They have difficulty with personal boundaries and fear abandonment and may express feelings of emptiness. They may obtain comfort from transitional objects (e.g., pets, stuffed animals, or other inanimate objects) and bring them into the hospital or to appointments. Patients with this disorder may either idealize or devalue others, illustrating the concrete way of viewing others as either all good or all bad. This is referred to as "splitting" when staff or others are pitted against one another. They may also become manipulative and claim that "you are the only person who truly understands me," or similar claims, to the clinician. Relationships are usually intense and short-lived. Suicidal gestures or self-mutilating behaviors including cutting or burning can occur frequently in borderline personality disorder.

Histrionic personality disorder presents with attention-seeking behaviors and excessive emotionality. Individuals may be dramatic or flirtatious, and like to be the center of attention. They may also exhibit seductive or provocative behaviors. Individuals with histrionic personality disorder may display behaviors that are exaggerated or theatrical. Child-like temper tantrums can also occur. Patients with this disorder often consider relationships to be more intimate than they are. They become bored with a routine, project, or relationship and can be easily influenced.[122,126] There is also a strong association between histrionic personality disorder and somatic symptom disorders (Somatoform disorders).

Narcissistic personality disorder patients exhibit arrogant, grandiose behaviors, a need for admiration, and an absence of empathy. Individuals feel entitled and that they are superior to others, often leading to exploitive behaviors. They may boast about their abilities or accomplishments. Those with the disorder may be preoccupied with success, power, or beauty, and require excessive admiration. Patients may demand only the "best" care and may not wish to associate with those who are perceived to be beneath them. They may also exhibit an overly sensitive response to criticism or defeat and have an underlying fragile state of self-esteem.[122,126]

18.8C CLUSTER C PERSONALITY DISORDERS

SIGNS AND SYMPTOMS

Avoidant personality disorder is characterized by inhibition, feeling inadequate, and sensitivity to criticism. Individuals feel inferior and are timid, avoiding new activities or taking risks. They may be shy or quiet in an attempt to remain invisible, and will avoid forming relationships for fear of criticism, disapproval, or rejection.[122] Those with the disorder will rarely speak up in public settings and are often employed in vocations where they can remain on the periphery. A history of social phobia is common.[122,127] In contrast to schizoid personality disorder, those with avoidant personality disorder would prefer relationships but need much reassurance of acceptance.

Dependent personality disorder presents as a pattern of submissive and clinging behavior due to an excessive need to be taken care of, or fear of separation. Individuals with this disorder feel that they cannot function without the help of others and have great difficulty making simple decisions. They feel helpless when alone. They are often pessimistic and filled with self-doubt, even seeking dominance or overprotection to avoid being alone.[122] Individuals may have difficulty initiating projects and will avoid leadership positions or become anxious if asked to do so.[126]

Obsessive-compulsive personality disorder shows a pattern of preoccupation with orderliness, perfectionism, and control.[122] It is not to be confused with OCD, discussed elsewhere in this chapter (Section 18.1D), which is characterized by obsessions and compulsions and patients maintain insight into their behaviors. In obsessive-compulsive personality disorder, much attention is paid to details, lists, rules, and schedules. They have difficulty understanding the perspectives of others and have high standards and moral principles. They work to control situations and may be reluctant to delegate tasks due to believing they need to be done a certain way. Additionally, they may spend excessive time on tasks, which can interfere with completion. Patients with this disorder may also be conscientious and inflexible, stingy, and stubborn. They may have difficulty discarding objects, becoming a "pack rat." There is similarity to "type A" personality traits in that those with this personality disorder display excessive devotion to work and productivity, time urgency, and competitiveness.[122]

MENTAL STATUS EXAMINATION

The MSE of a patient with a personality disorder will vary depending upon the specific disorder(s). The behavior of patients with Cluster A personality disorders may be guarded, detached, or odd. The behavior and appearance of a patient with histrionic personality disorder may be attention seeking and flamboyant. Those with narcissistic personality disorder may be arrogant or entitled.

Speech patterns or phrasing could be unusual in schizotypal personality disorder. Speech can be theatrical in histrionic personality disorder.

Mood and affect may be inappropriate in schizotypal personality disorder. In schizoid personality disorder, the affect could be diminished in range. A patient with antisocial personality disorder might display an angry or charming demeanor. Those with borderline personality disorder may exhibit labile mood and affect. An anxious mood might be apparent in the avoidant or schizotypal patient.

Concerning psychotic symptoms, paranoia may be present in paranoid personality disorder. Brief periods of paranoia may also occur in borderline personality disorder when the individual is under stress. Perceptual disturbances or ideas of reference may occur in schizotypal personality disorder.

Insight into the personality disorder and maladaptive behaviors is typically poor. Cognition is not significantly impaired unless there is a comorbid delirium, dementia, or substance intoxication or withdrawal.

DIFFERENTIAL DIAGNOSIS

The differential diagnosis for personality disorders can include psychotic disorders, depression, anxiety, SUD, or another personality disorder within the same cluster (Box 18.3).[122,126] Ensure that the symptoms of the personality disorder have been present since at least early adulthood and do not occur solely during the course of another psychiatric condition. For example, paranoia only occurring during exacerbations of schizophrenia would rule out paranoid personality disorder, or labile mood only occurring during a manic episode would rule out borderline personality disorder.

BOX 18.3 Differential Diagnosis for Personality Disorders

Psychotic disorders
Depression
Anxiety
Substance use disorder
Autism spectrum disorder
Personality disorder in the same cluster
Personality change due to another medical condition

DIAGNOSTIC STUDIES

There are no confirmatory diagnostic tests for psychiatric disorders; therefore, the *DSM-5* criteria are utilized in making the diagnosis.[122] In antisocial personality disorder, abnormal EEGs and other neurologic soft signs indicative of minimal brain damage are sometimes seen.[126]

It is also important to order appropriate toxicology screens and diagnostic tests to evaluate for comorbid medical conditions. Examples include a CBC, CMP, thyroid function studies, and potentially brain imaging. Other diagnostic tests may be ordered if appropriate to a specific medical diagnosis.

EVALUATION

The evaluation of a patient with a personality disorder should include a thorough psychiatric and medical history along with an MSE. A physical examination should be completed to assess for comorbid medical conditions. Diagnostic studies should be ordered as needed to rule out other conditions or to establish baseline functioning (e.g., CBC, renal or hepatic status) before initiating treatment.

Evaluate for long-standing impairment in thoughts, behavior, and functioning. Note whether the pattern of behavior is persistent in a variety of settings. The pattern should be able to be traced back at least to adolescence or early adulthood.[122] Additional history from other sources may be needed as well, due to the lack of insight and ego-syntonic nature of personality disorders. Clinicians should also consider the cultural background of the patient in order to determine whether symptoms are an expected component of the individual's cultural norms. For example, gender roles differ greatly in certain cultural, ethnic, or social communities. Additionally, religious beliefs or rituals as part of cultural norms may need to be distinguished from the magical beliefs of schizotypal personality disorder.

TREATMENT

- Psychotherapy is the recommended treatment for most personality disorders.[126]
  - Dialectical behavior therapy (DBT) is recommended for borderline personality disorder.[126]
    - DBT derives from several other techniques, including behavioral therapy. It has demonstrated efficacy in improving interpersonal skills and decreasing self-destructive behavior. There is a group skills component, as well as individual therapy. Therapists can be available for telephone consultations as needed if patients find themselves in a crisis that could result in injurious behavior to themselves or others.[126]
  - Patients with antisocial personality disorder may not respond as well to therapy and may be involved with the legal system due to their criminal behaviors.[126]
  - Avoidant personality disorder may benefit from assertiveness therapy.[126]
  - Those with obsessive-compulsive personality disorder may be more open to treatment in comparison to the other personality disorders, as they are more aware of their impairments.[126]
- Medications cannot be utilized to treat personality dysfunctions, but treating symptoms such as mood lability, depression, or anxiety is appropriate.[126]
  - Using mood stabilizers for patients with borderline or antisocial personality disorder can assist in decreasing impulsive or aggressive behaviors.
  - The use of SSRIs would be appropriate for the anxious features of Cluster C disorders.
  - Antipsychotics may be utilized for Cluster A disorders or for mood stabilization in Cluster B.

PATIENT EDUCATION

- PAs should educate patients that personality disorders are chronic, but treatment is available to assist the patient in recognizing and altering maladaptive thoughts and behaviors.
- Education should be provided about the diagnosis and other potential comorbid conditions. Knowledge can assist in compliance and motivation for treatment. Involving family members or others in the support system is imperative as well.
- Encourage patients to maintain a healthy support system and avoid becoming or remaining isolated.
- Patients should avoid illicit drugs, prescription drugs of abuse, and alcohol. These substances can exacerbate symptoms and interfere negatively with treatment.
- Encourage support groups for those with personality disorders.
- Educate patients on the benefits of keeping a journal as a way to express emotions.
- Encourage relaxation and stress reduction techniques such as meditation, mindfulness, yoga, positive imagery, and deep breathing exercises.
- Provide education on the importance of exercise, physical activity, and proper sleep, which can help improve symptoms of depression and anxiety and contribute to overall well-being.
- Maintain preventive medical care and recommended screenings.

18.9 PSYCHOTIC DISORDERS

MICHAEL HIGBEE

OVERVIEW

Schizophrenia and other psychotic disorders are some of the most perplexing, misunderstood, and undertreated mental health conditions. Often portrayed incorrectly in popular culture, psychotic disorders cause immense suffering of the individual, the family, and the community at large. Comorbid substance use, metabolic abnormalities, poor self-care and a multitude of other unwanted branches grow off the tree of schizophrenia. While great strides have been made in the knowledge and treatment of psychotic disorders, there remains much to learn about these complex diseases. Schizophrenia, the most thought about psychotic disorder, is postulated to be caused by the interaction of genes with an adverse environment. Experts estimate that genetics contribute about 80% to the disorder[127] with the other 20% coming from biologic factors such as birth complications, intrauterine infections/malnutrition, and psychosocial factors including adverse family interactions and growing up in an urban environment. The economic cost of schizophrenia in the United States is estimated between $94 million and $102 billion per year including indirect costs.[128]

While psychotic disorders are the focus of this section, schizophrenia will be given special consideration as most clinicians will encounter this disorder throughout their career. Of utmost importance is that not all disorders involving delusions and hallucinations necessitate a diagnosis of schizophrenia. This point cannot be overstated. Organic disorders, substance intoxication, and other psychotic disorders must be ruled out before a diagnosis of schizophrenia is given.

EPIDEMIOLOGY

Psychotic disorders are estimated to affect 1 in 150 individuals at some point in their lifetime worldwide[129]; however, other studies show a lifetime prevalence rate between 3.06% and 3.48%.[130] In the United States, the prevalence of schizophrenia is about 1%. Approximately half of those affected receive treatment. Access to care as well as misconceptions about these disorders remain barriers to adequate treatment.

Gender and Age

The prevalence ratio of schizophrenia is 1.4 to 1 male predominance.[131] The peak of onset of schizophrenia is between 15 and 30 years old; however, the first episode in men tends to occur from the teens to mid-20s and in females from the teens to late 20s. Earlier onset tends to predict a poor prognosis. Onset before age 10 and after age 45 is extremely rare. Late-onset schizophrenia is characterized by the first episode occurring after age 45. Men tend to have a worse prognosis than women.[132] Factors when comparing outcomes of males versus females included number/length of hospitalizations, periods of recovery, global functioning, and percentage of psychotic activity.

Risk Factors

Multiple risk factors contributing to the development of schizophrenia have been identified, though many have yet to be discovered. The following risk factors have been implicated in the etiology of schizophrenia:

- Increased paternal age at the time of conception[133]
- Higher number of children born to parents with schizophrenia; thought to reflect deinstitutionalization and subsequent community focus of treatment. Of note, fertility rate of persons with schizophrenia is close to that of the general population. There's a 10-fold greater risk of schizophrenia in offspring compared with the general population.
- Living in an urban area may increase psychosocial stressors.[134]
- Obstetric complications
- Winter or early spring birth is postulated to reflect increased incidence of maternal infection during these months.[135]
- Inflammation
- Cannabis use—THC is thought to be psychotomimetic while cannabidiol may have potential psychotolytic properties.

PATHOPHYSIOLOGY

The pathophysiology of psychotic disorders is multifactorial in nature. While these disorders are of immense complexity, there have been great strides in understanding these disease processes with the aid of neuroimaging, knowledge of genetics, and increased availability of information. The various factors contributing to the onset of psychotic disorders—most notably schizophrenia—are summed up below.

- Neurochemical factors
  - **Dopamine:** The most prominent neurochemical implicated in schizophrenia is dopamine. Most antipsychotics work by antagonizing dopamine type 2 receptors (D2). Drugs that increase dopamine activity, most notably cocaine and amphetamines, are thought of as psychotomimetics (i.e., psychosis inducing). With dopamine, it is important to consider which tracts in the brain are affected and how.
    - Too much dopamine in the mesolimbic dopamine pathway is thought to mediate positive symptoms, which include delusions and hallucinations
    - Too little dopamine in the mesocortical dopamine pathway mediates the negative and cognitive symptoms of schizophrenia including disorganized speech, diminished emotional expression, and avolition or lack of initiative to accomplish purposeful tasks (e.g., brushing teeth, bathing).
  - **Serotonin:** Second-generation antipsychotics (SGAs), also known as atypical antipsychotics, work by antagonizing both dopamine and serotonin. This is the defining difference between typical and atypical antipsychotics. Serotonin is thought to be involved in both positive and negative symptoms of schizophrenia.
  - **GABA:** Also known as gamma-aminobutyric acid, GABA is an inhibitory neurotransmitter that has a regulatory effect on dopaminergic neurons. Loss of this inhibitory effect may result in increased dopamine activity.
  - **Glutamate:** NMDA (N-methyl-D-aspartate) receptor antagonists such as PCP (phencyclidine) produce both positive and negative symptoms of schizophrenia.
  - **Nicotinic acetylcholine receptors:** Disruption may play a role in the cognitive symptoms of schizophrenia. These receptors respond to agonists such as nicotine and, as such, tobacco use may act as a form of self-medication.
- Neuroanatomic factors
  - **Decreased synaptic density:** Synaptic density is at its highest in the first 1 to 2 years of life. This density of synapses undergoes pruning during adolescence. A popular saying in neuroscience is that "neurons that fire together, wire together." Developmentally, the neurocircuits that do not fire often are eliminated during adolescence. Excessive pruning during this period is thought to underlie the development of schizophrenia[136]

  - **Cerebral ventricular changes:** Lateral and third ventricular enlargement has consistently been found in schizophrenia.
- Genetics
  - Concordance rate in monozygotic twins is about 40% whereas in dizygotic twins, the rate is about 10%.[137]
  - Increased expression of complement component 4 allele A, known as C4A, may be responsible for the excess synaptic pruning in adolescence and subsequent development of schizophrenia.[138]
  - In general, it is thought that a confluence of multiple genes, rather than a single gene, is responsible for the complex of symptoms that forms schizophrenia.

18.9A SCHIZOPHRENIA

MEDICAL HISTORY AND CLINICAL PRESENTATION

The signs and symptoms of patients with schizophrenia can be broken down into three stages: premorbid, prodromal, and eventual diagnosis. Premorbid signs and symptoms are nonspecific and typically include a delay in milestones such as sitting, standing, and walking.[139] Patients who eventually develop schizophrenia may also show delays in speech development and organizational skills. Increased clumsiness and slower reaction times have been noted. They tend to be more isolated, passive, and introverted. There have also been suggestions of differences in maternal bonding with a child who goes on to develop schizophrenia.[139] It has been postulated that the mother subconsciously perceives the child as "different" and this may affect maternal-child bonding.

Prodromal signs and symptoms are often recognized after a first psychotic break. These signs and symptoms may have been present for months or years prior to the diagnosis. Typically, the patient has shown progressively poorer functioning in family, occupational, and educational settings. The *DSM-5* has included attenuated psychosis syndrome under "conditions for further study." This was an effort to delineate subthreshold psychotic symptoms that may predict future psychotic disorders. While not an official diagnosis, this was an attempt at early identification and subsequent treatment with the hopes of mitigating the progression of schizophrenia and other psychoses. The presence of delusions, hallucinations, or disorganized speech must be present at least once a week for the last month to qualify.

Case Vignette

Mr. S, a 21-year-old male with no previous known psychiatric history, was brought to the local crisis center by police. He was found by police sitting on the median of a major highway wearing a heavy coat, boxers, and a pair of boots. Upon initial assessment, Mr. S presents with blunted affect and multiple tattoos on his face. He is guarded and dismissive with his answers. When asked why he decided to sit on the median of this major highway, he replies, "I just like to be spontaneous sometimes." He is further asked about the potential dangers of doing this, to which he is unable to say what these risks are. His urine drug screen is positive for THC and he has no past medical history. Collateral from his family reveals multiple run-ins with the law including one arrest that eventually led to 4 months in the county jail. His family states that he has become increasingly isolated and has been exhibiting bizarre behavior and angry outbursts. He initially denies delusions, hallucinations, or any other criteria for psychosis. On day 3 of admission, and with careful probing during assessment, Mr. S stands up and in an angry tone states, "I don't understand what's going on, I feel like people are controlling my movements, I feel like I'm controlling other people's movements. I just can't understand this! What the hell is going on with me!" He relates that this started 6 months prior and has progressed in intensity and frequency. He later endorses auditory hallucinations.

As the case above illustrates, patients often realize during the prodromal phase that something's "not quite right." Family members will notice differences in behaviors that represent a change from baseline. These prodromal signs and symptoms, however, are most often noticed in retrospect. The first psychotic break then follows and eventual diagnosis will depend on the timeline of signs and symptoms.

SIGNS AND SYMPTOMS

In the event that schizophrenia is eventually diagnosed, to qualify for a diagnosis, continuous signs must be present in some form for at least 6 months. The signs and symptoms can be broken down into three categories: positive, negative, and cognitive symptoms (Figure 18.8). A simple way to remember these domains is that positive symptoms add something that was not previously there (e.g., delusions and hallucinations). Negative symptoms present as deficits in something such as enjoyment or expressiveness. Cognitive symptoms include problems with working memory, attention, reasoning, etc. A common misperception among clinicians is that the positive symptoms should be the focus of interventions. However, patients and their families are equally bothered by the negative and cognitive symptoms. As such, all three domains need to be addressed.

- Positive symptoms
  - **Hallucinations:** Any of the five senses may be involved, though auditory hallucinations are the most prominent, followed by visual hallucinations. Tactile, gustatory, and olfactory hallucinations can occur but tend to be rare, and if present, consideration needs to be given to a possible medical or substance-induced cause.
    - **Auditory hallucinations:** Tend to be condescending in nature. Special attention needs to be given if command auditory hallucinations are present as these increase the risk of self-harm, suicide, and violent behavior. Auditory hallucinations may also present as sounds such as machines, music, etc. Voices can be multiple, single, loud, soft, intermittent, or

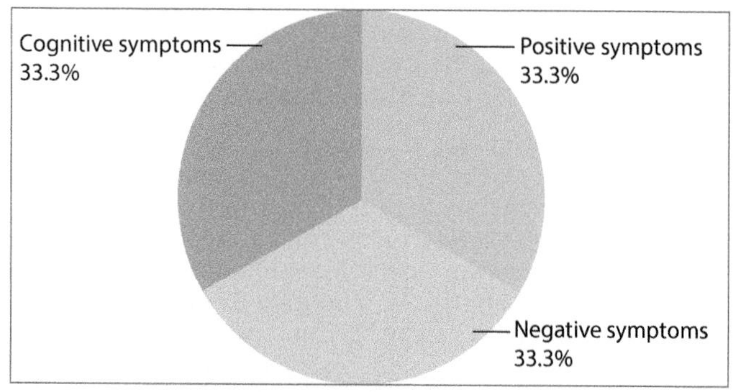

Figure 18.8 Theoretical percentage of consideration given to three domains of schizophrenia.

persistent. Specific descriptors can aid in gauging the effectiveness of treatment. Auditory hallucinations tend to respond well to medications.
    - **Visual hallucinations:** While less common than auditory hallucinations, visual hallucinations are a relatively common occurrence. In schizophrenia, they tend to present in the form of formless objects such as flashes of light, visual patterns, and shadows. When patients describe visual hallucinations as more detailed forms such as bugs or other humans, the differential diagnosis should include an underlying medical condition or substance-induced psychosis.
  - **Illusions:** In contrast to hallucinations, which are based on nonexistent images or sensations, illusions are distortions of real objects or sensations. An example would include a hand growing out of a doorknob or a face turning into a monster.
  - **Delusions:** Delusions are defined as fixed, false beliefs. Despite overwhelming evidence to the contrary, patients with delusions will continue to display an unwavering belief in these thoughts. Early in the disease, patients may have some insight that something is not quite normal. However, as schizophrenia progresses, the patient tends to show little or no insight to the delusional system. Medication tends to work well to improve this insight. A good practice to help gauge clinical response is to document the "distance" that the patient has from these delusions. Carefully worded questions to explore alternative explanations for these beliefs can be very useful (see techniques discussed in Diagnostic Studies section). Theoretically, delusions can be broken down into multiple themes; however, in clinical practice, they rarely fit into well-defined categories. A good practice to improve clarity is to describe the overall type of delusion with a comment on content (use of patient's own words in documentation is invaluable). For example, a patient who is receiving messages from God to influence the time of sunrise may be said to have delusions of grandiosity with religious content.
    - **Persecutory type:** Patients with persecutory delusions believe that entities such as the government, law enforcement, or even clinicians are plotting against them. In practice, this can hinder the therapeutic relationship or medication adherence. Patients may believe that the clinician is a government spy and, as such, they may refuse to provide applicable information. Delusions of persecution are some of the more common types seen in schizophrenia.
    - **Ideas of reference:** Defined as the belief that random events have personal significance, ideas of reference can take many forms. Some common themes include thoughts that characters on TV or lyrics in music are delivering special messages to the patient.
    - **Thought reading/thought broadcasting:** This is the belief that one can read other people's thoughts or that others can read their thoughts.
    - **Thought insertion/withdrawal:** This is the belief that a patient's thoughts are being withdrawn by an outside entity or that thoughts are being placed inside their mind.
    - **Erotomanic type:** Patients with this type falsely believe that they have a special relationship with someone. This person can be someone they know or someone of higher status such as an actor/actress or other public figure.
    - **Grandiose type:** Patients may believe that they have special powers such as the ability to control world events or that they are receiving messages directly from God.
    - **Somatic type:** In this type of delusion, patients may have a belief that an internal organ, such as their brain, is burning.
  - **Thoughts:** Often overshadowed by the emphasis on delusions and hallucinations, the characterization of schizophrenia as a thought disorder is commonly omitted. Disorders of thought can be assessed by observable behaviors and speech. With behaviors, the clinician can evaluate and comment on whether the patient is responding to internal stimuli (hallucinations). Regarding speech, certain characteristics can give clues to the clinician that a psychotic process is present such as increased speech latency, tangential speech, circumstantial speech, among others. Disruptions in thought processes are discussed below.
    - **Circumstantial speech:** When asked a question, the patient veers off topic but eventually returns.
    - **Tangential speech:** In contrast to circumstantial speech, when responding to a question, a patient with tangential speech never returns to the topic.
    - **Derailment (loosening of associations):** The patient abruptly switches topics. Distinguishing between derailment and tangentiality can be difficult. While confusing, derailment can be thought of as not following a logical progression of thoughts while tangential speech can be linear and logical, but the patient does not answer the question.
    - **Word salad:** Words are thrown together in a nonlinear, illogical manner.
    - **Neologisms:** This consists of nonsensical words that hold meaning to only the person using them.
    - **Poverty of thought:** Patients with poverty of thought may give short one-word answers. When asked to elaborate on answers during an assessment, they are often unable to.
    - **Thought blocking:** Patients with thought blocking will suddenly stop mid-sentence as if something interrupted their train of thought such as a hallucination.
- Negative symptoms:
  - **Can be broken into two categories:** Diminished expression and avolition-apathy. These can be primary or secondary (medication induced or other causes). By blocking dopamine, while decreasing positive symptoms, some medications may inadvertently induce negative symptoms. Whether primary or secondary, these signs and symptoms tend to endure throughout the illness while the positive symptoms typically respond to medications.
  - **Diminished expression**
    - **Affective flattening:** Patients may present with decreased facial expression (blunted or flat affect), decreased hand gestures, poor eye contact, and lack of vocal inflections. After being asked a question with high emotional valence such as the memory of a good time in their life, they may go on to describe it with concrete descriptors in a monotone voice with little to no facial expression and decreased hand gestures. Affect may also be inappropriate as in smiling when describing the death of a loved one.
    - **Speech:** Poverty of speech presents as short answers to open-ended questions. For example, when asked

"Tell me about the house you grew up in" the patient may answer "Just small." Increased speech latency due to internal stimuli or difficulty with cognition may be seen. When asked a question, the patient will show a brief pause before answering. They may appear to be looking behind the clinician or thinking about the question. As previously mentioned, thought blocking in which the patient stops midway through a sentence may be seen.

- **Avolition-apathy**
  - **Apathy:** The patient with schizophrenia with apathy appears disheveled and lacks emotional range. They appear with poor hygiene and may sit on the couch or lay in bed all day. They are indifferent to all things external, good or bad.
  - **Avolition:** Overlapping with apathy, avolition presents with the loss of motivation to perform even the smallest of daily activities. This is the aspect of the illness that is typically associated with medication noncompliance. Brushing teeth daily and other hygiene maintenance become difficult to perform. Poor cognition appears to be at the root of this as well as lack of motivation. Along with poor hygiene, patients with schizophrenia have decreased social drive and, as such, they typically have little to no meaningful social connections. As with the premorbid and prodromal phase, isolation becomes normal. Anhedonia, in which activities that once brought pleasure no longer do, is common in schizophrenia.

PHYSICAL EXAMINATION

Appearance

Patients with schizophrenia often appear disheveled and show abundant evidence of poor self-care, although occasionally they can appear obsessively groomed. They can appear older than their stated age. They may exhibit bizarre mannerisms as with catatonia. Echopraxia, in which the patient mimics the mannerisms of the interviewer, can be seen. Their behavior can range from catatonic stupor, in which the patient can seem lifeless, all the way to extreme agitation, usually in response to hallucinations. Eye contact is typically poor to nonexistent; however, at times they can have piercing eye contact as if they are staring through you. An important concept to keep in mind, no matter what the diagnosis is, is that the interview starts as soon as the patient is called to the office or interview room. In this manner, the patient's gait as well as any abnormal movements can be assessed as the patient walks back to the room. Patients may show shuffling gait, decreased arm swing or other evidence of medication side effects. For documentation purposes, objectivity is paramount. It is important to avoid using interpretations of the patient's appearance. As discussed earlier in the section on signs and symptoms, people with schizophrenia typically have trouble with activities of daily living and medication compliance secondary to cognitive symptoms. The following example should paint a good picture of a common appearance of a patient with schizophrenia.

The patient is a 25-year-old male, appearing older than his stated age. He appears to exhibit poor self-care as evidenced by unkempt, dirty hair, a long unshaven beard and poor dentition. Patient is also malodorous. He is dressed in multiple layers with a ripped heavy jacket despite temperatures in the 80s. He is noted to have decreased upper extremity movement. His eye contact is poor as he often looks off to the corner of the room. Patient is mostly cooperative.

Speech

In agitated states, patients with schizophrenia will often present with loud, rapid speech. In nonagitated states, patients can present with slowed speech or poverty of speech. Echolalia, in which the patient repeats the interviewer's comments, can be present. Speech latency is often increased. When asked simple questions, patients may appear to be pondering their answers for a long period of time before answering. They will also lack inflections of speech. See the example below on documentation continuing with our 25-year-old male.

Mr. S. exhibits poverty of content as evidenced by giving one-word answers to all questions. When asked to elaborate, he is usually unable to. Speech is soft in tone with a notable lack of inflection and speech latency is increased.

Thought Process

Thought process is typically assessed as linear versus nonlinear and logical versus illogical. Patients with schizophrenia often present with a nonlinear thought process. Tangential thought in which the patient starts to answer the question but then wanders off course, never to return to answer the question, can be seen. Though this is not necessarily nonlinear, this can give evidence of the cognitive symptoms. In contrast, loosening of associations or derailment, in which each succeeding sentence has no relation to the previous one, is often seen. The extreme end of loosening of associations is word salad in which the thought process is completely incoherent. Thought blocking in which the patient stops mid-sentence as if interrupted by something is commonly present. A common mistake made by clinicians is to characterize increased speech latency as thought blocking. Increased speech latency is usually, though not always, associated with cognitive symptoms, whereas thought blocking is associated with positive symptoms such as a hallucination or an influx of a bizarre belief.

Regarding illogical versus logical thought, patients with schizophrenia tend to show an illogical thought process. Again, as a thought disorder, patients with schizophrenia will have trouble arriving at a logical answer when asked a question. When asked why a car accident at an intersection happened, a patient with schizophrenia may answer that special forces were behind it. When presented with evidence that one of the drivers behind the wheel was impaired as a possible reason, a patient with schizophrenia may be unable to put this cause and effect together.

Mr. S's thought process was nonlinear as evidenced by mild loosening of associations. Thought blocking is present and thoughts are illogical.

Thought Content

Thought process can be thought of as "how" the patient arrives at answers, whereas thought content is the "what." Patients with schizophrenia typically present with delusions. These may be characterized as nonbizarre versus bizarre. An example of a nonbizarre delusion is the belief that the patient's spouse is cheating on them. Bizarre delusions, in contrast, are beliefs that have no basis in reality, such as the belief that a patient's organs are turning into plastic. An interviewing technique that can often help with eliciting thought content is "normalizing." An example of this when asking about paranoia would be as follows: "People often tell me that they feel that various gangs or the government is following them. Do you ever have feelings like this?" During this section of the MSE, it is very important to ask about the presence of suicidal or homicidal ideation.

Bizarre delusions are present as the patient believes that forces from another planet are controlling his thoughts.

Perception

As previously mentioned, auditory hallucinations are the most common and present in about 80% of patients with schizophrenia. Visual hallucinations present in about 50% of cases. On MSE, the only evidence of hallucinations may be an inappropriate laugh, a patient staring off intensely beyond the clinician or some other bizarre mannerism as patients often minimize or deny them. Again, using the technique of normalizing can help to elicit perceptual disturbances. It is also important to ask about the presence of command hallucinations as this can increase the risk of suicidal or homicidal ideation. When commenting on the presence of hallucinations, it is important to describe them (i.e., constant vs. intermittent, reassuring vs. condescending, loud vs. soft, multiple vs. single, blurry vs. vivid). Descriptors can be very helpful to document patient response to treatment.

Mr. S endorses command auditory hallucinations that voices coming from another planet are telling him to kill himself for his sins. He states that he intends to follow through on this as soon as the voice tells him how. He describes the voice as single, constant, and loud.

Mood and Affect

Mood is assessed by asking the patient. In schizophrenia, the patient's mood can be dependent on the presence or absence of delusions, hallucinations, and/or negative symptoms. Blunted affect can be present as a symptom of the illness or a side effect of medication. Affect can also be incongruent with the patient's reported mood.

Mr. S describes his mood as "happy." His affect is blunted, suspicious, and mood incongruent.

Sensorium

Patients with schizophrenia are typically alert and oriented, although when asked the typical questions to assess sensorium, they may give bizarre answers. Lack of orientation should prompt the clinician to consider other causes of psychosis. For example, a patient with unknown psychiatric history is brought by police to the crisis unit for acting bizarrely in the community. Upon initial assessment, he stared off into the distance and repeatedly got up from his seat and walked in a nonthreatening manner toward the door. He was subsequently sent for medical clearance where it was found that the patient had rhabdomyolysis. Treatment of this caused a resolution of his symptoms.

Mr. S is alert and oriented to time, city, state, season, and president. Sustained attention is impaired as evidenced by asking this provider to repeat questions frequently after he starts to answer them.

Judgment and Insight

Typically, patients with schizophrenia tend to have poor insight regarding the severity of their illness and their need for medication. This is another reason for poor medication adherence. They frequently blame family members or friends for "being the crazy ones" when they are forced to see a mental health clinician. Because of this lack of insight, collateral information from family and friends can be extremely helpful when assessing a patient.

Mr. S appears to have impaired judgment and insight. When asked about his recent medication noncompliance, he replies, "Nothing's wrong with me. My family just insists on me taking medicine."

DIFFERENTIAL DIAGNOSIS

The main categories of differential diagnosis of schizophrenia can be broken down into other psychiatric conditions, medical illness, and drug-induced psychosis. While most illicit substances are capable of producing signs and symptoms of schizophrenia, PCP, can cause a syndrome that most closely mimics the positive, negative, and cognitive picture of schizophrenia, though the use of this substance is not common. More commonly seen is stimulant intoxication, alcohol hallucinosis, or substance withdrawal. As a general rule, hallucinations that are caused by a substance tend to be more commonly visual or tactile, and if visual, they are usually more vivid. In contrast, with schizophrenia the hallucinations tend to be predominantly auditory and, if visual, they are typically not vivid. A simple UDS can be done to rule out drug-induced causes; however, a positive UDS cannot rule out underlying psychosis as patients frequently self-medicate with drugs and alcohol.

Multiple other psychiatric disorders must be considered before a diagnosis of schizophrenia is given. The signs and symptoms of schizophrenia are identical to those of other psychotic disorders including schizophreniform disorder and brief psychotic disorder. The differentiating factor in these disorders is the timetable. To arrive at a diagnosis of schizophreniform disorder, the signs and symptoms must be present for at least 1 month, but no more than 6 months. In brief psychotic disorder, signs and symptoms are present for at least 1 day, but no more than 1 month. Schizoaffective disorder, which requires the presence of a mood disorder and will be discussed later in Section 18.9B, should also be in the differential diagnosis. In delusional disorder, the delusions tend to be nonbizarre, whereas with schizophrenia they are more likely to present with bizarre delusions. Personality disorders that need to be considered include schizotypal, schizoid, paranoid, and borderline. In these personality disorders, micropsychotic episodes can occur. These symptoms tend to be milder in nature and patients will have difficulty identifying the date of onset. Mood disorders in the differential diagnosis include MDD with psychotic features and bipolar disorder with psychotic features. In these, the delusions are typically mood congruent. For example, a patient presenting in a manic state with psychotic features will usually have delusions of grandeur while a patient presenting in the midst of a depressive episode will tend to have delusions of a depressive nature. With mood disorders, the psychotic symptoms resolve along with the mood episode.

Nonpsychiatric medical causes of psychotic symptoms must be ruled out before a diagnosis of schizophrenia is given. Special attention should be paid to any disturbance in the patient's level of consciousness. Patients with schizophrenia are usually alert and oriented, though they may give bizarre answers to questions regarding orientation. Any disorientation or signs of clouded consciousness should alert the clinician to investigate for secondary causes. Delirium typically has an acute onset and causes confusion and inattention. Common causes of delirium include drug and alcohol withdrawal, hypoglycemia, hypoxia, hypercapnia, and fluid or electrolyte imbalances. Other common medical causes of psychotic features include a space-occupying lesion in the brain, temporal lobe epilepsy, dementia, vitamin B12 deficiency, thyroid disease, hepatic encephalopathy, Wernicke-Korsakoff syndrome, systemic lupus, multiple sclerosis, and various infections, including urinary tract infections (UTIs).

For differential diagnosis, consider factors such as onset of symptoms, family history, age of onset, and type of hallucinations.

- **Onset of symptoms:** Usually gradual with the presence of prodromal symptoms in schizophrenia. Medical causes tend to cause acute onset of symptoms with no prodrome.
- **Family history:** Presence of a psychiatric disorder in the family is suggestive of a psychiatric disorder, whereas no family history should prompt consideration of a secondary cause of psychosis.
- **Age of onset:** Primary psychiatric illnesses occur earlier in life, usually in the teens to mid-30s. Onset after 40 should prompt the clinician to investigate for a medical or drug-induced cause.
- **Type of hallucination:** Auditory hallucinations and nonvivid visual hallucinations are typical in schizophrenia. Vivid visual hallucinations and tactile and olfactory hallucinations should orient the clinician toward a medical or drug-induced cause.

DIAGNOSTIC STUDIES

While no diagnostic studies are available presently to diagnose schizophrenia, consideration should be given to assess for secondary causes of psychosis.

- CBC to assess for infectious causes
- Chemistry panel to assess for electrolyte abnormalities
- Hepatic panel to rule out liver disease
- UDS
- HIV screening
- Thyroid panel
- Vitamin B12
- Urinalysis
- Fluorescent treponemal antibody test to rule out tertiary syphilis
- Neuroimaging to rule out space-occupying lesions, demyelinating disorders, or cerebrovascular accident

The above tests do not necessarily need to be done with each patient; however, if there is reasonable suspicion, then these tests should be ordered to confirm or rule out a secondary cause.

EVALUATION

Obtaining a thorough history from a patient with schizophrenia can be limited, secondary to poor patient insight, the presence of paranoia, disorganized speech, or the stigma associated with it among many other reasons. As such, it can be immensely helpful to obtain collateral information from the patient's family and close associates. Questions should include the presence of family history, patient's previous level of functioning, rate of onset, behavior that deviates from patient's baseline, work history, any known use of illicit drugs, and any previous medical problems.

When taking a history and performing an MSE, careful attention should be paid to gently eliciting any suicidal ideation, violent ideation, and the presence of command hallucinations (again, collateral information can be immensely helpful here). As mentioned previously, the technique of normalizing can help to decrease the patient's defenses. When asking about auditory hallucinations, for example, the question can be phrased as "It's common for people to hear voices that others around them are unable to hear. Does this ever happen to you?" Another technique is gentle assumption where the clinician assumes that the patient hears the voices.

TABLE 18.12 Prognostic Factors to Consider in Patients With Schizophrenia

Good Prognosis	Poor Prognosis
Later onset	Early onset
Good premorbid social functioning	Poor premorbid social functioning
Married	Single
Good social support	Poor social support
No family history of schizophrenia	Family history of schizophrenia
Positive symptoms	Negative symptoms

This can be phrased as "When you hear the voices, what do they say?" This should be used cautiously as the patient with paranoid ideation can feel threatened that the interviewer "knows too much." If concern exists that the patient is a danger to themselves or others or they are unable to care for themselves, hospitalization may be warranted. Approximately 5% of patients with schizophrenia complete suicide.[140]

Other factors to consider during evaluation include the presence or absence of social supports. The presence of social supports is a good prognostic factor and can help with medication compliance as well as getting to appointments (Table 18.12). Living arrangements should be queried as a high proportion of patients with schizophrenia will experience homelessness at some point. A thorough history is imperative as it can help to discuss the prognosis and course with the patient and their family.

Assessment for comorbidities is of utmost importance as patients with schizophrenia have an innately higher risk of type 2 diabetes. Antipsychotic medication can further increase this risk; however, it should be discussed with the patient that the risk of metabolic abnormalities is higher in patients with schizophrenia who are medication naive versus the general population. As such, a baseline and ongoing body mass index (BMI) should be done. Consideration should be given to have a basic metabolic panel and lipids drawn every 3 to 6 months.

The course of the illness is one of many exacerbations and remissions. The usual course is characterized by a gradual onset culminating in a first psychotic break. If treated, the psychotic symptoms should respond to medication; however, residual symptoms will likely persist. With successful treatment, the patient should go into remission, but further exacerbations will typically follow. Despite the perception that most cases of schizophrenia have a poor outcome, studies show that approximately 50% of the cases of schizophrenia have a favorable prognosis.[141]

TREATMENT

Treating a patient with schizophrenia should be a process that involves the use of medications as well as nonmedical treatment approaches. This point cannot be overstated as medical professionals can sometimes neglect nondrug approaches. The goal of treatment therefore should focus on getting the patient as fully functional as possible.

Acute Psychosis

Treatment of acute psychosis requires immediate attention. This often requires hospitalization to prevent the patient from becoming a danger to themselves or others. This is best accomplished in the least restrictive manner possible, such as voluntary admission with the patient's consent. Unfortunately, however, involuntary hospitalization is often required as patients with schizophrenia exhibit poor insight. Typically, involuntary admission is allowed when the patient is an imminent danger to themselves or others or is unable to care for themselves; however, state laws vary.

The most common approach to deescalate the patient with acute psychosis is with the use of intramuscular (IM) haloperidol 5 mg/lorazepam 2 mg/diphenhydramine 50 mg, sometimes referred to in the ED or psychiatric hospital as "B-52" or "5-2-50." Other IM alternatives include fluphenazine, olanzapine, or ziprasidone. The advantage of these includes quick onset of action and reliable absorption.

The use of seclusion and/or restraint may need to be considered based on the level of dangerousness to self or others; however, medication and verbal deescalation should be employed before resorting to these measures.

Maintenance Phase

After an acute episode of psychosis has been adequately controlled, medication should be continued with the goal of returning the patient to the highest possible level of functioning, preventing relapse, and minimizing symptoms. Ongoing treatment with antipsychotics has been shown to decrease the incidence of relapse. Studies have shown that relapse rates of 27% of patients treated with ongoing antipsychotics versus 64% of those not treated.[142] At this point, there are no guidelines that have established the period of time that a patient needs to be on an antipsychotic. Rather than memorizing an exhaustive list of the various differences between antipsychotics, a few principles to guide treatment should suffice:

- First-generation, also known as conventional, antipsychotics block dopamine in multiple areas of the brain. While this mitigates positive symptoms, this can also increase the incidence of negative and cognitive symptoms and may increase the risk of side effects. In contrast, atypical or SGAs block both dopamine and serotonin in a more selective manner. In addition, they act as partial agonists thereby theoretically minimizing parkinsonism and worsening negative/cognitive symptoms. While an oversimplified example, if a first-generation antipsychotic blocks dopamine at 100%, a second-generation may block it at 70%.
- Low potency antipsychotics require a higher dose to achieve benefits whereas high potency ones require a lower dose.
- The choice of antipsychotics should not depend on efficacy as one antipsychotic has not been shown to have increased response over another (aside from clozapine, which has been shown to be more effective but carries the risk of severe and potentially fatal side effects). Instead, the choice of antipsychotic should be based on the side effect profile first and should be tailored to the patient profile second (first do no harm).
- An estimated 40% to 50% of patients are noncompliant. As such, consideration should be given to long-acting injectable preparations. Besides having the advantage of better compliance, plasma levels of drug tend to be more stable.
- The lowest possible dose of antipsychotic should be used to control symptoms.
- Patients who respond to a specific medication are likely to do so in the first 2 weeks. A trial period of 2 weeks should therefore be given before considering a switch to a different medication. If improvement is noticed in these 2 weeks, continued improvement may take several more weeks to months to occur.
- Low potency antipsychotics tend to cause more sedation whereas high potency ones can cause more movement disorders.
- Failure of two or more antipsychotics classifies a patient as a poor responder. In this case, consideration should be given to treatment with clozapine. Monitoring of absolute neutrophil count on CBC is mandatory as agranulocytosis, a potentially fatal complication, occurs in 1% to 2% of patients treated with clozapine.
- Although the response of positive symptoms to medications has been impressive, treatment of the cognitive and negative symptoms of schizophrenia has been disappointing. Newer medications are, however, showing promise for this.
- Owing to the high burden of side effects with antipsychotics, special care should be given to minimize and adequately manage them (discussed below). These side effects are responsible for a large proportion of patients discontinuing their medications.

Side Effects

When treating schizophrenia with antipsychotics, side effects may begin immediately while clinical improvement of symptoms may take days to weeks. As such, patients should be counseled about this to improve compliance. In general, low potency antipsychotics are more likely to cause sedation, postural hypotension, and anticholinergic side effects. High potency antipsychotics are more likely to cause extrapyramidal side effects (EPS). The most common side effects and their treatment are summarized below.

- **EPS:** These side effects are named for the extrapyramidal system, which regulates posture and muscle tone. This system does not travel through the pyramids of the medulla. When dopamine in this area is blocked, side effects can include dystonia, parkinsonism, bradykinesia, tardive dyskinesia (TD), tremor, and akathisia.
  - **Acute dystonia:** This side effect usually causes severe discomfort to the patient and should be treated promptly. Severe dystonia should be treated with 1 to 2 mg of benztropine or 50 mg of diphenhydramine IV or IM. In less severe cases, oral benztropine 1 to 2 mg can be used. Consideration should be given to decreasing the dose or switching to a different antipsychotic with less risk of dystonia.
  - **Parkinsonism:** This can be mild, moderate, or severe. Consideration to dose reduction or switching to another antipsychotic should be given. If not feasible, treatment can be started with benztropine 1 to 2 mg one to two times a day. Alternatively, if the patient cannot tolerate benztropine, amantadine 100 to 200 mg two to three times a day should be considered.
  - **Akathisia:** This can present as a mild subjective feeling of motor restlessness all the way to the objective inability of the patient to sit still. Severe akathisia can be extremely uncomfortable and anxiety provoking to the patient. First-line treatment should be with a beta blocker such as propranolol 40 to 60 mg twice a day or benztropine 1 to 2 mg twice daily. If these

first-line treatments are not feasible, treatment with a benzodiazepine can be considered; however, because of the risk of addiction as well as a possible association of benzodiazepine use and fatality in patients with schizophrenia, they are best avoided.[143]
  - **TD:** An involuntary movement disorder that can be a side effect of long-term antipsychotic use and can potentially permanent. This can be assessed using the AIMS (Abnormal Involuntary Movement Scale) test. If present, decreasing the dose or switching to an antipsychotic with a lower risk of TD is recommended as a first-line treatment. If this is not an option, treatment with a VMAT 2 (vesicular monoamine transporter type 2) inhibitor should be considered.
- **Prolactinemia:** Can present as galactorrhea or irregular menses in females and decreased libido and gynecomastia in men.
- **Metabolic side effects:** These include but are not limited to dyslipidemia, hypertension, insulin resistance, and obesity.
- **Anticholinergic side effects:** Urinary retention, constipation, blurry vision, dry mouth, and cognitive impairment.
- **Neuroleptic malignant syndrome (NMS):** NMS presents with fever, muscle rigidity, autonomic instability, and mental status changes. Although rare, this can be life threatening.
- **QT prolongation:** Patients at high risk of heart disease including the elderly and those with previous heart disease should have an EKG prior to starting an antipsychotic.

CONCOMITANT TREATMENT AND PATIENT EDUCATION

As previously mentioned, medication treatment should be one piece of the pie that makes up a holistic approach to the treatment of schizophrenia. Referral to a psychologist with experience in dealing with schizophrenia and other serious mental illness (SMI) can be very helpful to the patient. Due to the seriousness of schizophrenia, management at an SMI clinic (if the patient qualifies) can help immensely with coordination of care. At these clinics, patients are assigned a case manager who coordinates care with various professionals including psychiatric clinicians, social workers, and occupational therapists. For the most severe cases, assertive community treatment teams, also known as ACT teams, provide a higher level of care including assistance with housing, home delivery of medications, and skills training among other intensive services.

Another important aspect of treatment that can be overlooked is the engagement of the patient's social supports in the treatment of schizophrenia. In general, with the patient's permission, the course and prognosis of the disease should be discussed with the social supports of the patient. The National Alliance on Mental Illness (NAMI) provides resources for family and friends of those affected by schizophrenia and other mental illnesses.

When educating patients about the course and prognosis of schizophrenia, careful attention should be given to providing the patient with the proper balance of hope and reality. Although patients with schizophrenia often have poor insight into the need for treatment, it is important to involve the patient as much as possible in treatment decisions as these patients often feel that their sense of free will has been taken from them.

18.9B SCHIZOAFFECTIVE DISORDER

MEDICAL HISTORY AND CLINICAL PRESENTATION

According to the NAMI, the prevalence rate of schizoaffective disorder is 0.3%. Schizoaffective disorder comprises a period of concurrent psychotic symptoms including delusions, hallucinations, and/or disorganized speech or behavior with symptoms of a mood disorder, either depression or bipolar disorder. The psychotic symptoms, however, will persist when the symptoms of the mood disorder have resolved. In contrast, in bipolar disorder with psychotic features or MDD with psychotic features, the psychotic symptoms resolve along with the mood symptoms. Schizoaffective disorder can be broken down into depressive type or bipolar type depending on which mood symptoms are present.

Case Vignette

Mr. V, a 29-year-old Caucasian male with a history of schizophrenia, was admitted to the local psychiatric hospital with a complaint of increasing psychotic symptoms. Upon assessment, Mr. V. is agitated with rapid speech and flight of ideas. When asked about his recent sleep patterns, Mr. V states that over the last 2 weeks, he has been averaging about 2 to 3 hours per night. He reports increased energy, despite this decreased sleep. When asked about his mood, he states that it has been "Amazing." Collateral from his family reveals that Mr. V has become paranoid that the CIA has been following him and is trying to extract his thoughts. In addition, he has been acting bizarrely, often laughing inappropriately despite feeling like he is being followed.

After a week of hospitalization and a trial of valproic acid and risperidone, Mr. V's sleep has improved drastically and has been between 7 and 9 hours nightly. His speech is now of normal rate. His delusions of persecution and his bizarre behavior have decreased but are still moderate in severity. He is discharged and is seen at the clinic 2 weeks later. At this time, it was reported that his mood symptoms had continued to improve, however, his psychotic symptoms have persisted. Mr. V's differential diagnosis now would include schizoaffective disorder.

As seen in this patient vignette, the patient's manic episode was concurrent with his psychotic symptoms; however, when the mania was adequately treated with an antimanic agent, the psychotic symptoms continued to persist, making schizoaffective disorder a more likely diagnosis. Despite the clear diagnostic criteria for schizoaffective disorder, differentiating the negative symptoms of schizophrenia from mood symptoms that may be indicative of schizoaffective disorder clinically is a diagnostic challenge.

SIGNS AND SYMPTOMS

As with schizophrenia, psychotic symptoms include delusions, hallucinations, disorganized speech and/or behavior. These will run concurrently with mood symptoms of depression or bipolar disorder. The importance of differentiating between schizophrenia and schizoaffective disorder cannot be overstated. Differentiating between the two allows the clinician to determine which patients may benefit from the addition of a mood stabilizer. Leading experts suspect that schizophrenia and bipolar disorder share certain genotypes. As such, it has been suggested that bipolar disorder and schizophrenia may exist as a continuum of the same disease, rather than two separate entities.

PHYSICAL EXAMINATION

The MSE of patients with schizoaffective disorder is similar to the examination of a patient with schizophrenia. Patients will typically present with delusions, hallucinations, or bizarre behavior/disorganized speech. In addition, a patient with the bipolar subtype may present with rapid speech, flight of ideas, and psychomotor agitation, while patients with the depressive type may present with slowed speech and psychomotor retardation.

DIFFERENTIAL DIAGNOSIS

The differential diagnosis of schizoaffective disorder should include mood disorders with psychotic features, schizophrenia, schizophreniform disorder, brief psychotic disorder, drug-induced psychosis, and organic medical causes.

EVALUATION

In addition to the considerations given when a patient is diagnosed with schizophrenia, other important factors should be included when determining which medication may be warranted. For example, due to the high rate of noncompliance with medications as well as homelessness in this group, treatment with mood stabilizers that require close monitoring may be limited. Consideration regarding whether hospitalization is necessary is essential.

TREATMENT

First-line treatment of schizoaffective disorder mirrors that of schizophrenia. Use of an antipsychotic, such as quetiapine, can help with both the psychotic symptoms as well as the mood symptoms. Most of the second-generation agents are FDA approved for both bipolar disorder as well as schizophrenia. An advantage of these is that lab monitoring during use of these is not mandatory, though it is recommended. In the bipolar subtype, mood stabilizers such as lithium, valproic acid, and carbamazepine can be effective. These medications should be monitored closely. During an acute manic episode, mood stabilizers can be maintained at the moderate to high end of the therapeutic range. Once a manic episode has stabilized, these can then be adjusted to the low to middle range of therapeutic levels to minimize side effects.

For the depressive subtype, treatment with antidepressant medications can be used. An important point to remember when using these agents, however, is that antidepressants can induce mania if a patient has an undiagnosed bipolar subtype. As such, close monitoring for a manic switch is indicated. If initiating an antidepressant as an outpatient, follow-up in 1 to 2 weeks is prudent. In addition, patients should be counseled about this possibility.

PATIENT EDUCATION

Similar to patients with schizophrenia, patients with schizoaffective disorder should be educated about the remitting/relapsing nature of the disorder. Though the prognosis of schizophrenia and schizoaffective disorder closely mirror each other, some studies have suggested a slightly better outcome in patients with schizoaffective disorder.[144] Patients on mood stabilizers should be counseled on the importance of compliance with medication monitoring as well as potential side effects. Patients should also be given a referral for counseling as well as other ancillary services including assignment of a case manager and/or SMI evaluation.

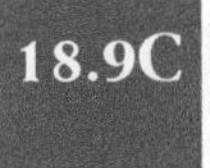

SCHIZOPHRENIFORM DISORDER

MEDICAL HISTORY AND CLINICAL PRESENTATION

Schizophreniform disorder is a condition in which the signs and symptoms are identical to those of schizophrenia, but two differences are noted. First, the timeline is briefer. For a patient to be diagnosed with schizophreniform disorder, the signs and symptoms must be present for at least 1 month, but <6 months (if >6 months, schizophrenia would be the diagnosis). The second difference is that in schizophreniform disorder, functional impairment may or may not be present, whereas in schizophrenia, functional impairment usually occurs. Typically, patients with schizophreniform disorder have a rapid onset and a shorter prodromal phase. Patients with this disorder will return to their baseline status when symptoms resolve. The presence of negative symptoms may portend a poor prognosis. Approximately two-thirds of patients diagnosed with schizophreniform disorder go on to develop schizophrenia.

SIGNS AND SYMPTOMS

The signs and symptoms of schizophreniform disorder are identical to those of schizophrenia; however, negative symptoms do not tend to be as prominent. As previously stated, the important difference is the time period of symptoms.

PHYSICAL EXAMINATION

The MSE will be almost identical to that of schizophrenia. One main difference is that patients with this disorder tend to be more perplexed and have better insight. It is almost as if the patient with schizophrenia, having a more gradual onset and a longer prodrome, has habituated to the symptoms. In contrast, the patient with schizophreniform disorder has not had time to "get used" to the symptoms. Blunted or flat affect may not be seen as often as in schizophrenia.

DIFFERENTIAL DIAGNOSIS

The differential diagnosis mirrors that of other psychotic disorders and should include other psychotic disorders, mood disorders, drug-induced psychosis, and medical conditions.

DIAGNOSTIC STUDIES

No diagnostic studies are specific to schizophreniform disorder; however, brain imaging has shown that the ventricular enlargement present in patients with schizophrenia is also present in schizophreniform disorder. Clinical suspicion for other causes of psychosis should be dictated by the patient's presentation and history.

EVALUATION

As with other psychotic disorders, patients must be carefully evaluated for the presence of suicidal or violent ideation and, if present, hospitalization may be warranted. When suspecting schizophreniform disorder, abrupt versus gradual onset may help to distinguish between the two. Family history and collateral information can aid in diagnosis.

TREATMENT

Treatment with a 3- to 6-month course of an antipsychotic medication should be started; however, consideration should be given to an indefinite time period as most patients will go on to develop schizophrenia. Patients with schizophreniform disorder may have a more rapid and complete response than those with schizophrenia. Psychotherapy can also help the patient to better understand and cope with their symptoms.

PATIENT EDUCATION

Patients and their families should be educated about the risk of progression to schizophrenia. As studies have shown decreased severity and frequency of symptoms in schizophrenic patients who are adequately treated, patients with schizophreniform disorder should be counseled about the importance of medication adherence.

18.9D BRIEF PSYCHOTIC DISORDER

MEDICAL HISTORY AND CLINICAL PRESENTATION

Brief psychotic disorder, a rare condition, is defined as the presence of psychotic symptoms including delusions, hallucinations, and/or disorganized thoughts for at least 1 day, but no more than 1 month. Typically, a clear association with a stressor can be identified. Stressors may include the loss of a relative or friend, a traumatic event, pregnancy, or childbirth, among others. Onset is usually abrupt.

SIGNS AND SYMPTOMS

The signs and symptoms of brief psychotic disorder are similar to the other psychotic disorders but may not encompass the entire picture of delusions, hallucinations, and disorganized speech/behavior. Negative symptoms may be present on rare occasions. In addition, patients with brief psychotic disorder will typically have had normal premorbid functioning.

PHYSICAL EXAMINATION

Patients with brief psychotic disorder will often present with normal hygiene. Bizarre behavior and emotional volatility may be noted. If hallucinations are present, patients may be seen responding to internal stimuli as evidenced by inappropriate laughter, delayed response to questions, or gazing beyond the clinician.

DIFFERENTIAL DIAGNOSIS

The differential diagnosis of brief psychotic disorder is similar to that for other psychotic disorders. Consideration should be given to psychosis-prone personality disorders including borderline personality, paranoid personality, and schizotypal personality disorders.

DIAGNOSTIC STUDIES

No specific diagnostic studies are available for brief psychotic disorder. As with other psychotic disorders, lab studies are used to rule out other causes of psychosis.

EVALUATION

Hospitalization should be considered as patients with brief psychotic disorder may be "unfamiliar" with their state of mind and therefore may theoretically be more prone to violent or suicidal ideation. In addition, hospitalization may allow the patient to regain their sense of reality.

TREATMENT

While some patients can be treated with supportive care alone, strong consideration should be given to starting an antipsychotic medication. In addition, psychotherapy can often help the patient to assimilate the experience. In addition, it can also guide the patient to process the triggering event and can reassure them of the expectation of normal premorbid functioning.

PATIENT EDUCATION

Of utmost importance, patients must be educated about the expectation that they are expected to make a full recovery. This experience can be frightening as the patient may develop anxiety about permanently "losing their mind."

18.9E DELUSIONAL DISORDER

MEDICAL HISTORY AND CLINICAL PRESENTATION

In contrast to other psychotic disorders, patients with delusional disorder tend to function normally in most areas of their lives. Whereas delusions are one of many symptoms of schizophrenia, in delusional disorder, they are the prominent symptom. Hallucinations are rarely present, but if they are, they tend to be congruent with the delusions. A patient who believes they are infested with parasites underneath the skin may experience tactile hallucinations of a crawling sensation. The bizarre behavior, disorganized thought process, and negative symptoms seen in schizophrenia are not present in delusional disorder. Delusions can take on many themes including erotomanic, grandiose, jealous, persecutory, or somatic, among others. Persecutory delusions are the most commonly encountered. The delusional system in delusional disorder tends to be of a nonbizarre nature. It has been postulated that delusional disorder involves the emotional limbic system while cognition remains intact. In schizophrenia, cognition is affected, which may hypothetically allow for the presence of bizarre delusions. If bizarre delusions are present, such as the belief that the patient's internal organs have been replaced by plastic, consideration that another psychotic process may be present should be given.

Whereas the incidence of schizophrenia is about 0.87%, the estimated incidence of delusional disorder stands at 0.2%. Family history of schizophrenia tends to be absent. In addition, delusional disorder does not tend to show any evidence of evolving to schizophrenia as it usually follows a stable course. Risk factors are summarized in Box 18.4.

BOX 18.4 Risk Factors for Delusional Disorder

Visual or hearing impairment
Family history of suspiciousness
Recent immigration
Interpersonal sensitivity

Delusional disorder has been thought to be a "purer" form of D2 receptor hyperfunction in contrast to schizophrenia, which involves other neurotransmitter systems including glutamate, GABA, and serotonin among others.[145] This may explain why antipsychotics that block this receptor treat positive symptoms more readily.

SIGNS AND SYMPTOMS

Delusions, defined as fixed false beliefs, are the prominent feature of delusional disorder. As previously mentioned, hallucinations are not typically present, but if present, they tend to be consistent with the delusion (e.g., a patient believing they are being followed may have auditory hallucinations of footsteps). The delusions are present for >1 month.

PHYSICAL EXAMINATION

The patient with delusional disorder is usually well groomed without any noticeable bizarre behavior. They may appear suspicious or grandiose depending on the content of the delusion. They may offer to show the clinician evidence backing up the delusion. A rather common occurrence in clinical practice is that of a patient with multiple excoriations on the skin who brings in a bottle filled with "dead bugs," which is often in reality scabs and other skin debris. Patients may also offer screenshots or recordings on their cell phone confirming the content of their delusions.

The patient's affect and mood are typically congruent with the delusional material. A patient believing their spouse is cheating on them may present with agitated or dysphoric affect.

MSE often reveals poor impulse control. As such, if the patient appears to be a danger to themselves or others, a careful risk assessment may reveal the depth of these intentions. MSE will almost always reveal poor insight to the delusion. As a result of this, patients with delusional disorder tend to be brought in by concerned family members, employers, or law enforcement.

DIFFERENTIAL DIAGNOSIS

A fact that cannot be overstated in the differential diagnosis of delusional disorder is that since the delusions are nonbizarre, the clinician needs to first establish that the belief is indeed a delusion. This may require collaboration with family members, law enforcement, or other individuals.

Once the presence of a delusion has been established, the differential diagnosis of delusional disorder mirrors that of other psychotic disorders. Neurologic abnormalities including epilepsy (particularly temporal lobe), CVA, space-occupying lesions (basal ganglia calcification), Huntington disease, early signs of Alzheimer disease, and delirium should be considered. Endocrinopathies can usually be ruled out with simple blood tests as can electrolyte abnormalities. UTIs should also be considered. Illicit substance use such as marijuana, amphetamines, cocaine, and hallucinogens can cause delusions and can be assessed with history and drug screening when warranted.

The psychiatric differential diagnosis of delusional disorder should include schizophrenia, schizophreniform disorder, brief psychotic disorder, bipolar disorder, and depression with psychotic features. If mood symptoms are present with delusions, delusional disorder can be safely ruled out. OCD and other anxiety disorders should be included. A patient with an anxiety disorder may respond that "I realize that the boss isn't conspiring to fire me but I can't help feeling that way" whereas the patient with delusional disorder may respond, "My boss has a meeting every day at 12 o'clock with his colleagues on how they will go about firing me." The patient with delusional disorder is convinced beyond a reasonable doubt and leaves no room for alternative explanations. Personality disorders such as narcissistic, borderline, paranoid, and schizotypal can also present with delusional thought process.

DIAGNOSTIC STUDIES

No specific diagnostic studies are presently available to confirm the diagnosis of delusional disorder. Studies should be ordered based on clinical suspicion of other causes of delusions.

EVALUATION

Evaluation of a patient with delusional disorder is a delicate art. Rather than an exhaustive list of questions to ask, several principles should be employed when exploring delusional material with patients.

- **First and foremost, do not refute the patient's belief.** Patients with delusional disorder have no insight to the false nature of their belief. Disputing these beliefs head on will immediately erode trust between the clinician and the patient. The clinician may miss an opportunity to elicit violent or suicidal ideation as this trust erodes.
- **Approach the assessment with interest and curiosity.** This can be done by simply asking questions and listening to answers nonjudgmentally.
- **The patient will typically ask the clinician "Do you believe me?"** Other common statements include "Everybody thinks I'm crazy, you probably think I'm crazy too! But I'm not." While not wanting to refute the delusion, the clinician needs to take great care not to reinforce it either. The therapeutic alliance can often be maintained by responding with statements such as "I need to get more information before I can decide" or "This sounds unusual but I'm hoping you can help me understand your situation more so I can see how I may help." Being deliberately vague can help to break the patient's defenses down.
- **Do not reinforce the delusion.** While this may immediately gain the patient's trust, it will not be therapeutic for the patient in the short term, and in the long term it may result in hostility toward the clinician. The patient who believes his spouse is engaged in an extramarital affair may ask the clinician "When I get a divorce, you'll tell my lawyer about this?"
- **Spend time establishing rapport with the patient before talking about medication treatment.** Patients often incorporate medical treatment into their delusional system so establishing trust before discussing medication is paramount. Keep in mind that poor insight is the rule. If a patient believes that nothing is wrong with them, why

would they agree to medical treatment? One approach may be to discuss medication treatment being aimed at treating the secondary symptoms of the delusion including anxiety and irritability.

TREATMENT

As with other psychotic disorders, treatment should include medication, psychotherapy, and potentially hospitalization. Regarding hospitalization, patients with delusional disorder commonly will need to be involuntarily hospitalized if they are determined to be a danger to themselves or others. Outside of extreme situations, hospitalization is best avoided.

Once trust has been established, medical treatment with an antipsychotic can be initiated. Antipsychotics can usually be effective in lower dosages in delusional disorder. Side effect profile should be a top consideration, especially in delusional disorder. A patient agreeing to take medication may incorporate the medicine into their delusion at the first sign of a side effect. For this reason, it is important to discuss side effects up front and use a start low, go slow approach. A 6-week trial should be given before switching to a different medication.

Individual psychotherapy, with the goal of helping the patient to gain distance between themselves and the delusions, can be immensely helpful.

PATIENT EDUCATION

Full remission of delusional disorder with ongoing treatment is seen in about one-third of patients. Mild impairment continued in about one-third of cases and moderate to severe impairment continued to occur in the other third.[146] Symptom fluctuation can vary with continuous symptomatology present in some cases and a more intermittent course in others. With the patient's permission, family should be educated about the diagnosis, illness course, and expectations of treatment.

18.10 PEDIATRIC PSYCHAITRY

Nathan Payne

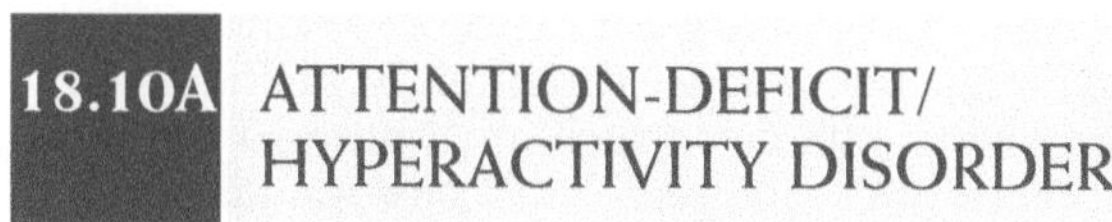

18.10A ATTENTION-DEFICIT/HYPERACTIVITY DISORDER

OVERVIEW

Attention-deficit/hyperactivity disorder (ADHD) is the most common neuropsychiatric disorder, affecting more than 10% of children and adolescents.[131,135] While inattention, fidgeting, and impulsivity are common aspects of everyday life in a healthy population, in ADHD symptoms are more pervasive and severe, interfering with learning, socialization, and vocational progress.[127] Nearly 80% of patients who are not treated to a point of amelioration develop comorbid conditions including anxiety, depression, and substance abuse. Even those who are appropriately managed may still find difficulties in their vocational and social endeavors.[143]

Historically, ADHD has been called many names including "hyperkinetic reaction of childhood," "minimal brain dysfunction," and "attention deficit disorder." Although in contemporary circumstances and among the lay population, ADD is a commonly used term, since 1994 the official name for the condition is "attention-deficit/hyperactivity disorder."[131]

EPIDEMIOLOGY

There is a high degree of variability in prevalence of ADHD throughout the world with rates varying from 0.1% up to 11% in their respectively studied populations.[135] ADHD affects males and females of all ages. Males are diagnosed more often, likely secondary to higher rates of observable, physiologic hyperactivity seen in male children and young adults.[140]

At least three quarters of adolescents with ADHD will continue to experience a degree of pervasive symptoms into adulthood. Particularly in the third and fourth decades, adult patients are more likely to experience comorbid anxiety and depression.[140]

Although environmental factors may exacerbate underlying ADHD, they are not causal. Rates are often lower in regions with lower socioeconomic standing, likely due to lack of resources including limited access to professional care.[128]

PATHOPHYSIOLOGY

ADHD has a strong genetic and neurobiologic etiology. Based on nearly 2 dozen studies over the past 30 years, there is a clear consensus that ADHD is a genetic condition wherein severity is based on a series of polygenic interactions.[139] Research funded by the National Institute of Health has repeatedly demonstrated anatomic anomalies in the brains of ADHD patients, including a significantly smaller right prefrontal cortex, caudate nucleus, and globus pallidus, "which suggests lack of connectivity of key brain regions that modulate attention, stimulus processing, and impulsivity."[133]

Multiple neurotransmitters, primarily dopamine and norepinephrine, play a crucial role in the pathophysiology of ADHD as well.[133] Dopamine is involved in modulation of risk-taking behaviors, impulsivity, and overall mood. Norepinephrine is involved in focus and concentration as well as mood. CNS stimulants (amphetamine and methylphenidate), which are considered first-line therapies for ADHD, are thought to directly and indirectly affect these neurotransmitters.[132]

For decades scientists have endeavored earnestly to link environmental factors to ADHD but have failed to point out a singular causal link. However, it is vitally important not to overlook the aggravating nature of environmental circumstances. Some studies have found strong correlations between early childhood exposure to heavy metals and pesticides and the development of ADHD. Premature birth, low birth weight, fetal exposure to drugs like acetaminophen, and brain injuries are other strong correlates.[137]

Despite a clear biologic basis for ADHD, it is equally clear that the condition results in mental health problems in almost all patients[142]; ergo, the term "neuropsychiatric." These co-occurring mental disorders are often thought to be a by-product of ADHD.[129] Over 60% of childhood cases have one or more comorbid disorders, including depression, anxiety, conduct disorder, oppositional defiant disorder, insomnia, addiction, Tourette syndrome, and autism.[145]

SIGNS AND SYMPTOMS

While clinical presentation of ADHD is highly variable, core characteristics of ADHD are inattention and/or hyperactivity/impulsivity. Factors including age, gender, culture, religion, and family history all impact presentation. There is also a significant difference in typical presentation between males and females with males having higher rates of predominantly hyperactive subtype classifications and females having primarily inattentive subtype.[141] The frequency and severity of symptoms are often variable depending on specific circumstances. For example, a child may be able to sit through an animated movie and accurately recall many details but cannot sit still or recall information from a short lesson in school; when a patient finds activity interesting, symptoms may be absent.

Objective findings in the hyperactive patient often include excessive fidgeting, restlessness, frequent postural changes, excessive talking, loudness, inappropriate running/climbing, pressured and/or rapid speech, interruptive or verbose communication, tangential or circumferential thought processes.[127] Inattentive findings may include frequent distraction (particularly by extraneous stimuli), losing items, missing appointments/deadlines, failing to turn in assignments (even when complete), avoiding tasks that require sustained mental effort, poor organizational skills, poor follow-through and task completion, procrastinating, making careless mistakes.

Hyperactive symptoms are more pronounced in childhood and often diminish with age. Inattentive findings are unnoticed at a young age and become more apparent into adulthood.[146]

Impaired function in multiple settings is a requisite for making a diagnosis. If a patient has symptoms consistent with a diagnosis, but reports no problems at work, with social contacts, or in academic settings, they should not be diagnosed or treated, and other causes should be considered.[134]

PHYSICAL AND MENTAL EXAMINATION

A comprehensive biopsychosocial evaluation should be completed with all patients. For pediatric evaluations, one or more third-party observers should be interviewed or complete a written assessment (e.g., Vanderbilt Assessment). For younger children, written assessments should be completed by the patient's primary guardian and a nonrelative teacher, therapist, or coach. Particularly in younger patients, it is prudent to seek several third-party observations as a child's ability to accurately convey symptoms may be limited. Subjective, self-report assessments are suitable for teenagers and adults.

The age of a patient at the time of evaluation correlates with the onset of symptoms. Hyperactivity and impulsivity are typically the first observable signs of ADHD, frequently seen as early as age 3. These core characteristics peak between age 7 and 9 and then begin to decline. Inattentive subtypes are typically diagnosed at a later age and their symptoms may decline slowly or not at all.[144]

DIFFERENTIAL DIAGNOSIS

It is prudent to rule out other diagnoses that may have overlapping signs and symptoms as there are conditions that are often misdiagnosed as ADHD. Owing to an abundance of overlapping symptoms, bipolar disorder, dyslexia, autism, substance abuse, and conduct disorder can be diagnosed as ADHD.[138]

DIAGNOSTIC STUDIES

Brain imaging and blood work are not necessary unless ruling out other conditions. EEG has been used in both diagnosis and treatment, via biofeedback, for decades. However, the benefits have not been demonstrated successfully in research[136] suggesting EEG is not currently a viable diagnostic tool. EKG is sometimes used for evaluation of cardiac risk factors prior to starting stimulant therapy in higher risk patients.

EVALUATION

The ADHD diagnosis is a clinical one and includes an interview with the patient as well as objective third-party observers (depending on age). Written assessments and quantitative testing should be documented prior to making a diagnosis. If symptoms occur with psychotic disorders like schizophrenia, personality disorders, or in substance misuse, other diagnoses should be considered.

Once a diagnosis is established, specify the presentation subtype and severity. A patient can be *predominately inattentive, predominately hyperactive/impulsive,* or *combined.* Severity is *mild, moderate,* or *severe.* In cases when ADHD criteria were met but have been reduced in severity for 6 months or longer, a patient is in *partial remission.*

TREATMENT

With the exception of preschool-age children, first-line therapy for ADHD is stimulant pharmacotherapy.[136] All patients should also be offered behavioral interventions, social skills training, and psychotherapy. In settings in which comorbidity is limited, pharmacotherapy alone many be sufficient.[122]

Although stimulant medication carries some inherent risk, the benefits typically outweigh the risks. The effective response to medication is considerably higher than its adjunct therapies[132,135] and shows a distinct therapeutic advantage over other treatment options. In primary care setting, clinicians should be capable of managing uncomplicated cases in school-age children and adults. A consultation with an experienced clinician may be prudent, particularly for ambiguous presentations or individuals with comorbid conditions.

Nonstimulant therapy, typically atomoxetine or bupropion, although empirically less effective than stimulants in large-scale studies are an alternative for those who cannot or should not use stimulants. High-risk populations include women of childbearing age, and those with a history of addiction, heart disease, and seizure disorders.

Behavioral therapy aims to reduce the symptoms of ADHD and often includes use of token-based economies and reward/consequence systems at home. The goal should be to positively reinforce good behavior and provide consistent, nonpunitive responses to bad behavior. Psychotherapy is a valuable tool primarily employed to combat comorbid mental health issues. If the individual denies anxiety, depression, mood lability, and behavioral issues and/or objective observers report no evidence thereof, psychotherapy is not necessary.[122]

In school-age children and adolescents, it often necessary to collaborate with their schools to facilitate accommodations. Common interventions may include extended exam time, private tutoring, decreased sensory environments, reward systems.

18.10B AUTISM SPECTRUM DISORDER

OVERVIEW

Autism spectrum disorder (ASD) is a neurodevelopment disorder that impairs a patient's communicative and interactive capacity resulting in pejorative social, vocational, and educational development. Symptoms can be mild, with very little objective signs of developmental delay. In severe cases, individuals may have markedly apparent signs of delay including pervasive limitations in speech, cognition, and motor function.[144]

In the primary care setting, the diagnostic and interventional role is limited to early detection and specialist referral. Existing developmental screening guidelines are typically sufficient for healthcare professionals to detect risk for ASD in young patients.

EPIDEMIOLOGY

Like many disorders that require a clinical diagnosis, ASD prevalence rates throughout the world are highly variable, ranging from 1 in 40 to 1 in 500, based on meta-analyses from Asia, Europe, and the United States.[129,140] In the United States, prevalence rates are 1 in 26 boys and 1 in 93 girls. These statistics are thought to be higher, compared to other countries, due to increased public awareness, professional training, and research investment in the United States.

Rates are three to four times higher in boys than girls based on an enormous study screening nearly 14 million patients in 2017.[143]

PATHOPHYSIOLOGY

The cause of ASD is unknown. It is generally accepted that ASD arises from genetic factors that disrupt expected neurodevelopment, particularly the way neurons connect anatomically and communicate chemically with one another.[122,138]

There are other statistically significant correlates of importance including advanced parental age (male and female), teratogenic exposure, perinatal trauma, and poor maternal health in pregnancy.[133]

SIGNS, SYMPTOMS, EXAMINATION

Early identification and referral are key in improving prognostic outcomes. The earliest symptoms typically present between 18 and 24 months.[139] The average patient will require more than 1 year to reach a definitive diagnosis.

ASD patients will have several persistent deficits related to language or communication, socialization, and behavior.[135] A professional evaluation should encompass screening for the following concerns:

- Trouble communicating, both verbally and abstractly
- Arbitrary or abnormally constructed language
- Poor social skills/delayed socialization
- Difficulty transitioning in routine tasks or schedules
- Abnormal behaviors (e.g., aggressive, hyperactive, anxious traits are common)

During a normal pediatric evaluation, clinicians may be informed about certain high-risk signs and symptoms. A list of common "red flag" symptoms is given in Box 18.5 along with a more comprehensive list of potential symptoms in preschool-age children.

EVALUATION AND TREATMENT

The goal for general clinicians, again, is early detection and specialist referral; ongoing evaluation and treatment will be dictated by the specialists. However, as patients with ASD may be on antipsychotic medications, general clinicians should be aware of and monitor for side effects. Patients with ASD commonly undergo physical, occupational, behavioral, and speech therapy. Treatment is tailored to the needs of both the child and the parent(s). Treatment can also include specialized schools, 24-hour supervisory living, and other community groups and interventions.

DIFFERENTIAL DIAGNOSIS

It is prudent to ensure the patient has ASD and not another condition. The differential diagnosis of ASD may include fetal alcohol syndrome, Rett syndrome, ADHD, hearing loss, OCD, tic disorders, lead toxicity, and other, less common, genetic conditions.[138,144,145]

18.11 SOMATOFORM DISORDERS

Dan Sturm

OVERVIEW

Somatoform disorders include somatoform disorder, illness anxiety disorder (IAD), functional neurologic deficit disorder, and factitious disorder (FD). This group of disorders is characterized by unexplained physical symptoms caused by emotional stress or difficult life situations. Because somatic disorders are not well understood, they have historically been viewed with skepticism by some clinicians. Nonetheless, these disorders have been described in the literature for over 150 years. Sigmund Freud was an early pioneer in describing how mental disturbances and emotions may be converted into physical symptoms. It is important for primary care clinicians to be familiar with these disorders because most of these patients present to their primary care clinicians. Their presentation varies widely. Some patients seem to ruminate on what appears to be a minor symptom. Others complain of multiple severe physical symptoms that may lead to disability. It is important to understand that these patients (except for those with FD) are not magnifying or exaggerating their discomfort, nor are they trying to mislead the clinician. To them, the physical pain or symptom(s) they feel is real. Somatoform disorder patients often develop excessive thoughts and behaviors related to their symptoms. These behaviors may vary, but often include frequent seeking of medical care or spending exorbitant amounts of time investigating their symptoms. Many excessively worry and become hyperfocused on their bodily sensations. The physical complaints associated with this disorder vary widely. Because of this, patients often have multiple physical complaints that may be vague or poorly connected. Office visits can become time consuming, and both the patient and the clinician often grow frustrated with one another. In addition, patients with somatic disorders may undergo unnecessary, expensive, and sometimes dangerous medical procedures in an effort to attribute their symptoms to a physical cause. Consider a somatoform disorder in patients who:

- Complain of multiple symptoms in different organ systems

BOX 18.5 Early Symptoms and Signs of Autism

Red flag signs

- Parental concerns about deficits in social skills
- Parental concerns about deficits in language skills or behavior
- Parental concerns about frequent tantrums or intolerance to change
- Delayed language and social/communication skills
- No babbling by 9 months
- No pointing or gestures by 12 months
- Lack of orientation to name by 12 months
- No single words by 16 months
- Lack of pretend or symbolic play by 18 months
- No spontaneous, meaningful (not repetitive or echolalic) two-word phrases by 24 months
- Any loss of language or social skills at any age

Impairments in social communication and interaction

- Lack of, delay, or regression in spoken language
- If present, spoken language may be atypical, for example:
    - Unusual intonations (monotone, sing-song)
    - Echolalia
    - Incorrect pronoun use (referring to self by name or as "you," "he," or "she," after age 3 years)
    - Non-speech-like vocalizations (e.g., grunting, squealing)
    - Limited to specific topics of interest
- Limited use of language for communication (e.g., using only single words even though capable of speaking in sentences)
- Reduced or absent nonverbal communication (gestures, facial expression)
- Little or no response to others' gestures or facial expression
- Lack of response or slow to respond when called by name (despite normal hearing)
- Reduced or absent interest in or attempts to share interest with another person (e.g., by pointing or monitoring the other's gaze), for example:
    - Lack of social smile or eye contact
    - Lack of imitation (e.g., clapping)
    - Limited or absent social bids
    - Lack of ability or interest in sustaining a social interaction
    - Resistance to being cuddled
- Lack of awareness of other people; appearing to be in his or her own world
- Preference for solitary play (lack of initiation or participation in social play with others)
- Lack of interest in other children or odd social approaches to other children (e.g., disruptive, aggressive)
- Lack of awareness of common social conventions (e.g., taking turns in a conversation, awareness of personal space)
- Lack of or minimal recognition or responsiveness to another's feelings (e.g., happiness, distress)
- Abnormal interactions with peers or adults (e.g., too friendly or too distant)
- Normal or even exaggerated level of motivation to socialize, with limited ability to infer the intentions or behaviors of others
- Motivated to socialize but not able to sustain a social interaction that is mutually enjoyable due to not respecting social conventions, due to an inability to anticipate the knowledge and interests of others, etc.
  For example, does not respect personal boundaries; may talk only about preferred interests and not engage in the social partner's interests.

Source: Data from Johnson CP, Myers SM. Identification and evaluation of children with autism spectrum disorders. Pediatrics. *2007;120:1183.*

- Complain of vague symptoms that exceed objective findings
- Avoid physical activity
- Have a history of other psychiatric disorders (depression, anxiety, OCD)
- Have a history of extensive diagnostic testing
- Complain of rejection from previous clinicians
- Display a high sensitivity to medication side effects
- See multiple clinicians for the same complaint
- Don't have relief from standard treatments

EPIDEMIOLOGY

Because of the way the psychiatric and medical communities have named and classified, then renamed and classified these disorders over the years, the true prevalence is unknown, but believed to affect around 4% to 6% of the general population.[147] Estimates are as high as 16% in primary care.[147] Onset is generally in adolescence or young adulthood and these disorders become chronic. Somatoform disorders affect people of all genders and cultures. However, as social roles have shifted over the years, the types of symptoms that men and women exhibit have changed as well. The stigmatization of depression or anxiety may lead to somatic complaints, particularly in older adults who grew up in an era in which the expression of negative emotions was discouraged.

PATHOPHYSIOLOGY

The mechanism in which the subconscious mind produces physical symptoms is not well understood. Psychosocial factors likely play a role. Risk factors for somatic symptoms may include:

- Childhood neglect
- History of any trauma (sexual or nonsexual; childhood or adult)
- History of depression or anxiety
- Alcohol and substance abuse
- Female sex
- Less than 12 years of education
- Low socioeconomic status
- Serious illness/injury to a close relative within the past 6 months
- Off work due to a medical illness

Biologic factors including the reactions between the CNS and the immune system are thought to play a role. The positive and negative feedback loops within the HPA axis help regulate the body's response to acute and chronic stress. Fluctuating levels of cortisol lead to the release of inflammatory cytokines, which may promote symptoms of fatigue, pain, and GI distress. In essence, the combination of psychosocial factors or environment and the body's physiologic response (biology) gives some support for a biopsychosocial model for explaining somatic symptoms.

18.11A SOMATIC SYMPTOM DISORDER

MEDICAL HISTORY AND CLINICAL PRESENTATION

Somatoform disorder is characterized by one or more chronic somatic complaints that causes dysfunction in a person's life. Often younger patients will complain of just one symptom, with pain being predominant. However, many patients with somatoform disorder will complain of multiple debilitating physical symptoms. These patients typically ruminate over their symptoms and spend disproportionate amounts of time worrying about the seriousness of their illness. Their obsessive thought processes about their symptoms cause significant disruptions in their quality of life and may lead to maladaptive behavioral changes, including frequent medical visits, lack of physical activity, or loss of employment.

SIGNS AND SYMPTOMS

Signs and symptoms vary by patient, but often, the chief complaint revolves around pain or discomfort. Examples include abdominal, back, or chest pain, headaches, shortness of breath, dizziness, sexual dysfunction, or urinary complaints. Fatigue may be a prominent complaint. These symptoms become chronic.

PHYSICAL EXAMINATION

Pertinent and reliable physical exam findings are absent, may be vague, or may not be anatomically explained.

DIFFERENTIAL DIAGNOSIS

Differential diagnosis varies depending upon the symptoms, but a thorough history and physical examination should be performed. The presentation for somatoform disorder most closely resembles that of IAD. A key distinction is that in somatoform disorder, the physical symptoms are usually multiple and become debilitating to the patient. If only one symptom is prominent, the symptom is likely to be pain. In IAD, the symptom(s) tend to be milder or vague in nature and it is the mental preoccupation with a relatively "minor" symptom that leads to psychological and/or behavioral dysfunction. Severe physical complaints are more noticeably absent in IAD.

DIAGNOSTIC STUDIES

No definitive diagnostic studies for somatoform disorder exist, but clinicians should perform a thorough history and physical examination followed by labs and diagnostic studies related to the symptoms. As always, clinicians should carefully weigh the risks, benefits, and costs of all diagnostic tests before ordering them.

EVALUATION

It may be helpful to consult with the patient's family, teachers, and other clinicians when pursuing a diagnosis of somatoform disorder. A psychosocial history should include new or recent stressors related to home, school, or occupation. Patients should be screened for comorbid conditions like depression and anxiety. Reassurance and empathy will be important in approaching this diagnosis so that patients do not feel discouraged or that their complaints are not being taken seriously.

TREATMENT

Clinicians should seek to minimize unnecessary diagnostic testing in this patient population. Simply reassuring patients that serious medical illness is not present is not likely to be effective. Explaining to patients about somatoform disorder requires a delicate approach. Some patients will simply reject the idea that their symptoms are being caused by emotional stress and may seek care elsewhere. Treating clinicians must continually reassure them that the symptoms they are feeling are real and there are legitimate biologic contributors (such as the HPA axis abnormalities mentioned above). The most effective treatment is for clinicians to set up regular visits with these patients. This allows the patient to feel they are being cared for, and helps the clinician monitor for any change in symptoms that may be alarming or related to physical illness. Developing treatment goals related to functional outcomes can be helpful. Assessing and treating for comorbid psychiatric illness is important, as is referral to a mental health specialist. A psychodynamic therapist who specializes in the mind-body connection is an option, as is CBT. Antidepressants alone or in combination with therapy may be helpful.

18.11B ILLNESS ANXIETY DISORDER

MEDICAL HISTORY AND CLINICAL PRESENTATION

As discussed previously, somatoform disorder and IAD are similar disorders in which somatic complaints lead to distressing symptoms and dysfunction in one's life. The somatic complaints in IAD tend to be less severe than in somatoform disorder, while the anxiety level is very high. Patients with IAD express excessive anxiety about having or acquiring a serious illness. IAD was formerly known as hypochondriasis.

As with somatoform disorder, patients with IAD are frequent visitors to primary care offices. Because IAD is also a chronic condition, many patients will have undergone extensive diagnostic testing. Maladaptive behavioral changes include having a low threshold for becoming alarmed about one's health, or self-checking for signs of illness. Patients are hyperaware of their bodily sensations and commonly misinterpret minor symptoms, such as abdominal bloating after a large meal, to be associated with something sinister like the presence of a malignancy. Other behaviors can include meticulous logging of symptoms or doctor shopping. Some patients begin a pattern of avoidance in which they will avoid doctors, hospitals, and others who are ill.

SIGNS AND SYMPTOMS

Symptoms will vary by patient, but the symptom itself is generally self-limiting or benign (e.g., tinnitus, bloating, globus sensation). The patient's reaction to the symptom causes significant preoccupation, anxiety, and behavioral changes.

PHYSICAL EXAMINATION

Physical examination will fail to demonstrate any signs of serious illness.

DIFFERENTIAL DIAGNOSIS

Please refer to somatoform disorder above to help differentiate between somatoform disorder and IAD. Comorbidity for IAD is high and includes:

- GAD
- Dysthymia
- Depression
- OCD
- Panic disorder
- SUD
- Personality disorders
- Body dysmorphic disorder

DIAGNOSTIC STUDIES

As with somatoform disorder, no definitive diagnostic studies for IAD exist but clinicians should perform a thorough history and physical examination followed by lab and diagnostic studies related to the symptoms.

EVALUATION

Similar to somatoform disorder, clinicians should show empathy when trying to understand any recent life stressors or possible triggers for the onset of symptoms. Gaining further information from family and friends can also be helpful.

TREATMENT

The treatment approach for IAD mimics that of somatoform disorder. The most effective treatment is for clinicians to set up regular visits with these patients. This allows the patient to feel they are being cared for, and helps the clinician monitor for any change in symptoms that may be alarming or related to physical illness. Developing treatment goals related to functional outcomes can be helpful. Assessing and treating for comorbid psychiatric illness is important, as is referral to a mental health specialist. A psychodynamic therapist who specializes in the mind-body connection is an option, as is CBT. Antidepressants alone or in combination with therapy may be helpful.

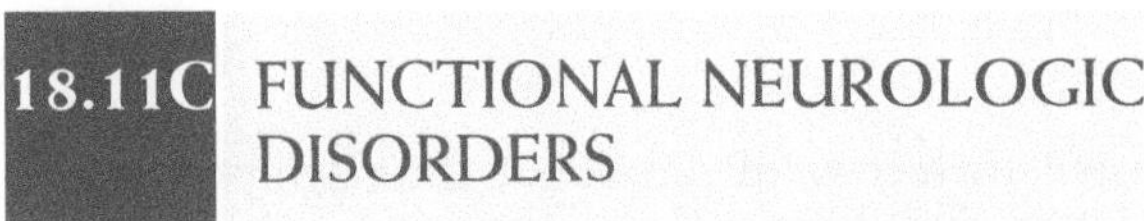

18.11C FUNCTIONAL NEUROLOGIC DISORDERS

MEDICAL HISTORY AND CLINICAL PRESENTATION

Functional neurologic disorders (FND) (formerly known as conversion disorder) is a type of somatoform disorder in which physical stress is converted into one or more neurologic symptoms. As with the above disorders, the patient is not intentionally faking the symptom. The biologic mechanism of how physical stress may affect the neurologic system is complex and not well understood, but imaging scans of the brain in these patients do support abnormally low areas of activation in the prefrontal cortex when they try to voluntarily move the corresponding body part. FND can be subclassified based upon the neurologic symptoms. Subtypes include motor, sensory, axial (gait and posture), speech, vision, and nonepileptic seizures. Women are affected more than men.

SIGNS AND SYMPTOMS

Symptoms will vary depending upon the subtype. Classically, patients with FND were thought to present after a precipitating life stressor or traumatic event. However, this is no longer felt to be true. Patients often have a history of prior unexplained symptoms or syndromes such as fibromyalgia or chronic fatigue. Some patients report dissociative symptoms (feelings disconnected from oneself).

PHYSICAL EXAMINATION

Clues to identifying a FND may include:

- Motor symptoms (weakness or paralysis) that begin abruptly and disappear with distraction
- Numbness or tingling that is equally split on the right and left half of the body
- Incongruence with the symptoms and the anatomic structure of the body
- Nonepileptic seizures may be identified by trying to open the eyelids during the event. In epileptic seizures, the eyelids will not resist being opened. Nonepileptic seizures also last longer (upward of several minutes) and most epileptic seizures are <1 minute.
- Inconsistencies on physical examination (e.g., a patient is unable to move his foot up and down when prompted, but then ambulates without a limp)
- Signature test—Difficulty signing their name in the presence of a visual FND. Blind individuals do not have difficulty signing their name.

DIFFERENTIAL DIAGNOSIS

Neurologic disorders that cause functional impairment consistent with the present symptoms should be ruled out.

EVALUATION

Evaluation should include a thorough history and physical examination, any pertinent laboratory tests, psychiatric history, and an MSE. Comorbidity is common and includes depression, GAD, and panic disorder. Patients may also have a secondary underlying neurologic disorder that is unrelated to FND. Neurology referral to help establish the diagnosis is important.

TREATMENT

Patients need to feel validated about their symptoms and disability. It should be stressed to the patient that the disorder is reversible with a multidisciplinary approach that includes both a neurologist and psychological interventions. CBT and/or psychotherapies should include components of education, trigger identification, and aspects of interpersonal functioning. Comorbid depression and anxiety should be treated with pharmacotherapy. Prognosis for FND remains poor due to delayed diagnosis, a lack of knowledgeable therapists, and ongoing psychosocial stressors in these patients' lives.

18.11D FACTITIOUS DISORDER

MEDICAL HISTORY AND CLINICAL PRESENTATION

Unlike the previously discussed disorders, patients with FD (formerly known as Munchausen syndrome) are purposely exaggerating, faking, or inducing symptoms of an illness. The illness may be physical or psychological in origin. In order to make the diagnosis, there must be evidence that the patient is providing false information or being deceptive. Additionally, the motivation for the deception must not include an external reward such as money, obtaining an insurance settlement, getting released from work, or avoiding jail time. Sympathy from family or healthcare workers and the attention from being "sick" form the key motivation that matters for patients with FD. Because of this, patients often request medical equipment that identifies them as being ill to the general public, such as the need for an oxygen tank or a wheelchair. The incidence of FD disorder is rare and accurate epidemiologic data on FD remains elusive because these patients typically flee to other practices when confronted with the diagnosis. Prevalence is thought to be higher in females and healthcare workers. In some situations, these actions are projected on another individual, typically a dependent. This is called FD by proxy.

SIGNS AND SYMPTOMS

Signs and symptoms vary considerably. However, common symptoms include:

- Chest pain
- Abdominal pain
- Hypoglycemia
- Diarrhea
- Seizures
- Weakness
- Skin wounds that do not heal

Symptoms may be self-induced by ingestion or injection of medications including insulin, thyroid hormone, laxatives, and feces. Some patients may even attempt to manipulate or tamper with their own laboratory specimens and medical records.

PHYSICAL EXAMINATION

The medical history will likely include an extensive list of medical problems. There will often be inconsistencies with physical examination findings related to the severity of the chief complaint. Overall, expect a lack of positive physical examination findings.

DIFFERENTIAL DIAGNOSIS

The main difference between malingering and FD is the motivation for the illness. A malingerer seeks a direct and immediate reward for their illness, such as a financial settlement, being excused from work/court/jail/childcare payments or obtaining narcotics. FD can be distinguished from other somatoform disorders and borderline personality disorder by the element of deception.

DIAGNOSTIC STUDIES

Clues to the diagnosis may include an extensive list of previous workups and invasive procedures performed without identifying any significant pathology or rationale for the symptoms. Other clues may include the onset of new symptoms prior to hospital discharge, poor responses to standard treatments, or a long list of allergies to known or effective therapeutics. Unlike most patients who avoid invasive procedures, those with FD seem overly enthusiastic about receiving them.

EVALUATION

An important aspect of evaluating patients with FD is obtaining the old medical records and searching them to look for inconsistencies or patterns. In order to continue the deception, patient intentionally avoid having their old medical records forwarded to their current clinicians.

TREATMENT

Avoiding unnecessary procedures and treatments is of paramount importance in patients with FD. All patients with suspected FD should have a psychiatric evaluation. Consultation with family members is important as well. Prognosis remains poor because most patients refuse psychiatric help and will often disappear from a practice once confronted. A multidisciplinary approach involving the family and other members of the healthcare team take an intervention-like approach. All treating clinicians should be notified so that unnecessary procedures and tests are not ordered without accompanying physical examination findings. Treating comorbid conditions including anxiety, depression, and SUD may be helpful.

18.12 SLEEP DISORDERS

Sarah Pryor

OVERVIEW

Sleep disorders are a common clinical problem and can lead to major effects on a patient's health, productivity, and quality of life. Typical complaints involve difficulty initiating or maintaining sleep, poor sleep quality, and/or early morning awakenings that lead to distress and impairment in daytime functioning.[148] Sleep complaints are often an acute issue with minor limitations and resolve quickly. When disturbances occur more regularly for a sustained period of time, then a diagnosis of insomnia should be considered. Not only do sleep disorders lead to significant stress, but they are also associated with an increased risk of coronary artery disease, heart failure, hypertension, diabetes, acute MI, and death.[148,149] Insomnia is now recognized as a disorder rather than a symptom and is classified by the *DSM-5* and *International Classification of Sleep Disorders,* 3rd edition (*ICSD-3*).[148,150]

EPIDEMIOLOGY

Insomnia disorder is one of the most common clinical complaints in primary care and poses a large economic burden and public health concern. Studies suggest that one-third of the population experiences some type of insomnia in a given year, with increased numbers seen in individuals who are female, older age or suffer from concurrent medical or mental disorders.[148,150–152] Of the patients who experience acute insomnia, approximately 50% go on to have a more chronic course.[152] The most common symptom is difficulty maintaining sleep (61%), followed by early-morning awakening (52%) and difficulty falling asleep (38%).[153] Insomnia is a risk factor for psychiatric disorders, with a close correlation with MDD, GAD and PTSD.[148,153,154]

PATHOPHYSIOLOGY

There is no universally accepted model for the pathophysiology of insomnia, and it is often multifactorial. For patients experiencing acute insomnia, sleep disturbances can often be linked to psychological factors, including stress, loss of a loved one, divorce, or domestic abuse. In addition, excessive caffeine intake, pain or discomfort, or compensatory factors including daytime napping or early bedtime, can result in cyclical sleep disturbances.

The most widely accepted theory for chronic insomnia is linked to hyperarousal, which is described as heightened physiologic, affective, or cognitive activity. This "heightened state" interferes with the natural disengagement from the environment, or ability to "turn off the brain," and leads to a decrease in the ability to sleep.[155] Individuals with insomnia often have complaints such as racing thoughts and excessive worry, which are manifested physiologically as an increase in whole-body metabolic rate, cortisol levels, whole-brain glucose consumption, elevated blood pressure, and high-frequency electroencephalographic activity during sleep.[155] Additional theories include an imbalance in sleep-promoting hormones (serotonin, melatonin) versus wake-promoting chemicals (orexin, histamine, and catecholamines).[148] Recent advances suggest a heritability and multigene involvement in insomnia with specific genes that can be linked to arousal regulation and sleep-wake processes.[155]

MEDICAL HISTORY AND CLINICAL PRESENTATION

The diagnosis of insomnia is made clinically; therefore, patients need a thorough medical history and physical examination. Clinicians should elicit a detailed sleep history that includes nocturnal and daytime sleep-related symptoms, their duration, and their association with psychological or physiologic stressors.[152] The "3 Ps" Model (Table 18.13) can be helpful in providing a framework for the assessment of insomnia. A sleep diary kept over a 2- to 4-week period maybe helpful to better understand an individual's sleep pattern, including total sleep time, wakefulness after sleep onset, and sleep efficiency.

Screening for any associated psychiatric or mood disorder and/or substance abuse is an important component of evaluation. Often individuals may self-medicate with alcohol or over-the-counter (OTC) medications as a means to initiate sleep, which leads to a reduction in rapid eye movement (REM) sleep and an increase in intermittent awakenings that decrease overall quality of sleep.

TABLE 18.13 The "3 Ps" Model for Evaluation of Insomnia

Factor	Description	Example
Predisposing factors	Factors that increase the risk for developing insomnia	Age, easy arousability, female sex, living alone, smoking, and various psychological disorders
Precipitating factors	Medical, environmental, or psychosocial stressors that initiate a pattern of poor sleep	Alcohol use, chronic pain, divorce, substance abuse, unemployment, stressful life events and comorbid conditions including diabetes, heart disease, thyroid disease, etc.
Perpetuating factors	Factors or behaviors that lead to a vicious cycle of continued sleep disturbances	Worrying about sleep, napping, chronic medication use

Source: *Data from Hein M, Senterre C, Lanquart J-P, et al. Hyperarousal during sleep in untreated, major depressed subjects with prodromal insomnia: a polysomnographic study.* Psychiatry Res. *2017;258:387–395. doi:10.1016/j.psychres.2017.08.061; Siddiqi N, House AO, Holmes JD. Occurrence and outcome of delirium in medical in-patients: a systematic literature review.* Age Ageing. *2006;35(4):350–364. doi:10.1093/ageing/afl005*

Ruling out other medical disorders associated with sleep disruption is imperative, including MDD, circadian rhythm disorders, restless legs syndrome, and obstructive sleep apnea. Some of the most common medical conditions associated with insomnia include chronic pain, pulmonary disease, heart failure, prostate problems, and gastroesophageal reflux disease (GERD).[156]

SIGNS AND SYMPTOMS

Patients have complaints of either difficulty initiating sleep, early morning awakening, or an inability to maintain sleep with trouble returning to sleep after awakening. Most patients report significant distress due to sleep disturbances that lead to an impairment in daytime functioning that can range from chronic fatigue, impaired attention, mood changes, and behavioral difficulties or change in academic performance or interpersonal relationships.[153] Often there is excessive worry during the bedtime hours surrounding sleep that only worsens the ability to initiate sleep.

The *DSM-5* utilizes a descriptive approach to classify insomnia based on duration of symptoms and frequency, whereas the ISD-3 categories insomnia into three types, Chronic Insomnia Disorder, Short-term Insomnia Disorder, and Other Insomnia Disorder. The major criteria for diagnosis by ISD-3 can be found in Box 18.6.

PHYSICAL EXAMINATION

There are no specific physical examination findings to support the diagnosis of insomnia. Patients may present with fatigue or malaise and can appear either anxious or depressed. A thorough examination should be done in order to rule out a number of other medical conditions that could cause sleep

BOX 18.6 ISD-3 Criteria for Diagnosis of Insomnia

Major criteria (all three required): difficulty falling asleep, difficulty staying asleep, early awakening

Daytime impairment manifested by at least one of the following: fatigue, malaise, poor attention or concentration, social or vocational/educational dysfunction, mood disturbance or irritability, daytime sleepiness, reduced motivation or energy, increased errors or accidents

Occurs at least three times per week for at least 1 month

Not related to inadequate opportunity, an inappropriate sleep environment, or another sleep disorder

Source: Data from Siddiqi N, House AO, Holmes JD. Occurrence and outcome of delirium in medical in-patients: a systematic literature review. Age Ageing. *2006;35(4):350–364. doi:10.1093/ageing/afl005*

TABLE 18.14 Differential Diagnosis for Insomnia

Diagnosis	Description
Pulmonary disorders	Chronic obstructive pulmonary disease, asthma, obstructive sleep apnea
Cardiovascular disorders	Congestive heart failure
Neurologic disorders	Migraine, seizure, or stroke
Endocrine disorders	Hypothyroidism or hyperthyroidism
Gastrointestinal disorders	Gastroesophageal reflux disease
Psychiatric disorders	Major depressive disorder, bipolar disorder, anxiety disorder, substance abuse disorder
Chronic pain disorders	Fibromyalgia, rheumatoid arthritis, osteoarthritis
Other sleep-related disorders	Restless legs syndrome

Source: Data from Momin RR, Ketvertis K. Primary insomnia. In: StatPearls. StatPearls Publishing; 2020. http://www.ncbi.nlm.nih.gov/books/NBK554516; Buysse DJ. Insomnia. JAMA. *2013;309(7):706–716. doi:10.1001/jama.2013.193; Hein M, Senterre C, Lanquart J-P, et al. Hyperarousal during sleep in untreated, major depressed subjects with prodromal insomnia: a polysomnographic study.* Psychiatry Res. *2017;258:387–395. doi:10.1016/j.psychres.2017.08.061*

disturbances. This includes a cardiovascular and pulmonary exam to assess for any infectious or inflammatory process, musculoskeletal exam to assess for pain, GI exam, and neurologic examination. A psychiatric examination should include examining the patient's mood, affect, thought process, perceptual disturbances, insight, and judgment.

DIFFERENTIAL DIAGNOSIS

The differential diagnosis for insomnia is summarized in Table 18.14.

DIAGNOSTIC STUDIES

There are no diagnostic studies required to make the diagnosis of insomnia. A polysomnography (i.e., sleep study) is not indicated for the routine assessment of insomnia, but can be used to rule out sleep apnea, periodic limb movement disorders, or parasomnias. Another sleep measuring modality is actigraphy, which involves a wearable device on the wrist or ankle. This tool gathers information about limb movement activity to provide patterns of wakefulness and sleep. Though helpful to provide multiple parameters (e.g., sleep latency, sleep efficiency, total sleep time, and wake after sleep onset), it is not required to make a diagnosis of insomnia.

Additional tools to aid in the diagnosis of insomnia consist of questionnaires, two of which are the Insomnia Severity Index (ISI) and the Pittsburgh Sleep Quality Index (PSQI). The ISI consists of seven questions that can be self-administered by patients, with the higher score correlating to the greater degree of insomnia. The PSQI helps to differentiate between various sleep-related disorders, taking into account different domains of sleep (quality, latency, duration, efficacy, medication use, daytime symptoms and disturbances) over a 4-week period.[150]

EVALUATION

Any patient who has complaints of acute or chronic insomnia should first be evaluated for any medical condition that could potentially warrant these symptoms. Individuals should be screened for medication and/or substance abuse disorders in addition to having a thorough psychiatric history. Screening for sleep disorders can be helpful in those patients who have experienced acute stress, including return from military service or loss of a loved one, as these individuals are at high risk for developing insomnia.

TREATMENT

Treatment includes both pharmacologic and nonpharmacologic options, which studies show have similar effectiveness and outcome.[150] Nonpharmacologic options are preferred due to side effect profile of medication and cost, as long as the patient is willing to engage in behavioral therapies.

- Nonpharmacologic options include the following:
  - **Sleep hygiene:** This includes limiting evening alcohol and caffeine, avoiding daytime naps, minimal use of smart devices prior to sleep, and creating a prebedtime ritual.
  - **CBT:** Addresses dysfunctional behaviors and beliefs about sleep that contribute to the perception of insomnia, which can be delivered in an individual or group setting.[153]
  - **Stimulus control:** Focuses on the association of bed and sleep, which involves limiting the bed to only sleep and sexual activity, as well as getting out of bed when awake and anxious at night.
  - **Sleep restriction therapy:** Limits the number of sleeping hours in order to increase sleep drive and stabilize circadian rhythm
  - **Relaxation therapy:** Includes regular exercise, muscle relaxation, and breathing exercises.
- Pharmacologic options should be limited to short-term use and combined with nonpharmacologic therapy.
  - Medication classes approved by the FDA include benzodiazepine receptor agonists, antihistamines, TCAs, and melatonin receptor agonists.
  - Side effects can be significant and include morning sedation, anterograde amnesia, impaired balance and increased falls, anxiety, and complex sleep-related behaviors (e.g., sleepwalking, sleep-related eating, driving, and sexual behavior).[157]
  - Long-term effects of pharmacologic management include potential tolerance, dependence, and addiction.

PATIENT EDUCATION

- Clinicians can help educate patients about the complexity of sleep and factors relating to their sleep disturbance. Acute stresses should be identified and managed before making a diagnosis of chronic insomnia. Patients should be educated that treatment of insomnia will take time and include changes in behavior, habits, and environment.[150]

18.13 DELIRIUM

Richard Bottner

MEDICAL HISTORY AND CLINICAL PRESENTATION

Delirium is a neurocognitive and psychiatric disturbance that primarily affects patients with medical comorbidities, especially those who require hospitalization.[157] Prevalence of delirium among hospitalized patients ranges from 3% to 42%.[158] In the hospital setting, risk factors for delirium include age, history of dementia or hypertension, recent mechanical ventilation, polytrauma, presence of metabolic acidosis, and end-organ damage or failure.[159] Delirium is associated with significant increase in morbidity and death.[157] There are two main etiologies of delirium. First, delirium can be caused by a medical condition such as disease of the CNS, metabolic derangements, infectious disease, fever, cardiac dysfunction, or systemic disease such as malignancy.[157] Second, delirium may result from specific medications or polypharmacy, or illicit substance use or withdrawal from such substances.[157] Several medication classes are considered deliriogenic including opioids, benzodiazepines, antihistamines, and anticholinergics.[160,161] The postoperative period also represents a high-risk time for developing delirium secondary to perioperative anesthetics administered.[162] The American Geriatrics Society Beers Criteria is an excellent reference for reviewing deliriogenic medications among geriatric patients.[163]

SIGNS AND SYMPTOMS

It is important to appreciate that the etiology of delirium is often multifactorial, and therefore there is a wide array of signs and symptoms associated with the diagnosis.[164] Delirium is represented by an altered degree of consciousness and decreased attention span.[157] Patients often exhibit impaired memory.[157] There is often a disassociation with time of day and disorientation to others; however, patients are typically aware of themselves.[157] Patients may report misperceptions affecting the auditory, visual, and tactile senses.[157] Delirium is often accompanied by either hyperactive or hypoactive components whereby patients may have dysregulated behavior or become lethargic.[157]

PHYSICAL EXAMINATION

The physical examination should focus on assessing possible etiologies. For example, presence of fever, diaphoresis, and tachycardia may represent sepsis secondary to an infectious cause. Careful attention should be paid to the patient's overall appearance including degree of alertness, presence of disheveled look, relationship of patient to their environment, general gait, and overall motor function, which may be hyperactive or hypoactive. A thorough neurologic examination should always be performed.

DIFFERENTIAL DIAGNOSIS

It is important to have a high index of suspicion for delirium as it is often misdiagnosed and underrecognized.[160] Delirium is an altered degree of awareness and perception coinciding with a reduced ability to concentrate or maintain focus.[157] Patients with delirium are often disoriented and have changes in memory or speech patterns.[157] Delirium must be distinguished from dementia.[165] Generally, this can be done by evaluating onset, duration, degree of change to attention, consciousness, and speech, and the underlying etiology.[165] Two key points may help differentiate the diagnoses: delirium is acquired in a relatively quick fashion, often within hours or days, whereas dementia develops over a much longer period of time.[157] In addition, delirium tends to have a "wax and wane" feature throughout the day and night whereas dementia represents a more static neurocognitive deficit.[157] It is helpful to consider the diagnosis of delirium in the context of the overall clinical picture keeping in mind the many etiologies that may contribute to delirium.

DIAGNOSTIC STUDIES

Depending on the clinical picture, assessment of underlying infectious disease may be warranted. This includes urine analysis and urine culture, blood cultures, rapid plasma reagin (RPR), and HIV. Metabolic abnormalities should be evaluated with a complete metabolic panel. Hematologic abnormalities may be assessed with a CBC. Diagnostic studies may include a chest x-ray, CT or MRI of the head and brain, EEG, or lumbar puncture.

EVALUATION

A thorough evaluation of previous clinical documentation and collecting collateral through discussion with family, friends, and cohabitants may reveal clues for a prior diagnosis of dementia.[160] A careful substance use history should be obtained and a complete review of medications performed. Specific comorbid medical conditions may raise suspicion for delirium including decompensated liver disease, uremia, untreated HIV, and SUDs. Several screening tools may contribute to the assessment of delirium. The most commonly used is the Confusion Assessment Method (CAM). Additional screening tools include the Delirium Rating Scale, the Nurses' Delirium Screening Checklist, and the Memorial Delirium Assessment Scale.[166] The Mini-Mental State Examination (MMSE) has low positive-predictive value in diagnosing delirium but may be helpful to rule out delirium for patients who perform well on the assessment.[167]

TREATMENT

Improving the physical environment is the first step in treating delirium.[157] Interventions include increasing familiarity of the environment by bringing in pictures of friends or family or other objectives that may have significance for the patient. Reestablishing a home routine may be helpful as well. Promoting sleep hygiene can help prevent and treat delirium. Patients should be encouraged to stay awake during the daytime hours and sleep during the overnight hours. For example, blinds should be kept open during the day, the television or radio turned on, and the clock in the room should show the correct time. During the overnight hours, checking of vital signs and other interruptions should be kept to a minimum as long as doing so does not pose any risk to the patient. Providing patients with ear plugs has been shown to prevent and treat delirium.[168] After surgery, patients should begin physical activity as soon as it is possible and safe.[160] Patients with acute medical pathologies should have those underlying conditions treated as quickly and effectively as possible.[157] Deliriogenic medications should be discontinued or dose-reduced.[157] For patients who are not improving, consultation with a psychiatrist is recommended.[157] Pharmacotherapies include antipsychotic medications. Haloperidol is considered first-line due to its reduced anticholinergic properties and relatively small chance of resulting in hypotension or excessive drowsiness.[157] Benzodiazepines are considered deliriogenic and should be avoided in the treatment of delirium unless the etiology is related to alcohol withdrawal.[157] The use of antipsychotics as a preventive measure in the hospital setting is not appropriate.[169] Delirium often fully resolves in <2 weeks but may continue for up to 30 days.[157] Careful evaluation of a patient's capacity to make their own medical decisions should take place in the setting of delirium.[157]

18.14 SUICIDAL IDEATION

Marci Contreras

OVERVIEW

Suicidality is complex and several factors should be considered when encountering a patient with suicidal ideation including biologic factors such as family history or comorbidities, environmental stressors, as well as history of mental illness. Suicidal patients may be seen in the ED. However, it is the primary care clinician who most commonly identifies risk factors for suicidal ideation and manages these patients. Patients may not disclose suicidal ideation unless directly asked. Therefore, it is important that clinicians feel prepared to screen these patients. The PA plays an important role in the screening and evaluation of the patient with suicidal ideation.

EPIDEMIOLOGY

Approximately 800,000 people die by suicide each year and estimates on the number of suicide attempts are at least 20 times higher.[170] Completed suicides are three times more common in males than females; however, suicide attempts are significantly more common in females than males. More than 50% of completed suicides involve firearms.

PATHOPHYSIOLOGY

There are complex structural and functional alterations at play in the brain when considering the pathophysiology of suicidal ideation. However, the brain regions most consistently implicated in mood disorders and suicidal behavior include the brainstem monoaminergic systems, the prefrontal cortex, the anterior cingulate cortex, the amygdala, and the hippocampus.[171]

MEDICAL HISTORY AND CLINICAL PRESENTATION

When eliciting a medical history, patients with suicidal ideation will often describe their *mental pain* (or psychological pain) as "unbearable." The most important question for the clinician to ask is "Do you have specific thoughts or behaviors toward suicide?" The patient may present with recent episodes of irritability or agitation, changes in mood, or a history of impulsivity. Clinicians should inquire about employment status, home environment, and relationship status. It is important for the clinician to gather information on the patient's history of substance use and whether they have a support system or participate in the community.

BOX 18.7 Risk Factors for Suicidal Ideation

Male
Poor coping skills
Major depressive disorder (anhedonia may play a large role)
Bipolar disorder
Other underlying mental illness
Comorbid physical illness
Substance use/abuse
Family history of suicidal behavior
Adolescents with emotional, behavioral, or mental health disorder
Trauma exposure (e.g., childhood trauma, abuse, or neglect)
Recent negative life event or psychosocial stressors (e.g., divorce, loss of job, loss of loved one); other source of shame, self-blame, humiliation
Poor support system, isolated, or feelings of rejection
History of previous suicide attempt
Self-destructive behavior
Anger or aggression
LGBTQ population
Military veterans with history of traumatic brain injury (TBI) or posttraumatic stress disorder (PTSD)

Simply having one of the risk factors (Box 18.7) may not necessarily put a patient at high risk for suicidal ideation but rather does make them susceptible especially in conjunction with feelings of hopelessness or helplessness. According to the interpersonal theory of suicide, individuals are at greatest risk of suicidal ideation when they feel a sense of burdensomeness to others, lack a sense of belonging, and feel hopeless that these states will not change.[172] Many of the risk factors are nonmodifiable. Therefore, it is important for the PA to ascertain what makes the patient *believe* their life is not worth living, rather than assessing a list of external factors that may or may not be changed. For example, an older White male with debilitating disease and history of substance misuse with access to firearms decides he is a burden to his adult children. The patient in this scenario might be considered high risk for suicidal ideation.

DIFFERENTIAL DIAGNOSIS

The differential diagnosis for suicidal ideation is outlined in Table 18.15.

TABLE 18.15 Differential Diagnosis for Suicidal Ideation

Diagnosis	Description
Suicide attempt	Potentially self-injurious behavior with some intent to die
Nonsuicidal self-injury	Self-injurious behavior with no intent to die

BOX 18.8 Determining Risk for Suicidal Ideation

Identify risk factors.

Does the patient have thoughts, plans, or suicidal intent?

"Tell me why you want to die."

"On a scale of 1 to 10, where would you rate your seriousness for wanting to die?"

"Have you taken any steps or preparation toward suicide?"

Identify protective factors. These include religious beliefs, good social support, married status, children in the home, and positive coping abilities. *(Note: Even in the presence of protective factors, acute risk factors may still exist and should be considered.)*

"Tell me your reasons for living."

"What or who do you rely on for support?"

"When you are having a difficult time, what keeps you going?

Determine patient risk for carrying through with suicide. Would you consider this patient to be at *high risk, moderate risk,* or *low risk*?

Example: Someone considered as *low risk* may present as a young, depressed female with a good support system, no history of mental illness or substance abuse and indicates that because of her religion she would never "seriously" consider ending her life.

EVALUATION

The first goal in evaluation of the patient with suicidal ideation is to establish whether the patient poses an imminent threat to self-harm (Box 18.8). Approach to the patient should be done in a calm and nonjudgmental way. The PA should establish trust and show compassion for the patient. Be an empathetic listener while letting the patient talk while not interrupting them. Patients with suicidal ideation feel as though they do not belong in the world, and the clinician spending time with them and taking an interest helps them to feel valued.

Patients with suicidal ideation usually feel they have no support and that life is "not worth living" and view suicide as the only way "out." These feelings of hopelessness, helplessness, and worthlessness play a central role. Patients may also describe feelings of emptiness, disconnect, and feel as though they do not matter. Some clinicians may fear that by asking a patient about suicidal ideation, this will increase the likelihood that they will take their own life. However, this is not true as most of these patients long for the opportunity to address these difficult questions.

- *Do not deny or neglect their feelings or downplay their emotions.*
- *Avoid placing emphasis on perceived support (e.g., "You have so much to live for!").*
- *Avoid interpreting their comments or behavior as "attention-seeking."*
- *Any signs or symptoms of distress should be taken seriously.*

During the visit, build a good rapport with the patient and avoid being rushed or interrupted. The patient already feels as though they are a "burden" and should not feel as though they are a burden to the clinician. Scanning social media posts may further help to establish risk and potentiate intervention. There are numerous instruments used to measure attitudes toward suicide and suicidal ideation. However, there is no gold standard. Other screening tools, such as those used for depression and anxiety, might be helpful in developing a treatment plan. It is important to keep in mind that these tools do not adequately predict whether a patient is at immediate risk for attempting suicide. All risk factors should be considered in assessment of the patient and the clinician should use their best judgment. There is no consensus on screening the general population for suicidal ideation. However, if a patient has one of the risk factors then further screening should be considered.

TREATMENT

The first priority in developing a treatment plan is *patient safety*. Treatment should not be "one-size-fits-all" but rather tailored to the specific patient and based on the assessment of risk level. The PA should provide all patients the phone number for the local crisis hotline and the national suicide prevention hotline and watch the patient put these numbers in their phone.

- Treat any underlying mental health disorders (e.g., depression).
- Reduce access to firearms (or other lethal means).
- Establish support through family and/or friends.
- Discuss ways to positively distract from unpleasant or suicidal thoughts.
- Provide written materials on warning signs.
- Establish emergency contacts.
- Discuss mechanisms for coping and direct the patient as to where they might seek help during times of crisis.
- Facilitate continuity of care. Set up a follow-up appointment and referral for a mental health clinician.

Dialectical behavioral therapy (DBT) is a type of CBT performed by a qualified mental health professional. DBT helps to regulate emotions, cope with triggers, and change unhealthy behaviors. Although it is unlikely that the primary care PA will provide psychotherapy, it is important to establish a therapeutic alliance. No-suicide contracts are no longer in favor because if the clinician suspects the patient might be in danger of self-harm then most likely the patient needs to be safe within an inpatient setting.

PATIENT EDUCATION AND ADDITIONAL RESOURCES

- Suicide Prevention Resource Center: www.sprc.org

- Suicide Assessment Five-step Evaluation and Triage (SAFE-T). Substance Abuse and Mental Health Services Administration; 2009. Available at: store.samhsa.gov/product/SAFE-T-Pocket-Card-Suicide-Assessment-Five-Step-Evaluation-and-Triage-for-Clinicians/sma09-4432?referer=from_search_result
- National Suicide Prevention Lifeline: suicidepreventionlifeline.org
- Crisis Text Line: crisistextline.org

18.15 PSYCHOPHARMACOLOGY

Samuel L. Gurevitz

ANTIDEPRESSANTS

There are several classes of antidepressants (Table 18.16). A primary indication for antidepressant agents is the treatment of major depressive disorders (MMDs). The use of antidepressants extends beyond MMD as these agents are used for the treatment of panic disorder, GAD, PTSD, OCD, social anxiety, and seasonal affective disorder. Additionally, antidepressants are commonly used to treat pain disorders such as neuropathic pain and the pain associated with fibromyalgia. Some antidepressants are used for treating PMDD, mitigating the vasomotor symptoms of menopause, and as an aid to smoking cessation.

All antidepressants have a warning for increasing the risk of suicidal thoughts and behavior in pediatric and young adult patients. Patients treated should be observed for clinical worsening and for emergence of suicidal thoughts and behaviors. In addition, any antidepressant that increases serotonin can be associated with serotonin syndrome.

Antidepressants inhibit several hepatic CYP450 isoenzymes and are primarily metabolized by the hepatic CYP450 isoenzymes (most often CYP2D6 and -3A4), making this class of medications a likely target for drug interactions when used with strong CYP450 inducers or inhibitors. Enzyme inhibition occurs rapidly, within 2 to 3 days, and enzyme induction is often a slower process that usually takes a number of days to a few weeks.

Selective Serotonin Reuptake Inhibitors—First-Line Treatment

MECHANISM OF ACTION

Selectively inhibits serotonin (5-HT) reuptake, resulting in an increase in intracellular serotonin and a greater availability of serotonin in the presynaptic axon terminal. Besides inhibiting 5-HT reuptake, vilazodone is a partial 5-HT_{1A} agonist and vortioxetine has activity at several 5-HT receptors.

CONTRAINDICATIONS

Avoid the use of MAOIs concurrently or within 14 days.

WARNINGS

When SSRIs are used in combination with serotonergic agents a potentially life-threatening serotonin syndrome may occur. Use SSRIs with caution in patients with a family history of bipolar disorder, mania, or hypomania. They may precipitate a mixed/manic episode. Use caution in patients with seizures. SSRIs may impair platelet aggregation, resulting in increased risk of bleeding events, particularly if used concomitantly with aspirin, NSAIDs, warfarin, or other anticoagulants.

ADVERSE EFFECTS

SSRIs are associated with nervousness, agitation, diarrhea, nausea, anorexia, sexual dysfunction, syndrome of inappropriate antidiuretic hormone secretion (SIADH), insomnia, and discontinuation syndrome (do not stop abruptly).

DRUG INTERACTIONS

Fluoxetine and paroxetine are moderate to strong inhibitors of CYP2D6. Fluvoxamine is both a strong CYP1A2 and CYP2C19 inhibitor.

TABLE 18.16 Classification of Antidepressants

SSRIs	SNRIs	TCAs	MAOIs	Atypical Antidepressants
Citalopram (Celexa)	Desvenlafaxine (Pristiq)	Amitriptyline (Elavil)	Isocarboxazid (Marplan)	Bupropion (Wellbutrin)
Escitalopram (Lexapro)	Duloxetine (Cymbalta)	Clomipramine (Anafranil)	Phenelzine (Nardil)	Mirtazapine (Remeron)
Fluoxetine (Prozac)	Levomilnacipran (Fetzima)	Desipramine (Norpramin)	Selegiline (Eldepryl)	Trazodone (Desyrel)
Paroxetine (Paxil)	Venlafaxine (Effexor)	Doxepen (Silenor)	Tranylcypromine (Parnate)	
Sertraline (Zoloft)		Imipramine (Tofranil)		
Vilazodone (Viibryd)		Nortriptyline (Pamelor)		
Vortioxetine (Trintellix)				

MAOIs, monoamine oxidase inhibitors; SNRIs, serotonin-norepinephrine reuptake inhibitors; SSRIs, selective serotonin reuptake inhibitors; TCAs, tricyclic antidepressants.

SSRIs have multiple routes of metabolism (primarily 2D6 and 3A4), enzyme inducers or inhibitors could increase or decrease SSRI plasma levels.

SPECIFIC INTERACTIONS

- **MAOIs:** Risk of serotonin syndrome
- **TCAs:** SSRIs inhibit metabolism, increasing TCA levels
- **Warfarin:** Inhibition of warfarin metabolism
- Phenytoin/Carbamazepine
- Beta blockers
- SSRIs, especially fluoxetine, inhibit conversion and leave opioids less effective

Serotonin-Norepinephrine Reuptake Inhibitors

MECHANISM OF ACTION

SNRIs selectively inhibit 5-HT and norepinephrine reuptake, resulting in an increased extracellular concentration of 5-HT and niacin equivalent (NE). In contrast to TCAs, these agents do not antagonize muscarinic, adrenergic, or histamine receptors, and produce few autonomic, sedative, or cardiovascular side effects.

SNRIs can cause a dose-dependent increase in blood pressure, presumably due to blocking reuptake of norepinephrine.

CONTRAINDICATIONS

Use of MAOIs concurrently with the SNRI or within 14 days of discontinuing the MAOI.

WARNINGS

SNRIs should be used cautiously in patients with narrow-angle glaucoma. When SNRIs are used in combination with serotonergic agents a potentially life-threatening serotonin syndrome may occur. In patients with bipolar disorder, used without a mood stabilizer, they may precipitate a mixed/manic episode. Use caution in patients with seizures. SNRIs may impair platelet aggregation, resulting in increased risk of bleeding events, particularly if used concomitantly with aspirin, NSAIDs, warfarin, or other anticoagulants. Abrupt discontinuation or interruption of therapy has been associated with a discontinuation syndrome.

ADVERSE EFFECTS

The most common adverse effects are nausea, headache, dizziness, fatigue, insomnia, and dry mouth. Other side effects include anxiety, blurred vision, urinary retention, sexual dysfunction, increased blood pressure and pulse, and SIADH.

DRUG INTERACTIONS

Duloxetine is a moderate inhibitor of CYP2D6.

Venlafaxine is metabolized by CYP2D6, duloxetine by CYPA12, and levomilnacipran metabolized by CYP3A4.

Tricyclic Antidepressants

MECHANISM OF ACTION

TCAs inhibit 5-HT and norepinephrine reuptake. They block muscarinic, α_1-adrenergic, and histaminic receptors, which relates to their adverse effects. These actions account for the major side effects of these drugs. Secondary amines, such as nortriptyline and desipramine, are less sedating and have fewer cardiovascular effects. Tertiary amines, such as amitriptyline and imipramine, are very sedating.

CONTRAINDICATIONS

Do not coadminister with or within 14 days of a MAOI.

WARNINGS

TCAs should be used cautiously in patients with conduction abnormalities; the risk of conduction abnormalities with these agents is elevated relative to other antidepressants. In addition, TCAs should be used cautiously in patients with narrow-angle glaucoma, in patients at risk of seizures, and in patients with bipolar disorders.

ADVERSE EFFECTS

The cholinergic blocking effect (anticholinergic) produces dry mouth, constipation, urinary retention, and blurred vision. The α-blocking effect produces orthostatic hypotension, and the H_1-antagonism produces sedation. The TCAs have been associated with SIADH. Adverse effects also include weight gain and decreased seizure threshold. Overdose can cause prolonged QT interval leading to torsades de pointes.

TCAs have adverse cardiovascular and anticholinergic effects and are particularly toxic in overdose, limiting their use. An overdose of these drugs can produce serious, life-threatening cardiac arrhythmias, delirium, and psychosis. As a group, they have a very narrow therapeutic index, which means that safety is an issue.

DRUG INTERACTIONS

TCAs are primarily metabolized by CYP2D6 and do not inhibit or induce CYP450 isoenzymes.

Monoamine Oxidase Inhibitors

MECHANISM OF ACTION

The MAOIs are classified according to their selectivity for the two main types of MAO enzymes. MAO-A preferentially metabolizes serotonin but will also metabolize norepinephrine and dopamine. MAO-B preferentially metabolizes dopamine and is used in the management of Parkinson disease. MAOIs inhibit the breakdown of serotonin, norepinephrine, and dopamine resulting in an increased concentration of serotonin, norepinephrine, and dopamine in the neuronal synapse.

CONTRAINDICATIONS

Do not use concurrently with buspirone, bupropion, dextromethorphan, SSRIs, SNRIs, sympathomimetics, TCAs, or foods high in tyramine.

WARNINGS

Since MAO is widely distributed throughout the body, MAOIs can be expected to cause diverse adverse effects. Some of the most serious adverse effects reported with MAOIs (e.g., hypertensive crisis, serotonin syndrome) have occurred when MAOIs were administered concomitantly with certain foods containing tyramine, or prescription or nonprescription (OTC) drugs.

MAOIs should be used with caution in patients with angle-closure glaucoma, bipolar disorder, seizures or at risk of seizures, and hyperthyroidism.

ADVERSE EFFECTS

Major adverse effects reported with MAOIs are orthostatic hypertension and the occurrence of a hypertensive crisis, which is sometimes fatal. Other common adverse effects are weight gain, sexual side effects, and urinary retention

DRUG INTERACTIONS

MAOIs should be avoided with foods containing high content of tyramine. This can cause a hypertensive crisis, a potentially serious and life threatening, but rare, adverse effect. In addition, many medications should be avoided: buspirone, cyclobenzaprine, decongestants, dextromethorphan, sympathomimetics, stimulants, and other antidepressants.

ATYPICAL ANTIDEPRESSANTS

Mirtazapine

MECHANISM OF ACTION

Mirtazapine blocks presynaptic α_2-adrenergic autoreceptors and heteroreceptors and thereby increases release of norepinephrine and serotonin, respectively. It is also a potent histamine H_1 receptor and an antagonist of 5-HT_2 and 5-HT_3 receptors.

CONTRAINDICATIONS

Do not coadminister with or within 14 days of a MAOI.

WARNINGS

Mirtazapine should be used cautiously in patients with narrow-angle glaucoma, bipolar disorder, and patients at risk for seizures. When used in combination with serotonergic agents a potentially life-threatening serotonin syndrome may occur. Agranulocytosis can occur with mirtazapine.

ADVERSE EFFECTS

Mirtazapine may cause sedation, constipation, dizziness, drowsiness, dry mouth, increased appetite, weight gain, hyponatremia, and increased serum cholesterol and triglyceride levels.

DRUG INTERACTIONS

Mirtazapine has no considerable inhibitory or inducing effects itself on CYP450 isoenzymes. Although it is metabolized by CYP2D6, -1A2, and -3A4. Therefore, inhibitors may increase, and inducers may decrease, mirtazapine concentration.

Bupropion

MECHANISM OF ACTION

Bupropion inhibits dopamine and norepinephrine reuptake.

CONTRAINDICATIONS

Bupropion should not be used in patients at risk for seizure disorders, such as bulimia or anorexia nervosa. The use with MAOIs concurrently or within 14 days should be avoided.

WARNINGS

Bupropion should be used cautiously in patients with narrow-angle glaucoma, bipolar disorder, and patients at risk for seizures. Bupropion may elevate blood pressure and cause delusions, hallucinations, and psychosis especially in patients with an underlying psychiatric illness. Can be stimulating; patients should take in the morning. May not be appropriate for patients with GAD or insomnia.

ADVERSE EFFECTS

Bupropion may cause agitation, dry mouth, insomnia, nausea, tremors, tachycardia, and weight loss. Hypertension may also occur so blood pressure should be regularly monitored.

DRUG INTERACTIONS

Bupropion is a moderate CYP2D6 inhibitor. It is metabolized by CYP2B6.

Trazodone

MECHANISM OF ACTION

This drug inhibits reuptake of serotonin, acts as a $5HT_{2a}$ receptor antagonist, and significantly blocks histamine (H_1) and α_1-adrenergic receptors.

CONTRAINDICATIONS

Trazodone should be not used with MAOIs.

WARNINGS

When trazodone is used in combination with serotonergic agents a potentially life-threatening serotonin syndrome may occur. Use trazodone cautiously in patients with narrow-angle glaucoma, bipolar disorder, and patients at risk for seizures. Trazodone may impair platelet aggregation, resulting in increased risk of bleeding events, particularly if used concomitantly with aspirin, NSAIDs, warfarin, or other anticoagulants.

ADVERSE EFFECTS

Most common adverse effects are drowsiness, dizziness, headache, nervousness, fatigue, dry mouth, nausea and vomiting, blurred vision. Other adverse effects associated with trazodone are priapism, orthostatic hypotension, and SIADH. Trazodone is more commonly used as a sleep aid than to manage depression.

DRUG INTERACTIONS

Trazodone is not a CYP450 isoenzyme inhibitor or inducer. Trazodone is mainly metabolized by CYP3A4, so inhibitors or inducers of CYP3A4 can influence trazodone's plasma concentration.

ATTENTION-DEFICIT/HYPERACTIVITY DISORDER MEDICATIONS

Dysfunction in the frontosubcortical pathways and imbalances in the dopaminergic and noradrenergic systems (norepinephrine) have been implicated in ADHD and form the basis for pharmacologic treatment. Pharmacologic agents used to treat ADHD can be divided into two main classes: stimulant and nonstimulant medications. Tables 18.17 and 18.18 list the two main classes and their mechanism of action. Tables 18.19 and 18.20 lists the contraindications, warnings, and adverse effects of the two main classes used to treat ADHD.

Amphetamines

CYP2D6 inhibitors may increase amphetamine levels, which is equivalent to increasing the dosage of amphetamines. Alcohol may increase plasma dextroamphetamine concentrations.

ATOMOXETINE

Poor metabolizers of CYP2D6 have better atomoxetine response, but also an increased risk of adverse effects.

Guanfacine

It is mainly metabolized by CYP3A4, which can be induced and inhibited, which can decrease or increase guanfacine concentrations, respectively.

Methylphenidate

Methylphenidate may be associated with important elevations in imipramine concentrations based on a case series study.

ANTIPSYCHOTICS

Antipsychotic medications were predominantly used in the treatment of schizophrenia; however, they are now used in a range of disorders and are evidence-based in the treatment of bipolar disorder, schizoaffective disorder and major depression (augmentation), autism (associated symptoms), and Tourette syndrome (associated symptoms) and are used off-label for other disorders.

Antipsychotic medications are broadly divided into typical (first-generation) and atypical (second-generation)

TABLE 18.17 Selected Stimulants for Attention-Deficit/Hyperactivity Disorder and Mechanism of Action

Generic Name	Brand/Trade Name	Mechanism of Action
Amphetamine	Adzenys XR	Increases the release of norepinephrine and dopamine from nerve terminals to boost norepinephrine and dopamine neurotransmission in the prefrontal cortex Amphetamines also have a peripheral sympathomimetic effect by stimulating β and α receptors
Amphetamine and dextroamphetamine	Adderall	See above
Dextroamphetamine	Dexedrine SR	See above
Lisdexamfetamine	Vyvanse	See above
Dexmethylphenidate	Focalin	Blocks the reuptake of dopamine and blocks the reuptake of norepinephrine to a much lesser degree to boost norepinephrine and dopamine neurotransmission in the prefrontal cortex
Methylphenidate	Concerta, Ritalin, Daytrana, Metadate, and Methylin	See above

TABLE 18.18 Nonstimulants for Attention-Deficit/Hyperactivity Disorder and Mechanism of Action

Generic Name	Brand/Trade Name	Mechanism of Action
Atomoxetine	Strattera	Selectively inhibits reuptake of norepinephrine
Clonidine extended release	Kapvay	Stimulates alpha-2 adrenoceptors in the brainstem activating inhibitory neurons, which results in reduced sympathetic outflow from the central nervous system (CNS) Increase norepinephrine in prefrontal cortex
Guanfacine extended release	Intuniv	See above

TABLE 18.19 Stimulants: Contraindications, Warnings, and Adverse Effects

Stimulant	Contraindications	Warnings	Adverse Effects
Amphetamines	During or within 14 days following monoamine oxidase inhibitor History of glaucoma Should be avoided in patients with symptomatic cardiovascular disease, hyperthyroidism, and moderate to severe hypertension	High potential for abuse and dependence Associated with serious cardiovascular events including sudden death in patients with preexisting structural cardiac abnormalities or other serious heart problems May increase heart rate and blood pressure Increased risk for seizure activity	Decreased appetite Weight loss Sleep difficulties Transient headaches Exacerbation of tics (rare) Increased heart rate or blood pressure Irritability or dysphoria Psychosis, euphoria, mania, severe depression
Methylphenidate	See above	See above	See above

antipsychotics although this distinction does not necessarily take into account the individuality in receptor profiles of the individual antipsychotic medications (Table 18.21).

MECHANISM OF ACTION

Schizophrenia involves a dysregulation of dopaminergic circuits with excess dopaminergic activity in the mesolimbic pathway (leading to positive symptoms of psychosis) and reduced dopaminergic activity in the mesocortical pathway (leading to negative symptoms). The antipsychotic drugs interact with multiple receptors affecting several neurotransmitter systems. The therapeutic effects of typical antipsychotics are believed to result from blockade of dopamine (D_2) receptors and the atypical antipsychotics result from the blockade of dopamine (D_2) receptors and serotonin ($5\text{-}HT_{2A}$) receptors. The alleviation of the positive symptoms of schizophrenia is due to the blockade of the D_2 receptors and the negative symptoms are alleviated by the blockade of the $5\text{-}HT_{2A}$ receptors. In addition, blockade of $5\text{-}HT_{2A}$ reduces extrapyramidal effects by increasing dopamine in the nigrostriatal areas and reduces hyperprolactinemia. The adverse effects are attributed to the blockade of a variety of

TABLE 18.20 Nonstimulants: Contraindications, Warnings, and Adverse Effects

Nonstimulants	Contraindications	Warnings	Adverse Effects
Atomoxetine	During or within 14 days following monoamine oxidase inhibitor or have a history of glaucoma; severe cardiac or vascular disorders in which the condition would be expected to worsen with increase in blood pressure or heart rate	Increased the risk of suicidal ideation; Hepatotoxicity Psychiatric effects Caution in comorbid bipolar disorder History of urinary retention CYP2D6 inhibitors or poor metabolizers	Abdominal pain, vomiting, decreased appetite Somnolence, fatigue, dizziness Elevation of heart rate and blood pressure Priapism Psychiatric symptoms, including suicidal thoughts or behaviors
Clonidine extended release	History of significant depression (may worsen depression symptoms)	Gradual withdrawal is needed Bradycardia Hypotension	Somnolence, fatigue, dizziness. dry mouth, sedation, headache, hypotension, bradycardia
Guanfacine extended release	See above	See above	See above

TABLE 18.21 Antipsychotic Medications

Typical Antipsychotics		Atypical Antipsychotics	
Generic Name	**Brand/Trade Name**	**Generic Name**	**Brand/Trade Name**
Chlorpromazine	Thorazine	Aripiprazole	Abilify
Fluphenazine	Prolixin	Brexpiprazole	Rexulti
Haloperidol	Haldol	Asenapine	Saphris
Perphenazine	Trilafon	Clozapine	Clozaril
Trifluoperazine	Stelazine	Olanzapine	Zyprexa
		Quetiapine	Seroquel
		Iloperidone	Fanapt
		Lurasidone	Latuda
		Paliperidone	Invega
		Risperidone	Risperdal
		Ziprasidone	Geodon
		Cariprazine	Vraylar
		Pimavanserin	Nuplazid

receptors such as α_1-receptors, muscarinic receptors, and H_1 receptors (in CNS).

Pimavanserin is noteworthy, it has no appreciable activity at the D_2 receptor but has antagonist activity at 5-HT_{2A} receptors. It is used to treat hallucinations and delusions associated with Parkinson disease psychosis. The other antipsychotic medications can worsen Parkinson disease symptoms.

WARNINGS

Older patients with dementia-related psychosis treated with antipsychotic drugs are at an increased risk of death. Most deaths are due to cardiovascular and infectious events. Antipsychotics may increase suicidality if they are used for depression.

ADVERSE EFFECTS

Blockade of α_1-receptors produces dizziness, orthostatic hypotension, and reflex tachycardia. Muscarinic receptor antagonism produces blurred vision, dry mouth, constipation, and urinary retention. Blocking the central nervous H_1 receptors produces drowsiness and weight gain. The blockade of 5-HT_{2A} is associated with anxiety and insomnia. The blockade of D_2 causes extrapyramidal effects (akathisia, dystonia, and pseudoparkinsonism) and elevated serum prolactin levels, which can lead to sexual dysfunction, gynecomastia, and menstrual irregularities. Other adverse effects include TD and NMS.

The atypical antipsychotics pose varying risks of QT prolongation, drug interactions, and metabolic adverse effects that may increase cardiovascular and cerebrovascular risks. These metabolic effects include hyperglycemia, dyslipidemia, and weight gain. Of the atypical antipsychotics, clozapine may be the most effective atypical antipsychotic for schizophrenia, but its use is limited due to the risk of agranulocytosis and myocarditis.

SPECIFIC MEDICATIONS

- **Chlorpromazine:** Anticholinergic effects, QT prolongation, postural hypotension, EPS common—"thorazine shuffle"
- **Haloperidol:** High likelihood for EPS
- **Clozapine:** Agranulocytosis (monitor CBC), postural hypotension, decreased seizure threshold
- **Olanzapine:** Similar to clozapine without agranulocytosis, EPS rare, excessive weight gain, increased incidence of hyperglycemia and diabetes ("Zyprexa diabetes")
- **Quetiapine:** Very sedating, few EPS, less prolactin effects
- **Ziprasidone:** Lowers seizure threshold
- **Risperidone:** Increases prolactin, effective for positive and negative symptoms

DRUG INTERACTIONS

Cigarette smoking is potent inducer of CYP1A2 enzymes which lower levels of clozapine, olanzapine, and trifluoperazine.

Several of the typical and atypical antipsychotics can interact with medications that inhibit or induce CYP1A2, CYP3A4 or inhibit CYP2D6. This will result in lower levels if induction occurs or higher levels if inhibition occurs leading to increase in levels of the antipsychotic involved.

ANXIOLYTICS

Benzodiazepines

Benzodiazepines are a large group of drugs (see Table 18.22). They share common pharmacologic effects. Some benzodiazepines are used in the management of anxiety disorders, insomnia, muscle spasms, spasticity, seizures, and alcohol withdrawal symptoms.

TABLE 18.22 Benzodiazepines

Generic Name	Brand/Trade Name
Alprazolam	Xanax
Chlordiazepoxide	Librium
Clonazepam	Klonopin
Clorazepate	Tranxene T-Tab
Diazepam	Valium
Estazolam*	Prosom
Flurazepam*	Dalmane
Lorazepam	Ativan
Oxazepam	Serax
Quazepam*	Doral
Temazepam*	Restoril
Triazolam*	Halcion

**Indicated for insomnia only.*

MECHANISM OF ACTION

Benzodiazepines facilitate the activity of GABA. The benzodiazepines bind to the α_1 and α_2 subunits of the $GABA_A$ receptors, while the nonbenzodiazepines (Z drugs) are selective for the α_1 subunits.

CONTRAINDICATIONS

Benzodiazepines are contraindicated in acute narrow-angle glaucoma, severe hepatic and respiratory impairment, and sleep apnea syndrome.

WARNINGS

Concomitant use of benzodiazepines and opioids may result in profound sedation, respiratory depression, coma, and death. Use with caution in patients with COPD or sleep apnea. Benzodiazepines are classified as schedule IV controlled substances; withdrawal, dependence, and abuse can occur. Their use should be limited to short-term treatment.

ADVERSE EFFECTS

Benzodiazepines may cause cognitive impairment, drowsiness, sedation, anterograde amnesia, ataxia, loss of inhibition, mood swings, and withdrawal symptoms after long-term treatment, and rebound anxiety after short-term treatment. Complex sleep-related behaviors with conscious awareness, such as sleepwalking, sleep eating, and sleep-driving has been associated with benzodiazepines.

DRUG INTERACTIONS

Medications that inhibit or induce CYP3A4 may increase or decrease the drug levels of alprazolam, clorazepate, clonazepam, diazepam, estazolam, flurazepam, quazepam, and triazolam, respectively.

AZAPIRONE DERIVATIVE

Buspirone

MECHANISM OF ACTION

The exact mechanism of action is unknown, but it is an agonist at 5-HT_{1A} autoreceptors and also has activity at 5-HT_{2A} and dopamine (D_2) receptors. Unlike the benzodiazepines, buspirone does not produce dependence. In addition, buspirone does not have anticonvulsant or muscle relaxant effects. It is only indicated for GAD.

CONTRAINDICATIONS

Buspirone should not be used together with MAOIs within 14 days.

WARNINGS

Potentially life-threatening serotonin syndrome has occurred with serotonergic agents. Use with MAOIs may result in hypertensive reaction.

ADVERSE EFFECTS

The most common effects are drowsiness and dizziness.

DRUG INTERACTIONS

Medications that inhibit or induce CYP3A4 may increase or decrease the drug levels of buspirone, respectively.

HYPNOTICS

There are several classes of medications used for insomnia besides benzodiazepines (see Table 18.23).

TABLE 18.23 Medications Approved for Insomnia

Class/Drug	Generic Name	Brand/Trade Name
Nonbenzodiazepines (Z drugs)	Eszopiclone Zaleplon Zolpidem	Lunesta Sonata Ambien, Ambien CR, Edluar, Intermezzo
Melatonin receptors agonist	Ramelteon	Rozerem
Orexin receptor antagonist	Suvorexant	Belsomra
Tricyclic antidepressant	Doxepin*	Silenor

**Low dose (3 to 6 mg).*

Nonbenzodiazepines (Z Drugs)

MECHANISM OF ACTION

Nonbenzodiazepines (Z drugs) facilitate the activity of GABA. The $GABA_A$ receptor has binding sites for the nonbenzodiazepines. The nonbenzodiazepines selectively bind to receptor of the α_1 subunit, while the benzodiazepines bind the α_1 and α_2 subunits. Because of their selective binding to the α_1 subunit the Z drugs produce sedative and hypnotic properties, while causing minimal anxiolytic, amnesic, and anticonvulsant effects compared to that of benzodiazepines.

CONTRAINDICATIONS

Patients who have experienced complex sleep behaviors should avoid nonbenzodiazepines.

WARNINGS

The nonbenzodiazepines may cause abnormal thinking and behavioral changes, worsening of depression or suicidal thinking, and risk of respiratory depression in patients with compromised function. In addition, lower doses are recommended for women and lower doses in men should be considered.

Nonbenzodiazepines are classified as schedule IV controlled substances; withdrawal, dependence, and abuse can occur.

ADVERSE EFFECTS
Common adverse effects associated with nonbenzodiazepines are headache, dizziness, drowsiness, nausea, nightmares, and agitation. Complex sleep-related behaviors with conscious awareness, such as sleepwalking, sleep-eating, and sleep-driving have been associated with nonbenzodiazepines.

DRUG INTERACTIONS
Eszopiclone, zaleplon, and zolpidem are metabolized by CYP3A4. Concurrent use with CYP3A4 inhibitors could increase their concentrations and CYP3A4 inducers could decrease their concentration.

Ramelteon

MECHANISM OF ACTION
Ramelteon is an agonist at the melatonin receptors MT_1 and MT_2. It is not a controlled substance.

CONTRAINDICATIONS
Concurrent use with fluvoxamine should be avoided.

WARNINGS
Ramelteon should be used cautiously in patients with depression and patients with COPD or sleep apnea.

ADVERSE EFFECTS
Common adverse reactions associated with ramelteon are somnolence, dizziness, fatigue, and nausea. Other adverse effects include increased prolactin level, hallucinations, agitation, mania, and complex sleep-related behaviors without conscious awareness.

DRUG INTERACTIONS
Ramelteon is metabolized by CYP1A2. Drugs that inhibit CYP1A2 could increase ramelteon's concentration and inducers can decrease the concentration.

Suvorexant

MECHANISM OF ACTION
Suvorexant is an antagonist at the OX1R and OX2R orexin receptors.

CONTRAINDICATIONS
Suvorexant should be avoided in patients with narcolepsy or strong CYP3A4 inhibitors, such as clarithromycin.

WARNINGS
Abnormal thinking/behavioral changes, sleep paralysis (inability to move or speak for up to several minutes during sleep-wake transitions), and mild cataplexy may occur with suvorexant. Should use with caution in patients with depression and in patients with a history of drug dependence. It is a schedule IV controlled substance.

ADVERSE EFFECTS
The most common adverse effects associated with suvorexant are somnolence, fatigue, and abnormal dreams. Complex sleep-related behaviors without conscious awareness have been reported.

DRUG INTERACTIONS
Suvorexant is metabolized by CYP3A4 so drugs that inhibit CYP3A4 will increase the suvorexant concentrations and inducers will reduce concentrations. Furthermore, suvorexant inhibits P-glycoprotein and, it can increase the concentration of other medications that are affected by P-glycoprotein.

Doxepen (Low Dose)

MECHANISM OF ACTION
Doxepen is a TCA. Doxepen at doses of 3 to 6 mg mainly inhibits histamine-1 (H_1) receptors, which causes sedation and hypnotic effect.

CONTRAINDICATIONS
Avoid use with MAOIs or within 14 days of stopping one, in patients with untreated narrow-angle glaucoma, or in those with severe urinary retention.

ADVERSE EFFECTS
Doxepen may cause residual next-day somnolence.

DRUG INTERACTIONS
Doxepen is metabolized by CYP2D6 and -2C19. Inhibitors of 2D6 or 2C19 will increase the concentration of doxepen.

MOOD STABILIZERS

The mainstays of treatment for bipolar disorders are lithium, anticonvulsants, carbamazepine, lamotrigine, valproate, and antipsychotics. The anticonvulsants and antipsychotics are discussed in other sections.

Lithium (Lithobid)

MECHANISM OF ACTION
Mechanism of action in treating bipolar disorders is unknown. It is postulated that lithium can modify sodium transport within nerve cells and can affect intraneuronal catecholamine metabolism.

CONTRAINDICATIONS
Patients with significant renal impairment, sodium depletion, dehydration, and significant cardiovascular disease. Although not a contraindication, the narrow therapeutic range makes monitoring difficult in noncompliant patients or those with extenuating life circumstances such as homelessness.

WARNINGS
Lithium can precipitate a potentially life-threatening serotonin syndrome and exacerbate psoriasis. Congenital cardiac anomalies are associated with lithium and should be used only when potential benefits outweigh potential risk during pregnancy.

ADVERSE EFFECTS
Common side effects of lithium include polydipsia, polyuria, weight gain, cognitive problems, sedation, tremor, ataxia, GI upset, acne, hypothyroidism, nephrogenic diabetes insipidus, leukocytosis, and flattened or inverted T waves. Lithium is also associated with decline in renal function and hypercalcemia.

DRUG INTERACTIONS
Medications that change renal function, salt balance, or water balance can alter the excretion and serum lithium concentrations so the clinician must monitor lithium levels in patients taking these medications. Medications increasing lithium levels are thiazide and loop diuretics, NSAIDs, angiotensin converting enzyme inhibitors, and angiotensin receptor blockers. Other notable drug interactions are with carbamazepine, which can increase the neurotoxicity of lithium without increasing lithium's concentration and increasing the risk of serotonin syndrome with antidepressants by enhancing their serotonergic effects.

COMMON CHIEF COMPLAINTS

Jennifer Simms Zorn

APPROACH TO FATIGUE

The differential diagnosis for fatigue is extensive, incorporating conditions from multiple organ systems. The first step in approaching a patient with fatigue is to rule out the presence of a general medical condition, as this is necessary for any psychiatric diagnosis. Patient age, length and rate of onset of symptoms, comorbidities, current medications, family history, and social history including drug and alcohol use must be established. The review of systems will provide additional details that can help narrow the differential diagnosis. When considering mental illness, questions regarding concentration, stress, sleep, life changes, and mood should be included. Common diagnoses and their associated symptoms are found in Table 18.24.

Physical exam should be directed at further differentiating the general medical conditions being considered (Table 18.25). Physical exam for mental illness will usually be normal; however, when mental illness is of concern, attention should be given to any signs of self-harm.

The physical exam evaluates the differentials, but additional lab work and testing would be of benefit. Hypothyroidism can be evaluated by assessing the patient's TSH and thyroxine (T4). Anemia can be evaluated by assessing a CBC count. In this case, all of the blood work would be within the normal ranges. In addition to evaluating blood work, the patient could complete an assessment screening for depression. There are several screening test that a clinician could utilize including the Zung or Beck Depression scales or the Patient Health Questionnaire-9 (PHQ-9).

Refer to Figure 18.9 when considering evaluation of a symptom that may be related to depression.

APPROACH TO CHEST PAIN IN THE CONTEXT OF POSSIBLE ANXIETY

Anxiety disorders frequently present with somatic symptoms including abdominal pain, headaches, or fatigue. In some instances of more severe or acute anxiety, patients may complain of chest pain, palpitations, or shortness of breath; these symptoms are frequently present in panic attacks. As with diagnosing any mental illness, the first step is differentiating the presence of a general medical condition. Patient history of mental illness, specifically anxiety and panic disorder, or similar symptoms in the past can be helpful in formulating a differential diagnosis (Table 18.26). Chest pain should always be worked up for a cardiac event, even if

TABLE 18.24 Differential Diagnosis Related to History of Patient With Fatigue

Diagnoses	Symptoms If Positive May Support Diagnosis
Anemia	Fatigue, palor of skin, blood in stool, dark tarry stools, heavy menses, diet vegetarian or low in red meat, personal or family history of anemias
Hypothyroid	Fatigue, weight gain, cold intolerance, personal or family history of endocrine disorder
Multiple sclerosis	Fatigue, visual disturbances, tingling or burning sensations, family history of neurologic disorders
Adjustment with depressed mood	Fatigue, known stressor, depressive symptoms (but would not meet criteria for major depression), personal or family history of depression or psychiatric diagnosis
Major depression	Fatigue, sleep issues, lack of pleasure, issues with focus and thinking, guilt or inadequate feelings, weight loss or gain, suidical thoughts, personal or family history of depression or psychiatric diagnosis
Substance-induced depression	Fatique, utilization of substances, depression symptoms related to use or withdrawal of substances, personal or family history of depression or psychiatric diagnosis

TABLE 18.25 Fatigue/Lack of Energy Differential Diagnosis Related to Physical Examination of Patient

Diagnoses	Positive Physical Exam Findings That Would Support the Diagnosis
Anemia	Cool skin temperature, pallor of skin, pallor of conjunctivae, hemoccult test positive
Hypothyroid	Dry skin, thyroid nodule or enlarged thyroid, presence of thyroid bruits, slow bowel sounds, Woltman sign (a delayed relaxation phase of the deep tendon reflexes)
Multiple sclerosis	Diminished sensation, decreased coordination, issues with rapid alternating movements, hyperreflexia with deep tendon reflexes
Adjustment with depressed mood	Flat effect, normal exam
Major depression	Flat effect, normal exam
Substance-induced depression	Decrease in alertness, lack of orentation, flat effect, track marks on skin

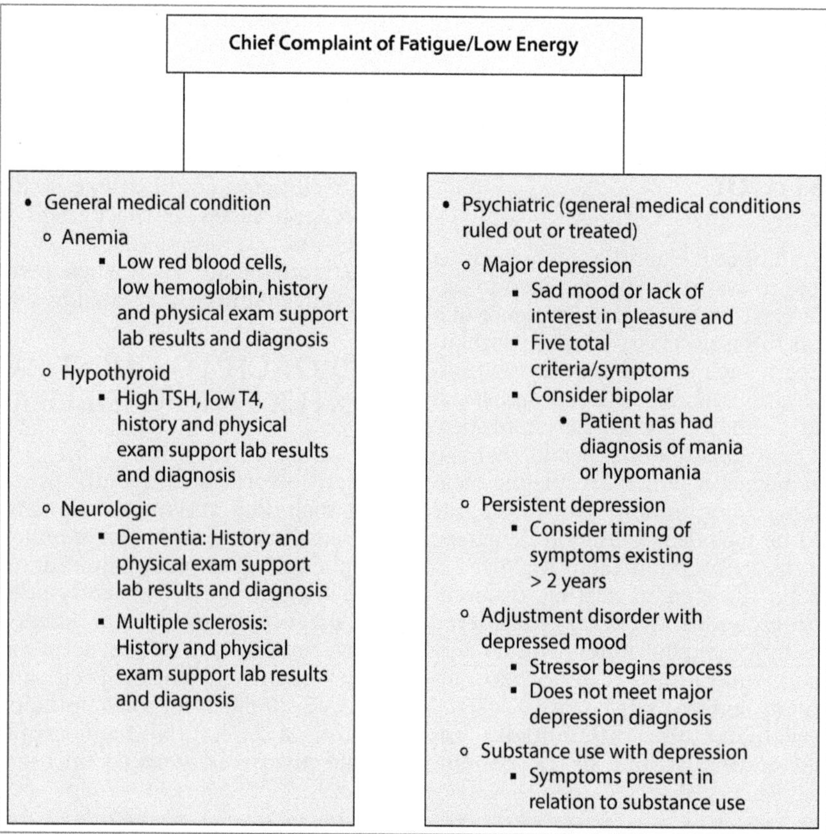

Figure 18.9 **Algorithm outlining recommended approach to fatigue/low energy as a chief complaint.** T4, thyroxine; TSH, thyroid-stimulating hormone.

TABLE 18.26 Differential Diagnosis Related to History of Patient With Chest Pain in the Context of Possible Anxiety

Diagnoses	Symptoms If Positive May Support Diagnosis
Angina	Chest pain, sharp pain, present with exertion, improves with rest
Costochondritis	Chest pain, reproducible with pressure on chest wall, history of trauma
Gastroesophageal reflux disease (GERD)	Pain in epigastric area and/or center chest, increased pain after meals, taking medication like TUMS relieves pain
Hyperthyroid	Weight loss, palpitations, heat intolerance
Generalized anxiety disorder	Worry about varity of things on most days, worry occurring >6 months, sleep issues, easy fatigue, irritable, restless
Panic attack	Chilling or hot feeling, sweating, chest pain, palpitations, nausea, choking, shortness of breath, shaking, feeling light-headed, numbness and tingling, fear of lost control and/or fear of dying
Panic disorder	Worry about the next attack or what could happen (for a month), symptoms as above related to panic attacks, more than one attack experience

anxiety is a leading differential. Anxiety-related chest pain can also mimic GI disorders such as GERD. History questions should include the presence of reflux and the relation of pain to eating or position.

Physical exam findings for anxiety will be normal but a focused physical exam remains important to rule out the presence of a general medical condition. Diagnoses that closely mimic the chest pain seen with anxiety, such as GERD and angina, will have specific physical exam findings (Table 18.27).

The physical exam evaluates the differentials, but additional lab work and testing would be of benefit in part due to cardiac risk. Hyperthyroidism can be evaluated by assessing the patient's TSH and T4. In this case, all of the blood work would be within the normal ranges. Cardiac risk could be evaluated with EKG to consider ischemia or arrhythmia. The EKG would not demonstrate ST segment elevation or depression and no arrhythmia. In addition to evaluating blood work, the patient could complete an assessment screening for anxiety like the GAD-7, but this is more for GAD, and the presentation is more consistent with panic disorder.

Refer to Figure 18.10 when considering evaluation of a symptom that can be related to anxiety.

TABLE 18.27 Differential Diagnosis Related to Physical Exam of Patient With Chest Pain in the Context of Possible Anxiety

Diagnoses	Positive Physical Exam Findings That Would Support the Diagnosis
Angina	Cool skin temperature, pallor of skin, pallor of conjunctivae, hemoccult test positive
Costochondritis	Pain with palpation of chest
Gastroesophageal reflux disease (GERD)	Pain with palpation in epigastric region
Hyperthyroid	Thyroid nodule or enlarged thyroid, presence of thyroid bruits, tachycardia, positive lid lag
Generalized anxiety disorder	Anxious/stressed mood, normal exam
Panic attack	Anxious/stressed mood, normal exam
Panic disorder	Anxious/stressed mood, normal exam

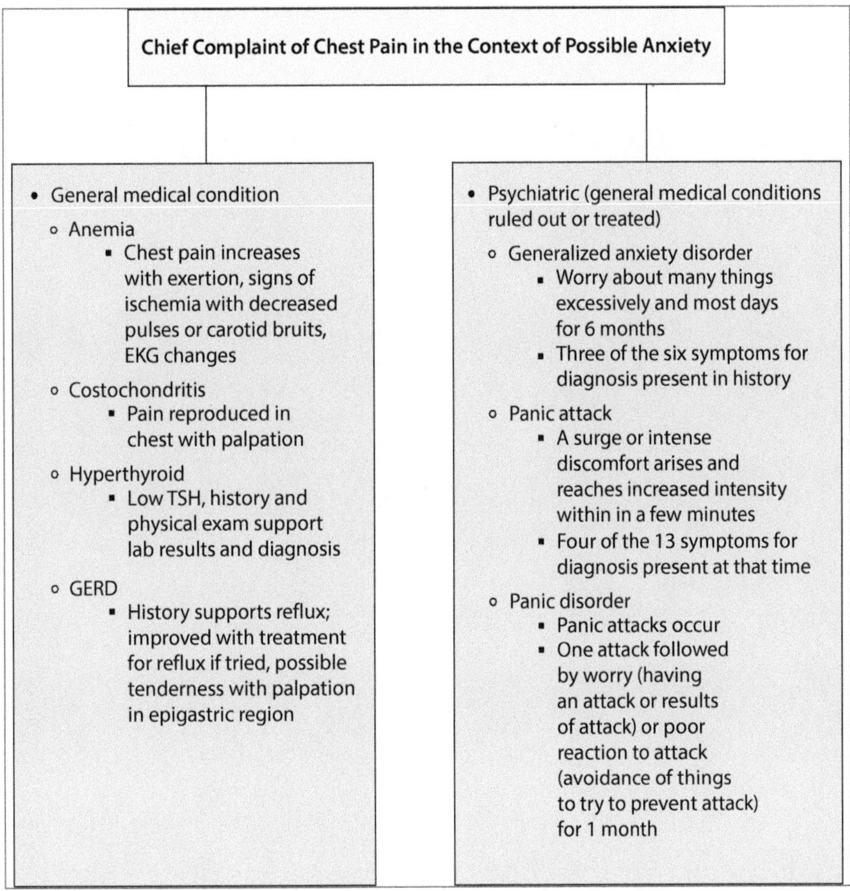

Figure 18.10 **Algorithm outlining recommended approach to chest pain as a chief complaint in the context of possible anxiety.** GERD, gastroesophageal reflux disease; TSH, thyroid-stimulating hormone.

KNOWLEDGE CHECKS

1. Discuss three medications that can be used in the treatment of opioid use disorder and the possible symptoms associated with opiate withdrawal.
2. Personality disorders are commonly divided into three clusters (A, B and C). Name the disorders in each cluster and the prototypical presentation for each disorder.
3. Complete a chart with the mechanisms of action and common side effects of the following antidepressant medication classes: SSRI, SNRI, TCA, MAOI.

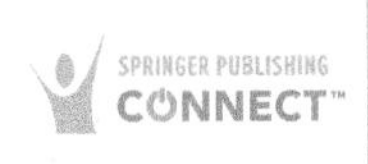

A robust set of instructor resources designed to supplement this text is located at **https://connect.springerpub.com/content/book/978-0-8261-8243-2.** Qualifying instructors may request access by emailing **textbook@springerpub.com.**

REFERENCES

The complete reference list for this chapter appears in the digital version of the chapter, accessible at https://connect.springerpub.com/content/book/978-0-8261-8243-2/chapter/ch18.

CHAPTER 19

CARE OF THE SEXUAL AND GENDER MINORITY PATIENT

DIANE BRUESSOW, JONATHAN BAKER, AND LAUREN EISENBEIS

LEARNING OBJECTIVES

1. Demonstrate the use of terminology and scientific constructs associated with sexual and gender minority (SGM) health.
2. Examine factors that influence health outcomes associated with sexual and gender diversity; the form taken by sex and gender; and the psychological well-being of SGM people.
3. Practice cultural humility and cultural awareness in patient interactions regarding sexual orientation, gender identity, and gender expression.
4. Formulate a broad and comprehensive definition of sex.
5. Employ an intersectional, syndemic approach to SGM health.
6. Integrate patient assessment and clinical decision-making strategies necessary for optimal SGM patient health.

INTRODUCTION

When practicing medicine with consideration for sexual orientation, gender identity (SOGI), and gender expression (SOGIE), the clinician's primary task is to eliminate assumptions that patients are heterosexual and cisgender. Sexual attraction, behavior, and identity—the three distinct constructs that together are referred to as sexual orientation—as well as gender identity, gender expression, and sex assigned at birth, are relevant in sexual and gender minority (SGM) health. LGBT identities represent only a portion of the individuals within the SGM domain. Though not intended to be all-encompassing, this chapter emphasizes high-value science-based concepts and topic areas that are foundational to SGM health and essential for SOGIE-inclusive patient-centered clinical medicine.

19.1 SEXUAL AND GENDER MINORITY HEALTH

OVERVIEW

Awareness of patient sexual orientation, gender identity (SOGI) and assigned sex at birth (ASAB), and the unique health needs of SGM patients, is an essential component of clinical practice. This chapter summarizes science-based definitions and concepts that are foundational to delivering patient-centered clinical medical care, including key historical events associated with SGM communities and cultures, as well as themes in clinical medicine that are considered essential in the care of SGM patients.

Best practices in clinical medicine have identified four instances when awareness of patient SOGI and ASAB should occur: during the patient intake, the PA-patient clinical interaction, and tracking of health outcomes and patient satisfaction.[1] Tools exist to support these recommended practices. Electronic health records (EHRs) must contain fields to document patient SOGI to comply with criteria to certify meaningful use.[2] When these data are collected at patient intake, they may inform the clinical encounter and may be utilized to track patient health outcomes and satisfaction. Providers of patient satisfaction scores also include variables relevant to SOGI and ASAB. Additionally, the U.S. Centers for Medicare and Medicaid Services (CMS) will reduce reimbursement fees for services for which patient satisfaction scores fall below a minimum threshold.[3,4]

Concepts

It is essential for PAs to understand what is meant by each of the constructs associated with SGM health and select the appropriate term for the correct use. Science-based concepts and terminology may not align with our patient's descriptions of themselves. When communicating with patients, always use the patient's preferred language, while medical records should reflect science-based terminology and quote their preferred language. Terms such as sexual preference and lifestyle have been used to deny civil rights to SGM people and thus have a distinctly negative connotation and should be avoided when speaking with patients.

Terminology

SGM populations refer to, but are not limited to, individuals who identify as lesbian, gay, bisexual, asexual, transgender, two-spirit, queer, and intersex. Individuals with same-sex or same-gender attractions or behaviors, those with a difference in sex development, and those with nonbinary constructs of SOGI and/or sex are also included.[5]

Sexual orientation is a catch-all term used only as a demographic descriptor and conceptualized by three distinct yet interrelated constructs with incomplete concordance among them: sexual attraction, behavior, and identity (Figure 19.1).[6,7] Consistency among these constructs is essential for psychological well-being, yet inconsistency is a common occurrence.

Sexual attraction refers to a neither tangible nor observable, latent, elusive, and nonquantifiable phenomenon of sexual or romantic desire that may be incongruent with the presentation of self and self-conception.[6] In other words, sexual attraction is not a measurable, scientific construct, and it may be inconsistent with sexual behavior or sexual identity. To normalize PA-patient rapport regarding human sexual development and allow sexual minority patients to be identified, affirmed, and supported prior to the debut of sexual behavior, it is uniquely important to discuss sexual attraction with adolescent patients during clinical encounters.

Sexual behavior refers to any consensual activity or patterns of activity—solitary, between two people, or in a group—that induces sexual arousal. There is significant variation in solitary and sociosexual behavior—beyond whether one's partner is of the same or another sex or gender—to include genital (explore whether the patient is an insertive or receptive partner as appropriate) and nongenital stimulation, and atypical sexual interests.

Most people with atypical sexual interests do not have a mental disorder. According to the *Diagnostic and Statistical Manual of Mental Disorders,* 5th edition (*DSM-5*), paraphilic disorders require the individual to have (1) feelings of distress about their (sexual) interests and not merely distress resulting from society's disapproval; or (2) a sexual desire or behavior that involves another person's psychological distress, injury, or death, or a desire for sexual behaviors involving unwilling persons or persons unable to consent.[8]

Sexual identity describes a conscious understanding of self and is akin to racial identity as both are influenced by society. Sexual identity is the appropriate construct for monitoring health disparities such as healthcare access, utilization, outcomes, and patient satisfaction, and may be included in patient intake forms. Sexual identity is often incorrectly conflated with sexual orientation.

Gender diversity is the expression of gender characteristics, including identities, that are not stereotypically associated with ASAB (Figure 19.2).[9] It is a common and culturally diverse human phenomenon that should not be judged as inherently pathologic or negative and is not in itself a mental disorder.[8,9] Gender diverse patients may feel that they have to choose between the psychological anguish of an inconsistent personal narrative resulting from hiding their gender identity, instead "performing" their socially expected gender role or the risk of discrimination and violence.[10–12]

Assigned sex at birth (ASAB) is based on phenotype. In the United States, newborns are either assigned male at birth (AMAB) or assigned female at birth (AFAB). Because it is possible to change sex markers on identity documents, including birth certificates, ASAB and legal sex may be different.

Gender identity describes a conscious understanding of self and is akin to racial identity as both are influenced by society. Self-awareness can occur at any age, although most gender diverse adults knew their gender identity was something other than their ASAB before puberty.[11,12] Concordance between gender identity and ASAB is described as cisgender, while transgender describes discordance. In the United States, gender identity is thought of in the binary male and female. However, in other countries and cultures, gender identity is recognized as bimodal, like a curve with two peaks, which accounts for the one-third of nonbinary transgender adults whose gender identity falls between the two peaks and whose gender identity is neither entirely male nor entirely female.[11] Gender markers that are recognized on official identity documents other than M/F may include X, T, I, E, O, or a blank.

Gender expression is separate and distinct from gender identity. It is vital to differentiate whether a patient's discordance is between their ASAB and gender identity or gender expression.[13] For example, a cisgender gay male patient may have a feminine gender expression and a gender identity that is solidly male has different healthcare needs than a patient with a female gender identity who was AMAB.[8]

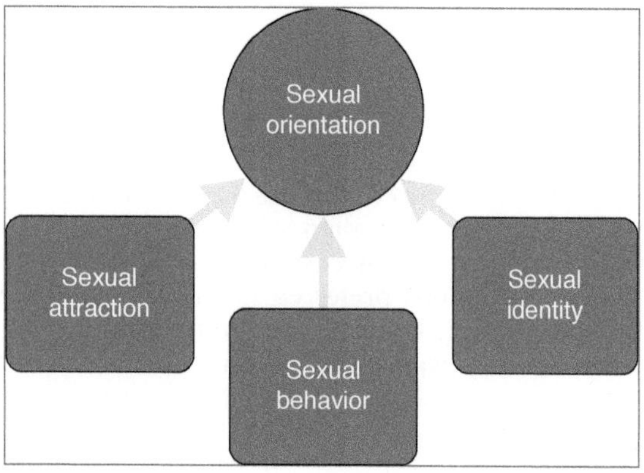

Sexual orientation
Sexual attraction
Sexual identity
Sexual behavior

Figure 19.1 **Sexual orientation is used as a demographic descriptor and conceptualized in terms of three distinct constructs: sexual attraction, sexual behavior, and sexual identity.**

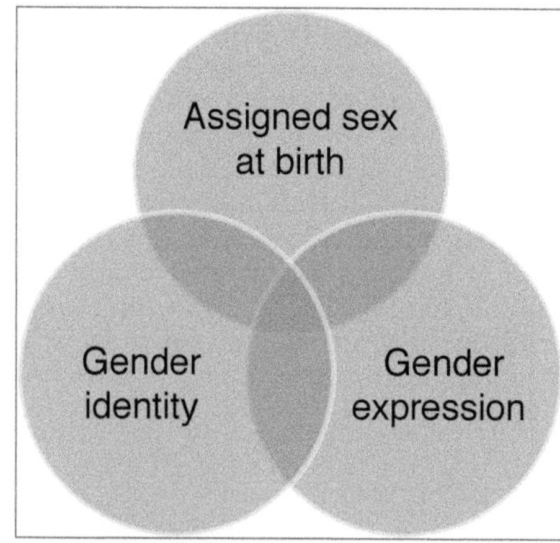

Figure 19.2 **Gender diversity.**

EPIDEMIOLOGY

Sexual Minority

As of 2020, 10.3 million U.S. adults identify as lesbian, gay, or bisexual (LGB).[14] However, significantly greater numbers of U.S. adults report same-sex attraction and behavior (19% [13.4% to 25.1%] of women and 7.9% [3.6% to 11.4%] of men report same-sex sexual attraction, and 17.4% [10.9% to 25%] of women and 6.2% [3.7% to 7.5%] of men report same-sex sexual behavior).[15] Adolescents are more heterogeneous in their definition and experience of their sexual attraction, behavior, and identity. Up to 20% of adolescent girls and 6% of adolescent boys report sexual minority identity as well as behavior. In addition, 66% of straight-identified girls and 10% of straight-identified boys report same-sex behavior.[16]

Gender Minority

In 2020 1.4 million, or 0.6% (0.3% to 0.8%, 2.77% in the District of Columbia), of U.S. adults, reported a gender identity that is something other than their ASAB.[14] An additional 149,750 or 0.73% (0.39% to 1.12%) of adolescents age 13 to 17 years have a gender identity other than their ASAB.[17] The socially restrictive environment within the United States may contribute to underreporting, whereas within more permissive environments, prevalence is reported closer to 4%.[18,19] Although the majority of transgender individuals identify as a male or female, in a survey (n = 27,715) of transgender adults across the United States, 31% identified as nonbinary. In addition, over 500 gender identities were captured, including culturally specific identities like aggressive (A) within the Black and African American community representing people AFAB with a masculine but not male gender identity, and travesti, fa'afafine, or mahu among South American, Samoan, or Hawaiian gender minority individuals, respectively.[11]

Context for Sexual and Gender Minority Health Status in the United States

To provide patient-centered clinical medical care to SGM patients across all ages, races, and ethnicities, religions, and social classes require a cultural and historical awareness of the factors that influence SGM communities within the United States (Exhibit 19.1).[20]

In the United States in 1957, homosexuality was criminalized, considered a sign of mental illness by the American Psychiatric Association (APA), and "treatments" of electroconvulsive, psychopharmacologic, and aversion therapies were standard practice. The same year, Dr. Evelyn Hooker's research on a small convenience sample of straight and gay men was published in which no psychological differences were identified in blind comparisons using standardized psychological tests.[21] This resulted in a widespread and incorrect assumption that sexual minorities experienced few psychological health disparities. The APA's removal of homosexuality from the *DSM* did not occur until 1973, preceding the initial decriminalization of homosexuality in the United States. However, it wasn't until researchers— who were themselves gay and lesbian-identified—collected data from the first general health surveys of sexual minorities in 1984–1985 for the National Lesbian Health Care Survey and 1996–1997 for the Urban Men's Health Study that a different picture began to emerge.[22] The data reflected high rates of intimate partner violence, very high rates of alcohol and other substance use, very high rates of depression and distress, very high rates of suicide attempts, and very high rates of HIV infection.[23–27]

EXHIBIT 19.1 Sexual and Gender Minority Aging

Sexual minority elders are a uniquely vulnerable population. Seniors who were alive during the era before depatholigization and decriminalization experienced a lifetime of discrimination and may bear the psychological scars of being institutionalized, living with a criminal record, or knowing others who were. The resulting distrust of medical and mental health professionals is among the many factors that contribute to delays in accessing care for disease prevention and early detection, leading to increased morbidity and mortality from later-stage diagnoses. Sexual and gender minority seniors are less likely to have spouses and children and may rely on families "of choice" comprising close friends and LGBT community-based organizations where they are available. Older adults who are dependent upon caregiving provided by assisted living, home health, or hospice staff are forced to choose between living authentically and disclosing their sexual attraction, behavior and identity, or in secrecy out of fear that they will be denied services or that they will experience verbal or physical abuse.

Source: Data from Choi SK, Meyer IH. *LGBT Aging: A Review of Research Findings, Needs, and Policy Implications.* The Williams Institute; 2016.

The initial body of health research on sexual minorities was mostly ignored by federal public health agencies. It wasn't until a meeting between lesbian health researchers and then-Secretary of the U.S. Department of Health and Human Services in 1993 that federal initiatives inclusive of sexual minorities were first initiated.[28] The research that followed had the effect of identifying additional disparities in health insurance coverage, access to quality health services, having a usual source of care, cancer, immunization, and infectious diseases, nutrition and weight, and public health infrastructure inclusion.[29,30] A research agenda was identified to advance understanding of sexual minority health through population-based data collection, methodologic research, research training, and policy on research participation.[7,29,31] In 2015, the National Institute of Health (NIH) established the SGM Research Office (SGMRO) to coordinate SGM-related research and activities by working directly with the NIH Institutes, Centers, and Offices.

Although many cultures have long recognized the variations within gender diversity, in 2010, the World Professional Association for Transgender Health (WPATH) was the first professional organization to consider the expression of gender characteristics, including identities, that are not typically associated with one's ASAB to be a common human phenomenon that occurs across all cultures and should not be judged as inherently pathologic or negative.[32] For context, other common, culturally diverse, and nonpathologic phenomena are homosexuality and left-handedness. It was not until 2013 that gender diversity was depathologized by the APA within their *DSM-5* stating "gender nonconformity is not in itself a mental disorder."[8,33] In 2018, the World Health Organization (WHO) sought to further depathologize gender diversity akin to how homosexuality and left-handedness are no longer considered a mental illness, introducing the term gender incongruence to the *International Statistical Classification of Diseases and Related Health Problems (ICD-11)*, and removing it from the mental health section of the publication.[34] Both the APA and WHO intentionally sought to maintain access to pharmacologic and nonpharmacologic interventions to resolve gender incongruence.[9]

Risk Factors

The higher prevalence of unhealthy behaviors and internalized disorders, including depression and anxiety experienced by SGM individuals noted above, is associated with a lack of affirmation or a consistent and stable personal narrative coherent with identity.[11,35–37] In other words, in individuals with an inconsistent personal narrative, for example, whose straight sexual identity is incongruent with their same-sex sexual attraction or behavior, a higher risk of multiple negative health outcomes is shown than in patients with a congruent lesbian, gay or bisexual identity and behavior.[10] Similar data exist regarding affirmed versus unaffirmed gender identity. Gender incongruent children who are affirmed in their gender in all domains (e.g., home, school, community) had have been shown to have developmentally normative levels of depression when compared with cisgender control subjects.[37] A lack of family acceptance results in up to eight times higher rates of suicidal behavior, substance use, and other unhealthy behaviors. Long-term negative psychosocial outcomes appear to result from a lack of affirmation in key developmental areas.[38]

Intersectionality and Syndemics

The SGM population in the United States is not homogeneous, thus approaching SGM patients with an intersectional lens is advised, considering all the factors that apply to an individual concurrently, rather than in isolation. A more advanced method would be to consider a syndemic approach. Unlike comorbid conditions, syndemic conditions describe the synergy between co-occurring epidemics experienced within a community. One illustration would be the syndemic relationship between depression and substance abuse among sexual minority men, or the disproportionate rates of new HIV infection among young, Black sexual minority men age 13 to 24 years, which are amplified by comorbidities of societal racism, sexism, and homophobia.[39,40]

Comprehensive Sexual History

A comprehensive sexual history will extend beyond reproductive health and sexually transmitted infection (STI) risk assessment, including sexual satisfaction and function. The U.S. Centers for Disease Control and Prevention (CDC)'s 5 "Ps" of sexual health, representing partners, practices, protection from STIs, past history of STIs, and pregnancy prevention, may be adapted to a more comprehensive 6 Ps to include pleasure, and performance.[19] A SGM-inclusive sexual history would replace questions like "do you have sex with men, women, or both?" with "what genders are your sexual partners?" and use gender-neutral anatomic terms such as genitals.

Areas for consideration during an SGM-inclusive comprehensive sexual history include a thorough reproductive history that includes the patient's interest in parenting, whether via assisted reproductive technologies, adoption or foster parenting, or other means; exploration of sexual function and dysfunction within the section representing pleasure and performance; as well as questions relevant to:

- Relationship status (considering living situations, legal rights)
- Relationship structure (i.e., monogamy, consensual non-monogamy, unilateral monogamy, polyamory)
- Sexual organ inventory of patient and their sexual partners
- Sexual organs use and sites of exposure (e.g., mouth, genitals, anus, fingers, hands, and others)
- Use and maintenance of sex toys and prosthesis
- STI risk reduction (including barriers/condoms and other methods discussed within the chapter)
- Recreational drug use associated with sex (e.g., illicit, prescription, sex-enhancement drugs, and alcohol)
- Transactional sex (e.g., sex for money, drugs, or housing)
- History of sexual abuse (particularly important to be aware of before physical examination)
- Safety during sex and within relationships[41]

Adequate information to understand our patients' sexual behaviors and associated healthcare needs should be obtained. Approaching patients without judgment and preconceptions is necessary. Sexual histories should be conversational, and as a patient reveals aspects of their sexual behaviors, a skilled clinician will build on that information. Consider that individuals who receive a fist into their anus during sex are at the highest sexual risk for acquiring hepatitis C. This complicated and potentially fatal disease often goes undetected for decades. Although exploring if patients engage in "anal fisting" without barrier protection seems like a radical and daunting task, a skilled clinician can obtain this information. It is unnecessary to ask every patient about anal fisting. However, it is relevant for PAs to develop the necessary skills required to decipher when more details are essential for a complete sexual history.

WHEN AND HOW TO ASK ABOUT SOGI

PAs should approach each patient with cultural humility.[1] Misgendering or deadnaming (using the name associated with the patient's ASAB rather than the name associated with the patient's gender identity) a gender diverse patient is not conducive to building PA-patient rapport or to the patient's psychological well-being as it can exacerbate gender dysphoria and trigger a reactive depression.[42] Many EHRs include fields for gender identity, ASAB, and preferred name, making it easier to know what name and pronouns the patient uses, their gender identity, and ASAB. However, research suggests PAs are unaware that this information may have been collected from the patient during intake.[43] In addition, poor EHR design places this information within the administrative pages along with demographics such as race and ethnicity instead of making it visible within the PA's workflow. Among PAs with experience working with SGM populations, some initiate their clinical encounters by concluding their introduction to the new patient with the question, "how would you like me to address you?"[44]

When working with pediatric populations, keep in mind that gender identity is understood by age 4. Retrospective studies of transgender adults find most were aware of their gender identity before puberty.[11] Young gender diverse patients benefit from a safe and nonjudgmental clinical environment and the opportunity to disclose their gender identity, specifically, whether they are a girl, a boy, both, neither, something else or allowing them to report they don't know. At puberty, sexual attraction may begin to be explored in a developmentally appropriate manner (i.e., "are you attracted to boys, girls, both, neither, or you don't know?") so that sexual minority adolescents can be identified, affirmed, and supported with appropriate preventive care and counseling.

When initiating a patient history pertaining to sex, always state why your patient's answers are pertinent to their healthcare and how their responses will be kept confidential and private. Be nonjudgmental, sensitive, and matter of fact. Consider what you are communicating nonverbally as well as verbally and avoid assumptions. Asking "are you sexually active" is often misunderstood. Oral and anal sex are not considered sexual activity among some adolescents and SGM patients who interpret the question to apply exclusively to penile-vaginal intercourse or coitus. Instead, ask open-ended questions and allow for answers other than those you might expect. Asking patients about their sexual behavior depends on whether the objective pertains to reproductive health, STI screening, sexual satisfaction, and function.

When exploring patient sexual identity, the CDC recommends three principles: do not to use labels that patients don't understand, such as homosexual and heterosexual, which may confuse people; use the labels that patients use to refer to themselves, like straight, gay, lesbian, and bisexual, which are better understood; and use follow-up questions to best categorize other responses.[6]

19.2 SPECIAL CONSIDERATIONS IN SEXUAL MINORITY HEALTH

19.2A SEXUAL MINORITY MEN AND MEN WHO HAVE SEX WITH MEN

The term men who have sex with men (MSM) has been used in the epidemiologic evaluation of a heterogeneous population that includes women and nonbinary individuals who were AMAB while often excluded sexual minority men and nonbinary individuals who were AFAB. When reviewing this section of the chapter, please keep in mind that the MSM classification obscures nuance pertaining to differences in sexual identity, sexual behaviors, and gender identity. This section will present data and recommendations related to behavior primarily but not exclusively associated with MSM, with the intent to consider how these data and guidelines can be applied to a diverse patient population that is inclusive of cisgender and heterosexual patients, as well as SGM.

SEXUAL BEHAVIORS

Many of the healthcare needs of MSM discussed in this chapter pertain to sexual activity involving the anus; however, it is essential to note that not all gay or bisexual-identified men engage in any or all of these behaviors (Table 19.1). For example, a gay-identified man AMAB may not engage in any sexual activity. Individuals may engage in nonpenetrative sexual behaviors or limit sexual behavior to the mouth and genitals (i.e., oral sex).

It is also important to note that straight-identified individuals often engage in sexual behaviors involving the anus. About a third of straight-identified individuals admit to engaging in anal sex, and barrier protection use rates are low (reportedly 20% to 30%). Straight-identified individuals commonly perceive barrier protection as pregnancy prevention rather than HIV/STI prevention, while lacking attention to the potential HIV/STI transmission risks from sexual behaviors involving the anus.[45]

TABLE 19.1 Sexual Behaviors of Men Who Have Sex With Men

Abbreviation	Medical Terminology	Lay Patient Language	Description
AI CLAI	Anal sex/ intercourse (condomless AI)	Anal sex Bareback	Sexual behavior involving the anus, typically penile insertive-anal receptive
RAI	Receptive anal sex/intercourse	Bottoming	Referring to the anal-receptive partner in anal sex
IAI	Insertive anal sex/intercourse	Topping	Referring to the penile-insertive partner in anal sex
–	Anilingus/ anal-oral sex/ intercourse	Rimming	Oral sex applied to the anus

PREVENTIVE MEDICINE AND EARLY DETECTION

Hepatitis Immunization

Hepatitis A virus (HAV) is transmitted through oral-fecal exposure, so individuals engaging in sexual behaviors involving the anus—especially oral-anal sex or anilingus—are at risk of acquiring the virus. HAV vaccination is recommended for all sexual minority men. Hepatitis B virus (HBV) is most commonly spread through sexual exposure. All patients without contraindication should be vaccinated for HBV. Consider obtaining titers to ensure immunity for all patients at increased risk, including sexual minority men. Among adults in the United States, MSM account for approximately 10% of HAV cases and 20% of cases of HBV infection.[46]

Human Papillomavirus

Human papillomavirus (HPV) infection of the anus can result in the development of condyloma acuminatum (anogenital warts), precancerous lesions, and persistent anal infection with oncogenic HPV may result in squamous cell carcinoma (SCC). While HPV-related SCC of the anus is rare in the general population, rates among MSM are reported around 40 cases per 100,000, similar to rates of colorectal and lung cancer in the general population.[47] HIV infection is another independent risk factor of anal SSC. MSM living with HIV infection have anal cancer rates reported as high as 140 cases per 100,000, rates higher than any cancer rate in the general population, including breast cancer.[47,48] Anal cancer is most commonly caused by HPV strains 16 and 18, which also cause the majority of HPV-related cancers of the cervix, head, and neck. Routine HPV vaccination is recommended for any individuals without contraindication through 26 years of age. Catch-up vaccination should be considered through age 45 if routine vaccination opportunities were missed. Populations most likely to benefit from catch-up vaccination include populations at increased risk such as MSM and any individuals engaging in sexual behaviors that transmit HPV.[49]

Anal Cytology and HPV Screening

Anal cytology can be used to screen for anal HPV related lesions. The test can be highly sensitive but has significantly lower specificity than cytologic screening for cervical cancer.[50] It does not require special equipment or training. A polyester tipped Dacron swab is moistened and then blindly inserted into the anal canal. Lateral pressure is applied in a circular motion while withdrawing the swab over 10 seconds. The swab is then vigorously agitated into a liquid-based cytology medium (the same medium used for cervical cytology) to dislodge the collected cells. The cytologic sample is evaluated using the Bethesda Criteria and reported like cervical cytology (i.e., benign, ASCUS, LSIL, ASC-H, HSIL).[51] HPV testing can be utilized to help improve the accuracy of the test.[52] At the time of publication, U.S. Preventive Services Task Force and CDC guidelines lack recommendations on cytologic screening and diagnosis of precancerous anal lesions.

All abnormal results from anal cytology should be followed with high-resolution anoscopy (HRA).[50] HRA is analogous to colposcopy and allows for visual detection of high-grade squamous intraepithelial lesions (HSIL). These lesions can be treated with topical therapies (e.g., imiquimod, 5-fluorouracil) or destructive therapies (surgery, electrocautery) while recognizing that recurrence is common.[51–53] Most precancerous lesions cannot be assessed by the naked eye, and only individuals with specific training in HRA should screen for, assess, and manage anal HSIL. In regions where HRA is not available, patients at high risk for anal cancer should be offered a quality digital anorectal exam (DARE) at least annually, and anorectal symptoms consistent with anal cancer (mass, pain, bleeding, discharge, itch) should be thoroughly evaluated.[54]

Populations at risk for anal dysplasia and subsequent development of anal cancer include:

- Individuals living with HIV
- Sexual minority men
- Individuals with iatrogenic immunosuppression (e.g., transplant recipients and individuals on immunosuppressive medication)
- Individuals with a history of other HPV-related disease (e.g., cervical/vaginal/vulvar dysplasia or cancer)[48]

HIV Burden

MSM account for about two-thirds of HIV diagnoses in the United States. Certain subpopulations, including young (25 to 34 years of age) Black and Brown MSM and MSM living in the South, are disproportionately affected.[55–57] Anal sex carries a higher risk of HIV transmission than oral or vaginal sex. Receptive anal intercourse (RAI) is up to 20 times more likely to transmit HIV than receptive vaginal sex. Insertive anal intercourse (IAI) also carries a higher risk of HIV acquisition than insertive or receptive vaginal sex.[58]

Antiretroviral (ARV) therapy effectively allows HIV to be managed similarly to other chronic diseases. ARV therapy suppresses viral load below the level of detection in a commercial laboratory setting (called undetectable viral load, or UVL). It is colloquially referred to as "U equals U" (U = U), meaning undetectable equals untransmittable because patients with an UVL do not transmit HIV to sexual partners. The persistence of an UVL reduces many of the comorbidities of HIV, including opportunistic infections.[59,60] The side effect profiles of ARVs are favorable to previously recommended pharmacologic regimens. Commercially available, fixed-dose, combination drugs containing multiple ARVs allow patients to suppress viral load with one tablet daily.

HIV, even when virally suppressed, causes chronic immune activation, dysfunction, and inflammation. These processes have shifted the cancer spectrum of people living with HIV from AIDS-defining cancers (e.g., Kaposi sarcoma and non-Hodgkin lymphoma) to non-AIDS-defining cancers (NADC), which are correlated with HIV infection but have increased rates among immunocompetent individuals living with HIV.[61,62] NADCs include Hodgkin lymphoma and cancers of the mouth, throat, liver, lung, and anus. In addition to HIV infection, factors including age, other viral infections (e.g., HPV and viral hepatitis), and other behavioral factors (e.g., alcohol or tobacco use) may increase the risk of developing NADCs. Although the medical management of HIV is similar to other chronic diseases, HIV infection continues to carry a greater burden of stigma. HIV transmission criminalization has been inconsistent with the scientific knowledge of HIV transmission for decades, and healthy sexual relationships can be especially difficult for people living with HIV.[63]

HIV Prevention

HIV prevention has evolved significantly. ARV medications, including daily emtricitabine/tenofovir-based regimens, are recommended for preexposure prophylaxis (PrEP) for certain indications (Box 19.1).[64–66] Injectable, implantable, and non-ARV-based regimens are under development. Daily oral emtricitabine/tenofovir disoproxil fumarate (F/TDF) was the first drug approved and recommended for PrEP and has demonstrated a 92% to 100% risk reduction for acquiring HIV.[67] A notable dosing caveat pertains to patients AMAB who are concurrently receiving feminizing hormone therapy (FHT). PrEP should be offered at once-daily dosing regimens while avoiding PrEP dosing regimens of less than continuous, daily frequency (such as on-demand or 2-1-1 PrEP dosing), as concurrent estradiol results in diminished serum PrEP levels similar to taking only 4 of 7 daily pills.[68]

Emtricitabine/tenofovir alafenamide (F/TAF) was approved after demonstrating similar effectiveness to F/TDF for reducing HIV transmission resulting from sexual behaviors involving the anus.[69] F/TAF is approved exclusively for individuals at risk of sexually transmitted HIV acquisition, and specifically excluding vaginal intercourse or intravenous drug use as it has not been adequately tested in this context.

Both F/TDF and F/TAF contain emtricitabine in a fixed combination with a prodrug of tenofovir-diphosphate (TFV-DP), the active drug that prevents HIV acquisition. Individual genetic differences result in different pharmacodynamics, pharmacokinetics, side effects, and adverse event profiles.[64,70]

HIV epidemiologic data and clinical research on PrEP often fail to address sexual and gender diversity. The literature particularly lacks robust data on gender diverse individuals who were AFAB. Regardless of SOGIE, the following risk factors for sexual transmission of HIV should be considered in all patients[41]:

- Residing in areas of high HIV incidence[55,65,66]
- Not using barrier protection consistently (unwilling, unable, or have barriers to negotiating use with partners)[55,65,66]
- Recent diagnosis of a bacterial STI[55,65,66,71]
- Engaging in anal sex[55,58,65,66]
- Engaging in transactional sex (i.e., sex for money, drugs, or housing)[55,65,66]
- Having sexual partners who are at high risk for unsuppressed HIV (i.e., partners with social and institutional barriers to HIV testing and treatment)[55,65,66]

BOX 19.1 Indications for Preexposure Prophylaxis

Sexually Active Sexual Minority Men, AMAB
A sexual relationship with a partner living with HIV
Multiple sex partners
AI with inconsistent condom use
STI with syphilis, gonorrhea, or chlamydia in the past 6 months
Commercial sex work
All Other Sexually Active Adolescents and Adults
A sexual relationship with a partner living with HIV
Multiple sex partners
History of inconsistent or no condom use
Commercial sex work
High HIV prevalence area or network
Intravenous Drug Users
HIV positive injecting partner
Sharing any injection equipment
Risk of sexual acquisition
Sexually and Gender Diverse Persons
The CDC recommends considering PrEP in all persons at risk of sexually acquiring HIV. Studies have been underpowered women and nonbinary individuals who were AMAB and have largely excluded men and nonbinary individuals assigned female at birth. At the time of publication, an exception pertains to the studies that support the FDA approval of emtricitabine/tenofovir alafenamide (F/TAF) in women AMAB.

AI, anal intercourse; AMAB, assigned male at birth; CDC, Centers for Disease Control and Prevention; FDA, Food and Drug Administration; PrEP, preexposure prophylaxis; STI, sexually transmitted infection.

Source: This chart is adapted from Descovy [package insert]. Gilead Sciences; December 2019. https://www.accessdata.fda.gov/drugsatfda_docs/label/2019/208215s012lbl.pdf; Owens DK, Davidson KW, Krist AH, et al. Preexposure prophylaxis for the prevention of HIV infection: U.S. Preventive Services Task Force Recommendation Statement. JAMA. *2019;321(22):2203–2213. doi:10.1001/jama.2019.6390; Smith DK, Van Handel M, Wolitski RJ, et al. Vital signs: estimated percentages and numbers of adults with indications for preexposure prophylaxis to prevent HIV acquisition—United States, 2015.* MMWR Morb Mortal Wkly Rep. *2015;64(46):1291–1295. doi:10.15585/mmwr.mm6446a4*

- Having more than one sexual partner[55,65,66]
- Individuals with partners with more than one sexual partner[55,65,66]

Patients must be tested for HIV before starting PrEP and regularly (quarterly in most cases) while taking PrEP. In the rare case of HIV seroconversion during PrEP use, PrEP dosing is inadequate to suppress HIV viral replication. It may result in the selection of resistant HIV, limiting future treatment options.

Renal function should be tested before and during PrEP. F/TDF can cause a reduction in glomerular filtration rate (GFR) and can rarely lead to renal failure. F/TAF should be considered in patients with preexisting renal disease.

F/TDF and F/TAF have anti-HBV activity. Patients should be tested for HBV infection and immunity at the time of PrEP initiation and should be vaccinated if lacking adequate immunity. If PrEP is discontinued in a patient with active HBV, appropriate HBV therapy must be considered to prevent viral rebound, which can progress to fulminant hepatic failure.[72] Three-site STI screening (oropharyngeal, genital, and rectal) should be considered based on sexual behavior. Increases in behavioral risk (i.e., increased number of sexual partners or increased frequency of sexual behaviors without barrier protection) is not an indication to withhold PrEP.[67,73,74]

HIV Risk Reduction

A risk reduction model allows patients to enjoy sex while reducing the risk of HIV transmission. The most effective risk reduction strategies are ARV-based PrEP and viral suppression of individuals living with HIV.[75] These strategies can and should be used in combination with others. Condoms are inexpensive and widely available but can reduce sexual enjoyment and can fail. Consistent condom use reduces the risk of HIV transmission by about 80%, but inconsistent condom use has little or no effect.[76] Withdrawal before ejaculation reduces exposure to infectious body fluids but does not eliminate it.[77] Mutual masturbation and nonpenetrative sex can be enjoyed without the risk of HIV transmission but often lead to penetrative sex. Nonoccupational postexposure prophylaxis (nPEP) using ARVs after potential exposure to HIV has limited efficacy data. It may help reduce the risk of seroconversion when initiated as soon as possible following HIV exposure.[78] STIs, especially herpes simplex virus (HSV), increase rates of HIV acquisition as inflammation recruits HIV target cells, and ulceration allows an ideal pathway for HIV infection.[79] Mixed data have been published on safer-sex counseling; a large randomized, clinical trial demonstrated that risk-reduction counseling by skilled counselors was unable to change individuals' sexual behaviors.[80]

SEXUALLY TRANSMITTED INFECTIONS

MSM are disproportionately affected by bacterial and viral STIs, including, but not limited to, infections with *Neisseria gonorrhoeae* (gonorrhea), *Chlamydia trachomatis*, and *Treponema pallidum* (syphilis). Obtaining an appropriately detailed sexual history is vital to genital and extragenital prevention, screening for, diagnosing, and treating STIs.

Gonorrhea and Chlamydia

Gonorrhea and chlamydia infections commonly affect the genitals, oropharynx, and rectum. These infections are localized, meaning each site must be tested based on its unique potential as a route of exposure. Positive rates of rectal bacterial STIs (gonorrhea and chlamydia) among MSM at STI clinics are reported around 10% to 25%. Rectal and oropharyngeal infections are frequently asymptomatic, so it is important that PAs follow screening guidelines, especially among MSM who may require more frequent screening. Rectal infections are most commonly asymptomatic but may cause proctitis symptoms, including bleeding, mucopurulent discharge, pain, and tenesmus (spasm). Extragenital testing for gonorrhea and chlamydia infection should be performed with polymerase chain reaction (PCR) based methods, which are significantly more sensitive and specific than traditional culture. Treatment guidelines must be followed to reduce bacterial resistance, which is increasingly recognized, especially among gonorrhea strains.[81]

Lymphogranuloma Venerum

Lymphogranuloma venerum (LGV) is a serovar of chlamydia and is predominantly recognized among MSM and people living with HIV. LGV is characterized by chlamydia infection with associated anogenital ulceration, inguinal lymphadenopathy, and proctitis, although a quarter of infections may be asymptomatic. Without a commercially available test specific for LGV, this diagnosis is clinically based on a positive chlamydia test in the context of a patient presentation consistent with LGV symptoms or failure of response to appropriate antibiotic treatment for uncomplicated chlamydia infection. Antibiotic treatment regimens for LGV are similar to those that treat chlamydia but are of longer duration.[82]

Syphilis

MSM account for most primary and secondary syphilis cases reported in the United States. It. is clinically important to determine a patient's most recent testing details (date and type of test), which testing methodology is appropriate, and how to interpret results. Treponemal testing detects antibodies specific to *T. pallidum*. This test remains positive after treatment, limiting utility in patients with prior infection and in populations with high baseline prevalence. Nontreponemal testing, such as the rapid plasma reagin (RPR) test, is not specific for *T. pallidum* but is used to detect reinfection and monitor response to treatment. False elevations in RPR titers have several causes, which include other STIs.[83]

Hepatitis C Virus

Sexual transmission of hepatitis C virus (HCV) is increasingly recognized among individuals engaging in RAI, especially among MSM living with HIV or using PrEP. RAI can cause trauma to the anorectal mucosa and inserted genitals or hands, allowing transmission of this bloodborne pathogen.[84] Anal fisting (the insertion of the hand into the anorectum) is particularly traumatic and is the riskiest sexual behavior for the transmission of HCV. Barrier protection (e.g., condoms and gloves) reduces the risk of sexual transmission of HCV. Individuals engaging in anal fisting should be educated on the risk, how to protect themselves, and regularly tested for HCV.[85] HCV reinfection is common in high-risk populations. PCR-based viral load testing can be used to check for reinfection once an individual is antibody positive.[86]

Sexually Transmissible Enteric Infections

Sexually transmissible enteric infections (STEIs), including *Giardia lamblia, Entamoeba histolytica*, and *Shigella* species, can be transmitted through anal sex, especially oral-anal sex. STEIs range from asymptomatic to causing a constellation of gastrointestinal symptoms such as diarrhea, bloating, and abdominal pain/cramping. Asymptomatic STEIs may go undetected while shedding occurs, perpetuating the spread of infection. Screening with stool samples is cumbersome for patients and clinicians; PCR-based testing is preferred. There are no routine screening recommendations; however, these infections should be considered within the differential diagnosis for the symptomatic patient with risk of sexual exposure.[87–89]

19.3 SPECIAL CONSIDERATIONS IN GENDER MINORITY HEALTH

This section presents recommendations pertaining to the clinical care of gender diverse patients after medical and surgical interventions. Quality of life is improved when distress is reduced, and function is improved through medically necessary and effective therapeutic interventions that improve congruence with gender identity (Table 19.2). Although considered primary care, criteria and dosing for feminizing and masculinizing hormone therapy (MHT) are beyond this chapter's scope.[9]

TABLE 19.2 Common Gender Affirming Medically Necessary and Effective Approaches

	Examples	Ages	Reversibility	Medical
Social transition	Gender-affirming hairstyles, clothing, name, gender pronouns, restrooms, etc.	Any	Completely reversible	No
Pubertal suppression	Gonadotropin-releasing hormone (GnRH) analogs (leuprolide/histrelin)	Tanner Stage G2/B2, not age	Completely reversible	Yes
Masculinizing/feminizing hormone therapy	Testosterone (for patients AFAB) Estradiol +/− an androgen inhibitor (for patients AMAB)	Adults, adolescents when appropriate	Partially reversible	Yes
Surgical interventions	"Top" surgeries (to create a male-typical chest shape or breast augmentation) "Bottom" surgeries (genitals or reproductive organs) Other: Facial feminization, chondrolaryngoplasty	Adults, adolescents when appropriate	Irreversible	Yes
Other interventions	Chest binding, electrolysis/laser hair removal, voice therapy, prosthetics	Varies	Varies	Sometimes
Legal transition	Changing name and gender on a birth certificate, school records, and other identity documents	Any	Reversible	Sometimes

AFAB, assigned female at birth; AMAB, assigned male at birth.

Source: Human Rights Campaign Foundation. Common steps in gender transition. In: Supporting and Caring for Transgender Children. *American Academy of Pediatrics; 2016:10. https://www.hrc.org/resources/supporting-caring-for-transgender-children*

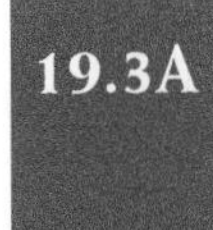

19.3A CLINICAL MEDICINE AFTER FEMINIZING/MASCULINIZING HORMONE THERAPY

The physical development of secondary sex characteristics initiated during puberty, whether triggered by endogenous or exogenous sex steroids and regardless of the age of initiation, is largely concluded after 5 years. Among patients, AFAB receiving MHT, specifically testosterone, deepening of the voice, and coarse facial and body hair are among the most noticeable secondary sex characteristics that develop. Among patients, AMAB receiving FHT, specifically estradiol with or without an antiandrogen, the most profoundly visible physical changes are breast development and a decrease in prostate and testicular size.

CANCER EARLY DETECTION

Regardless of hormone use, when a patient has an anatomic organ and has risk factors, screening according to guidelines is recommended.[90] Although guidelines do not specifically address when to initiate breast cancer screening among patients AMAB after the initiation of FHT, subject matter experts suggest following guidelines beginning 5–10 years after FHT was initiated.[90]

Studies suggest that the prevalence of breast cancer in patients AFAB on MHT, and prostate cancer in patients AMAB on FHT, are lower than among cisgender patients. However, there is not enough data to recommend whether breast and prostate cancer screening should be modified in any way. Therefore, PAs are advised to conduct an anatomic organ inventory and to follow cancer screening guideline recommendations. Among patients AFAB, in addition to the identification of androgen-sensitivity in a breast cancer case study, MHT is contraindicated in active estrogen-sensitive cancers as the liver aromatizes testosterone into estrogen. An active estrogen-sensitive cancer is an absolute contraindication to FHT.[90–93]

CLINICAL LAB VALUES

There are no specific recommendations on how to manage gendered clinical lab values. Subject matter experts will consider the total length of exposure to exogenous hormone therapy and the age at which exogenous hormone therapy was begun to inform whether natal sex, affirmed gender, or an average of the two is considered.[90]

BONE HEALTH

The risk of osteoporosis increases after gonadectomy when hormone therapy is subtherapeutic, though recommendations for screening initiation and interval are lacking. Subject matter experts propose following recommendations for agonadal or postmenopausal women.[90]

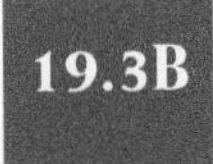

19.3B CLINICAL MEDICINE AFTER GENDER SURGERIES

Documentation in medical records should be placed under the past surgical history and identify the specific procedures (e.g., vaginoplasty, metoidioplasty with or without urethral lengthening, phalloplasty) rather than using outdated and ambiguous terms such as gender affirming surgery or sex reassignment surgery. Further, referring to a gender diverse patient in terms of their operative status (e.g., preoperative, postoperative, or nonoperative) is no longer advised.

Gender diverse patients who have undergone surgical modifications will have unique medical needs. An approach utilized in primary care practices inclusive of gender diverse patients is to solicit the anatomic organ inventory from a patient during intake to ensure each patient's unique anatomic circumstances are accounted for. By having an awareness of common surgical interventions, PAs can optimize patient satisfaction and health outcomes for their gender diverse patients.

TABLE 19.3 Facial Feminization Procedures

Procedure	Explanation
Frontal sinus setback	Contouring and flattening of the forehead to create a more feminine appearance
Orbital contouring	Reduction of the prominence of the superior orbital rims to reduce eyebrow hooding
Rhinoplasty/ septoplasty	Reshaping of the nose to create a more feminine appearance
Malar augmentation	Augmentation of the cheeks to enhance cheekbone prominence
Genioplasty	Reduction of the jaw and chin to reduce jaw width and chin projection to make a more slim and feminine face
Chondrolaryngoplasty	Reduction of the laryngeal prominence (Adam's apple)

TABLE 19.4 Facial Masculinization Procedures

Procedure	Explanation
Malar augmentation	Augmentation of the cheeks to create a more masculine appearance
Rhinoplasty/ septoplasty	Reshaping of the nose to create a more masculine appearance
Genioplasty	Augmentation of the jaw and chin to create a more prominent masculine jawline
Chondrolaryngoplasty	Creation of a laryngeal prominence (Adam's apple)

FACIAL GENDER SURGERY

The first area you look at when engaging with a new person is their face. When facial appearance is incongruent with gender identity, it can lead to misgendering resulting in the triggering of a reactive depression and other affectual disorders.[94] Facial gender surgery (FGS) allows for surgical alteration of a patient's native facial features to align with their gender identity.[95] FGS includes facial feminization surgery (FFS; Table 19.3) and facial masculinization surgery (FMS; Table 19.4). It encompasses a variety of different procedures listed below.

Postoperative care of patients undergoing FGS does not require any special considerations beyond what is consistent with other craniofacial surgeries. Patients are instructed to refrain from strenuous activity, use anti-inflammatory medications to reduce postoperative swelling, and maintain a balanced diet.

19.3C FEMINIZING AUGMENTATION MAMMOPLASTY

BACKGROUND

FHT, which may include exogenous estrogen and androgen blockers, will stimulate glandular breast tissue development. Despite this, approximately 60% to 70% of patients are unsatisfied with the degree of breast tissue present after beginning hormone therapy.[96] Feminizing augmentation mammoplasty is the placement of a silicone or saline implant to enhance breast size. This procedure allows patients to have a breast size proportional to their stature and frame. Among gender diverse patients, FHT is not a prerequisite for mammoplasty. For patients on FHT, subject matter experts recommend up to 3 years of hormone therapy to maximize hormonal breast development before mammoplasty. However, the literature has yet to recommend the ideal timing.[90]

CARING FOR PATIENTS AFTER FEMINIZING AUGMENTATION MAMMOPLASTY

Physical Examination

Breast implants can either be placed subpectorally, under the pectoralis major muscle or subglandularly, under the glandular breast tissue. When examining a patient and feeling for the breast implant's integrity, be sure to palpate around the entire circumference of the implant. If the implant placement is submuscular, ask the patient to contract their pectoralis muscles, this will allow you to see and feel the implant's location better. If the implant placement is subglandular, the implant's edges may be more palpable, and an implant ridge may be felt. Rippling or palpability of an implant is more common in thinner patients with less breast tissue.[97]

Most breast implants come in two forms: saline and silicone. Saline implants are filled with saline liquid, and the fluid inside can usually be easily palpated (Figure 19.3). In comparison, silicone implants are firmer to the touch and less pliable.[98]

Implant Care

It is important that patients know the type of implant they have when undergoing periodic surveillance screenings. Routine maintenance of silicone implants, per the U.S. Food and Drug Administration (FDA), recommends screening via MRI 3 years after the initial surgery and every 2 years thereafter.[99] If a patient has concern for a ruptured implant, such as sudden trauma to the chest, a saline implant will immediately deflate. In comparison, an MRI without contrast is required to determine if any trauma caused a tear or rupture of a silicone implant. It is important to remind patients that implants are not guaranteed to last forever, typically they last 5–20 years. However, implants do not need to be replaced every few years to be considered safe; implants can remain in place for life unless they are causing discomfort or harm to the patient.[100]

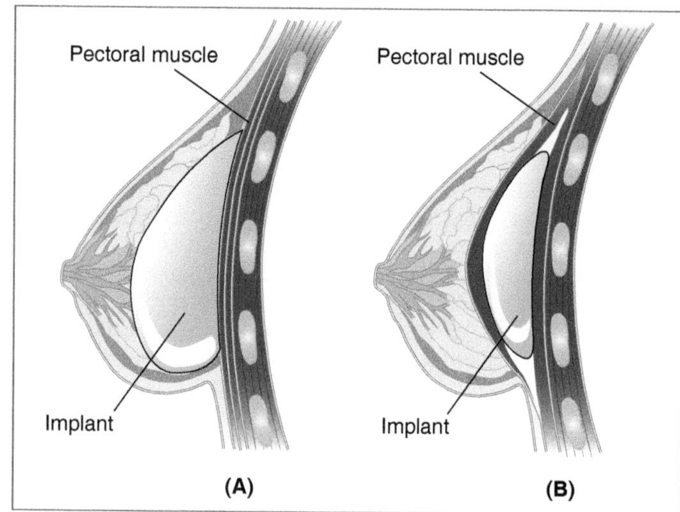

Figure 19.3 **Breast augmentation implant, subglandular (A) and subpectoral (B) options.**

Cancer Risks

Breast cancer risk in female and nonbinary patients AMAB is lower than cisgender females and higher than cisgender men. There is a lack of consensus on breast cancer screening recommendations in cisgender females, which contributes to the lack of consensus on recommendations for female and nonbinary patients AMAB. Patients AMAB undergoing FHT who are over 50 years of age do not meet the criteria for breast cancer screening until 5–10 years after initiation of FHT. Screening mammography is the recommended approach. For patients who meet these criteria and have breast implants, radiologists will adapt their views accordingly.[90]

An association has been identified between textured breast implants and breast implant-associated anaplastic large cell lymphoma (BIA-ALCL), a type of non-Hodgkin lymphoma.[101] While the risk for cancer is low, it is essential to discuss all associated risks associated with patients.

Other Considerations

The injection of unencapsulated liquid silicone freely into soft tissue to enhance cosmesis is colloquially referred to as "pumping." A lack of access to medically necessary transition-related care is often cited as the reason for pumping among patients. Industrial grade silicone products are often used due to easy accessibility and reduced cost compared to medical-grade silicone. Free silicone injections can lead to serious infections, deformities of the soft tissue at the injection site, difficulties with future reconstructions, pulmonary embolism, or death.[102] It is essential to talk to patients about safe surgical options, including formal breast augmentation mammoplasty with a licensed surgeon, rather than injecting silicone.

19.3D MASCULINIZING TOP SURGERY

BACKGROUND

For gender diverse patients who want to remove breast tissue and flatten their chest, a mastectomy or breast tissue removal is an available option. This procedure is often sought out by patients wishing to masculinize their appearance and is referred to as chest masculinization, or more colloquially as top surgery. MHT is not a requirement for masculinizing

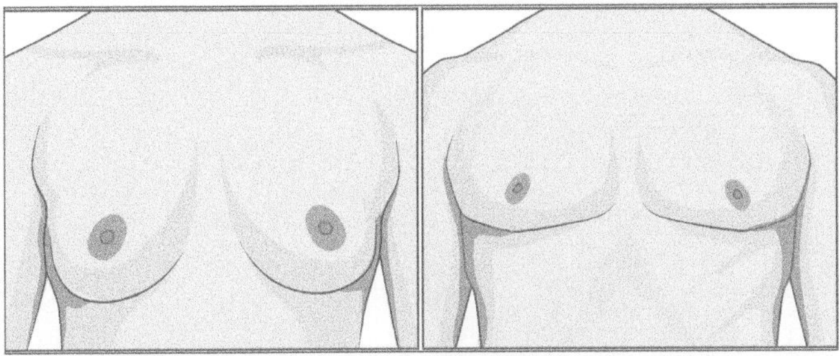

Figure 19.4 **Double incision with free nipple grafts.**

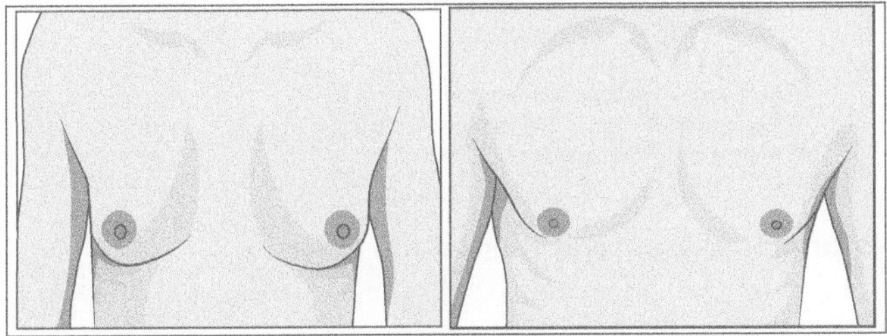

Figure 19.5 **Periareolar incision ("keyhole").**

top surgery for gender diverse patients AMAB. It is common for nonbinary patients AFAB to seek masculinizing top surgery without MHT. For male and nonbinary patients AFAB on MHT, histology reflects breast tissue atrophy at the cellular level, but gross atrophy is not appreciated.

Unlike a radical mastectomy, a common approach in the treatment of cancer in which all breast tissue and some lymph nodes are removed, top surgery seeks to contour existing chest tissue by removing most but not all breast tissue, as well as a reduction and translocation of the nipple-areola complex (NAC) to a more masculine location, and obliteration of the inframammary fold.[103] Surgical techniques include the double incision with free nipple graft (Figure 19.4) and periareolar (Figure 19.5), or "keyhole" approach (Table 19.5).[104] Indications for differentiating between various techniques include breast volume, whether the patient has a history of chest binding, and the surgeon's preference.

CARING FOR THE PATIENT AFTER TOP SURGERY

Physical Examination

When performing a physical examination in a male or nonbinary patient AFAB who has undergone chest masculinization surgery, PAs should palpate the entire chest wall from sternum to midaxillary line and assess the axillary lymph nodes. Any hard or palpable nodule should be notated with size and location. Where masses cannot be differentiated from scar tissue, a referral for MRI is necessary. Mammography is not recommended. Physical examination is reserved for new complaints due to the lack of evidence to support the inclusion of clinical breast examinations in breast cancer screening recommendations among female patients AFAB.[90]

Cancer Risks

For male and nonbinary patients AFAB who decide not to undergo surgery, the overall lifetime risk of developing breast cancer is approximately 12.4%.[105] PAs should following routine breast cancer screening guidelines for cisgender patients AFAB over the age of 40, referring patients with known or suspected *BRCA* mutations for genetic counseling. Referrals to gender-neutral radiology practices are preferred to

TABLE 19.5 Common Top Surgery Techniques

Surgical Technique	Technique Explanation	Benefits	Risks
Double incision with free nipple grafts	Breast tissue is removed through bilateral incisions strategically placed along the inferior pectoralis. The NAC is taken as a skin graft and moved to a masculine location on the chest wall.	The patient's former sagging skin can be placed taut against their chest for a flat appearance. Nipple size and location are changed to reflect a more masculine appearance.	Patients will have a loss of nipple sensation and larger, more prominent scars.
Periareolar incision ("keyhole")	A small incision is made below the NAC to remove breast tissue.	Little to no scarring occurs with this procedure, and nipple sensation is preserved.	Patients with excess breast tissue may have excess skin sagging or rippling after surgery, as well as no change in NAC size or location.

NAC, nipple areola complex.

women's pavilions, as masculine-identified patients' avoidance of women-centric settings has been documented to result in diagnoses at later, more dangerous stages.[90,105]

Following top surgery, routine screening mammography is not recommended. When diagnostic radiology is clinically indicated, MRI is the preferred exam.[90]

Of note, a case report describing androgen-receptive positive breast cancer in a patient AFAB on MHT has been published.[93]

19.3E FEMINIZING GENITAL SURGERY

BACKGROUND

Feminizing genital surgery, colloquially referred to as "bottom surgery," represents several procedures that may be used in varied combinations and may include a penectomy (removal of a penis), orchiectomy (removal of testicles), clitoroplasty (creation of a clitoris), urethroplasty (creation of a urethra), vulvoplasty (creation of vulva), and vaginoplasty (creation of a vaginal canal).

A clitoris is created using the dorsal penile nerves, artery, and veins so that clitoral sensation remains intact. A vaginal canal, when created, is located between the rectum and prostate; this is notable, as future digital prostate exams will be conducted via the vaginal canal rather than the rectum. Vaginoplasty creates a blind cuff that may be created from various autologous tissue grafts, or in some circumstances, may be graftless (Figure 19.6). Surgeons often require FHT to be discontinued before surgery to reduce deep vein thrombosis (DVT) risks. FHT regimens are modified after orchiectomy, antiandrogens are discontinued, and estradiol levels are reduced.

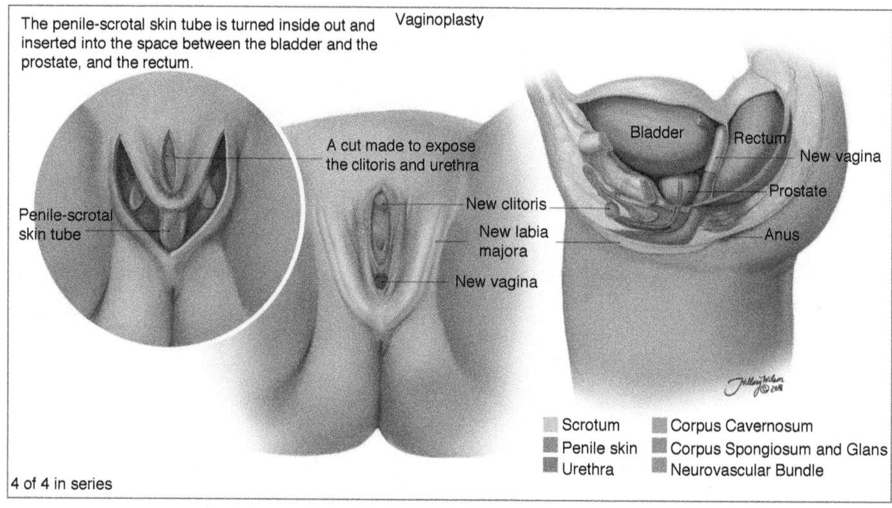

Figure 19.6 **Vaginoplasty. The penile-scrotal skin tube is turned inside out and inserted into the space between the bladder and the prostrate and the rectum.**
(Source: With permission from Hillary Wilson.)

PENILE INVERSION VAGINOPLASTY

The keratotic skin of the penis is inverted and used as an autologous graft to create a vaginal canal. If there is an inadequate penile skin length, additional tissue from the scrotum or abdomen may be used. If scrotal skin is used, patients must undergo electrolysis to remove all hair follicles before surgery.[106] Up to 18 months of electrolysis may be needed to take into consideration that at any given time, some hair will be in the dormant phase and may otherwise be missed with a shorter duration of hair removal, resulting in unwanted postoperative intravaginal hair growth.

PERITONEAL VAGINOPLASTY

For patients with inadequate penile skin, in place of using scrotal skin, the peritoneum can be harvested robotically or laparoscopically and added to the vaginal canal to increase vaginal depth.[107] Disadvantages include increased surgical time and time under anesthesia. Unlike the penile-inversion technique, a peritoneal graft does not have the cellular sloughing associated with keratinized skin or the odor associated with colon graft tissue.

Penile inversion vaginoplasty has a few specific complications compared to other surgical techniques, including an increased risk of vaginal infections among patients who do not undergo or have insufficient hair removal.

SIGMOID COLON VAGINOPLASTY

The sigmoid colon is the least common autologous graft for creating a vaginal canal, indicating limited penile and scrotal skin. One of the benefits of a laparoscopically harvested sigmoid colon vaginoplasty is that the colon tissue secretes mucus, resulting in a vaginal canal with natural lubrication. This mucus, however, may be perceived as unpleasant smelling vaginal discharge.[108]

Some of the complications associated with sigmoid colon vaginoplasty include, but are not limited to:

- **Diversion colitis:** Patients can develop inflammation of the bowel at the site of diversion from the original colon and the colon in the vagina. This can cause local infection and pain for the patient.[108]
- **Ulcerative colitis:** For patients with a history of ulcerative colitis, if the bowel is used, this condition will be transferred to the vaginal canal, and flare-ups can cause extreme discomfort and pain.[108]
- **Adenocarcinoma:** It is recommended that patients who have had a sigmoid colon vaginoplasty undergo yearly speculum exams with special consideration to screen for polyps or suspicious lesions, as cancer can occur inside the new vaginal canal.[109]
- **Colon prolapse:** In rare cases, the vaginal canal can prolapse outside the vaginal introitus. Prolapse leads to severe irritation and pain for the patient and typically requires a surgical procedure to fix.[108]

MINIMAL DEPTH VAGINOPLASTY

Some patients may not desire to have a vaginal canal but wish to have the external appearance of a vulva and a clitoris. Among the reasons cited, some patients do not want to have receptive vaginal sex. A minimal depth vaginoplasty refers to a feminizing genital surgery in which no vaginal canal is created.

There are no special considerations for patients who have undergone minimal depth vaginoplasty.

CARING FOR A POSTSURGICAL VAGINOPLASTY PATIENT

Physical Examination

Upon receiving the patient's consent, it is best to palpate to determine vaginal depth and width by performing a digital manual examination before dilation or speculum examination. This allows the PA to identify the appropriate size speculum or dilator. Each patient's postoperative anatomy is unique; it should never be assumed the same size dilator or speculum can be used for every patient. Speculum examination for visualization of the vaginal canal and bimanual exam may be conducted when appropriate.

The vaginoplasty procedure is limited to a vaginal canal that is either graftless or a blind cuff from an autologous graft. Cancer risks are associated with the cellular component of the graft tissue used: a penile-inversion procedure carries a risk of penile cancer; a colon tissue graft has the risk of colon cancer. At this time, allogenic graft tissue is not being utilized in transition-related surgical care. Cervical and ovarian cancer screenings are unnecessary, as the cervix, fallopian tubes, ovaries, and uterus do not exist.

Palpation of the prostate is conducted by digital vaginal examination rather than digital rectal examination due to the placement of the neovagina in the space between the prostate and the rectum. When clinically indicated, such as when signs or symptoms of prostatic hyperplasia or a personal or family history of prostate pathology, the prostate should be palpated through the superior vaginal wall. For patients who are undergoing FHT, the prostate is often small and difficult to palpate. Routine prostate exams are not recommended without concerning signs or symptoms.[110]

OTHER CONSIDERATIONS

Post-vaginoplasty: Sexually Transmitted Infections

Patients can contract STIs after vaginoplasty. HIV infection, genital and extragenital chlamydia infections, and gonorrhea are disproportionately elevated among gender diverse patients.[111] Furthermore, mucosal tissue, such as oral, anorectal, and sigmoid colon vaginoplasty, has an increased risk for acquisition of STIs.[108] A comprehensive sexual history should be explored with consideration for three-site (oropharyngeal, genital, rectal) STI screening.

Post-vaginoplasty: Dilation

An important part of vaginoplasty aftercare is maintaining an ongoing postoperative dilation schedule. Dilation refers to the technique of inserting a medical-grade dilator into the vagina to keep the canal patent. Dilation is initiated immediately after surgery, and dilators increase in depth and width until the vaginal canal is capable of receptive vaginal sex. Ongoing dilation maintains patency. The frequency and duration of each dilation session vary by surgeon's preference, starting with more than once a day until it is necessary only a few times a week. Vaginal dilation is a lifetime commitment without which a surgical revision may be required.[106]

Post-vaginoplasty: Urination and Foley Catheter Insertion

Patients may require a Foley catheter insertion at some point after surgery. Be sure to identify landmarks so the catheter may be inserted appropriately. The urethral opening may look different post-vaginoplasty, but it remains located between the clitoris and vaginal canal. The depth between the urethral meatus and bladder is only a few centimeters.

19.3F PHALLOPLASTY

BACKGROUND

Phalloplasty is a surgical procedure in which a penis is created. Each patient's surgical plan is individualized and customizable to their unique desires. Phalloplasty may also include a vaginectomy (removal of the vagina), urethral lengthening (lengthening of the native urethra so the patient can urinate while standing), insertion of an inflatable penile prosthesis to accommodate penile erections, or insertion of testicular implants. The tissue graft used within the phalloplasty can be created from a variety of different anatomic locations. The most common sites are the radial forearm free flap and anterolateral thigh flap.

The phalloplasty procedure is commonly performed in stages of two or three separate procedures, such as first creating the phallus and a second procedure to perform the urethral lengthening so the patient can urinate while standing. Each surgeon has their own unique surgical technique and plan.

RADIAL FOREARM PHALLOPLASTY

The radial forearm free flap phalloplasty involves taking a graft from the forearm skin and fat, radial artery, cephalic vein, and the antebrachial nerves to create the phallus (Figures 19.7 and 19.8). The neurovascular bundle from the radial forearm flap is attached to a neurovascular bundle in the groin. If a patient is undergoing urethral lengthening before surgery, patients must have permanent hair removal via electrolysis on a portion of their forearm, so the new urethra is hairless. As with preoperative preparation for vaginoplasty, hair removal must consider those hair follicles in the dormant phase at any given time.[112] One of the significant benefits to the radial forearm flap is the copious ability

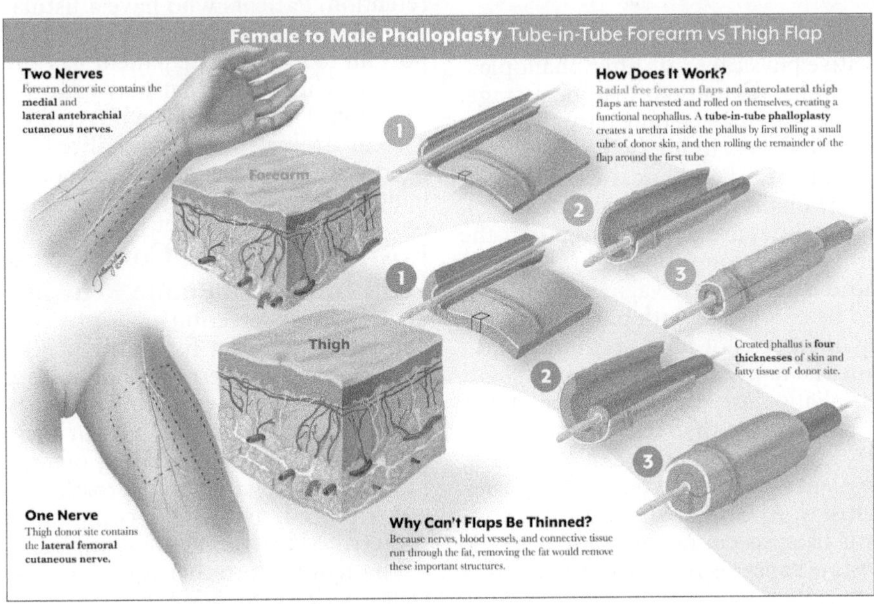

Figure 19.7 **Female to male phalloplasty. Tube-in-tube forearm versus thigh flap.**
(Source: With permission from Hillary Wilson.)

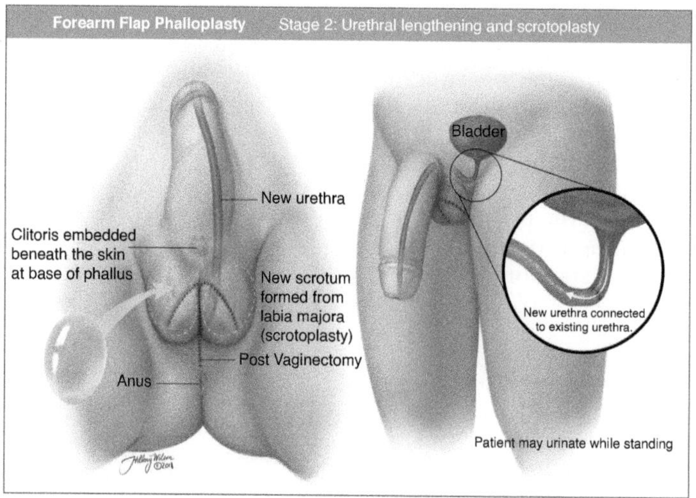

Figure 19.8 Forearm flap phalloplasty. Stage 2–urethral lengthening and scrotoplasty.
(Source: With permission from Hillary Wilson.)

of nerves in the forearm to be relocated and connected to nerves in the pelvis. The new phallus has sensation to touch. Additionally, in contrast to other graft sites, the forearm has increased sensation and is smaller.

ANTEROLATERAL THIGH PHALLOPLASTY

The anterolateral thigh flap involves taking the thigh skin and fat, superficial circumflex femoral artery, and typically the saphenous vein to create the phallus. This neurovascular bundle is attached to the groin. Like the radial forearm flap, if patients decide to have urethral lengthening, permanent hair removal is required before surgery, always considering those hair follicles in the dormant phase at any given time.[112] The anterolateral thigh has fewer available nerves, so sensation to touch may be more limited. This option is excellent for those patients who want a phallus with greater girth and length as the thigh has more fat than the forearm.

CARING FOR A POSTSURGICAL PHALLOPLASTY PATIENT

Physical Examination

When performing a sensitive physical exam after phalloplasty, it is important to consider the patient's surgical stage. Some patient's surgical processes may be only partially completed. Thus, it is important always to apply informed consent before examining a patient. The physical exam should include an inspection of the phallus, scrotum, and perineum to determine if any abnormalities are present. Inquire if the patient elected to have a vaginectomy or urethral lengthening. For patients who did not have a vaginectomy, routine pelvic exams should be conducted with patient consent when indicated. If the patient did not have urethral lengthening, be sure to examine the native urethral meatus.

Patients who are post-phalloplasty that keep their vagina should be assessed for risk factors that indicate screening for cervical cancer, HPV, and STI testing. When evaluating the patient, follow the patient's lead on the terminology they use to describe their anatomy. Always obtain informed consent before the insertion of a speculum or manual pelvic exam. Screening for prostate cancer is not warranted, as this organ is not present.

OTHER CONSIDERATIONS

Post-Phalloplasty: Insertion of Foley Catheter

The insertion of a Foley catheter in a postsurgical phalloplasty patient with urethral lengthening is very different from the insertion of a catheter in a natal phallus. The neourethra is tortuous and is often narrower than a natal urethra. Catheterization requires direct visualization with the use of a flexible cystoscopy and flexible guidewire. If your patient needs catheterization, it is essential to consult a urologist with experience in catheterizing a neophallus.

Post-Phalloplasty: Urinary Complications

Because of the complex nature of the newly constructed urethra, phalloplasty patients are prone to urinary complications. Even in the late stages after the phalloplasty, 25% to 50% of patients experience some type of complications such as a urinary stricture or fistula.[113] Patients experiencing a urinary stricture may complain of postvoid dribbling or feelings of bladder fullness, suggestive of a blockage, and retention. Patients who have a fistula will complain of leakage from an area other than their urethral meatus. It is important to assess if the patient has any signs or symptoms of a urinary infection that may exacerbate their current complication. Patients may be referred back to their surgeon or a local urologist with specialized skills.[114] Because of this procedure's complex nature, major complications should be handled by a specialist rather than in a primary care setting.

Post-Phalloplasty: Complications Associated With Inflatable Penile Prosthesis

To obtain an erection in a post-phalloplasty neophallus, patients require an inflatable penile prosthesis. Owing to the complex nature of a phalloplasty procedure, clinicians should ensure the penile prosthesis's integrity during routine exams. During the patient history, inquire if the patient has difficulties inflating or deflating their prosthesis. Examine the phallus and prosthesis to ensure erosion has not occurred, as this is a common complication following surgery.[115] If erosion or a complication should occur, refer the patient back to their surgeon as soon as possible to prevent a serious infection.

Post-Phalloplasty: Vascular Access

For patients who have undergone a radial forearm free flap, the radial artery is sacrificed to create the phallus. Radial pulses will not be present on physical examination, nor will vascular access be available from the donor site's radial artery.

19.3G METOIDIOPLASTY

BACKGROUND

Metoidioplasty, colloquially referred to by patients as a "meta," is the surgical creation of a microphallus from the natal clitoris after the patient experiences clitoromegaly resulting from MHT. As with a phalloplasty, a patient can elect to undergo a vaginectomy (removal of the vagina), urethral lengthening (lengthening of the native urethra so the patient can stand to pee), and the surgical insertion of testicular implants. The resulting microphallus is significantly shorter than a neophallus or natal phallus. It may be difficult for all patients to stand to pee or engage in penile insertive sex. Inflatable penile prosthetics currently on the market are not sized for patients who have undergone metoidioplasty. The primary benefit of metoidioplasty is the almost complete preservation of natal clitoral sensation.[116]

CARING FOR A POSTSURGICAL PATIENT

Before a physical examination, inquire if the patient had a vaginectomy or urethral lengthening. For patients who did not have a vaginectomy, pelvic exams should be conducted when appropriate. Upon receiving the patient's consent, this sensitive physical exam should include an inspection of the phallus, scrotum, and perineum to determine if any abnormalities are present. Post-metoidioplasty care mirrors that of the phalloplasty, without necessitating a graft site.

KNOWLEDGE CHECKS

- Create a plan to manage gender dysphoria/incongruence in the following patient scenarios. Include initial medications (formulation), monitoring (labs, physical examination), and any relevant patient education.
  1. A 10-year-old male, AFAB, Tanner Stage 2, without contraindications
  2. A 16-year-old female, AMAB, Tanner 5, without contraindications
  3. A 26-year-old male, AFAB, Tanner 5, without contraindications
  4. Present a science-based argument to support your recommendation for treatment of gender dysphoria/incongruence. Data and bioethics should be addressed.

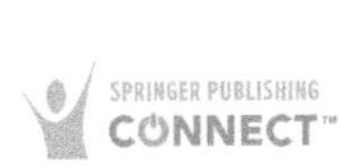

A robust set of instructor resources designed to supplement this text is located at **http://connect.springerpub.com/content/book/978-0-8261-8243-2.** Qualifying instructors may request access by emailing **textbook@springerpub.com.**

REFERENCES

The complete reference list for this chapter appears in the digital version of the chapter, accessible at https://connect.springerpub.com/content/book/978-0-8261-8243-2/chapter/ch19.

Chapter 20

PREVENTIVE MEDICINE

JOHN BASTIN, BRIGITTA CINTRON, AND COURTNEY WILKE

LEARNING OBJECTIVES

- Compare and contrast the primary domains of preventive medicine.
- Summarize the major health challenges patients face within each domain.
- Evaluate key measures of patient health and their ideal ranges for each domain.
- Assess a patient's risk profile given information about the patient.
- Create a plan to reduce a patient's risk within each domain and communicate this plan to the patient.

INTRODUCTION

The prevention of disease and injury is multifactorial and is the responsibility of every PA at every patient encounter. Prevention strategies range from patient education and counseling to prescribing medication to prevent or slow the progression of disease. These strategies will improve the patient's quality of life while also reducing the potential for unnecessary morbidity and mortality. This chapter provides recommendations and strategies for PAs to effectively counsel and educate patients in the prevention of disease and injuries.

20.1 PREVENTION OF CARDIOVASCULAR DISEASE

Despite advances in screening, early diagnosis, and treatment, atherosclerotic cardiovascular disease (ASCVD) remains the leading cause of morbidity and death throughout the world and the leading cause of death among minorities in the United States.[1]

20.1A PREVENTION STRATEGIES

EARLY INTERVENTION

Early intervention is the key to the prevention of ASCVD. This is accomplished by encouraging patients to adopt a healthy lifestyle, identifying those patients who are at risk for developing ASCVD and encouraging these patients to implement lifestyle modifications, and lastly implementing appropriate pharmacologic interventions as needed.

AGE-DRIVEN RISK ASSESSMENT

Age is a major risk factor for the development of ASCVD and all patients between the ages of 40 and 75 should meet with their clinician to undergo a 10-year ASCVD screening. This screening is especially important before starting a medication regimen for conditions such as hypertension, hyperlipidemia, or diabetes.

20.1B MODIFIABLE RISK FACTORS

HEART HEALTHY DIET

Patients should be encouraged to make healthy choices in their daily meal planning by increasing their consumption of vegetables, fruits, nuts, whole grains, and fish, and by including plant-based and lean animal protein. Conversely, patients should be counseled to reduce their intake of red meat and to avoid food and beverages that are high in trans fats, added sugars, and refined carbohydrates, which can contribute to the development of ASCVD.

ROUTINE EXERCISE

Adults should be encouraged to exercise on a regular basis. A good exercise prescription is to perform moderate intensity exercise for a total of 150 minutes per week or high intensity exercise for a total of 75 minutes per week. All patients, especially those with sedentary lifestyles, should undergo a complete medical evaluation prior to beginning any exercise regimen. Further information can be found in the exercise section of this chapter.

BODY MASS INDEX REDUCTION

Adults who are overweight (body mass index [BMI] 25–29.9 kg/m^2) or obese (BMI >30 kg/m^2) are at greater risk of developing ASCVD, heart failure, and atrial fibrillation. Patients who are classified as overweight or obese should implement weight management and reduction strategies, monitor food intake, and follow a regular exercise program. Keeping a log of food intake and exercise allows patients to better track their progress and they may be more successful in achieving their weight loss goals. Further information can be found in Section 20.5 Obesity.

TYPE 2 DIABETES MANAGEMENT

Patients diagnosed with type 2 diabetes should be encouraged at each office visit to implement healthy lifestyle changes such as improving their diet and exercising on a regular basis. If a patient's Hb A1c is 6.5% or greater, indicating glycemic control has not been achieved with lifestyle modifications alone, clinicians should then consider initiating or intensifying pharmacologic therapy at that time. Current recommendations suggest that individualized therapy based on a patient's comorbidities and lifestyle factors is important.[2] Initial management often involves a biguanide class of medications followed by the addition of a sodium-glucose cotransporter 2 (SGLT2) inhibitor or a glucagon-like peptide-1 (GLP1) receptor agonist if glycemic control is not achieved with monotherapy alone.

TOBACCO CESSATION

Patients should be screened for the use of all forms of tobacco products, including vaping and second-hand smoke exposure, at each office visit. Those patients who are found to use tobacco products should be encouraged to quit as well as offered smoking cessation counseling. Further information can be found in Section 20.6 Tobacco Cessation.

SCREENING AND MANAGEMENT OF HYPERLIPIDEMIA

Starting statin therapy (e.g., atorvastatin) is the first-line primary treatment strategy for the prevention of ASCVD. Statins should be started in patients who are found to have elevated low density lipoprotein (LDL) cholesterol levels (LDL >190 mg/dL), patients with diabetes, patients between 40 and 75 years of age, and those who are determined to be of significant risk for developing ASCVD.

BLOOD PRESSURE REGULATION

Attempts to lower blood pressure with nonpharmacologic interventions such as diet and exercise should be attempted first in all patients with an elevation in blood pressure. When pharmacologic therapy is started, the targeted goal of treatment should be a blood pressure that is <130/80 mm Hg.

20.2 OSTEOPOROSIS

Osteoporosis is a disease of the bone that is characterized by low bone mass and structural deterioration of the bone tissue. These factors may result in the bones becoming thin and fragile with a propensity for the development of fractures involving the hips, spine, and wrist.[3] Osteoporosis-related fractures can result in significant morbidity and even death, especially for older patients.

PATHOPHYSIOLOGY OF BONE LOSS

Bone has many diverse functions that include the protection of vital organs and the regulation of mineral homeostasis. As a continuation of these diverse functions, bone undergoes a constant cycle of remodeling. During remodeling, old bone is reabsorbed, and new, stronger bone is formed. During childhood, new bone is formed more quickly than it is absorbed, which results in stronger, denser bone tissue. Later in life, or as a result of menopause or secondary causes of bone resorption, bone loss may occur more quickly than the process of remodeling. This is encountered most commonly in women, especially right after the onset of menopause, and continues as the woman progresses into her postmenopausal years.[4]

RISK FACTORS FOR OSTEOPOROSIS

Risk factors for osteoporosis can be classified as modifiable or nonmodifiable. Modifiable risk factors are those that the patient can change through lifestyle modifications while nonmodifiable risk factors are inherent to the patient and cannot be changed.

Nonmodifiable Risk Factors

- **Sex:** Women are at a greater risk for developing osteoporosis, but men can also be affected.
- **Age:** As the patient ages, the risk for developing osteoporosis increases.
- **Body size:** Women with a small, thin body habitus are at greater risk of developing osteoporosis.
- **Ethnicity:** Women of Asian descent and Caucasian women are at a higher risk for developing osteoporosis. African American and Hispanic women have a lower, but still significant, risk for developing osteoporosis.
- **Family history:** Heredity may play a role in the development of osteoporosis.
- **Comorbidities:** Conditions such as premature ovarian failure and anorexia nervosa can expedite early bone loss.

Modifiable Risk Factors

- **Sex hormones:** Amenorrhea, low levels of estrogen in women, and low levels of testosterone in men can lead to the development of osteoporosis.
- **Calcium and vitamin D:** A diet low in calcium and vitamin D can predispose patients to the development of osteoporosis.
- **Medications:** Long-term use of medications, such as glucocorticoids and some anticonvulsants can lead to the development of osteoporosis.
- **Lifestyle:** An inactive lifestyle can lead to the development of osteoporosis. Regular physical activity is required for ongoing bone remodeling. In addition to regular physical activity, those who experience a sedentary lifestyle are much more likely to have minimal exposure to sunlight, inhibiting the body's production of vitamin D_3.
- Cigarette smoking and excessive alcohol and caffeine intake not only have a negative impact on a patient's overall health but can cause bone loss resulting in osteoporosis.[5]

SCREENING

According to the U.S. Preventive Services Task Force (USPSTF),[6] screening for osteoporosis should begin at age 65 or sooner for women who have risk factors for the development of osteoporosis.[6] A central dual-energy x-ray absorptiometry (DXA/DEXA) scan is the most commonly used screening tool to assess for the presence of osteoporosis. The DXA scan assesses the level of bone mineral density (BMD) at the hip and lumbar spine to define the presence of osteoporosis and guide treatment and prevention strategies.

PREVENTION

Adequate calcium intake, either through diet or nutritional supplements, can prevent the development of osteoporosis. Foods high in dietary calcium include milk, yogurt, cheese, and ice cream. Other dietary sources include green leafy vegetables, sardines, almonds, cereals, and bread and are essential in the prevention of the disease.

Calcium needs change throughout a patient's life, with a greater demand occurring during adolescence and early adulthood when rapid skeletal growth is occurring. Women who are pregnant, breastfeeding, or postmenopausal have a greater demand for calcium supplementation.

Vitamin D plays an important role in the absorption of calcium and bone health. Recommended daily intake for adults <70 years of age is 600 IU of vitamin D daily and 700 IU of vitamin D daily for adults age 70 years of age and older. While calcium and vitamin D are essential elements for overall bone health, recent evidence does not support either being used as a means of primary prevention of osteoporotic fractures in adults over age 65. Counseling on fall prevention should happen early on and risk should be regularly reassessed.

Exercise

Weight-bearing exercise such as jogging, walking, hiking, and climbing stairs contributes to development of strong bones.

Lifestyle Modifications

Stopping smoking and limiting excessive alcohol and caffeine intake will help to prevent bone loss.

Medications

A variety of medications can be used to prevent and treat osteoporosis. Medications such as bisphosphonates (Fosamax), calcitonin, estrogen, and estrogen agonist/antagonist (tamoxifen) work by inhibiting osteoclastic activity, thus preventing bone loss. Anabolic steroids (e.g., teriparatide) increase bone formation while reducing bone loss.[7]

SUMMARY

Osteoporosis can be prevented through healthy lifestyle choices, such as regular aerobic exercise, including calcium-rich foods in the daily diet, and taking calcium and vitamin D supplements. Avoidance of tobacco products and excessive amounts of caffeine and alcohol are also important lifestyle choices that aid in the prevention of osteoporosis. Screening and early detection are essential to prevent an osteoporosis-related fracture, which could result in significant morbidity and death.

20.3 CANCER SCREENING

No discussion on the topic of cancer screening is complete without first discussing the factors that put patients at risk for developing cancer. Breast cancer is the leading form of cancer in women and second leading cause of cancer-related deaths. Prostate cancer is the leading cancer in men and the third leading cause of cancer-related deaths. Cancer of the lung and bronchus top the list as the leading cause of cancer-related deaths in both men and women.[8]

AGE

As patients advance in age, they are at a greater risk of developing many types of cancer. According to the National Cancer Institute, advancing age is the most important risk factor for the development of cancer and the median age of cancer diagnosis is 66 years.[9] Cancer screening is an integral part of cancer prevention and clinicians should regularly discuss the importance of cancer screening for early detection with their patients. The American Cancer Society recommends the following screening.[9]

- Cervical cancer screening for human papillomavirus (HPV) in women starting at age 25 through age 65
- Colon cancer screening for patients at average risk starting at age 45
- Prostate cancer screening for men starting at age 45
- Breast cancer screening in women via annual mammograms starting at age 45
- Former or active smokers should be screened for lung cancer generally starting at age 55

ALCOHOL CONSUMPTION

Patients who regularly consume alcohol are at a greater risk of developing cancers involving the mouth, throat, esophagus, larynx, liver, and breasts. The risk is increased for patients who regularly drink alcohol in combination with tobacco use.

Prevention strategies should be directed at encouraging patients who drink alcohol to do so in moderation by limiting their daily consumption of alcoholic beverages to one drink per day for women and two drinks per day for men.

CANCER-CONTAINING SUBSTANCES

Cancer develops when changes occur in the DNA during cell replication. These changes may be related to a genetic predisposition, as is the case with family history of breast cancer. The development of cancer can also be related to environmental exposures that damage the DNA. Sun exposure and tobacco use are the two most widely known environmental exposures that can lead to the development of cancer. Other substances, classified as carcinogens, that are encountered in the environment or through occupational exposure can potentially put the patient at risk for development of cancer.

Prevention strategies should be directed at identifying the presence of carcinogens, avoiding exposure, or implementing controls such as wearing appropriate personal protective equipment to limit exposure.

HORMONAL THERAPY

While estrogen is beneficial in the treatment of pre- and postmenopausal symptoms in women, it is also classified as a carcinogen. There is an increased risk of breast cancer in women taking estrogen/progesterone combination hormone replacement therapy and an increased risk for the development of endometrial cancer in women who take unopposed estrogen.

Prevention strategies are centered around women who are considering starting hormone replacement therapy and include having a discussion with a clinician to understand the potential risks and benefits before starting estrogen therapy.

INFECTIOUS AGENTS

Infectious organisms, including viruses, bacteria, and parasites, can pose a cancer risk to those patients who are exposed to them. Viruses such as Epstein-Barr virus, hepatitis B virus, HPV, and HIV can be transmitted via contact with saliva, sharing needles, blood transfusions, or unprotected sexual intercourse. *Helicobacter pylori*, a bacterium that is spread through the consumption of contaminated food and water or through the fecal-oral route, has been implicated in the development of certain types of gastric cancers.[10] *Schistosoma haematobium*, a parasitic flatworm whose host is freshwater snails found in Africa and Middle East, can cause bladder cancer. Humans are infected when they are exposed to water contaminated with the flatworm, allowing it to burrow into the skin.

Prevention strategies are multifactorial and include avoiding contact with contaminated saliva and blood. Encouraging patients who are intravenous drug users to participate in needle exchange programs and avoiding unprotected sex by using a barrier form of contraception (e.g., condoms) can reduce risk of transmission.

OBESITY

Patients who are classified as obese, defined as a BMI >30 kg/m^2, are at greater risk for the development of postmenopausal breast cancer, as well as cancer of the colon, rectum, endometrium, esophagus, pancreas, and gallbladder.

Prevention should be directed at encouraging patients who are obese to lose weight through regular aerobic exercise and adhering to a healthy well-balanced diet.

MEDICAL RADIATION

Clinicians regularly incorporate the use of diagnostic imaging, such as CT scans and conventional radiographs to aid in the diagnosis of illnesses and injuries. Patients will often express concerns regarding the potential cancer risk from exposure to the radiation generated by one of these studies. While the risk is negligible for a patient to develop cancer from a single CT scan, the risk does increase with cumulative radiation exposure from multiple scans.[11,12]

Prevention efforts should be centered around reducing the cumulative radiation exposure by avoiding repetitive studies in patients with chronic medical conditions. This can be accomplished by obtaining a complete medical history and thorough review of the patient's medical records, especially for patients new to your practice or who you are not familiar with.

SUNLIGHT

UV radiation is emitted from the sun, sunlamps, and tanning beds and prolonged repetitive exposure can cause damage to the skin. This skin damage can subsequently lead to the development of skin cancer.

To prevent the development of skin cancer, patients should be encouraged to do the following:

- Wear a wide brim hat to protect the face, neck, and ears.
- Wear sunglasses to shield the eyes from the UV radiation.
- Wear long-sleeve shirts and long pants.
- Use a sunscreen that has a sun protective factor (SPF) of at least 15.

TOBACCO

The use of tobacco and tobacco products present the greatest risk of both developing cancer and dying from cancer. Exposure to the chemicals found in environmental cigarette smoke (also known as second-hand cigarette smoke) represents a greater risk of developing cancer than if that person were not exposed. Tobacco users are prone to developing cancers of the lung, larynx, mouth, esophagus, bladder, kidney, liver, stomach, pancreas, colon, and rectum.[13]

Prevention strategies are directed at encouraging patients who smoke to quit smoking during each clinical encounter and to also refer the patient to a trained tobacco treatment specialist (TTS) for counseling and nicotine replacement therapy (NRT).

20.4 PHYSICAL ACTIVITY

OVERVIEW

Until recently, regular physical activity had been a part of life throughout human history. However, a marked decrease in the amount of physical activity required for daily living has occurred in recent years, and with this there has been a concurrent reduction in total physical activity for most individuals. Unfortunately, this reduction in physical activity levels has had a harmful effect on both individual and public health. Evidence demonstrates that physical activity is effective as both primary and secondary prevention for a wide range of chronic medical conditions.[14] Because of this, globally there has been a push to encourage an increased level of physical activity to counter sedentary lifestyle trends. These efforts have had varying degrees of success, and there remains a strong need for continued progress in this direction.

EPIDEMIOLOGY

Although experts and public health officials have campaigned for the public to engage in greater physical activity, the adoption of such behavior has been limited. In 2018 only 24% of adults in the United States reported engaging in the recommended amount of aerobic and muscle-strengthening activity.[15] Similarly, just 20% of adolescents reported meeting this goal, a decrease of nearly 10% from just 6 years prior.[15]

EFFECTS OF EXERCISE

From a physiologic perspective, physical activity has many positive effects on the human body. Though the exact mechanisms are incompletely understood and continue to be explored with ongoing research, potential beneficial processes include improving vascular endothelial function in the heart, reducing insulin resistance, and promoting new neuron development in the brain.[16]

From a more epidemiologic perspective, the benefits of regular physical activity are undeniable. It reduces the risk of several chronic illnesses, including cardiovascular disease (CVD), hypertension, osteoporosis, diabetes mellitus, Alzheimer dementia, and colon and breast cancers, among other disease states.[17,18] Additionally, exercise improves symptoms of depression and anxiety.[17] It improves quality of life in a multitude of ways, including by reducing symptoms of chronic conditions such as osteoarthritis, multiple sclerosis, and dementia, and reduces the risk of premature death.[17,18] In the older patient population, it has been shown to reduce the risk of fall-related fractures, which can have a huge impact on quality of life.[19] Risk reduction for these adverse outcomes ranges from 20% to over 50%.[14]

GUIDELINES ON PHYSICAL ACTIVITY

The World Health Organization (WHO) and the Centers for Disease Control and Prevention (CDC) recommend that healthy adults engage in at least 150 minutes per week of at least moderate-intensity physical activity as well as twice weekly engagement in muscle strengthening.[14,17] These goals are thought to optimize the health benefits of increased physical activity and result in the health improvements noted above.

Unfortunately, achieving this amount of exercise can be challenging. Patients may be discouraged by the prospect of attempting to attain this level of activity, especially if they have comorbidities that affect their activity level. It is important to recognize that much smaller amounts of physical activity are clinically beneficial and reduce the risk of chronic disease and premature death.[18] Achieving just 50% or less of the activity goal prescribed by authorities improves an individual's health profile.[18] Even short episodes of light intensity physical activity, such as gentle walking, are beneficial. Walking is an ideal starting point for many individuals, as it is easy to do, requires no special equipment, and involves a relatively low degree of mechanical stress.

For individuals interested in starting to exercise, a clinician may be consulted to evaluate the patient's health. In general, in the absence of known CVD or symptoms or signs concerning for CVD, specific cardiac evaluation is not recommended. Conversely, those with known disease or symptoms concerning for it should be evaluated further with possible consideration for an EKG or stress testing, for example.[20]

For older adults who have higher risks of activity-related injury, the Exercise Assessment and Screening for You (EASY) Tool may be helpful.[21] This tool helps the clinician and the patient collaborate in identifying possible risks and the need for health screening related to ongoing symptoms, and it can also be used to develop a customized physical activity plan.

Large volumes of evidence demonstrate that from a public health perspective, the benefits of increased physical activity outweigh the risks. On an individual basis, the risk of harm is very small.[17] To reduce even this small risk, patients should consider the following[17]:

1. Slowly increase both the duration and intensity of the activity level. Most injuries related to increased activity are musculoskeletal (MS) and can be avoided by this simple method. Table 20.1 lists common activities and the intensity of activity associated with these.
2. Choose an activity that is appropriate given one's overall health. For example, if a patient is sedentary and has poor balance, in-line skating is likely to be a riskier endeavor than for someone with better overall physical fitness.
3. If a patient has comorbid conditions or symptoms with activity, they should follow up with their primary care clinician for monitoring and appropriate recommendations on activity.

TABLE 20.1 Exercise Intensity of Common Activities

Intensity Level	Exercise	Talk Test
Light	Walking slowly at 2 mph	Can talk comfortably
Moderate	Walking 3–4 mph	Can talk but not sing
Vigorous	Jogging	Can speak only few words without pausing for breath

Source: Piercy KL, Troiano RP, Ballard RM, et al. The physical activity guidelines for Americans. JAMA. *2018;320(19):2020–2028. doi:10.1001/jama.2018.14854*

ENCOURAGING BEHAVIORAL CHANGE

Lifestyle changes of any kind can be challenging, especially when a patient is attempting to change long-standing habits. It is important that when promoting increased physical activity, clinicians adopt an encouraging attitude with patients. Frequently individuals will be ambivalent about initiating substantial change in their lives, and it is likely that this conversation may be difficult. *Motivational interviewing* (MI) is a technique that may be useful. Clinicians increasingly employ MI as a valuable adjunctive tool in encouraging patients to exert more deliberate control over their own lifestyle choices. This method involves demonstrating empathy with the patient, helping the patient identify what is important to them, and reinforcing their commitment to change.[22] Evidence suggests that MI can be an effective tool in promoting increased physical activity.[23]

It is also important to consider a multimodal approach to behavior change. Communities often have programs available to encourage increased activity in their members, often through recreational outdoor or indoor activities. There may be structured programs that include small group support meetings and educational sessions. The benefits of technology should not be forgotten either, as step counters and fitness apps are used both as goal setting devices and as a means of providing regular coaching and encouragement.

Regardless of the methods employed, clinicians have a responsibility to encourage physical activity in their patients. The evidence for its value is overwhelming, and even incremental changes will yield clinical benefits.

20.5 OBESITY

OVERVIEW

When a person's weight is above what is considered healthy for their height, the person may be described as overweight or obese. These terms are designed to refer to the presence of excess adipose tissue and are useful as predictors of a patient's weight-related health risks. *Overweight* and *obesity* lie on a continuum, and although obesity is correlated with greater health risks, being overweight is also a risk factor for chronic weight-related diseases.

EPIDEMIOLOGY

In the United States, the prevalence of excess adipose tissue has risen substantially in the last several years. In the 1960s just 15% of Americans were classified as obese, by 2000 this had increased to 30.5% of Americans, and now more recently in 2016 this number had risen to nearly 40%.[24] An additional 32% of Americans meet the criteria for being overweight.[24]

EFFECTS OF OBESITY

Unfortunately, individuals who are overweight or obese face an elevated risk of many adverse health outcomes, including an increased risk of CVD, diabetes, hypertension, degenerative joint disease, obstructive sleep apnea, and some types of cancer including breast, prostate, and colon cancer.[25] In addition to its impact on potentially preventable causes of death and disability, it is also associated with an increased risk of mental illness such as depression and anxiety and an overall reduced quality of life.[25]

MONITORING WEIGHT

Because a person's weight can have significant long-term effects on their overall health and well-being, it is important that clinicians vigilantly monitor weight in their patients. BMI is useful as a screening tool to allow clinicians to evaluate a person's weight, though it does not directly measure adipose tissue. The BMI is calculated by dividing a person's weight in kilograms by the square of height in meters. The resulting ratio is used to categorize a patient's weight, as seen in Table 20.2. In general, BMIs above the normal range are correlated with higher risks of comorbid conditions, though this is not the case when the additional weight is due to muscle rather than adipose tissue.[25] Patients who are overweight or obese should be screened for common weight-related health complications, including depression, glucose intolerance, and cardiovascular conditions, among others.[25,26]

ETIOLOGY

Obesity develops as a result of multiple influences and involves a complex interplay between environmental and genetic factors. Genetic variations have been identified that affect the degree of adiposity in an individual, although these are thought to contribute far less to the prevalence of obesity in the United States compared to environmental factors.[25] Such environmental influences include decreased physical activity, increased caloric consumption, and more recently there is concern that alterations in gut flora play a role as well. Additionally, there are many medications in use today that can contribute to weight gain (see Table 20.3). Of course, in some cases a specific underlying disease process can be identified that contributes to excess weight, though this is relatively rare. Nonetheless, important treatable underlying causes of weight gain should be considered, such as Cushing syndrome and hypothyroidism.

TABLE 20.2 Body Mass Index Categories

BMI (kg/m^2)	Category
<18.5	Underweight
18.5 to <25	Normal
25 to <30	Overweight
≥30	Obese

BMI, body mass index.

TABLE 20.3 Common Medications Associated With Weight Gain

Drug Class	Examples
Antidepressants	Fluoxetine, paroxetine, citalopram
Antipsychotics	Risperidone, olanzapine, aripiprazole
Mood stabilizers	Lithium, carbamazepine
Corticosteroids	Prednisone, hydrocortisone
Insulin	Insulin isophane, regular insulin
Sulfonylureas	Glyburide, glimepiride
Antiepileptic drugs	Valproic acid, carbamazepine, divalproex

TREATMENT OF OBESITY

The goal of obesity treatment is to reduce the risk of weight-related health complications. A relatively small 5% to 10% reduction in weight can improve a patient's risk profile for chronic disease.[25,27] Lifestyle modifications that lead to weight loss, such as decreased caloric intake and increased physical activity, can be difficult to maintain on a long-term basis. Often the weight is regained over a relatively short-term time frame, in part due to the body's compensatory mechanisms.[25,27] This regained weight negates the long-term health benefits of the initial weight loss.

Current research suggests that lifestyle modification should be the basis of all weight loss endeavors.[24–29] A systematic multimodal approach that involves dietary education, behavior modification, and increased physical activity is most successful in promoting long-term lifestyle changes.[25,27] When such comprehensive weight loss maintenance programs involve regular healthcare visits, patients are more successful at maintaining a healthier weight over the long term.[27] Often this involves the engagement of multiple entities, including possibly dietitians, a community weight management group such as the National Diabetes Prevention Program, or even a commercial weight loss program.[27] The USPSTF recommends that all adult patients with a BMI ≥30 be referred to a program with a multimodal approach that includes behavioral counseling.[28]

Despite a patient's best efforts to initiate lifestyle changes, such changes are sometimes insufficient to achieve and maintain meaningful weight loss. If a patient has obesity (BMI ≥30) or has weight-related health problems, pharmacologic therapy may be considered as an adjunctive measure.[25] An individualized recommendation regarding the most appropriate treatment option can be made by considering such patient-specific factors as their underlying health conditions, level of motivation, and any specific contraindications to medical therapy. Examples of medications that can be used long-term to assist with weight loss include orlistat (a gastrointestinal lipase inhibitor), a phentermine and topiramate combination drug, and liraglutide (a GLP1 receptor agonist).

Even with the addition of pharmacotherapy to lifestyle changes, a patient may be unsuccessful in achieving meaningful weight loss. In patients with more severe obesity (BMI ≥40) and comorbid weight-related conditions, bariatric surgery may be considered.[25,27] These surgeries that promote weight loss do so by reducing the size of the stomach (leading to early satiety) and/or bypassing part of the intestines, thus reducing absorption of calories and nutrition. Surgery can be risky and may be associated with both short- and long-term complications, but in selected patients this more aggressive intervention has been shown to improve obesity-related comorbidities.[29]

PREVENTION OF OBESITY

Despite the many methods available to assist with weight loss, obesity remains a significant health risk for a large portion of the population. Even when weight loss is successfully achieved and maintained, evidence suggests that while quality of life and comorbid conditions may improve, long-term mortality may not.[27] The time-honored adage "an ounce of prevention is worth a pound of cure" succinctly summarizes the tactic most likely to be successful in defeating weight-related chronic diseases. Promotion of healthy lifestyle choices—whether through nutrition education, increased opportunity for physical activity, or a myriad of other interventions—can create an environment in which the healthy choice is an easier choice. Although many of these changes may require action at a community level, the clinician has a role in careful monitoring, appropriate interventions, and patient support. While maintaining a healthy weight can be challenging, the potential benefits are substantial.

20.6 TOBACCO CESSATION

It was 1964 when the first Surgeon General's report identified that smoking cigarettes was harmful to the human body.[30] At that time it is safe to presume that no one thought in the year 2020 there would still be discussion about smoking. Yet today statistics show approximately 14% of Americans are regular smokers. In the last 15 years, the United States has seen a substantial decline in smoking rates. In 2005, nearly 21% of Americans reported to be current smokers, defined as those who currently use cigarettes every day or nearly every day and have smoked at least 100 cigarettes over their lifetime.[31]

It is known that many people who do not consider themselves to be smokers do use other products such as electronic cigarettes or vapes or various forms of smokeless tobacco or smoke occasionally rather than daily. When assessing for tobacco use, it is important to ask about all potential forms of consumption and frequency of use.

The Brief Tobacco Intervention has been described as the most effective initial way to address tobacco use. All clinicians are busy and this method is beneficial as it only takes a few minutes to employ. Evidence has shown that even minimal interventions increase tobacco abstinence rates.[32]

Traditionally, the Brief Tobacco Intervention has been described as the 5 As. This can be further simplified as 2 As and an R. This stands for:

- Ask
- Advise
- Refer

ASK

It is a simple question, "Do you smoke, chew, or use any form of tobacco, vape, or e-cigarette?" The question is simple, but its value cannot be underestimated. What happens if the question is not asked each visit? A patient story will be used to illustrate.

Bill M. established with his primary care provider (PCP) 15 years ago. He was asked at his first visit if he smoked and he said yes. Bill has seen his PCP at least twice per year every year since and has not been asked about his smoking. Bill tells his family and friends that his doctor is OK with him smoking because his doctor knows he smokes, and he never discusses it with him.

As illustrated by the patient case, patients will assume a false sense of acceptance of their smoking behavior if it is not discussed. Often, clinicians do not discuss smoking due to time constraints, fear of confrontation, or thinking that the patient does not want to change. However, evidence proves otherwise. Nearly 80% of smokers want to quit at any given time, they may just not know how or where to start, and they need help. All clinicians have an obligation to help their patients become the healthiest possible and the health benefits of quitting smoking have been documented extensively. Clinicians must take the few minutes necessary to address tobacco use at every visit.

ADVISE

"Quitting smoking is the single most important thing you can do to improve your health and we have some resources to help you." If a patient's chief complaint can be linked to their smoking behavior it further increases the likelihood that they will make a quit attempt.

This is also the perfect opportunity for the clinician to discuss potential medications with the patient. The clinician should speak with them about the effectiveness of NRT. NRT is not a new drug for the patient. It is the one they have been using for however long they have been smoking minus all the tar and toxins that cause the most feared consequences of smoking. Their body has been used to having a dose of this drug multiple times per day. It is nearly physically impossible to go from some frequent use to none overnight. NRT allows the patient the opportunity to wean off the drug. This approach would be recommended with long-term use of any drug. NRT helps decrease cravings and withdrawal. NRT increases the chances of quitting by 60% compared to placebo.[33] This gives the patient more energy to deal with the psychological aspects of quitting without increasing their risk for side effects by trying a new medication.

Most patients may benefit from combination NRT. If they are smoking a pack per day or more, they will likely need more than one form of NRT. For instance, they can wear a patch that offers a slow, steady release of nicotine. Then when cravings get more intense, they can supplement with a fast-acting gum or lozenge. Patients need to be advised proper use of NRT, as often they will not read the directions on the box. If NRT is not used properly, it will not be effective.

NRT pearls:

- Nicotine gum is not like regular gum and it is not meant to be chewed continuously. It is to be broken open with the teeth and then parked between the cheek and gums. If constantly chewed the juices go to the stomach where the pH is too low for the nicotine to be absorbed properly.
- Do not cut patches. The medication is not uniformly distributed throughout the patch.
- Change patch the same time each day.
- Wear patch overnight to decrease morning cravings that tend to be the strongest.

- Having a "slip" and smoking a cigarette is not recommended but does occasionally occur. The average cigarette has 1 to 3 mg of nicotine and the patch is slow release with the strongest patch releasing 21 mg of nicotine over 24 hours. Smoking while wearing a patch is not recommended because it is preserving the "habit" of smoking behavior. A quit date should be set and NRT use should begin after the last cigarette has been smoked.

There are also prescription medications that can be discussed and recommended if appropriate. Varenicline and bupropion are the most common.

REFER

The average clinician is quite busy. The traditional 15 minute visit does not lend itself the opportunity to provide much tobacco cessation counseling. Refer your patient to someone who can spend the extra time with them that they need to be able to put this behind them for good. Look for a Certified Tobacco Treatment Specialist (CTTS) in your area. Many places offer free services for tobacco cessation. Here are some ideas on where to look for tobacco cessation help:

- The national quit line is 1-800-QUIT-NOW. It will help the patient identify resources in their local area as well as phone and internet services. Often, free NRT can be mailed to patients from many agencies providing phone and/or internet counseling.
- Check with your local hospital and county health department to see if counseling services are available.
- Consider pulmonary rehabilitation referral.
- Contact your local free clinic. Chances are they have already done the research and can tell you where your patients can go for tobacco cessation help.
- The National Cancer Institute's website: www.smokefree.gov
- The National Cancer Institute's text-messaging quit smoking program: Smokefree TXT: Text QUIT to 47848
- The Truth Initiative website: BecomeAnEX.org
- The Department of Health and Human Services website: BeTobaccoFree.gov
- The CDC Free Help to Quit Smoking website: www.cdc.gov/quit
- Substance Abuse and Mental Health Services Administration (SAMHSA) National Helpline: 1-800-662-HELP (4357)
- How to Quit Smoking at www.helpguide.org
- How to Quit Smoking or Smokeless Tobacco at www.cancer.org

20.7 VACCINATIONS/IMMUNIZATIONS

A vital part of preventive care is reviewing and recommending immunizations with patients on a regular basis. This brief section will focus on recommendations for adults age 19 and older. The content is based on the 2020 published work of the Advisory Committee on Immunization Practices (ACIP) and approved by the CDC along with many other physician organizations.[34] Please view www.cdc.gov for complete recommendations and contraindications. A few vaccines have been selected for discussion:

1. **Influenza vaccine, inactivated or recombinant:** One dose annually for all adults age 19 and older
2. **Tetanus, diphtheria, pertussis (Tdap or Td):** One dose Tdap for all adults age 19 and older and then Td or Tdap booster every 10 years
3. **Varicella (VAR):** Two doses for adults born 1980 or later; two doses for adults age 50 and older with an additional risk factor or another indication
4. **Zoster recombinant (RZV):** Two doses for adults age 50 and older
5. **Pneumococcal conjugate (PCV13):** One dose for adults age 19 and older with an additional risk factor or another indication; one dose for adults age 65 and older
6. **Pneumococcal polysaccharide (PPSV23):** One or two doses for adults age 19 to 64 depending on indication; one dose for adults age 65 and older

Risk factors, medical conditions, and other indications include pregnancy, immunocompromised state, HIV infection, asplenia, end-stage renal disease, hemodialysis, heart or lung disease, alcoholism, chronic liver disease, diabetes, healthcare personnel, and men who have sex with men.[35]

COMMON CHIEF COMPLAINTS

The goal of preventive medicine is to protect the individual from injury and illness while also promoting a healthy lifestyle. One primary means by which this is accomplished is to address those circumstances that lead to disability and death. A section on common chief complaints in preventive medicine would not be complete without a discussion on the Occupational Safety and Health Administration's "Fatal Four" leading causes of fatalities in the workplace.[36]

APPROACH TO CAUSES OF FATALITIES IN THE WORKPLACE

FALLS

Falls are responsible for 36.5% of all occupationally related deaths and are the leading cause of accidental deaths in the workplace. Falls typically occur when workers fall from a significant height, fall through holes, or have fallen off ladders, roofs, or scaffoldings.

STRUCK BY OBJECTS

Being struck by objects such as the failure of a rigging or the shifting of materials results in 10% of all occupationally related deaths.

ELECTROCUTIONS

Inadvertently coming into contact with overhead power lines, energized circuits, and improperly maintained extension cords and power tools result in 8.6% of accidental workplace deaths.

COMPRESSIVE INJURIES

Employees who are pinned or caught between heavy pieces of machines, devices, or tools account for 2.5% of accidental occupational deaths.

In addition to the fatal four discussed above, other common chief complaints in preventive medicine include:

EYE INJURIES

Eye injuries (Figure 20.1) occur in a variety of settings from homes to industrial laboratories, machine factories, and

INITIAL OCULAR INJURY ASSESSMENT

Identify

Identify the type of ocular injury:
- Penetrating
- Chemical splash
  - Type of chemical
- Exposure to welding arc

↓

Assessment

Assess visual acuity using a conventional Snellen chart.

Optional assessment tools include:
- Reading of newsprint at arms distance
- Finger count
- Perception of light and or color in severe ocular injuries

The assessment should be performed with and without glasses in patients who wear corrective lenses.

A pinhole test can be used to correct for the refractive error in patients with ocular injuries who do not have their glasses.

A pinhole test is performed by having the patient read the Snellen chart while looking through a small hole made in a piece of paper or cardboard. Consider using an 18 g needle to make the hole in the back of a prescription pad or other piece of thin cardboard.

↓

Initial Management

Chemical splash
- Assess ocular pH.
- Initiate ocular irrigation and continue until the pH is neutral.

Foreign body/exposure to welder's arc
- Evaluate with Wood's lamp and fluorescence stain to assess for damage to corneal epithelium.

Figure 20.1 **Algorithm for initial ocular injury assessment.**

agriculture settings. They occur most commonly in adult males between the ages of 20 and 40 years.[37]

Chemical Injuries to the Eyes

- Alkaline substances cause a more severe burn than acids and can rapidly penetrate the globe from the cornea to the retina.
- Despite the chemical, treatment centers around the copious irrigation of the patient's eyes with 1 to 2 L of normal saline until the pH in the conjunctival sac is between 7.0 and 7.3.

Corneal Foreign Bodies

- These injuries are commonly superficial but deep penetration into the globe can result in vision loss.
- Generally these foreign bodies are small pieces of metal, plastic, or wood that result from either not wearing or improperly fitting eye protection when cutting material.
- Tearing, photophobia, and a foreign body sensation will frequently be the patient's presenting complaints.

Ultraviolet Keratitis

- UV keratitis (UVK) results when there is damage to the epithelial layer of the cornea from exposure to UV light.
- UVK commonly occurs from an improper fitting of a welder's safety glasses or face shield that permits the UV light to strike the cornea obliquely.
- A foreign body sensation and photophobia develop 6 to 12 hours post exposure.
- The patient should also be cognizant if they detect UV light in their peripheral vision and promptly change their protective glasses.

Prevention of Eye Injuries

Prevention is centered around the wearing of properly fitting eye protection that is appropriate for the task being performed.

Be cognizant if the eye protection does not afford the proper level of protection required for the task (e.g., defective or poorly fitting).

Know the location of all eye wash stations.

MUSCULOSKELETAL INJURIES

MS injuries can be classified as any injury that affects the muscles, nerves, blood vessels, ligaments, and tendons. MS injuries can result from a variety of mechanism that include lifting heavy objects, bending, reaching overhead, pushing and pulling heavy loads, working in awkward positions, and repetitive motions. Common MS injuries include but are not limited to[38]:

- Carpal tunnel syndrome
- Tendinitis
- Rotator cuff injuries
- Lateral and medial epicondylitis
- Muscle strains and sprains

Prevention

- Use proper body mechanics when lifting.
- Do not attempt to lift heavy objects alone. Seek assistance of coworkers and use a lifting device to lift heavy objects.
- Reposition worktables to eliminate the need for long excessive reaching.
- Avoid activities or tasks that require frequent repetitive motion.
- Wear appropriate protective equipment (e.g., hard hats, steel toe boots).
- Avoid repetitive overhead work.

HEAT-RELATED INJURIES

A majority of heat-related injuries and fatalities occur within the first few days of heat exposure because the individual has not been given adequate time to acclimatize to the hot environment. Lack of acclimatization represents a major risk factor for fatal outcomes related to exposure in hot environments. Risk factors for a heat-related injury are[39]:

- Obesity
- Diabetes
- High blood pressure
- Heart disease
- Lower levels of physical fitness
- Certain medications such as diuretics, psychiatric, and high blood pressure medications
- Alcohol and illicit drug use

Prevention

- Provide for gradual exposure to the heat for those individuals who are not used to the hot climate
- Regular consumption of cool electrolyte-containing beverages.
- Frequent breaks in cool shady environments
- Wear light-colored nonrestrictive clothing

COLD-RELATED INJURIES

The development of cold-related injuries is dependent on the ambient temperature, length of time exposed to the temperature, and wind speed. Cold stress can present in a variety of ways.[40]

Hypothermia

Hypothermia is a progressive lowering of the body's core temperature. Shivering will be seen with mild hypothermia (core body temperature at 95 °F), whereas moderate to severe hypothermia is manifested by mental status changes, loss of consciousness, and eventually death.

Frostbite

Frostbite occurs when exposed parts of the body freeze from exposure to cold environment. This can occur with temperatures above freezing due to the wind chill. Symptoms progress from numbness and redness to the development of painful blisters when the affected body part has been rewarmed.

Trench Foot

Trench foot is a nonfreezing injury to the feet and is due to prolonged exposure to wet cold environments. Symptoms progress from wet macerated tissue to redness, swelling, and blister formation.

Prevention of Cold Stress

- Know the symptoms and monitor yourself and those around you.
- Dress in layers.
- Ensure your footwear is waterproof and insulated.
- Keep your head covered.
- If you become wet, change your clothes.
- Use moisture-wicking socks against the skin of your feet to direct sweat away from the skin.
- Change your socks if they become wet.

KNOWLEDGE CHECKS

1. Similar components can help with the prevention of cardiovascular disease, obesity, osteoporosis, and cancer. Discuss the similar components.
2. Smoking cessation can be the single most effective change that can improve one's health. How can clinicians help patients with smoking cessation?
3. Discuss where to find evidence-based recommendations regarding vaccinations and immunizations.
4. Discuss the Occupational Health and Safety Administration's "Fatal Four" injuries that result in fatalities in the workplace.
5. Discuss the nonmodifiable risk factors for osteoporosis.

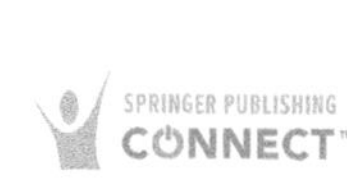

A robust set of instructor resources designed to supplement this text is located at **http://connect.springerpub.com/content/book/978-0-8261-8243-2.** Qualifying instructors may request access by emailing **textbook@springerpub.com.**

REFERENCES

The complete reference list for this chapter appears in the digital version of the chapter, accessible at https://connect.springerpub.com/content/book/978-0-8261-8243-2/chapter/ch20.

CHAPTER 21

ABUSE AND VIOLENCE IDENTIFICATION

THOMAS BALGA

LEARNING OBJECTIVES

- Distinguish between abusive injuries and accidental injury patterns in infants and children.
- Understand the concept of the sentinal injury and review common sentinel injuries.
- Review the inherent challenge to recognition of abusive injuries.

INTRODUCTION

The topic of abuse is something that cannot be confined to one organ system or patient visit type. Child abuse, domestic violence, elder abuse, and sexual abuse are serious and preventable public health problems that affect millions of people. Clinicians across all disciplines need to be well informed on the signs and symptoms of abuse in patients across the lifespan. The approach to the patient history and physical examination will vary based on the patient's age, type of abuse suspected, and practice setting. However, there are specific steps that clinicians can follow to ensure comprehensive and compassionate care to their patients when faced with these difficult situations.

21.1 CHILD MALTREATMENT

OVERVIEW

Child maltreatment includes all types of abuse and neglect of a child under the age of 18 by a parent, caregiver, or another person in a custodial role (e.g., clergy, coach, teacher) that results in harm, potential for harm, or threat of harm to a child.[1]

The U.S. Centers for Disease Control and Prevention (CDC) defines child maltreatment as "any act or series of acts of commission or omission by a parent or other caregiver that results in harm, potential for harm, or threat of harm to a child."[1] Child maltreatment refers to acts of *commission* (deliberate or intentional inflicted injury referred to as child abuse or nonaccidental trauma [NAT]) or *omission* (failure to provide for a child's needs resulting in harm or injury referred to as neglect) in children under 18 years of age.[1] The CDC's *Child Maltreatment Surveillance: Uniform Definitions for Public Health and Recommended Data Elements*[1] is recommended to enable more accurate incidence monitoring

More than 3 million children are estimated to be victims of abuse each year.[2] Child abuse takes many forms including neglect (61%), physical abuse (10.3%), sexual abuse (7.2%), emotional abuse (2.4%) and medical child abuse (0.9%), other threatened abuse, or parental substance use (2.7%).[3]

Clinicians are responsible for having a cognitive awareness of child abuse, maintaining this on their differential diagnosis, and reporting it to Child Protective Services (CPS) if suspected.

Child abuse has a significant lifelong impact on victims resulting in increased rates of depression, suicidal behaviors, and substance abuse.[4] Child abuse also has a significant impact for society, resulting in an increased use of social and healthcare services. Victims of child abuse have a lower quality of life and a higher risk of premature death.[5]

EPIDEMIOLOGY

Approximately 25% of children experience some form of child abuse or neglect in their lifetime. Approximately 40 million children worldwide are victims of abuse and neglect annually.[6] In the United States, an estimated 656,000 children were classified as victims of maltreatment in 2019, a rate of 8.9 victims per 1,000 children, resulting in an estimated 1,840 deaths from maltreatment, or a rate of five deaths each day. Boys have a higher child fatality rate than girls and the youngest of children are at the greatest risk, with 45.4% of deaths from child abuse occurring among infants and 70.3% of all child abuse fatalities occurring in children <3 years old (Figure 21.1).[3] Approximately 30% of children who sustained serious injuries or died had been previously seen and evaluated by a clinician, often in EDs.[7]

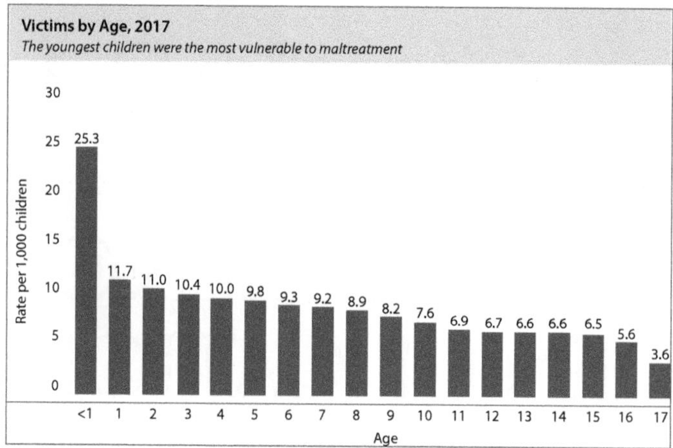

Figure 21.1 2017 Child Protective Services data.
(Source: U.S. Department of Health & Human Services, Administration for Children and Families, Administration on Children, Youth and Families, Children's Bureau. Child Maltreatment 2019. *U.S. Department of Health & Human Services; 2021:Exhibit 3–F. https://www.acf.hhs.gov/sites/default/files/documents/cb/cm2019.pdf*

DEFINITION OF PHYSICAL ABUSE

Physical abuse may be defined as any physical action ranging from those that leave no physical bruise on the child to those causing permanent disability, disfigurement, or death. Physical abuse is the use of physical force, such as hitting, kicking, shaking, burning, or other acts of force against a child. Even minor bruising should be taken seriously and further investigated by the clinician.

Infants are the highest risk group for physical abuse and their vulnerability is related to their small size, ability for infants to be hidden from society, and having disproportionally large heads (approximately one-fourth of the body length). Infants are at greatest risk injury from shaking, because they a have larger head size compared with the size of their body and poor neck strength. Rapid repetitive flexion, extension, and rotation cause greater movement of the large head resulting in possible rotational and impact injuries. When impact of the head occurs against an object, additional injuries such as bruising, lacerations, and fractures can result. Even impact against soft objects can result in significant injury.[8]

Another significant risk for abuse in infants is crying, which peaks at about 6 to 8 weeks of age. Additional pediatric risk factors include prematurity, disability, adoption, hyperactivity, and precociousness.

Triggering Events

Some triggering events for child abuse include crying, toileting, and soiling. Caretakers may have unrealistic adult expectations of the child's behavior and may lack understanding of children's needs and child development stages.

THE PERPETRATOR

Most child abuse occurs within the child's own home. A perpetrator is someone who is responsible for the abuse or neglect of a child. In the United States in 2019, over 525,000 perpetrators were reported; women accounted for more than half (53%) of perpetrators. The largest percentages of perpetrators are White (48.9%), African American (21.1%), or Hispanic (19.7%). The majority of perpetrators (83%) are in the age group of 18 to 44 years old and 77.5% of perpetrators are a parent of their victim.[3] There is no single profile of a child abuser; most child abuse results from a loss of impulse control and may be a one-time incident.

Confession

Confessions, or partial confessions with justification, made by the perpetrator are exceedingly rare. A perpetrator may say "I shook him, but it was to resuscitate him." A perpetrator may say "I did hit him, but it wasn't hard, and it was to discipline him."

INITIAL MEDICAL EVALUATION

Physical Abuse: Recognition

The approach to managing children with possible abuse is a cognitive challenge for clinicians. Unlike other disease processes that a clinician may manage in the pediatric patient, in cases of child abuse, the patient's caretakers may not necessarily act in the best interest of the child, even if they are not personally responsible for the injuries.

The chief complaints in physically abused children are often the usual medical complaints (80% of cases) such as alerted mental status, apnea, fussiness, vomiting, seizures, and BRUE.

BRUE (brief resolved unexplained event) is an episode the occurs in infants when the observer reports a sudden, brief resolved episode lasting <1 minute associated with at least one of the following: (1) pallor or cyanosis; (2) absent, decreased, or irregular breathing; (3) change in muscle tone; (4) altered level of responsiveness.

During the evaluation of a child with suspected maltreatment, the clinician must consider an alternative explanation such as an unintentional injury, NAT, or a medical cause. A careful and detailed history leading to the child's present condition is of utmost importance.

Electronic Medical Record Chart Review

It is important to use the electronic medical record (EMR) effectively and review the EMR for previous ED visits, social work notes, previous CPS involvement, frequent canceled appointments, or history of prior domestic violence.

History

When taking a medical history in these high-risk cases, it is important that the information obtained is accurate as being told and documented. A history should include a detailed story of what happened, who was present at the time of the event, and who witnessed the event. Additionally, history taking should include who decided to bring child for medical care and who was home when the event occurred. Another possibly insightful question to ask is, "Who called 911 and was there a delay?"

In general, concerning "red flag" histories for a patient with a serious injury include:

1. No history of trauma (e.g., "we do not know what happened," or "we just noticed the bruise")
2. Injuries that occur around toileting and around disciplinary events
3. An injury mechanism inconsistent with the infant's development and/or age
4. Changing or evolving history by the same source over time
5. Story discrepancies between different sources
6. An injury is attributed to the child (self-inflicted, e.g., "she hits her head in the crib at night"), a pet or sibling, or resuscitation or treatment efforts after the injury.
7. Mechanism does not match injury. For example, short vertical falls are defined as falls from approximately 1 to 4 feet; these falls rarely cause severe head trauma or multiple injuries.

8. Consider the evaluation of a 3-month-old who presents to the ED for evaluation of unexplained bruises. Historical questions to ask:

Key history:

- When was the child last behaving normally?
- Who were the caretakers at the time of injury?
- Who was home when the episode occurred?
- Who brought the patient to be seen?
- If 911 was called who placed the call?

It can be helpful to "create a mental video" by eliciting details of exactly what happened at the scene just before, during, and after the event.[9]

The past medical history (PMH) should also be reviewed including birth, underlying medical problems, and vaccination status. A prior history of an unexplained death of a child in the household is also risk factor for abuse.

In general, the clinician must exercise caution when using parental behavior as a factor during the evaluation of possible abuse. However, some suspicious parental behavior such as agitation and aggression may be taken in consideration. Other concerning behaviors may include an observed lack of emotional interaction between caretaker and child or an inappropriate response to a serious traumatic injury.[10]

When evaluating an injured child, it is imperative that the clinician hears what has occurred directly from the caretakers who witnessed the event. Clinicians should avoid interrupting caretakers as they present the given history of events leading to the child's injuries. Once the history has been obtained, clarifying questions may be asked. Asking caretakers to demonstrate what happened can be helpful and informative.

While the lack of appropriate explanation for a child's injury is concerning for abuse, a breakdown in communication can occur in several different ways. Inconsistent histories may be presented when different people ask questions in various ways. Occasionally, members of the healthcare team ask leading questions that encourage a desired answer. Other times, family members and caretakers may not fully understand the question secondary to language barriers. It is important to use interpreter services for non-English speaking families to ensure accurate understanding of questions.

Obtaining a careful social history is important when evaluating an injured child. Social history provides insight into the child's environment, which should be assessed for strengths and weaknesses. Social risk factors include domestic violence, substance abuse, psychiatric illness, criminality in household, young age of parents, and history of abuse in the household or prior CPS involvement; frequently, victims of fatal abuse were already known to CPS.

Interview of the Child

Children innately try to please adults. Consequently, clinicians should take steps to ensure they do not unintentionally influence the interview when having a discussion with the child. If at all possible, caregivers should step out of the room during this process as parents and other caregivers can easily influence the child with both nonverbal and verbal communication.

When interviewing school age children or older, the clinician should inform the child that it is okay for them to simply say "I don't understand the question" if they do not understand what they are being asked. The child should also be informed that that it is okay for them to simply say "I don't know" if they do not know the answer to a question. Additionally, children generally respond to positive body language, which can impact what the child discloses. Conversely, negative body language such as crossing one's arms or leaning back could have the opposite effect. It is best for the clinician to be aware of their body language and attempt to communicate neutral body language, particularly during the interview. If possible, each caretaker should be interviewed separately. While forensic evaluation can later be obtained by trained investigators, the data gathered during an initial visit generally guides and informs further investigation. It is important for the clinician to clearly state their role as the patient's advocate and to inform parents that abuse can occur without any physical findings.

Teamwork and Effective Communication

The process of evaluating and managing a child for suspected abuse is complicated and requires a multidisciplinary approach including emergency medical services (EMS), child abuse pediatricians (CAPS), social workers, radiologists, hematologists, surgeons, ophthalmologists, child abuse and neglect advocates, and other specialists.

Poverty, mental health, and substance abuse are the most common risk factors for child maltreatment and neglect; however, this can often cause bias and stereotyping by clinicians. It is important to remember that abuse can occur in any social or economic group and that clinicians must remain objective. Many abusers know what to say when prompted to mitigate suspicion; clinicians must be cognizant of this and aware that families that appear to be kind and loving can still cause harm. The clinician should remember the red flags and practice diligence when examining every patient.

PHYSICAL EXAMINATION

Recommend changing all children <6 years of age into gowns. Ensure proper lighting and an assistant if possible:

- Address airway, breathing, circulation (ABCs).
- **Signs of altered mental status:** Agitation, irritability, somnolence, evaluate verbal communication: slow response, repetitive questioning
- **Pediatric Glasgow coma scale (GCS) score:** Patients <2 years of age
- **GCS score:** Patients >2 years of age
- Vital signs on all children (rectal temperature under the age of 6 months)
- Evaluate for bulging fontanelles.
- Look for signs of basilar skull fracture such as retroauricular bruising (Battle sign), periorbital bruising (raccoon eyes), hemotympanum, cerebrospinal fluid otorrhea, or cerebrospinal fluid rhinorrhea.
- **Eye examination:** Eyelid injuries, subconjunctival hemorrhage, retinal hemorrhages
- Intraoral injuries, frenulum
- **Palpate for skull fractures:** Are there step-offs or crepitus of the skull? Are there any depressions of the skull?
- **Note any scalp hematomas:** Document swelling, size, location, and texture
- **Note any neurologic deficits:** Cranial nerves, sensation, reflexes[11]
- Chaperone for all genitourinary (GU) examinations
- Palpate all extremities, log roll the patient with your team, and palpate the entirety of the spine.

Bruising

Bruising is the most common manifestation of physical abuse and is often not appreciated or seen by the clinician.

Pre-mobile infants rarely sustain bruising.[12] Any bruising in an infant has high predictive significance and it is paramount to consider the developmental ability of the bruised child. More than three bruises from a single reported injury, bruising on opposite sides of the body, and associated petechiae should all increase suspicion. Careful inspection behind the head and neck including the postauricular and preauricular region is paramount. Examination should also include detailed inspection of the entire torso with a chaperone at the bedside.

Sentinel Injury

A sentinel injury is an injury that was reported to have been visible to at least one parent before the events leading to the current admission and was suspicious for abuse because the child was not mobile or there was an implausible explanation offered.[13] Sentinel injuries are otherwise relatively minor injuries that are suspicious for abuse and may serve as a warning to the clinician of subsequent abusive events. The following four questions can be used to screen children at risk for abuse:

1. **Location of bruising is important:** Is there bruising to the T-E-N (torso, ears, neck) or F-A-C-E-S (frenulum, angle of jaw, cheek [soft part], eyelids, sclera-subconjunctival) regions?
   i. **TEN-4-FACESp**
   ii. Any bruising in infants **4 months old and younger**
   iii. "FACES" bruising
   iv. **p** for patterned injuries in children 4 years of age and younger[14]
2. Is there bruising anywhere on an infant 4 months of age and younger?
3. Does the bruising or petechiae form any geometric shape or recognizable pattern?
4. Has a clear, developmentally consistent, and plausible story been provided that accounts for all of the child's injuries?

DIAGNOSTIC STUDIES

When evaluating concerns for physical abuse and bruising, laboratory analysis on the initial workup should include a complete blood count, platelet count, prothrombin time, partial thromboplastin time, von Willebrand factor antigen and factor VIII, factor IX, and liver function tests (LFTs). When preforming cardiopulmonary resuscitation on any child, especially in infants, consider trauma and toxicology causes. Toxicology levels should be obtained including fentanyl and Suboxone levels, which may need to be ordered separately.

21.1A ABUSIVE HEAD INJURY

Abusive head trauma (AHT) is the leading cause of fatal injuries in children <2 years of age. AHT is a revised nomenclature of "shaken baby syndrome," defining the cranial and brain pathology resulting from blunt trauma, shaking forces, or combined mechanisms.[15] AHT is a severe type of inflicted head injury that includes cranial, intracranial, and spinal injuries. Infant crying can lead to parental frustration and is the most common reported trigger by caregivers to shake an infant.[16] Infant crying peaks around 6 weeks, but AHT can occur at any stage of development. Children with a severe head injury and no history of trauma, a history of "low-impact" trauma, or severe head injury blamed on "home resuscitation efforts" or siblings should all raise suspicion for abuse.[17]

ETIOLOGY

Risk factors for AHT may include situations that involve the child, the family, and the caregiver. Abusive pediatric head trauma most often begins with anger and frustration over a screaming, inconsolable infant. Colic is a risk factor. Infant crying is greatest at 6 to 8 weeks of age and then declines. As a consequence, AHT peaks during this same period. The crying infants are at risk of a frustrated caregiver responding with violent shaking.

MEDICAL HISTORY AND CLINICAL PRESENTATION

The clinical manifestations of AHT vary with age, mechanism, and injury types. Clinical features may include an array of neurologic clinical signs including irritability, altered mental status, seizures, and coma. Clinician lack of confidence and overall discomfort with the evaluation of child abuse can contribute to the incorrect diagnosis. Up to one-third of AHT victims have evidence of a previous injury not initially recognized as inflicted; they may subsequently suffer a more severe or fatal injury.[18] Children with AHT may present with "occult symptoms" such as respiratory distress, emesis, poor feeding, macrocephaly, syncope.[19,20] AHT can cause other injuries of many other systems including integumentary, skeletal, and renal. Children with head injury, including small subdural hemorrhages (SDHs) or subarachnoid hemorrhages can be nontoxic appearing.

SIGNS AND SYMPTOMS

Clinicians may not recognize the signs and symptoms due to frequent lack of external signs of AHT (Box 21.1).

BOX 21.1 Signs and Symptoms of Abusive Head Trauma

- Apnea
- Altered mental status
- Bulging fontanel
- Bradycardia
- Cardiovascular collapse
- Decreased interaction
- Decreased level of consciousness
- Emesis
- Failure to thrive
- Hypothermia
- Irritability
- Increased sleeping
- Lack of a social smile
- Lethargy
- Microcephaly, Macrocephaly
- Poor feeding
- Respiratory distress and respiratory arrest
- Seizure

Skull Fractures

If available, three-dimensional (3-D) reconstruction of cranial CT images increase the likelihood of visualizing skull fractures and should be used whenever available. If a small skull fracture is noted on CT 3-D reconstruction that otherwise might not be seen on standard CT image, a skeletal survey may be necessary. Findings more consistent with an unintentional etiology include unilateral, linear skull fracture without intracranial injury or linear skull fracture with only a contact intracranial injury. Nonlinear skull fractures are more concerning for abuse as these fractures involve greater translational or linear forces.

Intracranial Injuries

Intracranial hemorrhage is one of the characteristic features of AHT. These hemorrhages can occur when the bridging veins are disrupted from angular (rotational) deceleration forces; infants are more vulnerable to these types of forces.

Subdural Hemorrhage

SDHs are the main feature of the AHT triad which includes retinal hemorrhage, encephalopathy, and SDH. SDH is described as the most common intracranial pathology in infants and toddlers; SDH appears in approximately 81% of cases of confirmed AHT.[21]

Subarachnoid Hemorrhage

Subarachnoid hemorrhages can be subtle and difficult to detect as they can be located on the interhemispheric region of the brain. Subarachnoid hemorrhages occur in nearly all fatal cases of inflicted head trauma. However, subarachnoid hemorrhages are also common in unintentional head trauma.

Epidural Hemorrhage

Epidural hemorrhage indicates bleeding in the space between the inner surface of the brain and the dura. Epidural hemorrhage is much more commonly associated with unintentional head trauma than AHT. Short falls (<4 feet) are the typical mechanism of injury.

DIAGNOSTIC STUDIES

Recognizing AHT in mild forms can be challenging and missing the diagnosis could have devastating consequences. The Pittsburgh Infant Brain Injury Score (PIBIS) developed by Dr. Rachel Berger may be able to assist clinicians in the evaluation of infants at increased risk for AHT that would benefit from a head CT scan (Table 21.1). Some of the findings that can be seen in traumatic brain injury (TBI) on CT neuroimaging include cerebral edema, traumatic infarction, diffuse axonal injury, shearing injury, and skull fractures. Midline shifts and signs of brain herniation can also be seen on CT imaging. Because of the frequency of spinal cord injuries in children with AHT, total spine MRI is recommended in patients with suspected abuse head trauma.

Table 21.1 Pittsburgh Infant Brain Injury Score for Abusive Head Trauma

Variable	Points
Abnormality on dermatologic examination	2
Age ≥3.0 mo	1
Head circumference > 85th percentile	1
Hemoglobin <11.2 g/dL	1

21.1B FRACTURES

MEDICAL HISTORY AND CLINICAL PRESENTATION

Fractures are a common finding in pediatrics; however, it is important to consider the mechanism of injury, timing, severity, and chronologic age of the child. Distinguishing NAT fractures from unintentional injury fractures can be challenging secondary to large variation in fracture type and location. Similar to any evaluation for traumatic injuries, a detailed presenting history is a key component. Fractures are the second most common type of sentinel injuries in physical abuse.

Fractures in any stage of healing are concerning for abuse. Several types of fracture have a higher specificity for physical abuse including rib fracture and classic metaphyseal lesions.[21]

PHYSICAL EXAMINATION

Rib Fractures

Rib fractures, especially posteromedial, are concerning for abuse in any age child, but especially infants. In cases of physical abuse, rib fractures occur as a result of the infant being squeezed by the perpetrator, generating anterior-posterior compressive forces. Accidental rib fractures in infants are uncommon. Clinicians should have a high index of suspicion for NAT in infants or young children without an accidental traumatic mechanism.

Classic Metaphyseal Lesions

Classic metaphyseal lesions (CMLs), also called bucket-handle fractures, are fractures around the growth plate and are generally considered diagnostic for child abuse when visualized in infants. CML fractures occur through the primary spongiosa of the distal metaphysis of long bones. CMLs occur from shearing and twisting forces and may involve the proximal humerus, distal radius, distal tibia, proximal tibia, and distal femur.

The timing of the skeletal survey is vital because CMLs will heal over time and may not be visualized on an x-ray. If a CML is noted on skeletal survey, a repeat focused skeletal survey should be obtained in 2 weeks to see if it has resolved. If it is no longer visualized on x-ray, that is concerning for CML and abuse. If a suspicious finding is appreciated again on the repeat skeletal survey, it is suggestive to be either congenital or a normal variant.

Other Fractures

Other fractures with a high specificity for abuse include scapular fractures, spinous process fractures, and sternal fractures.

Fractures with a moderate specificity for abuse include multiple fractures (especially bilateral), fractures of different ages, epiphyseal separations, vertebral body fractures, digital fractures, and complex skull fractures.

DIFFERENTIAL DIAGNOSIS

The differential diagnosis of fractures in young children includes accidental, abuse, birth injury, and increased bone fragility.

Laboratory analysis to consider for the evaluation of fractures includes level of calcium, phosphorus, alkaline phosphate, 25-hydroxyvitamin D, and parathyroid hormone levels.

DIAGNOSTIC STUDIES

A skeletal survey is mandatory for any patient under the age of 2 years when abuse is being considered. If the institution does not have a standardized approach to obtaining skeletal surveys, the child should be transferred to a facility that does. The skeletal survey includes chest anteroposterior and lateral, skull including lateral, upper arms, forearms, hands, pelvis, upper legs, lower legs, ankles, and feet. The skeletal survey should be performed by two pediatric radiologists who read the images individually and then review them together. A follow-up skeletal survey should be obtained 2 weeks after the first set. In cases concerning for physical abuse, complete skeletal survey is also recommended for all children under the age of 24 months in the household, especially on twin infants.

21.1C ABUSIVE ABDOMINAL INJURIES

MEDICAL HISTORY AND CLINICAL PRESENTATION

The evaluation for occult abdominal and pelvic injury is an integral part of any abuse evaluation. Children with inflicted abdominal injuries may have other findings of abuse including head injuries and fractures.

PHYSICAL EXAMINATION

Physical examination alone is unlikely to be adequate to detect abusive abdominal injuries as vomiting and fussiness maybe the only presenting features of acute abusive abdominal injuries. Inflicted blunt trauma to the abdomen may be caused by a perpetrator kneeling on a child, resulting in visceral injuries without cutaneous findings.[10]

DIAGNOSTIC STUDIES

Abdominal laboratory analysis, including LFTs, aspartate aminotransferase (AST), and alanine aminotransferase (ALT) in every child <5 years of age is recommended for evaluation of occult injury. Children who present with an elevated liver transaminase >80 IU/L should be evaluated by advanced imaging for possible occult abdominal trauma. These patients have a likelihood of about 20% of positive findings on CT scan. The focused assessment with sonography for trauma (FAST) examinations should be obtained in patients with possible trauma; however, pediatric FAST examinations do have a false negative rate of approximately 41.2%.[23] CT imaging remains the gold standard for a diagnosis of intra-abdominal injury, which should be used judiciously with consideration of risk secondary to radiation-induced malignancy later in life.[24]

21.1D BURN INJURIES

MEDICAL HISTORY AND CLINICAL PRESENTATION

Pediatric burns are a common type of physical abuse. The evaluation and management of pediatric burns can be complex, and children have a high risk of recurring abuse unless there is intervention. Many pediatric burns are a result of inadequate adult supervision; they can also result from child maltreatment. Worldwide, a child dies from burn accidental and abusive injuries every 5 minutes.[25,26] Nonfatal burns far outnumber fatal burns, and they area leading cause of morbidity often resulting in long-term physical, psychological, and financial repercussions.[26]

Approximately 20% of pediatric burn admissions are secondary to physical abuse. In the United States, scald burns are the leading cause of burn injury in small children, and scalds represent 70% of hospitalized burns in children <5 years of age.[27] Children are especially susceptible to burn injury due to their thin and delicate skin. Young children are also more at risk for accidental burns as they are mentally inquisitive and physically unstable and may sustain burn-related injuries after having applied downward traction on cords in the kitchen.

SIGNS AND SYMPTOMS

Burn Patterns

Inflicted burns often leave characteristic patterns that can distinguish them from accidental burns. These characteristic patterns include doughnut pattern in buttocks, burns that spare soles of feet, stocking glove pattern, and skin waterline mark. An isolated accidental cigarette burn can occur, and these tend to be superficial and not annular. Attention to detailed physical examination is important. Is the child able to give a detailed history consistent with the caretaker's explanation?

Purposeful inflicted "branding" usually reflects the objects that were used to cause the burn such as curling irons or cigarettes. Inflicted cigarette burns are usually deeper injuries, often in multiple locations, than accidental cigarette burns they also occur in areas of the body where accidental burns; would be unlikely. Cigarette burns may be confused with infectious processes such as impetigo. Cigarette lighters have a characteristic burn pattern.[28] It is important to remember that most modern lighters have a safety switch that may be difficult for young children to release resulting in a self-inflicted burn.

Splash Burns

Splash burns commonly involve liquid falling from any height onto the patient. This type of injury produces specific burn patterns. These burns tend to be irregular shapes and have various depths of injury. Hot liquid flows with gravity and cools as it travels down;[28] it is cooled by the relatively cool skin temperature. As the flow occurs, it may create an area that tapers down, resulting in an "arrow down" pattern. This pattern is more commonly seen in assaults on adults than in assaults on children.[28] Splash injuries can be accidental or intentional, and clothing can also greatly influence the specific of pattern of burns, so obtaining the article of clothing worn at the time of burn is helpful. For example, thick fabrics may retain heat, thus increasing the severity of injury.

Immersion Burns

Immersion burns are typically bilateral on upper or lower extremities and can have a sharp demarcation between the injured and the noninjured tissue. If a child has been held intentionally in hot water, the buttocks may have been spared as a result being held against an object such as the tub. In contrast, nonabusive immersion burns may have less sharply demarcated borders and may have accompanying splash marks.

It is important to work with the CPS team and ask if they would go to the scene and evaluate the home to see if the history provided is consistent with the dwelling. Reenactment of the event can be very informative and help determine if the history given is accurate.

21.1E SKIN CONDITIONS THAT MAY SIMULATE ABUSE

There are many skin conditions that may simulate abuse. Slate gray nevi, formally known as Mongolian spots, is common; however, they will not be associated with abrasions, swelling, edema, or erythema. Along with the absence of swelling and tenderness, the characteristic coloring and location of dermal melanoses help differentiate them from bruising.[29] Other conditions that may simulate abuse include staphylococcal scalded skin syndrome and phytophotodermatitis. Henoch-Schönlein purpura often presents with purpuric lesions and may at first be confused with bruises. These lesions will have the classic palpable purpura appearance and, unlike bruises, these lesions will be evenly purple.

Cupping and Cao Gio (Coining)

Some ethnic groups have cultural healing practices that can cause skin changes and marking. Two common practices are so-called "coining" and "cupping." Cupping, in which a small glass is heated and then applied to the patient's back, is used to treat various ailments. The process of cooling of the air inside the cup creates a vacuum that causes the cup to adhere to the skin leaving annular erythematous marks, petechiae, or bruises.[30] During the practice of coining, a coin lubricated with oil is rubbed vigorously over the chest and back to treat a fever. These marking will have a petechial appearance secondary to the microtrauma to the skin.

Documentation in Cases of No Concern for Abuse/Neglect

If, after considering the history, social history, physical examination, mechanism, timing, and severity of injury, there is no concern for abuse or neglect, documentation with the phrase "Abuse screen negative" can be completed.

21.1F SUDDEN UNEXPLAINED INFANT DEATH

Sudden unexplained infant death (SUID) can be defined as unexpected, sudden death of an infant that cannot be explained despite a comprehensive investigation including clinical evaluation, social factors, and complete forensic autopsy; SUID typically occurs in infants <6 months. Annually in the U.S, approximately 3,400 infants die suddenly without immediate apparent cause. Approximately half of these deaths are secondary to SUIDS, which is the leading cause of all infant deaths.[31]

With the concept of SUID there is a "triple-risk hypothesis," which offers that infants who die from SUID are born vulnerable with specific brainstem abnormalities and other factors that make them susceptible to sudden death.

SUID triple-risk hypothesis:

1. **Intrinsic risk:** 2 to 4 months critical development period
2. **Vulnerable infants:** Males, Black, exposure to substance abuse, children under CPS supervision, genetic factors
3. **Extrinsic factors:** Exogenous stressors, sleep environment

Some states require reporting all infant deaths to CPS. A prior family history of SUID should raise concern for abuse as the cause of death.

MEDICAL HISTORY AND CLINICAL PRESENTATION

It is commonly reported that the infant had been feeding and appearing well and died during sleep. When discovered by a caretaker, 911 is usually called immediately. Cardiopulmonary resuscitation is started by the caretaker or EMS on arrival and continued into the ED. Typically, there is no meaningful return to spontaneous circulation and the infant is pronounced dead.

If there is a return of spontaneous circulation (ROSC) then the etiology is abuse until ruled out. Infants who have been intentionally suffocated will usually not have any signs of oral facial trauma. In the presentation, pulmonary emphysema and conjunctival hemorrhage may be a sign of inflicted or accidental asphyxiation. In these cases, it is critical to work in collaboration with CPS, law enforcement, and the medical examiner to determine an accurate cause of death. CPS will evaluate the welfare of surviving siblings and create a safety plan for siblings.[32] Unfortunately, children may sustain an opioid ingestion accidentally. Children sometimes are purposely given an opioid or other agent resulting in death of a child. When performing cardiopulmonary resuscitation on any child, consider ingestions and toxicology causes.

PHYSICAL EXAMINATION

The physical examination of a deceased child must include a rectal temperature, which allows the Child Fatality Review Panel to determine estimated time of death. A detailed examination for sentinel injuries should be performed and the medical examiner notified about an infant death. The medical examiner may want to evaluate the infant in the ED directly to evaluate the skin. The process of freezing tissues distorts the appearance of ecchymosis and other important skin findings. In a timely manner, report to CPS any concerns for abuse or neglect and inquire about the welfare of other children in the home.

21.1G NEGLECT

The CDC defines neglect, the most common form of child abuse, as the failure to meet a child's basic physical and emotional needs.[33] These needs include housing, food, clothing, education, and access to medical care. Most state laws and CPS agency definitions focus on caregiver behaviors/omissions that result in actual or potential harm. Poverty, mental health, and substance abuse are the most common risk factors for child maltreatment and neglect. Children with a low socioeconomic status have rates of child abuse and neglect that are five times higher than those of children living in families with a higher socioeconomic status.[33,34]

Failure to attend to obvious signs of illness and failure to follow physician instructions are both types of medical neglect. In cases of pediatric failure to thrive, the differential diagnoses of both physical abuse and neglect should be considered. In children with failure to thrive, a careful, detailed history and comprehensive physical examination should be obtained. Careful detailed caloric intake measurements and direct feeding observations should be assessed. Home visits are essential and may reveal the cause of poor or failed growth.

The goal of the clinician during an encounter is to recognize neglect, clearly document concerns, and involve multidisciplinary teams to manage these complex cases, including CPS if indicated.

21.1H EMOTIONAL ABUSE

Emotional abuse is the deliberate behavior from a caretaker to a child that communicates to the child that they are unwanted, broken, and worthless. Examples include name calling, shaming, rejection, withholding love, and threatening. This may be harder to identify as there are no physical signs of mistreatment.

21.1I FICTITIOUS DISORDER IMPOSED ON ANOTHER

In fictitious disorder imposed on another, formerly known as Munchausen syndrome by proxy, a caregiver fabricates symptoms of an illness in the child, often resulting in complicated medical evaluations and workups. The child may be ill secondary to poisoning in order for the caregiver to assume the "sick role" by proxy.

MEDICAL HISTORY AND CLINICAL PRESENTATION

- **Most apparent:** Poisoning, strangulation, intentional infections
- **Less apparent:** Unnecessary exposure to acceptable risks associated with radiation, anesthesia, hospital infections; must consider necessity of any PORTs as well as possible intentional PORT contamination
- **Much less apparent:** Teaching sick role enactment as a coping strategy

KEY POINTS

- Although decision-making tools such as PECARN are helpful in pediatric head injury patients they should be used with caution in young infants.
- PECARN is a **head injury** prediction rule used to identify children who are very low risk of clinically significant traumatic brain injuries for whom advanced head CT imaging might be not be indicated.[12]
- Ophthalmologists consultation within 24 hours should be obtained.
- Lack of retinal hemorrhages does not exclude nonaccident trauma.

21.2 CHILD SEXUAL ABUSE

OVERVIEW

Sexual abuse may be defined as sexual violence against a child that occurs in the context of a caregiver relationship. It includes any attempted or completed sexual act with, sexual contact with, or exploitation of a child by a caregiver. Sexual abuse may involve inducing or coercing a child to engage in sexual acts. It includes behaviors such as fondling, penetration, and exposing a child to other sexual activities.[1]

During the evaluation for concerns of sexual abuse, the clinician should consider the possibility of false allegations. Family dynamics and child custody issues may need to be taken into consideration during the evaluation.

Sexual assault can occur when victims cannot consent or are incapable of understanding the consequences of their actions because of their age or intellectual capacity.[35]

EPIDEMIOLOGY

According to the U.S. Department of Health & Human Services, 60,927 children were victims of sexual abuse in 2019.[3] This number represents only a fraction of American children who were actually sexually abused. A survey of 1,200 middle and high school students identified that 18% of girls and 12% of boys had an unwanted sexual encounter during their adolescence.[36]

MEDICAL HISTORY AND CLINICAL PRESENTATION

The evaluation and investigation of pediatric sexual abuse include three important components: changes in behavior, medical findings, and disclosure by the child. Unlike other forms of child abuse, the determination of child sexual abuse relies primarily on the child's disclosure. The majority of children who are sexually abused will have no physical complaints related either to trauma or sexually transmitted infection. Most sexually abused children do not report any genital pain or complaints.[37]

Occasionally a child may disclose sexual abuse to a clinician; however, clinicians will much more commonly become aware of a child's disclosure or change in behavior secondhand from a caretaker. When this occurs, the clinician should obtain detailed facts directly from the caretaker regarding the child's behaviors that led to concern about sexual abuse and information about what this child disclosed to the caretaker. It is not usually necessary to obtain disclosure directly from the child. Children often do not disclose their abuse,[38] and physical findings are commonly absent or nonspecific.[39] Children who have been sexually abused are brought to the attention of clinicians usually when a child discloses to an adult that an uncomfortable event occurred.

It is generally recommended that clinicians refrain from questioning a child until they can be interviewed by a specially trained multidisciplinary team using forensic interviewing techniques. Sexual abuse disclosure regarding a child necessitates that a prompt report to CPS be made, even if the clinician is not certain that sexual abuse has occurred. Once reported to CPS, the investigation will be orchestrated by both CPS and local police in order to limit the number of times a child is questioned regarding the alleged sexual abuse. There should be only one coordinated forensic interview. When possible, children who are suspected to have been sexually abused should be evaluated at child advocacy centers or hospital-based child protection programs.

Children who have been sexually abused demonstrate an array of signs, symptoms, and behaviors. These may include sexualized behaviors, poor school performance, anxiety, and depression. One common medical finding presenting for evaluation of sexual abuse is vaginal discharge; however, vaginal discharge has a low likelihood of being secondary to sexual abuse. Sexual abuse of children is occasionally detected in clinical settings as children may present with anogenital findings including stooling issues, bleeding, inflammation, and vaginal discharge.[40]

When evaluating young children, open-ended questions should be used, and the clinician should avoid overinterpreting vague statements.

- Avoid multiple interviews.
- During the evaluation, minimal facts should be included:
  - If the parent reports the event and the child is age 3 or under, no further questioning of the child is necessary.
  - Who is/are the alleged perpetrator? What happened? Where did it happen? If you have this basic information, then it is not necessary to ask the child any questions on the initial evaluation; further information can be acquired during a multidisciplinary forensic interview.
  - If the child must be interviewed for minimal facts, the clinician should inform the parents that the child will be interviewed separately because the child may not discuss what happened in their presence.
  - Do not ask the child why the abuse occurred, as it implies to the child that they are to blame.
  - What are the next steps to protect the child or other victims?
  - Does the alleged perpetrator have access to siblings or other children?
  - Is immediate medical attention necessary? If the abuse took place within 120 hours, a medical examination is necessary to gather evidence. Whenever possible, the examination should be performed by a SANE (sexual assault nurse examiner).

PHYSICAL EXAMINATION

- Sexual assault is not limited to the anogenital region; it is imperative to perform a comprehensive head to toe examination, with detailed skin examination.
- Document any physical injuries including secure medical record photography.
- It is normal to be normal. It is common in sexual assault no have no physical findings. Some forms of abuse such as kissing and fondling do not cause physical injury. Both the hymen and the anus have the ability to stretch without visible injury.
- GU examination: The GU examination should always be chaperoned and documented in the EMR. Secured photos of any injuries can be critical pieces of evidence.
- In the evaluation of suspected sexual abuse, the clinician must be able identify abnormalities secondary to trauma due to sexual abuse versus normal anatomic variation. Anatomically, the hymen can have various normal shapes including annular and crescentic. Other normal variants include hymenal tags or bumps, thickening, or redundant hymen.[42] Nonspecific anogenital findings include anal fissures, vaginal discharge, erythema of vestibule, and perianal erythema.
- Anogenital finding suspicious for abuse include condyloma acuminatum in a child, acute labial abrasions or lacerations, and perianal lacerations.
- Findings suggestive of penetration include acute lacerations or scarring of the posterior fourchette.

21.2A ADOLESCENT SEXUAL ASSAULT

Sexual assault can be described as any nonconsensual sexual act. Sexual assault includes any situation in which nonvoluntary sexual contact occurs secondary to physical force, coercion, or impairment. Nonvoluntary sexual contact includes any nonconsensual touching of the anogenital region or breast.[37] Sexual assault also occurs when someone is impaired or incapacitated secondary to alcohol or drug use. Recreational drug use is common among adolescents and increases the risk for sexual abuse.[41] Alcohol use is the most common substance associated with sexual abuse. Substance abuse immediately before sexual assault has been reported to occur >40% of the time as reported by both adolescent victims and adolescent perpetrators.[42] Substances can also be used intentionally for sedating a victim or decreasing their inhibition. State laws generally define sexual activity as crime when an individual has been coerced or who has impaired decision-making capacity because of intoxication and is unable to consent.[43]

DIAGNOSTIC STUDIES

Clinicians should not force an adolescent to have a sexual assault evidence collection kit performed. Allowing patients to dictate what occurs to their body is humane and may assist in building trust. The forensic evidence collection is not needed medically. If the sexual assault occurred within the time frame to conduct a forensic examination (usually 72 hours to 96 hours following the assault) and the patent permits a forensic examination to be obtained, it may be completed when appropriate. The collection and transportation of specimens need to be coordinated with the sexual abuse response team, healthcare team, and law enforcement to ensure the integrity of the sexual assault kit chain of custody. Documentation of proper chain of custody for DNA evidence is critical to conviction. An attending physician or PA performs a medical screening examination.

TREATMENT

- Victims of sexual assault should be provided with sensitive and efficient care when being treated.
- Treatment goals should include medical care, emotional support, collection of evidence, and prevention of pregnancy and venereal disease in accordance with state statute.

21.2B DRUG-FACILITATED SEXUAL ASSAULT

Informed consent should be obtained when a toxicology collection is conducted. Poison control centers are an excellent resource and can be consulted regarding laboratory analysis and treatment recommendations. There are many different types of "date rape drugs," including ketamine and gamma-hydroxybutyrate (RHB), the most well known of which is a benzodiazepine sedative hypnotic named flunitrazepam (Rohypnol). Drugs such as RHB have short half-life; therefore, the toxicology screening should be performed in a timely manner, possibly even before completing the history and physical examination.[36]

21.2C SEXUALLY TRANSMITTED INFECTIONS

Sexually transmitted infections (STIs) are rare in sexually abused children and adolescents but may occur. When STIs are present, they can be paramount in making the diagnosis of sexual abuse and protecting children.[44] In children,

BOX 21.2 Indications for STI Testing in Possible Sexual Abuse

Child disclosure of sexual abuse
Genital-genital contact
Anal-genital contact
Oral-genital contact
Oral-anal contact
Urogenital discharge
Anal discharge
Unexplained urogenital or anal injury (acute or chronic)
Suspected sexual contact with a perpetrator or partner known to have a sexually transmitted infection
Sibling with a sexually transmitted infection and sexual abuse is a concern

the isolation of a sexually transmitted organism may be the first indicator and at time the only indicator that sexual abuse has occurred. STIs can be confirmed via hepatitis panel, serology for HIV/syphilis, urogenital swabs for *Chlamydia* and gonorrhea. If indicated, a throat swab may be obtained for gonorrhea. The interpretation of STI laboratory analysis can be challenging. *Trichomonas*, condyloma, and herpes simplex virus (HSV) are concerning and suspicious for abuse. However, HSV can be spread by direct contact with a caregiver that is not associated with sexual abuse. Such a caregiver with HSV can transmit to a child through usual direct contact. The human papillomavirus (HPV) causes anogenital warts, which can be diagnosed with detection of the lesion on physical examination. HPV infection can be caused by both sexual and nonsexual transmission.[44] The presence of *Chlamydia*, gonorrhea, syphilis, and HIV transmissible agents beyond the neonatal period is suggestive and concerning for sexual abuse.[44] The evaluation of sexual abuse solely on the basis of suspicion of an STI should proceed with caution until the STI diagnosis has been confirmed. Confirmation of an STI in children requires repeat testing to ensure the initial test result was not a false positive. Consideration should be made to treat for possible HIV exposure after sexual assault in both the prepubertal and adolescent population[44] (Box 21.2).

The CDC prophylactic treatment recommendations for pubertal victims includes ceftriaxone, azithromycin, metronidazole, HIV antiviral postexposure, and emergency contraception.

Sexual abuse can have a significant impact on the patient's mental health resulting in possible depression, suicide, substance abuse, posttraumatic stress disorder (PTSD), and repeat victimization.

21.2D STRADDLE INJURIES

Straddle injuries are the most common genital trauma in females and often cause anxiety because of the location and concern for future gynecologic and sexual development. Straddle injuries can be defined as an injury to the groin from falling on an object that is being straddled such as the bar of a bicycle. Straddle injuries occur when a child hits the perineal region on a solid object resulting in soft tissue injury between object and bony pelvis. When evaluating a child for a straddle injury, obtain detailed history including the beginning, middle, and end of the injury as there should be a consistent story. Girls usually sustain bruising or a laceration of the outer labia. The vagina and urethra are protected by the labia and not harmed. Hymenal injuries are rarely the result of unintentional injury such as accidental straddle injuries. The presence of a hymenal injury is suggestive of sexual abuse.[45]

When assessing straddle injuries, it is important to assess for an expanding hematoma. It is also important to determine if there is any anal or rectal involvement.

Avoid multiple examinations of children with genital trauma.

Most straddle injuries are minor and will heal without intervention.

21.2E SEX TRAFFICKING

There are many factors that contribute to the risk of sexual exploitation of minors (Figure 21.2). In one study of confirmed and suspected victims of domestic minor sex trafficking, 80% reported seeing a clinician within the year prior to their identification as victims. Most presented to EDs (63%), but a significant proportion (35%) presented to a variety of outpatient clinic settings.[46]

Children who are considered runaways are at increased risk of being trafficked and sex trafficking does not require force/fraud/coercion. Additionally, sex trafficking does not require the child be moved from one place to another nor does it require the involvement of a third party ("pimp"). Sex trafficking is when sex is exchanged for something of value.

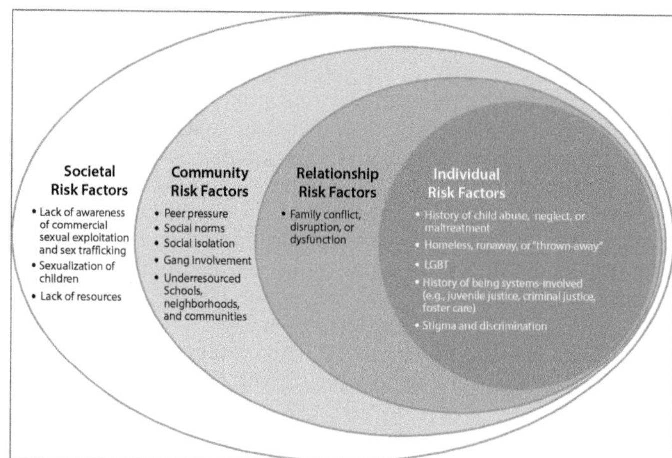

Figure 21.2 **Possible risk factors for commercial sexual exploitation and sex trafficking of minors.** LGBT, lesbian, gay, bisexual, or transgender.

(*Source: Institute of Medicine, National Research Council.* Confronting Commercial Sexual Exploitation and Sex Trafficking of Minors in the United States: A Guide for the Health Care Section. *National Academies Press; 2014. doi:10.17226/18886)*

HISTORY AND PHYSICAL EXAMINATION

Always use medical translators if there is a language barrier. Request that the person accompanying the patient leave to interview the patient alone; if the person refuses or gets angry when asked to leave, insist that it is standard practice. Provide trauma-informed care in a nonjudgmental fashion; remember that patients may not perceive themselves as victims. Commonly the trafficker has built strong bonds with the victim despite abuse so the relationship dynamics can be challenging to navigate.

Indicators of sex trafficking:

- Late presentation
- Poor or inconsistent story
- Signs that patient is being controlled
- Discrepancy between the verbal history and clinical findings
- Lack of official identification documentation
- Signs of physical injuries and abuse
- Avoiding eye contact
- Tattoos or branding that could be subtle or explicit with names or symbols indicating sale or property

If child sex trafficking is suspected, discuss the case with the treating team members before proceeding with the patient's evaluation so that delineation of medical, behavioral health, and safety issues can be done prior to evaluation. The case should be reported to CPS if the patient is <18 years of age and a social worker should be contacted. If the patient is in immediate danger, contact security and local law enforcement.

RISK FACTORS

Risk factors include the elements that entice the victim toward trafficking. Risk factors include young age (12–16 years old) females (at greatest risk), disability, lack of social supports, ethnic/racial minority status. Multiple studies suggest that a history of child abuse is a significant risk factor for later sexual exploitation.

Impact

Almost half of survivors have reported that they have attempted suicide. Victims of sex trafficking have reported infection rate of HIV of 30%–60%. Sex trafficking has significant impact on reproductive health including STIs, pregnancy, pregnancy terminations, and miscarriages. Victims of child sex trafficking are at high risk of numerous physical and behavioral health problems and are likely to seek medical attention. Clinicians are in a unique position to identify high-risk youth, address safety concerns, and offer critical services.[46]

Victim Identification Assessment and Evaluation

During the evaluation of a patient with concerns for trafficking, the clinician may ask direct questions, such as:

- Has anyone ever asked you to trade anything for sex: food, shelter, money, drugs, clothing, or anything else?
- Do you work, live, and sleep all in the same place?
- Do you make decisions for yourself or does someone else make decisions for you?
- Has anyone taken sexual photographs of you?

Obtaining a history from an exploited youth can be challenging. The patient may be evasive, hypervigilant, or hostile while attempting to protect the exploiter. Traffickers use various strategies to build and maintain total control of the victim.[47]

Barriers to disclosure:[48]

- Lack of trust
- Language/cultural translation
- Fear of retaliation
- Lack of trust
- Fear of law enforcement/arrest
- Shame
- Fear of deportation

General medical knowledge of common risk factors and indicators of child sex trafficking informs the clinicians of appropriate questions to consider, but this knowledge alone is insufficient to adequately identify, evaluate, and assist potential victims. Questions must be asked in a trauma-informed, culturally sensitive, victim-centered manner.[49] This "trauma-informed approach" requires skills not usually taught in health professional programs.[46]

TRAUMA-INFORMED CARE

Violent traumatic injuries are commonly treated by clinicians. Patients who are violently injured are disproportionately more likely to have a history of physical and psychological abuse. The adjunct to clinical care, taking into consideration how patients' past experiences affect how they may perceive and react to medical care, is a concept of "trauma-informed care."[50]

Trauma-informed care recognizes the impact of trauma and responds by integrating knowledge about trauma into principles, practices, and organizational culture change, to promotes a culture of safety, empowerment, and healing. The CDC outlines six principles for trauma-informed care:[51]

1. Safety
2. Trustworthiness and transparency
3. Peer support
4. Collaboration and mutuality
5. Empowerment, voice, and choice
6. Cultural, historical, and gender-based issues

The goal is to increase clinician awareness of the impact that trauma has on the patient and communities that they serve. Recognition of traumatic events along with proper intervention can assist in the prevention of lifelong consequences.

KEY POINTS

- It is normal to be normal: most children will have no signs or symptoms.
- Minimal facts must be obtained: Who? What? When?
- It is important to take care of the child medically and emotionally.
- Documentation:
  - What the victim or the perpetrator says should be accurately recorded.
  - Conclusions and general statements do not make good evidence for governmental agencies, law enforcement, or the courts.
  - Specific details of observations are useful. If there is physical evidence of abuse, photographs may be used as evidence. The size, color, and induration of lesions should be documented in the EMR, preferably with

an accompanying drawing when photographs are not possible.

- Sexual assault reporting and legal considerations:
  - Refer to the laws regarding the age of consent within the state where you are practicing. Specific sexual assault reporting requirements for caregivers, clinicians, and law enforcement vary state by state. The age of consent regarding sex also varies by state. Some states mandate that sexual contact between minors be reported if a certain age difference exists between the minor and the sexual partner even if the encounter was consensual.[36]
  - Clinicians who treat adolescents must be aware of the federal and state laws regarding adolescent consent and confidentiality. The way in which adolescents may consent for their own care and in which confidentiality is protected vary from state to state depending upon the adolescent's status as a minor or adult, the service involved, and the clinician's level of concern regarding harm to the patient or others. In some states, children of a given age can consent for medical treatment related to sexual heath without consent of a parent or caregiver.

21.3 ELDER ABUSE, NEGLECT, AND EXPLOITATION

OVERVIEW

Elder abuse is an intentional act, or failure to act, by a caregiver or another person in a relationship involving an expectation of trust that causes or creates a risk of harm to an older adult over the age of 59.[52] Elder abuse is commonly perpetrated by those who have an ongoing relationship that involves an expectation of responsibility toward the victim.

EPIDEMIOLOGY

Elder abuse is common both nationally and internationally, with approximately 5% to 10% of community-dwelling elders.[53] More than 20% of adults living in nursing homes each year are victimized.[54]

Approximately 1 in 20 individuals over the age of 65 experiences abuse or neglect. Abandonment, neglect, self-neglect, psychological abuse, and financial abuse/material exploitation are much more common than physical or sexual abuse. Patients are often victimized by different types of abuse at the same time.

MEDICAL HISTORY AND CLINICAL PRESENTATION

Risk factors for elder abuse include increasing age, functional disability, child abuse within a given population, frailty, social isolation, mental illness, substance abuse, and lower socioeconomic status.[55] Several studies demonstrate that older women are more likely to be victims of abuse than men.[56] Also, having a lower income has been associated with a higher likelihood of emotional, physical, and financial abuse.[56]

Caretaker risk factors for abuse include financial dependence on elder, mental illness, criminality, and substance abuse. Characteristics of perpetrator include being overly attentive to patients and aggressive behaviors, with the majority of perpetrators being spouses or caretakers.

SIGNS AND SYMPTOMS

Clinical signs of elder abuse include unexplained injuries, delays in seeking care, repeated fractures, bruising, and burns. Bruises over 5 cm or on the face, neck, and torso are particularly concerning. Spontaneous fractures can occur in the absence of abuse but should always be evaluated further.

EVALUATION

Patients should be screened individually, away from caregivers. The clinician should obtain a clear understanding of the living arrangements and care structure as well as ask directly about any abuse or maltreatment. Specific questions about the management and access to the patient's finances should also be reviewed.

The clinical presentation of elder abuse can be difficult to identify and varies by type of abuse. Signs may include inadequately explained or unusual locations for skin abrasions, lacerations, bruises, and burns. They could include spiral fractures of long bones and fractures at sites other than the wrist, hip, or vertebrae in a nonalcoholic elderly person. Patients may appear depressed or may note inadequate funds for food or medical care.

Barriers in Recognizing Elder Abuse

Recognizing elder abuse can be challenging. Some of the barriers include failure to recognize signs and symptoms of abuse, desire to trust caretakers, and personal bias. These barriers in recognizing elder abuse/neglect are usually a result of lack of knowledge and training to recognize abuse. Additionally, clinicians should always be aware of personal bias. Be aware of the "nice family"; as humans we have a difficult time understanding how someone who looks like us could do something horrible to an elder.

Neglect

Neglect can be defined as failure to provide for the need and protection of a vulnerable elderly person when such person has an ongoing relationship with the elder and a duty to protect and provide for those needs. Self-neglect is failure of a vulnerable elderly person to provide for their own needs, care and protection. Self-neglect is a failure of the elder to thrive in their environment.[57] This definition excludes elders who have decision capacity regarding self-care and protection who knowingly and freely choose not to provide adequately for such care and protection.[57]

Signs of neglect and abandonment:[58]

- Dehydration, malnutrition
- Untreated bed sores
- Poor personal hygiene
- Unattended or untreated health issues
- Hazardous or unsafe living conditions
- Unsanitary and unclean living condition
- Desertion of an older adult at a hospital, a nursing facility

Exploitation

Financial exploitation should be considered when there is an abrupt change of an elder to pay bills.[59] Another sign of financial exploitation is transfer of property by an elder who lacks decision-making capacity to make such a transfer.[60]

Indicators of financial exploitation:[58]

- Unpaid bills
- Unusual credit card purchases
- Missing money from accounts
- Missing possessions
- Language/cultural translation
- Abrupt changes in a will or other financial documents

Interventions

Elders with intact capacity to consent to protective services may accept or reject offered interventions from adult protection services (APS). If elder victims lack capacity to understand and provide consent, identify and contact the power of attorney (POA) as the court system may be petitioned for emergency or involuntary protective services.

Guardianship

Clinicians are often asked to make determinations of the need for guardianship in cases in which the elders have diminished capacity for self-care and protection. Six key factors are evaluated to determine the need for guardianship:

1. Presence of a medical condition that may produce functional disability
2. Cognitive impairment (short-term memory, communication, attention, executive function)
3. Difficulty involving everyday functioning (ability to provide nutrition, shelter, and safety)
4. Consideration of the individual's values and preferences
5. Risk of harm and level of supervision needed
6. Determination of whether less restrictive alternatives to guardianship are feasible

TREATMENT

Always address basic ABCs (airway, breathing, circulation) first. Similar to pediatric patients, adult patients are required to be in a hospital gown and a thorough physical examination is required. In addition to abuse, always address medical issues as elderly patients can be medically complicated. If an elderly patient declines intervention or treatment, then assess the patient to see if they have decision-making capacity. It may be necessary to contact the POA or family to help facilitate appropriate care. The safety of elderly patients is paramount: If the patient is in immediate danger, they should be admitted to the hospital to ensure patient safety, without visitation if family members are considered harmful.

Intervention

Victims of elder abuse have different situations and may require different types of interventions. One of the most promising responses to elder abuse cases has been the development of multidisciplinary teams. These teams may consist of PAs, nursing, social workers, adult protective services, and law enforcement.[56] These teams may also include ethicist, prosecutors, and civil attorneys.

Duty to Report

All territories and states of the United States including the District of Columbia have enacted laws providing protection of elders found to be neglected, abused, or financially exploited. Clinicians are mandated to report cases to state APS in which they have a reasonable suspicion for elder abuse of community-dwelling elder.[61] In all states and territories, elders in institutional settings are protected by state Long-Term Care Ombudsman Programs, which field complaints and advocate for long-term care elder residents.[62] Clinicians do not have to be certain that elder maltreatment has occurred before making a report to APS. The reporting requirements for elder abuse are not standardized among all states, but reporting is mandatory in most states. Mandatory reporting requires a clinician to report suspected abuse even if a competent elder patient specifically asks that the abuse not be reported.

KEY POINTS

- Elder abuse is very common, affecting 10% of older adult patients.
- Consider screening all elder patients for abuse.
- Elder patients may require admission if there are safety concerns.
- Documentation in the EMR:
  - What the victim and the perpetrator say should be accurately recorded.
  - Conclusions and general statements do not make good evidence for governmental agencies, law enforcement, or the courts.
  - Specific details of observations are useful. If there is physical evidence of abuse, photographs may be used as evidence. The size, color, and induration of lesions should be documented in the EMR, preferably with an accompanying drawing when photographs are not possible.

ADDITIONAL RESOURCES

- For complete list of anogenital findings, please refer to Table 1 of Adams JA, Harper K, Knudson S, Revilla J. Examination findings in legally confirmed child sexual abuse: it's normal to be normal. *Pediatrics.* 1994;94:310–317.
- Thomas Balga interviewing Dr. Andrea Asnes. Sentinel injuries in child abuse. March 28, 2017. https://soundcloud.com/yaleuniversity/thomas-balga-interviewing-dr-andrea-asnes
- Dr. Mary C. Pierce discusses infant bruising and child abuse. https://soundcloud.com/yaleuniversity/infant-bruising-and-child-abuse

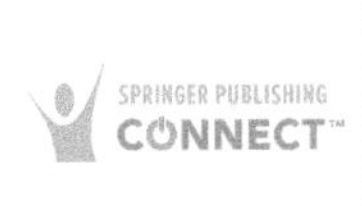

A robust set of instructor resources designed to supplement this text is located at **http://connect.springerpub.com/content/book/978-0-8261-8243-2.** Qualifying instructors may request access by emailing **textbook@springerpub.com.**

REFERENCES

The complete reference list for this chapter appears in the digital version of the chapter, accessible at https://connect.springerpub.com/content/book/978-0-8261-8243-2/chapter/ch21.

CHAPTER 22

SURGERY

KENNETH D. SHERRY AND CHRISTINE BRUCE

LEARNING OBJECTIVES

- Devise a preoperative plan for patients undergoing elective surgery.
- Order and interpret the diagnostic studies that should be done in the preoperative state in order to optimize patient outcomes.
- Design appropriate evaluation for patients with underlying conditions about to undergo elective surgery.
- Manage a patient with cardiovascular or pulmonary conditions planning to undergo elective surgery.
- Describe the presentation and surgical correction of patients with surgically related complaints.
- Differentiate between medical and surgical treatments of patients with various conditions.
- Develop a differential diagnosis for patients with various complaints that may have a surgical remedy.
- Evaluate and treat patients presenting with various complaints that may be addressed in a surgical setting.

INTRODUCTION

PAs play an integral role in the delivery of surgical services in the United States. In addition to serving as first and second assistants in the operating room, they are also highly involved with the preoperative management of patients going to the operating room. In the past, patients were "cleared" prior to going to the operating room but the emphasis today is on medical optimization prior to having the surgery performed. The care of the surgical patient by the PA can therefore occur both in the operating room but also in the preoperative and postoperative management of those patients.

22.1 PREOPERATIVE SURGICAL CARE

OVERVIEW

Preoperative assessment consists of optimizing the patient's medical status prior to undergoing surgical procedure. The extent of preoperative assessment and testing is based upon the patient's current medical condition, past medical history, planned surgical procedure, and the type of anesthesia that the patient will receive. Elective preoperative assessment should be done within 30 days of the planned surgical procedure to medically optimize the patient for the best outcome possible.

Perioperative medicine involves assessing the patient's preoperative risks and ordering and evaluating appropriate preoperative testing to optimize the patient for surgery. The Goldman Index is one such rating index assessing preoperative risk and potential surgical complications. This process also involves communicating with the surgical and anesthesia teams to ensure the patient has the best outcome. Comorbid conditions, risk factors, and potential surgical complications should be recognized and treated prior to surgical intervention. Preoperative planning does not need to be overly aggressive or involve additional cardiology consultations as many of these interventions prolong hospitalization without changing adverse effects.[1–3]

The intent of preoperative evaluation is to lower the risk for major adverse cardiac events (MACE), which increase the risk for morbidity and mortality in adult patients undergoing surgery. This includes the assessment of the functional capacity of the patient with referral for additional testing as needed.[2,3] Complete preoperative care also includes ensuring that patients receive appropriate preoperative antibiotics such as cefazolin, a first-generation parenteral cephalosporin, which provides sufficient antibiotic coverage as prophylactic antibiotics in low-risk for contamination cases.

The type of anesthesia that the patient is to receive is best determined by the anesthesiologist in consultation with the surgeon. There is no evidence that general anesthesia outperforms regional anesthesia in terms of patient outcomes so the type of anesthesia should be determined by the anesthesiologist who will be administering it.[4,5]

DIAGNOSTIC STUDIES

Table 22.1 summarizes preoperative diagnostic testing.

TABLE 22.1 Preoperative Diagnostic Testing

Diagnostic Test	Rationale
Hemoglobin/hematocrit	Obtain a baseline prior to surgery, if the patient has a history of anemia (chronic kidney disease), physical examination findings (pallor or tachycardia), or is anticipated to have a large amount of blood loss during the procedure.
Platelet count	Evaluates platelet quantity. Obtain a baseline if the patient has a history of thrombocytopenia (chronic liver disease) or thrombocytosis. General rule: platelet count <50,000 increases the risk for spontaneous bleeding. Platelet function analyzer better assesses platelet quality.
Coagulation studies	Prothrombin time (PT), activated partial thromboplastin time (aPTT), and international normalized ratio (INR). Patients taking warfarin or other vitamin K antagonists that work on the extrinsic clotting system should be assessed with the PT/INR. Direct oral anticoagulants (DOACs) do not affect the PT or INR and do not readily have laboratory testing to predict their activity. Heparin affects the intrinsic clotting system and is assessed by the aPTT or anti-Xa. Patients with known clotting factor disorders, such as hemophilia or von Willebrand disease (use ristocetin cofactor test), or advanced liver disease should be assessed through coagulation studies.
Comprehensive metabolic panel (CMP)	Provides an overall assessment of electrolytes, blood sugar, renal and liver function. Electrolytes can be abnormal because of underlying medical conditions or because of medications that the patient is taking. Patients with chronic kidney disease typically will have an elevation in potassium, which could predispose to cardiac problems during surgery if not corrected.
Creatinine	Provides an overall assessment of renal function but can be altered if the patient has a low body mass index. Interpretation should be based upon the patient's body habitus so a normal creatinine in an elderly frail patient may not truly indicate normal renal function. Consider evaluating with cystatin C if this is the case.
ALT (alanine transaminase, formerly SGPT) and AST (aspartate aminotransferase, formerly SGOT)	These are transaminases which will be increased in the setting of hepatitis, nonalcoholic fatty liver disease, or any other inflammatory process in the liver. In the setting of alcoholic hepatitis, the ratio of AST to ALT will be 2.0 or higher.
Alkaline phosphatase	Not specific for liver disease because it is also elevated in bone disease, bowel infarction, and cholelithiasis. Marker for cholestasis.
Direct (conjugated bilirubin)	Bilirubin is formed as a result of breakdown of hemoglobin (hemolysis) and is conjugated in the liver and excreted into the bile. Marker of hepatobiliary obstruction.
Indirect (unconjugated bilirubin)	Measurement of unconjugated bilirubin. Marker for hepatobiliary disease and hemolysis.
Urinalysis	Typically only performed when procedure is on the genitourinary system. Asymptomatic bacteriuria is not routinely treated unless it would be detrimental for an infection such as patients undergoing joint replacements or transplantation (to be clear of infection prior to immunosuppression).
Chest x-ray	Not routinely performed unless the patient has known COPD or if they have unexplained respiratory difficulty. Chest films add little value above what is obtained on the patient history and physical exam unless pneumonia is suspected preoperatively.
Electrocardiography (EKG)	Not routinely indicated in asymptomatic patients. Should be performed in patients with known CAD, and may be performed in patients with arrhythmias, peripheral vascular disease, previous stroke, or structural heart disease. EKGs should be compared against previous EKGs to ascertain whether any changes have occurred.
Echocardiography	Echocardiography assesses left ventricular function and calculates an ejection fraction, which is helpful in patients with a history of heart disease in order to categorize patients into preserved versus reduced cardiac function. It also evaluates heart valves and chamber function.
Cardiac stress testing	For patients with increased risk for major adverse cardiac events, stress testing may be performed as part of the evaluation especially if the results of this test alter the operative plan.
Polysomnography	Patients who are suspected of having obstructive sleep apnea should undergo polysomnography and have treatment established on CPAP prior to the elective surgery.
Spirometry	Spirometry could be used to plan a lung resection in order to find out whether the patient will be able to tolerate such an aggressive surgery. Should also be performed in patients with known lung disease (COPD or constrictive disease).

CAD, coronary artery disease; COPD, chronic obstructive pulmonary disease; CPAP, continuous positive airway pressure.

EVALUATION

Cardiovascular Risk

Cardiovascular risk must be assessed as part of the preoperative evaluation. Many cardiac risk indexes and prediction models are available to guide the assessment. As a general rule, the following surgeries increase the risk for major cardiac events: thoracic, abdominal, orthopedic, cancer-related and vascular surgery and patients with underlying ischemic heart disease, heart failure, diabetes mellitus, previous stroke or other cerebrovascular disease, and chronic kidney disease. The strongest predictor of high risk is recent coronary event regardless of whether this was treated with thrombolytics or percutaneous coronary intervention.[6]

Assessment of the patient's functional capacity is important for risk stratification. Patients who can walk 4 miles an hour on a flat surface, those who can climb two flights of stairs without stopping, and those who can perform vigorous housework such as mopping have, on average, a functional capacity of at least 4 metabolic equivalents (METs). Patients who are unable to perform these activities should undergo cardiac stress testing for optimization.[7]

Patients with coronary artery disease should be assessed for the stability of their symptoms; routine stress testing is not warranted. Elective surgery is delayed for at least 6 months following acute coronary event.

Patients with known heart failure should be optimized to the greatest extent possible prior to undergoing elective surgery.

Patients with cardiac arrhythmias such as atrial fibrillation may develop rapid ventricular response during and after surgery as a result of catecholamine release, fluid shifts, and stress of the operation. Patients with a history of malignant arrhythmias typically continue their antiarrhythmic medications throughout the operative period. Keep in mind that all antiarrhythmic medications have the potential to be proarrhythmic. Patients who have coronary disease and surgical indications for valvular heart disease may be able to undergo both procedures concurrently. If cardiac surgery is indicated, this should be performed before the elective surgery.

Pulmonary Conditions

Pulmonary conditions may complicate the perioperative state and can include pneumonia, respiratory failure, and worsening of underlying pulmonary disease. Assessment of the pulmonary system must be part of the overall evaluation. Pulmonary complications can result in patients with sleep apnea. Many patients with obstructive sleep apnea are undiagnosed; therefore, questioning should be done to assess for this condition. Patients with obstructive sleep apnea should be carefully monitored with continuous pulse oximetry for breathing difficulty. Patients can utilize a continuous positive airway pressure therapy (CPAP) machine in the postoperative recovery room.

Smoking complicates pulmonary management as does chronic obstructive pulmonary disease (COPD), obstructive sleep apnea, and cardiac asthma, which is caused by heart failure. The nutritional state of the patient also significantly impacts the pulmonary system. Lung function progressively declines with age so aging should be taken into consideration. The site of surgery also impacts pulmonary risk with surgery in the thoracic cavity having the most significant effect. Surgery performed on an emergent basis rather than an elective basis prohibits pulmonary optimization of these patients, putting them at higher risk for poor outcome. As a general rule, the longer the duration of surgery, the more significantly the pulmonary system is impacted. Patients with underlying COPD who undergo general anesthesia typically will have more difficulty being weaned from the ventilator due to their hypoxic drive to breathe.

Pulmonary indexes and risk calculators aid in predicting poor pulmonary outcomes. Risk calculators include Surgical Risk Preoperative Assessment System (SURPAS) and the National Surgical Quality Improvement Program (NSQIP) Surgical Risk Calculator (SRC) that are used to predict risks of common postoperative complications.[8] Patients with low oxygen saturation are at increased risk for pulmonary complications during surgery. Ascertaining patient history of shortness of breath or physical deconditioning informs pulmonary management of the surgical patient.

Patients who smoke should be discouraged from smoking with the optimal time frame for quitting being 6 to 8 weeks prior to surgery.[9]

Pulmonary Prevention Strategies

Pulmonary prevention strategies should be applied to lessen the risk for atelectasis. Incentive spirometry and deep breathing exercises are useful to prevent pulmonary complications and postoperative pneumonia.

Medication Reconciliation

Assessment of the patient's current medications should include prescribed medications, vitamin and mineral supplements, complementary medications, and over-the-counter medications. When medication reconciliation is performed, adverse medication combinations may be identified and altered prior to the patient having surgery. It is important that the dosing is accurate and pill identifier software can be used to help the patient identify exactly which dose of the medication is being taken.

Although beta blockers are known to lower cardiovascular mortality, they should not be started just prior to surgery. Beta blockers can interfere with sympathetic response that occurs if hypotension is encountered, blocking reflexive tachycardia pathways. Beta blockers taken on a regular basis, however, can be continued in the perioperative period. If starting a beta blocker for cardioprotection for surgery is necessary, it should be done >1 week prior to the planned procedure.[6]

Hypertensive patients do not necessarily need to have strict blood pressure control prior to surgery as anesthesia can naturally lower the blood pressure at the time of surgery. Patients taking chronic antihypertensive medications are typically instructed to take them the morning of surgery with just a sip of water. This does not include diuretics, which are typically held the morning of surgery because these agents can decrease intravascular volume and cause electrolyte disturbances.

Note that the body does not have a backup system for saving potassium. Since patients are typically not permitted oral intake prior to surgery, it is prudent that potassium supplementation be given as part of the intravenous (IV) fluid regimens as needed. This is especially important if the patient has some fluid overload and is treated with a loop diuretic, as this also causes further potassium loss from the body. On the other hand, hyperkalemia can cause life-threatening dysrhythmias and must be managed appropriately.

Certain surgeries may require unique medication adjustments. Patients undergoing cataract surgery who have a history of taking alpha$_1$ blockers are at increased risk for the development of intraoperative floppy iris syndrome. These patients are given phenylephrine and ketorolac intraoperatively in order to prevent this complication.[10] Clonidine, a centrally acting $alpha_2$ receptor agonist used as an antihypertensive agent, should be held preoperatively as this agent has been shown to increase perioperative hypotension and nonfatal myocardial infarction.[11]

On the morning of surgery, blood pressures should be taken prior to the patient taking the antihypertensive medication so as not to exacerbate an already low blood pressure.

Statin medications (HMG-CoA reductase agents) are typically given the night prior to surgery and continued on a nightly basis following surgery as there are benefits besides cholesterol-lowering with the use of these medications.

Aspirin should be held ideally for at least 5 days to prevent excessive bleeding. Aspirin irreversibly blocks cyclooxygenase so that the platelet will be affected for the life of the platelet. Nonsteroidal anti-inflammatory drugs (NSAIDs) other than aspirin should be held for 1 to 3 days as these agents reversibly block cyclooxygenase, allowing the platelet to regain its function. Acetaminophen can be continued as long as the patient's liver function is sufficient. Clopidogrel can be used for antiplatelet therapy or as part of dual antiplatelet therapy and increases the risk for bleeding. For emergent surgery such as fractured femoral neck, clopidogrel use should not delay surgery as delay in surgery will be associated with more complications than the increased risk for bleeding.[12]

As a general rule, complementary medications and vitamin and mineral supplements are not taken the morning of surgery. There is an increased risk for adverse perioperative effects with the use of St. John's wort, which patients may be taking for depression. This medication should be stopped for 2 weeks prior to receiving anesthesia.

Postoperative Pain Management

Postoperative pain management includes addressing the patient's pain and optimizing judicious use of narcotics to relieve the pain while not oversedating patients. Patient–controlled anesthesia allows the patient to administer pain medication in small amounts as needed, which can improve overall pain management. As narcotic medications cause constipation, patients should be given a liberal bowel regimen, in the appropriate setting. Docusate, a stool softener, is not sufficient to prevent narcotic-induced constipation. Patients should be given clear expectations for postoperative pain management with step down to non-narcotic analgesia occurring in a deliberate fashion.

Nutritional State

Nutritional state should be addressed to enhance the patient's ability to heal and recover postoperatively. Although total parenteral nutrition can supply appropriate calories, vitamins, and minerals, it should be a second-line treatment because gut atrophy can occur with long-term use and there are many problems that are encountered with refeeding of these patients after prolonged parenteral nutrition. Enteral nutrition can be given once abdominal peristalsis returns, so assessing the patient for return of peristalsis is an important part of the postoperative management. Percussing the abdominal cavity for increased air and distention may be a clue that the patient is not yet ready for oral intake.

Some studies have shown that chewing gum or sucking on hard candy postoperatively can help to restore peristalsis in order to stimulate cephalic-vagal reflex and bowel peristalsis.[13] This gum should not be sugar-free gum as artificial sweeteners used in sugar-free gum act as an osmotic agent and can lead to diarrhea. Mobilization of the patient may also help to restore the peristalsis postoperatively. The diet should be gradually advanced from clear to full liquids and, if tolerated, a soft diet can be instituted but this largely depends on the type of surgery the patient underwent.

Careful measurements of input and output are also reviewed in order to ensure that sufficient intravascular volume is present. Patients with underlying chronic heart failure and chronic renal failure should also be weighed on a daily basis and clinically assessed to ensure the volume overload is not occurring.

Prevention of Venous Thromboembolic Disease

Mobilizing the patient soon after surgery is essential to prevent venous stasis and deep vein thrombosis (DVT). Use of intermittent compression devices both intraoperatively and postoperatively can also lessen the risk for thrombosis. Low-molecular-weight heparin can pharmacologically be utilized to lessen the risk for clot formation.

Deep Vein Thrombosis Prophylaxis

DVT prophylaxis can be done with intermittent pneumatic compression devices, low-dose unfractionated heparin, low-molecular-weight heparin, and direct oral anticoagulants (DOACs) that are non-vitamin K antagonists such as dabigatran, rivaroxaban, and apixaban. Venous thromboembolism prophylaxis is indicated for abdominal, pelvic, and orthopedic surgery. There is little reason to not use the intermittent pneumatic compression devices. The Caprini Score assesses the thromboembolism risk with assignment of points based upon patient age, underlying medical conditions, past medical history, presence of malignancy, and type, location, and duration of surgery.

Hip fracture surgery and total knee and hip arthroplasties are high-risk procedures for thromboembolic disease and these patients require intermittent pneumatic compression devices along with pharmacologic prophylaxis. The medication of choice for these patients is low-molecular-weight heparin initially followed by DOACs or warfarin.[14] This prophylaxis continues for up to 35 days postoperatively for those who are low risk for bleeding.

Routine placement of inferior vena cava filters for venous thromboembolic (VTE) prophylaxis is not recommended as these devices do not prevent the formation of venothrombotic disease and have no effect on mortality. There is no routine preoperative assessment via venous compression ultrasound or Doppler studies prior to the patient undergoing surgery.[15]

Patients taking anticoagulants to prevent VTE have an increased risk for perioperative bleeding. Minor surgery such as skin lesion removal, dental surgery, and cataract extraction can be performed while the patient is anticoagulated. When vitamin K antagonist such as warfarin are discontinued prior to surgery, they should be stopped 5 days prior to surgery to a goal international normalized ratio (INR) of <1.5. DOACs are typically stopped 2 to 3 days prior to surgery as long as the patient has normal liver and kidney function as these agents have a very short half-life.

Bridging Anticoagulation

Bridging anticoagulation involves stopping of the oral vitamin K antagonist and giving short-term IV heparin. If the patient cannot continue to take these medications, short-term use of heparin is indicated. Restarting anticoagulation following surgery is dependent upon clotting risk versus the potential for bleeding. It will typically take 4 to 5 days for warfarin to have therapeutic benefit, so patients are started on heparin—which has an immediate anticoagulant effect—and warfarin may be started with the understanding that the INR will take several days to become therapeutic. Additionally, during the initiation of warfarin therapy, patients are actually prothrombotic due to decreased levels of protein C and S, which occur prior to diminished thrombin levels.

Anticoagulation can begin within 24 hours after the procedure; if the risk of bleeding is high, it can be delayed for 2 to 3 days, but this must be discussed with the surgeon prior to resumption of anticoagulation. DOACs have activity within 1 to 3 hours, eliminating the need for heparinization as long as the patient is able to take oral medications. One potential issue with the DOACs is that once given, they cannot readily be reversed if the patient starts to bleed.

Patients with atrial fibrillation who are at high risk for the development of thromboembolism may need to have bridging performed. When bleeding risk for the procedure is high, bridging with heparin after stopping warfarin is typically warranted. Patients with valvular disease are at much greater risk for poor outcomes, especially if there is a mechanical valve replacement. The current practice is for less frequent utilization of bridging as comparison trials have shown that lack of bridging did not increase adverse events while bridging that was done increased the risk for bleeding.

Patients taking antiplatelet medications require special consideration when undergoing surgery. Dual antiplatelet therapy with aspirin and a $P2Y_{12}$ inhibitor such as clopidogrel, ticagrelor, or prasugrel should consider whether the patient has a bare-metal stent or a drug-eluting stent, the time since the stent placement, and the indication for the dual antiplatelet therapy. Patients with a drug-eluting stent should have anticoagulation for at least 1 year. Patients with bare-metal stents should have continuation of the dual antiplatelets for 30 days without missing any dosing followed by 6 months of additional therapy. If it can be avoided, elective surgery should not be done within these time frames. Patients with acute coronary syndrome should have dual antiplatelet therapy for at least 1 year even if no stent was placed. Aspirin should be continued for all of these patients.

Transfusion Considerations

Most patients can handle postoperative anemia with crystalloid fluid infusion as long as the hemoglobin is maintained at a level of 8 mg/dL and the patient does not have significant underlying cardiac or pulmonary disease. Transfusions are considered for hemoglobin levels of 7 mg/dL or lower or active, uncontrolled bleeding. Platelet transfusion can be considered if the platelet count falls below 50,000 as spontaneous bleeding can occur with platelet counts at this level or lower. If the patient's platelet count is below 50,000 due to immune thrombocytopenia, platelet transfusions might result in further platelet destruction, which would mandate stabilization of the platelets with glucocorticoids. Patients with a falling platelet count who are receiving heparin should be evaluated for possible heparin-induced thrombocytopenia, which is complicated by paradoxic clot arterial or venous clot formation rather than bleeding.

Underlying Medical Conditions and Perioperative Management

Diabetic patients should have reasonable control of their blood sugar prior to undergoing surgery because uncontrolled hyperglycemia interferes with the healing process. Oral medications used to manage diabetes are usually held the morning of surgery while metformin is typically held several days prior to surgery because of the risk of lactic acidosis. Since the oral agents are not used preoperatively, insulin is used for short-term therapy. Patients taking basal insulin should continue this perioperatively because the liver continues to make sugar even when oral intake does not occur. Patients with type 1 diabetes will get the same dose of basal insulin while patients with type 2 diabetes who are not eating can have the basal insulin dose reduced 25% to 50%.

Patients with hypothyroidism should continue taking levothyroxine the morning of surgery with a sip of water. Patients who are poorly controlled for hypothyroidism should have elective surgery delayed until better control is achieved to prevent myxedema coma. Patients with hyperthyroidism should continue their antithyroid medication and thyroid-stimulating hormone (TSH) can be checked to ascertain that adequate control for hyperthyroidism has been obtained prior to the patient undergoing surgery. Patients with uncontrolled or untreated hyperthyroidism are at risk for the development of thyroid storm.

Patients with adrenal insufficiency who do not receive lifesaving cortisol have an increased risk for both morbidity and mortality. Patients with uncorrected adrenal insufficiency cannot mount a cortisol response and therefore cannot maintain vascular tone. The amount of corticosteroid replacement is higher than the amount of steroids that the patient traditionally takes as stress doses of steroids are needed. This mirrors what happens to people undergoing surgery as they have an increased catecholamine release during surgery, which requires glucocorticoid support for these patients.

22.2 GASTROINTESTINAL SURGERY

22.2A ANAL FISSURE

OVERVIEW

An anal fissure is a linear superficial tear or denuded epithelial lining of the anus typically located at the posterior midline.

Anal fissures can occur either spontaneously or after the passage of a large, hard stool; constipation; muscular spasm; or trauma. Patients taking long-term narcotics and pregnant patients are at increased risk for the development of anal fissures.

SIGNS AND SYMPTOMS

Anal fissures can be painful and can cause bright red rectal bleeding during and after a bowel movement. Other symptoms may include burning or itching in the anal region. Severe pain occurs during defecation. Even following passage of a bowel movement, the pain can continue for up to 2 hours.

PHYSICAL EXAMINATION

Inspection of the anus will reveal a visible tear in the lining exterior (typically in the posterior midline at 6 o'clock) to the anal verge. Pain and spasm may occur during digital rectal examination. Examination of the anus may show spasm of the sphincter muscles. There may be a skin tag or small lump from fibrotic skin (pile). Palpation of the area reveals tenderness, which may preclude a digital rectal examination from being performed (Figure 22.1).

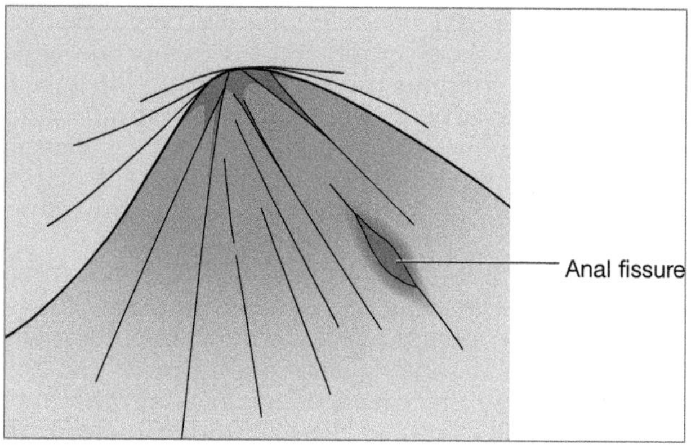

Figure 22.1 **Anal fissure.**
(Source: Small A. Advanced health assessment of the abdomen, rectum, and anus. In: Myrick KM, Karosas LM, eds. Advanced Health Assessment and Differential Diagnosis: Essentials for Clinical Practice. *Springer Publishing Company; 2021: Fig. 8.32.)*

TABLE 22.2 Differential Diagnosis for Anal Fissure

Condition	Description
Anal fistula	Abnormal connections between two epithelial surfaces. Perianal fistula allows drainage of fecal material with possibility of some of the drainage occurring through other epithelial surface such as the vagina. Extraintestinal manifestation of Crohn disease.
Crohn disease	May affect the perianal area. Anal fistulas rather than fissures are more common with Crohn disease and these tend to appear lateral to the site of a typical fissure. Condition is typically associated with abdominal pain and other extraintestinal manifestations.
Anal cancer	Related to infection with human papillomavirus especially genotypes 16 and 18. Squamous cell is the most common cell type of anal cancer while colorectal cancer most commonly is caused by adenocarcinoma.
Sarcoidosis	Associated with anal fissures but these occur laterally as opposed to midline location.
Syphilis	Suspect in patients who have anal fissures that failed to heal. Men having sex with men is the highest risk category.

The typical anal fissure occurs along the midline. Fissures that are off the midline require further investigation.[16] Even though anal fissures can be associated with rectal bleeding, the identification of one should not preclude investigation of new-onset rectal bleeding for patients at risk for other conditions that can cause GI bleeding.

DIFFERENTIAL DIAGNOSIS

Table 22.2 summarizes the differential diagnosis for anal fissure.

DIAGNOSTIC STUDIES

Anal fissure is a clinical diagnosis and is diagnosed with the history and physical examination.

TREATMENT

In most cases a small anal tear spontaneously heals in 6 to 8 weeks. Prolonged healing taking longer than 8 weeks defines a chronic anal fissure. Treatment should include stool softeners, warm sitz baths, topical steroids, topical diltiazem or topical nitroglycerin, and anesthetic ointments applied to the affected area Topical diltiazem has been demonstrated to promote healing with fewer adverse reactions than the topical nitroglycerin.[17] Botulinum toxin type A can be administered if topical treatment fails. This agent will relax the anal sphincter and prevent further spasm.

Surgical treatment is indicated for intolerable pain or lack of healing. Surgical methods may include excision of the sentinel pile, and lateral internal sphincterotomy.

PATIENT EDUCATION

Anal fissures are common conditions that are associated with perirectal pain and bleeding during defecation. Topical diltiazem and topical nitroglycerin may be utilized for medical therapy and these agents should be used for up to 8 weeks to ensure that healing takes place.

22.2B APPENDICITIS

OVERVIEW

Appendicitis is inflammation of the vermiform appendix that can lead to abscess, peritonitis, ileus, and even death from overwhelming sepsis if not diagnosed and treated in a timely fashion. It is the most common surgical procedure performed in every decade of life.[18] Although many patients have imaging performed to confirm the diagnosis of acute appendicitis, this diagnosis remains a clinical one. Laparoscopic or open appendectomy remains the treatment of choice for adults with acute appendicitis, but surgery versus antibiotic therapy remains controversial for pediatric patients with acute appendicitis.

EPIDEMIOLOGY

The lifetime risk of appendicitis is 8.6% in men and 6.7% in women with an annual incidence of 9.38 per 100,000 persons.[18]

PATHOPHYSIOLOGY

The cause of appendicitis is not fully understood, but various explanations have been developed. Luminal obstruction of the appendix interferes with the release of the goblet cell secretion resulting in an increase in intraluminal pressure which leads to increased ischemia of the appendiceal wall. Translocation of bacteria across the lumen leads to transmural inflammation of the appendix.[18] Hyperplasia of lymphoid tissue can cause obstruction of the lumen of the appendix. Fecaliths can also block the appendix leading to obstruction and acute appendicitis.

Appendicitis can be caused by closed loop obstruction of the lumen of the appendix, such as a fecalith, lymphoid hypertrophy, intestinal worms, traumatic injury, or tumors. Intraluminal blockage of the appendix allows bacteria to multiply inside the hollow viscus leading to swelling, purulence, and pain.

MEDICAL HISTORY AND CLINICAL PRESENTATION

Pain initially may begin in the epigastrium and typically migrates to the right lower quadrant (RLQ). Patients are usually anorexic. Fever and chills may or may not be present.

Nausea and vomiting can occur. Diarrhea can also be seen, particularly with a retrocecal appendix. The presence of abdominal pain, rigidity, and loss of bowel sounds can indicate perforation and signify an acute surgical abdomen.

SIGNS AND SYMPTOMS

Symptoms typically develop and worsen over 1 to 2 days following onset. Recent viral illness may precede acute appendicitis. Appendicitis during later trimester of pregnancy may cause the gravid uterus to position the appendix higher and more lateral in location, sometimes mimicking cholecystitis. Signs and symptoms of acute appendicitis can vary widely depending on the age of the patient.[19]

PHYSICAL EXAMINATION

The hallmark of appendicitis is pain with palpation of the RLQ over McBurney's point, which is located one-third the distance from the anterior superior iliac spine of the pelvis to the umbilicus. RLQ pain with palpation in the left lower quadrant (LLQ) is called Rovsing sign. Pain elicited with extension of the right hip is called a positive psoas sign and may indicate a retrocecal appendix. Obturator sign is reproduction of pain with internal rotation of the patient's thigh, which will stretch the obturator muscle and cause pain if an inflamed retrocecal appendix overlies the area. Involuntary guarding and rebound tenderness will usually be present on exam. Low-grade fever is common.

DIFFERENTIAL DIAGNOSIS

Table 22.3 summarizes the differential diagnosis for appendicitis.

DIAGNOSTIC STUDIES

Appendicitis is predominantly a clinical diagnosis, although no single individual sign or symptom is fully reliable to diagnose or exclude this condition. Complete blood count (CBC) usually shows mild elevations of the white blood cell (WBC) count. Higher range of leukocytosis may indicate appendiceal rupture. Urinalysis (UA) may be abnormal showing ketones in the urine from the patient's inability to eat. UA may also exclude a urinary tract infection in the differential diagnosis. Acute inflammation can cause the C-reactive protein (CRP) to be elevated.

Hematuria might be seen with cystitis, ureteral and kidney stones, or retrocecal appendicitis. Because ectopic pregnancy can present similarly to appendicitis a pregnancy test should be performed in woman of childbearing age. Ultrasound of the abdomen demonstrates wall thickening of the appendix, luminal distention, and lack of appendix compressibility (Figure 22.2). Transvaginal ultrasound can identify ovarian pathology such as an ovarian torsion or cyst or ectopic pregnancy. Ultrasound is preferred in children and pregnant women in order to avoid radiation exposure from CT scan imaging, but this type of imaging is operator dependent.[20] CT scan of the abdomen and pelvis, with or without contrast, provides the most reliable diagnostic confirmation of acute appendicitis.

TREATMENT

In most cases, appendectomy is indicated in acute appendicitis. Surgery is performed to prevent complications from untreated appendicitis. Laparoscopic appendectomy is most

TABLE 22.3 Differential Diagnosis for Appendicitis

Condition	Description
Crohn disease	Most common location of the GI tract is the terminal ileum, which is located in the right lower quadrant. Patients may have fever, nausea and vomiting, diarrhea, and right lower quadrant pain. Stricture may be seen on CT of the abdomen. Extraintestinal manifestations may also be seen.
Gallbladder colic	Right upper quadrant pain radiating between the scapulae. Positive Murphy sign showing inspiratory stoppage and pain with palpation in the right upper quadrant. Abdominal ultrasound shows thickening of the gallbladder wall, pericholecystic fluid, gallstones, dilated cystic duct.
Meckel diverticulum	Pediatric diagnosis with right lower quadrant abdominal pain. Ectopic gastric mucosal tissue can become inflamed. Hard clinical differentiation from appendicitis. Technetium scan may show this ectopic gastric tissue.
Mesenteric adenitis	Inflammation of the mesenteric lymph nodes, which can occur in the setting of acute streptococcal infection or following upper respiratory tract infection. Lymphocytosis may be seen. Ultrasound will show a normal appendix.
Viral gastroenteritis	Nausea, vomiting, diarrhea are common symptoms and precede abdominal pain. Abdominal pain may be described as cramping. Does not cause localization of pain into the right lower quadrant.
Intussusception	Telescoping of the intestine with barium enema showing a coiled spring sign where the bowel invaginates. Examination may have palpable sausage-shaped mass. Intermittent colicky pain with symptom-free periods between the colicky pain.
Ureteral stone	Right-sided flank pain that can radiate into the anterior upper and lower abdomen including the scrotum and vagina. May be associated with hematuria. Noncontrast CT preferred image to make this diagnosis.
Spontaneous bacterial peritonitis	Occurs in the setting of cirrhosis with ascites. Gram-negative rods are typical pathogen. Rebound tenderness, abdominal distention, and increased neutrophil count.
Ectopic pregnancy	Consideration for all women with childbearing potential. Lower pelvic pain classic. History may be consistent with missed menses. Transvaginal ultrasound can demonstrate condition.
Ovarian torsion	Abrupt onset pain in either lower quadrant. Ultrasound demonstrates torsion.
Pelvic inflammatory disease	Salpingitis and endometritis can have referred pain into the right lower quadrant. May be associated with cervical discharge. Highest occurrence is soon after menses.

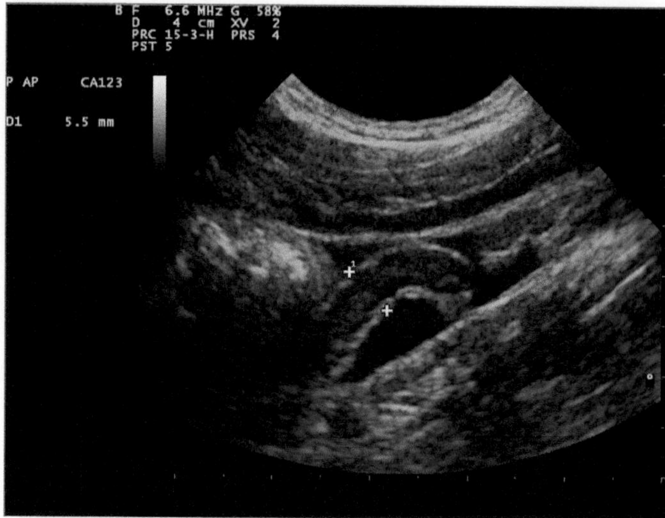

Figure 22.2 Ultrasound image of appendicitis. Note distended and curved appendix with periappendiceal fluid.
(Source: Nevit Dilmen.)

commonly performed and is associated with a lower rate of postoperative wound infection compared to the open appendectomy.[19] There is ongoing debate about the role of antibiotics alone being appropriate therapy for acute appendicitis in the pediatric population.[20]

Patients with appendiceal abscess formation can be managed nonoperatively with intravenous antibiotics and CT-guided percutaneous drainage with interventional radiology (IR) followed by interval appendectomy. Treating uncomplicated acute appendicitis with antibiotics alone results in higher recurrence and hospital readmission. Intravenous antibiotic selection may include piperacillin/tazobactam, ceftriaxone and metronidazole, and ciprofloxacin or levofloxacin with metronidazole.

Perforation of the appendix can be life threatening if unrecognized. Interval appendectomy following perforation can be performed 1 to 2 months following nonoperative treatment with IV antibiotics and percutaneous IR drainage, especially in the pediatric population with uncomplicated appendicitis.

Complicated appendicitis diagnoses necessitate the patient having a visible hole in the appendix or a fecalith located in the abdomen. In the absence of either condition, the patient is classified as having uncomplicated appendicitis. Subsets of complicated appendicitis include necrotic or gangrenous portions of the appendix and patients with an abscess as a complication from their appendicitis.[21]

A modest delay in performing appendectomy has not been proved to cause significant adverse outcomes provided that antibiotics are given in a timely fashion. Delaying appendectomy does not appear to increase complications but the longer the time to appendectomy, the lengthening of the duration of hospital stay resulting in increased cost.[22]

Interval appendectomy involves the removal of the appendix after resolution of a previously perforated appendicitis that has an associated appendiceal mass or abscess. Interval appendectomy may also be performed for patients who have uncomplicated, nonperforated appendicitis who later decide to have an elective appendectomy. The rate of recurrent appendicitis after nonoperative management of uncomplicated appendicitis ranges from 24% to 38%. Interval appendectomy may be preferable when a fecalith is identified. The decision to perform interval appendectomy is an individual one and based upon multiple factors including the experience of the surgeon recommending this treatment.[23]

PATIENT EDUCATION

The majority of patients with appendicitis fully recover. Antibiotics should be taken until completion of the course. Nonsurgical patients may later have an interval appendectomy after treatment with antibiotics and experience full recovery; this is still a controversial option and these decisions are individualized in order to have the best outcome for each patient.

22.2C BILIARY DYSKINESIA

OVERVIEW

Gallbladder dyskinesia may be caused by gallbladder spasm or chronic acalculous cholecystitis. Biliary dyskinesia occurs when there is an abnormal movement of bile through biliary tract. Because of lack of effective gallbladder contraction in response to ingestion of food—which should induce release of bile into the common duct and duodenum—the right upper quadrant abdominal pain associated with biliary dyskinesia usually occurs postprandially. No obstructing gallbladder or common bile duct (CBD) stones are demonstrated on diagnostic imaging studies. This pain associated with biliary dyskinesia can also be associated with sphincter of Oddi dysfunction or spasm.

SIGNS AND SYMPTOMS

Typically, pain occurs in the epigastrium and right upper quadrant after ingesting high fat content meals. Pain can radiate into the right scapula. Symptoms can last several minutes to hours and often recur after meals. The symptoms may mirror biliary colic or pain caused by gallstones. Nausea, vomiting, and anorexia can accompany symptoms. Fever and chills are not typically seen.

PHYSICAL EXAMINATION

Abdominal examination may be entirely normal. Palpation of the right upper quadrant may or may not elicit discomfort. Murphy sign is usually negative, as the gallbladder is typically not distended to cause irritation with palpation upon deep inspiration. A right upper quadrant mass is not palpable. Murphy sign is positive when the patient is unable to fully inspire when the clinician palpates the right upper quadrant. Murphy sign is not related to just the patient having right upper quadrant pain with palpation.

DIFFERENTIAL DIAGNOSIS

Table 22.4 summarizes the differential diagnosis for biliary dyskinesia.

DIAGNOSTIC STUDIES

For patients with convincing symptoms consistent with gallbladder dysfunction, ultrasound of the gallbladder is initially performed. If the ultrasound fails to identify gallstones or pericholecystic fluid collection, a scintigraphy with hepatobiliary iminodiacetic acid (HIDA) scan may be performed along with calculation of the gallbladder

TABLE 22.4 Differential Diagnosis for Biliary Dyskinesia

Condition	Description
Acute cholangitis	Fever, chills, jaundice, and abdominal pain located primarily in the right upper quadrant. Acute infection affecting the gallbladder can be demonstrated on MRI. Antibiotics indicated until surgery can be performed.
Chronic cholecystitis	Repeated attacks of intermittent abdominal pain consistent with gallbladder colic. Ultrasound can show thickened gallbladder wall and possibly calcifications from the recurrent bouts (porcelain gallbladder).
Acute pancreatitis	Epigastric or periumbilical pain radiating straight through to the back. Elevations of amylase and lipase. Can occur in the setting of gallstones or following heavy alcohol intake.
Sickle cell crisis/gallstone formation	Can be associated with gallstone disease as patients with sickle cell have chronic hemolysis leading to the production of black pigment stones.
Appendicitis	Pain in the periumbilical area localizing in the right lower quadrant with anorexia, nausea and vomiting. Clinical diagnosis. May be right upper quadrant pain for pregnant women due to migration of appendix into the right upper quadrant.
Pneumonia	Right lower lobe pneumonia can have radiation of pain into the right upper abdomen mimicking gallbladder disease.
Biliary colic	Steady right upper quadrant pain, which can radiate to the right scapula. Can be associated with diaphoresis, nausea, and vomiting. Pain can last for several hours in total and then dissipates.

ejection fraction (EF). This nuclear imaging study injects a radiotracer to allow circulation in the liver with eventual accumulation in the gallbladder over time, typically several hours. Ingestion of a high fatty meal or administration of intravenous cholecystokinin (CCK) can be used to provoke replication of the patient's symptoms by trying to induce gallbladder contraction and bile secretion into the duodenum. EF calculates the amount of bile that empties into the duodenum. Because of the inconsistency of the evaluation of those with a gallbladder dyskinesia the role of scintigraphy is not fully defined.[24] Patients presenting with signs and symptoms consistent with gallbladder disease but no organic pathology demonstrated on ultrasound are diagnosed with biliary dyskinesia if gallbladder EF is <35%.[25]

An esophagogastroduodenoscopy (EGD) can be done to visualize the appearance of the esophagus, stomach, and duodenum in the evaluation for other causes such Barrett esophagus, peptic ulcer disease, erosive gastritis, hiatal hernia, or duodenitis. A gastric emptying study can determine if the patient's symptoms may be caused by gastroparesis, which can be seen in patients with long-standing diabetes mellitus.

TREATMENT

Laparoscopic cholecystectomy is the recommended surgical approach following diagnosis Nonsurgical treatment may include dietary restriction of high fat content meals, use of antacids, or a trial of proton pump inhibitors (PPIs).

Patients without surgical indications for laparoscopic cholecystectomy based upon ultrasound findings who were found to have a gallbladder EF of <35% following HIDA screening experienced better pain relief and significant improvement in quality of life after undergoing laparoscopic cholecystectomy rather than being treated with medical management for biliary dyskinesia.[26] The advantage of laparoscopic cholecystectomy in the pediatric population is less convincing for surgical benefit but this may be due to wider overlap between biliary dyskinesia and functional dyspepsia in the pediatric population.[27]

Surgery is usually recommended for continuation of the patient's symptoms in the setting of proven biliary dyskinesia. Long-term follow-up of patients who underwent laparoscopic cholecystectomy in the setting of proven biliary dyskinesia shows continued improvement of abdominal symptoms for as long as 10 years after laparoscopic surgery.[28]

PATIENT EDUCATION

Patients with biliary dyskinesia can attempt conservative medical management but evidence now shows that there are long-term advantages for undergoing elective laparoscopic cholecystectomy. Laparoscopic cholecystectomy will not improve functional or nonulcer dyspepsia symptoms.

22.2D CARCINOID SYNDROME

OVERVIEW

Carcinoid syndrome is the most common of the neuroendocrine tumors that secrete ectopic hormones. It is most commonly seen in the small bowel and it is most likely to secrete serotonin. It appears that the incidence of this tumor is actually increasing.

Carcinoid syndrome comprises neuroendocrine tumors that secrete vasoactive substances, such as serotonin, which subsequently is broken down in the liver and excreted in the urine as the metabolite 5-HIAA (5-hydroxyindoleacetic acid).[29] Patients may have ongoing symptoms for some time that do not appear to be related to one another, leading to a delay in diagnosis. Occult primary lesions usually do not cause systemic effects as serotonin (5-hydroxytryptamine) is metabolized by the liver. Metastatic disease involving the liver usually will present as carcinoid syndrome. The most common location is the appendix but it can also involve the ileum, jejunum, rectum, and duodenum. The tumor can also be found in the lungs, pancreas, and biliary tract. All carcinoid tumors are considered malignant because of their likelihood of invasion and metastasis.

PATHOPHYSIOLOGY

Carcinoid heart disease is caused by the development of fibrotic plaques on the right-sided cardiac valves with tricuspid regurgitation being most commonly affected. Right-sided heart failure ensues causing dyspnea and fatigue, elevated jugular venous pulse, pleural effusions, ascites, and edema.[30] These carcinoid plaques are caused by the proliferative effects of elevated levels of serotonin on valve tissue producing thickened and stiffened leaflets.[30]

MEDICAL HISTORY AND CLINICAL PRESENTATION

The classic presentation of carcinoid syndrome includes diarrhea, cutaneous flushing, wheezing or asthma-like symptoms, and hyperkeratosis and hyperpigmentation.[31] Heart–related manifestations can include tricuspid regurgitation.

Clinical presentation of patients with carcinoid tumors depends on the tumor location. Signs and symptoms typically do not present until late in the disease process, and complaints may include vague abdominal pain or bloating, diarrhea, constipation, nausea, difficulty with breathing, wheezing, and weight loss.

Risk factors include older age, sex (women > men), race (higher in African Americans), and family history of multiple endocrine neoplasia, type I (MEN I).

PHYSICAL EXAMINATION

Small bowel obstructions from the tumor can cause severe abdominal pain, distention, nausea, and vomiting. These tumors can cause local fibrosis of the bowel resulting in kinking or twisting, which leads to obstruction. Other presenting findings include intussusception of the intestine, weight loss, GI bleed, abnormal or excessive hair growth on the face or body, and a palpable abdominal mass. Carcinoid syndrome may indicate hepatic metastasis and presents with flushing of the skin, diarrhea, sweating, and wheezing. This is caused by the systemic effects caused by secretion of vasoactive substances when venous drainage from a tumor escapes hepatic metabolism.

DIFFERENTIAL DIAGNOSIS

Table 22.5 summarizes the differential diagnosis for carcinoid syndrome.

DIAGNOSTIC STUDIES

Laboratory studies include plasma and urine analysis to check for elevated serum serotonin levels and presence of 5-HIAA in the urine. Barium contrast studies can detect carcinoid tumors. Lesions of the large intestine and rectum can be demonstrated with barium enema. Small bowel follow-through imaging may show a discrete lesion. Capsule endoscopy should be avoided if narrowing from a stricture is suspected. CT scan of the abdomen with contrast can be performed for evaluation of suspected hepatic metastasis.

Upper GI endoscopy and colonoscopy are performed to obtain a specimen for biopsy and pathologic diagnosis. MRI can provide a clear picture of the extent of involvement and tumor size. A radionuclide scan can be used to determine metastatic spread throughout the body.

TABLE 22.5 Differential Diagnosis for Carcinoid Syndrome

Diagnosis	Description
Asthma	Causes wheezing, which can also be seen with carcinoid syndrome. Asthma is typically a long-standing disease starting in childhood especially in the atopic child. Asthma is not associated with flushing or diarrhea.
Irritable bowel syndrome	Can be associated with diarrhea but without heart problems or wheezing.
Crohn disease	Affects the terminal ileum most commonly, which approximates the most likely site of carcinoid syndrome, which is the appendix. There is abdominal pain and diarrhea, which may be bloody, but no wheezing. Extraintestinal manifestations may also be seen with Crohn disease.

TREATMENT

Surgery is indicated for a primary carcinoid tumor. Laparotomy requires adequate resection of the bowel and adequate mesenteric margins. Surgical resection is largely dependent on the size of the tumor. Small primary lesions can be treated with simple local excision. Larger tumors with metastatic spread require wide en bloc resection performed. Symptomatic palliative relief in patients with carcinoid syndrome can be provided by daily subcutaneous injections of the somatostatin analog octreotide. Other nonoperative treatments include radioembolization and chemoembolization, beam radiation or implantation of radioactive seedings near the tumor, chemotherapy, hormone therapy, and gene targeted therapies.

Carcinoid tumors of the appendix are unlikely to metastasize. Lesions of the jejunum and ileum are frequently multicentric. Carcinoid syndrome is most likely to occur when the tumor involves the ileum. Prognosis is related to the size of the tumor and presence of metastasis; muscle wall spread and lymph node involvement contribute to a poorer prognosis. Survival rates decrease as the tumor size increases. Induction of general anesthesia in carcinoid patients may provoke a life-threatening crisis causing hypotension, flushing, tachycardia, and arrhythmias from serotonin release. These symptoms can be rapidly reversed with administration of intravenous octreotide. Carcinoid lung tumors may be removed by segmental lung resection of the airway above and below the tumor, known as a sleeve resection. Larger lung tumors may require a lobectomy and removal of involved lymph nodes. Liver resection is performed for tumors with hepatic metastasis; however, multiple liver lesions may be considered unresectable with a corresponding poor prognosis.

Right-sided heart disease is a known complication of carcinoid syndrome. Patients with metastatic carcinoid disease to the liver may benefit from surgical resection of both the primary tumor and its metastasis. Postoperatively, these patients may also benefit from somatostatin analogs in order to protect the heart from further damage for any micrometastasis that was not removed during surgery.[32]

There have been improvements noted in patient's quality of life when somatostatin analogs are given for the medical treatment of this condition[33] even after resection of the primary tumor. Long-acting somatostatin analogs can alleviate symptoms and act as antiproliferative agents to reduce the progression of carcinoid heart disease.[30]

Monitoring includes an ongoing evaluation of the use of serotonin inhibitor whose mechanism of action is to interfere with the formation of serotonin by this tumor.[31]

PATIENT EDUCATION

Long-term control of symptoms caused by carcinoid syndrome can be achieved. There is a role for medical and surgical therapy with this condition, and long-term follow-up for recurrence of the tumor is needed for optimal results.

TABLE 22.6 Differential Diagnosis for Cholangiocarcinoma

Condition	Description
Hepatocellular carcinoma	Associated with cirrhosis and therefore jaundice, ascites, and caput medusa. Tends to occur in the periphery rather than central portion of the liver.
Cholangitis	Charcot triad of fever, jaundice, and right upper quadrant pain. Acute infection within the gallbladder and associated with gallstones.
Ampullary carcinoma	Jaundice, pruritus, anorexia, and distended palpable gallbladder. ERCP used for biopsy to confirm the diagnosis.
Pancreatic cancer	Weight loss, epigastric and back pain, which are not features of cholangiocarcinoma.
Choledocholithiasis	Gallstones lodged in the common bile duct leads to jaundice, may be associated with enlarged cystic duct.

ERCP, endoscopic retrograde cholangiopancreatography.

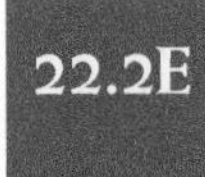

22.2E CHOLANGIOCARCINOMA (BILE DUCT CANCER)

OVERVIEW

Cholangiocarcinoma is a primary GI malignancy arising from the bile duct epithelium that is typically not diagnosed until late in the disease process resulting in a universally poor outcome. Three anatomic locations occur: intrahepatic, perihilar, and distal bile duct. Biliary obstruction is a common thread in all three locations. Liver transplantation is curative only in the setting of perihilar cholangiocarcinoma.[34]

Cholangiocarcinoma is the second most common primary hepatic neoplasia and has a rising incidence. Risk factors include chronic biliary tract inflammation. Chronic liver disease from hepatitis C or hepatitis B, alcoholic liver disease, and ulcerative colitis complicated by primary sclerosing cholangitis increase the risk for development of this condition. The only curative therapy is surgical resection or liver transplantation.[35]

EPIDEMIOLOGY

Cholangiocarcinoma is considered a rare type of cancer. The condition typically occurs in patients older than age 50, but it can occur at any age. Patients with advanced disease typically complain of right upper quadrant pain. Prognosis of cholangiocarcinoma is 90% mortality rate at 5 years.

Biliary tract cancer accounts for <1% of all cancers and affects chiefly the older male population. Treatment is based on surgery if possible, radiation, and possibly chemotherapy. Early palliative care may be appropriate for patients with this type of cancer.[36]

PATHOPHYSIOLOGY

This cancer arises from the bile duct epithelium. It can be intrahepatic or extrahepatic and can involve the bifurcation of the ducts. Cell type is typically adenocarcinoma. These tumors can either be infiltrating nodular or diffusely infiltrating type.

MEDICAL HISTORY AND CLINICAL PRESENTATION

Abdominal pain, jaundice, pruritus, clay-colored stools, fatigue, and unintended weight loss may be the presenting symptoms. Because these symptoms are not specific for this condition, late diagnosis is the rule rather than the exception.

PHYSICAL EXAMINATION

Abdominal examination may show a palpable, distended gallbladder in the right upper quadrant due to the inability of the gallbladder to drain. Jaundice can be seen if the tumor obstructs the biliary tree.

DIFFERENTIAL DIAGNOSIS

Table 22.6 summarizes the differential diagnosis for cholangiocarcinoma.

DIAGNOSTIC STUDIES

Blood work includes liver transaminase and cholestatic testing. Tumor marker to check the level of cancer antigen CA 19-9 is performed. Ultrasound of the abdomen and CT scan imaging will show the tumor if biliary obstruction presents with the disease. Percutaneous transhepatic cholangiography (PTC) can be performed. Endoscopic retrograde cholangiopancreatography (ERCP) can identify and biopsy the tissue or perform FISH (fluorescence in situ hybridization) testing on the brush biopsy. IR can be used to perform a needle-guided biopsy of the lesion under ultrasound or CT guidance. Magnetic resonance cholangiopancreatography (MRCP) can visualize the lesion but is limited in that no tissue biopsy can be obtained.

TREATMENT

The staging of the disease is determined by the extent of the disease, prognosis, and treatment options. Cholangiocarcinoma treatment may include surgical resection, biliary drainage via a surgical bypass procedure or biliary stenting, liver transplantation, chemotherapy, radiation therapy, or photodynamic therapy. Participation in clinical trials and palliative care may be options for patients with poor prognosis, as the disease can be difficult to treat and is usually fatal.

Surgical resection depends on the location of the tumor. Tumors confined within the bile ducts have better outcomes. Distal CBD cancers are treated with a Whipple procedure (pancreaticoduodenectomy). Biliary bypass can be palliative to offer improved symptomatic relief of biliary obstruction. Surgical treatment for cholangiocarcinoma can be technically challenging and is best performed in a tertiary medical facility that specializes in advanced surgical procedures. Patients who had fine needle aspiration for biopsy performed for bile duct cancer may be ineligible for liver transplantation due to the potential for metastatic seeding of the tumor.

PATIENT EDUCATION

Mortality risk is related to cholangiocarcinoma is related to liver failure and recurrent sepsis caused by biliary obstruction. Even in the setting of radical surgery and complete resection, there is a high incidence of local and regional recurrence and distant metastasis.[37]

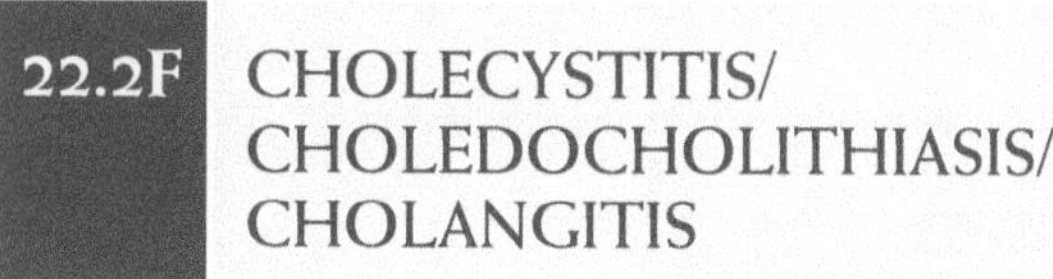

22.2F CHOLECYSTITIS/ CHOLEDOCHOLITHIASIS/ CHOLANGITIS

OVERVIEW

Cholecystitis is an acute or chronic infection of the gallbladder, typically from to gallbladder infection from impacted gallstones interfering with gallbladder release of bile.

Choledocholithiasis refers to the presence of a gallstones in the CBD leading to obstruction of bile into the duodenum. The condition can cause jaundice and liver damage. Stone formation can also be caused by bile stasis in the bile ducts rather than just a gallstone that lodges in the common duct. Patients may spontaneously pass a gallstone into the CBD without cholecystitis being present. Gallstone pancreatitis occurs when a stone in the CBD passes through the ampulla of Vater, allowing bile to reflux into the pancreatic ducts. Primary CBD stone formation can be seen after cholecystectomy.

Acalculous cholecystitis is a condition that occurs in critically ill patients. It can be related to trauma, surgery, shock, burns, sepsis, total parenteral nutrition, or prolonged fasting. Patients have right upper quadrant pain, fever, leukocytosis, and abnormal liver tests. Although there are no specific findings making this diagnosis, abdominal ultrasound and HIDA scan can confirm this diagnosis. The definitive therapy for acalculous cholecystitis is cholecystectomy. Cholecystostomy or percutaneous drainage can also be done and may be lifesaving if the patient is unable to tolerate traditional cholecystectomy.[38]

The majority of people with gallstones never become symptomatic. If gallstones are found incidentally, elective cholecystectomy is not indicated due to the high number of people with gallstones who never become symptomatic.

EPIDEMIOLOGY

Cholecystitis is the most prevalent surgical condition in industrialized countries. The most common cause of cholecystitis and biliary colic is cholelithiasis; 1% to 2% of people who have cholelithiasis develop symptoms or complications per year. Complications include biliary colic, acute or chronic cholecystitis, choledocholithiasis, cholangitis, pancreatitis, and gallbladder cancer.[39] It is estimated that 20% of individuals with gallstones will develop biliary colic. Biliary colic occurs when the gallbladder contracts against an obstruction, typically a gallstone that is lodged in the gallbladder neck.

PATHOPHYSIOLOGY

Gallstones are composed of cholesterol, calcium bilirubinate, or both. Choledocholithiasis is a condition of having gallstones that are located in the CBD. Black pigmented gallstones form from increased bilirubin levels in the bile, typically the result of ineffective erythropoiesis or hemolysis,[40] while brown pigmented stones occur in the setting of bacterial or parasitic infection.[41]

MEDICAL HISTORY AND CLINICAL PRESENTATION

Biliary colic worsens with oral intake. Right upper quadrant or epigastric pain may last several hours. Complaints of pain radiating to the back or shoulder are seen. Nausea and vomiting are often present. Jaundice may be seen with choledocholithiasis and cholangitis. Patients with choledocholithiasis report dark urine or clay-colored stools, which are caused by the inability of bile pigments to reach the stools.

SIGNS AND SYMPTOMS

Pain is typically located in the right upper quadrant of the abdomen or epigastrium and can radiate to the scapular area of the back. Gallbladder colic is described as sharp and steady until full resolution of the pain occurs. Nausea and vomiting can be present. Acute cholecystitis implies infection and symptoms of jaundice, fever, chills, and severe vomiting can be seen in patients with suspected cholangitis. Epigastric pain radiating to the back can also indicate acute pancreatitis.

PHYSICAL EXAMINATION

Pain elicited on palpation of the right upper quadrant may indicate acute cholecystitis. Patients who have asymptomatic gallstones will usually have normal examination findings. Cholecystitis may be associated with fever and signs of peritoneal irritation, including rebound tenderness and guarding. Murphy sign is the replication of pain when the clinician palpates under the liver edge and the patient ceases deep inspiration because of painful contact of the palpating hand. This occurs because the inflamed or distended gallbladder descends as the thoracic girth of the thorax pushes the liver and gallbladder lower.

The degree of tenderness in the right upper quadrant or epigastrium on abdominal exam may vary. Courvoisier sign (a palpable, nontender gallbladder on physical examination) may be seen when gallbladder dilation develops because of an obstruction of the CBD typically caused by cancer located at the head of the pancreas. Right upper quadrant abdominal pain, fever, and jaundice is referred to as Charcot triad and indicates cholangitis. The addition of hypotension and altered mental status defines Reynold pentad.

DIAGNOSTIC STUDIES

Only 10% to 15% of gallstones can be seen on plain abdominal x-rays. Ultrasound of the gallbladder is the gold standard for detecting gallstones (Figure 22.3). Findings on

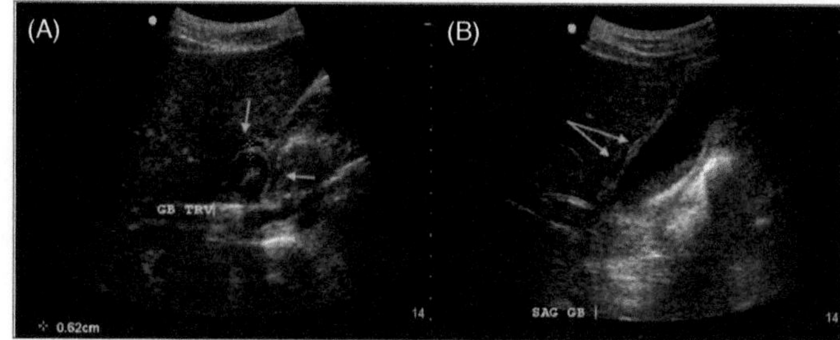

Figure 22.3 Acute cholecystitis. (A) Transverse gallbladder view with thickened wall measuring 6.2 mm. (B) Longitudinal gallbladder view. Green arrows indicate hypoechoic pericholecystic fluid outside the gallbladder wall.

(Source: *Kanter C. Introduction to diagnostic ultrasound. In: Campo TM, Lafferty KA, Costantino TG, Ufberg JW, Wilbeck J, eds.* Essential Procedures for Emergency, Urgent, and Primary Care Settings. *3rd ed. Springer Publishing Company; 2022: Fig. 5.61.)*

ultrasound for acute cholecystitis include fluid around the gallbladder, a thickened gallbladder wall, and gallbladder distention. CBD stones should be suspected if ultrasound shows dilation of the CBD >4 mm and corresponding liver transaminitis and hyperbilirubinemia are seen on metabolic blood profile. ERCP or endoscopic ultrasound (EUS) can be used to determine the presence of choledocholithiasis. Patients with symptoms of biliary colic and no identifiable gallstones on imaging should have a HIDA scan performed where nonvisualization of the gallbladder can indicate acute cholecystitis. Failure of the gallbladder to take up the radiotracer within 4 hours is consistent with blockage of the cystic duct.[42] Patients can receive an intravenous administration of CCK to stimulate gallbladder wall contraction and bile flow during the test and calculate an EF of the gallbladder. Reproduction of biliary colic pain is consistent with acute cholecystitis. Gallstones can also be evaluated with CT scan of the abdomen but ultrasound is the preferred test.

Ultrasound is not as useful to detect gallstones within the CBD; however, it can demonstrate intrahepatic biliary dilation. CT scan can reveal the presence of cholelithiasis and cholecystitis and is also useful to detect CBD dimension. The gold standard for the diagnostic evaluation of the biliary tree and choledocholithiasis is an MRCP; however, the study is expensive and cannot be performed in patients with metal implants, extreme body mass index, or claustrophobia. EUS and MRCP have largely replaced ERCP for the diagnosis of choledocholithiasis in patients at intermediate risk for choledocholithiasis. EUS is less invasive than ERCP, and MRCP is also noninvasive. These tests are highly sensitive and specific for choledocholithiasis.[43] ERCP has the advantage of being able to remove the stone but has the disadvantage of also possibly causing cholangitis or pancreatitis. Abdominal CT and percutaneous cholangiopancreatography are alternative methods for diagnosing choledocholithiasis. PTC is typically performed in patients who are not candidates for ERCP, who have failed ERCP, who have surgically altered anatomy preventing endoscopic access to the biliary tree, or who have intrahepatic stones.[44]

Intraoperative cholangiography is highly reliable for diagnosing choledocholithiasis at the time of cholecystectomy, but it is highly operator dependent and is not routinely performed by many surgeons as laparoscopic surgery has largely replaced open surgery as the preferred method for cholecystectomy.[45] Another intraoperative approach for detecting choledocholithiasis is intraoperative ultrasonography. During laparoscopy, an ultrasound probe is inserted into the peritoneal cavity though a 10-mm trochar and is used to scan the bile ducts.

Laboratory testing usually includes a CBC and comprehensive metabolic profile (CMP) in patients with suspected acute cholecystitis. Leukocytosis is often present with an acute attack. Increased serum bilirubin and alkaline phosphatase levels may indicate cholestasis, cholangitis, or choledocholithiasis. Total bilirubin levels >3 mg/dL are associated with choledocholithiasis.[42] Elevated serum amylase and lipase levels can accompany gallstone pancreatitis.

DIFFERENTIAL DIAGNOSIS

Table 22.7 summarizes the differential diagnosis for cholecystitis, choledocholithiasis, and cholangitis.

TREATMENT

Patients who are asymptomatic with gallstones do not require surgical treatment unless these stones become symptomatic. Diet for these patients should include avoiding foods high in fat, greasy foods cooked in oils, unrefined white foods (such as bread and pasta), and processed foods. Symptomatic gallstone patients should receive surgical referral and treated with cholecystectomy or some other form of intervention to relieve the pain associated with the acute attack and risk of worsening infection. Early operative treatment for acute cholecystitis decreases overall length of stay in the hospital and avoids complications. Operating early also decreases the rate of conversion from laparoscopic to open procedures and actually reduces risk of mortality.[42] Complications of gallstones include recurrent or worsening biliary colic, acute and chronic cholecystitis, gallstone pancreatitis, and cholangitis.

The mainstay of the management of choledocholithiasis is removal of the CBD stone either endoscopically or surgically. The approach to stone removal depends on when the stone is discovered. If the stone is detected before or after cholecystectomy, the stone should be removed with ERCP. The choice of treatment for patients with choledocholithiasis found during surgery includes intraoperative ERCP, intraoperative CBD exploration (laparoscopic or open), or postoperative ERCP.

TABLE 22.7 Differential Diagnosis for Cholecystitis, Choledocholithiasis, and Cholangitis

Condition	Description
Acute cholangitis	Fever, chills, jaundice, and abdominal pain located primarily in the right upper quadrant. Acute infection affecting the gallbladder, which can be demonstrated on MRI. Antibiotics indicated until surgery can be performed.
Chronic cholecystitis	Repeated attacks of intermittent abdominal pain consistent with gallbladder colic. Ultrasound can show thickened gallbladder wall and possibly calcifications from the recurrent bouts (porcelain gallbladder).
Acute pancreatitis	Epigastric or periumbilical pain radiating straight through to the back. Elevations of amylase and lipase. Can occur in the setting of gallstones or following heavy alcohol intake.
Sickle cell crisis	Can be associated with gallstone disease as patients with sickle cell have chronic hemolysis leading to the production of black pigment stones. Sickle cell crisis can occur anywhere in the body, including the gallbladder.
Appendicitis	Pain in the periumbilical area localizing in the right lower quadrant with anorexia, nausea and vomiting. Clinical diagnosis. May be right upper quadrant pain for pregnant women due to migration of appendix into the right upper quadrant.
Pneumonia	Right lower lobe pneumonia can have radiation of pain into the right upper abdomen mimicking gallbladder disease.

Patients with suspected acute cholangitis should be admitted to the hospital with monitoring for and treating sepsis, providing intravenous antibiotic coverage, and establishing biliary drainage. The choice of antibiotics should take into consideration whether the infection is community-acquired or healthcare-associated, as well as individual risk factors for infection with resistant bacteria. Empiric antibiotic regimens for intra-abdominal infections include antimicrobials with activity against enteric streptococci, coliforms, and anaerobes.[46] Blood cultures must be obtained prior to initiation of antibiotics, allowing therapy to be tailored. Once the source of infection is controlled, antibiotic therapy for patients with acute cholangitis is continued for an additional 4 to 5 days.

Biliary drainage is required in all patients with acute cholangitis. The timing of biliary drainage depends on disease severity. In patients with mild to moderate cholangitis, biliary drainage should be performed within 24 to 48 hours. Patients with mild to moderate cholangitis that fails to respond to conservative management for 24 hours and patients with severe (suppurative) cholangitis require urgent (within 24 hours) biliary decompression. Endoscopic sphincterotomy with stone extraction and/or stent insertion for establishing biliary drainage in the setting of acute cholangitis should be performed rather than treatment with antibiotics alone.

The risk of surgery increases two- to threefold for acute cholecystitis performed on an emergency basis. Laparoscopic cholecystectomy has become the gold standard of surgically removing the gallbladder as a safe and effective procedure. Patients with biliary colic or nonacute cholecystitis can usually have the surgery performed on an outpatient basis.

Treatment for patients with acute cholecystitis usually requires hospitalization. Intravenous fluids should be administered because vomiting and infection can cause dehydration. Broad-spectrum antibiotics are given including intravenous ciprofloxacin and metronidazole, piperacillin/tazobactam, or ampicillin/sulbactam.

Laparoscopic cholecystectomy is considered safe in patients with acute cholecystitis. Intraoperative cholangiogram should be performed in patients with suspected choledocholithiasis. In patients who are not medically stable who undergo surgery with general anesthesia, a percutaneous cholecystostomy tube can be inserted by IR for decompression of the distended gallbladder and pain relief. Patients with cholangitis or gallstone pancreatitis require NPO (nothing by mouth) diet status, fluid resuscitation, treatment with broad-spectrum antibiotics, and gastroenterology consultation for possible ERCP and sphincterotomy of the ampulla of Vater to decompress the bile ducts.

CBD stones should be removed to prevent complications such as jaundice, cholangitis, or pancreatitis. Laparoscopic CBD exploration, open CBD exploration, and ERCP with stone removal are all options for the removal of CBD stones. CBD stones identified by preoperative ERCP are removed by ERCP. When ERCP is not available or not feasible (due to surgically altered anatomy such as previous Roux-en-Y gastric bypass), surgical CBD exploration (either laparoscopic or open) becomes the only option. CBD stones that are identified by preoperative MRCP, by EUS, or by intraoperative cholangiography entails both surgical CBD exploration or ERCP removal of stones.[47]

PATIENT EDUCATION

Patients who have asymptomatic gallstones should not have surgery. Patients with acute cholecystitis have improved outcomes if the procedure is done early rather than late. There is a lower rate of conversion from laparoscopic to open cholecystectomy when the surgery is performed within the first 24 hours of symptoms due to acute cholecystitis. Patients with acalculous cholecystitis should have either laparoscopic removal of the gallbladder or percutaneous drainage. Patients should avoid high fat intake following cholecystectomy until the liver's intrahepatic ducts are able to sufficiently store enough bile for release after high fat intake. High fat intake post cholecystectomy may result in malabsorption of this food.

22.3 VASCULAR SURGERY

22.3A ABDOMINAL AORTIC ANEURYSM

OVERVIEW

Abdominal aortic aneurysm (AAA) is a common and potentially life-threatening condition. Approximately 7,000 deaths per year are attributed to ruptured AAA in the United States.[48] Of the 50% of patients with ruptured AAA who reach the hospital for treatment, between 30% and 50% will die in the hospital.[49] Ruptured AAA is universally fatal without immediate surgical intervention. Most patients with AAA are asymptomatic; therefore, screening plays an important role to identify these patients to prevent aneurysmal rupture as risk of rupture is primarily related to the size of the aneurysm. Elective surgery has a significantly better outcome than repair after rupture.

An aneurysm is an abnormal dilation of an artery. The abdominal portion of the aorta lies between the diaphragm and the iliac arteries. A diameter >3 cm is considered aneurysmal. Saccular aneurysm occurs when a portion of the artery forms an outpouching, or mushroom-like appearance on imaging studies. Fusiform aneurysms involve growth of the entire arterial dimension similar to the length of a link of sausage.

EPIDEMIOLOGY

Branches off the abdominal aorta include the celiac, superior mesenteric, inferior mesenteric, renal, and gonadal arteries. Most AAAs begin distal to the renal arteries. Men are affected 10-fold more frequently than women, with age of onset between 50 and 70 years. Risk factors of developing an aortic aneurysm include smoking, atherosclerosis, hypertension, hypercholesterolemia, collagen vascular disease (such as Marfan syndrome and Ehlers-Danlos syndrome), family history, and obesity. Patients with arterial atherosclerosis can also have peripheral artery disease, carotid artery disease, and occlusive coronary artery heart disease.

PATHOPHYSIOLOGY

True aneurysm of an artery is transmural and involves all three layers of the arterial wall (adventitia, media, and intima). Pseudoaneurysms involve only the adventitial layer. An aortic dissection occurs from a defect in the intima when blood flows between the weakened layers of the arterial wall, causing a serious potential for life-threatening rupture. An aortic dissection can progress to vascular compromise of the coronary circulation and ostia of the visceral arterial blood supply.

MEDICAL HISTORY AND CLINICAL PRESENTATION

Patients may be asymptomatic with the aneurysm being found incidentally on physical examination or seen on an abdominal image. Patients may notice a sensation that their heart is beating in their abdomen. Development of severe abdominal pain radiating to the back or flank, a palpable pulsatile mass in the abdomen, and hypotension are considered the classic triad for AAA rupture and can be ominous signs. Claudication at rest with sudden unremitting severe leg pain can occur if the aneurysm includes the iliac arteries or if an embolic event occurs.

Unlike other vasculopathies, there is an inverse relationship that has been found between diabetes and AAA development and enlargement.[50] In the setting of diabetes, however, there is higher operative mortality rate and lower long-term survival rate for the diabetic patient who undergoes surgical repair.

SIGNS AND SYMPTOMS

An abdominal pulsatile mass can be palpable on examination. The abdominal aorta is an abdominal vascular structure that bifurcates at the level of the umbilicus. An abdominal bruit may be present and indicates vascular turbulence. An abdominal lift or heave may be felt. Examination findings of abdominal tenderness, hypotension, and tachycardia suggest progression in aneurysmal size, rupture, or vascular compromise. Distal lower extremity pulses can be diminished or unequal. In addition, skin pallor or coolness to touch can suggest limb-threatening ischemia. Most common presentation is in men with lower back pain age 50 to 70 years, especially if the patient has smoked or has atherosclerosis.[51]

DIFFERENTIAL DIAGNOSIS

Table 22.8 summarizes the differential diagnosis for AAA.

DIAGNOSTIC STUDIES

Abdominal ultrasound is routinely used for screening in asymptomatic patients and is recommended as a one-time screen for men older than age 65, especially if they have ever smoked or have a family history of AAA. It is a noninvasive and cost-effective method to assess size and the presence of thrombus within the arterial lumen. The key measurement is an abdominal aortic width of 5 cm or greater, posing a greater risk of aneurysmal rupture.[52] AAA below a dimension of 5 cm can be serially monitored with ultrasound scans performed every 6 to 12 months.[53] An aortogram with contrast is helpful for surgical planning, as it can identify involvement of other blood vessels with runoff into the renal, mesenteric, and iliac arteries. Abdominal plain radiographic films (cross-table lateral view) will outline the AAA if it is calcified. CT angiography (CTA) or MRI can also provide greater anatomic detail of the aneurysm location.

TREATMENT

Evaluation and workup of asymptomatic patients can be performed electively as an outpatient. Treatment depends on the size of the aneurysm, which is directly proportional to the likelihood of growth, leakage, or rupture. The larger the size of the aneurysm, the higher the tensile stress on the vessel and the higher the likelihood of rupture. Once an AAA reaches a dimension >5 cm, vascular surgical referral is indicated. Medical management of AAA must include blood pressure control and smoking cessation.

Repair of asymptomatic AAA is generally indicated for asymptomatic AAA ≥5.5 cm, rapidly expanding aortic aneurysms, AAA associated with peripheral arterial aneurysm (such as iliac or popliteal), or symptomatic peripheral artery disease (including iliac occlusive disease). The primary goals of aneurysm repair are to prevent rupture while minimizing morbidity and mortality associated with repair. Two

TABLE 22.8 Differential Diagnosis for Abdominal Aortic Aneurysm

Condition	Description
Acute aortic dissection	Life-threatening vascular emergency typically presenting with back pain that is classically described as a tearing sensation. Involves the rapid development of a false, blood-filled channel within the tunica media of the aorta rather than interfering with all three layers of the aorta.[51] Although the pain is felt in the back, it can also be felt in the chest, abdomen, or groin. Dissection can occur anywhere along the length of the aorta including the chest; extension of the arterial dissection can go all the way into the abdominal cavity. Patient may develop weakness and paresthesias in the lower extremities, which are red flag symptoms for aortic dissection.
Diverticulitis	Can cause left lower quadrant abdominal pain along with obstipation. Patients may have leukocytosis and CT scan of abdomen will show thickening bowel wall along with inflammation of the pericolic fat. Abscess surrounding the involved area may also be noted.
Ureteral colic	May cause flank pain radiating to the anterior abdominal wall; pain is intermittent and interferes with the patient getting into a comfortable position ("renal colic"). If abdominal aortic aneurysm (AAA) is a missed diagnosis it will be life-threatening. Patients with ureteral colic may have hematuria that can be microscopic or gross. Crystals may be seen in the urine and radiopaque stone could be visualized in the kidney or ureter.
Ovarian torsion	Can cause continuous pelvic pain and pain in the lower abdomen along with nausea and vomiting. Adnexal mass may be palpated. AAA is not as common in women.
Inflammatory bowel disease	Can cause abdominal pain with or without diarrhea that may be bloody. Tenesmus and fecal urgency can occur. Extraintestinal manifestations may also be seen and can include erythema nodosum and pyoderma gangrenosum, perianal fistulas, or uveitis.
Appendicitis	Considered to be the most common surgical emergency in every decade of life. Periumbilical pain radiating to the right lower quadrant may occur. AAA should be considered especially in the setting of an older male who may have a history of smoking as missing AAA rupture is life-threatening.

methods of aneurysm repair are available: traditional open surgery with intrapositional graft placement and endovascular aneurysm repair (EVAR). EVAR can be performed for infrarenal aortic aneurysms in patients with adequate access through patent femoral and iliac arteries. An individualized approach when choosing the type of AAA repair should consider anatomic factors, patient age, gender, risk for rupture, and risk for perioperative morbidity and mortality[54]:

1. EVAR may be preferred in patients with favorable anatomy who are at increased perioperative risk.
2. EVAR may be appropriate in patients with favorable anatomy but who do not have a high surgical risk.
3. Open surgical repair may be preferred for younger patients who have a low or average perioperative risk.

Diagnosis of aneurysmal leakage or rupture requires aggressive intravenous fluid resuscitation, blood pressure support, heart rate control, type and cross-match for blood transfusion, and immediate EVAR or open operative intervention. Open repair is reserved for patients with anatomy not amenable to endovascular graft deployment (such as suprarenal aneurysms or extension below the aortic bifurcation). Postoperative management in the ICU setting is required.

22.3B CAROTID ARTERY DISEASE

OVERVIEW

Carotid artery disease refers to narrowing, or stenosis, of the carotid artery from the development of atherosclerosis caused by a buildup of plaque comprising fatty substances and cholesterol deposits. High-grade carotid artery stenosis means stenosis of at least 70% occlusion of the internal carotid artery, which may be a marker of increased risk for not only stroke but all-cause mortality. Patients with carotid artery stenosis who undergo successful surgical intervention with either carotid endarterectomy (CEA) or endovascular repair with or without stenting remain at high risk for stroke and cardiovascular disease as it is difficult to maintain optimal medical therapy in these patients on a long-term basis.[55]

The common carotid artery arises from the brachiocephalic artery (branch off the aorta) on the right and the aortic arch on the left. It then bifurcates to form the internal and external carotid arteries. The internal carotid artery has a proximal branch into the ophthalmic artery then continues to the circle of Willis, which supplies the brain.

EPIDEMIOLOGY

Atherosclerotic occlusive disease of the carotid artery is a major cause of thromboembolic stroke. Stroke is a major cause of disability and death in the United States. Atherosclerotic plaque in the carotid artery, especially the internal carotid artery, leads to both plaque disruption and embolization of this plaque into the intracranial circulation, causing a stroke.

PATHOPHYSIOLOGY

Atherosclerosis can lead to plaque rupture, ulceration, hemorrhage, thrombosis, and low flow states of carotid blood flow. The cerebral circulation is served by a rich flow of collateral blood supply. The low flow state of this system may contribute to thrombosis of the carotid artery and may be asymptomatic. Plaque debris that becomes dislodged into the cerebral blood flow can cause a thromboembolic event and subsequent stroke, with the potential for permanent neurologic disability. Cerebral vascular accidents (CVAs) are the third most common cause of death in the United States.

MEDICAL HISTORY AND CLINICAL PRESENTATION

Patients may not present with any symptoms until they have a stroke. Occurrence of motor weakness, clumsiness, or expressive or cognitive aphasia may be temporary. Resolution of symptoms within 24 hours may indicate a reversible neurologic deficit known as a transient ischemic attack (TIA). Amaurosis fugax is referred to as transient monocular blindness due to occlusion of a branch of the ophthalmic artery and a characteristic symptom of carotid artery disease. TIAs are considered a warning sign for strokes.

PHYSICAL EXAMINATION

A carotid bruit may be auscultated over the carotid arteries, which can indicate turbulence in the carotid blood flow. The presence of a carotid bruit does not always indicate a hemodynamically significant stenosis exists. Patients who are asymptomatic will not exhibit any fixed neurologic weakness on exam. Cranial nerves remain intact and symmetric. A delay of the carotid artery pulse upstroke on the affected side can be sometimes found or may be equivocal with bilateral carotid stenosis. Fundoscopic examination may reveal the presence of Hollenhorst plaques on the retina as evidence of previous emboli to the retina.

DIFFERENTIAL DIAGNOSIS

Table 22.9 summarizes the differential diagnosis for carotid artery disease.

DIAGNOSTIC

Carotid artery stenosis is usually diagnosed by carotid color flow duplex ultrasound scan, typically the only diagnostic tool needed in the clinical investigation to make the diagnosis. Carotid ultrasound screening can be used to identify patients at high risk for stroke in the setting of asymptomatic carotid artery stenosis. Not only can patients be identified

TABLE 22.9 Differential Diagnosis for Carotid Artery Disease

Condition	Description
Carotid artery dissection	Seen more frequently in a younger rather than the older population. Patients may present with neck pain. Can be associated with trauma, significant neck motion such as that which occurs with motor vehicle accident, or even vigorous exercise. Intimal flap and intramural thrombus can be demonstrated on CT angiography or magnetic resonance angiography.
Plaque rupture leading to carotid artery thrombosis	Seen in patients with long-standing carotid artery stenosis. Stenosis can occur to the point where little blood flow is passed through the stenosis or acute plaque rupture can lead to downstream occlusion.
Fibromuscular dysplasia of carotid artery	Progressive narrowing of vessel wall. More common in females, Asians, and patients younger than age 50. Intramural lesions are seen without calcifications as this occurs from muscular overgrowth and not from atherosclerosis.

who are high risk for stroke but it can also help to risk stratify patients for more intensive management of carotid disease especially patients who have peripheral arterial disease.[56] CTA with contrast or MRI also may be helpful; however, duplex ultrasound is more cost effective, rapidly performed, and widely available.

Screening for Asymptomatic Stenosis

The U.S. Preventive Services Task Force recommends against screening for asymptomatic carotid artery stenosis in the general adult population assigning it as D recommendation.[57]

TREATMENT

The type of treatment for carotid disease depends on the clinical history, degree of stenosis, and characteristics of the plaque formation (such as location and appearance on imaging). Nonoperative therapy includes various lifestyle modifications including tobacco cessation, dietary improvements through cholesterol and sodium reduction, weight loss, and increasing daily exercise. Medications to achieve blood pressure control and reduction of elevated lipid levels are important. Statin medications are effective for their cholesterol-lowering action, reduction of intimal wall inflammation, and plaque stabilization. Antiplatelet therapy with daily aspirin and clopidogrel is effective to prevent neurologic events. Antiplatelet therapy is preferred over vitamin K antagonists or direct oral anticoagulants in the setting of carotid artery disease. During an acute cerebrovascular event, consideration for initiation of intravenous heparin therapy can be done after is the patient is ruled out for having hemorrhage-related stroke.

Patients treated medically instead of surgically for asymptomatic carotid artery stenosis do have an increased risk for the development of neurologic symptoms including stroke. Best medical therapy for carotid stenosis includes aspirin as the antiplatelet of choice along with statins and appropriate blood pressure medications to normalize the blood pressure.[58] Continued lifestyle changes to improve health poses is important for lowering risk for stroke.

Indications for surgery include >70% to 99% unilateral stenosis, evidence of bilateral disease, or >50% stenosis with recurring TIAs despite aspirin therapy. Carotid artery endarterectomy for carotid artery stenting (CAS) plus medical therapy is the best way to treat asymptomatic patients with 60% to 99% carotid stenosis.[59] Surgical intervention can produce lifelong protection against stroke-related death and disability for patients with asymptomatic carotid stenosis. After significant carotid stenosis has occurred, the risk for stroke continues until the stenosis is cleared. CEA with patch angioplasty remains the preferred treatment for most patients with symptomatic internal carotid artery atherosclerosis. More recently, the use of CAS has gained popularity with improved technology and physician skills. The procedure is less invasive than CEA and may offer equivalent or better outcomes with continued technical advances, particularly in some patients who may be at increased risk for poor outcomes with CEA Patients with asymptomatic carotid stenosis may benefit from CEA over CAS.[60]

Endovascular treatment of carotid artery stenosis caused by atherosclerotic plaque is a viable alternative to carotid artery endarterectomy. Outcomes from both of these surgeries have shown no significant difference between the two treatments with regard to stroke or death.[61] There is no surgical consensus for recommending one surgical procedure over the other at this time. Age has been identified as increasing the risk for adverse outcomes in patients with carotid artery stenosis regardless of the surgical procedure with patients age 75 or higher being the most at risk for adverse outcomes.[62]

For patients with recently symptomatic carotid stenosis of 70% to 99% who have a life expectancy of at least 5 years, CEA is recommended rather than medical management alone. CAS rather than CEA is chosen for select patients with recently symptomatic carotid stenosis of 70% to 99% who have any of the following conditions[63,64]:

- A carotid lesion that is not suitable for surgical access
- Radiation-induced stenosis
- Restenosis after endarterectomy
- Clinically significant cardiac, pulmonary, or other disease that greatly increases the risk of anesthesia and surgery
- Contralateral carotid occlusion

An interesting situation occurs when patients have both asymptomatic carotid artery stenosis and coronary artery disease. Patients may undergo a staged carotid angioplasty and stenting prior to undergoing coronary artery bypass and have low risk for perioperative complications. Patients undergoing carotid intervention prior to surgery have low risks for death, stroke, and myocardial infarction.[65]

Transcarotid artery revascularization (TCAR) is a new procedure for treatment of carotid artery disease for those who are at risk for open surgery, such as the older adult and those who have undergone previous CEA. TCAR involves temporarily reversing the carotid blood flow, preventing debris from migrating antegradely into the cerebral blood circulation, and implantation of a carotid stent to stabilize the plaque in attempt to prevent future cerebrovascular events.

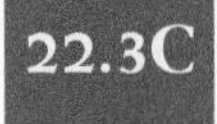

22.3C MESENTERIC ISCHEMIA/ MESENTERIC INFARCTION

OVERVIEW

Mesenteric ischemia is caused by transient reduction in perfusion to the bowel needing urgent intervention. It continues to be a condition associated with high rates of morbidity and mortality. Even when surgical or radiologic intervention is able reperfuse the affected segment of the bowel, there continues to be a complex cascade inflammatory event with the release of chemical mediators triggered by mesenteric ischemia/reperfusion that will need to be addressed by decreasing cardiovascular risk factors after resolution of the acute problem.[66] Three types of mesenteric ischemia exist: acute mesenteric ischemia, chronic mesenteric ischemia, and colonic ischemia.

Acute mesenteric ischemia can occur as a result of an embolism, thrombosis, or venous mesenteric ischemia. There may be transient reversible ischemia, chronic reversible ischemia, or acute widespread significant ischemia. The blood supply of the intraperitoneal portion of the gut is received from the celiac artery, superior mesenteric artery (SMA), and inferior mesenteric artery (IMA). The intraperitoneal organs are divided into the foregut, which includes the stomach and duodenum; the midgut extends from the proximal jejunum to the proximal descending colon; and the remainder of the intraperitoneal colon constitutes the hindgut.

TABLE 22.10 Pathophysiology of Mesenteric Ischemia/Mesenteric Infarction

Vascular Insult	Cause	Explanation
Arterial	Embolism	Embolism originating from the left side of heart thrombus or from rupture of an aortic atherosclerotic plaque or aneurysm. Iatrogenic cause may be from interventional radiologic procedures.
Arterial	Thrombosis	Progression of atherosclerosis at the origin of the superior mesenteric artery. Atherosclerotic plaque rupture may also occur in the setting of acute thrombosis of the vessel.
Arterial	Vasculitis	Several rheumatologic conditions such as rheumatoid arthritis, lupus, polymyositis, dermatomyositis, and polyarteritis nodosum can result in ischemia of the bowel. External compression typically involves the celiac axis from a nerve plexus causing external compression. Other masses within the bowel can also result in compression to the celiac axis.
Venous	Thrombosis	Involves the superior mesenteric vein when it occurs. Condition may be associated with portal hypertension and cirrhosis, hypercoagulable states, using oral contraceptives, and high-risk prothrombotic states such as postoperatively.
Venous	Hypoperfusion	Occurs as a result of lower blood pressure with blood being shunted away from the intestine. Seen with shock, heart failure, dialysis, medications promoting thrombosis such as oral contraception, surgery and trauma, polycythemia, and pancreatitis.

EPIDEMIOLOGY

Colonic ischemia typically appears in patients who have atherosclerosis. Factors that increase risk for mesenteric ischemia include atrial fibrillation, acute myocardial infarction, and generalized atherosclerosis. Patients hospitalized in the ICU and who are bedbound have a higher incidence of mesenteric ischemia. Mesenteric ischemia is not an uncommon cause for the acute abdomen. This condition is much more likely to occur in the older patient who has multiple comorbidities.

PATHOPHYSIOLOGY

Compromise of the arterial blood supply to the gut can lead to intestinal ischemia and can be acute or chronic in nature. Vascular occlusion to the major blood vessels of the gut can result from intrinsic thrombotic or embolic events, such as mural cardiac thrombus formation from atrial fibrillation or a hypercoagulable state such as that from polycythemia. In addition, vasopressor agents can produce acute ischemia to the gut due to their vasoconstrictive effect. Extrinsic causes of mesenteric arterial occlusion can also occur from extraluminal compression of blood vessels as seen with a strangulated intestinal hernia or by an intra-abdominal mass. Sudden occlusion of the SMA from an embolus is the most common cause of acute intestinal ischemia and can rapidly result in infarction of the midgut because of the absence of well-developed collateral blood circulation. Intestinal ischemia with a single vessel thrombosis following progression of atherosclerotic occlusive disease is less commonly seen because of the development of a rich supply of collateral circulation prior to vascular occlusion. Nonocclusive vascular ischemia can be initiated by systemic hypoperfusion and is compounded by vasoconstriction within the vascular mesenteric bed. Chronic intestinal ischemia is usually the end stage of atherosclerotic vascular disease and usually involves all three of the visceral blood supplies to the gut. Chronic ischemic disease increases with age with risk factors including hypertension, smoking, diabetes mellitus, and hypercholesterolemia.

Table 22.10 summarizes the pathophysiology of mesenteric ischemia/mesenteric infarction.

MEDICAL HISTORY AND CLINICAL PRESENTATION

Sudden onset of severe abdominal pain, nausea, vomiting, and diarrhea can be seen in patients with mesenteric ischemia suggesting an acute embolus of the SMA. Patients with suspected chronic mesenteric ischemia may present with crampy abdominal pain after eating which is known as abdominal angina. Chronic disease results in decreased oral intake over time and weight loss is typical. Nausea, vomiting, constipation, or diarrhea may also occur. Chronic mesenteric ischemia can be mistaken for malignant disease or biliary colic associated with gallstones.

PHYSICAL EXAMINATION

A classic finding with acute mesenteric ischemia is pain out of proportion to physical findings on clinical examination. Patients tend to be restless and in agonizing discomfort but the physical examination of the abdomen does not show excessive tenderness. Rectal examination can identify hemoccult positive blood. Cardiac examination may reveal irregular rate and rhythm consistent with atrial fibrillation. Physical exam in patients with chronic mesenteric ischemia may reveal the presence of abdominal bruits. Evidence of peripheral vascular or coronary artery disease is commonly found in these patients.

DIFFERENTIAL DIAGNOSIS

Table 22.11 summarizes the differential diagnosis for mesenteric ischemia/mesenteric infarction.

DIAGNOSTIC STUDIES

Although the history and physical examination may suggest mesenteric ischemia, imaging is usually warranted as part of the evaluation process. If bowel necrosis is suspected, the patient should proceed to the operating room without delay for lifesaving measures. Fluids and volume are needed en route to prevent ischemia from progressing. Early diagnosis is critical for planning appropriate management and obtaining the best clinical outcomes. CT and MRI with angiographic imaging are the preferred tests for the initial evaluation of suspected mesenteric ischemia. These tests are

TABLE 22.11 Differential Diagnosis for Mesenteric Ischemia/Mesenteric Infarction

Diagnosis	Description
Large bowel obstruction	Abdominal pain, distention, hypoactive bowel sounds, nausea and vomiting, and obstipation. CT of the abdomen can identify the etiology of the obstruction such as volvulus, tumor, or internal hernia.
Infectious colitis	Presents similarly to mesenteric ischemia. Colonoscopy identifies the area of ischemia, pathology can reveal microscopic colitis. Pseudomembranes are seen in the setting of *Clostridioides difficile* infection. Stool studies can identify the pathogen.
Acute pancreatitis	Heralded by passage of a gallstone or patient having a history of high intake of alcohol. Pain occurs at the epigastrium boring straight through to the back. Amylase and lipase levels may be elevated. CT can show pancreatic edema from inflammation. Flatplate of the abdomen can show pancreatic calcifications in the setting of chronic pancreatitis.
Ulcerative colitis	Affects the rectum extending proximally. Notable symptoms include bloody diarrhea with pain. There may be associated fecal urgency and extraintestinal manifestations such as pyoderma gangrenosum.
Crohn disease	Affects the entire length of the gastrointestinal tract from mouth to anus. Notable symptoms are more pain and diarrhea, although bloody diarrhea may occur. Predilection for the terminal ileum so may be confused with acute appendicitis. Extraintestinal manifestations such as uveitis, anal fistula, aphthous ulcers of the mouth, or erythema nodosum may be seen.
Diverticulitis	Left lower quadrant abdominal pain, fever, elevated white blood cell count with a shift to the left. CT can show colonic thickening with fat stranding and possible abscess formation.
Gastroenteritis	Can be bacterial or viral in etiology. Nausea and vomiting typically precede abdominal pain. Anorexia common. CT fails to show signs of ischemia or infarction.

able to identify both acute and chronic mesenteric ischemia and provide visualization of anatomy, pathogenesis, and clinical features.[67]

An elevated WBC count and elevated hematocrit result from hemoconcentration as fluid is sequestered in the area of bowel infarction. Elevated lactic acid levels are commonly encountered leading to metabolic acidosis as colonic tissue dies. Emergent arteriography may be diagnostic when acute intestinal ischemia occurs as it can identify the area of blockage. CTA with contrast of the abdomen and pelvis is reliable and provides the fastest evaluation.

Abdominal radiographs are often normal in the early phase of the presentation. As the intestinal wall becomes inflamed and edematous, a characteristic "thumbprinting" of the intestinal wall can occur on abdominal films from air in the bowel wall, which is known as pneumatosis. Evaluation of patients with chronic ischemic disease can include selective visceral angiography to identify the site of involvement. Duplex scanning with color flow analysis can provide noninvasive evaluation to provide both anatomic and physiologic information about the celiac and superior mesenteric arteries and this is usually the initial study in patients with suspected chronic mesenteric ischemia.

TREATMENT

Acute mesenteric ischemia is a surgical emergency; resection of any infarcted bowel must occur immediately. Despite aggressive treatment in the acute setting, the condition of acute mesenteric ischemia carries a high mortality rate. Patients with chronic ischemia require diagnostic evaluation with angiogram to define the involvement and provide mapping for surgical planning.

The appropriate management of an acute embolus of the SMA will usually include embolectomy. Assessment of bowel viability within 30 minutes after reperfusion will determine the need for resection of the infarcted bowel segment. Management of visceral ischemia from thrombotic occlusion is often the end stage of progressive atherosclerotic occlusion. Thrombectomy alone is often not sufficient to restore mesenteric blood flow requiring vascular bypass, endarterectomy, or resection of the distal end of the diseased vessel. Bowel viability is reassessed to determine if surgical resection must be performed; 50 to 100 cm of viable small bowel is required to provide enough surface area in order to sustain adequate nutrition. When bowel viability remains in question and massive bowel resection is detrimental to maintaining nutritional status, a second-look operation should be planned to follow in 12 to 24 hours to reassess the appearance of the bowel. The salvaged area of remaining small bowel is critical to avoiding the patient's lifelong dependence on parental nutrition after surgery.

Argatroban, a direct thrombin inhibitor given intravenously, may have a role in the medical management of acute venous thrombosis. The use of Argatroban led to the resolution of the thrombus, rapid improvement of symptoms, low incidence of bowel resection and bleeding complications, and low mortality rate.[68]

PATIENT EDUCATION

Mesenteric ischemia is not a common entity, but when this condition occurs, it is life-threatening. Atherosclerosis is the primary risk factor for the development of mesenteric ischemia, so management of lipids and other cardiovascular risk factors is essential. Patients who have atrial fibrillation should be appropriately anticoagulated either with traditional oral vitamin K antagonists such as warfarin or by DOACs.

22.4 SURGICAL EMERGENCIES

22.4A NECROTIZING FASCIITIS

OVERVIEW

Necrotizing fasciitis (NF) is a serious infection of the deep soft tissues that results in progressive destruction of the muscle fascia and overlying subcutaneous fat. In lay terms, it can be referred to as a flesh-eating disease. This infection typically spreads along the muscle fascia due to its relatively poor blood supply while muscle tissue is frequently spared because of its generous blood supply. The process progresses rapidly over several days, with changes in skin color from reddish purple to patches of blueish gray. It commonly involves the extremities and perineum. Within 3 to 5 days after onset, skin breakdown with bullae (containing thick pink or purple fluid) and frank cutaneous gangrene can be seen. The disease is characterized clinically by fulminant tissue destruction, systemic signs of toxicity, and high mortality rate.

Bacteria may enter the body through a break in the skin, such as a cut or burn, which sets up a patient for developing this condition. NF may be divided into three microbiologic categories: polymicrobial infection (type 1), monomicrobial infection (type 2), and infection associated with *Vibrio vulnificans* after contact with fish or other marine organisms (type 3).[69] Polymicrobial (type 1) NF (caused by aerobic and anaerobic bacteria) usually occurs in older adults and/or in individuals with underlying comorbidities. Diabetes is a significant risk factor, especially in the setting of peripheral vascular disease. Monomicrobial (type 2) NF (most commonly group A streptococcus [GAS]) may occur in any age group and in individuals without underlying comorbidities.

EPIDEMIOLOGY

In the United States, there are an estimated 3.5 cases of invasive GAS infections per 100,000 persons; necrotizing infections make up approximately 6% of these cases. Methicillin-resistant *Staphylococcus aureus* (MRSA) is involved in up to a third of all cases of NF and community outbreaks have occurred, especially in areas in which this pathogen is endemic.[70] *Streptococcus* and Enterobacteriaceae are the most common pathogens identified with polymicrobial infection. The most common comorbidity for this condition is diabetes mellitus. Outcome is worse when a delay in diagnosis occurs for patients with advanced age. Early surgical intervention may improve morbidity and mortality risks.[71]

MEDICAL HISTORY AND CLINICAL PRESENTATION

Risk factors for developing this condition include poor immune function (chemotherapy, corticosteroid use, radiotherapy, HIV/AIDS, or prior organ or bone marrow transplantation), diabetes mellitus, obesity, cancer, intravenous drug use, alcoholism, and peripheral artery disease. NF most commonly affects the extremities but it can occur in any area of the body.[69]

Fournier gangrene—NF of the perineum—is a form of polymicrobial (type 1) infection typically beginning abruptly with severe pain that may spread rapidly to the anterior abdominal wall and the gluteal muscles. Men are more commonly affected than women and involvement in men can include the scrotum and penis. Involvement in women may include the labia.

SIGNS AND SYMPTOMS

Clinical manifestations of necrotizing infection include skin erythema (without sharp margins), edema that extends beyond the visible erythema, severe pain (out of proportion to examination findings in some cases), fever (102–105 °F), crepitus overlying the affected skin, and the formation of skin bullae, necrosis, or ecchymosis. Patients may complain of severe burning or throbbing pain that occurs suddenly and does not respond well to opiates.[69] Lack of specific signs and symptoms of NF can lead to missed or delayed diagnosis in 85% to 100% of the cases.[72] This condition may be confused with both abscess and cellulitis.

PHYSICAL EXAMINATION

Early in the disease, skin changes occur such as simple superficial skin infection, cellulitis, or abscess, and diagnosis may be difficult. Early presenting clinical features include fever, swelling, pain, and redness.[73] Hardening of the skin and surrounding soft tissues of the affected area develops. The overlying skin may appear shiny, warm, red, and tense along with exquisite tenderness.[74]

Clues to making this diagnosis includes pain out of proportion to what the clinical presentation looks like, lack of response to antibiotic therapy, bullae in the skin, and x-rays showing gas in the soft tissues.[73]

As the disease progresses, formation of bullae and blisters occur. Skin necrosis due to thrombosis of blood vessels is seen with the skin turning from red to blue and black indicating skin death. Crepitus of the skin indicates the presence of gas in the soft tissues. Palpation over the skin often will show decreased or absent sensation to touch. The subcutaneous tissue may be firm and indurated, such that the underlying muscle groups cannot be palpated distinctly. Marked edema may produce a compartment syndrome with complicating myonecrosis requiring urgent surgical fasciotomy. Fever, leukocytosis, and tachycardia can lead to system toxicity and cardiovascular collapse.

DIAGNOSTIC STUDIES

Plain x-ray examination of the affected area may show gas present in the subcutaneous tissue suggesting necrotizing changes. CT scan may demonstrate fascial thickening, edema, subcutaneous gas, and abscess formation. MRI with contrast injection provides better enhancement of fluid collection and deep fascial thickening. Ultrasound is limited in use to show superficial abscess formation but not sensitive enough to make the diagnosis of NF. The laboratory evaluation includes CRP, total WBC count, hemoglobin, serum sodium, creatinine, and blood glucose. Abnormalities may include leukocytosis with left shift, acidosis, coagulopathy, hyponatremia, elevated inflammatory markers (CRP and/or erythrocyte sedimentation rate), and elevations in serum creatinine, lactate, creatine kinase (CK), and aspartate aminotransferase (AST) concentrations. Elevations in serum CK or AST concentrations suggest deep infection involving muscle or fascia. Blood cultures (two sets) should be obtained prior to administration of antimicrobial therapy.

TREATMENT

Treatment of necrotizing infection consists of early and aggressive surgical exploration and debridement of necrotic tissue, together with broad-spectrum empiric antibiotic therapy and hemodynamic support. Administration of antibiotic therapy in the absence of debridement is associated with a mortality rate approaching 100%. Empiric treatment of necrotizing infection should consist of broad-spectrum antimicrobial therapy, including activity against gram-positive, gram-negative, and anaerobic organisms. Antibiotic therapy must be initiated promptly after obtaining blood cultures. A carbapenem or beta-lactam-beta-lactamase inhibitor plus an agent with activity against MRSA (such as vancomycin or daptomycin), plus clindamycin, for its antitoxin and other effects against toxin-elaborating strains of streptococci and staphylococci. Antibiotic treatment should be tailored to findings on Gram stain, culture, and sensitivity results when available. Hemodynamic instability may require aggressive supportive care with fluids and vasopressors. Intravenous fluid requirements may be high, and albumin replacement may be required in the setting of capillary leak syndrome associated with streptococcal toxic shock syndrome (TSS). Hyperbaric oxygen therapy, administration of IV immunoglobulin (IVIG) and supportive therapy can be useful. Other treatments include intravenous hydration, prevention of thromboembolic events, pain control, and local wound care. IVIG is part of this treatment if streptococcal superantigens are identified in order to destroy this bacteria. This leads to an overall decrease in the release of cytokines in the proliferation of T cells and tumor necrosis factor.[75]

Hyperbaric oxygen can be effective if anaerobes are part of this infection. Hyperbaric oxygen is toxic to these anaerobes and can also enhance the activity of leukocytes while promoting formation of granulation tissue. This treatment also can boost the action of antibiotics.[69] NF is a surgical emergency. Prompt aggressive wound debridement must be performed as soon as the diagnosis is suspected. Radiographic imaging studies should not delay surgical intervention when there is crepitus on examination or rapid progression of clinical manifestations. The areas of skin extending beyond the induration must be debrided and the entire necrotic tissue completely excised. The goal of operative management is to perform aggressive debridement of all necrotic tissue until healthy, viable (bleeding) tissue is reached. Inspection and debridement in the operating room should be continued every 1 to 2 days until the necrotic tissue is no longer present. For severe necrotizing infection involving the extremities, amputation may be needed to control the infection. Adequate wound coverage with sterile dressings over exposed tendons, ligaments, and bones must be maintained. Wound care and debridement in patients with Fournier gangrene can be difficult because of soiling of the wound with urine or feces of the perineum. Regular dressing changes and a fecal management system and/or urinary catheter placement are usually required to assist with wound healing. A diverting colostomy may be necessary to keep the perineal area free of fecal contamination.

22.4B PNEUMOTHORAX

OVERVIEW

A pneumothorax is the presence of air in the pleural space of the thoracic chest cavity. The lung is covered by visceral pleura, whereas the thorax is covered with parietal pleura. Pneumothorax can occur spontaneously or secondary to other causes such as direct or indirect trauma to the chest.

EPIDEMIOLOGY

Approximately 17 to 23 cases of pneumothorax occur per 100,000 people per year and are more common in men than women.[76] Some patients with mild or chronic pneumothorax may be asymptomatic and discovered incidentally. A primary spontaneous pneumothorax most commonly occurs in young, thin males in the absence of significant lung disease. Secondary spontaneous pneumothorax typically occurs in patients with existing lung disease. Risk factors for the development of a secondary pneumothorax include COPD, cigarette smoking, and tuberculosis. Emphysema is a major risk factor due to rupture of a bleb that occurs in the setting of emphysema.

PATHOPHYSIOLOGY

Patients with bullous emphysema (COPD) can develop air in the pleural space from rupture of the thin wall of the bullous bleb formations that occur in the setting of chronic air trapping. Patients requiring high inspiratory pressures on mechanical ventilation can develop iatrogenic pneumothorax. Infections such as tuberculosis or *Pneumocystis jirovecii* are also factors. Other iatrogenic causes of a pneumothorax can include placement of central venous catheters, thoracocentesis, needle biopsy, or operative trauma from an unintentional opening in the pleural space (such as during open heart procedures or open nephrectomy).[76] There are four common types of pneumothoraces (Table 22.12).[77,78]

MEDICAL HISTORY AND CLINICAL PRESENTATION

Patients usually present with sudden onset of shortness of breath and pleuritic chest pain. Since pneumothorax is usually unilateral, the pain is usually felt on the ipsilateral side, but may be central or can be bilateral in the setting of bilateral pneumothorax.

PHYSICAL EXAMINATION

In patients with a small pneumothorax, physical examination findings may be normal. When a large pneumothorax is present, characteristic findings include decreased chest excursion and enlarged hemithorax on the affected side, diminished breath sounds, absent tactile or vocal fremitus, and hyperresonant percussion. Subcutaneous emphysema is rarely seen. Evidence of labored breathing or use of accessory muscles suggests a sizeable pneumothorax. Tracheal

TABLE 22.12 Four Types of Pneumothoraces

Type	Description
Simple	Without mediastinal shift to the contralateral side. Patients are clinically and hemodynamically stable.
Tension	Air in the pleural space builds up enough pressure to interfere with venous return, leading to hypotension, tachycardia, and severe dyspnea. Tension pneumothorax may be seen in approximately 1% to 2% of patients,[77] higher in patients with trauma and patients receiving mechanical ventilation; in the latter group, patients who develop initial signs of pneumothorax are more likely to rapidly progress to cardiovascular collapse than those who are not on mechanical ventilation.[78]
Open	Defect in the chest wall allows continuous air entry into the thorax from outside. Open pneumothorax is usually caused by blunt force trauma to the chest (such as a fall, occupational injury, or motor vehicle accident).
Catamenial	Occurs within 1–2 days after menstruation as the result of pelvic or thoracic endometriosis; tends to recur if not treated.[45]

deviation away from the affected side is a late sign but it does not always indicate the presence of a tension pneumothorax. Hemodynamic compromise (such as tachycardia or hypotension) is an ominous sign and suggests a tension pneumothorax and/or impending cardiopulmonary collapse.

DIAGNOSTIC STUDIES

The diagnosis of pneumothorax is a radiologic one. Initial imaging typically includes chest radiography (CXR) that is performed in the upright position with the pneumothorax demonstrated in the apical or apicolateral position. CXR will reveal absence of lung markings on the affected side usually in the apex of the lung. Expiration films can highlight the differences between the normal and affected lung. The first rib and clavicle can sometimes interfere with detection of a small pneumothorax in the upright position. Tension pneumothorax may show mediastinal shift or tracheal deviation displaced away from the affected side.

The choice of imaging modality is dependent upon the stability of presentation, the availability of bedside ultrasonography, and the degree of suspicion for competing diagnoses. In general, while those who are unstable should have rapid bedside imaging with pleural ultrasonography, those with a stable presentation can wait for confirmation by plain CXR. Occasionally, chest CT is required for those in whom the diagnosis is uncertain, those suspected to have a loculated pneumothorax, or stable trauma patients who require CT to assess the extent of other injuries. Incidental pneumothorax may also be found on chest CT.

Chest CT is the best modality for determining the presence, size, and location of intrapleural gas.[76] Small amounts of air in the pleural space and pleural pathology including pleural effusions and adhesions as well as loculations can be better appreciated by CT compared with plain radiographic imaging. Based upon its superior resolution and observational studies, chest CT is considered more accurate than either CXR or ultrasonography for the diagnosis of pneumothorax.[79]

Laboratory findings of pneumothorax are nonspecific but may reveal a mild leukocytosis without left shift. Most patients who present with pneumothorax have routine laboratories performed including D-dimer level and troponin levels to investigate the cause of dyspnea and chest pain. Peripheral oxygen saturation (Spo_2) may be normal in those without underlying lung disease in whom the pneumothorax is small. Patients with sizeable pneumothorax or preexisting lung disease typically will have evidence of oxygen desaturation. Electrocardiographic findings are also nonspecific and may reveal sinus tachycardia. A more serious rhythm disturbance (such as bradycardia) may be associated with severe hypoxemia or indicate tension pneumothorax and impending cardiovascular collapse.

TREATMENT

Simple pneumothorax of <20% can be observed and treated with supplemental oxygen followed by repeat CXR examination for comparison. Chest tube insertion through a thoracostomy offers the most definitive treatment for a pneumothorax. These are inserted under local anesthesia at bedside in an area referred to as the "safe triangle" to avoid injury to internal organs. This area is located under the axilla of the affected side and is delineated by a horizontal line of the nipple and borders of the latissimus dorsi and pectoralis major muscles. A chest tube remains attached to a negative pressure suction system (typically low pressures of −10 to −20 cm H_2O pressure). Any open chest wound should be immediately covered with a dressing that allows an airtight seal to prevent the development of a tension pneumothorax.

Tension pneumothorax is a surgical emergency. Needle thoracostomy should be performed, usually in the midclavicular line of the second intercostal space on the affected side of the chest. This decompresses the air within the pleural space and allows blood return to the heart. Tube thoracostomy is inserted as soon as possible and attached to a closed water-seal suction canister system. Chemical pleurodesis through an existing chest tube (using talc, tetracycline, minocycline, or doxycycline) promotes adhesion of the lung to the inside of the chest wall. Pleurectomy, scraping of the pleura to encourage continual expansion of the lung, can be done through open thoracotomy, or less invasive approach with video-assisted thoracoscopic surgery (VATS). Chemical pleurodesis can help the lung to adhere to the chest wall. Open pneumothorax will require surgical closure of the chest wall defect and subsequent chest tube placement.

COMMON CHIEF COMPLAINTS

APPROACH TO ABDOMINAL PAIN

Patients who present with pain may need surgical intervention to treat this pain. The location of pain can be a clue to the anatomic location producing the pain. Abdominal pain is a common location for pain to occur and the differential diagnosis is vast due to the high number of structures contained in the abdominal cavity.

The abdomen is divided into quadrants that contain visceral organs. The right upper quadrant of the abdomen primarily contains the liver, gallbladder, and pancreatic head. The left upper quadrant of the abdomen consists primarily of the spleen, stomach (also midline location), and left kidney. The RLQ consists of the appendix, cecum, and right ovary, and right fallopian tube. The LLQ contains the sigmoid colon, rectum, left ovary, and left fallopian tube.

Abdominal pain radiating to the back is consistent with pancreatitis. Abdominal pain radiating to the right scapula suggests biliary colic. Flank pain that radiates to the anterior abdominal area is classically associated with renal colic secondary to ureteral lithiasis. Left upper quadrant abdominal pain radiating to the left shoulder is consistent with splenic rupture and Kehr sign.

Abdominal pain that is described as a gnawing, hunger-like pain that improves with food intake is consistent with duodenal ulcer. Food making pain worse is consistent with biliary tract disease and gastric ulceration.

In patients with ascites, a change in mental status or acute abdominal pain can be consistent with spontaneous bacterial peritonitis.

Pelvic pain can be associated with salpingitis, ruptured ectopic pregnancy, and endometritis in the setting of sexually transmitted infection. Cervicitis can also occur as a result of a sexually transmitted infection accompanied by vaginal discharge.

Testicular pain can occur as a result of testicular torsion, torsion of the appendix testis of the epididymis, and acute epididymitis. Patients with acute epididymitis may have relief of pain with elevation of the testicle, which is known as Prehn sign. The cremasteric reflex is typically absent in the setting of acute testicular torsion.

KNOWLEDGE CHECKS

1. Develop an evaluation strategy for a 45-year-old female who is seen in the office with steady right upper quadrant abdominal pain that occurred 1 hour after having a banana split at her local ice cream parlor.
2. Determine what complaints and physical exam findings would be consistent with acute appendicitis.

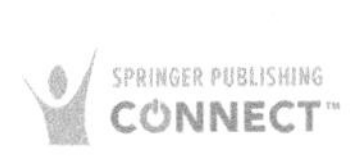

A robust set of instructor resources designed to supplement this text is located at **http://connect.springerpub.com/content/book/978-0-8261-8243-2.** Qualifying instructors may request access by emailing **textbook@springerpub.com.**

REFERENCES

The complete reference list for this chapter appears in the digital version of the chapter, accessible at https://connect.springerpub.com/content/book/978-0-8261-8243-2/chapter/ch22.

Chapter 23

GENETIC DISORDERS

NGUYEN H. PARK

LEARNING OBJECTIVES

- Describe the cellular and molecular mechanisms underlying human inheritance.
- Define the role of genetic variation in health and disease.
- Describe the use of molecular, biochemical, and chromosomal tests in the diagnosis of genetic disorders.
- Understand the epidemiology, pathophysiology, subtypes, variable presentations, and diagnostic and therapeutic modalities for the most commonly seen genetic conditions.

INTRODUCTION

Genetic disorders present unique challenges for PAs in diagnosis, evaluation, differential diagnosis, and treatment, as they can affect patients along the entire life spectrum and can present with signs and symptoms that may be difficult to interpret without insight into the underlying genetic pathophysiology. In addition, they often impact multiple organ systems, and many times have far-reaching consequences for consideration within families and across generations. With the culmination of the Human Genome Project, the tantalizing promise of personalized medicine gave hope to clinicians that treatments could be found for previously diagnosable, but untreatable genetic disorders. The rate of growth of information regarding our knowledge of genetics and genomics since then has been exponential, leading to new understandings of disease, new avenues for pharmacogenomics, and new questions to explore. This chapter begins with an overview of the basic knowledge regarding genetics/genomics needed to care for patients with genetic disorders, as well as touching on the unique ethical considerations of genetic disease, based upon the outline from the PA Genetic/Genomic Guidelines (2016).[1] It then highlights a few of the many genetic diagnoses researchers, scientists, and clinicians are learning more about daily, from cystic fibrosis (CF), a disease long known for its sweat chloride test, now treatable with CF modulator drugs that target the CFTR protein, to acute intermittent porphyria (AIP), a disease first described in 1889 by a Swedish physician, now treatable with an interference RNA therapeutic approved by the U.S. Food and Drug Administration (FDA) in November 2019.[2,3] PAs working in varied branches of medicine from nephrology to pulmonology to specialized genetics clinics authored this chapter and work across the country caring for patients with genetic disorders on a daily basis.

23.1 GENETIC DISORDERS BASICS

Nguyen H. Park

OVERVIEW

Regardless of clinical specialty, it is important for PAs to understand basic genetics concepts in order to best evaluate, diagnose, screen, test, treat, and refer patients with genetic disorders, especially with the rise of direct-to-consumer testing. Genetic and genomic competencies for PAs were established first in 2007,[4] then updated again in 2016,[1] though familiarity with and understanding of numerous genetic disorders have been part of PA education since its inception. In each iteration of the PA genetic and genomic competencies, the medical knowledge for practice competency emphasized the need for fluency in the basic vocabulary of the cellular and molecular mechanisms underlying human inheritance and an understanding of the role of variation in genetic disorders and health. The depth and breadth of genetic and genomic knowledge cannot be covered in the limited space available here, however, this section will provide the most basic knowledge necessary to help PAs care for their patients, interpret physical examination and laboratory findings, and refer patients for appropriate testing, evaluation, and treatment by medical geneticists and genetic counselors.

Basic Genomic Terminology

To understand the pathophysiology behind genetic disorders, facility with the basic physiology of our genes and genome is paramount. These definitions and explanations are derived from the U.S. National Library of Medicine's Genetics Home Reference and the National Human Genome Research Institute's Introduction to Genomics, where modules for more in-depth information can be found.[5] The central aspect of molecular genetics that informs our understanding of genetic disorders is the process of transformation from DNA to RNA to the assembly of proteins, which are the foundation of the human body's structure and functions.

- **DNA:** Deoxyribonucleic acid (DNA) is the hereditary material in humans and almost all other organisms and is usually found in the cell nucleus of nearly every cell in the body. It is structured as a double helix, made up primarily of four chemical bases: adenine (A), guanine (G), cytosine (C), and thymine (T) that pair up predictably, A with T, and C with G. DNA replicates itself during the process of cell division to ensure that each new cell has an exact copy of the DNA in the original cell. DNA is also found in the mitochondria, passed from mother to offspring.
- **RNA:** Ribonucleic acid (RNA) is also made up of nucleotide bases, of which there are several types. Messenger RNA (mRNA) carries the information from DNA out of the cell nucleus into the cytoplasm and interacts with a ribosome, which reads the mRNA's sequence of bases. Three bases make up a codon, each sequence coding for a unique amino acid. From these amino acids, transfer RNA (tRNA) builds each protein.
- **Chromosome:** Chromosomes are thread-like structures found in a cell's nucleus and are made up of DNA tightly coiled around proteins called histones. Chromosomes are normally seen only when the cell is dividing. Humans have 23 pairs of chromosomes: 22 pairs of autosomes, and 1 pair of sex chromosomes, with females having two X chromosomes and males having one X and one Y chromosome.
- **Genes:** Genes are the basic physical and functional unit of heredity. In humans, they can vary in size from a few hundred DNA bases to more than 2 million bases. Humans have approximately 20,000–25,000 genes. Every person has two copies of each gene, one from each parent.
- **Genetics:** Genetics is the study of genes.
- **Allele:** Alleles are forms of the same gene with small differences in their sequence of DNA bases. These small differences contribute to each person's unique physical features.
- **Genome:** The genome is an organism's complete set of DNA, including all genes within cell nuclei and within mitochondrial DNA (mDNA). Each genome contains all information needed to build and maintain that organism. In humans, a copy of the entire genome—more than 3 billion DNA base pairs—is contained in all cells that have a nucleus.
- **Genomics:** Genomics is the study of all of a person's genes, including interactions of those genes with each other and with the person's environment.
- **Exons:** Exons are the regions of genes that code for proteins, not including mDNA. Only about 1% of DNA is made up of protein-coding genes; however, the majority of genetic diseases arise from mutations in the exons.
- **Introns:** Introns are the regions of genes that do not code for proteins, and which have been found to serve multiple regulatory functions. For example, some are located within protein-coding genes but are removed before a protein is made. Regulatory elements, such as enhancers, can be located in introns.
- **Variant:** Each human genome contains variants, not all of which are clinically significant. When a clinically significant variant occurs, it can be caused by a mutation. A mutation can create changes to base pairs in a genetic sequence that may render the gene's protein/product/action as inactive, leading to loss of function (LOF) or may cause erroneous activity, leading to gain of function (GOF).
- **Single nucleotide polymorphism (SNP):** A SNP is a change of one base pair in a genetic sequence.

The next basic terminology set for PAs to understand underpins heritability and thus inheritance.

- **Proband:** A proband is an individual being studied or reported on and is usually the first affected individual in a family who brings a genetic disorder to the attention of the medical community.
- **Mendelian inheritance:** Mendelian inheritance refers to patterns of inheritance that are characteristic of organisms that reproduce sexually, usually understood as the consequence of a single gene first described by Gregor Mendel. Examples include types of inheritance such as autosomal dominant, X-linked, and autosomal recessive.
- **Autosomal dominant inheritance:** This type of inheritance refers to a gene found on a non-sex chromosome (an autosome). Dominant inheritance means that only a single copy of the disease-associated mutation is needed to cause the disease.
- **Autosomal recessive inheritance:** This type of inheritance refers to a gene found on a non-sex chromosome (an autosome). Recessive inheritance requires the presence of two abnormal copies of the gene.
- **Sex-linked inheritance:** Sex-linked diseases are passed down through families through one of the X or Y chromosomes.
- **X-linked recessive inheritance:** This type of inheritance is caused by mutations in genes on the X chromosome. In males (who have only one X chromosome), one altered copy of the gene in each cell is sufficient to cause the condition. In females (who have two X chromosomes), a mutation would have to occur in both copies of the gene to cause the disorder.
- **Carrier:** An individual who carries one abnormal and one normal copy of a gene without any associated phenotypic changes is a carrier. However, researchers have noted that some carriers—such as those with fragile X syndrome—may have milder or associated disorders. The abnormal copy can be passed on to future generations leading to genetic disorder.
- **Mosaicism:** Mosaicism refers to the presence of two or more populations of cells with different genotypes in one individual; it is described as either somatic (secondary to postzygotic mutations), which may affect only a portion of the body and may not be transmitted to progeny, or germ-line mosaicism, which is usually only discovered when it leads to inherited conditions in multiple offspring.

EPIDEMIOLOGY

The incidence of disease caused by genetic disorders is difficult to calculate. Monogenic diseases, resulting from changes in a single gene—which make up just a small portion of genetic disorders—are believed to affect 10/1,000 births globally. Cancer, which can be attributed to inherited genetic mutations in 5–10% of cases, was reported to be responsible for 1 in every 6 deaths worldwide.[6] Increased incidences of certain genetic disorders may be noted in populations with more intermarriage, such as those isolated geographically or

Table 23.1 Common Mutation Types

Mutation Type	Example
Deletion: Changes the number of DNA bases by removing a piece of DNA. Small deletions may remove one or a few base pairs within a gene, while larger deletions can remove an entire gene or several neighboring genes. The deleted DNA may alter the function of the resulting protein(s).	22q11.2 deletion syndrome
Duplication: Consists of a piece of DNA that is abnormally copied one or more times. This type of mutation may alter the function of the resulting protein.	Fragile X syndrome
Frameshift: Occurs when the addition or loss of DNA bases changes a gene's reading frame. A reading frame consists of groups of 3 bases that each code for one amino acid. A frameshift mutation shifts the grouping of these bases and changes the code for amino acids. The resulting protein is usually nonfunctional.	Insertions, deletions, and duplications can all be frameshift mutations.
Insertion: Changes the number of DNA bases in a gene by adding a piece of DNA. As a result, the protein made by the gene may not function properly.	Huntington disease
Missense: Point mutation in which the change of a single base pair causes the substitution of a different amino acid in the resulting protein. This amino acid substitution may have no effect, or it may render the protein nonfunctional.	Progeria syndrome
Nonsense: Point mutation in which the substitution of a single base pair leads to the appearance of a stop codon where previously there was a codon specifying an amino acid. The presence of this premature stop codon results in the production of a shortened, and likely nonfunctional, protein.	Neurofibromatosis, type 1
Repeat expansion: A mutation that increases the number of times that a short DNA sequence is repeated. This type of mutation can cause the resulting protein to function improperly.	Myotonic dystrophy

through self-selection such as among certain ethnic groups, for example, with Ashkenazi Jewish ancestry.

PATHOPHYSIOLOGY

Genetic disorders can be caused by mutation or malfunction anywhere within the entire genome or anywhere along the sequence from DNA to RNA to proteins (Table 23.1). However, not all mutations cause genetic disorders. The presence of numerous variants of unknown significance (VUS) found in genomic analysis are frequently seen in patients without any specific health problems. As more testing is done, the physiologic expression of these these VUS are identified and classified.

MEDICAL HISTORY AND CLINICAL PRESENTATION

When a high index of suspicion for genetic disease is noted in childhood, medical history and clinical presentation frequently reveal dysmorphic features and developmental delays. Newborn screening (NBS), though based upon a standard Recommended Uniform Screening Panel (RUSP),[7] differs from state to state as some may have added conditions for which they screen. For patients born outside the hospital or outside the United States, such screening may not have been performed. Whether NBS was performed and the results, if completed, should be noted.

As genetic disorders may affect multiple systems throughout the body, signs and symptoms in several organ systems should predispose clinicians to consider evaluation by medical geneticists. Many times, patients may present with nonspecific findings that may not fit perfectly within one specific genetic disorder or diagnosis. Within known genetic disorders such as Down syndrome, characterized by trisomy, or three copies, of chromosome 21, clinical presentation may vary along a wide spectrum depending upon which genes and critical regions have been affected. For instance, some individuals with Down syndrome may have significant memory and learning challenges while others are able to maintain gainful employment.

SIGNS AND SYMPTOMS

Signs and symptoms will vary according to each particular condition.

PHYSICAL EXAMINATION

- Careful plotting and study of growth charts can assist in assessment of growth patterns or developmental delay in infants and children.
- Observation of muscle tone can be an important indicator of the presence of genetic disorders, especially in infants and children.

DIFFERENTIAL DIAGNOSIS

While close physical examination of each system is important, a general observation of the patient can allow a gestalt sense of a syndrome or constellation of findings. The consideration of notable findings—for example, an unusually tall patient with long limbs, cardiac murmur, and pectus excavatum—can aid in building a differential diagnosis, in this case Ehlers-Danlos versus Marfan syndrome.[8]

DIAGNOSTIC STUDIES

Appropriate diagnostic tests for significant signs and symptoms should be ordered, such as echocardiogram for cardiac murmur appreciated in marfanoid-appearing patients. However, with significant wait times for appointments with medical geneticists, it is important to refer patients to genetic services in a timely fashion while other testing is ongoing.

Table 23.2 Common Genetic Tests

Diagnostic Test	Description
Fluorescence in situ hybridization (FISH)	Helps identify where a particular gene falls within an individual's chromosomes using short sequences of single-stranded DNA that match a portion of the gene the researcher is examining called probes. Assists in the search for genetic deletions or duplications by detecting if specific DNA sequences are present. Largely replaced by microarrays.
High-resolution karyotype analysis	Chromosomal analysis, which can detect chromosome abnormalities like trisomies, translocations, deletions as small as 3-5 Mb and duplications larger than ~5 Mb, thus less diagnostic yield than CMA.
Chromosomal microarray (CMA)	Used to detect copy number variants (CNVs): deletions or duplications of chromosome material that range in size from approximately 1 kilobase (kb) to multiple megabases (Mb), with the largest CNVs resulting in a loss or gain of an entire chromosome.
Multigene panel testing	*Off the shelf:* designed by a laboratory to include genes commonly associated with a broad phenotype or a recognizable syndrome with genetic heterogeneity *Custom-designed:* includes genes selected by a clinician for analysis by clinical sequencing. Results for each gene on the custom multigene panel are reported to the ordering clinician, whereas the results from the remaining genes sequenced (but not requested by the clinician) are not analyzed or included in the final laboratory report.
Whole exome testing	Used to identify and analyze the sequence of all protein-coding nuclear genes in the genome.
Whole genome sequencing (WGS)	Used to identify and analyze the sequence of all coding and noncoding nuclear DNA. Mitochondrial DNA is part of the genome; however, mitochondrial sequencing is often ordered as a separate laboratory test.

In addition, PAs should understand the difference between screening and genetic testing. Screening is a general tool for patient populations such as newborns or athletes undergoing physical examinations for sports. Genetic testing for a suspected condition or diagnosis is more focused and may involve several different modalities. Table 23.2 is a partial list of the most common types of testing.

EVALUATION

The primary tool for PAs when evaluating patients suspected of genetic disorders is a carefully obtained multigenerational family and medical history. This aids in the creation of a pedigree, which also includes any behavioral or environmental risk factors, such as tobacco use or radiation exposure. Frequently, a pattern of inheritance may suggest further workup. PAs should ascertain if a patient's family background might include "genetic islands," which describe literal and/and or figurative islands in which a group might be more likely to marry within their group for either geographic, religious, or cultural reasons. In these cases, the likelihood of a founder mutation, in which one mutation is seen more often within an associated group, may be increased.

Physical examination should not exclude any systems, as genetic disease can manifest across multiple systems, from ophthalmic to orthopedic. However, physical examination is most often guided by the history, which can lead to an index of suspicion for varying syndromes, allowing for targeting of specific systems. In children, assessment of growth patterns, achievement of developmental milestones, and a comprehensive head-to-toe examination will assist in diagnosis. Careful documentation will allow for observation of progression of symptomatology.

For most patients with genetic disease, lifetime monitoring and repeat evaluation of associated systems will be required, such as annual echocardiograms for congenital cardiac defects.

TREATMENT

- For those trained before the age of genomics, testing for genetic conditions was largely thought of as useful only for understanding management of the condition, and thus not always necessary. As costs decrease for genetic testing, determining the exact nature of genetic diseases is recommended for two key reasons. First, treatments now exist for conditions, such as CF, for which symptom management was the sole therapeutic option; second, genetic testing may reveal a more accurate and treatable diagnosis for patients previously misdiagnosed with a condition believed to be untreatable. For genetic conditions termed "actionable," quickly ascertaining a diagnosis and beginning intervention, especially in infants or children, can prevent irreversible sequelae, and/or further impairment.
- For genetic conditions termed "unactionable," such as Down syndrome, early intervention with speech, occupational, or physical therapy can significantly enhance quality of life.
- There are currently over 600 genetic conditions with practice resources/recommendations from the American College of Medical Genetics and Genomics.[9]
- Evaluation by a clinical geneticist or genetic counselor is important to determine extent of disease in family members and potential for heritability.

PATIENT EDUCATION

- Patients with genetic conditions should be counseled that offspring may inherit a mutation, though actual risk is highly dependent on each condition and each individual.
- Clinicians should be aware of and be able to refer patients to patient support groups as well as local, state, and federal resources.

- Knowledge about genetic variants and genes is increasing, so patients should see their medical geneticists/genetic counselors regularly as new information may arise that could impact treatment and monitoring.

SPECIAL CONSIDERATIONS

Genetic conditions present unique ethical, legal, and social issues (ELSI) for clinicians, patients, and patients' families. Issues of privacy and duty to warn are more complex when dealing with genetic conditions. Because genetic disorders often involve generations of family members, a patient's decision-making may differ from other medical conditions. For example, a patient may elect not to undergo testing for early-onset Alzheimer dementia, though review of family history supports a high risk. The principles of beneficence, autonomy, nonmaleficence, and justice should be observed at all times, with the PA's role as one of providing nondirective counseling, excellent care, and referral to any necessary specialty care.

PAs should promote informed decision-making by being aware of resources within the patient's health system, city/town, state, or within the federal system. PAs should inform patients of the Genetic Information Nondiscrimination Act,[10] passed in 2008, which protects patients from discrimination regarding employment or health insurance coverage based on an individual's genetic information. This protection does not, however, apply to life insurance, disability insurance, and long-term care insurance.

Additionally, though cultural competence is always considered in medical discussions, careful consideration of patients' understanding of statistical and genetic literacy should also be factored into any discussions regarding genetic conditions.

KEY POINTS

- The central aspect of molecular genetics that informs our understanding of genetic disorders is the flow of information from DNA to RNA to proteins.
- Patients may present with multiple complaints across multiple organ systems, which may be nonspecific in nature.
- PAs should be aware that ELSI can play a significant role at every stage of care.
- Patients suspected of having a genetic condition should be referred to a medical geneticist or genetic counselor for proper diagnosis, management, and treatment, if possible.
- Referral to a genetic counselor will be helpful for patients in understanding their disorder, prenatal planning, and risk assessment of family members.

23.2 CYSTIC FIBROSIS

Daniel Goldstein

OVERVIEW

CF is an autosomal recessive genetic disease that involves mutations of the CF transmembrane regulator (*CFTR*) gene. A person with CF has two copies of a *CFTR* mutation, one from each parent. People with a single copy of the mutated gene are considered carriers and are unlikely to be symptomatic. If both parents are carriers, there is a 25% chance with each pregnancy that a child will inherit one mutation from each parent and be affected, a 50% chance the child will inherit just one copy and be a carrier, and a 25% chance the child will not inherit a mutation. CF carriers are found in every ethnic group. More than 10 million Americans are asymptomatic carriers with a CF gene mutation.[12]

EPIDEMIOLOGY

According to the CF Foundation, >1,700 mutations have been identified in the *CFTR* gene.[11] An estimated 30,000 children and adults in the United States have CF.[12] One in 2,500 Caucasian newborns in the United States are diagnosed with CF.[12] A patient with CF in the United States born today is expected to survive >40 years and progress in treatment options have improved the prognosis over the past few decades.[13] The median survival age is higher in males than in females.[13]

PATHOPHYSIOLOGY

The *CFTR* gene is translated via mRNA into a protein and is then transported to the cell membrane. The cytogenetic location of the gene is 7q31.2, which is the long (q) arm of chromosome 7 at position 31.2.[14] The CFTR protein functions as a channel to allow sodium and chloride ions to enter and exit the cell. This movement of ions leads to a balance of salt and water and secretory cells to produce thin, watery mucus. When the CFTR protein is absent or not functioning properly, thick and sticky mucus can build up on the cell surface and accumulate in various organs including the lungs, pancreas, digestive tract, and reproductive organs. For males with CF, the vas deferens is missing or blocked by thick mucus, leading to infertility. Reproductive problems are less common in females. Thickening of cervical mucus can affect movement of sperm and make it difficult to reach the egg. With depletion of liquid on the airway surface in the lungs, the cilia in the bronchioles do not function well, and thick secretions get trapped in the airways instead of being naturally cleared out with a cough and breathing. The trapped mucus leads to increased risk of pulmonary infections and inflammation, which leads to bronchiectasis.

23.2A RESPIRATORY INVOLVEMENT

MEDICAL HISTORY AND CLINICAL PRESENTATION

For the majority of patients with CF, the disease affects the lungs. The clinical presentation, age at diagnosis, severity of symptoms, and rate of disease progression in the organs involved varies widely. Patients diagnosed with CF as adults are less likely to have pancreas involvement but will present with pulmonary symptoms.

SIGNS AND SYMPTOMS

A common symptom of CF is a chronic cough, either dry or with sputum production. Other pulmonary symptoms include chest congestion, pleuritic chest pain, wheezing, hemoptysis, dyspnea on exertion, and fatigue. Sinusitis is commonly seen in CF, and sinus pain is a common complaint.

PHYSICAL EXAMINATION

Sinuses may be tender to percussion. On lung examination, there may be inspiratory crackles, squeaks, or pops, and expiratory wheezes and rhonchi. Digital clubbing is sometimes seen.

DIFFERENTIAL DIAGNOSIS

Over time, most CF patients will develop bronchiectasis, which is an irreversible, abnormal dilation and thickening of the airways causing structural lung damage. Prior to bronchiectasis and CF diagnosis, patients with chronic cough are sometimes told they have asthma, allergic rhinitis, gastroesophageal reflux disease, pneumonia, tuberculosis, allergic bronchopulmonary aspergillosis, and chronic obstructive pulmonary disease (COPD). Patients will be poorly controlled with inhaled corticosteroids and long-acting bronchodilator medications and get recurrent lung infections, prompting an expansion of the differential diagnosis.

DIAGNOSTIC STUDIES

Ordering a high-resolution computed tomography (HRCT) of the chest is key for diagnosing bronchiectasis. Chest CT is more accurate and sensitive than chest radiography (CXR) in detecting bronchiectasis and parenchymal and airway lesions. Imaging shows increased bronchoarterial ratio manifested by signet ring sign, lack of bronchial tapering, bronchial wall thickening, air trapping, and centrilobular nodularity.[15] Bronchiectasis findings are more commonly seen in the upper lobes with CF.[15] Chest CT also shows dilated scarred airways and mucus plugging of small airways described as tree-in-bud findings. A CXR is often normal for CF patients, but in patients with advanced bronchiectasis there may be "tram-tracks," which are parallel line opacities on the CXR indicating bronchial wall thickening.[15] Sinus disease is also common because of trapped mucus creating a favorable environment for bacterial growth.

EVALUATION

Monitoring of lung function with spirometry is done several times per year for CF patients. A drop in the forced expiratory volume in 1 second (FEV_1) indicates worsening lung function and often indicates acute or worsening lung infections. Worsening findings on chest CT and a rise in nonspecific inflammatory markers, such as high sensitivity C-reactive protein, can also be associated with exacerbations in bronchiectasis and lung infection. The primary goals for CF patients are to maintain or improve lung function and raise the FEV_1 and prevent lung infections.

TREATMENT

- *Pseudomonas aeruginosa* is a commonly found gram-negative bacteria cultured in the bronchoalveolar lavage (BAL) with bronchoscopy or with a sputum culture in CF patients. Chronic infection can lead to greater decline in lung function, more frequent lung exacerbations, and reduced quality of life.
- Quinolones are the only oral class of antibiotics effective in eradicating *Pseudomonas*, but often the bacteria form biofilms making it very difficult to eradicate.
- Several weeks of intravenous (IV) antibiotics are often needed if quinolone drugs are ineffective for clearing the *Pseudomonas*.
- Many patients will need suppressive therapy for *Pseudomonas* refractory to eradication and rely on inhaled antibiotics, such as tobramycin and aztreonam, to prevent clinical exacerbations.

PATIENT EDUCATION

- The hallmark of treatment for pulmonary CF patients consists of airway clearance methods to remove trapped mucus in the bronchiectatic airways of the lungs. Theoretically, effective daily airway clearance reduces the risk of developing lung infections.
- One airway clearance measure is wearing a high-frequency chest wall oscillation device called a percussion vest. Also, blowing into a handheld positive expiratory pressure (PEP) device and doing chest physiotherapy (PT) can be equally effective in facilitating airway clearance.
- Inhaling hypertonic saline can be beneficial by triggering the patient to cough deeply allowing trapped mucus to be coughed out of the lungs.
- Dornase alfa, a DNAse enzyme, is an effective mucolytic making it less dense and easier to cough out.
- All patients with CF and bronchiectasis can improve airway clearance by engaging in aerobic exercise on a regular basis.

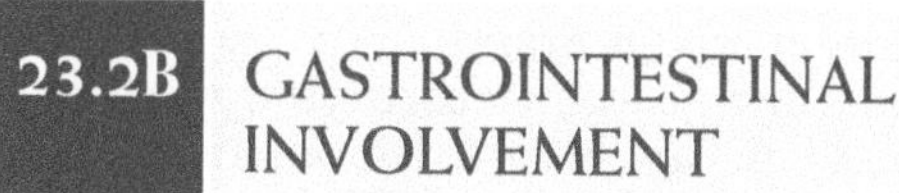

23.2B GASTROINTESTINAL INVOLVEMENT

MEDICAL HISTORY AND CLINICAL PRESENTATION

Many CF patients will have buildup of mucus in the gastrointestinal (GI) tract causing blockages, especially in the newborn and infants, leading to meconium ileus. The mucus can block ducts to the pancreas preventing the secretion of enzymes to help with normal digestion. The blocked enzymes lead to impaired absorption, especially with fats and proteins.

SIGNS AND SYMPTOMS

CF patients with GI involvement will often complain of abdominal pain, diarrhea that does not resolve, and foul-smelling, bulky, greasy stools. Infants and young children with CF commonly exhibit poor growth and low body weight despite a good appetite.

PHYSICAL EXAMINATION

A blockage in the small intestine in a newborn with thicker-than-normal meconium causing meconium ileus should raise suspicion of a CF diagnosis. Pancreatitis and gallstones are commonly seen in untreated CF patients with GI involvement.

DIFFERENTIAL DIAGNOSIS

It may not be obvious that common GI symptoms may be secondary to CF. Other conditions to consider in addition to meconium ileus secondary to CF include Hirschsprung disease and bowel atresia. Failure to thrive and poor weight gain could be secondary to celiac disease, and there are many causes of pancreatitis.

DIAGNOSTIC STUDIES

A contrast barium enema is often used for confirming a diagnosis of meconium ileus suspected based on clinical and diagnostic evidence. Checking serum levels for immunoreactive trypsinogen (IRT), an enzyme precursor made in the pancreas, is an NBS test for CF performed in the United States and other Western developed countries. Elevated IRT levels may reflect the severity of pancreatic function and of the *CFTR* gene defect.[16] If the NBS is positive with elevated IRT levels, the patient should undergo a sweat chloride test, which is considered the gold standard for helping to diagnose CF. A positive sweat test >60 mmol/L means a CF diagnosis is likely, and a test result of <40 mmol/L means the diagnosis is unlikely. The CFTR protein is found in the skin, and there is more salt content in the sweat for a person with a defective CFTR protein. If the sweat chloride test is high, a confirmatory genetic test to check for mutations of the *CFTR* gene is done by collecting DNA from the blood, saliva, or tissue sample from inside the cheek. Complete fatty replacement of the pancreas and pancreatic cysts are common findings seen in CF patients. Ultrasound, CT of the abdomen, and MRI are all beneficial for diagnosis.

EVALUATION

Pancreas enzyme supplements need to be taken before each meal and snacks, and sometimes supplemental nutrition is required via gastrostomy tube feedings overnight to provide additional calories. Fat-soluble vitamin intake (A, D, E, K) is needed because of difficulty in absorption. Insulin may be needed for CF-related diabetes.

TREATMENT

- A major revolution in treatment for patients with CF is the development of CF modulator drugs, targeted to allow the CFTR protein to function better. Ivacaftor (trade name Kalydeco), approved by the FDA in January 2012, was the first CF modulator drug to directly address the underlying defect in CF. One known mutation causes a gating defect, preventing the protein from opening correctly to enable salt and water to flow in and out of cells like it should. Ivacaftor is a CFTR potentiator and works by keeping the gate open longer at the cell surface allowing better flow of mucus and hydration. Although ivacaftor only benefited a small number of patients with CF, the developmental pathway established by ivacaftor led to other CFTR modulator drugs that could benefit many more CF patients.[17]
- Approximately 90% of patients with CF have at least one copy of F508del, which is the most common CF gene mutation.[12,18] The F508del mutation affects protein folding, resulting in low amounts of protein to be translated from the DNA. The low quantity of CFTR protein means less is available on the cell surface. Orkambi is a combination of a corrector (lumacaftor) and potentiator (ivacaftor), approved by the FDA in July 2015, and was the first approved modulator to treat patients homozygous for the F508del mutation.[19] Lumacaftor helps the CFTR protein to fold correctly into its three-dimensional shape to allow it to reach the cell membrane surface. Tezacaftor and ivacaftor (Symdeko) is a second combination corrector and potentiator modulator drug that was approved by the FDA in February 2018. Symdeko was reported to improve pulmonary function at least as well as Orkambi with less reported side effects.[20]
- Trikafta (elexacaptor-tezacaftor-ivacaftor) is a new triple therapy modulator approved by the FDA in October 2019 which may help up to 90% of patients with CF age 12 and older that is approved for patients with at least one F508del mutation. Elexacaptor and tezacaftor work by allowing more protein to reach the cell surface and ivacaftor helps the proteins stay open longer once they get to the surface.[11] Clinical studies showed Trikafta improved patient-reported respiratory symptoms, better lung function via spirometry, and lower sweat chloride concentration in patients with a single F508del allele.[18]

PATIENT EDUCATION

- CF modulator drugs have the potential to allow CF patients to live longer and improve their quality of life.

SPECIAL CONSIDERATIONS

Patients with CF are also at increased risk of becoming infected with pulmonary nontuberculous mycobacteria (NTM), which, like *Pseudomonas*, can be quite difficult to eradicate. The most common pathogenic NTM species seen in CF patients is *Mycobacterium avium* complex (MAC), followed by *Mycobacterium abscessus*.[21] Patients with NTM infection are usually on treatment for a minimum of 18 months, which includes a combination of oral, inhaled, and intravenous antibiotics.[22] Often patients with CF will be prescribed a macrolide antibiotic such as azithromycin 250 mg daily or 500 mg three times weekly for anti-inflammatory and immunoprotective benefits to prevent growth of bacteria leading to lung infections. Patients with CF should stop azithromycin monotherapy as part of their regimen if they have a positive culture for NTM; monotherapy with a macrolide may place the patient at greater risk of resistant mycobacteria infection.[21]

KEY POINTS

- CF is an autosomal recessive genetic disease that occurs because of mutations in the *CFTR* gene. There are >1,700 mutations that have been identified with the most common one being F508del.
- The most common areas of the body affected by CF are the lungs and GI tract. Patients are prone to chronic, recurrent lung infections and pancreatic insufficiency due to mucus blockage in the airways and pancreatic ducts.
- Most patients with CF will develop bronchiectasis in the lungs, which is best diagnosed via HRCT of the chest. *Pseudomonas* is one of the most common bacteria organisms cultured in the sputum or via bronchoscopy.
- Many patients with CF are required to take pancreatic enzyme supplements before each meal to aid in digestion. Most patients with CF require daily airway clearance measures to prevent mucus plugging in the lungs and minimize the risk of developing lung infections.
- CF modulator drugs allow the CFTR protein to function better by addressing the underlying defect in CF. Trikafta is a new triple therapy drug approved by the FDA in October 2019 for patients with at least one F508del mutation that may help up to 90% of patients with CF 12 years and older.

23.3 DOWN SYNDROME

Wesley Patterson

OVERVIEW

Down syndrome is a genetic disorder in which an individual has an extra copy of chromosome 21. Down syndrome is the most common genetic cause of intellectual disability and the most common autosomal aneuploidy condition compatible with life. This disorder can affect individuals of any gender or race. The diagnosis of Down syndrome is made or confirmed through a chromosome analysis (karyotype). General management for individuals with Down syndrome includes monitoring growth, development, and behavior closely as well as annual monitoring of hearing, vision, hemoglobin, and thyroid function. In infancy, an echocardiogram is recommended as well as early intervention services such as speech therapy, occupational therapy, and physical therapy.[23,24]

EPIDEMIOLOGY

Down syndrome is observed in 1:800 live births.[25] Advanced maternal age (defined as a woman 35 years or older at the time of delivery) is associated with an increased risk of having a child with Down syndrome because older eggs have an increased risk of improper chromosome division.[26,27] However, it is important to note that most children with Down syndrome are born to women under the age of 35 as more women are having children during this stage of life.[26,27] There are three types of Down syndrome:[23,24]

- **Trisomy 21:** About 95% of individuals with Down syndrome have a full extra copy of chromosome 21, meaning each cell in the body has 3 copies of chromosome 21. This typically occurs spontaneously by nondisjunction in either the sperm or egg prior to fertilization. Trisomy 21 is not inherited. The recurrence risk for trisomy 21 is 1% but may be higher in mothers of advanced maternal age.
- **Translocation Down syndrome:** Unbalanced translocations account for about 3% of individuals with Down syndrome (also known as familial Down syndrome). This results from the fusion of an extra chromosome 21 with another acrocentric chromosome (usually chromosome 14 or 21). Parental chromosome analyses would be beneficial to determine if a parent is a balanced translocation carrier. If the mother is a balanced translocation carrier the recurrence risk is 10% to 15%, and if the father is a balanced translocation carrier the recurrence risk is 2% to 5%. If a parent carries a 21;21 translocation the recurrence risk is 100%.
- **Mosaic Down syndrome:** Mosaicism accounts for about 2% of individuals with Down syndrome. These individuals have the normal 2 copies of chromosome 21 in some cells and 3 copies of chromosome 21 in other cells. Mosaic Down syndrome is not inherited. These individuals typically have milder phenotypes.

PATHOPHYSIOLOGY

Down syndrome is caused by an extra copy of chromosome 21.[23–29] There are approximately 300 genes located on chromosome 21, 215 of which are protein-coding genes.[26] Different genes and critical regions on chromosome 21 contribute to the unique phenotype. A strong candidate gene for the intellectual disability associated with Down syndrome is the *DYRK1A* gene.[26,28] This gene encodes an enzyme that is essential in the development of the nervous system.[26,28] When this gene is overexpressed, it can lead to learning difficulties and memory issues.[26,28]

MEDICAL HISTORY AND CLINICAL PRESENTATION

Down syndrome is associated with multisystem involvement. The medical history and clinical presentation can vary among affected individuals; however, the majority of individuals with Down syndrome will have some degree of intellectual disability, short stature, congenital heart defects (50%), GI issues, transverse/single palmar creases (50%), and distinct facial features.[23–29] The degree of intellectual disability may be mild, moderate, and, less frequently, severe.[23,24,26–29] Some individuals may be considered high functioning and be able to maintain a job and live independently.[28] The most common congenital heart defect is an atrioventricular canal defect, but ventricular septal defects are also common.[26,28] GI issues may include celiac disease, Hirschsprung disease, and intestinal defects such as atresia or obstruction.[23,25,27,29] Other manifestations include frequent upper respiratory tract infections, frequent ear infections, iron deficiency anemia, hypothyroidism, and obstructive sleep apnea.[23–29] Vision issues and hearing loss are also common.[23–29] Individuals with Down syndrome are also at an increased risk for leukemia and Alzheimer disease.[23–29]

SIGNS AND SYMPTOMS

Box 23.1 summarizes the signs and symptoms of Down syndrome.[23–29]

PHYSICAL EXAMINATION

Box 23.2 summarizes the common physical examination findings in patients with Down syndrome. Characteristic features can be seen in Figure 23.1.[23–29]

DIFFERENTIAL DIAGNOSIS

Down syndrome can typically be differentiated from other genetic disorders due to the unique facial features and physical examination findings (Table 23.3).[29] Individuals with Down syndrome, congenital hypothyroidism, 49,XXXXY syndrome, and Zellweger syndrome may present with intellectual disability, hypotonia, poor feeding and weight gain,

BOX 23.1 Signs and Symptoms of Down Syndrome

Intellectual disability
Developmental delay
Distinctive features
Microcephaly
Atlantoaxial instability
Short stature
Congenital heart defects
Gastrointestinal issues
Poor muscle tone (hypotonia)

BOX 23.2 Common Physical Examination Findings in Down Syndrome

Distinctive facies: flat and round face, epicanthal folds with upslanting palpebral fissures, flat nasal bridge, small and low-set ears with overfolded helices, and small mouth with protruding tongue
Brachycephaly and/or microcephaly
Poor muscle tone (hypotonia)
Short stature
Short neck
Small hands and feet
Transverse palmar crease (single crease)
Short and incurved fifth finger (clinodactyly)
Gap between first and second toes (sandal gap)
Speckling on iris (Brushfield spots)

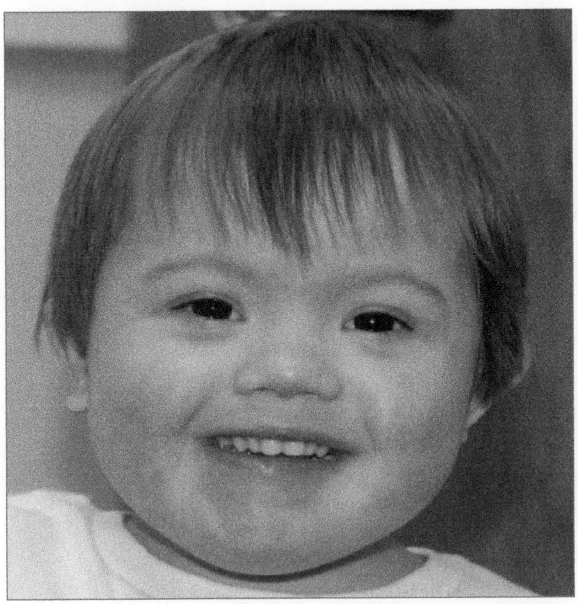

Figure 23.1 A toddler with Down syndrome, illustrating characteristic features: microcephaly, fine hair, flat and round facies, epicanthal folds with upslanting palpebral fissures, flat nasal bridge, and small, low-set ears with overfolded helices and upturned ear lobes (hypotonia).

and distinctive facies. Individuals with congenital hypothyroidism typically have coarse facial features, large fontanelles, and umbilical hernias, which are not present in Down syndrome. In the United States, congenital hypothyroidism is detected through NBS programs. However, it is important to note that infants with Down syndrome may also have low thyroid hormone levels. Individuals with Down syndrome and 49,XXXXY syndrome have similar features (upslanting palpebral fissures, epicanthal folds, and clinodactyly), but individuals with 49,XXXXY syndrome may have wide spaced eyes (hypertelorism) and normal head, nose, and ear size. This syndrome only affects males. Also, at an older age, males develop sparse body hair and breast enlargement

Table 23.3 Differential Diagnosis for Down Syndrome

Diagnosis	Description
Congenital hypothyroidism	Low thyroid hormone at birth, coarse facial features, large fontanelle, poor feeding and weight gain, hypotonia
49,XXXXY syndrome and other high-order multiple X chromosome disorders	Only in males, intellectual disability, distinctive facial features, articulation issues, defiant behavior, hypotonia
Zellweger syndrome or other peroxisomal disorders	Peroxisomal disorder, intellectual disability, distinctive facial features, skeletal abnormalities, hypotonia, poor feeding, seizures, hearing loss, vision loss

(gynecomastia). Down syndrome and Zellweger syndrome can also have similar features (microcephaly, upslanting palpebral fissures, flattened facies, and hypotonia), but individuals with Zellweger syndrome may also have skeletal abnormalities and seizures as well as develop life-threatening issues with the heart, liver, and kidneys. This condition can be lethal in infancy. Individuals with Zellweger syndrome also have elevated very long chain fatty acids (VLCFAs), and an individual with Down syndrome would have normal VLCFAs. Each of the disorders may also be differentiated with a simple chromosome analysis. An individual with Down syndrome would have an extra chromosome 21, an individual with 49,XXXXY syndrome would have three extra X chromosomes, and an individual with congenital hypothyroidism or Zellweger syndrome would have normal chromosomes.

DIAGNOSTIC STUDIES

Fluorescence in situ hybridization (FISH) and a chromosome analysis can also be performed via prenatal diagnostic tests: chorionic villus sampling (CVS), amniocentesis, and cell-free DNA.[24,27,29] Prenatal screening may be performed indirectly by measuring different biochemical levels in the mother's blood along with ultrasound.[24,27,29] However, the diagnosis should be confirmed through FISH or a chromosome analysis.[24,27,29] While FISH testing is sufficient to make the diagnosis of Down syndrome, it will not elucidate which type of Down syndrome is present. Therefore, a high-resolution chromosome analysis is the recommended test for diagnosis. If mosaic Down syndrome is suspected, a specific mosaic chromosome analysis should be ordered, where the lab will examine more cells to determine if mosaicism is present.[24,27,29]

EVALUATION

General management for individuals with Down syndrome includes monitoring growth, development, and behavior closely as well as annual monitoring of hearing, vision, and thyroid function. In infancy, an echocardiogram is recommended as well as early intervention services such as speech therapy, occupational therapy, and physical therapy.[23]

TREATMENT

There is no cure for Down syndrome. Treatment is focused on the specific, individualized concerns of each patient. Specialists may include audiology for hearing issues, cardiology for congenital heart defects, developmental-behavioral pediatrics for intellectual disability and learning difficulties, gastroenterology for feeding issues and/or GI issues, ophthalmology for visual concerns, and otolaryngology for frequent ear infections. Individuals with Down syndrome usually start early intervention, speech therapy, occupational therapy, and physical therapy early in life.[23]

PATIENT EDUCATION

- Genetic counseling is needed to discuss the recurrence risk for the family. This will depend on the type of Down syndrome as well as the maternal age.
- Annual eye examinations and hearing screenings; monitoring of hemoglobin and thyroid-stimulating hormone level.
- Females with Down syndrome have reduced fertility and have an overall chance of having a child with Down syndrome of 35% to 50%. Males are typically infertile.
- For a complete list of recommendations and anticipatory guidance broken down by age, the Committee on Genetics of the American Academy of Pediatrics has created *Health Supervision for Children with Down Syndrome*, which is updated periodically.[23]

KEY POINTS

- The most common genetic cause of intellectual disability is Down syndrome.
- Most cases of Down syndrome occur sporadically due to nondisjunction (95%).
- Every individual suspected of having Down syndrome should have a chromosome analysis to determine the family's recurrence risk.
- Advanced maternal age is associated with an increased risk of having a child with Down syndrome; however, most children with Down syndrome are born to women under the age of 35.

23.4 ACUTE INTERMITTENT PORPHYRIA

Laura D. Buch

OVERVIEW

AIP is a metabolic genetic disorder caused by a mutation of the *HMBS* gene on chromosome 11. If an acute attack does occur, it is commonly triggered by ingestion of certain medications, alcohol, or catalyzed by another stressor. Often an acute attack will first present with abdominal pain, progress to psychiatric manifestations, and finally peripheral neuropathy. Acute attacks should be managed with human hemin and symptomatic treatments, and recurrent attacks can be managed with givosiran or liver transplant.

AIP is the most prevalent and severe form of acute porphyria, a group of metabolic diseases, and is caused by a mutation in the *HMBS* gene located on the long arm of chromosome 11 (11q24.1-q24.2). AIP is an autosomal dominant condition with an onset of symptoms frequently occurring after puberty.[30]

EPIDEMIOLOGY

AIP is present in about 1/2,000 Europeans and is found in even higher rates among the Northern European population. AIP exhibits low penetrance with only 10% to 20% of heterozygotes becoming symptomatic in their lifetime. Though inheritance is equal in both sexes, AIP is more likely to manifest in women than in men.[30]

PATHOPHYSIOLOGY

Deficient enzyme hydroxymethylbilane synthase (HMBS), necessary for the synthesis of heme, a fundamental component of hemoglobin, leads to accumulation of neurotoxic porphyrin precursors delta-aminolevulinic acid and porphobilinogen (PBG). Acute attacks of AIP can be life-threatening and are commonly precipitated by alcohol, steroid hormone changes, infection, fasting, and various drugs, including several antibiotics, antipsychotics, and antiepileptics.[30,31] These catalysts exacerbate the already deficient HMBS, resulting in an acute attack. Recurrent attacks can lead to chronic kidney disease and increased risk for hepatocellular carcinoma.[32]

SIGNS AND SYMPTOM

Exhibit 23.1 summarizes signs and symptoms consistent with AIP.

PHYSICAL EXAMINATION

In a patient experiencing an acute attack, evaluation of the abdomen is crucial, and may reveal distention and decreased bowel sounds. Abdominal tenderness is unlikely. Muscle weakness may be observed proximally in the lower extremities and may involve the upper extremities or distal portions of the arms and legs. Evaluation of the cranial nerves should be performed, as these may also be affected. Complete paralysis or seizure activity may be observed. Patients may appear confused, restless, agitated, have an altered affect, or range from somnolent to comatose.[33]

Exhibit 23.1 Signs and Symptoms Consistent With Acute Intermittent Porphyria

Symptoms of an acute attack progress from abdominal pain, psychiatric symptoms, then peripheral neuropathy:

- Abdominal pain: severe, epigastric, colicky
- Psychiatric manifestations: depression
- Peripheral neuropathy: ascending weakness, autonomic neuropathies (may lead to hypertension and tachycardia)

Other symptoms of an acute attack can include:

- Central nervous signs: delirium, weakness, quadriplegia, respiratory failure, cortical blindness, coma
- Reddish brown urine: darkens with exposure to air, warmth, light

Attacks last for about 1 week and, unlike many other porphyrias, does not present with a skin rash.

Source: Data from Whatley SD, Badminton MN. Acute intermittent porphyria. In: Adam MP, Ardinger HH, Pagon RA, et al, eds. *GeneReviews*. University of Washington; 2005. https://www.ncbi.nlm.nih.gov/books/NBK1193

DIFFERENTIAL DIAGNOSIS

Table 23.4 summarizes the differential diagnoses for AIP. Of note, there are many causes of abdominal pain that may be confused with AIP (appendicitis, ischemic bowel disease, diverticulitis). And while a urinary PBG may be elevated and indicate an acute attack of AIP, these conditions may precipitate an attack and cannot be excluded solely based on elevated urinary PBG.[34]

DIAGNOSTIC STUDIES AND EVALUATION

If an individual is having symptoms consistent with AIP, they should be tested for elevated urinary PBG. If this is positive, then begin treatment immediately. Once elevated urinary PBG is established, determine the type of acute porphyria by performing biochemical testing. Confirmatory testing should consist of *HMBS* gene sequencing, and blood relatives can then be assessed for the known gene change.[34]

TREATMENT

- Avoid precipitating factors and recommend a diet with consistent ingestion of carbohydrates.
- For those with confirmed acute attack, immediately administer 10% dextrose in 0.45% saline IV and human hemin IV at 3–4 mg/kg once daily for 4 days.
- Pain should be managed with parenteral opiates, nausea/vomiting with antiemetics and IV fluids, and anxiety/insomnia with short-acting benzodiazepines.
- The only curative treatment for recurrent attacks is liver transplantation.
- To reduce the rate of occurrence and reduce PBG levels, once monthly injections of givosiran may be used.[35] Givosiran is an interference RNA therapeutic that represses production of hepatic delta-aminolevulinic acid synthase and was approved by the FDA in November 2019.[33]

Table 23.4 Differential Diagnosis for Acute Intermittent Porphyria

Diagnosis	Examples	How to Differentiate from Acute Intermittent Porphyria (AIP)
Other causes of neuropathy	Guillain-Barré syndrome, lead poisoning	AIP causes elevated urinary porphobilinogen (PBG)
Other causes of neuropsychiatric symptoms	Neurodegenerative disease, substance use, encephalitides	Both may cause hyponatremia and abnormalities on neuroimaging; AIP causes elevated urinary PBG
Other causes of seizures	Hypoglycemia, uremia, hypocalcemia	AIP causes elevated urinary PBG
Other acute porphyrias	Hereditary coproporphyria (HCP)	Both cause elevated urinary PBG, AIP more than HCP; HCP with increased fecal porphyrins, rare blistering photosensitivity
	Variegate porphyria (VP)	High plasma porphyrin with fluorescent peak
	5-Aminolevulinic acid dehydratase porphyria	5-Aminolevulinic acid dehydratase porphyria causes elevated urinary aminolevulinic acid (ALA) instead of PBG

PATIENT EDUCATION

- AIP is a genetic disorder that affects how the body makes heme, which is used to help carry oxygen, leading to a buildup of chemicals in the body.
- Patients having an attack may experience belly pain, muscle weakness, a fast heartbeat, reddish brown urine, and mental symptoms. These symptoms usually go away after an attack.
- To treat these attacks, patients will receive hemin, which will help the body stop making the chemicals that are causing their symptoms. There are other treatment options available.
- Patients with AIP should avoid things that are known to trigger attacks, like certain medicines and alcohol, and should eat plenty of carbohydrates.

KEY POINTS

- AIP is an autosomal dominant disorder that is characterized by a pathogenic change in the *HMBS* gene.
- Alterations in the *HMBS* gene lead to decreased synthesis of the HMBS enzyme and accumulation of porphyrin precursors.
- Acute attacks are preceded by physiologic stressors, hormonal changes, and ingestion of porphyrinogenic substances.
- Signs and symptoms of acute attacks include progression from abdominal pain to psychiatric manifestations then peripheral neuropathy.
- Acute attacks of AIP should be managed with hemin and symptom control; recurrent attacks may be treated with givosiran or liver transplantation. Avoidance of exacerbating factors is crucial in the prevention of an acute attack.

23.5 KLINEFELTER SYNDROME

Amy Maurer

OVERVIEW

Klinefelter syndrome (KS) is the most common sex chromosome aneuploidy and the most common cause of male primary hypogonadism.

EPIDEMIOLOGY

The prevalence of KS is approximately 1 in 660 male births. Caused by the presence of at least one additional X chromosome in an XY male, 80% to 90% of males with KS have a karyotype of 47,XXY. The presence of additional X chromosomes is much rarer and these are often considered "variants" of KS. About 10% of affected males have the milder mosaic form in which some tissues have a 47,XXY karyotype and others are 46,XY (46,XY/47,XXY).

In 47,XXY KS, the additional X chromosome originates from a random nondisjunction during gametogenesis in either parent. Mosaic KS results from random postzygotic mitotic nondisjunction. Maternal age over 35 mildly increases the risk of KS. No other definitive risk factors are known. It affects all races, ethnicities, and socioeconomic statuses equally. At least partly due to KS's nonspecific features, the detection rate is low and up to 70% of affected males are not diagnosed during their lifetime.

PATHOPHYSIOLOGY

During puberty, the presence of the additional X chromosome causes progressive fibrotic destruction of the Leydig cells and the seminiferous tubules of the testes resulting in a decrease in sperm and testosterone (T) production. Sperm production is affected earlier and more severely than T production.

MEDICAL HISTORY AND CLINICAL PRESENTATION

Men with KS are diagnosed at a mean age of 30 years. Clinical features vary based on developmental stage and KS severity with only the most severe phenotypes recognized prior to puberty. In a neonate, KS may be suspected due to genital anomalies such as hypospadias, small phallus (micropenis), or cryptorchidism. Prepubertal boys with KS may present with difficulties in learning, socialization, behavior, and/or language. Rate of KS detection increases during the typical pubertal ages since affected males may present due to failure to begin or complete puberty. In adulthood, an affected male typically complains of infertility or symptoms of T/androgen deficiency.

SIGNS AND SYMPTOMS

KS may affect the endocrine and the musculoskeletal systems and neurodevelopment. During infancy, males with KS may exhibit speech and motor delays, hypotonia, and motor planning difficulties. Prior to puberty, most boys lack obvious features, but hypertelorism may be present. Puberty may begin when expected, but testes do not reach the typical adult male size and secondary sexual characteristics may be slow to appear. During puberty, the boy with KS is likely to grow taller than expected. Despite variations in growth rates, it is rare for a boy with 47,XXY to have a height below the 25th percentile. Adult males with untreated KS may have small testes and truncal obesity.

PHYSICAL EXAMINATION

Affected pubertal boys may have gynecomastia, cryptorchidism, increased growth and tall stature, low muscle mass, increased fat mass, scoliosis, kyphosis, ligamentous laxity, wide hips, narrow shoulders, and/or truncal hypotonia.

Affected men may demonstrate the same findings noted in pubertal boys, and generally have testes that are very small and firm. The testes may approach or reach normal size in patients with mosaic KS. A small prostate may also be noted.

DIFFERENTIAL DIAGNOSIS

Differential diagnoses for KS include gonadotropin deficiency (Kallmann syndrome), hypopituitarism, and Marfan syndrome.

DIAGNOSTIC STUDIES

One or more redundant X chromosomes noted on karyotyping is considered definitively diagnostic for KS. A minimum of 20 metaphase cells should be assessed to decrease the risk of a false negative result in the case of mosaic KS. An adult male presenting with classic features of KS and primary hypogonadism can be given a presumptive diagnosis of KS without karyotyping if the man is not interested in conceiving a child. In contrast, males with gonadotropin deficiency, hypopituitarism, or Marfan syndrome have a 46,XY karyotype.

Advances in genetic testing have increased incidental prenatal detection of KS during routine prenatal screening or via noninvasive prenatal testing (NIPT). These tests are not diagnostic and must be confirmed via amniocentesis, CVS, or a postnatal karyotype.

EVALUATION

During infancy, patients with KS should be evaluated for hormonal abnormalities at 3 months of age since males with KS may have abnormal levels of T and other hormones. A pediatric endocrinologist can guide parents as they consider T treatment. The infant should be monitored for speech and motor delays.

In a prepubertal child with KS, height (sitting and standing) should be measured annually and bone age assessed every 2 to 3 years. Two DEXA scans are recommended during childhood. A pediatric endocrinologist can discuss issues related to fertility preservation with the patient and his parents.

Boys and men with KS are not intellectually impaired but may have difficulty with language-based learning and motor planning and evaluation is recommended.

Typically, postpubertal males and men have low serum free and total T. Rarely, a male with KS will have normal T levels, but levels will usually fall as the normal testicular tissue is destroyed. Affected men also typically have elevated levels of follicle-stimulating hormone and luteinizing hormone.

Underscoring the importance of routine preventive care, KS is related to multiple co-occurring conditions including dentofacial abnormalities, behavioral problems, cardiovascular disease, increased risk of COPD and pneumonia, increased risk of osteoarthritis, osteoporosis, chronically low muscle mass and strength, learning and developmental disabilities, personality disorders, and tremor. When compared with men without KS, those with KS have a higher absolute risk of most cancers and autoimmune diseases, but it remains small. Their absolute risk of breast cancer is up to 50 times higher than men without KS, but their lifetime risk remains <1%. KS patients appear to have a slightly lower lifetime risk of prostate cancer.

TREATMENT

There is no cure for KS. Although most KS management recommendations are based upon small clinical trials and clinical expert experience, a multidisciplinary approach to the care of patients with KS is widely accepted as the gold standard to optimize health and quality of life in patients with KS regardless of when the patient is diagnosed. Collaborating with a medical geneticist, genetic counselor, and an endocrinologist may help expedite evaluation and treatment while providing additional resources for the patient and his family. Treatment generally focuses on T supplementation and fertility preservation, which is generally managed by endocrinology. The optimal approach to fertility preservation and T therapy is under debate. As specific needs are identified, appropriate specialists, therapists, and counselors can be recruited to address them.

Appropriate surveillance and preventive care can decrease the risk of adverse sequelae of KS. Unfortunately, the lifespan of males with KS is decreased by 5 to 6 years when compared to their unaffected male peers. An earlier age at diagnosis due to a more severe phenotype may indicate an even shorter lifespan.

PATIENT EDUCATION

Affected patients (and their parents) should be advised that they did not cause the boy's diagnosis by anything they did or neglected to do. The genetic basis of KS and a review of the patient's own karyotype should be discussed with him and his family. They should be advised that there is no cure for KS and that signs and symptoms are highly variable. Education is likely to be an ongoing process throughout the lifespan with new questions arising as the patient matures.

KEY POINTS

- KS is the most common sex chromosome aneuploidy and is caused by the presence of one or more supernumerary X chromosomes in males.
- Most males with KS have a 47,XXY karyotype.
- Over 50% of males with KS are not diagnosed during their lifetime.
- There is no cure for KS.
- Treatment and management of KS depend on syndrome severity and age at diagnosis.

23.6 MARFAN SYNDROME

Melissa Murfin

OVERVIEW

Marfan syndrome is an inherited, connective tissue disorder that shows considerable variability in presentation. The most common manifestations occur in the skeletal muscles and joints, cardiovascular system, and ophthalmic system.[36] Patients with Marfan syndrome are often noted to be taller than average with long extremities, joint laxity, and scoliosis. These patients may also be nearsighted, requiring vision correction, and may suffer from cardiac valvular disorders.[36] With appropriate diagnosis and medical care, patients can expect to achieve a normal life span.[36]

EPIDEMIOLOGY

Marfan syndrome is estimated to occur in 2 to 3 people per 1,000.[37] The disease is related to a mutation in the *FBN1* gene, which codes for the fibrillin 1 protein that is important in connective tissue formation. The genetic mutation is inherited in an autosomal dominant pattern; however, as many as 25% of cases are thought to be a result of a new mutation.[37] The disease affects both males and females equally and is distributed across all races.[37]

PATHOPHYSIOLOGY

In Marfan syndrome, mutations in the *FBN1* gene lead to changes in production of fibrillin 1. Patients may be idiopathic, or have decreased fibrillin 1 production, decreased fibrillin 1 secretion, inability to incorporate fibrillin 1 molecules into the extracellular matrix.[38] Similar defects are found in families that carry the mutation.

MEDICAL HISTORY AND CLINICAL PRESENTATION

Marfan syndrome affects multiple systems throughout the body. The most common manifestations of the disease are noted in the skeletal system and are related to increased bone growth. Patients often appear tall and thin with arm span 1.5 times greater than the patient's height and elongated fingers and toes.[38] Joint hypermobility is also often present and may be identified in pediatric patients.[38] Patients may exhibit the wrist sign, an overlap of the thumb and fifth fingers when encircling them about their opposite wrist.[38]

Cardiovascular manifestations of Marfan syndrome range from mild to severe. Aortic dissection is the most common cardiac cause of death in patients with Marfan syndrome. Murmurs may be present and associated with mitral valve regurgitation or prolapse or tricuspid regurgitation.[38] Pediatric patients with severe defects may present with heart failure while the risk of cardiomyopathy increases with age.

Myopia is common, often leading to vision correction at a young age. Additional issues may occur with age including glaucoma, cataracts, and retinal detachment. Skin manifestations are uncommon and may help differentiate Marfan syndrome from Ehlers-Danlos syndrome and other connective tissue disorders.[38]

SIGNS AND SYMPTOMS

Signs and symptoms include[39]:

- Above average height
- Arachnodactyly (i.e., abnormally long fingers and toes)
- Mitral valve murmur
- Severe myopia
- Height is typically 1.5× above average (although not formal diagnostic criteria)
- Reduced upper to lower segment ratio
- Increased arm span to height ratio

PHYSICAL EXAMINATION

Common physical examination findings of Marfan syndrome include:

- Arachnodactyly: + wrist and thumb signs
- Anterior chest wall deformities: pectus carinatum or pectus excavatum
- Flat foot
- Joint hypermobility
- Scoliosis
- Skin striae
- Mitral valve prolapse

- Aortic root enlargement
- Ectopia lentis
- Early cataracts
- Increased intraocular pressure consistent with glaucoma

DIFFERENTIAL DIAGNOSIS

Table 23.5 summarizes the differential diagnosis for Marfan syndrome.

DIAGNOSTIC STUDIES

Table 23.6 summarizes the diagnostic testing for Marfan syndrome.

EVALUATION

Patients require an echocardiogram, fundoscopic examination, and genetic testing. Family history information is important to collect.

TREATMENT

- Evaluation by a clinical geneticist or genetic counselor is important to determine extent of disease in family members and potential for inheritability.
- Cardiology evaluation is needed to determine extent of cardiac abnormalities. Beta blockers or angiotensin receptor blockers (ARBs) may be useful in decreasing stress on a heart with an aortic root enlargement.[36]
- Ophthalmology evaluation to address myopia and possible lens dislocation is essential.[36]
- Orthopedic evaluation to address presence of scoliosis and assist with joint fatigue may be useful.[36]

PATIENT EDUCATION

- Patients with Marfan syndrome should be aware that offspring have a 50% chance of inheriting the mutation in the *FBN1* gene.[36]
- Annual eye examination is needed to assess for cataracts, glaucoma, and ectopia lentis.
- Contact sports, high intensity exercise, and heavy lifting should be avoided.

Table 23.5 Differential Diagnosis for Marfan Syndrome

Diagnosis	Description
Ehlers-Danlos syndrome	Skin with widened atrophic scars vs. striae Progressive congenital scoliosis or scoliosis that develops within first year of life. Facial appearance: thin lips and nose, small chin, large eyes
Ectopia lentis syndrome	Dislocation of lens, skeletal abnormalities present Aortic root enlargement generally not present
Familial thoracic aortic aneurysm and dissection (FTAAD)	Aortic root enlargement present Skeletal findings, ocular finding generally not present

Source: Data from Kanakis GA, Nieschlag E. Klinefelter syndrome: more than hypogonadism. Metabolism. *2018;86:135–144. doi:10.1016/j.metabol.2017.09.017*

Table 23.6 Diagnostic Testing for Marfan Syndrome

Diagnostic Test	Findings
FBN1 gene	70%–90% of patients with clinical indications of Marfan syndrome expected to carry a mutation
Echocardiogram	Evaluate aortic root and mitral valve. Aortic root dilatation with a Z score ≥2 for patients 20 years of age and older; >3 for patients under 20 years of age

Source: Data from Marfan syndrome—FBN1. GTR: Genetic Testing Registry. https://www.ncbi.nlm.nih.gov/gtr/tests/502890; Genetic and Rare Diseases Information Center. Marfan syndrome. https://rarediseases.info.nih.gov/diseases/6975/disease

- For patients with potential pneumothorax, SCUBA and other positive pressure breathing should be avoided. Playing musical brass wind instruments such as a trumpet or a tuba should also be avoided.

KEY POINTS

- Marfan syndrome is inherited in an autosomal-dominant fashion; however, 25% of cases arise from idiopathic mutations.
- Patients may present with multiple complaints including ocular, cardiovascular, and musculoskeletal symptoms.
- Common signs and symptoms include above-average height, long fingers and limbs, heart murmurs, and vision issues.
- A genetic counselor should be utilized for prenatal consultation.

23.7 TAY-SACHS DISEASE

RENA GODFREY

OVERVIEW

Tay-Sachs disease (TSD) is a neurodegenerative disorder that is one of over 500 inherited metabolic diseases, and more specifically, one of more than 70 lysosomal storage diseases.[40,41] The symptoms emerge as a result of impaired capacity to degrade the ganglioside sphingolipid GM2 due to absent or markedly reduced beta-hexosaminidase A activity in lysosomes.[42] The severity and speed of progression of TSD is primarily dependent on levels of residual enzyme activity. It is a rapidly fatal disease in infancy, where enzyme activity is virtually undetectable, though juvenile and late-onset forms have slower progression in the presence of some residual enzyme activity.[42,43]

EPIDEMIOLOGY

While TSD has traditionally been considered a disease of the Ashkenazi Jewish population, carrier screening in this group has resulted in a disease prevalence closer to that of the general population.[44] Historically, individuals of French Canadian descent in southeastern Quebec and the Cajun region of Louisiana have also had an increased incidence of TSD.[44] Inheritance is autosomal recessive and affects males and females equally. In the general population, 1 in 250 to 300 individuals is a carrier, and the incidence of disease is

1:100,000.[42,44] Carrier screening is performed by measuring beta-hexosaminidase A activity, though there is a small risk of false positive results.[44] With recent development of cost effective molecular methods targeting disease-causing mutations, a combination of both tests is the most comprehensive approach.[44] Screening may be performed preconception or during pregnancy.

PATHOPHYSIOLOGY

TSD is a recessive disease caused by a mutation in the *HEXA* gene located on chromosome 15 (15q23-24).[45] More than 130 different mutations of the *HEXA* gene have been identified.[42] This gene encodes the alpha subunit of the lysosomal enzyme beta-hexosaminidase A, responsible for breaking down the GM2 gangliosides into GM3 by removing a GalNac (N-acetyl-galactosamine) molecule. Gangliosides are complex glycosphingolipids present on the cell membrane and are continuously synthesized and degraded. Deficiency of this enzyme leads to accumulation of GM2 gangliosides within the lysosome that results in cell dysfunction and eventual cell death.[45] Since GM2 gangliosides are most abundant in neurons in the brain and spinal cord, neurologic manifestations dominate the presentation.[42]

MEDICAL HISTORY AND CLINICAL PRESENTATION

Disease development is characterized by progressive neurodegeneration. The classic form of TSD presents in infancy, progression is rapid, and the child dies before age 5. The infants appear normal at birth, then develop initial symptoms between 3 and 6 months. Parents often first notice decreased visual awareness prompting a concern for blindness. Other symptoms include hypotonia, muscle weakness, failure to meet milestones, an exaggerated startle response to loud noise, spasticity, seizures, and deafness.[42]

Juvenile onset TSD presents between 2 and 10 years of age. These children generally live until late childhood or adolescence. While disease in infancy is marked by lack of skill development, juvenile onset disease is characterized by a loss of skills. Previously normal, initial symptoms include clumsiness, ataxia and weakness, followed by dysarthria, dysphagia, behavioral problems, and cognitive decline.[42]

Late-onset TSD manifests between adolescence and the mid-30s, is a less severe form, progresses more slowly, and has a more heterogeneous presentation. These patients may live a relatively full life, though with disability. Affected individuals may experience clumsiness, progressive muscle weakness and wasting, tremors, ataxia, dysarthria, dysphagia, dystonia, and spasticity.[42] Behavioral changes are not uncommon in this group, and include bipolar episodes, paranoia, and hallucinations.[42]

SIGNS AND SYMPTOMS

Signs and symptoms include failure to meet milestones in infancy, blindness in infancy, developmental regression in infancy or early childhood, progressive muscle weakness, and ataxia in adolescence or adulthood.[43]

PHYSICAL EXAMINATION

Physical examination should be comprehensive and include referral to ophthalmology and neurology. Delays in growth and development, neuromuscular abnormalities, cardiopulmonary abnormalities, presence of organomegaly, and skin changes should be evaluated. The presence of a cherry red spot on the macula is suggestive of infantile TSD, though it may or may not be present in juvenile TSD. This finding is secondary to thinning of the macular cells exposing the underlying choroid.[42] Any infant presenting with hypotonia and weakness should be evaluated for possible infection, trauma, congenital cardiac disease, endocrine disorders, and toxic exposures.

DIFFERENTIAL DIAGNOSIS

Differential diagnoses for TSD include Sandhoff disease, Leigh syndrome, spinal muscular atrophy, adrenoleukodystrophy (ALD), adult neuronal ceroid lipofuscinosis, and amyotrophic lateral sclerosis (ALS).

DIAGNOSTIC STUDIES

Concern for TSD, or related disorders should include an enzyme assay for lysosomal storage diseases, molecular analysis of the *HEXA* gene, mDNA sequencing, and possibly whole exome analysis. Diagnostic studies may also include a brain MRI, EMG, echocardiogram, EKG, swallow study, abdominal ultrasound, and other pertinent studies based on symptom presentation.

TREATMENT

There is no therapy for TSD at this time, and management is limited to supportive care. Medications to manage symptoms may be indicated and may include anticonvulsants for seizure disorders and psychotropic medications for psychiatric disorders. A gene therapy trial is currently ongoing. Please visit clinicaltrials.gov for more information.

KEY POINTS

- Long-term carrier screening in the Ashkenazi Jewish population has resulted in disease prevalence that is closer to that of the general population.
- The severity of disease and speed of progression are dependent upon the level of residual enzyme activity in lysosomes.
- Infantile onset disease is fatal within 2 to 3 years of diagnosis. Those with adult onset TSD may live for several decades with their disorder.
- The ophthalmologic finding of a cherry red spot on the macula is not present in late onset disease.
- Behavioral changes may occur in late onset TSD.

23.8 FRAGILE X SYNDROME

Anne M. McRae

OVERVIEW

Fragile X syndrome (FXS) is an X-linked trinucleotide repeat disorder classically associated with cognitive and behavioral impairment, although variable manifestations can occur depending on underlying genotype.

FXS is characterized by intellectual and behavioral impairment as well as some characteristic dysmorphic craniofacial features.

Table 23.7 Genotype-Phenotype Correlations with FMR1 CGG Repeat Lengths

Variant Type	FMR1 CGG Repeat Length	Methylation Status	Clinical Status	
			Male	Female
Gray zone	45–54 repeats	Unmethylated	Unaffected Offspring are at risk for premutation	Unaffected Offspring are at risk for premutation
Premutation	~55–200 repeats	Unmethylated	At risk for FXTAS	At risk for FXTAS and FXPOI
Full mutation	200 repeats	Methylated	100% symptomatic	50% with intellectual deficits

FMR1, fragile X mental retardation 1; FXPOI, fragile X-associated primary ovarian insufficiency; FXTAS, fragile X-associated tremor/ataxia syndrome.
Source: Adapted from Hunter JE, Berry-Kravis E, Hipp H, Todd PK. FMR1 *disorders. In: Adam MP, Ardinger HH, Pagon RA, et al, eds.* GeneReviews. *University of Washington; 1998. https://www.ncbi.nlm.nih.gov/books/NBK1384*

EPIDEMIOLOGY

The estimated incidence of full mutation is approximately 1 in 5,000 males. Females are also affected to varying severities with reported penetrance of 50% to 60% in those who harbor a full mutation.[46]

PATHOPHYSIOLOGY

FXS is due to haploinsufficiency of the FMR1 protein (FMRP), a widely expressed protein that is important in normal neuronal functioning.

MEDICAL HISTORY AND CLINICAL PRESENTATION

FXS is an X-linked form of cognitive and behavioral impairment that was first described in 1943 by Martin and Bell.[47] Cardinal features include intellectual disability and a characteristic neurobehavioral profile. Significant behavioral and emotional disturbances are commonly described; nearly half of males and 20% of females with FXS meet clinical criteria for autism spectrum disorder.[48]

SIGNS AND SYMPTOMS

In addition to typical cognitive and neurobehavioral features, mild hypotonia, joint laxity, gastroesophageal reflux, otitis media, and mitral valve prolapse are seen at increased frequency. Seizures may also be noted and may occur at a higher rate in those with autism spectrum disorders.[48,49] Family history may demonstrate additional members with FXS; other supportive features include ovarian insufficiency in females and a tremor-ataxia disorder in both sexes consistent with X-linked inheritance.

PHYSICAL EXAMINATION

While physical features may not be striking in younger patients, associated findings to investigate on examination include macrocephaly (relative or frank) with long facies, prominent chin, prominent forehead, and large ear size. Peripubertal macroorchidism is also considered a classical feature. Less specific features may include mild hypotonia and joint hyperextensibility.[49]

DIFFERENTIAL DIAGNOSIS

The scope of physical and neurologic features in FXS is relatively nonspecific. Differential diagnoses include nonsyndromic autism spectrum disorder and X-linked cognitive impairment. An entity referred to as fragile XE syndrome presents with less pervasive neurologic manifestations and absence of FXS facial features. Similar craniofacial gestalt and delays may also be signs of Soto syndrome, although generalized overgrowth and higher frequency of congenital anomalies are expected in that disorder.

EVALUATION

It is recommended by the American College of Medical Genetics that all males with autism spectrum disorder or supportive neurobehavioral findings be tested for FXS. Testing for FXS should be performed in females if there is a strong clinical suspicion and/or supportive family history findings.[50]

DIAGNOSTIC STUDIES

Historically, the diagnosis of FXS was made at the cytogenetic level by culturing chromosomes with folic acid deficient medium, resulting in the expression of the namesake "fragile site" on Xq27.[51] It is now known that the disorder is a result of haploinsufficiency of the FMRP. The *FMR1* gene contains a stretch of repeated CGG nucleotides (termed trinucleotide repeats) that can become unstable and elongate during meiosis; after a threshold of approximately 200 repeats is surpassed, silencing of gene transcription occurs due to hypermethylation.[52,53] Increased repeat lengths that have not yet reached the threshold for methylation (termed "premutations") are responsible for primary ovarian insufficiency and tremor-ataxia disorders in females. *FMR1* CGG repeat analysis is the initial diagnostic test of choice. Similar to other trinucleotide repeat disorders, meiotic instability can result in progressive expansion between generations. Clinical and reproductive risks based on repeat size have been delineated (Table 23.7).[54]

TREATMENT

There is currently no specific treatment for FXS. Supportive therapy for affected individuals includes formal developmental/neuropsychiatric evaluations; psychologic evaluation with consideration of pharmalogic intervention for behavioral disturbances; screening and standard intervention for gastroesophageal reflux disease (GERD), recurrent otitis media; and regular auscultation for mitral valve prolapse.[49]

PATIENT EDUCATION

Formal genetic counseling is indicated. Referral to a dedicated multidisciplinary fragile X clinic is ideal. Families should be provided resources from support organizations and social programs, as well as anticipatory guidance regarding lifelong care needs.

KEY POINTS

- All males with autism spectrum disorder should be tested for FXS.
- Females can be affected to a variable degree.
- Family history may be positive for primary ovarian insufficiency and movement disorders.
- Complex X-linked trinucleotide repeat inheritance warrants genetic counseling.

23.9 ANGELMAN SYNDROME

ANNE M. MCRAE

OVERVIEW

Angelman syndrome (AS) is a rare genetic neurodevelopmental disorder characterized by happy demeanor, global developmental delays, cognitive impairment, and especially pervasive expressive speech impairment. The molecular underpinnings of this disorder are complex and involve disturbances in DNA imprinting.

EPIDEMIOLOGY

The prevalence of AS is estimated to be 1/12,000–24,000 in the general population.[55]

PATHOPHYSIOLOGY

AS is caused by deficient expression of the maternal *UBE3A* gene. Abnormal *UBE3A* expression disrupts a post-translational modification system that is important for several critical cellular processes.

MEDICAL HISTORY AND CLINICAL PRESENTATION

AS is a neurodevelopmental disorder named for the physician who in 1965 first described patients with the classical scope of features including severe cognitive and language impairments and unique behaviors including persistent happiness and excitability.[56] He described the landmark cases as "puppet children" given their demeanor in conjunction with stereotypic and stiff hand movements. Additional key findings included postnatal onset microcephaly and development of seizures in the first few years of life.

SIGNS AND SYMPTOMS

While some early nonspecific features such as gastroesophageal reflux, hypotonia, or poor feeding may be present, developmental delays may not be obviously noted until 6 to 12 months of age. Features of the pathognomonic AS demeanor may be recognized in the first years of life. Development of meaningful language is almost uniformly absent, although receptive language is typically advanced as compared to expressive skills. Ambulation is significantly delayed. Strabismus and refractive errors are common.[57,58]

PHYSICAL EXAMINATION

Physical examination findings are subtle but may progress over time. Attention to growth trajectory of head circumference is important. Facial features include broad mouth, prognathism, and frequent drooling. Neurologic examination may include brisk reflexes and tremulous movement in limbs; if ambulatory, a wide-based ataxic gait is classic.[59] Paroxysms of laughter may be appreciated throughout clinical assessment.[57]

DIFFERENTIAL DIAGNOSIS

Several disorders may mimic AS. Rett syndrome is also associated with acquired microcephaly, essentially absent speech, and epilepsy; however, frank regression is expected in Rett syndrome. Mowat-Wilson syndrome can present with cognitive impairments, seizures, and similar craniofacial features as AS; in contrast, congenital anomalies are prevalent. Pitt-Hopkins syndrome presents with global delays and acquired microcephaly; however, paroxysmal hyperventilation episodes and absence of characteristic facial features can differentiate from AS.[60,61] Screening for inborn errors of metabolism should be considered in the setting of developmental delays, epilepsy, and absence of congenital anomalies.

EVALUATION

History and physical examination are often sufficient to raise suspicion for AS. Prenatal/perinatal history and growth parameters are normal, and absence of congenital anomalies is expected. Other evaluations that may support the diagnosis include essentially normal brain MRI and characteristic EEG findings.[62] Family history of similar findings is improbable but not impossible depending on underlying genetic mechanism.

DIAGNOSTIC STUDIES

AS is a prototypical imprinting disorder. DNA imprinting is a mechanism by which gene expression is altered without changing gene sequence. Methylation is a common form of DNA imprinting. Imprinting results in variable gene expression based on parent of origin, as imprinting patterns differ in male and female gametes. Therefore, pathogenic variants of the same imprinted region can have distinctive clinical manifestations depending on whether maternal or paternal copies of the genetic information are altered. AS is caused by deficient expression of the maternal *UBE3A* allele. Abnormal maternal expression is most commonly secondary to a recurring deletion within the maternal copy of 15q11.2q13. Additional etiologies include paternal uniparental disomy of chromosome 15 (both copies of chromosome 15 coming from father), maternal imprinting center disturbance, or pathogenic variants within the maternal *UBE3A* gene itself.[63,64] Methylation analysis can detect all of these except the latter. Initial diagnostic strategy includes methylation analysis of the AS critical region. If the methylation pattern confirms AS, further studies to determine the underlying mechanism are warranted. If methylation pattern is normal, targeted *UBE3A* genetic analysis should be considered if suspicion for AS remains high.

TREATMENT

No specific treatment exists. Standard supportive therapies and developmental programs are a mainstay. While expressive language is profoundly impaired, augmentative communication devices should be pursued to optimize outcomes.[65] It is important that epilepsy is treated by clinicians familiar with AS, as some anticonvulsants are contraindicated.[66]

Pharmacologic treatment for behavioral manifestations can also be considered.[67] Scoliosis occurs at an increased rate and should be screened for regularly.[68]

PATIENT EDUCATION

Clinicians should offer families anticipatory guidance regarding expected developmental outcomes and need for lifelong support. Counseling regarding epilepsy risks is important. Genetic counseling is extremely important given molecular complexities and variable recurrence risks.

KEY POINTS

- AS results in global developmental delays, most notably in speech.
- A unique neurobehavioral profile including paroxysmal laughter and overall happy demeanor is typical.
- Seizures are the most prominent medical concern.
- Complex molecular underpinnings and variable recurrence risks warrant genetic counseling.

23.10 NEUROFIBROMATOSIS

Ashley Taylor

OVERVIEW

Neurofibromatosis encompasses three separate conditions including neurofibromatosis 1 (NF1), neurofibromatosis 2 (NF2), and schwannomatosis.[69] The neurofibromatoses primarily affect cells in the nervous system and each disorder has different manifestations.[69] NF1 mainly affects nerve sheath cells in the peripheral nervous system.[70] Two of the main features of NF1 include café-au-lait macules and neurofibromas.[69] NF2, which primarily affects the central nervous system, has the main feature of bilateral schwannomas that grow on the vestibular nerve.[69] Schwannomatosis causes schwannomas to grow anywhere except the vestibular nerve.

NF1, NF2, and schwannomatosis are autosomal dominant genetic conditions. These conditions are caused by pathogenic variants in known specific genes. NF1 is caused by pathogenic variants in the *NF1* gene,[71] NF2 is caused by pathogenic variants in the *NF2* gene,[72] and schwannomatosis is caused by pathogenic variants in the *LZTR1* and *SMARCB1* genes.[72]

EPIDEMIOLOGY

NF1 is the most prevalent of the neurofibromatoses with an incidence of 1 in 3,000 to 4,000 in the population.[69] The incidence of NF2 is 1 in 40,000 and schwannomatosis has a similar incidence to that of NF2.[69]

PATHOPHYSIOLOGY

NF1, NF2, and schwannomatosis are caused by gene mutations. NF1 is caused by a pathogenic variant in the *NF1* gene located on chromosome 17. Both the *NF1* and *NF2* genes are large and are prone to mutations.[69] The *NF1* gene has one of the highest mutation rates of all genes and more than 500 mutations have been identified.[69] Both the *NF1* and *NF2* genes function as tumor suppressors.[69]

MEDICAL HISTORY AND CLINICAL PRESENTATION

NF1 is an autosomal dominant genetic condition that primarily involves the peripheral nervous system and the skin.[70] NF2 is also autosomal dominant and primarily involves the central nervous system.

SIGNS AND SYMPTOMS

Diagnosis of NF1 requires two clinical criteria.[70] Clinical criteria include six or more café-au-lait macules (>5 mm in prepubertal patients and >15 mm in postpubertal patients); two or more neurofibromas or one plexiform neurofibroma; freckling in the axillary or inguinal regions; optic pathway glioma; two or more iris hamartomas (Lisch nodules); a distinctive osseous lesion such as sphenoid wing dysplasia or long-bone dysplasia (with or without pseudoarthrosis); and a first-degree relative with NF1 according to above-mentioned criteria.[70]

Diagnosis of NF2 in children requires two or more of these findings: a schwannoma at any location including intradermal, skin plaques present at birth, a meningioma, a cortical wedge cataract, a retinal hamartoma, a mononeuropathy (particularly causing a facial nerve palsy, foot or wrist drop, or third nerve palsy).[72] Diagnosis of NF2 in adults requires bilateral vestibular schwannomas; unilateral vestibular schwannoma accompanied by any two of the following: meningioma, schwannoma, glioma, neurofibroma, or cataract in the form of subscapular lenticular opacity or cortical wedge; or multiple meningiomas accompanied by either unilateral vestibular schwannoma or any two of the following: schwannoma, glioma, neurofibroma, or cataract in same form as previously listed.[72]

PHYSICAL EXAMINATION

For patients with NF1, a neurologic physical examination is important to identify any neurologic signs or symptoms that may warrant further imaging. An examination by an ophthalmologist is recommended to look for optic pathway glioma and Lisch nodules.[71] Developmental assessment in children is important due to the risk for learning disability found in 50% of individuals with NF1.[71]

For patients with NF2, hearing evaluation and complete eye examination are important parts of the physical examination. Annual MRI is also recommended starting at age 10 to 12 years.[72]

DIFFERENTIAL DIAGNOSIS

Table 23.8 summarizes the differential diagnosis for neurofibromatosis.

DIAGNOSTIC STUDIES

NF1 and *NF2* gene testing are both available to help with diagnostic purposes and to assist with genetic counseling and family planning.[71,72] Other studies are indicated based on clinically apparent signs or symptoms.[71,72] Brain MRI is important for diagnosing the brain lesions of NF2.[72] Brain MRI is ordered for patients with NF1 based on clinical assessment.[70]

Table 23.8 Differential Diagnosis of Neurofibromatosis 1 and 2

Diagnosis	Description
Legius syndrome	Café-au-lait macules similar to neurofibromatosis 1, mild freckling, no neurofibromas or optic pathway glioma, learning problems
Schwannomatosis	Multiple schwannomas of cranial, spinal or peripheral nerves, usually without vestibular ocular or cutaneous features of neurofibromatosis 2
McCune-Albright syndrome	Jagged coast of Maine café-au-lait macules, polyostotic fibrous dysplasia with fracture, precocious puberty, no neurofibromas
Noonan syndrome	Fewer café-au-lait macules, lentigines, pulmonic valve stenosis, short stature, pectus excavatum

Source: Data from Miller DT, Freedenberg D, Schorry E, et al. Health supervision for children with neurofibromatosis 1. Pediatrics. *2019;143:e20190660. doi:10.1542/peds.2019-0660 ; Friedman JM. Neurofibromatosis 1. In: Adam MP, Ardinger HH, Pagon RA, et al, eds.* GeneReviews. *University of Washington; 1998. http://www.ncbi.nlm.nih/NBK1109*

EVALUATION

Evaluation consists of clinical examination, imaging, and the option of genetic testing.

TREATMENT

Treatment involves evaluation by appropriate specialists regarding abnormalities of the eye, central or peripheral nervous system, spine or long bones, cardiovascular system, or endocrine system.[71] Surgeons or oncologists can treat tumors with appropriate intervention.[71]

PATIENT EDUCATION

- Patients should have annual physical examination by a clinician familiar with neurofibromatosis.[71]
- Annual ophthalmology examination is recommended in childhood for patients with NF1 and annually for patients with NF2.[72]
- Regular developmental assessment is recommended in childhood for patients with NF1.[71]
- Regular blood pressure monitoring is important due to the risk for renal artery stenosis and pheochromocytoma for patients with NF1.[71]
- NF1 and NF2 are both autosomal dominant and there is a 50% chance of passing on the condition during each future pregnancy.[71,72]
- Regular hearing evaluation and annual brain MRI is important for patients with NF2.[72]

KEY POINTS

- NF1 is the most prevalent of the neurofibromatoses with an incidence of 1 in 3,000–4,000. NF2 and schwannomatosis have a similar incidence of 1 in 40,000.
- Both the *NF1* and *NF2* genes are tumor suppressor genes.
- NF1 and NF2 are both autosomal dominant genetic conditions.

23.11 EHLERS-DANLOS SYNDROME

JINA STEPHEN

OVERVIEW

Ehlers-Danlos syndrome (EDS) is a term used to describe a group of connective tissue disorders that are caused by genetic mutations that result in defective or decreased collagen.[73] Collagen is a protein that is vital to providing strength and elasticity to our connective tissues such as our skin, joints, skeleton, and blood vessels. The main signs and symptoms related to this group of disorders include joint hypermobility, skin hyperextensibility, and fragile blood vessels. There are 13 subtypes of EDS that are differentiated based on the inherited mutation and associated symptoms.

EDS disorders are related to genetic mutations that affect collagen structure, processing, or production. These abnormalities can result in lack of collagen or decreased strength of collagen. EDS is classified based on underlying genetic mutations and characteristics of each subtype. The most recent classification of the syndrome includes 13 subtypes. Most of the symptoms related to EDS involve the skin, muscles, skeleton, and blood vessels.

EPIDEMIOLOGY

The combination of the various forms of EDS occurs in 1 in 5,000 individuals. Hypermobile and classical EDS are the most common forms of EDS with hypermobile affecting 1 in 5,000 and classical type occurring in 1 in 20,000 to 40,000.[74]

PATHOPHYSIOLOGY

EDS can be inherited in an autosomal dominant or autosomal recessive manner; however, in some cases, EDS can be the result of a de novo mutation. At least 19 genes have been identified as causes of the various subtypes of EDS, except for the hypermobility type for which the genetic cause is still unknown. The genes that have been identified are responsible for encoding various subtypes of collagen while others encode proteins associated with collagen processing.[75]

MEDICAL HISTORY AND CLINICAL PRESENTATION

Depending on the subtype, EDS has a variable presentation. Some subtypes are identifiable at birth if newborns present with hip dislocations, hypotonia, or clubfoot. However, patients often present to their primary care offices or the ED for evaluation of issues related to the joints—such as pain and dislocations—or for skin manifestations such as major bleeding from minor trauma, poor wound healing, or severe bruising. In the vascular subtype, patients may present with life-threatening symptoms such as organ rupture, arterial aneurysm, or recurrent pneumothorax.[73,75]

SIGNS AND SYMPTOMS

Many of the subtypes of EDS have some degree of classical features including skin hyperextensibility, joint hypermobility, and connective tissue fragility. Each subtype can be further differentiated based on the presence or absence of these features, the level of variability in these common features, as well as a few distinguishing signs and symptoms.[73,74]

Common skin findings include soft, velvety/doughy skin, elastic "snap back" skin, easy bruising, severe scarring even from minor trauma, and/or poor wound healing. Joint hypermobility may result in frequent subluxations, dislocations, delays in ambulation, and osteoarthritis. Fragile blood vessels may be associated with deformities of the heart such as weakening of the bicuspid valve, dilation of the aorta, or mitral valve prolapse.

Some of the distinguishing features of each type are specified in Table 23.9.

PHYSICAL EXAMINATION

Ocular features such as deformities of the cornea or blue sclerae may be evident.

Skin findings may include bruising, varicose veins, atrophic scarring, delayed wound healing, molluscoid pseudotumors, subcutaneous spheroids, and soft, thin, or very stretchy skin.

Musculoskeletal features may include excess joint laxity and joint hypermobility, kyphoscoliosis, short stature, or talipes.

Table 23.9 Distinguishing Features of Ehlers-Danlos Syndrome

Type	Distinguishing Features
Classical	Molluscoid pseudotumors, spheroids
Classical-like	No atrophic scarring
Cardiac-valvular	Progressive cardiac valve involvement
Vascular	Arterial dissection and rupture, intestinal perforation, uterine rupture, arteriovenous malformations, early varicose veins, pneumothoraces
Hypermobility	Hypermobility of small and large joints, chronic pain
Arthrochalasia	Congenital bilateral hip dislocation, hypotonia, osteopenia
Dermatosparaxis	Delayed fontanelle closure, blue sclerae, short stature
Kyphoscoliotic	Bilateral hip dislocation, progressive kyphoscoliosis, hypotonia, possible hearing loss or ocular and scleral fragility, marfanoid habitus
Brittle cornea syndrome	Microcornea, early-onset keratoconus and keratoglobus
Spondylodysplastic	Short stature, limb bowing, osteopenia
Musculocontractural	Progressive kyphoscoliosis, adducted thumbs, congenital talipes
Myopathic	Congenital hypotonia or muscle atrophy that improves with age
Periodontal	Periodontitis, premature tooth loss, pretibial plaques

Source: Data from Genetic and Rare Diseases Information Center. Ehlers-Danlos syndromes. https://rarediseases.info.nih.gov/diseases/6322/ehlers-danlos-syndromes; National Institutes of Health. Ehlers-Danlos syndrome—Genetics Home Reference. U.S. National Library of Medicine; 2014. http://www.lb7.uscourts.gov/documents/2-13-CV-126.1-PRC.pdf

Cardiac signs may include murmur suggestive of mitral valve prolapse.

Some subtypes have a characteristic facies:

- In vascular EDS, that includes large eyes, small chin, sunken cheeks, thin nose and lips, and lobeless ears.
- Dermatosparaxis EDS has a characteristic appearance that may involve loose skin of the face, full eyelids, blue tinged sclerae, epicanthal folds, palpebral fissures, and micrognathia.
- Periodontitis
- Rupture of intestines, uterus, or eyeball[75]

DIFFERENTIAL DIAGNOSIS

Table 23.10 summarizes the differential diagnosis for EDS.[76]

DIAGNOSTIC STUDIES

Table 23.11 summarizes diagnostic testing for EDS.

EVALUATION

EDS is primarily a clinical diagnosis. Various major and minor criteria have been established to aid in diagnosis. Some of the subtypes can be identified and/or confirmed via genetic testing and skin biopsies can reveal some characteristic abnormalities in collagen structure. Routine studies such as CT scans, MRI, ultrasound, or angiography may aid in identifying some of the manifestations of the various subtypes. Some subtypes can be diagnosed via CVS and amniocentesis in the prenatal setting.[73,77]

TREATMENT

Treatment of EDS is often symptomatic and prophylactic against serious or life-threatening complications. Depending on subtype, EDS requires a multidisciplinary approach to treatment and may involve a team of dermatologists, cardiologists, cardiothoracic surgeons, plastic surgeons, physical therapists, pain management specialists, ophthalmologists, dentists, geneticists, genetic counselors, hematologists, and/or psychologists.[73]

Table 23.10 Differential Diagnosis of Ehlers-Danlos Syndrome

Diagnosis	Description
Marfan syndrome	Can be differentiated based on pathologic genetic variation in *FBN1*, presence of ectopia lentis, bone overgrowth, skin findings of Ehlers-Danlos syndrome not present in Marfan syndrome
Loeys-Dietz syndrome	Can be differentiated based on pathogenic variant in *SMAD2, SMAD3, TGFB2, TGFB3, TGFBR1*, or *TGFBR2*. May also have symptoms such as hypertelorism, cleft palate or bifid uvula, not common in Ehlers-Danlos syndrome.
Cutis laxa	Cutaneous features differ slightly: lacks "snap back" after stretched, no easy bruising or scarring. Differentiated via skin biopsy findings

Table 23.11 Diagnostic Tests for Ehlers-Danlos Syndrome

Diagnostic Test	Rationale
Next generation sequencing	Specific mutations help to differentiate the type of Ehlers-Danlos syndrome (EDS) Classical (cEDS): *COL5A1 or COL5A2, COL1A1* Classical-like (clEDS): *TXNB* Cardiac-valvular (cvEDS): *COL1A2* Vascular (vEDS): *COL3A1, COL1A1* Hypermobility (hEDS): Unknown Arthrochalasia (aEDS): *COL1A1 or COL1A2* Dermatosparaxis (dEDS): *ADAMTS2* Kyphoscoliotic (kEDS): *PLOD1 or FKBP14* Brittle cornea syndrome (BCS): *ZNF469 or PRDM5* Spondylodysplastic (spEDS): *SLC39A13, B4GALT6 or B4GALT7* Musculocontractural (mcEDS): *CHST14 or DSE* Myopathic (mEDS): *COL12A1 or FKBP14* Periodontal (pEDS): *C1R*
Echocardiogram	Can help to identify aortic dilation, mitral valve prolapse, or other valve abnormalities present in certain subtypes
CT, MRI, angiograms, ultrasounds	May help to identify vascular abnormalities and skeletal abnormalities
Chorionic villus sampling (CVS) and amniocentesis	May reveal deficiencies in specific types of collagen related to particular subtypes
Beighton Score	Score of 5 or higher defines generalized joint hypermobility

Source: Data from National Institutes of Health. Ehlers-Danlos syndrome—Genetics Home Reference. U.S. National Library of Medicine; 2014. http://www.lb7.uscourts.gov/documents/2-13-CV-126.1-PRC.pdf; National Organization for Rare Disorders. Ehlers Danlos Syndromes. https://rarediseases.org/rare-diseases/ehlers-danlos-syndrome; Pauker SP, Stoler JM. Overview of the management of Ehlers-Danlos syndrome In: Post TW, ed. UpToDate. *UpToDate; 2021. https://www.uptodate.com/contents/overview-of-the-management-of-ehlers-danlos-syndromes*

PATIENT EDUCATION

Patient education varies based on subtype; however, general recommendations should include[78]:

- **Skin precautions:** Sunscreen, mild soaps, specialized suture and wound care, use of protective gear, vitamin C.
- **Musculoskeletal precautions:** Physical therapy, utilize braces, avoid lifting, high impact exercise, and contact sports.
- **Cardiac precautions:** Prophylactic antihypertensives and monitoring.
- It is important that patients who are diagnosed with EDS establish care with a genetics specialist for a discussion regarding reproductive implications.
- Obstetric patients should be managed by high risk and specialty centers.

KEY POINTS

- EDSs are a group of inherited disorders that are inherited in an autosomal dominant or autosomal recessive pattern. EDS can sometimes also be the result of a de novo mutation. These mutations cause issues with collagen.
- EDS presentation is varied among subtypes, but the most common symptoms are related to joint hypermobility, skin hyperextensibility, and connective tissue fragility.
- EDS diagnosis is primarily clinical; however, it can be confirmed with genetic testing and skin biopsies.
- EDS management is multidisciplinary and often involves several types of specialists to aid in prophylaxis and to prevent life-threatening complications.

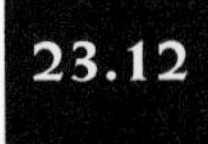

23.12 X-LINKED ADRENOLEUKODYSTROPHY

LAURA D. BUCH

OVERVIEW

X-linked adrenoleukodystrophy (X-ALD) is the most common peroxisomal disorder and is due to a mutation of the *ABCD1* gene on the X chromosome. X-ALD is a devastating condition and can present as cerebral adrenoleukodystrophy (cerebral ALD), adrenomyeloneuropathy (AMN), adrenocortical insufficiency (Addison-only), or in females with a presentation similar to AMN. There may be a higher incidence of X-ALD than is currently observed as NBS efforts expand. In X-ALD, the transporter responsible for bringing VLCFAs into the peroxisome does not function properly, and VLCFAs build up in the body's tissues. Demyelination in the brain may occur, and sensory and motor neurons may be affected. Adrenal function is negatively impacted as well. To prevent these effects, hematopoietic stem cell transplantation (HSCT) should occur prior to neurologic symptom onset. Supportive care is encouraged, and gene therapy trials are currently underway.

There are two main X-ALD phenotypes: cerebral ALD and AMN. Cerebral ALD presents in childhood and is characterized by rapidly progressive inflammatory demyelination within the brain, resulting in severe neurologic and cognitive decline. Without treatment, those with cerebral ALD quickly progress to a vegetative state, followed by death.[79] AMN is a noninflammatory axonopathy affecting the ascending sensory and descending motor spinal tracts, resulting in a gradually worsening spastic paraplegia.[79,80] Other presentations include adrenocortical insufficiency (Addison-only) and an AMN-like presentation in female carriers.

EPIDEMIOLOGY

X-ALD is observed in 1/14,700 births, though data vary and X-ALD may be observed at a higher incidence with an increase of states participating in X-ALD NBS.[81]

PATHOPHYSIOLOGY

The *ABCD1* gene is responsible for encoding a transporter that brings VLCFAs into the peroxisome. When this transporter does not function properly, VLCFAs build up in all tissues of the body, resulting in ALD. VLCFAs predominantly accumulate in the myelin of the brain and spinal cord, adrenal cortex, and the Leydig cells of the testes.[81]

SIGNS AND SYMPTOMS

Exhibit 23.2 summarizes signs and symptoms consistent with X-ALD.[82,83]

Exhibit 23.2 Signs and Symptoms Consistent with X-Linked Adrenoleukodystrophy

Symptoms present in 90% to 95% of affected individuals:

- **Cerebral ALD:** childhood onset of behavioral issues, hyperactivity, declining school performance, seizures, vomiting, dysphagia, auditory/visual impairment, fatigue, ataxia
- **AMN:** adult onset of lower extremity pain/weakness, peripheral neuropathy, sphincter dysfunction, impotence, adrenal problems
- **Adrenocortical insufficiency (Addison-only):** childhood or adult onset of adrenal insufficiency with symptoms of dark skin, anorexia, vomiting, muscle weakness

Symptoms present in 5% to 10% of affected individuals: headache, increased intracranial pressure, hemiparesis, dementia, paralysis

Females with X-ALD: Previously thought to be asymptomatic carriers, middle-age women may develop symptoms consistent with AMN. Female carriers typically have normal adrenal function.

ALD, adrenoleukodystrophy; AMN, adrenomyeloneuropathy; X-ALD, X-linked adrenoleukodystrophy.

Source: Data from Genetic and Rare Diseases Information Center. X-linked adrenoleukodystrophy. https://rarediseases.info.nih.gov/diseases/5758/x-linked-adrenoleukodystrophy#ref_14049; Engelen M, Kemp S, de Visser M, et al. X-linked adrenoleukodystrophy (X-ALD): clinical presentation and guidelines for diagnosis, follow-up and management. *Orphanet J Rare Dis.* 2012;7:51. doi:10.1186/1750-1172-7-51

PHYSICAL EXAMINATION

In a patient with X-ALD, evaluation of the eyes and ears can reveal decreased visual acuity, visual field deficits, and hearing loss. Examination of the musculoskelet and neurologic system shows decreased strength, muscle wasting, extremity stiffness/limited range of motion, ataxic gait, lack of coordination, decreased sensation, impaired vibratory sense, memory loss, and focal neurologic deficits. Hair on the scalp may appear scanty, and skin may be hyperpigmented. Rectal examination may reveal decreased sphincter tone. Other observations may include inattentiveness, hyperactivity, or active psychoses.[79,82,84]

DIFFERENTIAL DIAGNOSIS

Table 23.12 summarizes the differential diagnosis for X-ALD.

Table 23.12 Differential Diagnosis for X-Linked Adrenoleukodystrophy

Diagnosis	Examples	How to Differentiate from X-ALD
Other leukodystrophies	Krabbe disease, metachromatic leukodystrophy	MRI findings may be similar; use family history, clinical course, gene sequencing, and VLCFA levels
Other causes of spinal cord dysfunction	Multiple sclerosis, amyotrophic lateral sclerosis, vitamin B12 deficiency, other spastic paraplegias	Rate of progression can be helpful in differentiating X-ALD from these causes
Other causes of behavior problems or poor academic performance	Attention deficit hyperactivity disorder (ADHD), autism spectrum disorder, other psychiatric, developmental, or learning disorders	These are not commonly seen in association with focal neurologic deficits and can be differentiated from X-ALD with brain MRI
Other causes of adrenal insufficiency	Autoimmune adrenalitis, infectious adrenalitis, cancer, adrenal hemorrhage or infarction, drugs, congenital adrenal hypoplasia	A patient's medical history can reveal past infections, medications, or other causes of adrenal insufficiency

VLCFA, very long chain fatty acid; X-ALD, X-linked adrenoleukodystrophy.

EVALUATION AND DIAGNOSTIC STUDIES

Make an accurate diagnosis of X-ALD and rule out other potential causes of symptoms with the following diagnostic studies: Plasma total lipid VLCFAs, gene sequencing of the *ABCD1* gene, plasma ACTH and cortisol level to evaluate adrenal function, brain MRI to assess for progressive white matter changes in cerebral ALD, and a vitamin B12 level.

TREATMENT

- If completed prior to onset of neurologic symptoms, HSCT can halt demyelination.
- Symptoms related to adrenal insufficiency should be managed with corticosteroids.
- Current experimental treatments include Lorenzo's oil and gene therapy. Lorenzo's oil is a combination of oleic and erucic acid triglycerides and is not FDA approved, nor shown to slow disease progression. Gene therapy trials are underway and have shown promise.
- Physical therapy and supportive care are other important aspects of care.[81]

PATIENT EDUCATION

- X-ALD is a rare genetic disease that destroys the myelin sheath, or fatty covering, of the nerve cells in the brain.
- X-ALD also causes adrenal dysfunction, which can lead to symptoms that are consistent with Addison disease.
- There are several forms of ALD, which differ in their presentation, severity, and rate of progression.
- Treatment options are available for X-ALD, and there are several clinical trials currently in progress.

KEY POINTS

- X-ALD is a disorder that mainly affects males and is characterized by a pathogenic alteration of the *ABCD1* gene.
- Alterations in the *ABCD1* gene cause problems with peroxisomal β-oxidation and lead to accumulation of VLCFAs in all tissues of the body.
- Accumulation of VLCFAs results in impaired adrenal and nervous system functions.
- Signs and symptoms that may aid in the diagnosis of X-ALD include behavioral disturbances, seizures, ataxia, and hyperpigmented skin.
- Once diagnosed, X-ALD requires treatment, which can include HSCT, corticosteroids, and supportive care.

COMMON CHIEF COMPLAINTS

APPROACH TO GENETIC DISORDERS

Though genetic disorders are by nature heterogeneous, common chief complaints should raise the index of suspicion in clinicians. These complaints can be seen at any stage of development from infancy to adulthood, depending on the severity of dysfunction. Because of the nature of genetic disorders, chief complaints will frequently span across multiple organ systems, and may be accompanied by cognitive impairments. Patients with milder forms of the genetic disorder or who are carriers may demonstrate only a few of the common chief complaints, and frequently, these may be noted on obtaining a thorough family history. Family history is key to risk assessment determination. The more first-degree relatives who exhibit signs/symptoms of the disorder and an earlier age of onset of the signs/symptoms, the greater the suspicion for genetic influences.

Common chief complaints include failure to thrive, skin changes such as hyper- or hypopigmentation and thin scalp hair, visual and hearing changes, developmental delays or reversal/loss of milestones, hypotonia and muscle weakness, microcephaly, intellectual disability, seizures, frequent joint dislocations, infertility, easy bruising, and abnormal growth patterns or pubertal development.

In infants and children, tracking of changes in growth and achievement of developmental milestones with growth charts will be paramount for monitoring progression of disease and to assist with diagnosis. The ongoing presence of a pattern of a chief complaint should increase the index of suspicion that a genetic abnormality is the cause, after ruling out acute

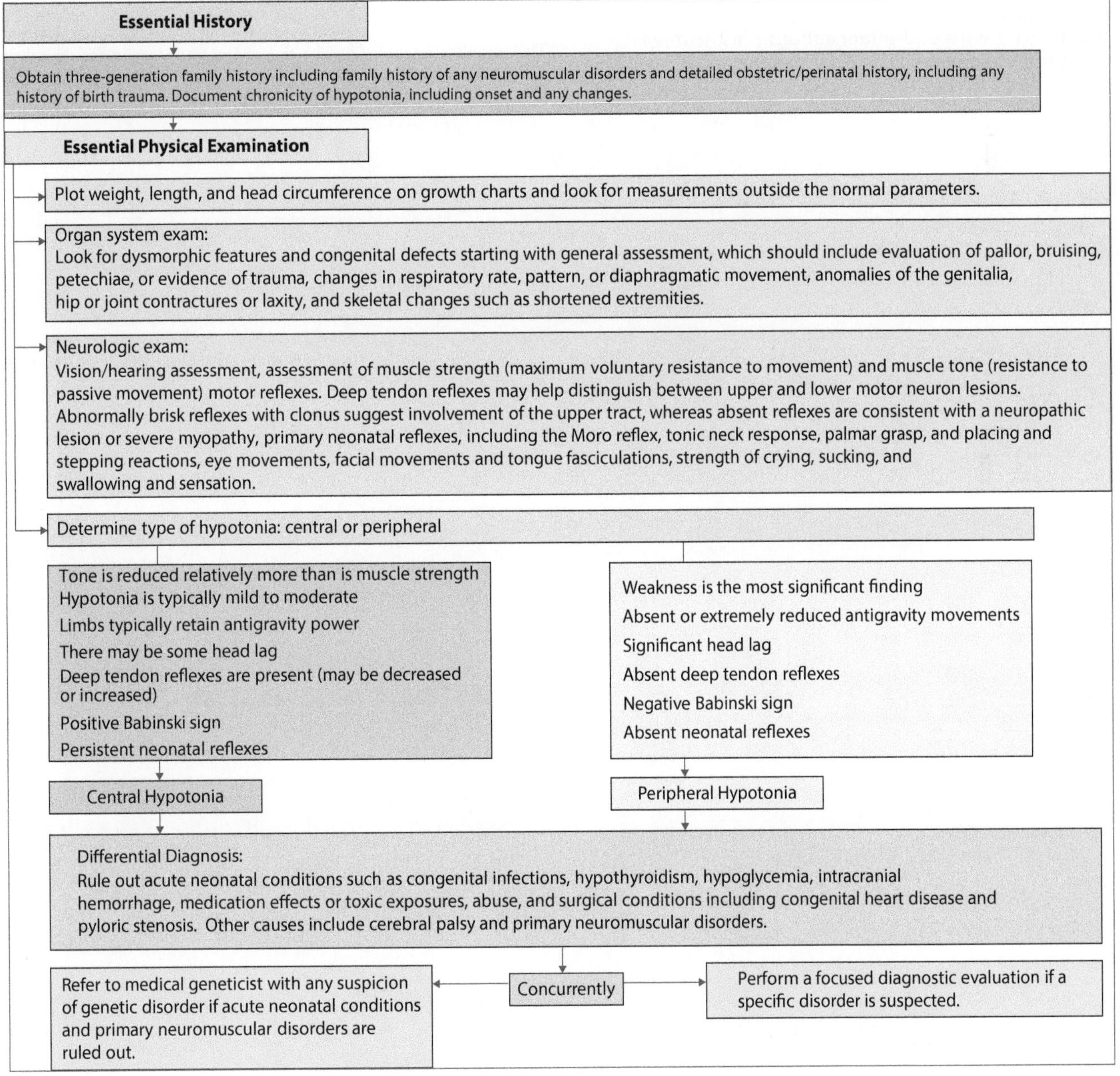

Figure 23.2 **Approach to hypotonia in infants.**

causes such as infection, hypothyroidism, hypoglycemia, medication/drug effects, and intracranial hemorrhage.

The algorithm presented in Figure 23.2 will give an example of evaluation for hypotonia in infants, a chief complaint often noted in genetic disorders, including Down syndrome, X-ALD, and inborn errors of metabolism. On physical exam, a hypotonic infant will have a frog-like position when supine, with decreased spontaneous activity and decreased muscle resistance to stretch. For the primary care PA, referral to a medical geneticist and genetic counselor at the earliest suspicion of a genetic disorder for chief complaints such as hypotonia will decrease morbidity.

KNOWLEDGE CHECKS

1. Understanding the pathophysiology behind each of the most common mutation types is central to diagnosis and treatment of genetic disorders. Define and give an example of each of the following types of mutations: deletion, duplication, frameshift, insertion, missense, nonsense, and repeat expansion.
2. Familiarity with and understanding of the most common diagnostic tests used in genetics allows a clinician to order the appropriate test based upon a differential diagnosis based upon a thorough history and physical examination. Create a table that lists the most common diagnostic tests and their utility.
3. Awareness of unique ELSI is paramount when clinicians are caring for patients with genetic disorders. Give examples of how these may differ when compared to other medical disorders and what clinicians can do to assist their patients when dealing with genetic disorders.

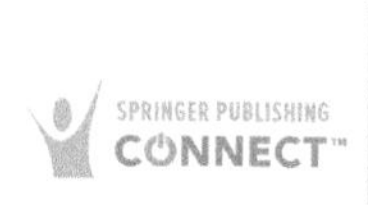

A robust set of instructor resources designed to supplement this text is located at **http://connect.springerpub.com/content/book/978-0-8261-8243-2.** Qualifying instructors may request access by emailing **textbook@springerpub.com.**

REFERENCES

The complete reference list for this chapter appears in the digital version of the chapter, accessible at https://connect.springerpub.com/content/book/978-0-8261-8243-2/chapter/ch23.

INDEX